tenth edition

Maingot's

ABDOMINAL
OPERATIONS

Volume I

tenth edition

Maingot's

ABDOMINAL
OPERATIONS

Volume I

Editors

Michael J. Zinner, MD, FACS
Moseley Professor of Surgery
Harvard Medical School
Surgeon-in-Chief
Brigham and Women's Hospital
Boston, Massachusetts

Seymour I. Schwartz, MD
Distinguished Alumni Professor and Chair
Department of Surgery
University of Rochester School
  of Medicine and Dentistry
Rochester, New York

Harold Ellis, CBE, DM, MCh, FRCS
Clinical Anatomist
Department of Anatomy
United Medical and Dental School
University of London
Emeritus Professor of Surgery
University of London
London, United Kingdom

Assistant Editors

Stanley W. Ashley, MD
Senior Surgeon
Brigham and Women's Hospital
Associate Professor of Surgery
Harvard Medical School
Boston, Massachusetts

David W. McFadden, MD
Professor of Surgery
Chief, Division of General Surgery
University of California Los Angeles
  School of Medicine
Los Angeles, California

McGraw-Hill
Medical Publishing Division

New York Chicago San Francisco Lisbon London Madrid Mexico City Milan
New Delhi San Juan Seoul Singapore Sydney Toronto

McGraw-Hill

*A Division of The **McGraw·Hill** Companies*

Maingot's Abdominal Operations, Tenth Edition

3 4 5 6 7 8 9 0   KGP/KGP   0 9 8 7 6 5 4 3 2 1

ISBN: 0-8385-6106-3 (set, domestic)

Notice

Managing Editor, Development: Kathleen McCullough
Production Service: York Production Services
Design: Libby Schmitz

ISBN: 0-8385-0627-5 (set, international)

CONTRIBUTORS

Robin Abel, BSc, MB, BS, FRCS
Research Fellow
Department of Pediatric Surgery
Institute of Child Health
University of London
London, United Kingdom

Jack Abrahamson, MB, ChB, FRCS, FACS
Chairman of Surgery
Carmel Hospital
Haifa, Israel

Steven A. Ahrendt, MD
Assistant Professor of Surgery
The Johns Hopkins University School of Medicine
Baltimore, Maryland

John Alexander Williams, MD, FRCS
Consultant Surgeon
Birmingham, Nuffield, and Priory Hospitals
Professor of Gastrointestinal Surgery
University of Birmingham
Birmingham, United Kingdom

Stanley W. Ashley, MD
Senior Surgeon
Brigham and Women's Hospital
Associate Professor of Surgery
Harvard Medical School
Boston, Massachusetts

Stephen A. Barnes, MD
Chief Resident, Department of Surgery
The Johns Hopkins Hospital
Fellow, Department of Surgery
The Johns Hopkins University School of Medicine
Baltimore, Maryland

Robert W. Beart, Jr., MD
Professor of Surgery
Chairman, Colorectal Surgery
University of Southern California
Los Angeles, California

R. Daniel Beauchamp, MD
Associate Director of Clinical Programs
Vanderbilt Cancer Center
Associate Professor of Surgery and Cell Biology
Vanderbilt University School of Medicine
Nashville, Tennessee

Robert S. Bennion, MD
Associate Professor of Surgery
University of California Los Angeles School of Medicine
Los Angeles, California

Jonathan S. Berek, MD
Vice Chair, Department of Obstetrics and Gynecology
Chief, Gynecology and Gynecologic Oncology
Professor
Jonsson Comprehensive Cancer Center
University of California Los Angeles School of Medicine
Los Angeles, California

Scott M. Berry, MD
Surgery Chief Resident
University of Cincinnati School of Medicine
Cincinnati, Ohio

Elisa H. Birnbaum, MD
Assistant Professor of Surgery
Washington University School of Medicine
St. Louis, Missouri

Kirby I. Bland, MD
Executive Surgeon-In-Chief
Brown University Affiliated Hospitals
J. Murray Beardsley Professor and Chairman
Department of Surgery
Brown University School of Medicine
Providence, Rhode Island

Leslie H. Blumgart, MD, FACS, FRCS
Chief, Hepatobiliary Surgical Section
Director, Hepatobiliary Disease Program
Enid A. Haupt Chair
Memorial Sloan Kettering Cancer Center
Professor of Surgery
Cornell University Medical College
New York, New York

Scott J. Boley, MD, FACS
Chief of Pediatric Surgical Service
Montefiore Medical Center
Professor of Surgery and Pediatrics
Albert Einstein College of Medicine
Bronx, New York

David C. Brooks, MD, FACS
Surgeon
Brigham and Women's Hospital
Assistant Professor of Surgery
Harvard Medical School
Boston, Massachusetts

L. Michael Brunt, MD
Staff Surgeon
Barnes-Jewish Hospital
Assistant Professor of Surgery
Washington University School of Medicine
St. Louis, Missouri

John M. Burch, MD
Chief, General Surgery
Denver General Hospital
Professor of Surgery
University of Colorado Health Sciences Center
Denver, Colorado

Agustin A. Burgos, MD
Resident in Surgery
Tulane University School of Medicine
New Orleans, Louisiana

Ronald W. Bussutil, MD, PhD
Director, Dumont–UCLA Transplant Center
Professor of Surgery
Dumont Chair in Transplantation Surgery
University of California Los Angeles School of Medicine
Los Angeles, California

John L. Cameron, MD
Surgeon-in-Chief
The Johns Hopkins Hospital
Professor of Surgery
Chairman, Department of Surgery
The Johns Hopkins University School of Medicine
Baltimore, Maryland

Helena R. Chang, MD, PhD
Staff Surgeon
Roger Williams Hospital
Associate Professor in Surgery and Pathobiology
Brown University
Providence, Rhode Island

Nicholas J. W. Cheshire, MD, FRCS
Lecturer in Surgery
St. Mary's Hospital
Imperial College of Medicine
London, United Kingdom

Alfred Cushierei, MD, ChM, FRCS(Ed), FRCS(Eng), FRCS(Glas[Hon]), FRCSI(Hon)
Consultant Surgeon
Dundee Teaching Hospital
NHS Trust
Ninewalls Hospital and Medical School
Professor and Head
Department of Surgery
University of Dundee
Dundee, United Kingdom

John M. Daly, MD
Surgeon-in-Chief
New York Hospital
Lewis Atterbury Stimson Professor and Chairman
Cornell University Medical College
New York, New York

Haile T. Debas, MD
Dean, School of Medicine
The Mauric Galante Distinguished Professor of Surgery
University of California San Francisco
San Francisco, California

Malcolm M. DeCamp, Jr., MD
Associate Surgeon
Division of Thoracic Surgery
Brigham and Women's Hospital
Assistant Professor of Surgery
Harvard Medical School
Boston, Massachusetts

Tom R. DeMeester, MD
Professor and Chairman, Department of Surgery
University of Southern California School of Medicine
Los Angeles, California

Harold Ellis, CBE, DM, MCh, FRCS
Clinical Anatomist
Department of Anatomy
United Medical and Dental School
University of London
Emeritus Professor of Surgery
University of London
London, United Kingdom

S. T. Fan, MBBS, MS, FRCS(Glasg), FACS
Professor of Surgery
Division of Hepatobiliary Surgery
Department of Surgery
The University of Hong Kong
Queen Mary Hospital
Hong Kong

Douglas G. Farmer, MD
Fellow, Transplantation Surgery
Division of Pancreas and Liver Transplantation
Dumont–University of California Los Angeles
    Transplant Center
Los Angeles, California

Victor W. Fazio, MD
Rupert Turnbull Chairman
Department of Colorectal Surgery
Cleveland Clinic Foundation
Professor of Surgery
Ohio State University School of Medicine
Cleveland, Ohio

Carlos Fernandez-del Castillo, MD
Assistant Surgeon
Massachusetts General Hospital
Assistant Professor of Surgery
Harvard Medical School
Boston, Massachusetts

Aaron S. Fink, MD
Chief, Surgical Service
Atlanta Veterans Administration Medical Center
Decatur, Georgia
Associate Professor of Surgery
Emory University School of Medicine
Atlanta, Georgia

Josef E. Fischer, MD
Surgeon-in-Chief
University of Cincinnati Hospital Group
Christian R. Holmes Professor
Chairman, Department of Surgery
University of Cincinnati
Cincinnati, Ohio

James W. Fleshman, MD
Associate Professor of Surgery
Washington University School of Medicine
St. Louis, Missouri

Manson Fok, MBBS, FRCS(Edin)
Senior Lecturer
Department of Surgery
The University of Hong Kong
Queen Mary Hospital
Hong Kong

Eric W. Fonkalsrud, MD
Chief of Pediatric Surgery
University of California Los Angeles Medical Center
Professor of Pediatric Surgery
University of California Los Angeles School of
    Medicine
Los Angeles, California

Robert D. Fry, MD
Chief, Division of Colon and Rectal Surgery
Professor of Surgery
Thomas Jefferson University
Philadelphia, Pennsylvania

Geoffrey Glazer, MS, FRCS, FACS
Consultant Surgeon
St. Mary's Hospital
Honorary Senior Lecturer in Surgery
Imperial College of Medicine
London, United Kingdom

Steven L. Glorsky, MD
Attending Surgeon
Lower Florida Keys Health System

Key West, Florida
Former Clinical Instructor of Surgery
University of Southern California School of Medicine
Los Angeles, California

Jay L. Grosfeld, MD
Surgeon-in-Chief
J. W. Riley Hospital for Children
Lafayette Page Professor and Chairman
Department of Surgery
Indiana University School of Medicine
Indianapolis, Indiana

J. Michael Henderson, MD
Staff Surgeon
Chairman, General Surgery
The Cleveland Clinic Foundation
Cleveland, Ohio

Oscar J. Hines, MD
Resident in Surgery
University of California Los Angeles School of
    Medicine
Los Angeles, California

Darryl T. Hiyama, MD
Assistant Professor of Surgery
Division of General Surgery
University of California Los Angeles School of
    Medicine
Los Angeles, California

Edward R. Howard, MS, FRCS
Department of Surgery
King's College Hospital
Denmark Hill
London, England

Bernard M. Jaffe, MD
Professor and Vice-Chairman
Department of Surgery
Tulane University School of Medicine
New Orleans, Louisiana

David Johnston, MBChB, MD, ChM, FRCS
Consultant Surgeon
Leeds General Infirmary
Professor of Surgery
University of Leeds
Leeds, United Kingdom

Barbara M. Kadell, MD
Clinical Professor and Chief, Gastrointestinal
    Radiology
University of California Los Angeles Medical Center
Vice Chair, Department of Radiological Sciences
University of California Los Angeles School of
    Medicine
Los Angeles, California

Kim U. Kahng, MD
Associate Professor of Surgery
Vice Chairman, Administrative Affairs
Medical College of Pennsylvania
Hahnemann University
Philadelphia, Pennsylvania

Ronald N. Kaleya, MD
Associate Professor of Surgery
Montefiore Medical Center
Albert Einstein College of Medicine
Bronx, New York

Joseph A. Karam, MD
Research Fellow
Instructor in Surgery
The Medical College of Pennsylvania
Hahnemann University
Philadelphia, Pennsylvania

Seiji Kawasaki, MD
Professor and Chairman
First Department of Surgery
Shinshu University School of Medicine
Matsumoto, Japan

Keith A. Kelly, MD, FACS
Chair, Department of Surgery
Mayo Clinic Scottsdale
Scottsdale, Arizona
Professor of Surgery
Mayo Medical School
Rochester, Minnesota

Ira J. Kodner, MD
Chief, Section of Colon and Rectal Surgery
Jewish Hospital and Barnes Hospital
Professor of Surgery
Washington University School of Medicine
St. Louis, Missouri

Han C. Kuijpers, MD, PhD
Associate Professor of Gastroenterologic Surgery
University Hospital Nymegen
Nymegen, Netherlands

Keith D. Lillemoe, MD, FACS
Active Staff
The Johns Hopkins Hospital
Associate Professor of Surgery
The Johns Hopkins University School of Medicine
Baltimore, Maryland

Pamela A. Lipsett, MD
Co-Director, Surgical Intensive Care Unit
Attending Surgeon
Johns Hopkins Hospital
Associate Professor of Surgery, Anesthesia, Critical Care
    Medicine
Johns Hopkins University School of Medicine
Baltimore, Maryland

Michael Liptay, MD
Fellow in Thoracic Surgery
Brigham and Women's Hospital
Harvard Medical School
Boston, Massachusetts

Carson D. Liu, MD
Surgical Resident
University of California Los Angeles School of
    Medicine
Los Angeles, California

Edward H. Livingston, MD
Attending Surgeon
University of California Los Angeles School of
    Medicine
Assistant Chief, Surgical Service
Veterans Medical Center, West Los Angeles
Assistant Professor of Surgery
Assistant Dean
University of California Los Angeles School of
    Medicine
Los Angeles, California

David S. K. Lu, MD, CM
Attending Radiologist
University of California Los Angeles Medical Center
Assistant Professor of Radiology
University of California Los Angeles School of
    Medicine
Los Angeles, California

Masatoshi Makuuchi, MD, PhD
Chairman, Second Department of Surgery
Tokyo University Hospital
Professor of Hepatobiliary Pancreatic Surgery
    Divisionand of Artificial Organs and
    Transplantation Division
University of Tokyo, Faculty of Medicine
Tokyo, Japan

Iain Martin, MBChB, MD, FRCS
Consultant Surgeon
Leeds General Infirmary
Senior Lecturer
Leeds University
Leeds, United Kingdom

Miguel E. Martinez Noack, MD
Postdoctoral Fellow in Surgery
Tulane University School of Medicine
New Orleans, Louisiana

Jeffrey B. Matthews, MD
Associate Chief of General Surgery
Beth Israel Hospital
Associate Professor of Surgery
Harvard Medical School
Boston, Massachusetts

Emeran A. Mayer, MD
Director, Center for Functional Bowel and Motility
  Disorders
University of California Los Angeles Center for Health
  Sciences
Professor of Medicine and Physiology
University of California School of Medicine
Los Angeles, California

David W. McFadden, MD
Professor of Surgery
Chief, Division of General Surgery
University of California Los Angeles School of Medicine
Los Angeles, California

Howard R. Mertz, MD
Assistant Professor of Medicine
Division of Gastroenterology
Vanderbilt University School of Medicine
Nashville, Tennessee

J. Michael Millis, MD
Co-Director, Liver Transplant Program
University of Chicago Hospitals
Assistant Professor of Surgery
University of Chicago
Chicago, Illinois

Fredrick J. Montz, MD
Attending Surgeon
Gynecologic Oncology Service
University of California Los Angeles Center for Health
  Sciences
Associate Professor
Department of Obstetrics and Gynecology
University of California Los Angeles School of Medicine
Los Angeles, California

Ernest E. Moore, MD
Chief, Department of Surgery
Denver General Hospital
Professor and Vice Chairman of Surgery
University of Colorado Health Sciences Center
Denver, Colorado

Frederick A. Moore, MD
Director, General Surgery and Trauma and Critical
  Care
Hermann Hospital
Professor and Vice Chairman of Surgery
University of Texas–Houston Medical School
Houston, Texas

Sean J. Mulvihill, MD
Chief, Division of General Surgery
Associate Professor of Surgery
University of California San Francisco
San Francisco, California

Robert J. Myerson, MD
Associate Professor of Radiology
Radiation Oncology Center

Washington University School of Medicine
St. Louis, Missouri

David L. Nahrwold, MD
Surgeon-in-Chief
Northwestern Memorial Hospital
Loyal and Edith Davis Professor and Chairman
Department of Surgery
Northwestern University Medical School
Chicago, Illinois

L. K. Nathanson, FRACS
Consultant Surgeon
Royal Brisbane Hospital
Associate Professor of Surgery
University of Queensland
Brisbane, Queensland, Australia

Santhat Nivatvongs, MD, FACS
Consultant in Colon and Rectal Surgery
Mayo Clinic
Professor of Surgery
Mayo Medical School
Rochester, Minnesota

Jeffrey A. Norton, MD
Attending Surgeon
Barnes Hospital
Professor of Surgery
Chief of Endocrine and Oncologic Surgery
Washington University School of Medicine
St. Louis, Missouri

Marshall J. Orloff, MD
Professor of Surgery
University of California San Diego Medical Center
University of California San Diego School of Medicine
San Diego, California

Mark S. Orloff, MD
Associate Professor of Surgery
Section of Solid Organ Transplantation
Strong Memorial Hospital
University of Rochester
Rochester, New York

Thomas George Parks
Consultant surgeon
Belfast City Hospital
Professor of Surgical Science
Queen's University of Belfast
Belfast, Ireland

Edward Passaro, Jr., MD
Chief, Surgical Service
Veterans Administration Medical Center West Los
  Angeles
Professor of Surgery
University of California Los Angeles School of Medicine
Los Angeles, California

Carlos A. Pellegrini, MD
Professor of Surgery
Chairman, Department of Surgery
University of Washington School of Medicine
Seattle, Washington

Gary R. Peplinski, MD
Resident in Surgery
Barnes Hospital
Washington University School of Medicine
St. Louis, Missouri

Jeffrey H. Peters, MD
Chief, Section of General Surgery
University of Southern California University Hospital
Associate Professor of Surgery
University of Southern California School of Medicine
Los Angeles, California

Jack Pickleman, MD
Chief, Division of General Surgery
Loyola University Medical Center
Dr. and Mrs. John Igini Professor of Surgery
Loyola University Stritch School of Medicine
Maywood, Illinois

Henry A. Pitt, MD
Professor and Vice Chairman
Department of Surgery
Johns Hopkins University School of Medicine
Baltimore, Maryland

John H. C. Ranson, MD*
S. Arthur Localio Professor of Surgery
New York University
New York, New York

David W. Rattner, MD
Associate Visiting Surgeon
Massachusetts General Hospital
Associate Professor of Surgery
Harvard Medical School
Boston, Massachusetts

Robert A. Read, MD
Surgical Consultants
Denver, Colorado

Howard A. Reber, MD
Chief of Surgery
Sepulveda Veterans Administration Medical Center
Sepulveda, California
Professor and Vice Chairman
Department of Surgery
University of California Los Angeles School of Medicine
Los Angeles, California

John J. Ricotta, MD
Chairman, Department of Surgery
Millard Fillmore Hospital

Professor of Surgery
State University of New York at Buffalo
Buffalo, New York

Rolando H. Rolandelli, MD
Associate Professor of Surgery
Medical College of Pennsylvania
Hahnemann University
Philadelphia, Pennsylvania

Steven Rose, MD
Associate Professor of Radiology
University of California San Diego School of Medicine
Los Angeles, California

R. David Rosin, MS, FRCS, FRCS (Edin)
Chief Gastro-Intestinal and Soft Tissue Tumor Service
St. Mary's Hospital
Imperial College of Medicine
University of London
London, United Kingdom

Joel J. Roslyn, MD
Professor and Chairman
Department of Surgery
The Medical College of Pennsylvania
Hahnemann University
Philadelphia, Pennsylvania

Seymour I. Schwartz, MD
Distinguished Alumni Professor and Chair
Department of Surgery
University of Rochester School of Medicine and
    Dentistry
Rochester, New York

Mika N. Sinanan, MD, PhD
Attending Surgeon
University of Washington Medical Center
Assistant Professor of Surgery
University of Washington School of Medicine
Seattle, Washington

Peter W. Soballe, MD, FACS
Assistant Professor of Surgery
Head, Surgical Oncology
National Naval Medical Center
Bethesda, Maryland
Uniformed Services University of Health Sciences
Washington, DC

Nathaniel J. Soper, MD
Staff Surgeon
Barnes Hospital
Associate Professor of Surgery
Washington University School of Medicine
St. Louis, Missouri

*Deceased

David I. Soybel, MD
Associate in Surgery
Brigham and Women's Hospital
Associate Professor of Surgery
Harvard Medical School
Boston, Massachusetts

Lewis Spitz, MB, ChB, PhD, FRCS
Nuffield Professor of Pediatric Surgery
Consultant Surgeon
Great Ormond Street Hospital for Children
Professor
Institute of Child Health
University of London
London, United Kingdom

Bruce E. Stabile, MD
Chairman, Department of Surgery
Harbor–University of California Los Angeles Medical
   Center
Torrance, California
Professor of Surgery
University of California Los Angeles School of
   Medicine
Los Angeles, California

Michael J. Stamos, MD
Chief, Section of Colon and Rectal Surgery
Harbor–University of California Los Angeles Medical
   Center
Torrance, California
Assistant Professor of Surgery
University of California Los Angeles School of Medicine
Los Angeles, California

David J. Sugerbaker, MD
Chief, Surgical Services
Dana Farber Cancer Institute
Chief, Division of Thoracic Surgery
Brigham and Women's Hospital
Associate Professor of Surgery
Harvard Medical School
Boston, Massachusetts

Harvey J. Sugerman, MD
Vice Chairman, Department of Surgery
Virginia Commonwealth University
David M. Hume Professor of Surgery
Medical College of Virginia
Richmond, Virginia

James C. Thompson, MD
Surgeon, The University of Texas Medical Branch
   Hospitals
Ashbel Smith Professor of Surgery
The University of Texas Medical Branch
Galveston, Texas

Ronald K. Tompkins, MD, MSc
Chief, Section of Gastrointestinal Surgery
University of California Los Angeles Medical Center
Professor of Surgery
University of California School of Medicine
Los Angeles, California

Andrew L. Warshaw, MD
Chief, General Surgery
Massachusetts General Hospital
Harold and Ellen Danser Professor of Surgery
Harvard Medical School
Boston, Massachusetts

Karen W. West, MD
Associate Professor
Section of Pediatric Surgery
Indiana University School of Medicine
Indianapolis, Indiana

Edward E. Whang, MD
Assistant Resident, General Surgery
Department of Surgery
University of California Los Angeles
Los Angeles, California

**John Wong, MBBS, PhD, MD(Hon), FRACS,
   FRCS(Edin), FACS (Hon)**
Professor and Head
Department of Surgery
The University of Hong Kong
Queen Mary Hospital
Hong Kong

Charles J. Yeo, MD
Attending Surgeon
The Johns Hopkins Hospital
Professor of Surgery
Associate Professor of Oncology
The Johns Hopkins University School of Medicine
Baltimore, Maryland

Peter T. Zimmerman, MD
Assistant Clinical Professor of Radiology
University of California Los Angeles School of
   Medicine
Los Angeles, California

Michael J. Zinner, MD, FACS
Moseley Professor of Surgery
Harvard University Medical School
Surgeon-in-Chief
Brigham and Women's Hospital
Boston, Massachusetts

CONTENTS

PREFACE

It is an honor and a privilege to be given the opportunity to edit *Maingot's Abdominal Operations*. In the past five decades and through nine editions, this text has become the standard for all general surgeons and surgeons-in-training. The new edition of this textbook is a complete revision—a completely new book. We have expanded the focus of the book to include more operative procedures as well as new concepts in diagnosis and new management of diseases. As in past editions, we have drawn on internationally recognized groups of contributors who share their contemporary experience with the readers. This book is an up-to-date text on current diagnostic procedures and surgical techniques related to the management and care of patients with all types of abdominal disease and injury.

An extensive artwork program was undertaken for this 10th edition. More than 700 line drawings have been redone. They depict the chapter authors' preferred method for performing certain surgical procedures. Approximately 80% of all the illustrations in this edition are new, giving the book a more modern and consistent look.

Section I, Diagnostic and Interventional Procedures, deals with the symptoms and conditions that bring the patient to the surgeon. These include gastrointestinal bleeding, functional gastrointestinal syndromes, nausea and vomiting, constipation and diarrhea, and abdominal pain. The contributors bring newer concepts and treatment to these areas.

Many sections have been added, including contemporary endoscopic and laparoscopic techniques, since these are becoming an increasingly important operative tool for the practicing surgeon. In many sections of the book there are deliberate duplications to bring more than one perspective to an important disease entity. For example, in the section on peptic disease of the stomach and duodenum, two perspectives are given—one by David Johnston and Iain Martin, one by Bruce Stabile and Edward Passaro. This book is the work of distinguished international authors, and is intended to represent a complete and explicit account of the diseases and techniques for their treatment as are currently practiced in the world's finest teaching hospitals, large general hospitals, and surgical clinics.

In addition to adding new chapters, we have expanded old chapters. For example, we have extended the topic of operations on the esophagus into Benign Disorders of the Esophagus (Chapter 24) and Surgical Procedures to Resect or Replace the Esophagus (Chapter 26). We have added chapters on the Surgical Management of Ascites (Chapter 56), as well as on Gynecological Pelvic Procedures (Chapter 82) as they relate to the surgeon dealing with gastrointestinal disease. In each chapter, where appropriate, laparoscopic procedures have been added as they become more established in the practice of abdominal surgery.

In the preface to his sixth edition, Rodney Maingot noted: "As all literature is personal, the contributors have been given a free hand with their individual sections. A certain latitude in style and expression is stimulating to the thoughtful reader." Similarly, in this edition, we have tried to maintain consistency for the reader; however, the contributors have been given a free hand in their contributions.

I give my appreciation and grateful thanks to my co-editors, Seymour Schwartz and Harold Ellis for their assistance in the preparation of this edition. Without their support and cooperation, we would not have been able to publish this edition. I am also intensely grateful for the contributions of Stanley Ashley and David McFadden. They played an essential role in organizing early components of the text. They have generously given their time and made important contributions, not only as chapter contributors, but also as section editors.

At Appleton & Lange, I would like to thank Edward H. Wickland, Jr. for his unwavering support during the lengthy time of this project development. His support and the support of the publisher was critical to the success of this textbook. Also at Appleton & Lange, the support and help of Kathleen McCullough, Managing Editor of Development, and Cynthia Shepard, developmental editor, were invaluable in finally putting all this work into a single comprehensive textbook. Their suggestions and attention to detail made it possible to overcome the innumerable problems that occur in publishing such a large textbook.

I have had the good fortune to deal with outstanding illustrators during the development of this book. These include Gwynne Gloege, who was our in-house illustrator at the University of California, Los Angeles, as well as Philip Ashley, medical illustrator extraordinaire, who, in addition to creating quality illustrations, maintained a consistent stylistic theme throughout the entire book by coordinating a group of outstanding medical illustrators, including Tracie Aretz, Jessica Buchman, Juan Garcia, Nicole Mock, and Lynn Reynolds. A special thanks goes to Jessica Buchman for her commitment, professionalism, and tireless efforts throughout the entire project.

Finally, I owe a great debt of gratitude to my three assistants who have survived the trials of this book, Carole Dool, Karen Tyler, and Patrina Tucker. They have helped me with every step of the work, from helping type manuscripts, to reading and editing proof, and for their encouragement during the prolonged dry periods and preparation of this textbook.

To all of those who contributed, thank you very much.

Michael J. Zinner, MD, FACS

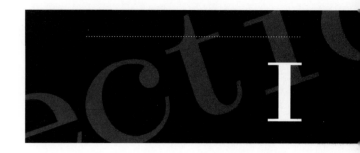

I

DIAGNOSTIC AND INTERVENTIONAL PROCEDURES

1

Radiology of the Abdomen

Barbara M. Kadell ▪ *Peter Zimmerman* ▪ *David S.-K. Lu*

Radiology of the abdomen has progressed rapidly in the nearly 100 years since the discovery of the x-ray in 1895. Each new diagnostic modality has expanded the radiologist's ability to offer more accurate diagnoses and, with interventional techniques, has increased treatment options. It is now rare for a surgical patient not to have some imaging work-up done either preoperatively, in the immediate postoperative period, or in the course of follow-up.

Plain abdominal films and barium contrast studies of the gastrointestinal tract were the earliest imaging methods used to evaluate the abdomen and are still the modalities of choice in many clinical situations. Advances in equipment design such as image intensification and digital spot filming have decreased radiation exposure to the patient and have increased resolution. Technical refinements such as double contrast techniques and improved contrast agents have enhanced accuracy. Finally, the use of adjunctive medication such as glucagon and metoclopramide to alter bowel motility have improved the quality of gastrointestinal contrast examinations.

Nuclear medicine studies are being used increasingly for their functional imaging capabilities rather than their ability to search for focal organ defects. Quantification of gastrointestinal motility is possible using radioactive isotope–labeled meals. Isotope studies are used to locate inflammation and infection and are used routinely in the evaluation of patients with biliary and gallbladder disease.

In patients with colonic and ovarian carcinoma, commercially available radiolabeled monoclonal antibodies permit the visualization of distant tumor sites. In the future, this technique may become routine for evaluation of patients with other neoplasms.

In most medical centers, *ultrasound* is now a routine diagnostic examination as well as an excellent method of guiding interventional procedures in the abdomen. Sonography has virtually replaced cholecystography in the initial work-up of the patient suspected of having gallbladder disease. Because of its ability to differentiate tissue characteristics, sonography has become a valuable technique for evaluating solid organs such as the liver, pancreas, and spleen. Doppler techniques are widely used for assessing blood flow. Endoscopic ultrasound is performed to assess extent of extramucosal disease in patients with esophageal, gastric, and colonic pathology, and intraoperative ultrasound is used to search for small neoplasms of the liver and pancreas.

Computed tomography (CT) has become a standard procedure of evaluation in the patient with suspected abdominal pathology. Rapid scanning and high resolution have become possible because of refinements in equipment and technique. Newer, safer contrast agents are available as are optimal rates of contrast delivery with power injectors. Evaluation of the solid organs, the bowel, mesentery, peritoneum, lymph nodes, bones, and major blood vessels is now possible. CT is commonly used in the emergency room, especially in patients with acute abdominal pain or blunt abdominal trauma. In the postoperative patient, it is used to determine the presence of fluid collections, abscesses, and hematomas. CT is also used to guide interventional procedures such as biopsies or drainages of fluid collections.

Magnetic resonance imaging (MRI) has multiplanar imaging capabilities and is capable of differentiating small differences in soft tissue characteristics. However, its use in the abdomen is limited compared to its use in other portions of the body, such as the central nervous system and musculoskeletal system, owing to continued problems with motions artifacts, examination time, standardization of bowel and intravenous contrast, uniformity of scanning sequences, and spatial resolution. Rapid advancements in the field will undoubtedly make MRI increasingly useful in abdominal surgery and exploration. In some institutions, it is already the imaging modality of choice for evaluation of the liver and pancreas. MRI angiography also is being used in an increased number of applications in the abdomen.

The large and diverse number of imaging tools used for evaluation of the abdomen make it possible to answer the same clinical question with several different modalities. These are all equally reliable, with no one single correct method. The choice of which method to use depends on such factors as equipment availability, cost, technical expertise, patient status, and the physician's and radiologist's confidence and comfort with a particular algorithm.

In the following sections, we outline the approach taken at our institution. Other equally acceptable approaches may be used in other centers.

■ RADIOLOGY OF THE ESOPHAGUS

Radiologic evaluation of the esophagus is accomplished primarily by the use of a radiopaque contrast esophagram. Newer imaging modalities such as CT, MRI, and endoscopic ultrasound are used in patients with suspected trauma or tumor, often to answer specific questions raised by the esophagogram. Nuclear medicine techniques help to quantify esophageal emptying and may reveal reflux in the pediatric patient.

PLAIN FILMS

Esophageal pathology may be discovered incidentally on the most frequently requested radiographic examination, the chest film.[1,2]

Trauma

In the patient who has sustained trauma to the chest or trauma to the esophagus as a result of instrumentation, foreign body perforation, or Boerhaave's syndrome, plain film findings may include mediastinal widening, subcutaneous and/or mediastinal emphysema, pleural effusions, pneumothorax, or hydropneumothorax (Fig 1–1).

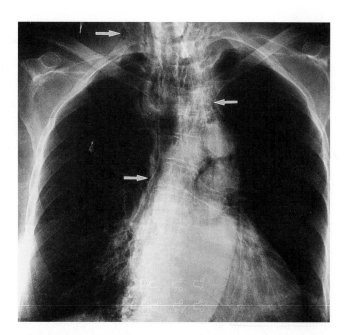

Figure 1–1. Esophageal perforation during endoscopy. Mediastinal and subcutaneous emphysema is evident (arrows).

Motility Disorders

In patients with esophageal motility disorders such as achalasia, scleroderma, or pseudo-obstruction, chest films may be positive only in advanced phases of the diseases. Chest radiographs taken in the erect position may reveal an air-fluid level in a dilated esophagus, widening of the paraspinous stripe, or obliteration of the posterior heart border as seen on a lateral film. Pulmonary infiltrates may occur if aspiration complicates the motility disorder (Fig 1–2).

Neoplasms

A large esophageal neoplasm, such as a carcinoma or, rarely, a leiomyoma, may cause a retrotracheal, subcarinal or retrocardiac mass on a chest radiograph. If the mass causes obstruction, the esophagus will be dilated and fluid filled.

Diverticula and Hernias

Esophageal diverticula and large duplication cysts may appear on chest radiograph as a mass, with or without an air-fluid level. A large Zenker's diverticulum may produce a superior mediastinal mass. An epiphrenic diverticulum may cause a retrocardiac mass, whereas a midesophageal diverticulum will cause a subcarinal mass. A large hiatal hernia may produce a retrocardiac mass often containing an air-fluid level.

Varices

Rarely, large distal esophageal varices may produce a retrocardiac or posterior mediastinal lobulated mass sil-

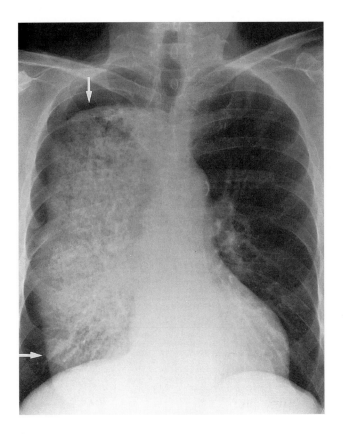

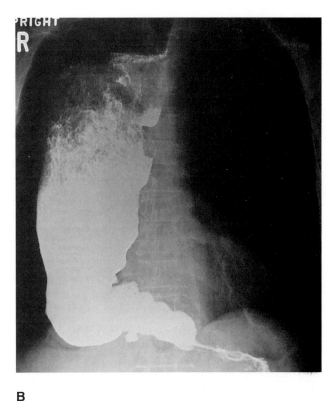

Figure 1–2. **A.** Large right thoracic "pseudomass" is the result of markedly distended esophagus in a patient with achalasia (arrows). **B.** Barium esophagram shows markedly dilated esophagus.

houetting the descending aorta, as seen on a chest radiograph.

Postoperative

Patients who have had surgical procedures such as esophagogastrectomy with esophageal pull-up, esophagectomy with colonic interposition, or hiatal hernia repair with fundal plication often have indicative findings on a chest radiograph. These include an air/fluid–filled intrathoracic stomach or interposed colonic segment. A fundal plication produces a smooth masslike defect in the medial aspect of the gastric air bubble (Fig 1–3).

CONTRAST ESOPHAGOGRAPHY

Double-Contrast Barium Esophagogram

When esophageal disease is suspected clinically, a contrast examination is indicated. This examination has evolved into a highly accurate method of showing even very small mucosal lesions. A biphasic barium esophagogram is the imaging procedure of choice for morphologic examination of the esophagus. A complete barium study of the esophagus consists of upright (air

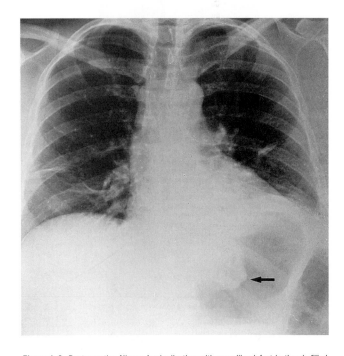

Figure 1–3. Postoperative Nissen fundoplication with masslike defect in the air-filled gastric fundus (*arrow*).

contrast), prone (full column), and supine examinations (mucosal relief; reflux evaluation).[3–5]

Upright. The patient is given high-density barium to coat the esophageal mucosa. Effervescent granules in a small amount of water also are given to produce gas which distends the barium-filled lumen, thereby allowing an excellent view of the esophageal mucosa (Fig 1–4). The mucosa of the distended esophageal lumen will appear smooth and featureless in the normal patient.

Reflux esophagitis may appear as thickened or nodular mucosa, granular mucosa, or a combination of both conditions (Fig 1–5). Ulceration and inflammatory polyps and strictures may be present (Fig 1–6).[6]

Barrett's esophagus occurs when the normal squamous epithelium of the esophagus is replaced by columnar epithelium. This condition is thought to result from long-standing gastroesophageal reflux and is a premalignant condition.

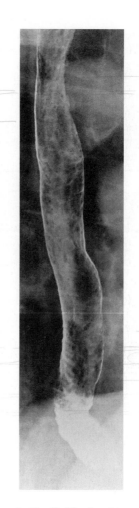

Figure 1–5. Reflux esophagitis with diffusely nodular mucosa pattern of the entire esophagus.

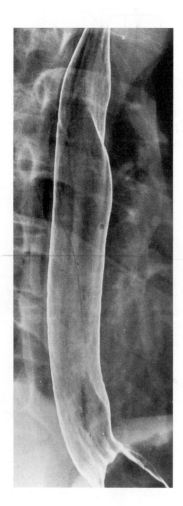

Figure 1–4. Normal air contrast esophagram showing a smooth and featureless mucosa.

Radiographic findings may include those mentioned for reflux esophagitis, plus a high esophageal stricture (Fig 1–7). Ulcers and strictures may occur at a distance from the gastroesophageal junction. However, most strictures that occur in patients with Barrett's esophagus occur in the more common distal esophageal location. A reticular mucosal pattern seen on air contrast views occasionally has been described in these patients. Contrast esophagography may be helpful in determining patient risk for Barrett's esophagus. Patients with a high stricture or ulcer and a reticular mucosal pattern are considered high risk and should undergo endoscopy.[4]

Infectious esophagitis may result from *Candida*, herpes, cytomegalovirus (CMV), or the HIV virus. On double-contrast views, *Candida* infections appear as discrete, plaquelike lesions or with an overall shaggy appearance and an irregular contour with ulcerations. Rarely, a mass lesion consisting of necrotic material and abundant fungis (fungus ball) may be present. Herpes may appear as clusters of small ulcerations on an otherwise normal mucosal background. Advanced esophageal

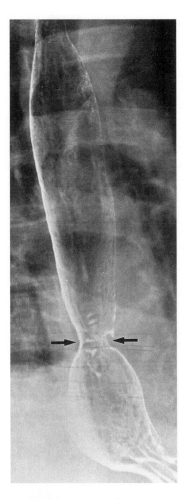

Figure 1–6. Reflux esophagitis with ulcerations (*arrows*) and stricture.

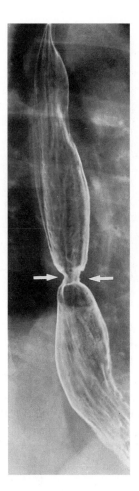

Figure 1–7. Barrett's esophagus with stricture (*arrows*) at junction of the middle and distal thirds of the esophagus.

herpes infection may be difficult to differentiate radiologically from severe candidiasis. CMV may produce discrete ulcerations similar to those seen in herpes infection. A more distinctive finding is the presence of one or more flat, large ulcerations.

Abnormalities on esophagography also may be present with other esophagitides such as those due to Crohn's disease, radiation, drugs, or those associated with dermatologic disorders; for example, epidermolysis bullosa dystrophica, bullous pemphigoid, or pemphigus vulgaris. Clinical history is therefore important, since some of these lesions produce similar radiographic changes.[7]

Neoplasms. Benign esophageal neoplasms are often submucosal and have a smooth surface. They are significantly less common than malignant esophageal tumors. Leiomyomas are the most common benign neoplasm and are found mostly in the middle third of the esophagus (Fig 1–8). These smooth, submucosal lesions may contain calcification. In profile, they have a smooth surface and the upper and lower borders form either right or obtuse an-

gles with the adjacent esophageal wall. A small number may cause annular lesions. Other benign masses of the esophagus include papillomas, adenomas, inflammatory esophagogastric polyps, and duplication cysts.[8]

Esophageal carcinoma. Squamous cell esophageal carcinoma is the most common esophageal neoplasm. Early lesions appear as small polypoid masses on air contrast view. A superficial tumor may appear radiographically as multiple, small mucosal nodules. Advanced tumors may appear as infiltrating, polypoid, ulcerative, or varicoid lesions. Infiltrating tumors usually cause luminal narrowing, nodular mucosa, and an abrupt transition between normal esophagus and tumor (Fig 1–9). Polypoid tumors often ulcerate and may produce obstruction due to their bulk. Varicoid carcinoma, the most unusual radiographic presentation, appears as markedly thickened mucosal folds and may be confused with esophageal varices. Dysphagia is rarely present with this variety.

Esophageal adenocarcinoma frequently arises in Barrett's mucosa. Early tumors may appear radiographi-

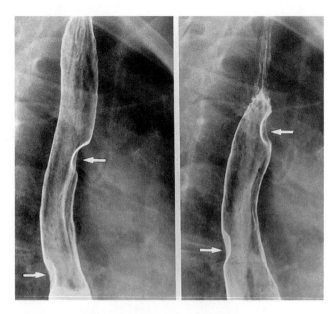

Figure 1–8. Esophageal leiomyomas (*arrows*) in the midthoracic esophagus. Note smooth contour, typical of submucosal lesions.

cally as polypoid lesions or as a straightening and rigidity of a portion of the wall of a stricture. Advanced lesions frequently narrow or obstruct the lumen and cause mucosal nodularity. Ulceration may be present.[9]

Varices. Varices may appear on air contrast views as serpiginous filling defects that change with respiration and patient position. Care must be taken to rule out the possibility of a varicoid esophageal carcinoma, an uncommon carcinoma that may diffusely involve the mucosa without causing significant obstruction. Respiration rarely changes the appearance of these tumor masses.

Prone–full column views. Prone esophageal views are taken as the patient swallows a large bolus of barium to distend maximally the esophagus and gastroesophageal junction. Webs, strictures, diverticula, and hiatal hernias are optimally demonstrated with this view.

Webs. Esophageal webs are seen in the anterior aspect of the proximal cervical esophagus. They appear as thin, smooth, linear defects in the barium column, but occasionally may be circumferential. Most occur without an underlying disease. However, some webs also may occur with dermatologic diseases involving the esophagus; for example, bullous pemphigoid, or epidermolysis bullosa dystrophica, and Plummer-Vinson syndrome. Webs may cause partial esophageal obstruction and aspiration.

Strictures. Esophageal strictures may result from postoperative scarring, reflux esophagitis, Crohn's disease, radiation, caustic ingestion, dermatologic diseases, infiltrat-

ing metastases, and as a complication of nasogastric intubation. The clinical history is important in determining the cause of strictures. Benign strictures usually produce a smooth tapered luminal narrowing (Fig 1–10).

Esophageal diverticula. Zenker's diverticulum, occurring at the pharyngoesophageal junction, is the most common esophageal diverticulum. Midesophageal diverticulum is the second most common diverticulum, and epiphrenic diverticulum is the least common. Most are produced by pulsion, but some midesophageal diverticula may be caused by traction owing to prior mediastinal inflammation or as a result of an underlying motility disorder. On barium esophagram, these diverticula appear as smooth outpouchings from the esophageal lumen and usually have a narrower neck than base. They may retain contrast after the remainder of the esophagus has emptied (Fig 1–11).

Hiatal hernia. Hiatal hernias are the most common abnormality seen on the full-column esophagogram. Most are of the sliding type, and the cardia may be seen above the

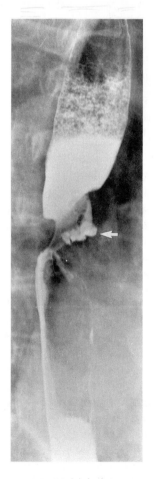

Figure 1–9. Short, abrupt, infiltrating lesion with mucosal ulceration (*arrow*) in esophageal carcinoma.

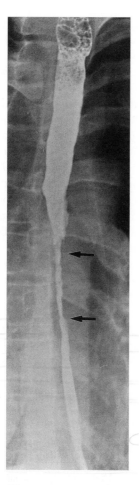

Figure 1–10. Long esophageal strictures due to lye ingestion (*arrows*).

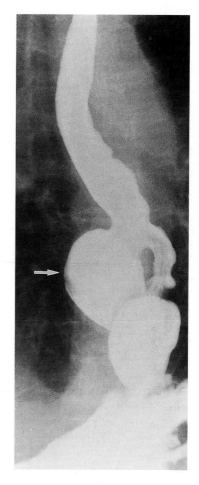

Figure 1–11. Large epiphrenic diverticulum.

diaphragm only when the patient is examined in the prone position. When upright, the hernia may reduce or be more difficult to distend. A hiatal hernia should be suspected if a mucosal ring is seen 2 cm or more above the diaphragm or if gastric folds are present above the diaphragm (Fig 1–12). A Schatzki ring is a thin, weblike circumferential constriction that may occur at the cardioesophageal junction. The hernia is inferior to this ring. If the diameter of the lumen at the level of the ring is less than 13 mm, there is a high correlation with dysphagia. Prone full-column views best demonstrate these.

A paraesophageal hernia is significantly less common than an axial hiatal hernia. It occurs when the cardioesophageal junction is in its normal subdiaphragmatic location, but a portion of the stomach herniates alongside the distal esophagus through the esophageal hiatus. These hernias are usually asymptomatic. However, with large hernias, a risk of incarceration and strangulation exists (Fig 1–13).[4]

Supine view. Mucosal relief films show the partially collapsed lumen of the esophagus and are performed with the patient in a supine position. The normal barium-coated, collapsed esophageal lumen shows straight, parallel, fine mucosal folds that are only a few millimeters apart. Esophageal varices appear as thick and serpiginous filling defects. The gastric fundus is filled with barium and the patient is evaluated for the presence of reflux. The presence of gastroesophageal reflux may be demonstrated with the understanding that reflux may be an intermittent phenomenon and not always documented during the brief period of radiographic examination.[6]

Single-Contrast Esophagogram

Single-contrast esophagogram, without air contrast technique, is used in patients suspected of having a foreign body impaction. After the foreign body has been removed or has spontaneously passed, a full repeat esophagogram should be performed to rule out the presence of a partially obstructing lesion such as a web, stricture, Schatzki ring, tumor, or dysmotility. A single-contrast study also may be performed to determine whether displacement or effacement of the esophagus as a result of an extrinsic process is present.

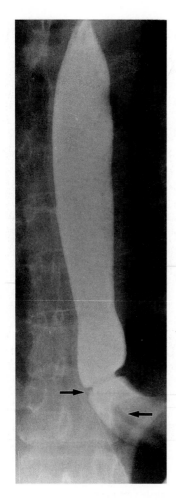

Figure 1–12. Hiatal hernia on full column esophagram. Both mucosal ring (*arrow*) and gastric folds (*arrow*) are seen above the diaphragm.

Esophagography Using Water-Soluble Iodinated Contrast

Esophagography with iodinated contrast material is used in patients suspected of having esophageal perforation due to posttrauma, instrumentation, violent retching or vomiting (suspected Boerhaave's syndrome), or, postoperatively, to demonstrate anastomotic integrity. If the clinical suspicion is aspiration or a tracheoesophageal fistula, barium is the preferred contrast agent, since the hypertonic properties of iodinated contrast in the tracheobronchial tree may cause inflammation and pneumonitis.

Videotaped Esophagography

Videotaped esophagography is performed to evaluate esophageal mortility. It is an excellent method by which to differentiate between patients who have motility disorders and those who have normal motility. Esophageal manometry may be necessary in a number of patients to subclassify the motility disorder.[5,10,11]

The patient is examined in the prone position. Up-

right views are not useful because gravity contributes to esophageal emptying. The patient is observed through a number of swallows, and the entire esophagus is viewed from the top of the barium column as it passes distally.

In normal patients, the upper esophageal sphincter relaxes on swallowing, allowing the bolus to enter the esophagus. Primary peristaltic or contraction waves, initiated by swallowing, move the bolus distally. A secondary peristaltic wave is a propulsive contraction that occurs when a portion of the bolus remains in the thoracic esophagus and causes distention. The wave clears the esophagus. The lower esophageal sphincter relaxes as these peristaltic waves approach. Tertiary contractions are nonpropulsive waves and are seen more commonly in older patients and in those with motility disorders.

Characteristic patterns of abnormal motility are seen with many diseases. In patients with diffuse esophageal spasm (DES), lumen-obliterating tertiary contraction waves may be present (Fig 1–14). In achalasia, swallowing is normal, but the usual esophageal primary stripping wave does not progress through the esophagus and the lower esophageal sphincter does not relax. The esophagus demonstrates varying degrees of dilatation, depending on severity, with a tapered narrowing ("rattail" deformity) at the level of the cardioesophageal junction (Fig 1–15). Nonpropulsive, tertiary contrac-

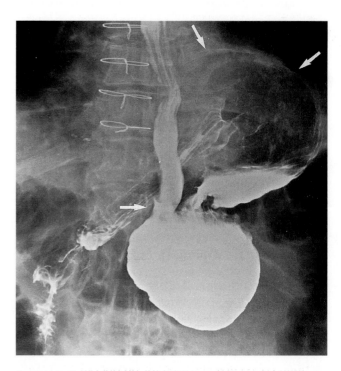

Figure 1–13. The gastroesophageal junction is below the diaphragm (*arrow*) and the gastric body (*arrows*) has herniated through the esophageal hiatus resulting in an "upside-down" stomach.

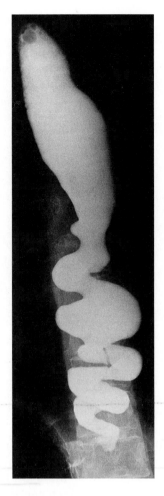

Figure 1–14. Diffuse esophageal spasm. Esophageal dilatation and deep tertiary contractions are present.

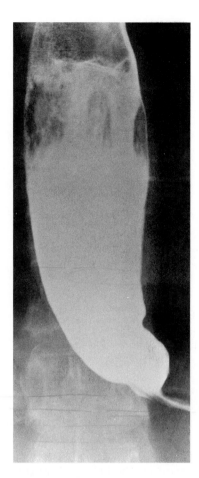

Figure 1–15. Achalasia. The esophagus is dilated and there is marked, tapered narrowing at the cardioesophageal junction (rat-tail deformity) (*arrows*).

tions may be present. In the patient with scleroderma, swallowing is normal, and motility appears normal in the proximal one-third of the esophagus (striated muscle) but dissipates in the lower two-thirds of the esophagus (smooth muscle). Varying degrees of esophageal dilatation may be present. Relaxation of the lower esophageal sphincter enables reflux to occur. Mucosal changes are often present. Hiatal hernias, ulcerations, and strictures may appear as complications.

In the final phase of motility evaluation, the patient is placed in the supine position and evaluated for reflux.

CT AND MRI

Cross-sectional imaging techniques are not only useful in outlining the esophagus but also to demonstrate the relationship between the esophagus and the structures around it. CT is currently used for preoperative staging of esophageal carcinoma (Fig 1–16). However, it is not a universally accepted procedure for this purpose.[12–15]

It is used to evaluate esophageal involvement and displacement by disease in surrounding organs such as thyroid, lung, vascular rings, lymphoma, and mediastinal masses. Additionally, CT can be used to explain extrinsic pressure defects seen on a barium esophagography. Finally, CT is used to determine the extent of mediastinal involvement in esophageal trauma. Findings in esophageal perforation include periesophageal fluid, extraluminal air, esophageal thickening, and pleural effusion.[16] CT is also used to determine if a tumor has recurred in the postoperative patient.[17]

The study is optimized by giving the patient barium paste to coat the esophageal mucosa and intravenous iodinated contrast to improve delineation of vessels and fat planes. The scan extends from the thoracic inlet through the liver.

Involvement of the trachea, aorta, and pericardium can be accurately assessed, but assessment of mediastinal involvement decreases owing to the variability of fat planes in different patients.

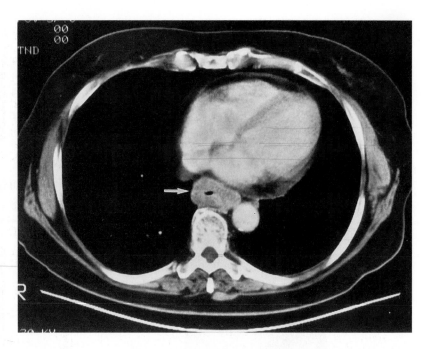

Figure 1–16. Esophageal carcinoma on CT. Arrow indicates markedly thickened esophageal wall due to carcinoma. No extension beyond esophageal wall is present.

The criteria on CT for abnormal lymph nodes is enlargement or low attenuation due to necrosis. Accuracy in assessing lymph node involvement is compromised because of the frequency of tumor-involved but normal-sized lymph nodes.

The cardioesophageal junction, a region where carcinoma frequently occurs, is often difficult to evaluate on CT because of suboptimal distention. Such distention may produce a pseudotumor as a result of either a collapsed hiatal hernia or gastric fundus.

MRI currently has limited use in the investigation of esophageal disease. It is primarily used for evaluating the extent of mediastinal disease in lesions involving the esophagus, either primarily or secondarily. Limitations include long scan times. However, because of its multiplanar reconstruction capabilities and superior tissue-contrast sensitivity, MR may eventually prove to be a superior modality.[17]

SONOGRAPHY

In recent years, endoscopic sonography has offered hope of more accurate assessment of the esophageal wall and surrounding mediastinum, and is performed most frequently in cases of neoplasm evaluation. It is also helpful is assessing an esophagogastric anastomosis is cases of suspected tumor recurrence and in differentiating achalasia from pseudoachalasia, which is a smooth narrowing of the distal esophagus produced by submucosally infiltrating tumor that appears similar on esophagography to achalasia.

Endoscopic sonography also may prove useful in assessing the extent of mediastinal tumor involvement and in evaluating diseased but normal-sized lymph nodes. Many lesions visualized also may be biopsied.[18,19] This procedure requires a team approach by an expert endoscopist and radiologist.

The normal endoscopic sonogram of the esophagus shows five alternating hyperechoic and hypoechoic layers of the esophageal wall: the superficial mucosa, deep mucosa, interface between the submucosa and muscularis, muscularis propria, and the adventitia (Figs 1–17 and 1–18). Tumor invasion disrupts these normal layers. A major pitfall of this method is the inability of the endoscope to traverse many stenotic esophageal lesions.

Conventional sonography may be helpful in infants to assess the presence of gastroesophageal reflux after the ingestion of barium or milk. This procedure may also be used in follow-up, after antireflux surgical procedures have been performed.

NUCLEAR MEDICINE

Nuclear medicine techniques in the esophagus afford quantification of the volume of retained foods or liquids. It is a simple, noninvasive technique and can be used as a screening test for dysmotility. Sensitivity is low in disorders where peristalsis is preserved but manometry shows high-amplitude contractions (nutcracker esophagus).

The patient is given technetium pertchnecate (^{99m}Tc)–containing liquid and is studied in a supine position. A gamma camera covering the whole esophagus is used for imaging.[20] The patient performs several dry swallows after swallowing the radiolabeled liquid. In the

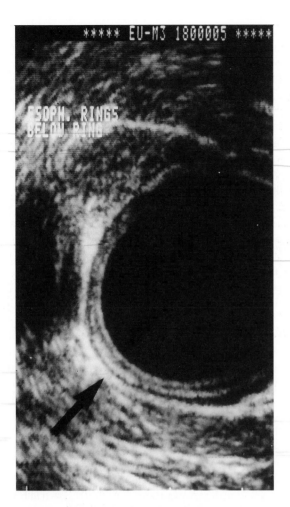

Figure 1–17. Normal endoscopic sonogram of the esophagus demonstrating five alternating hyperechoic and hypoechoic layers of the esophageal wall (*arrow*).

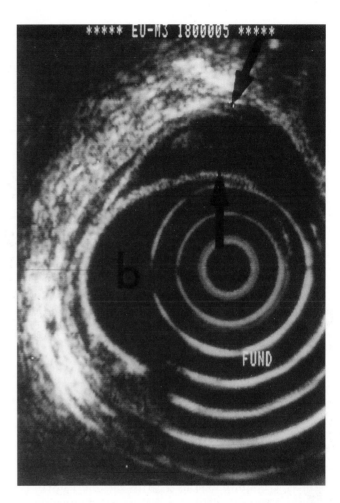

Figure 1–18. Carcinoma of the esophagus on sonogram. The normal esophageal wall is disrupted by the infiltrating tumor (*arrow*).

normal patient, activity decreases rapidly with no activity remaining after 5 to 10 seconds. The role of this technique is somewhat controversial. Some investigators find it to be worthwhile in assessing response after treatment, especially in patients with achalasia.

Scintigraphic methods to determine gastroesophageal reflux have shown low sensitivity. They involve administering a liquid containing ⁹⁹ᵐTc–sulfur colloid and imaging the patient in the supine position, and also using a gamma camera.

■ RADIOLOGY OF THE STOMACH AND DUODENUM

Radiographic evaluation of the stomach and duodenum is accomplished primarily by an upper gastrointestinal series (UGI) using barium as the contrast agent. Important refinements, such as the double contrast technique, have improved the quality of the examina-

tion as well as the detection of lesions. This method permits detailed examination of the lumen of the bowel. The use of CT now permits evaluation of the lumen, evaluation of the bowel wall, and evaluation of the relationship of adjacent organs, major blood vessels, lymph nodes, and peritoneum to the stomach and duodenum.

PLAIN FILMS

Plain abdominal films still have diagnostic value when evaluating the stomach.[21,22] Most patients have a small amount of gas, the gastric air bubble, present in the gastric fundus on an upright radiograph. Distortion of the gastric bubble may signify gastric pathology (Table 1–1). Gastric distention may arise from many causes, including air swallowing, diabetes, immobilization, drug side effects, and gastric outlet obstruction.

Absence of the gastric air bubble may indicate esophageal obstruction due either to tumor or motility disor-

TABLE 1–1. GASTRIC PATHOLOGY ON PLAIN RADIOGRAPHS

Distended stomach
Absent gastric air bubble
Displaced gastric air bubble
Double gastric air bubble
Intraluminal defects in air bubble
Air in gastric wall
Calcification
Pneumoperitoneum

der. Displacement of the air bubble may result from enlargement of surrounding organs such as the spleen, pancreas, or liver. The most common cause of gastric displacement is splenomegaly. A large hiatal hernia may cause the gastric air bubble to be in an abnormal left retrocardiac position, and gastric volvulus may produce a plain radiograph with the appearance of two gastric fluid levels, one above and one below the diaphragm.

Intraluminal defects in the gastric bubble may be produced by foreign bodies, mucosal or submucosal neoplasms, enlarged rugal folds, varices, hiatal hernia sacs, or postoperative states, such as with a Nissen fundoplication. Fold thickening may suggest neoplasm, gastritis, or a gastric hypersecretory state.

An uncommon but important sign to look for on plain films is the appearance of air in the wall of the stomach. Emphysematous gastritis may be caused by caustic ingestion, alcohol abuse, or gastric infarction, and has a 60% to 80% mortality rate.

On occasion, mucinous gastric neoplasms may be suggested on plain films by the fine, stippled calcifications often present in the tumor.

UPPER GASTROINTESTINAL SERIES

Mucosal detail is best evaluated by a double-contrast or biphasic barium examination of the stomach and duodenum. This is performed as part of a UGI series and also includes double-contrast examination of the esophagus.[23,24]

The patient should be given nothing by mouth 8 to 12 hours prior to the examination. Some examiners recommend administration of small quantities of IV glucagon (0.1 mg) to produce short-term hypotonia.

A small amount of high-density barium is used to coat the mucosa of the esophagus and stomach. Effervescent granules (sodium bicarbonate mixed with a small amount of H_2O to release CO_2) are added to distend the lumina of these areas. The patient is placed in the supine, prone, and oblique positions. Small mucosal lesions and ulcers should be detectable with optimal mucosal coating, compression spot radiographs, and luminal distention. Additional barium of a lower density

then is given to distend the stomach further and to determine if there are defects in the contrast-distended lumen.

The patient should be reasonably mobile and compliant for an optimal examination. When the patient is compromised, the examination should be tailored and possibly abbreviated. If a gastric perforation is suspected, an iodinated water-soluble contrast agent should be substituted for barium.[25]

Position

The gastric position may be altered by changes in surrounding organs such as the liver, spleen, pancreas, or diaphragm. The most common abnormality of gastric position is in a hiatal hernia where a portion of the gastric fundus herniates above the diaphragm through the esophageal hiatus. If the hernia is large, an air-fluid level in a left retrocardiac density may be seen on chest radiograph.

Torsion of the stomach may occur from laxity of its suspensary ligaments, diaphragmatic paralysis, or diaphragmatic defects, usually hiatal. Organoaxial volvulus occurs when the stomach rotates around an axis connecting the cardia and the pylorus. Mesenteroaxial volvulus indicates a rotation around an axis between the midlesser to midgreater curvature. This creates an "upside-down stomach" where the gastric body is in a position superior to the fundus. A double bubble may be seen on plain films with the superior air-fluid level above the diaphragm (air and fluid in the gastric body), and the inferior air-fluid level below the diaphragm (air and fluid in the gastric fundus). If no vascular compromise or obstruction is present, the patient may be asymptomatic and this anatomic aberration will be discovered incidentally. With vascular occlusion, acute symptoms of pain and vomiting will be present. Mortality rates are high unless the lesion is recognized and treated urgently (Fig 1–19).

Size and Shape

The "normal" range for gastric size is variable. The stomach may be abnormally small as a result of prior surgery, caustic ingestion, or neoplasms encroaching on the lumen. It may be abnormally large as a result of outlet obstruction, diabetes, the effects of certain medications, or immobilization.

Gastric shape or contour is also variable. Abnormalities may result from prior surgery, scarring from ulcer disease, neoplasms, or extrinsic compression from enlargement of surrounding organs.

Barium-Filled Contour

The barium-filled contour is normally smooth on the lesser curve and demonstrates a "regular irregularity" along the greater curvature from the orientation of the

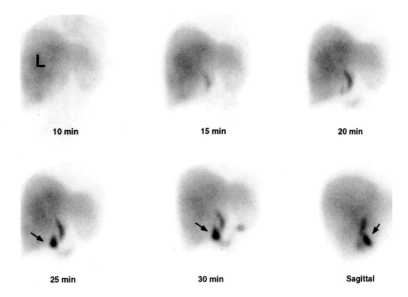

Figure 1–84. Normal ^{99m}Tc-HIDA hepatobiliary scan. Note tracer activity outlining the liver by 10 minutes, and excretion into the biliary tree with visualization of the gallbladder (*arrows*) by 20 minutes.

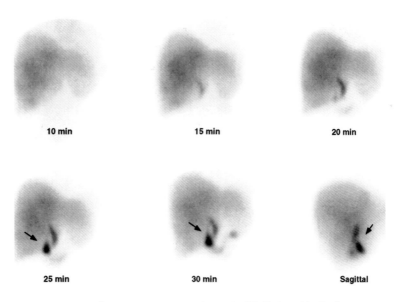

Figure 1–105. Normal ^{99m}Tc-HIDA scan. Note visualization of gallbladder (*arrow*) by 25 minutes.

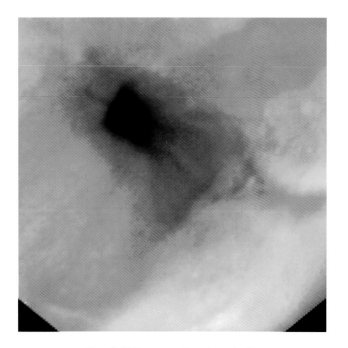

Figure 3–1. Biopsy-proven Barrett's esophagitis.

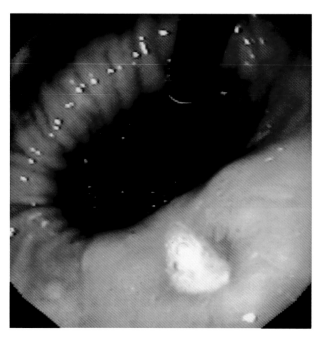

Figure 3–2. A proximal gastric ulcer noted with the endoscope in the retroflexed position.

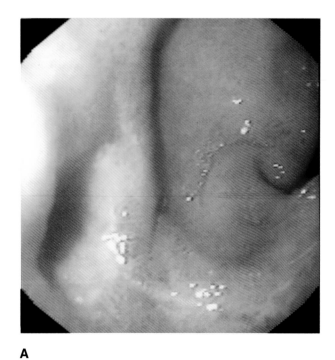

A

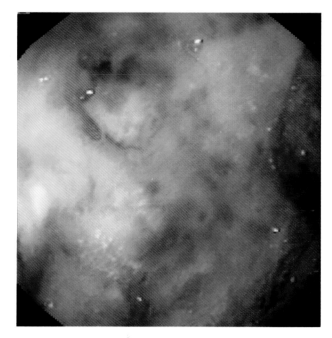

B

Figure 3–5. A. This duodenal ulcer was noted during upper gastrointestinal endoscopy in a patient with persistent epigastric abdominal pain.
B. Endoscopic image of an acute duodenal ulcer associated with surrounding duodenitis.

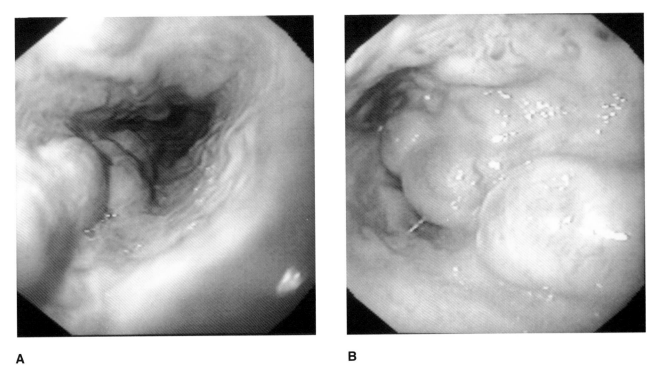

A

B

Figure 3–6. **A** and **B**. Two endoscopic images of esophageal varices.

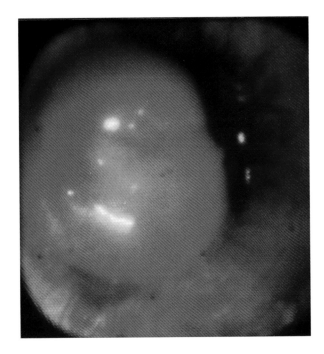

Figure 3–7. B. Photograph demonstrating a recently banded esophageal varix. (Courtesy of Dr. Greg Stiegmann).

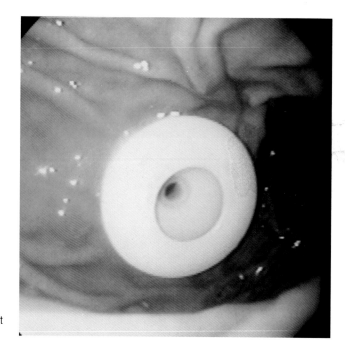

Figure 3–8. Endoscopic view of percutaneous endoscopic gastrostomy tube seated against the gastric wall and loosely opposing the gastric wall to the anterior abdominal wall.

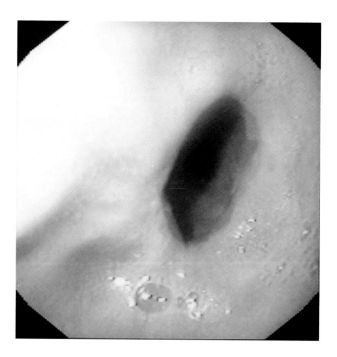

Figure 3–9. A benign peptic esophageal stricture which was treated with endoscopic dilatation.

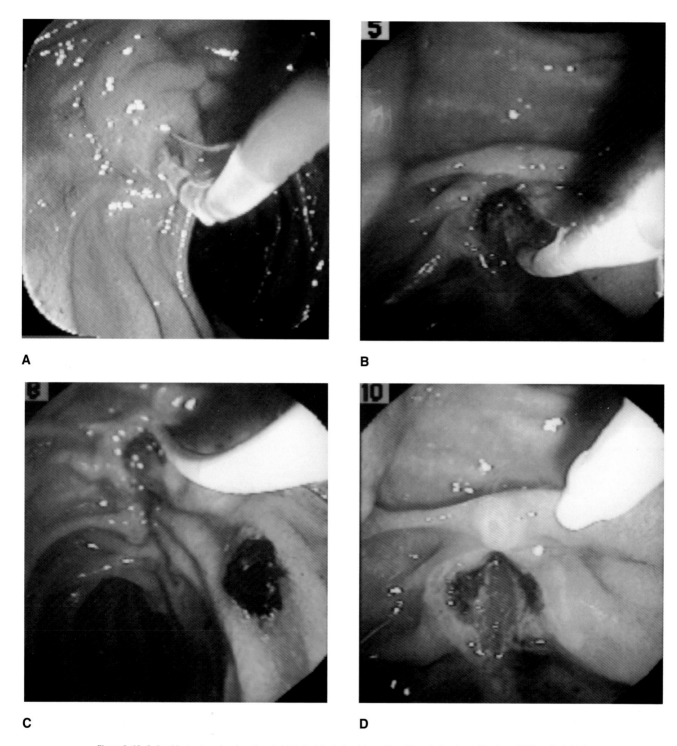

Figure 3–16. A. A sphincterotome has been inserted into the bile duct and is positioned for spincterotomy. (Courtesy of Wilson-Cook Medical, Winston-Salem, NC). **B**. The sphincterotomy is nearing completion. (Courtesy of Wilson-Cook Medical, Winston-Salem, NC). **C**. The bile duct is being swept with a balloon catheter after completing the sphincterotomy. Note the previously removed common bile duct stone lying free in the duodenum. (Courtesy of Wilson-Cook Medical, Winston-Salem, NC). **D**. View of the sphincterotomy after clearing the common bile duct. Note that the choledochal epithelium is seen readily. (Courtesy of Wilson-Cook Medical, Winston-Salem, NC).

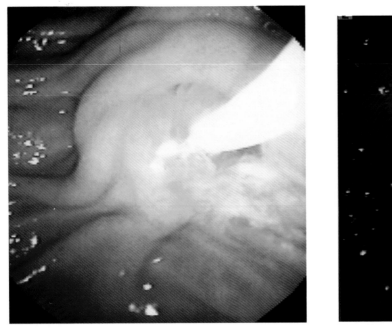

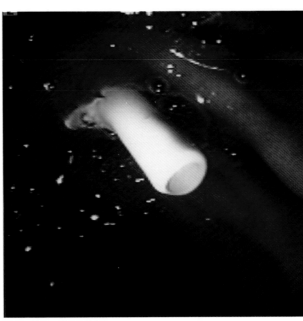

A

B

Figure 3–20. A. Purulent bile streams from the ampulla in this patient with suppurative cholangitis. **B**. An endoprosthesis has been inserted for biliary drainage.

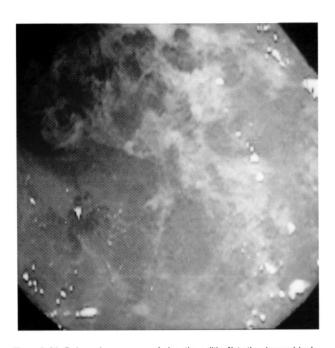

Figure 3–24. Endoscopic appearance of ulcerative colitis. Note the abnormal background mucosa.

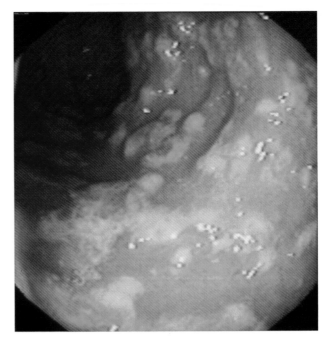

Figure 3–25. Endoscopic appearance of pseudomembranous colitis.

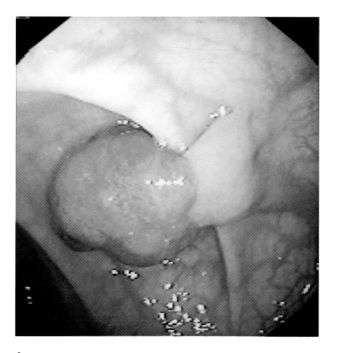

A

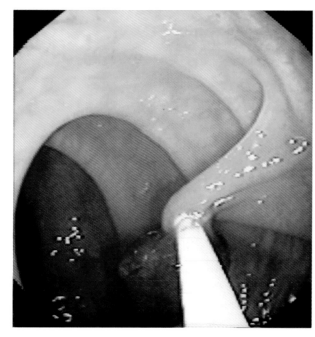

B

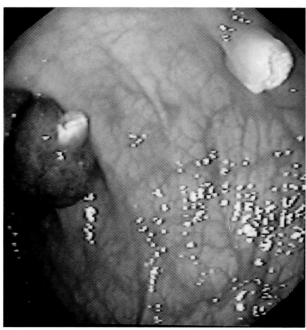

C

Figure 3–26. A. A pedunculated sigmoid colon polyp. **B**. The polyp has been snared with a polypectomy snare. **C**. The polyp has been successfully transected with the snare. Note the transected polyp head, as well as the hemostatic polypectomy site on the stalk.

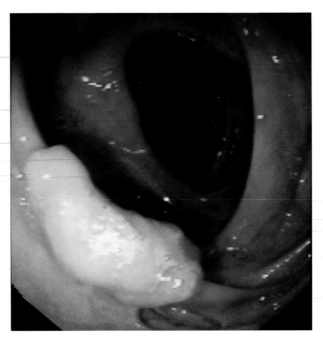

Figure 3–27. A sessile colonic polyp. These can often be removed with a snare, either by creation of a pseudo-stalk or in piecemeal fashion.

mucosal folds. Projections of barium outside of this contour include gastric diverticula, most commonly seen arising from the posterior gastric fundus. These should not be confused with gastric ulcers, which are unusual in that location. A less common gastric diverticulum arises from the greater curvature aspect of the gastric antrum.

Other projections or outpouchings from the lumen include ulcerations and perforations. Ulcerations are usually well-marginated compared with perforations.

Duodenal diverticula occur more frequently than gastric diverticula and arise from the medial aspect of the second portion of the duodenum. They may be multiple and rarely cause symptoms (Fig 1–20). However, occasionally the common bile duct and pancreatic duct may enter into a duodenal diverticulum with resultant stasis and possible biliary or pancreatic symptomatology.

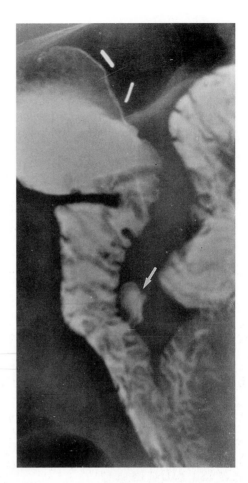

Figure 1–20. Small duodenal diverticulum arising from the medial aspect of the second duodenum (*arrow*).

Mucosal Evaluation
The lumen is examined to determine if rugal folds are of normal size and if any abnormal filling defects are present.

Mucosal fold pattern. Gastritis may cause an abnormal mucosal pattern and may have multiple etiologies including drugs, radiation, uremia, Crohn's disease, and infectious agents. Radiographic findings include thickened rugal folds and small collections of barium, which represent shallow ulcers or erosions surrounded by a halo of edema, and gastric irritability.[26]

Abnormally large gastric folds may be present in many disease states (Table 1–2). These include gastritis, Menetrier's disease, lymphoma, gastric varices, pancreatitis, and Zollinger-Ellison syndrome.[27]

INFLAMMATORY LESIONS

Gastric Ulcers
Gastric ulcers are examined both in profile and en face. Diagnostic criteria are applied to determine whether an

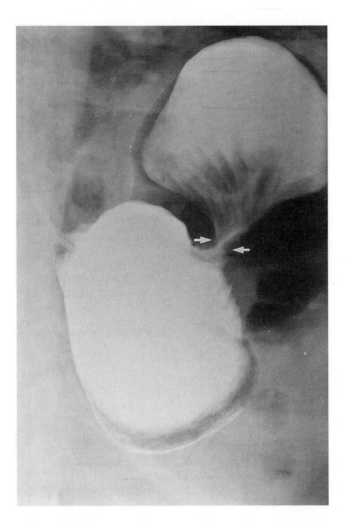

Figure 1–19. Mesenteroaxial volvulus with torsion. Arrows indicate the point of twisting in the gastric body.

TABLE 1–2. LARGE GASTRIC RUGAL FOLDS

> Idiopathic
> Gastritis
> Menetrier's disease
> Lymphoma
> Zollinger-Ellison Syndrome
> Pancreatitis
> Gastric varices
> Pneumoperitoneum

ulcer is benign or has occurred as a result of gastric malignancy.[28] Most gastric ulcers are benign. Radiographic signs supporting a benign state include

1. Penetrating sign—when seen in profile, the ulcer crater should project from the contrast-filled lumen and erode into the stomach wall rather than into a mass in the stomach wall (Fig 1–21).
2. Radiating mucosal folds—when the crater is seen en face, mucosal folds should radiate to the crater's edge without any mucosal nodularity.

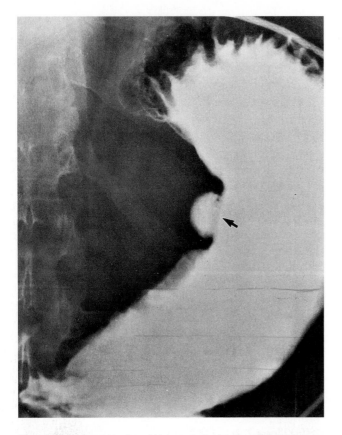

Figure 1–21. Benign gastric ulcer which is penetrating into the gastric wall and projecting from the contrast-filled lumen. Arrow indicates lucent-ulcer collar at the base of the crater.

3. Crater margin
   a. Hampton's line—a smooth thin line at the ulcer neck is seen in profile and is due to the overhanging edge of gastric mucosa as a result of slight undermining of the ulcer into the submucosa.
   b. Ulcer collar—a thickened or edematous mucosal line at the neck of the ulcer (Fig 1–21).
   c. Ulcer mound—tends to be more edematous than a collar or line, the ulcer remains in the center of the mound, and no mucosal nodularity is present.
   d. Test of healing—gastric ulcers should be followed to complete healing. Often they will heal without any residua, although occasionally a scar may persist.

Malignant gastric ulcers. Radiographic signs supporting malignancy include

1. Intraluminal crater—when seen in profile, the crater may not extend beyond the line of the barium-filled lumen but rather, erodes into a mass within the gastric wall (Fig 1–22).
2. Nodular crater margins—tumor nodules may be seen at the margins of the crater, with the ulcer located extrinsically within a mass.
3. Carman's sign (see ulcerating gastric carcinoma)—presents as a meniscus-shaped gastric ulcer with its convexity pointed toward the gastric lumen.

Differentiation between a benign and malignant gastric ulcer will occasionally be difficult to make by radiographic criteria alone. This is especially true in the case of certain benign ulcers that have significant edema and inflammation in the surrounding mucosa, producing nodular folds or a mass effect.

Giant ulcers. Giant ulcers are those greater than 3 cm in size. Although most of these are benign, complications such as perforation or bleeding are more likely than with smaller lesions.

Duodenal Ulcers

Duodenal ulcers are usually located in the duodenal bulk (95%) and are postbulbar in only 5%.[28] Ulcers in other atypical locations should raise the possibility of Zollinger-Ellison syndrome. Duodenal ulcers may be seen en face as a discrete puddle of contrast material with mucosal folds radiating to its edge, or in profile, as a projection from the duodenal lumen (Fig 1–23). Deformity of the bulb, giving it a cloverleaf appearance, may occur and may persist from scarring after the ulcer crater has healed. Giant duodenal ulcers are those mea-

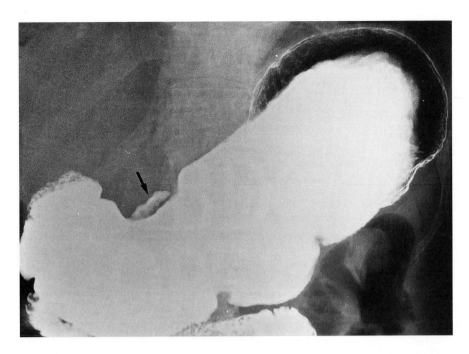

Figure 1–22. Intraluminal ulcer crater (*arrow*). The ulcer crater is recessed into the lumen in this ulcerating gastric malignancy.

suring more than 2 cm in diameter and are more likely to develop complications. Duodenal ulcers are nearly always benign.

Perforation

If an UGI is performed for suspected ulcer perforation, the use of iodinated water-soluble contrast is suggested, since extravasated contrast may flow freely from an ulcer crater into the peritoneal cavity or may fill a walled-off cavity.

CT may be performed in patients with abdominal pain and unsuspected perforation.[29,30] Small amounts of extraluminal air and extravasated contrast are more easily appreciated on CT than on plain films or conventional UGI contrast examination. CT may also reveal fluid collections formed as a result of a perforation that has already sealed or as a result of penetration. The actual ulceration, however, may be difficult to discern.

Aortoduodenal fistula. An uncommon cause for duodenal erosion or perforation is aortoduodenal fistula. This condition occurs as a result of erosion of either an aortic graft or aneurysm into the third portion of the duodenum. CT may show extravasation of ingested contrast around the graft, extraluminal gas, duodenal mural thickening, thickening of soft tissues around the graft, or aneurysm-indicating inflammation. Prompt recognition of these findings is important in the diagnosis of this potentially fatal condition.[31,32]

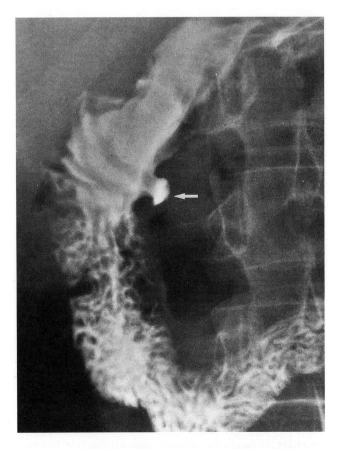

Figure 1–23. Postbulbar duodenal ulcer (*arrow*).

Zollinger-Ellison Syndrome

Gastrinoma, a nonbeta, islet cell tumor may cause the Zollinger-Ellison syndrome. Patients with this syndrome have recurrent and often refractory peptic ulcer disease and marked gastric acid hypersecretion. A constellation of radiographic features may strongly suggest this diagnosis. These abnormalities include a large amount of gastric fluid causing barium dilution, large gastric rugal folds, ulcers which occasionally are found in atypical locations such as postbulbar or in the jejunum, and thickened rugal folds in the small bowel caused by the chemical enteritis produced by the large outpouring of gastric acid (Fig 1–24).[33]

GASTRIC MASSES

Polyps

Most gastric polyps are hyperplastic polyps and are not true neoplasms. They occur randomly in the stomach and are usually less than 1.5 cm in diameter. On rare occasions, gastric polyps may be very large in size.[34,35]

Gastric adenomas are true neoplasms. They are more likely to be single and are most often located in the antrum where, if pedunculated, they may prolapse into the duodenal bulb. On single examination the movable polyp may be seen in two locations.

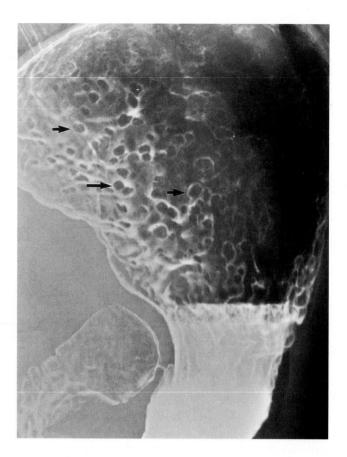

Figure 1–25 Multiple hamartomatous polyps in a patient with Gardner's syndrome (*arrows*).

Multiple syndromes that include gastric polyps have been described.[36] In Peutz-Jeghers syndrome, the polyps are hamartomas and almost always benign. In Canada-Cronkhite syndrome, the inflammatory polyps, which usually carpet the stomach, are also benign. Patients with familial polyposis and Gardner's syndrome often have gastric polyps that may be either hamartomas or adenomas. Adenomas have malignant potential (Fig 1–25).

Gastric Carcinoma

The radiographic appearance of gastric carcinoma, responsible for 90% to 95% of gastric tumors, is variable. Polypoid, ulcerating, or infiltrating features may predominate.[37] Polypoid tumors appear on contrast UGI as lobulated intraluminal masses that may contain barium collections as a result of ulcerations on the colon's surface (Fig 1–26).

Ulcerated carcinomas occur when much of the tumor has ulcerated. The Carman-Kirklin complex is a sign described for a specific flat, ulcerating carcinoma straddling the lesser curvature and involving both the anterior and posterior gastric walls.[27,38] The convex border of the meniscus-shaped ulcer is directed toward

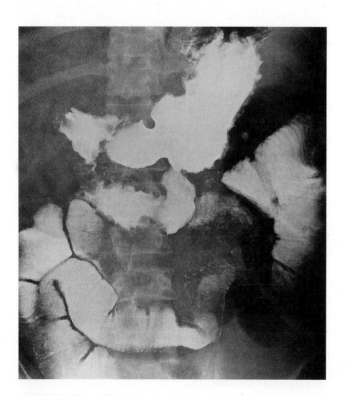

Figure 1–24. Zollinger-Ellison syndrome with thickened gastric rugal folds, small bowel dilatation, and barium dilution in the small bowel.

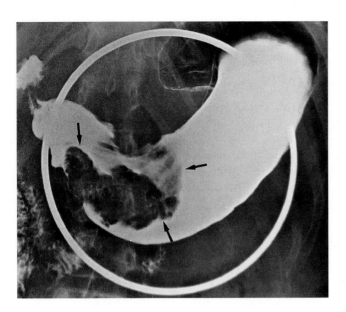

Figure 1–26. Polypoid gastric carcinoma (*arrows*).

the gastric lumen, and a lucent rim is formed around the ulcer by heaped-up tumors. Although valuable, this sign is rare.

Infiltrating carcinomas, also referred to as scirrhous or linitus plastica–type carcinomas, cause a narrow, rigid appearance of the gastric lumen and may involve a portion, usually distal, or all of the stomach.

CT may be helpful in evaluating patients with gastric carcinoma, since it will show the contrast-filled lumen and also the actual gastric wall thickening caused by the

tumor.[39] Optimal gastric distention with contrast, gas, or H_2O is helpful for accurate evaluation of wall thickening.[40] The small calcifications sometimes seen in mucinous tumors may be more apparent when using CT than when using plain films or barium studies.[41] CT is most often used to assess the presence of extragastric spread when surgical intervention is anticipated, since knowledge of the routes of spread is important. Evaluation of surrounding organs is possible with CT. The liver and both local and distant lymph nodes must be examined for metastatic lesions and intraperitoneal seeding. "Drop" metastases to the pelvis or ovaries (Kruckenberg's tumors) must also be sought. There is a wide discrepancy in the literature regarding the accuracy of CT in assessing tumor extent preoperatively. Recent reports appear more favorable, probably as a result of improved technology and techniques that enhance resolution (Fig 1– 27).[42–46]

Gastric Remnant Carcinoma
Patients who have had partial gastrectomies, often for benign disease, are at increased risk for developing gastric carcinoma in the gastric remnant as much as 15 to 25 years after surgery. Bile reflux into the remnant has been postulated as a causative factor.[47]

Gastric Lymphoma
Gastric lymphoma occurs less frequently than gastric carcinoma. The ratio is approximately 1:20. The radiographic appearance can be quite different than carcinoma. Lymphoma often causes large lesions, with large ulcerations and large mucosal folds (Fig 1–28).[48]

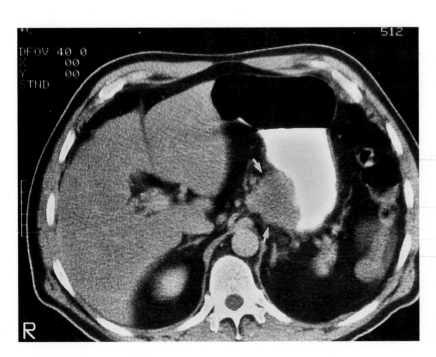

Figure 1–27. Infiltrating gastric carcinoma in the gastric fundus involving the gastroesophageal junction (*arrows*).

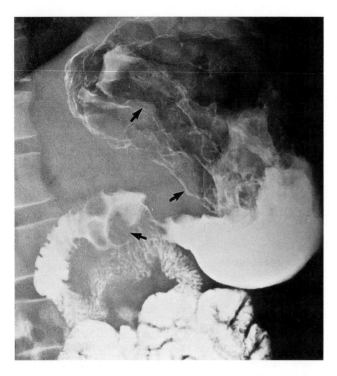

Figure 1–28. Gastric lymphoma. Large, nodular, gastric folds are present throughout the stomach (*arrows*) without significant luminal narrowing. The tumor also involves the duodenal bulb (*arrows*).

Marked gastric wall thickening, as well as evidence of lymphoma in surrounding organs and lymph nodes, may be present on CT. Gastric lymphoma will occasionally be difficulty to differentiate radiographically from an extensive carcinoma (Fig 1–29).[39,48]

Leiomyomas

Leiomyomas account for approximately 2.5% of gastric neoplasms and are the most common benign gastric tumor.[49] They are often less than 3 cm in size and are submucosal in location. When viewed in profile, they have a smooth surface with the borders of the mass forming either obtuse or right angles with the wall of the stomach (Figs 1–30 and 1–31). When viewed en face, normal mucosa may course over the lesion. These lesions are often incidental findings. When symptomatic, it is often due to the ulceration of the overlying mucosa. In such cases, the lesion will appear like a "bull's-eye" owing to barium in the central ulcer crater.

Other small submucosal lesions occurring in the stomach include lipomas, aberrant pancreas, neurofibromas, and hemangiomas. These are radiographically similar to leiomyomas.

Leiomyosarcoma

Leiomyosarcomas account for 1% to 3% of malignant gastric tumors, with most of these occupying the gastric fundus and body. They often present as large lesions containing large ulcerations with the mass projecting outside of the stomach and a small portion visualized as encroaching on the gastric lumen. This "iceberg" phenomenon and complete visualization of a mostly exogastric mass is best appreciated using CT.[50]

Metastatic Disease

Metastases to the stomach may occur via direct invasion of tumors in adjacent organs or as a result of hematoge-

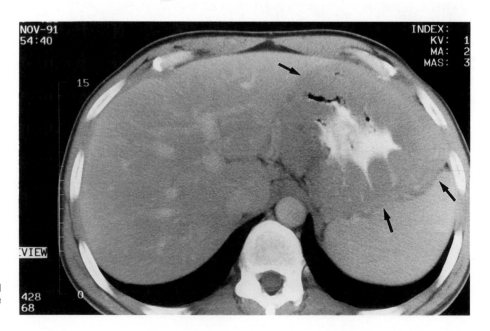

Figure 1–29. Gastric lymphoma causing marked thickening of the gastric wall (*arrows*) and large mucosal folds (CT).

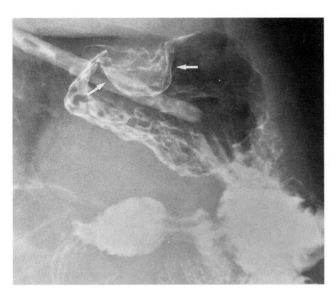

Figure 1–30. Gastric leiomyoma causing a smooth submucosal fundal mass (*arrows*).

nous spread.[51-53] Tumors in organs surrounding the stomach that may invade are colonic, via the gastrocolic ligament, and pancreatic, via the transverse mesocolon. The most common hematogenous metastatic lesions to the stomach are from malignant melanoma and breast cancers. Metastatic breast cancer may also cause this bull's-eye type of lesion or a scirrhous infiltration of the wall similar to that seen with a linitis plastica type of gastric carcinoma. Lung and kidney cancer and Kaposi's

sarcoma may also cause submucosal, ulcerating (bull's-eye) metastatic neoplasms.

Bezoars

Bezoars are masses of ingested material formed in the stomach. They may be composed mainly of vegetable fibers (phytobezoars), hair (trichobezoars), or a mixture of both (trichophytobezoars). They are found in patients with unusual dietary habits and in patients who have had prior gastric surgery or diabetes, probably resulting from altered motility (Fig 1–32).

Duodenal Neoplasms

Most polyps occurring in the duodenum are adenomatous and frequently are discovered as incidental findings. Multiple polyps may be present in patients with a polyposis syndrome.[36]

Villous polypoid tumors often are found in the descending duodenum and are often larger than the usual adenomatous polyp. These have a frond-covered surface (cauliflower appearance) with barium trapped in the interstices of the mass. The risk of malignancy in these lesions is high (80% in lesions >4 cm in size).[54]

Carcinoma of the duodenum occurs distal to the duodenal bulb. It may appear as a polypoid, ulcerating or annular (napkin-ring) lesion with an abrupt transition from normal mucosa to lesion and a narrowed lumen. Thickening of the duodenal wall or a mass may be seen (Fig 1–33).[55]

Periampullary carcinomas frequently are polypoid and cause symptoms by obstructing the pancreatic and

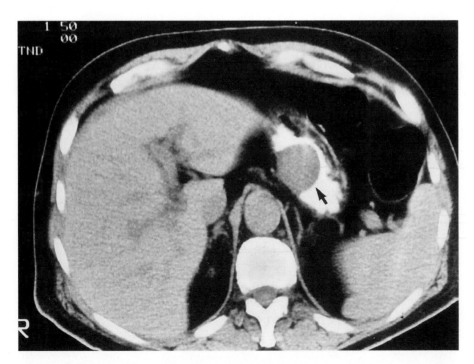

Figure 1–31. Gastric leiomyoma on CT (*arrows*).

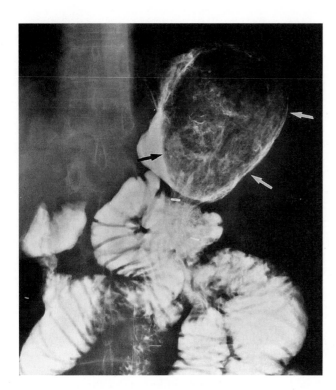

Figure 1–32. Gastric bezoar (phytobezoar) (*arrows*) in a patient who has undergone a subtotal gastrectomy with a Billroth II anastomosis.

common bile duct. Radiographically, they appear as a polypoid mass in the duodenum on UGI study. More likely, biliary dilation to the level of the ampulla and pancreatic ductal dilatation will suggest the diagnosis even though the actual neoplasm is rarely seen.

In addition to occurring in the stomach, submucosal duodenal lesions can occur in Brunner's gland hyperplasia. The latter is most often seen on barium study as multiple nodules in the duodenal bulb.[56]

Tumors in surrounding organs such as the pancreas, kidney, or colon may also invade the duodenum. Tumor involvement of para-aortic lymph nodes may cause duodenal displacement and obstruction. These changes are best seen on CT.

GASTRIC MOTILITY

Nuclear Medicine Studies

Gastric emptying studies are of value in quantifying gastric motility in a variety of clinical problems, including postoperative gastric dysfunction. The patient is given a ^{99m}TC labeled–sulfur colloid test meal and is imaged immediately after the meal and at regular intervals thereafter. Values are plotted on a curve and compared to normal curves available for that particular meal.[57–59]

POSTOPERATIVE STOMACH

The postoperative stomach is evaluated in the immediate postoperative period to assess emptying, anastomosic integrity, or for late complications such as recurrent ulceration or tumor, dysmotility, fistula formation, dumping, or obstruction.[60] Accurate information regarding the surgical procedure performed is helpful. Additionally, knowledge of common gastric surgeries and their radiographic appearances is helpful. These include hiatal hernia repairs, pyloroplasty, partial gastrectomy with Billroth I and Billroth II anastomoses, gastro-

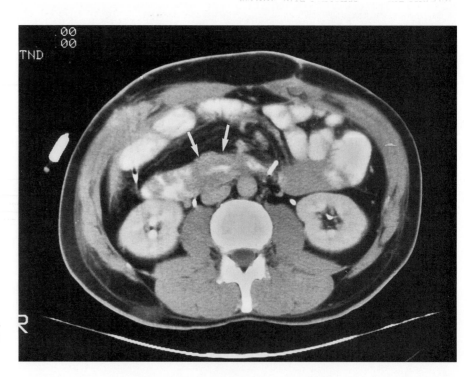

Figure 1–33. Carcinoma of the duodenum on CT. *Arrows* indicate wall thickening in the region of the tumor of the third portion of the duodenum.

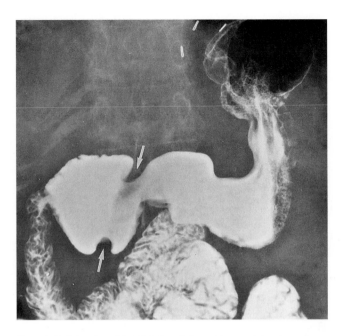

Figure 1–34. Pyloroplasty defect. Note the pyloric canal is now patulous (*arrows*).

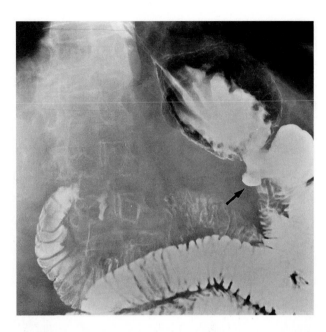

Figure 1–35. Subtotal gastrectomy with Billroth II anastomosis. *Arrow* indicates anastomotic ulcer.

jejunostomy, and gastric restrictive procedures (Figs 1–34 and 1–35). A scout radiograph, taken before contrast is given, helps to show orientation of staples, clips, and drainage tubes. Water-soluble contrast is often used in the immediate postoperative period, especially if extravasation is anticipated. Observation of the direction of flow of the first swallow of contrast will reveal important information, particularly in patients who have undergone gastric restrictive procedures.

Plication defects such as those seen after a hiatal hernia repair may cause a "masslike" projection into the gastric lumen. Radiographically, postoperative changes may resemble ulcers or masses or, conversely, ulcers or tumor may be masked by significant postoperative deformity.

In patients who have undergone gastrojejunostomy, filling of the afferent limb often is not possible on GI studies. If afferent limb obstruction is suspected, CT is helpful for outlining a dilated, fluid-filled limb when obstruction exists.

■ RADIOLOGY OF THE SMALL BOWEL

Radiology of the small bowel is primarily performed by plain film and barium studies.

PLAIN FILMS

Plain abdominal films are often the first means by which small bowel disease is suggested. An adequate abdominal plain film series consists of a supine radiograph, taken with the bottom of the film at the symphysis pubis and the x-ray beam centered at the iliac crest; an erect abdominal film, which helps to assess gas and fluid in distended bowel; and an erect chest film, by which small amounts of air may be seen under the diaphragm and unsuspected chest disease, possibly contributing to abdominal symptoms, may be uncovered. If the patient cannot be examined in the erect position, decubitus film, taken with the left side down, may be performed.[61–63]

Small Bowel Obstruction

Swallowed air and intestinal secretions cause dilatation of the bowel in patients with small bowel obstruction (Fig 1–36). Dilated small bowel loops (>3 cm) with air-fluid levels present may be seen on upright or decubitus views. Some gas may be present in the colon, but the small bowel distention will be greater than any seen in the colon. Serial radiographs may show progressive small bowel distention with decreasing colonic gas. With a high degree of obstruction, the bowel may occasionally be completely filled with fluid, giving the appearance of a "gasless" abdomen. Upright radiographs may show very small air collection trapped between the plicae of the small bowel. This finding has been described as resembling a "string of pearls" (Fig 1–37).

Except in very few instances, plain radiographs will not reveal the cause of a small bowel obstruction. In a patient with gallstone ileus, the diagnosis is suggested by the findings of a small bowel obstruction accompanied by air in the biliary tree and a calcified gallstone in an ectopic location. The presence of a loop of bowel in an

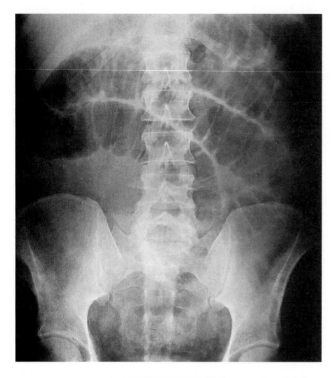

A

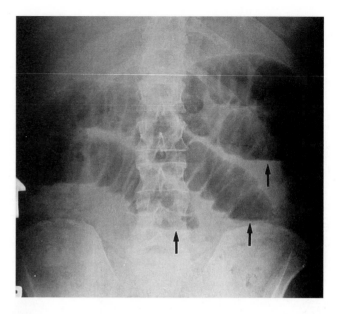

B

Figure 1–36. Small bowel obstruction. **A.** Supine radiograph shows marked small bowel dilatation with no significant colon gas. **B.** Upright film shows multiple air-fluid levels present in the small bowel (*arrows*).

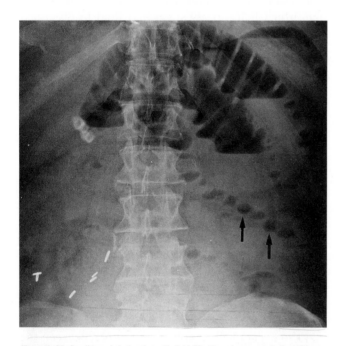

Figure 1–37. Small bowel obstruction with fluid-filled bowel segments in the left lower quadrant showing only a small amount of gas on an erect film. These short air-fluid levels resemble a string of pearls (*arrows*).

abnormal position, below the pubic ramus for example, may suggest an incarcerated hernia as the cause of obstruction (Fig 1–38).

Tangles of linear air collections and other evidence of a bowel obstruction may suggest the cause to be due to a mass of parasites.[62–63]

Ileus

The terms *adynamic ileus, paralytic ileus,* and *nonobstructive ileus* all represent the same clinical situation in which motility is diminished and the small bowel is dilated without an obstruction being present. This may occur after trauma, peritonitis, surgery, or with electrolyte disturbances. Dilated loops of small bowel with varying amounts of colon gas, but without progression of dilatation on serial radiographs, are the predominant findings.[62]

Pneumatosis

Linear streaks of gas paralleling the small bowel wall, as seen on plain radiographs, may indicate pneumatosis, or air, in the bowel wall. The presence of ischemic or gangrenous bowel must be ruled out. Other conditions associated with pneumatosis include collagen vascular diseases, steroids, postendoscopy, and postjejunoileal bypass.

Pneumoperitoneum

Pneumoperitoneum may be present as a result of small bowel perforation. History may suggest causes such as ischemia, tumor, trauma, or inflammatory bowel disease. On a plain film, other extraluminal gas collections,

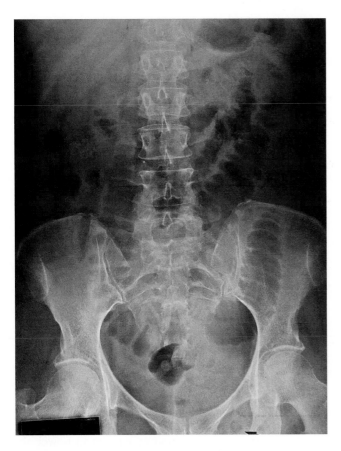

Figure 1–38. Small bowel obstruction due to an incarcerated left inguinal hernia. *Arrow* indicates bowel in an abnormal position below the pubic ramus.

which may appear bubbly or mottled, may result from abscess formation often due to inflammatory bowel disease.

SMALL BOWEL SERIES

A small bowel series with barium as the contrast agent is the primary method by which the small bowel mucosa and lumen are examined (Table 1–3). A conventional small bowel series can provide a great deal of information, if done in a meticulous manner. The patient is

TABLE 1–3. INDICATIONS FOR SMALL BOWEL SERIES

Suspected inflammatory bowel disease
Small bowel obstruction—to determine site and etiology
Systemic disease with suspicion of small bowel involvement
Search for small bowel tumor, either primary or metastatic
Search for small bowel fistula
Trauma
Hemorrhage
Ischemia
Malabsorption

given 16 ounces of barium by mouth and radiographs are taken at regular intervals until the barium column has reached the cecum. Compression spot radiographs of suspicious areas are taken.[64,65]

An alternative method is enteroclysis, or small bowel enema. The patient is orally or nasally intubated, and a small bowel tube is positioned with its tip beyond the Ligament of Treitz. A high-density barium is injected into the tube (200 to 250 cc), followed by injection of methylcellulose or water as the double-contrast agent. The barium coats the mucosa and the methylcellulose distends the bowel lumen, giving the bowel a translucency that affords a clear view of the mucosa. Another advantage of this method is that the entire small bowel is filled at once (Fig 1–39). Spot radiographs and overhead radiographs are taken. Disadvantages of enteroclysis include tube discomfort and the time and radiation necessary to position the tube. Since the bowel is visualized only distal to the Ligament of Treitz, there is no examination of the esophagus, stomach, or duodenum as is available with an UGI and small bowel series.[65,66]

Enteroclysis is indicated in patients

1. With obscure GI bleeding after negative routine diagnostic studies
2. To determine the full extent of bowel involve-

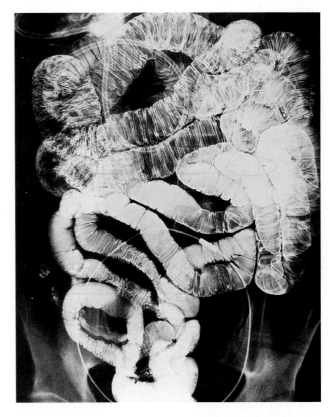

Figure 1–39. Normal enteroclysis. Note the presence of a jejunal tube.

ment in a patient with Crohn's disease when surgery is anticipated

3. When looking for an offending site and the cause in a patient with multiple episodes of small bowel obstruction
4. When searching for small bowel neoplasms in a patient with a polyposis syndrome

Water-Soluble Iodinated Contrast Agent Small Bowel Examination

Barium is used as the contrast agent in most cases that include small bowel obstruction, after it is determined that no obstruction exists in the colon. Water-soluble iodinated contrast agents should be used in patients who are suspected of having spontaneous or postoperative bowel perforation. Patients with fistulas should also be examined with water-soluble, iodinated contrast.

Despite the fact that a site of extravasation may not be identified on water-soluble contrast small bowel examination, contrast in the renal collecting system and bladder may indicate extravasation with subsequent absorption from the peritoneal cavity and excretion into the urinary tract.

Water-soluble agents are not recommended unless extravasation is suspected, since most of these agents are hypertonic and cause fluid to be drawn into the small bowel, resulting in contrast dilution. This dilution significantly diminishes the quality of the examination.[65]

Small Bowel Obstruction

Contrast studies of the small bowel are not always necessary, particularly in patients who have had prior abdominal surgery and therefore may have obstruction owing to adhesions. Contrast studies may be of value in patients with no prior surgery or in patients with suspected tumor recurrence. These studies may also be helpful to confirm that an obstruction exists, to outline the site of obstruction, and to determine from bowel configuration at the site of obstruction what the cause might be. A transition zone from dilated-to-decompressed bowel should be sought. Once the colon is ruled out as a site of obstruction and there is no suspicion of perforation, danger of administering barium by mouth is no longer present, since there is no inspissation of the contrast above a small bowel obstruction. Enteroclysis can also be used. Barium in the bowel may be unwelcomed if the patient is to have immediate surgery. Water-soluble contrast agents may be helpful in cases of high small bowel obstruction. They are not as useful in distal small bowel obstruction because of the hyperosmolar nature of these agents. The large outpouring of fluid into the bowel lumen that these agents produce causes marked contrast dilution and obscures detail in the distal small bowel.[63–67]

CT in Bowel Obstruction. CT in patients with suspected bowel obstruction can be very helpful in differentiating whether an obstruction exists by easily identifying a caliber discrepancy between proximal obstructed and distal nonobstructed small bowel without the necessity of administering oral contrast (Table 1–4) (Fig 1–40). CT has the ability to show thickened bowel wall in a patient with obstruction, which may suggest strangulation. Thickened bowel wall, enhancing bowel wall, and submucosal edema all may be suggestive of vascular compromise. CT is especially helpful in patients with a history of malignancy and symptoms of bowel obstruction, and it often may show whether recurrent or metastatic tumor is the cause of obstruction. It is also helpful in patients with no prior surgery or history of malignancy and may reveal infarction, mass, or infection as a result of inflammatory bowel disease, diverticulitis, or appendicitis. CT is not as useful in patients with a history of prior surgery and in whom adhesions are the most likely cause of obstruction, since adhesions are not clearly seen on CT and only the presence of an obstruction will be confirmed.[68–72]

Intussusception

Intussusception occurs when a segment of the bowel, the intussusceptum, invaginates into a more distal segment, the intussuscipiens, and may result in bowel obstruction. There are multiple factors that can cause intussusception, including polypoid tumors, duplications, Meckel's diverticulum, adhesions, and dysmotility. It may be seen evanescently in a normal patient and most commonly is caused by polypoid lesions. The radiographic appearance of a "coiled spring" is due to the distended intussuscipiens and the double intestinal mucosa folds of both intussusceptum and intussuscepiens.

Findings on CT may include those of a small bowel obstruction, with dilated fluid/air–filled proximal loops and nondilated loops distal to the intussusception. These may appear as locally distended segments of bowel with a "crescent-target" mass appearance from the low density mesenteric fat surrounding the intussusceptum (Fig 1–41).[72–74]

TABLE 1–4. CT OF BOWEL OBSTRUCTION

To conform or exclude diagnosis of obstruction
To determine site
To diagnose cause:
    tumor
    intussusception
    afferent loop obstruction
    gallstone ileus
    bowel ischemia or infarction
    hernia
    abscess

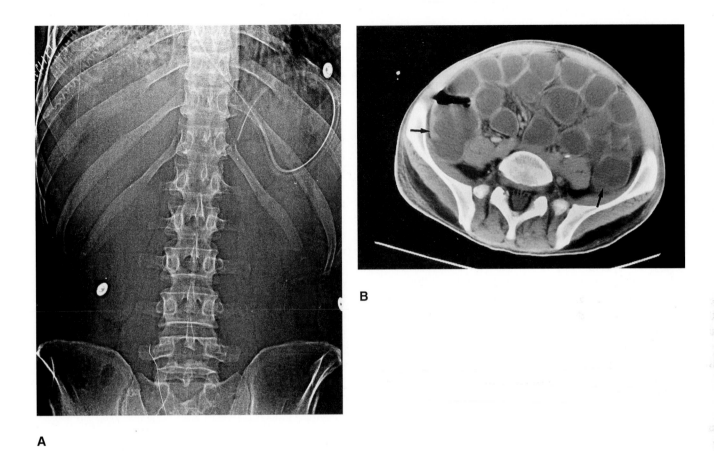

A

B

Figure 1–40. Ileus seen on abdominal CT. **A.** Supine abdominal radiograph shows a gasless abdomen. **B.** CT shows fluid-filled small and large bowel indicating an ileus (*arrows* point to ascending and descending colon).

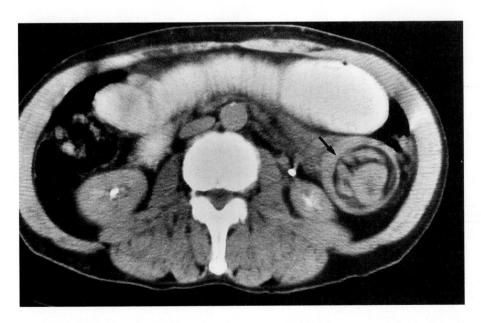

Figure 1–41. Small bowel obstruction due to intussusception of a hamartoma in a patient with Peutz Jegher syndrome. *Arrow* points to intussusceptum. Note dilated proximal small bowel.

INFLAMMATORY BOWEL DISEASE

The majority of patients with Crohn's disease have involvement of the terminal ileum either as the sole site or with multiple sites in the small and large bowel (Fig 1–40). The extent of diseased bowel may be from 10 to 30 cm proximal to the ileocecal valve with milder changes present 10 to 20 cm proximal to the more clearly involved area.[75–78]

The earliest detectable radiographic findings are aphthous ulcers. When these are the sole abnormality, differentiation from infectious processes such as *Yersinia, Salmonella,* tuberculosis, or *Candida* may be difficult. Mucosal folds may be thickened. The bowel lumen is often markedly narrowed, hence the term "string sign" (Fig 1–42).[77] Longitudinal and transverse ulcerations may give the mucosal surface a "cobblestoned" appearance. In some patients severe ulceration and edema may present as a bowel segment that is devoid of mucosa. Contrast-filled bowel loops may be separated owing to thickening of the involved bowel wall and fibrofatty proliferation of the mesentry.[78]

With transmural disease, tracts into the wall of the bowel may occur. These may progress to fistulae between loops of bowel or between the bowel and bladder, urethra, prostate, vagina, or skin—frequently in the perineal area. The most common fistulous communication

is between diseased ileum and cecum or ascending colon (Fig 1–43). Skip areas of disease are frequent as is asymmetric involvement of the bowel. The mesenteric side of the bowel tends to show greater involvement than the antimesenteric side. Pseudodiverticula occur when uninvolved bowel segments distend in otherwise restricted, asymmetrically diseased bowel loops.

Stenotic segments are evident when fibrosis occurs and may lead to obstruction. Plain radiographs may show markedly distended bowel loops proximal to chronically obstructed segments. In patients with long-standing chronic obstruction, distention appears in bowel loops near the obstructed segment rather than uniformly throughout the small bowel. On plain radiographs, the degree of proximal chronic small bowel distention may be so great as to be confused with colonic dilatation. Occasionally, enteroliths will be seen proximal to an obstructing lesion or in a pseudo-diverticulum.[79,80] These enteroliths are formed when, because of stasis, ingested foreign material remains in the bowel and acts as a nidus for the development of a concretion or enterolith. The precipitation of calcium salts in the alkaline medium of the distal small bowel may cause these to calcify, making them visible on plain radiographs. Perforation of the bowel has been reported and is an unusual complication of Crohn's disease.

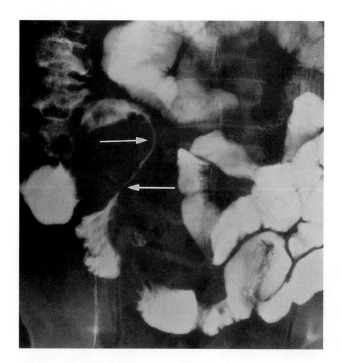

Figure 1–42. Crohn's disease of the terminal ileum. There is marked narrowing of the lumen (string sign) with loss of the normal mucosal pattern (*arrows*). The segment is separated from proximal segments owing to fibrofatty proliferation of the mesentery.

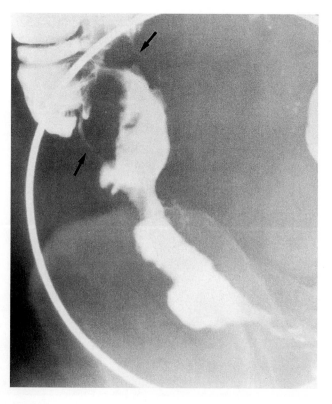

Figure 1–43. Crohn's disease of the terminal ileum. Sinus tracts into the bowel wall are present, and fistulous tracts between the terminal ileum and ascending colon are present (*arrows*).

Ultrasound may show the thickened wall of involved bowel segments. These may have a target appearance if the segment is scanned transversely with the narrowed lumen demonstrated as the center of the target. Distended fluid-filled loops proximal to a stricture may be demonstrated as well as an irregular fluid-filled collection, when an abscess is present.[81,82]

Abdominal CT findings include thickening of the wall of diseased segments, often with a target appearance, if viewed in cross-section, owing to the narrowing of the contrast-filled lumen and thick wall, separation of bowel loops due to fibrofatty proliferation of the mesentery, and lymphadenopathy (Fig 1–44). Fistulous tracts may be outlined, and sometimes a very small amount of air or contrast present in the bladder or other abnormal location may be the first sign of a sinus tract, or fistula. This evidence of a fistula may sometimes be seen on CT without clear findings on either conventional contrast or plain-film radiography. Bladder wall thickening seen on CT may be caused by the direct extension of inflammation from an adjacent involved bowel loop. An abscess may appear as a well-defined zone of low attenuation with a thick wall. Air bubbles may be present within the abscess. CT-guided aspiration or catheter drainage of a fluid collection is often possible.[83–85]

Once the inflammatory disease is established in the small bowel, it may become more severe and stenotic in the involved areas, although it is unusual for it to spread either distally or proximally in the absence of surgery.[77] Also, regression of the radiographic changes of Crohn's disease in the upper gastrointestinal tract and small bowel is rare.[86,87] Findings on imaging studies often correlate poorly with the clinical status of the patient. Thus, once the diagnosis is established, frequent follow-up radiographic examinations of the patient are unnecessary unless a complication is suggested by the patient's clinical condition (eg, obstruction, perforation, abscess, or fistula).

Postoperative recurrence and progression of disease occur with an incidence as high as 80%. It is almost always at an anastomosis, mostly on the ileal side of an ileocolic anastomosis but occasionally on the colonic side. Mucosal fold thickening and ulceration are suggestive of recurrent disease, which may progress from being nonstenotic to stenotic. The previously mentioned complications of Crohn's disease may occur within the areas of recurrence.[77,78,86]

INFECTIOUS DISEASE

Since the bowel can respond in only a limited number of ways, several infectious diseases will produce similar radiographic findings. *Giardia*, hookworm, and tapeworm may cause proximal small bowel mucosal fold thickening and excessive small bowel fluid. Ascaris may appear as a coiled filling defect with a fine internal line of contrast representing the gastrointestinal tract of the worm. Tuberculosis involving the small bowel also involves the ileum and ascending colon and may be radiologically indistinguishable from Crohn's disease. A high percentage of patients with intestinal tuberculosis develop strictures and subsequent obstruction.[88]

In immunosuppressed patients, infectious diseases such as cryptosporidium, *Mycobacterium avium intracellulare*, CMV, and *Isospora belli* may cause abnormal small bowel studies with mucosal fold thickening and distortion, bowel irritability, and excessive bowel secretions.[89–91]

CT may be valuable in showing bowel distention, mucosal fold and wall thickening, fluid, adenopathy, and mesenteric thickening.

SMALL BOWEL PERFORATION

Small bowel perforation may result from trauma, ischemia, inflammatory bowel disease, obstruction, and tumor. Pneumoperitoneum may be seen on plain radiographs along with ileus and/or ascites. Water-soluble contrast small bowel series are used to demonstrate the extravasation site. While small perforations may be difficult to detect, the appearance of contrast in the renal collecting system indicates extravasation into and absorption from the peritoneal cavity. CT may show very small amounts of extraluminal air and contrast material.[72]

SMALL BOWEL TRAUMA

The small intestine is the fourth most common site of injury following the liver, spleen, and kidney. Blunt trauma to the GI tract may be difficult to diagnose. CT is presently the most reliable imaging modality. Oral con-

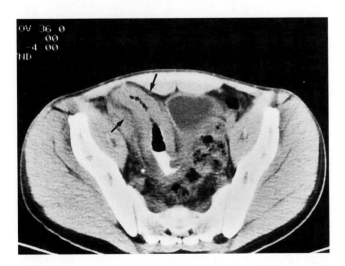

Figure 1–44. Crohn's disease of the distal ileum on CT. Bowel segment viewed longitudinally shows marked mural thickening (*arrows*).

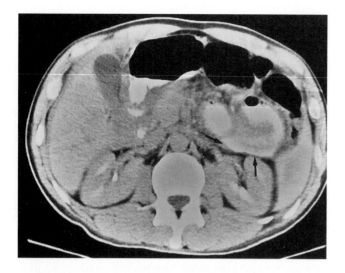

A

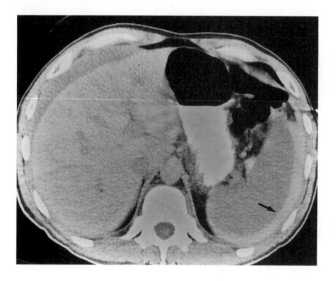

B

Figure 1–45. Small bowel perforation due to blunt abdominal trauma. **A.** Fluid (blood) is present in the peritoneal cavity. The high density (*arrows*) of the perisplenic blood suggests extravasation of oral contrast in the area. **B.** *Arrows* indicate contrast extravasation in the proximal jejunum.

trast is administered (250 to 400 cc water-soluble iodinated) and peritoneal lavage should be restricted until after CT is done so that no iatrogenic air or fluid is present in the abdomen. Diagnostic findings on CT include free air and extravasation of contrast, bowel wall and/or mesenteric hematoma, and free abdominal fluid. If findings are not diagnostic on an early CT scan, but clinical symptoms suggest bowel injury, a repeat scan should be performed, since significant radiographic changes may not be manifest shortly after injury (Fig 1–45).

The duodenum and proximal jejunum are the most frequent sites of injury.[72,92,93]

SMALL BOWEL HEMORRHAGE AND ISCHEMIA

Bleeding into the wall of the small bowel may occur as a result of anticoagulation, bleeding disorders, trauma, or vascular lesions. On contrast examination, thickening of the valvuli conniventes with a spikelike configuration described as a "stacked coin" can be seen. If the hemorrhage is localized, it may give the appearance of a submucosal mass.

Ischemia of the small bowel may occur as a result of thrombosis, embolus, compression, vasculitis, infiltration, or trauma. The severity of radiographic changes correlates with the degree of compromise. Thickening of valvuli and separation of bowel loops may be seen on plain radiographs and barium studies. Bowel wall thickening and the extent of involvement will be evident with CT. Submucosal hemorrhage and/or edema may occur along the mesenteric margin of an involved bowel loop and appear as "thumbprints" indenting the lumen (Fig 1–46). This thumbprint may be seen on plain films or contrast studies. Air in the bowel wall or portal venous system may be present if gangrene should occur. Hyperenhancement of the bowel wall and vascular congestion of the mesentery also may occur. Early findings may be visible on CT before there are any significant plain film abnormalities.

With venous thrombosis, a thrombus may be visualized in the superior mesenteric vein as well as thicken-

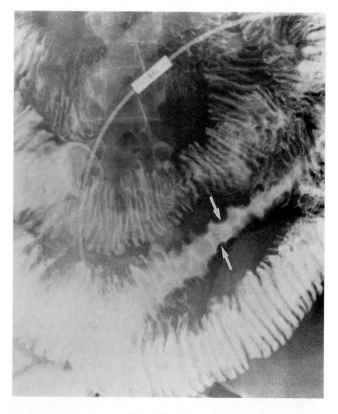

Figure 1–46. Small bowel ischemia. Multiple filling defects or thumbprints, are the result of submucosal hemorrhage and edema (*arrows*).

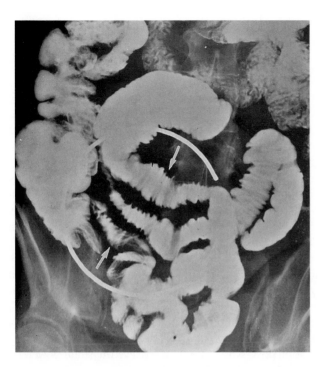

Figure 1–47. Radiation changes of the small bowel. Ileal segments are narrowed, separated, and have thickened valvuli conniventes (*arrows*).

ing and enhancement of the bowel wall of the involved segments.[72,94–97]

RADIATION

Radiation changes seen in the small bowel are usually due to the vasculitis caused by the effects of radiation on the patient. Radiation doses that produce significant change are generally in the 5000 to 6000 R range. Acutely, there may be mucosal ulceration, irritability with thickened mucosal folds, and, possibly, thumbprinting of the bowel. Later changes, which may occur 5 to 6 years after radiation, include thickening of the valvuli, luminal narrowing, and stenoses with proximal dilatation from partial obstruction by the narrowed segments and angulation due to adhesions (Fig 1–47). CT shows the marked mural thickening and extent of bowel involvement (Fig 1–48). Fistulae may arise from bowel damaged by radiation.[98–100]

MALABSORPTION

A large number of small bowel diseases may cause clinical malabsorption. Among them are sprue, Whipple disease, lymphangiectasia, and amyloidosis, scleroderma, and nodular lymphoid hyperplasia. They may result in varying degrees of bowel dilatation, prominence or nodularity of mucosal folds, and hypersecretion.[65,91]

SMALL BOWEL DIVERTICULA

Duodenal diverticula occur with great frequency but are rarely symptomatic. The common bile duct may insert into an ampulla located in a duodenal diverticulum and the patient may have biliary and/or pancreatic symptoms. Jejunal diverticula occur on the mesenteric border of the bowel and are usually asymptomatic. If numerous, they may act as multiple blind loops and produce malabsorption from bacterial overgrowth. Pseudodiverticula may occur in scleroderma and Crohn's disease. In scleroderma, muscle atrophy causes asymmetric distention of the bowel, resulting in a diverticular outpouching. In Crohn's disease, asymmetrical scar-

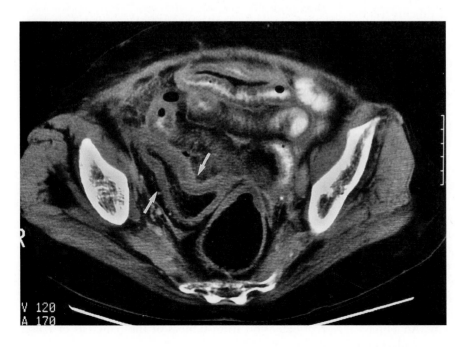

Figure 1–48. Radiation changes of the small bowel on CT. Mural thickening is marked in the distal ileum (*arrows*).

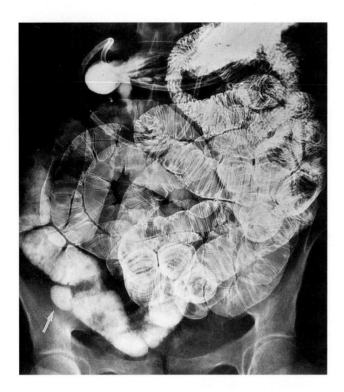

Figure 1–49. Meckel's diverticulum on enteroclysis. *Arrow* points to diverticulum.

ring causes the normal segment of bowel to form an out-pouching.

Meckel's diverticula occur in approximately 1% to 3% of the population. They are typically on the antimesenteric border of the ileum and within 2 ft of the ileocecal valve. Symptoms result from bleeding caused by ectopic gastric mucosa in the diverticulum or to intussusception. If obstruction or inflammation occurs, symptoms may be similar to those of appendicitis. Technetium pertechnecate (^{99m}Tc) nuclear medicine scans are helpful in diagnosing Meckel's diverticula with ectopic gastric mucosa. Otherwise, Meckel's diverticula will be difficult to demonstrate unless ileal loops are separated by fat or inflammation. Enteroclysis is probably indicated if a Meckel's diverticulum is clinically suspected (Fig 1–49).[101,102]

SMALL BOWEL FISTULAE

Fistulae communicating with the small bowel may arise from Crohn's disease, neoplasms, diverticulitis, pancreatitis, radiation enteritis, or as a postoperative complication. They may be demonstrated on contrast bowel examinations by using CT or by performing a fistulogram if the fistula has a cutaneous communication. A combined fistulogram and CT scan may provide additional information. A catheter is inserted into the cutaneous opening and water-soluble iodinated contrast is injected under fluoroscopic observation. An enterovaginal fistula may be demonstrated best by placing a balloon catheter in the vagina and injecting contrast under fluoroscopic guidance.

SMALL BOWEL NEOPLASMS

Carcinoid tumors, usually found in the appendix or ileum, are the most common primary bowel neoplasms. The primary tumor grows into the wall of the bowel and may produce a strong desmoplastic reaction. Radiographically, separation and angulation of bowel segments in a patient with no reason to have adhesions should suggest this diagnosis. Ischemia may occur if vessels are compromised by the scarring and fibrosis that occurs. CT will help to fully outline the extent of tumor involvement of both bowel and mesentery (Fig 1–50). Benign small bowel tumors occur with greater frequency. Adenomas (including villous adenomas) are mucosal lesions, while leiomyomas, neurogenic tumors, and lipomas are all submucosal lesions. Lipomas are often soft and compressible and may have the characteristic low density of fat on CT scan.

Polyposis syndromes may involve the small bowel. In Peutz-Jeghers' syndrome the polyps are histologically hamartomas and usually are found in the small bowel but also may be found in the stomach and colon. Patients with both familial polyposis and Gardner's syndrome may have adenomatous small bowel polyps. In Cronkhite-Canada's syndrome the inflammatory polyps known to occur may appear in the small bowel but are found more regularly in the stomach and colon.

Adenocarcinoma is not a common small bowel neoplasm and occurs predominantly in the duodenum and jejunum. On barium studies it will appear as an abrupt annular lesion often accompanied by ulceration. Proximal dilatation may occur owing to obstruction caused by the tumor.[103–107]

Lymphoma may be primary in the small bowel or may be a manifestation of widespread disease. Non-Hodgkin's lymphoma is more common than Hodgkin's lymphoma.[106,108] Radiographically, multiple nodules, bowel infiltration with diffuse wall thickening, or aneurysmal dilatation of a segment secondary to partial replacement of the bowel wall due to tumor, may occur. An ulcerating mass with fistulae to other bowel segments also may be seen.

Metastatic Disease

The most common neoplasms to metatasize to small bowel are melanoma, breast, kidney, and Kaposi's sarcoma. Most are hematogenous metastases and, when ulcerated, may have a "bull's eye" or target appearance. Mesenteric metastatic lesions may cause serosal involvement of the bowel with mucosal tethering, angulation, and separation of bowel loops. Metastatic carcinoma of the breast may produce scirrhous infiltrating lesions. Direct extension from tumors of the pancreas or colon may occur.[106,107,109–112]

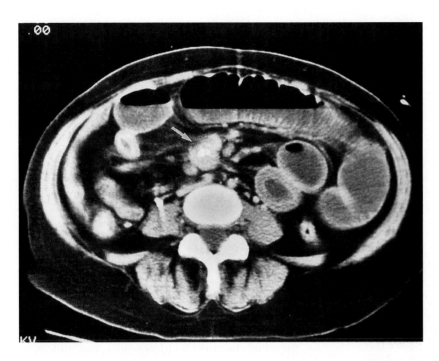

Figure 1–50. Carcinoid tumor causing small bowel ischemia. A mass in the mesentery (*arrow*) was found to encase the superior mesenteric vein at surgery. Note thickened bowel wall due to ischemia.

POSTOPERATIVE RADIOLOGY

Postoperative investigation of the small bowel is performed to investigate complications such as obstruction or anastomotic leaks.[113]

AFFERENT LOOP SYNDROME

Obstruction of an afferent limb after a Billroth II surgical gastrojejunostomy or a Roux-en-Y limb may be due to anastomotic stricture, adhesions, ulceration, recurrent tumor, or kinking of the bowel. Plain abdominal films are often inconclusive, and the afferent limb may not opacify on an UGI study.

CT is the preferred method of visualizing a dilated afferent or Roux-en-Y limb, and it will demonstrate a dilated, sometimes cysticlike structure in the region of the duodenum. Pressure resulting from obstruction may also cause biliary and gallbladder distention. Ultrasound may also be used to show the dilated afferent limb.

SHORT BOWEL

If necessary, contrast studies of the bowel are useful in assessing the length of bowel for further surgery and for nutritional evaluation.

JEJUNOILEAL BYPASS

Evaluation of patients having undergone these procedures, usually for morbid obesity, may be difficult. Large segments of small bowel may not be filled either via antegrade or retrograde contrast studies. If the bypassed segments are not visualized with routine contrast studies, CT may be helpful in showing these segments.

ILEOSTOMY ENEMA

In a patient with an ileostomy and suspected distal small bowel disease or obstruction, a catheter can be placed in the ileostomy and contrast (either barium or water soluble, depending on the indication) may be injected under fluoroscopic observation. A dose of 1 mg glucagon given intravenously enhances the amount of retrograde filling possible.

CONTINENT ILEOSTOMY

Koch's continent ileostomy consists of a reservoir consisting of distal ileal segments, with an inverted nipple valve fashioned to aid continence. Complications include incontinence caused by leaking of and around the nipple, internal fistulae and "pouchitis," an inflammation of the mucosa of the pouch. Radiographic examination is possible by intubating the pouch and injecting contrast and air. This can also be done using CT by first filling the pouch with dilute contrast material by catheter.

ILEOANAL POUCHES

The ileoanal reservoir has become a frequently used method for creating a continent ileostomy. Several different surgical procedures have been described using this theory (J-pouch, S-pouch, W-pouch). The procedure is performed as a staged operation with creation of an ileostomy to allow healing of the reservoir. The pouch can be imaged by doing a contrast enema using a small catheter in the rectum or ileostomy, or by CT.[114] Immediate postoperative complications include anastomotic leaks, obstruction, abscesses, or inflammation of the pouch (pouchitis). Late complications include pouchitis and stricture at the ileonanal anastomosis (Fig 1–51).[115]

■ RADIOLOGY OF THE COLON

Evaluation of the colon can be accomplished by plain abdominal radiograph, contrast enema, delayed antegrade barium examination, abdominal CT, angiography, defecography, endoscopic ultrasound, radionuclide immunoscintigraphy, and with radiopaque markers.

PLAIN FILMS

Plain films of the abdomen often given the first indication of colonic pathology.

Obstruction

Films should be taken in the supine, erect, or left lateral decubitus positions. Small amounts of colon gas are normally seen in healthy patients. In patients with colonic obstruction, dilated air-filled loops of colon (with air-fluid levels on upright films) are seen proximal to the area of obstruction with little or no gas present in the decompressed bowel distal to the narrowed segment. If the ileocecal valve is competent, little or no gas may be present in the small bowel. With an incompetent ileocecal valve, dilated air-filled small bowel may make the diagnosis more difficult. Perforation may occur, often with large amounts of free air.[116–118]

Volvulus

Sixty to seventy-five percent of large bowel volvulus involves the sigmoid colon. Plain radiographs are often diagnostic. The classic appearance is a dilated, inverted U-shaped gas-filled structure, in the midabdomen or right upper quadrant, representing the obstructed sigmoid colon. The volvulus can resemble three flexures: the hepatic, splenic, and dilated sigmoid colon in its aberrant location in the upper abdomen (Fig 1–52). A single-column contrast enema will confirm this diagnosis by showing a smooth tapered "beaked" appearance of the bowel at the site of torsion (Fig 1–53). The enema may help to reduce the volvulus. Although rare, volvulus of the transverse colon and splenic flexure may occur.[119]

Cecal volvulus occurs less commonly than sigmoid volvulus and only in those patients where the right colon is not completely fixed to the posterior parietal peritoneum. The site of torsion is in the ascending colon since it is distal to the ileocecal valve. Plain films may show a large gas-filled bowel segment either in the midabdomen or in the right upper quadrant (Fig 1–54). A single-column enema may show a "beaked" appear-

ance at the ascending colon twist point, with some or little contrast, passing proximally to the cecum which is in an ectopic position. The enema may help reduce the obstruction.[116–118]

Pseudo-obstruction

Marked colonic distention without mechanical obstruction may occur as a result of pharmacologic, endocrine, neural, and myopathic factors. The term *primary intestinal pseudo-obstruction* may be used if no etiology is determined. Other terms used for this distention include *idiopathic megacolon* and *Olgivie's syndrome* (Fig 1–55).[117,118]

Inflammatory Bowel Disease

Gas in the colon can be an effective contrast agent, particularly when the bowel is moderately dilated. Thickened haustra may indicate colonic edema and suggest inflammatory bowel disease. A number of clinical conditions including idiopathic inflammatory bowel disease, pseudomembranous enterocolitis, and infectious colitis of numerous etiologies, will have this presentation.

A narrowed, tubular, air-filled lumen may indicate chronic ulcerative colitis, and a nodular gas-filled lumen may suggest inflammatory bowel disease and pseudopolyposis (Fig 1–56). In a patient with abdominal pain, fever, and diarrhea, a dilated colon on plain film may suggest toxic megacolon. The transverse colon is often the portion of bowel that appears most dilated, probably because the patient is supine and colonic gas rises to this level. Although toxic megacolon occurs most frequently in ulcerative colitis, it can also be seen in Crohn's colitis, amebiasis, ischemic colitis, and pseudomembranous colitis. Serial plain film radiographs should be carefully examined for evidence of pneumatosis or free air, which would indicate colonic perforation. Contrast enemas are contraindicated in the patient suspected of having a toxic megacolon.[120,121]

Ischemia

Plain radiographs may show thickening of haustra in the involved area and large filling defects (thumbprints) owing to submucosal hemorrhage and edema. These findings are most common in the splenic flexure region. Evidence of pneumatosis or free air may be present in patients where ischemia has progressed to bowel necrosis.

Neoplasms

On rare occasion, a colon neoplasm can be seen in the gas-filled colonic lumen. A contrast enema or endoscopy is usually necessary to confirm the diagnosis (Fig 1–57).

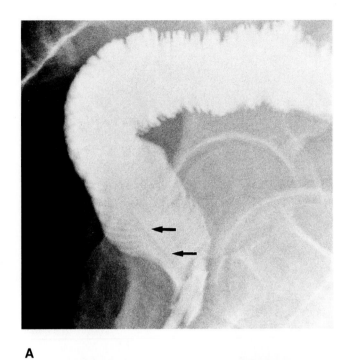

A

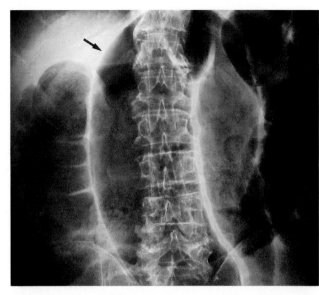

Figure 1–52. Sigmoid volvulus. Supine radiograph showing inverted U-shaped dilated sigmoid colon in the midabdomen (*arrows*) interposed between the hepatic and splenic flexures.

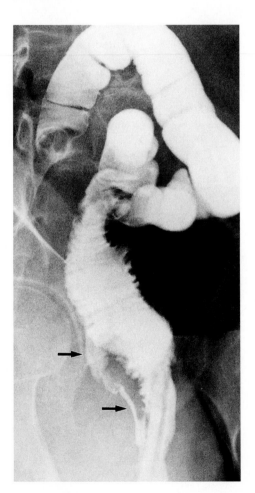

B

Figure 1–51. Ileoanal reservoirs. A. Normal ileoanal reservoir. Arrows indicate anastomotic line. B. Sinus tract arising from distal anastomotic disruption.

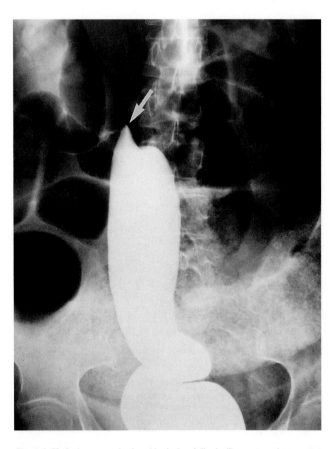

Figure 1–53. Barium enema in sigmoid volvulus. A "beaked" appearance is present at the site of torsion (*arrows*).

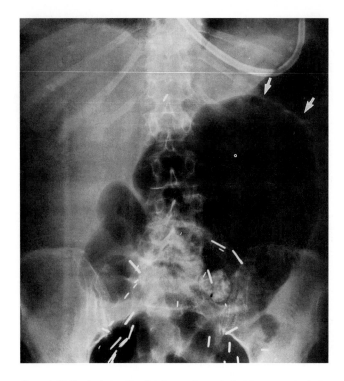

Figure 1–54. Cecal volvulus. The dilated cecum is seen in the left upper quadrant. *Arrows* indicate the cecal tip.

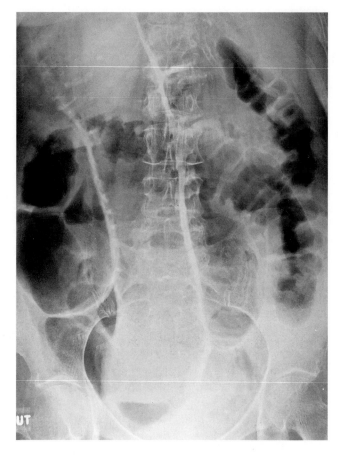

Figure 1–55. Colonic pseudo-obstruction. Markedly dilated colon in a patient, proven by endoscopy to have no obstruction.

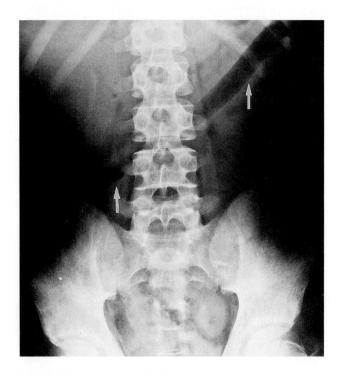

Figure 1–56. Chronic ulcerative colitis. Plain film shows a tubular ahaustral transverse colon (*arrows*).

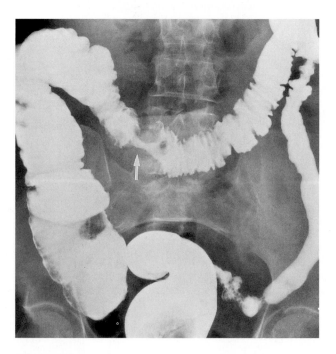

Figure 1–57. Colonic carcinoma. Barium enema confirms the presence of an annular carcinoma (*arrow*).

TABLE 1–5. CAUSES OF PNEUMATOSIS

Pneumatosis Coli
Mesenteric vascular occlusion
Acute necrotizing enterocolitis
Intestinal obstruction
Caustic ingestion
Peptic ulcer
Postendoscopy
Steroid therapy
Immunosuppression
Collagen disorders
Perforated diverticula
Trauma
Postsurgical bowel anastomosis
Pneumatosis cystoides intestinalis

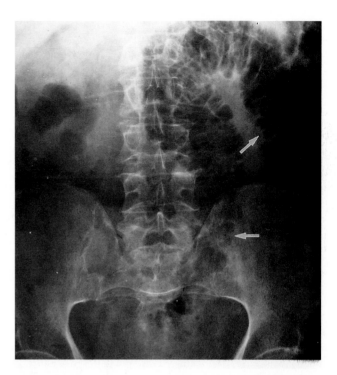

A

Pneumatosis

Air in the wall of the colon may be seen with varied clinical entities that range in clinical importance from incidental and benign to life threatening (Table 1–5) (Fig 1–58). The radiographic appearance may be that of bubbles in the bowel wall or linear stripes of air paralleling the lumen.[118]

CONTRAST EXAMINATIONS

Contrast enemas are the principal radiographic technique for studying the colonic lumen. The current procedure of choice when looking for mucosal disease is double contrast barium enemas which use a small amount of high-density barium to coat the lumen and insufflated air to advance the barium and distend the lumen. A dose of 1 mg glucagon given intravenously, immediately prior to the examination, promotes smooth muscle relaxation, thereby enhancing the quality of the examination. Meticulous bowel preparation involving a liquid diet, a regimen of laxatives, and a rectal suppository given the morning of the examination contributes to a technically high-quality examination.[122–124]

Single-column studies may be indicated in cases of suspected obstruction, diverticulitis, ischemia, or fistula. Single-column technique utilizing water-soluble iodinated contrast material is preferred in patients with suspected colonic perforation due to trauma, tumor perforation, or leaking surgical anastomoses. Additionally, this technique is indicated to insure that barium artifacts are eliminated, if subsequent abdominal CT is to be performed.[123,124]

Colostomy

Colostomy enemas may be performed using commercially available devices designed for this purpose (EZ-EM, Westbury, NY). A catheter tip with a closely fitting cone around it is inserted into the colostomy, and the cone is positioned so that a seal occurs. The patient holds the device in place as the study is performed.[124]

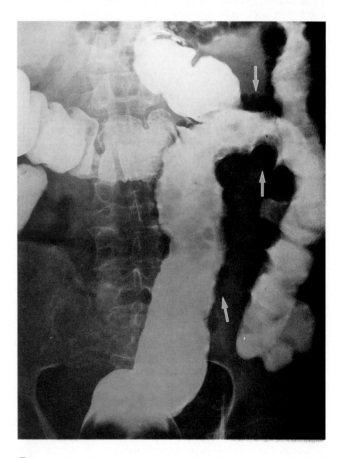

B

Figure 1–58. *Pneumatosis cystoides intestinalis.* **A.** Plain film shows multiple air bubbles in the wall of the sigmoid colon (*arrows*). **B.** Barium enema shows the contrast-filled lumen indented by gas-filled cystic structures (*arrows*).

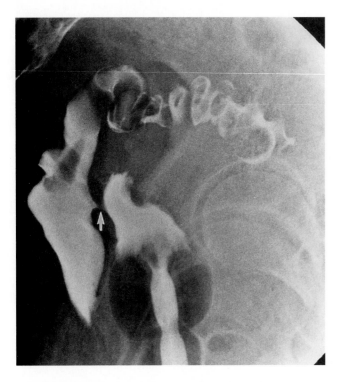

Figure 1–59. Vaginogram demonstrating rectovaginal fistula. A balloon catheter occludes the vagina and injected contrast outlines the fistulous tract (*arrow*) between the anterior rectum and posterior vaginal wall.

Sinography

If a fistula from the colon communicates with another bowel segment, it may be visualized by contrast enema. If a cutaneous communication is present, a catheter may be inserted into the skin opening and contrast injected under fluoroscopic observation. CT is also useful to outline a fistulous tract and contrast can be given via a cutaneous opening at the same time. If a rectovaginal fistula is suspected, it may be outlined by contrast enema or vaginography using a balloon catheter (Fig 1–59).

Complications

Complications of barium enema infrequently occur; the most dangerous is colonic perforation. This occurs in .02% to .04% of cases and has a 50% mortality rate, especially if the perforation is in the intraperitoneal portion of the colon. The cause is usually a combination of factors such as enema tip, rectal balloon, over distention, and, possibly, diseased bowel mucosa. Prompt recognition of this complication is critical, since it constitutes a surgical emergency. Soilage of the peritoneal cavity by barium and bowel contents causes a nidus for infection and peritonitis, adhesions, and granuloma formation. Rare allergic reactions to barium preparations and latex enema balloons have been reported.[125]

Delayed Antegrade Barium Examination

In a patient with severe inflammatory bowel disease, contrast enema may be contraindicated, although information regarding gross estimate of colonic disease is still necessary. Giving the patient a large quantity of barium orally and taking delayed radiographs when contrast has reached the colon may help in approximating colonic involvement.

Colon Evaluation by Barium Enema

The mucosa of the normal colon, when examined by air contrast technique, has a smooth, featureless appearance. The colon is evaluated by several standards such as position, size or distensibility, contour of the luminal margin, and mucosal appearance.

Position

The position of the colon may be abnormal as a result of congenital rotational anomalies, diaphragmatic hernias, or from acquired lesions such a volvulus or displacement by surrounding organs.

Diverticular Disease

Diverticulosis. Diverticulosis is the most common contour-altering abnormality in patients past middle age. The sigmoid colon is the zone most frequently involved, but diverticula can be diffuse. When viewed in profile, a diverticulum is a smooth, ovoid outpouching with a neck slightly narrower than the base. En face, it appears as a puddle or circle of barium (Fig 1–60).

Diverticulitis. Diverticulitis occurs when a microperforation or macroperforation of a diverticulum has occurred. Radiographic findings include extravasation of contrast material on enema examination, evidence of a pericolic extraluminal air collection indicating an abscess, or evidence of a paracolic soft tissue mass, also suggestive of an abscess. The portion of bowel involved also lacks normal distensibility. When there is marked irritability, the narrowed segment may be difficult to differentiate from a colonic cancer. Fistulae to the bladder, vagina, adjacent bowel, or skin may occur. Complete obstruction to the retrograde flow of barium also may occur.[126,127]

The accuracy in diagnosing diverticulitis has improved significantly with CT (Table 1–6). Not only is the lumen of the bowel visible, but so is wall thickness, inflammation in the surrounding fat and evidence of fistulae to adjacent organs. Filling of the colon with low density contrast at the time of examination and the administration of intravenous and oral contrast will help optimize findings by filling of the small bowel, bladder, and kidneys. CT findings associated with diverticulitis are listed in Table 1–6 and include air in the bladder or vagina, or a tract to the skin suggesting a fistula (Fig 1–61).[127–130]

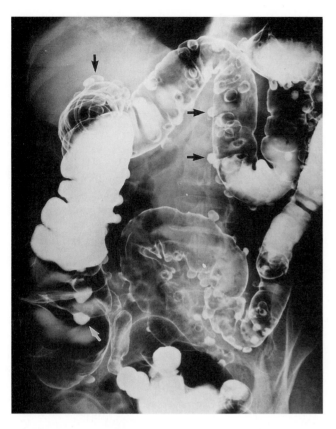

Figure 1–60. Diverticulosis on double-contrast barium enema. Diverticula are scattered throughout the colon (*arrows*).

TABLE 1–6. CT FINDINGS IN DIVERTICULITIS

Presence of diverticula
Inflammatory infiltration of periodic fat
Thickened colonic wall (> 4 mm)
Fluid or contrast within colonic wall indicating an intramural tract
Pelvic abscess and inflammatory changes of the colon
Peritonitis with inflammatory changes of the colon
Any of the above and air in the bladder, vagina, or a tract to the skin suggesting a fistula[12-15]

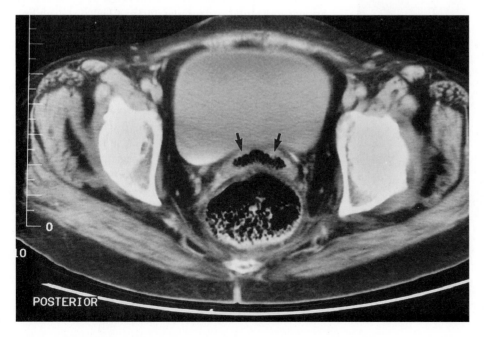

Figure 1–61. Diverticulitis with sigmoid vaginal fistula on CT. Air in the vagina (*arrows*) owing to sigmoid-vaginal fistula.

Ulcerating Lesions of the Colon

Ulcerative colitis. Double-contrast barium enema techniques allow the earliest changes of the colonic mucosa to be imaged. The normally featureless pattern assumes a fine granularity that is likened to frosted glass. With larger erosions, a coarser granular appearance may be seen. With deeper ulcerations, ulcers may appear as collar-button outpouchings from the luminal margin. The disease may involve only the rectum, the rectum and sigmoid colon, or the entire colon (pancolitis) (Fig 1–62). An increase in the retrorectal space, normally about 1 cm, may occur. The bowel is involved in continuity and symmetrically. The terminal ileum is spared except in cases of pancolitis where the terminal ileum may be dilated and smooth, and the ileocecal valve is patulous. These ileal changes have been referred to as "backwash ileitis."[131–133]

Mucosal filling defects or psuedopolyps may be present and are the result of either edematous mounds of nonulcerated mucosa or regenerating mucosa. These

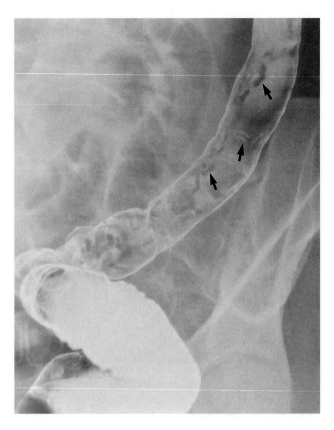

Figure 1–63. Ulcerative colitis with filiform pseudopolyps. Multiple filiform pseudopolyps are indicated by (*arrows*).

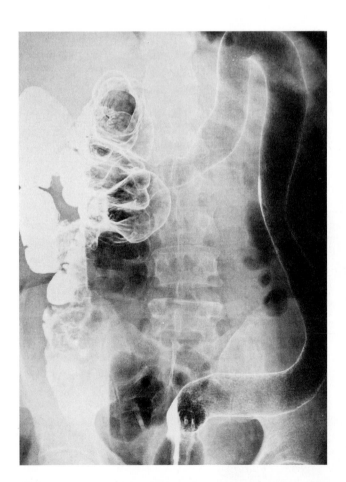

Figure 1–62. Ulcerative colitis involving only the left colon. There is a granular mucosal pattern, loss of haustration, and loss of distensibility from the midtransverse colon distally. The right colon is normally distensible.

may be sessile, polypoid, or filiform (Fig 1–63). Large masses pseudopolyps may be present and may simulate a neoplasm.[134]

Narrowing of the colonic lumen and loss of haustration are common radiographic findings. The colon may appear shortened and tubular and may lack distensibility. Strictured zones owing to hypertrophy of the musculous mucosa may be present and may be difficult to differentiate from an infiltrating carcinoma. Radiographic remissions may accompany clinical remissions.[135,136] Complications may be due to disease in the colon or its numerous extracolonic manifestations.

Toxic megacolon usually is suggested by the clinical course and plain abdominal radiographs. Contrast enemas are not necessary and follow-up imaging with plain films is adequate (see section on plain film colon).[137,138]

Carcinoma of the colon is a complication of ulcerative colitis that is prevalent in patients with long standing disease.[139,140] Diagnosis may be difficult since lesions may be atypical in appearance. In contrast to the abrupt annular lesions seen in noncolitis carcinoma, ulcerative colitis carcinoma may have the appearance of a stricture or may be multicentric. Flat, ulcerating lesions may be difficult to detect radiographically.[141]

CT

The bowel wall may be thickened and of low density because of either edema or fat infiltration. The increase in the retrorectal space may be due to contraction of the rectum and proliferation of pelvic fat (Fig 1–64). Irregularly thickened bowel wall and infiltration of pericolic fat may be seen with the complication of colon carcinoma.[142–144]

Colectomy is generally performed for ulcerative colitis. It is generally accompanied by creation of a continent ileal-anal pouch. Complications include anastomotic leaks, obstruction, abscesses, and pouchitis. The pouch is best imaged either via contrast enema or retrograde via ileostomy before the ileostomy is taken down.[145,146]

Sclerosing cholangitis is a common extraintestinal manifestation of ulcerative colitis and is seen in 5.5% of patients. In a patient with ulcerative colitis and abnormal biliary function, imaging of the biliary tree may be accomplished using endoscopic retrograde cholangiopancreatography (ERCP) or transhepatic cholangiogra-

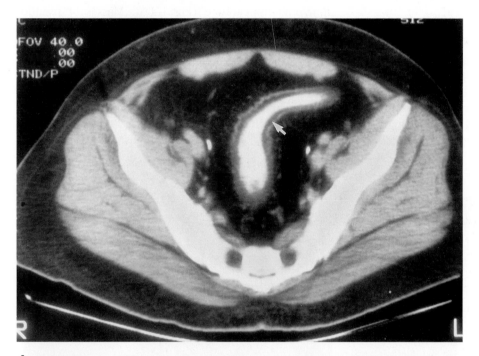

A

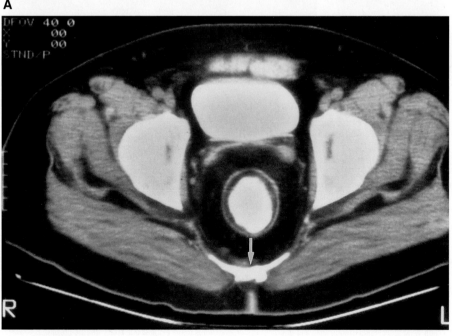

B

Figure 1–64. Ulcerative colitis on CT. **A.** The bowel is ahaustral with a thickened wall that contains a zone of fat density (*arrow*) **B.** The rectum also has a thickened wall containing a zone of fat density. There is a large amount of perirectal fat that causes an increase in the retrorectal space (*arrow*).

phy. Short multifocal structures of both the extrahepatic and/or intrahepatic ducts may occur (Fig 1–65). Bile duct carcinoma also develops in this patient population and may be difficult to differentiate radiographically from sclerosing cholangitis. The changes described include an annular constricting lesion with proximal dilatation of the biliary tree, diffuse infiltration of the bile ducts, or an intraluminal polypoid mass lesion. CT may show discontinuous intrahepatic biliary dilatation and thickening of the walls of the extrahepatic ducts.[147,148]

CROHN'S COLITIS

The earliest changes are seen in the mucosa and are best imaged using double-contrast techniques. These changes are aphthous lesions, which are shallow ulcerations surrounded by a lucent halo of edema on a background of normal mucosa. Large, deep, undermined ulcers may occur as the disease progresses, and if oriented longitudinally and transverse, the bowel may assume a cobble-

stoned appearance (Fig 1–66). The tracts extending into the bowel wall may extend beyond the wall and into other organs, thus producing fistulae.[149–151]

Unlike ulcerative colitis, Crohn's colitis is often discontinuous, producing skip areas of disease that may be asymmetric in its involvement of a bowel segment. Pancolitis may occur. Bowel strictures are not uncommon and often are accompanied by obstructive symptoms.

Pseudopolyps may be "cobblestones" of nonulcerated tissue remaining after longitudinal and transverse ulcerations occur, or they may have a filiform or sessile polypoid appearance (Fig 1–66). Masses of pseudopolyps may be large enough to cause obstructive symptoms.[134,152] Perirectal disease is common. Fistulas and sinus tracts may be imaged on contrast enema but are more likely to be seen on pelvic CT.[153]

Radiographic remissions are unusual in Crohn's colitis, and the patient's clinical status often will correlate poorly with the radiographic picture. Remissions may occur in the earliest stages of the disease but have not been

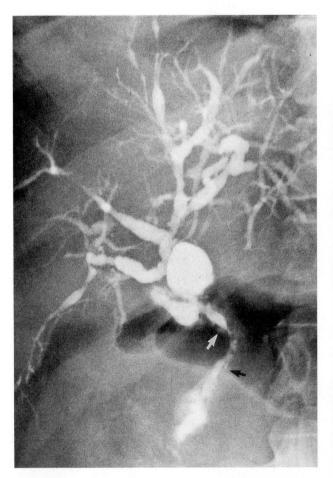

A

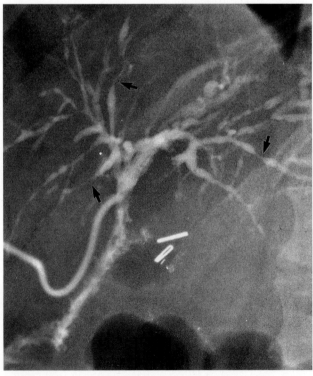

B

Figure 1–65. Sclerosing cholangitis in ulcerative colitis. **A.** Multiple mural irregularities and diverticulalike outpouchings of the extrahepatic biliary tree are present. **B.** Numerous intrahepatic ductal strictures are present (*arrows*). Patient has undergone a choledochojejunostomy for extensive extrahepatic sclerosing cholangitis.

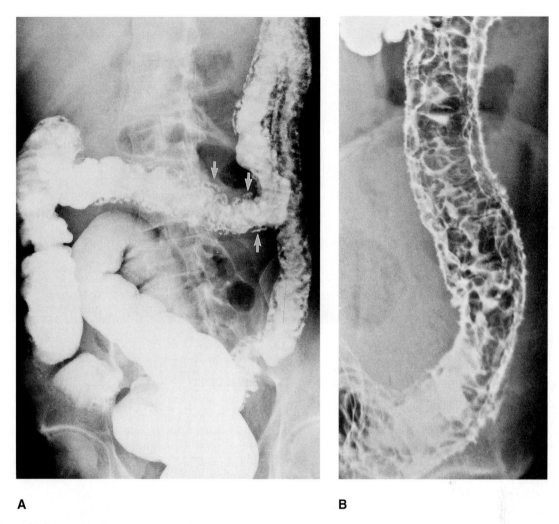

A   **B**

Figure 1–66. Crohn's colitis with extensive ulceration. **A.** *Arrows* indicate longitudinal ulceration of the transverse colon. **B.** Longitudinal and transverse ulcerations give a cobblestoned appearance to the bowel. *Arrows* indicate tract into the bowel wall.

reported in advanced stages. Recurrence after surgery occurs frequently, often on the ileal side of an ileocolic anastomosis. Fistulae may appear in other bowel loops, bladder, skin, vagina, or urethra. Abscesses also may be found. Toxic megacolon occurs, although it is less likely than in patients with ulcerative colitis. Plain films are adequate to follow patients with pancolitis.[120]

Carcinoma occurs with greater frequency in patients with Crohn's colitis than in noncolitic patients. It occurs more commonly in fistulous tracts, around the rectum, and in bypassed segments. Preoperative diagnosis is unusual since these regions are difficult to image.[139,154]

Extracolonic manifestations include arthritis, urinary calculous disease, and obstruction due to an inflammatory mass and fistulae involving the bladder. Gallstones are common.[147,148]

A great deal of information can be gained from abdominal CT in Crohn's disease that involves the colon; the full extent of bowel wall thickening and involvement can be appreciated, as can abscesses and fistulae (Fig 1–67). Fistulae in the perianal region cannot be imaged by any other means. Enterovesical fistulae are notoriously difficult to document. However, CT enables visualization of a few air bubbles in the bladder and also will show adjacent bowel inflammation, thereby securing the diagnosis. Extracolonic manifestations such as gallstones, renal stones, sacroiliitis, and the rare complication of osteomyelitis also may be diagnosed.[142–144,155,156]

OTHER COLITIDES

With amebiasis, the cecum and rectosigmoid are the frequent sites of radiographic involvement since these organisms commonly pool in areas of stasis. The cecum is most frequently involved and may be cone shaped. Collar-button ulcers may occur in areas of involved bowel and large masses of granulation tissue, called amebomas, occur. Strictures may also develop.

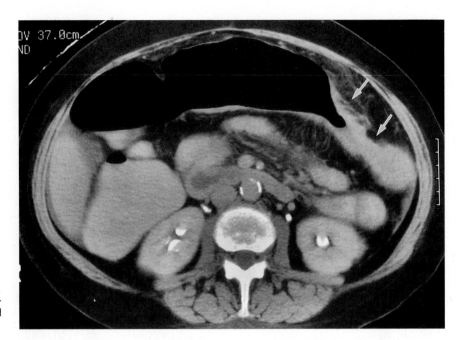

Figure 1–67. Crohn's colitis on CT. Splenic flexure stricture due to Crohn's colitis with thickened bowel wall and infiltration of the pericolic fat (*arrows*).

Tuberculosis involving the colon also may involve the cecum and right colon. Distal ileal disease and marked colonic stricturing may occur.

Other infectious colitides are those as a result of *Campylobacter* (indistinguishable from ulcerative colitis), *Shigella,* or *Yersinia* organisms. These organisms may produce changes such as irritability, thickened or lost haustra, or ulceration. Gonorrhea, herpes, infection, and lymphogranuloma venereum (LGV) produce inflammation that is often limited to the rectum.[157,158]

OTHER

Pseudomembranous colitis is frequently seen in the postsurgical patient following antibiotic therapy. The organism *Clostridium difficile* overgrows and liberates an enterocolitis-producing toxin. Radiologically, plaque-like lesions that are pseudomembranes are seen on single-contrast examination. These are composed of sloughed mucosa and inflammatory cells. The mucosa may have a shaggy appearance and haustra may be thickened owing to colonic edema. Ulceration is uncommon. CT is of value in showing marked wall thickening in the appropriate patient.[159]

Typhlitis

Typhlitis occurs in patients with neutropenia. The condition may be a complication of leukemia, lymphoma, or immunosuppression. A combination of infection, ischemia, and neoplastic cell infiltration may lead to bowel perforation. The cecum may show marked wall thickening, pericolic fat infiltration, and extraluminal fluid. CT is the least invasive method of imaging this lesion (Fig 1–68).[160,161]

Ischemic Colitis

Ischemic colitis may occur because of thrombosis, embolism, or low blood flow due to hypotension or vasculitis, which causes inadequate bowel perfusion.

Plain films may show thumbprints indenting the gas-filled lumen because of submucosal hemorrhage and edema. Contrast examination may show mucosal ulcers or perforation, if bowel necrosis has occurred. The splenic flexure of the colon is the site most frequently involved, although any portion of the colon may be involved. The bowel may heal with no radiographic sequelae, with stricture formation, or it may progress to gangrene and perforation (Figs 1–69 and 1–70).[162]

Radiation Colitis

Radiation changes may be either acute or chronic. Acute changes are in the periradiation period. Submucosal hemorrhage, edema, and mucosal ulceration may occur. Chronic changes may be seen, since the effects of radiation cause vascular changes (pathogenesis similar to that of vasculitis) and may not be manifest from months to years following radiation. These changes include strictures and fistulas. Clinical history is essential in making this diagnosis since similar radiographic findings may be seen in other conditions such as ulcerative proctitis, Crohn's disease, and diverticulitis (Fig 1–71).

Colonic Masses

Luminal defects. Since polypoid adenomas are considered to have malignant potential, the search for early colon cancer has become a search for colonic polyps (Fig 1–72).[163,164] When evaluating a polypoid colonic lesion,

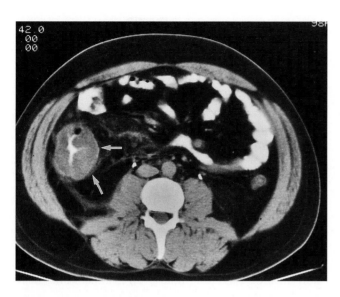

Figure 1–68. Typhlitis. Cecal wall thickening and infiltration of the pericolic fat is present in this patient with acute leukemia (*arrows*).

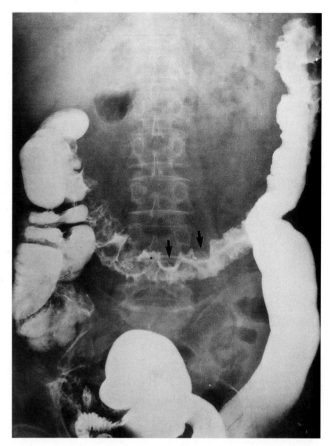

Figure 1–69. Ischemic colitis. Barium enema shows thumbprintlike indentations of the transverse colon and splenic flexure due to submucosal hemorrhage and edema (*arrows*).

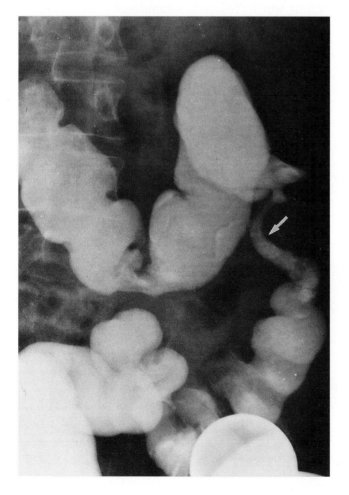

Figure 1–70. Stricture due to ischemic colitis (*arrow*).

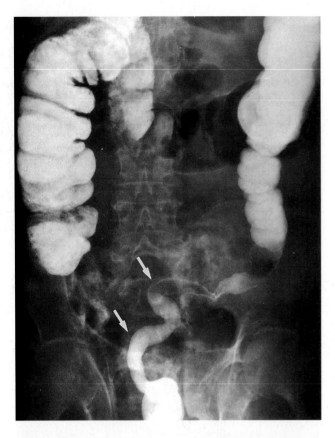

Figure 1–71. Radiation changes of the colon. Marked narrowing of the sigmoid colon is the result of the late changes of radiation colitis (*arrows*). Areas of increased bone density in the sacrum are caused by radiation osteitis.

the criteria for determining whether it is benign or malignant are

1. Size—lesions >2 cm in size have a 25% likelihood of malignancy, whereas lesions <1 cm in size have a 1% likelihood.
2. Sessile lesions are more likely to be malignant.
3. Rapid growth indicates malignancy, as does indentation of the colonic wall at the site of the lesion.[118]

Villous adenomas are adenomatous polyps covered with multiple excrescences. Barium may be trapped in the crevices of the lesion, giving it a cauliflowerlike appearance on barium enema examination. Most of these are larger than 2 cm when discovered and therefore have a high likelihood of being malignant. The most likely location is rectosigmoid, with the cecum the next most frequent site.[165]

Other neoplasms presenting as colonic filling defects include lipomas. These soft, smooth mucosal lesions are found most frequently in the right colon and may change in shape when a compression paddle is applied to them. This ability to change shape has been called the "squeeze sign."

Other neoplastic polypoid lesions involving the colon are neurofibromas, leiomyomas, and carcinoid tumors, which are usually submucosal in the rectum.

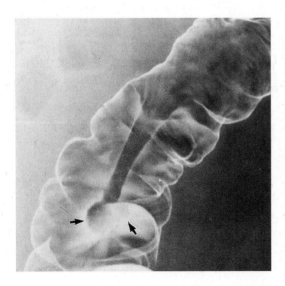

A

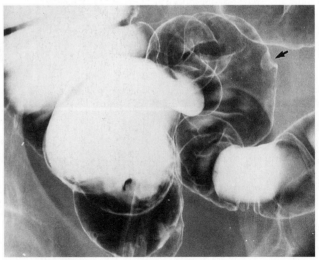

B

Figure 1–72. Adenomatous colonic polyps. **A.** Pedunculated polyp (*arrows*) on a long stalk. **B.** Sessile polyp (*arrow*).

TABLE 1–7. POLYPOSIS SYNDROMES INVOLVING THE COLON

Malignant	Polyps	Potential
Familial polyposis	adenomas	high
Gardner's syndrome	adenomas	high
Turcot's syndrome	adenomas	high
Peutz-Jeghers syndrome	hamartomas	low
Cronkhite-Canada syndrome	harmartomatous resembling juvenile	none

Polyposis Syndromes

Polyposis syndromes involving the colon include familial polyposis, Gardner's syndrome, Turcot's syndrome, Peutz-Jeghers' syndrome, Cowden's syndrome (multiple hamartoma syndrome, MHS) and Candida-Cronkhite's syndrome (Table 1–7) (Fig 1–73). Familial polyposis, Gardner's syndrome, and Turcot's syndrome are considered by some investigators to be part of the same disease spectrum referred to as familial adenomatous polyposis syndrome (FAPS). In both familial polyposis and Gardner's syndrome, the polyps are adenomas. Patients have a 100% risk of developing carcinoma if these are left untreated.[166–169]

Lymphoid hyperplasia, colonic urticaria, and *Pneumatosis cystoides intestinalis* may occasionally resemble colonic polyps (Fig 1–58).[168]

Colonic Cancer

Adenocarcinoma of the colon constitutes 95% of colonic malignancies. In recent years, there has been a shift in distribution from predominantly left-sided tumors to a more equal distribution between the right and left sides. Tumors may appear annular or polypoid on contrast enema. Additionally, they may be scirrhous and may appear radiographically similar to inflammatory bowel disease. High-risk patients include those with a polyposis syndrome, a family history of carcinoma, a history of inflammatory bowel disease, or those who have had prior colonic malignancy. There is a 3.5% incidence of synchronous carcinomas, and patients who have had one colon cancer are more likely to develop a metachronous lesion. Patients who have colon cancer are also more likely to have polyps elsewhere. Because of the possibility of synchronous cancers and polyps, the colon must be thoroughly examined even if only a single lesion has been discovered. Unusual first presentations of colon carcinoma are metastatic liver mass, bowel obstruction or perforation, or multiple pulmonary metastases.[163]

Enthusiasm for CT as the ultimate modality for presurgical staging is tempered by accuracy rates of only 69% to 88%. In a patient with rectal carcinoma, information regarding the lower and upper margins of the lesion and its relationship to the levator ani, anal sphincter, and pelvic muscles is needed. Evidence of metastatic disease should also be sought.[170–173] Errors in sensitivity are the result of the inability to detect microscopic invasion of pericolonic fat and to the inability to assess the presence of metastases in normal-sized lymph nodes. Small metastases to the peritoneal cavity may not be visible even on an optimal scan. Currently, routine staging using CT is not recommended for primary colorectal tumors because of its inaccuracy. However, it should be used for patients in whom locally extensive or widespread disease is suggested, especially for those in whom radiation therapy alone or in combination with later surgery is anticipated.

In patients who are being evaluated for recurrent colorectal carcinoma, the imaging criteria are similar to those for the primary lesion: thickening of the bowel wall, a soft tissue mass, and any evidence of tumor in the liver, lungs, lymph nodes, or peritoneum. A frequent problem in the postoperative patient is that granulation tissue, hemorrhage, or edema may also produce the soft tissue mass seen with recurrent tumor. Thus, these benign postoperative changes are radiologically indistinguishable from those produced by recurrent tumor; they may persist as long as 2 years, particularly in the pelvis, in patients who have undergone abdominoperineal or low anterior resection. Any enlargement of a known mass may, however, signal tumor recurrence. Despite its faults, CT is currently the best modality for the detection of recurrent tumor and distant metastases, especially if the recurrence develops extraluminally (Fig 1–74).[170,171] Additionally, it is a good modality for image-guided percutaneous biopsy.

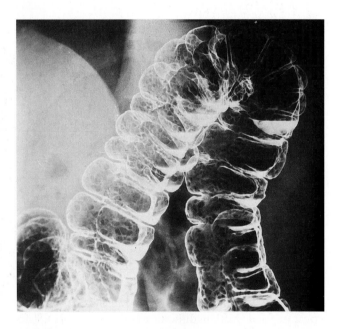

Figure 1–73. Familial polyposis. The colonic mucosa is carpeted with adenomatous polyps.

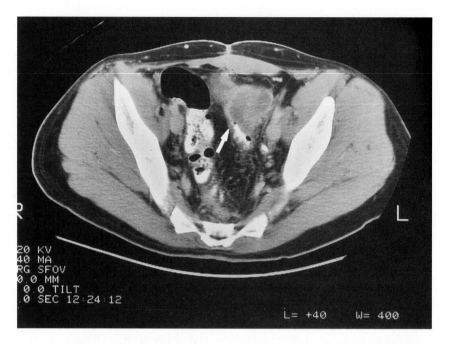

A

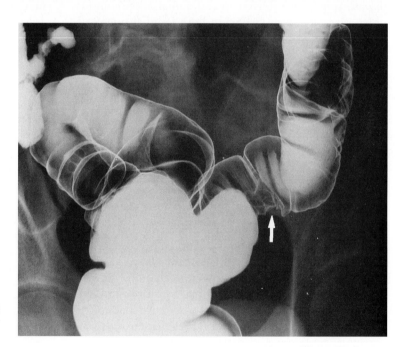

Figure 1–74. Recurrent colonic carcinoma. **A.** CT reveals a mixed-density left pelvic mass (*arrows*). **B.** Double-contrast enema shows a serosal lesion in this same region (*arrows*).

B

MRI

Because of differences in scanners, scanning protocols, and the lack of standardization of bowel and intravenous contrast used, MRI is difficult to compare with CT in evaluating the patient with colon carcinoma. Limitations for accuracy in initial staging are similar to those noted for CT. These include the inability to determine if microscopic invasion of pericolonic fat has occurred and to detect metastases in normal-sized lymph nodes. Differentiation of benign postoperative inflammatory masses from recurrent tumor is also difficult. The multiplanar capability of MRI may be useful when determining if colonic tumor has invaded bone or muscle.[163,171,173]

SONOGRAPHY

Transabdominal sonography may be useful in evaluating the liver in a patient with colon carcinoma; however, transrectal sonography has added advantages since the layers of the bowel can be distinguished and the depth of tumor invasion can be assessed. Sensitivities have been reported ranging from 67% to 90% for perirectal spread to only 50% to 57% for regional node metastases. Another limitation is that the endoscope may not be able to traverse a stenotic lesion, which is a frequent finding in colonic carcinoma.[172]

NUCLEAR MEDICINE

Radiolabeled monoclonal antibodies directed toward tumor-associated antigens is a promising method being used for the evaluation of patients with colorectal carcinoma. Indium III ([III]In)-labeled satumomab pendetide (Onco Scint Cytogen Corp, Princeton, NJ) is the first approved agent for imaging colorectal lesions. Imaging with this agent may supplement the information currently available from CT and barium studies and may help detect tumor sites in the pelvis and extrahepatic abdomen. This information may alter surgical approach or preoperative systemic therapy.[174,175]

Primary Colonic Lymphoma

Primary lymphoma of the colon is rare but may occur in 6% to 12% of patients with disseminated disease. Most of these patients have non-Hodgkin's lymphoma. Radiographically, the lesion may resemble an annular carcinoma or may appear as a cavitated mass or multiple polyps. The polypoid form is almost always disseminated and the colon is carpeted with polyps. This appearance may be indistinguishable from some of the polyposis syndromes.[176]

Endometriosis

Ectopic implants of endometrial tissue on the serosa of the colon may cause smooth muscle hyperplasia. The most frequent location is the anterior rectosigmoid region in the area of the cul de sac, although any portion of the bowel may be involved (Fig 1–75). Serosal implants of endometriosis may cause mucosal pleating or spiculation of the bowel wall. Annular lesions due to endometriosis may be radiologically indistinguishable from colon carcinoma.[177,178]

Metastatic Disease

Metastatic disease to the colon may occur by three routes. First, direct invasion of the colon by tumors in the pancreas, stomach, kidney, prostate, gallbladder, and ovary may occur. Bowel angulation, mucosal pleating or nodularity, or annular narrowing may be seen on contrast enema. Second, intraperitoneal seeding is a common route by which ovarian, gastric, or pancreatic cancer metastasizes to the colon. Pleating of the colonic mucosa or mass effects displacing colon are seen as a result of serosal involvement and peritoneal metastatic masses. Drop metastases to the pelvis (Blumer's shelf) from a proximal bowel lesion may be confused with a rectosigmoid tumor. Finally, tumors of the breast, lung, and melanoma may metastasize to the colon hematogenously. Lesions can have a scirrhous appearance not unlike inflammatory bowel disease or may resemble ulcerated submucosal masses, the target or bull's-eye appearance.[179,180]

Postoperative Colon

The colon may need to be evaluated postoperatively for complications such as leaks and strictures or for evidence of tumor recurrence. An accurate assessment of the postoperative state is facilitated by detailed information about the surgical procedure performed.[181]

FUNCTIONAL RADIOGRAPHIC EVALUATION OF THE COLON

Defecography, or evacuation proctography, is a radiographic method used for evaluation of anorectal functional disorders. Patients usually have severe constipation or incontinence. The rectum is filled with a barium paste that has the consistency of stool. Commercial preparations are available (Evac-U-Paste, EZ-EM, Anatrast). The patient is examined fluoroscopically while sitting in the lateral position on a commode. Evacuation is videotaped and spot radiographs are obtained. Measurements are made on the films obtained of the anorectal angle at rest, while instructed to lift, and during defecation. These measurements are compared to available normals. Morphologic abnormalities such as rectoceles, rectal prolapse, enteroceles, and intussusception may be visualized, as well as functional abnormalities such as puborectalis dysfunction and the descending perineum syndrome (Fig 1–76).[182,183]

RADIOPAQUE MARKET STUDIES

Radiopaque marker studies are used in patients with chronic constipation where an estimate of transit time is desired. The patient swallows capsules containing a known quantity of radiopaque markers (Sitzmarks Radiopaque Markers, Konsyl Pharmaceuticals, Fort Worth, TX). Abdominal radiographs are taken on day 4 and day 7 and the markers are counted. The numbers and site are compared with normal controls, giving an approximation of transit time.[184,185]

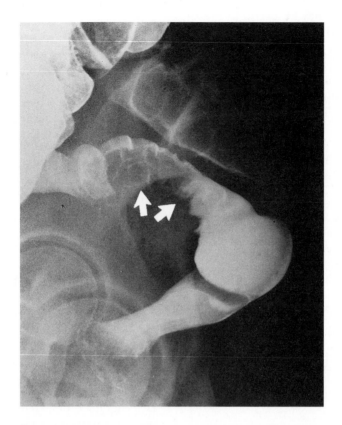

A

B

Figure 1–75. Endometriosis. **A.** A large serosal mass as a result of endometriosis causing an impression on the anterior aspect of the rectosigmoid (*arrows*). **B.** Endometriosis on CT. A serosal implant due to endometriosis on the sigmoid colon is indicated by *arrows*. The large left pelvic mass is an endometrioma.

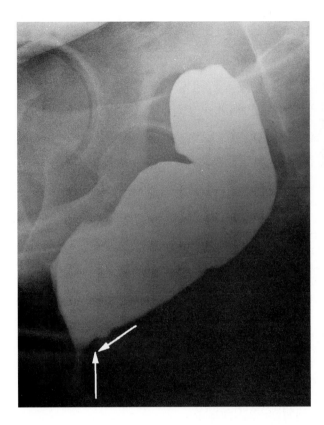

A

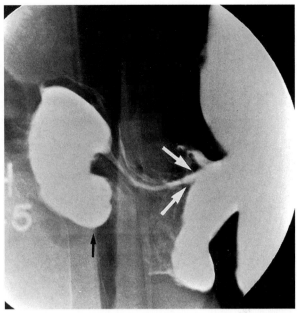

B

Figure 1–76. Defecography. **A.** Junction of arrows indicates a normal anorectal angle seen on evacuation. **B.** Anorectal intussusception. *Arrows* indicate point at which invagination occurs. A tetrocele is also present (*black arrow*).

■ RADIOLOGY OF THE APPENDIX

Although the appendix is only a very small portion of the gastrointestinal tract, disease of this structure is probably the most frequent cause of abdominal surgical emergency.[186]

The diagnosis can be made on the basis of clinical history and physical examination, but, in approximately 20% of patients with appendicitis, the findings are atypical. This is the group that may undergo imaging studies. Obstruction of the lumen of the appendix followed by inflammation is the usual course of events. Radiologic findings are based on this inflammation.[187]

PLAIN FILMS

Plain film abnormalities include a calcific density (appendicolith) in the right lower quadrant, a right lower-quadrant mass, cecal ileus, loss of the psoas margin, or distortion of the right flank stripe. Extraluminal gas in the right lower or upper quadrants or frank pneumoperitoneum may also be present (Table 1–8). These radiologic findings are variable. An appendicolith is the most diagnostically reliable sign, although it is only found in 10% of patients. When present, the likelihood of complicated appendicitis, such as perforation or abscess, is nearly 50%.[187]

TABLE 1–8. PLAIN FILM FINDINGS OF APPENDICITIS

Calcified appendicolith
Right lower quadrant mass
Cecal ileus
Loss of right psoas margin
Distortion of right flank stripe
Extraluminal gas collections
Pneumoperitoneum

TABLE 1–9. CONTRAST ENEMA FINDINGS OF APPENDICITIS

Mass defect—medial wall cecum or ascending colon
Irritability or mucosal spiculation cecum, ascending colon or terminal ileum
Lack of filling or incomplete filling appendix

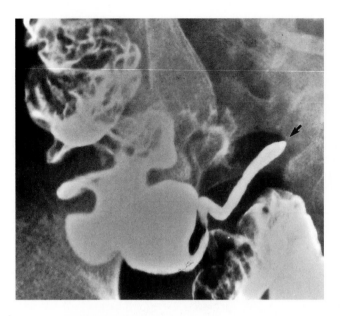

Figure 1–77. Normal appendix filled on barium enema. *Arrows* indicate cobra-head appendiceal tip.

Prior to the use of CT and ultrasound, contrast enema using either barium or water-soluble contrast was the only other radiographic technique available to confirm the diagnosis of appendicitis (Table 1–9). A full-column technique is employed and no preparation of the patient is necessary. If the entire appendix fills, either during the study or as seen on a postevacuation film, appendicitis does not exist (Fig 1–77). The filled tip, a "cobra-head" configuration, should be sought. On occasion the lumen may fill only partially and an abscess or perforation will be present at the tip. Other important findings include an extrinsic mass defect on the medial wall of the cecum or ascending colon (Fig 1–78). Nonfilling of the appendix without any signs of a mass is an unreliable sign, since many normal appendices do not fill on contrast enema examinations.[188]

CT

CT is a significantly more direct and accurate way of confirming the diagnosis of appendicitis (Table 1–10). Severity of disease and complications can also be evaluated. Also, other disease processes may be diagnosed in the patient with an acute abdomen and no radiographic signs of appendicitis. Good bowel filling with contrast material prior to the examination is helpful (Fig 1–79).

Findings on CT include a distended, thick-walled appendix that may enhance when intravenous contrast is given (Fig 1–80). Streaking of the periappendiceal fat is an important sign of inflammation. Fluid collections owing to abscess formation and poorly defined soft tis-

sue masses may be present. A calcified appendicolith may be seen in the appendiceal lumen or free in an abscess cavity. A thickened cecal wall and/or terminal ileal wall and thickening of the anterior renal and lateral conal fascia are also frequent findings. Even if the appendix is in an atypical location such as retrocecal, it will maintain a constant relationship to the cecum. In most cases the position of the cecum can be appreciated readily on CT.

With complicated appendicitis, peritonitis with ascites and thickening of the peritoneum, a large inflammatory mass, phlegmon, or an appendiceal abscess may exist.

The differential diagnosis includes cecal diverticulitis, mucocele of the appendix, perforation of a cecal neoplasm, tubo-ovarian abscess, and Crohn's disease. Pitfalls in the diagnosis may include bowel loops that are poorly filled with contrast material and calcifications that are not appendicoliths, such as pills or lymph nodes.[187–192]

ULTRASOUND

Graded compression sonography was described by Puylaert in 1986 and has increased the value of sonography

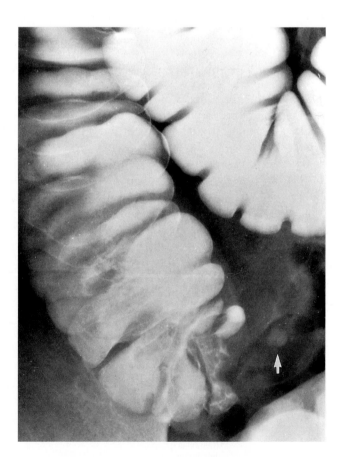

Figure 1–78. Nonfilling of cecal tip and appendicolith (*arrows*).

TABLE 1–10. APPENDICITIS

UNCOMPLICATED APPENDICITIS
    Periappendiceal or pericecal inflammation
    Abnormal thick walled appendix
    Thickening of the medial cecal wall
    Thickened wall of the distal small bowel
    Thickened anterior renal and lateral conal fascia
    Appendicolith

COMPLICATED APPENDICITIS
    Peritonitis
    Phlegmon
    Abscess

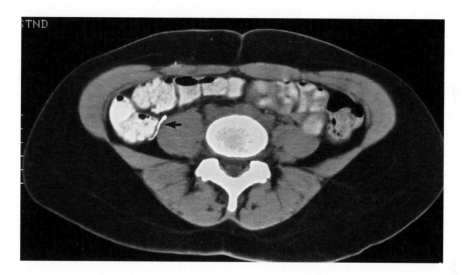

Figure 1–79. Normal appendix seen on CT (*arrow*).

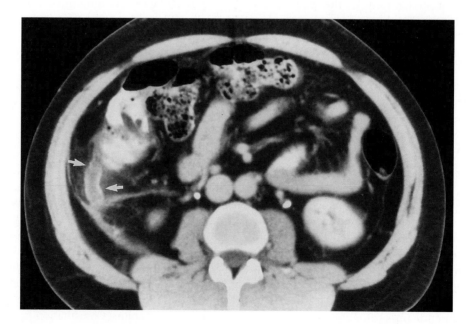

Figure 1–80. Acute appendicitis on CT showing distended thick walled appendix with inflammatory streaking of periappendiceal fat (*arrows*).

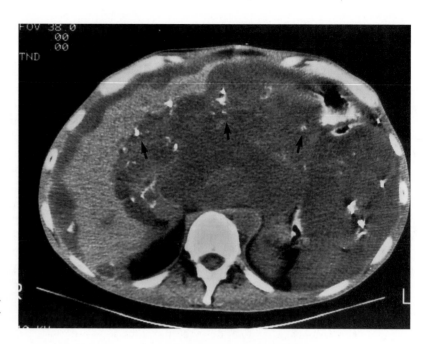

Figure 1–81. *Pseudomyxoma peritoneii* secondary to ruptured cystadenocarcinoma of the appendix on CT. *Arrows* point to calcifications scattered throughout gelatinous collections.

in the patient being evaluated for appendicitis.[193–195] Gentle pressure is applied with the transducer over the area of discomfort. This pressure helps displace bowel, gas, and fecal material. A normal appendix may be seen in 10% to 15% of individuals, providing evidence against the diagnosis of appendicitis. In a patient with appendicitis, the appendix appears tubular, is not compressible, has no peristalsis, and measures >6 mm in its transverse diameter. An appendicolith with posterior shadowing may be present. Complicated appendicitis with an abscess may show as a hypoechoic mass in the cecal region.

The advantage of sonography in the patient suspected of appendicitis is that there is no radiation, thus making it preferable for children and pregnant women. Additionally, no contrast material is used, and it is quicker and less expensive than CT. Sonography is limited in obese patients and those in whom pain is too great to permit graded compression. Sonographic evaluation is also user-dependent and may be useless in the hands of an inexperienced sonographer. The technique is not as accurate as CT for evaluating severity of appendicitis.

NEOPLASMS

Appendiceal mucoceles may be caused by mucosal hyperplasia, mucinous cystadenoma or mucinous cystadenocarcinoma. Preoperative diagnosis is important. Leaking or rupture at the time of surgery may lead to *Pseudomyxoma peritonei*. If a cystadenoma is present, the appendiceal ostia may become occluded, leading to inflammation and appendicitis.

Plain film findings may be a right lower quadrant mass that may have a rimlike calcification. If *Pseudomyxoma peri-*

tonei is present, there may be an overall hazy density of the abdomen similar to that seen in ascites, separation of bowel loops, and faint scattered calcification.

A well-marginated fluid or soft tissue mass is present on CT examination. Bowel loops are displaced without thickened bowel walls. With superimposed appendicitis, streaking of the periappendiceal fat and bowel wall thickening may be present.

Scalloped fluid-density lesions, often containing streaks of calcification throughout the abdomen, are noted when *Pseudomyxoma peritonei* is present (Fig 1–81).

On MRI examination, mucoceles may have a low signal on T1-weighted images and a high signal on T2-weighted images, if they primarily contain fluid. If they contain mucin, they may be bright on both T1- and T2-weighted images.[187,196] Malignant neoplasms such as carcinoid are usually found incidentally at surgery.

■ RADIOLOGY OF THE LIVER

EXAMINATION TECHNIQUES

Ultrasound, CT, and MRI have supplanted nuclear scintigraphy and angiography since the 1970s and 1980s. Nevertheless, the choice of the appropriate test can be confusing. In addition, specific diseases and indications also require different protocols for ultrasound, CT, and MRI. The appropriate test depends on the specific clinical indication, knowledge of the sensitivity, specificity, and limitations of the different tests available; and the patient's body habitus. Consultation between the referring physician and the radiologist therefore can optimize the imaging strategy and obviate unnecessary tests.[197–199]

The inferior outline of the liver is often visible on plain radiographs, and therefore it is sometimes possible to diagnose hepatomegaly on plain films. Ultrasound is a noninvasive, low cost, and readily available test that has good accuracy in delineating haptic disease. Piezoelectric crystals in the ultrasound transducer are stimulated to send sound waves through the body and then listen for the echoes as the sound is reflected by tissue interfaces. The reflected echoes can then be reconstructed by computer to form an image. However, it is suboptimal in obese patients and those in whom the rib cage and overlying bowel gas obscure the liver. Nevertheless, it is superior to other modalities in its ability to differentiate between cystic and solid lesions. Its Doppler capability is particularly suited for assessment of the hepatic vasculature.[199]

CT is currently the hepatic imaging modality of choice.[197] It is more reliable than ultrasound in consistent visualization of the entire liver. Optimal technique requires intravenous contrast and therefore is limited to use in patients who do not have renal insufficiency or significant contrast allergies. In such patients, ultrasound or MRI may be preferable. Many protocols exist for hepatic CT. Slice thickness, volume, rate of intravenous contrast administration, and scan time need to be altered depending on the clinical indication, in order to optimize the study. For routine hepatic evaluation, incremental bolus dynamic scan is the preferred technique. Scanning is performed during optimal contrast enhancement of the liver, usually between approximately 45 seconds and 3 minutes after initiation of bolus contrast infusion (Fig 1–82). When evaluation of a possible hemangioma is required, a single-level bolus dynamic scan is performed. Multiple scans are obtained at a single level through the lesion at different time intervals and after contrast infusion to determine the enhancement profile of the lesion. CT arterial portography, obtained during contrast infusion into the splanchnic circulation by an angiographic catheter placed in the superior mesenteric or splenic vein, is the most sensitive form of invasive CT and is used for detection of hepatic lesions. It is performed in select patients who are being considered for hepatic tumor resection.[200] A CT arterial portogram often requires a delayed CT for joint interpretation, usually obtained after 4 to 6 hours, because of possible confusing perfusion defects that may be seen on the first CT.

One remarkable advance in CT technology is *spiral CT*.[201,202] The new generation of CT scanners can produce higher resolution images without motion artifact because of their increased speed and ability to scan through the entire liver in one single breath-hold. The X-ray tube and detectors actually spin around the patient as the table moves through the scanner; thus the term *spiral* or *helica*. With the capability of acquiring motion-free, high-resolution data through a volume of tis-

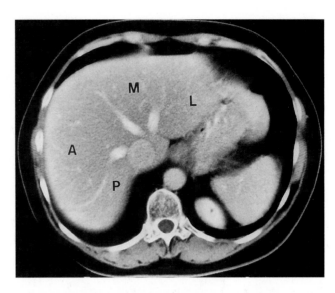

Figure 1–82. Normal CT through the upper part of the liver. Note the good opacification of the three hepatic veins which, at this level, marks the division of the liver into the anterior (A) and posterior (P) segments of the right lobe and the medial (M) and lateral (L) segments of the left lobe.

sue, good 3-dimensional displays of data are now possible, including spiral CT angiography. This technique involves high-rate injection of intravenous contrast and precise timing to spiral scan through the region of interest during optimal vascular opacification. The technique is excellent for visualization of large- and medium-sized vessels such as the portal vein and hepatic veins. However, the patient must be able to breath-hold, therefore limiting its use for uncooperative, unconscious, or very sick patients.

MRI is still evolving. Inherent advantages of MRI include lack of radiation, better contrast resolution, multiplanar capability (Fig 1–83), and the diminished allergic reactions and renal toxicity of its intravenous contrast agent, gadolinium. Disadvantages include suboptimal spatial resolution, susceptibility to motion artifacts, length of time required for a complete study (between 30 and 60 minutes), and higher cost. At its current stage of development, MRI has already surpassed routine CT in both detection and characterization of liver lesions, especially in the evaluation of hepatic metastasis and hemangiomas. Again, depending on the specific clinical indication, different imaging sequences are required and the examination must be tailored to the question at hand. Contraindications include claustrophobia and metallic foreign bodies. Further developments in fast imaging techniques and MRI contrast agents are promising and may enable MRI to become more accurate and routine.[198,203–207]

Although ultrasound, CT, and MRI have, in most instances, replaced radionuclide imaging of the liver, nuclear scintigraphy remains important in the diagnosis of specific disorders.[199,204] A pharmaceutical agent is la-

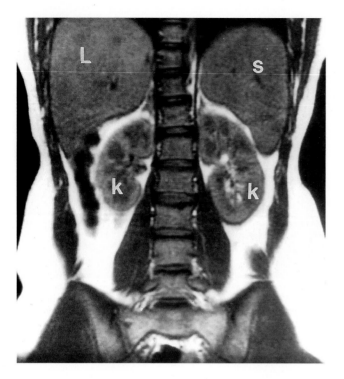

Figure 1–83. Coronal T1-weighted MRI image of abdomen. L: liver, S: spleen, K: kidney.

beled with a radionuclide and then injected into the patient. The radiopharmaceutical agent then is distributed in the body according to its pharmaceutical properties. The radionuclide enables detection and imaging of this distribution by emitting gamma photons detectable by a gamma camera. The liver-spleen scan used to be the only noninvasive imaging modality available for the detection of hepatic lesions. In this test, the pharmaceutical sulfur colloid is labeled with ^{99m}Tc, the radionuclide. Sulfur colloid is avidly taken up by the body's reticuloendothelial system, including the spleen and Kupffer cells in the liver; hence the name liver-spleen scan. Hepatic lesions that do not contain Kupffer cells show up as "cold spots." This property can be used to differentiate between hepatic lesions with differential amounts of Kupffer cells such as hepatic adenomas and focal nodular hyperplasia (FNH). The sulfur colloid scan is also sensitive in the detection of early or mild hepatic dysfunction such as early cirrhosis, before anatomic and detectable changes occur on other imaging modalities. Another common test is labeled RBC scanning for the confirmation of suspected hemangiomas.[204] An image is formed based on body blood pool distribution of ^{99m}Tc-labeled RBCs. The hepatobiliary scan is performed primarily for evaluation of biliary function but is also useful for assessment of hepatic function. ^{99m}Tc-labeled iminodiacidic acid derivatives, such as IDA, HIDA, and DISIDA, are taken up by hepa-

tocytes and excreted into the biliary tree. Global hepatic function can be monitored and is useful, for example, in the assessment of hepatic function in liver transplant patients (Fig 1–84).

Diagnostic angiography and venography are performed seldomly except in conjunction with potential interventional procedures. Nevertheless, hepatic arteriography can be important in preoperative evaluation of hepatic resection and is currently the gold standard for diagnosis of hepatic artery thrombosis and stenosis post-liver transplantation (Fig 1–85).

HEPATIC TUMORS AND TUMORLIKE CONDITIONS

Some general principles apply to all imaging modalities in the differentiation between benign and malignant tumors.[198,208–214] Poorly defined margins, heterogeneity, necrosis, invasion of vasculature, and biliary obstruction all suggest malignancy.

Malignant tumors

Of the malignant hepatic tumors, metastasis outnumbers, by far, the primary tumors. When evaluating for the presence of hepatic metastasis, ultrasound is a simple and cheap method for screening.[210] However, many patients will need additional imaging because of poor sonographic visualization. One therefore may elect to screen with CT. Both noncontrast and contrast-enhanced images are important for detection of liver metastasis. Most metastases are hypovascular relative to the liver and therefore will appear as hypodense defects after contrast enhancement. However, some metastases tend to be vascular, such as melanoma, islet cell tumors, carcinoid tumors, and some breast carcinomas. These metastases may not be visible on contrast-enhanced images, and often can be more obvious on noncontrast images. Metastases that calcify, such as mucinous carcinomas of the colon, are also more obvious on noncontrast images. Information about the site of the primary tumor is important so that a precontrast scan of the liver is obtained when necessary.

When metastasis to the liver is discovered without a known primary site, certain findings possibly may help to indicate them. For example, calcification occurs with mucinous metastasis; in the elderly male patient it will most likely result from a colonic mucinous carcinoma. Cystic metastasis raises the possibility of cystadenocarcinoma of the ovary, pancreas, colon, and sarcomas and metastasis that are hyperechoic on ultrasound or isodense to hyperdense on contrast-enhanced CT tend to result from hypervascular primaries.

While MRI is slightly more sensitive than contrast CT for detection of hepatic metastasis,[205,207] it is more expensive and in most patients is not more advantageous than contrast CT. Nevertheless, it is useful if more sensitivity is desired. In patients with proven hepatic metastasis amenable to surgical resection, MRI may detect ad-

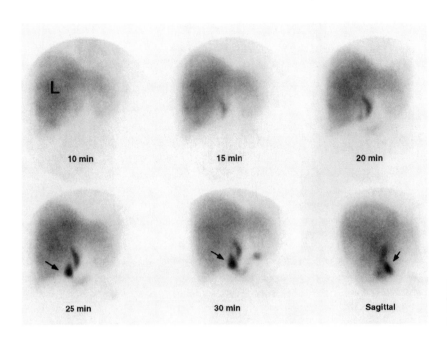

Figure 1–84. Normal ^{99m}Tc-HIDA hepatobiliary scan. Note tracer activity outlining the liver by 10 minutes, and excretion into the biliary tree with visualization of the gallbladder (*arrows*) by 20 minutes. (See color insert.)

ditional lesions which may preclude operation (Fig 1–86). If even more sensitivity is desired, CT arterial portography is the best preoperative imaging technique.[206] Intraoperative ultrasound is probably the most sensitive technique, but it would be preferable to make the operative decision without having to resort to laparotomy.[198]

Primary malignant tumors of the adult liver comprise hepatocellular carcinoma (HCC), fibrolamellar carcinoma, bile duct malignancies, and rare mesenchymal tumors such as angiosarcoma. HCC can present as a single large lesion, multiple nodules throughout the liver, or in a diffuse infiltrative state. Any mass in a cirrhotic liver must be viewed with suspicion. Both ultrasound and CT (precontrast and postcontrast) are sensitive for the focal form of HCC. Some tumors may show a capsule, which is important for therapeutic decisions. Portal venous invasion is common and should be sought. MRI can be helpful in evaluating for HCC and is useful for differentiating HCC from regenerating nodules.[215,216] It may also show additional, otherwise undetected, lesions. Again, CT arterial portography is more sensitive for lesion detection and often is performed in conjunction with arterial chemoinfusion and embolization techniques.

Fibrolamellar carcinoma, a variant of HCC occurring predominantly in young women, has a good prognosis after surgical resection. A minority of patients will have

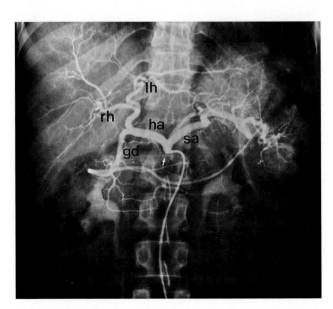

Figure 1–85. Normal hepatic arteriogram. Note catheter tip in celiac artery (*arrow*). ha: hepatic artery, sp: splenic artery, rh: right hepatic artery, lh: left hepatic artery, gd: gastroduodenal artery.

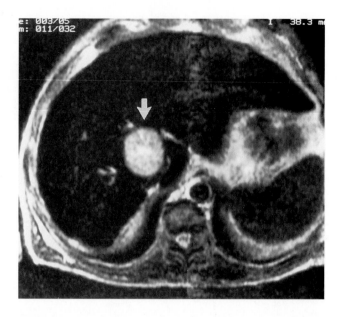

A

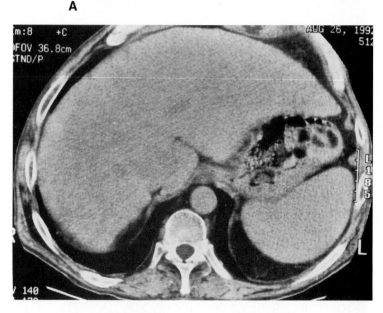

Figure 1–86. Liver MRI showing lesion not seen on conventional CT. **A.** T2-weighted MR image showing hepatocellular carcinoma (*arrow*), clearly demarcated from surrounding liver that is very hypointense owing to hemachromatosis. Corresponding CT image **B**. failed to show the lesion.

B

underlying cirrhosis. Alpha-fetal protein levels are usually normal. On imaging, it is usually a well-defined hypervascular mass with a central scar. The scar is usually best shown on contrast-enhanced CT as a central low-density region corresponding to the nonvascular fibrous nature of the scar. The major differential for this tumor is FNH, a benign tumor which also contains a central scar. MRI can be helpful in differentiating between the two,[214] although there is no single pathognomic finding.

The second most common primary hepatic malignancy is the intrahepatic form of cholangiocarcinoma. It tends to be a firm, fibrous, hypovascular tumor that is hyperechoic on ultrasound and heterogeneous on con-

trast-enhanced CT. Calicification is common since the tumors may be mucin-secreting.

Both primary and secondary involvement of the liver may be seen in Hodgkin's and non-Hodgkin's lymphoma. In early Hodgkin's disease, the infiltration of the liver is microscopic and not usually detectable by any imaging modality. Later stages of the disease may manifest as larger nodules detectable by ultrasound, CT, or MRI. Non-Hodgkin's lymphoma also may be diffusely infiltrative or nodular, the former difficult to detect except for the presence of hepatomegaly. Hepatic lymphoma, which develops in immunosuppressed patients with AIDS or organ transplants, tends to be nodular and easier to detect. Lymphoma arising from the porta hepatis also has been described in liver transplant patients. The masses are hypoechoic on ultrasound, hypodense on contrast CT, and T1 hypointense and T2 hyperintense on MRI, which is nonspecific and cannot be distinguished from other tumors.[197]

Biliary cystadenoma and cystadenocarcinoma are rare tumors of bile duct origin with characteristic imaging appearances. They are considered together because there is evidence to suggest transformation from the benign to the malignant form. These tumors characteristically appear as large, multilocular cystic masses. While ultrasound is better at visualizing the thinner septae within the tumors, CT is better for overall view of the tumor owing to their large size. Solid papillary components should raise the possibility of malignancy. The main differential for these tumors on imaging is the hydatid cyst.[209]

Angiosarcoma of the liver is extremely rare. The key to this diagnosis is thorotrast exposure. Imaging findings can be variable depending on the degree of hemorrhage and, rarely, may mimic the appearance of benign hemangioma.

Benign Tumors

Hemangioma is the most common benign primary tumor of the liver. It is more common in women and may be multiple. Autopsy series have shown an incidence as high as 20%. Because of their high incidence, liver imaging is dedicated to differentiating hemangiomas from other lesions.[198,203,204,209] Conventional CT usually shows a hypodense lesion precontrast and peripheral nodular type of enhancement postcontrast (Fig 1–87). Although this is very suggestive of the diagnosis of hemangioma, it is not definitive. On ultrasound, the typical hemangioma is a well-defined, homogeneously hyperechoic lesion.

When such a lesion is found incidentally in a patient without history of malignancy, follow-up with ultrasound may be sufficient. However, if there is a history of malignancy or atypical features present on ultrasound, further imaging is necessary for confirmation. Several possible choices are available in this setting. A dedicated single-level dynamic CT through the lesion of interest can be definitive in up to 50% to 60% of patients. However, the two modalities of choice are MRI or RBC scintigraphy. The size and location of the lesion will determine which of these modalities to use. Tumors >2.5 cm and not adjacent to large vessels should undergo RBC scan, since the test accuracy approaches 100%. The diagnosis hinges on the demonstration of persistence of activity within the lesion on delayed images, which physiologically correspond to the pooling of blood within dilated vascular spaces of the hemangioma. Smaller tumors and those located near large vessels should undergo MRI because of its superior spatial resolution. T2-weighted images show the lesion to be very hyperintense, similar to the signal intensity of other fluid structures. Even though one cannot distinguish a hemangioma from a cyst based on MRI alone, this is rarely a clinical concern because MRI is almost always performed to characterize a known solid lesion. Despite its specificity, angiography rarely is performed because of its invasiveness. A biopsy should be avoided when hemangioma is suspected. Although usually safe, significant hemorrhagic complications have been reported. Also, the diagnostic accuracy of biopsy specimens is unacceptably poor for hemangiomas.

FNH is the second most common benign hepatic tumor. It is composed of hyperplastic hepatocytes and bile ductules surrounding a vascular central fibrous scar. Other than the presence of a central scar, the lesion has

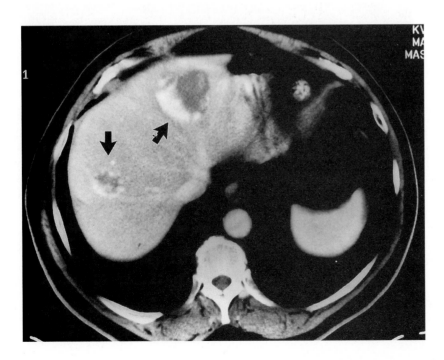

Figure 1–87. CT of hemangioma. Note the nodular peripheral enhancement pattern of the two lesions (*arrows*).

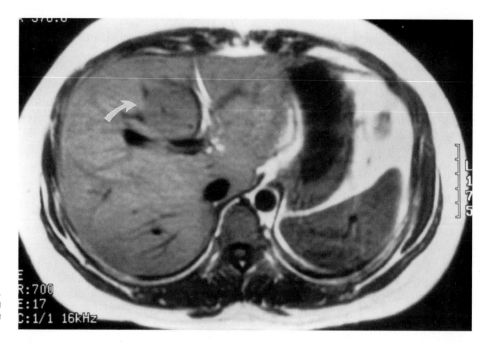

Figure 1–88. Focal nodular hyperplasia on MRI. T1-weighted image shows hypointense lesion (*curved arrow*) with an even more hypointense central scar.

nonspecific features on ultrasound or CT (Fig 1–88). The signal intensity of the lesion is variable on MRI but the central scar has distinctive signal characteristics that may help in differentiating it from other tumors. Angiography also shows a distinctive pattern of vascularity but is not pathognomonic. Sulfur colloid scintigraphy is probably the most helpful test when FNH is suspected. In most cases, the FNH contains normal or an increased number of Kupffer cells that take up the sulfur colloid (Fig 1–89), which rarely occurs with other hepatic tumors.[197,203,209,214,217]

Hepatocellular adenoma is a rare benign tumor with an increased incidence in the last two decades because of the prevalence of birth control pill (BCP) usage. It occurs primarily in women on BCP but also may occur in men on anabolic steroids. It is typically a large lesion (average 8 to 19 cm) that presents with areas of hemorrhage and necrosis. Their amount and distribution determines tumor appearance on imaging (Fig 1–89).[197,209] If hemorrhage and necrosis are not present, the tumor tends to be hyperechoic on ultrasound, hypodense on precontrast CT with heterogenous peripheral enhancement

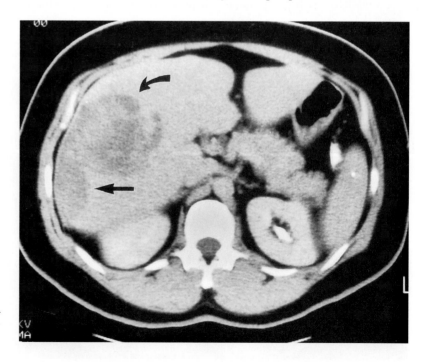

Figure 1–89. Hepatocellular adenoma. CT shows lesion (*curved arrow*) with high-density material corresponding to intratumoral hemorrhage. There is also an adjacent subcapsular hematoma (*arrow*).

postcontrast, and hyperintense on both T1- and T2-weighted images. On sulfur colloid scintigraphy, most of the tumors will not demonstrate uptake, although it may occur in up to 20% of cases. Most adenomas are single; vary rarely, however, multiple adenomas may be present in multiple hepatocellular adenomatosis.

Tumorlike Conditions

In cirrhotic livers, it is often difficult to evaluate for hepatocellular carcinoma because of the underlying distortion of normal hepatic architecture. This is compounded by the occurrence of regenerative and hyperplastic nodules in cirrhosis that can simulate HCC. Many regenerative nodules are not visible because of their small size and similar histology. However, they may show up as hypoechoic nodules on ultrasound or as hypodense or hyperdense nodules on CT. MRI is the most sensitive and specific technique for evaluating these nodules. Unlike most tumors, regenerative nodules tend to be isointense or hyperintense on T1-weighted images and hypointense on T2-weighted images, the latter being very specific for regenerating nodules. However, one must be careful with the larger hyperplastic nodules that may contain dysplastic features. These are known as adenomatous hyperplasia, and there is evidence that these nodules are premalignant. Recent work has shown the possibility of the usefulness of MRI in identifying early malignant change in these large nodules by demonstrating hyperintense foci within the hypointense nodule on the T2-weighted image.[203,209,212,215,216,218]

True hepatic cysts are common and have been found in up to 14% of patients on autopsy series. They are of congenital or developmental origin and are lined by a thin layer of bile duct epithelium. Their significance lies in the fact that small cysts, <1 cm in size, often cannot be consistently distinguished from solid tumors. Ultrasound is often the most reliable test for evaluation of cysts, if they can be visualized. Ultrasound criteria for a simple cyst are (1) an echoic structure, (2) imperceptibly thin, smooth wall, and (3) through-transmission of sound. If any of these criteria cannot be met, one cannot reliably distinguish these lesions from cystic tumors, abscesses, hematomas, or even solid tumors when they are small. Cysts are hypodense and do not enhance with contrast on CT. When they are smaller than 1 cm, CT may not be definitive due to partial volume-averaging effects. In this situation, either follow-up or ultrasound may be appropriate, although ultrasound also may not be definitive, depending on the patient's body habitus and overall impedance to sound transmission. MRI shows the lesions to be very hyperintense on T2-weighted images, as are other fluid structures.[199,209]

FOCAL HEPATIC INFECTIONS

Pyogenic abscesses

Pyogenic liver abscesses most commonly develop from ascending cholangitis, pyelophlebitis (portal vein septicemia), diverticulitis, appendicitis, and bacteremia from such sources as bacterial endocarditis. Direct extension and penetrating injuries are less common etiologies. Abscesses of bilary tract origin tend to be multiple. Those of portal venous origin tend to be solitary and most often are located in the right lobe.[219]

Hepatic abscesses are best detected by ultrasound. Early, small lesions can be echogenic, but most established abscesses are primarily heterogeneous cystic structures with through-transmission of sound. A well-defined capsule may be present. Abscesses containing air may show extremely echogenic reflectors with variable shadowing which, if large amounts of air are present, may compromise evaluation of the lesion.

In most situations where abscesses are suspected, the clinical findings are seldom specific enough to point to the liver as the location. It is common practice, therefore, to request a test that evaluates the entire abdomen. In this situation CT is definitely the test of choice. Sensitivity of CT is as high as 97% for detection of pyogenic hepatic abscesses. Contrast enhancement is essential not only for increased sensitivity but also for precise delineation and assessment for therapeutic drainage. Most abscesses are well defined and may show an enhancing rim. Some are multiloculated collections that may or may not communicate. None of these findings are specific, and they may be seen in hematomas and tumors. However, presence of air is highly indicative of infection (Fig 1–90).

Scintigraphy with gallium or labeled leukocytes may be useful in select patients for detection of hepatic abscesses. Usually it is performed in patients in whom other imaging techniques have failed to reveal the source of infection and in whom a continued search throughout the entire body is mandated. Abscesses appear as "hot lesions." The appearance of abscesses on MRI corresponds to heterogeneous cystic lesions.

Cholangiography is useful in identifying abscesses of biliary origin by virtue of their communication with the biliary tree. Biliary drainage is a natural extension of cholangiography when biliary source of sepsis is established.

Amebic, Echinococcal, and Schistosomal Infections

Some nonpyogenic hepatic infections may have distinctive features on imaging. These include amebic, echinococcal, and schistosomal infections.[197,219]

Amebic infection is common worldwide; up to 7% of infected patients develop hepatic abscesses. The organisms gain access to the liver from the colon through the portal venous circulation. However, lymphatic in-

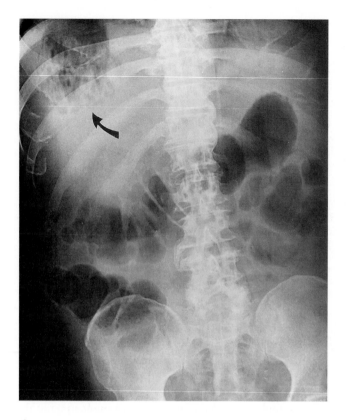

A

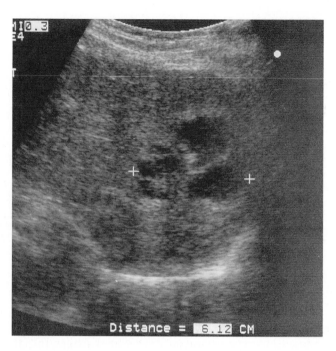

B

Figure 1–90. Hepatic abscess. **A.** Plain film showing gas collection (*curved arrow*) over the liver from a gas-forming bacterial abscess. **B.** Ultrasound in another patient showing confluent fluid loculations (*between cursers*) with ill-defined and thick walls in the left lobe of the liver as well as an abscess.

fection and direct extension from the colon also can occur. On ultrasound and CT, the abscess is located in the right lobe, is usually solitary, and abuts the liver capsule. Lesions tend to be round or oval in shape, sharply defined by an enhancing rim on CT, and may be unilocular or multilocular (Fig 1–91). On gallium scan and labeled leukocyte scan, the lesion will appear as "cold" nodules surrounded by "hot" rims. Secondary

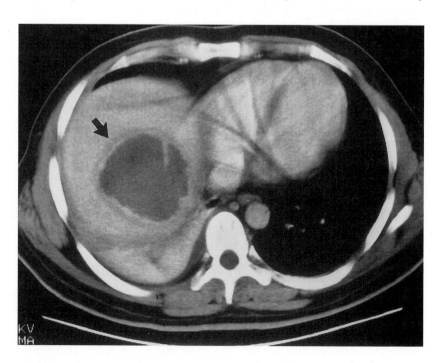

Figure 1–91. Amebic abscess on CT (*arrow*). Note the irregular, thick, enhancing wall and classic location at the dome of the liver.

findings must be sought in suspected liver amebic abscess. The chest plain film is abnormal in the majority of patients and findings may consist of elevation of the right hemidiaphragm, right pleural effusion, and right basal atelectasis. In fact, amebic infection extends directly into the right thoracic cavity through the diaphragm in 20% to 25% of patients and can lead to pulmonary consolidation, abscess, and empyema. Peritoneal fluid and inflammation may be indicative of peritoneal amebiasis.

Confirmation of amebic infection may be difficult. Aspiration of the amebic abscess yields a characteristic reddish-brown viscous material often described as "anchovy paste." However, this material is a mixture of destroyed hepatocytes and blood and only rarely are the organisms themselves identified. The organisms are more commonly found in the tissues immediately surrounding the abscess. Nevertheless, aspiration and drainage are important to rule out superinfection by other bacteria and for therapy.

Hydatid disease results from larval infection by the parasites *Echinococcus granulosus* or *Echinococcus multilocularis*. The former is much more common and is prevalent in areas such as South America, Australia, New Zealand, and Mediterranean countries where dogs, the definitive host, are used in sheep and cattle raising. The latter is more prevalent in Alaska and western Canada, where wolves act as the definitive host. *Echinococcus granulosus* infection is acquired through ingestion of contaminated food or other particles. The larvae penetrate the blood stream from the gut and are carried to the liver, although they may also settle in other parts of the body where the infection takes the form of hydatid cysts. The appearance of the hepatic cyst depends on the stage of development and on complications. It often presents as a large, well-defined, peripherally calcified lesion on plain films. On ultrasound, CT, or MRI, the characteristic lesion consists of a well-defined, often calcified, thick- or thin-walled "mother" cyst, with multiple smaller "daughter" cysts usually arranged in the periphery within the mother cyst (Fig 1–92). The daughter cysts may be free floating and may rupture and form membranes and debris within the mother cyst. Complications include bacterial superinfection and abscess formation, and rupture into the biliary tree, where it can lead to biliary obstruction and cholangitis. *Echinococcus multilocularis* infection is more aggressive and often takes the form of an infiltrative masslike lesion. This infection has a propensity to spread to the liver hilum. Amorphous calcification and necrotic areas may be present.

Schistosoma infection is prevalent worldwide. *S. japonicum* is endemic in Southeast Asia, *S. mansoni* in Africa, the Middle East, and Caribbean, and *S. hematobium* in the Mediterranean region. Humans are infected through contact with contaminated fresh water such as irrigation canals and streams where the organisms are

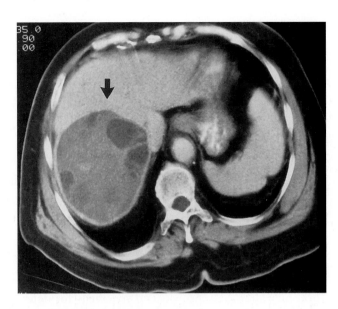

Figure 1–92. Hydatid cyst from *E. granulosus* infection, CT demonstrates typical, well-demarcated cyst (*arrow*) containing several smaller peripheral or daughter cysts (cyst-in-cyst appearance).

shed by the snail, its intermediate host, and penetrate through the skin or mucous membrane. The organisms then travel through the blood stream and eventually settle in the portal venous circulation where they incite chronic granulomatous inflammation leading to periportal fibrosis and portal hypertension. *S. hematobium* tends to infect the urinary tract more than the liver. On imaging, the liver may appear cirrhotic due to the hepatic fibrosis and portal hypertension. The hallmark of *S. japonicum* infection on CT is a network of calcific bands radiating through the liver but especially involving the liver capsule, producing a "turtle-back" appearance. The same bands can be seen on ultrasound as echogenic structures. In *S. mansoni* infection, the bands are hypodense and fibrotic and do not usually calcify, but may show contrast enhancement.

Opportunistic Infections in AIDS and the Immunocompromised Hosts

A variety of common fungal, mycobacterial, parasitic, and viral infections occur in immunocompromised patients, and their incidence has increased with the AIDS epidemic.[220,221] In the liver, many of these infections share the same imaging findings including *Candida*, the most common fungal infection, cytomegalovirus, the most common viral infection, *Mycobacterium tuberculosis* and *Avium intracellularae*, and extrapulmonary *Pneumocystis carinii*. All of these infections commonly present as microabscesses. On ultrasound, these foci may be tiny hyperechoic dots with or without shadowing, larger hypoechoic masses, or hyperechoic lesions with hypoechoic rims (bull's-eye). On CT, they are often nonspecific hypodense lesions, although many calcify and present as myriad hyperdense foci. Other abdominal organs such as spleen, kidneys, and pancreas may be involved in the same fashion. The aim of imaging is not to make a specific etiologic diagnosis but to determine whether opportunistic hepatic infection is present.

DIFFUSE LIVER DISEASES

Fatty Infiltration

Fatty infiltration of the liver is seen in many conditions including obesity, diabetes mellitus, alcoholic liver disease, malnutrition, total parenteral nutrition, hyperlipidemia, and hepatitis. The pattern of deposition is extremely variable and may be diffuse, geographic, or focal, with the diffuse form presenting as areas of focal sparing. It is extremely important to recognize this entity because the focal fatty infiltration or sparing may mimic tumors and other focal lesions, and the diffuse form may alter the sensitivity and specificity for detection of focal disease. Location of the abnormality may be a clue to its nature. Focal fat deposition, for example, has a predilection for the medial segment of the left lobe anteriorly adjacent to the falciform ligament (Fig 1–93), and focal fatty sparing has a predilection for the subcapsular regions, adjacent to the gallbladder fossa, interlobar fissure, and porta hepatis. Another clue is the absence of mass effect so that no displacement of adjacent structures is evident and vessels travel through the lesion without altering course.[222]

On ultrasound, diffuse fatty infiltration raises the echogenicity of the liver and precludes good transmission of sound to the deep structures, thus rendering evaluation of the deep parenchyma suboptimal. Focal lesions appear as echogenic lesions and may simulate hemangiomas. CT is the study of choice for visualization of the fatty deposition. Noncontrast CT images are more accurate than contrast images, in which the intrinsic density of the liver is a sensitive reflector of the degree of fatty infiltration and fat lowers the parenchymal density. When a tumor or other focal lesion cannot be differentiated from fatty deposition or focal sparing, MRI can, in most cases, be definitive in excluding a tumor.[212,216] Otherwise, follow-up studies may confirm resolution of the abnormality since fat can be mobilized in a matter of weeks.

Hepatitis

Acute or chronic inflammation of the liver occurs most commonly with viral infection and alcohol abuse, but also may be seen with toxicity to a variety of agents including acetaminophen, isoniazid, amiodarone, chlorpromazine, carbon tetrachloride, halothane, oral contraceptives, alpha-methyldopa, methotrexate, azathioprine, 6-mercaptopurine, and radiation. The diagnosis is based on clinical and biochemical findings. The role of imaging is to exclude focal abnormalities and biliary obstruction and to document vascular patency. In acute disease, the liver is usually enlarged. On ultrasound, there may be a diffuse decrease in the liver echogenicity that enhances the brightness of the portal triads, referred to as the "starry sky pattern." There also may be a diffuse increase in echogenicity from fatty infiltration which occurs especially in alcoholic hepatitis. Nonspecific gallbladder wall thickening and portal and gastrohepatic ligament adenopathy also may be present. On CT, hepatomegaly, gallbladder wall thickening, and adenopathy are also well appreciated. Also, one may see nonspecific diffuse peri-

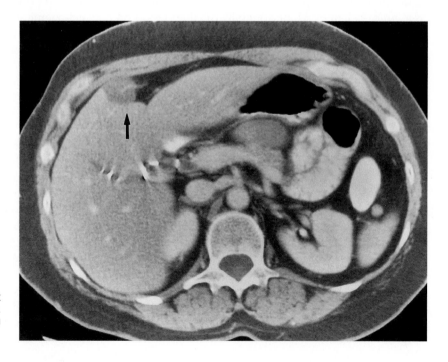

Figure 1–93. Classic location for focal fatty deposition in the left lobe medial segment adjacent to the falciform ligament (*arrow*). Note vessel coursing through it without deviation, suggesting the correct diagnosis.

portal lucency, probably as a result of edema or lymphedema. Hepatic parenchymal density usually is decreased from edema or fatty infiltration.

In chronic hepatitis, depending on the severity and duration of the inflammation, the liver may be atrophic, with cirrhotic change. Amiodarone toxicity results in a characteristically high-density liver from metabolic accumulation of iodine. Radiation hepatitis occurs when a part of the liver is unavoidably included in the radiation portal. The area of injury manifests as a hypoechoic region on ultrasound and as a hypodense region on CT, with a tell-tale straight margin corresponding to the limit of the radiation beam.

Infiltrative Disorders

A variety of diffuse hepatic diseases result from abnormal accumulation or deposition of specific metals or metabolites. These include hemachromatosis, Wilson's disease, glycogen storage diseases, amyloidosis, and Gaucher's disease.

Hemachromatosis refers to abnormally increased iron stores in the body accompanied by parenchymal damage of the involved organs. The liver is the primary organ involved in both primary and secondary hemachromatosis. CT shows increased attenuation of the liver in proportion to the degree of iron deposition; analysis of hepatic density can be used to quantitate the amount of iron and to follow the efficacy of therapy. Other causes of diffuse, increased hepatic density include amiodarone toxicity, Wilson's disease, glycogen storage disease, and intravenous gold therapy for rheumatoid arthritis. Analysis of the pattern of visceral involvement within the abdomen also may differentiate between primary and secondary hemachromatosis. MRI also will show sensitivity in detection of iron stores; ultrasound will not.

Glycogen storage disease, amyloidosis, and Gaucher's disease all manifest with nonspecific hepatomegaly. When fatty infiltration occurs, the liver is echogenic on ultrasound and lower in density on CT. However, glycogen itself may increase hepatic density. One must search carefully for focal lesions in glycogen storage disease since there is an increased incidence of hepatic adenomas.

Cirrhosis and Portal Hypertension

In most cases the diagnosis of cirrhosis can be made on the basis of clinical and laboratory data, but imaging techniques provide an excellent depiction of the status of the liver. Imaging is also invaluable in the evaluation of possible hepatocellular carcinoma.[215,216,218]

The liver parenchyma is coarsely echogenic on ultrasound, whereas it is hypodense and often heterogeneous on CT, depending on the degree of fibrosis and fatty infiltration. On MRI, the parenchyma usually show mild increased signal on T2-weighted images. All imaging modalities show the gross morphologic changes that consist of hepatomegaly in the early stages and a shrunken, nodular liver in the later stages. There often is a characteristic relative atrophy of the right lobe or hypertrophy of the left or caudate lobes. Secondary findings often are present in the rest of the abdomen, many of which are related to portal hypertension. These include ascites, mesenteric edema, splenomegaly, and multiple varices including esophageal, gastric, and perisplenic (Fig 1–94). A re-canalized umbilical vein also may be present. Enlargement of the portal vein above 13 mm is diagnostic of portal hypertension. The portal vein may thrombose with resultant collateral vessels in the porta hepatis (cavernous transformation of the portal vein). Doppler ultrasound and MRI with special angiographic sequences are capable of determining di-

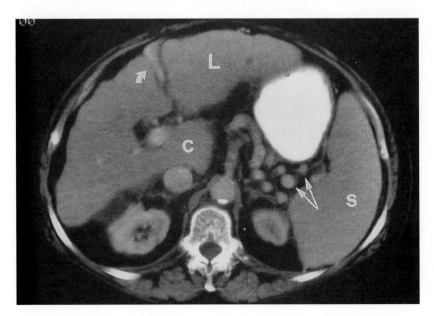

Figure 1–94. CT findings in cirrhosis. Note nodular surface of liver, hypertrophy of the left (L) and caudate (C) lobes, splenomegaly (S), recanalized paraumbilical vein (*curved arrow*), and perisplenic varices (*arrows*).

rection of flow in the portal vein, with reversal of flow diagnostic of portal hypertension.

The heterogenous, nodular parenchyma can pose problems for the detection of hepatocellular carcinoma. In fact, the infiltrative form of HCC often is not detectable by imaging. Often a tumor may be evident on only one modality; however, it is impossible to predict which modality would be the optimal one. Another confounding factor is the presence of regenerating nodules that must be differentiated from a small carcinoma. Regenerating nodules may have varied appearances on ultrasound and CT but have a characteristically low signal on T2-weighted images on MRI, enabling their differentiation from HCC, which is almost always T2-hyperintense.

Vascular Disorders

Budd-Chiari syndrome. Occlusion of hepatic venous outflow may be primary or secondary to a variety of disorders. The etiology of the primary form is controversial but is characterized by the presence of a partially or completely obstructive membranous lesion in the inferior vena cava at or above the hepatic venous confluence. Secondary obstruction occurs as a result of thrombosis in hypercoagulable states and mass lesions. The liver is typically enlarged because of congestion with signs of portal hypertension, such as ascites.

Imaging plays a vital role in the diagnosis of this disorder.[197,199] Caval and hepatic venography has been and still remains the gold standard. However, in most cases, CT, Doppler sonography, especially with color, and MRI with angiographic sequences have replaced invasive venography. Duplex sonography is an excellent initial screening modality in suspected Budd-Chiari syndrome, readily identifying acute thrombus and stenotic lesions. The affected veins may show very thick echogenic walls with proximal dilatation or may be obliterated completely, in chronic cases. Collateral draining veins also may be seen. Reversal of flow in the hepatic veins or inferior vena cava is diagnostic and also may be demonstrated. However, one must be careful in acute cases where the liver is edematous and the hepatic veins are compressed and difficult to visualize. CT shows the same morphologic changes but also shows a characteristic heterogeneous patchy enhancement pattern, sparing usually the caudate and inferior part of the left lobe medial segment (Fig 1–95). With its multiplanar capability and ever improving vascular sequences, MRI also may depict obstructive lesions. Angiography and venography should be reserved for problematic cases and for demonstrating thin membranes that may be difficult to visualize on cross-sectional imaging.

Portal vein thrombosis. Portal vein thrombosis usually occurs as a complication of other disorders in the upper abdomen. It leads to splenomegaly, varices, and ascites. In most cases, the diagnosis is made easily with cross-sectional imaging. Angiography may not be as good as cross-sectional imaging in depicting the portal vein, unlike most other vascular structures in the body. The inability to visualize the portal vein may be due to the fact that the technique involves injection of contrast into the superior mesenteric or splenic artery. Thus, the portal vein is visualized only indirectly in the venous phase, where the contrast is diluted. The main portal vein is a large structure that should be easily identified on ultra-

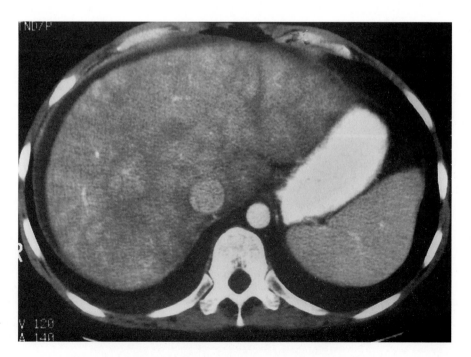

Figure 1–95. Budd-Chiari Syndrome. CT shows heterogeneous enhancement throughout the liver.

sound, CT, or MRI. Nonvisualization should always raise the possibility of thrombosis. Intrahepatic portal venous branches are less consistently seen but can be easily evaluated in the great majority of patients.

Ultrasound is the primary screening modality due to its duplex and color Doppler capabilities. In acute thrombosis, the thrombus may be seen as an echogenic clot filling, distending, or partially obstructing the portal vein. In cases where a bland thrombus needs to be differentiated from tumor thrombus, Doppler evidence of arterial signal from within the thrombus is diagnostic of tumor.

CT may show the thrombus to be a hyperdense clot on noncontrast scans and a hypodense filling defect on contrast studies (Fig 1–96).

In the smaller portal vessels, MRI may be more sensitive than ultrasound or CT in detecting thrombi.[223,224] In chronic portal venous thrombosis, the portal vein may be obliterated and not visible on any imaging modality. There also may be multiple collateral vessels present in the porta hepatitis to compensate for the portal vein, known as "cavernous transformation of the portal vein."

Hepatic infarction. Infarction of liver parenchyma is uncommon due to the dual-hepatic blood supply. Nevertheless, it may occur in any hypercoagulable state and as a result of arterial emboli. The ischemic segment is typically an area of hypoperfusion on contrast-enhanced CT and may be characteristically peripheral and wedged-shaped (Fig 1–97). The degree of hypoperfusion depends on the degree of ischemia. With severe infarction, the parenchyma may become necrotic and gas may be seen without infection. Over time, the diseased region will atrophy. The infarcted regions are hypoechoic on ultrasound and T2 hyperintense on MRI due to edema.

Hepatic Trauma

In blunt abdominal trauma, the liver is the second most commonly injured organ. Because of its large size it ranks first in penetrating abdominal injuries. CT is the imaging modality of choice in all abdominal trauma and is highly accurate in evaluating injury throughout the abdomen. However, it has no role in evaluating hemodynamically unstable patients for whom laparotomy should be performed immediately.

On CT, lacerations appear as non-enhancing clefts extending centrally from the liver capsule. Intrahepatic hematomas are hyperdense regions on noncontrast scans and hypodense regions on contrast-enhanced scans. Contusions may be more subtle but have a similar appearance to hematomas; however, they are usually less defined. Subcapsular hematomas consist of a crescent-shaped hypodense structure at the liver periphery indenting the normally enhancing liver margin (Fig 1–98). The mass effect on normally enhancing liver is the differentiating feature from subphrenic or perihepatic fluid or hematoma. The density of the hematoma varies depending on the age of the hemorrhage. Immediately after trauma the nonclotted blood is similar in density to normal flowing blood. With time, as clot formation takes place, density increases. Imaging is usually performed at this time. Chronic hematomas may be very low density from lysis and liquefaction of the clot. Another common finding in liver trauma is a zone of periportal lucency which likely represents blood tracking along the portal triads. In some patients, this may be the only sign of hepatic trauma.

Findings associated with poor prognosis include injury to the vascular pedicle or hepatic venous confluence, deep perihilar lacerations, large hemoperitoneum

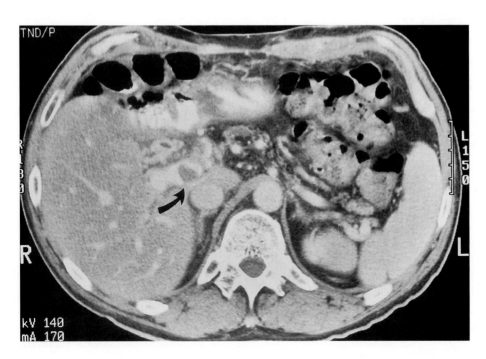

Figure 1–96. CT demonstration of a clot in the portal vein (*arrow*). CT demonstration.

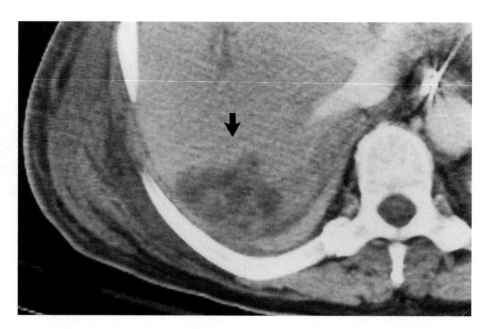

Figure 1–97. Hepatic infarct on CT (*arrow*) Note the characteristic peripheral, wedge-shaped configuration.

or failure of normal resorption of hemoperitoneum within one week, and rapid progression of any injury. Occasionally, severe hemorrhage can be investigated by angiography with possible therapeutic embolization. However, angiography is frequently more useful for delayed posttraumatic vascular complications.

Most posttraumatic complications develop within the first month after trauma. These include hepatic artery pseudoaneurysm (Fig 1–99), arteriovenous fistula, abscess, and biloma. Serial CT scans over this time period therefore should be performed. Aspiration of fluid col-

lections may be required for diagnosis. When biloma is suspected, hepatobiliary scintigraphy may be useful in identifying leaks. With suspected hepatic pseudoaneurysm or arteriovenous fistula, angiography should be performed.

Ultrasound may be useful as an adjunctive technique in trauma. In children, it is especially desirable because radiation is avoided. Most significant hepatic injury is readily identified by ultrasound. Blood is anechoic immediately after hemorrhage; with time and clotting, the hematoma becomes echogenic. After several days the

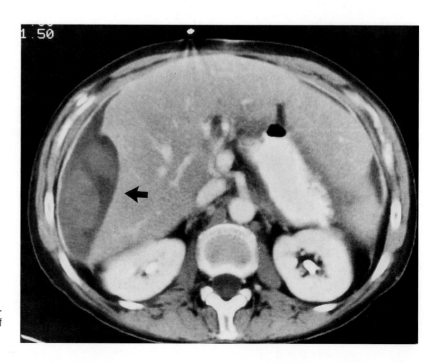

Figure 1–98. Subcapsular hematoma on CT (*arrow*). Note the indentation of the liver margin, and the heterogeneous appearance of the organizing hematoma with hyperdense areas.

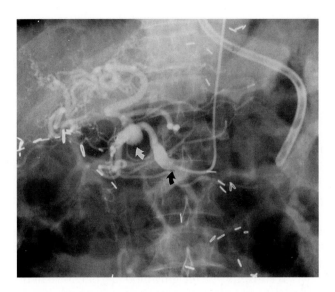

Figure 1–99. Hepatic artery pseudoaneurysm. Hepatic arteriogram showing rounded contrast-filling structure (white arrow) arising from the junction of the proper hepatic, common hepatic, and gastroduodenal arteries. Note catheter tip (black arrow) in the hepatic artery.

hematoma usually becomes anechoic, with liquefaction. Large hematomas may have a characteristic whorllike pattern with alternating hypoechoic and hyperechoic bands.

MRI is extremely sensitive to blood products and their evolution after acute hemorrhage. Consequently, it can be very useful in differentiating hematomas from other fluid collections, although it is still contraindicated in the acute setting.

LIVER TRANSPLANTATION

Imaging is an integral part of pretransplant evaluation of potential candidates and of posttransplant evaluation for potential complications.[225–230] In pretransplant assessment, it is essential for determining the status of the portal vein. In most patients, size, patency, and direction of flow of the portal vein are established easily by duplex sonography. Occasionally, CT, MR, and even angiography may be needed. A portal vein diameter of 4 mm has been used as a minimum for liver transplant candidacy. Evidence of portal vein thrombosis and cavernous transformation alerts the surgeon to the need for reconstruction with donor venous grafts. In patients with hepatocellular carcinoma or other liver malignancies, sonography and CT are important in excluding those with extrahepatic disease.

After successful transplantation, different imaging modalities help monitor the patient for possible complications. In adults with primary choledochocholedochostomy and T tube placement, T tube cholangiograms help determine leaks and strictures. All patients should be on antibiotics for the procedure. The contrast is administered by slow gravity infusion to prevent

biliary sepsis and pressure disruption of the fresh anastomosis. Most leaks occur at the site of anastomosis of T tube insertion. Strictures may be anastomotic or nonanastomotic. If they are nonastomotic, hepatic arterial ischemia should be considered.

In the first weeks posttransplantation, duplex sonography is used to monitor the patency of the hepatic vasculature and the hepatic artery for potential risk of thrombosis. Documentation of intrahepatic arterial signal is taken as evidence of patent hepatic artery in adults. However, nonvisualization of the hepatic artery may be due to technical factors and the difficulty of performing satisfactory examinations in the immediate postoperative patient because of overlying wound, bandage, drains, and other limiting factors. In these patients, angiography is indicated if clinical suspicion for hepatic artery thrombosis exists. After the initial few weeks posttransplantation, other vascular complications may occur, such as hepatic artery anastomotic stenosis. Duplex sonography may suggest the diagnosis, but angiography is the gold standard. Current investigation into MRI angiography and CT angiography may prove these novel techniques to be useful in the future.

With hematomas, bile leaks, intrahepatic or extrahepatic abscesses, or other fluid collections, CT is the imaging modality of choice. Although ultrasound has the advantage of portability, examinations are often unsatisfactory for reasons already stated. Needle aspirations and drainages may be performed by either ultrasound or CT guidance, and the choice depends on their accessibility and visualization.

Transplant rejection cannot be determined by imaging. On duplex sonography, abnormal diastolic flow patterns in the hepatic artery are nonspecific. The small hepatic arterial branches often are pruned and splayed on angiography. However, this is also nonspecific, since it merely reflects hepatic edema.

Imaging plays an important role in the diagnosis of posttransplant malignancies. There is an increased incidence of lymphomas and sarcomas in these patients as a result of chronic immunosuppression. Lymphomas in this population are unusually manifested as extranodal disease, including focal lesions within the liver and the portahepatis.

■ RADIOLOGY OF THE SPLEEN

Detailed radiographic examination of the spleen was not possible prior to the use of CT and ultrasound. Plain films could document splenomegaly or splenic calcification but little else (Fig 1–100). Nuclear medicine scintigraphy made the diagnosis of focal splenic defects possible, but suboptimal resolution precluded identification of small lesions.

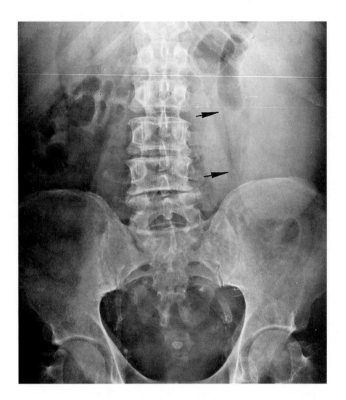

Figure 1–100. Splenomegaly (*arrows*).

The normal spleen may have clefts, notches or lobulations and, in approximately 10% of the population, one or more accessory spleens may be present (Fig 1–101). These are often small (1 to 1.5 cm in diameter) and located in the region of the splenic hilum.

Positional abnormalities of the spleen may occur in patients with left diaphragmatic hernias containing bowel and spleen, in syndromes which include cardiac defects and intermediate situs, and in cases of "wandering spleen." In the latter congenital variation, the dorsal gastric mesentery may remain unfused with the dorsal peritoneum and persist as a long mesentery. In these cases a mobile spleen may present as an anterior abdominal mass. Complications include torsion and ischemia. CT, ultrasound, and radionuclide scanning may assist in the diagnosis.[231,232]

CT is currently the imaging modality of choice in the evaluation of patients with suspected splenic lesion.[233,234] Lesions are often discovered incidentally. The upper limit of normal length for the spleen is 13 cm. This measurement, however, does not take into account splenic width. Radiographic experience and judgment regarding size usually preclude the need for measurement.

INFLAMMATORY LESIONS

Splenic abscesses are not common lesions. Patients with this finding are often immunosuppressed and have generalized infection. Aerobic organisms are more common than anaerobic, and fungi are a common cause.

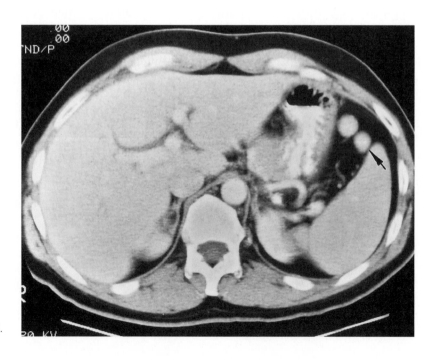

Figure 1–101. Two accessory spleens (*arrow*).

If single, an abscess may appear on CT as a low-density collection with a rim that enhances with IV contrast administration. Septa may be present. Rarely, air bubbles are seen. Ultrasound may show debris and mural nodularity within the lesions. There is often a left pleural effusion. The defect, if greater than 2 cm in diameter, should be visible on a ^{99m}Tc nuclear medicine liver spleen scan. To confirm its infectious nature, a gallium 67 (Ga^{67}) or ^{III}In leukocyte scan may be useful. Fine-needle aspiration and biopsy, using CT or ultrasound guidance, may be done when necessary to obtain material for culture or to differentiate between abscess and tumor.

Microabscesses usually occur in immunosuppressed patients. They are often small and multiple and are caused by fungus. Similar lesions are frequently present in the liver. The most common organism is *Candida albicans,* although other agents may also be responsible. Additionally, microabscesses of nonfungal origin, such as *Aspergillus* organisms, *Cryptococcocus* organisms, *Mycobacterium avium intercellulare, Mycobacterium tuberculosis,* and *Pneumocystic carinii,* also occur.

A bull's-eye lesion has been described on sonographic examination and is due to a cluster of inflammatory cells surrounded by a zone of fibrosis. Another sonographic description is the "wheel within wheel" caused by tissue containing necrotic fungus surrounded by inflammation. Splenomegaly often accompanies this lesion.

CT will show multiple lesions, each of which is <1 cm in diameter and well defined. Multiple calcifications may develop with *Pneumocystic carnii.*

Ecchinococcus disease involving the spleen is shown well by CT and ultrasound. The typical presentation is a finely demarcated, multilocular lesion with calcification in its wall.[233–235]

SPLENIC CYSTS

Cystic lesions occurring in the spleen may be congenital, parasitic (usually of *echinococcus* etiology), posttraumatic, postinfectious, or due to pancreatitis (pseudocysts), hematomas, or postinfarction. CT is the imaging modality of choice.

True epithelial-lined cysts are rare. Eighty percent of splenic cysts are not true cysts and are posttraumatic. CT appearance is that of thin-walled, hypoattenuating lesions that do not enhance when IV contrast is given (Fig 1–102).

SPLENIC NEOPLASMS

Benign

The most common benign splenic neoplasms are hemangiomas, hamartomas, and lymphangiomas. Splenic hemangiomas are usually small lesions of low density on noncontrast scans that enhance after IV contrast administration and occasionally may contain calcifications. Hamartomas are more likely to be single than lymphangiomas which may be single or multiple. Both appear as low-density splenic lesions on CT.

Malignant

Angiosarcoma, a rare tumor, is the most common primary malignant neoplasm of the spleen. It occurs in

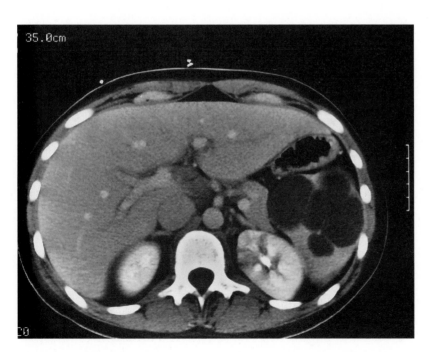

Figure 1–102. Multiloculated splenic cyst.

TABLE 1–11. CT OF SPLENIC LYMPHOMA

Homogeneous enlargement with no focal masses
Military lesions
Large solitary mass
Multiple 2 to 10 cm masses
Normal despite presence of tumor cells

older patients, most of whom have had thoratrast injection years prior to development of the tumor. Splenomegaly with hypodense, often enhancing, lesions may be seen. Low-density zones resulting from hemorrhage also may be seen.

Lymphoma is the most common malignant neoplasm to involve the spleen (Table 1–11). Unfortunately, most imaging studies may evaluate inaccurately the full extent of splenic involvement. Focal lesions can be seen more clearly than diffuse infiltration. Marked splenomegaly suggests involvement, but splenomegaly is by no means a pathognomonic sign of lymphomatous infiltration. The radiographic appearance of splenic lymphoma covers a wide spectrum.[236–238] At times, it might appear normal despite the presence of tumor cells.

Splenic metastases are relatively uncommon and usually are due to melanoma, ovarian, lung, breast, or stomach carcinoma. On CT, metastases are usually of lower density than the surrounding spleen. Occasionally, they may appear cystic. Sonographically they may also be variable in appearance. The radiographic appearance of the splenic metastases and the primary do not correlate well.

Splenic displacement or direct invasion may occur from tumors in surrounding organs such as the stomach, colon, pancreas, or kidney. Soft tissue sarcomas may also involve the spleen.[236]

SPLENIC INFARCTION

Splenic infarction can accompany a number of systemic diseases. These usually fall into the categories of hematologic, embolic, traumatic, or obstructive and most often are the result of the effects of a pancreatic tumor or pancreatitis on splenic vessels.

CT with intravenous contrast infusion is currently the most reliable imaging modality for the delineation of splenic infarction. Classic findings are one or more hypodense, wedge-shaped peripheral lesions. Similar lesions may occur in other organs such as the kidneys or liver. However, an infarct may cause poorly defined hypodense zones or a mottled density. With time the defect may disappear completely or leave a scar that causes a contour defect.

In patients who sustain repeated episodes of infarction, the spleen may appear very small and calcified. This is a common finding in patients with sickle cell anemia. In hemoglobin sickle cell disease, episodes of infarction may cause calcification in the subcapsular zone.[233–235]

TRAUMA

The spleen is the organ most frequently injured in patients who have sustained blunt abdominal trauma. CT of the abdomen with IV contrast is currently the preferred imaging modality in the radiographic work-up of

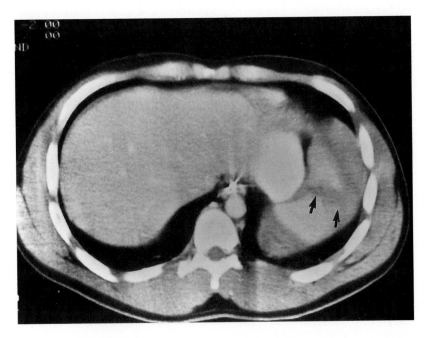

Figure 1–103. Splenic laceration (*arrows*) with perisplenic hematoma.

this type of patient.[239] Grading systems have been described in the radiology literature to quantitate the degree of injury, but these have not proven accurate in determining the need for surgical intervention. Treatment choices ultimately are based on the patient's hemodynamic status and on clinical evaluation.[240–242]

Findings on CT include subcapsular hematomas, intrasplenic hematomas, splenic lacerations, and, occasionally, infarction. A subcapsular hematoma has the appearance of a crescentic low-density collection hugging the lateral splenic margin. A laceration is an irregular linear defect that should not be confused with a splenic cleft, which is a sharp, smooth, linear defect (Fig 1–103). Blood is usually present around the spleen and in the pelvis. With episodes of intermittent bleeding, the hematoma may have an "onion skin" appearance.

Even if a clear splenic defect is not visualized, high-density fluid around the spleen is an important sign of injury. This is owing to the density of the blood and also to extravasation of iodine-laden blood during the period of examination.

The initial CT may appear normal even though the spleen has been lacerated or fractured because significant bleeding may not occur immediately. If clinical evidence of bleeding occurs after the initial scan, the patient should be rescanned in order to search for delayed splenic rupture. CT is also a good method to follow healing in the patient who is treated conservatively. Healing time will depend on the severity of the injury.[242]

■ RADIOLOGY OF THE GALLBLADDER

Many techniques are available for gallbladder imaging. The examination of choice depends on the clinical indication. In general, ultrasound is the preferred method for first-time screening. Because the gallbladder is relatively superficial in location and is inferior to the liver that serves as an acoustic window, it is an easily visualized structure that is seldom obstructed from view by intervening bowel gas or overlying rib cage. It is important to examine the gallbladder after a 6 to 8 hour fast since a contracted gallbladder may not be visible and internal pathology such as stones may be missed. The normal gallbladder should appear as an ovoid, fluid-containing, subhepatic structure measuring no more than 4 to 5 cm in width, with a smooth wall measuring no more than 3 to 4 mm in thickness. Ultrasound is the most sensitive test for detection of gallstones and is superior to other modalities in differentiating gallbladder wall thickening from pericholecystic fluid.[243–246]

The gallbladder can also be examined by CT and MRI. The same anatomic principles apply as on sonography. CT is excellent in depiction of gross pathology such as invasive gallbladder carcinoma and also can be diagnostic in acute cholecystitis. However, CT is limited by its inherent lack of flexibility in imaging planes, and it is not ideal for imaging an organ that can be twisted and folded upon itself. Although MRI can visualize the gallbladder well, there is little indication for its use when the gallbladder is the only organ of interest.[244]

Oral cholecystography is seldom performed now, although it remains a tool in gallbladder imaging for special situations. The patient is instructed to take the contrast agent orally the night before. The oral contrast agent is taken up by the liver and excreted into the biliary tree where it becomes concentrated by the gallbladder. When the gallbladder fills normally, this is the best test for imaging of the hyperplastic cholecystoses, in other words, adenomyomatosis and cholesterolosis (see below), and it is superior to sonography in counting the number of gallstones and in measuring their size. Although not commonly necessary, this may be useful in special circumstances such as in percutaneous radiologic interventions in the gallbladder (Fig 1–104).[247]

Functional information may be obtained by performing the biliary nuclear medicine scan with radiolabeled HIDA derivatives which are intravenously injected, absorbed by hepatocytes, and excreted into the bile. Normally, the tracer is in the common bile duct within 10 to 15 minutes, fills the normal gallbladder in 90% of patients by 30 minutes, in 95% of patients by 45 minutes, and in 100% of patients by 60 minutes (Fig 1–105). Gallbladder visualization establishes cystic duct patency and excludes acute cholecystitis. However, to be specific, confirmation of acute cholecystitis requires further scanning. This further delay in diagnosis now can be avoided by pharmacological intervention. Morphine is injected intravenously at 60 minutes, constricting the sphincter of Oddi and diverting bile into the gallbladder. Persistent nonvisualization of the gallbladder is evidence for cystic duct obstruction.[244,245,248]

CHOLELITHIASIS

Ultrasound is the most sensitive modality for detection of gallstones and should be the first screening study whenever this is the primary imaging objective. Calculi appear as gravitationally dependent, mobile, echogenic foci within the gallbladder lumen, with sharp, clean shadowing owing to obstruction of sound propagation. Occasionally, a stone may be adherent to the wall of the gallbladder, and tiny stones <5 mm may not be accompanied by a consistent shadow despite optimizing the scanning parameters. Therefore these stones often can be confused with polyps. Sludge normally appears as sandlike material layering within the gallbladder without shadowing. Occasionally, sludge is viscous enough to form echogenic masses known as umefactive sludge, simulating calculi or even polypoid tumors. Rigorous

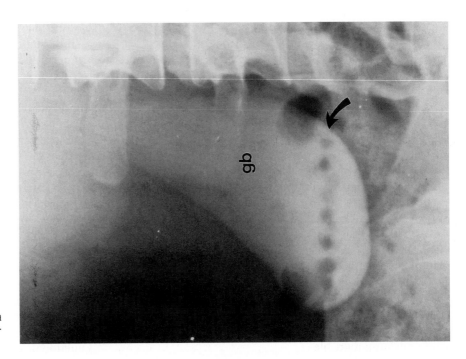

Figure 1–104. Oral cholecystogram. This patient has a layer of multiple stones (*curved arrow*). Note the clear delineation of each stone useful for size measurements.

scanning techniques with multiple transducers and scanning from different windows and multiple positions of the patient is needed for proper differentiation of these entities.[243–246]

Approximately 15% to 20% of calculi are radiopaque on plain film, and the numbers are higher for CT. Gallstones characteristically have multiple facets and rim calcification, and occasionally a fissure containing nitrogen gas may be visible in the center of the stone. This is important for their differentiation from renal calculi on abdominal plain films. On CT, pure cholesterol stones may be hypodense to bile, but often the stones are isodense and therefore not visible. CT can never exclude the presence of gallstones.[245]

Oral cholecystography may be helpful in gallstone imaging in the special but rare situation of planning percutaneous extraction or dissolution of gallstones in patients unfit for surgery when it is necessary to know precisely how many stones are present and how big they are (Fig 1–104).[247]

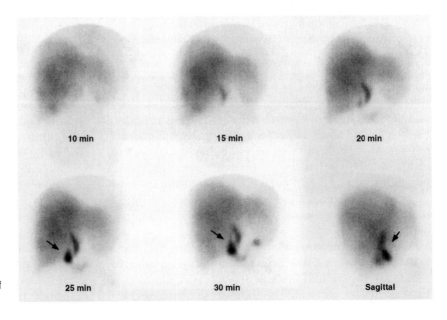

Figure 1–105. Normal ^{99m}Tc-HIDA scan. Note visualization of gallbladder (*arrow*) by 25 minutes. (See color insert.)

ACUTE CALCULUS CHOLECYSTITIS

Imaging is seldom necessary in the patient with classic symptoms and physical signs of acute cholecystitis; timely surgery should not be delayed for radiologic evaluation. However, several tests are helpful in increasing the level of confidence for diagnosis in special cases. The choices between ultrasound and scintigraphy is a matter of institutional preference and availability. The radiolabeled HIDA-derivative scintigram is the best test to exclude the possibility of acute cholecystitis with near 100% negative predictive value. With pharmacologic enhancement, it is also very sensitive and has a good positive predictive value. However, pharmacologically enhanced studies are not consistently available, and the test takes longer to perform than an ultrasound. Sonography, on the other hand, is simpler to perform and is more widely and readily available. It has a reported sensitivity of between 76% to 96% and a specificity that is between 60% to 100% for acute cholecystitis and, most importantly, is capable of detecting other potential causes of abdominal pain.[246,248,249]

On nuclear scintigraphy, filling of the gallbladder excludes acute cholecystitis. A positive scan consists of nonvisualization of the gallbladder despite pharmacologic enhancement (Fig 1–106). On sonography, the two most important signs are the presence of gallstones and maximal tenderness over the gallbladder (sonographic "Murphy's" sign). The presence of gallstones may be the only information necessary for a decision to perform a cholecystectomy; the sonographic Murphy's sign alone is a very specific sign for acute cholecystitis (reported to be 85%).[246] Another specific sign is the presence of pericholecystic fluid (Fig 1–107), but other findings such as wall thickening and distention are nonspecific by themselves, although useful in conjunction with other signs. Gallbladder wall thickening, for example, may be seen in chronic cholecystitis, congestive heart failure, hypoalbuminemia, hepatitis, and allergic reactions to drugs.

CT is not the primary imaging modality of choice because of its suboptimal sensitivity for stone detection. However, if fluid stranding is seen in the fat adjacent to the gallbladder, this is a very specific sign for acute

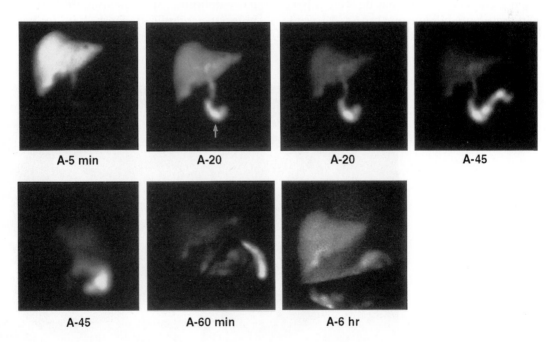

^{99m} Tc DISHIDA SCAN

ACUTE CHOLECYSTITIS

A-5 min   A-20   A-20   A-45

A-45   A-60 min   A-6 hr

UCLA 0963358 10/4/93

Figure 1–106. Positive ^{99m}Tc-HIDA scan in patient with acute cholecystitis. No gallbladder visualization was achieved. Note activity within duodenum (*arrow*) by 20 minutes.

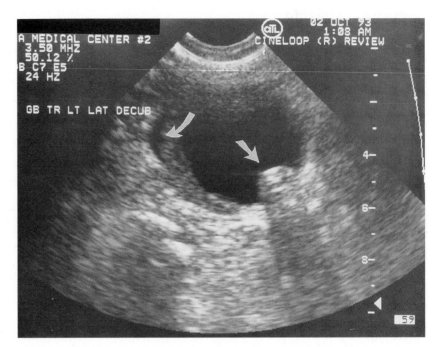

Figure 1–107. Acute cholecystitis on sonography. This patient exhibited the sonographic Murphy's sign. Sonogram shows gallstones (*arrow*), wall thickening (>4 mm), and pericholecystic fluid (*curved arrow*).

cholecystitis (Fig 1–108). Unfortunately, it is not a very sensitive sign.

Multiple complications may arise from acute cholecystitis, and they should be sought on every imaging study. Irregular wall thickening and intraluminal membrane formation may be seen in gangrenous cholecystitis; pericholecystic fluid may be seen in perforation, with resultant biloma or abscess. Mirizzi's syndrome occurs when stone impaction of the gall-bladder neck or cystic duct leads to inflammatory stricture of the adjacent common bile duct. It should be suspected whenever biliary dilatation occurs proximal to the cystic duct insertion, in acute cholecystitis. Although ultrasound is excellent for the screening of uncomplicated acute cholecystitis, CT is more definitive in delineating the extent of any pericholecystic complication, especially for bilomas and abscesses.

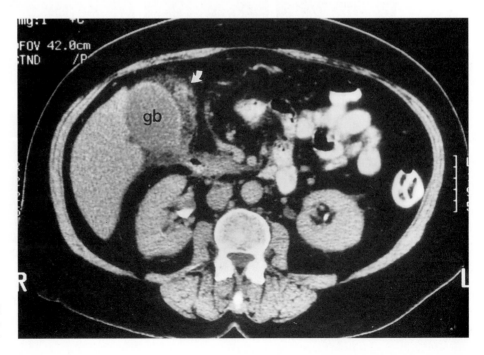

Figure 1–108. CT of acute cholecystitis. Note fluid stranding in the pericholecystic fat (*curved arrow*), a good sign of acute cholecystitis (gb: gallbladder).

ACALCULOUS CHOLECYSTITIS

Acute acalculous cholecystitis is a difficult diagnosis to make, both clinically and radiologically. Clinical and biochemical parameters such as fever, leukocytosis, and liver enzyme elevation are all nonspecific, and pain and tenderness are difficult to elicit when the patient is unconscious. Similarly, sonographic and CT parameters such as distention, wall thickening, sludge formation, and the presence of stones are almost useless by themselves because they are common findings in a patient population with multiple factors such as hypoalbuminemia, prolonged fasting, parenteral nutrition, and multiple transfusions. More helpful signs, such as pericholecystic fluid, sonographic Murphy's sign, and stranding in the adjacent fat on CT (Fig 1–108), may be specific but, unfortunately, are insensitive. Nuclear scintigraphy with HIDA derivatives may be helpful if gallbladder filling is achieved, thereby excluding cholecystitis. However, many patients without cholecystitis will demonstrate gallbladder nonvisualization despite pharmacologic enhancement because of their intercurrent infection, hepatic failure, fasting state, and parenteral nutrition. Thus, this finding is rendered nonspecific, and extreme caution is needed in their interpretation.[245,249–251]

Despite the suboptimal performance of imaging in making a definitive diagnosis of acalculous cholecystitis, imaging is nevertheless useful in excluding cholecystitis in those gallbladders that appear normal or sonography, CT, or scintigraphy. The combination of multiple imaging characteristics, although nonspecific by themselves, also increases the positive predictive value, especially when they are correlated with clinical and biochemical findings. When all else fails, another approach may be a diagnostic and therapeutic percutaneous cholecystostomy. Although bile analysis will yield positive cultures in a small number of cases, draining of the gallbladder will have one of two possible outcomes: (1) the patient improves and therefore had acalculous cholecystitis or (2) does not improve, and whenever unexplained pepsis occurs the gallbladder is removed from diagnostic consideration, even if there was no cholecystitis.[252]

One form of acalculous cholecystitis deserves special mention: that which occurs in patients with AIDS. Pathogens that have been implicated include CMV, *Cryptosporidium,* and other opportunistic infections. On imaging, the appearance of the gallbladder is nonspecific and looks like any acalculous cholecystitis. However, since infection affects the entire biliary tree, thickening of the bile duct wall may be present.[243,245]

CHRONIC CHOLECYSTITIS

Chronic inflammation of the gallbladder is seen histologically in virtually all patients with gallstones. Nonspecific ultrasound and CT findings include cholelithi-

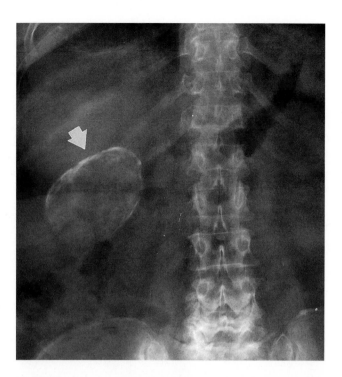

Figure 1–109. Porcelain gallbladder. Plain film shows ovoid calcification corresponding to the gallbladder wall (*arrow*).

asis, sludge, milk of calcium bile, and gallbladder wall thickening. On HIDA scintigraphy, there may be delayed visualization of the gallbladder. It is important to recognize calcification in the gallbladder wall, the porcelain gallbladder (Fig 1–109), which has a 20% to 25% association with the development of gallbladder carcinoma.[253] Another complication of chronic cholecystitis and cholelithiasis, which usually occurs in elderly women, is "gallstone ileus" caused by gallstone erosion through the gallbladder and duodenal wall. This diagnosis can be made on the abdominal plain film whenever classic signs of small bowel obstruction are seen in association with air in the biliary tree (Fig 1–110).

ADENOMYOMATOSIS AND CHOLESTEROLOSIS

Adenomyomatosis and cholesterolosis are part of a group of benign conditions also known as hyperplastic cholecystoses. These conditions have thickening of the gallbladder wall in common[245,254,255] and they both may be the cause of symptoms in some patients. Adenomyomatosis consists of proliferation of mural smooth muscle and is characterized histologically by the presence of small diverticular invaginations of the epithelium into the thickened smooth muscle, also known as Rokitansky-Aschoff sinuses. On sonography and CT, gallbladder wall thickening may be diffuse, segmental, or fundal (also known as adenomyoma) in location. Another specific sign present only on ultrasound is a "ring-down"

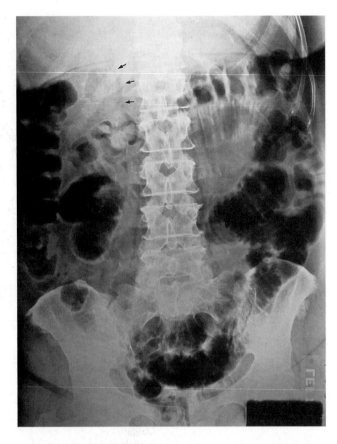

Figure 1–110. Gallstone ileus. Note the dilated small bowel loops due to obstruction. There is air outlining the biliary tree (*small arrows*) owing to fistulization between the gallbladder and the duodenum. The obstructing calculus could not be identified on this plain film.

artifact caused by cholesterol crystals trapped in the Rokitansky-Aschoff sinuses. The best test for this condition is the oral cholecystogram, which will show the pathognomonic diverticular outpouchings.

Cholesterolosis is caused by subepithelial accumulation of cholesterol-laden histiocytes. This is now recognized as an incidental finding on sonography that manifests as a small, echogenic polyp without shadowing. When the inner wall of the gallbladder is carpeted by myriad tiny polyps, the condition is known pathologically as strawberry gallbladder.

GALLBLADDER NEOPLASMS

Malignancies such as lymphoma and metastasis are extremely rare. Melanoma accounts for 50% of metastases. Gallbladder carcinoma presents most commonly as a mass replacing the gallbladder, usually with liver invasion (Fig 1–111) and less commonly as either a polypoid lesion or focal or diffuse gallbladder wall thickening. Other important findings include the presence of gallstones (seen in 80% to 90% of cases) and gallbladder wall calcification (porcelain gallbladder). Ultrasound is better for definition of the smaller lesions, but in the advanced cases, CT would be required to delineate the entire extent of the tumor, including adjacent liver invasion or metastasis, invasion of portal structures, and adenopathy. Distant metastasis is rare in gallbladder carcinoma.[243,245,256]

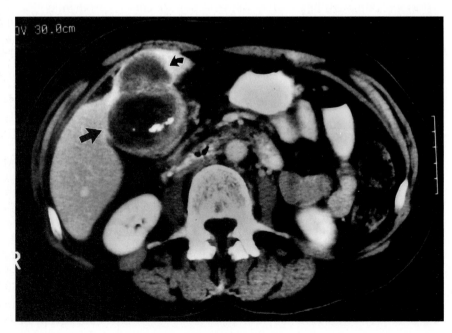

Figure 1–111. Gallbladder carcinoma. CT shows mass replacing gallbladder (*arrow*) engulfing the gallstones and invading into the adjacent liver parenchyma (*curved arrow*).

Benign tumors of the gallbladder are extremely rare. Most are adenomas and present as polypoid lesions. The difficulty with these lesions is that they cannot be differentiated from polypoid carcinomas on imaging. Therefore, any polyp that is not small (<5 mm) and is not uniformly echogenic should raise the suspicion of a carcinoma.

■ RADIOLOGY OF THE BILE DUCTS

EXAMINATION TECHNIQUES

Choosing the best imaging study for the biliary tree can be confusing, given the multitude of tests available. Understanding the capabilities and limitations of the available modalities is essential for deciding on the optimal test for a particular clinical indication. Ultrasound and CT have equal sensitivity and specificity for identifying biliary dilatation, but ultrasound should be the first screening test in suspected biliary obstruction because it is simpler and cheaper to perform. CT is better at delineating extrabiliary extent of pathology. The new generation of helical CT scanners with their thin-section capability is expected to improve detection of small lesions such as distal common bile duct stones. Cholangiography, on the other hand, is the gold standard for defining intrabiliary disease but is invasive and should be reserved for diagnostic information not otherwise obtainable, or combined with interventional procedures in the biliary tree. The HIDA scintigram is yet another useful tool since it provides functional information regarding bile flow and is especially valuable in detection of postoperative bile leaks.[257–260]

Proper sonographic technique involves imaging through multiple acoustic windows to find the best possible images of the bile ducts. Different techniques may be required for the various hepatic segments. Visualizing the intrahepatic ducts or the common hepatic duct is rarely problematic, but the distal common bile duct is often obscured by overlying bowel gas. The normal common hepatic duct is less or equal to 6 mm but may be larger in elderly patients. The common duct may be up to 10 mm in diameter in postcholecytectomy patients. In equivocal cases, a fatty meal challenge test may be performed. In this test, the common hepatic duct is first measured at a reliable and reproducible location. The patient then is given a fatty meal and rescanned 45 minutes later to obtain another measurement at the same location. An unobstructed dilated duct should decrease in size by 2 mm, whereas a truly obstructed duct may either increase of not change in size.[261]

On CT, normal peripheral intrahepatic ducts are not visible unless thin sections are obtained. If they are larger than the corresponding peripheral portal venous

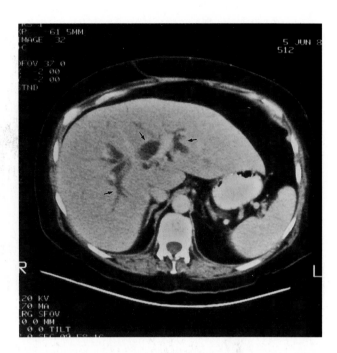

Figure 1–112. Dilated intrahepatic bile ducts on CT. Note low-density tubular structures (*small arrows*) adjacent to the portal venous branches. Normally these are not visible on conventional 10 mm thick CT sections.

branches, then biliary obstruction is assumed (Fig 1–112).[262] CT also has the advantage of visualizing the distal common bile duct, making it better than ultrasound for pancreatic carcinoma, common bile duct stones, and ampullary tumors.

Cholangiography may be done percutaneously, through an existing T tube, or by ERCP. The THC is nearly 100% successful for opacifying the biliary tree in the setting of intrahepatic biliary dilation, and 85% successful for nondilated ducts. The only true contraindication is severe coagulopathy. The complication rate is minimal at 3.5% and includes hemorrhage, cholangitis, and bile leaks. ERCP is also very successful and may be the procedure of choice when there are no dilated intrahepatic ducts. Patients with Billroth II or Roux-en-Y gastroenterostomies are not eligible for ERCP, and for them THC is the only choice.[258,259]

IMAGING PRINCIPLES IN BILIARY OBSTRUCTION

When imaging is performed for possible biliary obstruction, the following questions must be addressed: (1) Is there obstruction? (2) Where is the obstruction? and (3) What is the cause of the obstruction?

On ultrasound and CT, the diagnosis of biliary obstruction rests on the visualization of abnormally dilated ducts. Intrahepatic biliary dilatation is very specific but only 77% sensitive for biliary obstruction. Extrahepatic biliary dilatation is very sensitive (may occur before a

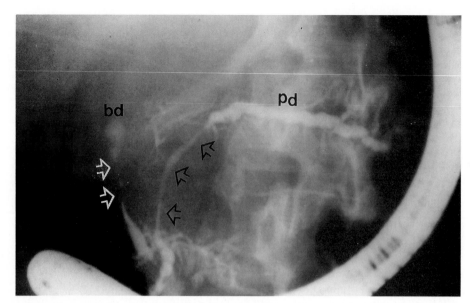

Figure 1–113. Double-duct sign on cholangiography in pancreatic carcinoma. Note the adjacent strictures (*open arrows*) in the common bile duct (bd) and pancreatic duct (pd).

rise in bilirubin) but less specific. Also, although uncommon, obstruction cannot be excluded totally on the basis of a normal ultrasound and CT, and if clinical and biochemical parameters continue to suggest biliary obstruction, cholangiography may be needed.

On cholangiography, the appearance and pattern of the obstructive lesion may indicate the likely diagnoses. Luminal filling defects indicate stones, with a differential diagnosis of air bubbles and blood clots. Multiple strictures implicate sclerosing cholangitis and AIDS cholangitis. Extrinsic compression suggests liver tumors intrahepatically and portal adenopathy extrahepatically. Concurrent, adjacent strictures involving both the distal common bile duct and pancreatic duct are classic signs of pancreatic carcinoma (Fig 1–113).

CONGENITAL ANOMALIES

Choledochal cysts refer to a spectrum of congenital or developmental biliary abnormalities. The pathogenesis is believed to arise from mural weakening of the bile duct secondary to aberrant common bile duct–pancreatic duct junction and chronic reflux of pancreatic secretions into the biliary tree. Choledochal cysts are classified into types 1 through 5. A type 1 cyst consists of fusiform dilatation of the extrahepatic common duct (Fig 1–114) and is the most common, accounting for 80% to 90% of all choledochal cysts. Type 2 cysts are saccular outpouchings from the common duct. Type 3 choledochal cysts, also known as choledochoceles, and are dilatations of the intramural ampullary portion of the distal common duct which may protrude into the duodenal lumen. Type 4 cysts are multiple extrahepatic and/or intrahepatic cysts. Type 5 choledochal cysts also

are known and Caroli's disease and consist of multiple segmental intrahepatic ductal cystic dilatations.

Radiologically, although cholangiography is the gold standard for diagnosis, ultrasound and CT can be suggestive. There is an increased incidence of stones, cholangitis, and cholangiocarcinoma in this condition. Biliary obstruction is also commonly present, with more proximal bile duct dilatation. Caroli's disease also is associated with renal cysts.[259,263]

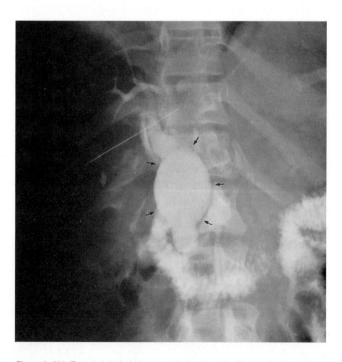

Figure 1–114. Type 1 choledochal cyst on cholangiography. Note the fusiform dilatation of the extrahepatic duct (*arrows*).

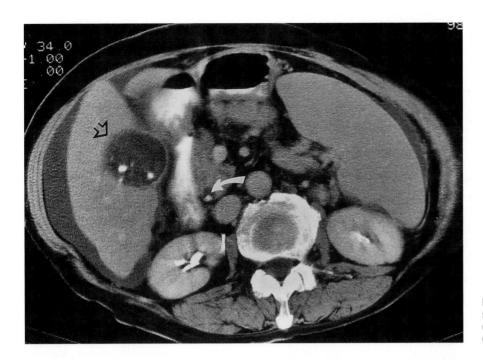

Figure 1–115. Calcified distal CBD stone on CT. Axial section through the pancreatic head shows calcified density (*curved arrow*) within the distal CBD. Note also calcified gallstones within gallbladder (*open arrow*).

CHOLEDOCHOLITHIASIS

The diagnosis of common duct stones can be difficult.[264–266] Ultrasound can be up to 80% sensitive but requires prolonged dedicated technique, since the distal common duct is a relatively blind spot for ultrasound because of adjacent bowel gas. CT is excellent for visualizing calcified stones (Fig 1–115), and newer breath-hold thin section helical CT holds promise for significantly increasing sensitivity of CT for detection of small and noncalcified ductal stones. Cholangiography is the gold standard, but even cholangiograms can be difficult to interpret since air bubbles, mucus, clot, and debris can all mimic calculi. It is also important not to mistake sphincter of Oddi spasm for an impacted ampullary stone (Fig 1–116).

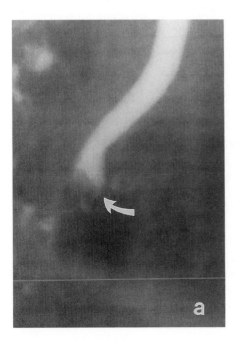
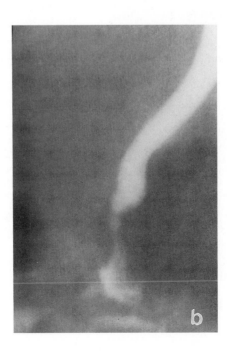

Figure 1–116. Pseudocalculus sign of ampullary spasm. **A.** Cholangiogram shows abrupt ending to the contrast column at the ampulla (*curved arrow*), mimicking an impacted stone. **B.** With fluoroscopic monitoring, the ampulla opens up 10 seconds later allowing contrast to flow into the duodenum. No calculus is present.

INFLAMMATORY DISORDERS

Sclerosing Cholangitis

Cholangiography is useful for diagnosing sclerosing cholangitis in the correct clinical setting.[259,267] The findings include strictures, which can be long or bandlike, and are commonly multiple and arranged in series (leading to "beading" of the ducts). The peripheral ducts may appear pruned, and there may be diverticular outpouchings, a finding that is nearly pathognomonic. In 85% to 90% of cases both the intrahepatic and extrahepatic ducts are involved. Extrahepatic duct–only involvement occurs in 5% to 10%, and intrahepatic duct–only involvement is rare (Fig 1–117). Secondary findings on imaging, due to complications, include stones, cholangitic abscesses, and cholangiocarcinoma. The latter can be difficult to detect in the background of preexisting strictures. However, any rapidly developing stricture, marked bilary dilatation owing to obstruction, or mass seen on ultrasound or CT should be viewed with suspicion (Fig 1–118). On ultrasound and CT, the segmental biliary strictures are difficult to appreciate because of the diffusely thickened and fibrosed ducts that do not dilate despite obstruction.

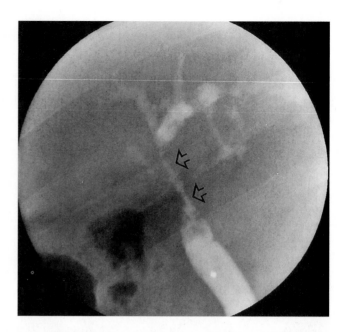

Figure 1–118. Cholangiocarcinoma in patient with sclerosing cholangitis. Note high-grade stricture (*open arrows*) in proximal common hepatic duct that was malignant on brush biopsy. Note also the irregularly dilated intrahepatic ducts from sclerosing cholangitis.

High-resolution sonograms of the common duct may demonstrate the actual thickened bile duct walls.[257] Gallbladder abnormalities include wall thickening, which may be focal or diffuse.

Bacterial Cholangitis

The role of ultrasound and CT in bacterial cholangitis is primarily to determine the presence of bile duct dilatation suggestive of a biliary source for sepsis. Often, this is the presenting symptom for a patient with previously unknown biliary disease. Once biliary obstruction is diagnosed, it is also important to determine the level and cause to determine the optimal method of drainage. Most obstructions occur in the distal common duct and are easily accessible through ERCP. Higher level obstructions and those that fail ERCP may require transhepatic percutaneous drainage. It is important to decide before the procedure whether a right, left, or combined approach would be optimal, depending on the information ultrasound or CT has provided.

Recurrent Pyogenic Cholangitis (Oriental Cholangiohepatitis)

This rare entity is seen almost exclusively in the Asian population. Etiology is controversial, but there appears to be an association with *Clonorchis* species and other parasites. Radiologically, the disease is characterized by multiple intrahepatic segmental biliary strictures with dilated proximal segments filled with stones or casts of sludge. There is also a predilection for the left lobe, es-

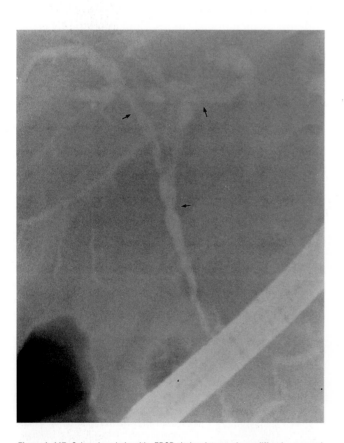

Figure 1–117. Sclerosing cholangitis. ERCP cholangiogram shows diffusely narrowed CBD along with multiple short strictures involving both the intrahepatic and extrahepatic ducts (*arrows*).

pecially the lateral segmental ducts. Recurrent bacterial infections may result in abscess formation.[259,268]

AIDS-related Cholangitis

In patients with AIDS, cholangitis results in scarring and fibrosis of the bile ducts that appear very similar to the scarring seen in sclerosing cholangitis. Multiple organisms have been implicated, including *Cryptosporidium* and CMV. Sonography may demonstrate thickened bile duct walls, along with diffuse gallbladder wall thickening due to HIV-related cholecystitis. Cholangiography may show multiple strictures in both the intrahepatic and extrahepatic ducts. There is a predilection for the ampulla, which may distinguish it from sclerosing cholangitis.[258,269]

Parasitic Infestations

Ascariasis is the most common helminth infestation of the bile ducts. Diagnosis is by cholangiography, which demonstrates the moving worm, often several inches along (*A. lumbricoides*), within the biliary tree.

Clonorchiasis is endemic to Asia and is caused by the liver fluke, *Clonorchis sinensis,* which is transmitted by ingestion of infected raw fish. The intrahepatic ducts are the organisms' natural habitat, where they cause obstruction, periductal inflammation, and fibrosis. They may manifest as elliptical filling defects within obstructed, dilated segmental ducts. The extrahepatic ducts are usually spared. Complications include stones, abscess, and cholangiocarcinoma, the latter tending to occur peripherally, corresponding to the peripheral distribution of the infection.[258,270]

NEOPLASMS

Cholangiocarcinoma

Cholangiocarcinoma is the most important primary tumor of the bile ducts.[258,271] Predisposing conditions include sclerosing cholangitis, choledochal cyst, clonorchiasis, and Thorotrast exposure. Radiologically, three distinct patterns may be seen: intrahepatic mass, hilar tumor (Klatskin's tumor), and distal duct form. The liver mass presentation comprises 20% to 30% of cholangiocarcinomas. Calcifications may be present. Ultrasound may show a hypoechoic or hyperechoic or mixed echogenicity mass. CT typically shows a low-density, heterogeneous, and often peripherally enhancing mass. The hilar Klatskin's tumor is the most common type of cholangiocarcinoma. Ultrasound and CT characteristically show intrahepatic biliary dilatation with a normal common duct and often a subtle hint of the hilar mass. There also may be segmental or lobar atrophy present. Portal and retroperitoneal adenopathy are also common. Cholangiography is diagnostic, with a stricture seen straddling the bifurcation (Fig 1–119) and isolated left and right systems. The distal duct form of cholan-

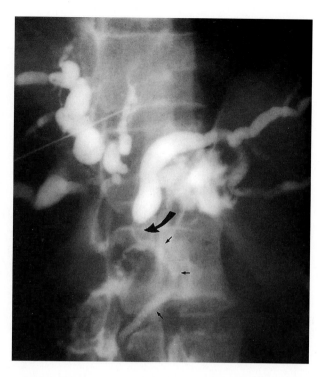

Figure 1–119. Hilar Klatskin tumor. Cholangiogram showing stricture at the bifurcation (*curved arrow*), isolating the right and left ducts. The common bile duct (*small arrows*) is nondilated.

giocarcinoma usually presents as a stricture and, less commonly, as a polypoid filling defect. The stricture may be irregular with overhanging edges suggestive of a malignant stricture, or it may be smooth and indistinguishable from benign strictures. Brush biopsy through ERCP or transhepatic route may be helpful for cytological diagnosis.

Periampullary Carcinoma

Malignant lesions causing obstruction at the ampulla may be duodenal or biliary in origin. They are often amenable to curative surgery. Ultrasound, CT, or cholangiography all show obstruction at the ampulla, although the actual lesion may be small and not visualized.

Cystic Bile Duct Tumors (Biliary Cystadenoma/Cystadenocarcinoma)

These are rare mucin-secreting tumors that often reach a large size by the time they are discovered. The tumors rarely are malignant but are considered to have malignant potential. On ultrasound and CT they are typically large, thin-walled cystic lesions with fine septations (Fig 1–120). Thick walls or septations and mural nodules indicate possible malignancy.

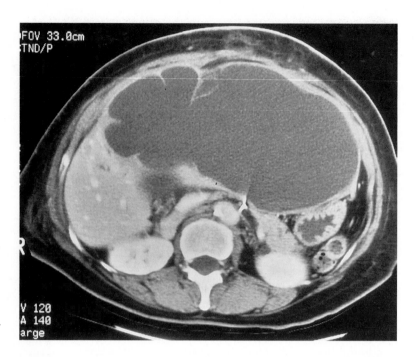

Figure 1–120. Biliary cystadenoma. CT shows cystic lesion with septations.

Adenoma and Granular Cell Tumors

Adenomas and granular cell tumors are rare polypoid benign tumors found primarily in the extrahepatic common duct. Adenomas are usually asymptomatic and only occasionally cause bile duct obstruction. Granular cell tumors are typically 1 to 2 cm in size and probably of Schwann cell origin. These tumors occur in young black women. Surgical resection is curative for both tumors.

POSTSURGICAL CONDITIONS

Postcholecystectomy Injuries

Injury to the biliary tree may occur during cholecystectomy. The incidence has increased since the introduction of laparoscopic cholecystectomy.[272–274] Traumatic strictures and complete ligation of the common bile duct may occur (Fig 1–121). Bile leaks may occur at the cystic duct stump, common bile duct, or from a variant duct of Luschka that drains directly into the gallbladder from the right lobe of the liver. These small ducts are transected during dissection of the gallbladder away from the liver. Ultrasound and CT are the primary imaging modalities to screen for biliary injuries. HIDA nuclear medicine scan may also be helpful for detecting bile leaks. Cholangiography, usually via ERCP, is the definitive test, if the screening modalities are positive.

Bile Duct Injuries in Liver Transplantation

After liver transplantation, the end-to-end biliary anastomosis or the choledochoenteric anastomosis is a frequent site of bile leakage. Another common place for bile leakage is the T tube insertion site. With a T tube in

place, a routine diagnostic cholangiogram can be performed easily. The patient should always be on antibiotics during the cholangiogram, and the contrast should be administered with slow infusion, preferably by gravity, because of the risks of biliary sepsis and increased pressure against a fresh surgical anastomosis.

Liver transplant patients also are prone to developing bile duct strictures. These may be anastomotic strictures or ischemic strictures secondary to hepatic artery

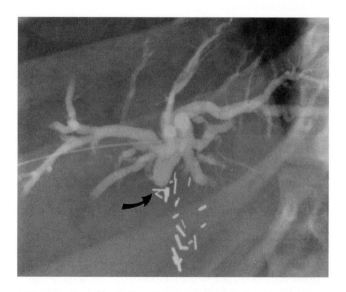

Figure 1–121. Ligation of CBD at cholecystectomy. Cholangiogram shows complete obstruction at mid CBD (*curved arrow*), corresponding to the level of cholecystectomy staples.

thrombosis or stenosis. If biliary dilatation occurs and nonanastomotic strictures are identified, the hepatic artery must be investigated for possible stenosis or thrombosis.[275,276]

Biliary-Enteric Anastomosis

On plain film, ultrasound, and CT, it is normal to see air in the bile ducts in patients with biliary-enteric anastomoses. In fact, lack of visualization of pneumobilia may be a sign of obstruction. As with any anastomosis, failure can result in bile leaks and strictures. Reflux of bowel contents into the bile ducts also predispose to stone formation, especially if narrowing is present at the anastomosis. Since ERCP usually is not possible in these patients, diagnostic cholangiography can be performed only by the percutaneous transhepatic route. Balloon dilatation of the anastomotic stricture also may be done through the transhepatic approach.[259]

■ RADIOLOGY OF THE PANCREAS

Prior to CT, ultrasound, MRI, and ERCP, imaging of the pancreas was indirect and radiographic diagnosis of pancreatic disease was dependent on changes produced in surrounding organs, as seen on plain films or barium studies. Visualization of the pancreatic parenchyma, ductal system, and surrounding vasculature, as well as changes affecting surrounding organs, is now possible.

Plain films of the abdomen are often taken in the patient with an acute abdomen. Findings in pancreatic disease are usually those of large masses, calcifications, or abnormal gas patterns.

CT is currently the imaging modality of choice for visualizing the pancreas.[277] High-resolution sequential bolus dynamic scanning is used for the evaluation of both inflammatory and neoplastic pancreatic pathology. Significant pancreatic work is being done in MRI; its place in evaluating pancreatic transplants and small islet cell tumors has been well documented. Improvements in MRI bowel and intravenous contrast agents, and standardization of MRI sequences may eventually make it the superior technique.

Using new helical CT scanners, the entire pancreas can be scanned in a single breath-hold and a bolus of IV contrast may be maintained during the entire time of scanning. Oral contrast is used to define the surrounding bowel. Artifacts due to respiratory motion are not a problem. Rapid scanning is especially helpful in the seriously ill patient.[278]

ERCP has become increasingly useful for both its diagnostic and interventional capabilities. Endoscopy permits visualization and biopsy, if necessary, of any portion of the bowel. Both the biliary tree and pancreatic ductal system may be visualized on a single examination.

Diagnosis of inflammatory, congenital, and neoplastic diseases can be made and interventional procedures such as sphincterotomy, dilatation of strictures, stone removal, and stent placement are possible.[279]

The use of angiography has decreased as CT and ERCP studies increase. It is still of value in the work-up of islet cell tumors, the investigation of the occasional vascular complications of pancreatitis, the determination of operability of some pancreatic carcinomas, and to outline anomalous vasculature. Its potential for intervention may be of value in patients with hemorrhage due to trauma or pancreatitis.

CONGENITAL ANOMALIES

Congenital anomalies of the pancreas include pancreas divisum, annular pancreas, and ectopic pancreas.

Pancreas Divisum

Pancreas divisum occurs as a result of failure of fusion of the dorsal and ventral pancreatic anlage. The pancreatic head and uncinate process are drained by the duct of Wirsung via the major papilla, and the body and tail of the pancreas are drained through the duct of Santorini via the minor papilla. This anomaly is demonstrated best by ERCP and is shown in 3% to 4% of ERCPs. Cannulation of the major papilla fills the duct of Wirsung, which is short, and shows terminal branching in the pancreatic head. It is important that this be differentiated from a duct that is truncated because of tumor encasement. In the latter case, the duct ends abruptly without branching. The duct of Santorini is filled via the minor papilla (Fig 1–122).[280]

Annular Pancreas

Annular pancreas occurs when the ventral pancreatic bud, which usually atrophies in pancreatic development, persists and encircles the duodenum. Symptoms may occur in infancy or middle age and are related to duodenal obstruction. In adults, chronic duodenal obstruction may lead to peptic ulcer disease.[281]

In the pediatric patient with duodenal obstruction from annular pancreas, the classic plain film sign is the "double bubble." This is due to the dilated stomach and duodenal bulb proximal to the obstructing annular pancreas. In adults, plain film findings are not significant unless marked duodenal obstruction develops. An upper GI plain film may show narrowing of the second duodenum and possibly the presence of a peptic ulcer. ERCP may show the pancreatic duct in the head of the pancreas as encircling the duodenum.

Ectopic Pancreas

Ectopic pancreas or pancreatic rests are common anomalies that are usually small (<1.5 cm in diameter) sub-

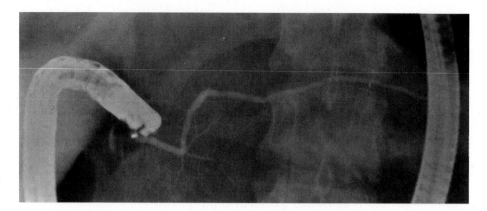

Figure 1–122. Pancreas divisum. The dorsal duct is filled by cannulating the minor papilla.

mucosal lesions with a central collection of contrast, as seen on UGI. The collection represents a rudimentary pancreatic duct. Their location is usually the gastric antrum or duodenum. They are most often incidental findings on UGI studies.[282]

PANCREATIC INFLAMMATORY DISEASE

Plain abdominal films are the first examination performed in a patient with suspected pancreatitis (Table 1–12). Findings on plain film include gallstones, a gasless abdomen, or a localized ileus confined to the duodenum or proximal jejunum. This latter finding is called a sentinel loop and indicates inflammation in the surrounding area. The transverse colon may be dilated with an abrupt transition to narrowed colon distal to the splenic flexure. This "colon cut-off sign" is either due to spasm and/or spread of inflammation via the phrenicocolic ligament from the pancreas to the descending colon. Separation of the greater curvature of the stomach and transverse colon may occur as a result of inflammation and/or fluid collections. Air bubbles in this area may signify abscess formation (Fig 1–123). Other mottled lucencies may be due to fat necrosis. Elevation of the hemidiaphragm and a left pleural effusion are frequently present.[283,284]

TABLE 1–12. PLAIN FILM FINDINGS IN PANCREATITIS

Gasless abdomen
Sentinel loop
Gallstones
Pancreatic calcifications
Colon cut-off sign
Separation of great curve stomach and transverse colon
Extraluminal air bubbles—abscess
Extraluminal mottled density—fat necrosis
Elevation of left hemidiaphragm
Left pleural effusion

Barium studies may show markedly coarsened gastric rugal folds, elevation of the greater curvature of the stomach, and widening of the duodenal loop with coarsened duodenal mucosal folds and an enlarged papilla of Vater. A reverse 3 sign of the duodenal sweep may be present and is caused by the enlarged pancreas creating an extrinsic pressure defect above and below the ampulla, which is fixed by the entrance of pancreatic duct (Table 1–13). This sign may also be seen with pancreatic carcinoma. Extravasation of contrast from the duodenum or colon may be seen secondary to the inflammatory process eroding into the bowel.[284]

CT and ultrasound allow the clinician to visualize the pancreas itself rather than only the surrounding structures. Sonographic examination often is limited in these patients because of overlying bowel gas. The pancreas is evaluated best with good contrast filling of the surrounding bowel and IV-iodinated contrast administration. The normal pancreas enhances homogeneously and has either a smooth or slightly undulating margin (Fig 1–124). The size varies in different people with elderly people often having smaller, more lobulated appearing glands. The head measures about 3 to 4 cm, the body 2 to 3 cm, and the tail about 1 to 2 cm with gradual tapering between segments. The tail may have bulbous configuration that may be confused with a mass (Fig 1–125). With modern scanners, the normal thin, tubular, smooth pancreatic duct may be seen, on occasion. The fat surrounding the pancreas is homogeneous and of low density.[277,284–287]

Indications for Imaging

The diagnosis of pancreatitis is made on clinical evaluation based on history, physical findings, and laboratory tests. Imaging often is not needed for diagnosis. CT appearance of the pancreas may be normal in up to 30% of patients with acute pancreatitis.

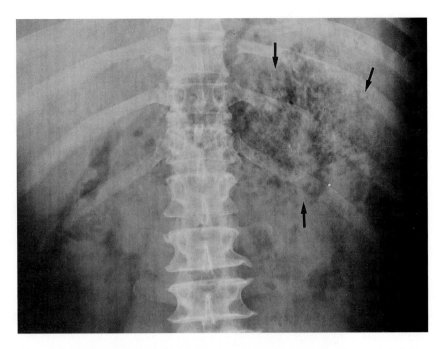

Figure 1–123. Pancreatic abscess due to pancreatitis. *Arrows* indicate multiple extraluminal left upper quadrant air bubbles as a result of pancreatic necrosis and abscess.

TABLE 1–13. CONTRAST STUDIES OF PANCREATITIS

Coarse gastric rugal folds
Widening of the duodenal sweep
Reverse 3 sign
Coarsened duodenal folds
Enlarged ampulla of Vater
Bowel fistula

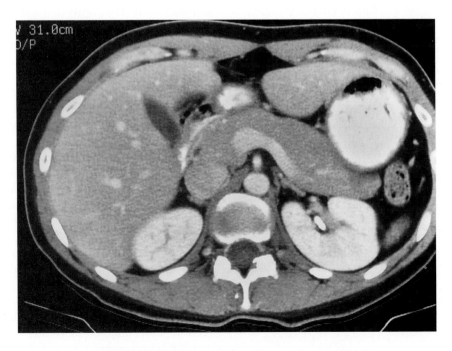

Figure 1–124. CT showing a normal smooth pancreas in a young person.

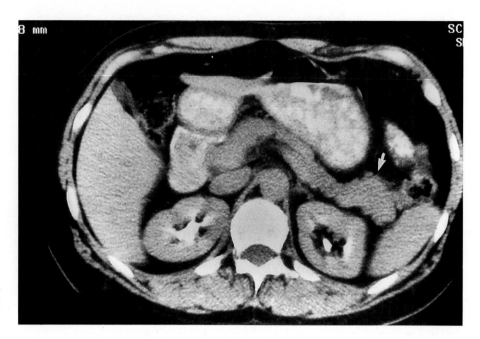

Figure 1–125. CT of a normal pancreas in an elderly patient. The pancreas has an undulating margin, and the bulbous tail (*arrows*) is a normal variant.

The goals of imaging are

1. To exclude other abdominal disorders that may clinically mimic pancreatitis
2. To confirm the diagnosis of pancreatitis
3. To evaluate the extent in order to stage severity
4. To define presence or extent and nature of complications
5. As image guidance for radiologic intervention

Although not completely accurate, CT can group patients into those having low- or high-risk likelihood for developing complications (Table 1–14). In many patients, disease progression and complications may develop after the initial scan, especially those with severe pancreatitis who may require serial scans. With mild pancreatitis, a slight to moderate increase in the size of the gland may result (Fig 1–126). Moderate pancreatitis will produce diffuse glandular enlargement with some fluid around the gland. The normally homogeneous black peripancreatic fat becomes hazy and streaked (Fig 1–127). Severe pancreatitis will produce marked pancreatic enlargement and total loss of normal-appearing peripancreatic fat. Poorly defined inflammatory masses (phlegmons) or fluid collections may be seen. CT can also provide information related to bowel, biliary, and vascular involvement. Pancreatic ascites may be present and pleural effusions are a frequent finding (Fig 1–128). Peripancreatic fluid collections may resolve spontaneously. CT- or ultrasound-guided fine-needle aspiration is helpful in determining when fluid collections are infected.

With rapid scanning and IV bolus CT technique, estimates of pancreatic necrosis and prediction of patients at risk for abscess development can be made. Nonenhancement of the pancreas with this technique signals pancreatic necrosis and the probability of supervening infection (Fig 1–128).[288]

Complications of acute pancreatitis include pancreatic abscess, either within the gland or the peripancreatic area. Abscesses are the result of infection of pancreatic or peripancreatic fluid or a necrotic portion of pancreas. They usually appear as a low-density fluid collection that may contain air bubbles (20%) (Fig 1–129). When extraluminal air is seen in a patient with pancreatitis, erosion into the bowel also must be con-

TABLE 1–14. CT FINDINGS IN ACUTE PANCREATITIS

Mild	Moderate	Severe
Slight to moderate enlargement of pancreas	Diffuse pancreatic enlargement	Marked pancreatic enlargement
	Peripancreatic fluid	Peripancreatic fat
	Peripancreatic fat streaking	Inflammatory masses (phlegmons)
	Pleural effusions	Peripancreatic fluid collections
		Extrapancreatic fluid collections
		Nonenhancement of pancreas (necrosis)
		Ascites
		Pleural effusions
		Vascular complications
		Splenic vein thrombosis
		Pseudoaneurysms
		Hemorrhage (due to vascular erosion)
		Biliary obstruction

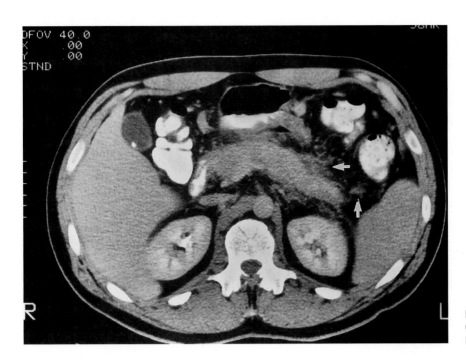

Figure 1-126. Acute pancreatitis with mild radiographic changes. The gland is enlarged with streaking of the peri-pancreatic fat (*arrows*). Note gallstone.

sidered. Some abscesses may be treated using CT guidance and percutaneous drainage, but surgery is often required.

If a persistent collection of fluid due to pancreatitis forms a fibrous wall, it has become a pseudocyst. Although usually located in the lesser sac, pseudocysts may dissect to other areas including the pelvis, liver, spleen, mediastinum, or psoas muscle. They appear on CT as round or oval fluid density masses with a well-defined wall. The pseudocyst may decompress spontaneously or may be treated by image-guided catheter drainage or surgical intervention.

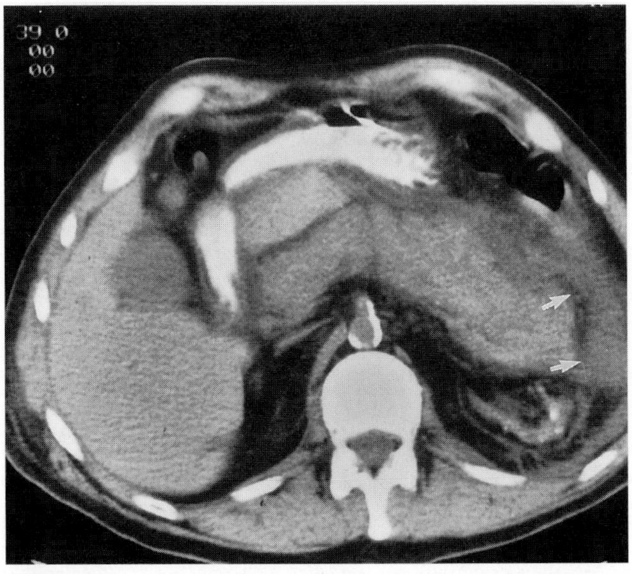

Vascular complications of pancreatitis include vascular occlusion, hemorrhage due to vascular erosion, or pseudoaneurysm formation. Splenic vein thrombosis can be readily seen on contrast-enhanced CT examination. With hemorrhage due to vascular erosion, angiography and therapeutic embolization may be necessary.[277,284,288]

Biliary involvement usually causes distal bile duct obstruction with intrahepatic and proximal extrahepatic dilatation, as seen on CT or sonogram. Biliary obstruction is, however, a more frequent complication of chronic pancreatitis.[284]

Chronic Pancreatitis

The classic plain film finding is pancreatic calcification. The calcifications may be diffuse or localized, and size is variable.

In the patient with chronic pancreatitis, CT findings include parenchymal and pancreatic ductal calcifications, ductal dilatation, texture inhomogeneity, and contour irregularities. Splenic vein thrombosis and varices may be present. Portions of the gland may atrophy. Dilatation of the intrahepatic and proximal extrahepatic biliary tree with tapered narrowing of the distal CBD may be seen.

Ductal dilatation, size alterations, and contour irregularities can be seen on sonographic examination.

Figure 1-127. Acute pancreatitis with more marked radiographic changes on CT. **A.** The gland is markedly enlarged with peripancreatic fluid present (*arrows*).

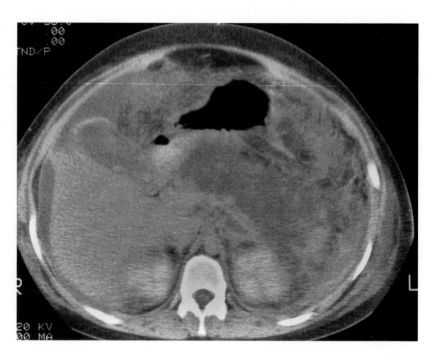

Figure 1–128. Severe pancreatitis on CT. There is no vascular enhancement of the pancreas. Pancreatic necrosis was found at surgical exploration. Pancreatic ascites is present.

Doppler techniques may confirm obstruction of the portal venous system.

ERCP is the most useful imaging technique in establishing the diagnosis of chronic pancreatitis (Fig 1–130). Early changes involving ductal side branches may become irregular and clubbed. The main pancreatic duct may be dilated and may have areas of stricture or occlusion, as well as intraductal calculi. This beaded appearance has been described as a "chain of lakes."[277,284]

PANCREATIC NEOPLASMS

Ductal adenocarcinoma is the most common pancreatic neoplasm. Ninety percent of pancreatic tumors are a result of ductal carcinoma, with the head of the pancreas being involved in 60% to 70% of cases.

Sonographic examination is often the first imaging study obtained in a patient with abdominal pain and/or jaundice. A hypoechoic pancreatic mass relative to nor-

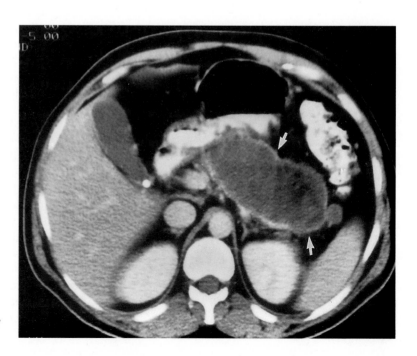

Figure 1–129. Pancreatic abscess. Acute pancreatitis with surgically confirmed pancreatic abscess (*arrows*).

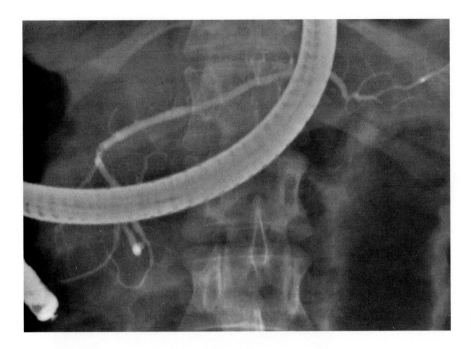

Figure 1–130. Normal ERCP. Note smooth, tapering duct and fine, thin side branches.

mal portions of the gland may be seen. Accompanying findings are dilatation of the pancreatic duct, biliary dilatation, and a dilated (Courvoisier) gallbladder.

CT remains the imaging method of choice when pancreatic carcinoma is clinically suspected (Table 1–15).[277,289–291] Rapid pancreas scanning protocols with IV and oral contrast should be used. The use of helical scanners increases the likelihood of visualizing small lesions. An inhomogeneous pancreatic head mass with biliary dilatation may be seen. The ductal dilatation may be both intrahepatic and extrahepatic, and the dilated duct may abruptly end at the level of the mass where it is encased by tumor. A dilated pancreatic duct and dilated gallbladder are often present. An advantage of CT is that it may also reveal, when present, hepatic and nodal metastases, local extension into the peripancreatic fat or surrounding organs, ascites and invasion, en-

TABLE 1–15. CT FINDINGS IN CARCINOMA OF THE HEAD OF THE PANCREAS

Biliary dilatation—extrahepatic and intrahepatic stopping at the pancreatic head
Gallbladder distention (Courvoisier gallbladder)
Dilated pancreatic duct
Splenic vein and portal vein thrombosis
Encasement of superior mesenteric vessels with loss of fat rim surrounding the SMA
Extension into peripancreatic fat
Hepatic and/or nodal metastases
Ascites

casement, or thrombosis of blood vessels in the area of tumor. Occasionally, the pancreatic neoplasm will not be visible despite excellent imaging technique. However, its presence will be inferred by the ancillary findings of biliary, gallbladder, and pancreatic ductal dilation (Fig 1–131).

Tumors of the body of the pancreas may produce dilatation of the pancreatic duct proximal to the tumor, a pancreatic contour abnormality, and a low-density mass. Invasion of blood vessels, especially the superior mesenteric artery, and/or thrombosis of the splenic vein may be present (Figs 1–132 and 1–133).

Tumors of the pancreatic tail principally show enlargement of this area by a low-density mass that is inhomogeneous as compared with the remainder of the pancreas.

Radiographic signs that indicate unresectability are hepatic and distant metastases, peripancreatic extension of tumor, invasion of contiguous organs, vascular encasement or invasion, and local adenopathy (Figs 1–132 and 1–133).[292]

ERCP is an excellent method for establishing the diagnosis of pancreatic ductal adenocarcinoma. Since the tumor arises from the duct, opacifying the duct will often reveal a lesion. Also, ERCP permits some interventional procedures, such as biliary stent placement, in the severely jaundiced patient.

The classic finding on ERCP of a carcinoma of the pancreatic head is the double duct sign, with either complete or partial obstruction, or displacement of both the distal pancreatic and distal common bile duct

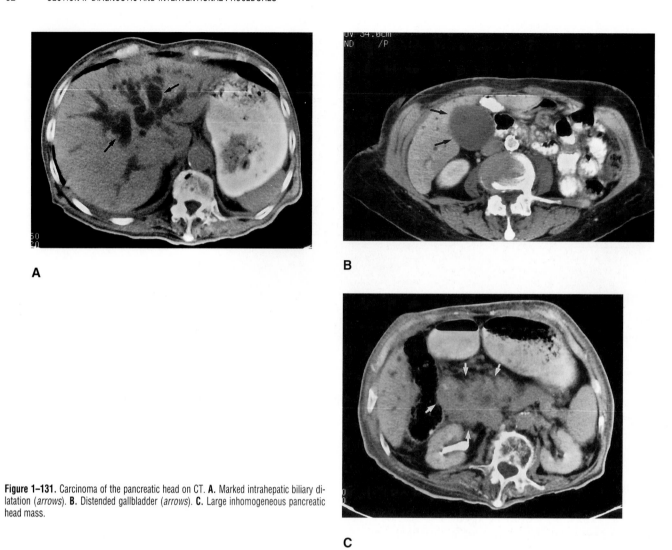

A

B

C

Figure 1–131. Carcinoma of the pancreatic head on CT. **A.** Marked intrahepatic biliary dilatation (*arrows*). **B.** Distended gallbladder (*arrows*). **C.** Large inhomogeneous pancreatic head mass.

Figure 1–132. Carcinoma of the body of the pancreas. An inhomogeneous mass in the body of the pancreas is present on CT. *Arrow* indicates a dilated proximal pancreatic duct. The splenic vein is occluded.

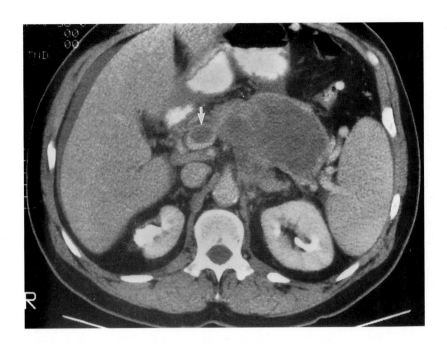

Figure 1–133. Mucinous ductal adenocarcinoma in the body and tail of the pancreas on CT. *Arrow* indicates thrombosis of the portal vein. The splenic vein is occluded and ascites are present. Posterior extension of the tumor on the left is present.

in the area of the tumor. If contrast passes proximal to the obstruction, dilatation of the ducts may be seen. Chronic pancreatitis and ampullary carcinoma may occasionally produce a double duct sign.

Transhepatic cholangiography now is used rarely as a diagnostic modality for pancreatic head tumors but may be employed when decompression of an obstructed biliary tree is desired via a transhepatic biliary tube. The usual finding is an abrupt narrowing or com-

plete obstruction of the distal common bile duct at the level of the tumor (Fig 1–134).

MRI on T1-weighted, fat-suppressed images may be helpful in cases where there are small pancreatic tumors, but the outline of the gland is preserved. Oral and IV contrast materials are used. Many different oral bowel agents have been tried, including Kaopectate (Upjohn), superparamagnetic iron oxide particles with silicone coating (AMI121 Advanced Magnetics, Cambridge, MA), and in-

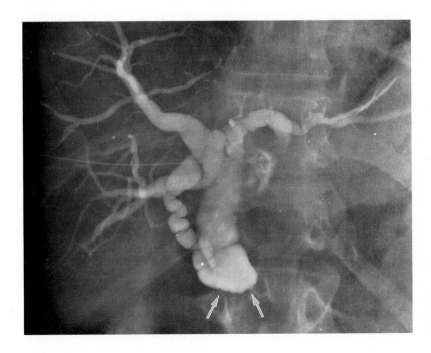

Figure 1–134. Transhepatic cholangiogram in carcinoma of the pancreatic head. There is marked dilatation of the cystic duct, extrahepatic, and intrahepatic bile ducts with complete obstruction of the distal duct (*arrow*).

travenous agents such as Gadolinium (Gd-DTPA-Mag-nevist, gadopentate dimeglumine, Berlex Laboratories, Wayne, NJ). Their use causes diffuse homogeneous contrast enhancement of the normal pancreas and increases the conspicuity of a mass.[293–297]

Islet Cell Tumors

These neoplasms are often small and hard to define, and imaging is often critical in guiding the surgeon. Suspicion often is aroused by abnormal laboratory tests, although on occasion a nonfunctioning islet cell tumor may be found incidentally.

Excellent bolus technique and rapid CT scanning are helpful in detecting these neoplasms. Small tumors in the wall of the duodenum are the most difficult to image. Nonfunctioning tumors may be quite large when first discovered, since, in the early stages, they do not produce the biochemical changes that attract attention.

Insulinomas are found equally in the head, body, and tail of the pancreas. Typical lesions are small (90% are <2 cm in diameter) hypervascular masses that may be solitary (85%) or multiple. A small lesion in the pancreatic tail may be difficult to differentiate from a tortuous splenic vein. MRI is a promising technique for localizing small neoplasms, if optimum technique and equipment are used.[277,298] Intraoperative ultrasound has been shown to be useful for the detection of small lesions not visible by other diagnostic techniques.[299]

Gastrinomas appear as a focal contrast-enhanced mass that may contain foci of calcification. The average tumor size is 3.5 cm. Half occur as solitary in the pancreatic head or tail and 10% present as diffuse pancreatic hyperplasia. Metastases, often in the form of liver or nodal lesions, are vascular in nature and may be present in 60% of patients at the time of diagnosis.[277,300,301] On angiography, they appear as a dense homogeneous blush.

Nonfunctioning tumors may be large and will enhance with intravenous contrast, as does the remainder of the pancreas. They are diagnosed mainly by their pancreatic contour–altering effects.

CYSTIC PANCREATIC LESIONS

Congenital pancreatic cysts may be solitary or multiple and may occur in conjunction with diseases that cause cysts in other organs, such as cystic fibrosis, adult polycystic kidney disease, and von Hippel-Lindau disease. Imaging studies such as ultrasound and CT will demonstrate pancreatic cysts as well as cysts in other involved organs. Patients with von Hippel-Lindau disease may also have renal cell carcinomas and microcystic adenomas of the pancreas (Table 1–16).

Other cystic-appearing lesions include pseudocysts and abscesses (described under pancreatitis), and *Echinococcus* cyst, which usually has a characteristic ap-

TABLE 1–16. CYSTIC PANCREATIC LESIONS

Congenital cystic masses
  Single true cyst—rare
  Multiple true cysts
  Adult polycystic kidney disease
  von Hippel-Lindau disease
  Cystic fibrosis
Inflammatory cystic lesions
  Pseudocyst
  Abscess
  Echinococcus disease
Neoplasms
  Serous cystadenoma
  Mucinous cystadenoma or cystadenocarcinoma
  Solid and papillary epithelial neoplasm
May mimic cystic lesions
  Cholecdochal cyst
  Postoperative, eg, post-Puestow procedure

pearance of daughter cysts and a calcified wall. A choledochal cyst in the pancreatic head may be confused with a pancreatic cystic lesion.[302]

Cystic Neoplasms

Only 5% of pancreatic tumors are cystic neoplasms, and these are generally of two types.

The microcystic adenoma, or glycogen-rich serous cystadenoma, usually occurs in elderly female patients and is almost always benign. It has a characteristic appearance on CT. In 20% of cases, foci of calcification are present, as are a cluster of small cystic spaces each usually <2 cm in size and >6 in number.[302–304]

Mucinous cystadenomas or macrocystic adenomas are potentially malignant neoplasms occurring more frequently in female patients. They are usually located in the pancreatic body or tail. On CT, a large hypovascular mass with a definite wall, a few septations, and often mural nodules may be seen (Fig 1–135). On MRI, the lesion may be of varying signal intensity depending on the presence of hemorrhage and the protein content of the fluid. Each compartment, as marked by septation, is >2 cm in diameter with usually less than six compartments.

Solid and papillary epithelial neoplasms are rare, low-grade malignancies that occur most often in young female patients (<40 years of age). They may have a cystic appearance, if hemorrhage has occurred. They appear on imaging studies (CT, MRI, ultrasound) as large, sharply marginated lesions. The internal architecture varies from solid to a combination of a thick, irregular wall with a fluid-filled interior (Fig 1–136).[304,305]

METASTATIC DISEASE

Metastatic disease to the pancreas occurs more frequently as direct extension from a lesion in a contigu-

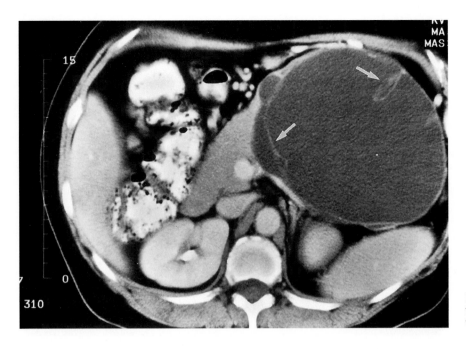

Figure 1–135. Macrocystic adenoma (mucinous cystadenoma) of the pancreatic tail on CT. Large, thinwall lesion with few septations (*arrows*) are present.

ous organ than as hematogenous spread. Radiologic findings are usually that of a mass to be differentiated from a primary pancreatic neoplasm.

Pancreatic lymphoma with involvement of the gland occurs, on occasion, in non-Hodgkin's lymphoma, histocystic, and Burkett's lymphoma. Glandular involvement is rare in Hodgkin's disease. Peripancreatic adenopathy and intrinsic pancreatic disease may be difficult to differentiate on imaging studies. When glandular involvement does occur, it can be differentiated from carcinoma by its large size and marked adenopathy.[306]

PANCREATIC TRAUMA

The pancreas is infrequently involved in blunt abdominal trauma. Findings may be subtle and hard to demonstrate immediately after trauma. When clinical suspicion of pancreatic involvement exists despite an initial unrevealing scan, serial scans should be done with high contrast bolus, thin sections, and rapid scanning techniques. Findings mimic pancreatitis, with gland swelling, fascial thickening, and fluid collections. Portions of the gland that have been devascularized will not

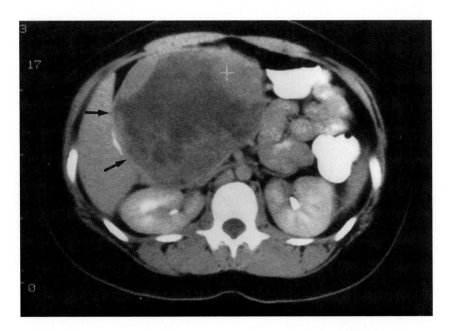

Figure 1–136. Solid and papillary epithelial neoplasm in a 17-year-old female (*arrows*) on CT. Cystic appearance is due to central hemorrhage.

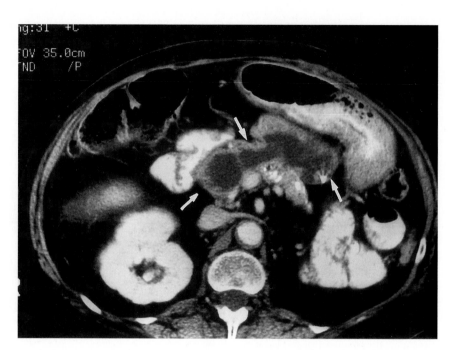

Figure 1–137. Post-Puestow procedure for chronic pancre-atiitis scan on CT. A fluid-filled segment of small bowel is anastomosed to the pancreatic duct (*arrows*). Note pancre-atic calcifications.

enhance with IV contrast and occasionally a linear de-fect due to fracture or laceration may be seen.[307,308]

POSTOPERATIVE PANCREAS

Complications of pancreatic surgery include anasto-motic leaks, strictures, abscesses, and pseudocyst forma-tion. A diagram of the operation is often helpful to the radiologist.

Common procedures are

1. Sphincterotomy—air may be present in the bil-iary tree on plain films, and barium may be seen to reflux into the common duct on an UGI.
2. Pancreatic ductal drainage (Puestow proce-dure)—a Roux-en-Y limb is anastomosed to the opened pancreatic duct. Barium or air may fill this bowel loop. Obstruction of the loop with di-latation is seen best using CT (Fig 1–137).
3. Whipple procedure—if a distal gastrectomy has been performed, an UGI may show a gas-trojejunostomy and possibly contrast refluxing into the biliary tree. On CT, the jejunal limb anastomosed to the biliary tree and pancreatic duct may fill with contrast or fluid. If the radi-ologist is not aware that this surgical procedure has been performed, this segment of bowel may be confused with either mass or extralu-minal fluid collection. CT is the best method for investigating possible jejunal limb obstruc-tion.[308]

■ RADIOLOGY OF THE MESENTERY, OMENTUM, AND PERITONEUM

Prior to the advent of cross-sectional imaging, radiologic evaluation of the peritoneum, mesentery, and omentum was limited to plain films and analysis for extrinsic effects on contrast-opacified bowel. Cross-sectional imaging modalities allow direct visualization of the peritoneum, mesentery, and omemtum, and have thereby revolu-tionized radiologic evaluation of this region. CT is the preferred technique in most institutions owing to tech-nical limitations of MRI and ultrasound that are particu-larly relevant in the mesentery and omentum.

There are several factors that make CT an excellent modality for imaging the peritoneum, mesentery, and omentum. These include the abundance of fat in the mesentery in all but the most asthenic individuals, rapid scan time that minimizes artifacts from physiological motion in the abdomen, and the ability to opacify bowel reliably and easily. Adipose tissue on CT is of very low (−100 to −160 Hounsfield Units [HU]) attenuation, providing excellent contrast to solid viscera, bowel, blood vessels, lymph nodes, and abnormal tissue, the latter generally being of similar attenuation to muscle and viscera (approximately +30 to +80 HU).

MRI of the mesentery and omentum is currently lim-ited by the lack of a reliable bowel contrast agent, arti-facts consequent to the physiologic motion in the ab-domen, and the long scan times required for many pulse sequences.

Optimal sonographic evaluation of a region requires the presence of an "acoustic window" (region through which sound is not significantly attenuated) such as a homogeneous solid organ like the liver, or a fluid composition structure such as the urinary bladder or large volume ascites. Sound waves are attenuated significantly by fat and are reflected by air. Therefore the peritoneal cavity, with the exception of the solid viscera-containing upper quadrants and the pelvis adjacent to the urinary bladder, is not ideally suited for sonographic evaluation.

Because of the above considerations, the majority of the discussion of radiologic findings in this section will involve CT. It should be noted that despite the above described limitations regarding imaging of the peritoneum, omentum, and mesentery, MRI and US are extremely effective modalities for evaluation of the solid abdominal and pelvic organs, and may be equal or superior to CT for certain clinical indications. In addition, MRI and US do not emply ionizing radiation and both possess unique capabilities to evaluate blood vessels and blood flow without the use of intravenous contrast agent.

CT ANATOMY

The CT appearance of the normal small bowel mesentery is a fat-containing area central to the small bowel loops which contains mesenteric vessels and occasionally small (<1 cm) lymph nodes.[309] The greater omentum appears as a homogeneous fat attenuation structure anterior and lateral to the transverse colon and small bowel.[310] The attenuation of normal mesenteric and omental fat is approximately −100 to −160 HU, similar to that of normal subcutaneous fat.

GENERAL CT PATHOLOGIC FEATURES

CT depicts tissues as a continuum of attenuations, measured by HU, with only certain ranges of attenuations being specific for a given tissue or substance. Tissues or substances that have specific CT attenuations include fat, air, calcification, and usually water, which is designated as zero HU. Unfortunately, the attenuation of viscera, muscle, and most nonfatty, nonfluid lesions is not sufficiently different to allow lesion characterization by this parameter. This fact, in conjunction with the limited number of ways the peritoneum, mesentery, and omentum can respond to pathologic insults, renders the CT appearance of many abnormalities in this region nonspecific. However, despite its nonspecificity, detection or sensitivity is excellent in patients with an adequate amount of intra-abdominal fat. In addition, although the CT appearance of the lesion per se is nonspecific, assessment for the presence or absence of abnormalities in other organs in conjunction with clin-

ical data yields a narrow differential diagnosis or specific diagnosis in many cases. If the imaging and clinical data do not provide a sufficiently specific diagnosis, imaging-guided biopsy or aspiration can be performed.

The general CT features of peritoneal, mesenteric, and omental disorders include increased attenuation of mesenteric or omental fat ("dirty" fat), obscuration of mesenteric vessel margins, thickening of mesenteric vascular bundles ("stellate" mesentery), thickening of peritoneal surfaces, nodules, masses, and rigidity of mesenteric leaves.[309]

■ INFLAMMATORY DISORDERS

LOCALIZED INFLAMMATION FROM CONTIGUOUS ORGANS

Inflammatory conditions can involve the mesentery, omentum, or peritoneum in a local or generalized manner. Localized inflammation can occur secondary to extension from contiguous inflamed organs such as in appendicitis, diverticulitis, and cholecystitis. CT findings include wall thickening of the primary inflamed organ, increased attenuation, inflammatory mass (phlegmon), or fluid in adjacent mesenteric fat, and abscess (Fig 1–138). Since appendicitis and diverticulitis often have significant perienteric inflammatory components, CT is very useful in imaging these entities and their complications. Pancreatitis can extend from its retroperitoneal origin into the mesentery and omentum. CT can demonstrate mesentric and omental abnormalities similar to those described above, in addition to imaging the pancreas and assessing gland viability and patency of adjacent vasculature with intravenous contrast. CT of Crohn's disease may demonstrate fistulization and fibrofatty proliferation of the mesentery, in addition to perienteric abnormalities similar to those in appendicitis or diverticulitis. Fibrofatty mesenteric proliferation ranges in appearance from an increase in the amount of normal-appearing mesenteric fat to increased attenuation of mesenteric fat. CT is very helpful in differentiating this cause of small bowel loop separation from mesenteric abscess.[309,311–313]

INTRAPERITONEAL ABSCESS

Intraperitoneal abscess remains a serious clinical problem with significant morbidity and mortality, despite advances in surgical technique, antibiotic therapy, and supportive care. The most common cause in recent decades is postsurgical, as opposed to the first half of the 20th century when intestinal perforation and inflammation were more common.[309,311] Prompt diagnosis and institution of therapy are essential, and both can be achieved by radiologic means. Debate still exists concerning the imaging approach of the suspected abdominal abscess, but in our institution, as in many others, CT has become the primary modality. Ultrasound can be very effective in the detection of abdominal abscess, particularly in regions with an acoustic window such as the right upper quadrant, left upper quadrant, and pelvis (near a full bladder), with accuracies being reported as high as 96%.[314,315] Some of the studies reporting very high accuracies do not specify abscess location (eg, hepatic, peritoneal cavity), and it is probable that accuracies may be lower in areas lacking an acoustic window. Ultrasound is limited by operator dependency, obesity, and issues attendant to postoperative status, including ileus, bandages, open wounds, drains, and abdominal tenderness. Nuclear scintigraphy (indium-labeled leukocytes, Gallium-67 scan) is also very accurate in abscess detection,[314,315] but the delay in diagnosis (up to 48 hours with gallium scan) and the lack of anatomic and spatial delineation limit its utility in acutely ill patients. Plain films may suggest the presence of an abscess by the presence of mass effect or extraluminal air, but sensitivity is low (50%) and confirmatory cross-sectional imaging is necessary.[316] Computed tomography has none of the above limitations, is more accurate than ultrasound, and provides the anatomic information required for interventional radiologic or surgical therapy.[314–318] However, ultrasound does possess certain unique characteristics, including relatively low cost, rapidity, real-time imaging (helpful for certain interventional cases), Doppler capability, unlimited imaging planes (may distinguish subpulmonic from subphrenic fluid using sagittal plane), portability, and lack of ionizing radiation, and therefore it may be preferred in certain situations.

The CT appearance of an abscess is variable and depends on its stage of evolution and location. In its early stage, when neutrophils accumulate in the infected tissue, an abscess may appear as a mass of soft tissue attenuation.[309,319] As liquefactive necrosis occurs, the center or entire lesion attains waterlike attenuation, with most abscesses having attenuations between 15 and 35 HU (Fig 1–138).[319,320] A later stage abscess occasionally can have a soft tissue, high-attenuation appearance as a result of high-attenuation pus or necrotic material.[321] Most abscesses are discrete, oval, spherical, or biconvex lesions, although they may be ill defined, and those adjacent to organs may be crescentic in shape.[309,320] The most specific CT feature is the presence of intralesion gas, which is seen in one-third to one-half of abscesses (Fig 1–138).[314,320] A thick, enhancing wall composed of vascular connective tissue may be present and, when seen in conjunction with a fluid density center, indicates a mature, chronic abscess.[311] Ancillary CT findings include thickening of adjacent fascia and increased attenuation of adjacent fat. Occasionally, features suggestive of abscess etiology are present, such as a calcific density or appendicolith in a right lower quadrant

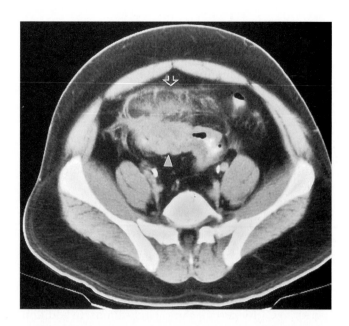

A

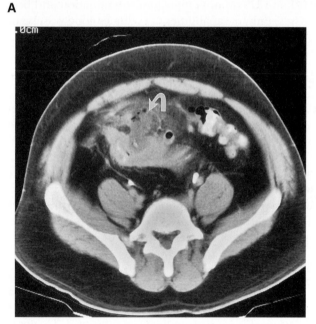

B

Figure 1–138. Diverticulitis; sigmoid colon. **A.** There is wall thickening of the sigmoid colon (*arrowhead*) and increased attenuation of the pericolonic fat (*open arrow*). **B.** Discrete fluid collection with air bubbles consistent with small abscess (*curved arrow*), is present.

appendiceal abscess, or a high-attenuation object in a postoperative foreign body abscess.[309]

Although CT is extremely sensitive for detection of intra-abdominal abscess, the CT appearance is nonspecific. Other low-attenuation masses include hematoma (not acute), biloma, pseudocyst, lymphocele, and necrotic neoplasm.[317] Gas within a mass can be seen in noninfected necrotic or bowel-communicating neoplasm.[317] However, in the proper clinical setting, a mass/fluid collection having the CT criteria of an abscess is likely to be an abscess. If confirmation is required, CT- or ultrasound-guided aspiration can be performed, often as the first step in percutaneous drainage.

The sonographic appearance of an abscess is variable, ranging from an anechoic mass with through transmission to a complex echogenic mass. Gas within an abscess appears as echogenic foci with or without acoustic shadowing. A thick, echogenic wall may be present.[317]

DIFFUSE PERITONITIS

Diffuse peritonitis can result from many causes, including bacterial, granulomatous, and chemical. Diffuse peritonitis may develop secondary to extension of localized inflammatory processes (appendicitis, diverticulitis), hollow viscus perforation, or abdominal surgery. The CT findings include increased attenuation of mesenteric and omental fat, peritoneal thickening and enhancement, and ascites.[309] Abdominal tuberculosis (TB) occurs in 6% to 38% of those with pulmonary TB, and 4% of these individuals develop TB peritonitis. CT findings include thickening and nodularity of peritoneal surfaces, high-attenuation (20 to 45 HU) ascites due to high protein and cell count, mesenteric/omental lymphadenopathy (40% low attenuation), hepatosplenomegaly, and focal hepatic or splenic lesions.[310] The CT findings of peritonitis are nonspecific, since peritoneal carcinomatosis, lymphoma, and malignant mesothelioma may have a similar appearance.

INTRA-ABDOMINAL PANNICULITIS

Intra-abdominal panniculitis is a benign, idiopathic process of lipocytic degeneration, inflammation, and fibrosis of the adipose tissue of the mesentery, omentum, and retroperitoneum, resulting in ill-defined or masslike fatty lesions.[322–324] Alternative etiologies of fat inflammation, such as pancreatitis, Weber-Christian disease, or inflammatory bowel disease must be excluded before this diagnosis can be made. This process has a variable and confusing nomenclature, and the multiple (at least 11) terms proposed to designate it probably reflect different points along a single pathologic and clinical continuum.[322] The nomenclature is dependent on the predominant histopathology, with mesenteric lipodystrophy, mesenteric panniculitis, and retractile mesenteritis implying lipocyte degeneration, inflammation, and fibrosis predominance, respectively.

Barium studies may show extrinsic mass effect, narrowing, fixation, and dilatation of bowel loops. In the fibrotic form of this disease, mass effect and evidence of serosal involvement (tethering, spiculation) may mimic serosal involvement by carcinoid tumor or other metastases.[310] The CT findings are variable, ranging from ill-defined areas of increased attenuation of fat to single or multiple inhomogeneous (soft tissue/fat/fluid attenuation) masses with occasional calcifications. In contrast to neoplasms, blood vessels are displaced and surrounded but rarely invaded. The nodular form of this disease may mimic a teratoma, liposarcoma, or any soft tissue mass if the fat component is minimal.[309,310,326]

■ NEOPLASMS

Neoplastic involvement of the mesentery, omentum, and peritoneum is predominantly secondary to metastatic disease, especially carcinomatosis and lymphoma.[327] Primary neoplasms are rare and usually of mesenchymal origin.

PRIMARY NEOPLASMS

Primary tumors in the peritoneal cavity include desmoid tumors, lipomatous tumors, mesothelioma (malignant and cystic), and miscellaneous extremely rare neoplasms. Desmoid tumors are benign, locally aggressive fibroblastic lesions, most often seen in patients with Gardner's syndrome who have undergone surgery, and which occasionally arising sporadically. The CT appearance of intra-abdominal desmoid tumor is an enhancing or nonenhancing soft tissue attenuation mass occurring in the mesentery, pelvis, or retroperitoneum. Abdominal wall desmoid tumors also occur, usually in Gardner's syndrome. The tumor may be locally invasive, involving bowel, blood vessels, and ureters.[328,329]

Lipomatous tumors include the benign lipoma, infiltrating lipomatosis, and several types of liposarcoma. The lipoma is a homogeneous, encapsulated, fat attenuation mass that may have several thin, linear soft-tissue components representing fibrous tissue. Lipogenic liposarcomas are inhomogeneous lesions of fat and soft-tissue attenuation, with the soft-tissue components being thicker and more ill defined than those present in a lipoma. Myxoid liposarcoma, which contains a large component of mucinous matrix (myxoid), has an attenuation intermediate between fat and muscle. The pleiomorphic liposarcoma is composed of undifferentiated cells and consequently is of nonspecific soft-tissue attenuation rather than fat or fluid. Infiltrating lipomatosis is a condition of extensively infiltrating, histologically benign, mature fat involving the abdomen and/or pelvis and the lower extremity.[330]

Abdominal mesothelioma exists in two forms: malignant peritoneal mesothelioma and benign cystic mesothelioma. Malignant peritoneal mesothelioma is a rare, asbestos-related neoplasm of mesothelial cell origin. CT findings include nodular, irregular thickening of the peritoneal surfaces, mesenteric rigidity and stellate appearance (thickened perivascular tissue), sheetlike masses, and ascites.[331] The differential diagnosis on CT findings include metastases, lymphoma, and granulomatous peritonitis. Cystic mesothelioma is a rare, benign neoplasm of mesothelial cell origin with no asbestos association and occurs in a younger age group (mean age 37) than does malignant mesothelioma. The CT appearance is a uni-loculated or multiloculated cystic mass which may occur anywhere in the peritoneal cavity, although a pelvic location is most common.[327]

SECONDARY NEOPLASMS

The most common cause of neoplastic involvement of the mesentery, omentum, and peritoneum is metastatic disease, most often due to lymphoma or carcinoma. CT can detect implants 1 cm or smaller, particularly if adequate intra-abdominal fat is present.[310] Rigorous attention to technique, especially bowel opacification and vascular enhancement, is important in maximizing lesion detection. CT peritoneography, which entails intraperitoneal instillation of water-soluble contrast agent, further improves the detection of small peritoneal implants, but is rarely employed due to its invasive nature.[310]

There are four modes of dissemination of metastatic neoplasm through the peritoneal cavity: (1) direct spread along mesenteric and ligamentous structures, (2) intraperitoneal seeding, (3) lymphatic spread, and (4) hematogenous dissemination.[309,327,332,333] This classification emphasizes the predominant mode of spread for a neoplasm, but more than one mechanism can be operative in a given individual. *Direct spread* occurs when the tumor extends outside the border of the organ of origin, extending along peritoneal surfaces to involve other structures. Examples of direct spread include gastric, colonic, and pancreatic carcinomas spreading via the transverse mesocolon and involving the connected organs, biliary neoplasms spreading via the gastrohepatic and hepatoduodenal ligaments, and ovarian carcinoma spreading along all adjacent peritoneal surfaces.[309] The CT appearance depends on the stage and degree of spread. The early stage of extension is manifest as increased attenuation in the mesenteric or ligamentous fat adjacent to the primary neoplasm, while more advanced spread produces a mass with its epicenter at the organ of tumor origin, traversing the contiguous ligaments or mesentery. Further extension results in peritoneal surface thickening and nodularity, and infiltration of the mesentery and omentum resulting in increased attenuation, rigidity, and masses. Confluent masses in the omentum, often due to ovarian carci-

noma, are the cause of "omental cakes." Direct spread of carcinoid tumor to the small bowel mesentery (or lymph nodes) often produces a characteristic CT appearance. The metastatic lesion may be evident as a soft-tissue mass in the right lower quadrant mesentery, with surrounding radiating soft tissue stranding, the latter due to reactive desmoplasia incited by the metastatic focus. Liver metastases (80% if the primary lesion is >2 cm) and lymphadenopathy may or may not be present, and the typically small, mural lesion rarely is detected on CT. Barium studies may reveal a small submucosal (actually deep mucosa) lesion, but more frequently demonstrate extrinsic mass effect or effects of desmoplasia incited by the metastasis in the form of mucosal tethering and/or bowel fixation and angulation.[310,334] The differential diagnosis of mesenteric carcinoid tumor on CT includes desmoplastic metastases (breast, pancreatic carcinoma primaries), lymphoma, and retractile mesenteritis.[334]

Intraperitoneal seeding is the result of tumor cell dissemination via flow of ascitic fluid and subsequent deposition and growth of an implant. The location of implant deposition is dependent upon the natural flow of intraperitoneal fluid, which is governed by multiple factors, including peritoneal compartmentalization, gravity, and changes in intra-abdominal pressure due to respiration.[333] Consequent to these factors, the retrorectal pouch of Douglas, the small bowel mesentery in the ileocecal region, the superior aspect of the sigmoid mesocolon, and the right paracolic gutter are the most common sites for seeded tumor implants.[333] The primary neoplasms that typically spread by this route (and also via direct spread) are adenocarcinomas of the ovary, stomach, colon, and pancreas.[309] The CT appearance of intraperitoneal seeding is soft-tissue masses, often associated with ascites, at one or more of the usual sites of pooling and, occasionally, peritoneal thickening.[309] Calcified implants are sometimes present and suggest ovarian or mucinous colonic carcinoma primary lesions.[310] A rare form of intraperitoneal seeding, *Pseudomyxoma peritonei,* can produce a distinctive radiologic appearance. This condition results from the rupture of a mucinous cystadenocarcinoma or cystadenoma, usually of the ovary or appendix, causing large volume gelatinous ascites. Characteristic CT appearances include low-attenuation masses or diffuse intraperitoneal low-attenuation material with septations, often causing scalloping of the liver margin due to mass effect. Occasionally, the septations or lesion walls contain calcification.[335]

Lymphatic extension is the primary mode of intraperitoneal dissemination of lymphoma (non-Hodgkin's more commonly than Hodgkin's), but plays a minor role for dissemination of carcinomas.[309,333] Mesenteric lymphadenopathy on CT is evident as round or oval masses, >1 cm in size, in the mesenteric fat, although early lymphadenopathy may appear as an increased number of nonenlarged (<1 cm) lymph nodes. Large, confluent nodal masses surrounding the mesenteric vessels may produce a "sandwichlike" appearance.[336] Mild mesenteric lymphadenopathy is a nonspecific finding and may be present in a variety of nonneoplastic diseases, such as Crohn's disease, sprue, Whipple's disease, sarcoidosis, AIDS, tuberculous peritonitis, and giardiasis.[309] Low-attenuation lymphadenopathy is occasionally present, and the differential diagnosis for this includes TB, Whipple's disease, treated lymphoma, metastases, and pyogenic infection.[310]

Hematogenous dissemination occurs via the mesenteric arteries where cells implant on the antimesenteric side of bowel and subsequently grow into intramural nodules. CT findings include focal bowel wall mass or thickening, or thickening of the mesenteric leaves.[309,332]

MESENTERIC CYSTS

Mesenteric and omental cysts are imprecise terms that have been applied to a variety of rare lesions that have similar gross morphology but are histologically distinct.[337–339] The lesions generally occur in children and young adults and include lymphangioma, enteric duplication cyst, nonpancreatic pseudocyst (probably postinfectious or posttraumatic etiology), enteric cyst, and mesothelial cyst.[337] The general imaging appearance of these lesions is a cystic, uniloculated or multiloculated, noncalcified mass in the mesentery or omentum. The lesions vary with regard to wall thickness and presence or absence of fat content (chyle), loculations, septations, or internal debris. Sonography delineates the internal nature of fluid-filled structures better than CT and is therefore better suited to assess the presence of internal debris, septations, or thin loculations. CT and MRI are capable of demonstrating fat content and the presence of chylous material.[337]

Although overlap may exist in the imaging appearance of these lesions, a thick enhancing wall suggests enteric duplication cyst or nonpancreatic pseudocyst, and fat content has only been described in lymphangiomas and enteric duplication cysts. The latter two lesions alternatively may contain serous or hemorrhagic fluid and therefore may not be of fat attenuation. Mesenteric and enteric cysts are usually simple, unilocular cysts; lymphangioma is usually multilocular; nonpancreatic pseudocysts may be unilocular or multilocular; and an enteric duplication cyst is usually unilocular. Other lesions that may have a similar imaging appearance include cystic (necrotic or degenerated) smooth muscle tumor, cystic mesothelioma, abscess, cystic metastasis, and teratoma.[337]

INTRAPERITONEAL FLUID

Intraperitoneal fluid is found in a large number of conditions. The fluid may be transudative (protein less than 2.5 gm/dL, specific gravity <1.016) or exudative in nature, the latter usually the result of infectious, inflammatory, hemorrhagic, or neoplastic conditions.[340] Imaging studies are usually requested for confirmation, quantification, localization, and determination of etiology of the ascites. Plain films are insensitive for the detection of ascites, requiring over 500 cc of intraperitoneal fluid to be present, while ultrasound and CT are both highly sensitive.[340,341] Owing to its relatively low cost, the lack of ionizing radiation, rapidity, and high sensitivity (routinely detects 5 to 10 cc of fluid), ultrasound is an excellent primary modality for this clinical indication.[340,341] A normal ultrasound excludes the presence of significant intraperitoneal fluid. If the ultrasound is equivocal or is positive for fluid but the etiology is still unknown, a CT study may be helpful. In a patient with exudative ascites and a history suggestive of neoplasm, CT is probably the best initial study.[340]

Simple transudative ascites has the sonographic appearance of a homogeneous, mobile, anechoic collection with deep acoustic enhancement, and a CT appearance of a low-attenuation (0 to 30 HU) collection.[341] Simple ascites tends to insinuate between organs rather than displace them. Small amounts of fluid tend to collect in the right perihepatic space, the posterior subhepatic space (Morrison's pouch), and the pouch of Douglas. As the volume of ascites increases, fluid can be identified in the paracolic gutters and by its insinuation between mesenteric leaves, sometimes causing the small bowel loops to float.[341]

Definitive characterization of ascites as transudate or exudate is not possible by CT, ultrasound, or MRI; however, features exist that are suggestive of the nature of the fluid.[342–344] Sonographic features of exudative ascites include internal echoes, septations, loculations, and the matting of bowel loops. However, absence of these features does not exclude an exudate.[342] The attenuation of ascitic fluid on CT usually increases with increasing protein content, but the differences are not sufficient to permit reliable differentiation.[311,343] Fluid with attenuation less than zero HU is suggestive of chylous ascites.[340] Recent hemoperitoneum (less than 48 hours) can often be distinguished from other fluid collections owing to its high attenuation (>30 HU) and the occasional presence of the hematocrit effect.[340] However, the attenuation of intraperitoneal blood decreases rapidly with time, consequent to rapid clot lysis from respiratory and peristaltic motion in the abdomen.[345] The appearance of a transudate on MRI is low-signal intensity on T1-weighted images and high-signal intensity on T2-weighted images. With increasing protein content, the signal intensity of the fluid on T1-weighted images increases. Subacute hemorrhage has a high-signal intensity on T1-weighted images owing to the paramagnetic effects of methemoglobin.[344] Despite the unique physical principles utilized to create images on MRI, the signal intensities of fluids are not sufficiently specific to allow definitive fluid characterization. In addition, the long scan times, artifacts from physiological motion, and lack of reliable bowel contrast agents render MRI detection of small amounts of ascites and lesser sac fluid problematic.[340]

Several other imaging features, independent of fluid appearance, have been described as indicators of malignant ascites. These include the tethering of small bowel loops along the posterior peritoneum,[346] and concordant, proportional amounts of fluid in the greater and lesser sacs. In patients with benign ascites, fluid is predominantly in the greater sac.[340] A normal (<3 mm) gallbladder wall thickness in patients with ascites is suggestive of malignant ascites, in contrast to mural thickening (>3 mm) which is associated with be-

nign ascites in 82% of cases. This association is reflective of the benign ascites that often accompanies cirrhosis and portal hypertension.[347] Other manifestations of metastatic disease such as hepatic and splenic lesions, lymphadenopathy, peritoneal implants, and detection of a likely primary tumor are all highly suggestive of a malignant etiology of ascites.

■ FREE INTRAPERITONEAL AIR

Most patients with gastrointestinal tract perforation and pneumoperitoneum will be diagnosed by clinical findings and plain radiographs, but in some patients with early perforation, other acute abdominal disorders may be simulated. These patients may undergo a CT scan of the abdomen and unsuspected free intraperitoneal air may be demonstrated. Intraperitoneal air appears on CT as extraluminal air, devoid of haustral or small bowel folds, often nondependent in position, and anterior to the liver or subjacent to the anterior abdominal wall (Figs 1–139, 1–140).[348] CT also may suggest the source of perforation, evidenced by abnormality in the perforated segment of bowel and/or air bubbles, extravasated oral contrast, fluid, or increased attenuation in the fat adjacent to the site of perforation.[348] CT can detect minute amounts of pneumoperitoneum and is superior to abdominal or upright chest radiographs in this regard.[349,350]

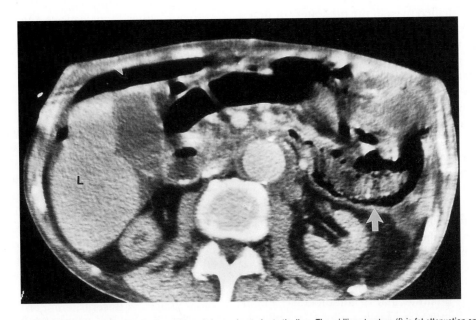

Figure 1–139. Pneumoperitoneum. There are two small collections of free air (*arrows*) anterior to the liver. The midline structure (f) is fat attenuation and, with different windows, would be easier to identify as fat.

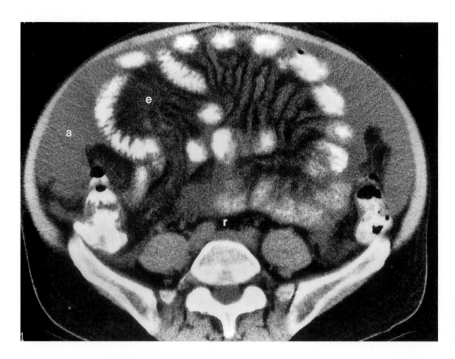

Figure 1–140. Pneumatosis intestinalis and pneumoperitoneum due to ischemic small bowel. There is intramural air in a jejunal loop (*arrow*), and free intraperitoneal air (*arrowhead*) anterior to the liver (1).

■ MESENTERIC VENOUS THROMBOSIS

Mesenteric venous thrombosis is the cause of 5% to 15% of cases of acute mesenteric ischemia; the other causes are SMA embolus (50%), nonocclusive ischemia (30%), and SMA thrombosis.[351] Mesenteric vascular thrombosis may not result in ischemia if it is subacute or chronic in nature, since this allows time for development of collateral vessels.[348] Etiologies of superior mesenteric vein (SMV) thrombosis, which is involved in 95% of all cases of mesenteric venous thrombosis, include portal hypertension, hypercoagulable states, abdominal inflammatory and neoplastic processes, primary (idiopathic), abdominal surgery, and trauma.[351]

The CT appearance of SMV thrombosis is a low-attenuation filling defect in the vessel lumen with peripheral enhancement, the latter due to enhancing vasa vasorum.[352] The sonographic appearance of SMV thrombosis is a dilated vein filled with echogenic material with no detectable flow upon Doppler interrogation.[351] MRI has potential for evaluating the mesenteric vasculature by virtue of the inherent contrast of flowing blood (producing a signal void on spin-echo images and high-signal intensity on gradient-echo images) to surrounding solid tissues. However, the clinical utility of MRI for this indication remains uncertain.

In patients with bowel ischemia or infarction of any cause, CT may reveal relatively specific findings such as intramural, mesenteric or portal venous gas, and focal bowel wall thickening, or less specific signs such as diffuse bowel wall thickening, bowel dilatation, mesenteric edema, and ascites (Fig 1–140).[351,353–355] These findings are all nonspecific, but their presence in the proper clinical setting, particularly but not necessarily in conjunction with an occluding lesion in the SMA or SMV, are highly suggestive of bowel ischemia. Although mesenteric angiography is probably the modality of choice in suspected acute ischemia, this disorder often simulates other acute abdominal entities, and consequently a CT scan is frequently obtained. CT can suggest the diagnosis of ischemia and exclude other disorders, but its sensitivity for ischemia is unimpressive. In two separate retrospective studies of 23 patients with proven bowel ischemia, CT enabled a specific prospective diagnosis in only 26%[354] and 39%[355] of patients.

■ MESENTERIC EDEMA

Diffuse mesenteric edema is most commonly secondary to hypoalbuminemia, the latter usually due to cirrhosis or nephrotic syndrome. Often as a result mesenteric venous or lymphatic obstruction and mesenteric ischemia are less common causes. The CT findings characteristic of mesenteric edema include diffuse increased attenuation of mesenteric fat, indistinct mesenteric vessels, relative sparing of the retroperitoneal fat, and occasional association of bowel wall thickening and subcutaneous edema. Malignant infiltration of the mesentery may cause thickening of the mesenteric leaves, but this is usually distinguished from edema by mesenteric leave rigidity and less diffuse involvement.[310,356]

■ MESENTERIC HEMORRHAGE

Mesenteric hemorrhage is uncommon, and usually is due to blunt trauma, bleeding diathesis, or aneurysm rupture.[310] A small hematoma may be manifest on CT as streaky soft-tissue infiltration of the mesentery, whereas a larger hematoma may appear as a masslike lesion or an interspersed density between mesenteric leaves. The attenuation of a hematoma on CT varies with time, being of high attenuation (50 to 60 HU) acutely, decreasing with time, and approaching water attenuation (0 to 20 HU) by 2 weeks.[348,357]

■ INTERNAL HERNIA

An internal hernia is defined as protrusion of a viscus through a peritoneal or mesenteric orifice within the confines of the abdominal cavity. The hernia apertures may be congenital or acquired defects, or preexisting anatomic structures such as the foramen of Winslow.[358] Generally, the content of the hernia is mobile segments of small or large intestine, but the greater omentum or other viscera are occasionally included.[359] Internal hernias may be clinically silent if easily reducible, but larger ones may cause symptoms and eventuate in a small bowel obstruction.

The autopsy incidence of internal hernias is reported to be 0.2% to 0.9%.[358] Typical locations and relative frequencies are as follows: paraduodenal (53%), pericecal (13%), foramen of Winslow (8%), transmesenteric (8%), pelvis and supravesical (7%), intersigmoid (6%), and retroanastamotic (5%) (usually after partial gastrectomy and gastrojejunostomy).[358,360] Paraduodenal hernias are the most common type, with approximately 75% occurring on the left via the paraduodenal fossa of Landzert.[359]

Each type of internal hernia has specific radiologic features, the description of which is beyond the scope of this chapter. There are general features on barium studies and CT that are shared by most internal hernias including abnormal location of an intestinal segment in a susceptible region, encapsulation of small bowel loops, and dilatation and stasis within, and fixation of, herniated loops.[358,359] The likelihood of radiologic diagnosis of an internal hernia is maximized by performance of the study during a symptomatic period, rather than at a time when spontaneous reduction may have occurred. In general, a small bowel series demonstrates the most useful diagnostic findings of internal hernia, but CT also may be of value.[358]

ABDOMINAL WALL

The anterior abdominal wall is composed of multiple layers, and CT, MRI, and ultrasound (high frequency, short focus) all provide excellent delineation of the anterior abdominal wall. Most adults have sufficient body fat to visualize individual muscles (Fig 1–141). The primary muscles composing the posterior abdominal wall are the latissimus dorsi and the paraspinal muscle groups.[309]

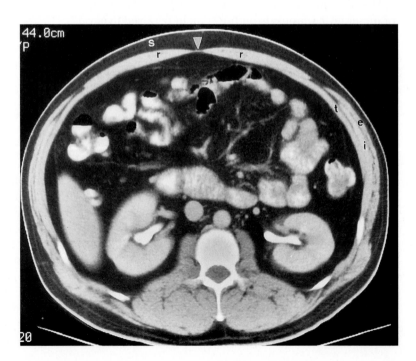

Figure 1–141. CT of the normal anterior abdominal wall. The individual muscle groups and subcutaneous fat (s) layers are well delineated. The paired rectus muscles (r) are joined in the midline by the linea alba (*arrowhead*); (e) external and (i) internal oblique muscles, (t) transversus abdominis muscle.

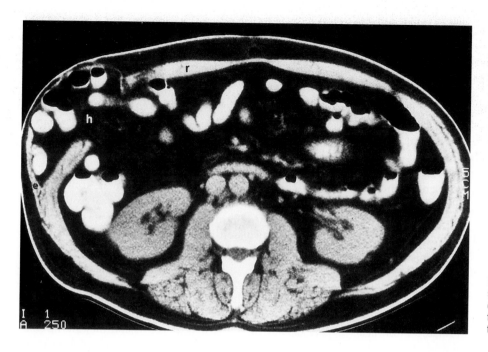

Figure 1–142. Spigelian hernia. Herniation of small bowel loops and mesentery (h) through a defect along the semilunar line, lateral to the rectus abdominus muscle (r), beneath an intact external oblique muscle (e).

External Hernia

An external hernia is caused by prolapse of an intestinal segment or other intra-abdominal structure through a defect in the wall of the abdomen or pelvis. CT can detect small defects in the peritoneum and abdominal wall fascial layers, directly visualize the hernia and its contents, and diagnose bowel obstruction and ischemia secondary to incarceration, manifest by segmental bowel dilatation, and bowel wall thickening, respectively.[359]

Barium studies will demonstrate hernias containing bowel and bowel-related complications. MRI and ultrasound also may be helpful, but the evaluation of an intestinal component and potential complications is achieved better by CT. The role of imaging in hernias includes confirmation of equivocal hernias, delineation of the content of a known hernia, and diagnosis of complications such as bowel obstruction and ischemia resulting from incarceration.

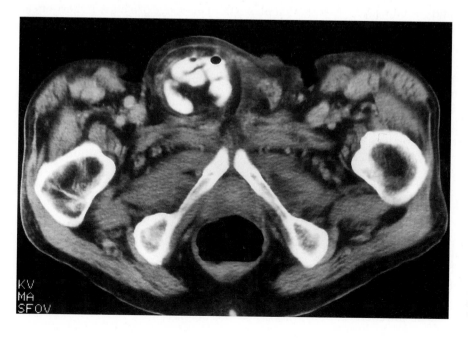

Figure 1–143. Inguinal hernia. Small bowel has herniated into right inguinal canal. The bowel caliber and wall thickness are normal.

An additional radiologic technique for diagnosis of hernias is herniography, which entails intraperitoneal injection of water-soluble contrast agent to assess for hernia sac presence, particularly in the pelvis and groin areas. The indications in adults have included groin pain with equivocal clinical findings and evaluation for inguinal hernia recurrence after surgical repair. In children, herniography has been used to evaluate for contralateral inguinal hernia prior to surgical repair. A patient suspected of having an incarcerated hernia should not undergo herniography, since the neck of the hernia would be obstructed, and the sac will not be demonstrated.[361]

The various types of abdominal wall hernias include umbilical, ventral, incisional, lumbar, and Spigelian, while pelvic hernias include inguinal (most common), femoral, obturator, sciatic, and peroneal. The nomenclature for specific hernia types refers to the anatomic location of the orifice.[359] Barium studies will demonstrate bowel involvement and bowel-related complications in a hernia, whereas CT will demonstrate hernia contents, complications, and the defect itself, particularly in abdominal wall hernias where the structure to be imaged is orthogonal to the scan plane (Figs 1–142 and 1–143). Plain films may diagnose an inguinal hernia by the presence of a mass or gas-containing structure overlying the obturator foramen, and the presence of bowel incarceration by dilated bowel loops converging towards a finding suggestive of a hernia.[359]

Hematoma

Abdominal wall hematoma most commonly occurs in the sheath of the rectus abdominus muscle and also may occur laterally. Etiologies include anticoagulant therapy, trauma, iatrogenic (percutaneous procedures), surgery, spontaneous (idiopathic), and straining.[362] The CT appearance of an abdominal wall hematoma is an inhomogeneous, masslike lesion, often elliptical or spindle shaped, within one or more layers of the abdominal wall. The CT attenuation of an acute hematoma is usually high (greater than muscle) and decreases with time, approaching water attenuation in 2 to 4 weeks.[309] The MRI appearance of blood is variable depending upon the age of clot, patient hematocrit, and the field strength of the magnet.

Inflammation

Inflammatory processes of the anterior abdominal wall can result from surgery, trauma, extension from intra-abdominal processes, and altered host immunity.[362] Imaging is particularly useful for evaluating fluid components to distinguish cellulitis or phlegmon from an abscess, and CT and ultrasound are both generally effective in this regard. CT may be the preferable modality owing to its ability to delineate associated intraperi-

toneal and retroperitoneal processes and may provide a more global depiction for treatment planning.

The CT findings of abdominal wall cellulitis/phlegmon are nonspecific and include streaky soft-tissue densities, loss of fat planes, muscle enlargement, and ill-defined masses of varying attenuation.[309,362] An abscess appears as a mass, often ovoid or spindle shaped, with a central low-attenuation zone or a localized fluid collection.[309,362] Intralesion gas occasionally may be present, but this may be also caused by a fistula or an open wound. As in the peritoneal cavity, the imaging appearance of an abdominal wall abscess is not specific, but the above findings are highly suggestive in the proper clinical setting and may be confirmed via needle aspiration.

Neoplasms

Neoplasms of the abdominal wall are uncommon and may be primary or secondary. Benign primary neoplasms are usually mesenchymal in origin and include lipoma, neurofibroma, and desmoid tumor. An endometrioma can occur rarely in a surgical scar, typically after a Cesarean section. Primary malignant neoplasms include sarcomas, lymphoma, and urachal carcinoma.[362]

Metastases may involve the abdominal wall via a hematogenous route or by direct spread. Hematogenous lesions may involve either the subcutaneous fat or the abdominal wall muscles. Subcutaneous metastases appear as soft-tissue attenuation nodules and are usually secondary to melanoma, lung, renal, and ovarian cancer primary lesions.[362] Involvement of the muscles is manifest as muscle enlargement or mass, often with a nonmuscle attenuation.[309] Direct spread from intra-abdominal malignancies such as colon carcinoma can occur and manifests as muscle thickening, loss of fat planes, and presence of a mass.[309] Peritoneal dissemination of tumor such as gastric, ovarian, or colonic carcinoma can result in an isolated metastasis near the umbilicus.[309,362] Rarely, an implant in the abdominal wall may occur as result of seeding from percutaneous biopsy of an intra-abdominal malignancy or by tracking of tumor cells via an indwelling drain for malignant biliary obstruction.[362] As in the peritoneal cavity, the CT appearance of abdominal wall neoplasms is nonspecific, with the exception of lipomatous tumors.

REFERENCES

1. Cole TJ, Turner MA. Manifestations of gastrointestinal disease on chest radiographs. *Radiographics* 1993;13:1013–1034

2. Stark P, Thordarson S, McKinney M, et al. Manifestations of esophageal disease on plain chest radiographs. *AJR Am J Roentgenol* 1990;155:719–734

3. Laufer I. Technique and Normal Anatomy. In: Levine MS (ed), *Radiology of the Esophagus*. Philadelphia, PA: WB Saunders; 1989:1

4. Levine MS, Rubeson SE, Oh DJ, et al. Update on esophageal radiology. *AJR Am J Roentgenol* 1990;155:933–941

5. Low VHS, Rubesin SE. Contrast evaluation of the pharynx and esophagus. *Radiol Clin North Am* 1993;31:1265–1292

6. Chen MYM, Ott DJ, Sinclair JW, et al. Gastroesophageal reflux disease: correlation of esophageal pH testing and radiographic findings. *Radiology* 1992;185:483–486

7. Levine MS. Infectious Esophagitides. In: Gore RM, Levine MS, Laufer I (eds), *Textbook of Gastrointestinal Radiology*. Philadelphia, PA: WB Saunders; 1994:403

8. Levine MS. Benign Tumors. In: Levine MS (ed), *Radiology of the Esophagus*. Philadelphia, PA: WB Saunders, 1989:113

9. Levine MS, Halvorsen RA. Esophageal Carcinoma. In: Gore RM, Levine MS, Laufer I (eds), *Textbook of Gastrointestinal Radiology*. Philadelphia, PA: WB Saunders;1994:446

10. Ott DJ. Motility Disorders. In: Gore RM, Levine MS, Laufer I (eds), *Textbook of Gastrointestinal Radiology*. Philadelphia, PA: WB Saunders, 1994:346

11. Ott DJ, Abernethy, WB. Radiologic evaluation of esophageal motility: results in 170 patients with chest pain. *AJR Am J Roentgenol* 1990;155:983–985

12. Halvorsen, RA, Thompson, WM. CT of esophageal neoplasms. *Radiol Clin North Am* 1989;27:667–685.

13. Halvorsen, RA, Jr., Magruder-Habib K, et al. Esophageal cancer staging by CT: long term follow-up study. *Radiology* 1986;161:147–151

14. Trenkner SW, Halvorsen RA, Jr., et al. Neoplasms of the upper gastrointestinal tract. *Radiol Clin North Am* 1994;32:15–24

15. Rankin S. The role of computerized tomography in the staging of oesophageal cancer. *Clin Radiol* 1990;42:152–153

16. White CS, Templeton PA. Esophageal perforation: CT findings. *AJR Am J Roentgenol* 1993;160:767–770

17. Takashima S, Takeuchi N, et al. Carcinoma of the esophagus: CT vs MR imaging in determining resectability. *AJR Am J Roentgenol* 1991;156:297–302

18. Botet JF, Lightdale CJ, et al. Preoperative staging of esophageal cancer: comparison of endoscopic ultrasound and dynamic CT. *Radiology* 1991;181:419–425

19. Liu J-B, Miller LS, et al. Transnasal ultrasound of the esophagus: preliminary morphologic and function studies. *Radiology* 1992;184:721–727

20. Malmud LS, Fisher RS. Scintigraphic evaluation of esophageal transit, gastroesophageal reflux and gastric emptying. In: Gotschalk A, Hoffer PB, Potchen EJ (eds), *Diagnostic Nuclear Medicine*. Baltimore, MD: Williams & Wilkins; 1988:663

21. Gurney JW, Olson DL, Schroeder BA. The gastric bubble: roentgen observations. *Radiographics* 1989;9:467–485

22. Cole TJ, Turner MA. Manifestations of gastrointestinal disease on chest radiographs. *Radiographics* 1993;13:1013–1034

23. Laufer I. *Double Contrast Gastrointestinal Radiology with Endoscopic Correlation*. Philadelphia, PA: WB Saunders, 1983

24. Levine MS, Rubesin SE, Herlinger H, et al. Double-contrast upper gastrointestinal examination: technique and interpretation. *Radiology* 1988;168:593–609

25. Gedgaudas-McClees RK. Radiology of the stomach. In: Gedgaudas-McClees RK (ed), *Handbook of Gastrointestinal Imaging*. London, England: Churchill-Livingstone; 1987:41

26. Eisenberg RL. Stomach. In: Eisenberg RL (ed), *Gastrointestinal Radiology*. Philadelphia, PA: JB Lippincott; 1990:179

27. Nelson SE. The discovery of gastric ulcers and the differential diagnosis between benignancy and malignancy. *Radiol Clin North Am* 1969;7:5–25

28. Levine MS. Peptic ulcers. In: Gore RM, Levine MS, Laufer I (eds), *Textbook of Gastrointestinal Radiology*. Philadelphia, PA: WB Saunders; 1994:562

29. Fultz PJ, Skucas J, Weiss SL: CT in upper gastrointestinal tract perforations secondary to peptic ulcer disease. *Gastrointest Radiol* 1991;17:5–8

30. Jeffrey RB, Jr. Gastrointestinal perforation and obstruction. In: Jeffrey RB Jr (ed), *CT and Sonography of the Acute Abdomen*. New York, NY: Raven Press; 1989:214

31. Jeffrey RB, Jr. Aortoenteric Fistula. In: Jeffrey RB, Jr. (ed), *CT and Sonography of the Acute Abdomen*. New York, NY: Raven Press; 1989:281

32. Higgins RSD, Steed DL, Zajko AB, Sumkin J, Webster MW. Computed tomographic scan confirmation of paraprosthetic enteric fistula. *Am J Surg* 1991;162:36–38

33. McGuigan JE. The Zollinger-Ellison Syndrome. In: Sleisinger MH, Fordtran JS, (eds), *Gastrointestinal Disease*. Philadelphia, PA: WB Saunders; 1989:909

34. Feczko PJ, Halpert RD, Ackermann LV. Gastric polyps: radiological evaluation and clinical significance. *Radiology* 1985;155:581–584

35. Smith HJ, Lee EL. Large hyperplastic polyps of the stomach. *Gastrointest Radiol* 1983;8:19–23

36. Dodds WJ. Clinical and roentgen features of the intestinal polyposis syndromes. *Gastrointest Radiol* 1976;1:127–142

37. Levine MS, Megebow AJ. Carcinoma. In: Gore RM, Levine MS, and Laufer I (eds), *Textbook of Gastrointestinal Radiology*. Philadelphia, PA: WB Saunders 1994:660

38. Kirklin BR. The value of the meniscus sign in the roentgenologic diagnosis of ulcerating gastric carcinoma. *Radiology* 1934;22:131–135

39. Scatarige JC, DiSantis DJ. CT of the stomach and duodenum. *Radiol Clin North Am* 1989;27:687–706

40. Gassios KJ, Tsianos EV, et al. Use of water or air as oral contrast media for computed tomographic study of the gastric wall. *Gastrointest Radiol* 1991;16:293–297

41. Hwang HY, Choi BI, et al. Calcified gastric carcinoma: CT findings. *Gastrointest Radiol* 1992;17:311–315

42. Rasch L, Brenoe J, Olesen KP. Predictability of esophagus- and cardiotumor resectability by preoperative computed tomography. *Eur J Radiol* 1990;II:42–45

43. Botet JF, Lightdale CJ, Zauber AG, et al. Preoperative staging of gastric cancer: comparison of endoscopic US and dynamic CT. *Radiology* 1991;181:426–432

44. Hori S, Tsuda K, Murayama S, et al. CT of gastric carcinoma: preliminary results with a new scanning technique. *Radiographics* 1992;12:257–268

45. Halpert RD, Feczko PJ. Role of radiology in the diagnosis

and staging of gastric malignancy. *Endoscopy* 1993;25: 39–45

46. Munami M, Kawauchi N, Itai Y, et al. Gastric tumors: radiologic-pathologic correlation and accuracy of staging with dynamic CT. *Radiology* 1992;185:173–178

47. Goodman P, Levine MS, Gohil MN. Gastric carcinoma after gastrojejunostomy for benign disease. *Gastrointest Radiol* 1992;17:211–213

48. Brady LW. Malignant lymphoma of the gastrointestinal tract. *Radiology* 1980;137:291–298

49. Levine MS: Benign Tumors. In: Gore RM, Levine MS, Laufer I (eds), *Textbook of Gastrointestinal Radiology*. Philadelphia, PA: WB Saunders; 1994:640–644

50. Navert TC, Zornoza J, Ordonez N. Gastric leiomyosarcomas. *Am J Roentgen* 1982;139:291–297

51. Meyers MA, McSweeney J. Secondary neoplasms of the bowel. *Radiology* 1972;105:1–11

52. Joffe N. Metastatic involvement of the stomach secondary to breast carcinoma. *Am J Roentgen* 1975;123: 512–521

53. Goldstein HM, Beydonn MT, Dodd GD. Radiologic spectrum of metastatic melanoma to the gastrointestinal tract. *Am J Roentgen* 1977;129:605–612

54. Miller JH, Gisvold JJ, Weiland LH, et al. Upper gastrointestinal tract: villous tumors. *Am J Roentgen* 1980; 134:933–936

55. Farah MC, Jafri SZ, Schwab RE, et al. Duodenal neoplasms: role of CT. *Radiology* 1987;162:839–843

56. Merine D, Jones B, Ghahremani GG, et al. Hyperplasia of brunner glands: the spectrum of its radiographic manifestations. *Gastrointest Radiol* 1991;16:104–108

57. Siegel JA, Krevsky B, Maurer AH, et al. Scintigraphic evaluation of gastric emptying: are radiolabeled solids necessary? *Clin Nucl Med* 1988;14:40–46

58. Malmud LS, Vitti RA. Gastric emptying. [Editorial] *J Nucl Med* 1990;31:1499–1500

59. Camilleri M. Zinsmeister AR, Greydanus MP, et al. Towards a less costly but accurate test of gastric emptying and small bowel transit. *Dig Dis Sci* 1991;36:609–615

60. Smith C, Deziel DJ, Kubicka RA. Evaluation of the postoperative stomach and duodenum. *Radiographics* 1994; 14:67–86

61. Williams SM. Technique and normal anatomy. In: Gore RM, Levine MS, Laufer I (eds), *Textbook of Gastrointestinal Radiology*. Philadelphia, PA: WB Saunders; 1994:152

62. Baker SR. *The Abdominal Plain Film*. Stanford, CT: Appleton & Lange; 1990:155–242

63. Eisenberg RL. Small bowel obstruction. In: Eisenberg RL (ed), *Gastrointestinal Radiology: A Pattern Approach*. Philadelphia, PA: JB Lippincott; 1990:411

64. Herlinger H. Small Bowel. In: Laufer I (ed), *Double Contrast Gastrointestinal Radiology with Endoscopic Correlation*. Philadelphia, PA: WB Saunders; 1979:423–494

65. Feczko, P, Halpert R, et al. Radiology of the Small Bowel. In: Gedgaudas-McClees RK (ed), *Gastrointestinal Imaging*. New York, NY: Churchill-Livingstone; 1987:99

66. Herlinger H, Maglinte DDT. The small bowel enema with methylcellulose. In: Herlinger H, Maglinte D (eds), *Clinical Radiology of the Small Intestine*. Philadelphia, PA: WB Saunders; 1989:119

67. Goldberg HI, Dodds W. Roentgen evaluation of small bowel obstruction. *Dig Dis Sci* 1979;24:245–248

68. Megibow AJ, Balthazar EJ, et al. Bowel obstruction: evaluation with CT. *Radiology* 1991;180:313–318

69. Fukuya T, Hawes DR, et al. CT diagnosis of small-bowel obstruction: efficacy in 60 patients. *AJR Am J Roentgenol* 1992;158:765–769

70. Frager D, Medwid SW, et al. CT of small-bowel obstruction: value in establishing the diagnosis and determining the degree and cause. *AJR Am J Roentgenol* 1994;162: 37–41

71. Gazelle GS, Goldberg MA, et al. Efficacy of CT in distinguishing small-bowel obstruction from other causes of small bowel dilatation. *AJR Am J Roentgenol* 1994;162: 43–47

72. Jeffrey RB Jr. *The Gastrointestinal Tract, CT and Sonography of the Acute Abdomen*. Raven Press, New York, NY, 1989:201

73. Gourtsoyiannis NC, Papakonstantinou O. Adult enteric intussusception: additional observations on enteroclysis. *Abdom Imaging* 1994;19:11–17

74. Agha F. Intussusception in adults. *AJR Am J Roentgenol* 1986;146:527–531

75. Kadell BM. *Radiologic Features of Ulcerative Colitis and Crohn's Disease*. In: Targan SF, Shanahan F (eds), *Inflammatory Bowel Disease*. Baltimore, MD: Williams & Wilkins; 1994:366

76. Nelson SW. Some interesting and unusual manifestations of Crohn's disease ("regional enteritis") of the stomach, duodenum and small intestine. *AJR Am J Roentgenol* 1969;107:86–101

77. Marshak RH. Granulomatous disease of the intestinal tract (Crohn's disease). *Radiology* 1975;114:3–22

78. Glick SN. Crohn's disease of the small intestine. *Radiol Clin North Am* 1987;25:25–45

79. Javors BR, Wecksell A, et al. Crohn's disease: Less common radiographic manifestations. *Radiographics* 1988;8: 259–275

80. Brettner A, Euphrat EJ. Radiological significance of primary enterolithiasis. *Radiology* 1970;94:283–288

81. Yeh HC, Rabinowitz JG. Granulomatous enterocolitis: findings by ultrasonography and computed tomography. *Radiology* 1983;149:253–259

82. Kaftori JK, Pery M, et al. Ultrasonography in Crohn's disease. *Gastrointest Radiol* 1984;9:137–142

83. Gore RM, Marn CS, Kirby DF, et al. CT findings in ulcerative, granulomatous and indeterminate colitis. *AJR Am J Roentgenol* 1984;143:279–284

84. Gore RM. Cross-sectional imaging of inflammatory bowel disease. *Radiol Clin North Am* 1987;25:115–131

85. Fishman EK, Wolf EJ, Jones B, et al. CT evaluation of Crohn's disease: effect on patient management. *AJR Am J Roentgenol* 1987;184:537–540

86. Goldberg HI, Caruthers SB Jr, Nelson JA, et al. Radiographic findings of the national cooperative Crohn's disease study. *Gastroenterol* 1979;77:925–937

87. Ekberg O, Fork F-T, et al. Predictive value of small bowel radiography for recurrent Crohn disease. *AJR Am J Roentgenol* 1980;135:1051–1055

88. Eisenberg RL. *Gastrointestinal Radiology: A Pattern Approach*. Philadelphia, PA: JB Lippincott; 1990:475

89. Ekberg O, Jones B, et al. Infections and other inflammatory conditions. In: Gore RM, Levine MS, Laufer I (eds), *Textbook of Gastrointestinal Radiology*. Philadelphia, PA: WB Saunders; 1994:845

90. Jones B, Fishman EK. CT of the gut in the immunocompromised host. *Radiol Clin North Am* 1989;27:763–772

91. Goldberg HI, Sheft DJ. Abnormalities in small intestine contour and calibre. A working classification. *Radiol Clin North Am* 1976;14:461

92. Mirvis SE, Gens DR, et al. Rupture of the bowel after blunt abdominal trauma: Diagnosis with CT. *AJR Am J Roentgenol* 1992; 159:1217–1221

93. Nghiem HV, Jeffrey RB Jr. CT of blunt trauma to the bowel and mesentery. *AJR Am J Roentgenol* 1993;160:53–58

94. Lund EC, Han SY, et al. Intestinal ischemia: comparison of plain radiographic and computed tomographic findings. *Radiographics* 1988;8:1083–1108

95. Federle MP, Chan G, et al. Computed tomographic findings in bowel infarction. *AJR Am J Roentgenol* 1984;142: 91–95

96. Smerud MJ, Johnson CD. Diagnosis of bowel infarction: a comparison of plain films and CT scans in 23 cases. *AJR Am J Roentgenol* 1990;154:99–103

97. Klilnani MT, Marshak RH, et al. Intramural intestinal hemorrhage. *AJR Am J Roentgenol* 1964;92:1061–1071

98. Mandelson RM, Nolan DJ. The radiological features of radiation enteritis. *Clin Radiol* 1985;36:141–148

99. Rishman EK, Zinreich ES, et al. Computed tomographic diagnosis of radiation ileitis. *Gastrointest Radiol* 1984;9: 149–152

100. Mason GR, Dietrich P, et al. The radiological findings in radiation-induced enteritis and colitis: a review of 30 cases. *Clin Radiol* 1970;21:232–247

101. Glick SN, Maglinte DDT, et al. Association of Meckel's diverticulum and Crohn's disease. *Gastrointest Radiol* 1988;13:67–71

102. Maglinte DDT, Elmore MF, et al. Meckel's diverticulum: radiologic demonstration by enteroclysis. *AJR Am J Roentgenol* 1980;134:925–932

103. Bessette JR, Maglinte DDT, et al. Primary malignant tumors in the small bowel: a comparison of the small-bowel enema and conventional follow-through examination. *AJR Am J Roentgenol* 1989;153:741–744

104. Laureat F, Reynaud M, et al. Diagnosis and categorization of small bowel neoplasms: role of computed tomography. *Gastrointest Radiol* 1991;16:115–119

105. McCarthy S, Stark DD, et al. Computed tomography of abdominal carcinoid tumors. *J Comput Assist Tomogr* 1984;8:846–850

106. Maglinte DDT. Malignant Tumors. In: Gore RH, Levine MS, Laufer I (eds), *Textbook of Gastrointestinal Radiology*. Philadelphia, PA: WB Saunders; 1994:900

107. Levine MS, Droos AT, et al: Annular malignancies of the small bowel. *Gastrointest Radiol* 1987;12:53–58

108. Megibow AJ, Balthazar EJ, et al. Computed tomography of gastrointestinl lymphoma. *AJR Am J Roentgenol* 1983; 141:541–547

109. Fishman EK, Kuhlman JE, et al. CT of malignant melanoma in the chest, abdomen and musculoskeletal system. *Radiographics* 1990;10:603–620

110. Chang SF, Burrell MI, et al. The protean gastrointestinal manifestations of metastatic breast carcinoma. *Radiology* 1978;126:611–617

111. Marshak RH, Khilnani MT, et al. Metastatic carcinoma of the small bowel. *AJR Am J Roentgenol* 1965;94:385–394

112. Feczko PF, Collins DD. Metastatic disease involving the gastrointestinal tract. *Radiol Clin North Am* 1993;31: 1359–1373

113. Smith C, Deziel DJ. Appearances of the postoperative alimentary tract. *Radiol Clin North Am* 1993;31:1235–1254

114. Kremers PW, Scholz FJ, et al. Radiology of the ileoanal reservoir. *AJR Am J Roentgenol* 1985;145:559–567

115. Theoni RF, Fell SC, et al. Ileoanal pouches: comparison of CT, scintigraphy, and contrast enemas for diagnosing post surgical complications. *AJR Am J Roentgenol* 1990; 154:73–78

116. Eisenberg RL. Large Bowel Obstruction. In: Eisenberg RL (ed), *Gastrointestinal Radiology. A Pattern Approach*. Philadelphia, PA: JB Lippincott; 1990:722

117. Gore RM, Eisenberg RL. Large bowel obstruction. In: Gore RM, Levine MS, Laufer I (eds), *Textbook of Gastrointestinal Radiology*. Philadelphia, PA: WB Saunders; 1994:1247

118. Caroline DF, Maglinte DDT. Radiology of the colon. In: Gedgaudas-McClees RK (ed), *Gastrointestinal Imaging*. New York, NY: Churchill-Livingstone; 1987:107

119. Mindelzun RE, Stone JM. Volvulus of the splenic flexure: radiographic features. *Radiology* 1991;181:221–223

120. Rice RP. Plain abdominal film roentgenographic diagnosis of ulcerative diseases of the colon. *AJR Am J Roentgenol* 1968;104:544–550

121. Prantera C, Lorenzetti R, et al. The plain abdominal film accurately estimates extent of active ulcerative colitis. *J Clin Gastroenterol* 1991;13:231–234

122. Gelfand DW, Chen MY, Ott DJ. Preparing the colon for the barium enema examination. *Radiology* 1991;178: 609–613

123. Theoni RF, Margulis AR. The state of radiographic technique in the examination of the colon: a survey in 1987. *Radiology* 1988;168:7–12

124. Laufer I. Barium studies. In: Gore RM, Levine MS, Laufer I (eds), *Textbook of Gastrointestinal Radiology*. Philadelphia, PA: WB Saunders; 1994:1028

125. Gelfand DW. Complications of gastrointestinal radiologic procedures. 1. Complications of routine fluoroscopic studies. *Gastrointest Radiol* 1980;5:293–315

126. Wolf BS, Khilnani et al. Diverticulosis and diverticulitis: roentgen findings and their interpretation. *AJR Am J Roentgenol* 1957;77:726–743

127. Balthazar EJ. Diverticular disease. In: Gore RM, Levine MS, Laufer I (eds), *Textbook of Gastrointestinal Radiology*. Philadelphia, PA: WB Saunders; 1994:1072

128. Hulnick DH, Megibow AJ, et al. Computed tomography in the evaluation of diverticulitis. *Radiology* 1984;152: 481–495

129. Jeffrey RB Jr. The gastrointestinal tract. In: Jeffrey RB, Jr (ed), *CT and Sonography of the Acute Abdomen*. New York, NY: Raven Press; 1989:234–260

130. Cho CK, Morehouse HT. Sigmoid diverticulitis: diag-

nostic role of CT—comparison with barium enema studies. *Radiology* 1990;176:111–115

131. Laufer I. The radiologic demonstration of early changes in ulcerative colitis by double contrast technique. *Can Assoc Radiol J* 1975;26:116–121

132. Laufer I, Hamilton J. The radiological differentiation between ulcerative and granulomatous colitis by double contrast radiology. *Am J Gastroenterol* 1976;66:259–269

133. Kadell BM. Radiologic features of ulcerative colitis and Crohn's disease. In: Targan SF, Shanahan F (eds), *Inflammatory Bowel Disease.* Baltimore, MD: Williams & Wilkins; 1994:366

134. Lichtenstein JE. Radiologic-pathologic correlation of inflammatory bowel disease. *Radiol Clin North Am* 1987; 25:3–24

135. Gore RM. Colonic contour changes in chronic ulcerative colitis: reappraisal of some old concepts. *AJR Am J Roentgenol* 1992;158:59–61

136. Keeley F, Gohel VK. A roentgenologic remission in ulcerative colitis. *AJR Am J Roentgenol* 1961;86:906–910

137. Diner WC, Barnhard HJ. Toxic megacolon. *Semin Roentgenol* 1973;5:433–436

138. Halpert RD. Toxic dilatation of the colon. *Radiol Clin North Am* 1987;25:147–155

139. Pezco PJ. Malignancy complicating inflammatory bowel disease. *Radiol Clin North Am* 1987;25:157–174

140. James EM, Carlson HC. Chronic ulcerative colitis and colon cancer: can radiographic appearance predict survival patterns? *AJR Am J Roentgenol* 1978;130:825–830

141. Hooyman JR, MacCarty RL, et al. Radiographic appearance of mucosal dysplasia associated with ulcerative colitis. *AJR Am J Roentgenol* 1987;149:47–51

142. Gore RM, Marn CS, et al. CT findings in ulcerative, granulomatous and indeterminate colitis. *Am J Radiol* 1984; 143:279–284

143. Gore RM, Fezco PJ, et al. CT of inflammatory bowel disease. *Radiol Clin North Am* 1989;27:717–741

144. Gore RM. Cross sectional image of inflammatory bowel disease. *Radiol Clin North Am* 1987;25:115–131

145. Kremers PW, Scholz FJ, et al. Radiology of the ileoanal reservoir. *AJR Am J Roentgenol* 1985;145:559–567

146. Theoni RF, Fell SC, et al. Ileoanal pouches: Comparison of CT, scintigraphy and contrast enemas for diagnosing post surgical complications. *AJR Am J Roentgenol* 1990; 154:73–78

147. Fezco PJ. Intestinal and extraintestinal complications of inflammatory bowel disease. *Radiol Clin North Am* 1987; 25:145–146

148. Williams SM, Harned RK. Hepatobiliary complications of inflammatory bowel disease. *Radiol Clin North Am* 1987;25:175–188

149. Laufer I, Costopoulos L. Early lesions of Crohn's disease. *AJR Am J Roentgenol* 1978;130:307–311

150. Ni X-YU, Goldberg H. Aphthoid ulcers in Crohn's disease: radiographic course and relationship to bowel appearance. *Radiology* 1986;158:589–596

151. Goldberg HI. Focal ulcerations of the colon in granulomatous colitis. *AJR Am J Roentgenol* 1967;101:296–300

152. Bernstein JR, Ghahremani G, et al. Localized giant pseudopolyposis of the colon in ulcerative and granulomatous colitis. *Gastrointest Radiol* 1976;3:431–435

153. Yousem DM, Fishman EK, et al. Crohn's disease: perirectal and perianal findings at CT. *Radiology* 1988;167:331–334

154. Miller TL, Skucas J, et al. Bowel cancer characteristics in patients with regional enteritis. *Gastrointest Radiol* 1987; 12:45–52

155. Goldberg HI, Gore RM, et al. Computed tomography in the evaluation of Crohn's disease. *AJR Am J Roentgenol* 1983;140:277–282

156. Yeh HC, Rabinowitz JG. Granulomatous enterocolitis: findings by ultrasonography and computed tomography. *Radiology* 1983;149:253–259

157. Eisenberg RL, Infectious ulcerative lesions of the colon. In: Eisenberg RL (ed), *Gastrointestinal Radiology: A Pattern Approach.* Philadelphia, PA; JB Lippincott; 1990:585

158. Glick SN. Other inflammatory conditions. In: Gore RM, Levine MS, Laufer I (eds), *Textbook of Gastrointestinal Radiology.* Philadelphia, PA: WB Saunders; 1994:1142

159. Fishman EK, Kavuru M, et al. Pseudomembranous colitis: CT evaluation of 26 cases. *Radiology* 1990;180:57–60

160. Taylor AJ, Dodds WJ, et al. Typhlitis in adults. *Gastrointest Radiol* 1985;10:363–369

161. Frick MP, Maile CW, et al. Computed tomography of neutropenic colitis. *AJR Am J Roentgenol* 1984;143:763–765

162. Wolf EL. Ischemic disease of the gut. In: Gore RM, Levine MS, Laufer I (eds), *Textbook of Gastrointestinal Radiology.* Philadelphia, PA: WB Saunders; 1994:2694

163. Theoni RF, Laufer I. Polyps and cancer. In: Gore RM, Levine MS, Laufer I (eds), *Textbook of Gastrointestinal Radiology.* Philadelphia, PA: WB Saunders; 1994:1160

164. Collier BD, Foley WD. Current imaging strategies for colorectal cancer. *J Nucl Med* 1993;34:537–540

165. Iida M, Iwashita A, et al. Villous tumor of the colon: correlation of histologic, macroscopic and radiographic features. *Radiology* 1988;167:673–677

166. Harned RK, Buck JL. Polyposis syndromes. In: Gore RM, Levine MS, Laufer I (eds), *Textbook of Gastrointestinal Radiology.* Philadelphia, PA: WB Saunders, 1994;1228

167. Bartram CL, Thornton A. Colonic polyp patterns in familiar polyposis. *AJR Am J Roentgenol* 1984;142:305–308

168. Eisenberg RL. Multiple filling defects in the colon. In: Eisenberg RL (ed), *Gastrointestinal Radiology: A Pattern Approach.* Philadelphia, PA: JB Lippincott, 1990;692.

169. Dodds WJ. Clinical and roentgen features of the intestinal polyposis syndromes. *Gastrointest Radiol* 1976;1:127–142

170. Freeny PC, Marks WM, et al. Colorectal carcinoma evaluation with CT: preoperative staging and detection of postoperative recurrent. *Radiology* 1986;158:347–356

171. Theoni RF. Colorectal cancer: cross sectional imaging for staging of primary tumor and detection of local recurrence. *AJR Am J Roentgenol* 1991;156:909–915

172. Selfkin MD, Ehrlich SM, et al. Staging of rectal carcinoma: prospective comparison of endorectal US and CT. *Radiology* 1989;170:319–322

173. Thompson WM, Trenker SW. Staging colorectal carcinoma. *Radiol Clin North Am* 1994;32:25–37

174. Ryan JW. Immunoscintigraphy in primary colorectal cancer. *Cancer* 1993;71:4217–4224

175. Neal CE, Abdel-Naby H. Clinical immunoscintigraphy of recurrent colorectal carcinoma. *Appl Radiol* 1994;23:32–39

176. O'Connell DJ, Thomson AJ. Lymphoma of the colon. The spectrum of radiologic changes. *Gastrointest Radiol* 1978;2:377–380

177. Gordon RL, Evers K, et al. Double-contrast enema in pelvic endometriosis. *AJR Am J Roentgenol* 1982;138:544–552

178. Arrive L, Hricak H, et al. Pelvic endometriosis MR imaging. *Radiology* 1989;171:687–692

179. Meyers MW. Distribution of intra-abdominal malignant seeding: dependency on dynamics of flow of ascitic fluid. *AJR Am J Roentgenol* 1973;119:198–206

180. Rubesin SE, Furth EE. Other tumors. In: Gore RM, Levine MS, Laufer I (eds), *Textbook of Gastrointestinal Radiology*. Philadelphia, PA: WB Saunders, 1994:1220

181. Scholz FJ. Postoperative colon. In: Gore RM, Levine MS, Laufer I (eds), *Textbook of Gastrointestinal Radiology*. Philadelphia, PA: WB Saunders; 1994:1342

182. Goei R. Anorectal function in patients with defecation disorders and asymptomatic subjects: evaluation with defecography. *Radiology* 1990;174:121–123

183. Kelvin FM, Maglinte DT, et al. Pelvic prolapse assessment with evacuation proctography (defecography). *Radiology* 1992;184:547–551

184. Ogorek CP, Reynolds JC. Chronic constipation: diagnosis and treatment. *Endoscopy Review*, Nov/Dec 1987.

185. Bouchoucha M, Devroede G, et al. What is the meaning of colorectal transit time measurement? *Dis Colon Rectum* 1992;35:773–782

186. Gedgaudas-McClees RK. Radiology of the colon. In: Gedgaudas-McClees RK (ed), *Handbook of Gastrointestinal Imaging*, Churchill-Livingstone, 1987:163

187. Balthazar EJ. Disorders of the appendix. In: Gore RM, Levine MS, Laufer I (eds), *Textbook of Gastrointestinal Radiology*. Philadelphia, PA: WB Saunders; 1994;1310

188. Rice RP, Thompson WM, Fedyshin PJ, et al. The barium enema in appendicitis: spectrum of appearances and pitfalls. *Radiographics* 1984;4:393–409

189. Jeffrey RB, Jr. The gastrointestinal tract. In: Jeffrey RB, Jr (ed), *CT and Sonography of the Acute Abdomen*. New York, NY: Raven Press; 1989:234

190. Chambers TP, Federle MP. CT of the acute abdomen. *Appl Radiol* 1992;65–72

191. Shapiro MP, Gale ME, Gerzuf S. CT of appendicitis: diagnosis and treatment. *Radiol Clin North Am* 1989;27(4):753–762

192. Malone AJ, Wolf CR, et al. Diagnosis of acute appendicitis. Value of unenhanced CT. *AJR Am J Roentgenol* 1993:160:763–766

193. Puylaert JBCM. Acute appendicitis: ultrasound evaluation using graded compression. *Radiology* 1986;185:355–360

194. Jeffrey RB, Laing FC, Lewis FR. Acute appendicitis: high-resolution real-time ultrasound findings. *Radiology* 1987;163:11–14

195. Balthazar EJ, Birnbaum BA, et al. Acute appendicitis: CT and ultrasound correlation in 100 patients. *Radiology* 1994;190:31–35

196. Madwed D. Mindelzun R, Jeffrey RB. Mucocele of the appendix: imaging findings. *AJR Am J Roentgenol* 1992;159:69–72

197. Baron R, Freeny PC, Moss AA. The liver. In: Moss AA, Gamsu G, Genant HK (eds), *Computed Tomography of the Body*, 2nd ed. Philadelphia, PA: WB Saunders; 1992

198. Birnbaum BA, Weinreb JC, Megibow AJ, et al. Definitive diagnosis of hepatic hemangiomas: MR imaging versus Tc-99m-labeled red blood cell SPECT. *Radiology* 1990;176:95–101

199. Dalan K, Day DL, Ascher NL, et al. Imaging of vascular complications after hepatic transplantation. *AJR Am J Roentgenol* 1988;150:1285–1290

200. deLange EE, Mugler JP, III, Bosworth JE, et al. MR imaging of the liver: breath-hold T1-weighted MP-GRE compared with conventional T2-weighted SE imaging-Lesion detection, localization, and characterization. *Radiology* 1994;190:727–736

201. Ferrucci JT. Liver tumor imaging: current concepts. *AJR Am J Roentgenol* 1990;155:473–484

202. Flint EW, Sumkin JH, Zajko AB, et al. Duplex sonography of hepatic artery thrombosis after liver transplantation. *AJR Am J Roentgenol* 1988;151:481–483

203. Gore RM. Normal anatomy and examination techniques, diffuse liver disease, and vascular disorders of the liver and splanchnic circulation. In: Gore RM, Levine MS, Lauffer I (eds), *Textbook of Gastrointestinal Radiology*, Philadelphia, PA: WB Saunders, 1993

204. Hamm B, Thoeni RF, Gould RG, et al. Focal liver lesions: characterization with nonenhanced and dynamic contrast material-enhanced MR imaging. *Radiology* 1994;190:417–423

205. Jeffrey RB. Abdominal imaging in the immunocompromised patient. *Radiol Clin North Am* 1992;30:579–596

206. Jones EC, Chezmar JL, Nelson RC, et al. The frequency and significance of small (<15 mm) hepatic lesions detected by CT. *AJR Am J Roentgenol* 1992;158:535–539

207. Karhunen PJ. Benign hepatic tumors and tumor-like conditions in men. *J Clin Path* 1986;39:183–188

208. Koslin DB, Mulligan SA, Berland LL. Duplex assessment of the portal venous system. *Semin Ultrasound CT MR* 1992;13(1):22–33

209. Lee JKT, Dixon WT, Ling D, et al. Fatty infiltration of the liver: demonstration by proton spectroscopic imaging. *Radiology*, 1984;153:195–201

210. Lomas DJ, Britton PD, Farman P, et al. Duplex doppler ultrasound for the detection of vascular occlusion following liver transplantation in children. *Clin Radiol* 1992;46:38–42

211. Mahfouz A-E, Hamm B, Taupitz M, et al. Hypervascular liver lesions: differentiation of focal nodular hyperplasia from malignant tumors with dynamic Goadlinium-enhanced MR imaging. *Radiology* 1993;186:133–138

212. Mahfouz A-E, Hamm B, Wolf K-J. Peripheral washout: a sign of malignancy on dynamic gadolinium-enhanced MR images of focal liver lesions. *Radiology* 1994;190:49–52

213. Mitchell DG. Focal manifestations of diffuse liver disease at MR imaging. *Radiology* 1992;185:1–11

214. Moody AR, Wilson SR, Greig PD. Non-Hodgkin's lymphoma in the porta hepatis after orthotopic liver transplantations: sonographic findings. *Radiology* 1992;182:867–870

215. Murakami T, Kuroda C, Marukawa T, et al. Regenerating nodules of liver cirrhosis: MR findings with pathologic correlation. *AJR Am J Roentgenol* 1990;155:1227–1231

216. Outwater EK, Mitchell DG, Vinitski S. Abdominal MR imaging: evaluation of a fast spin-echo sequence. *Radiology* 1994;190:425–429

217. Rappacini GL, Pompili M, Caturelli E, et al. Focal ultrasound lesions in liver cirrhosis diagnosed as regenerating nodules by fine needle biopsy: follow-up of 12 cases. *Dig Dis Sci* 1990;35:422–427

218. Ros PR, Barreda, P, Gore RM. Focal hepatic infections. In: Gore RM, Levine MS, Lauffer I (eds), *Textbook of Gastrointestinal Radiology*, Philadelphia, PA: WB Saunders; 1993.

219. Ros PR. Benign and malignant liver tumors. In: Gore RM, Levine MS, Lauffer I (eds). *Textbook of Gastrointestinal Radiology*, Philadelphia, PA: WB Saunders; 1993

220. Rummeny EJ, Wernecke K, Saini S, et al. Comparison between high-field-strength MR imaging and CT for screening of hepatic metastases: a receiver operating characteristic analysis. *Radiology* 1992;182:879–886

221. Segel MC, Zajko AB, Bowen AD, et al. Hepatic artery thombosis after liver transplantation: radiologic evaluation. *AJR Am J Roentgenol* 1986;146:137–141

222. Silverman PM, Patt RH, Garra BS, et al. (eds). MR imaging of the portal venous system: value of gradient-echo imaging as an adjunct to spin-echo imaging. *AJR Am J Roentgenol* 1991;157(2):297–302

223. Soyer P, Laissy J-P, Sibert A, et al. Focal hepatic masses: Comparison of detection during arterial portography with MR imaging and CT. *Radiology* 1994;190:737–740

224. Soyer P. Segmental anatomy of the liver: utility of a nomenclature accepted worldwide. *AJR Am J Roentgenol* 1993;161:572–573

225. Spouge AR, Wilson SR, Gopinath N, et al. Extrapulmonary pneumocystis carinii in a patient with AIDS: sonographic findings. *AJR Am J Roentgenol* 1990;155:76–78

226. Vilgrain V, Flejou J-F, Arrive L, et al. Focal nodular hyperplasia of the liver: MR imaging and pathologic correlation in 37 patients. *Radiology* 1992;184:699–703

227. Weisleder R, Stark D. Magnetic resonance imaging of the liver. *Semin Ultrasound CT MR* 1989;10:63–77

228. Wellings RM, Olliff SP, Olliff JFC, et al. Duplex doppler detection of hepatic artery thrombosis following liver transplantation. *Clin Radiol* 1993;47:180–182

229. Wernecke K, Vassallo P, Bick U, et al. The distinction between benign and malignant liver tumors on sonography: value of a hypoechoic halo. *AJR Am J Roentgenol* 1992;159:1005–1009

230. Wheeler DA, Edmondson HA. Cystadenocarcinoma with mesenchymal stroma CMS in the liver and bile ducts. A clinicopathologic study of 17 cases, 4 with malignant change. *Cancer* 1985;56:1434–1445

231. PreKarski J, Federle MP, et al. Computed tomography of the spleen. *Radiology* 1980;135:683–689

232. Dodds WJ, Taylor AJ. Radiologic imaging of splenic anomalies. *AJR Am J Roentgenol* 1990;155:805–810

233. Freeman JL, Jafri SZ, et al. CT of acquired abnormalities of the spleen. *Radiographics* 1993;13:597–610

234. Taylor AJ, Dodds WJ. CT of acquired abnormalities of the spleen. *AJR Am J Roentgenol* 1991;157:1213–1219

235. Kawashima A, Fishman EK. Benign splenic lesions. In: Gore RM, Levine MS, Laufer I (eds), *Textbook of Gastrointestinal Radiology*. Philadelphia, PA: WB Saunders; 1994:2251

236. Kawashima A, Fishman EK. Malignant splenic lesions. In: Gore RM, Levine MS, Laufer I (eds), *Textbook of Gastrointestinal Radiology*. Philadelphia, PA: WB Saunders; 1994:2276

237. Shirkhoda A, Ros PR, et al. Lymphoma of the solid abdominal viscera. *Radiol Clin North Am* 1990;28:785–799

238. Fishman EK, Kuhlman JJE, et al. CT of lymphoma: Spectrum of disease. *Radiographics* 1991;11:647–669

239. Jeffrey RB Jr. The spleen. In: Jeffrey RB Jr (ed). *CT and Sonography of the Acute Abdomen*. New York, NY: Raven Press; 1989:77

240. Mirvis SE, Whitley NO, et al. Blunt splenic trauma in adults: CT-based classficiation and correlation with prognosis and treatment. *Radiology* 1989;171:33–39

241. Jeffrey RB Jr. CT diagnosis of blunt hepatic and splenic injuries: a look to the future. *Radiology* 1989;171:17–18

242. Do HM, Cronan JJ. CT appearance of splenic injuries managed nonoperatively. *AJR Am J Roentgenol* 1991;175:757–760

243. Laing FC. The gallbladder and bile ducts. In: Rumack CM, Wilson SR, Charboneau JW (eds), *Diagnostic Ultrasound*, St. Louis, MO: Mosby Year Book; 1991

244. Turner MA. Examination techniques and normal anatomy (of the gallbladder and biliary tract). In: Gore RM, Levine MS, Lauffer I (eds), *Textbook of Gastrointestinal Radiology*. Philadelphia, PA: WB Saunders; 1993

245. Zeman RK, Burrell MI. *Gallbladder and Bile Duct Imaging: A Clinical Radiological Approach*. New York, NY: Churchill-Livingstone; 1987

246. Laing FC, Federle MP, Jeffrey RB, et al. Ultrasonic evaluation of patients with acute right upper quadrant pain. *Radiology* 1981;140:449–451

247. Simeone JF, Mueller PR, Ferricci JT Jr. Non-surgical therapy of gallstones: implications for imaging. *AJR Am J Roentgenol* 1989;152:11–17

248. Krishnamurthy GT, Turner FE. Pharmacokinetics and clinical application of technetium 99m-labeled hepatobiliary agents. *Sem Nucl Med* 1990;20:130–149

249. Zeman RK. Cholelithiasis and cholecystitis. In: Gore RM, Levine MS, Lauffer I (eds), *Textbook of Gastrointestinal Radiology*. Philadelphia, PA: WB Saunders; 1993

250. Shulman WP, Rogers JV, Rudd TG, et al. Low sensitivity of sonography and cholescintigraphy in acalculous cholecystitis. *AJR Am J Roentgenol* 1984;142:531–534

251. Mirvis SE, Vainright JR, Nelson AW, et al. The diagnosis of acute acalculous cholecystitis. A comparison of sonography, scintigraphy and CT. *AJR Am J Roentgenol* 1986;147:1171–1175

252. Lee MJ, Saini S, Brink JA, et al. Treatment of critically ill patients with sepsis of unknown cause: value of percutaneous cholecystostomy. *AJR Am J Roentgenol* 1991;156: 1163–1166

253. Berk RN, Armbruster TG, Salzstein SL. Carcinoma in the porcelain gallbladder. *Radiology* 1973;106:29–31

254. Lichtenstein JE. Adenomatosis and cholesterolosis: the "hyperplastic cholecystoses." In: Gore RM, Levine MS, Lauffer I (eds), *Textbook of Gastrointestinal Radiology*, Philadelphia, PA: WB Saunders; 1993

255. Raghavendra BN, Subramanyam BR, Blathazar EJ, et al. Sonography of adenomyomatosis of the gallbladder: radiologic-pathologic correlation. *Radiology* 1983;146:747–752

256. Ward EM, Stephens DH. Neoplasms (of the gallbladder and biliary tract). In: Gore RM, Levine MS, Lauffer I (eds), *Textbook of Gastrointestinal Radiology*, WB Saunders, Philadelphia, 1993

257. Laing FC. The gallbladder and bile ducts. In: Rumack CM, Wilson SR, Charboneau JW (eds), *Diagnostic Ultrasound*. St Louis, MO: Mosby Year Book; 1991

258. Turner MA. Examination techniques and normal anatomy (of the gallbladder biliary tract.) In: Gore RM, Levine MS, Lauffer I (eds), *Textbook of Gastrointestinal Radiology*. Philadelphia, PA: WB Saunders; 1993

259. Zeman RK, Burrell MI. Gallbladder and bile duct imaging: a clinical radiological approach. New York, NY: Churchill-Livingstone; 1987

260. Rosenthal SJ, Cox GG, Wetzel LH, Batnitzky S. Pitfalls and differential diagnosis is biliary sonography. *Radiographics* 1990;10:285–311

261. Darweesh RMA, Dodds WJ, Hogan WJ, et al. Fatty-meal sonography for evaluating patients with suspected partial common duct obstruction. *AJR Am J Roentgenol* 1988; 151:63–68

262. Liddell RM, Baron RL, Ekstrom JE, et al. Normal intrahepatic bile ducts: CT depiction. *Radiology* 1990;176: 633–635

263. Critten SJ, McKinley MJ. Choledochal cyst-clinical features and classification. *Am J Gastroenterol* 1985;80:643–648

264. Laing FC, Jeffrey RB Jr. Choledocholithiasis and cystic duct obstruction: Difficult ultrasonographic diagnosis. *Radiology* 1983;146:475–479

265. Cronan JJ. US diagnosis of choledocholithiasis: a reappraisal. *Radiology* 1986;161:133–134

266. Cronan JJ. The imaging of choledocholithiasis. *Semin Ultrasound CT MR* 1987;8:75–84

267. McCarty RL, LaRusso NF, Weisner RH, et al. Primary sclerosing cholangitis: findings on cholangiography and pancreatography. *Radiology* 1983;149:39–44

268. vanSonnenberg E, Casola G, Cubberley DA, et al. Oriental cholangiohepatitis: diagnostic imaging and interventional management. *AJR Am J Roentgenol* 1986;146: 327–331

269. Dolmatch BL, Laing FC, Federle MP, et al. AIDS-related cholangitis: radiographic findings in nine patients. *Radiology* 1987;163:313–316

270. Choi BI, Park JH, Kim YI, et al. Peripheral cholangiocarcinoma and clonorchiasis: CT findings. *Radiology* 1988; 169:149–153

271. Ward EM, Stephens DH. Neoplasms (of the gallbladder and biliary tract). In: Gore RM, Levine MS, Lauffer I (eds), *Textbook of Gastrointestinal Radiology*. Philadelphia, PA: WB Saunders; 1993

272. Ghahremanin GG. Postsurgical and traumatic lesions of the biliary tract. In: Gore RM, Levine MS, Lauffer I (eds), *Textbook of Gastrointestinal Radiology*. Philadelphia, PA: WB Saunders; 1993

273. Ghahremani GG, Crampton AR, Berstein JR, et al. Iatrogenic biliary tract complications: radiologic features and clinical significance. *Radiographics* 1991;11:44–45

274. Deziel DJ, Millikan KW, Economou SG, et al. Complications of laparoscopic cholecystectomy: a national survey of 4,292 hospitals and an analysis of 77,604 cases. *Am J Surg* 1993;165:9–14

275. Evans RA, Raby ND, O'Grady, JG, et al. Biliary complications following orthotopic liver transplantation. *Clin Radiol* 1990;41:190–194

276. Gomes AS. Diagnosis and radiologic treatment of biliary complications of liver transplantation. *Semin Interv Radiol* 1992;9:283–289

277. Theoni RF, Blankenberg F. Pancreatic imaging: computed tomography and magnetic resonance imaging. *Radiol Clin North Am* 1993;31:1085–1113

278. Gore RM. Pancreas: normal anatomy and examination techniques. In: Gore RM, Levine MS, Laufer I (eds), *Textbook of Gastrointestinal Radiology*. Philadelphia, PA: WB Saunders; 1994:2096

279. Dupuy DE, Costello P, Ecker CP. Spiral CT of the pancreas. *Radiology* 1992;183(3):815–818

280. Agha FP, Williams KD. Pancreas divisum: incidence, detection and clinical significance. *Am J Gastroenterol* 1987; 82:315–320

281. Glazer GM, Margulis AR. Annular pancreas: etiology and diagnosis using endoscopic retrograde cholangiopancreatography. *Radiology* 1979;133:303–306

282. Gore RM, Fernbach SK, Ghahremani GG. Pancreas: anomalies and anatomic variants. In: Gore RM, Levine MS, Laufer I, (eds), *Textbook of Gastrointestinal Radiology*, Philadelphia, PA: WB Saunders, 1994:2122

283. Gedgaudas-McClees RK. Radiology of the pancreas. In: Gedgaudas-McClees RK (ed), *Gastrointestinal Imaging*. New York, NY: Churchill-Livingstone; 1989:237

284. Balthazar EJ. Pancreatitis. In: Gore RM, Levine MS and Laufer I (eds), *Textbook of Gastrointestinal Radiology*. Philadelphia, PA: WB Saunders; 1994:2132

285. Moulton JS. The radiologic assessment of acute pancreatitis and its complications. *Pancreas* 1991;6(1):S13–S22

286. Hill MC, Huntington DK. Computed tomography and acute pancreatitis. *Gastroenterol Clin North Am* 1990;19: 811–842

287. Galthazar EJ. CT diagnosis and staging of acute pancreatitis. *Radiol Clin North Am* 1989;27:19–38

288. Freeny PC. Angio-CT: diagnosis and detection of complications of acute pancreatitis. *Hepatogastroenterol* 1991; 38:109–115

289. Freeny PC. Radiologic diagnosis and staging of pancreatic ductal adenocarcinoma. *Radiol Clin North Am* 1989; 27:121–128

290. Niederou C, Grendell JH. Diagnosis of pancreatic carcinoma: imaging techniques and tumor markers. *Pancreas* 1992;7:66–86

291. Balthazar EJ, Chako AC. Computed tomography of pancreatic masses. *Am J Gastroenterol* 1989;85:343–349

292. Nghiem HV, Freeny PC. Radiologic staging of pancreatic adenocarcinoma. *Radiol Clin North Am* 1994;32:71–80

293. Mitchell DG, Shapiro M, et al. Pancreatic disease: findings on state-of-the-art MR images. *AJR Am J Roentgenol* 1992;159:533–538

294. Reimer P, Sarni S, et al. Techniques for high-resolution echo-planar MR imaging of the pancreas. *Radiology* 1992; 182:175–179

295. Torres GM, Erquiaga E, et al. Preliminary results of MR imaging with superparamagnetic iron oxide in pancreatic and retroperitoneal disorders. *Radiographics* 1991; 11:785–791

296. Vellet AD. Characterization of pancreatic adenocarcinoma by magnetic resonance imaging. *Can Assoc Radiol J* 1991;42:180–184

297. Vellet AD, Romano W, et al. Adenocarcinoma of the pancreatic ducts: comparative evaluation with CT and MR imaging. *Radiology* 1992;183:87–95

298. Pavone P, Mitchell DG, et al. Pancreatic B-cell tumors: MRI. *J Comput Assist Tomogr* 1993;17:403–407

299. Doherty GM, Doppman JL, et al. Results of a prospective strategy to diagnose, localize and resect insulinomas. *Surgery* 1991;110:989–997

300. Rossi P, Allison DJ. Endocrine tumors of the pancreas. *Radiol Clin North Am* 1989;129–162

301. Coppman JL, Shawker TH, Miller DL. Localization of islet cell tumors. *Gastroenterol Clin North Am* 1989;18: 793–804

302. Ross PR, Hamrick-Turner JE, et al. Cystic masses of the pancreas. *Radiographics* 1992;12:673–686

303. Mathieu D, Guigui B. Pancreatic cystic neoplasms. *Radiol Clin North Am* 1989;27:163–176

304. Rugazzola C, Procacci C. Cystic tumors of the pancreas: evaluation by ultrasonography and computed tomography. *Gastrointest Radiol* 1991;16:53–61

305. Ohtomo K, Furui S. Solid and papillary epithelial neoplasm of the pancreas: MR imaging and pathologic correlation. *Radiology* 1992;184:567–570

306. Friedman AC. Pancreatic neoplasms. In: Gore RM, Levine MS, Laufer I (eds), *Textbook of Gastrointestinal Radiology*. Philadelphia, PA: WB Saunders; 1994:2161

307. Jeffrey RB Jr. The pancreas in CT and sonography of the acute abdomen. In: Jeffrey RB Jr (ed), Raven Press; 1989

308. Gore RM, Nahrwold DL. Pancreatic trauma and surgery. In: Gore RM, Levine MS, Laufer I (eds), *Textbook of Gastrointestinal Radiology*. Philadelphia, PA: WB Saunders, 1994:2193

309. Heiken J. Abdominal wall and peritoneal cavity. In: Lee JKT, Sagel SS, Stanley RJ (eds), *Computed Body Tomography with MRI Correlation*. New York, NY: Raven Press; 1989:661–705

310. Silverman PM, Cooper C. Mesenteric and omental lesions. In: Gore RM, Levine MS, Laufer I (eds), *Textbook of Gastrointestinal Radiology*, Vol 2. Philadelphia, PA: WB Saunders; 1994:2367–2381

311. Jeffrey RB. The Peritoneal cavity and mesentery. In: Moss AA, Gamsu G, Genant HK (eds), *Computed Tomography of the Body with Magnetic Resonance Imaging*, Vol 3: *Abdomen and Pelvis*. Philadelphia, PA: WB Saunders; 1992:1139–1181

312. Goldberg HI, Gore RM, Margulis, AR, et al. Computed tomography in the evaluation of Crohn's disease. *AJR Am J Roentgenol* 1983;140:277–282

313. Frager DH, Goldman M, Beneventano TC. Computed tomography in Crohn's disease. *J Comput Assist Tomogr* 1983;7:819–824

314. Knochel JQ, Koehler PR, Lee TG, Welch DM. Diagnosis of abdominal abscesses with computed tomography, ultrasound, and ¹¹¹In leukocyte scans. *Radiology* 1980;137: 425–432

315. Korobkin M, Callen PW, Filly RA, et al. Comparison of computed tomography, ultrasonography and Gallium-67 scanning in the evaluation of suspected abdominal abscess. *Radiology* 1978;129:89–93

316. Halber MD, Daffner RH, Morgan CL, et al. Intraabdominal abscess: current concepts in radiologic evaluation. *AJR Am J Roentgenol* 1979;133:9–13

317. Mueller PR, Simeone JF. Intraabdominal abscesses: Diagnosis by sonography and computed tomography. In: CT and ultrasonography in the acutely ill patient. *Radiol Clin North Am* 1983;21(3):425–444

318. Wolverson MK, Jagannadharao B, Sundaram M, et al. CT is a primary diagnostic method in evaluating intraabdominal abscess. *AJR Am J Roentgenol* 1979;133:1089–1095

319. Callen PW. Computed tomographic evaluation of abdominal and pelvic abscesses. *Radiology* 1979;131:171–175

320. Schneckloth G, Terrier F, Fuchs WA. Computed tomography of intraperitoneal abscesses. *Gastrointest Radiol* 1982;7:35–41

321. Balthazar EJ. Disorders of the appendix. In: Gore RM, Levine MS, Laufer I (eds), *Textbook of Gastrointestinal Radiology*. Philadelphia, PA: WB Saunders; 1994;1310–1342

322. Hartz R, Stryker S, Sparberg M, Poticha SM. Mesenteric tumefactions. *Am Surg* 1980;46:525–529

323. Kipfer RE, Moertl CG, Dahlin DC. Mesenteric lipodystrophy. *Ann Int Med* 1974;80:582–588

324. Handelsman JC, Shelly WM. Mesenteric panniculitis. *Arch Surg* 1965;91:842–850

325. Katz ME, Heiken JP, Glazer HS, Lee JKT. Intraabdominal panniculitis: clinical, radiographic, and CT features. *AJR Am J Roentgenol* 1985;145:293–296

326. Mata JM, Inaraja L, Martin J, et al. CT features of mesenteric panniculitis. *J Comput Assist Tomogr* 1987;11(6): 1021–1023

327. Hamrick-Turner JE, Chiechi MV, Abbitt PL, Ros PR. Neoplastic and inflammatory processes of the peritoneum, omentum, and mesentery: diagnosis with CT. *Radiographics* 1992;12:1051–1068

328. Baron RL, Lee JKT. Mesenteric desmoid tumors. *Radiology* 1981;140:777–779

329. Kawashima A, Goldman SM, Fishman EK, et al. CT of intraabdominal desmoid: is the tumor different in patients with Gardner's disease. *AJR Am J Roentgenol* 1994;162: 339–342

330. Waligore MP, Stephens DH, Soule EH, McLeod RA. Lipomatous tumors of the abdominal cavity: CT appearance and pathologic correlation. *AJR Am J Roentgenol* 1981;137:539–545

331. Whitley ND, Brenner DE, Antman KH, et al. CT of peritoneal mesothelioma. *AJR Am J Roentgenol* 1982;183:531–535

332. Meyers MA, McSweeney J. Secondary neoplasms of the bowel. *Radiology* 1972;105:1–11

333. Meyers MA. *Dynamic Radiology of the Abdomen,* 4th Ed, New York, NY: Springer-Verlag; 1994:115–219

334. Cockey BM, Fishman EK, Jones B, Siegelman SS. Computed tomography of abdominal carcinoid tumor. *J Comput Assist Tomogr* 1985;9:38–42

335. Seshul MB, Coulan CM. Pseudomyxoma peritonei: computed tomography and sonography. *AJR Am J Roentgenol* 1981;136:803–806

336. Mueller PR, Ferruci JT, Harbin WP, et al. Appearance of lymphomatous involvement of the mesentery of ultrasonography and body computed tomography: the "sandwich sign." *Radiology* 1980;134:467

337. Ros PR, Olmstead WWM, Moser RP, et al. Mesenteric and omental cysts: histologic classification with imaging correlation. *Radiology* 1987;164:327–332

338. Vanek VW, Phillips AK. Retroperitoneal, mesenteric, and omental cysts. *Arch Surg* 1984;119(7):830–842

339. Nakamura H, Hashimoto T, Akashi H, Mizumoto S. Distinctive CT findings of unusual mesenteric cysts. *J Comput Assist Tomogr* 1987;11:1024–1025

340. Gore RM. Ascites and peritoneal fluid collections. In: Gore RM, Levine MS, Laufer I (eds), *Textbook of Gastrointestinal Radiology,* Vol 2. Philadelphia, PA: WB Saunders; 1994:2352–2365

341. Gooding GAW, Cummings SR. Sonographic detection of ascites in liver disease. *J Ultrasound Med* 1984;3:164–172

342. Edell SL, Gefter WB. Ultrasonic differentiation of types of ascite fluid. *AJR Am J Roentgenol* 1979;133:111–114

343. Bydder GM, Kreel L. Attenuation values of fluid collections within the abdomen. *J Comput Assist Tomogr* 1980;4:145–150

344. Terrier F, Revel D, Pajannen H, et al. MR imaging of body fluid collections. *J CAT* 1986;10:953–962

345. Federle MP, Jeffrey RB. Hemoperitoneum studied by computed tomography. *Radiology* 1983;148:187–192

346. Seltzer SE. Analysis of the tethered-bowel sign on abdominal CT as a predictor of a malignant ascites. *Gastrointest Radiol* 1987;12:245–249

347. Tsujimoto F, Miyamoto Y, Tada S. Differentiation of benign from malignant ascites by sonographic evaluation of gallbladder wall. *Radiology* 1985;157:503–504

348. Jeffrey RB. *CT and Sonography of the Acute Abdomen.* New York, NY: Raven Press; 1989:201–261

349. Stapakis JC, Thickman D. Diagnosis of pneumoperitoneum: abdominal CT vs. upright chest film. *J Comput Assist Tomogr* 1992;16:713–716

350. Jeffrey RB, Federele MP, Wall S. Value of computed tomography in detecting occult gastrointestinal perforation. *J Comput Assist Tomogr* 1983;7:825–826

351. Wolf EL. Ischemic Disease of the Gut. In: Gore RM, Levine MS, Laufer I (eds), *Textbook of Gastrointestinal Radiology,* Vol 2. Philadelphia, PA: WB Saunders; 1994:2694–2706

352. Rosen A, Korobkin M, Silverman PM, et al. Mesenteric vein thrombosis: CT identification. *AJR Am J Roentgenol* 1984;143:83–86

353. Federele MP, Chun G, Jeffrey RB, Rayor R. Computed tomograhic findings in bowel infarction. *AJR Am J Roentgenol* 1984;142:91–95

354. Alperin MB, Glazer GM, Francis IR. Ischemic or infarcted bowel; CT findings. *Radiology* 1988;166:149–152

355. Smerud MJ, Johnson CD, Stevens DH: Diagnosis of bowel infarction: a comparison of plain films and CT scans in 23 cases. *AJR Am J Roentgenol* 1990;154:99–103

356. Silverman PM, Baker ME, Cooper C, Kelvin FM. CT appearance of diffuse mesenteric edema. *J Comput Assist Tomogr* 1986;10:67–70

357. Riso MJ, Federele MP, Griffiths BG. Bowel and mesenteric injury following blunt abdominal trauma, evaluation with CT. *Radiology* 1989;144:143–148

358. Meyers MA. *Dynamic Radiology of the Abdomen,* 4th ed. New York, NY: Springer-Verlag; 1994:519–549

359. Ghahremani GG. Abdominal and pelvic hernias. In: Gore RM, Levine MS, Laufer I (eds), *Textbook of Gastrointestinal Radiology,* Vol 2. Philadelphia, PA: WB Saunders; 1994:2382–2400

360. Ghahremani GG, Meyers MA: Internal abdominal hernias. *Curr Probl Radiol* 1975;5:1–30

361. Ekberg O. Herniography. In: Gore RM, Levine MS, Laufer I (eds), *Textbook of Gastrointestinal Radiology,* Vol. 2. Philadelphia, PA: WB Saunders; 1994:2321–2327

362. Marn C. Anterior abdominal wall. In: Gore RM, Levine MS, Laufer I (eds), *Textbook of Gastrointestinal Radiology,* Vol 2. Philadelphia, PA: WB Saunders; 1994:2401–2411

2

Diagnostic Angiography and Interventional Radiology

Steven C. Rose

■ HISTORICAL PERSPECTIVE

The rapidly expanding specialty of diagnostic angiography and interventional radiology has been dependent upon convergence of an array of technical developments from many diverse fields. As a result of these innovations, the invasiveness of a wide range of diagnostic and therapeutic procedures can be minimized using radiologic imaging modalities to guide small-caliber devices through natural conduits and soft tissue planes within the body.

Milestones in radiologic imaging include the discovery of X-rays in 1895 by Roentgen, followed by the development of fluoroscopy, image intensifiers, and rapid film changers in the 1930s and 1940s, and digital subtraction angiography in the 1980s. Static grayscale ultrasound was introduced in 1974. During the late 1970s, the advent of real-time scanning devices permitted sonographic guidance for needle biopsy and drainage of fluid collections. Since the introduction of computed tomography (CT) in 1973, profound advances in image resolution and scan speed have made CT an essential modality for assessment of abdominal disease and have allowed CT guidance for percutaneous biopsy and drainage of fluid collections.

The first use of *intravascular radiopaque contrast media* was made by Haschek and Lindenthal in 1896 when they injected Teichman's mixture into the vessels of an amputated hand.[2] In 1923 Berberich and Hirsh described strontium bromide contrast studies of the arteries and veins in living human subjects.[3] The era of less toxic intravascular organic iodide contrast media was ushered in by Swick in 1929.[4]

Although *intravascular access* has been recorded as early as 1665 by Christopher Wren, the modern hypodermic needle was first developed and used by Alexander Wood circa 1850. In 1928 Moniz and colleagues described direct-injection carotid angiography.[5] During the same year Forssman passed a urethral catheter transvenously into his own right atrium.[6] Transfemoral aortography was first described by Farinas in 1941.[7] The era of modern angiography and subsequently, interventional radiology was issued in by Seldinger's technique of percutaneously introducing an angiographic catheter into an artery that was larger than the vascular access needle.[8] Seldinger accomplished this exchange over a relatively atraumatic guidewire. Extruded radiopaque angiographic catheters were developed in the 1950s. Continued improvement in both catheter and guidewire technology has radically expanded diagnostic and therapeutic capabilities.

Vascular interventional radiology dates to 1964 when Dotter and Judkins reported dilation of stenotic superficial femoral arteries with coaxial Teflon dilators.[9] Widespread acceptance of percutaneous transluminal angioplasty (PTA) did not occur until 1974 when Gruntzig developed, and demonstrated the efficacy of, double-lumen balloon dilation catheters for use in arterial stenoses.[10] Milestones in abdominal transcatheter vascular intervention include the use of intra-arterial vasopressin for control of variceal upper gastrointestinal hemorrhage,[11] the use of autologous clot for embolization of upper gastrointestinal bleeding sites,[12] the initial development of transcatheter expandable metallic intravascular stents,[13] the conceptualization of transjugular intrahepatic portosystemic shunt (TIPS) placement to remedy portal hypertension,[14] and the advancement of percutaneous treatment of abdominal malignancies by using various transcatheter and transneedle regimens in the 1980s.

Important advances in the development of *abdominal nonvascular interventional radiology* include the introduction of percutaneous transhepatic cholangiography by Huard in 1937,[15] percutaneous biliary drainage by Molnar in 1974,[16] percutaneous drainage of fluid collections by Gronvall and others in 1977,[17] balloon dilation of biliary-enteric strictures by Molnar in 1978,[18] and percutaneous feeding gastrostomy by Sacks and associates in 1983.[19] Genitourinary interventional radiologic advances are outside the scope of this chapter.

■ DIAGNOSTIC ANGIOGRAPHY

OVERVIEW

Vascular access for angiographic procedures usually is achieved with a modified Seldinger technique.[8] Typically, a thin-walled 18-gauge arterial needle is used to puncture the common femoral artery. The transfemoral route is generally both simpler and safer than others.[20] Should the transfemoral arterial access be nonusable owing to aortoiliac occlusive disease, alternate routes include the transbracheal arterial and translumbar aortic routes. A floppy-tipped guidewire (typically 0.035 to 0.038 inch in diameter) is passed through the needle and positioned under fluoroscopic guidance within the abdominal aorta. The needle is removed and an angiographic catheter (usually 4 to 7 French [Fr]) is advanced over the stationary guidewire. If flush aortography (near-simultaneous opacification of the abdominal aorta and the regional branch vessels) is desired, iodinated contrast media is rapidly injected (eg, 20 to 25 mL/sec for 2 seconds) via a multiple side-hole catheter with a pigtail-shaped tip. If opacification of a single arterial bed is desired (selective arteriography), then a catheter with a tip shaped to reflect the anatomic configuration of the branch artery and its relationship to the aorta is positioned such that the tip is in the proximal portion of the target vessel. The rate of contrast media injection in selective arteriography should reflect the arterial caliber and estimated rate of blood flow (eg, 4 to 10 mL/sec).

Images may be acquired with conventional-cut film or digital acquisition. Digital acquisition of images either may be subtracted (a photographic manipulation to remove the noncontrast-filled background image information and to leave only images of the opacified artery) or nonsubtracted. Filming parameters (eg, rate and timing) are generally set to acquire images during (1) the arterial phase of contrast filling, (2) the capillary or parenchymal phase, and (3) the late or venous phase. Portal venous opacification may be optimized by administration of a potent regional vasodilator to speed arteriovenous transit. Commonly, 25 mg of tolazoline is injected via the angiographic catheter just prior to injection of the contrast material into the superior mesenteric artery (SMA).

When the examination is completed, the angiographic catheter is removed and hemostasis is obtained by compression of the arteriotomy site for at least 10 to 15 minutes. In uncomplicated angiography, a patient is kept in bed with the involved extremity held relatively immobile for 6 to 8 hours.

PATIENT PREPARATION

Oral fluids should be encouraged to assure adequate hydration and to minimize the risk of contrast-induced nephropathy. An intravenous line is necessary to administer intraprocedural fluid and drugs. In most patients, serum creatinine should be measured to screen for occult renal insufficiency, a risk factor for contrast-induced renal failure. If either a disease- or drug-induced coagulopathy is suspected, evaluations of the platelet count, prothrombin time, and possibly partial thromboplastin time or bleeding time is suggested.

In patients with a documented history of prior contrast reaction, prophylactic administration of adrenocorticosteroids (eg, Prednisone, 20 mg po 13 hours, 7 hours, and 1 hour prior to angiography) diminishes the risk of recurrent reactions.[21] If prior reactions have been severe, intravenous cimetidine (300 mg) and diphenhydramine (25 to 50 mg) may be added to the prophylactic regimen. The use of nonionic contrast media may be indicated.

Continuous or frequent periodic monitoring of the patient's blood pressure, pulse, EKG tracing, and arterial oxygen saturation should be standard operating procedure. Additionally, equipment and trained personnel must be immediately available to manage cardiopulmonary resuscitation.

COMPLICATIONS

Complications are infrequent, but do occur. The sources of mortality and morbidity are somewhat predictable and therefore partially preventable.

Access site complications generally are the result of inadequate hemostasis with resultant hemorrhage or pseudoaneurysm formation and, infrequently, arteriovenous fistualization. In Hessel's classic study of angiographic complications, puncture-site complications requiring intervention or complicated patient care were significantly lower for the transfemoral route (0.47%) than for the translumbar (0.58%) or transaxillary route (1.7%).[20] Since hemorrhage into the axillary sheath may lead to irreversible brachial plexus injury, the transaxillary route generally has been abandoned for the safer, more peripheral, high brachial approach. Because compression of the aortic puncture site is not possible with the translumbar route, suboptimally controlled hypertension and coagulopathic states constitute contraindications to this route. Risk factors for puncture-site bleeding and pseudoaneurysm formation include hypertension, coagulopathy (including anticoagulation), use of large-diameter catheters, brittle arteries, puncture-site cephalad to the inguinal ligament, improper arterial compression technique and patient motion. Preventative measures include optimized blood pressure control and hemostatic function, careful placement of the puncture site over the femoral head (for compression), use of the smallest catheters feasible, enforced patient immobilization, and careful observation for bleeding or hematoma at the puncture site. Sandbag compression and most pressure dressings are ineffective and may obscure an expanding hematoma. Should an expanding hematoma, pseudoaneurysm, or arteriovenous fistula form in spite of these precautions, ultrasonically directed arterial compression has been shown to be an effective noninvasive treatment in the majority of these cases.[22]

A problem peculiar to the pediatric population involves intense arterial spasm near the puncture site with secondary femoral arterial thrombosis. Preventative measures include liberal patient sedation, hydration and warmth, gentle use of small atraumatic needles, guidewires and catheters, frequent administration of intra-arterial nitroglycerine, consideration of systemic anticoagulants, and possible weight-adjusted doses of calcium channel–blocking agents. Should the femoral pulse be lost, expectant management or thrombectomy is preferred to operative reconstruction, in most cases.[23]

Local intra-arterial complications include subintimal passage of guidewire catheter or injected contrast material, causing an arterial dissection that encroaches on the arterial lumen, perforation of the artery (0.4%),[22] local arterial thrombosis (0.1%), and distal embolization (0.1%)[20] of either fibrinoplatelet material or cholesterol crystals. Risk factors include catheter diameter, the duration of the procedure, stiffness and design of

the guidewires and catheters, arterial tortuosity, aneurysm formation or advanced occlusive disease, advancement of the catheter selectively into more peripheral small-caliber vessels, and operator inexperience.[20,24] Recent technical advances have allowed passage of small-diameter steerable catheters over highly visible, steerable, atraumatic guidewires into small-caliber peripheral superselective arterial branches with negligible risk. In selected cases, anticoagulation calcium channel–blocking agents and vasodilators are warranted to prevent catheter-induced thrombosis.

Contrast-induced nephrotoxicity primarily affects the renal tubules and occurs as a result of angiography in approximately 1% of procedures.[25–27] The onset, manifested as oliguria, usually occurs within 48 hours; renal function peaks at 4 to 5 days and usually returns to the preangiographic baseline in 10 to 14 days. Risk factors include preexistent renal insufficiency, diabetes mellitus (particularly if azotemic), congestive heart failure, and multiple myeloma (if dehydrated). Possible risk factors include dehydration, advanced age, large volumes of contrast media, and hyperuricemia. Preventative measures include screening for occult renal insufficiency (serum creatinine), hydration, and optimization of cardiac function. The value of using nonionic contrast media to prevent contrast-induced nephrotoxicity remains controversial. If available and feasible for the given study, CO_2-angiography represents a technique that avoids all risk of contrast-related nephropathy.[28] Digital-subtraction angiography permits the use of smaller volumes of contrast.

Systemic reactions to contrast media are idiosyncratic, occur rapidly (94% within 20 minutes of contrast injection) and range from the common, mild reactions that occur in approximately 1 of 15 to 30 examinations and require no treatment (eg, urticaria) to the rare, life-threatening severe reactions that occur in approximately 1 of 1,000 to 4,000 examinations (eg, laryngeal edema or anaphylactoid cardiopulmonary collapse).[29] Contrast reactions are fatal in approximately 1 of 15,000 to 90,000 examinations. Risk factors include a history of atopy (4-fold risk), prior contrast reactions (10-fold risk), age over 50 years, and preexistent heart disease (5-fold risk). Preventative measures include prophylactic regimens of steroids (at least 12 hours before contrast injection) and H_1- and H_2-antihistamine therapy.[21] Two recent large surveys indicate that nonionic contrast media significantly diminishes the risk of contrast reactions relative to ionic contrast media, particularly severe reactions in high-risk patients.[30,31] Universal usage of nonionic contrast media currently is made impractical because of the 8- to 10-fold increase in cost.

SPECIFIC APPLICATIONS

Hepatic Angiography

The role of angiography for evaluation of liver diseases has been altered radically by technologic advances. Whereas angiography was once a mainstay for detection and characterization of liver masses, current noninvasive techniques such as ultrasound, computed tomography (CT), magnetic resonance imaging (MRI) and, occasionally, nuclear medicine have been shown to have superior sensitivity, less risk, and a lower cost. Additionally, percutaneous biopsy under ultrasound or CT guidance has been proven safe and provides a tissue-specific diagnosis.

On the other hand, angiography still has an important role because increasingly sophisticated advances in hepatobiliary surgery such as transplantation, various portosystemic shunts, and multisegmental liver resection have mandated a preoperative knowledge of individual vascular anatomy, vascular involvement by the disease process (eg, arterial encasement or portal vein thrombosis), and hemodynamic status (eg, portal venous pressure and direction of flow).

Arterial anatomy. The celiac trunk provides arterial inflow to the foregut structures. Most commonly, the first-order branches are the common hepatic, left gastric, and splenic arteries, although many variant patterns of arterial supply have been described.[32] Angiography is useful in preoperative detection of these normal variants.

Venous anatomy. The portal vein, formed by the confluence of the splenic and the superior mesenteric veins just ventral to the inferior vena cava, provides approximately two-thirds of the vascular inflow to the liver. Intrahepatically, the portal vein branches travel with the

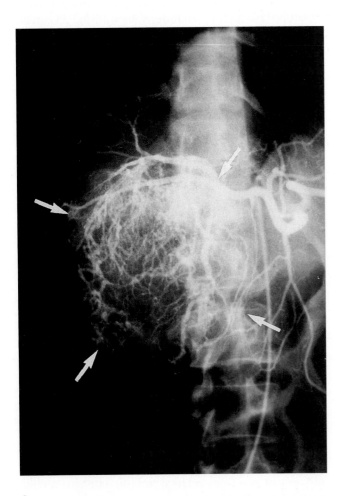

A

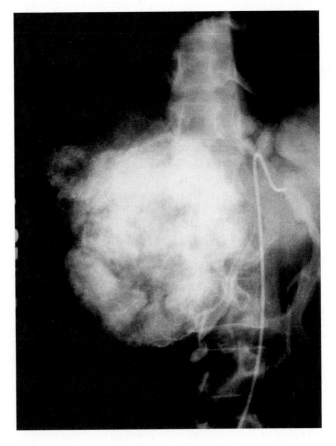

B

Figure 2–1. Angiographic manifestations of neovascularity in a middle-aged female with fibrolamellar-hepatocellular carcinoma of the liver. **A.** Arterial-phase anteroposterior view, celiac angiogram documents bizarre arterial course, caliber and branching pattern of the tumor (*between white arrows*). Adjacent normal, large-caliber arteries have been displaced around the tumor. **B.** Parenchymal phase, same injection demonstrates an intense inhomogeneous hypervascular contrast stain of the tumor.

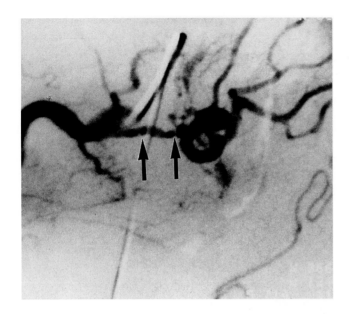

A

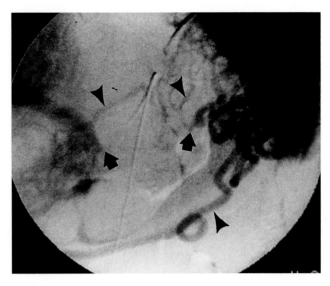

B

Figure 2–2. Arterial encasement and venous occlusion by a hypovascular scirrhous malignancy in a patient with pancreatic adenocarcinoma of the tail of the pancreas. **A.** Arterial phase, anteroposterior view, digital-subtraction angiogram of the celiac trunk shows an irregular segment of splenic artery narrowing due to serrated encasement (*black arrows*). **B.** Venous phase of the same injection demonstrates occlusion of the splenic venous segment between the black arrows; collateral drainage (*arrowheads*) of the spleen occurs via the gastroepiploic and short gastric/left gastric venous arcades.

branches of the hepatic artery and the bile ducts within the hepatic segments.

The hepatic veins course between hepatic segments and are, therefore, useful surgical landmarks. The right hepatic vein courses in the intersegmental fissure between the anterior and posterior segments of the right lobe, the middle hepatic vein in the interlobar fissure between the right and left lobes, and the left hepatic vein in the intersegmental fissure between the medial and lateral segments of the left lobe.

Normally, small communications occur at the sinusoidal level between adjacent hepatic-venous branches, portal venous branches, hepatic artery–to–portal venous branches, and portal vein–to–hepatic venous branches. In some pathologic states (eg, cirrhosis or Budd-Chiari syndrome) these shunts may enlarge.

Hepatic neoplasia and masses.

Overview. Depending on the biology and the growth characteristics of a mass, the angiogram may manifest a variety of vascular alterations. As they grow, neoplasms (particularly if malignant) generate a system of internal vascular channels termed *neovascularity or vascular neoformation* that typically are devoid of endothelium and media. Tumoral neovascularity is characterized angiographically by a cluster of vessels that have a serpiginous

course, irregular caliber, a bizarre branching pattern, and nonhomogeneous capillary or parenchyma stain (Fig 2–1). Intratumoral necrosis may be evidenced angiographically by collections of contrast known as *pools* or *lakes*. As tumors or masses expand, surrounding native vessels are involved secondarily. Simple mass expansion results in displacement of vessels from the normal course. Infiltration or invasion of a tumor around a native vessel may cause *vascular encasement:* narrowing of the lumen and/or focal deviation in the vessel course. *Serrated encasement* refers to fine, jagged margination of the lumen caused by direct tumoral invasion and is specific for malignancy (Fig 2–2). *Serpiginous encasement* manifests as a sharply angulated, irregular course to vessels distorted locally by disordered growth within a tumor and is suggestive for, but not diagnostic of, malignancy. *Smooth* encasement, a gradual tapered narrowing of the vessel caliber, is a nonspecific angiographic finding that may be seen with malignant tumors, chronic inflammation, or fibrosis (Fig 2–3). Ultimately, any encasing process may occlude a vessel, especially thinwalled, easily compressed veins (Fig 2–2 and 2–4). Additional venous findings include *arteriovenous shunting* (early, dense opacification of the veins) and direct *intraluminal tumoral extension* (Fig 2–4 and 2–5), both of which are strongly suggestive of malignancy. Intraluminal extension most often occurs with hepatocellular car-

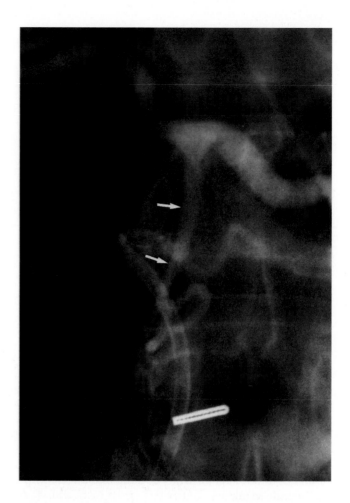

Figure 2–3. Smooth encasement of the gastroduodenal artery (*arrows*) owing to chronic pancreatitis. Magnified anteroposterior view of the celiac arteriogram. Same case as Figure 2–19.

cinoma but also may be seen with cholangiocarcinoma, renal cell carcinoma, and adrenal carcinoma.

In general, the dominant angiographic findings of highly vascular malignancies such as hepatocellular carcinoma are neovascularity with a dense capillary (parenchymal)–phase stain, whereas hypovascular scirrhous tumors such as cholangiocarcinoma or pancreatic carcinoma primarily demonstrate vascular encasement.

Benign tumors and masses. *Cavernous hemangiomas* are focal areas of arrested vascular development that contain ectatic vascular spaces lined by endothelium supported by a fibrous stroma without normal organ parenchyma. Blood flow through the sinusoidal spaces is sluggish. Angiographically, feeding arteries and draining veins are of normal caliber and arteriovenous shunting is not present. Smaller hemangiomas typically are well defined (Fig 2–6), whereas large hemangiomas may have indistinct margins. The ectatic vascular channels fill sluggishly from the periphery toward the center and retain the hypervascular stain very late into the venous phase (Fig 2–6). Occasionally, the central portions of large hemangiomas fail to fill because of in situ thrombosis. Either bolus-enhanced dynamic CT or tagged red

blood cell (RBC) nuclear medicine studies are the preferred modalities for diagnosis of cavernous hemangiomas. These tests are noninvasive, more specific diagnostically, and less expensive than angiography (Fig 2–7). Distinction of hemangiomas from hemangioendotheliomas, angiosarcomas, vascular metastases, or hepatocellular carcinomas may be difficult. Careful skinny-needle biopsy of areas of the mass not in contact with the liver capsule may be necessary for definitive diagnosis (Fig 2–7).[33] This is inadvisable, however, if the mass extends to the capsule, since cavernous hemangiomas may bleed massively. In the case of giant cavernous hemangiomas of infancy, transcatheter embolization may permit stabilization of congestive heart failure until spontaneous involution occurs within the initial year or so of life.[34]

Hemangioendotheliomas are vascular dysplasias in young children, and they usually manifest as an upper abdominal mass associated with high-output congestive heart failure. Similar to cavernous hemangiomas, sinusoids trap contrast until late in the venous phase. However, as a result of the hyperdynamic state, feeding arteries and draining veins are dilated, and arteriovenous shunting usually is present. Owing to potential malig-

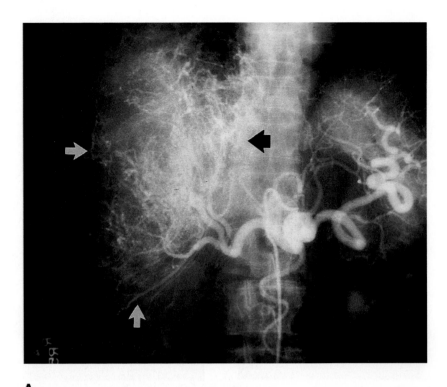

A

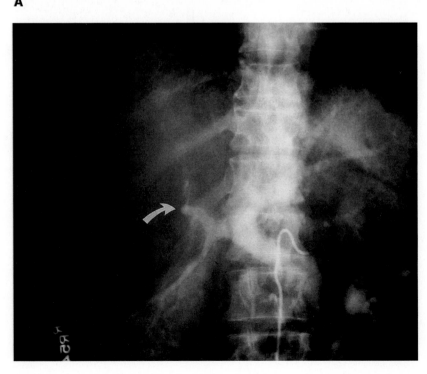

B

Figure 2–4. Portal invasion by hepatoma. **A.** Arterial-phase anteroposterior view, celiac angiogram demonstrates neovascularity of a large mass (*arrows*) occupying nearly the entire right lobe of the liver. **B.** Venous phase, same injection shows occlusion (*curved white arrow*) of the right portal vein.

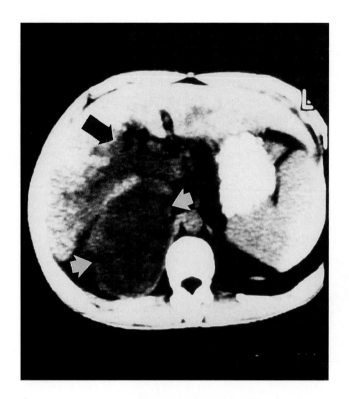

A

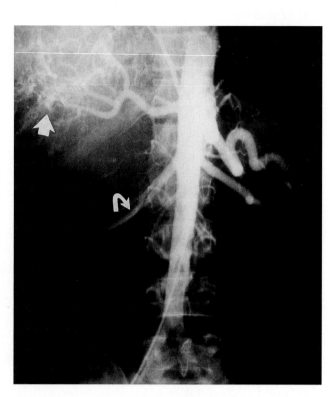

B

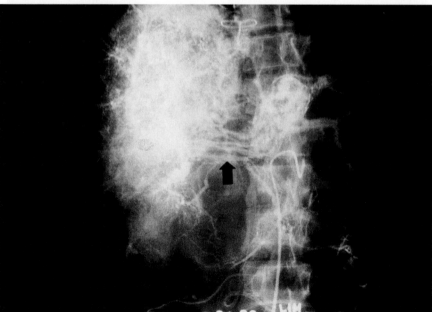

C

Figure 2–5. Venous invasion by hepatoma. **A.** Contrast-enhanced CT scan at the level of the liver documents a nonenhancing mass (*black arrow*) within the posterior aspect of the right hepatic lobe with a large extension (*white arrows*) into the retroperitoneum posteriorly. **B.** Arterial phase; anteroposterior view, flush abdominal aortogram demonstrates hypervascular liver mass (*straight arrow*) and caudal displacement of the right renal artery (*curved arrow*). **C.** Venous phase; anteroposterior view celiac arteriogram shows a large intraluminal-filling defect (tumor thrombus) within the portal vein (*black arrow*) *Continued*

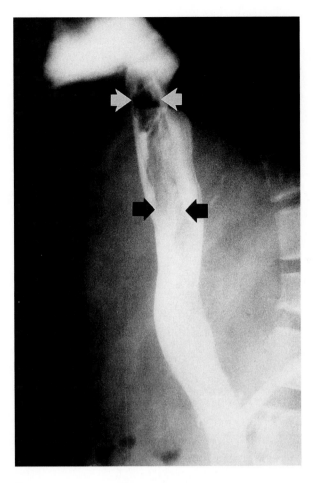

Figure 2–5, cont'd. D. Lateral view; inferior vena cavagram defines a large tumor thrombus (*arrows*) within the inferior vena cava. The patient's head is to the top of the illustration, and ventral surface to the reader's left.

D

nant degeneration, hemangioendotheliomas require resection. Preoperative transcatheter embolization may be a useful surgical adjunct to optimize the child's cardiac status, allow growth to a more favorable age, and minimize intraoperative blood loss.[35]

Hepatic adenomas are benign neoplasms that consist of hepatocytes, are found primarily in women of reproductive age, and are associated with use of oral contraceptives. The tumors are usually large, solitary, and well defined. Surrounding arteries and veins are displaced by the mass; thus, the vascular supply courses inward from the periphery. The parenchymal phase is marked by a hypervascular stain without pooling or other stigmata of malignancies. Since these tumors present a risk of life-threatening hemorrhage and spontaneous involution is rare, excision is often recommended.

Focal nodular hyperplasia consists of a central stellate fibrotic scar surrounded by a mass of hepatocytes, Kupfer cells, and proliferating bile ducts. These tumors are found in both men and women of all ages. Similar to the angiographic appearance of an adenoma, focal nodular hyperplasia is frequently a well-marginated hypervascular mass (or masses) with a nodular texture to the stain

and is fed via peripherally placed arteries. Angiographic clues that may allow distinction of focal nodular hyperplasia from an adenoma include finding a portion of the arterial supply that penetrates centrally before branching out into the mass ("spoke-wheel" appearance), or identifying bands of nonstaining fibrous septae within the mass. Since many of these tumors contain Kuppfer cells, accumulation of technetium pertchenate 99m (^{99m}TC)–sulfur colloid on a liver-spleen scan may allow a definitive diagnosis to be made.

Regenerating nodules represent foci of hepatocellular proliferation stimulated by hepatocyte loss from cirrhosis, liver resection, or trauma. Surrounding vessels are displaced by the expanding mass and feeding arteries tend to be scarce. The parenchymal stain is usually homogeneous, similar to adjacent regions of normal liver. The angiographic stigmata of malignancy are absent.

Cysts, abscesses, and other *nonneoplastic masses* are angiographically manifest by vascular displacement and an absence of parenchymal stain within the mass. Occasionally, a hypervascular stain may surround the mass because of compression of normal parenchyma.

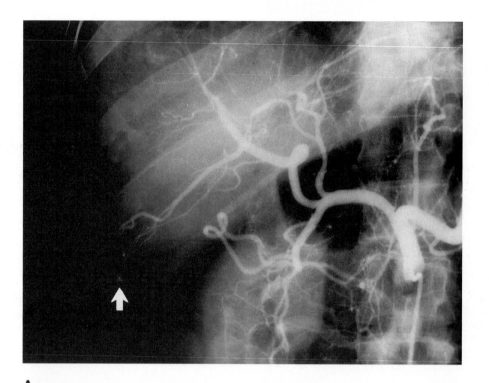

A

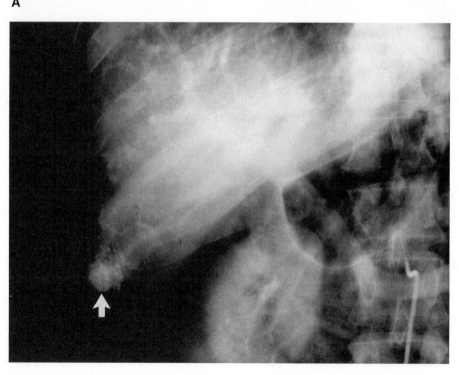

B

Figure 2–6. Angiographic appearance of a small hepatic hemangioma. **A.** Arterial phase; anteroposterior view, celiac angiogram shows early filling of the hemangioma (*white arrow*) in the caudal aspect of the right lobe. The feeding hepatic artery is normal and no early draining veins are present. **B.** Venous phase; same injection documents persistent contrast stain within the hemangioma (*white arrow*).

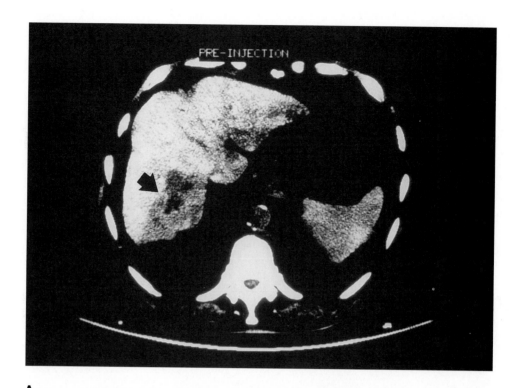

Figure 2–7. Hepatic cavernous hemangioma. **A.** Noncontrast CT scan of the abdomen at the level of the liver shows a hypodense mass (*black arrow*) in the posterior segment of the right lobe. **B.** Repeat CT scan 28 minutes following a bolus injection of contrast media documents homogeneous contrast enhancement of the entire mass. *Continued*

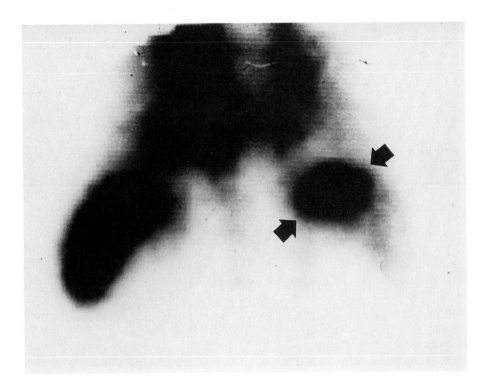

C

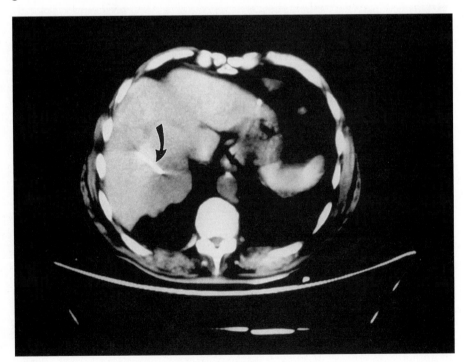

D

Figure 2–7, cont'd. C. Posterior view; 99mTc-RBC nuclear medicine scan confirms that the mass is radiointense (*black arrows*). **D.** Owing to an atypical early-draining vein seen angiographically (not shown), a skinny-needle (20 gauge) biopsy (*black arrow*) was performed to rule out malignancy. Note that the needle route was selected to traverse normal hepatic parenchyma prior to entering the subcapsular mass.

Malignant masses. Hepatocellular carcinoma (hepatoma) is usually found in patients with cirrhosis and/or hepatitis B exposure. Three morphologic patterns are found: (1) solitary, (2) multicentric, and (3) diffuse infiltrating. Angiographically, solitary hepatomas are usually well-defined hypervascular masses with tumor neovascularity fed via enlarged hepatic arteries (Fig 2–1). Hepatic artery–to–portal vein shunting or portal venous invasion by tumor is a relatively specific angiographic finding for hepatoma. The less differentiated, multicentric, and diffuse infiltrating hepatomas are more ill-defined, less vascular, and present a greater diagnostic challenge, particularly in the setting of liver cirrhosis (Fig 2–4).

When feasible, the preferred treatment of solitary hepatomas is surgical resection. Therefore, the goals of preoperative angiographic evaluation are to define the anatomy of the feeding arteries, localize the tumor within a specific hepatic lobe or segment, and exclude portal-vein invasion or additional foci of tumor. A useful adjunct to routine angiography for preoperative planning of hepatomas (and other hypervascular malignancies) is CT arteriography. In this procedure, the angiographic catheter is placed within the celiac trunk in the angiography suite and the patient is transferred to the CT scanner. Diluted contrast is power injected (eg, 260 mL of 15% strength contrast at a rate of 1.5 mL/sec), and a dynamic CT (eg, 1 slice every 6 seconds) of the liver is performed and followed by a repeat delayed scan (eg, 4 hours) to assess possible flow-related artifacts (Fig 2–8E). CT arteriography is superior to routine angiography and standard contrast-enhanced CT for definition of the extent of tumor, location relative to vascular landmarks, and detection of supernumerary tumors.[36] In patients with a right hepatic artery re-placed to the superior mesenteric artery, the right hepatic lobe is not adequately assessed by CT arteriography; thus, CT portography (discussed below under metastases) is probably a more appropriate procedure.

Cholangiocarcinomas are infiltrating scirrhous adenocarcinomas of the bile ducts, tend to be hypovascular, and manifest themselves angiographically with arterial encasement. Diagnosis and staging is primarily performed by CT, endoscopic retrograde cholangiopancreatography (ERCP), and transhepatic cholangiography.

Metastases generally reflect the biologic behavior and angiographic appearance of the primary tumor. Hypervascular metastases are usually multiple well-defined masses of varying size that are detected in the parenchymal phase as areas of intense contrast staining (Fig 2–9). Examples include choriocarcinoma, renal cell carcinoma, leiomyosarcomas, endocrine tumors, carcinoid, and some gastrointestinal-tract tumors. In contrast, both hypovascular and hypervascular metastases may be evident angiographically as foci with a dearth of contrast during the portal venous or late phase, when the normal liver parenchyma maximally enhances (the "Swiss-cheese" appearance) (Fig 2–9); examples include metastases from primary carcinoma of the lung, pancreas, and many gastrointestinal malignancies. In patients with potentially resectable hepatic metastases, the preoperative angiographic evaluation is similar to that employed for hepatomas. In general, CT arteriography (described above) best defines hypervascular tumors, whereas CT portography functions best for hypovascular metastases. In the latter, the angiographic catheter is placed into the superior mesenteric artery (beyond any replaced hepatic arteries, if present) using minimal contrast. In the CT scan, relatively dense contrast is power injected into the superior mesenteric artery (eg, 200 mL of a 60% strength solution of contrast injected at 1.3 mL/sec), followed by a short delay (eg, 15 sec), a dynamic CT of the liver, then a delayed (eg, 4 hours) repeat scan.[37] Because abnormalities are not histologically specific and occasionally represent flow-related artifacts, corroboration with biopsy or other imaging modalities is suggested.[38,39]

Preoperative to liver transplantation or portosystemic shunts. Technically demanding and potentially morbid surgical procedures performed to remedy endstage liver failure and/or portal hypertension (and in the case of liver transplantation, utilizing scarce resources) are becoming more common. It is imperative to evaluate patients thoroughly to ensure the advisability of the operation and to plan the optimal surgical approach. A complete angiographic evaluation includes assessment of arterial anatomy; patency, direction of flow, and approximate pressure of the portal venous system; the presence and extent of varices; and the patency and pressure of the hepatic veins, inferior vena cava, and, potentially, the left renal vein. Arterial anatomy and antegrade evaluation of the portal venous system, including assessment of varices, is accomplished via separate celiac and superior mesenteric arterial contrast injections (arterial portography).

The status of the hepatic veins is assessed via transvenous selective catheterization and contrast injection into the hepatic veins (free-hepatic venography). Wedged-hepatic venography is accomplished by either advancing a standard angiographic catheter peripherally in the hepatic venous system until it is impacted, or by inflating a balloon catheter until it occludes the hepatic venous branch, followed by contrast injection. Normally, homogeneous staining of the surrounding hepatic sinusoids

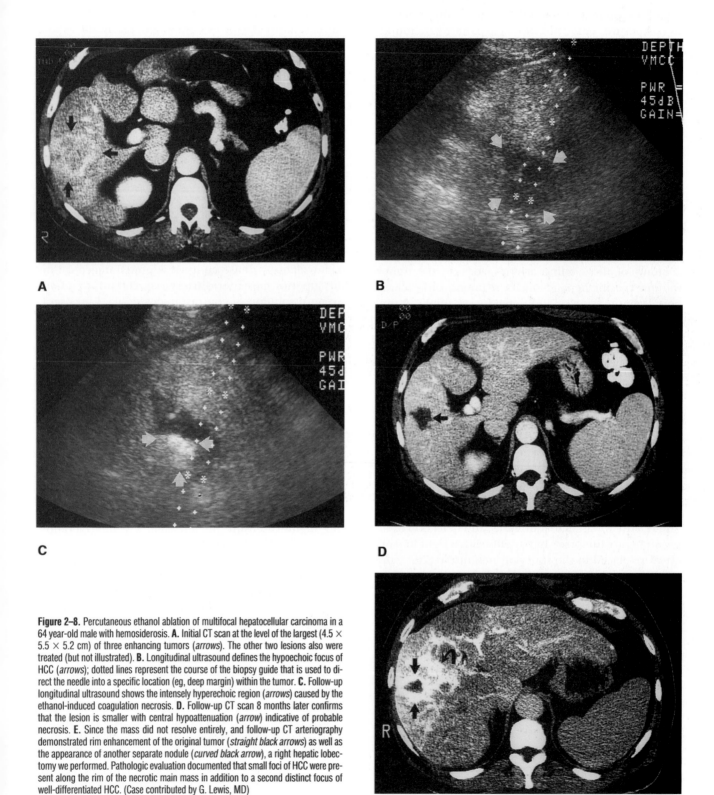

Figure 2–8. Percutaneous ethanol ablation of multifocal hepatocellular carcinoma in a 64 year-old male with hemosiderosis. **A.** Initial CT scan at the level of the largest (4.5 × 5.5 × 5.2 cm) of three enhancing tumors (*arrows*). The other two lesions also were treated (but not illustrated). **B.** Longitudinal ultrasound defines the hypoechoic focus of HCC (*arrows*); dotted lines represent the course of the biopsy guide that is used to direct the needle into a specific location (eg, deep margin) within the tumor. **C.** Follow-up longitudinal ultrasound shows the intensely hyperechoic region (*arrows*) caused by the ethanol-induced coagulation necrosis. **D.** Follow-up CT scan 8 months later confirms that the lesion is smaller with central hypoattenuation (*arrow*) indicative of probable necrosis. **E.** Since the mass did not resolve entirely, and follow-up CT arteriography demonstrated rim enhancement of the original tumor (*straight black arrows*) as well as the appearance of another separate nodule (*curved black arrow*), a right hepatic lobectomy we performed. Pathologic evaluation documented that small foci of HCC were present along the rim of the necrotic main mass in addition to a second distinct focus of well-differentiated HCC. (Case contributed by G. Lewis, MD)

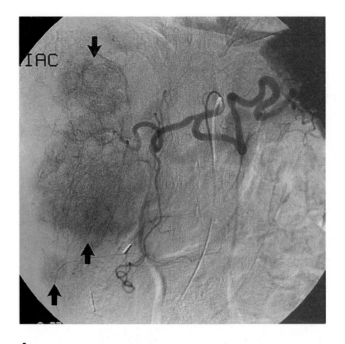

A

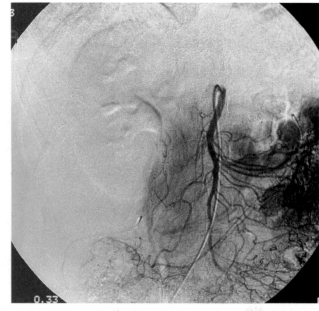

B

C

Figure 2–9. Preferential hepatic arterial supply to hypervascular liver metastases in a 72 year-old female with a primary adenocarcinoma of the colon. **A.** The tumors (*arrows*) stain intensely during arterial phase of a celiac digital subtraction angiogram (antero-posterior view). **B.** On arterial portography, contrast was injected into the SMA in order to opacify the portal venous structures. **C.** While the liver parenchyma stains with contrast on the portal venous phase, the tumors (*arrows*) do not, creating the Swiss-cheese appearance.

occurs followed by drainage through the hepatic vein–to-hepatic vein connections (Fig 2–10). With increasing degrees of cirrhosis and portal hypertension, an increasing proportion of the contrast flows from the occluded hepatic venules, via the sinusoids, into the portal venous system (Fig 2–11). In cases of nonopacification of the portal vein after arterial portography, wedged-hepatic venography is a useful technique to opacify the portal vein in a retrograde fashion. Retrograde portal venous

opacification permits distinction of portal vein occlusion from reversed (hepatofugal) portal venous blood flow.

With the hepatic venous catheter in a wedged position, portal venous pressure can be estimated transsinusoidally. Normal portal venous pressure ranges from 4 to 15 cm saline. Pressures greater than 15 cm saline are indicative of portal hypertension. Hemorrhage from gastroesophageal varices generally does not occur unless portal venous pressure is at least 20 to 25 cm saline.

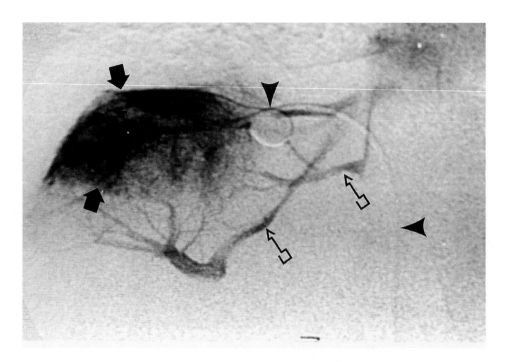

A

Figure 2–10. Normal hepatic vein hemodynamic study in a patient with portal hypertension. **A.** Anteroposterior view; digital subtraction wedged hepatic venogram. Contrast injected by a transfemoral venous balloon catheter (*black arrowsheads*) causes a regional stain of the hepatic parenchyma (*closed black arrows*). Normal communication with neighboring hepatic veins is seen (*open black arrows*). The communicating hepatic veins drain centrally into the right hepatic vein. **B.** Anteroposterior view; digital subtraction inferior vena cavagram reveals a normal appearance to the suprarenal inferior vena cava. *Continued*

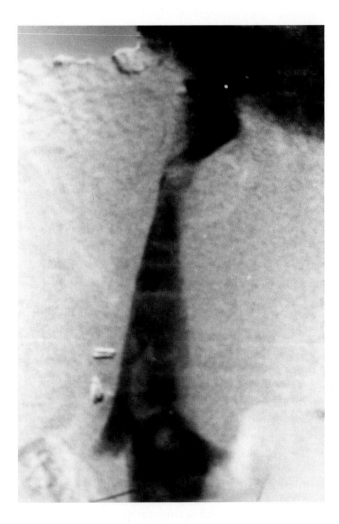

B

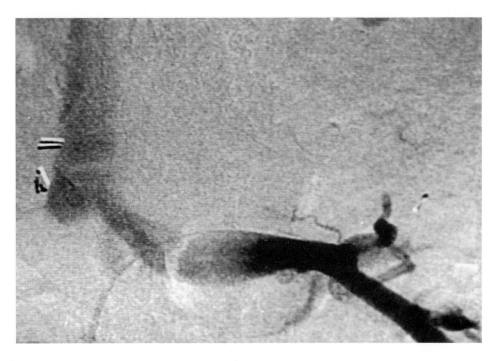

C

Figure 2–10, cont'd. C. Anteroposterior view; digital subtraction left renal venogram is normal. The wedged hepatic venous pressure was 18/16 mm Hg; the free hepatic venous pressure was 15/3 mm Hg; the right atrial pressure was 12/6 mm Hg; and the infrarenal IVC pressure was 15/14 mm Hg for a corrected sinusoidal pressure of 3 mm Hg (normal). The cause of portal hypertension was portal venous occlusion due to invasion by hepatocellular carcinoma. The above study excluded cirrhosis as the cause of portal hypertension; therefore the patient underwent a decompressive splenorenal bypass rather than a TIPS procedure.

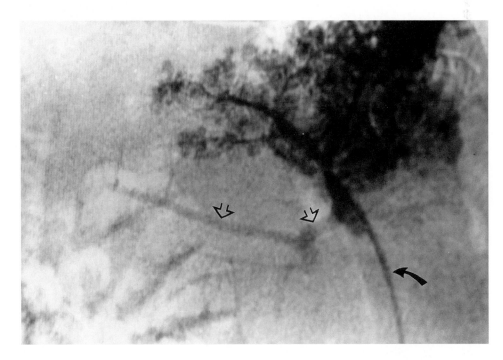

Figure 2–11. Portal venous filling on wedged hepatic venography in a 72 year-old male with portal hypertension as a result of alcoholic cirrhosis. Anteroposterior view; digital subtraction wedged hepatic venogram via a purposely impacted angiographic catheter (*curved arrows*) demonstrates the typical hepatic parenchymal stain as well as filling of peripheral branches of the right portal vein (*open arrows*). The direction of portal venous blood flow is hepatopetal (normal).

Wedged-hepatic venous pressures reflect the severity of sinusoidal and postsinusoidal fibrosis, as is seen in cirrhosis. Alternatively, angiographic evidence of portal hypertension in the face of a normal wedged hepatic–venous pressure suggests a presinusoidal etiology such as portal venous thrombosis (Fig 2–10). Wedged-hepatic venous pressure reflects the portal venous pressure generated to overcome the combination of obstruction to transsinusoidal blood flow and the pressure within the inferior vena cava. The component caused by obstruction to the transsinusoidal blood flow is termed the corrected sinusoidal pressure and is obtained by subtracting the measured pressure within the inferior vena cava from the hepatic vein wedge pressure. Normal corrected sinusoidal pressure is less than 10 cm saline. Wedged-hepatic venous pressure may be artificially elevated by regional intrahepatic arterioportal communications and artifactually depressed by hepatic vein-to-hepatic vein collateral channels; hence, measurements need to be taken in more than one location. Alternatively, infrequently employed techniques to image and obtain pressure recordings of the portal vein include direct transhepatic portal vein puncture, splenoportography (direct needle punc-

ture into the splenic pulp), and open cannulation of the umbilical vein by minilaparotomy.

Since anatomic variants may occur, and hepatic fibrosis or hepatomegaly may obstruct flow or distort the inferior vena cava, inferior vena cavography usually is included in the preoperative angiographic evaluation. Owing to potential anatomic variants of the left renal vein, left renal venography is warranted in patients who are candidates for splenorenal-type portosystemic shunts (Fig 2–10).

In patients with preexisting but potentially failing portosystemic shunts, systemic transvenous access usually permits selective catheterization of the shunt, if patent, in order to measure pressure gradients, perform angiography, and dilate stenoses. If direct cannulation is unsuccessful, transarterial portography, supplemented with image subtraction, will usually allow assessment of shunt patency.

The *Budd-Chiari syndrome* refers to a constellation of diseases that result in obstruction of hepatic-venous drainage. The classical triad of clinical findings are right upper-quadrant pain, hepatosplenomegaly, and rapidly progressive ascites. The anatomic levels of involvement

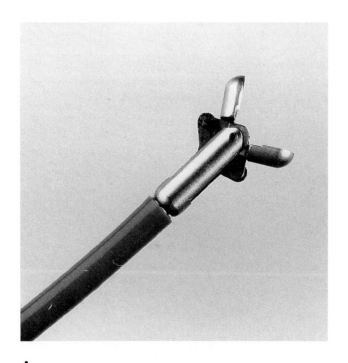

A

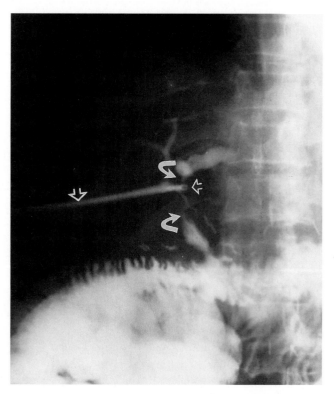

B

Figure 2–12. A. Close-up view of the working end of a transvenous myocardial biopsy forceps. This device may be used for either transvenous liver biopsy or transcatheter biopsy of endoluminal masses. **B.** Anteroposterior radiograph demonstrating the above myocardial biopsy forceps (*open arrows*) being used, via a transhepatic route, to biopsy a long bile-duct stricture (*curved arrows*) suspected to be malignant. The biopsy was of high quality and diagnostic of cholangiocarcinoma. The patient had had a prior choledochojejunostomy.

may include (1) the inferior vena cava (eg, congenital webs or invasive renal cell carcinoma), (2) the hepatic veins (eg, tumoral invasion by hepatoma or thrombosis, either idiopathic or related to hypercoagulable states), and (3) the hepatic venules (eg, in situ thrombosis seen in patients after bone-marrow transplantation). Inferior vena cavography is used to assess inferior vena caval patency. If the inferior vena cava is patent, selective wedged-hepatic venography is performed in at least two of the three hepatic veins. Venographic findings may include direct visualization of hepatic venous tumor or thrombus, the "spider web" appearance of numerous hepatic venous and systemic collateral channels, and portal venous opacification which may, in severe cases, demonstrate hepatofugal flow. In patients with hepatic venule thrombosis, angiographic findings are usually nondiagnostic, thus necessitating biopsy. Because most of these patients have considerable ascites and are coagulopathic, direct percutaneous hepatic biopsy is contraindicated. Transvenous hepatic biopsy can be performed safely with acquisition of histologically satisfactory samples using myocardial biopsy forceps (Fig 2–12).[40,41] Recent reports indicate that duplex ultrasound may represent an acceptable noninvasive technique to diagnose, stage, and follow patients with suspected Budd-Chiari syndrome.[42]

Visceral Angiography

Arterial anatomy. Vascular inflow to the intra-abdominal viscera is via the celiac trunk, the SMA, IMA, and paired internal iliac arteries that roughly supply the foregut, midgut, hindgut, and pelvic viscera, respectively. Variant patterns of arterial supply are common and are detailed in the references.[32]

Vascular interconnections are common in the mesenteric watershed and serve as important collateral blood supplies. The liver intrinsically has a dual vascular inflow: the hepatic artery and the portal vein. Supernumary arterial supply may be present if portions of the left hepatic artery are replaced to the left gastric artery, or portions of the right hepatic artery are replaced to the SMA. Intraparenchymally, innumerable small hepatic artery–to-hepatic artery communications exist. The stomach is fed by multiple-named arteries including the right and left gastric, right and left gastroepiploic, branches of the left inferior phrenic, gastroduodenal, and multiple short gastric arteries. These inflow arteries intercommunicate via a rich submucosal plexus of unnamed small arteries. In addition to the splenic artery, the spleen may be served by arcades involving the short gastric or gastroepiploic arteries. The pancreas is supplied via the dorsal pancreatic artery, multiple pancreatic tail branches from the splenic artery, and the pancreaticoduodenal arcades from both

the hepatic and superior mesenteric arteries, all of which interconnect by an intraparenchymal network. Because of the large and small vessel communications, the foregut is relatively resistant to ischemia.

The celiac and SMA circulations communicate via the pancreaticoduodenal arcades and, occasionally, the dorsal pancreatic artery or arc of Buhler. Within the mesentery, numerous unnamed arterial loops connect the multiple arteries that feed the jejunum and ileum. Unlike the foregut angioarchitecture, the intramural small-caliber arteries of the midgut (vasa recta) have sparce intercommunications and therefore function similarly to end arteries. Because of the paucity of small vessel interconnection, the bowel between the ligament of Treitz and the rectosigmoid junction is at higher risk of infarction, particularly with embolization, either spontaneous or iatrogenic.

The angioarchitecture of the colon to the rectosigmoid junction is typified by the named branch artery (eg, right colic artery) coursing through the mesentery. At the colonic margin, the artery bifurcates into two branches: one passes antegrade, relative to the fecal stream, along the bowel wall; the other passes retrograde. Each branch anastomoses with the corresponding branch from the neighboring colonic artery to form an arcade along the entire course of the colonic wall. This arcade is termed the *marginal artery of Drummond* (Fig 2–13). The innumerable vasa recta arise from the marginal artery to penetrate the colonic wall. Arterial communication between the SMA and IMA circulations is made via a portion of the marginal artery (connecting

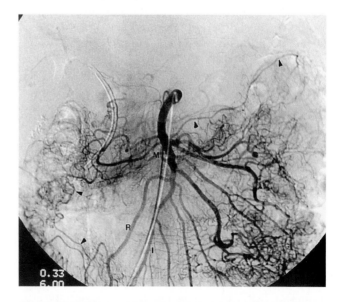

Figure 2–13. Marginal artery of the colon. Selective injection into the SMA demonstrates the marginal artery (*arrowheads*) supplied by the iliocolic (I), right colic (R), and middle colic (M) arteries.

the left branch of the middle colic artery and the ascending branch of the left colic artery) and/or the *arc of Riolan* (an intramesenteric branch connecting the middle and left colic arteries more centrally).

The rectum is supplied via the superior hemorrhoidal arteries from the IMA circulation as well as the middle and inferior hemorrhoidal arteries from the internal iliac arteries bilaterally. The rich submucosal arterial plexus renders the rectum relatively resistant to ischemia and provides an important source of collateral supply between the systemic and mesenteric circulations.

Gastrointestinal hemorrhage. Angiography plays an important role in both the diagnostic evaluation of gastrointestinal (GI) hemorrhage, and its nonoperative management (see section on vascular intervention). The role of angiography differs depending on whether the GI hemorrhage is acute and massive (defined as 600 mL/24 hours) or chronic and recurrent. In the former clinical scenario, the dominant angiographic abnormality is extravasation of contrast material from the bleeding artery, which requires active hemorrhage of at least 0.5 mL/minute at the time of angiography.[43] Alternatively, the dominant angiographic findings in the setting of chronic GI hemorrhage are the vascular abnormalities (eg, tumor neovascularity, angiodysplasia, or pseudoaneurysm) that are predisposed to recurrent bleeding; active hemorrhage at the time of angiography is not a prerequisite. Based on the presence or absence of hematemesis or return of blood through the nasogastric tube, acute massive GI hemorrhage may be divided further into upper (proximal to the ligament of Treitz) and lower (distal to the ligament of Treitz) sources. In virtually all cases of acute GI hemorrhage, barium studies are to be avoided assiduously; the diagnostic yield is low due to the presence of intraluminal blood. Additionally, barium obscures visualization both endoscopically and angiographically.

In patients with *acute massive upper GI hemorrhage* refractory to conservative management (gastric lavage, bedrest, and blood replacement), endoscopy is the preferred initial invasive diagnostic and interventional modality. In most patients, endoscopic evaluation can distinguish arteriocapillary from variceal bleeding, locate the source, identify the etiology, and often provide hemostasis. Angiography is indicated for suspected arteriocapillary bleeding in the setting of failed endoscopic management, particularly if hemostatic transcatheter methods, such as intra-arterial vasopressin infusion or transcatheter embolization, are being considered. The angiographic technique usually commences with selective contrast injection into the celiac trunk with anterioposterior (AP) film acquisition. Filming should be continued sufficiently late to identify extravascular contrast accumulated within the bowel lumen after contrast dis-

sipation from the overlaying vessels (Fig 2–14). If no contrast extravasation is identified, then selective studies are performed sequentially in the SMA, the left gastric artery, and the gastroduodenal artery. If no contrast extravasation is found in spite of all of the above selective studies, and the evidence for arteriocapillary hemorrhage of the upper GI tract is strong, then a therapeutic trial of vasopressin infusion into the left gastric artery may be warranted. Support for this approach is derived from the knowledge that the source of 85% of gastric bleeding is from the left gastric artery,[44] and that GI hemorrhage is often evanescent.

Acute massive lower GI hemorrhage typically presents as bright red- or maroon-colored blood from the rectum, with nasogastric aspirate negative for blood. In contradistinction to bleeding from the upper GI tract, endoscopy often is limited in lower GI hemorrhage because of obscuration by intraluminal blood. Since the time lapse between active bleeding at the hemorrhage site and the appearance of blood from the rectum may vary considerably, it is imperative to document active bleeding by a radionuclide scan prior to angiography. Radionuclide bleeding scans, which most commonly utilize ^{99m}Tc-labeled RBCs, may detect GI hemorrhage with a bleeding rate as low as 0.1 mL/min.[45] Transfer of the patient to the angiography suite as soon as the radionuclide bleeding scan is positive for hemorrhage further improves the likelihood of angiography being diagnostic. The angiographic technique includes selective contrast injection into the SMA and the IMA with AP film acquisition. Frequently, at least two angiographic series are necessary to study the entire vascular watershed: one with filming of the upper abdomen, a second centered over the lower abdomen and pelvis. Patients should have a urinary catheter placed in the bladder prior to angiography, since contrast media cleared by the kidneys collects in the bladder and may obscure a pelvic bleeding site.

The hallmark of *chronic recurrent GI hemorrhage* is intermittent bleeding. The quantity of blood loss may or may not be massive. Unlike the situation with acute massive hemorrhage, the evaluation of chronic GI hemorrhage should make thorough use of noninvasive techniques, including both upper and lower GI barium and/or endoscopic studies, prior to angiographic assessment. In this small but enigmatic group of patients, conventional angiography has been shown to detect the source of bleeding in approximately 50% of patients.[48] The etiology most commonly discovered is a vascular malformation, especially an angiodysplasia, or vascular ectasia. Most angiodysplasias occur in the right or transverse colon but may occur anywhere in the gut. The triad of angiographic findings are (1) early draining veins, (2) dense, persistent draining veins, and (3) a hypervascular capillary stain (Fig 2–15). In extensive angiodysplasias, the feeding arteries may enlarge. Historically, preferred treatment of

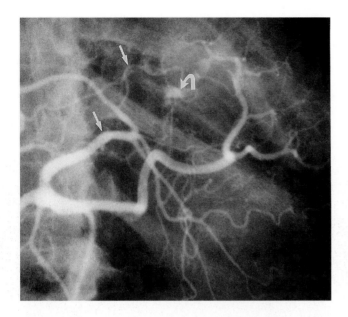

A

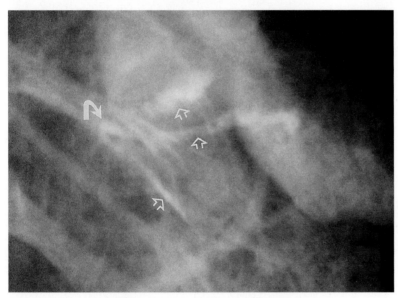

B

Figure 2–14. Active, acute, massive upper GI hemorrhage in a 42 year-old alcoholic male. **A.** Anteroposterior view, arterial phase of the celiac arteriogram; contrast is extravasated (*curved white arrow*) from small branches derived from the left gastric artery (*straight white arrows*). **B.** Magnified view; venous phase of the same injection demonstrates extravacated contrast material both pooled within the ulcer crater (*curved white arrow*) and spilled over into the surrounding radiating gastric mucosal folds (*open arrows*).

localized angiodysplasia has been surgical resection. Owing to the sessile, submucosal nature of angiodysplasas, operative detection and evaluation of the extent of these lesions is frequently difficult. Intraoperative localization, particularly in the cases of small-bowel lesions or failed prior resection, may be assisted considerably by injection of 1 mL of methylene blue through a preoperatively placed angiographic catheter superselectively positioned with the tip lying within the immediate vascular supply to the affected segment of bowel.[47] In those patients with negative conventional angiography, provocative angiography may be warranted. Specifically, the angiographic

catheter is placed within the SMA or other candidate circulation, transcatheter pharmacologic agents are administered to promote bleeding, and angiography is repeated. Agents employed include intra-arterial vasodilators such as nitroglycerine, 25 to 50 µg, tolazoline, 25 to 50 mg; or papaverine, 30 mg, systemic heparinization, and/or intra-arterial thrombolytic agents (urokinase, 1 million units administered during a period of 30 to 35 minutes.[48,49] The availability of blood replacement and access to the operating room should be arranged in advance. Heparin may be reversed with intravenous protamine sulfate in a ratio of 1 mg of protamine for every

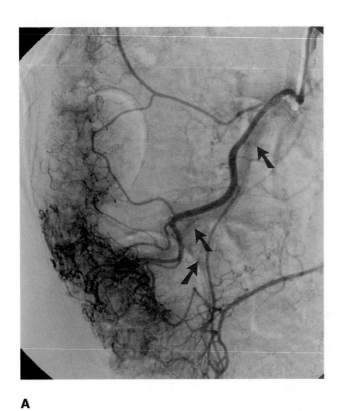

A

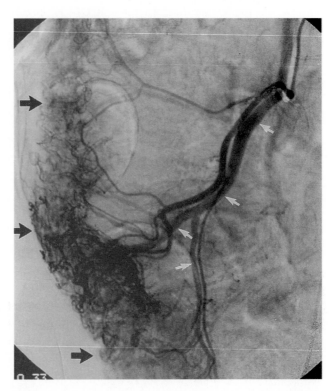

B

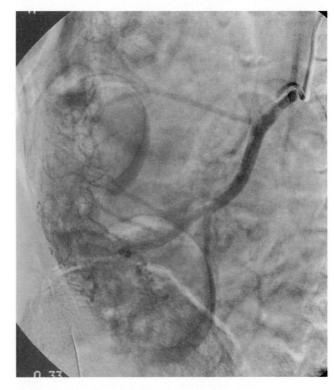

C

Figure 2–15. Right colonic angiodysplasia in a 57 year–old male with chronic recurrent episodes of maroon-colored blood per rectum requiring blood transfusion on three occasions. **A.** During the early arterial-phase film of the subselective right colic artery contrast injection (anteroposterior view, digital subtraction angiogram), faintly opacified early draining veins are identified (*black arrows*). **B.** In the capillary-phase film, an abnormally dense region of contrast opacification of small-caliber dysplastic vessels is present (*black arrows*) as well as abnormally dense draining veins (*white arrows*). **C.** During the venous phase of filming, the veins draining the angiodysplasia remain both abnormally dense and persistent.

90 units of heparin; typically only 50% to 66% of the heparin dose is reversed. If bleeding is massive, intra-arterial vasopressin may be infused emergently via the indwelling angiographic catheters.

Bowel ischemia. Bowel ischemia has a wide range of potential presentations. The time course may be acute with infarcted or potentially infarcted bowel or it may be chronic with postprandial abdominal pain and malnutrition. The mechanism may be arterial occlusive disease (central or peripheral), venous occlusive disease, or poor perfusion (nonocclusive ischemia) caused by congestive heart failure or digitalis toxicity.

The angiographic evaluation begins with a flush aortogram in a lateral projection to visualize the origins of the celiac trunk, SMA, and IMA; all are common sites of arterial occlusive disease. If patent, then the SMA, and often the celiac trunk and IMA are selectively injected, with AP filming performed to evaluate small-caliber arterial detail and venous drainage. In order not to obscure the findings in nonocclusive mesenteric ischemia, intra-arterial vasodilators should not be used in the initial SMA injection.

Angiographic findings in the case of atherosclerotic arterial occlusive disease are typically high-grade stenosis and/or occlusion of the juxtaostial portions of the mesenteric arteries (Fig 2–16). Although flow-limiting lesions are generally required in at least two of the three mesenteric arteries for the clinical syndrome to manifest, the status of the aforementioned collateral pathways has a profound impact on the degree of ischemia.[50,51] If poorly collateralized, symptoms may occur with single-vessel disease.[51] Alternatively, if collateral supply is well developed, a patient may remain asymptomatic or minimally symptomatic despite occlusion in all three vessels. Less common etiologies for a similar angiographic pattern include fibromuscular dysplasia, Takayasu's arteritis, and midaortic syndrome. Eccentric narrowing along the cephalad margin of the juxtaosteal portion of the celiac trunk by portions of the diaphragmatic crura is relatively common and termed the *median arcuate ligament syndrome* (Fig 2–17). The association of vascular insufficiency with the median arcuate ligament syndrome is controversial.

Although acute arterial embolism may cause proximal arterial occlusion indistinguishable from arteriosclerosis-related thrombosis, fragmentation and distal embolization commonly cause associated small-artery occlusion with filling defects or a trailing edge of embolus that identifies the embolic etiology (Fig 2–18). Bowel ischemia, related to small-branch artery narrowing or occlusion, may be seen with radiation, carcinoid-induced elastic vascular sclerosis, peritoneal carcinomatosis, operative ligation, vasculitis, and ergot toxicity.

Mesenteric venous occlusive disease is relatively rare.

Angiographic diagnosis is made by the lack of opacification of a normal major venous conduit (eg, superior mesenteric vein) and the appearance of multiple mesenteric varices.

Nonocclusive mesenteric ischemia is found in patients with low cardiac output and/or poor perfusion states. The angiographic manifestations are most prominent in the SMA and are (1) a patent but diffusely constricted mainstream SMA, (2) focal narrowing at more peripheral arterial branch points, and (3) superimposed beaded appearance with areas of severe narrowing alternating with areas of near-normal caliber. The diffuse vasoconstrictive pattern to the SMA may also be seen as a normal physiologic response (vascular redistribution) to hypotension or as a pharmacologic response to infusion of vasopressors. In the clinical setting of probable nonocclusive mesenteric ischemia that is corroborated angiographically, improved gut perfusion may be attempted with an intra-arterial papaverine infusion of 3 mg/min for 20 minutes followed by a 30-mg bolus, followed by repeat SMA angiography.[52] If the angiogram documents improved SMA blood flow, continuance of the papaverine infusion at 0.75 mg/min. for 24 hours is warranted.

Pancreatic neoplasia. Angiography has largely been supplanted by other noninvasive modalities, particularly CT, for the evaluation of pancreatic neoplasms.[53] Occasionally, angiography is useful to (1) establish nonoperability owing to vascular invasion in a patient with pancreatic adenocarcinoma,[54] (2) identify potentially operable patients with cystic pancreatic masses, and (3) detect and localize endocrine tumors.

Arteriographic technique includes superselective injection into the gastroduodenal artery, the splenic artery (to include evaluation of the splenic vein), and, if feasible, the dorsal pancreatic artery, with magnification filming. Recent literature indicates that angiography rarely adds staging information not available by high quality CT in patients with potentially resectable pancreatic adenocarcinomas.[53] Alternatively, preoperative vascular mapping appears to be warranted for these patients (see discussion under prepancreaticoduodenectomy). In patients with relatively well-defined pancreatic masses containing cystic spaces determined by CT, the differential diagnosis includes necrotic pancreatic adenocarcinoma (probably not resectable), pancreatic pseudocyst (a candidate for conservative treatment or percutaneous drainage), and cystadenoma or cystadenocarcinoma, (a likely candidate for operative resection). Since the cystoadenoma/cystoadenocarcinomas are usually hypervascular, whereas adenocarcinomas and pseudocysts are not, angiography is useful to determine which patients would likely benefit from excision.

The peptide-producing adenomas derived from embryonic neural-crest tissue share the biochemical amine

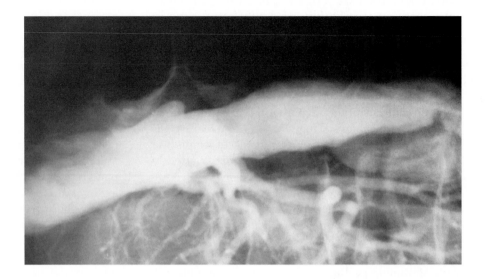

A

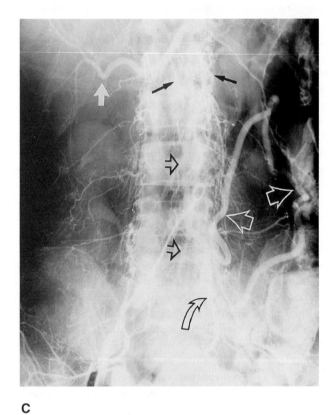

B

C

Figure 2–16. Chronic mesenteric ischemia due to atherosclerosis in a 67 year–old female with a 1 year history of postprandial abdominal pain and a 25 lb weight loss. **A.** Lateral view (patient's head to the reader's left); abdominal aortogram demonstrates no antegrade flow in any vessel coursing ventrally from the aorta; diagnostic for proximal occlusion of the celiac trunk, SMA, and IMA. **B.** Anteroposterior view; arterial-phase abdominal aortogram confirms absence of antegrade mesenteric blood flow. Of note, a small infrarenal abdominal aortic aneurysm and moderate stenosis of the left renal artery are present. **C.** Late-phase film from aortogram (anteroposterior view) documents reconstitution of the hepatic artery (*solid white arrow*) from innumerable unnamed retroperitoneal collateral arteries (*solid black arrows*), and the SMA (*open straight black arrows*) and IMA (*open curved arrow*) from internal iliac artery sources via the hemorrhoidal complex and an enlarged marginal artery of Drummond (*open white arrow*). An operative aortoceliacomesenteric bypass graft relieved her symptoms.

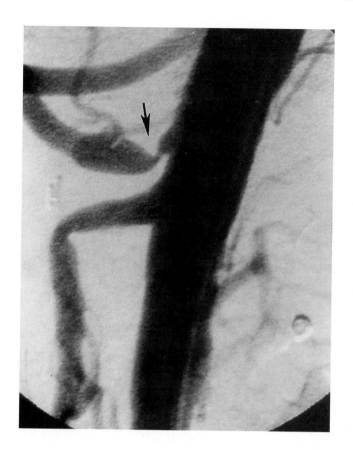

Figure 2–17. Median arcuate ligament syndrome in a 73 year–old female with atypical postprandial abdominal fullness and a 45 lb weight loss over a 3 month period. Lateral view digital-subtracted abdominal aortogram documents a typical nonostial eccentric stenosis (*black arrow*) of the proximal celiac trunk typically due to extrinsic compression by the median arcuate ligament of the diaphragm. This patient's symptoms were improved on an oral regimen of metoclopromide and were most likely due to gastroparesis documented by endoscopy and nuclear medicine gastric-emptying study.

precursor uptake and decarboxylation (APUD) pathway and, hence, are known as APUDomas. APUDomas, such as insulinomas and gastrinomas, manifest symptoms while the tumors are relatively small (<3 cm) and difficult to locate by CT, MR, and transabdominal ultrasound. Since most APUDomas are hypervascular relative to the pancreas, superselective pancreatic angiography is useful for localization. However, some islet cell tumors are either very small and surgically nonpalpable or hypovascular. Historically, transhepatic portal venous hormonal sampling of the venous tributaries draining the pancreas was utilized to localize the tumor before a partial pancreatectomy.[55] Currently, sterile intraoperative ultrasound has been shown to be effective in the detection of small pancreatic adenomas and is currently the procedure of choice for small tumor localization.[56]

Prepancreaticoduodenectomy. Pancreaticoduodenectomy (the Whipple procedure), performed for both neoplastic and inflammatory disease, involves extensive dissection and requires an intact biliary vascular supply for healing. Routine preoperative angiography–detected vascular abnormalities mandates modification of surgical technique in approximate 30% of cases (Fig 2–19).[57] Cited examples include (1) asymptomatic celiac trunk occlusion or stenosis requiring arterial bypass grafting (3%), (2) replaced hepatic arterial supply coursing dorsal to the portal vein and bile ducts necessitating arterial preservation procedures (22%), and (3) arterial pseudoaneurysms (5%), arteriovenous fistulae (5%), or splenic vein thrombosis (8%) owing to chronic pancreatitis, which may mandate splenectomy or preoperative transcatheter embolization.

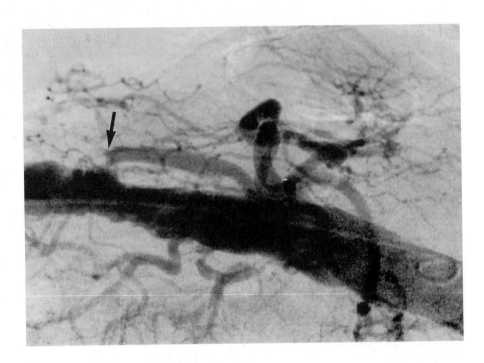

A

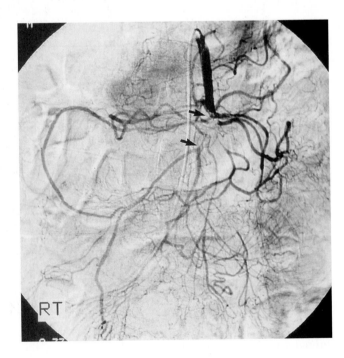

B

Figure 2–18. Mesenteric ischemia caused by an embolus in a 76 year–old female with an abrupt onset of intermittent abdominal pain 2 weeks previously. **A.** Lateral-view; digital subtraction abdominal aortogram (patient's head is to the reader's right) shows the origins of both the celiac trunk and SMA to be normal although the latter vessel is abruptly occluded (*black arrow*) approximately 8 cm beyond its origin. **B.** Anteroposterior view; arterial phase of a digital-subtraction angiogram confirmed a short segment occlusion (*between black arrows*) owing to the embolus, with reconstruction of the distal branches via small bowel arcades and the marginal artery of the right colon.

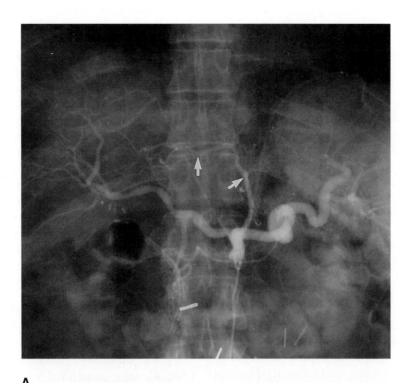

A

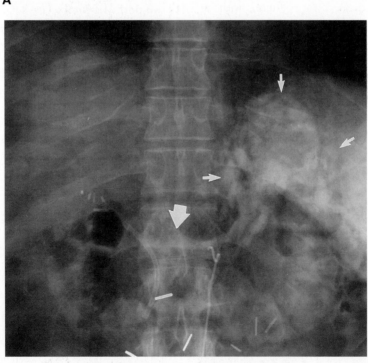

B

Figure 2–19. Pre-Whipple angiogram in a 38 year–old male with chronic pancreatitis. **A.** Anteroposterior view; arterial-phase film of the celiac arteriogram demonstrates a replacement of the left hepatic artery to the left gastric artery (*arrows*). **B.** On the venous phase of the celiac angiogram, the splenic vein is nearly occluded (*large arrow*) near the portal vein confluence, with multiple associated gastric varices (*small arrows*).

■ VASCULAR INTERVENTIONAL RADIOLOGY

PORTAL HYPERTENSION

The *TIPS procedure* in its current form using expandable metallic stents was first described in humans in 1990.[58] In the short interval since, the TIPS procedure has gained widespread acceptance, although its role in relation to conservative management including endoscopic sclerotherapy and to operative portosystemic shunts remains to be defined. Most commonly, TIPS procedures are performed for variceal hemorrhage, although other indications include treatment of intractable ascites, hepatorenal syndrome, and preoperative decompression of abdominal varices.[59] Because of the prohibitive mortality rate for operative portosystemic shunting, TIPS is the portal decompression procedure of choice in patients with Child's-Pugh class C. Since the TIPS procedure, unlike operative portosystemic shunts, neither incites right upper-quadrant fibrosis nor alters the extrahepatic portal or systemic venous system, it is also the preferred portal decompressive "bridge" procedure prior to liver transplantation. Because the TIPS procedure is significantly less invasive when compared to operative portosystemic shunting and peritoneal-venous shunting, it may be indicated for patients with intractable ascites and good hepatic functional reserve (Child's-Pugh class A). Owing to apparent suboptimal primary patency rate of 17% to 67% at 1 year following the TIPS procedure, the results of long-term studies (5 year follow-up) are required to establish its role in many patients with variceal bleeding and Child's-Pugh class A or B hepatic function.

The in-hospital mortality rate for patients who undergo a TIPS procedure urgently for variceal hemorrhage has been reported to range from 56% to 62% as opposed to 5% to 18% for patients with nonurgent TIPS procedure.[60,61] Clearly, preprocedural aggressive medical management to obtain hemostasis, including vasoconstrictive treatment, balloon tamponade, and endoscopic sclerotherapy, is essential for optimal outcome from a TIPS procedure. Additionally, color-flow duplex ultrasound is useful to assure portal vein patency, since portal-vein occlusion is the most common cause of initial technical failure of TIPS.[59,60] Prophylactic antibiotics to prevent *Staphylococcus epidermidis bacteremia* infection has been recommended.[59]

Venous access is obtained via the right internal jugular vein, often assisted with ultrasound guidance. If necessary, the left internal jugular vein, or either external jugular vein, may be utilized. A long (40 cm) 9- to 10-F vascular sheath is inserted and passed to the intrahepatic portion of the inferior vena cava where baseline systemic venous pressure is recorded. Coaxially, an angiographic catheter is used selectively to catheterize a hepatic vein, usually the right hepatic vein. Currently, two portal-venous access sets are commercially available that differ in specific components but share similar functions.[59,62] A coaxial needle and catheter combination is thrust, under fluoroscopic guidance, anteriorly 3 to 4 cm into the liver parenchyma (Fig 2–20). The needle then is removed and aspiration performed as the

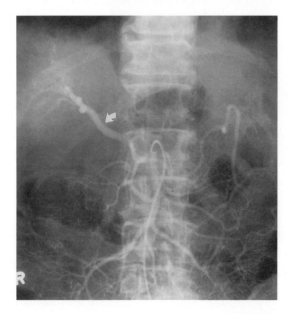

A

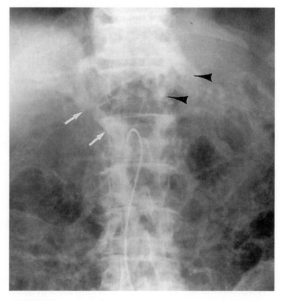

B

Figure 2–20. TIPS procedure in a 70 year–old male with intractable acities. The transarterial portogram (**A** and **B**) demonstrates evidence of portal hypertension. **A.** During the arterial phase of the SMA injection, a replaced right hepatic artery (*arrow*) is noted which has "corkscrewing" of the intrahepatic arterial branches owing to hepatic cirrhosis. **B.** On the venous phase, the portal vein (*white arrows*) is shown to be patent with hepatopetal flow, poor filling of the intrahepatic branches as a result of portal hypertension, and opacification of gastric and esophageal varices (*black arrowheads*). *Continued*

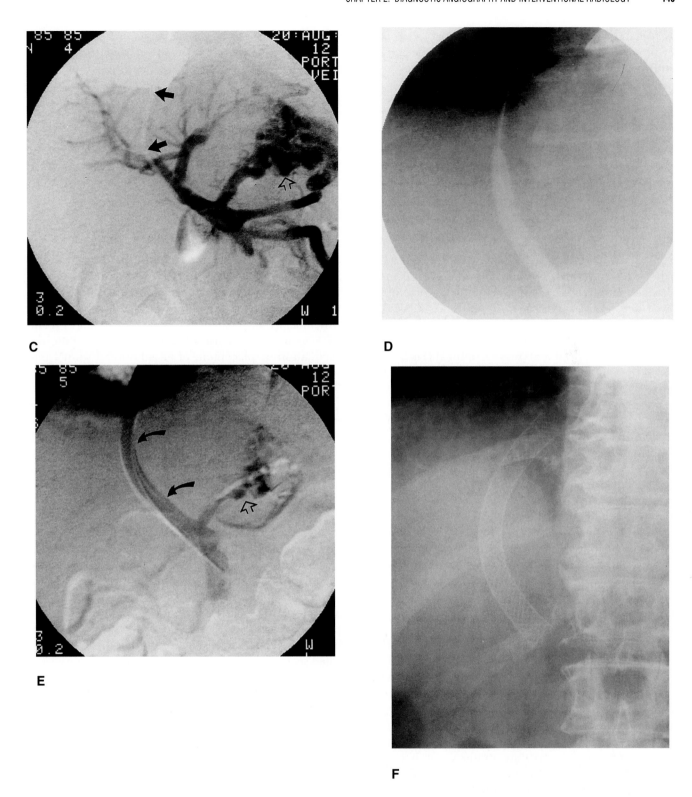

Figure 2–20, cont'd. C. After the needle/catheter combination (*black arrows*) has been passed from the right hepatic vein to the right portal vein, a direct portogram confirms the intraportal catheter position and filling of gastroesophageal varices (*open arrow*). **D.** An 8-mm balloon catheter is used to dilate the transhepatic tract. **E.** After a deployment of two Wallstents within the single TIPS tract followed by balloon dilation to 10 mm, a repeat direct portogram shows brisk flow within the stent (*black arrows*), lack of filling of intrahepatic portal venous branches (hepatofugal flow), and minimal filling of the varices (*open arrow*). **F.** Plain anteroposterior radiograph of the upper abdomen displays the appearance of the Wallstents within the intraparenchymal tract.

combination is withdrawn toward the hepatic vein. After blood is aspirated, contrast material is injected to confirm an appropriate position within the portal vein, ideally between the portal vein bifurcation and the first-order branches of either the right or left portal vein. A heavy-duty guide wire is passed and seated within either the splenic or superior mesenteric vein. The parenchymal tract is predilated with the coaxial catheter and cannula combination. Via the catheter, portal venous pressures are recorded and a portal venogram obtained to document varices, determine the direction of portal venous flow, and estimate the length of parenchymal tract to be stented. The tract is dilated with a balloon catheter to 8 mm diameter. Through the vascular sheath and over the guidewire, a metallic expandable stent is deployed and expanded to 8 mm. Most commonly, a Wallstent wire-mesh endoprosthesis (Scneider, Minneapolis, MN) is used. Its relatively small-caliber (7 Fr), supple delivery system, and capacity to conform to curved or angulated tracts between the hepatic and portal veins make it optimal (Fig 2–21). Portal venography and portal venous pressures are repeated. Angiographically, if flow is brisk through the stent, varices are diminished, and the portal vein–systemic venous gradient is less than 15 mm Hg, the TIPS procedure is completed. If not, the stented tract is dilated to 10 mm diameter and portal venography and pressures are repeated. If the pressure gradient is <15 mm Hg but esophagogastric varices still fill, or variceal hemorrhage has occurred within the past 24 hours, transcatheter embolization of the coronary vein may be indicated. If the portal-systemic venous gradient pressure remains above 15 mm Hg, options include dilation of the stents to 12 mm diameter or placement of a second TIPS conduit parallel to the first. Termination portal venography and pressures within the portal vein and inferior vena cava or right atrium are obtained as a baseline for future reference.

In order to detect tract stenosis, usually due to intimal hyperplasia, recommended postprocedural follow-up includes assessment, at approximately 3 month intervals, of the TIPS stent and portal-venous hemodynamics with color-flow duplex ultrasound. This may be supplemented with transvenous catheterization of the TIPS stent to obtain portal venography and portal vein–systemic venous pressure gradients at 6 to 12 month intervals if asymptomatic, and sooner if symptoms of portal-venous hypertension recur. Ultrasound findings suggestive for TIPS stenosis or occlusion include absence of flow in the stent (specificity 87%), slowed flow in the stent by 50%, flow velocity greater than 250 cm/sec, or conversion of intrahepatic portal-venous flow from hepatofugal to hepatopetal.[63–65]

The TIPS results of reported large series to date are summarized in Table 2–1.[59,60,66–71] TIPS can be per-

formed with a high rate of technical success (93% to 100%), is effective in lowering portal-venous pressure, usually provides short-term hemostasis (86% to 100%) and improvement of ascites (83% to 95%), and has a low rate of procedural complications (<10%).[72] The 30 day (3.6% to 25%) and long-term mortality rates of 11% to 27% over 7 to 15 months tend to reflect the severity of liver dysfunction, hemodynamic stability of the patient, and the presence or absence of multiorgan failure but, nevertheless, compare favorably to the mortality rates encountered with operative portosystemic shunts. The primary problem with TIPS procedures is the incidence of rehemorrhage (4.5% to 31% with approximately 50% due to variceal bleeding) and restenosis or occlusion of the portal vein to inferior vena cava tract. In the subset of patients who have been meticulously followed with screening color-flow duplex ultrasound and/or transvenous portography, the primary patency rate at 1 year ranges from 17% to 51%. With use of percutaneous techniques (redilation or placement of an additional stent), improved secondary patency rates can reach 83% to 97%.[73–75]

New or worsened encephalopathy occurs at a rate between 9% and 24%, similar to operative portal venous decompression procedures. Fortunately, in nearly all cases, encephalopathy can be managed medically. Risk factors include age >60 years and Child's-Pugh class C cirrhosis in younger patients.[76] In 25% of patients, liver function may worsen as a result of portal-vein shunting. However, in 33% of patients undergoing TIPS procedures prior to scheduled liver transplantation, liver function may improve to the degree that transplantation is no longer necessary.[59,77] TIPS procedures in patients with cirrhosis and portal hypertension have been shown to induce significant hemodynamic changes including an increase in cardiac output of 17% to 50%, increase in pulmonary artery pressure of 33% to 100%, diminution in systemic vascular resistance of 10% to 33%, and elevated splanchnic blood flow.[78,79] For these reasons, caution should be used when considering TIPS procedures for patients with severe cardiopulmonary insufficiency.

Percutaneous dilation of stenosed, failing, operative portosystemic shunts can be safely and effectively accomplished via a transfemoral venous route (Fig 2–22).[80] Alternatively, *transcatheter embolization* of shunts may be employed to close portosystemic shunts with associated hepatic encephalopathy resistant to medical therapy.[80,81]

Partial splenic embolization may be utilized in patients with hypersplenism in whom retention of some functioning splenic tissue is desired.[82,83] Alternatively, if splenectomy is desired, but rendered risky due to massive splenomegaly or thrombocytopenia, *preoperative splenic artery embolization* may minimize operative blood loss.[84]

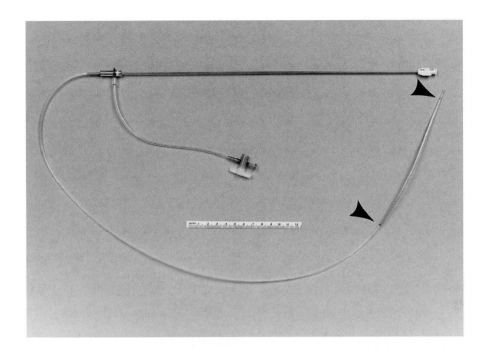

A

B

Figure 2–21. One type of expandable metallic stent (Wallstent, Schneider, Inc. Minneapolis, MN) useful for TIPS procedures or internal biliary reconstruction. **A.** The delivery set which is passed over a guidewire. The stent (*between arrowheads*) is compressed over the shaft of the delivery system and constrained by an outer membrane. **B.** Close-up view with the constraining membrane incompletely retracted allowing partial deployment of the metallic stent. *Continued*

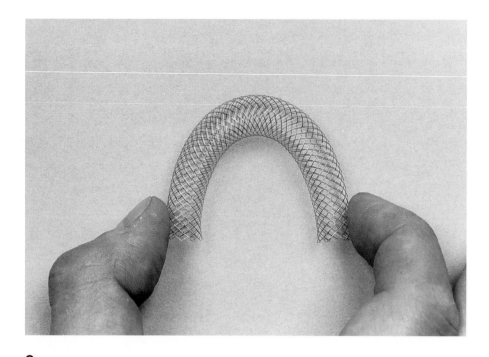

C

Figure 2–21, cont'd. C. Fully deployed stent, purposely bent to illustrate the ability of the device to adapt to curved structures.

HEPATIC MALIGNANCY

Until recently, the sole modality available for potential cure in patients with either primary or metastatic hepatic malignancy has been surgical removal. The anticipated improvement in survival rates from tumor excision has been offset in part by perioperative mortality rates that approximate 10%. The role for external-beam radiation or systemic chemotherapy has been limited by suboptimal tumoricidal effect, systemic side effects, and/or hepatic toxicity. Recent advances that offer promise for both cure and palliation of primary or metastatic hepatic malignancy include regional chemotherapy infusion, transcatheter arterial embolization, chemoembolization, and direct tumoral ablation via percutaneous ethanol injection or thermal necrosis. The transcatheter techniques (regional chemoinfusion, transcatheter embolization, and chemoembolization) take advantage of the unique hepatic vascular supply. Specifically, the dominant vascular supply to the hepatic parenchyma is via the portal vein, whereas the primary tumoral vascular supply is the hepatic artery (Fig 2–23). This duality of vascular supply permits selective delivery of a high dose of chemotherapy to the tumor while minimizing systemic toxicity, or selectively causing tumoral infarction through arterial embolization while simultaneously preserving hepatocytic vascular supply.

Regional transcatheter hepatic-arterial chemotherapy infusion has been utilized for treatment of both primary and metastatic hepatic malignancies, since the early 1960s. The effect of regional infusion is maximized when the chemotherapeutic agent has (1) a steep tumoricidal dose–response curve with higher drug doses resulting in greater tumoricidal effect, and (2) a high proportion of the drug being cleared from circulation on the initial pass through the liver. Currently, regional infusion is generally achieved through surgically implanted pumps with delivery of the agent through a catheter placed into the gastroduodenal artery and the tip placed in the proper hepatic artery. The gastroduodenal artery is ligated to prevent inadvertent backwash of drug to the enteric and pancreatic circulation. The primary role of angiography is to detect vascular anomalies that would affect drug delivery, such as a right hepatic artery replaced to the SMA (Fig 2–24). Large-vessel transcatheter embolization may be used to either (1) protect nontarget organs from accidental perfusion (eg, right gastric artery occlusion) (Fig 2–24) or (2) redistribute the vascular supply so that the entire hepatic arterial infusion is through a solitary artery (eg, embolization of a replaced right hepatic artery origin in order to develop intrahepatic transarterial collaterals so that a solitary common hepatic catheter can infuse the entire liver).[85] Long-term indwelling percutaneous catheter infusion of the hepatic arteries has been limited by infection, catheter migration, catheter-induced complications, and lifestyle considerations. Nevertheless, short-term infusion by small-caliber catheters inserted via the transbrachial ap-

TABLE 2–1. SUMMARY OF PATIENT PROFILES, CLINICAL INDICATIONS, TYPE OF STENTS, TECHNICAL SUCCESS, COMPLICATIONS AND OUTCOME OF EIGHT REPORTED SERIES OF TIP'S PROCEDURES

	LaBerge	Helton	Zemel	Bilbao	Barton	Richter	Darcy	Hauenstein
NO. OF PATIENTS	100	59	55	84	60	120	50	262
CHILD'S–PUGH CLASSIFICATION								
A	10	4		9				27%
B	35	22		35				51%
C	55	33		40				22%
INDICATION								
Variceal Hemorrhage	94 (94%)	57 (97%)		50 (66%)	60 (100%)			
Intractable Ascites	3 (3%)	2 (3%)		22 (26%)				
Hepato Renal Sd	2 (2%)							
Preop Decompression	1 (1%)							
PREEXISTENT CONDITIONS								
Ascites	78 (78%)	46 (71%)	41					
Encephalopathy	39 (39%)	29 (49%)						
Portal Vein Thrombosis	10 (10%)	at least 1						
Hepatic Vein Thrombosis	1 (1%)							
TYPE OF STENT	WALLSTENT	WALLSTENT	PALMAZ	WALLSTENT	Z STENT & WALLSTENT	PALMAZ	PALMAZ	PALMAZ & WALLSTENT
Coronary Vein Embolization	34%	32%						
RESULTS								
Initial Technical Success	96 (96%)	55 (93%)	55 (100%)	82 (98%)		111 (93%)	48 (96%)	98%
Portosystemic Gradient (mm Hg)								
Pre-TIPS	20.4	18.1±5.6		21±2.0		29±5	23.3	
Post-TIPS	10.4±0.9	10.5±3.6		5.7±1.2		12±4	11.5	≤12 in 93%
Follow-Up Duration (Mean)	7.6 mo	7 mo	7.6 mo		6.5 mo	15 mo	5 mo	19 mo
STATUS								
OLT (Orthotopic Liver Transplantation)	22 (22%)			20 (24%)				
Non-OLT, Survival	48 (48%)			41 (49%)				
Non-OLT, Died	26 (26%)		6 (11%)	23 (27%)	13 (22%)	13 (12%)		
COMPLICATIONS								
30 day Mortality	13 (13%)	15 (25%)	2 (3.6%)		13 (21.6%)	6 (5.3%)	10 (19.6%)	3%
NONFATAL								
Worsened Encephalopathy	18 (18%)	10 (17%)	5 (9.1%)			2 (2.2%)	5 (9.1%)	25%
Liver Dysfunction	24 (24%)							
Fever	10 (10%)							
Intra-Abdominal Bleed	1 (1%)	2 (3%)						
Myocardial Infarction	1 (1%)	1 (2%)						
Renal Insufficiency	3 (3%)							
Other	1 (1%)	5 (8%)	3 (6%)					
EFFECTIVENESS								
Hemostasis	88/94 (94%)	53/55 (96%)	NR[a]	NR	60 (100%)	NR	12/14 (86%)	NR
Rebleed	17/88 (19%)	17/55 (31%)	3 (5%)	NR	NR	5 (4.5%)	NR	1 (107%)
Variceal	NR	11/55 (19%)	NR	NR	11 (20%)	NR	3 (6.5%)	NR
Improved Ascites	49/59 (83%)	NR	39/41 (95%)					
Renal Insufficiency Improved	6/9 (67%)							
Thrombocytopenia Improved	6/13 (46%)							
Liver Function Improved	2 (27%)							
Encephalopathy Improved		7 (12%)						

[a]Not reported.

proach may offer a cost effective, less invasive alternative to operatively placed infusate pumps. Prospective trials demonstrate that regional chemoinfusion via surgically placed infusate pumps improves tumoral response (42% to 68%) when compared to systemic chemotherapy (10% to 21%), but affords no improvement in overall survival.[86] Most likely, this seeming contradiction is explained on the basis of perioperative mortality and drug-induced gut ulceration, or biliary sclerosis (inadvertent perfusion of the gastric or duodenal vascular supply).

Transcatheter arterial embolization of small-caliber intrahepatic arteries has been effective in reducing overall tumoral burden with diffuse liver metastases. Commonly utilized agents include Gelfoam (a biodegradable gelatin sponge) powder or small pledgets and polyvinyl alcohol (Ivalon) particles (a permanent agent; 150 to 250 μm diameter). Lipiodol, an oily liquid–radiographic contrast agent, has been shown to have a proclivity for hepatocel-

lular carcinoma while being spontaneously cleared from the normal liver parenchymal via the lymphatics. In order to minimize the risk of hepatic necrosis, the patency of the portal vein should be documented, and sufficient hepatocytic reserve should remain. A serum bilirubin > 5 mg/dL or Child's-Pugh class C are relative contraindications to transcatheter embolization. Superselective catheterization should be performed, when feasible, to prevent accidental embolization of the cystic, right gastric, or gastroduodenal arteries. Transcatheter embolization has been most commonly employed for palliation of (1) hormonally active tumors such as metastatic carcinoid, and (2) local symptoms, such as pain, from tumor growth. Transcatheter arterial embolization has been reported to result in a temporary objective response of smaller tumor size and lower level of serum hormones in 72% to 80% of patients with carcinoid or islet cell tumors.[84] Subjective improvement has been reported to oc-

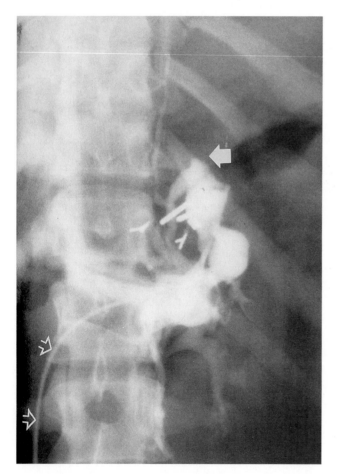

A

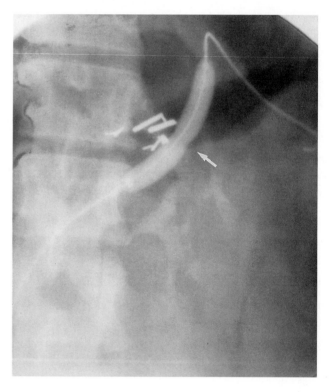

B

Figure 2–22. Transcatheter restoration of function of a failing distal splenorenal (Warren) shunt in a 43 year-old alcoholic female with recurrent variceal hemorrhage. **A.** Anteroposterior view; splenorenal shuntogram via a transfemoral venous angiographic catheter (*small open white arrows*) demonstrates occlusion of the splenorenal vein anastomosis (*large solid white arrow*). Contrast drains into the left renal vein and inferior vena cava. **B.** After probing with an angiographic catheter, a guidewire was passed into the distal splenic vein and an 8-mm diameter balloon catheter was used to dilate the anastomosis. Note the residual waist on the balloon (*arrow*) which demarcates the level of the anastomosis. *Continued*

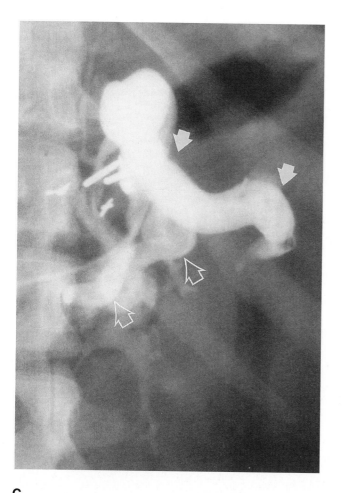

C

Figure 2–22, cont'd. C. Following PTA, contrast injection into the splenic vein (*solid arrows*) drains via the splenorenal shunt into the left renal vein (*open arrows*).

cur in 94% to 100% of patients. Approximately 50% of patients develop a postembolization syndrome manifested by pain, fever, leukocytosis, nausea, and occasionally, ileus.[85] Infectious complications occur in 8% of cases, manifested as either a hepatic abscess or septicemia. In addition to meticulous sterile technique, antibiotic prophylaxis is recommended and should provide coverage for both skin and gut pathogens. In patients with APUDomas, including carcinoid, arterial embolization may precipitate release of vasoactive amines. Cardiopulmonary instability may be minimized by prophylactic administration of pharmacologic antagonists such as somatostatin analogues.

Transcatheter chemoembolization (TCE) is a relatively new technique that mixes chemotherapeutic drugs with embolic agents (Fig 2–25). As well as causing tumor ischemia and infarction, the addition of embolic agents results in prolonged chemotherapeutic contact with the tumor cells and may increase drug intake from anoxia-induced altered tissue permeability. Typically, the chemo-

therapeutic agent is emulsified with Lipiodol. The emulsification fills portal venous channels at the tumor periphery via arterioportal communications to improve tumoricidal effects on marginal tumor and "daughter" nodules. Epinephrine may be injected intra-arterially prior to embolization in order to vasoconstrict normal arteries and divert flow to tumor. Gelfoam pledgets or other particulate emboli often are embolized at the completion of the procedure to further promote stasis of blood flow.

TCE generally has been reserved for palliative treatment of patients who are not candidates for operative resection. Patients with small, solitary hepatocellular carcinomas (HCC) have a significantly improved survival rate in comparison to patients with large, multifocal or diffuse tumors, particularly if the chemoembolic agents can be delivered into subsegmental arteries (Tables 2–2 and 2–3).[87–93] The results of TCE in both patients with small solitary tumors and widespread disease compare favorably to patients with nonoperable hepatoma with no specific treatment (mean survival 4 to 6 months) and those with systemic chemotherapy (20% response rate, 25% mortality rate attributable to chemotherapy).

In general, contraindications to TCE include extrahepatic metastases, portal vein occlusion, poor hepatorenal reserve (total bilirubin >3 mg/dL, prothrombin time >15 seconds, serum albumin under 3.0 mg/dL, or serum creatinine >2 mg/dL), and inadequate bone marrow reserve (platelet count <50,000/mm^3, white blood count <2000/mm^3). Most patients experience pain, low grade fever, and transient (<5 days) elevation of liver enzymes. Rarely, liver abscess, cholecystitis, and Lipiodal pneumonitis may occur. When HCC recurs following chemoembolization, it is most often in a different segment, or along the tumoral margin that is supplied by the portal vein.

The experience using TCE for non-*HCC liver metastases* is limited. Initial results of TCE for palliation of hormonally active liver metastases are given in Table 2–4, and suggest that, in nonoperative candidates, it is highly effective in providing symptomatic relief (100%) and diminishing hormonal secretion (by at least 90%) with minimum morbidity.[94,95]

Percutaneous ethanol injection therapy (PEI) uses ultrasonic guidance to pass skinny (21 to 22 g) needles directly into and adjacent to a hepatic tumor (Fig 2–8), with 2 to 8 ml of absolute ethanol injected per session, and 1 to 3 sessions performed each week on an outpatient basis. Depending on the number and size of tumors, the total number of injections may range from 3 to 20. Major complications are rare. Contraindications include intractable ascites and severe coagulopathy. Most work with this technique has been in patients with HCC (Table 2–5).[96,99] Of note, in cases with advanced cirrhosis, patients tend to die of cirrhotic sequelae rather than of tumor progression.[96,98]

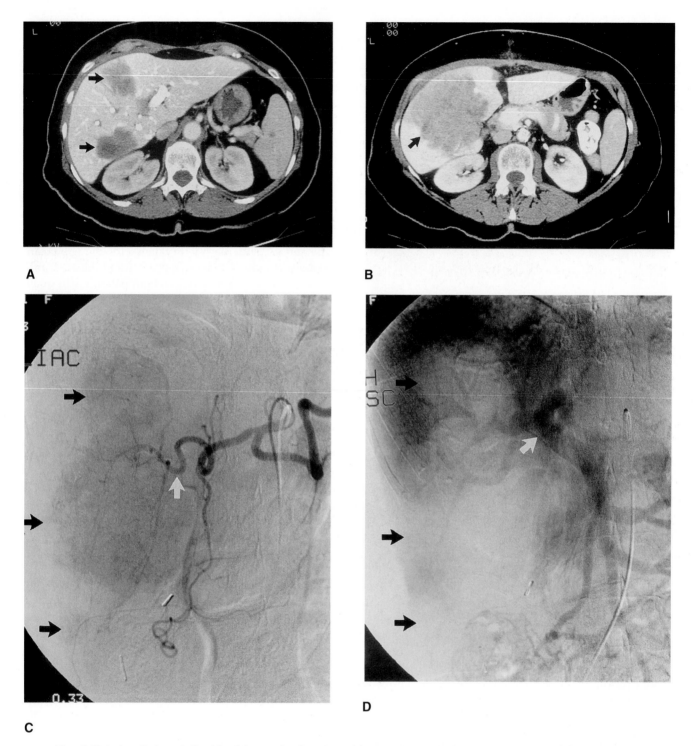

Figure 2–23. Angiographic demonstration of the relative separation of vascular supply between an intrahepatic malignancy (hepatic artery) and the uninvolved hepatic parenchyma (portal vein) in a 72 year-old woman with metastatic colon carcinoma. **A.** and **B.** Contrast-enhanced CT scans at two levels of the liver demonstrate multiple nonenhancing masses (*black arrows*) within the brightly enhancing liver. **C.** On the arterial phase of the celiac angiogram (anteroposterior view, digital-subtraction angiogram), the tumors are fed by hepatic arterial branches (*white arrow*) and have an intense parenchymal stain (*black arrows*); no stain of the liver parenchyma is evident. **D.** On the venous phase of the SMA angiogram, portal venous inflow (*white arrow*) feeds the normal liver parenchyma, whereas the tumors (*black arrows*) appear as regions of absent contrast stain (Swiss-cheese appearance).

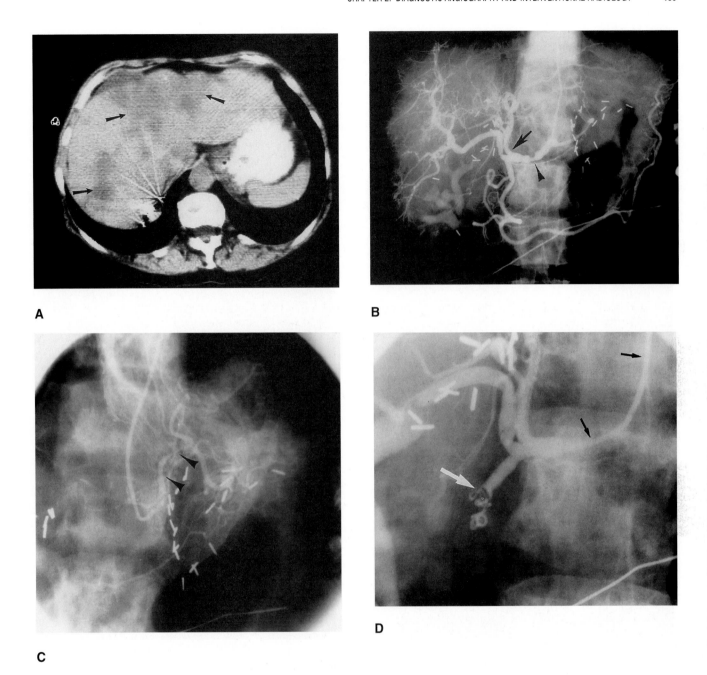

Figure 2–24. An example of angiographic evaluation and intervention in a 59 year–old female with right upper-quadrant pain and a history of breast carcinoma treated 23 years earlier with a radical mastectomy. **A.** Contrast-enhanced CT scan at the level of the liver demonstrates multiple hypoattenuating intrahepatic masses (*arrows*) which were biopsy-proven to be metastatic breast carcinoma. **B.** Anteroposterior view of a transbrachial celiac angiogram detects an early bifurcation of the hepatic artery (*black arrow*); incidentally noted guidewire-induced common hepatic artery vasospasm (*black arrowhead*). **C.** Anteroposterior view; selective left gastric arteriogram proved classic anatomy, specifically no replaced left hepatic arterial supply (*black arrowsheads*; guidewire-induced vasospasm). **D.** Magnified anteroposterior view; common hepatic arteriogram. Transcatheter stainless steel–coil embolization of the gastroduodenal artery (*white arrow*) has been performed in order to prevent inadvertent perfusion of the duodenum by chemotherapeutic drugs. A 5 day course of chemotherapy was infused via the angiographic catheter (*black arrows*) placed in the common hepatic artery. The early bifurcation of the hepatic artery forced placement of the catheter tip upstream from the gastroduodenal artery in order to perfuse all portions of the liver.

Regardless of the mode of local therapy (PEI, TCE, or surgical resection), hepatoma commonly recurs, usually as a new tumor at a separate, nontreated site (84% of recurrences in Shiina's series).[98] The primary role of PEI is in nonoperative candidates with Child's-Pugh class A or B cirrhosis. These patients should have no more than 3 tumors that are less than 4 to 5 cm diameter which are approachable with ultrasound guidance. Potentially, all approachable solitary HCCs less than 3 cm in diameter may be optimally treated

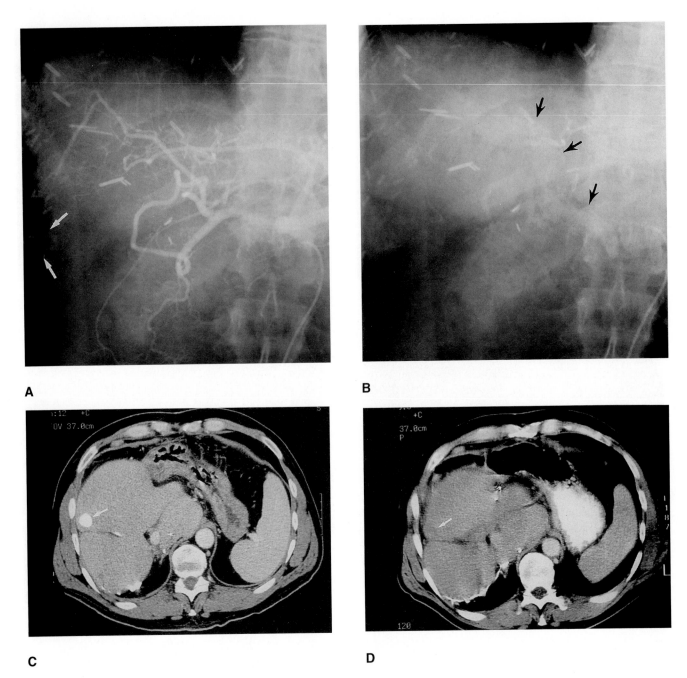

Figure 2–25. Hepatic chemoembolization of a recurrent metastatic spindle cell sarcoma (primary colon tumor) in a 50 year-old male who had previously undergone a hepatic right lobectomy. **A.** Celiac trunk arteriogram; anteroposterior view demonstrates a hypervascular 2.8-cm mass (*arrows*) fed via the middle hepatic artery. Multiple right upper-quadrant clips are from prior right lobectomy. **B.** Venous-phase celiac angiogram confirms portal vein patency (*black arrows*). Chemoembolization of the liver was performed in 2 sittings using a combination of polyvinyl alcohol, contrast, mitomycin, and cis-platinum. **C.** CT scan performed on the same day following the second episode of chemoembolization; documents retained (static) contrast within the hypervascular lesion (*arrow*). **D.** Repeat CT scan at approximately the same level, 6 weeks later, demonstrates virtual disappearance of the previously hypervascular mass, and a small residual focus of presumptive scar (*arrow*). [Case contributed by E. Hauptmann, M.D.].

with PEI, since the likelihood of complete tumor necrosis in very small tumors is high and the patient is spared surgical resection.[95,98] Transcatheter embolization may be best reserved for those patients with multiple or recurrent tumors, or tumors located in areas not readily accessible to ultrasound-directed needle puncture such as those anteriorly adjacent to the diaphragm.

Use of PEI for non-HCC metastatic malignancy is unproven. Other image-guided, locally destructive techniques are being developed for potential treatment of metastatic disease. These include percutaneous thermal

TABLE 2–2. RESULTS OF CHEMOEMBOLIZATION OF SMALL (<5 CM), SOLITARY OR LIMITED (<3) HEPATOCELLULAR CARCINOMAS

Series	Number of Patients	Regimen	Response (Necrosis)		Survival (Yrs)(%)				
			Complete	*Partial*	*1*	*2*	*3*	*4*	*5*
Yamada, Subset	66	Nonselective; Gelfoam + Doxorubicin + Mitomycin C	—	—	72	55	47	—	—
Matsui	100	Subsegmental; Lipidol + Doxorubicin + Mitomycin C + Gelfoam	7/11 (64%)	—	100	92	78	67	—
Park	14	Segmental; ETOH + Lipiodol	3/5 (60%)	2/5 (40%)	—	—	—	—	—
Matsuo	12	Segmental; Lipiodol + Doxorubicin + Gelfoam	10/12 (83%)	2/12 (17%)	—	—	—	—	—

TABLE 2–3. CHEMOEMBOLIZATION OF LARGE, NONOPERABLE HEPATOCELLULAR CARCINOMAS

Series	Number of Patients	Regimen	Survival (Yrs)(%)				
			1 Yr	*2 Yr*	*3 Yr*	*4 Yr*	*5 Yr*
Yamada	739	Nonselective; Gelfoam & Doxorubicin + Mitomycin C	51	28	13	8	6
Clouse	30	Selective; epinephrine + Lipiodol + Doxorubicin	61	36	—	—	—
Uflacker	33	Nonselective; Lipiodol + Mitomycin C + Ivalon	50	—	—	—	—

TABLE 2–4. THE RESULTS OF CHEMOEMBOLIZATION OF HORMONALLY ACTIVE HEPATIC METASTASES

Series	Number of Patients	Type of Tumor	Symptom Relief(%)	Hormonal Response(%)	Tumor Ablation(%)		Survival (Yrs)(%)				
					Complete	*Partial*	*1*	*2*	*3*	*4*	*5*
Therasse	23	Carcinoid	100	91	11	24	70	55	43	33	33
Stokes	20	Carcinoid; Islet Cell	100	100	—	—	—	—	—	—	—

TABLE 2–5. THE RESULTS OF PERCUTANEOUS ETOH FOR HEPATOCELLULAR CARCINOMA

Series	Number of Patients	Necrosis		Survival (Yrs)(%)					Comments
		Complete	*Partial*	*1*	*2*	*3*	*4*	*5*	
Livraghi	35	30/35 (86%)	5/35 (14%)	100	—	80	—	—	Smaller than 5 cm diameter
Salmi	27	—	—	87	—	63	—	—	
Shiina									
All patients	146	15/21 (71%)	6/21 (29%)	79	64	46	38	38	98 included TCE
"Cure"	98	—	—	85	70	62	52	52	Fewer than 3 lesions, 3 cm diameter
Solinas	45	35/45 (78%)	10/45 (22%)	95	87	75	70	—	PEI + TCE

ablation (laser or microwave probes) and operative ultrasound-guided cryotherapy.[100]

TRAUMA

In most patients with blunt trauma to the abdomen and
selected patients with penetrating injuries, peritoneal
lavage and a CT scan are excellent complimentary techniques to detect hemoperitoneum and to assess the integrity of the abdominal solid viscera, respectively.[101] In
patients who are candidates for nonoperative management of hepatic or splenic injuries and who manifest evidence of continued hemorrhage (hypotension, dropping
hematocrit, hemobilia, or enlarging fluid collections), angiography is definitive for diagnosis of hepatic and splenic
arterial injuries. Transcatheter embolization has been
demonstrated to be both safe and efficacious for treatment of arterial injury of the liver (88%) and spleen
(94%).[101,102] In the liver, small-particulate material
(Gelfoam pledgets, Ivalon particles, or microcoils) is
placed as close to the site of arterial injury as possible. Distal placement of emboli lessens the likelihood of continued bleeding owing to collateral supply and minimizes
the amount of liver tissue at risk for potential necrosis.
Portal venous inflow generally protects the liver from infarction after hepatic arterial blockade. In the spleen,
larger stainless steel coils are placed in the main splenic
artery to lower the intrasplenic blood pressure and preserve splenic perfusion via the collaterals. Transcatheter
embolization has also been widely used for treatment of
renal, retroperitoneal, and pelvic hemorrhage.

PANCREATITIS-ASSOCIATED ARTERIAL INJURY

Autodigestion and inflammation may cause arterial wall
disruption in patients with pancreatitis (5% to 10%) or
pancreatic pseudocysts (15% to 20%).[103] Clinical manifestations are classically abdominal pain and/or hemorrhage, especially gastrointestinal hemorrhage. Clinically
silent hemorrhagic pseudocysts occasionally may be detected on cross-sectional imaging studies. Angiography is
used to make the specific diagnosis. Confirmation, localization, and characterization of the arterial injury is made
angiographically. These angiographic findings include
pseudoaneurysm formation (possibly associated with a
pseudocyst); extravasation into the gut, retroperitoneum,
pancreatic duct, or biliary tree; or arteriovenous fistulization. The vessels most commonly affected are the splenic
(42%), gastroduodenal (22%), and small pancreatic arteries (25%).[102] Subselective particulate transcatheter embolization has been shown to be safe and effective for immediate hemostasis. Unfortunately, recurrent bleeding
has been reported in 37% of successfully embolized cases;
thus, either repeat embolization or surgical resection may
be necessary for definitive treatment.[103]

GASTROINTESTINAL HEMORRHAGE

The two transcatheter techniques available to achieve
hemostasis in patients with acute, massive arteriocapillary GI hemorrhage are intra-arterial infusion of vasopressin and particulate embolization. Transcatheter
techniques may be definitive in cases in which the etiology of bleeding is either self-limited and unlikely to rebleed (eg, colonic diverticular hemorrhage) or
amenable to medial therapy (eg, peptic ulcer disease).
Alternatively, transcatheter techniques are useful for
converting surgical treatment from emergent to elective
when the source of bleeding is associated with a high
likelihood of rehemorrhage (eg, colonic angiodysplasia), or is due to resectable malignancy.

Vasopressin therapy is administered via a catheter
placed in the main trunk of the artery supplying the
bleeding site (celiac trunk, SMA or IMA) (Fig 2–26).
The infusion is initiated at 0.2 U/min for 20 to 30 minutes, followed by a repeat angiogram. If bleeding has
ceased, the infusion is continued at 0.2 u/min; if bleeding continues, the rate is increased to 0.4 U/min, the
maximum allowable rate without excessive complications, and the angiogram repeated in 20 to 30 minutes.
If bleeding persists, vasopressin is likely to fail, and
transcatheter embolization or operative resection or repair is mandated. As long as the patient manifests hemostasis (negative NG aspirate, no transfusion requirement, etc) the vasopressin infusion is slowly decreased
to 50% every 6 to 12 hours until the infusion has been
maintained at 0.1 U/min for 6 to 12 hours. The vasopressin infusion then is replaced with saline infusion for
an additional 6 to 12 hours. If no bleeding is evident after this period of observation, the transarterial infusion
catheter is removed.

Since vasopressin is a potent vasoconstrictor, potential complications include regional (mesenteric) as well
as distant (coronary, lingual) ischemia or infarction as
well as systemic hypertension, cardiac dysrrhythmias,
and hyponatremia. Vasopressin has a disproportionately intense effect on gut arterioles and capillaries as
compared to either large-caliber arteries or visceral arteries. Therefore, vasopressin infusion is most effective
on diffuse mucosal processes (eg, gastritis) or bleeding
from small-caliber arteries (eg, Mallory-Weiss tears or diverticular hemorrhage). Bleeding due to either large
caliber arteries associated with transmural inflammation (eg, penetrating duodenal ulcers) or tumor neovascularity generally responds poorly to vasopressin.

Owing to the multiple arterial loops and the submucosal plexes of small-caliber arteries, transcatheter embolization is safe in the foregut and probably the hindgut (rectum), provided collateral vascular supply has
not been disrupted by prior surgery or embolization.
The midgut (distal duodenum to the rectosigmoid junc-

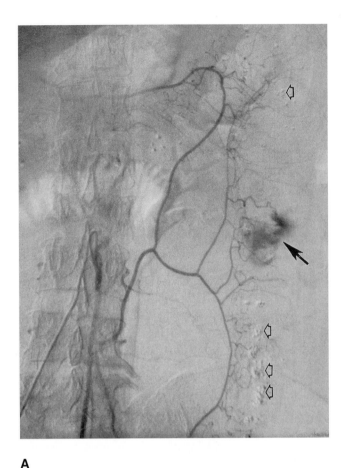

A

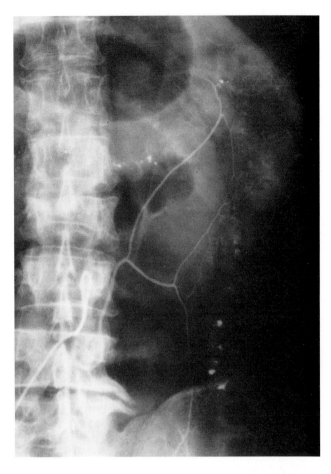

B

Figure 2–26. Vasopressin infusion from massive lower GI hemorrhage as a result of a bleeding diverticulum in a 51 year-old male. **A.** Anteroposterior view; arterial-phase IMA angiogram (subtracted film) shows extravasated contrast (*solid black arrow*) from the bleeding site in the middescending colon. Of note are multiple misregistered foci caused by barium inspissated from a prior diagnostic enema within other diverticuli (*open black arrows*). **B.** Anteroposterior view (unsubtracted) of a repeat IMA angiogram performed 1/2 hour following the initiation of a vasopressin infusion at 0.2 units per minute. No contrast extravacation is present, and diffuse pharmacologically caused vasospasm, particularly of small-caliber arteries, is evident. By clinical parameters, he ceased to bleed and was successfully managed nonoperatively.

tion) is at high risk of bowel infarction or development of ischemic strictures owing to the microvascular architecture.

The goal of embolization is to achieve hemostasis by decreasing the arterial pressure at the bleeding site. At the same time, tissue viability and eventual healing must be assured by allowing tissue perfusion to occur from preserved collateral supply. Ideally, the feeding artery will eventually recanalize. Gelfoam typically is resorbed over several days to 3 weeks; therefore, it is frequently utilized for initial attempts at arterial blockade. Permanent agents, such as stainless steel coils and Ivalon particles, are reserved for subsequent embolizations if recurrent bleeding occurs. Agents which occlude the microvasculature or are cytotoxic (eg, powders, ethanol or other liquid agents) are contraindicated since they are designed to cause tissue necrosis.

Owing to the arterial arcades of the foregut, refractory hemorrhage may occasionally mandate either embolization of more than one supplying artery, or adjunctive vasopressin infusion of arterial trunks that provide collateral supply.[104] In patients who have midgut hemorrhage that is nonresponsive to vasopressin infusion and who are poor operative risks, careful subselective transcatheter embolization may be warranted. Design advances in very small diameter catheters (2.5 to 3.0 Fr) permit delivery of small Gelfoam particles or readily controlled microcoils to the specific bleeding artery, thus limiting the risk of bowel infarction.[105]

MESENTERIC ISCHEMIA

Vasodilator therapy has been advocated to reverse the vasoconstrictive components of acute mesenteric ischemia.[105]

The greatest experience has been obtained using transcatheter infusion of papaverine at 30 to 60 mg/hr into the SMA for 12 to 24 hours. Infusion of prostaglandin E$_1$ at 0.6 to 1.5 mg/hr, has also been described. The primary role of vasodilator therapy has been to prevent ischemic bowel (usually small bowel) from progressing to infarction during the period in which any underlying compromised hemodynamic factors, such as congestive heart failure or digitalis toxicity, are corrected, or the patient is being prepared for, or is recovering from, operative revascularization. Support for this practice is derived from survival rates of 45% to 60% in patients with nonocclusive acute mesenteric ischemia who were given vasodilator therapy[106,107] as compared to the historical survival rates of approximately 10% for untreated patients.[108] Of note, however, is that patient populations were not similar and the infusion series were reported more than a decade after the noninfusion series.

Although surgical embolectomy and/or bowel resection has been the standard treatment for proximal SMA embolism and mesenteric venous thrombosis, limited experience using thrombolysis has been described. Schoenbaum and colleagues recently reported four patients with acute abdominal pain and no peritoneal signs who had emboli in the proximal SMA with reconstitution of distal SMA branches, primarily via the IMA, and who were successfully treated with intra-arterial urokinase.[109] Infusion duration tended to be long (30 to 40 hours) and two patients required laparotomy (exploration only, in one; resection of a small segment of infarcted bowel in the other). Patients with peripheral SMA emboli, intact distal vessels, and no peritoneal signs may require only transcatheter papaverine infusion with or without systemic anticoagulation.[110] One case of successful transcatheter thrombolysis via the transhepatic route has been reported for superior mesenteric venous thrombosis[111]; transarterial infusion (via the SMA) does not seem to be effective.[112]

Traditional techniques for operative revascularization of patients with *chronic mesenteric ischemia* have been transaortic endarterectomy and aortomesenteric bypass grafting. Use of *percutaneous transluminal angioplasty* (PTA) has been reported by several authors (Table 2–6).[113–117] Of note, PTA has a high technical success rate (over 86%) for dilation of nonostial stenoses of both the SMA and celiac trunks, but is relatively ineffective for dilation of ostial stenoses and extrinsic compression of the celiac trunk by the median arcuate ligament. Complication rates for PTA are acceptably low (0% to 25% clinically significant, with no procedure-related deaths). Rapid relief of abdominal pain occurs in nearly all patients with technically successful mesenteric PTA. Unfortunately, restenosis rates are very high. Primary patency at two years appears to be no greater than 25%, although repeat PTA may improve the secondary patency. Recent surgical revascularization series (Table 2–7) report 3 to 4 year primary patency rates of 70% to 93%.[118–120] This author believes that because of great durability of results, operative revascularization is indicated for patients who are surgical candidates and have convincing clinical symptoms and confirmatory angiographic abnormalities. PTA is probably best reserved for those patients who have either unacceptable surgical risk factors or limited life expectancy. In patients with atypical clinical symptoms or angiographic findings, a therapeutic trial of PTA may be warranted to determine if mesenteric ischemia is the cause of pain prior to embarking on operative revascularization.

TABLE 2–6. RESULTS OF PERCUTANEOUS TRANSLUMINAL ANGIOPLASTY FOR TREATMENT OF CHRONIC MESENTERIC ISCHEMIA

Series	Year	Number of Patients	Number of Vessels	Technical Success	Sx[a] Relief	Major Complications	In Hospital Mortality	% Primary Patency				% Secondary Patency			
								1	2	3	4	1	2	3	4
Golden	1982	7	7 (SMA)	6/7 (86%)	6/6 (100%)	NR[b]	0 (0%)	33	17	—	—	33	17	—	—
Roberts	1983	4	4 (SMA)	4/4 (100%)	4/4 (100%)	1 (25%) Brachial Artery occlusion	0 (0%)	50	25	—	—	100	50	—	—
Odurny/ Sniderman	1988/ 1991	10	19 12 (SMA) 7 (Celiac)	8/10 (80%); (nonosteal 100%)	8/8 (100%)	0 (0%)	1 (10%) unrelated	30	20	10	10	50	30	30	30
Rose	1994	8	9 7 (SMA) 1 (Celiac) 1 (Both)	7/9 (78%)	5/7 (71%)	2/8 (25%) Bowel infarction due to cholesterol emboli; Arm hematoma	1 (11%) Congestive heart failure	33	0	—	—	33	0	—	—

[a]Symptoms.
[b]Not related.

TABLE 2–7. RECENT RESULTS OF SURGICAL REVASCULARIZATION FOR TREATMENT OF CHRONIC MESENTERIC ISCHEMIA

Series	Year	Number of Patients	Number of Vessels	Type of Surgery	Initial Sx[a] (Survivors) (%)	Major Complications (%)	In Hospital Mortality (%)	Primary Patency (%)	Mean Follow-up Period (months)
Hollier	1981	56	2-3 = 77% 1 = 23%	Vein graft 36% Dacron 30% Endart 20% Reimpl. 10% PTFE 4%	96	NR	9	73	38
Rapp	1986	67	2-3 = 94%	Transaortic endart = 47 Antegrade aortomesenteric graft = 20	100	21	7.5	93	53
Beebe	1987	10	2-3 = 100%	Antegrade aortomesenteric graft = 24	100	20	0	70	43

[a]Signs.
[b]Not related.

■ NONVASCULAR INTERVENTION

BILIARY SYSTEM

Percutaneous transhepatic cholangiography (THC) has been described as long ago as 1937,[15] and external *percutaneous biliary drainage* (PBD) as long ago as 1956.[120] However, it was not until the mid to late 1970s that PBD became a widely accepted procedure for nonoperative treatment of obstructive jaundice. This followed the development of skinny-needle access for THC and coaxial exchange systems to allow passage of heavy-duty guidewires.

The *technique of PBD* begins with intravenous antibiotic prophylaxis (primarily for coverage of gram-negative rods), monitored conscious sedation and analgesia, and sterile preparation. The two usual approaches are from the right midaxillary line caudal to the tenth rib using fluoroscopic guidance to traverse the right hepatic lobe or from the epigastrium using combined ultrasound and fluoroscopic guidance to traverse the left hepatic lobe. A skinny (21 or 22 gauge) needle is used to find a usable bile duct: ipsilateral, intrahepatic, sufficiently large to accept the drain, and at least several centimeters proximal to the level of biliary obstruction. This usually is confirmed by injecting small quantities of contrast media (Fig 2–27). Once a suitable bile duct has been entered, a small amount of bile (eg, 10 mL) is aspirated to minimize the risk of PBD-related bacteremia. Sufficient contrast media is injected gently to provide a crude cholangiogram. A guidewire is passed through the needle into the biliary tree, the needle is removed and replaced with a coaxial exchange catheter set, which allows passage of a working guidewire. An angiographic catheter is passed over the working guidewire and the catheter/guidewire combination is used to probe the site of biliary obstruction. If the obstructive site is easily negotiated, the tract is dilated and an inter-

nal/external biliary drain (usually 8- to 10-Fr diameter) is placed so that side holes are within the biliary system above and below the level of obstruction. If the obstruction cannot be passed easily, an external drain is left above the obstruction for initial biliary decompression. The obstructed site usually can be transversed safely on a subsequent attempt a couple of days later.

Three fundamental types of drainage are possible. *External biliary drainage* refers to placement of the catheter so that the tip and side holes are entirely upstream from the site of obstruction. Advantages are (1) maximally efficient biliary decompression with gravity drainage (particularly important in patients with sepsis or cholangitis), (2) the ability to flush the catheter to maintain patency, and (3) simple replacement over a guidewire. Disadvantages include (1) less secure catheter anchorage, (2) loss of bile salts, electrolytes and fluid, and (3) the need for a drain exiting the body as well as for a drainage bag for collection.

Internal/external (or universal) drainage refers to percutaneous transhepatic passage of the catheter across the obstruction with side holes placed upstream as well as downstream (Fig 2–28). Bile, as well as duodenal contents, may be drained externally, if left to dependent drainage, or internally into the alimentary tract, if the catheter is capped. Advantages include (1) the versatility of type of drainage including elimination of the drainage bag and (2) the ability to flush or exchange the drain easily. Internal/external drainage is probably slightly less effective for biliary decompression and more likely to become occluded by duodenal mucus than pure external drainage. Additionally, a drain continues to exit the patient.

Internal drainage refers to placement of an intrabiliary conduit (endoprosthesis) which extends from above the biliary obstruction to either the downstream bile duct or small bowel. Endoprostheses may be introduced either percutaneously (usually for obstruction in the porta he-

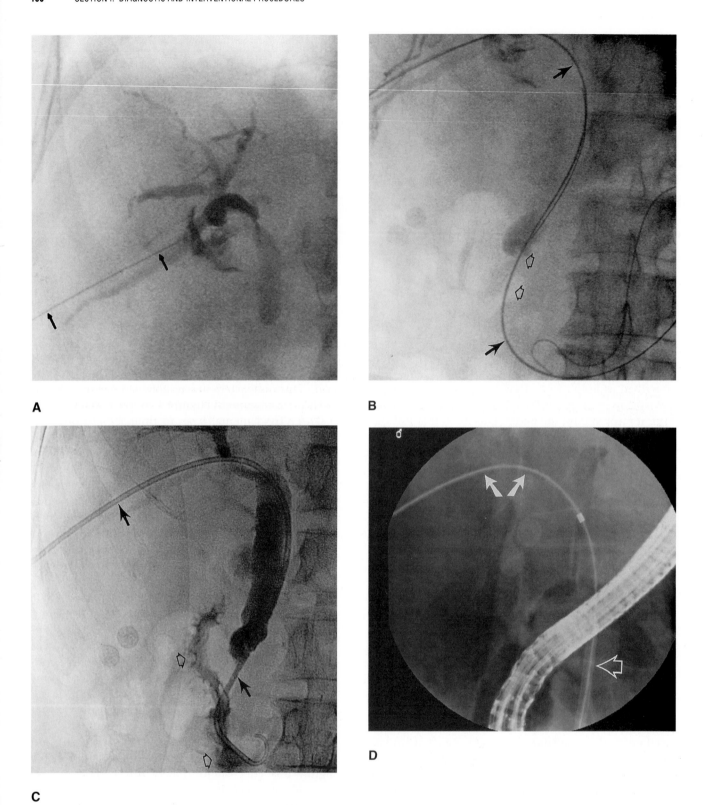

Figure 2–27. Technique for internal/external percutaneous biliary drainage and rendezvous procedure in a 76 year-old male with obstructive jaundice owing to ampillary carcinoma. Initial endoscopy proved the diagnosis with a biopsy, but attempts to cannulate the biliary duct failed. **A.** A 22-gauge needle (*black arrows*) has been placed into a right-sided bile duct, and a small amount of contrast injected to provide a crude working cholangiogram. **B.** A heavy-duty guidewire (*solid arrows*) has been passed beyond the tumor (*open arrows*) into the duodenum. **C.** After tract dilation, an 8.3-Fr internal/external biliary drainage catheter (*solid arrows*) has been positioned so that the side holes above the tumor permit bile to pass the obstruction and flow into the duodenum (*open arrows*). **D.** Two days later, a 400 cm–long guidewire (*solid white arrows*) was passed via the drain and retrived endoscopically. After removal of the percutaneous drain, an 11 Fr plastic endoprosthesis (*open white arrow*) was passed transendoscopically into the bile duct above the level of the tumor. *Continued*

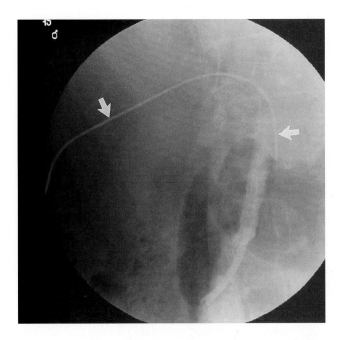

E

Figure 2–27, cont'd. E. A 6-Fr temporary external percutaneous biliary drain (*white arrows*) has been replaced above the endoprosthesis. Contrast injection via the external biliary drain demonstrates that the endoprosthesis is properly positioned with brisk flow of contrast into the duodenum.

patic region) or transendoscopically (usually for distal common bile duct obstruction). The advantages include (1) no external devices and (2) preservation of bile salts, electrolytes, and fluids. However, patency cannot be prolonged by flushing, and exchange is an option only for plastic endoprostheses which are endoscopically placed.

The results of several large published series (Table 2–8) indicate that PBD can be performed with a high degree of technical success (94% to 97% of procedures).[121-124] Major periprocedural complication rates range from 4% to 8% and are due primarily to hemorrhage and infection (sepsis, suppurative cholangitis, and/or hepatic abscesses). Procedure-related mortality rates range from 1% to 6%; minor periprocedural complications range from 20% to 30%. Delayed complications occur most often as a result of catheter occlusion, drain dislodgment, or suppurative cholangitis.[121] Both mortality rates and major complication rates for drainage of benign biliary obstruction tend to be one-third to one-half the rate for drainage of most common malignant strictures.[124,125] This difference probably results from the longer duration of intubation and the poorer overall health of patients with malignant biliary obstruction.

Sochendra originally described the transendoscopic placement of internal biliary endoprostheses in 1980.[126] In centers with skilled interventional endoscopists, endoscopic placement of biliary stents has replaced percutaneous delivery as the initial nonoperative biliary de-

compressive procedure of choice for nonresectable malignant biliary obstruction. Advantages include decreased pain and complications associated with the establishment of the transhepatic tract.[127,128] Endoscopic success rates are highest (approximately 95%) and mortality and major morbidity rates lowest (approximately 2% and 10%, respectively) for lesions of the distal common bile duct (CBD).[129] Mid CBD malignancy as a result of cholangiocarcinoma is most amenable to attempted operative resection, with operative biliary diversion if the tumor is nonresectable.[130] With endoscopic drainage alone, proximal (high) CBD, hilar, and intrahepatic malignant strictures have a lower success rate (67%) and a higher mortality and morbidity rate (8% and 17%, respectively).[129] Hilar and intrahepatic malignant stenosis can be decompressed successfully via bilateral internal/external PBDs or reconstructed with flexible metallic expandable stents.[131-134] In cases of failed transendoscopic drainage, radiologic percutaneous transhepatic placement of a small-caliber biliary catheter allows for a combined radiologic-endoscopic approach (rendezvous procedure) to internal biliary drainage (Fig 2–27).[135] A long (400 to 500 cm) guidewire is passed coaxially through the small PBD into the duodenum and is retrieved via the endoscope. A transendoscopic stent then is placed over the guidewire in a retrograde fashion. A temporary angiographic catheter is left above the internal stent for 24 to 48 hours to guarantee adequate internal drainage prior to removal of the transhepatic access.

The recent development of metallic expandable stents allows deployment of large-caliber, flexible conduits (8 to 10 mm) through a small-caliber tract (7 to 10 Fr) (Fig 2–21). Metallic stents may be delivered either percutaneously or transendoscopically. Unlike plastic endoprostheses, they generally cannot be removed. Stent occlusion can occur due to accumulation of mucinous debris or tumor overgrowth. Recanalization procedures available to restore stent function include balloon extraction of debris,[136] thermal coagulation of tumor,[136] placement of additional stents for tumoral overgrowth, and coaxial placement of either a plastic endoprosthesis or internal/external PBD. Initial results suggest that primary patency rates are not significantly different between metallic and plastic endoprostheses.[137] In patients with hepatic or renal dysfunction, 30 day mortality rates may be improved with metal stents as compared to plastic endoprostheses (18% vs 33%). There appears to be no difference in 30 day mortality rates in patients with normal hepatic and renal function (8%).[137] The primary disadvantage of metallic stents is the substantially higher cost (approximately $1000 per stent) compared to plastic drains ($60 to $160 per drain).

Percutaneous transhepatic techniques allow for adjunctive options relevant specifically to cholangiocarcinoma. This route allows cytologic analysis of bile sam-

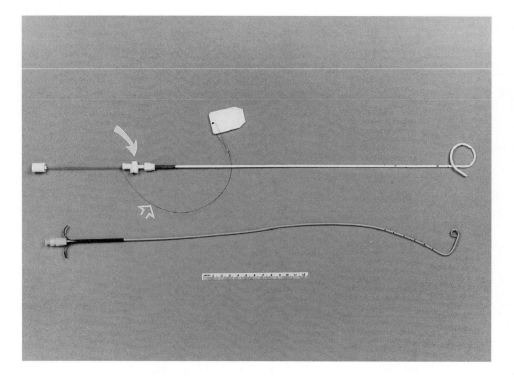

A

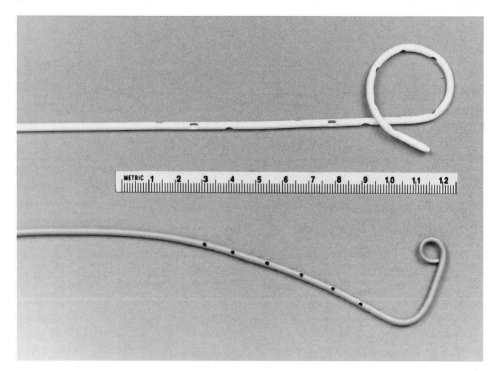

B

Figure 2–28. Two examples of internal/external biliary drainage catheters. **A.** The upper drain is a Cope-type locking-pigtail catheter (10-Fr PBD, Meditech, Inc., Watertown, MA) in which the cinch line (*open white arrow*) keeps the pigtail loop closed and is secured by the locking hub (*solid white arrow*). The lower drain (8.3-Fr biliary ring, Cook, Inc, Bloomington, IN) is a more rigid nonlocking system often used as the initial PBD to traverse the biliary stricture. **B.** Close-up view of the distal end of both internal/external PBD devices illustrated in **A.** Note that the side holes extend up the catheter shaft in order for bile to enter the drain above the stricture and be delivered via the pigtail into the small bowel. Additional side holes can be added in order to customize the drain to match the patient's anatomy.

TABLE 2–8. RESULTS OF PERCUTANEOUS BILIARY DRAINAGE

Series	Year	Number of Patients	Success	Major Complications (Acute)			Minor		Late
				Death	*Bleeding*	*Infection*	*Bleeding*	*Infection*	
Mueller	1982	200	188/200 (94%)	3 (1.5%)	6 (3%)	7 (3.5%)	18 (9%)	21 (10.5%)	22%
Carasco	1984	161	—	9 (6%)	—	—	—	—	—
Hamlin	1986	118	114/118 (97%)	3 (2.5%)	3 (2.5%)	2 (1.6%)	19 (16%)	16 (14%)	35
Yee	1984	217	—	4 (1%)	1 (0.5%)	8 (4%)	—	—	—

ples[138] or brush biopsy,[139] as well as definitive histologic evaluation of suspected cholangiocarcinoma using either myocardial biopsy forceps (Fig 2–12)[140] or a Simpson atherectomy device.[141] If internal/external PBD catheters are in position, transcatheter brachytherapy, typically with iridium 192 seeds or wire, permits high-dose endoluminal radiotherapy. At least two reports suggest prolonged survival in patients with hilar cholangiocarcinoma who undergo brachytherapy with or without external beam or radiation (13 to 17 months in treated patients, 2 months in controls).[142,143]

BENIGN BILIARY STRICTURES

Benign biliary strictures are caused most commonly by iatrogenic events, especially cholecystectomy. They also may be due to inflammatory conditions such as sclerosing cholangitis, choledocholithiasis, or pancreatitis. Initial surgical biliary drainage procedures afford acceptable long-term results for extrahepatic strictures. Operative restenosis rates generally range from 10% to 25%. Restenosis rates following subsequent operative repairs are much higher. Operative repair of benign intrahepatic biliary strictures is technically difficult.

Published reports of percutaneous cholangioplasty (balloon dilation) report success rates ranging from 67% to 85% and restenosis rates ranging from 22% to 34% at 2 to 3 years (Fig 2–29).[144–148] Patency rates relate to the site of stricture: intrahepatic (100%), extrahepatic and suprapancreatic (92%), biliary-enteric anastomoses (75%), and intrapancreatic (33%).[148] Patency rates at 3 years also depend on the etiology of stricture: iatrogenic (76%), biliary-enteric anastomoses (67%) and sclerosing cholangitis (42%).[146]

Transendoscopic sphincterotomy is the initial modality of choice for treatment of benign periampullary strictures. Operative biliary-enteric bypass is the preferred treatment for extrahepatic bile duct strictures not caused by sclerosing cholangitis. In patients with extrahepatic benign strictures due to sclerosing cholangitis, recurrent strictures after operative repair, or complicating factors such as portal hypertension or right upper quadrant scarring, repeated balloon dilation either via a percutaneous or transendoscopic route is an attractive modality (Fig 2–30).[149] Plastic endoprostheses, although valuable as

temporary postprocedural stents, are not advisable for long-term use because of their inevitable occlusion by debris. Expandable metallic endoprostheses have been deployed in some patients with benign strictures[149,150]; however, the long-term natural history is unknown, prolonged patency is not assured, and the presence of a permanent indwelling foreign body may complicate subsequent operative and nonoperative intervention. Furthermore, mucosal hypertrophy has been reported in the canine model.[151] Thus, the role of metallic stents for treatment of benign strictures has not yet been established.[150]

Intrahepatic strictures, especially if multifocal, are generally most amenable to percutaneous cholangioplasty either via a transhepatic route or T tube tract. In patients with primary sclerosing cholangitis, maintenance of continuous biliary access is desirable.[152,153] In patients requiring repeated biliary access and who undergo hepaticojejunostomy, fixation of the Roux-en-Y loop to the anterior abdomen allows fluoroscopically guided puncture with retrograde catheter passage to the biliary system.[154,155]

Percutaneous extraction of retained bile duct stones via a T tube tract under radiologic guidance has been widely practiced since the early 1970s (Fig 2–31). In one large series of 661 patients, percutaneous extraction was successful in 95% of cases.[156] In patients without T tube access, transendoscopic papillotomy and stone extraction using retrieval baskets or occlusion balloons is effective in approximately 90% of cases, with minimal morbidity. Alternatively, transhepatic stone removal is an excellent nonoperative option for patients with failed endoscopic retrieval. Mechanical extraction using wire baskets or occlusion balloons, first to fragment the stones, then to deliver the pieces into the duodenum, is successful in over 90% of cases with morbidity rates of 12% to 14% and 30 day mortality rates of 3% to 4%.[157,158] For very large stones (>15 mm), transhepatic fragmentation can be accomplished with electrohydraulic lithotripsy, ultrasonic lithotripsy, or tunable dye lasers.[159]

Chemodissolution of bile duct stones with methyl tert-butyl ether is limited by toxicity if the drug passes into the duodenum, suboptimal effectiveness (works only on cholesterol stones), and lack of FDA approval for intrabiliary usage.

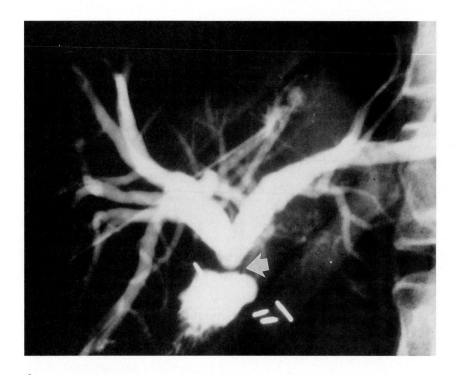

A

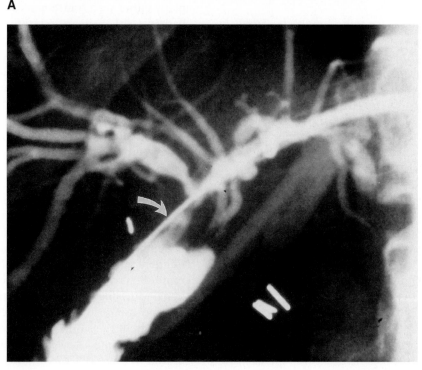

B

Figure 2–29. Balloon dilation of a biliary-enteric anastomic stricture. **A.** Anteroposterior view of a transhepatic cholangiogram demonstrates dilation of the intrahepatic bile ducts due to a high grade benign stricture at the hepaticojejunostomy anastomosis. **B.** Following establishment of a left-sided percutaneous biliary-drainage access route, a guidewire (*white arrow*) has been negotiated past the stricture into the jejunal limb. *Continued*

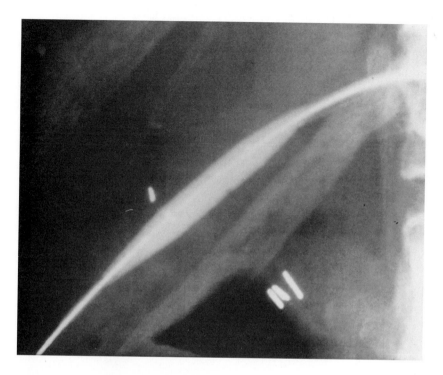

C

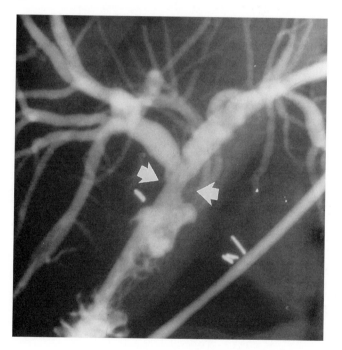

D

Figure 2–29, cont'd. C. Over the guidewire, a balloon dilation catheter has been passed across the stricture and expanded to 10 mm diameter with disappearance of the balloon waist. **D.** Following balloon dilation and placement of an internal/external biliary drain as a stent, repeat cholangiography documents improvement in the anastomotic diameter and free drainage of contrast from the biliary tree into the Roux limb. *White arrows* define the level of the biliary-enteric anastomosis.

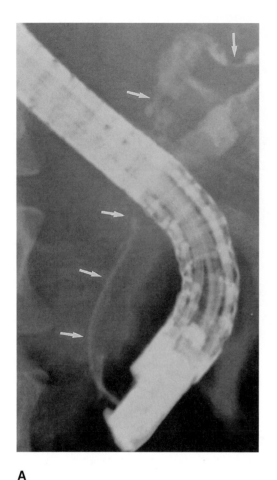

A

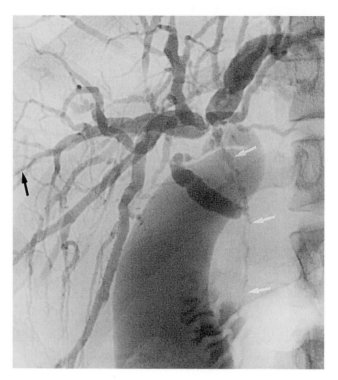

B

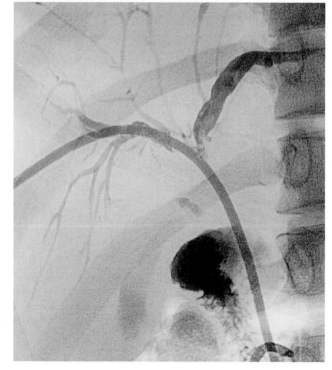

C

Figure 2–30. Percutaneous management of primary sclerosing cholangitis in an 18 year–old male with obstructive jaundice and fever. **A.** ERCP with patients in a prone position documents the diagnosis manifest as both extrahepatic and intrahepatic strictures (*arrows*). The intrabiliary filling defects were noted fluoroscopically to represent air bubbles. The extrahepatic stricture was too fibrotic to allow retrograde passage of a transendoscopic stent. **B.** Transhepatic cholangiogram via right-sided PBD (*black arrow*) confirms the diagnosis and severity of the extrahepatic biliary strictures (*white arrows*). **C.** Following transbiliary guidewire passage, the common hepatic and bile ducts were dilated with a 7-mm diameter balloon, which in turn allowed placement of a chronic indwelling internal/external PBD. Postprocedurally the patient was rendered asymptomatic. Note the diminished caliber of the intrahepatic bile ducts on the final cholangiogram.

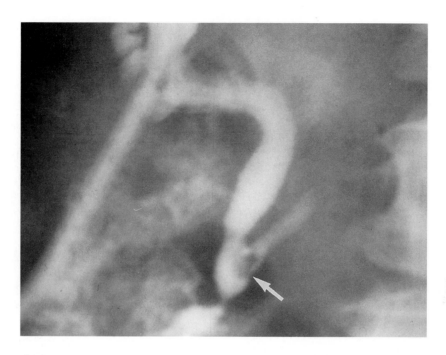

A

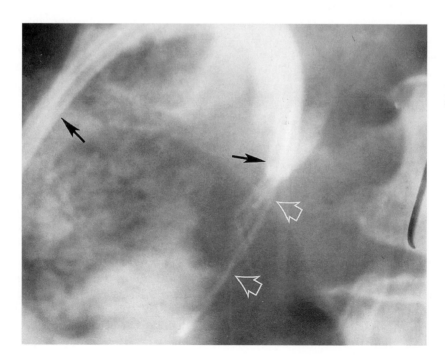

B

Figure 2–31. Percutaneous T tube tract extraction of a retained common bile duct calculus in a patient 6 weeks, after open cholecystectomy and common bile duct exploration. **A.** Anteroposterior view of a postoperative T tube cholangiogram documents a faceted filling defect (*solid white arrow*) consistent with a calculus at the junction of the distal common bile duct and pancreatic duct. **B.** After removal of the T tube over a guidewire, a steerable catheter (*solid black arrows*) was directed into the distal common bile duct. A Dormia stone basket (*arrowheads*) was passed coaxially and used to entrap the radiolucent calculus which was delivered into the duodenum. A new T tube was then advanced into the biliary tree. *Continued*

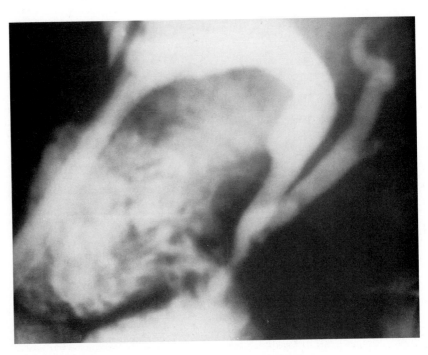

Figure 2–31, cont'd. C. A repeat T tube cholangiogram 2 days later confirms the absence of the biliary calculus.

C

Biliary injury is usually iatrogenic and occurs as a result of biliary tract surgery, especially laparoscopic cholecystectomy. Patients commonly present weeks to months postoperatively with fever, abdominal pain, jaundice, and/or sepsis. Most injuries involve either a leak (eg, dislodged cystic duct clip) or stricture. The initial step in management is to obtain a cholangiogram (either transhepatically or transendoscopically) and cross-sectional imaging, usually a CT scan, to confirm the diagnosis and to establish the extent of injury. Next, biliary diversion or decompression is provided either with transendoscopic sphincterotomy and retrograde stent placement or internal/external PBD.[160–163] Associated fluid collections (bilomas, abscesses, biliary ascites) are drained percutaneously. In selected cases of biliary strictures, balloon dilation (cholangioplasty) may be performed, although biliary-enteric bypass is used more commonly. In the case of operative repair, the biliary drainage catheter provides a valuable guide for surgical dissection of the inflamed and scarred postoperative right upper quadrant. In patients with biliary leaks without associated strictures, the above regimen is sufficient to avoid reoperation in 48% to 67%.[160–162] Mortality rates range from 2% to 5%.

Percutaneous access into the gallbladder has been shown to be both safe and practical for a range of diagnostic and therapeutic purposes.[164–166] Although direct transperitoneal puncture of the gallbladder fundus can be performed, access is achieved most commonly via the right transhepatic route because only 17% of patients have neither right colon nor liver between the gallbladder and abdominal wall[167] and the risk of free peritoneal spillage of bile is minimized. In patients who have failed endoscopic and transhepatic cholangiography, percutaneous cholecystography is an alternate technique used to perform cholangiography.[164,168] Although the intrahepatic bile ducts tend to be underfilled, images of the distal common bile duct can be expected to be sufficient to diagnose causes of obstruction.

Percutaneous cholecystostomy (PC) is a low-risk modality that is both diagnostic and therapeutic in critically ill patients with acute cholecystitis.[166,169,170] Noninvasive imaging techniques are rarely definitive. Ultrasound abnormalities such as gallbladder distention, wall thickening, and pericholecystic fluid collections are common, but nonspecific. Radionuclide hepatobiliary scanning is often falsely positive in chronically or critically ill bedridden patients. In patients with acute calculus cholecystitis, PC allows clinical stabilization so that cholecystectomy can be performed electively rather than urgently. In patients with acalculous cholecystitis, PC is usually definitive, and cholecystectomy can be avoided unless gallbladder necrosis has occurred.

Percutaneous gallbladder access affords adjunctive methods to remove gallstones in nonoperative candidates. Techniques include contact dissolution with monooctanoin or methyl tert butyl ether[171,172] and mechanical fragmentation and extraction.[173,174] In patients with failed endoscopic and transhepatic biliary drainage, PC, although not ideal, can be used to provide biliary decompression if the obstruction involves the distal CBD.[164]

THE ALIMENTARY TRACT

Esophagus

Removal of esophageal foreign bodies. Fluoroscopically guided retrieval of blunt esophageal foreign bodies has been shown to be very effective, safe, simple, and inexpensive. In a survey of the Society of Pediatric Radiology, 64 institutions performed removal, using a Foley catheter, of blunt, usually radiopaque (eg, coins) esophageal foreign bodies in over 2500 children.[175] Foreign body extraction was successful in 95% of these cases. No deaths or major complications occurred and minor complications occurred in 0.4% of cases.

The child is placed in a prone-oblique position on the fluoroscopic table. A Foley catheter is passed, either orally or nasally, beyond the foreign body. The balloon is gently inflated and the catheter retracted under fluoroscopic observation. During extraction of the foreign body, the fluoroscopic table is tilted head down to avoid any risk of aspiration. Variance of the technique includes use of a Dormia stone basket (eg, radiolucent or round structures) or a magnet-imbedded catheter for removal of esophageal or gastric nickel-cadmium batteries. Radiologic techniques should not be used in cases with sharp foreign bodies and only with great caution in patients with known underlying esophageal disease.

Esophageal stricture. Esophageal strictures both benign and malignant, are frequently amenable to nonoperative outpatient treatment. Guidance may be fluoroscopic, endoscopic, or a combination of both. Endoscopy affords visualization of the mucosal surface with the option of diagnostic biopsy. Radiologic evaluation and guidance permits assessment of the stricture length and lumen of the gut beyond the strictured site.[176] The most common etiologies of benign esophageal strictures include postoperative anastomotic (eg, esophagoesophageal or esophagogastric), peptic due to gastroesophageal reflux, caustic agent ingestion, achalasia, and webs. The traditional approach to nonoperative management of benign strictures has been bougienage, either blind or over a guidewire. Although clinical response rates have been high, the risk of esophageal perforation approximates 8%.[176] Additionally, bougienage accomplishes radial dilation at the expense of generating considerable shear force as the tapered dilator tip advances across the strictures.[177] Alternatively, balloon dilation provides the force for radial dilation with negligible creation of shear forces. In one series, balloon dilation resulted in a more durable result than bougienage (9.3 months vs 2.3 months).[178]

Fluoroscopically guided techniques of balloon dilation of esophageal strictures involve either transnasal or transoral passage of an angiographic catheter (or an amputated nasogastric tube) to just above the stricture, followed by passage of a torquable angiographic guidewire across the stenosis. The guiding catheter is removed and replaced with a balloon-dilating catheter (Fig 2–32). In general, the targeted diameter of dilation is 20 mm in adults (proportionately smaller in children), although up to 40 mm diameter may be necessary in patients with achalasia.[178] In patients with corrosive stricture, dilation beyond 15 mm is probably not warranted because of the high risk of esophageal rupture.[179] Initially, many patients can be dilated to 20 mm; however, if severe chest pain is noted, multiple sessions (2 to 4) may be required to reach the targeted diameter safely.

Technical success rates and rates of initial clinical improvement both approximate 100% for balloon dilation of benign esophageal strictures.[178–182] Perforation rates in general are low (0% to 8%), although they are substantially higher in patients with corrosive strictures (32%) as a result of the extensive fibrosis. Esophageal leaks with fistula formation related to esophagogastric or esophagocolic anastomoses have been nonoperatively managed by dilation of the anastomosis.[184] Recurrence of symptoms due to restenosis with mean onset between 9 to 28 months is common (20% to 40%) and is amenable to repeat dilation.[176,178,179,182] Balloon dilation of malignant strictures is reported to yield initial symptomatic improvement, but of unacceptably short durability.

In patients with nonresectable esophageal malignant strictures, multiple transendoscopic modalities have been developed to provide palliative relief of dysphagia, including laser therapy, thermal ablation, and placement of nonexpandable plastic stents.[184] More recently, metallic expandable stents have been developed that can be deployed under fluoroscopic or combined endoscopic-fluoroscopic guidance. Although limited to selected investigational sites, initial results suggest that nearly all patients receive initial palliation of symptoms with negligible complications.[185–187] Most stents remain patent for the remainder of the patient's life. Symptoms may recur as a result of food impaction (may be removed with a stone basket or balloon catheter) or tumor overgrowth (treated with either an additional stent or laser therapy). Improved stent designs make stent migration relatively rare.

Stomach

Balloon dilation. Benign strictures causing gastric outlet obstruction are most commonly antropyloric in location owing to peptic ulcer disease or are found at gastrojejunal anastomoses as a result of postoperative scarring. Gastric distention as a result of obstruction, combined with the difficult angles and unpredictable lumenal course within the strictured segments, makes gastric stricture intubation more difficult in these locations than most other sites in the GI tract. Technical

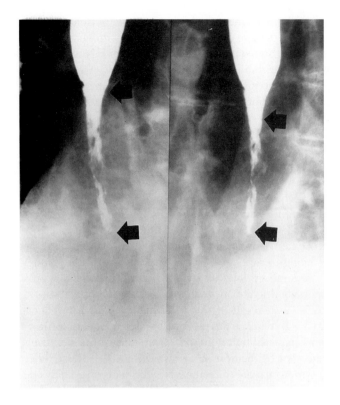

A

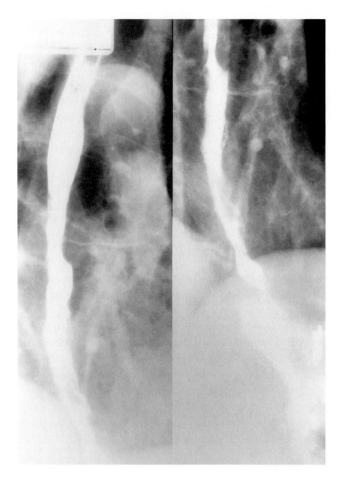

B

Figure 2–32. Balloon dilation of an esophagojejunal anastomotic stricture in an elderly female with incapacitating dysphasia after a total gastrectomy for Zollinger-Ellison syndrome. **A.** Two step oblique views of an upright barium esophagram document a high-grade stricture (*black arrows*) of the distal esophagus, with no significant barium passing into the jejunum. **B.** Following dilation to 15-mm diameter, the luminal diameter is improved and barium passes readily into the jejunum.

failure to intubate the strictures occurs in approximately 33% of cases.[180] Combined radiologic and endoscopic guidance likely improves the eventual technical success rate.[176] In adults, the target diameter for dilation is usually 15 mm, but to prevent dumping syndrome in morbidly obese patients with gastroenteric anastomoses, the target diameter is lessened to 12 mm.[180] Balloon dilation results in initial symptomatic relief of gastric outlet obstruction in approximately 67% to 80% of patients.[176,188] The reported results of long-term symptomatic improvement are variable, but may be as high as 83% at 1 year and 69% at 2 years.[189] Balloon dilation of anastomotic strictures seems to have a more durable result than in nonanastomotic strictures.[189] As expected, malignant strictures have much poorer long-term patency than benign strictures. Gastric outlet obstruction arising shortly after gastrojejunostomy may be due to kinks of the efferent jejunal limbs or to unfavorable movement through the transverse mesocolon. These functional causes of obstruc-

tion do not respond to balloon dilation and require surgical revision.

Percutaneous gastrostomy and percutaneous gastroenterostomy.
Enteric access for nutritional support or alimentary decompression of chronic bowel obstruction historically has been performed operatively (procedure-related mortality rates 1.8% to 6.0%; major complication rates 13% to 23%) or transendoscopically (procedural mortality rates 0% to 2%; major complication rates 10% to 20%). Recently, the fluoroscopically guided radiologic technique of placement of percutaneous gastrostomy (PG) and percutaneous gastroenterostomy (PGE) tubes has been developed. The results of several large series are presented in Table 2–9 and this technique compares favorably to surgically and endoscopically placed PG and PGE tubes.[190–194] Additionally, radiologic placement is frequently feasible in situations where endoscopic placement is not, such as patients with esophageal or head and neck malignancies. A PG

TABLE 2–9. THE RESULTS OF RADIOLOGICALLY GUIDED PLACEMENT OF PERCUTANEOUS GASTROSTOMY AND GASTROENTEROSTOMY TUBES

Author	Year	Number of Patients	Success	Mortality	Morbidity (%)	
					Major	*Minor*
O'KEEFFE	1989	100	100	0	0	25
HALKIER	1989	252	99	0.8	1.6	4.4
HICKS	1990	158	100	0	6	12
SAINI	1990	125	99	0	1.6	9.5
DEUTSCH	1992	68	100	0	4.7	7.8

tube is sufficient for feeding or decompression in most patients (Fig 2–33). PGE tubes, which can be more complex in construction, more expensive, and technically more demanding to place, may be reserved for patients with symptomatic gastroesophageal reflux, documented aspiration, gastric outlet obstruction, or gastroparesis (Fig 2–34 and 2–35).

The two most important structures to avoid in radiologic placement of PG tubes are the left lobe of the liver and the transverse colon. The liver edge can be mapped out with ultrasound or percussion. The transverse colon usually can be visualized by the presence of intraluminal gas but may be identified definitively if a cup of barium is administered orally or via nasogastric tube the previous evening (Figs 2–33 and 2–34). If feasible, a nasogastric tube or angiographic catheter is advanced into the

stomach. After administration of intravenous glucagon, the stomach is distended with air via the nasogastric tube. If a large bore (>16 to 18 Fr) gastric tube is anticipated, percutaneous gastropexy can be performed by placement of 3 to 4 T fasteners delivered via an 18 gauge slotted needle (Fig 2–35). Gastropexy, by securely fixing the anterior wall of the stomach to the anterior abdominal wall, permits single-session placement of large bore tubes without the risk of access loss or peritoneal spillage during tract dilation.[193] Under fluoroscopic guidance, an 18 gauge needle is passed through the anterior wall of the midbody of the stomach and directed toward the pylorus. Ideally, a heavy-duty guidewire is passed intralumenally and directed into the duodenum. The needle is removed and the tract is dilated. If gastropexy is not employed, a Cope-loop type nephrostomy catheter is used for PG feeding[194] and a Carey-Alzate-Coons tube is used for PGE feeding.[195] With gastropexy, large-bore (20 to 24 Fr) balloon-retention feeding tubes can be placed into the stomach, which affords a wider selection of administered feedings (eg, blenderized foods) and medications. Additionally, recently developed systems permit coaxially placed jejunal feeding tubes (Fig 2–34 and 2–35). The primary advantages to these systems are (1) the ability simultaneously to decompress the stomach while feeding transjejunally (eg, in patients with gastroparesis or GE reflux), and (2) simple replacement of the jejunal component over a guidewire while maintaining the transgastric access. Feedings may begin after 1 day or with the onset of bowel sounds in patients with PG tubes, and may begin immediately in patients with PGE tubes.

The potential major complications include hemorrhage requiring transfusion, peritonitis, tube dislodgement, sepsis, gastrocolic fistula, and aspiration.[190–193] Minor complications include superficial wound infections, transpyloric (distal) migration of the tube, minor skin-site bleeding, cellulitis, leakage of ascites, and pneumoperitoneum.

Colon

Colonic stricture dilation. Similar to anastomotic strictures of the proximal gastrointestinal tract, colorectal anastomotic strictures respond well to balloon dilation, with reported technical success rates ranging from 80% to 100% (Fig 2–36).[176] Balloon dilation may be beneficial for treatment of ischemic colonic strictures in infants previously afflicted with necrotizing enterocolitis. Ball and associates reported dilation of 9 nonobstructing, radiographically proven colonic strictures distal to an enterostomy in 5 infants.[196] Subsequent enterostomy closure, usually on the next day, was successful in all 5 infants.

Percutaneous cecostomy. In patients with adynamic ileus involving the colon (Ogilvie's syndrome) with cecal dilation >12 cm diameter, the initial decompressive treat-

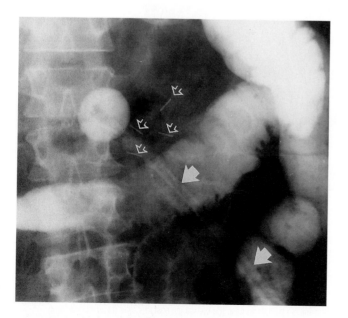

Figure 2–33. Percutaneous gastrostomy; 47 year–old male status-post radical neck dissection and irradiation for hypopharyngeal carcinoma, was unable to swallow either solids or liquids. The edge of the left lobe of the liver was identified by ultrasound. Barium given via a nasogastric tube the evening prior opacified the colon. Fluoroscopically placed T fasteners (*open arrows*) fixed the anterior wall of the stomach to the anterior abdominal wall. A 22-Fr gastrostomy tube (*solid arrows*) was placed between the T fasteners, and secured by inflation of the balloon.

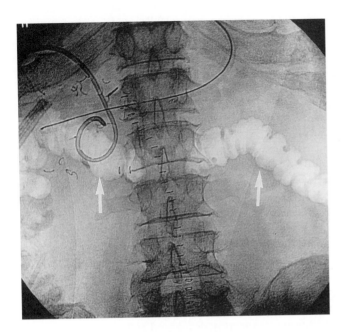

A

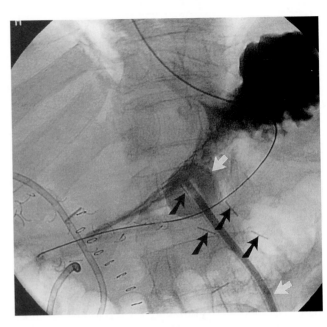

B

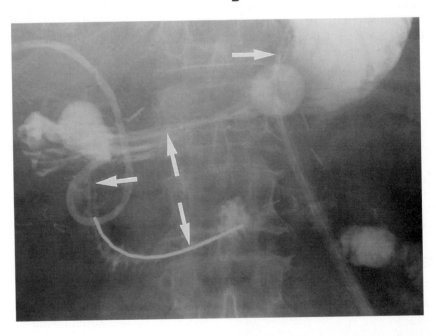

C

Figure 2–34. Percutaneous gastroenterostomy in a 65 year-old male with gastric outlet obstruction caused by massive antral, pyloric, and duodenial edema due to a bile leak (the reason for the PBD). He had undergone a prior cholecystectomy for gangrenous cholecystitis. Attempted endoscopic gastrostomy failed because of the gross distortion of the anatomy. The left lobe of the liver was defined by ultrasound. On the initial anteroposterior radiography, the course of the transverse colon is marked by the bowel gas pattern (*white arrows*). Note the nasogastric tube that allows subsequent gastric insufflation in order to provide a large, easy-to-define, some-what turgid gastric target. **B.** Four T fasteners (*black arrows*) were placed for gastropexy. Following establishment and dilation of the gastric access, a 22-Fr bal-loon–tipped percutaneous gastrostomy tube (*white arrows*) was positioned at approximately the junction of the gastric body and antrum. Contrast pooled in the gas-tric fundus was injected intraprocedurally to confirm intragastric position of the needles. Initial attempts to pass the coaxial jejunostomy tube under fluoroscopic guidance were unsuccessful. **C.** Subsequent combined endoscopic and fluoroscopic placement succeeded in passing the weighted jejunal feeding tube (*white arrows*) into the distal duodenum.

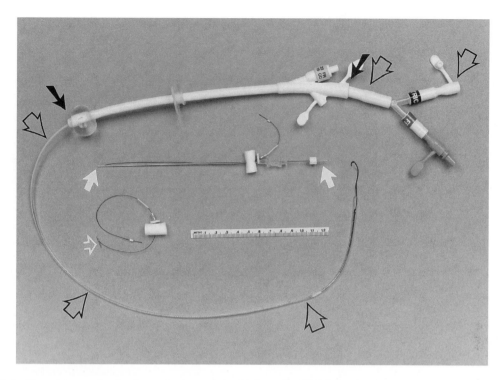

Figure 2–35. Coaxial percutaneous gastroenterostomy and gastropexy devices. The large-caliber (22 Fr) balloon-tipped gastrostomy tube (*between angled solid black arrows*) permits coaxial passage of a smaller caliber (9 Fr) jejunostomy feeding tube (*open black arrows*). The weighted distal end of the jejunostomy tube would normally be cut off in order to allow passage over a guidewire. The jejunostomy device has two ports; one is to permit gastric decompression while the other is used for enteral feeding. The slotted gastropexy delivery needle with a loaded T fastener is displayed between the *solid white arrows*, and a free T fastener is indicated by the *open white arrow*.

ment is conservative. In those cases which fail conservative therapy, colonoscopic decompression is usually successful. In cases of colonoscopic failure, percutaneous cecostomy is a nonoperative option for colonic decompression.[197] Most commonly, a trocar technique is used, via an anterior approach, to place an approximate 12 Fr self-retaining catheter. In order for a tract to form and prevent peritoneal leakage, the catheter should be left in place for at least 2 weeks prior to removal.

DRAINAGE OF INTRA-ABDOMINAL FLUID COLLECTIONS

Pancreatitis-associated Fluid Collections

Pancreatic and peripancreatic inflammatory tissue without a defined fluid collection may represent either pancreatic phlegmon or necrosis. If intervention is indicated, surgical debridement is the procedure of choice. Percutaneous aspiration may be helpful to determine if a phlegmon is infected.[198] In contrast, patients with defined pancreatitis-associated fluid collections (eg, pseudocysts) may be managed expectantly, operatively, or via percutaneous drainage. Patients with asymptomatic, noninfected, small (<4 cm) nonenlarging pseudocysts may be treated conservatively since many will resolve spontaneously. Patients with painful (or otherwise symptomatic) and/or enlarging noninfected pseudocysts may be drained percutaneously, usually on an elec-

tive basis. Alternatively, patients with infected pseudocysts or pancreatic abscesses must be drained urgently to treat the associated sepsis.

Since most patients with either infected or noninfected pseudocysts will have solitary collections, single drains are most often sufficient.[199] Reported nonoperative cure rates range from 66% to 100%.[200] The mean duration of drainage ranges from 20 to 29 days in patients with isolated pseudocysts.[199,201] If communication to the pancreatic duct or GI tract is present, much longer drainage time is required (96 to 104 days).[201] In patients in whom percutaneous drainage fails, endoscopic retrograde cholangiopancreatography (ERCP) is often valuable for preoperative planning. Success rates for aspiration alone approximate 30%.[198] However, patients with advanced, multifocal or multiloculated ill-defined pancreatic abscesses usually require multiple catheters to provide effective drainage[198,202] and, additionally, nonoperative cure rates are lower in these patients (32% to 70%, depending on severity). Most patients with complex pancreatic abscesses eventually requiring operative debridement and drainage were satisfactorily stabilized so that these operative procedures could be performed safely on a nonemergent basis.[198,202]

CT scan is the optimal modality for establishing the diagnosis of pancreatitis-associated fluid collections. It

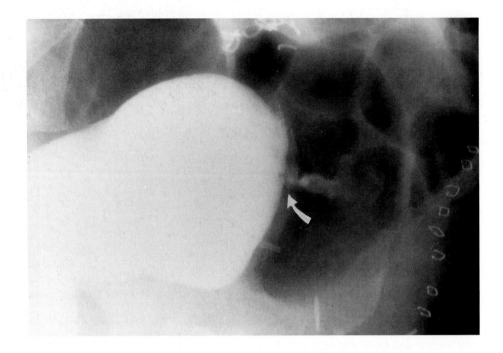

A

B

Figure 2–36. Balloon dilation of a colonic anastomic stricture in an elderly male 2 years after a sigmoidectomy diverticulitis with a progressive mechanical, small-bowel obstruction due to an anastomic colorectal stricture. **A.** Lateral view; limited water-soluble contrast enema with contrast from the filled rectum trickling through the pinpoint anastomic lumen (*white arrow*) into the air-filled descending colon. **B.** Triple-lumen balloon–dilation catheter partially expanded, with a narrowed waist (*white arrows*) indicating a level of anastomosis. *Continued*

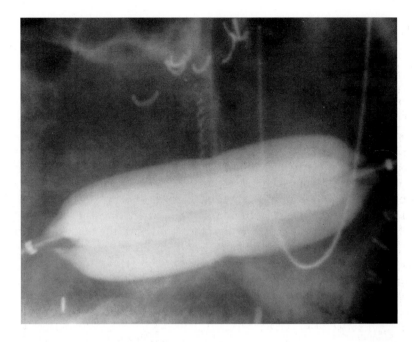

C

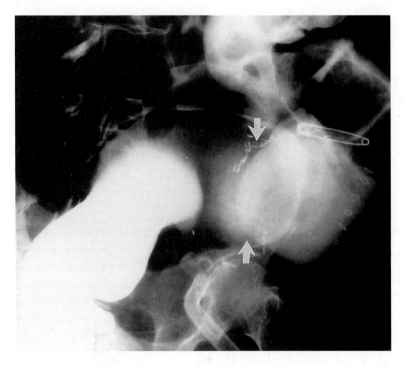

Figure 2–36, cont'd. C. The balloon catheter is fully expanded to 27 mm, with virtual obliteration of the balloon waist. **D.** Repeat contrast enema demonstrates rapid retrograde flow of contrast into the descending colon (*arrows* define the level of the anastomosis). Postprocedurally, the patient's symptoms of bowel obstruction abated.

D

also accurately characterizes the collections as to number, size, location, loculations, and margin characteristics, and permits planning of the percutaneous drainage access. Documented relatively safe access routes include transperitoneal, retroperitoneal, transgastric, transhepatic, and transduodenal.

Intraperitoneal and Enteric-associated Abscesses

Diagnosis and management of intra-abdominal fluid collections are dependent upon high-quality imaging techniques. Although ultrasound can frequently diagnose the presence of intra-abdominal fluid collections inexpensively, quickly, noninvasively, and, if necessary, at the bedside, CT provides a more thorough map of the number, location, and size of the collections and qualitative characteristics such as loculations, fluidity, and extensions, and the location of structures to be avoided during percutaneous access. As a result, CT is usually the preferred modality for preintervention planning.

The most common method used for catheter introduction is the Seldinger technique. CT or ultrasound is used to guide an 18 to 22 gauge needle into the abscess (or other fluid collection) while avoiding other structures such as bowel and blood vessels (Fig 2–37). Once entry into the fluid collection is confirmed by aspiration of a small quantity of the contents, a guidewire is inserted, the needle withdrawn, the tract dilated, and a drainage catheter placed. Fluoroscopy may be useful during tract dilation to ensure that the guidewire position remains constant and the drain is positioned optimally. The size of the drain selected depends mostly on the viscosity and nature of the fluid to be drained.

Larger drain diameters (12 to 20 Fr) are utilized for collections of viscous or necrotic contents. The catheter position may be secured with both a locking pigtail loop (Cope-type loop) and skin fixation (skin suture or adhesive discs). The drain should be placed to either a closed-system gravity drain bag or low-wall suction. Additionally, the drain should be flushed 2 to 3 times daily with sterile saline (typically 10 cc, although more may be used for large cavities if lavage is desired).

Adequacy of abscess drainage is accessed by both a salutory clinical response (afebrile, normal white blood count, and resolution of pain) and by diminution of drainage to <10 mL/day (corrected for flush volumes). Prior to drain removal, resolution of the abscess cavity should be confirmed by CT or ultrasound; fluoroscopy is generally not helpful because injected contrast media artifactually may distend a collapsed cavity.

If the clinical response is incomplete or the daily drainage persistently elevated, one must suspect (1) an

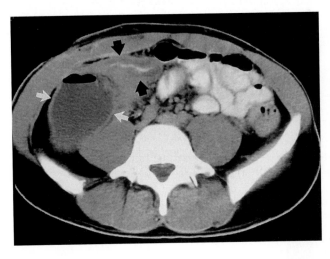

A

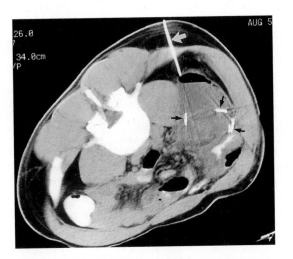

B

Figure 2–37. Percutaneous drainage of an intra-abdominal abscess. Eight days following an appendectomy, this 36 year–old male presented with right lower quadrant pain and fever. **A.** Initial CT scan demonstrated an approximate 6 cm × 7 cm air-containing fluid collection (*white arrows*) in the pericecal region. Note that the cecum (*black arrows*) has been displaced anteriorly and manifests profound bowel-wall thickening. **B.** The patient was rolled over on the CT table and placed in a prone oblique position. An 18 gauge needle (*white arrow*) followed by a 0.038 inch guidewire (*black arrows*) was introduced into the cavity. A large amount of purulent material was aspirated via the percutaneous drainage catheter. **C.** A CT scan two days later confirms that the cavity (*white arrows*) has nearly disappeared.

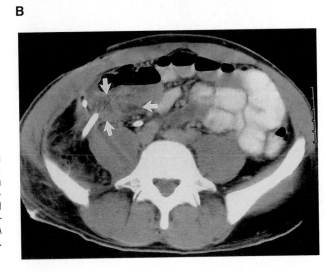

C

incompletely drained cavity (eg, due to loculations or septae), (2) a fistulous communication to the bowel, bile ducts, pancreatic ducts or urinary tract, or (3) additional undrained fluid collections. Fluoroscopic evaluation by injection of contrast media is helpful to evaluate the internal architecture of the cavity (eg, loculation) and to detect fistulae (Fig 2–38). Cross-sectional imaging (CT, ultrasound) is necessary to find separate undrained collections. Cure may require additional drain placement, replacement of existing drains if plugged with debris, or repositioning of indwelling drain into undrained pockets of fluid.

Abscesses arising from bowel or biliary fistulae are frequently related to prior gastrointestinal surgery.[203] The experience has been the only 17% of fistulae have

been identified at the time of the initial drainage procedure; the remainder were proven on subsequent fluoroscopic-tube checks performed for protracted excessive drainage (75 to 100 mL/day) (Fig 2–38). Successful treatment requires effective drainage of both the abscess cavity and the site of the leak. In approximately 33% of patients, multiple catheters are necessary. Prolonged drainage may be necessary, typically requiring 2 to 5 weeks with success rates of approximately 80%.[203] Causes of treatment failure include prior regional irradiation, underlying malignancy, or suboptimal positioning of drains. Percutaneous drainage has been shown to successfully treat most patients with abscesses secondary to diverticulitis,[204,205] appendicitis,[206–208] and Crohn's disease.[209] Generally, the purpose

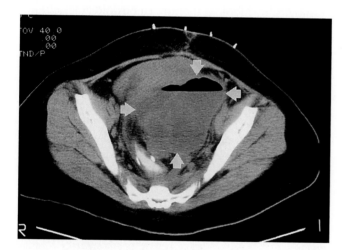

A

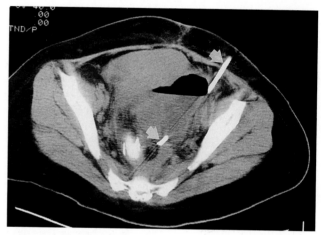

B

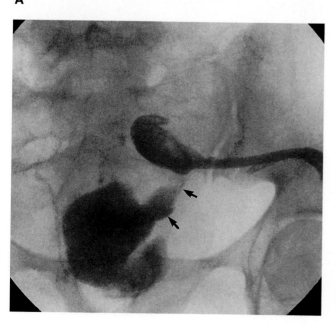

C

Figure 2–38. Percutaneous drainage of a postoperative abscess in a 30 year-old patient with Gardner's syndrome. She was febrile after a total colectomy with ilioanal pull-through. **A.** On CT scan, a 10-cm diameter gas-containing left pelvic fluid collection (*arrows*) was found. The small opacities on the anterior abdomen were pieces of angiographic catheter taped to the skin to assist with access planning. **B.** Using CT guidance, a 12-Fr percutaneous locking–pigtail drain (*arrows*) was placed. **C.** An abscessogram obtained after 1 month of protracted drain output documented a communication (*arrows*) to the ilioanal pouch that was not seen at the time of initial drain placement, in spite of being suspected. After 3 months of continued drainage, the bowel communication closed, the abscess collapsed, the drain was removed and the patient was cured.

of percutaneous drainage is to eliminate the need for operative drainage in most patients, to permit surgery, if necessary, to be performed on an elective basis, and to allow primary bowel resection and repair. Nevertheless, urgent operative drainage is necessary in most patients with extensive, poorly defined abscesses, particularly if the abscesses extend between bowel loops.[208] Abscesses smaller than 3 cm and phlegmons tend to respond to antibiotics alone and require neither percutaneous nor operative drainage.[208]

Hematomas that are large, symptomatic, and/or infected may be drained effectively with percutaneous drainage.[208] If the hematoma has lysed spontaneously, simple tube drainage is sufficient. If the hematoma consists of organized clot, intracavitary thrombolysis has been safe and effective in promoting clot lysis and affording percutaneous drainage.[210] Additionally, intracavitary urokinase has been documented to decrease fluid viscosity and break down septae in complicated abscesses.[211-212]

Lymphoceles

Lymphoceles, caused by operative disruption of small lymphatics, are amenable to percutaneous drainage. As a result of continued lymphatic leak, drainage typically is prolonged (months) and frequently requires intracavity sclerosis using agents such as Betadine, tetracycline, alcohol and Bleomycin.[200] Eventual cure rates are reported to approximate 85% to 90%.

Intrahepatic Fluid Collections

Pyogenic hepatic abscesses may be due to hematogenous seeding, biliary obstruction, or superinfection of preexistent bilomas, tumors, or cysts. Percutaneous drainage allows successful nonoperative resolution in approximately 85% of cases.[213] Either CT or ultrasound may be used to guide access to avoid pleura, bowel, and vascular structures (Fig 2–39). Complications are relatively infrequent (approximately 4%) but include sepsis, bleeding (including hemobilia), peritoneal spillage, pneumothorax and empyema. In patients with an abscess in communication with the biliary tree, a search should be made for possible downstream biliary obstruction. If present, biliary decompression should be provided by the percutaneous, endoscopic, or operative methods already described.

The diagnosis of amebic abscess may be confirmed serologically. Medical therapy (metronidizole, chloroquine) is effective treatment in nearly all patients.[214] Diagnostic aspiration may be indicated in patients with negative serologic titers or suspected superimposed pyogenic infection. Percutaneous drainage is probably warranted in patients with pyogenic superinfections, very large abscesses causing compression of surrounding structures, or large abscesses that abut the diaphragm and are at risk of intrapericardial rupture.

Echinococcal cysts carry a potential risk of anaphylactic reaction if spillage occurs during drainage; thus, surgical resection is usually the preferred method of treatment.

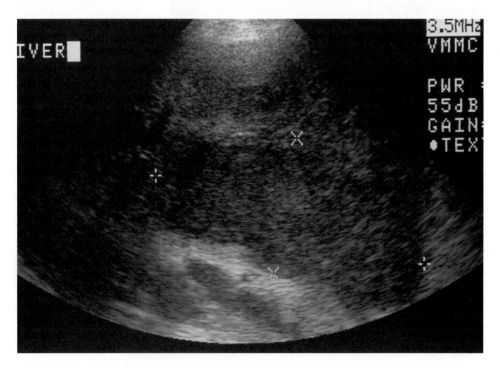

Figure 2–39. Drainage of two pyogenic liver abscesses in a 57 year–old male with constitutional symptoms, fever, and weight loss. A CT scan at the outside hospital reportedly demonstrated two intrahepatic masses thought to represent metastatic disease. **A.** Ultrasound examination defined one 6.4 × 13.5 × 3.3-cm hypoechoic mass (the second mass was identified but not illustrated). *Continued*

A

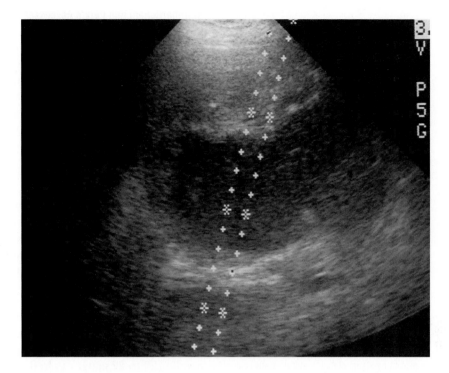

B

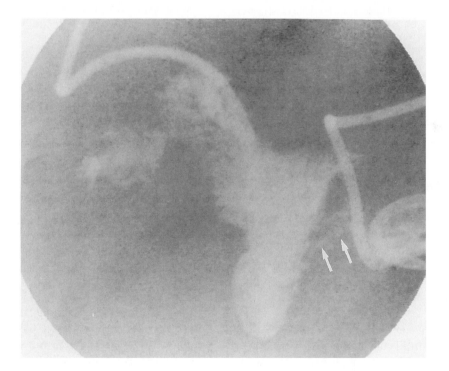

C

Figure 2–39, cont'd. B. The biopsy guide markers describe the anticipated course of the access needle. Two abscess drains were placed, one into each cavity. **C.** The abscessogram delineated the inner architecture of the larger cavity, and documented a communicating tract (*arrows*) to the second cavity. Two weeks later the drains were removed and the patient was cured.

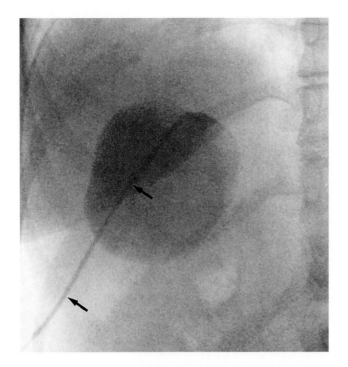

Figure 2–40. Trial of hepatic cyst aspiration in a 50 year–old female with increasing right upper–quadrant pain. Ultrasound documented a large anechoic intrahepatic cyst. The remainder of the work-up was negative. Using ultrasound guidance, an 18 gauge needle was advanced into the cyst and was exchanged for a 6-Fr vascular dilator (*arrows*). The cyst was drained completely, yielding 125 ml of straw-colored fluid, followed by removal of the dilator. Cytologic and bacteriologic evaluations were negative. The patient was rendered asymptomatic. The referring surgeon subsequently performed a successful cyst marsupialization.

Nevertheless, one author reported successful drainage and sclerotherapy in 13 patients with ecchinococcal cysts, with no occurences of anaphylaxis.[215]

Although most noninfected benign hepatic cysts are asymptomatic, large cysts can, on occasion, cause pain or biliary obstruction. If a trial of cyst aspiration provides symptomatic improvement, percutaneous cyst drainage and ethanol sclerosis may be attempted (Fig 2–40). Success rates are as high as 88% with acceptably low complication rates of 12% reported.[216] Symptomatic cysts refractory to intracavitary sclerotherapy may require operative resection or decompression.

Splenic Fluid Collections

Symptomatic splenic fluid collections are relatively rare. Etiologies include pseudocysts, abscesses, hematomas, necrotic tumors, or cysts. These are easily detected by either CT or ultrasound. Diagnostic aspiration may be helpful to prove infection or render a cytological diagnosis. Most of these fluid collections are treated with splenectomy and antibiotics. Percutaneous drainage has been performed in a limited number of patients and is curative in approximately 70% (96% if a unilocular abscess).[200,217,218]

Retroperitoneal and Pelvic Abscesses

Percutaneous drainage has been shown to be effective and relatively safe for drainage of renal, perinephric, subphrenic, iliopsoas, tubo-ovarian and perirectal abscesses.[200] In addition to traditional extraperitoneal approaches, access may be obtained via CT-directed transgluteal, transciatic, or transperoneal approaches. Ultrasound-guided transrectal or transvaginal routes are also available.

PERCUTANEOUS BIOPSY

Radiologically guided percutaneous biopsy has become widely accepted for providing tissue-specific diagnosis of focal lesions in the liver, pancreas, kidneys, adrenal glands, spleen, and retroperitoneal lymph nodes, as well as other retroperitoneal structures, including the musculoskeletal system. Relative to operative open-biopsy techniques, percutaneous techniques are, in general, less expensive and less morbid. With intrahepatic masses, they are the only reasonably feasible techniques.

Cytologic evaluation usually is performed using a fine needle (20 to 22 gauge) passed to and fro within the lesion while aspirating with an attached syringe.[219,220] Histologic evaluation is provided using larger-bore needles (16 to 20 gauge).[220,221] Recently developed automated, spring-loaded biopsy guns have yielded improved pathologic specimens (less blood and crush artifact) and are probably less painful for patients than previous large-bore core needles.[220,222] Fine-needle aspiration, in general, provides a high degree of sensitivity (70% to 90%) for detection of malignancy. However, it frequently is not possible to obtain tumor-specific details such as differentiation of lymphoma type or determination of the tissue of origin of metastases. Malignant tissue may be missed as a sampling error, so malignancy cannot always be excluded.

Histologic evaluation with large-bore needles, although less sensitive for detection of malignancy than fine-needle sampling, does, in fact, occasionally detect tumors not found by the latter technique. More importantly, histologic evaluation of tissue architecture permits determination of specific malignant tumor characteristics and better diagnosis of benign processes.[220] Some authors recommend performing only a fine-needle aspirate initially, reserving large-bore biopsy for cases where cytology is either negative or not sufficiently definitive.[223] Other authors recommend obtaining both cytologic and histologic evaluation of the initial setting, since both sensitivity (approximately 90%) and specificity (approximately 95%) are improved with the combination. This also may be appropriate in a medical center that does not have a highly skilled cytopathologist. With this approach, however, there is a modestly increased risk of bleeding because of the larger needles.[220–222,224] In patients at risk of bleeding complications (eg, coagulopathy), Gelfoam embolization of the biopsy tract through an outer guiding needle or cannula may be performed.[220] In essence, cytologic and histologic examination are complimentary techniques for tissue evaluation of masses.

Depending on tumor size and location, patient habitus and ability to cooperate, and in combination with operator experience, either CT or ultrasound may be used for biopsy guidance. An access route that avoids bowel and vascular structures is preferable. If unavoidable, bowel (including colon) can be safely traversed with fine needles (20 to 22 gauge).[221] If a hepatic lesion is subcapsular in location, a route should be planned that traverses hepatic parenchyma in order to allow tamponade if the lesion proves to be a mass predisposed to hemorrhage, such as a hemangioma or angiosarcoma (Fig 2–7).[33] In patients with large tumors, the biopsy should be obtained near the periphery to minimize the likelihood of sampling necrotic tissue.

Surveys have documented fine-needle biopsy to be relatively safe.[33] Procedurally related deaths occur in approximately 1 of 3,000 to 15,000 biopsies. Most deaths are due to either hemorrhage from liver biopsies (particularly hemangiomas and angiosarcomas) or to pancreatitis from pancreatic biopsies (presumably due to puncture of the pancreatic duct). Neuroendocrine tumors present unique risks related to the potential release of the vasoactive amines; fatal carcinoid crisis has been reported following biopsy of a carcinoid liver metastasis. Therefore, one may need to premedicate such patients with a somatostatin analogue.[225] Additionally, biopsy of a pheochromocytoma theoretically carries a risk of precipitating a hypertensive crisis that requires management with phentolamine and/or propanlol.

Although it is likely that tumor cells are shed along the tract in most biopsies of malignancies, actual tumor seeding in humans is rare and has been documented in between 1 of 1,000 to 1 of 20,000 biopsies.[33,226] It is most common to see this phenomenon with pancreatic adenocarcinoma, renal cell carcinoma, transitional cell carcinoma, and retroperitoneal sarcomas and may manifest itself approximately 3 to 4 months following the biopsy. Most patients with potentially resectable pancreatic or renal malignancy should *not* have a preoperative percutaneous biopsy. In patients who have undergone percutaneous biopsy of a resectable mass that has proven to be malignant, operative resection should attempt to include the biopsy tract.

Nonfocal processes in the liver generally may be biopsied at the bedside using large-bore needles in low-risk patients who have neither ascites nor a significant coagulopathy. In patients with sufficient ascites to interfere with body-wall tamponade of capsular bleeding and/or an impaired coagulation system, either transvenous liver biopsy (discussed under vascular intervention) or direct percutaneous biopsy through a cannula followed by tract

embolization are reasonably safe techniques to obtain tissue for histologic examination.[41,227] Diffuse diseases involving either native kidneys (eg, glomerulonephritis) or transplant kidneys (eg, rejection) may be evaluated histologically using ultrasonically guided large-bore needle biopsy. Transcatheter techniques available for biopsy of endoluminal biliary masses are discussed in the section on biliary intervention.

ACKNOWLEDGEMENTS

I wish to express my gratitude for the assistance of Cynthia L. Zarilla, RN; Edmond L. Raker, MD; Raymond V. Rose, MD; and Carla Talley in the preparation of this manuscript.

REFERENCES

1. Roentgen WC. On a New Kind of Rays. *Erste Mitt Sitzber Phys-Med Ges* (Wurzburg) 1895;137
2. Haschek E, Lindenthal OT. A contribution to the practical use of the photography according to roentgen. *Wien Klin Wochenschr* 1896;9:63
3. Berberich J, Hirsch S. Die rontgenographische darstellung der arterien und venun am lebenden. *Munchen Klin Wochenschr* 1923;49:2226
4. Swick M. Darstellung der niere und harnwege im röntgenbild durch intravenöse einbringung eines neuen kontraststoffes, des uroselectans. *Klin Wochenschr* 1929;8:2087–2089
5. Moniz E, Diaz A, Lima A. La radioarteriographie et la topographie cranioencephalique. *J Radiol Electrol Med Nucl* 1928;12:72
6. Forssman W. Ueber kontrastdarstellung der höhlen des lebenden rechten herzens und der lungenschlagader. *München Med Wchnschr* 1931;78:489–492
7. Farinas PL. A new technique for the arteriographic examination of the abdominal aorta and its branches. *Am J Roent Radium Therapy* 1941;46:641–645
8. Seldinger SI. Catheter replacement of the needle in percutaneous arteriography. A new technique. *Acta Radiol (Stockh)* 1953;39:368–376
9. Dotter CT, Judkins MP. Transluminal treatment of arteriosclerotic obstruction. Description of a new technique and a preliminary report of its applications. *Circulation* 1964;30:654–670
10. Gruntzig A, Hopff H. Perkutane rekanalization chronischer arterieller verschlusse mit einem neuen dilatations - katheter. *Dtsch Med Wochenschr* 1974;99:2502–2511
11. Nusbaum M, Baum S, Kuroda K, Blakemore WS. Control of portal hypertension by selective mesenteric arterial infusion. *Arch Surg* 1968;97:1005–1013
12. Rosch J, Dotter CT, Brown MJ. Selective arterial embolization: a new method for control of acute gastrointestinal bleeding. *Radiology* 1972;102:303–306
13. Dotter CT. Transluminally placed coilspring endarterial tube grafts: long-term patency in canine popliteal artery. *Invest Radiol* 1969;4:329–332

14. Rosch J, Hanafee WN, Snow H. Transjugular portal venography and radiologic portocaval shunt: an experimental study. *Radiology* 1969;92:1112–1114

15. Huard P, Do-Xuan-Hop: La ponction transhepatique des canaux biliares. *Bull Soc Med Chir de l'Indochine.* 1937;15:1090–1100

16. Molnar W, Stockum AE. Relief of obstructive jaundice through percutaneous transhepatic catheter: a new therapeutic method. *AJR Am J Roentgenol* 1974;122:356–367

17. Gronvall J, Gronvall S, Hegedus V. Ultrasound-guided drainage of fluid-containing masses using angiographic catheterization techniques. *AJR Am J Roentgenol* 1977;129:997–1002

18. Molnar W, Stockum AE. Transhepatic dilatation of choledochoenterostomy strictures. *Radiology* 1978;129:59–64

19. Sacks BA, Vine HS, Palestrant AM, et al. A nonoperative technique for establishment of a gastrostomy in the dog. *Invest Radiol* 1983;18:485–487

20. Hessel SJ, Adams DF, Abrams HL. Complications of angiography. *Radiology* 1981;138:273–281

21. Cohan RH, Dunnick NR, Bashore TM. Treatment of reactions to radiographic contrast material. *AJR Am J Roentgenol* 1988;151:263–270

22. Fellmeth BD, Roberts AC, Bookstein DG, et al. Postangiographic femoral artery injuries: nonsurgical repair with US-guided compression. *Radiology* 1991;178:671–675

23. Smith C, Green RM. Pediatric vascular injuries. *Surgery* 1981;90:20–31

24. Mani RL. Computer analysis of factors associated with post catheterization arterial thrombosis. *Invest Radiol* 1975;10:378–384

25. Eisenberg RL. Renal failure after major angiography can be avoided with hydration. *AJR Am J Roentgenol* 1981;136:859–861

26. Kumar S. Low incidence of renal failure after angiography. *Arch Int Med* 1981;141:1262–1270

27. DeElia JA. Nephrotoxicity from angiographic contrast material. *Am J Med* 1982;72:719–725

28. Weaver FA, Pentecost MJ, Yellin AE, et al. Clinical applications of carbon dioxide/digital subtraction arteriography. *J Vasc Surg* 1991;13:266–273

29. Ansell G. An epidemiologic report on adverse reactions in urography: ionic and nonionic media. *Diagn Imaging* 1987;9:6–10

30. Palmer FJ. The RACR survey of intravenous contrast media reactions final report. *Australas Radiol* 1988;32:426–428

31. Katayama H, Yamaguchi K, Kozuka T, et al. Adverse reactions to ionic and nonionic contrast media. A report from the Japanese Committee on the Safety of Contrast Media. *Radiology* 1990;175:621–628

32. Kadir S, Lundell C, Saeed M. Celiac, superior, and inferior mesenteric arteries. In: Kadir S (ed.), *Atlas of Normal and Variant Angiographic Anatomy.* Philadelphia, PA: WB Saunders; 1991;298–300

33. Smith EH. Complications of percutaneous abdominal fine-needle biopsy. Review. *Radiology* 1991;178:253–258

34. Tumors. In: Reuter SR, Redman HC, Cho KJ (eds), *Gastrointestinal Angiography, 3rd ed.* Philadelphia, PA: WB Saunders; 1986;162

35. Burrows PE, Rosenberg HC, Chuang HS. Diffuse hepatic hemangiomas: percutaneous transcatheter embolization with detachable silicone balloons. *Radiology* 1985;156:85–88

36. Sitzmann JV, Coleman JA, Pitt HA, et al. Preoperative assessment of malignant hepatic tumors. *Am J Surg* 1990;159:137–143

37. Heiken JP, Weyman PJ, Lee JKT, et al. Detection of focal hepatic masses: prospective evaluation with CT, delayed CT, CT during arterial portography, and MR imaging. *Radiology* 1989;171:47–51

38. Peterson MS, Baron RL, Dodd GD III, et al. Hepatic parenchymal perfusion defects detected with CTAP: imaging-pathologic correlation. *Radiology* 1992;185:149–155

39. Harned RK II, Chezmar JL, Nelson RC. Imaging of patients with potentially resectable hepatic neoplasms. *AJR Am J Roentgenol* 1992;159:1191–1194.

40. Gamble P, Colapinto RF, Stronell RD, et al. Transjugular liver biopsy: a review of 461 biopsies. *Radiology* 1985;157:589–593

41. Lipchik EO, Cohen EB, Mewissen MW. Transvenous liver biopsy in critically ill patients: adequacy of tissue samples. *Radiology* 1991;181:497–499

42. Millener P, Grant EG, Rose S, et al. Color Doppler-imaging findings in patients with Budd-Chiari syndrome: correlation with venographic findings. *AJR Am J Roentgenol* 1993;161:307–312

43. Nusbaum M, Baum S. Radiographic demonstration of unknown sites of gastrointestinal bleeding. *Surg Forum* 1963;14:374–375

44. Kelemouridis V, Athanasoulis CA, Waltman AC. Gastric bleeding sites: an angiographic study. *Radiology* 1983;149:643–648

45. Alavi A, Ring EJ. Localization of gastrointestinal bleeding: superiority of ^{99m}Tc Sulfur colloid compared with angiography. *AJR Am J Roentgenol* 1981;137:741–748

46. Sheedy PF II, Fulton RE, Atwell DT. Angiographic evaluation of patients with chronic gastrointestinal bleeding. *AJR Am J Roentgenol* 1975;123:338–347

47. Athanasoulis CA, Moncure AC, Greenfield AJ, et al. Intraoperative localization of small bowel bleeding sites with combined use of angiographic methods and methylene blue injection. *Surgery* 1980;87:77–84

48. Rosch J, Keller FS, Wawrukiewicz AS, et al. Pharmacoangiography in the diagnosis of recurrent massive lower gastrointestinal bleeding. *Radiology* 1982;145:615–619

49. Glickerman DJ, Kowdley KV, Rosch J. Urokinase in gastrointestinal tract bleeding. *Radiology* 1988;168:375–376

50. Rapp JH, Reilly LM, Qvarfordt PG, et al. Durability of endarterectomy and antegrade grafts in the treatment of chronic visceral ischemia. *J Vasc Surg* 1986;3:799–806

51. McCollum CH, Graham JM, DeBakey ME. Chronic mesenteric arterial insufficiency: results of revascularization in 33 cases. *So Med J* 1976;69:1266–1268

52. Vascular Diseases. In: Reuter SR, Redman HC, Cho KJ (eds), *Gastrointestinal Angiography,* 3rd ed. Philadelphia, PA: WB Saunders; 1986;111

53. Freeny PC, Traverso LW, Ryan JA. Diagnosis and staging of pancreatic adenocarcinoma with dynamic computed tomography. *Am J Surg* 1993;165:600–606

54. Dooley W, Cameron J, Pitt H, et al. Is preoperative angiography useful in patients with periampullary tumors? *Ann Surg* 1990;211:649–655

55. Ingemansson S, Lunderquist A, Lunderquist I, et al. Portal and pancreatic vein catheterization with radioimmunologic determination of insulin. *Surg Gynecol Obstet* 1975; 141:705–711

56. Gorman B, Charboneau JW, James EM, et al. Benign pancreatic insuloma: preoperative and intraoperative sonographic localization. *AJR Am J Roentgenol* 1986;147:929–934

57. Biehl TR, Traverso LW, Hauptmann E, Ryan JA Jr. Preoperative visceral angiography alters intraoperative strategy during the Whipple procedure. *Am J Surg* 1993;165:607–612

58. Richter GM, Noeldge G, Palmaz JC, et al. Transjugular intrahepatic portacaval stent shunt: preliminary clinical results. *Radiology* 1990;174:1027–1030

59. LaBerge JM, Ring EJ, Gordon RL, et al. Creation of transjugular intrahepatic portosystemic stents with Wallstent endoprosthesis: results in 100 patients. *Radiology* 1993; 187:413–420

60. Helton WS, Belshon A, Althaus S, et al. Critical appraisal of the angiographic portocaval shunt (TIPS). *Am J Surg* 1993;165:566–571

61. Granger DR, Dodra G, Matalon TA, et al. Transjugular portal systemic shunt stent (TIPS): factors influencing outcome. *Hepatology* [Abstr] 1993;18:280A

62. Rosch J, Uchida BT, Baton RE, Keller FS. Coaxial catheter-needle system for transjugular portal vein entrance. *J Vasc Intervent Radiol* 1993;4:145–147

63. Feldstein VA, Wall SD, Gordon RL, et al. Accuracy of Doppler sonography in assessing patency of transjugular intrahepatic portosystemic shunts. *Radiology* [Abstr] 1993; 189(P):181

64. LaFortune M, Pomier-Layrargues G, Dauzat M, et al. Short- and long-term hemodynamic effects of transjugular intrahepatic portosystemic shunt creation: Doppler imaging - manometric correlation. *Radiology* [Abstr] 1993;189(P):181

65. Longo JM, Bilbao JI, Rousseau HP, et al. Transjugular intrahepatic portosystemic shunt: evaluation with Doppler sonography. *Radiology* 1993;186:529–534

66. Richter GM, Roeren T, Noeldge G, Brado M. Five-year results of TIPS: technical standards and long-term clinical efficacy *J Vasc Intervent Radiol* [Abstr] 1993;4:38.

67. Zemel G, Brown J, Becker GJ, et al. TIPS: Long-term follow-up *J Vasc Intervent Radiol* [Abstr] 1993;4:44

68. Bilbao JI, Rousseau H, Longo JM, et al. Percutaneous portacaval shunt with wallstent endoprosthesis. *J Vasc Intervent Radiol* [Abstr] 1993;4:44

69. Barton RE, Saxon RR, Keller FS, et al. Clinical efficacy of TIPS with self-expandable Z stents and Wallstents. *J Vasc Intervent Radiol* [Abstr] 1993;4:45

70. Darcy MD, Picus D, Vesely TM, et al. Efficacy and complications of transjugular intrahepatic portosystemic shunts. *Radiology* [Abstr] 1993;189(P):227

71. Hauenstein KH, Haag K, Ochs A, et al. Transjugular Intrahepatic portosystemic shunts: technical and early clinical complications. *Radiology* [Abstr] 1993;189(P):229

72. Freedman AM, Sanyal AJ, Tisnado J, et al. Complications of transjugular intrahepatic portosystemic shunt: a comprehensive review. *Radiographics* 1993;13:1185–1210

73. Saxon RR, Barton RE, Petersen BD, et al. Transjugular intrahepatic portosystemic shunt: middle-term shunt patency. *Radiology* [Abstr] 1993;189(P):227

74. Malisch TW, Mazer MJ, Meranze SG, et al. Life-table analysis of middle-term patency of transjugular intrahepatic portosystemic stent. *Radiology* [Abstr] 1993;189(P):227

75. Peron JM, Rousseau H, Vinel JP, et al. Long-term follow up study of transjugular intrahepatic portosystemic shunts (TIPS). *Hepatology* [Abstr] 1993;18:102A

76. Sellinger ML, Ochs AG, Haag K, et al. Hepatic encephalopathy in patients with transjugular intrahepatic portosystemic shunts. *Radiology* [Abstr] 1993;189(P):229

77. Somberg KA, Lake JA, Doherty MM, et al. The clinical course following transjugular intrahepatic portosystemic shunts (TIPS) in liver transplant candidates. *Hepatology* [Abstr] 1993;18:103A

78. Huonker M, Schumacher O, Ochs A, et al. Acute hemodynamic effects of TIPS. *Hepatology* [Abstr] 1993;18:281A

79. Lotterer E, Wengert A, Moosmuller A, et al. Effects of transjugular intrahepatic portal systemic shunt (TIPS) on hepatic and systemic hemodynamics in patients with alcoholic cirrhosis. *Hepatology* [Abstr] 1993;18:102A

80. Ruff RJ, Chuang VP, Alspaugh JP, et al. Percutaneous vascular intervention after surgical shunting for portal hypertension. *Radiology* 1987;164:469–474

81. Uflacker R, Silva AO, d'Albuquerque LAC, et al. Chronic portosystemic encephalopathy: embolization of portosystemic shunts. *Radiology* 1987;165:721–725

82. Kumpe DA, Rumack CM, Pretorius DH, et al. Partial splenic embolization in children with hypersplenism. *Radiology* 1985;155:357–362

83. Brandt C, Rothbarth L, Kumpe D, et al. Splenic embolization in children: long-term efficacy. *J Pediatr Surg* 1989; 24:642–645

84. Hickman MP, Lucas D, Novak Z, et al. Preoperative embolization of the spleen in children with hypersplenism. *J Vasc Intervent Radiol* 1992;3:647–652

85. Wallace S, Carrasco CH, Charnsangavej C, et al. Hepatic artery infusion and chemoembolization in the management of liver metastases. *Cardiovasc Intervent Radiol* 1990; 13:153–160

86. Pentecost MJ. Transcatheter treatment of hepatic metastases. *AJR Am J Roentgenol* 1993;160:1171–1175

87. Allison DJ, Booth A. Arterial embolization in the management of liver metastases. *Cardiovasc Intervent Radiol* 1990;13:161–168

88. Yamada R, Kishi K, Sonomura T, et al. Transcatheter arterial embolization in unresectable hepatocellular carcinoma. *Cardiovasc Intervent Radiol* 1990;13:135–139

89. Matsui O, Kadoya M, Yoshikawa J, et al. Small Hepatocellular Carcinoma: Treatment with subsegmental transcatheter arterial embolization. *Radiology* 1993;188:79–83

90. Park JH, Han JK, Chung JW, et al. Superselective transcatheter arterial embolization with ethanol and iodized oil for hepatocellular carcinoma. *J Vasc Intervent Radiol* 1993;4:333–339

91. Matsuo N, Uchida H, Nishimine K, et al. Segmental transcatheter hepatic artery chemoembolization with iodized oil for hepatocellular carcinoma: antitumor effect and influence on normal tissue. *J Vasc Intervent Radiol* 1993;4:543–549

92. Clouse ME, Stokes KR, Kruskal JB, et al. Chemoembolization for hepatocellular carcinoma: epinephrine followed by a doxorubicin-ethiodized oil emulsion and gelatin sponge powder. *J Vasc Intervent Radiol* 1993;4:717–725

93. Uflacker R, Silva AO, d'Albuquerque LA. Transarterial chemoembolization for the treatment of primary and secondary neoplasms of liver: long-term follow-up. *Radiology* [Abstr] 1993;189(P):145

94. Therasse E, Breittmayer F, Roche A, et al. Transcatheter chemoembolization of progressive carcinoid liver metastasis. *Radiology* 1993;189:541–547

95. Stokes KR, Stuart K, Clouse ME. Hepatic arterial chemoembolization for metastatic endocrine tumors. *J Vasc Intervent Radiol* 1993;4:341–345

96. Livraghi T, Vettori C. Percutaneous ethanol injection therapy of hepatoma. *Cardiovasc Intervent Radiol* 1990;13:146–152

97. Salmi A. Percutaneous alcohol injection of hepatocellular carcinoma [Letter]. *Ann Intern Med* 1989;110:494

98. Shiina S, Tagawa K, Niwa Y, et al. Percutaneous ethanol injection therapy for hepatocellular carcinoma: results in 146 patients. *AJR Am J Roentgenol* 1993;160:1023–1028

99. Solinas A, D'Agostino HB, Morelli A. Percutaneous management of hepatocellular carcinoma: the Perugia experience. *Radiology* [Abstr] 1993;189(P):117–118

100. Onik GM, Percutaneous ablation of liver malignancy. *Soc Cardvasc Intervent Radiol* [Annual Meeting Program] 1993:78–82

101. Sclafani SJA, Weisberg A, Scalea TM, et al. Blunt splenic injuries: nonsurgical treatment with CT, arteriography, and transcatheter arterial embolization of the splenic artery. *Radiology* 1991;181;189–196

102. Schwartz RA, Teitelbaum GP, Katz MD, Pentecost MJ. Effectiveness of transcatheter embolization in the control of hepatic vascular injuries. *J Vasc Intervent Radiol* 1993;4:359–365

103. Boudghene F, L'Hermine C, Bigot J-M. Arterial complications of pancreatitis: diagnostic and therapeutic aspects in 104 cases. *J Vasc Intervent Radiol* 1993;4:551–558

104. Ring EJ, Oleaga JA, Freiman D, et al. Pitfalls in the angiographic management of hemorrhage: hemodynamic considerations. *AJR Am J Roentgenol* 1977;129:1007–1013

105. Garten AJ, Mitty HA, Gendler R, et al. Changing role of coil embolization in the treatment of renal lesions and gastrointestinal hemorrhage. *Radiology* [Abstr] 1993;189(P):146

106. Boley SJ, Sprayregen S, Siegelman SS, Veith FJ. Initial results from an aggressive roentgenological and surgical approach to acute mesenteric ischemia. *Surgery* 1977;82:848–855

107. Clark RA, Gallant TE. Acute mesenteric ischemia: angiographic spectrum. *AJR Am J Roentgenol* 1984;142:555–562

108. Herr FW, Silen W, French SW. Intestinal gangrene without apparent vascular occlusion. *Am J Surg* 1965:110:231–238

109. Schoenbaum SW, Pena C, Koenigsberg P, Katzen BT. Superior mesenteric artery embolism: treatment with intraarterial urokinase. *J Vasc Intervent Radiol* 1992;3:485–490

110. Boley SJ, Feinstein FR, Sammartano R, et al. New concepts in the management of emboli of the superior mesenteric artery. *Surg Gyn Obstet* 1981;153:561–569

111. Yankes JR, Uglietta JP, Grant J, Braun SD. Percutaneous transhepatic recanalization and thrombolysis of the superior mesenteric vein. *AJR Am J Roentgenol* 1988;151:289–290

112. Morse SS, Clark RA. Management of nonocclusive and occlusive mesenteric ischemia. In: Kadir S (ed), *Current Practice of Interventional Radiology*. Philadelphia, PA: BC Decker; 1991;394–400

113. Golden DA, Ring EJ, McLean GK, Freiman DB. Percutaneous transluminal angioplasty in the treatment of abdominal angina. *AJR Am J Roentgenol* 1982;139:247–249

114. Roberts L, Wertman DA Jr, Mills SR, et al. Transluminal angioplasty of the superior mesenteric artery: an alternative to surgical revascularization. *AJR Am J Roentgenol* 1983;141:1039–1042

115. Odurny A, Sniderman KW, Colapinto RF. Intestinal angina: percutaneous transluminal angioplasty of the celiac and superior mesenteric arteries. *Radiology* 1988;167:59–62

116. Sniderman KW. Angioplasty for treatment of chronic mesenteric ischemia. In: *Current Practice of Interventional Radiology*, Kadir S, (ed.), Philadelphia, PA: BC Decker 1991;400–407

117. Rose SC, Quigley TM, Raker EJ. Revascularization for chronic mesenteric ischemia: comparison of operative arterial bypass grafting and percutaneous transluminal angioplasty. *J Vasc Intervent Radiol* 1995;6:339–349

118. Hollier LH, Bernatz PE, Pairolero PC, et al. Surgical management of chronic intestinal ischemia: a reappraisal. *Surgery* 1981;90:940–946

119. Beebe HG, MacFarlane S, Raker EJ. Supraceliac aortomesenteric bypass for intestinal ischemia. *J Vasc Surg* 1987;5:749–754

120. Remolar J, Katz S, Rybak B, et al. Percutaneous transhepatic cholangiography. *Gastroenterology* 1956;31:39–46

121. Mueller PR, van Sonnenberg E, Ferrucci JT Jr. Percutaneous biliary drainage: technical and catheter-related problems in 200 procedures. *AJR Am J Roentgenol* 1982;138:17–23

122. Carrasco CH, Zounoza J, Bechtel WJ. Malignant biliary obstruction: complications of percutaneous biliary drainage. *Radiology* 1984;152:343–346

123. Hamlin JA, Friedman M, Stein MG, Bray JF. Percutaneous biliary drainage: complications of 118 consecutive catheterizations. *Radiology* 1986;158:199–202

124. Yee ACN, Ho C-S. Complications of percutaneous biliary drainage: benign *vs* malignant diseases. *AJR Am J Roentgenol* 1987;148:1207–1209

125. Cohan RH, Illescas FF, Saeed M. Infectious complications of percutaneous biliary drainage. *Invest Radiol* 1986;21:705–709

126. Sochendra N, Reynders-Frederix V. Palliative bile duct drainage: a new endoscopic method of introducing a transpapillary drain. *Endoscopy* 1980;12:8–11

127. Speer AG, Cotton PB, Russel RCG, et al. Randomized trial of endoscopic *versus* percutaneous stent insertion in malignant obstructive jaundice. *Lancet* 1987;2:57–62

128. Stanley J, Gobien RP, Cunningham J, Andriole J. Biliary decompression: an institutional comparison of percutaneous and endoscopic methods. *Radiology* 1986;158:195–197

129. Deviere J, Cremer M. Endoscopic approach to malignant biliary obstruction. *Cardiovasc Intervent Radiol* 1990;13:223–230

130. Ring EJ. Radiologic approach to malignant biliary ob-

struction: review and commentary. *Cardiovasc Intervent Radiol* 1990;13:217–222

131. LaBerge JM, Doherty M, Gordon RL, Ring EJ. Hilar malignancy: treatment with an expandable metallic transhepatic biliary stent. *Radiology* 1990;177:793–797

132. Lammer J, Klein GE, Kleinert R, Hauseggar K, Einspieler R. Obstructive jaundice: use of expandable metallic endoprosthesis for biliary drainage: work in progress. *Radiology* 1990;177:789–792

133. Lameris JS, Stoker J, Nijs HGT, et al. Malignant biliary obstruction: percutaneous use of self-expandable stents. *Radiology* 1991;179:703–707

134. Becker CD, Glattli A, Maibach R, Baer HV. Percutaneous palliation of malignant obstructive jaundice with the Wallstent endoprosthesis. Follow-up and reintervention in patients with hilar and nonhilar obstruction. *J Vasc Intervent Radiol* 1993;4:597–604

135. Chespak LW, Ring EJ, Shapiro HA, et al. Multidisciplinary approach to complex endoscopic biliary intervention. *Radiology* 1989;170:995–997

136. Lee MJ, Dawson SL, Mueller PR, et al. Palliation of malignant bile duct obstruction with metallic biliary endoprostheses: techniques, results, and complications. *J Vasc Intervent Radiol* 1992;3:665–671

137. Hausegger KA, Wildling R, Flueckiger F, et al. Plastic *versus* expandable metal biliary endoprostheses: final report of a randomized trial. *Radiology* [Abstr] 1993; 189(P):307

138. Harrell GS, Anderson MF, Berry PF. Cytologic bile examination in the diagnosis of biliary duct neoplastic strictures. *AJR Am J Roentgenol* 1981;137:1123–1126

139. Mendez G Jr, Russell E, Levi JU, et al. Percutaneous brush biopsy and internal drainage of biliary tree through endoprosthesis. *AJR Am J Roentgenol* 1980;134:653–659

140. Terasaki K, Wittich GR, Lycke G, et al. Percutaneous transluminal biopsy of biliary strictures with a bioptome. *AJR Am J Roentgenol* 1991;156:77–78

141. Kim D, Porter DH, Siegel JB, et al. Common bile duct biopsy with the Simpson atherectomy catheter. *AJR Am J Roentgenol* 1990;154:1213–1215

142. Nunnerly HB, Karani JB. Intraductal radiation. *Radiol Clin N Am* 1990;28:1237–1240

143. Hayes JK Jr, Sapozink MD, Miller FJ. Definitive radiation therapy in bile duct carcinoma. *J Radiat Oncol Biol Phys* 1988;15:735–744

144. Williams HJ, Bender CE, May GR. Benign postoperative biliary strictures: dilation with fluoroscopic guidance. *Radiology* 1987;163:629–634

145. Gallacher DJ, Kadir S, Kaufman SL, et al. Nonoperative management of benign postoperative biliary strictures. *Radiology* 1985;156:625–629

146. Mueller PR, van Sonnenberg E, Ferrucci JT Jr, et al. Biliary stricture dilatation: multicenter review of clinical management in 73 patients. *Radiology* 1986;160:17–22

147. Moore AV Jr, Illescas FF, Mills SR, et al. Percutaneous dilation of benign biliary strictures. *Radiology* 1987;163:625–628

148. Citron SJ, Martin LG. Benign biliary strictures: treatment with percutaneous cholangioplasty. *Radiology* 1991;178:339–341

149. Rossi P, Salvatori FM, Bezzi M, et al. Percutaneous man-

agement of benign biliary strictures with balloon dilation and self-expanding metallic stents. *Cardiovasc Intervent Radiol* 1990;13:231–239

150. Ivancev K, Petersen BD, Uchida BT, et al. Long-term results of Gianturco-Rosch Z stents for treatment of benign biliary strictures. *J Vasc Intervent Radiol* [Abstr] 1993;4:53

151. Vorwerk D, Kissinger G, Handt S, Gunther RW. Long-term patency of Wallstent endoprostheses in benign biliary obstructions: experimental results. *J Vasc Intervent Radiol* 1993;4:625–634

152. May GR, Bender CE, LaRusso NF, Wiesner RH. Nonoperative dilation of dominant strictures in primary sclerosing cholangitis. *AJR Am J Roentgenol* 1985;145:1061–1064

153. Skolkin MD, Alspaugh JP, Casarella WJ, et al. Sclerosing cholangitis: palliation with percutaneous cholangioplasty. *Radiology* 1989;170:199–206

154. Russell E, Yrizarry JM, Huber JS, et al. Percutaneous transjejunal biliary dilatation: alternate management for benign strictures. *Radiology* 1986;159:209–214

155. Maroney TP, Ring EJ. Percutaneous transjejunal catheterization of Roux-en-Y biliary-jejunal anastomoses. *Radiology* 1987;164:151–153

156. Burhenne JH. Percutaneous extraction of retained biliary tract stones: 661 patients. *AJR Am J Roentgenol* 1980;134:888–898

157. Stokes KR, Falchuk KR, Clouse ME. Biliary duct stones: update on 54 cases after percutaneous transhepatic removal. *Radiology* 1989;170:999–1001

158. Gandini G, Righi D, Regge D, et al. Percutaneous removal of biliary stones. *Cardiovasc Intervent Radiol* 1990;13:245–251

159. Picus D, Weyman PJ, Marx MV. Role of percutaneous intracorporeal electrohydraulic lithotripsy in the treatment of biliary tract calculi: work in progress. *Radiology* 1989;170:989–993

160. Kaufman SL, Kadir S, Mitchell SE, et al. Percutaneous transhepatic biliary drainage for bile leaks and fistulas. *AJR Am J Roentgenol* 1985;144:1055–1058

161. van Sonnenberg E, Casola G, Wittich GR, et al. The role of interventional radiology for complications of cholecystectomy. *Surgery* 1990;107:632–638

162. van Sonnenberg E, D'Agostino HB, Easter DW, et al. Complications of Laparoscopic cholecystectomy: coordinated radiologic and surgical management in 21 patients. *Radiology* 1993;188:399–404

163. Brandabur JJ, Kozarek RA. Endoscopic repair of bile leaks after laparoscopic cholecystectomy. *Sem Ultrasound CT MRI* 1993;14:375–380

164. van Sonnenberg E, Wittich GA, Casola G, et al. Diagnostic and therapeutic percutaneous gallbladder procedures. *Radiology* 1986;160:23–26

165. Vogelzang RL, Nemcek AA. Percutaneous cholecystostomy: diagnostic and therapeutic efficacy. *Radiology* 1988;168:29–34

166. van Sonnenberg E, D'Agostino HB, Goodacre BW, et al. Percutaneous gallbladder puncture and cholecystostomy: results, complications, and caveats for safety. *Radiology* 1992;183:167–170

167. Warren PL, Kadir S, Dunnick NR. Percutaneous cholecystostomy: anatomic considerations. *Radiology* 1988;168:615–616

168. Garel LA, Belli D, Grignon A, Roy CC. Percutaneous cholecystography in children. *Radiology* 1987;165:639–641

169. Lee MJ, Saini S, Brink JA, et al. Treatment of critically ill patients with sepsis of unknown cause: value of percutaneous cholecystostomy. *AJR Am J Roentgenol* 1991;156:1163–1166

170. Browning PD, McGahan JP, Gerscovich EO. Percutaneous cholecystostomy for suspected acute cholecystitis in the hospitalized patient. *J Vasc Intervent Radiol* 1993;4:531–538

171. van Sonnenberg E, Casola G, Zakko SF, et al. Gallbladder and bile duct stones: percutaneous therapy with primary MTBE dissolution and mechanical methods. *Radiology* 1988;169:505–509

172. Mueller PR, Lee MJ, Saini S, et al. Percutaneous contact dissolution of gallstones: complexity of radiologic care. *Radiographics* 1991;11:759–770

173. Picus D, Marx MV, Hicks ME, et al. Percutaneous cholecystolithotomy: preliminary experience and technical considerations. *Radiology* 1989;173:487–491

174. Miller FJ, Rose SC, Buchi KN, et al. Percutaneous rotational contact biliary lithotripsy: initial clinical results with the Kensey Nash lithotrite. *Radiology* 1991;178:781–785

175. Campbell JB, Condon VR. Catheter removal of blunt esophageal foreign bodies in children. Survey of the Society For Pediatric Radiology. *Pediatr Radiol* 1989;19:361–365

176. McLean GK, Meranze SG. Interventional radiologic management of enteric strictures. *Radiology* 1989;170:1049–1053

177. McLean GK, LeVeen RF. Shear stress in the performance of esophageal dilation: comparison of balloon dilatation and bougienage. *Radiology* 1989;172:983–986

178. Starck E, Paolucci V, Herzer M, Crummy AB. Esophageal stenosis: treatment with balloon catheters. *Radiology* 1984;153:637–640

179. Song H-Y, Han Y-M, Kim H-N, et al. Corrosive esophageal stricture: safety and effectiveness of balloon dilation. *Radiology* 1992;184:373–378

180. McLean GK, Cooper GS, Hartz WH, et al. Radiologically guided balloon dilation of gastrointestinal strictures, Part I: technique and factors influencing procedural success. *Radiology* 1987;165:35–40

181. Dawson SL. Mueller PR, Ferrucci JT Jr, et al. Severe esophageal strictures: indications for balloon catheter dilatation. *Radiology* 1984;153:631–635

182. deLange EE, Shaffer HA Jr. Anastomotic strictures of the upper gastrointestinal tract: results of balloon dilation. *Radiology* 1988;167:45–50

183. deLange EE, Shaffer HA Jr, Daniel TM, Kron IL. Esophageal anastomotic leaks: preliminary results of treatment with balloon dilation. *Radiology* 1987;165:45–47

184. Jaffe MH, Fleischer D, Zeman RK, et al. Esophageal malignancy: imaging results and complications of combined endoscopic-radiologic palliation. *Radiology* 1987;164:623–630

185. Cwikiel W, Stridbeck H, Tranberg K-G, et al. Malignant esophageal strictures: treatment with a self-expanding nitinol stent. *Radiology* 1993;187:661–665

186. Song H-Y, Choi K-C, Cho B-H, et al. Esophagogastric neoplasms: palliation with a modified Gianturco stent. *Radiology* 1991;180:349–354

187. Song H-Y, Choi K-C, Kwon H-C, et al. Esophageal strictures: treatment with a new design of modified Gianturco stent: work in progress. *Radiology* 1992;184:729–734

188. Kozarek RA. Hydrostatic balloon dilation of gastrointestinal stenoses: a national survey. *Gastrointest Endosc* 1986;32:15–19

189. McLean GK, Cooper GS, Harz WH, et al. Radiologically guided balloon dilation of gastrointestinal strictures, Part II: results of long-term follow-up. *Radiology* 1987;165:41–43

190. O'Keeffe F, Carrasco CH, Charnsangavej C, et al. Percutaneous drainage and feeding gastrostomies in 100 patients. *Radiology* 1989;172:341–343

191. Halkier BK, Ho C-S, Yee ACN. Percutaneous feeding gastrostomy with the Seldinger technique: review of 252 patients. *Radiology* 1989;171:359–362

192. Hicks ME, Surratt RS, Picus D, et al. Fluoroscopically guided percutaneous gastrostomy and gastroenterostomy: analysis of 158 consecutive cases. *AJR Am J Roentgenol* 1990;154:725–728

193. Saini S, Mueller PR, Gaa J, et al. Percutaneous gastrostomy with gastropexy: experience in 125 patients. *AJR Am J Roentgenol* 1990;154:1003–1006

194. Deutsch L-S, Kannegieter L, Vanson DT, et al. Simplified percutaneous gastrostomy. *Radiology* 1992;184:181–183

195. Alzate GD, Coons HG, Elliott J, Carey PH. Percutaneous gastrostomy for jejunal feeding: a new technique. *AJR Am J Roentgenol* 1986;147:822–825

196. Ball WS Jr, Kosloske AM, Jewell PF, et al. Balloon catheter dilatation of focal intestinal strictures following necrotizing enterocolitis. *J Pediatr Surg* 1985;20:637–639

197. Casola G, van Sonnenberg E. Percutaneous cecostomy. In: *Current Practice of Interventional Radiology*, Kadir S, ed. Philadelphia, PA; BC Decker: 1991;450–452

198. van Sonnenberg E, Wittich GR, Casola G, et al. Complicated pancreatic inflammatory disease: diagnostic and therapeutic role of interventional radiology. *Radiology* 1985;155:335–340

199. van Sonnenberg E, Wittich GR, Casola G, et al. Percutaneous drainage of infected and noninfected pancreatic pseudocysts: experience in 101 cases. *Radiology* 1989;170;757–761

200. van Sonnenberg E, D'Agostino HB, Casola G, Halasz NA, et al. Percutaneous abscess drainage: current concepts. *Radiology* 1991;181:617–626

201. Freeny PC, Lewis GP, Traverso LW, Ryan JA. Infected pancreatic fluid collections: percutaneous drainage. *Radiology* 1988;167:435–441

202. Steiner E, Mueller PR, Hahn PF. Complicated pancreatic abscesses: problems in interventional management. *Radiology* 1988;167:443–446

203. Papanicoulaou N, Mueller PR, Ferrucci JT Jr, et al. Abscess-fistula association: radiologic recognition and percutaneous management. *AJR Am J Roentgenol* 1984;143:811–815

204. Neff CC, van Sonnenberg E, Casola G, et al. Diverticular abscesses: percutaneous drainage. *Radiology* 1987;163:15–18

205. Mueller PR, Saini S, Wittenburg J. Sigmoid diverticular abscesses: percutaneous drainage as an adjunct to surgical resection in 24 cases. *Radiology* 1987;164:321–325

206. Nunez D Jr, Huber JS, Yrizarry JM, et al. Nonsurgical

drainage of appendiceal abscesses. *AJR Am J Roentgenol* 1986;146:587–589

207. van Sonnenberg E, Wittich GR, Casola G, et al. Periappendiceal abscesses: percutaneous drainage. *Radiology* 1987;163:23–26

208. Jeffrey RB Jr, Federle MP, Tolentino CS. Periappendiceal inflammatory masses: CT-directed management and clinical outcome in 70 patients. *Radiology* 1988; 167:13–16

209. Casola G, van Sonnenberg E, Neff CC, et al. Abscesses in Crohn disease: percutaneous drainage. *Radiology* 1987; 163:19–22

210. Vogelzang RL, Tobin RS, Burstein S, et al. Transcatheter intracavitary fibrinolysis of infected extravascular hematomas. *AJR Am J Roentgenol* 1987;148:378–380

211. Park JK, Kraus FC, Haaga JR. Fluid flow during percutaneous drainage procedures: an *in vitro* study of the effects of fluid viscosity, catheter size, and adjunctive urokinase. *AJR Am J Roentgenol* 1993;160:165–169

212. Lahorra JM, Haaga JR, Stellato T, et al. Safety of intracavitary urokinase with percutaneous abscess drainage. *AJR Am J Roentgenol* 1993;160:171–174

213. Bret PM, Ritchie RG. Percutaneous drainage of liver abscesses and fluid collections. In: *Current Practice of Interventional Radiology*, Kadir S, (ed.) Philadelphia, PA; BC Decker: 1991;481–486

214. Ralls PW, Barnes PF, Johnson MB, et al. Medical treatment of hepatic amebic abscess: rare need for percutaneous drainage. *Radiology* 1987;165:805–807

215. Bret PM, Fond A, Bretagnolle M, et al. Percutaneous aspiration and drainage of hydatid cysts in the liver. *Radiology* 1988;168:617–620

216. van Sonnenberg E, Wroblicka JT, D'Agostino HB, et al. Symptomatic hepatic cysts: percutaneous drainage and sclerosis. *Radiology* 1994;190:387–392

217. Tikkakoski T, Siniluoto T, Paivansalo M, et al. Splenic abscesses. Imaging and intervention. *Acta Radiol* 1992;33: 561–565

218. Gleich S, Wolin DA, Herbsman H. A review of percutaneous drainage in splenic abscess. *Surg Gynecol Obstet* 1988;167:211–216

219. Kinney TB, Lee MJ, Filomena CA. Fine-needle biopsy: prospective comparison of aspiration *versus* nonaspiration techniques in the abdomen. *Radiology* 1993;186: 549–552

220. Moulton JS, Moore PT. Coaxial percutaneous biopsy technique with automated biopsy devices: value in improving accuracy and negative predictive value. *Radiology* 1993;186:515–522

221. Brandt KR, Charboneau JW, Stephans DH, et al. CT- and US-guided biopsy of the pancreas. *Radiology* 1993;187: 99–104

222. Parker SH, Hopper KD, Yakes WF, et al. Image-directed percutaneous biopsies with a biopsy gun. *Radiology* 1989; 171:663–669

223. Baker ME. CT-guided percutaneous biopsy of focal hepatic lesions. In: *Current Practices of Interventional Radiology*, Kadir S, ed. Philadelphia, PA; BC Decker: 1991; 486–492

224. Gazelle GS, Haaga JR, Rowland DY. Effect of needle gauge, level of anticoagulation and target organ on bleeding associated with aspiration biopsy: work in progress. *Radiology* 1992;183:509–513

225. Bissonnette RT, Gibney RG, Berry BR, Buckley AR. Fatal carcinoid crisis after percutaneous fine-needle biopsy of hepatic metastasis: case report and literature review. *Radiology* 1990;174:751–752

226. Lundstedt C, Stridbeck H, Anderson R, et al. Tumor seeding occurring after fine-needle biopsy of abdominal malignancies. *Acta Radiol* 1991;32:518–520

227. Chuang VP, Alspaugh JP. Sheath needle for liver biopsy in high-risk patients. *Radiology* 1988;166:261–262

3

ENDOSCOPY

Aaron S. Fink

The earliest endoscopes were rigid, open-ended devices that allowed inspection and biopsy of the proximal 40 cm[1] or the distal 25 cm of the gastrointestinal tract. Although rigid sigmoidoscopy continues to be employed, the instruments used for this procedure afford limited examinations that often prove uncomfortable for both patient and endoscopist. Semi-flexible lensed gastroscopes were introduced in the 1930s 1940s[2]; these instruments also proved difficult to use. A major advance occurred when fiberoptic technology was coupled with gastrointestinal endoscopy in the late 1960s. The fully flexible endoscopes that resulted from this union became the primary diagnostic tools for evaluation of the upper and lower gut,[3–7] as well as for the evaluation of the pancreaticobiliary system.[8–11] Soon thereafter, therapeutic interventions were introduced, allowing snare excision of polypoid masses,[12] hemostasis of bleeding lesions,[13–16] incision of the biliary sphincter,[17,18] and dilatation of strictures.[19]

Applications and use of gastrointestinal endoscopy have continued to expand. Indeed, a recent survey sponsored by the British Society of Gastroenterology suggested that in the near future, as many as 1% of the population will undergo upper gastrointestinal endoscopy annually.[20] Undoubtedly, this technology will continue to play a primary role in diagnosis and treatment of gastrointestinal disorders.

■ INSTRUMENTATION

In all flexible endoscopic systems, light is transmitted down the endoscope shaft in order to illuminate the surface to be examined. The reflected image is conveyed back to the endoscopist via one of two different modalities: fiberoptics or electronics. In fiberoptics, a fixed lens at the end of the instrument shaft focuses the image on internal fiberoptic bundles. The image then is carried to an adjustable lens on the instrument head through which it is viewed directly. The fiberoptic bundle is 2 to 3 mm wide and is composed to 20000 to 40 000 individual fine glass fibers, each approximately 10 μm in diameter. The image undergoes a series of internal reflections within each fiber as it is transmitted up the bundle. It is then faithfully transmitted back to the viewer by ensuring identical orientation (coherent) of the fibers at each end of the bundle. This process requires that each fiber be coated with low optical–density glass to prevent the escape of light. This "packing material" creates the characteristic meshed image seen in fiberoptic endoscopes. As a result, fiberoptic endoscopic images will never achieve the resolution of rigid lens systems; however, the fiberoptic endoscope is extremely flexible and reasonably portable.

In video endoscopes, the image is reflected on a charged coupled device (CCD) chip mounted on the end of the instrument shaft. These chips are charge-

189

coupled devices with thousands of light-sensitive points (pixels); the greater the number of pixels, the better the resolution. Chips contain from 30 000 (approximately the resolution of fiberoptic endoscopes) to 150 000 pixels. The image then is transmitted through electronic wires to additional electronics in the instrument head. The electronic wires and switches in the video endoscope replace the light bundle and adjustable lens found in the fiberoptic endoscope.

There are two types of color CCD chips. The earliest devices utilized a mosaic chip, which contains extra pixels and allows primary-color filters to be overlaid on the black and white image. These chips can be used with standard xenon light sources. Newer color video endoscopes use sequential chips, in which all pixels are sequentially illuminated with the light of the three primary colors, alternating each color 20 to 30 times per minute. Each colored image is stored transiently in the image processor before being fed to the electron guns in the television monitor. Sequential chips are smaller and can be mounted on smaller diameter endoscopes. Although they offer better resolution, sequential chips require larger, more expensive light source/processor units.

In other developments, automatic endoscope cleaners are being used more often. Guidelines for acceptable endoscope disinfection, including use of automatic disinfectors, have recently been published.[21,22] However, as emphasized in these guidelines, these automatic cleaners cannot substitute for adequate manual cleaning of the endoscope.

Finally, attempts to improve endoscopic training have resulted in creation of computer simulators for teaching endoscopic skills.[23,24] Simulators have been developed for flexible sigmoidoscopy,[25] gastroscopy,[26,27] ERCP,[26,28,29] and colonoscopy.[29]

■ MONITORING

Even though gastrointestinal endoscopy performed by a trained endoscopist is a safe procedure, complications do occur. In many series, cardiopulmonary complications are the most frequently reported.[30] These complications include aspiration, oversedation, hypotension, hypoventilation, arrhythmia, bradycardia (vasovagal), and airway obstruction. Many of the airway obstruction complications are associated with the use of intravenous-conscious sedation,[31] defined as decreased consciousness associated with preservation of protective reflexes.[32] Elderly patients or those with preexisting cardiopulmonary conditions are at increased risk for these complications,[31,33,34] as are those undergoing more extensive endoscopic interventions.[30,34,35]

Monitoring the status of the patient before, during, and after the procedure is a critical component of safe

patient care. Ideally, such monitoring will detect signs of patient distress prior to the compromise of vital functions. Signs that are usually monitored include the level of consciousness and comfort, vital signs, and ventilatory status of the patient. Usually, oxygenation status and cardiac electrical activity are also monitored; the latter requires electronic monitoring devices such as pulse oximeters. The use of such devices reduces manual labor associated with monitoring and frequently will document arterial oxygen desaturation or altered pulse rate.[34,36] Further, in a darkened endoscopy room, pulse oximetry will enhance assessment of the ventilatory status of a patient. Although automated monitoring devices have not been demonstrated to alter clinical outcome, routine pulse oximetry is still recommended.[37] However, it must be emphasized that the use of monitoring devices must not replace a dedicated assistant.

Supplemental nasal oxygen decreases the frequency of desaturation during endoscopic procedures. Its use is recommended in high-risk patients, including those with significant cardiopulmonary disease and those undergoing complex, prolonged procedures.[38–41] Patients with advanced obstructive pulmonary disease are at particular risk of hypoxemia and hypercapnia. Freeman and associates[42] recently demonstrated that repeat desaturation following administration of supplemental oxygen predicts hypoventilation and justifies careful consideration before further administration of sedatives.

■ ENDOSCOPY OF THE UPPER GASTROINTESTINAL TRACT

INDICATIONS

Upper gastrointestinal endoscopy is one of the most frequently performed flexible endoscopic procedures. Current indications recommended by the American Society for Gastrointestinal Endoscopy are outlined in Table 3–1.

In certain conditions, it has been proposed that upper gastrointestinal endoscopy be performed periodically in screening for esophageal or gastric malignancies. While there are no well designed, long-term studies demonstrating the efficacy of such an approach, certain recommendations can be made.

Esophageal conditions claimed to be predisposed to the development of malignancy include achalasia, lye ingestion, Plummer-Vinson syndrome, and Barrett's esophagitis (Fig 3–1). In achalasia, although the risk remains undefined, recent studies suggest that approximately 2% to 7% of patients will ultimately develop esophageal carcinoma.[43–45] Most of these tumors are

TABLE 3–1. INDICATIONS FOR UPPER GASTROINTESTINAL ENDOSCOPY

DIAGNOSTIC EVALUATION
Upper abdominal pain unresponsive to appropriate therapy
Upper abdominal pain associated with constitutional changes (eg, anorexia, weight loss)
Dysphagia or odynophagia
Esophageal reflux symptoms unresponsive to appropriate therapy
Persistent unexplained vomiting
Other system disease in which upper GI pathology will alter management
    eg, peptic ulcer in organ transplant candidate or arthritis patient; aerodigestive cancer of head and neck
Familial adenomatous polyposis
Confirmation and tissue diagnosis of radiologic abnormalities
    Suspected neoplasm
    Gastric or esophageal ulcer
    Stricture or obstruction
Gastrointestinal bleeding
    Most active or recent bleeds
    When surgical intervention is considered
    Rebleeding after acute self-limited bleed
    Suspicion of portal hypertension or aortoenteric fistula
    Chronic blood loss or iron deficiency anemia with negative colonoscopy
Required sample of duodenal or jejunal tissue
Evaluate acute injury after caustic ingestion

PERIODIC SURVEILLANCE
Barrett's esophagus
Familial adenomatous polyposis
Prior adenomatous gastric polyps

FOLLOW-UP
Selected ulcers (esophageal, gastric, or stomal)
Previously treated esophageal varices

THERAPY
Bleeding lesions (eg, ulcers, tumors, vascular malformations)
Sclerotherapy or banding of esophageal varices
Removal of foreign bodies
Selected polypectomy
Insertion of feeding tubes (eg, PEG, PEJ)
Dilatation of stenotic lesions
Palliation of stenosing neoplasms

(Adapted from Standards of Practice Committee. *Appropriate Use of Gastrointestinal Endoscopy.* Manchester, MA: American Society of Gastrointestinal Endoscopy; 1992)

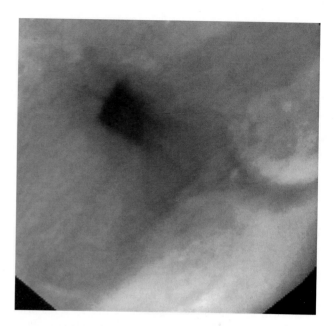

Figure 3–1. Biopsy-proven Barrett's esophagitis. (See color insert.)

squamous cell lesions which, unfortunately, present in a relatively advanced state, resulting in poor 5-year survivals.[46] Surveillance may be appropriate in those patients with untreated disease or persistent dilation and stasis.[47]

Carcinoma is also a significant long-term (approximately 40 years) risk (increased 1000-fold) in those patients with esophageal injury secondary to caustic ingestion, with most lesions occurring in the midesophagus.[48–50] Since these lesions present at an early stage, resectability and cure frequently are possible.[48–50] Thus, endoscopic screening is probably appropriate even >30 years after earlier caustic injury, especially following onset of symptoms.

Plummer-Vinson syndrome is an extremely rare condition characterized by postcricoid esophageal webs and iron-deficiency anemia. Proximal esophageal carcinoma is reported to develop in 12% of individuals with this disorder,[51,52] suggesting a possible role for surveillance endoscopy.

Barrett's esophagitis (Fig 3–1) is characterized by replacement of normal esophageal squamous epithelium with specialized columnar epithelium. Reported prevalence of this condition varies, depending on the diagnostic method used and the population surveyed. The reported incidence varies between 2% and 20% of patients, with the highest incidence occurring in those with gastroesophageal reflux, scleroderma, or dysphagia.[53] Although it is clear that Barrett's esophagitis is a premalignant condition, the degree of risk remains unclear. Longer segments (>8 cm) and high-grade dysplasia are associated with greater risk of malignant degeneration.[54,55] Aggressive surveillance programs can distinguish high-grade dysplasia from early adenocarcinoma[56,57]; such programs are probably most appropriate for patients considered to be good surgical candidates.[56,58] The finding of cancer or high-grade dysplasia without associated inflammation is an indication for surgical resection in the "good-risk" patient.[56]

Certain gastric conditions are also claimed to be predisposed to malignant degeneration, prompting consideration of endoscopic surveillance. These conditions include previous adenomatous polyps, polyposis syndromes, postgastrectomy surgery, and pernicious anemia.

Recommendations for follow-up of gastric epithelial polyps parallel those for patients with colonic polyps. Hyperplastic gastric polyps are found most commonly and have little malignant potential.[59,60] In contrast, adenomatous polyps are premalignant lesions, and their risk of malignant transformation is size dependent.[61,62] Surveillance for gastric adenomatous polyps should probably follow recommendations similar to those for adenomatous colonic polyps.

Polyposis syndromes also merit consideration of endoscopic surveillance, since 33% to 100% of patients with these disorders harbor upper gastrointestinal polyps, many of which are adenomatous.[63–65] Indeed, the risk of duodenal and ampullary carcinoma is increased in these disorders.[63,66,67] Surveillance with both end- and side-viewing instruments is indicated in this setting.

Previous gastric surgery for benign disease imposes a 2- to 4-fold increased risk of development of carcinoma in the residual gastric stump, beginning 15 years after gastric surgery.[68–71] The incidence varies between 5% to 6% and appears to be preceded by development of dysplasia.[72] Although debated,[73,74] selected surveillance is probably indicated beginning 15 years after surgery for benign disease, particularly for symptomatic patients or those with previously identified mucosal dysplasia.[70,75]

Currently, surveillance is not recommended for patients with pernicious anemia, given the relatively low risk (2 fold) for development of gastric carcinoma.[76–79] However, at the time of the initial diagnosis, it would seem appropriate to biopsy the gastric mucosa, seeking other risk factors associated with malignant degeneration (eg, dysplasia or polyps).

PATIENT PREPARATION

Minimal preparation is usually required for upper gastrointestinal endoscopy. Patients should fast for at least 4 to 6 hours before the examination, although a longer time may be required in the presence of esophageal or gastric outlet obstruction. Occasionally, a gastric outlet obstruction will mandate preendoscopic passage of a large-bore tube for esophageal aspiration or gastric lavage. Before the study, dentures and eyeglasses should be removed. Intravenous access should be obtained if sedation is planned or if the patient is actively bleeding.

Prophylactic antibiotics are rarely indicated; the most compelling indications include performance of esophageal sclerotherapy or dilatation in patients with prosthetic heart valves, previous endocarditis, systemic-pulmonary shunts, or recent vascular or orthopedic prostheses.[80–82] In addition, a randomized prospective trial has demonstrated that intravenous cephalosporins decrease the rate of skin infection when given prior to percutaneous endoscopic gastrostomy (PEG).[83] Appro-

priate blood bank support should also be available for patients with major gastrointestinal bleeding.

Many endoscopists spray topical pharyngeal anesthesia onto the posterior pharyngeal wall in order to suppress the gag reflex. This practice, as well as the use of a small-diameter endoscope, is particularly helpful if minimal or no intravenous sedation is to be used. The patient then is placed in the desired position, usually the left lateral decubitus, with the head slightly elevated on a pillow (supine for PEG). Next, sedation is administered, if desired. Combinations of benzodiazapines (eg, diazepam, midazolam) and narcotics (eg, fentanyl, meperidine) are used most commonly. Since routine diagnostic upper gastrointestinal endoscopy can usually be performed quite rapidly, short-lived agents (eg, fentanyl) offer greater utility. It should be remembered that older patients often require less intravenous sedation than younger patients.

DIAGNOSTIC AND THERAPEUTIC TECHNIQUES

Diagnostic Technique

The 120-cm forward-viewing endoscope is preferred for routine diagnostic endoscopy. Smaller diameter pediatric endoscopes (both fiberoptic and video) currently are available for use in small children or patients with strictures.

It is vital that a well-trained assistant stand at the patient's head throughout the examination. This assistant must protect the patient's airway (with suction) at all times. In addition, the assistant can hold or manipulate the endoscope when desired and maintain the position of the mouth piece.

After adequately preparing the patient and confirming that the equipment is in proper working order, the endoscope tip is lubricated and then inserted directly into the esophagus. Intubation is accomplished best under direct vision by advancing the endoscope over the tongue, past the uvula and epiglottis, and then posterior to the cricoarytenoid. This maneuver will place the endoscope tip at the cricopharyngeal sphincter, which will relax and allow entry into the cervical esophagus if the patient swallows. Alternatively, the endoscope can be introduced blindly, guiding the tip into the midline of the patient's pharynx with previously inserted second and third fingers of the left hand. Once the endoscope is in the proper position, the fingers are removed, the mouth piece slid into position, and the patient instructed to swallow, allowing the endoscope to be advanced into the esophagus. This latter technique is more dangerous for both patient and endoscopist.

Once in the esophagus, the instrument is advanced under direct vision to the desired endpoint (usually the proximal duodenum), taking care to survey the mucosa both during insertion and withdrawal. Inspection is often better during withdrawal when the viscera are well distended with air; this is often the best time to pursue detailed examination and/or sampling of lesions noted during insertion. During insertion, the endoscopist should note the distance from the incisors of the primary anatomic landmarks: the cricopharyngeal and lower esophageal sphincters, the incisura, the pylorus, and the superior duodenal angle. The endoscope should never be advanced without vision and should always be withdrawn when in doubt.

It is usually possible to perform much of the upper gastrointestinal endoscopy by using the "single-handed" technique. This technique utilizes the left hand to control the up-down knob as well as the air/water and suction buttons, while the right hand inserts, withdraws, or rotates the instrument shaft. When required, the right hand is taken off the shaft and used to manipulate the left/right control knob.

The endoscope is rapidly advanced to the esophagogastric (EG) junction, noting the "Z-line", where the white squamous esophageal mucosa meets the red columnar gastric epithelium. This line should be within 2 cm of the diaphragmatic "pinch zone", which marks the diaphragmatic esophageal hiatus. This point can be accentuated by asking the patient to sniff while the area is visualized. The gastric cardia is intubated by advancing through the EG junction under direct vision; left tip deflection may be needed to maintain proper orientation.

After aspirating any gastric contents, the four gastric walls are surveyed using combinations of tip deflection and shaft rotation, insertion, or withdrawal. The endoscope is next advanced parallel to the longitudinal gastric folds along the greater curve; entry into the antrum usually requires "corkscrewing" around the vertebral column. This affords an end-on view of the pylorus. Usually, passage through the pylorus can be seen as well as felt, and the maneuver is facilitated by use of the single-handed technique. Entry into the duodenal bulb is recognized by its typical granular, pale mucosa. Finally, the second portion of the duodenum is entered by advancing to the superior duodenal angle, and then simultaneously deflecting the tip and rotating the shaft to the right. Paradoxically, withdrawal of the endoscope at this point usually advances the endoscope down the duodenum as the tip is corkscrewed around the superior duodenal angle. All areas should be carefully surveyed again as the endoscope is withdrawn.

With a forward-viewing endoscope in the stomach, it is particularly difficult to visualize the cardia, proximal fundus, and the lesser curve. Thus, when in the antrum, either prior to entering or after withdrawing from the duodenal bulb, the endoscope should be retroflexed by simultaneously flexing the tip up 180° while advancing the shaft (Fig 3–2). In this position, the tip then can be rotated through 180° in either direction in order to visualize the cardia and fundus. In the retroflexed position, the endoscope can be withdrawn to inspect the cardia.

Techniques of Tissue Sampling

When desired, tissue samples are most frequently obtained by directed biopsy. These are taken with cupped forceps (Fig 3–3) passed through the therapeutic channel of the endoscope. Ideally, lesions should be biopsied from an en face position. However, spiked biopsy forceps (Fig 3–3) may facilitate biopsy of lesions that must be approached tangentially (eg. esophagus). In either case, the forceps are applied with open jaws; once properly located, they are closed gently and withdrawn. Multiple biopsies usually should be obtained. For ulcers (Fig 3–2), one should biopsy the rim in all four quadrants, as well as the base. Standard biopsy rarely penetrates the muscularis mucosa. Deeper biopsy can be obtained by using the "jumbo" forceps or with a diathermy snare loop.[84,85]

Lesions can also be sampled by brush cytology. In this technique, a sleeved brush (Fig 3–4) is passed through the therapeutic channel towards the lesion. Once over the lesion, the brush head is advanced out of the sleeve and rubbed repeatedly over the lesion; the brush then is pulled back into the sleeve, and both are withdrawn together. When convenient, the brush head is extended and wiped across several glass slides. These are rapidly fixed and sent for cytologic processing. Often, it is recommended that when using disposable cytology brushes,

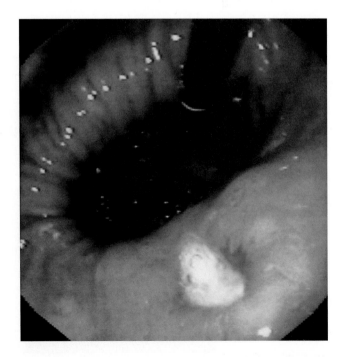

Figure 3–2. A proximal gastric ulcer noted with the endoscope in the retroflexed position. (See color insert.)

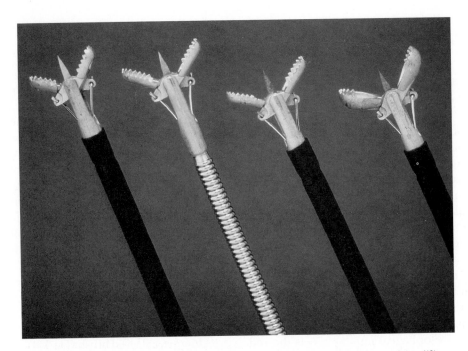

Figure 3–3. Magnified image of disposable biopsy forceps (Courtesy of Wilson-Cook Medical, Winston-Salem, NC).

the brush head should be transected and dropped into fixative. Analysis of this fluid often provides a good cytology specimen.

Various staining techniques are described to improve visualization of mucosal abnormalities.[86] Most involve spraying with dyes (eg, methylene-blue, indigo-carmine, Congo-red) which stain or react with the mucosa.[86]

Hemostasis—Nonvariceal

Despite recent advances, mortality from upper gastrointestinal bleeding has changed little during the past 30 years.[87] Endoscopy plays a critical role in evaluation and treatment of the disorder and should be performed soon after the patient has become stable. Upper gastrointestinal endoscopy will accurately identify the

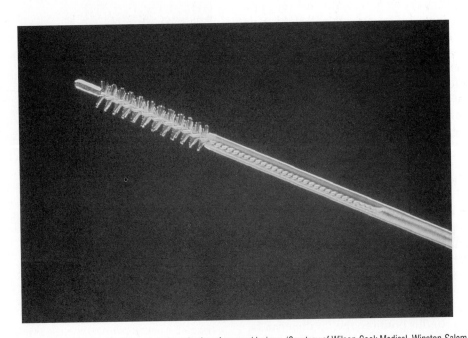

Figure 3–4. Disposable cytology brush allows cytologic evaluation of mucosal lesions. (Courtesy of Wilson-Cook Medical, Winston-Salem, NC).

bleeding source in 80% to 95% of patients.[88,89] If possible, the upper gastrointestinal tract first should be lavaged free of all blood and clots. The endoscopic examination is then performed, seeking active bleeding or stigmata of recent hemorrhage such as clot, black spots, or a visible vessel. Attempts should be made to obtain complete visualization of the esophagus, EG junction, fundus, antrum, pylorus, and proximal duodenum.

Decisions to use hemostatic therapy are complicated in that 70% to 85% of patients stop bleeding on their own and require no further intervention.[90] However, therapy would seem appropriate for those lesions that readily are treated endoscopically and in which factors are identified that predict rebleeding with its associated poor prognosis.[90] These factors include actively bleeding lesions (usually ulcers) (Figs 3–2 and 3–5) or those with a nonbleeding visible vessel or a sentinel clot.[91–94] A sentinel clot is associated with a smaller risk of rebleeding in comparison to the first two factors.[92,93] Mallory-Weiss tears and Dieulafoy's disease[95] are less common nonvariceal lesions that may be treated with endoscopic intervention. Two types of hemostatic treatments are available: injection and thermal therapy.

Injection therapy is performed with a 4-mm 23-gauge needle passed through the operating channel of the endoscope. The sclerosant is injected submucosally at three or four sites surrounding a bleeding vessel and at an additional three or four sites 1 to 2 cm from the vessel. The amount injected varies with different agents, but it should be small enough to avoid extension or damage to surrounding tissues, yet large enough to induce tamponade (and possibly sclerosis) by compressing adjacent tissue. Agents available include epinephrine (alone or with normal or hypertonic saline), absolute alcohol, thrombin in normal saline, sodium tetradecyl sulfate, and polidiocanol. These agents all appear to be effective (85% to 95%) when properly used in appropriate settings.[96–99] In addition, all agents appear safe, with complications occurring in no more than 1% to 2% of patients.[95–99] No prospective clinical trial currently demonstrates superiority of any one of the available agents.

Thermal therapies use heat to control hemorrhage by inducing tissue coagulation, collagen contraction, and vessel shrinkage.[100] The two main types of thermal energy have either light or electricity as their energy source.

Monopolar electrocoagulation transfers electric current from a generator to the tissues and then to the patient's ground plate. Because of the high energy density, the electric current is converted to heat at the small area of contact between the electrode and the tissue. The current is applied circumferentially around the artery until the bleeding stops. The heat generated, which can reach several thousand degrees, is sufficient to cause

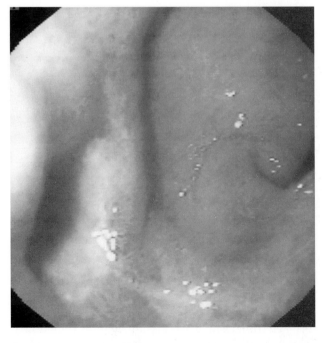

A

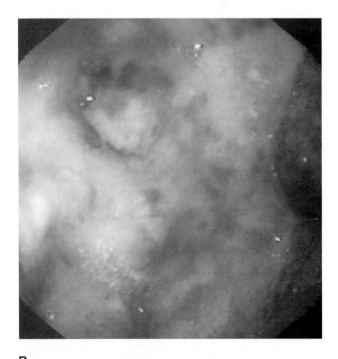

B

Figure 3–5. A. This duodenal ulcer was noted during upper gastrointestinal endoscopy in a patient with persistent epigastric abdominal pain. **B.** Endoscopic image of an acute duodenal ulcer associated with surrounding duodenitis. (See color insert.)

full-thickness tissue damage.[100] Therefore, the technique should be performed only by an endoscopist experienced with this modality.

Bipolar probes use two active electrodes to concentrate current density close to the probe tip. This allows effective coagulation at lower temperatures (100°C).[101] The probe is placed against the bleeding site, tamponading the bleeding. Current (50W) is then passed in several 2 second pulses. This will bond intimal surfaces (coaptation) of the bleeding vessels. The heater probe applies heat to the vessel by conduction. Coaptation is achieved by tamponading the vessel with the probe and applying three or four sequential pulses of 20 to 30 J each.

The laser generates heat as light is absorbed by the tissues. Two types of lasers currently are used for hemostasis: the argon and the neodymium-yttrium aluminum garnet (Nd: YAG) lasers. The argon laser is of limited use in the severely bleeding patient since the light is absorbed by red blood cells, decreasing the amount of energy applied to the vessel. Disadvantages of laser therapy include extreme heat (Nd:YAG laser has a greater risk of full-thickness injury), expense, and lack of portability.

Thermal-type therapies are successful in 80% to 95% of cases with a rebleeding rate of 10% to 20%.[100,102] They are easy to use and safe, with a perforation rate of 0.5%.[100,102]

Results of individual trials of nonvariceal (ulcer) bleeding have failed to demonstrate outcome benefit of endoscopic therapy. Recently, two large meta-analyses of multiple randomized prospective trials were published.[103,104] Although the two reports differed in number of the studies reviewed and their analytic methods, both clearly demonstrated that endoscopic laser treatment significantly decreased the rate of continued or recurrent bleeding, the need for urgent surgery, and patient mortality. Similarly, injection and thermal therapies were demonstrated to decrease the rate of rebleeding and the need for surgical intervention. It should be noted that the benefit of endoscopic therapy was predominantly confined to patients with high-risk stigmata (ie, active bleeding or visible vessels). These findings further support the role of endoscopic hemostasis for nonvariceal bleeding, especially in those lesions found to have poor prognostic features.

Hemostasis—Variceal

Bleeding esophageal varices (Fig 3–6) remain a significant clinical problem with hospital mortality rates approaching 30%.[87] Without some form of intervention, two-thirds of patients who survive an initial episode of bleeding will rebleed.[105] Although controlled clinical trials have demonstrated that acute sclerotherapy reduces transfusion requirements compared with conven-

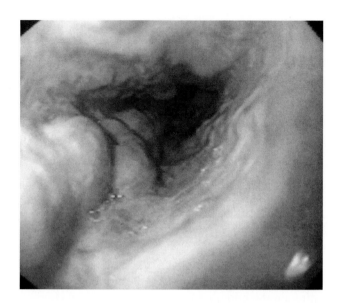

A

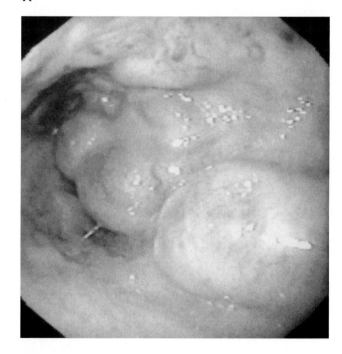

B

Figure 3–6. A and **B**. Two endoscopic images of esophageal varices. (See color insert.)

tional medical treatment,[106] long-term survival is probably not altered.[107]

The condition of the patient should be optimized before sclerotherapy. This should include repletion of volume and coagulation factors. The stomach also should be lavaged to clear blood clots. In the presence of massive bleeding, it may be necessary to begin an intravenous vasopressin infusion or pass a Senstaken-Blakemore or similar tube for 12 to 24 hours before attempting sclerotherapy. If possible, however, sclerotherapy without prior tamponade is favored, since this approach is equally effective, and lessens blood requirement and major complication rates.[108]

As yet, there is no universally accepted sclerosant.[109] The most commonly used sclerosants in the United States are 0.7% to 3.0% sodium tetradecyl sulfate and 5% sodium morrhuate.[110] In Europe, ethanolamine is more commonly used. All of these agents can cause tissue damage and inflammation; controlled clinical data demonstrating superiority of any one agent are lacking.

Sclerosants can be injected either intravariceally or paravariceally. Intravariceal injection is preferred, since it controls acute variceal bleeding more effectively (91% vs 19%).[111] Injections are begun just above the gastroesophageal junction. Once the needle is placed into a varix, a test dose of 0.5 mL of sclerosant is given to ensure intravariceal placement. After placement is confirmed, an additional 1.5 mL is injected at that site. This technique is repeated in a circular fashion until all varices at this level have been treated. Injections are continued by moving proximally, injecting at 2- to 3-cm intervals until small-caliber vessels are encountered. The total amount of sclerosant used varies with the agent used, but in general should not exceed 20 mL per session. If active variceal bleeding is encountered, injections are begun just proximal to the bleeding site and continued until bleeding subsides. A second session of sclerotherapy should be performed 5 days later. Sclerotherapy is usually repeated at 1 to 3 week intervals until varices are ablated.

Sclerotherapy controls acute variceal hemorrhage in at least 85% of episodes and probably lowers the rate of recurrent bleeding.[107] Propranolol may decrease the rate of recurrent bleeding while awaiting variceal obliteration.[112] Although portacaval shunting is significantly more effective than sclerotherapy in preventing rebleeding, it is associated with a greater incidence of encephalopathy and has a questionable survival benefit.[113–117] Further, in patients who are candidates for transplant, shunt surgery may compromise future transplantation surgery.

Recent reports have focused attention on endoscopic ligation as an alternative method for variceal eradication. In this technique, varices are ligated with elastic bands similar to those used during hemorrhoidal ligation (Fig 3–7). When compared to schlerotherapy, endoscopic ligation appears to be as effective.[118,119] In addition, it may improve morbidity and mortality.[118]

Prophylactic scherotherapy has been suggested as a method of preventing initial bleeding episodes and improving survival in cirrhotics. However, recent results cast doubt on the benefit of this approach.[120,121] Indeed, the Veterans Affairs Cooperative study was terminated prematurely owing to increased mortality in the prophylactic sclerotherapy group.[120]

Percutaneous Endoscopic Gastrostomy and Jejunostomy

PEG is now the preferred method for long-term feeding in patients who are unable to swallow or who require supplemental nutrition or chronic gastric decompression.[122] PEG has supplanted surgical gastrostomy, since it is as safe[123,124] and is less expensive.[124] PEG and percutaneous endoscopic jejunostomy (PEJ) are contraindicated in patients with total esophageal obstruction, massive ascites, or intra-abdominal sepsis.

Prior to the procedure, a single dose of prophylactic cephalosporin (or equivalent) is given intravenously.[83] The patient is placed in the supine position, and the abdomen is prepared and draped using sterile technique. The endoscope then is passed into the stomach, which is distended with air insufflation. The assistant then presses on the abdomen with a finger at the point where transillumination is observed. Ideally, this point should be approximately two-thirds or three-quarters of the distance from the umbilicus to the midpoint of the left costal margin. It is critical that the assistant's finger be observed clearly to indent the stomach.

A polypectomy snare is passed through the endoscope channel; the wire loop is opened and placed over the bulge created by the assistant's finger. The selected site on the abdominal wall then is infiltrated with local anesthesia. If desired, the fine needle used to anesthetize the skin can be inserted into the abdomen at the gastrostomy site; observation of the clean entry of the needle into the stomach suggests that the position is adequate. After making a small incision (approximately 5 mm) in the skin, the assistant then inserts an intravenous cannula through the incision which must be seen to enter the stomach. The snare then is tightened around the cannula and the inner stylet is removed. In the "pull technique,"[125–127] a heavy silk suture is placed through the cannula and firmly grasped with the polypectomy snare. The cannula is withdrawn, and the endoscope with the tightened snare is removed, bringing the suture out of the patient's mouth. The suture is tied to a well-lubricated gastrostomy tube with a specialized tapered external end. The assistant then pulls on the suture until the attached tube exits the abdominal wall. The endoscope is reinserted and used to view the inner bolster of the tube as the stomach is loosely seated against the abdominal wall (Fig 3–8). The endoscope then is removed, and the tube is secured in place on the abdominal wall, usually with an external bolster.

Two other techniques can be used: In the "push technique,"[128] a guidewire, in lieu of a suture, is inserted through the cannula and pulled out of the patient's mouth. The gastrostomy tube then is pushed over the

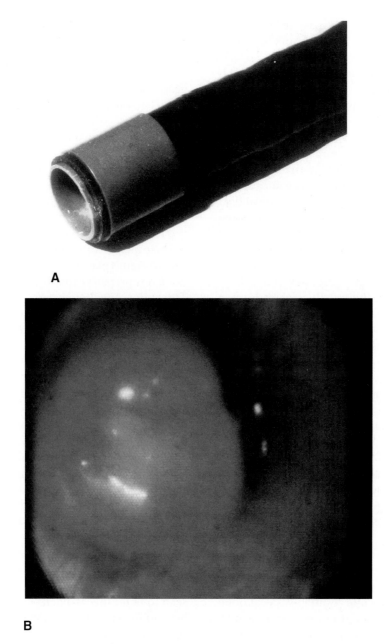

A

B

Figure 3–7. A. The endoscopic variceal band ligator which is mounted on the end of a standard endoscope. The device is activated after drawing the varix within the ligating device using the endoscope's suction. **B.** Photograph demonstrating a recently banded esophageal varix. (See color insert.)

wire until it exits the abdominal wall. This technique offers several technical advantages.[129] Finally, in the "introducer technique,"[130] the stomach is inflated, the site of insertion is selected, and the intravenous cannula is introduced into the stomach as described above. A J-tipped guidewire then is passed through the cannula into the stomach, and the cannula is removed. Next, an introducer with a peel-away sheath is passed over this wire, allowing removal of the wire and introducer. A Foley catheter or other similar gastrostomy tube then is placed through the sheath, its balloon is inflated, the sheath is removed, and the catheter is secured to the abdominal wall.

The procedure can be extended to include PEJ in patients who fail to tolerate gastric feedings owing to severe gastroesophageal reflux or gastric atony. This is achieved by passing a jejunal feeding tube through the PEG lumen. The jejunal feeding tube then can be placed into the duodenum or jejunum under endoscopic or fluoroscopic guidance. Endoscopically, the je-

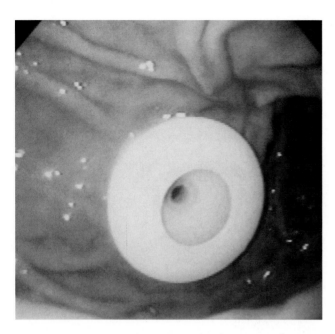

Figure 3–8. Endoscopic view of percutaneous endoscopic gastrostomy tube seated against the gastric wall and loosely opposing the gastric wall to the anterior abdominal wall. (See color insert.)

junal tube is grasped with the foreign-body forceps and is guided into the duodenum under direct vision. Alternatively, the tube is pulled into the duodenum with the endoscope. A simplified method for PEJ insertion, using a nasobiliary catheter as a jejunal tube, has recently been described.[131] Although PEJ is claimed to decrease the incidence of aspiration following PEG,[132,133] this claim is disputed.[134,135]

Foreign Body Extraction

Foreign bodies are ingested predominantly by two groups of patients: children (ages 1 to 5 years) who accidentally swallow an object, and adults who are obtunded, inebriated, have a psychiatric disorder, or are prisoners.[136,137] Most objects (80% to 90%) will pass spontaneously, but 10% to 20% must be removed endoscopically,[138] and approximately 1% require surgical intervention.[139] Removal is usually necessary if the object has failed to move within 48 to 72 hours. Objects wider than 2 cm or longer than 5 cm rarely will pass and usually require endoscopic intervention. Signs of respiratory compromise or inability to handle secretions constitute a true emergency and require immediate extraction of the object.

When performing endoscopic extraction, protection of the airway is of vital importance. Thus, the procedure should be performed with the patient in the Trendelenburg position to prevent the object from falling into the trachea during removal. Endotracheal intubation is

rarely required. An endoscopic overtube should be considered when removing sharp objects or multiple fragments. It often is helpful to rehearse extraction ex vivo, using a similar foreign body.[140]

Coins are the most common object swallowed by children. Although a coin can lodge in the trachea or esophagus, its location can be readily ascertained with cervical radiography. If in the trachea, the edge of the coin seen in the anteroposterior view and its flat surface in the lateral view. The opposite is seen with a coin in the esophagus.[141] These films should be repeated if more than an hour has passed since the last films or if the symptoms suddenly disappear. Coins lodged in the esophagus should be removed promptly, since the risk of pressure necrosis and fistula formation increases progressively.

Endoscopic extraction is accomplished after adequate sedation with the patient in the Trendelenburg position. The coin is localized and grasped with a polypectomy snare or a rat-tooth or tenaculum forceps. A Foley catheter is not recommended, since it does not control the object well during removal. The coin usually will pass if it reaches the stomach.

In the adult population, meat impaction represents the most common foreign body. These impactions should be removed if they remain longer than 12 hours. If the bolus should pass, esophagoscopy is still required, since an obstructing esophageal lesion will be found in 70% to 95% of patients.[137] Papain therapy is not indicated.[141]

Sharp objects such as toothpicks, fish or chicken bones, needles, and razor blades should be removed promptly because of the small, but real, risk of perforation. Use of an overtube may greatly facilitate the removal of sharp objects. If the object has a single sharp end (eg, an open safety pin) and is directed orad, it can be pushed into the stomach, rotated to point the sharp end distally, and then removed. Surgical removal is probably best with items for which endoscopic extraction appears to carry an excessive risk. If the object has passed beyond endoscopic access, a trial of spontaneous passage is reasonable, with daily radiographic monitoring. If the object fails to progress after 2 to 3 days, or if the patient becomes symptomatic, surgical removal may be in order.

Ingested button batteries can injure the esophagus by direct, corrosive action. In the stomach, they can erode and release toxic components.[142,143] These batteries usually pass readily in other parts of the gastrointestinal tract without causing harm. After endoscopically removing a battery from the esophagus, it is important to inspect the esophagus for possible damage.

When encountered, cocaine-filled packets should never be removed endoscopically because of the risk of breakage.[144] Recent studies suggest a possible role for

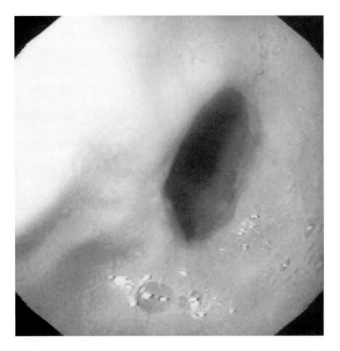

Figure 3–9. A benign peptic esophageal stricture which was treated with endoscopic dilatation. (See color insert.)

expectant management in this situation.[141] Patients managed in this way should be monitored closely since they may require surgery for bowel obstruction.

Stricture Dilatation

Most commonly, a patient with an esophageal stricture (Fig 3–9) complains of dysphagia or odynophagia. A barium swallow is initially obtained to demonstrate the structure and length of the obstructing lesion. Endoscopy should then be performed to identify the nature and severity of the stricture. Multiple biopsies and cytologic brushing of the area should always be obtained before and/or after dilatation.

Esophageal strictures have multiple causes, the most common of which is benign peptic stenosis secondary to gastroesophageal reflux. Most peptic and many radiation strictures are amenable to dilation therapy, which is a relatively safe procedure that is usually performed on an outpatient basis. Overall success rates approaching 90% are reported for benign strictures.[145] Although each therapeutic intervention should aim to eliminate dysphagia, many suggest that no more than three dilators of successive size should be used at each session. Treatment should be continued until a diameter of 14 to 15 mm (approximately 45 French [Fr]) is achieved. The frequency of dilation will depend on the severity of the stricture and the patient's symptoms.

Several types of dilators are currently available (Fig 3–10). These include the push type (either mercury-filled or guidewire-driven), which applies both axial and radial forces, and the balloon type, which applies only

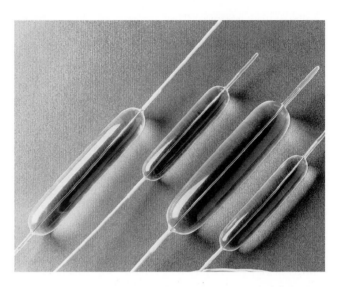

A

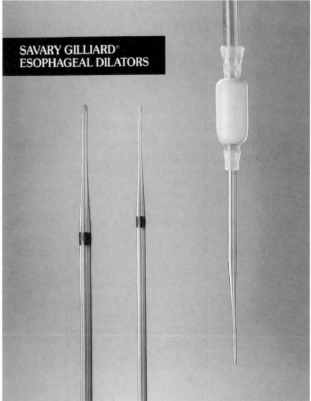

B

Figure 3–10. A. Balloon dilators used during endoscopic dilatation (Courtesy of Microvasive, Boston Scientific Corporation, Watertown, MA). **B.** Modified Savary Gilliard esophageal dilators that can also be used during endoscopic dilatation. These dilators are guidewire driven. Note that esophageal prostheses can be inserted over the dilators (Courtesy of Wilson-Cook Medical, Winston-Salem, NC).

radial forces. Guidewire-driven dilators are easy to pass and offer the added safety of the guidewire; balloon dilators can be monitored endoscopically. As such, these new dilators (guidewire and balloon) have relegated the use of mercury-filled dilators to those patients with mild to moderate chronic strictures in a relatively straight esophagus.

Guidewire-driven dilators are suitable for use with tight strictures or when other dilators cannot be used. These are fairly rigid devices made of polyvinyl chloride (Savory; Wilson-Cook Medical, Winston Salem, NC). Each dilator has a hollow core and can be passed over an endoscopically or fluoroscopically placed guidewire.[146,147] Although there are no controlled trials, some endoscopists maintain that fluoroscopic control increases the safety and effectiveness of dilatation.[148,149] Guidewire-driven, metal-olive dilators (Eder-Puestow) are rarely, if ever, used anymore.

Balloon dilators are used for short strictures, stenotic stomas, and achalasia.[150–153] These dilators can be passed over a guidewire or through the therapeutic channel of the endoscope. Balloon dilation of achalasia provides long-term success in approximately 75% of cases, although several sessions are required frequently.[154] Results may be improved by use of newly introduced balloon dilators that provide a more reproducible dilatation.[155] Balloon dilatation for achalasia will need to be reevaluated as laparoscopic esophageal myotomy is developed.[156,157] While balloon dilatation also has been utilized for treatment of corrosive strictures, the perforation rate may be increased in this setting.[158,159]

Endoscopic intervention frequently is required for malignant esophageal strictures. Patients with unresectable tumors or tracheoesophageal fistula may require palliative dilation and, occasionally, placement of an esophageal prosthesis.[160] Placement of these devices requires initial esophageal dilation followed by endoscopic assessment of tumor location and length. Under fluoroscopic guidance, the prosthesis is placed so that the distal end is 3 to 5 cm beyond the tumor or fistula. Laser ablation[161–163] and electrocoagulation therapy[164] also may provide reasonable palliation. Recent reports suggest that laser ablation and endoprosthesis insertion are complementary techniques that should be considered along with radiation therapy in seeking palliation of unresectable esophageal malignancy.[165–167]

COMPLICATIONS

Diagnostic upper gastrointestinal endoscopy is a remarkably safe procedure with complications reported in approximately 0.1% of cases.[168] Cardiopulmonary problems are the most common complications and are usually attributable to oversedation (see Monitoring).

Diagnostic upper endoscopy is rarely associated with mortality (<0.01%).[168]

Procedure-related complications are also unusual following upper gastrointestinal endoscopy. Perforation is of greatest concern and occurs more frequently following emergency interventions and therapeutic procedures such as dilation,[154,169,170] sclerotherapy,[171] or thermal hemostasis.[100] When dilating or laser ablating esophageal malignancies, perforation may occur in as many as 10% of cases.[161,165] Intensive medical treatment is being used with greater frequency in managing iatrogenic esophageal perforations.[172,173] This approach is acceptable in clinically stable patients with rapidly detected, well-contained perforations.[173]

Other unique complications include ulceration and stricture following esophageal sclerotherapy[107]; these are treated as described above. Finally, local wound infection (including necrotizing fasciitis) can follow PEG, especially if the incision is too small or the tube is pulled too tight against the gastric wall.[174] Rarely, PEG is complicated by separation from the abdominal wall with resultant peritonitis or by colonic injury with resultant gastrocolonic fistula.[174]

■ ENDOSCOPY OF THE PANCREATICOBILIARY TREE

INDICATIONS

In 1968, McKune[8] introduced endoscopic retrograde cholangiopancreatography (ERCP) when he described endoscopic guidance of a catheter into the ampulla of Vater. Following improvements in this revolutionary diagnostic technique, it became possible to image the pancreatic ductal system without surgical intervention. Approximately 5 years later, German[17] and Japanese[18] physicians described endoscopic sphincterotomy. This therapeutic extension of ERCP greatly expanded one's options: certain pancreaticobiliary disorders not only could be diagnosed, but could also be treated and often cured via endoscopic access. Our therapeutic options continue to expand as ancillary therapeutic maneuvers (eg. endoprosthesis insertion, dilatation, lithotripsy) continue to be described.

As outlined in Table 3–2, diagnostic and therapeutic endoscopic intervention may be indicated for numerous biliary and pancreatic disorders. It must be emphasized, however, that diagnostic information and therapeutic outcomes frequently can be achieved via several alternative mechanisms. Thus, in addition to the patient's clinical situation and prognosis, consideration also must be given to locally available radiologic and surgical expertise. When choosing between transhepatic and endoscopic access for evaluating biliary disorders, ERCP is usually selected, given its lower morbidity rate,[175] as well

TABLE 3–2. INDICATIONS FOR PANCREATICOBILIARY ENDOSCOPY

DIAGNOSTIC EVALUATION
Jaundice due to suspected biliary obstruction (if endoscopic therapy is concurrently available)
Suspected biliary or pancreatic disease
Recurrent or moderate to severe pancreatitis of unknown etiology
Chronic pancreatitis and/or pseudocyst (preoperative)
Sphincter of Oddi manometry

THERAPY
Endoscopic sphincterotomy
 Choledocholithiasis
 Papillary stenosis
 Sphincter of Oddi dysfunction
 Prior to biliary endoprosthesis insertion or balloon dilatation
 Sump syndrome
 Choledochocele
 Ampullary carcinoma in patients unfit for surgery
Biliary endoprosthesis insertion
 Benign or malignant strictures
 Biliary fistula
 Postoperative bile leak
 Large, unremovable common duct stones (High-risk patients)
Nasobiliary drain insertion
 Prevention or treatment of acute cholangitis
 Chemical dissolution of common duct stones
 Decompression of obstructed common bile duct
 Post-operative bile leak (if endoprosthesis insertion fails/unavailable)
Balloon dilatation of biliary strictures

Adapted from Standards of Practice Committee. *Appropriate Use of Gastrointestinal Endoscopy.* Manchester, MA: American Society of Gastrointestinal Endoscopy; 1992

as the opportunity to intervene therapeutically. It is evident that relative indications and contraindications will continue to evolve in this rapidly expanding field.

PATIENT PREPARATION

Patient preparation for pancreaticobiliary endoscopy is similar to that for upper gastrointestinal endoscopy. Thus, prior to ERCP, patients should fast for a minimum of 6 to 8 hours (usually overnight). Although iodine allergy appears to impose minimal risk, most endoscopists will premedicate "contrast-allergic" patients with intravenous steroids and occasionally, with antihistamines. In addition, a nonionic contrast agent may be appropriate in this circumstance.

Intravenous access is required for administration of analgesia, intestinal paralytics, and other medications. Since the procedure is performed with the patient in the prone position, the intravenous cannula is preferred in the right arm so that the intravenous tubing is accessible and does not lie under the patient. Coagulation profiles, and type and screen may be indicated preoperatively, especially if therapy is contemplated for established obstructive jaundice.

The patient's dentures and eyeglasses should be removed. Prophylactic antibiotics are not universally required. However, as mentioned above, they should be administered to any patient with an appropriate history (eg, artificial cardiac valves, valvular heart disease). Additional indications for antibiotic prophylaxis include a significant question of biliary and/or pancreatic ductal stasis (especially if therapeutic intervention is not available), sphincterotomy for stones with gallbladder in situ, suspected pancreatic pseudocyst, acute pancreatitis, and possible or planned therapy (eg. endoprosthesis insertion).

The patient's oropharynx is anesthetized with local anesthesia, usually cetacaine or xylocaine sprays. While some endoscopists initiate the procedure with the patient in the prone position on the x-ray table, most use the left lateral decubitus position with the left arm behind the back, anticipating conversion to the prone position once the endoscope is appropriately located in the descending duodenum. The patient should be adequately sedated prior to insertion of the endoscope; incremental doses of intravenous midazolam and meperidine are utilized most frequently. Most endoscopists do not favor administration of preoperative analgesia for fear of complicating safe administration of intravenous analgesia immediately before and during the examination.

DIAGNOSTIC AND THERAPEUTIC TECHNIQUES

Endoscopic Retrograde Cholangiopancreatography

ERCP is a sophisticated procedure requiring the cooperation of a skilled endoscopist and an interested radiologist. Indeed, it is essentially a radiologic procedure "driven" by an endoscopist. After the patient is appropriately prepared, the long side-viewing endoscope is passed into the upper esophagus through the cricopharyngeus. The scope is passed rapidly into the proximal stomach where any residual secretions are aspirated. The gastric mucosa can be surveyed rapidly, although valuable cannulation time should not be wasted. As the scope is passed towards the pylorus, it is vital to keep it within the central axis of the antrum; such a position is ensured by maintaining the scope perpendicular to the incisura. Because of the location of the lens of the endoscope, the pylorus is only minimally visualized (if at all) when intubated. Passage into the duodenal bulb is felt rather than seen.

If indicated, the duodenal bulb is rapidly surveyed, and then the endoscope is passed into the descending duodenum. This maneuver requires corkscrewing the endoscope around the superior duodenal angle. The endoscope usually is withdrawn during this maneuver, ideally leaving the scope in the short-scope position, 60 to 70 cm from the incisors, facing the medial duodenal wall (Fig 3–11A). If the endoscope is passed into the duodenum by continually advancing, steering, and

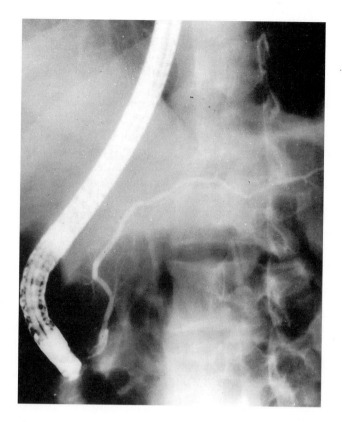

A

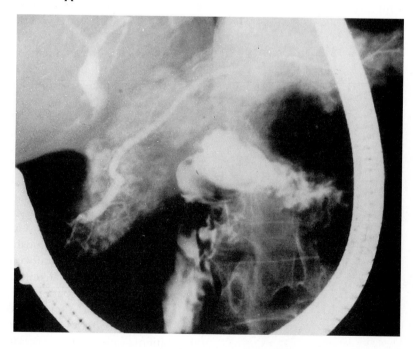

B

Figure 3–11. A. Duodenoscope in the short-scope position in the descending duodenum, facing the ampulla. The endoscopic pancreatogram is normal. **B**. The long-scope position is not preferred because it is more uncomfortable to the patient and it reduces control at the endoscope tip. However, this position may be required for cannulation of the accessory papilla, as in this example. Note that in this case of pancreas divisum, excessive contrast injection has caused "acinarization" of the dorsal pancreas.

rotating, the long-scope position usually results (Fig 3–11B). This position is not preferred; it is not only uncomfortable to the patient, but it also reduces control of the endoscope tip.

If in the short-scope position, the papilla frequently will be directly in view along the medial duodenal wall. If not, the papilla usually can be located at the apex of one or several longitudinal folds arising from the inferior duodenal angle. Once located, intermittent boluses of glucagon (0.25 mg) should be administered to induce and maintain duodenal paralysis. A scout radiograph is obtained to verify adequate radiologic technique, as well as to identify calcifications or other findings present before contrast injection. The papilla then is cannulated using one of the various types of catheters that are available (Fig 3–12). Catheters with radiopaque tips are often preferred since the radiologic marker facilitates radiologic identification of the catheter tip. Once the papilla has been cannulated successfully, contrast is injected under radiologic control so as to avoid overfilling the biliary and/or the pancreatic ductal systems. If dilated ducts are encountered, use of diluted (half-strength) contrast may prevent obscuring small stones. Attention to radiologic technique is critical since diagnostic information is only as good as the quality of the radiologic images obtained.

Selective cannulation of the biliary and pancreatic ducts is the key to successful ERCP, as well as to therapeutic intervention. Although various maneuvers are available (eg, cannulation with taper-tipped catheters, guidewires, sphincterotomes), all aim to manipulate the catheter into the correct ductal axis. The pancreatic duct tends to enter the papilla in a relatively perpendicular fashion. In contrast, the bile duct runs towards the 11 o'clock position from the lower right aspect of the papilla.

Persistent failure to obtain a pancreatogram should raise the possibility of pancreatic divisum (Fig 3–13) or other ductal anomalies. Identification of these anomalies may require cannulation of the minor (accessory) papilla. Accessory papillary cannulation usually requires repositioning the endoscope into a long position, use of thin (0.018 inch) guidewires and special catheters, and intravenous secretin injection to render the accessory papilla more prominent.

As mentioned above, attention to proper radiologic technique is critical to obtaining interpretable radiographs. Artifacts such as air bubbles, streaming and layering of contrast, and contrast spillage into the duodenum should be recognized and corrected with proper technique. With the expertise currently available, the greatest risk that ERCP poses may well be misinterpretation.[176] Further, while surgeons are relatively familiar with cholangiograms, pancreatograms remain more difficult to interpret.[177] This task has been facilitated with recent agreement on the endoscopic classification of chronic pancreatitis (Table 3–3).[178] Other abnormalities such as neoplasms (Fig 3–14), chronic inflammatory changes (Fig 3–15), and anatomic anomalies should become more familiar as experience increases.

When indicated, therapeutic options now allow concurrent management of both biliary and pancreatic disorders. Such a philosophy is appropriate, since septic complications occur almost exclusively in the presence of untreated biliary and pancreatic ductal stasis.[179,180] Therefore, in patients with known biliary strictures or stones or pancreatic pseudocysts, unless endoscopic therapy is contemplated, ERCP should be done only as a preoperative study prior to planned surgical or radiologic intervention.

Even when utilized exclusively as a preoperative maneuver, ERCP may be of considerable benefit to patients with pancreatic pseudocysts. Nealon and associates[181] prospectively evaluated the role of routine preoperative ERCP in patients with pancreatic pseudocysts who were referred for operative intervention. Over a 36-month period, ERCP was attempted in 41 consecutive patients with pseudocysts. Twenty-four of the forty-one patients were believed to be recovering from acute pancreatitis. Successful ERCP was obtained in 39 of the 41 patients and revealed unsuspected chronic pancreatitis in 9 of the patients originally believed to have acute disease. Dilated pancreatic and common bile ducts were observed in 23 and 12 patients, respectively;

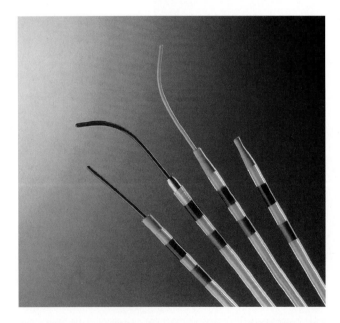

Figure 3–12. Selection of ERCP catheters demonstrating several of the different tips available. Many of the catheters' tips are radioopaque which facilitates location of the catheter during fluoroscopic imaging. Note that most of the catheters allow passage of 0.035-inch guidewires. (Courtesy of Microvasive, Boston Scientific Corporation, Watertown, MA).

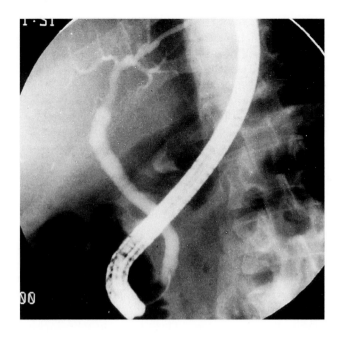

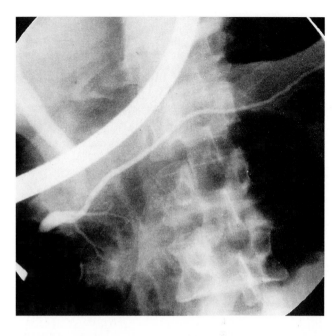

A   **B**

Figure 3–13. A. In this example of pancreas divisum, contrast injection at the main ampulla only fills the common bile duct. **B**. Opacification of the dorsal pancreatic duct via accessory papillary cannulation proves pancreas divisum.

these abnormalities were seen only in patients with chronic pancreatitis. Most importantly, ERCP findings led to alteration of the operative plan in 24 of the 41 patients, 22 of whom had chronic pancreatitis. In early retrospective studies, Sugawa and Walt[182] and O'Connor and associates also suggested similar benefit for preoperative ERCP in patients with pseudocysts.

TABLE 3–3. CAMBRIDGE CLASSIFICATION OF ENDOSCOPIC PANCREATOGRAPHIC CHANGES IN CHRONIC PANCREATITIS

Terminology	Main pancreatic duct	Abnormal main pancreatic duct branches	Additional features
Normal	Normal	None	None
Equivocal	Normal	<3	None
Mild	Normal	≥3	None
Moderate	Abnormal	≥3	None
Severe	Abnormal	≥3	One or more: large cavity, obstruction, filling defects, severe dilation, or irregularity

Adapted from Fink AS. Endoscopic intervention for pancreatic disorders. In: Hunter JG, Sackier J (eds), *High Tech Surgery: New Approaches to Old Diseases*, New York, NY: McGraw-Hill; 1993:245–254.

Ahearne and associates[184] have further suggested that preoperative ERCP can be used as the basis for an algorithm with which to select the appropriate therapeutic modality for patients with pancreatic pseudocysts. In their algorithm, it is assumed that pseudocysts associated with pancreatic duct obstruction or pancreatic ductal communication require surgical intervention. Thus, in elective cases, if preoperative ERCP reveals either pancreatic duct obstruction or pseudocyst communication, surgery is necessary; lack of both findings allows percutaneous drainage. Among 102 patients with pseudocysts seen over a six year period, adequate preoperative ERCP had been obtained in 40 to 69 electively treated patients. Retrospective application of the algorithm to these 40 patients revealed that in 26 of them, treatment course followed the algorithm; in 14 patients, the selected therapy differed from the algorithm. In the group that followed the algorithm, there was one treatment failure and two complications (3/26 = 12%); in the group that did not follow the algorithm, 6 of 14 (43%) experienced either treatment failure or complication. The authors propose prospective testing of their algorithm to prove its validity.

Endoscopic Sphincterotomy

If endoscopic sphincterotomy (Fig 3–16) is indicated, the diagnostic cannula is removed and replaced with a sphincterotome (Fig 3–17). The latter consists of a stan-

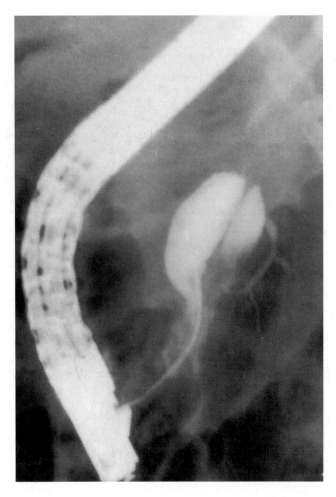

Figure 3–14. The double-duct sign which is diagnostic of pancreatic carcinoma.

dard cannula containing a continuous wire loop, 20 to 30 mm of which is exposed near the tip. Initially, the tip is inserted well into the bile duct (Fig 3–16A); sphincterotomy must not be attempted until the sphincterotome has been clearly demonstrated to be within the bile duct and not the pancreatic duct. With guidewire-driven sphincterotomes (Fig 3–17), the bile duct is deeply cannulated with an 0.035-inch guidewire that is introduced via the diagnostic cannula. The sphincterotome then is exchanged for the catheter over the guidewire. Use of an insulated guidewire allows the wire to remain in place (and maintains deep biliary cannulation) while the sphincterotomy is performed.

Once proper ductal cannulation is verified, the sphincterotome is withdrawn until approximately half of the wire is visible outside of the papilla, pointing toward the 11 or 12 o'clock position. The wire is then tightened, bowing it against the papillary roof. Current is then applied in short bursts while maintaining gentle upward force on the wire (Fig 3–16B); thus, the incision is made in small increments. Since complications (see below) appear to be related to incision length, it is important to ensure that the sphincterotomy length is adequate, but not excessive. Thus, only a small (eg, 5 mm) incision is needed to facilitate subsequent therapeutic interventions (eg, endoprosthesis insertion), while larger incisions usually are made when dealing with choledocholithiasis (based on the size of the largest stone). Inability to cannulate the bile duct deeply, anatomic factors (eg, Billroth II gastrectomy, duodenal diverticulum), and operator inexperience all may con-

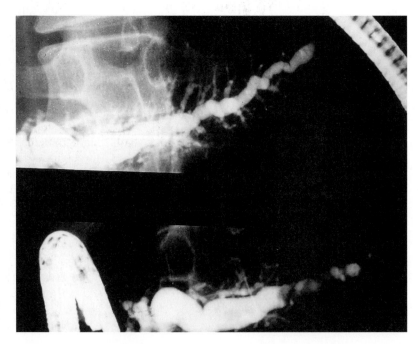

Figure 3–15. This endoscopic pancreatogram demonstrates severe chronic pancreatitis. Note the dilated main duct with its chain-of-lakes appearance, as well as the grossly abnormal side branches.

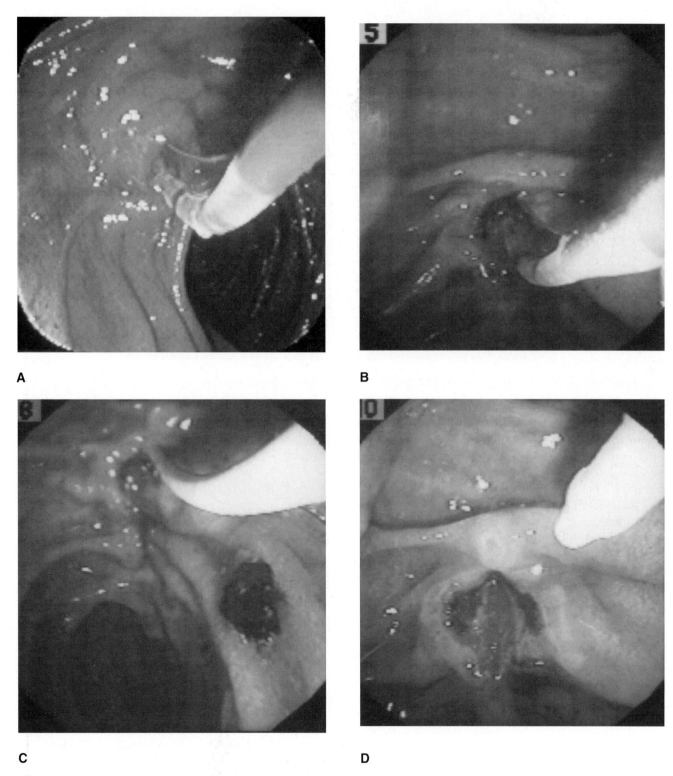

Figure 3–16. A. A sphincterotome has been inserted into the bile duct and is positioned for spincterotomy. **B**. The sphincterotomy is nearing completion. **C**. The bile duct is being swept with a balloon catheter after completing the sphincterotomy. Note the previously removed common bile duct stone lying free in the duodenum. **D**. View of the sphincterotomy after clearing the common bile duct. Note that the choledochal epithelium is seen readily. (See color insert.) (Courtesy of Wilson-Cook Medical, Winston-Salem, NC).

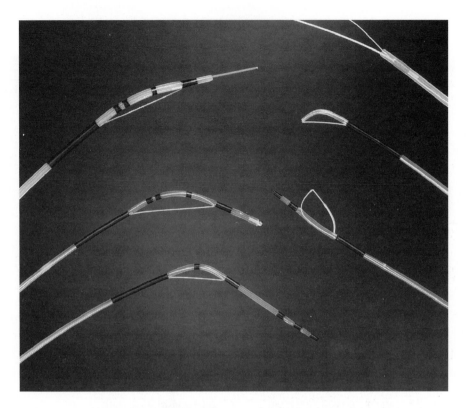

Figure 3–17. Examples of the different types of endoscopic sphincterotomes currently available (Courtesy of Wilson-Cook Medical, Winston-Salem, NC).

tribute to sphincterotomy failure. Several more common indications for endoscopic sphincterotomy are discussed below.

Choledocholithiasis. Retained or recurrent common bile duct stones represent the most common indication for endoscopic sphincterotomy (Fig 3–18). Large series from expert centers consistently report that sphincterotomy is successful in approximately 95% of cases.[185–187] In these expert centers, over 90% of bile ducts can be subsequently cleared of calculi with balloon catheters or Dormia baskets, resulting in an overall ductal clearance rate that approximates 85%.[185–187] Stone size is often a limiting factor; stones >2 cm in diameter often require fragmentation prior to removal.[188] Since these results come from expert centers, a 65% ductal clearance rate may be more realistic for inexperienced endoscopists.

It is recommended that ductal clearance be attempted at the time of endoscopic sphincterotomy, since relying upon spontaneous stone passage increases the risk of cholangitis, pancreatitis, and stone impaction, as well as increasing the need for repeated endoscopic interventions.[189] Adequate ductal drainage must be ensured if all stones cannot be removed. The latter can be accomplished with nasobiliary drainage[190] or endoprosthesis insertion[191]; the choice depends on the clinical setting (eg, need for repeat cholangiogram, planned solvent infusion, residual stone burden, patient risk factors).

In addition to treating retained or recurrent common bile duct stones, endoscopic sphincterotomy has been utilized extensively in elderly patients with symptomatic choledocholithiasis and a gallbladder in situ.[192,193] Provided patients are treated with prophylactic antibiotics, the risk of acute cholecystitis in this setting is <2%.[192–194] In addition, if such patients are followed for a period of several years, <20% will require elective or semi-elective cholecystectomy.[195,196] Even if these patients do require cholecystectomy, the common bile duct is usually found to be clear of stones.[195,196]

Although endoscopic sphincterotomy with the gallbladder in situ is acceptable therapy for elderly, high-risk patients, its use in younger patients is controversial. Certainly, routine preoperative endoscopic sphincterotomy is not warranted in patients undergoing biliary operations for symptomatic cholelithiasis.[197,198] However, the advent of laparoscopic cholecystectomy has created uncertainty regarding the role of preoperative ERCP.[199] As techniques for laparoscopic management of choledocholithiasis become more reliable and more available, it is likely that the role of preoperative ERCP will become less of an issue. Until that time, these decisions will probably be influenced most by the locally available

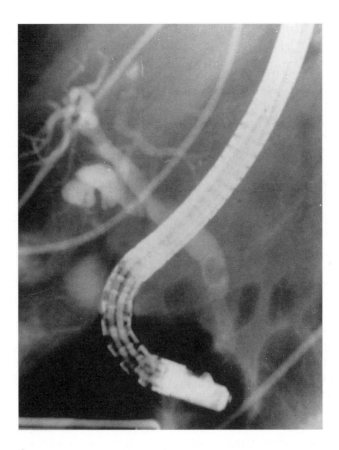

A

B

Figure 3–18. A. Endoscopic cholangiogram demonstrating choledocholithiasis. Note the sphincterotome, radiologically demonstrated within the common bile duct prior to sphincterotomy. **B**. The common bile duct subsequently was cleared endoscopically using Dormia baskets as illustrated in this figure. (Courtesy of Wilson-Cook Medical, Winston-Salem, NC)

endoscopic expertise as well as by individual patient preference.[199]

Sphincter of Oddi Dysfunction. Sphincter of Oddi dysfunction must be considered in patients with unexplained biliary colic or acute pancreatitis. Multiple noninvasive tests have been evaluated in this disorder (eg, ultrasonography, scintigraphy), but all appear to lack adequate sensitivity or specificity. The development of endoscopic manometric techniques now allows direct measurement of motility and intraluminal pressures (Fig 3–19) within both the biliary and pancreatic segments of the sphincter of Oddi,[200] although not without a moderate risk of pancreatitis.[201,202] This risk may be lessened by using an aspirating catheter during sphincter of Oddi manometry.[201,203,204]

A classification system has been developed by enthusiasts who claim that patients can be categorized into one of three groups based on their clinical history, laboratory evaluation, and results of diagnostic ERCP (Table 3–4).[205,206] Indeed, the proponents of this system maintain that manometry is optional in type I patients (definitive sphincter of Oddi dysfunction).[205,206]

Although the importance of much of this data continues to be debated, elevated basal pressure appears to be the major manometric abnormality. It is present in most patients with organic disease and abnormal motility and it may predict short-term response to endoscopic sphincterotomy. Thus, in a prospective randomized study of type II (presumptive sphincter of Oddi dysfunction) postcholecystectomy patients, Geenen and associates[207] noted that 94% of patients with an elevated basal sphincter pressure ($\geq$40 mm Hg) experienced a benefit from sphincterotomy in contrast to only 42% of patients with a normal sphincter pressure. However, only 61% of such patients exhibited symptomatic improvement in Roberts-Thomson's and Toouli's series[208]; further, improvement in the latter study failed to correlate with manometric results. Since sphincterotomy for sphincter of Oddi dysfunction is associated with an increased complication rate compared to sphincterotomy for other conditions[209,210] in type II patients, it would seem inappropriate to recommend this procedure based on sphincter of Oddi pressure alone.

Acute Cholangitis. As suggested by several retrospective studies,[211–213] urgent endoscopic intervention has been clearly shown to be the procedure of choice for patients with acute suppurative cholangitis (Fig 3–20).[214] In these patients, it is especially prudent to aspirate bile before performing cholangiography; cholangiography, in turn, should be performed with minimal contrast injection. After abnormalities have been identified, sphincterotomy and stone extraction can be attempted in stable patients. In critically ill patients, simple nasobiliary drainage or stenting without sphincterotomy should be performed, reserving sphincterotomy and duct clearance for a later session when the patient is more stable.

Lai and associates[215] randomized 82 of 96 patients with acute cholangitis to emergency ERCP followed by either surgical decompression or endoscopic drainage using a 7 Fr nasobiliary tube. All patients had common bile duct stones that were removed following the resolution of cholangitis. When compared to ERCP plus surgical drainage, exclusive endoscopic management significantly decreased both mortality (10% vs 32%) and morbidity (34% vs 66%). The retained stone rate was also lower in the group treated with endoscopy alone (7% vs 29%).

Acute Gallstone Pancreatitis. Since laparotomy and duodenotomy are not required, endoscopic sphincterotomy would seem to be an ideal alternative to early surgical intervention in gallstone pancreatitis. Several uncontrolled reports[216–222] have demonstrated the relative safety and potential benefit of urgent endoscopic sphincterotomy for selected cases (usually severe) of acute gallstone pancreatitis.

Randomized prospective data regarding this critical issue are also available. Neoptolemos and associates[223] compared early (<72 hours) ERCP and endoscopic sphincterotomy with conservative management in patients with acute gallstone pancreatitis. All patients underwent ultrasound and biochemical testing within 24 hours and severity prediction within 48 hours of admission. After screening, if gallstones were suspected, patients were randomized to early ERCP and sphincterotomy (59 patients) or conservative management (62 patients). Overall complications were significantly decreased in patients treated endoscopically (17% vs 34%). As illustrated in Table 3–5, the results were particularly striking in those patients in whom a severe attack of pancreatitis was predicted.

In a more recent study, Fan and associates[224] randomly assigned 195 patients with acute pancreatitis to either early (<24 hrs) endoscopic intervention (n = 97) or initial conservative treatment (n = 98) with endoscopic intervention only if their condition deteriorated. One hundred twenty-seven (65%) of their patients were ultimately found to have biliary stones. Early endoscopic intervention significantly decreased the incidence of biliary sepsis (0% vs 12%). In addition, overall morbidity was significantly decreased (16% vs 33%) by early endoscopic intervention in those ultimately proven to have biliary stones. Early ERCP also decreased mortality in these patients (2% vs 8%), although this difference was not statistically significant.

Consideration of the above data suggests that on admission, pancreatitis severity should be assessed using one of the objective prognostic factor systems.[225–230] Ur-

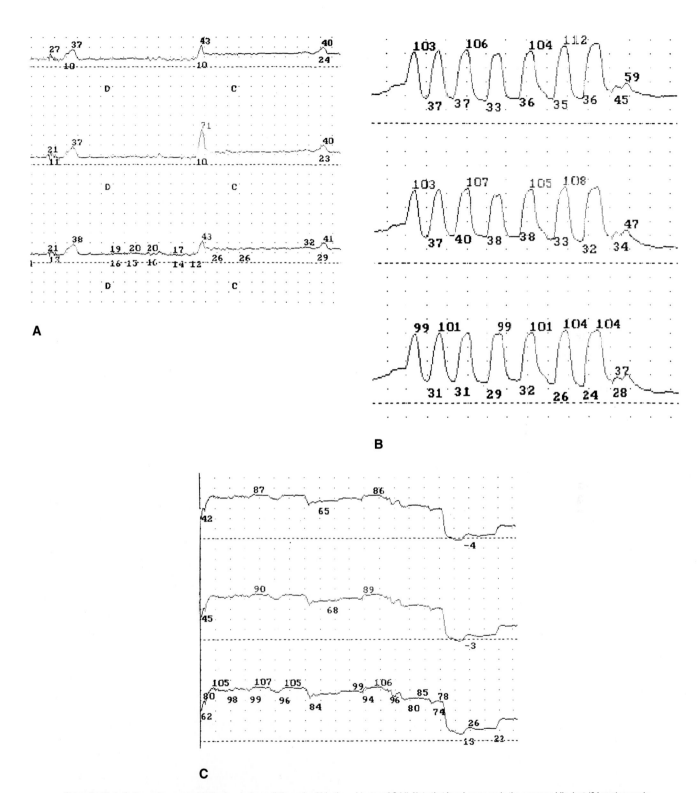

Figure 3–19. A. Endoscopic manometric tracing during pull-through within the sphincter of Oddi. Note that basal pressure in the common bile duct (24 mm) exceeds that within the duodenum (10 mm). **B.** Compressed analysis from the same study reveals normal phasic wave pressures (normal = 130 ± 16 mm) and activity. **C.** Abnormal study demonstrating elevated basal pressure (65 to 68 mm) in this patient with definitive (type I) sphincter of Oddi dysfunction. (Courtesy of Dr. Joseph Geenen, Racine, WI).

TABLE 3–4. CLASSIFICATION OF SUSPECTED SPHINCTER OF ODDI DYSFUNCTION

	Type I	Type II	Type III
	Definite	*Probable*	*Possible*
Biliary-type Pain	+	+	+
Abnormal Liver Function Tests[a]			
(SGOT, Alk Phos >2 × nl)	+	±[b]	−
Abnormal ERCP			
Dilated CBD (>12 mm)	+	±[b]	−
Delayed Drainage (>45 min)	+	±[b]	−
Sphincter of Oddi Manometry	Not Necessary	Especially Useful	Essential

[a]Documented on two or more occasions
[b]Only one or two of these criteria are present
(Adapted from Geenan JE, Hogan WJ, Dodds WJ. Sphincter of Oddi. In: MV Sivak Jr (ed), *Gastroenterologic Endoscopy*. Philadelphia, PA: WB Saunders; 1987.

gent ultrasonographic evaluation should be obtained to seek gallstones. If **experienced** endoscopic support is available, urgent ERCP and sphincterotomy should be considered for patients with severe disease and definite gallstones, especially if clinical deterioration continues or rapid resolution fails to occur. Urgent ERCP also should be considered in patients with severe disease and equivocal ultrasonographic examinations if gallstones are likely, as judged by clinical and biochemical crite-

ria.[231–233] If choledocholithiasis is demonstrated, then endoscopic sphincterotomy should be performed.

Fortunately, most patients with biliary pancreatitis can be managed conservatively. Following improvement, laparoscopic cholecystectomy should be performed prior to discharge.[234] Recently, elective endoscopic sphincterotomy without cholecystectomy has been proposed as a therapeutic alternative for high-risk patients who are deemed unfit for surgery and have recovered from an attack of gallstone pancreatitis.[235–237]

Endoprosthesis Insertion

Descriptions of biliary endoprosthesis insertion rapidly followed introduction of endoscopic sphincterotomy. Currently available endoprostheses vary in their composition, shape, size, length, and method of anchorage. The small-caliber (6 to 7 Fr) pig-tailed endoprostheses initially used were associated with a high incidence of early occlusion from sludge, resulting in recurrent jaundice and/or cholangitis.[238,239] Subsequent improvements led to development of straight 10 and 11.5 Fr endoprostheses with side flaps for retention,[240,241] as well as self-expandable metal stents.[242] Although the ideal endoprosthesis is yet to be developed, both in vitro[243,244] and in vivo[245] studies support the use of large-bore (10 Fr or larger) stents.

The large-caliber plastic stents are inserted using a three-layer technique (Fig 3–21). Initially, a diagnostic

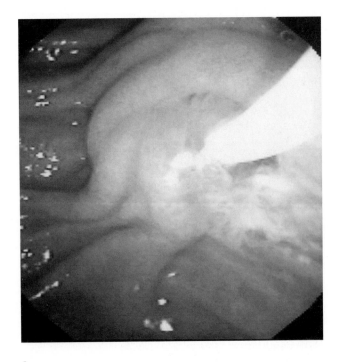

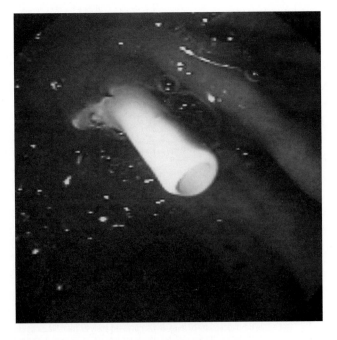

A

B

Figure 3–20. A. Purulent bile streams from the ampulla in this patient with suppurative cholangitis. **B.** An endoprosthesis has been inserted for biliary drainage. (See color insert.)

TABLE 3–5. ENDOSCOPIC VERSUS CONSERVATIVE TREATMENT OF SEVERE ACUTE GALLSTONE PANCREATITIS

	Endoscopic Treatment	Conservative Treatment
Complications	6/25 (25%)[a]	17/28 (61%)
Hospital Stay (days)	9.5[a]	17
Mortality	1/25 (2%)	5/28 (18%)

[a]p<0.05 versus conservative treatment.
Adapted from Fink, AS. Endoscopic intervention for pancreatic disorders. In: Hunter JG, Sackier J. (eds), *High Tech Surgery: New Approaches to Old Diseases*. New York, NY: McGraw-Hill; 1993:245–254.

cholangiogram or pancreatogram is obtained to identify the extent of the lesion and to determine what length of endoprosthesis is required. If desired, a small sphincterotomy then can be performed to facilitate subsequent manipulations; this maneuver is often unnecessary. An atraumatic guidewire and an overlying Teflon catheter (Fig 3–21) are passed well up the desired duct, passing any stricture. Various independent manipulations of the guidewire and catheter may be required to obtain the desired position. Once these accessories are in the proper location, the endoprosthesis is pushed into place using a pusher tube. Ideally, the endopros-

thesis will be located with its upper flap above the stricture and its lower flap just outside the papilla.

A special delivery system is used to insert self-expanding metal stents in a collapsed state (9 Fr in diameter). After release, the stent shortens in length and expands to 8 to 10 mm in diameter (30 Fr). While the delivery system can be cumbersome,[246] the experienced endoscopists in the European Wallstent study group reported successful insertion in 97% of cases.[247] In addition, the total number of endoscopic interventions is reported to be decreased by use of self-expanding metal stents,[247] suggesting some economic justification for utilizing these more expensive devices.

Self-expanding stents appear to be significantly less prone to sludge occlusion and, therefore, longer-lived than straight plastic stents.[248] Despite their longer patency, however, self-expanding metal stents clearly have problems. Thus, shortly after insertion (2 to 7 days), these stents become nonremovable owing to resultant tissue reaction and fibrosis; indeed, some become completely incorporated into the bile duct wall.[249] Furthermore, these stents are plagued by tumor ingrowth, which is usually treated by subsequent insertion of a plastic stent through the metal stent.[249]

Biliary endoprostheses have been utilized for multiple indications. The location of the lesion is the primary determinant of technical difficulty and success rate. Ma-

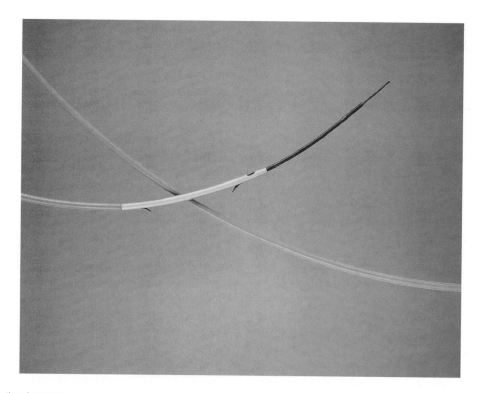

Figure 3–21. The three-layer component system for endoprosthesis insertion, consisting of an inner 0.035-inch guidewire, a Teflon overtube, the large caliber stent (10 or 11.5 Fr) and the pusher tube. (Courtesy of Wilson-Cook Medical, Winston-Salem, NC).

lignant strictures below the bifurcation (Figs 3–14, 3–22, and 3–23) can be stented successfully in as many as 90% of cases, with morbidity and mortality rates approximating 2% to 5% each.[250] Success rates fall rapidly and morbidity rates progressively increase as the location of the stricture climbs above the bifurcation.[251–253] Lesions at the hilum or above may require insertion of more than one endoprosthesis.[251–253]

In addition to malignant obstruction, endoscopically inserted endoprostheses have been used increasingly in treating benign biliary disorders, including strictures. Since most benign strictures follow penetrating or operative trauma, the review of Binmoeller and associates[254] was well received. These authors reported that 95% of 77 postoperative biliary leaks could be managed successfully using a variety of endoscopic techniques, including endoscopic sphincterotomy alone or in conjunction with nasobiliary catheter or endoprosthesis insertion. The advent of laparoscopic cholecystectomy has been associated with an increased incidence of major biliary ductal injury.[255–257] Fortunately, endoscopic treatment also has proven successful for many of these injuries.[256,258,259] Thus, the Amsterdam group[258] reported that their technique of dilation followed by staged insertion of two 10 Fr stents was successful in 94% of 70 such injuries. Of particular note, the stents have been removed from 46 of their patients; after a mean follow-up of 42 months, only 17% have restrictured. The long-term results are awaited anxiously.

Similar endoscopic maneuvers have proven useful in other benign biliary conditions including sclerosing cholangitis,[260] choledochoceles,[261] pancreas divisum,[262,263] and complications following orthotopic liver transplantation.[264] Several preliminary reports even describe endoscopic access to the gallbladder via the cystic duct, allowing diagnosis and treatment of gallbladder disorders.[265,266]

In addition to biliary disorders, several groups have also published preliminary reports describing endoscopic intervention in the management of benign pancreatic disorders.[267–269] Temporary decompression has been used to decompress the pancreatic ductal system after potentially traumatic endoscopic intervention,[270] after extracorporeal lithotripsy of pancreaticolithiasis (see below), or as a means of selecting patients best suited for more permanent drainage procedures. An example of the latter was published by Roman and associates.[271] These authors proposed that patients with pancreas divisum might be best selected for surgical intervention based on their response to temporary endoscopic stenting of the minor papilla.

Other reports suggest that permanent endoscopic pancreatic drainage (achieved by combining sphincterotomy, stone extraction, stricture dilatation, and stenting) might offer long-term benefit in patients with chronic pancreatitis. Thirty such patients were treated with a combination of pancreatic sphincterotomy and endoprosthesis insertion by Huibregste and associates.[272] Seventeen of the twenty-one patients with chronic relapsing pancreatitis improved. Furthermore, 7 of 10 patients with chronic pain improved, six of whom became pain-free during a 10- to 34-month follow-up period. These promising results were not obtained without complication. Pancreatic abscess developed in two patients, and pancreatic ductal disruption occurred in one patient, who subsequently died. The authors indicate that patients with a dominant main-duct stricture were most likely to respond favorably to endoscopic therapy. Similar results in 14 patients were reported by McCarthy and associates,[262] who also noted the favorable prognosis for patients with dominant main-duct stricture.

Grimm and associates[273] report a larger experience with endoscopic therapy for chronic pancreatitis. Endoscopic intervention using a combination of pancreatic sphincterotomy, stone extraction, and stenting was successful in 61 of 70 patients with intractable pain. One-third of the patients developed mild pancreatitis that resolved with supportive therapy. In addition, two patients (3%) died following treatment of septic complications. Fifty of the sixty-one (82%) successfully treated patients were initially relieved of their pain; however, on follow-up, only 35 (57%) remained pain-free.

Extracorporeal shock wave lithotripsy (ESWL) has been reported to facilitate endoscopic management of pancreaticolithiasis.[273–278] The largest experience comes from Brussels,[278] where 123 patients have been treated with a combination of ESWL and endoscopic intervention. ERCP with endoscopic pancreatic sphincterotomy and other ancillary procedures (eg, nasopancreatic drainage, Fogarty or balloon extraction, stenting) was undertaken several hours after ESWL. Pancreatic stones were fragmented successfully in all but one patient. Although the main pancreatic duct was completely cleared in only 59% of patients, most patients (90%) experienced a decrease in main pancreatic duct diameter. While no procedure-related mortalities occurred, 34% of patients developed sepsis of pancreatic origin, which the authors claimed were "relatively minor and not life-threatening." Many patients developed complete or partial pain relief, although frequency of pain relief decreased with the length of follow-up.

Pancreatic pseudocysts also have been approached endoscopically. Nasopancreatic drains[279,280] or endoprostheses[272] have been used to drain these cysts when they communicate with the main pancreatic duct. If the mature cyst impinges on the stomach or duodenum, endoscopically created cystoenterostomies have been cre-

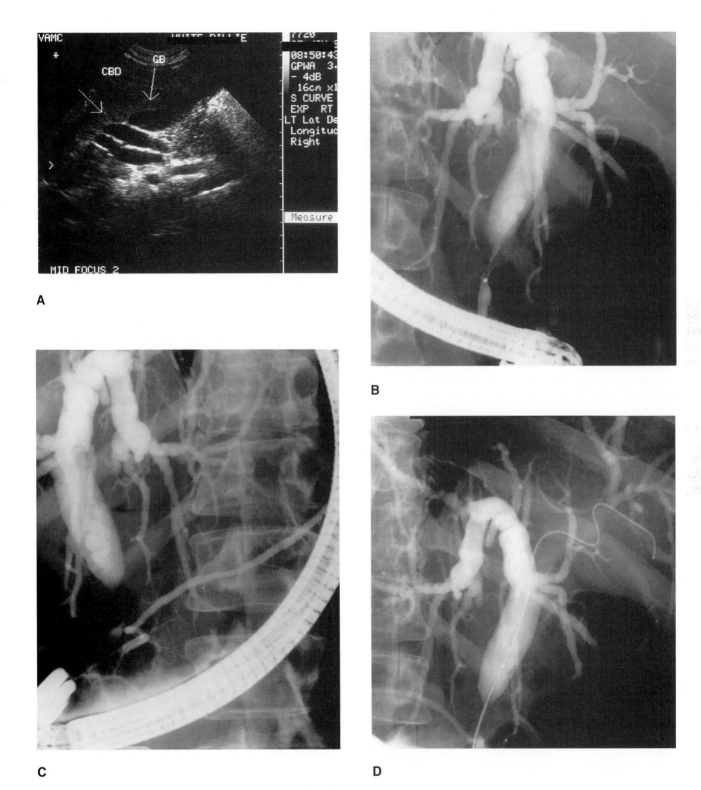

Figure 3–22. A. A right upper-quadrant ultrasound obtained in a deeply jaundiced patient. Note the dilated gallbladder (GB) as well as the dilated extrahepatic common bile duct (CBD). **B**. ERCP demonstrates a tight distal common bile duct structure, suggestive of pancreatic cancer or cholangiocarcinoma. **C**. Repeat injection now visualizes a normal pancreatic duct, confirming the diagnosis of cholangiocarcinoma. **D**. A guidewire has been passed across the stricture in preparation for endoprosthesis insertion.

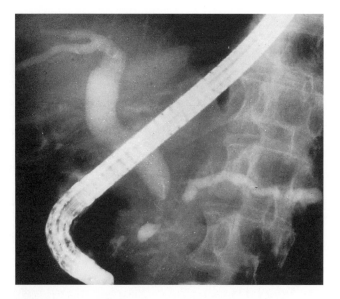

A

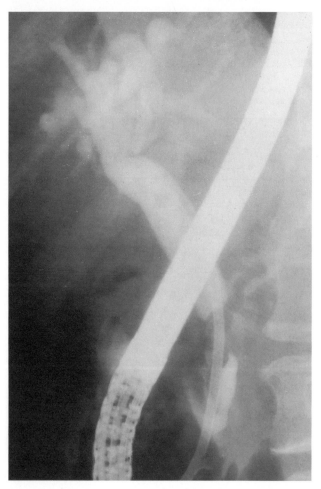

B

Figure 3–23. A. Endoscopic cholangiogram demonstrating obstruction of the distal common bile and pancreatic ducts, characteristic of pancreatic carcinoma. **B**. Successful endoscopic stenting bypassed the stricture and relieved the obstructive jaundice.

ated for drainage.[281,282] Cremer and associates[282] reported 22 endoscopic cystoduodenostomies that were successful in 96% of patients, with only a 9% recurrence rate. Pain relief was obtained in 20 of the 22 patients. This group also reported 11 endoscopic cystogastrostomies with 100% success rate, 19% relapse rate, and pain relief in 9 of 11 patients. Even though these results are promising, complication rates, especially bleeding, have been high. Thus, the role of endoscopically created cystoenterostomy remains to be established.

The choice of therapeutic modality (operative, percutaneous, or endoscopic) depends on multiple factors including the general status of the patient, the location and extent of the lesion, and the local expertise available. Obviously, in appropriate circumstances, surgical resection offers the only possibility for cure. However, in patients unfit for surgery or with unresectable lesions, it can be difficult to determine the optimal palliative modality.

Palliation of unresectable malignant biliary obstruction in elderly, high-risk patients appears to be one of the most significant indications for biliary endoprostheses. In these circumstances, randomized prospective trials have demonstrated that endoscopically inserted stents are superior to percutaneous stents and at least as good as biliary enteric bypass.[283–286] Furthermore, endoscopic intervention is less expensive, requires a shorter hospital stay, and incurs less patient discomfort. These results are discounted somewhat, but not completely, by the subsequent need to replace occluded stents or to bypass duodenal obstruction in those patients (approximately 10% to 15%) who survive long enough to develop these complications.[286]

COMPLICATIONS

Although generic endoscopic complications (eg, medication reaction, cardiopulmonary events [see Monitoring]) can occur after ERCP, the complications specifically associated with pancreaticobiliary cannulation include pancreatitis and sepsis. Post-ERCP pancreatitis is associated with multiple forceful pancreatic duct injections, usually while struggling during a difficult bile duct cannulation. While the reported incidence of this complication is definition-dependent, it probably occurs in no more than 2% to 3% of ERCPs.[287] Although most cases are mild, severe, life-threatening pancreatitis can occur. Randomized prospective trials have not demonstrated any beneficial effect of prophylactic somatostatin in decreasing the incidence of ERCP-induced pancreatitis.[288–290]

Since bacteremia occurs in approximately 15% of patients undergoing diagnostic ERCP,[291] it is not surprising to learn that sepsis can follow ERCP. The risk of cholangitis or septicemia, particularly, is increased following attempted endoscopic therapy in the presence of infected bile.[292] Techniques that may decrease post-ERCP sepsis include administering antibiotics in cases with suspected bacterobilia (eg, cholangitis), minimizing injection volume and pressure (vide supra), and ensuring adequate drainage at the completion of the procedure preferably via concurrent endoscopic intervention (eg, sphincterotomy and stone extraction, endoprosthesis).[291,293]

Contaminated equipment or wash water can lead to avoidable sepsis, especially in the presence of ductal obstruction.[180,294] Such a source should be strongly considered in the presence of *Pseudomonas* infection and should lead to a review of disinfection procedures.

Following endoscopic sphincterotomy, serious complications can occur and may require surgical intervention. These complications include hemorrhage, perforation, cholangitis, and pancreatitis. Although experienced centers report morbidity and mortality rates of 6.5% and 1.0%, respectively,[186,189,295] less experienced centers have reported disturbingly high failure and morbidity rates.[189,296] Approximately 75% to 80% of complications can be managed without surgery.

Hemorrhage is the most common complication seen after endoscopic sphincterotomy and can be avoided by slow, controlled incisions. Epinephrine injection or balloon tamponade[297] may be useful if endoscopic vision is not obscured by the bleeding. If surgical intervention is necessary, it is probably best to include ligation of the feeding vessel.

Perforation, the least common complication, most often leads to surgical intervention and mortality.[189] The diagnosis usually is made upon discovering air or contrast in the retroperitoneal space. CT scan also may be helpful if differentiation from postsphincterotomy pancreatitis proves difficult.[298] If diagnosed early, and the bile duct has been cleared, many patients can be managed with nasobiliary decompression, nasogastric suction, and intravenous antibiotics.[189] However, if stones remain in the common bile duct, or if the patient deteriorates after attempted conservative management, surgical intervention is indicated and should include clearance and decompression of the bile duct and retroperitoneal drainage.

Pancreatitis and cholangitis also can follow endoscopic sphincterotomy. Pancreatitis may be decreased by minimizing trauma during cannulation and avoiding coagulation near the pancreatic duct. Cholangitis should be extremely uncommon if adequate biliary drainage has been achieved.

Since sphincterotomy complications are related to incision length, and since only a small incision (if any)

is necessary prior to stent insertion, it is most unusual to see postsphincterotomy complications after placing endoprostheses. Indeed, early after insertion, sepsis should not occur if adequate drainage has been achieved. However, the median patency period for 10- and 11.5-Fr plastic endoprostheses is 6 months.[245] Thus, stent occlusion is inevitable and usually is heralded by recurrent cholangitis, unless stents are routinely changed before onset of sepsis. Most cases of endoprosthesis occlusion can be successfully treated with antibiotics and stent replacement.

■ ENDOSCOPY OF THE SMALL INTESTINE

Endoscopic access to the small bowel is limited: the third portion of the duodenum can be reached during standard upper gastrointestinal endoscopy and the most distal ileum can be accessed via the ileocecal valve during colonoscopy. If necessary, the distal duodenum and very proximal jejunum can be reached by oral passage of a long (160 cm) colonoscope.[299] However, this approach is technically demanding and may inflict moderate patient discomfort.

Obscure gastrointestinal bleeding is the most frequent indication for small bowel endoscopy. The latter is best performed at laparotomy, since nonoperative "push" endoscopy utilizing long endoscopes will make a diagnosis in only 50% of patients.[299]

For intraoperative endoscopy, a long colonoscope is inserted per os or per anus. The endoscope is then advanced down from the duodenum or up from the colon into the small bowel. This is performed under endoscopic vision, taking care to minimize air insufflation. The surgeon guides the endoscope tip, telescoping the bowel over the endoscope and applying pressure to reduce loops in the stomach or colon. Intraoperative endoscopy has also been recommended for other indications, including selection of the appropriate extent of intestinal resection.[300]

Although intraoperative endoscopy is considered the "gold standard" for endoscopic evaluation of the small bowel,[300–304] nonsurgical endoscopic alternatives have been proposed. The Sonde-type enteroscope is specifically designed to allow small bowel visualization on an ambulatory basis.[305,306] This long, flexible enteroscope is passed through the nose into the stomach where its terminal-weighted balloon is inflated. Peristalsis then is allowed to carry the enteroscope distally into the ileum. Concerns have been raised about diagnostic capability of this passive instrument, since it lacks tip deflection.[307,308] Furthermore, it offers no therapeutic capabilities owing to the lack of an appropriate channel. Sonde-type small bowel endoscopy is claimed to be reasonably comparable to interoperative endoscopy in depth of insertion and ability to detect small bowel vascular ectasias.[309] It has been suggested that demonstration of diffuse vascular ectasias at small bowel endoscopy should preclude intraoperative endoscopy or surgical exploration.[309]

■ ENDOSCOPY OF THE LOWER GASTROINTESTINAL TRACT

INDICATIONS

Endoscopic evaluation of the lower gastrointestinal tract can be performed using anoscopy, rigid or flexible sigmoidoscopy, and colonoscopy. This section will focus on the latter two techniques, which constitute the majority of lower gastrointestinal endoscopic procedures.

The modality selected will depend on the indications involved (Tables 3–6 and 3–7). While multiple indications are listed for flexible sigmoidoscopy (Table 3–6), the majority of examinations are performed to screen for rectosigmoid neoplasia in asymptomatic patients. The American Cancer Society,[310,311] the National Cancer Institute,[312,313] and the American College of Physicians[314] recommend that every patient over 50 years of age should undergo annual fecal occult–blood tests and screening flexible sigmoidoscopy at three to five year intervals. The cost effectiveness of these recommendations has been questioned.[315–318] Flexible sigmoidoscopy studies have discovered numerous polyps and cancers.[319,320] However, although suggested,[321] controlled trials have failed to demonstrate that these discoveries translate into decreased mortality from colorectal cancer.[322]

Equally confusing is the ability of sigmoidoscopic screening to predict the status of the proximal colon. The conventional view is that there is minimal risk of proximal colonic neoplasia (and hence, no need for further investigation) if sigmoidoscopy is negative or

TABLE 3–6. INDICATIONS FOR FLEXIBLE SIGMOIDOSCOPY

DIAGNOSTIC EVALUATION
Screening asymptomatic patients for colorectal neoplasia
Suspected distal colonic disease (without indication for colonoscopy)
Evaluation of the colon in conjunction with barium enema
Evaluation for anastomotic recurrence in rectosigmoid carcinoma

THERAPY
All colonoscopic procedures under special circumstances:
    Polypectomy following subtotal colectomy
    Laser treatment of rectal carcinoma

Adapted from Standards of Practice Committee. *Appropriate Use of Gastrointestinal Endoscopy.* Manchester, MA: American Society for Gastrointestinal Endoscopy; 1992.

TABLE 3–7. INDICATIONS FOR COLONOSCOPY

DIAGNOSTIC EVALUATION
Evaluation of clinically significant abnormality on barium enema
Evaluation of unexplained gastrointestinal bleeding:
    Hematochezia without obvious anorectal source
    Melena without upper GI etiology
    Fecal occult blood
Unexplained iron deficiency anemia
Surveillance for colorectal neoplasia:
    Possible synchronous lesion in patient with treatable neoplasm
    Possible recurrent lesion following resection of colorectal neoplasm (Planned follow-up)
    Hereditary predisposition for colorectal neoplasm
    Chronic ulcerative colitis
Chronic inflammatory bowel disease (if pertinent to clinical management)
Clinical significant, unexplained diarrhea
Intraoperative identification of nondiscernible lesion

THERAPY
Hemostasis
Foreign body removal
Polypectomy
Decompression:
    Acute non-toxic megacolon
    Sigmoid volvulus
Dilatation of stenotic lesions
Palliation of stenotic or bleeding neoplasm
Marking neoplasm for surgical localization

Adapted with permission from Standards of Practice Committee. *Appropriate Use of Gastrointestinal Endoscopy.* Manchester, MA: American Society for Gastrointestinal Endoscopy; 1992.

only reveals hyperplastic polyps. However, recent colonoscopic studies[319,323,324] have found proximal colonic adenomas in 20% to 51% of patients without neoplasms within reach of the flexible sigmoidoscope. In addition, other studies[325–327] have found an equivalent number of proximal adenomas when a hyperplastic (as opposed to adenomatous) polyp was found in the distal colon. Subsequent prospective studies concluded that distal hyperplastic polyps had no predictive value.[328,329] Thus, the role of flexible sigmoidoscopy in screening for colorectal neoplasia remains unclear.

Other indications for flexible sigmoidoscopy include hematochezia and bloody diarrhea. In the former circumstance, etiologies most frequently are discovered if the procedure is performed soon after passage of the bright-red bloody stool. The proximal colon does not need to be examined if a fissure or hemorrhoid is discovered in association with fresh blood in the perianal area. When evaluating bloody diarrhea, flexible sigmoidoscopy may reveal characteristic findings in immunocompromised patients (viral colitis) or in patients who have recently received antibiotics (*C. Difficile* colitis).

Table 3–7 describes indications for colonoscopy that are recommended by the American Society for Gastrointestinal Endoscopy. Several guidelines have been previously published,[330,331] seeking to decrease the overuse of this arduous and occasionally morbid procedure.

As with flexible sigmoidoscopy, the role of colonoscopy in cancer surveillance remains unsettled. The high accuracy and therapeutic potential of colonoscopy render it superior to flexible sigmoidoscopy and barium enema. Owing to cost issues, however, the latter combination has been recommended in lieu of colonoscopy, even in high-risk patients.[332,333] Indeed, the definition of high-risk patients who merit screening is unclear. It is clear that first-degree relatives of patients with colorectal cancer are at increased risk for neoplasia.[334,335] However, the only hereditary indications currently agreed upon are the cancer-family syndrome and three first-degree relatives with colon cancer.[336–338]

Ulcerative colitis (Fig 3–24) is another high-risk condition in which the optimal frequency of colonoscopic screening is debated.[339–344] While dysplasia is accepted as a premalignant lesion, variable actions are proposed, depending on the severity of the dysplasia.[342,343] Recent studies suggest that the finding of DNA aneuploidy may predict future development of dysplasia,[345,346] thereby facilitating decisions regarding screening regimens. Despite a recent report to the contrary,[347] a severe attack of ulcerative colitis is usually considered a contraindication to colonoscopy.

Finally, surveillance is indicated following polypectomy or resection of colon cancer. While the optimal fre-quency of surveillance is yet to be defined in controlled trials, previous regimens demanded significant resource utilization.[348] Thus, in estimating the expense incurred in serial colonoscopic follow-up of 50 year–old men following polypectomy, Ransohoff and associates[349] estimated that it would cost between $82,000 and $330,000 to save one life, depending upon the efficiency and safety of the surveillance program. Current recommendations suggest that patients with single, or only a few, adenomas should have colonoscopy within three years after polypectomy.[350] After one negative three year follow-up examination, subsequent colonoscopy can be repeated at five year intervals.[350] Follow-up endoscopies may be necessary at one and four years in those patients with multiple polyps or with suboptimal initial clearing examination.[350] Following resection of colorectal carcinoma, similar surveillance regimens have been proposed, with the exception of an initial clearing examination one year after resection.[338]

PATIENT PREPARATION

Most endoscopic evaluations of the lower gastrointestinal tract can be done as outpatient procedures. For flexible sigmoidoscopy of the nonstrictured colon, limited preparation is all that is necessary. This can usually be accomplished by administration of one or two phosphate enemas (eg, Fleet) 20 to 30 minutes before the examination; no dietary restrictions are required. If the procedure is performed promptly, the colon is usually clean up to the level of the transverse colon or even hepatic flexure in young patients. In the presence of severe diverticular disease or other narrowing, antispasmotics (eg, glucagon) may be required during enema administration. Alternatively, the patient may be prepared with oral lavage, as described below.

For colonoscopy, all iron-containing medications should be stopped at least 3 days prior to the procedure since these compounds produce a dark, sticky stool that interferes with inspection and is difficult to clear. The patient should begin a light diet (preferably clear liquids) the day before the examination.

The colon can be cleared with one of two techniques: purgatives with or without enemas, and oral lavage. Currently, the most frequently used purgative is Fleet Phospho-Soda, which is taken in 1.5 ounce doses the evening before and the morning of the exam. Ideally, each dose should be mixed in 4 ounces of water and followed by at least three 8-ounce glasses of clear liquids. The last dose should be completed no less than three hours before the examination. It must be remembered that Fleet Phospho-Soda contains significant sodium and phosphate, and is, therefore, contraindicated in patients with congestive heart failure or renal failure. If properly followed, this regimen rarely requires subsequent ene-

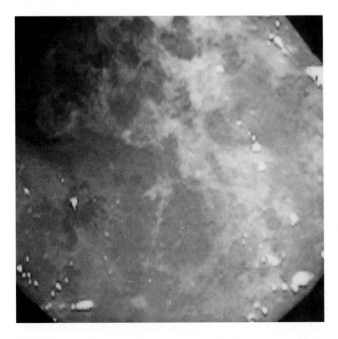

Figure 3–24. Endoscopic appearance of ulcerative colitis. Note the abnormal background mucosa. (See color insert.)

mas, as are usually administered in combination with other laxatives (eg, bisacodyl, castor oil).

Oral lavage regimens are popular for colonic cleansing owing to their ease, rapidity, and effectiveness. Although they rarely cause significant cramping, they require ingestion of large fluid volumes that can cause bloating, as well as nausea and vomiting. The most popular solution (Golytely) is a mixture of polyethylene glycol and electrolytes (sodium sulfate, potassium chloride, and bicarbonate) that is dispensed as a powder and reconstituted in 4 liters of water. The use of sodium sulfate in lieu of sodium chloride markedly reduces intestinal absorption of sodium.[351] The solution is rendered isomotic by the addition of a nonabsorbable solute (polyethylene glycol). The use of polyethylene glycol, in lieu of mannitol, prevents generation of hydrogen by colonic bacteria, thereby avoiding the risk of explosion during electrocautery. The solution is ingested during a period of two to three hours, beginning late in the afternoon, if colonoscopy is scheduled early the next morning; for a late afternoon colonoscopy, it can be taken early the same day. These solutions have a salty, unpleasant taste which may limit patient compliance. Although low sodium solutions have been developed, these new solutions are equivalent to standard solutions in terms of patient acceptance, compliance, and cleansing quality.[352]

While transient bacteremia occurs during colonoscopy, prophylactic antibiotics usually are not required. Exceptions to this include patients with prosthetic heart valves, vascular grafts, or recent orthopedic implants.

DIAGNOSTIC AND THERAPEUTIC TECHNIQUES

Flexible Sigmoidoscopy

There are several general principles that should be remembered whenever performing flexible sigmoidoscopy or colonoscopy. These include (1) insufflate as little as possible and aspirate excess air, (2) push as little as possible so as to avoid unnecessary loops, (3) withdraw the endoscope frequently in order to shorten the colon, (4) correlate the shaft length inserted with the anticipated location (eg, 50 cm should be at the splenic flexure), and (5) respond to patient discomfort, which usually indicates excessive looping or insufflation.[353]

Endoscopic examination of the lower gastrointestinal tract should always be preceded by digital rectal examination. This procedure both lubricates and relaxes the anus. Thereafter, having verified that all functions (especially air insufflation) are working properly, the endoscope is introduced either by pressing it sideways into the rectum until the sphincter relaxes or by pushing the tip alongside the forefinger as the latter is withdrawn. Insertion should always be done gently, since this is the most sensitive area of the colorectum.

It must also be remembered that only limited maneuvers of the endoscope are possible and include insertion, withdrawal, or twisting (with or without tip deflection). In addition, the patient's abdomen can be compressed or their position can be changed. Empiric trials of various manipulations often are necessary to maximize insertion.

The initial view obtained usually reveals a "red-out." This is remedied by withdrawing the scope and insufflating air until the lumen is visualized. The endoscope then is progressively advanced into the bowel until the maximum desired insertion is achieved. Given the relatively short length of the flexible sigmoidoscope, insertion can usually be performed using the single-handed technique, (see Endoscopy of the Upper Gastrointestinal Tract). Various combined manipulations usually allow the endoscope to be advanced well into the descending colon and occasionally beyond the splenic flexure; clockwise torque may prove helpful in passing the sigmoid–descending colon junction.

Therapeutic interventions, including biopsy, hemostasis, dilatation, and polypectomy (see below) can be performed through the flexible sigmoidoscope. Some endoscopists maintain that polypectomy should only be done after formal colonic preparation, in lieu of simple enemas.[354]

Colonoscopy

The technical principles described for flexible sigmoidoscopy are equally germane for colonoscopy.[355] Colonoscopy is distinctly more difficult, given the length of colon to be examined as well as the need to pass both the splenic and hepatic flexures. Despite this fact, most experienced endoscopists also utilize the single-handed technique during colonoscopy. However, it is occasionally helpful to have an assistant advance and withdraw the colonoscope.

Upon reaching the splenic flexure, the colonoscope should be straightened (usually by withdrawal combined with torque) prior to continued insertion. This not only increases the mechanical efficiency of the endoscope, but also facilitates deeper insertion. Again, combined manipulations are utilized until the splenic flexure is passed and the transverse colon is entered. Application of external pressure on the sigmoid loop by an assistant may be needed to enter the transverse colon. The transverse colon then is passed, usually with little difficulty; repeated in-and-out maneuvers as well as external pressure are required occasionally.

Passage of the hepatic flexure and deep intubation of the ascending colon may prove difficult. Again, several empiric trials of various combined maneuvers usually are required to accomplish this goal. Deflation, withdrawal, external pressure, and change of the patient's position may prove useful. Once the ascending colon is intubated, one should not conclude that insertion is complete until the ileocecal valve or the appendiceal orifice is identified; transillumination or palpation in the right iliac fossa also may be helpful in this regard.

Numerous disorders can be both diagnosed and treated during lower gastrointestinal endoscopy. Depending on the specific circumstances, therapy can be performed before or after completing the diagnostic examination.

Hemostasis

There are multiple causes of lower gastrointestinal bleeding (eg, Fig 3–25). Patients present with three different clinical scenarios: chronic bleeding, recent severe bleeding, and active bleeding. The nature of the presentation will influence the diagnostic and therapeutic interventions used.

Patients with chronic bleeding present with a history of melena, hematochezia or blood-streaked stools, or are found to have occult fecal blood, with or without anemia. Flexible endoscopy will diagnose the source of bleeding in most of these patients. Although sigmoidoscopy often will identify the cause, the remaining colon usually needs to be cleared, either radiologically or endoscopically. Therefore, it may be desirable to proceed directly to colonoscopy, especially if colonic neoplasm is a significant risk. Some investigators have sug-

gested use of fiberoptic sigmoidoscopy followed by barium enema in patients with fecal occult blood.[356] However, colonoscopy has been shown to offer greater diagnostic yield and to be less expensive than sigmoidoscopy plus barium enema.[357] For these reasons, colonoscopy is recommended as the procedure of choice for the patient with occult fecal blood.[358,359] If colonoscopy is negative in this setting, many would recommend upper gastrointestinal endoscopy. However, Thomas and Hardcastle[360] followed 283 patients with occult bleeding and negative colonoscopic examinations over five years and concluded that upper gastrointestinal studies were not needed if the patient remained asymptomatic.

Colonoscopy is indicated in the patient with a recent severe, but currently inactive bleed. The patient should be adequately resuscitated, coagulation parameters should be corrected, and the colon should be prepared as described above. During colonoscopy, stigmata of recent hemorrhage are sought: active bleeding, adherent clot in a single diverticulum or on an ulcerated lesion, or a nonbleeding visible vessel in an ulcer. If the site of bleeding is found, it may be treated directly (see Endoscopy of the Upper Gastrointestinal Tract).

Management of active, severe lower gastrointestinal bleeding remains controversial. Flexible sigmoidoscopy should probably be the initial procedure in most patients with active lower gastrointestinal bleeding. If the source of bleeding remains obscure, colonoscopy then should be performed. Some investigators believe that colonoscopy can be performed safely in actively bleeding patients without preparation, since blood is a good cathartic and will prepare the bowel adequately. Other investigators, however, raise the concern about hampered visibility, which limits therapeutic options and potentially increases the risk of perforation; most recommend urgent lavage, followed by colonoscopy.[361] This approach will frequently identify angiodysplasia as the source of the colonic hemorrhage.[361] Caution is appropriate when using thermal techniques (monopolar or bipolar electrocautery, heater probe, laser) to treat angiodysplasias, since they tend to occur in the thin-walled proximal colon.

Polypectomy

Most colonic polyps are asymptomatic (Fig 3–26 and 3–27) and are discovered on screening or diagnostic barium radiographs or endoscopic examination. While colonic polyps can ulcerate and bleed, or rarely cause partial bowel obstruction, neoplastic polyps (adenomas) are of primary clinical import due to their malignant potential. Nonneoplastic polyps (hyperplastic, hamartomas, lymphoid aggregates, and inflammatory polyps) have no malignant potential and only need to be distinguished from their neoplastic counterparts.

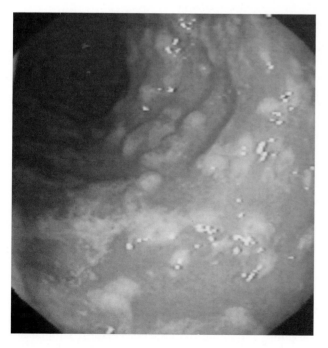

Figure 3–25. Endoscopic appearance of pseudomembranous colitis. (See color insert.)

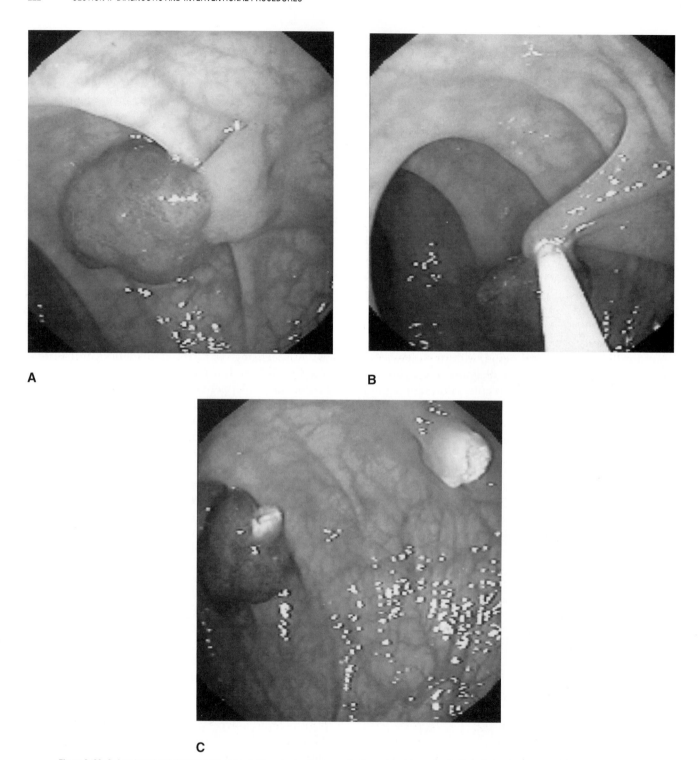

A

B

C

Figure 3–26. A. A pedunculated sigmoid colon polyp. **B**. The polyp has been snared with a polypectomy snare. **C**. The polyp has been successfully transected with the snare. Note the transected polyp head, as well as the hemostatic polypectomy site on the stalk. (See color insert.)

Adenomas occur in a variety of shapes, sizes, and histologic patterns. Polyps are described as pedunculated or sessile, depending on whether they contain a discrete stalk. According to the World Health Organization,[362] neoplastic polyps can be classified as tubular (<25% vil-lous tissue), tubulovillous (25% to 75% villous tissue), or villous adenomas (>75% villous tissue). Tubular adenomas are the most common (80%), while tubulovillous (15%) and villous adenomas (5%) are encountered much less frequently. Some degree of dysplasia

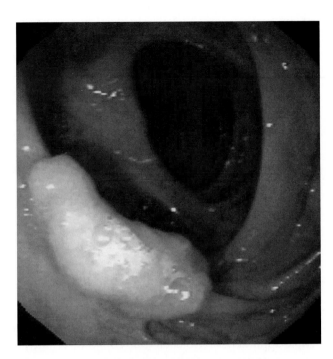

Figure 3–27. A sessile colonic polyp. These can often be removed with a snare, either by creation of a pseudo-stalk or in piecemeal fashion. (See color insert.)

occurs in all polyps and low-grade and high-grade (severe) descriptors are recommended.[362] Increasing dysplasia correlates with increasing adenoma size, extent of villous component, and patient age.[363] The risk of invasive cancer also increases with increasing polyp size.[363]

Although most polyps >1 cm can be detected by double-contrast but not single-contrast barium enema,[364,365] colonoscopy is preferred since it allows biopsy and removal of most of these lesions with minimal morbidity (1% to 2%) and mortality (0.03%).[366,367] Recent studies attest to the diagnostic reliability of colonoscopy for polyp detection.[368,369] Further, several studies suggest that colonoscopic polypectomy will reduce subsequent cancer mortality.[370,371]

After appropriate preparation and visualization of the polyp, the endoscopist must decide whether and how to treat the lesion. Therapeutic options include hot biopsy, electrocoagulation, and excision. Regular biopsy forceps should not be used since they will leave residual adenomatous fragments which can lead to polyp recurrence. In contrast, hot biopsy will conduct thermal energy to the polyp base, destroying any remaining polypoid tissue. Hot biopsy should not be used on lesions >6 mm, since excessive thermal energy is required.[372] Ulcerated, indurated sessile lesions may be malignant and it is best to remove them surgically.

Polypectomy technique has become reasonably standardized,[372] such that most pedunculated polyps can be removed endoscopically in one piece (Fig 3–26). If safe,

most polyps should be removed when visualized, since they may not be as easily located upon withdrawing the endoscope. However, the import of completing the colonoscopic examination must be remembered in order not to miss synchronous lesions. Further, most polyps over 1 cm in diameter can usually be relocated, allowing polypectomy to be deferred until instrument withdrawal.

A snare (Fig 3–28) is placed around the head of the polyp and then maneuvered down the stalk, taking care to place the catheter tip at the desired transection site (Fig 3–26B). When the snare is in proper position, the polyp is transected by progressively closing the snare while applying continuous coagulation current. Sessile polyps (Fig 3–27) less than 2 cm in diameter can usually be removed in one piece. The snare is placed around the polyp, with the wire directly on the mucosa. The snare then is closed as the polyp is lifted, entrapping the mucosa and minimal submucosa. One can often create a pseudostalk in this manner. Electrocautery then is applied while the polyp is continuously lifted away from the colonic wall. Larger polyps may require piecemeal removal in 1- to 1.5-cm segments.[373] Following successful endoscopic resection of a large sessile polyp, follow-up colonoscopy should be done in 3 to 6 months to verify completeness of the resection. Extremely large polyps may require more than one endoscopic session or an operation for complete removal.

It is important to move the polyp during excision so as to avoid conducting current into, and thus injuring, the opposite colonic wall. It is also important to retrieve resected polyps for pathological examination. While some small polyps can be suctioned into a specimen

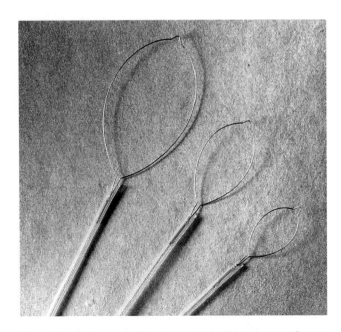

Figure 3–28. Selection of polypectomy snares demonstrating various sizes. (Courtesy of Microvasive, Boston Scientific Corporation, Watertown, MA).

trap, large polyps must either be lassoed with the snare or retrieval basket, or sucked against the endoscope tip; the latter techniques require endoscope removal.

Polypectomy is definitive treatment of polyps with carcinoma in situ or for moderately or well-differentiated invasive cancer distant from the excisional margin without vascular or lymphatic invasion.[350,374–377] Assuming acceptable surgical risk, colectomy is usually indicated following endoscopic resection of malignant polyps that do not meet these criteria.[378,379] Colonoscopy should be done three months following endoscopic resection of a polyp with favorable criteria, in order to verify the absence of residual tissue. Thereafter, surveillance can revert to the schedule outlined above.

Colonic Decompression

Acute pseudo-obstruction of the colon, first described by Ogilvie in 1948,[380] is characterized by acute massive dilation of the cecum and right colon without organic obstruction. If untreated, the distension can lead to perforation, peritonitis, and death.

Conservative treatment is indicated in patients with cecal diameters <9 to 10 cm, since perforation is a minimal risk. Nothing should be given by mouth, and nasogastric suction should be initiated; gentle enemas and insertion of a rectal tube may also prove beneficial.[381] Fluid and electrolyte abnormalities should be corrected, narcotics should be stopped, and any infections or associated conditions treated as possible. Serial abdominal examinations and repeat abdominal radiographs should be performed every 12 to 24 hours. If the cecal diameter continues to increase and exceeds 12 or 13 cm, or if there is no improvement in 48 to 72 hours, the colon should be decompressed.

Decompression can be a tedious procedure, requiring patience and experience. Air insufflation should be kept to a minimum; frequent irrigation through the suction channel may be necessary to clear the channel and maintain visibility. Although the cecum is the optimal endpoint, successful decompression has been achieved with passage to the hepatic flexure. The colonic lumen should be collapsed by applying intermittent suction as the endoscope is withdrawn. If desired, a decompressive tube can be left in the ascending colon.[382] Colonoscopy will prove successful in 80% to 85% of patients with Ogilvie's syndrome.[381–384] However, if a second decompression is required, 40% of these patients will experience yet another recurrence of colonic dilation.[385] Bloody colonic contents or dark-blue or black mucosa suggests ischemia or necrosis; if seen, the procedure should be terminated and the patient taken to the operating room. Operative intervention is also indicated if colonoscopy is unavailable or unsuccessful, or if dilation recurs after two previous endoscopic decompressions.

Colonic volvulus is another potential indication for colonoscopic decompression. Although a relatively uncommon cause of intestinal obstruction, colonic volvulus is not uncommon in elderly, institutionalized patients. Colonoscopic decompression of a sigmoid volvulus can be a useful temporizing measure, allowing the colon to be prepared for elective operative treatment.[383,386] Colonoscopy also can provide assessment of bowel viability, the most important prognostic indicator; visualization of ischemic mucosa mandates operative intervention. Although colonoscopy will decompress the volvulus in most patients, recurrence is frequent (50% to 70%) without operative treatment.[387] While colonoscopic decompression of cecal volvulus may be of benefit, it is often unsuccessful and may only delay operative treatment.[387]

Stricture Dilatation

In hopes of avoiding surgical resection, nonoperative treatment of colonic strictures is being pursued with increasing frequency.[388,389] Both radiologic and endoscopic approaches have been utilized; however, the endoscopic approach is technically easier and allows visual inspection and histologic evaluation of the stricture. While strictures of diverse etiology have been addressed endoscopically, anastomotic strictures appear to offer the best results.[390]

Once the stricture has been identified, it is the responsibility of the endoscopist to determine its cause. This may require biopsies and/or mucosal brushing. The pediatric colonoscope may aid in visualizing the colon proximal to the stricture.

The dilators used for these procedures are the same or similar to those used in the upper gastrointestinal tract. Balloon dilators are most commonly used, since they can be placed anywhere in the colon, access permitting. Ideally, they are positioned under direct vision via the colonoscope, once the latter is correctly positioned distal to the stricture. Silicone lubrication is usually necessary in order to pass the dilating catheter through the scope. Longer (8 cm) and wider (diameters greater than 51 Fr) balloons are associated with improved results.[388] If angulation precludes through-the-scope insertion, the balloon dilators can be positioned under fluoroscopic guidance via a colonoscopically placed guidewire. In the left colon, hollow-core rigid dilators also can be inserted under fluoroscopic control over previously inserted guidewires. Several preliminary reports suggest that balloon dilatation may be a reasonable option in patients with recurrent Crohn's strictures that are within reach of the colonoscope.[391,392]

Endoscopic Nd:YAG lasers have been used to relieve malignant obstruction, allowing luminal recanalization and bowel preparation prior to resection[393,394] or providing palliation in over 85% of patients with advanced disease.[395–397] Prior to attempting this procedure, the endoscopist should have experience with laser therapy elsewhere in the gastrointestinal tract.

COMPLICATIONS

While infrequent, significant complications can occur in association with diagnostic or therapeutic colonoscopy. Fluid and electrolyte imbalance can occur during bowel preparation; dehydration and hypovolemia are more common than fluid overload. The risk of these complications has been decreased by the introduction of oral purge solutions containing sodium sulfate and nonabsorbable solutes (eg, polyethylene glycol).

Cardiopulmonary complications also can occur following analgesia administration. These reactions have been previously discussed (see Monitoring).

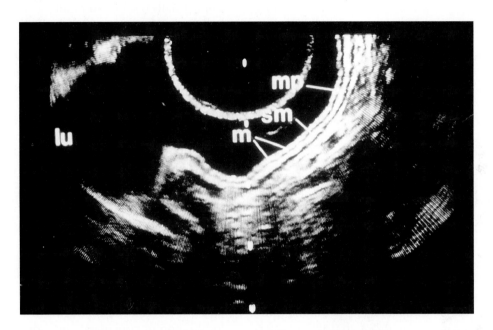

A

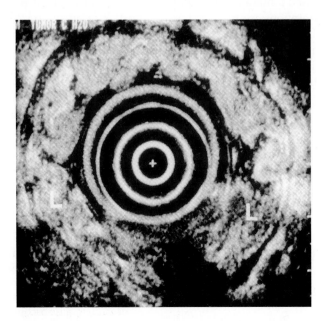

B

Figure 3–29. A. Endoscopic ultrasonographic image of the gastrointestinal tract demonstrating the five layers typically seen (m = mucosa; sm = submucosa; mp = muscularis propria; lu = lumen). **B**. An esophageal cancer as seen with endoscopic ultrasound. (Courtesy of Dr. Clive Albert, Atlanta, GA).

Complications specifically related to colonoscopy include hemorrhage and perforation. The former is most unusual following diagnostic colonoscopy, occurring in 0% to 0.07% of cases.[398–401] Hemorrhage in this setting is usually intra-abdominal, resulting from excessive force during manipulation. Serosal or mucosal tears are the most common sources.[402,403]

Although still uncommon, hemorrhage is seen more often following polypectomy (0.77% to 3.3%).[398–401] Postpolypectomy bleeding can be immediate or delayed. Most hemorrhage occurring immediately following polypectomy is due to inadequate coagulation of the nutrient vessel; this complication can usually be handled during colonoscopy either by resnaring and recoagulating the polypectomy stump[404] or by standard hemostatic techniques.[401] Approximately 2% of polypectomies are complicated by delayed bleeding that usually stops without need for transfusion.[401] This complication can be managed expectantly with supportive therapy.

Perforation is the most common complication of diagnostic colonoscopy, occurring in 0% to 0.26% of cases.[398–401] These injuries are caused by mechanical or pneumatic pressure and are most common at the rectosigmoid or sigmoid–descending colon junctions. While surgery is often required, patients with limited, confined perforations may be managed conservatively with bowel rest, intravenous fluids, and antibiotics, and close observation.[405]

Therapeutic colonoscopy, including polypectomy or hemostasis, can also be complicated by perforation. Reported incidences range from 0.29% to 0.42% of interventions[398–401]; the risk is increased following removal of sessile polyps.[399,401] These perforations are managed as described above.[406,407] Following polypectomy, patients occasionally develop localized peritoneal irritation, fever, tachycardia, and leukocytosis without overt perforation. This syndrome has been labeled "transmural burn", "postpolypectomy coagulation syndrome", or "serositis" and is probably attributable to a transmural electrocoagulation injury. Patients with this unusual complication can also be treated conservatively with uneventful recovery expected within 48 to 72 hours.[401,405,407]

■ ENDOSCOPIC ULTRASOUND

Fiberoptic endoscopes with small ultrasound probes mounted on their distal ends are now available. Current technology allows high-resolution ultrasonographic visualization of the gastrointestinal tract as well as nearby organs and structures.

Characteristic images are now well documented.[408,409] Individual layers of the gastrointestinal wall are visualized as five distinct layers of alternating hyperechogenicity and hypoechogenicity (Fig 3–29A). The first two layers correspond to the interface and the mucosa, the third layer represents the submucosa, the fourth layer represents the muscularis mucosa, and the fifth layer represents the adventitia/serosa.[408,409] Endoscopic ultrasonography can distinguish structures as small as 2 mm in diameter.[410]

The procedure is performed much like routine diagnostic endoscopy. Preparation, medication, and endoscope passage are performed in the usual fashion. Once the endoscope is in the desired position, acoustic coupling usually is achieved by filling both the lumen and a balloon on the endoscope tip with deaerated water. Ultrasonographic scanning then can be performed and recorded. Newer endoscopic ultrasound instruments offer both 7.5 MHz (resolution = 1 mm; depth of field ≈ 5 to 7 cm) and 12-MHz transducers (resolution ≈ 0.5 mm; depth of field ≈ 3 cm).[411]

This technique has a steep learning curve[410,412] and requires significant initial capital investment. Despite these concerns, preliminary studies suggest that endoscopic ultrasonography may improve diagnostic capability as well as the ability to assess tumor resectability. This modality more accurately stages depth of esophageal tumor invasion (Fig 3–29B), but not distant metastases, when compared to dynamic CT scan.[409] Further, overall staging of esophageal carcinoma was improved by combined use of endoscopic ultrasound plus dynamic CT scanning, compared to CT alone.[409] Endoscopic ultrasonography provided even better results when compared to CT scanning for staging of gastric carcinoma,[409] localization of pancreatic endocrine tumors,[410,413] and evaluation of small peripancreatic masses.[412,414] Snady and associates[414] further noted that endoscopic ultrasound aided patient management in 75% of patients with small (<5 cm) peripancreatic masses by providing more details about the disease, and changed management in 32% by achieving a diagnosis or correcting an errant diagnosis. Endoscopic ultrasonography has also proven beneficial in evaluation of extrahepatic bile duct cancer,[415] colorectal carcinoma,[416] anorectal Crohn's disease,[417] and the response of esophageal cancer to combined radiation and chemotherapy.[418]

REFERENCES

1. Schindler R. *Lehrbuch und Atlas der Gastroskopie.* Munich, Germany: IF Lehmann; 1923
2. Schindler R. Ein vollig ungefahrliches flexibles gastroskkop. *München Med Wochenschr* 1932;79:1268–1269
3. Hirschowitz BI, Curtiss LE, Peters CW, et al. Demonstration of a new gastroscope, the "fiberscope." *Gastroenterology* 1958;35:50–53
4. Lemire S, Cocco AE. Visualization of the left colon with the fiberoptic gastroduodenoscope. *Gastrointest Endosc* 1966; 13:29–30

5. Overholt BF. Clinical experience with the fibersigmoidoscope. *Gastrointest Endosc* 1968;15:27

6. Oshiba S, Watanabe A. Endoscopy of the colon. *Gastroenterol Endosc (Tokyo)* 1965;7:440–442

7. Niwa H: Endoscopy of the colon. *Gastroenterol Endosc (Tokyo)* 1965;7:402–408

8. McCune WS, Shorb PE, Moscovitz H. Endoscopic cannulation of the ampulla of Vater: a preliminary report. *Ann Surg* 1968;85:693–697

9. Oi I. Fiberduodenoscopy and endoscopic pancreatocholangiography. *Gastrointest Endosc* 1970;17:59–62

10. Kasugai T, Kuno N, Kobayashi S, Hattori K. Endoscopic pancreatocholangiography, I: the normal endoscopic pancreatocholangiogram. *Gastroenterology* 1972;63:217–226

11. Vennes JA, Silvis SE. Endoscopic visualization of bile and pancreatic ducts. *Gastrointest Endosc* 1972;18:147–152

12. Wolff WI, Shinya H. Colonofiberoscopy. *JAMA* 1971;217:1509–1512

13. Crafoord C, Frenckner P. Nonsurgical treatment of varicose veins of the esophagus. *Acta Otolaryngol* 1939;27:422–429

14. Moersch HJ. Further studies on the treatment of esophageal varices by injection of a sclerosing solution. *Ann Otol Rhinol Laryngol* 1941;50:1233–1244

15. Patterson CO, Rouse MO. Injection treatment of esophageal varices. *JAMA* 1946;130:384–386

16. Koch H, Pesch HJ, Bauerle H, et al. Experimentelle untersuchungen und klinische erfahrungen zur electrokoagulation blutende lasionen im oberen gastrointestinaltrakt. *Fortschr Endoskop* 1972;10:67–71

17. Classen M, Demling L. Endoskopishe sphinkterotomie der papilla vateri und steinextraktion aus dem ductus choledochus. *Dtsch Med Wochenschr* 1974;99:496–497

18. Kawai K, Abasaka Y, Murakami K, et al. Endoscopic sphincterotomy of the ampulla of Vater. *Gastrointest Endosc* 1974;20:148–151

19. den Hartog Jager FC, Bartelsman JF, Tytgat GN. Palliative treatment of obstructing esophagogastric malignancy by endoscopic positioning of a plastic prosthesis. *Gastroenterology* 1979;77:1008–1014

20. Working Party of the Clinical Services Committee of the British Society of Gastroenterology: provision of gastrointestinal endoscopy and related services for a district general hospital. *Gut* 1991;32:95–101

21. Axon ATR. Working party report to the World Congresses of Gastroenterology, Sydney, 1990. Disinfection and endoscopy: summary and recommendations. *J Gastroenterol Hepatol* 1991;6:23–24

22. Bottrill PM, Axon ATR. Cleaning and disinfection of flexible endoscopes and ancillary equipment: use of automatic disinfectors. *J Gastroenterol Hepatol* 1991;6:45–47

23. Noar MD, Soehendra N. Endoscopy simulation training devices. *Endoscopy* 1992;24:159–166

24. Baillie J, Evangelou H, Jowell P, Cotton PB. The future of endoscopy simulation: a Duke perspective. *Endoscopy* 1992;24(suppl 2):542–543

25. Baillie J, Jowell P, Evangelou H, et al. Use of computer graphics simulation for teaching flexible sigmoidoscopy. *Endoscopy* 1991;23:126–129

26. Noar MD. Robotics interactive endoscopy simulation of ERCP/sphincterotomy and EGD. *Endoscopy* 1992;24 (suppl 2):539–541

27. Beer-Gabel M, Delmotte JS, Muntlak L. Computer assisted training in endoscopy (C.A.T.E.): from simulator to a learning station. *Endoscopy* 1992;24(suppl 2):534–538

28. Baillie J, Gillies DF, Cotton PB, Williams CB. A computer simulation for teaching basic ERCP techniques. *Gastrointest Endosc* 1988;34:302

29. Williams CB, Baillie J, Gillies DF, et al. Teaching gastrointestinal endoscopy by computer simulation: a prototype for colonoscopy and ERCP. *Gastrointest Endosc* 1990;36:49–54

30. Silvis SE, Nebel O, Rogers G, et al. Cardiopulmonary complications are more common than bleeding or perforation during diagnostic procedures. *JAMA* 1986;235:928–930

31. Lieberman DA, Wuerker CK, Katon RM. Cardiopulmonary risk of esophagogastroduodenoscopy: role of endoscope diameter and systemic sedation. *Gastroenterology* 1985;88:468–472

32. Shane SM. *Conscious sedation for ambulatory surgery.* Baltimore, MD: University Park Press; 1983

33. Bell GD, Spickett GP, Reeve PA, et al. Intravenous midazolam for upper gastrointestinal endoscopy: a study of 800 consecutive cases relating dose to age and sex of patient. *Br J Clin Pharmacol* 1987;23:241–243

34. DiSario JA, Waring JP, Talbert G, Sanowski RA. Monitoring of blood pressure and heart rate during routine endoscopy: a prospective, randomized, controlled study. *Am J Gastroenterol* 1991;86:956–960

35. Reiertsen O, Skjoto J, Jacobsen CD, et al. Complications of fiberoptic gastrointestinal endoscopy—five years' experience in a central hospital. *Endoscopy* 1987;19:1–6

36. McKee CC, Ragland JJ, Myers JO. An evaluation of multiple clinical variables for hypoxia during colonoscopy. *Surg Gynecol Obstet* 1991;173:37–40

37. Council on Scientific Affairs, AMA. The use of pulse oximetry during conscious sedation. *JAMA* 1993;270:1463–1468

38. Bell GD, Bown S, Morden A, Coady T, Logan RFA. Prevention of hypoxaemia during upper gastrointestinal endoscopy by means of oxygen via nasal cannulae. *Lancet* 1987;1:1022–1024

39. Griffin SM, Chung SCS, Leung JWC, LI AK. Effect of intranasal oxygen on hypoxia and tachycardia during endoscopic cholangiopancreatography. *Br Med J* 1990;300:83–84

40. Jaffe PE, Fennerty MB, Sampliner RE, Hixson LJ. Preventing hypoxemia during colonoscopy: a randomized controlled trial of supplemental oxygen. *J Clin Gastroenterol* 1992;14:114–116

41. Standards of Practice Committee, American Society of Gastrointestinal Endoscopy. Conscious sedation and monitoring of patients undergoing gastrointestinal endoscopic procedures. *Gastrointest Endosc* 1990;37:120–121

42. Freeman ML, Hennessy JT, Cass OW, Pheley AM. Carbon dioxide retention and oxygen desaturation during gastrointestinal endoscopy. *Gastroenterology* 1993;105:331–339

43. Chuong JJH, DuBovik S, McCallum RW. Achalasia as a risk for esophageal carcinoma. A reappraisal. *Dig Dis Sci* 1984;29:1105–1108

44. Peracchia A, Segalin A, Bardini R, et al. Esophageal carcinoma and achalasia: prevalence, incidence, and results of treatment. *Hepatogastroenterol* 1991;38:514–516

45. Aggestrup S, Holm JC, Sorenson HR: Does achalasia predispose to cancer of the esophagus? *Chest* 1992;102:1013–1016

46. Wychulis AR, Woolman GL, Anderson HA, Ellis FH, Jr. Achalasia and carcinoma of the esophagus. *JAMA* 1971;215:1638–1641

47. Richter JE. Motility disorders of the esophagus. In: Yamada T, Alpers DH, Owyang C (eds), *Textbook of Gastroenterology*. Philadelphia, PA: J.B. Lippincott, 1991;1083–1122

48. Leape LL, Ashcraft KW, Scarpelli DG, et al. Hazard to health—liquid lye. *N Engl J Med* 1971;248:232–235

49. Appleqvist P, Salmo M. Lye corrosion carcinoma of the esophagus. *Cancer* 1980;45:2655–2658

50. Hopkins RA, Postlethwait RW. Caustic burns and carcinoma of the esophagus. *Ann Surg* 1982;194:146–148

51. Chisholm M. The association between webs, iron and post-cricoid carcinoma. *Postgrad Med J* 1974;50:215–219

52. Geerlings SE, Statins van Eps LW. Pathogenesis and consequences of plummer-vinson syndrome. *Clin Invest* 1992;70:629–630

53. Hameeteman W, Tytgat GNJ, Houthoff HJ, Van den Tweel JG. Barrett's esophagus: development of dysplasia and adenocarcinoma. *Gastroenterology* 1989;96:1249–1256

54. Miros M, Kerlin P, Walker N. Only patients with dysplasia progress to adenocarcinoma in Barrett's esophagus. *Gut* 1991;32:1441–1446

55. Iftikhar SY, James PD, Steele RJC, et al. Length of Barrett's esophagus: an important factor in the development of dysplasia and adenocarcinoma. *Gut* 1992;33:1155–1158

56. Reid BJ, Weinstein WM, Lewin KJ, et al. Endoscopic biopsy can detect high-grade dysplasia or early adenocarcinoma in Barrett's esophagus without grossly recognizable neoplastic lesions. *Gastroenterology* 1988;94:81–90

57. Levine DS, Haggitt RC, Blout PL, et al. An endoscopic biopsy protocol can differentiate high-grade dysplasia from early adenocarcinoma in Barrett's esophagus. *Gastroenterology* 1993;105:40–50

58. Spechler SJ. Endoscopic surveillance for patients with Barrett's esophagus: does the risk justify the practice? *Ann Intern Med* 1987;106:902–904

59. Hattori T. Morphological range of hyperplastic polyps and carcinomas arising in hyperplastic polyps of the stomach. *J Clin Path* 1985;38:622–630

60. Hughes R. Diagnosis and treatment of gastric polyps. *Gastrointest Endosc Clin N Am* 1993;2:457–467

61. Seifert E, Gail K, Weismuller J. Gastric polypectomy. *Endoscopy* 1985;15:8–11

62. Harju E. Gastric polyposis and malignancy. *Br J Surg* 1986;73:632–633

63. Shemesh E, Bat L. A prospective evaluation of the upper gastrointestinal tract and periampullary region in patients with Gardner syndrome. *Am J Gastroenterol* 1985;80:825–827

64. Sabre RG, Frost AG, Jagelman DG, et al. Gastric and duodenal polyps in familial adenomatous polyposis: a prospective study of the nature and prevalence of upper gastrointestinal polyps. *Gut* 1987;28:306–314

65. Johan G, Offerhaus A, Giardiello M. The risk of upper gastrointestinal cancer in familial adenomatous polyposis. *Gastroenterology* 1992;102:1980–1982

66. Beckwith PS, van Heerden JA, Dozois RR. Prognosis of symptomatic duodenal adenomas in familial adenomatous polyposis. *Arch Surg* 1991;126:825–828

67. Offerhaus GJA, Giardiello FM, Krush AJ, et al. The risk of upper gastrointestinal cancer in familial adenomatous polyposis. *Gastroenterology* 1992;102:1980–1982

68. Schafer LW, Larson DE, Melton LJ III, et al. The risk of gastric cancer after surgical treatment for benign disease. *N Engl J Med* 1983;309:1210–1213

69. Schuman BM, Waldbaum JR, Hiltz SW. Carcinoma of the gastric remnant in a US population. *Gastrointest Endosc* 1984;30:71–73

70. Greene FL. Gastroscopic screening of the post-gastrectomy stomach. Relationship of dysplasia to remnant cancer. *Am Surg* 1989;55:12–15

71. Stalnikowicz R, Benbassat J. Risk of gastric cancer after gastric surgery for benign disorders. *Arch Intern Med* 1990;150:2202–2206

72. Stael-von-Holstein C, Hammar E, Eriksson S, Huldt B. Clinical significance of dysplasia in gastric remnant biopsy specimens. *Cancer* 1993;72:1532–1535

73. Stael-von-Holstein C, Eriksson S, Huldt B, Hammar E. Endoscopic screening during 17 years of gastric stump carcinoma: a prospective clinical trial. *Scand J Gastroenterol* 1991;26:1020–1026

74. Offerhaus GJA, Tersmette AC, Giardiello FM, et al. Evaluation of endoscopy for early detection of gastric-stump cancer. *Lancet* 1992;340:33–35

75. Greene FL. Neoplastic changes in the stomach after gastrectomy. *Surg Gynecol Obstet* 1990;171:477–480

76. Schafer LW, Larson DE, Melton LJ III, et al. Risk of development of gastric carcinoma in patients with pernicious anemia: a population based study in Rochester, Minnesota. *Mayo Clinic Proc* 1985;60:444–448

77. Brinton, LA, Gridley G, Hrubec Z, et al. Cancer risk following pernicious anemia. *Br J Cancer* 1989;59:810–813.

78. Sjoblom SM, Sipponen P, Jarvinen H. Gastroscopic follow up of pernicious anemia patients. *Gut* 1993;34:28–32

79. Hsing AW, Hansson LE, McLaughlin JK, et al. Pernicious anemia and subsequent cancer: a population based cohort study. *Cancer* 1993;71:745–750

80. Cohen L, Korsten M, Scherl, et al. Bacteremia after endoscopic injection sclerosis. *Gastrointest Endosc* 1983;29:198–200

81. Botoman VA, Surawicz CM. Bacteremia with gastrointestinal endoscopic procedures. *Gastrointest Endosc* 1986;32:342–346

82. Ho H, Zuckerman M, Wassen C. A prospective controlled study of the risk of bacteremia in emergency sclerotherapy of esophageal varices. *Gastroenterology* 1991;101:1642–1648

83. Jain N. Larson D, Schroeder K, et al. Antibiotic prophylaxis for percutaneous endoscopic gastrostomy. *Ann Int Med* 1987;107:824–828

84. Bjork JT, Geenen JE, Soergel KH, et al. Endoscopic evaluation of large gastric folds: a comparison of biopsy techniques. *Gastrointest Endosc* 1977;24:22–23

85. Dekker W, Tytgat GN. Diagnostic accuracy of fiberendoscopy in the detection of upper intestinal malignancy: a follow-up analysis. *Gastroenterology* 1977;73:710–714

86. Ida K, Tada M: Chromoscopy. In: Sivak MV Jr (ed), *Gastroenterologic Endoscopy*. Philadelphia, PA: WB Saunders; 1987:203–220

87. Silverstein F, Gilbert DA, Tedesco FJ, et al. The national ASGE survey on upper gastrointestinal bleeding, II: clinical prognostic factors. *Gastrointest Endosc* 1981;27:80–93

88. Morris DW, Levine GM, Soloway RD, et al: Prospective, randomized study of diagnosis and outcome in acute upper gastrointestinal bleeding: endoscopy versus conventional radiography. *Am J Dig Dis* 1975;20:1103–1109

89. Peterson WL, Barnett CC, Smith HJ, et al. Routine early endoscopy in upper gastrointestinal bleeding. *N Engl J Med* 1981;304:925–929

90. Fleischer D. Etiology and prevalence of severe persistent upper gastrointestinal bleeding. *Gastroenterology* 1983;84:538–543

91. Wara P. Endoscopic prediction of major rebleeding—A prospective study of stigmata of hemorrhage in bleeding ulcer. *Gastroenterology* 1985;88:1209–1214

92. Storey DW, Bown SG, Swain CP, et al. Endoscopic prediction of recurrent bleeding in peptic ulcers. *N Eng J Med* 1981;305:915–916

93. Swain CP, Storey DW, Bown SG, et al. Nature of the bleeding vessel in recurrently bleeding gastric ulcers. *Gastroenterology* 1986;90:595–608

94. Starlinger M, Becker HD. Upper gastrointestinal bleeding—Indications and results in surgery. *Hepatogastroenterol* 1991;38:216–219

95. Stark ME, Gostout CJ, Balm RK. Clinical features and endoscopic management of Dieulafoy's disease. *Gastrointest Endosc* 1992;38:545–550

96. Breuer RI, Craig RM. Injection therapy and topical agents in the treatment of gastrointestinal bleeding. In: Silvis SE Jr (ed), *Therapeutic Gastrointestinal Endoscopy*, 2nd ed. New York, NY: Igaku-Shoin Medical Publishers; 1990:212–222

97. Rajgopal C, Palmer KR. Endoscopic injection sclerosis: effective treatment for bleeding peptic ulcer. *Gut* 1991;32:727–729

98. Chung SCS, Leung JWC, Sung JY, et al. Injection or heat probe for bleeding ulcer. *Gastroenterology* 1991;100:33–37

99. Oxner RBG, Simmonds NJ, Gertner DJ, et al. Controlled trial of endoscopic injection treatment for bleeding from peptic ulcers with visible vessels. *Lancet* 1992;339:966–968

100. Jiranek G, Auth D, Silverstein F. Endoscopic thermal hemostasis for peptic ulcer bleeding. In: Silvis SE Jr (ed), *Therapeutic Gastrointestinal Endoscopy*, 2nd ed. New York, NY: Igaku-Shoin Medical; 1990:175–193

101. Laine L. Determination of the optimal technique for bipolar electrocoagulation treatment. An experimental evaluation of the BICAP and gold probes. *Gastroenterology* 1991;100:107–112

102. Chung SCS, Leung JWC, Sung JY, et al. Injection or heat probe for bleeding ulcer. *Gastroenterology* 1991;100:33–37

103. Sacks HS, Chalmers TC, Blum AL, et al. Endoscopic hemostasis: an effective therapy for bleeding peptic ulcer. *JAMA* 1990;264:494–499

104. Cook DJ, Guyatt GH, Salena BJ, Laine LA. Endoscopic therapy for acute nonvariceal upper gastrointestinal hemorrhage: a meta-analysis. *Gastroenterology* 1992;102:139–148

105. Christensen E, Fauerholdt L, Schlichting P, et al. Aspects of the natural history of gastrointestinal bleeding in cirrhosis and the effect of prednisone. *Gastroenterology* 1981;81:944–952

106. Clark AW, Westaby D, Silk DBA, et al. Prospective controlled trial of injection sclerotherapy in patients with cirrhosis and recent variceal hemorrhage. *Lancet* 1980;2:552–554

107. Sivak MV Jr, Blue MG. Endoscopic sclerotherapy of esophageal varices. In: Silvis SE Jr (ed), *Therapeutic Gastrointestinal Endoscopy*, 2nd ed. New York, NY: Igaku-Shoin Medical; 1990:42–97

108. Lo G-H, Lai K-H, Ng W-W, et al. Injection sclerotherapy preceded by esophageal tamponade versus immediate sclerotherapy in arresting active variceal bleeding: a prospective randomized trial. *Gastrointest Endosc* 1992;38:421–424

109. Jensen DM, Silpa ML, Tapia JI et al. Comparison of different methods for endoscopic hemostasis of bleeding canine esophageal varices. *Gastroenterology* 1983;84:1455–1461

110. McClave SA, Kaiser SC, Wright RA, et al. Prospective randomized comparison of esophageal variceal sclerotherapy agents: sodium tetradecyl sulfate versus sodium morrhuate. *Gastrointest Endosc* 1990;36:567–571

111. Sarin SK, Nanda R, Sachdev G, et al. Intravariceal versus paravariceal sclerotherapy: a prospective, controlled, randomized trial. *Gut* 1987;657–662

112. Vinel J-P, Lamouliatte H, Cales P, et al. Propranolol reduces the rebleeding rate during endoscopic sclerotherapy before variceal obliteration. *Gastroenterology* 1992;102:1760–1763

113. Cello JP, Grendell JH, Crass RA, et al. Endoscopic sclerotherapy versus portacaval shunt in patients with severe cirrhosis and acute variceal hemorrhage: long-term follow-up. *N Engl J Med* 1987;316:11–15

114. Teres J, Bordas JM, Bravo D, et al. Sclerotherapy vs distal splenorenal shunt in the elective treatment of variceal hemorrhage: a randomized clinical trial. *Hepatology* 1987;7:430–436

115. Burroughs AK, Hamilton G, Phillips A, et al. A comparison of sclerotherapy with staple transection of the esophagus for the emergency control of bleeding from esophageal varices. *N Engl J Med* 1989;321:857–862

116. Henderson JM, Kutner MH, Millikan WJ Jr, et al. Endoscopic variceal sclerotherapy compared with distal splenorenal shunt to prevent recurrent variceal bleeding in cirrhosis. *Ann Intern Med* 1990;112:262–269

117. Planas R, Boix J, Broggi M, et al. Portacaval shunt versus endoscopic sclerotherapy in the elective treatment of variceal hemorrhage. *Gastroenterology* 1991;100:1078–1086

118. Steigmann GV, Goff JS, Michaletz-Onody PA, et al. Endoscopic sclerotherapy as compared with endoscopic ligation for bleeding esophageal varices. *N Engl J Med* 1992;326:1527–1532

119. Gimson AES, Ramage JK, Panos MZ, et al. Randomized trial of variceal banding ligation versus injection scle-

rotherapy for bleeding oesophageal varices. *Lancet* 1993;342:391–394

120. The Veterans Affairs Cooperative Variceal Sclerotherapy Group. Prophylactic sclerotherapy for esophageal varices in men with alcoholic liver disease: a randomized, single-blind, multicenter clinical trial. *N Engl J Med* 1991; 324:1779–1784

121. van Ruiswyk J, Byrd JC. Efficacy of prophylactic sclerotherapy for prevention of a first variceal hemorrhage. *Gastroenterology* 1992;102:587–597

122. Herman LL, Hoskins WJ, Shike M. Percutaneous endoscopic gastrostomy for decompression of the stomach and small bowel. *Gastrointest Endosc* 1992;38:314–328

123. Ho C, Yee ACN, McPherson R. Complications of surgical and percutaneous gastrostomy: review of 233 patients. *Gastroenterology* 1988;95:1206–1210

124. Stiegmann GV, Goff JS, Silas D, et al. Endoscopic versus operative gastrostomy: final results of a prospective randomized trial. *Gastrointest Endosc* 1990;36:575–578

125. Ponsky JL, Gauderer MWL. Percutaneous endoscopic gastrostomy: a nonoperative technique for feeding gastrostomy. *Gastrointest Endosc* 1981;27:9–11

126. Larson DE, Burton DD, Schroeder KW, DiMagnio EP. Percutaneous endoscopic gastrostomy: indications, success, complications and mortality in 314 consecutive patients. *Gastroenterology* 1987;93:48–52

127. Ponsky JL, Gauderer MWL. Percutaneous endoscopic gastrostomy: indications, limitations, and results. *World J Surg* 1989;13:165–170

128. Sacks BA, Vine HS, Palestrant AM, et al. A nonoperative technique for establishment of a gastrostomy in the dog. *Invest Radiol* 1987;18:485–487

129. Hogan RB, Demarco DC, Hamilton JK, et al. Percutaneous endoscopic gastrostomy—to push or pull: a prospective randomized trial. *Gastrointest Endosc* 1986; 32:253–258

130. Russell TR, Brotman M, Norris F. Percutaneous endoscopic gastrostomy: a new simplified and cost-effective technique. *Am J Surg* 1984;148:132–137

131. MacFadyen BV, Catalano MF, Raijman I, Ghobrial R. Percutaneous endoscopic gastrostomy with jejunal extension: a new technique. *Am J Gastroenterol* 1992;87: 725–728

132. Mamel JJ. Percutaneous endoscopic gastrostomy. *Am J Gastroenterol* 1989;84:703–710

133. Lewis BS. Perform PEJ, not PEG. *Gastrointest Endosc* 1990; 36:311–313

134. DiSario JA, Foutch PG, Sanowski RA. Poor results with percutaneous endoscopic jejunostomy. *Gastrointest Endosc* 1990;36:257–260

135. Kadakia SC, Sullivan HO, Starnes E. Percutaneous endoscopic gastrostomy or jejunostomy and the incidence of aspiration in 79 patients. *Am J Surg* 1992;164: 114–118

136. Spitz L. Management of ingested foreign bodies in childhood. *Br Med J* 1971;4:469–472

137. Vizcarrondo FJ, Brady PG, Nord JH. Foreign bodies of the upper gastrointestinal tract. *Gastrointest Endosc* 1983; 29:208–210

138. Davidoff E, Towne JB. Ingested foreign bodies. *NY State J Med* 1975;75:103–107

139. Ziter FMH. Intestinal perforations in adults due to ingested opaque foreign bodies. *Am J Gastroenterol* 1976; 66:382–385

140. Webb WA. Management of foreign bodies of the upper gastrointestinal tract. *Gastroenterology* 1988;94:204–216

141. Brady PG. Endoscopic removal of foreign bodies. In: Silvis SE Jr (ed), *Therapeutic Gastrointestinal Endoscopy*, 2nd ed. New York, NY: Igaku-Shoin Medical; 1990:8–125

142. Temple DM, McNeese MC. Hazards of battery ingestion. *Pediatrics* 1983;71:100–103

143. Votteler TP, Nash JC, Rutledge JC. The hazard of ingested alkaline disk batteries in children. *JAMA* 1983;249:2504–2506

144. Suarez CA, Arango A, Lester JL III. Cocaine-condom ingestion: surgical treatment. *JAMA* 1977;238:1391–1392

145. The Standards of Training and Practice Committee, American Society for Gastrointestinal Endoscopy: Esophageal dilation: guidelines for clinical application. *Gastrointest Endosc* 1991;37:183–187

146. Monnier PH, Hsieh V, Savary M. Endoscopic treatment of esophageal stenosis using Savary-Gilliard bougies: technical innovations. *Acta Endoscopia* 1985;15:1–5

147. Dumon J, Meric B, Sivak MV, Fleischer D. A new method of esophageal dilation using Savary-Gilliard bougies. *Gastrointest Endosc* 1985;31:379–382

148. Tulman AB, Boyce HW. Complications of esophageal dilation and guidelines for their prevention. *Gastrointest Endosc* 1981;27:229–234

149. McClave SA, Wright RA, Brady PA. Prospective randomized study of Maloney esophageal dilation-blinded versus fluoroscopic guidance. *Gastrointest Endosc* 1990;36: 272–275

150. Lindor KD, Ott BJ. Balloon dilation of upper digestive strictures. *Gastroenterology* 1985;89:545–548

151. Graham DY, Tabibian N, Schwartz JT, Smith JL. Evaluation of the effectiveness of through-the-scope balloons as dilators of benign and malignant strictures. *Gastrointest Endosc* 1987;33:432–435

152. Chen P-C. Endoscopic balloon dilation of esophageal strictures following surgical anastomoses, endoscopic variceal sclerotherapy, and corrosive ingestion. *Gastrointest Endosc* 1992;38:586–589

153. Yamamoto H, Hughes Jr RW, Schroeder KW, et al. Treatment of benign esophageal stricture by Eder-Puestow or balloon dilators: a comparison between randomized and prospective nonrandomized trials. *Mayo Clin Proc* 1992; 67:228–236

154. Vantrappen G, Hellemans J. Treatment of achalasia and related motor disorders. *Gastroenterology* 1980;79: 144–145

155. Cox J, Buckton GK, Bennett JR. Balloon dilation in achalasia: a new dilator. *Gut* 1986;27:986–989

156. Vantrappen G, Janssens J. To dilate or to operate. *Gut* 1983;24:1013–1019

157. Kessler RM. Modern diagnostic and therapeutic thoracoscopy. In: Hunter JG, Sackier JM (eds), *Minimally invasive surgery*. New York, NY: McGraw-Hill; 1993:329–338

158. Chen P-C. Endoscopic balloon dilation of esophageal strictures following surgical anastomoses, endoscopic variceal sclerotherapy, and corrosive ingestion. *Gastrointest Endosc* 1992;38:586–589

159. Song H-Y, Han Y-M, Kim H-N, et al. Corrosive esophageal stricture: safety and effectiveness of balloon dilation. *Radiology* 1992;184:373–378

160. Loizou LA, Rampton D, Bown SG. Treatment of malignant strictures of the cervical esophagus by endoscopic intubation using modified endoprostheses. *Gastrointest Endosc* 1992;38:158–164

161. Bown SG, Hawes R, Matthewson K, et al. Endoscopic laser palliation for advanced malignant dysphagia. *Gut* 1987;28:799–807

162. Siegel HI, Laskin KJ, Dabezies MA, et al. The effect of endoscopic laser therapy on survival in patients with squamous-cell carcinoma of the esophagus. Further experience. *J Clin Gastroenterol* 1991;13:142–146

163. Mathus-Vliegen EMH, Tytgat GNJ. Palliation by laser photoablation: a multidisciplinary quality assessment. *Gastrointest Endosc* 1992;38:365–368

164. Jensen DM, Machicado G, Randall G, et al. Comparison of low power YAG laser and BICAP tumor probe for palliation of esophageal cancer strictures. *Gastroenterology* 1988;94:1263–1270

165. Loizou LA, Grigg D, Atkinson M, et al. A prospective comparison of laser therapy and intubation in endoscopic palliation for malignant dysphagia. *Gastroenterology* 1991;100:1303–1310

166. Reed CE, Marsh WH, Carlson LS, et al. Prospective, randomized trial of palliative treatment for unresectable cancer of the esophagus. *Ann Thorac Surg* 1991;51:522–526

167. Bown SG. Palliation of malignant dysphagia: surgery, radiotherapy, laser, intubation alone or in combination? *Gut* 1991;32:841–844

168. Mandelstam P, Sugawa C, Silvis SE et al. Complications associated with esophagogastroduodenoscopy and with esophageal dilation. *Gastrointest Endosc* 1976;23:16–19

169. Tulman AB, Boyce HW. Complications of esophageal dilation and guidelines for their prevention. *Gastrointest Endosc* 1981;27:229–234

170. Miller RE, Tiszenkel HI. Esophageal perforation due to pneumatic dilation for achalasia. *Surg Gynecol Obstet* 1988;166:458–460

171. Sivak MV Jr. Endoscopic injection sclerosis of esophageal varices: ASGE survey. [letter] *Gastrointest Endosc* 1982;28:41

172. Anderson JR: Oesophageal injury, part 1: the changing face of the management of instrumental perforations *Gullet* 1990;1:10–15

173. Shaffer HA, Valenzuela G, Mittal RK. Esophageal perforation: a reassessment of the criteria for choosing medical or surgical therapy. *Arch Intern Med* 1992;152:757–761

174. Strodel WE, Ponsky JL: Complications of percutaneous gastrostomy. In: Ponsky JL (ed), *Techniques of Percutaneous Gastrostomy*. New York, NY: Igaku-Shoin; 1988:63

175. Bilbao MK, Dotter CT, Lee TG, Katon RM. Complications of endoscopic retrograde cholangiopancreatography (ERCP): a study of 10,000 cases. *Gastroenterology* 1976;70:314–320

176. Fink AS, Valle PA, Chapman M, Cotton PB. Radiological pitfalls in endoscopic retrograde pancreatography. *Pancreas* 1987;1:180–187

177. Reuben A, Johnson AL, and Cotton PB. Is pancreatogram interpretation reliable? A study of observer variation. *Br J Radiol* 1978;51:956–962

178. Axon ATR, Classen M, Cotton PB, et al. Pancreatography in chronic pancreatitis: international definitions. *Gut* 1984;25:1107–1112

179. Zimmon DS, Falkenstein DB, Riccobaon C, et al. Complications of endoscopic retrograde cholangiopancreatography: analysis of 300 consecutive cases. *Gastroenterology* 1975;69:303–309

180. O'Connor HJ, Axon ATR. Gastrointestinal endoscopy: infection and disinfection. *Gut* 1983;24:1067–1077

181. Nealon WH, Townsend CM, Thompson JC. Preoperative endoscopic retrograde cholangiopancreatography (ERCP) in patients with pancreatic pseudocyst associated with resolving acute and chronic pancreatitis. *Ann Surg* 1989;209:532–540

182. Sugawa C, Walt AJ. Endoscopic retrograde cholangiopancreatography in the surgery of pancreatic pseudocysts. *Surgery* 1979;86:639–647

183. O'Connor M, Kolars J, Ansel H, et al. Preoperative endoscopic retrograde cholangiopancreatography in the surgical management of pancreatic pseudocysts. *Am J Surg* 1986;151:18–24

184. Ahearne PM, Baillie JM, Cotton PB, et al. An endoscopic retrograde cholangiopancreatography (ERCP)-based algorithm for the management of pancreatic pseudocysts. *Am J Surg* 1992;163:111–116

185. Cotton PB. Endoscopic management of bile duct stones (apples and oranges). *Gut* 1984;25:587–597

186. Leese T, Neoptolemos JP, Carr-Locke DL. Successes, failures, early complications and their management following endoscopic sphincterotomy: results in 394 consecutive patients from a single centre. *Br J Surg* 1985;72:215–219

187. Vaira D, D'Anna L, Ainley C. Endoscopic sphincterotomy in 1000 consecutive patients. *Lancet* 1989;2:431–434

188. Chung SCS, Leung JWC, Leong HT, Li AKC. Mechanical lithotripsy of large common bile duct stones using a basket. *Brit J Surg* 1991;78:1448–1450

189. Cotton PB, Lehman G, Vennes J, et al. Endoscopic sphincterotomy complications and their management: an attempt at consensus. *Gastrointest Endosc* 1991;37:383–393

190. Leung JWC, Cotton PB. Endoscopic nasobiliary catheter drainage in biliary and pancreatic disease. *Am J Gastroenterol* 1991;86:389–394

191. Cotton PB, Forbes A, Leung JWC, Dineen L. Endoscopic stenting for long-term treatment of large bile duct stones; a 2-5 year follow up. *Gastrointest Endosc* 1987;33:401–412

192. Escourrou J, Cordon JA, Lazarthes F, et al. Early and late complications after endoscopic sphincterotomy for biliary lithiasis with and without gallbladder in situ. *Gut* 1984;25:598–602

193. Neoptolemos JP, Carr-Locke DL, Fraser I, Fossard DP. The management of common bile duct calculi by endoscopic sphincterotomy in patients with gallbladder in situ. *Br J Surg* 1984;71:69–71

194. Siegel JH, Safrany L, Ben-Zvi JS, et al. Duodenoscopic sphincterotomy in patients with gallbladders in situ: re-

port of a series of 1272 patients. *Am J Gastroenterol* 1988;83:1255–1259

195. Hill J, Martin DF, Tweedle DG. Risks of leaving the gall-bladder in situ after endoscopic sphincterotomy for bile duct stones. *Br J Surg* 1991;78:554–557

196. Ingoldby CJH, el-Saadi J, Hall RI, Denyer ME. Late results of endoscopic sphincterotomy for bile duct stones in elderly patients with gall bladders in situ. *Gut* 1989;30:1129–1131

197. Neoptolemos JP, Carr-Locke DL, Fossard DP. Prospective randomized study of preoperative endoscopic sphincterotomy versus surgery alone for common bile duct stones. *Br Med J* 1987;294:470–474

198. Stain SC, Cohen H, Tsuishoysha M, Donavan AJ. Choledocholithiasis. Endoscopic sphincterotomy or common bile duct exploration. *Ann Surg* 1991;213:627–634

199. Fink AS. Current dilemmas in the management of common bile duct stones. *Surg Endosc* 1993;7:285–291

200. Silverman WB, Ruffolo TA, Sherman S, et al. Correlation of basal sphincter pressures measured from the bile duct and the pancreatic duct in patients with suspected sphincter of Oddi dysfunction. *Gastrointest Endos* 1992; 38:440–443

201. Sherman S, Troiano FP, Hawes RH, Lehman GA. Sphincter of Oddi manometry: decreased risk of clinical pancreatitis with use of a modified aspirating catheter. *Gastrointest Endos* 1990;36:460–466

202. Rolny P, Anderberg B, Ihse I, et al. Pancreatitis after sphincter of Oddi manometry. *GUT* 1990;31:821–824

203. Sherman S, Hawes RH, Troiano FP, Lehman GA. Pancreatitis following bile duct sphincter of Oddi manometry: utility of the aspirating catheter. *Gastrointest Endosc* 1992;38:347–350

204. Gilbert DA, DiMarino AJ, Jensen DM, et al. Status evaluation: sphincter of Oddi manometry. *Gastrointest Endosc* 1992;38:757–759

205. Hogan WJ, Geenen JE. Biliary dyskinesia. *Endoscopy* 1988;20:179–188

206. Hogan WJ, Geenen JE, Dodds WJ. Dysmotility disturbances of the biliary tract: classification, diagnosis, and treatment. *Semin Liver Dis* 1987;7:302–310

207. Geenen JE, Hogan WJ, Dodds WJ, et al. The efficacy of endoscopic sphincterotomy after cholecystectomy in patients with sphincter of Oddi dysfunction. *N Engl J Med* 1989;320:82–87

208. Roberts-Thomson IC, Toouli J. Is endoscopic sphincterotomy for disabling biliary-type pain after cholecystectomy effective? *Gastrointest Endosc* 1985;31: 370–373

209. Krims PE, Cotton PB. Papillotomy and functional disorders of the sphincter of Oddi. *Endoscopy* 1988;20:203–207

210. Sherman S, Ruffolo TA, Hawes RH, Lehman GA. Complications of endoscopic sphincterotomy: a prospective series with emphasis on the increased risk associated with sphincter of Oddi dysfunction and nondilated bile ducts. *Gastroenterology* 1991;101:1068–1075

211. Gogel HK, Runyon BA, Volpicelli NA, Palmer RC. Acute suppurative cholangitis due to stones: treatment by urgent endoscopic sphincterotomy. *Gastrointest Endosc* 1987;33:210–213

212. Leung JWC, Chung SCS, Sung JY, et al. Urgent endo-scopic drainage of acute suppurative cholangitis. *Lancet* 1989;1:307–309

213. Lai ECS, Paterson IA, Tam PC, et al. Severe acute cholangitis: The role of emergency nasobiliary drainage. *Surgery* 1990;107:268–272

214. Leung JWC, Venezuela RR. Cholangiosepsis: endoscopic drainage and antibiotic therapy. *Endoscopy* 1991;23: 220–223

215. Lai ECS, Mok FPT, Tan ESY, et al. Endoscopic biliary drainage for severe acute cholangitis. *N Engl J Med* 1992;326:1582–1586

216. Safrany L, Cotton PB. A preliminary report: urgent duodenoscopic sphincterotomy for acute gallstone pancreatitis. *Surgery* 1991;89:424–428

217. van der Spuy S. Endoscopic sphincterotomy in the management of gallstone pancreatitis. *Endoscopy* 1981;13:25

218. Rosseland AR, Solhaug JH. Early or delayed endoscopic papillotomy (EPT) in gallstone pancreatitis. *Ann Surg* 1984;199:165–167

219. Ligoury CI, Meduri B, DiGiulio E, Conard JM. Endoscopic treatment of acute pancreatitis. In: Banks PA, Bianchi Porro G (eds), *Acute pancreatitis: Advances in pathogenesis, diagnosis, and treatment.* Milan, Italy: Masson Italia Editori; 1984:151–160

220. Tulassay Z, Farkas IE. Endoscopic sphincterotomy in acute gallstone pancreatitis. *Lancet* 1988;2:1314

221. Neoptolemos JP, London N, Slater ND, et al. A prospective study of ERCP and endoscopic sphincterotomy in the diagnosis and treatment of acute gallstone pancreatitis. *Arch Surg* 1986;121:697–702

222. Delmotte JS, Pommelet P, Houcke P, et al. Initial duodenoscopic sphincterotomy in patients with acute cholangitis or pancreatitis complicating biliary stones. [abstract] *Gastroenterology* 1982;82:1042

223. Neoptolemos JP, Carr-Locke DL, London NJ, et al. Controlled trial of urgent endoscopic retrograde cholangiopancreatography and endoscopic sphincterotomy versus conservative treatment for acute pancreatitis due to gallstones. *Lancet* 1988;2:979–983

224. Fan S-T, Lai ECS, Mok FPT, et al. Early treatment of acute biliary pancreatitis by endoscopic papillotomy. *N Engl J Med* 1993;328:228–232

225. Blamey SL, Imrie CW, O'Neill J, et al. Prognostic factors in acute pancreatitis. *Gut* 1984;25:1340–1346

226. Ranson JHC, Rifkind KM, Roses DF, et al. Prognostic signs and the role of operative management in acute pancreatitis. *Surg Gynecol Obstet* 1974;139:69–81

227. Dammann HG, Dreyer M, Walter TA, et al. Prognostic indicators in acute pancreatitis: clinical experience and limitations. In: Beger HG, Buchler M (eds). *Acute Pancreatitis.* Berlin, Germany: Springer-Verlag; 1987:181–197

228. Mayer AD, McMahon MJ. The diagnostic and prognostic value of peritoneal lavage in patients with acute pancreatitis. *Surg Gynecol Obstet* 1985;160:507–512

229. Bank S, Wise L, Gersten M. Risk factors in acute pancreatitis. *Am J Gastroenterol* 1983;78:637–640

230. Agarwal N, Pitchumoni CS. Simplified prognostic criteria in acute pancreatitis. *Pancreas* 1986;1:69–73

231. Blamey SL, Osborne DH, Gilmour WH, et al. The early identification of patients with gallstone associated pan-

creatitis using clinical and biochemical factors only. *Ann Surg* 1983;198:574–578

232. Davidson BR, Neoptolemos JP, Leese T, Carr-Locke DL. Biochemical prediction of gallstones in acute pancreatitis: a prospective study of three systems. *Br J Surg* 1988; 75:213–215

233. Mayer AD, McMahon MJ. Biochemical identification of patients with gallstones associated with acute pancreatitis on the day of admission to hospital. *Ann Surg* 1985; 201:68–75

234. Pelligrini CA. Surgery for gallstone pancreatitis. *Am J Surg* 1993;165:515–518

235. Davidson BR, Neoptolemos JP, Carr-Locke, DL. Endoscopic sphincterotomy for common bile duct calculi in patients with gall bladder in situ considered unfit for surgery. *Gut* 1988;29:114–120

236. Neoptolemos JP and Rowley S. Advantages of nonsurgical treatment of bile duct stones: *Hepatogastroenterology* 1989;36:313–316

237. May GR and Shaffer EA. Should elective endoscopic sphincterotomy replace cholecystectomy for the treatment of high-risk patients with gallstone pancreatitis? *J Clin Gastroenterol* 1991;13:125–128

238. Laurence BH, Cotton PB. Decompression of malignant biliary obstruction by duodenoscopic intubation of bile ducts. *Br Med J* 1980;280:522–523

239. Zimmon DS, Clemett AR. Endoscopic stents and drains in the management of pancreatic and biliary duct obstruction. *Surg Clin NA* 1982;62:837–844

240. Huibregtse K, Haverkamp HJ, Tytgat GNJ. Transpapillary positioning of a large 3.2 mm biliary endoprosthesis. *Endoscopy* 1981;13:217–219

241. Huibregtse K, Tytgat GNJ. Palliative treatment of obstructive jaundice by transpapillary introduction of large bore bile duct endoprosthesis. *Gut* 1982;23:371–375

242. Gilliams A, Dick R, Dooley JS, Wallsten H, El-Din A. Self-expandable stainless steel braided endoprosthesis for biliary strictures. *Radiology* 1990;174:137–140

243. Leung JWC, Del Favero G, Cotton PB. Endoscopic biliary prosthesis: a comparison of materials. *Gastrointest Endosc* 1985;31:93–95

244. Rey JF, Maupetit P, Greff M. Experimental study of biliary endoprosthesis efficiency. *Endoscopy* 1985;17:145–148

245. Speer AG, Cotton PB, MacRae KD. Endoscopic management of malignant biliary obstruction: stents of 10 French are preferable to stents of 8 French gauge. *Gastrointest Endosc* 1988;34:412–417

246. Bethge N, Wagner HJ, Knyrim K, et al. Technical failure of biliary metal stent deployment in a series of 116 applications. *Endoscopy* 1992;24:395–400

247. Huibregtse K, Carr-Locke DL, Cremer M, et al. Biliary stent occlusion: a problem solved with self-expanding metal stents? *Endoscopy* 1992;24:391–394

248. Davids PHP, Groen AK, Rauws EAJ, et al. Randomised trial of self-expanding metal stents versus polyethylene stents for distal malignant biliary obstruction. *Lancet* 1992;340:1488–1492

249. Hausegger KA, Kleinert R, Lammer J, et al. Malignant biliary obstruction: Histologic findings after treatment with self-expanding stents. *Radiology* 1992;185:461–464

250. Huibregtse K, Katon RM, Coene PP, Tytgat GNJ. Endoscopic palliative treatment in pancreatic cancer. *Gastrointest Endosc* 1986;32:334–338

251. Deviere J, Baize M, DeToeuf J, Cremer M. Long-term follow-up of patients with hilar malignant stricture treated with endoscopic internal biliary drainage. *Gastrointest Endosc* 1988;34:95–101

252. Polydorou AA, Cairns SR, Dowsett JF, et al. Palliation of proximal malignant biliary obstruction by endoscopic endoprosthesis insertion. *Gut* 1991;32:685–689

253. Ducreux M. Liguory CI, Lefebvre MD. Management of malignant hilar biliary obstruction by endoscopy: results and prognostic factors. *Dig Dis Sci* 1992;37:778–783

254. Binmoeller KF, Katon RM, Shneidman R. Endoscopic management of postoperative biliary leaks: review of 77 cases and report of two cases with biloma formation. *Am J Gastroenterol* 1991;86:227–232

255. Meyers WC, Southern Surgeons Club. A prospective analysis of 1518 laparoscopic cholecystectomies. *N Engl J Med* 1991;324:1073–1078

256. Kozarek R, Gannan R, Baerg R, et al. Bile leak after laparoscopic cholecystectomy: diagnostic and therapeutic application of endoscopic retrograde cholangiopancreatography. *Arch Intern Med* 1992;152:1040–1043

257. Deziel D, Millikan KW, Economou SG, et al. Complications of laparoscopic cholecystectomy: a national survey of 4,292 hospitals and an analysis of 77,604 cases. *Am J Surg* 1993;165:9–14

258. Davids PHP, Rauws EAJ, Coene PPLO, et al. Endoscopic stenting for post-operative biliary strictures. *Gastrointest Endosc* 1992;38:12–18

259. Liguory C, Vitale GC, Lefebre JF, et al. Endoscopic treatment of postoperative biliary fistulae. *Surgery* 1991; 110:779–784

260. Cotton PB, Nickl N. Endoscopic and radiologic approaches to therapy in primary sclerosing cholangitis. *Semin Liver Dis* 1991;11:40–48

261. Martin RF, Biber BP, Bosco JJ, Howell DA. Symptomatic choledochoceles in adults. Endoscopic retrograde cholangiopancreatography recognition and management. *Arch Surg* 1992;127:536–539

262. McCarthy J, Geenen JE, Hogan WJ. Preliminary experience with endoscopic stent placement in benign pancreatic diseases. *Gastrointest Endoscopy* 1988;34:16–18

263. Lans JI, Geenen JE, Johanson JF, Hogan WJ. Endoscopic therapy in patients with pancreas divisum and acute pancreatitis: a prospective, randomized, controlled clinical trial. *Gastrointest Endos* 1992;38:430–434

264. Wolfsen HC, Porayko MK, Hughes RH, et al. Role of endoscopic retrograde cholangiopancreatography after orthotopic liver transplantation. *Am J Gastroenterol* 1992; 87:955–960

265. Soehendra N. Access to the cystic duct: a new endoscopic therapy of gallbladder diseases? *Endoscopy* 1991;23:36–37

266. Tamada K, Seki H, Sato K, et al. Efficacy of endoscopic retrograde cholecystoendoprosthesis (ERCCE) for cholecystitis. *Endoscopy* 1991;23:2–3

267. Burdick JS, Hogan WJ. Chronic pancreatitis: selection of patients for endoscopic therapy. *Endoscopy* 1991;23:155–160

268. Malfertheiner P, Buchler M. Indications for endoscopic or surgical therapy in chronic pancreatitis. *Endoscoy* 1991;23:185–190

269. Ammann RW. A critical appraisal of interventional therapy in chronic pancreatitis. *Endoscopy* 1991;23:191–193

270. Geenen JE. A/S/G/E distinguished lecture—endoscopic therapy of pancreatic disease: a new horizon. *Gastrointest Endosc* 1988;34:386–389

271. Siegel JH, Ben-Zvi JS, Pullano W, Cooperman A. Effectiveness of endoscopic drainage for pancreas divisum; endoscopic and surgical results in 31 patients. *Endoscopy* 1990;22:129–133

272. Huibregtse MD, Schneider B, Vrij AA, Tytgat GNJ. Endoscopic drainage in chronic pancreatitis. *Gastrointest Endosc* 1988;34:9–15

273. Grimm H, Meyer W-H, Ch Nam V, Soehendra N. New modalities for treating chronic pancreatitis. *Endoscopy* 1989;21:70–74

274. Kerzel W, Ell C, Schneider T, Matek W, et al. Extracorporeal piezoelectric shockwave lithotripsy of multiple pancreatic duct stones under ultrasonographic control. *Endoscopy* 1989;21:229–231

275. Sauerbruch T, Holl J, Sackmann M, Paumgartner G. Extracorporeal shock wave lithotripsy of pancreatic stones in patients with chronic pancreatitis and pain: a prospective follow up study. *Gut* 1992;33:969–972

276. Neuhaus H. Fragmentation of pancreatic stones by extracorporeal shock wave lithotripsy. *Endoscopy* 1991;23:161–165

277. Cremer M, Deviere J, Delhaye M, et al. Stenting in severe chronic pancreatitis: results of medium-term follow-up in seventy-six patients. *Endoscopy* 1991;23:171–176

278. Delhaye M, Vandermeeren A, Baize M, Cremer M. Extracorporeal shock-wave lithotripsy of pancreatic calculi. *Gastroenterology* 1992;102:610–620

279. Kozarek RA, Patterson DJ, Ball TJ, Traverso LW. Endoscopic placement of pancreatic stents and drains in the management of pancreatitis. *Ann Surg* 1989;209:261–266

280. Kozarek RA, Ball TJ, Patterson DJ, et al. Endoscopic transpapillary therapy for disrupted pancreatic duct and peripancreatic fluid collections. *Gastroenterology* 1991;100:1362–1370

281. Sahel J, Bastid C, Pellat B, et al. Endoscopic cystoduodenostomy of cysts of chronic calcifying pancreatitis: a report of 20 cases. *Pancreas* 1987;2:447–453

282. Cremer M. Deviere J, Engelholm L. Endoscopic management of cysts and pseudocysts in chronic pancreatitis: long-term follow-up after 7 years of experience. *Gastrointest Endoscopy* 1989;35:1–9

283. Shepard HA, Royle G, Ross APR, et al. Endoscopic biliary endoprothesis in the palliation of malignant obstruction of the distal common bile duct: a randomized trial. *Br J Surg* 1988;75:1166–1168

284. Anderson JR, Sörensen SM, Kruse A, et al. Randomised trial of endoscopic endoprothesis versus operative bypass in malignant obstructive jaundice. *Gut* 1989;30:1132–1135

285. Smith AC, Dowsett JF, Hatfield ARW. A prospective randomised trial of by-pass surgery versus endoscopic stenting in patients with malignant obstructive jaundice [abstract]. *Gut* 1989;30:A1513

286. Dowsett JF, Russell RCG, Hatfield ARW. Malignant obstructive jaundice, a prospective randomized trial of bypass surgery vs endoscopic stenting. [abstract] *Gastroenterology* 1989;96:A128

287. Cotton PB. Progress report. ERCP. *Gut* 1977;18:316–341

288. Binmoeller KF, Harris AG, Dumas R, et al. Does the somatostatin analogue octreotide protect against ERCP-induced pancreatitis? *Gut* 1992;33:1129–1133

289. Persson B, Slezak P, Efendic S, Häggmark A. Can somatostatin prevent injection pancreatitis after ERCP? *Hepatogastroenterol* 1992;39:259–261

290. Sternlieb JM, Aronchick CA, Retig JN. A multicenter, randomized, controlled trial to evaluate the effect of prophylactic octreotide on ERCP-induced pancreatitis. *Am J Gastroenterol* 1992;87:1561–1566

291. Kullman E, Borch, Lindström E. et al. Bacteremia following diagnostic and therapeutic ERCP. *Gastrointest Endosc* 1992;38:444–449

292. Keighley MRB. Micro-organisms in the bile. A preventable cause of sepsis after biliary surgery. *Ann R Coll Surg Engl* 1977;59:328–324

293. Devière J, Motte S, Dumonceau JM, et al. Septicemia after endoscopic retrograde cholangiopancreatography. *Endoscopy* 1990;22:72–75

294. Classen DC, Jacobson JA, Burke JP, et al. Serious pseudomonal infections associated with endoscopic retrograde cholangiopancreatography. *Am J Med* 1988;84:590–596

295. Lambert ME, Betts CD, Hill J, et al. Endoscopic sphincterotomy: the whole truth. *Br J Surg* 1991;78:473–476

296. Cotton PB, Baillie J, Pappas TN, Meyers WS. Laparoscopic cholecystectomy and the biliary endoscopist. *Gastrointest Endosc* 1991;37:94–97

297. Staritz M, Ewe K, Goerg K, et al. Endoscopic balloon tamponade for conservative management of severe hemorrhage following endoscopic sphincterotomy. *Z Gastroenterol* 1984;22:644–646

298. Sarr M, Fishman EK, Milligan FD, et al. Pancreatitis or duodenal perforation after peri-Vaterian therapeutic endoscopic procedures: diagnosis, differentiation, and management. *Surgery* 1986;100:461–466

299. Foutch PG, Sawyer R, Sanowski RA. Push-enteroscopy for diagnosis of patients with gastrointestinal bleeding of obscure origin. *Gastrointest Endosc* 1990;36:337–341

300. Lau WY. Intraoperative enterscopy—indications and limitations. *Gastrointest Endosc* 1990;36:268–271

301. Greenberg G, Phillips M, Tovee E, Jeejeebhoy KN. Fiberoptic endoscopy during laparotomy in the diagnosis of small intestinal bleeding. *Gastroenterology* 1976;71:133–135

302. Bowden T, Hooks V, Marnsberger A. Intraoperative gastrointestinal endoscopy. *Ann Surg* 1980;191:680–687

303. Strodel W, Eckhauser F, Knol J, et al. Intraoperative fiberoptic endoscopy. *Am Surg* 1984;50:340–344

304. Mathus-Vliegen E, Tytgat G. Intraoperative endoscopy: Technique, indications, and results. *Gastrointest Endosc* 1986;32:381–384

305. Tada M, Shimizu S, Kawai K. A new transnasal sonde-type fiberscope (SSIF VII) as a pan-enteroscope. *Endoscopy* 1986;18:121–124

306. Lewis B, Waye J. Total small bowel enteroscopy. *Gastrointest Endosc* 1987;33:435–438

307. Lewis B, Waye J. Chronic gastrointestinal bleeding of obscure origin: The role of small bowel enteroscopy. *Gastroenterology* 1988;94:1117–1120

308. Lewis B, Waye J. Small bowel enteroscopy in 1988: pros and cons. *Am J Gastroenterol* 1988;83:799–802

309. Lewis BS, Wenger JS, Waye JD. Small bowel enteroscopy and intraoperative enteroscopy for obscure gastrointestinal bleeding. *Am J Gastroenterol* 1991;86:171–174

310. American Cancer Society. Cancer of the colon and rectum. *CA* 1980;30:208–215

311. Summary of Current Guidelines for the Cancer-Related Checkup: Recommendations. New York, NY: American Cancer Society; 1989

312. Working Guidelines for Early Cancer Detection: Rationale and Supporting Evidence to Decrease Mortality. Bethesda, MD: National Cancer Institute; 1987

313. Smart CR. Critique of the early cancer detection guidelines of the US Preventive Services Task Force and the National Cancer Institute. *Mayo Clin Proc* 1990;65:892–898

314. Clinical Efficacy Assessment Project. Screening for Colorectal Cancer. Philadelphia, PA: American College of Physicians: 1990

315. Neugut AI and Pita S. Role of sigmoidoscopy in screening for colorectal cancer: a critical review. *Gastroenterology* 1988;95:492–499

316. England WL, Halls JJ, Hunt VB. Strategies for screening for colorectal carcinoma. *Med Decis Making* 1989;9:3–13

317. Selby JV, Friedman GD. Sigmoidoscopy in the periodic health examination of asymptomatic adults. *JAMA* 1989;261:595–601

318. Ransohoff DF, Lang CA. Screening for colorectal cancer. *N Engl J Med* 1991;325:37–41

319. Foutch PG, Mai H, Pardy K. Flexible sigmoidoscopy may be ineffective for secondary prevention of colorectal cancer in asymptomatic, average-risk men. *Dig Dis Sci* 1991;36:924–928

320. Foley DP, Dunne P, Dervan PJ, et al. Left-sided colonoscopy and haemoccult screening for colorectal neoplasia. *Eur J Gastroenterol Hepatol* 1992;4:925–936

321. Selby JV, Friedman GD, Quesenberry, Jr CP, Weiss NS. A case-control study of screening sigmoidoscopy and mortality from colorectal cancer. *N Engl J Med* 1992;326:653–657

322. Selby JV, Friedman GD, Collen MF. Sigmoidoscopy and mortality from colorectal cancer: the Kaiser Permanente Multiphasic Evaluation Study. *J Clin Epidemiol* 1988;41:427–434

323. DiSario JA, Foutch PG, Mai HD, et al. Prevalence and malignant potential of colorectal polyps in asymptomatic, average-risk men. *Am J Gastroenterol* 1991;86:941–945

324. Rex DK, Lehman GA, Hawes RA, et al. Screening colonoscopy in asymptomatic average-risk persons with negative fecal occult blood tests. *Gastroenterology* 1991;100:64–67

325. Achkar E, Carey W. Small polyps found during fiberoptic sigmoidoscopy in asymptomatic patients. *Ann Intern Med* 1988;109:880–883

326. Provenzale D, Martin ZZ, Holland KL, Sandler RS. Colon adenomas in patients with hyperplastic polyps. *J Clin Gastroenterol* 1988;10:46–49

327. Blue MG, Sivak MV Jr, Achkar E, et al. Hyperplastic polyps seen at sigmoidoscopy are markers for additional adenomas seen at colonoscopy. *Gastroenterology* 1991;100:564–566

328. Provenzale D, Garrett JW, Condon SE, Sandler RS. Risk for colon adenomas in patients with rectosigmoid hyperplastic polyps. *Ann Intern Med* 1990;113:760–763

329. Rex DK, Smith JJ, Ulbright TM, Lehman GA. Distal colonic hyperplastic polyps do not predict proximal adenomas in asymptomatic average-risk subjects. *Gastroenterology* 1992;102:317–319

330. American Society of Gastrointestinal Endoscopy. Appropriate use of gastrointestinal endoscopy. *Gastrointest Endosc* 1989;34(Suppl 8S):5–11

331. Health and Public Policy Committee, American College of Physicians. Clinical competence in colonoscopy. *Ann Intern Med* 1987;107:772–774

332. Eddy DM, Nugent FW, Eddy J, et al. Screening for colorectal cancer in a high-risk population. *Gastroenterology* 1987;92:682–692

333. Eddy DM. Screening for colorectal cancer. *Ann Intern Med* 1990;113:373–384

334. Sauar J, Hausken T, Hoff G, et al. Colonoscopic screening examination of relatives of patients with colorectal cancer, I: a comparison with an endoscopically screened normal population. *Scand J Gastroenterol* 1992;27:661–666

335. Sauar J, Hoff G, Hausken T, et al. Colonoscopic screening examination of relatives of patients with colorectal cancer. II. Relations between tumour characteristics and the presence of polyps. *Scand J Gastroenterol* 1992;27:667–672

336. Love RR, Morrissey JF. Colonoscopy in asymptomatic individuals with a family history of colorectal cancer. *Arch Intern Med* 1984;144:2209–2211

337. Lanspa SJ, Lynch HT, Smyrk TC, et al. Colorectal adenomas in the Lynch Syndromes. *Gastroenterology* 1990;98:1117–1122

338. Fleischer DE, Goldberg SB, Browning TH. Detection and surveillance of colorectal cancer. *JAMA* 1989;261:580–585

339. Löfberg R, Broström O, Karlén P, et al. Colonoscopic surveillance in long-standing total ulcerative colitis—a 15-year follow-up study. *Gastroenterology* 1990;99:1021–1031

340. Lennard-Jones JE, Melville DM, Morson BC, et al. Precancer and cancer in extensive ulcerative colitis: findings among 401 patients over 22 years. *Gut* 1990;31:800–806

341. Gyde S. Screening for colorectal cancer in ulcerative colitis: dubious benefits and high costs. *Gut* 1990;31:1089–1092

342. Nugent FW, Haggitt RC, Gilpin PA. Cancer surveillance in ulcerative colitis. *Gastroenterology* 1991;100:1241–1248

343. Woolrich AJ, DaSilva M, Korelitz BI. Surveillance in the routine management of ulcerative colitis: the predictive value of low-grade dysplasia. *Gastroenterology* 1992;103:431–438

344. Langholz E, Munkholm P, Davidson M, Binder V. Colorectal cancer risk and mortality in patients with ulcerative colitis. *Gastroenterology* 1992;103:1444–1451

345. Löfberg R, Broström O, Karlén P, et al. DNA aneuploidy in ulcerative colitis: reproducibility, topographic distribution, and relation to dysplasia. *Gastroenterology* 1992;102:1149–1154

346. Rubin CE, Haggitt RC, Burmer GC, et al. DNA aneuploidy in colonic biopsies predicts future development

of dysplasia in ulcerative colitis. *Gastroenterology* 1992;103:1611–1620

347. Alemayehu G, Järnerot G. Colonoscopy during an attack of severe ulcerative colitis is a safe procedure and of great value in clinical decision making. *Am J Gastroenterol* 1991;86:187–190

348. The Role of Colonoscopy in the Management of Patients with Colonic Polyps. American Society of Gastrointestinal Endoscopy. Manchester, MA: Publication 1014, 1986.

349. Ransohoff DF, Lang CA, Sung Kuo H. Colonoscopic surveillance after polypectomy: considerations of cost-effectiveness. *Ann Intern Med* 1991;114:177–182

350. Bond JH. Polyp guideline: diagnosis, treatment, and surveillance for patients with nonfamilial colorectal polyps. *Ann Intern Med* 1993;119;836–843

351. Davis GR, Santa Ana CA, Morawski SG et al. Development of a lavage solution associated with minimal water and electrolyte absorption or secretion. *Gastroenterology* 1980;78:991–995

352. Froehlich F, Fried M, Schnegg JF, Gonvers JJ. Low sodium solution for colonic cleansing: a double-blind, controlled, randomized prospective study. *Gastrointest Endosc* 1992;38:579–581

353. Cotton PB, Williams CB. *Practical Gastrointestinal Endoscopy.* Oxford, England: Blackwell Scientific; 1990

354. Bond JH, Levitt MD: Colonic gas explosion—is a fire extinguisher necessary? [editorial]. *Gastroenterology* 1979; 77:1349–1350

355. Webb WA. Colonoscoping the "difficult" colon. *Am Surg* 1991;57:178–182

356. Irvine EJ, O'Connor JO, Frost RA, et al. Prospective comparison of double contrast barium enema plus flexible sigmoidoscopy versus colonoscopy in rectal bleeding: barium enema versus colonoscopy in rectal bleeding. *Gut* 1988;29:1188–1193

357. Rex DK, Weddle RA, Lehman GA, et al. Flexible sigmoidoscopy plus air contrast barium enema versus colonoscopy for suspected lower gastrointestinal bleeding. *Gastroenterology* 1990;98:855–861

358. Standards of Training and Practice Committee, American Society of Gastrointestinal Endoscopy. The role of endoscopy in patients with lower gastrointestinal bleeding. *Gastrointest Endosc* 1988;34(suppl): S23–S25

359. Health and Public Policy Committee, American College of Physicians. Clinical competence in colonoscopy. *Ann Intern Med* 1987;107:772–774

360. Thomas WM, Hardcastle JD. Role of upper gastrointestinal investigations in a screening study for colorectal neoplasia. *Gut* 1990;31:1294–1297

361. Jensen DM, Machicado GA. Diagnosis and treatment of severe hematochezia. *Gastroenterology* 1989;96:299–306

362. Morson BC, Sobin LH. Histological typing of intestinal tumours. In International Histological Classification of Tumours. No. 15. Geneva, Switzerland: World Health Organization; 1976

363. Fenoglio CM, Pascal RR. Colorectal adenomas and cancer: pathologic relationships. *Cancer* 1982;50:2601–2608

364. de Roos A, Hermans J, Shaw PC, Kroon H. Colon polyps and carcinomas: prospective comparison of the single- and double-contrast examination in the same patients. *Radiology* 1985;154:11–13

365. Jensen J, Kewenter J, Asztely M, et al. Double contrast barium and flexible rectosigmoidoscopy: a reliable diagnostic combination for detection of colorectal neoplasm. *Br J Surg* 1990;77:270–272

366. Knutson CO, Max MH: Diagnostic and therapeutic colonoscopy. A critical review of 663 examinations. *Arch Surg* 1979;114:430–435

367. Shinya H, Wolff WI. Morphology, anatomic distribution and cancer potential of colonic polyps: analysis of 7000 polyps endoscopically removed. *Ann Surg* 1979;190:679–683

368. Hogan WJ, Stewart ET, Geenen JE, Doggs WJ, et al. A prospective comparison of the accuracy of colonoscopy vs air-barium contrast exam for detection of colonic polypoid lesions. [abstract] *Gastrointest Endosc* 1977;23:230

369. Hixson LJ, Fennerty MB, Sampliner RE, Garewal HS. Prospective blinded trial of the colonoscopic miss-rate of large colorectal polyps. *Gastrointest Endosc* 1991;37:125–127

370. Gilbertsen VA, Nelms JM. The prevention of invasive cancer of the rectum. *Cancer* 1978;41:1137–1139

371. Winawer SJ, Zauber AG, Ho MN, et al. Prevention of colorectal cancer by colonoscopic polypectomy. The National Polyp Study Workgroup. *N Engl J Med* 1993;329:2020–2029

372. Waye JD. Endoscopic treatment of adenomas. *World J Surg* 1991;15:14–19

373. Walsh RM, Ackroyd FW, Shellito PC. Endoscopic resection of large sessile colorectal polyps. *Gastrointest Endosc* 1992;38:303–309

374. Morson BC, Whiteway JE, Jones EA, et al. Histopathology and prognosis of malignant colorectal polyps treated by endoscopic polypectomy. *Gut* 1984;25:437–444

375. Cranley JP, Petras RE, Carey WD, et al. When is endoscopic polypectomy adequate therapy for colonic polyps containing invasive carcinoma? *Gastroenterology* 1986;91:419–427

376. Eckardt VF, Fuchs M, Kanzler G, et al. Follow-up of patients with colonic polyps containing severe atypia and invasive carcinoma. *Cancer* 1988;61:2552–2557

377. Muto T, Sawada T, Sugihara K. Treatment of carcinoma in adenomas. *World J Surg* 1991;15:35–40

378. Coverlizza S, Risio M, Ferrari A, Fenoglio-Preiser CM, Rossini FP. Colorectal adenomas containing invasive carcinoma: pathologic assessment of lymph node metastatic potential. *Cancer* 1989;64:1937–1947

379. Nivatvongs S, Rojanasakul A, Reiman HM, et al. The risk of lymph node metastasis in colorectal polyps with invasive adenocarcinoma. *Dis Colon Rectum* 1991;34:323–328

380. Ogilvie H. Large intestinal colic due to sympathetic deprivation: a new clinical syndrome. *Br Med J* 1948;2:671

381. Gosche JR, Sharpe JN, Larson GM. Colonoscopic decompression for pseudo-obstruction of the colon. *Am Surg* 1989;55:111–115

382. Harig JM, Fumo DE, Loo FD, et al. Treatment of acute nontoxic megacolon during colonoscopy: tube placement versus simple decompression. *Gastrointest Endosc* 1988;34:23–27

383. Strodel WE, Brothers T. Colonoscopic decompression of pseudo-obstruction and volvulus. *Surg Clin NA* 1989;69:1327–1335

384. Marcon NE. Endoscopic colonic decompression. *Can J Gastroenterol* 1990;4:542–545

385. Vanek VW, Al-Salti M. Acute pseudo-obstruction of the colon (Ogilvie's syndrome): an analysis of 400 cases. *Dis Colon Rectum* 1986;29:203–210

386. Starling JR. Initial treatment of sigmoid volvulus by colonoscopy. *Ann Surg* 1979;190:36–39

387. Tejler G, Jiborn H. Volvulus of the cecum: report of 26 cases and review of the literature. *Dis Colon Rectum* 1988;31:445–449

388. Kozarek RA. Hydrostatic balloon dilation of gastrointestinal stenoses: a national survey. *Gastrointest Endosc* 1986;32:15–19

389. Oz MC, Forde KA. Endoscopic alternatives in the management of colonic strictures. *Surgery* 1990;108:513–519

390. Dinneen MD, Motson RW. Treatment of colonic anastomotic strictures with 'through the scope' balloon dilators. *J Royal Soc Med* 1991;84:264–266

391. Blomberg B, Rolny P, Järnerot G. Endoscopic treatment of anastomotic strictures in Crohn's disease. *Endoscopy* 1991;23:195–198

392. Breysem Y, Janssens JF, Coremans G, et al. Endoscopic balloon dilation of colonic and ileo-colonic Crohn's strictures: long-term results. *Gastrointest Endosc* 1992;38: 142–147

393. Kiefhaber P, Keifhaber K, Huber F. Preoperative neodymium: YAG laser treatment of obstructive colon cancer. *Endoscopy* 1986;18:44–46

394. Eckhauser ML. Laser therapy of colorectal carcinoma. *Surg Clin N Am* 1992;72:597–607

395. Mathus-Vliegen EMH, Tytgat GNJ. Laser ablation and palliation in colorectal malignancy. *Gastrointest Endosc* 1986;32:393–396

396. Brunetaud JM, Maunoury V, Ducrotte P. Palliative treatment of rectosigmoid carcinoma by laser endoscopic photoablation. *Gastroenterology* 1987;92:663–668

397. Daneker GW Jr, Carlson GW, Hohn DC, et al. Endoscopic laser recanalization is effective for prevention and treatment of obstructions in sigmoid and rectal cancer. *Arch Surg* 1991;126:1348–1352

398. Rogers BHG, Silvis SE, Nebel OT, et al. Complications of flexible fiberoptic colonoscopy and polypectomy. An analysis of the 1974 ASGE survey. *Gastrointest Endosc* 1975;22:73–77

399. Smith LF. Symposium. Fiberoptic colonoscopy: complications of colonoscopy and polypectomy. *Dis Colon Rectum* 1976;19:407–412

400. Fruhmorgen P, Demling L. Complications of diagnostic and therapeutic colonoscopy in the Federal Republic of Germany: results of an inquiry. *Endoscopy* 1979;11: 146–150

401. Waye JD, Lewis BS, Yessayan S. Colonoscopy: a prospective report of complications. *J Clin Gastroenterol* 1992;15: 347–351

402. Hunt RH. Towards safer colonoscopy. *Gut* 1983;24: 371–375

403. Livstone EM, Cohen GM, Troncale FJ, Touloukian RJ. Diastatic serosal lacerations: an unrecognized complication of colonoscopy. *Gastroenterology* 1974;67:1245–1247

404. Spencer RJ, Coates HL, Anderson MJ Jr. Colonoscopic polypectomies. *Mayo Clinic Proc* 1974;49:40–43

405. Kavin H, Sinicrope F, Esker AH. Management of perforation of the colon at colonoscopy. *Am J Gastroenterol* 1992;87:161–167

406. Christie JP, Marrazzo J III. "Mini-perforation" of the colon—not all postpolypectomy perforations require laparotomy. *Dis Colon Rectum* 1991;34:132–135

407. Waye JD. The postpolypectomy coagulation syndrome. *Gastrointest Endosc* 1981;27:184–186

408. Kimmey MB, Martin RW, Haggitt RC, et al. Histologic correlates of gastrointestinal ultrasound images. *Gastroenterology* 1989;96:433–441

409. Botet JF, Lightdale CJ, Zauber AG, et al. Preoperative staging of esophageal cancer: comparison of endoscopic US and dynamic CT. *Radiology* 1991;181:419–425

410. Rösch T, Lightdale CJ, Botet JF. Localization of pancreatic endocrine tumors by endoscopic ultrasound. *N Engl J Med* 1992;326:1721–1726

411. Botet JF, Lightdale CJ, Zauber AG, et al. Preoperative staging of gastric cancer: comparison of endoscopic US and dynamic CT. *Radiology* 1991;181:426–432

412. Rösch T, Braig C, Gain T, et al. Staging of pancreatic and ampullary carcinoma by endoscopic ultrasonography. Comparison with conventional sonography, computed tomography, and angiography. *Gastroenterology* 1992; 102:188–199

413. Lightdale CJ, Botet JF, Woodruff JM, Brennan MF. Localization of endocrine tumors of the pancreas with endoscopic ultrasonography. *Cancer* 1991;68:1815–1820

414. Snady H, Cooperman A, Siegel J. Endoscopic ultrasonography compared with computed tomography with ERCP in patients with obstructive jaundice or small peripancreatic mass. *Gastrointest Endosc* 1992;38: 27–34

415. Tio TL, Wijers OB, Sars PRA, Tytgat GNJ. Endosonographic TNM staging of extrahepatic bile duct cancer: comparison with pathological staging. *Gastroenterology* 1991;100:1351–1361

416. Tio TL, Coene PPLO, van Delden OM, Tytgat GNJ. Colorectal carcinoma: Preoperative TNM classification with endosonography. *Radiology* 1991;179:165–170

417. van Outryve MJ, Pelckmans PA, Michielsen PP, van Maercke YM. Value of transrectal ultrasonography in Crohn's disease. *Gastroenterology* 1991;101:1171–1177

418. Nousbaum JB, Robaszkiewica M, Cauvin JM, et al. Endosonography can detect residual tumour infiltration after medical treatment of oesophageal cancer in the absence of endoscopic lesions. *Gut* 1992;33:1459–1461

4

Laparoscopic Surgery

L. Michael Brunt ■ *Nathaniel J. Soper*

Laparoscopy is a technique in which the peritoneal cavity and abdominal contents are examined using an endoscope inserted directly through the abdominal wall. At the time of the publication of the last edition of this textbook in 1990, laparoscopic applications in general surgery were limited primarily to diagnostic procedures, which were being performed by a minority of practicing surgeons. However, two subsequent events have dramatically altered the nature of laparoscopic surgery: (1) the attachment of a miniature television camera to the eyepiece of the laparoscope has allowed visualization of the operative field on a video monitor, and (2) the development and widespread acceptance of laparoscopic cholecystectomy. As a result, general surgery has undergone an unprecedented revolution that has required the retraining of surgeons and the reequipping of operating rooms worldwide for the performance of laparoscopic surgery.

The benefits of laparoscopic or minimally invasive surgery over traditional open abdominal surgery are most evident from series comparing laparoscopic to open cholecystectomy.[1-3] These series have demonstrated that the laparoscopic approach leads to a reduction in postoperative pain and diminished postoperative hospitalization and disability. The advantages of laparoscopic cholecystectomy have quickly led to its acceptance as a standard therapy for the treatment of patients with symptomatic cholelithiasis.[4] Consequently, techniques have rapidly developed for minimally invasive surgical approaches to other organs within the abdomen. This chapter begins with a review of the principles of laparoscopic techniques, equipment, instrumentation, and other aspects of basic laparoscopy. The technical features of specific laparoscopic procedures along with the clinical indications and results using a minimally invasive approach also are reviewed.

■ HISTORICAL BACKGROUND

Several of the landmark contributions to the development of surgical laparoscopy in the 20th century are shown in Table 4–1. The first endoscopes were crude instruments that were limited by their poor optics and the risks of thermal injury from the light. Two important technologic advances in the late 19th century that allowed the development of viable endoscopes were the invention of the incandescent light bulb by Edison in 1880 and improved optical systems developed in Germany in the 1890s. In 1897, Nitze[5] reported his experience with the first modern cystoscope. In 1901, Kelling[6] used the cystoscope to perform the first laparoscopic examination of the abdominal cavity in a canine model. Kelling created a pneumoperitoneum by injecting the abdominal cavity with air and inserting a cystoscope through the abdominal wall. Since Kelling was able to view the peritoneal cavity and its contents through the endoscope, he termed this new procedure *celioscopy*. In 1911, Jacobeus[7] performed the first endoscopic examinations of the abdominal and thoracic cavities in humans and is credited with coining the terms *laparoscopy*

TABLE 4–1. HISTORICAL MILESTONES IN LAPAROSCOPIC SURGERY

Year	Investigator	Contribution
1901	Kelling	1st laparoscopic exam of the abdominal cavity
1911	Jacobeus	1st laparoscopic exam in humans
1929	Kalk	Dual trocar technique
1938	Veress	Spring-loaded obturator needle for pneumoperitoneum
1966	Hopkins	Development of the rod lens optical system
1960's & 1970's	Semm	Development of automatic CO_2 insufflator and numerous laparoscopic instruments
Early 1980's	—	Development of miniature TV camera chip
1987	Mouret	1st laparoscopic cholecystectomy

and *thoracoscopy*. Jacobeus carried out 115 laparoscopic examinations over a period of 1 year, with only one major complication that required open laparotomy. However, because of limitations in exposure and laparoscopic instrumentation, these early laparoscopic procedures were diagnostic only. In 1929, Kalk[8] reported the use of a dual trocar technique which allowed simultaneous insertion of operating instruments and improved the diagnostic and therapeutic capabilities of laparoscopic surgery. Early laparoscopists frequently introduced their trocars and laparoscopes directly into the abdominal cavity without first creating a pneumoperitoneum. In 1938, Veress[9] developed a spring-loaded obturator needle for inducing therapeutic pneumothorax in patients with tuberculosis. This needle subsequently was adapted for establishing pneumoperitoneum in a safer manner and remains in use today.

In spite of these improvements in laparoscopic technique and instrumentation, laparoscopy was performed infrequently in the ensuing two decades because it was considered a blind procedure with an increased risk of serious injury to intraperitoneal organs. However, in the 1960s, further technologic advances and surgical innovations led to the increased acceptance of laparoscopy. In 1966, the Hopkins rod lens system was developed for rigid endoscopes that greatly improved image clarity and brightness. Kurt Semm, a German gynecologist and engineer, also pioneered many new techniques and technological advances in laparoscopic surgery in the 1960s.[10] One of his most significant contributions was the development of an automatic insufflator that precisely controlled gas flow and monitored intra-abdominal pressures during laparoscopy. Semm also developed a variety of laparoscopic surgical instruments and performed the first laparoscopic appendectomy in 1983.[11] For his many contributions, Semm is recognized as one of the fathers of modern laparoscopic abdominal surgery.

Although these advances led to the widespread use of laparoscopy for diagnostic and sterilization procedures in gynecologic surgery, few general surgeons used it in their surgical practice. The exceptions were pioneering individuals such as George Berci and Alfred Cushieri, who used diagnostic laparoscopy for evaluating and staging patients with abdominal malignancies.[12,13] In the early 1980s, a miniature television camera was developed that attached directly to the laparoscope. Coupled with high resolution video monitors, it provided a video endoscopic view of the abdominal cavity. With this technologic breakthrough, it was possible to coordinate movements by the surgeon and assistants, enabling them to carry out more complex laparoscopic tasks and procedures. Subsequently, in 1987, Phillipe Mouret,[14] in France, performed the first laparoscopic cholecystectomy in a human. Almost simultaneously McKernan and Saye[15] performed the first laparoscopic cholecystectomy in the United States in 1988. The procedure was quickly popularized in the United States by Reddick and Olsen,[16] who are credited with the first report of laparoscopic cholecystectomy in the English literature.[17] The widespread acceptance of laparoscopic cholecystectomy by the public[18] and the surgical community has expanded surgical laparoscopy into most areas of general surgery and other surgical disciplines.

■ EQUIPMENT AND INSTRUMENTATION

LAPAROSCOPES

Modern laparoscopes come in a variety of sizes and configurations (Fig 4–1). The most commonly used laparoscopes are rigid instruments that employ the Hopkins rod lens system of optics. The basic components of the rod lens system include a series of quartz rod lenses and image reversal system, optical fibers for the transmission of light, an objective lens, and an eyepiece.[19] These features allow enhanced light transmission and image resolution, as well as superior color reproduction. Rigid laparoscopes come in sizes ranging from 3 to 10 mm in diameter and a variety of viewing angles. The 0° or end/forward viewing laparoscope is the easiest to use, and its use results in the least amount of image distortion, as well as the brightest image. Angled (30°, 45°) scopes provide greater versatility by allowing the operator to look around corners and over the surfaces of solid structures (eg, the liver). Although oblique viewing scopes are more difficult to operate because the orientation axis of both the telescopic lens and video camera must be maintained, they are preferred by most experienced laparoscopists for performing advanced procedures. Recently, flexible laparoscopes have been developed that use fiberoptic bundles for visualization and that provide even greater flexibility in the viewing angle (Fig 4–1B).

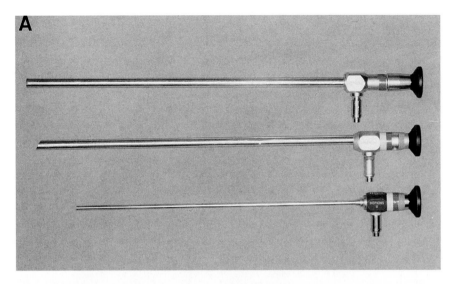

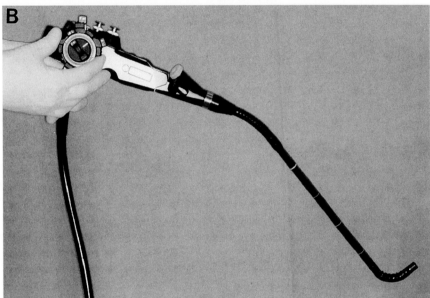

Figure 4–1. Laparoscopes. **A**. Standard laparoscopes are the 10 mm straight (0°) scope (top), 10 mm 30° laparoscope (middle) and 5 mm 0° scope (bottom). **B**. Flexible 10 mm laparoscope (Fujinon, Inc).

The laparoscopic field may be viewed directly through the eyepiece or through an attached video camera that projects the image onto a video monitor. The image seen directly through the eyepiece is generally sharper and truer in color than the video image, but coordinated movements by different members of the surgical team are nearly impossible to perform. The use of a video camera therefore is required for most laparoscopic surgical procedures other than simple diagnostic examinations. Another limitation of most rigid laparoscopes is repetitive fogging of the lens due to condensation from high temperature and humidity within the peritoneal cavity. Use of an antifog solution or pre-

warming of the laparoscope in hot water is required to counteract this problem.

VIDEO IMAGING SYSTEMS

The single most important technologic advance in the field of laparoscopic surgery has been the development of high-quality video imaging systems that allow surgeons to work together while watching a video monitor. The basic components required for video laparoscopy include the laparoscope, a light source, a video camera, a camera control unit, and a video monitor (Fig 4–2). A high-intensity light source (usually xenon) is necessary

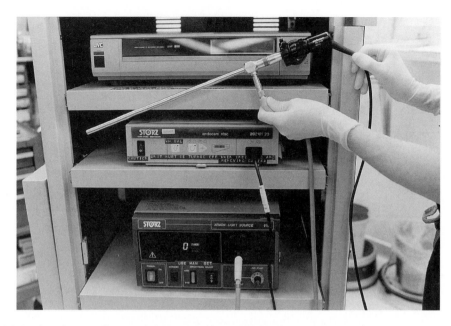

Figure 4–2. Video unit for laparoscopic surgery. Shown are the laparoscope with attached light cable and camera that are connected to the light source and camera control unit, respectively. A videocassette recorder also is connected to the system. Not shown is a videomonitor positioned on top of the videocart.

to provide adequate illumination of the peritoneal cavity. The light source is connected to the laparoscope by either a fiberoptic cable or a fluid-filled cable. The fiberoptic cables consist of an inner core of glass that has a high refractive index which absorbs much of the light input but which is subject to maintenance difficulties owing to breakage of individual fiberoptic glass rods. Fluid-filled cables consist of plastic fluid-filled tubes, the ends of which are sealed by quartz plugs. Compared to the fiberoptic cables, these fluid-filled cables have less light absorption and improved natural color display. The transmission of heat, generated by the light source, to the end of the laparoscope was a major problem with earlier light sources and had the potential for causing burns internally, or fires externally. However, modern light sources are equipped with a heat shield that reduces the amount of heat transmitted through the cable to minimize this risk. Nonetheless, thermal damage is still possible if the end of a laparoscope is left in contact with an object for a prolonged period of time.

The video camera is attached directly to the eyepiece of the laparoscope and contains both a manual focus mechanism and a zoom capability. The essential electronic component of the video camera is a solid-state chip sensor or a charged coupled device (CCD). The CCD functions as an electronic retina that transmits light received from the laparoscope into an electronic signal and then is transduced into a video image. The CCD itself comprises numerous light-sensitive photodiodes, or pixels.[20] Light activation of an individual pixel results in the generation of an electronic signal that is conducted via cable to the camera control unit housed on the video cart. The camera control unit then processes this signal and reconstructs the image on the video monitor using conventional horizontal scanning.

The quality of the video image depends on several technical factors, including resolution, color, light sensitivity, signal to noise ratio, and image size.[20,21] The degree of resolution of the video camera is determined by the number of pixels in the CCD. The minimal resolving power required of the video camera for operative laparoscopy should be 400 lines of resolution per inch. Most laparoscopic cameras currently in use have a single-chip sensor that provides a 450 horizontal lines/inch of resolution. Newer three-chip cameras also have been developed that provide up to 700 lines/inch of resolution and improve chromatic accuracy.

High-resolution video monitors are required for suitable reproduction of the endoscopic image. In general, the resolution capability of the monitor should match that of the video camera such that a one-chip camera is best coupled with a monitor that provides at least 400 lines of resolution/inch. Three-chip cameras require more expensive monitors with 700 lines of resolution to realize the improved resolution of the extra chip sensors.

Two separate video monitors, placed on each side of the operating table, are commonly used for most laparoscopic cases, allowing all members of the surgical team an unobstructed view of the operation. Additional monitors may be useful for some advanced laparoscopic procedures. The screen size of the video monitor ranges from 13 to 21 inches. The use of special video carts for housing the monitors and other video components allows greater flexibility (Fig 4–3).

Several new technologies under development have the potential to enhance video imaging capabilities in laparoscopic surgery. These include three-dimensional videolaparoscopes, robotics, and high-definition television. The considerable expense of many of these new technologies, however, currently limits their application to investigational centers.

INSUFFLATORS

The creation of a working space for laparoscopic surgery within the abdominal cavity generally is accomplished using CO_2 delivered to the patient via an automatic, high-flow, pressure-regulated insufflator. A variety of gases have been used in the past to obtain pneumoperitoneum, including room air, oxygen, nitrous oxide, and carbon dioxide. Room air and oxygen are no longer used because they support combustion and carry an increased risk of gas embolism. Nitrous oxide has unpredictable absorption characteristics and may support combustion, limiting its clinical utility. Carbon dioxide is currently the agent of choice because of the low risk of gas embolism, lack of toxicity to peritoneal tissues, rapid rate of reabsorption, low cost and ease of use. It also suppresses combustion, making it safe for use with the electrocautery or laser.

Ideally, the insufflator should be able to deliver CO_2 at a flow rate of up to 8 to 10 L/min with a minimum acceptable flow rate of 6 L/min. At lower maximal flow rates, loss of pneumoperitoneum and laparoscopic visualization can occur from small gas leaks and repeated removal and reinsertion of the laparoscopic instruments. In addition to regulating gas flow, the insufflator monitors intra-abdominal pressure and stops delivery of CO_2 whenever the pressure exceeds a predetermined level. This pressure limit usually is set at 12 to 15 mm Hg because of the risk of hypercarbia, acidosis, and adverse hemodynamic and pulmonary effects at higher pressures.[22,23] The insufflator also should be equipped with an alarm that sounds whenever the pressure limit is exceeded. A variety of high-flow insufflators are available for clinical use.

TROCARS AND INSUFFLATION NEEDLES

Two types of instruments are used to gain access to the peritoneal cavity for laparoscopic surgery: the Veress needle and the laparoscopic trocar-sheath assemblies (laparoscopic ports). The Veress needle is designed to achieve pneumoperitoneum prior to inserting laparoscopic trocars in a "closed" fashion. It consists of an outer sharp cutting needle and an inner blunt spring-loaded obturator. As the Veress needle is inserted into the peritoneal cavity, resistance at the muscle fascia causes the blunt tip to retract backwards (Fig 4–4). Once the cutting needle has penetrated freely into the

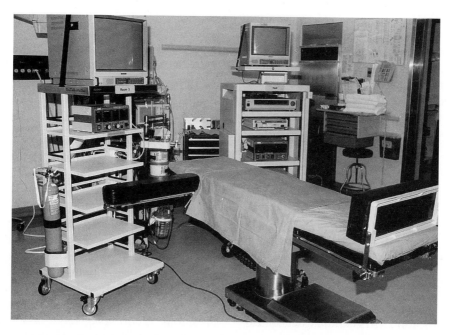

Figure 4–3. Operating room set up for laparoscopic surgery. The two carts on either side of the operating room table house videomonitors, a CO_2 insufflator, light source, camera control unit and videocassette recorder.

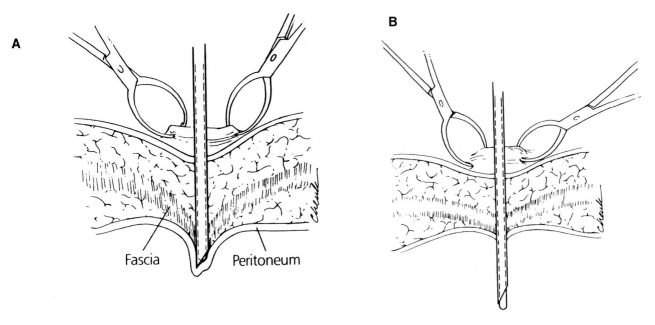

Figure 4–4. Veress needle insertion. **A**. As the sharp edge of the needle penetrates the muscle fascia, the blunt tip retracts into the needle sheath. **B**. Once the needle has penetrated freely into the peritoneal cavity, the blunt stylet springs forward beyond the cutting needle. (Modified from Soper NJ, et al (eds), *Essentials of Laparoscopy*. St. Louis, MO: Quality Medical; 1993:39.

peritoneal cavity, the blunt stylet springs beyond the cutting needle, thereby reducing the risk of injury to intraperitoneal structures. The inner stylet is hollow, with a side hole at its tip to allow instillation of liquid or gas. Both reusable and disposable varieties of Veress needles are available.

The basic laparoscopic port consists of an outer hollow sheath or cannula that has a valve to prevent CO_2 gas from escaping, a side port for instillation of gas, and a portal for instrument access. An inner removable trocar fits through the outer sheath and is used only while inserting the port through the abdominal wall. The most commonly used trocars are 5 mm and 10 mm in diameter, although ports ranging from 3 to 18 mm in diameter are available for specialized procedures. The principal choice of trocars is between reusable versus disposable (Fig 4–5). Reusable trocars are radiopaque and equipped with rotational trumpet valves and gaskets to prevent air leaks. They have the advantage of lower costs, but they require careful maintenance to keep the trocar tips sharp and the unit airtight. A variety of disposable trocars are available commercially from a number of different manufacturers. Disposable trocars may be equipped with a retractable safety shield that sheaths the trocar tip upon entry into the peritoneal cavity, possibly decreasing the risk of organ injury. The single-use trocar tip also guarantees sharpness with each insertion. Disposable trocars contain flapper valves to prevent gas leaks and are generally radiolu-

cent. Special gripping devices can be attached to many of the disposable trocars to prevent their inadvertent displacement during the laparoscopic procedure. Both types of trocars come with reducer sheaths that allow insertion of smaller instruments through the larger port while preventing gas leakage.

The Hasson cannula is used for gaining initial access to the abdominal cavity with an open cutdown technique. It has a conical blunt tip which is fitted into the cutdown site and buttressed in place with fascial sutures attached to the wings of the cannula (Fig 4–6).

SURGICAL INSTRUMENTS

Many instruments have been designed specifically for laparoscopic surgery. These instruments are modifications of standard open-surgical instruments and are 30 to 40 cm in length with shaft diameters of 3 to 10 mm. The shafts of these instruments may be insulated with nonconductive material, and the working tips are metal to allow use with electrocautery and to provide durability. These instruments are more delicate than their open-surgical counterparts and are more likely to break or malfunction if handled improperly. Reusable and disposable variations of most of these instruments are available. The principal advantage of the reusable instruments is cost savings; the disadvantages are the associated maintenance costs, deterioration in function during the period of time they are in use or with im-

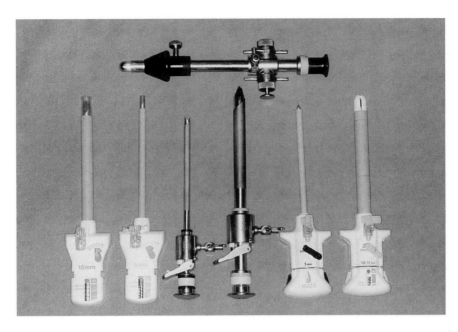

Figure 4–5. Laparoscopic trocars. The trocars shown across the lower panel can be inserted using either an open or closed technique. The Hasson cannula (*top*) requires an open insertion method exclusively.

proper use, and potential difficulties with cleaning and sterilization. Disposable instruments have the advantage of guaranteed sharpness and sterility with each use. They also have improved capabilities for shaft rotation, usually allowing 360° rotation with fingertip control. Potentially, these benefits are offset by both purchasing and waste-disposal costs. Most operating rooms currently utilize a core of reusable instruments supplemented with disposable items, according to the needs or demands of a particular procedure.

A representative assortment of the various laparoscopic dissecting and grasping instruments are shown in Fig 4–7. Most laparoscopic dissecting forceps are equipped with atraumatic (blunt or pointed) tips that can be used to dissect or spread tissues bluntly. Forceps with either a gentle curve or right-angle configuration are particularly useful for dissecting around corners and encircling structures. Grasping instruments come with either atraumatic or toothed jaws. The handles often have a ratchet mechanism for locking onto the tissue being grasped. Large grasping forceps such as the claw forceps can be used for tissue extraction. Fan-shaped retractors are designed for retracting tissues, especially solid organs such as the liver. Laparoscopic cautery probes come with a variety of tips, including spatula, hook, and right-angle configurations. Most cautery probes have additional channels for suction and irrigation. Representative types of laparoscopic scissors are shown in Fig 4–8. The hook scissors have tips that approximate before the jaws cut, thereby making it easier

and safer to cut tubular structures. They also allow one to grasp the tissue and pull it away from adjacent structures before cutting. However, dulling of the blades with erratic cutting is a frequent problem. Microscissors are useful for more delicate incisions, such as those required during cystic duct cholangiography. Scissors with a Metzenbaum-type configuration of the tip with

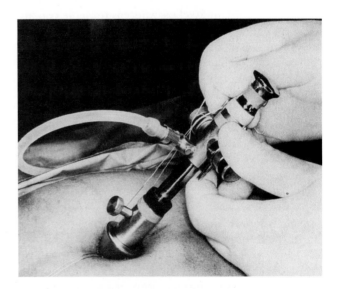

Figure 4–6. Hasson cannula inserted at the umbilicus. The conical tip is wedged into the incision and secured in place with fascial sutures that are looped over the suture wings on the cannula. (From Soderstrom RM. Basic operative technique. In: Soderstrom RM (ed), *Operative Laparoscopy.* New York, NY: Raven Press; 1993:30)

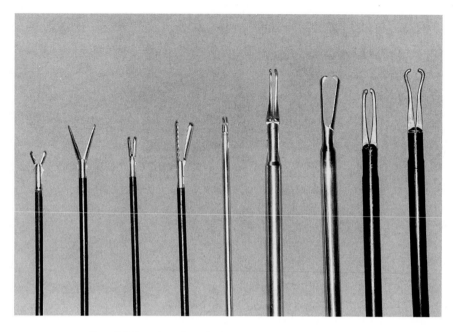

Figure 4–7. Dissecting and grasping instruments for laparoscopic surgery.

cautery capability are useful for performing more complex maneuvers, such as adhesiolysis. The slightly curved jaws of the scissors allow better visualization of the tips and make it easier for cutting to be focused at the instrument tip. The 360° rotational shaft of the cautery scissors facilities dissection at different angles and from different positions.

Clip appliers are the primary modality for ligating blood vessels and other tubular structures. Disposable clip appliers contain 20 clips, whereas reusable clip appliers carry only a single clip at a time, thus requiring the instrument to be removed and reinserted with each application. The clips are made of titanium and range from 7 to 11 mm in length. Disposable clip appliers are generally preferred for use in procedures that require multiple clips.

Ligation of hollow structures also may be accomplished with specialized pre-tied ligating loop sutures. These devices (Fig 4–9) consist of a suture (plain, chromic catgut or polydioxanone material) that has been threaded through a plastic push rod and pre-tied with a slip knot (Roeder knot). The push rod and suture loop are inserted laparoscopically via a hollow reducing sleeve; the suture then is looped around the structure to be ligated, and the knot is slid down to close the loop. The disadvantage of this technique is that the structure to be ligated must be divided prior to applying the pre-tied loop. As laparoscopic general surgery has advanced, a variety of other laparoscopic suturing instruments and suture techniques also have been described.[24] A number

of laparoscopic needle holders have been designed for laparoscopic suturing (Fig 4–10) with either spring-loaded (Castro-type) or ratcheted-handle mechanisms. Sutures may be tied with the laparoscopic instruments, using totally intracorporeal techniques similar to instrument ties. Alternatively, the knots may be tied extracorporeally using either a hand-tied slip knot or standard square knots advanced into position by using a knot-pusher device (Fig 4–11).

Irrigation/aspiration probes are essential for most laparoscopic procedures in order to maintain a clear operative field. Irrigation and aspiration channels may be incorporated into surgical instruments (eg, cautery), but the working channels are small and subject to frequent clogging. Specialized fenestrated suction tips are better for removing large amounts of fluid and blood. Irrigation systems can be driven by gravity, by a pressurized bag, or by a pneumatic pump. The pneumatic pump provides more forceful irrigation (300 to 700 mm Hg pressure) for removal of clots and particulate debris. The addition of heparin (5000 U/L) to the irrigation bag may inhibit clotting and fibrin formation and reduce problems with removal of large clots.

Removal of tissue laparoscopically has become a greater challenge as larger structures and solid organs are being approached with minimally invasive techniques. Specialized entrapment bags for removing tissue have been developed that have a variety of operational and strength characteristics. The type of bag used depends both on the size of the structure being re-

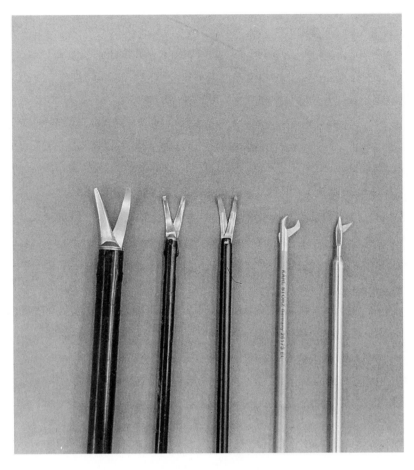

Figure 4–8. Laparoscopic scissors.

moved and on the need for absolute integrity of the bag. Tissue morcellation devices have been described for fragmenting solid organs, such as the kidney or spleen, into smaller sizes that can then be removed through small incisions.[25]

STAPLING DEVICES

The technical difficulty of extensive suturing has provided the impetus for the development of endoscopic stapling devices. Laparoscopic staples are modifications of the stapling devices used in open surgery and have been used to perform gastrointestinal resections and anastomoses (Fig 4–12). The endoscopic linear cutting stapler fires six rows of staples and cuts between the 3rd and 4th staple lines. Other endoscopic staplers (e.g., TA-type, US Surgical Corp) fire three rows of staples and do not have a cutting blade. Three sizes of instruments are available that fire staple lines that are either 30 mm, 35 mm, or 60 mm in length. The 30 mm and 35-mm staplers fit through 12-mm laparoscopic ports, whereas 15 to 18-mm ports are required for the larger staplers. A range of staple lengths is available depending on the thickness of the tissue to be divided. Endoscopic linear and TA (tracheal anastomosic) staplers have been used to perform intestinal resections, gastric resections, and appendectomy. The linear cutting staplers also have been used to ligate and divide mesentery and other vascular structures, including the lateral pelvic ligaments during hysterectomy and oophorectomy, and the renal vein. Each of these staplers is a single-patient use item, but may be reloaded up to three times before disposal.

Laparoscopic hernia staplers are actually tissue-approximating staplers that fire a single titanium staple with either a B-shaped or box configuration. These staplers require an 11- or 12-mm laparoscopic port for insertion and have a fully rotational shaft; some models bear an articulating tip. The articulating tip is especially helpful for the fixation of mesh to the inguinal floor during laparoscopic hernia repair. Besides laparoscopic hernia repair, these staplers have other applications such as re-approximating the peritoneum after retroperitoneal dissections or closure of mesenteric defects after intestinal resections.

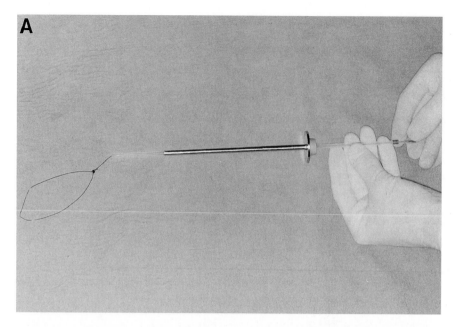

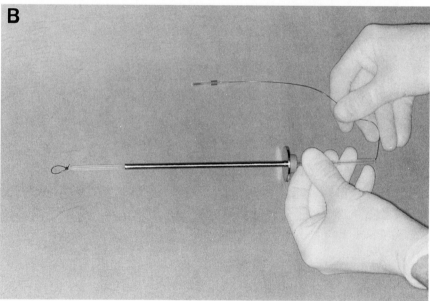

Figure 4–9. Laparoscopic pre-tied ligating loop suture (Endoloop). **A.** The loop is loaded through a hollow introducer tube. **B.** The plastic push rod at the end of the instrument is broken and the knot is tightened as the tip of the pushrod is advanced. (Courtesy of Ethicon Endosurgery, Inc.)

THERMAL INSTRUMENTS

The two modalities used for coagulation and hemostasis laparoscopically are the laser and the electrocautery. Detailed discussions of the operational characteristics of these modalities can be found in recent reviews.[26–28] Electrocautery exerts its tissue coagulation and cutting effects by either vaporization, dessication, or fulguration. Electrocautery may be utilized in a monopolar or bipolar mode. With monopolar cautery, the cautery probe itself serves as one electrode. The current passes through the cautery tip into the tissue being coagulated and then flows back to the ground plate on the patient's skin. The patient, therefore, becomes the conducting medium for passage of current from the delivery site to the return plate. The current path taken to the target tissue back to the patient-return electrode is no different for laparoscopic surgery than with open surgical use of monopolar cautery.[28] Bipolar cautery isolates the electrical circuit from the rest of the patient by using two contact points. One point is the source of the current and the other serves as the return electrode. The only tis-

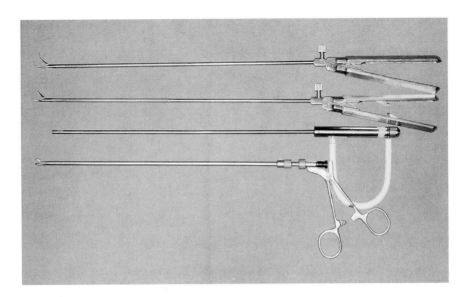

Figure 4–10. Laparoscopic needle holders. A variety of shaft and instrument tip configurations are shown. A spring loaded or ratcheted mechanism for locking onto the needle usually is employed.

sue through which current is conducted is between the two contact tips. While bipolar cautery is highly effective for coagulating tissues or vessels locally, it is less effective than monopolar cautery for cutting or dessicating tissues.

Several precautions must be taken when using electrocautery during laparoscopic surgery. The shafts and handles of the cautery instrument must be well insulated to avoid inadvertent burns to the patient or operating surgeon. The entire tip of the cautery instrument must be well visualized endoscopically to avoid contact with other structures that could be cauterized or injured. Concerns have been expressed that possible injury to remote sites could occur owing to capacitive coupling effects from the laparoscopic trocars and other laparoscopic instruments present within the abdominal cavity.[29] It has been estimated that 5% to 40% of the power that the electrocautery is set to deliver can be coupled or transferred into a standard 10-mm trocar sheath.[28] Theoretically, energy transferred into these instruments or sheaths could burn adjacent organs and tissues. Many injuries believed secondary to a capacitive coupling effect

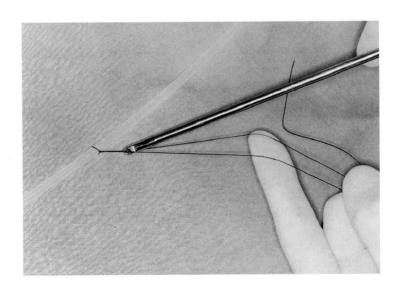

Figure 4–11. Laparoscopic knot pusher. After the suture has been placed laparoscopically, the knot is tied extracorporeally. Each throw in the knot is then slid securely into position with the knot pusher.

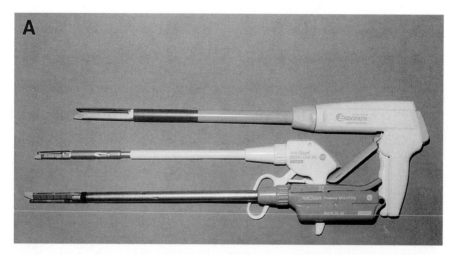

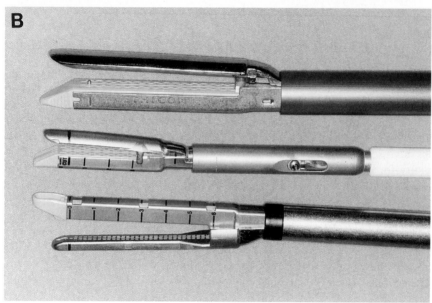

Figure 4–12. Endoscopic staplers for laparoscopic surgery. **A**. Full view demonstrating straight or pistol grip handles. **B**. Close-up of stapler tip and cartridge. Shown from top to bottom (in figure **A** and **B**) are the 1.60 mm linear cutter (Courtesy of Ethicon Endosurgery, Inc), 2.30 mm Endo GIA (Courtesy of US Surgical Corp) and 3.60 mm Endo TA (Courtesy of US Surgical Corp) staplers.

were more likely from unrecognized trocar injuries or direct cautery burns.[30] In the modern era of laparoscopic surgery, it is acknowledged that most laparoscopic cautery injuries are the result of direct burns from the cautery probe tip. In over 1000 laparoscopic cholecystectomies performed at out institution, there has not been a single case of cautery injury that could be attributed to a capacitive coupling effect. Nonetheless, it is recommended that the energy wattage of the electrosurgery unit for laparoscopic procedures be set at the lowest power level ($\leq$30 watts) to eliminate the potential for capacitive coupling or arcing from spark-gap sources.

Several types of lasers (argon, CO_2, KTP = potassium thionyl chloride, YAG = yttrium aluminum garnet) are available for use in laparoscopic surgery. Laser energy may be delivered to a tissue site either via quartz fibers as a free beam or by using a direct contact tip (sapphire tip and sculpted fiber devices). Contact tips operate by direct energy transfer similar to electrocautery. Free-beam lasers depend on radiation transfer and absorption by tissue to generate heating and coagulation effects. The use of a free-beam laser requires the selection of an appropriate "back stop" for the beam (eg, the abdominal wall or liver) to prevent injury to other viscera.

A major disadvantage associated with the use of lasers in laparoscopic surgery is cost. Electrocautery units are available in all operating rooms, and cautery probes and scissors are standard components of laparoscopic instrument sets. Laser units are expensive ($60,000 to $150,000 purchase costs), often requiring an additional patient charge. Recently, the use of laser versus electro-cautery was compared in a randomized, prospective trial of 100 patients undergoing laparoscopic cholecystectomy.[31] Blood loss was significantly less in the electrocautery group and in several cases, intraoperative laser malfunction resulted in completion of the dissection with cautery. Given the additional expense associated with laser use, it would appear that it is not warranted for routine use during laparoscopic cholecystectomy.

■ BASIC PRINCIPLES OF LAPAROSCOPY

PNEUMOPERITONEUM AND TROCAR INSERTION

The first step in performing laparoscopic surgery is to create a pneumoperitoneum. The pneumoperitoneum may be achieved using either a closed technique with the Veress needle or by an open minilaparotomy technique. The preferred site for insertion of the Veress needle is at the umbilicus, where the abdominal wall is thinnest and is well away from fixed internal organs. If the patient has had prior abdominal surgery in the vicinity of the umbilicus, an alternative site for insertion of the Veress needle may be chosen, or an open insertion technique may be used. Alternative insertion sites for Veress needle placement include the right or left midsubcostal regions, right and left iliac fossae, and supraumbilical region along the linea alba.

Regardless of the method of initial access to the peritoneal cavity, the patient should be in the supine position on the operating room table and strapped securely in place. This is done to avoid patient movement during the frequent repositioning that is necessary for laparoscopic surgery. A Foley catheter usually is inserted to drain the urinary bladder and to reduce the risk of bladder injury by the Veress needle or trocar. Decompression of the stomach with an oral gastric tube also is advisable, both to avoid inadvertent puncture of a distended stomach and to provide better exposure and access to the upper abdomen.

The patient is placed in the Trendelenburg position to allow bowel loops to ascend into the upper abdomen. A small incision (vertical or horizontal) is made at the inferior aspect of the umbilicus. The incision should be just large enough to accommodate the desired trocar; if the incision is too large, the trocar is more likely to slip out of the puncture site while the laparoscope repeatedly is moved. The subcutaneous tissue is bluntly dissected away until the umbilical fascia is palpable. The abdominal wall inferior to the umbilicus then is lifted with one hand while the Veress needle is inserted through the fascia at the base of the umbilicus. The needle (and subsequent trocar) should be inserted at a 45° angle toward the pelvis and away from the aorta and in-

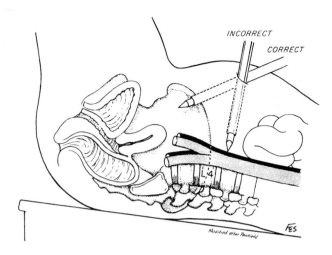

Figure 4–13. Angle of trocar insertion. The trocar should be inserted at a 45° angle toward the pelvis and away from the aorta and inferior vena cava. (From Cali RW. Laparoscopy. *Surg Clin N Amer* 1980;60:407)

ferior vena cava (Fig 4–13). One can frequently appreciate two clicks of the spring-loaded Veress needle as it penetrates first the fascia and then the peritoneum. Several maneuvers should be carried out to confirm the free intraperitoneal position of the needle. First, the needle is aspirated and irrigated to demonstrate the absence of return of blood or bowel contents and a free flow of fluid. Second, a saline drop test is performed in which the needle is filled with saline and fluid is demonstrated to flow freely by gravity into the peritoneal cavity as negative pressure is generated by lifting the abdominal wall. Finally, the needle is moved back and forth, which indicates that the tip is free within the peritoneal cavity.

The needle is connected to the insufflator and CO_2 is instilled at a rate of 1 L/min. The opening pressure recorded on the insufflator should be ≤10 mm Hg. Initial pressures of 10 mm Hg or higher may indicate placement of the needle in the preperitoneal or other closed space. A low flow rate for CO_2 should be used initially to avoid gas embolism or vagal stimulation from sudden stretching of the peritoneum. Upon insufflating approximately 1L of CO_2, increased tympany in all four quadrants of the abdomen is confirmed, and the flow rate may be increased. Although high-flow insufflators are designed to deliver flow rates of up to 8 to 10 L/min, the maximum flow rate through the small-caliber Veress needle is approximately 2.5 L/min. Preperitoneal insufflation of CO_2 is characterized by tympany isolated to the abdominal wall near the needle and by higher insufflation pressures. If at any point during insertion or insufflation there is uncertainty about the intraperitoneal location of the needle, it should be removed and reinserted. Once intra-abdominal pressure has reached

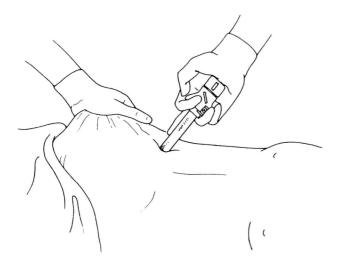

Figure 4–14. Abdominal wall lift technique for closed insertion of the initial trocar. The abdominal wall should be elevated and stabilized with the nondominant hand. (From Soper NJ, et al (eds), *Essentials of Laparoscopy.* St. Louis, MO: Quality Medical; 1993:56)

15 mm Hg, generally requiring 3 to 6 L of CO_2, the Veress needle is removed, and the trocar is inserted through the same site.

If one suspects adhesions near the site of Veress needle placement or if an alternative insertion site is chosen, it is advisable to begin by inserting a 5-mm trocar and laparoscope first to confirm position and freedom of the site. The trocar is grasped firmly in the palm of one hand and inserted using gentle, firm pressure while elevating the abdominal wall with the other hand or with towel clips (Fig 4–14). Control is paramount throughout insertion of the first trocar; sudden forward movement upon entry of the trocar into the peritoneal cavity accounts for most trocar injuries to retroperitoneal vascular structures. Once the port is in, the inner trocar is removed, leaving the outer cannula and sheath is place. Return of CO_2 gas is confirmed by opening either the stopcock or flapper valve on the port and then connecting the insufflation line to the sheath. The videotelescope is inserted and a general inspection of the peritoneal cavity, including underlying viscera and retroperitoneum, is carried out to assess for visceral injury. Additional trocars then are inserted under direct endoscopic vision.

In the open approach to insertion of the laparoscope, the umbilical fascia and peritoneum are incised under direct vision. The dissection should be kept close to the umbilicus, where there is less tissue between the fascia and peritoneal cavity and where all layers of the abdominal wall are fused. It is helpful to grasp the base of the umbilicus with a Kocher clamp, elevate it, and then incise the fascia with Mayo scissors. The amount of preperitoneal fat varies, but some dissection may be

required before one encounters the peritoneum. Blunt-finger dissection within the preperitoneal space should be minimized, since it separates the peritoneum from the fascia and makes identification and opening of the peritoneum more difficult. Once the peritoneum has been opened, digital palpation confirms that the adjacent peritoneal space is free. The laparoscopic port must be secured at the fascial site of entry in an airtight manner to prevent escape of CO_2 gas and loss of pneumoperitoneum. Two methods have been used for this purpose, as shown in Fig 4–15. One may place concentric purse-string sutures of O-gauge monofilament suture in the umbilical fascia. These sutures are used to cinch the fascia around a standard 10-mm laparoscopic port using a Rumel tourniquet technique. An alternative approach uses the Hasson trocar/cannula, which was designed specifically for an open insertion method (Figs 4–6 and 4–15E). The Hasson cannula requires placement of simple sutures in either side of the fascia. The cannula tip then is inserted through the fascial/peritoneal opening, and the nose of the conical sleeve is fitted into the umbilical opening and locked onto the cannula. The fascial sutures are pulled up tightly around the suture wings of the cannula, wedging it into the umbilical fascia and providing an airtight seal.

Following open insertion of the initial trocar, the port is connected to the CO_2 insufflator and the abdomen is inflated to 15 mm Hg pressure. Insufflation may be carried out at a higher flow rate with the open method than with the Veress needle because the risk of trocar insertion into a blood vessel or closed space has been eliminated. However, rapid expansion of the peritoneum in some patients may be associated with an increased vagal response, bradycardia, and postoperative shoulder pain.

The potential for trocar-related complications exists with both closed and open methods for establishing pneumoperitoneum. All surgeons who perform laparoscopic surgery should be adept at both methods and well versed in the expeditious recognition and management of complications. The true incidence of such complications is difficult to ascertain because the injuries are rare and rarely are reported. In one study from Europe, the incidence of serious vascular injury from either the Veress needle or trocar was 0.03% to 0.1%.[32,33]

The incidence of such complications should be reduced, if not eliminated, using an open insertion technique. Liberal use of an open insertion technique is also advisable in patients with previous abdominal surgery who have an incision near the umbilicus. In patients with long midline incisions in whom one would expect to have adhesions along the entire length of the incision, the use of an alternative insertion site with a closed technique may pose less risk than the open insertion method. An additional advantage of the open technique is that it provides a larger incision for removal of tissue at the conclusion of the case. Disadvantages of the open method include problems with CO_2 leak and loss of pneumoperitoneum from an incomplete seal.

ANESTHESIA

General anesthesia is the preferred anesthetic method for patients undergoing most therapeutic laparoscopic surgical procedures. The advantages of general anesthesia as compared to other types of anesthesia are twofold: (1) it allows for complete control of the patient's ventilation, which might otherwise be compromised by systemic absorption of CO_2 and increased diaphragmatic pressure from the pneumoperitoneum and (2) it enables complete relaxation of the abdominal wall muscles necessary for adequately maintaining pneumoperitoneum. Regional (epidural) anesthesia has been used for selected cases in which general anesthesia is contraindicated. For laparoscopic cholecystectomy, this necessitates a thoracic epidural at the T2-L1 level. The initial insufflation of the peritoneal cavity must be slow and at a lower pressure than that used with general anesthesia. Shoulder pain from irritation of the diaphragm by CO_2 occurs frequently. An additional risk of performing laparoscopic surgery under epidural anesthesia is that ventilation may be compromised owing to the effects of increased diaphragmatic pressure, and the patient may not be able to increase ventilation sufficiently to prevent the development of hypercarbia. Therefore, the amount of sedation with intravenous medications one can use to supplement the effects of the epidural is limited. In selected patients, local anesthesia has been used for performing laparoscopic procedures of short duration. These are usually diagnostic procedures in which only one or two small laparoscopic ports are needed.

The pulmonary and hemodynamic changes that occur during laparoscopy should be familiar to both surgeons and anesthetists. The CO_2 pneumoperitoneum causes an increase in total peripheral resistance and central venous pressure.[34] An increase in entidal $PaCO_2$ may occur due to increased intra-abdominal pressure and absorption of CO_2.[22] The reverse Trendelenburg position may further decrease venous return and lower cardiac output and blood pressure. These changes are insignificant in most individuals but could lead to serious hemodynamic consequences in patients with depleted intravascular volume, underlying cardiac disease, or compromised pulmonary function (eg, chronic obstructive pulmonary disease). Consequently, close intraoperative monitoring of patients is essential, regardless of the method of anesthesia. All patients should have continuous monitoring of EKG, blood pressure, and O_2 saturation. Patients under general anesthesia should be intubated to complete both protection of the airway and capnometric monitoring of end-tidal CO_2. An esophageal stethoscope should be used for frequent monitoring of the heart sounds. Pulmonary atelectasis, decreased functional residual capacity, and high-peak airway pressures may also be seen.[35]

CO_2 embolism is a potentially lethal complication of laparoscopic surgery that should be detected by careful intraoperative monitoring. Gas embolism may occur as a result of trocar or needle penetration of a blood vessel or from gas embolism into venous channels cut during laparoscopic surgery.[36] Gas embolism may be heralded by the sudden hemodynamic collapse of the patient. There may be associated dysrhythmias, a mill wheel–type heart murmur, cyanosis, and pulmonary edema. End-tidal CO_2 initially increases, but may fall abruptly if there is severe right ventricular dysfunction.[22] Prompt recognition and management of CO_2 embolism is critical for patient survival. The pneumoperitoneum should be deflated immediately, and the patient should be placed in the left lateral decubitus position with the head down (Durant position). Insertion of a central venous cathether with aspiration of the right ventricle also should be carried out. It is important that one exclude other causes for hemodynamic collapse, such as bleeding, for which prompt recognition and treatment is required.

PATIENT SELECTION

The success of any laparoscopic operation depends on both proper patient selection and the technical skill and experience of the laparoscopist. As surgeons have gained experience and techniques have become more advanced, the number of absolute contraindications to laparoscopy has decreased (Table 4–2). Uncorrectable coagulopathy is an absolute contraindication. Laparoscopy may be attempted successfully in some patients who have had multiple previous abdominal operations. However, if the patient has been known to have a "frozen abdomen" or prior episodes of peritonitis, the success rate in developing a working space to obtain pneumoperitoneum is markedly diminished. Such patients also may have an increased risk of intestinal injury from a trocar or from attempts at laparoscopic adhesiolysis. Intestinal obstruction with massive abdominal distension contraindicates a laparoscopic approach because of the absence of a working space within the peritoneal cavity. Patients with hemorrhagic shock or severe cardiac dysfunction should not be approached laparoscopically because of the likelihood of further cardiac compromise. Finally, the advantages of laparo-

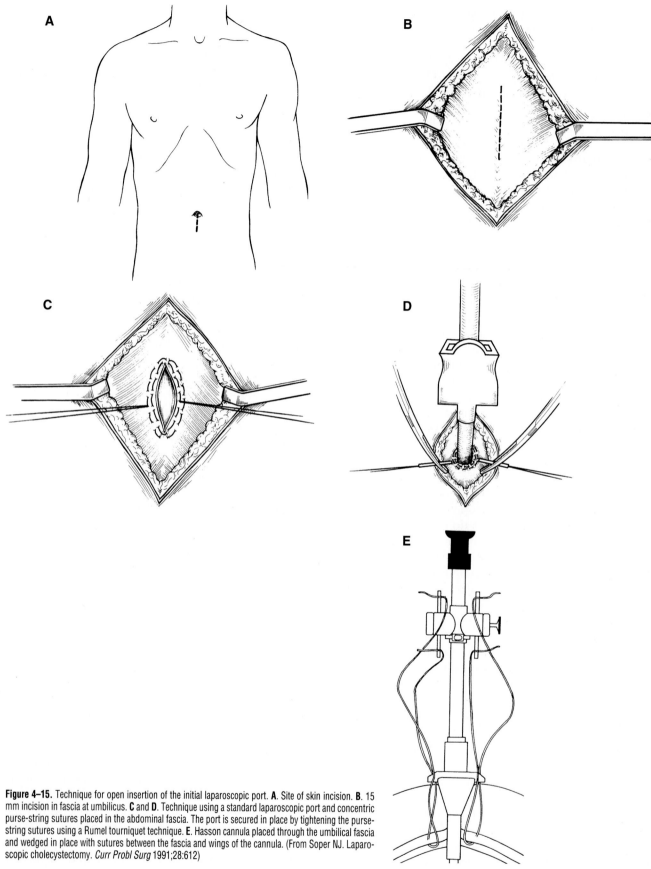

Figure 4–15. Technique for open insertion of the initial laparoscopic port. **A**. Site of skin incision. **B**. 15 mm incision in fascia at umbilicus. **C** and **D**. Technique using a standard laparoscopic port and concentric purse-string sutures placed in the abdominal fascia. The port is secured in place by tightening the purse-string sutures using a Rumel tourniquet technique. **E**. Hasson cannula placed through the umbilical fascia and wedged in place with sutures between the fascia and wings of the cannula. (From Soper NJ. Laparoscopic cholecystectomy. *Curr Probl Surg* 1991;28:612)

TABLE 4–2. CONTRAINDICATIONS TO LAPAROSCOPIC SURGERY

Absolute	Relative
Uncorrectable coagulopathy	Inability to tolerate general anesthesia
"Frozen" abdomen from adhesions	
Intestinal obstruction with massive abdominal distension	Abdominal sepsis/peritonitis
	[a]Intra-abdominal malignancy
Hemorrhagic shock	Pregnancy
Severe cardiac dysfunction	Morbid obesity
Concomitant disease requiring laparotomy	Multiple previous abdominal operations
	Severe COPD[b]
	Diaphragmatic hernia

[a]Excluding colon carcinoma
[b]Chronic obstructive pulmonary disease

scopy are lost in patients who have other diseases that require open laparotomy.

Experience with laparoscopic cholecystectomy has demonstrated that laparoscopic procedures can now be carried out successfully in many patients who formerly were thought to have contraindications to this approach. Abdominal sepsis with generalized peritonitis is usually an indication for open laparotomy, although patients with peritonitis from perforated ulcer[37] and perforated appendicitis[38] have been managed successfully in selected cases. Laparoscopy may be indicated in the diagnosis and staging of intra-abdominal malignancies and in selected therapeutic procedures such as laparoscopic colon resection. However, at this time the diagnosis of malignancy in the biliary tract or other site should remain a relative contraindication to the laparoscopic approach owing to the potential for incomplete resection and cutaneous and intra-abdominal seeding of the tumor.[39] Pregnancy once was considered an absolute contraindication to laparoscopy because of the unknown effects of CO_2 pneumoperitoneum on the fetus. However, several reports have demonstrated successful laparoscopic cholecystectomy in patients with severe biliary symptoms during the second trimester of pregnancy, without untoward effects on either the mother or fetus.[40,41] Morbid obesity is no longer a contraindication to laparoscopic procedures, provided adequate pneumoperitoneum can be established and the abdominal wall thickness does not exceed the length of the trocars. Although the procedure may be technically more difficult in obese patients, the success rate of laparoscopic cholecystectomy in the morbidly obese has been no different than in nonobese patients[42–44] and has been associated with less complications than open surgery.[42] The management of patients with severe chronic obstructive pulmonary disease remains problematic. In some cases, it may be possible to carry out the procedure under regional or local anesthesia. However, the increased diaphragmatic pressure and CO_2 absorption from the pneumoperitoneum and intravenous sedation required may further compromise the pulmonary condition of the patient. However, the advantage of a minimally invasive approach in such patients is that there is less impairment of postoperative pulmonary function than there is with conventional open surgery.[45,46] Advanced age, by itself, is not a contraindication to laparoscopy, and many patients have undergone successful laparoscopic procedures in the eighth and ninth decades of life with the same benefits as in younger individuals.

COMPLICATIONS

Laparoscopy is associated with unique risks and complications that do not exist with open surgery. The most important of these complications are major vascular injuries, intestinal injuries, and CO_2 embolism, any one of which is potentially lethal. The true incidence of major complications due to laparoscopy itself has been difficult to ascertain, since complications happen infrequently and most occurrences are unreported. The mortality from several large series of diagnostic gynecologic laparoscopy has averaged 0.05% with a range of 0.014% to 0.13%.[47,48] Major complications have occurred in 0.15% to 0.6% of cases with an average rate of 0.38%. Most data on morbidity and mortality in the field of laparoscopic general surgery come from large series of laparoscopic cholecystectomy. The mortality rate for laparoscopic cholecystectomy has ranged from 0% to 0.8%.[4,49–52] Major technical complications occurred in 0.6% to 2.4% of cases. However, these data reflect outcomes in specialized centers that have developed considerable expertise in the technique and probably underestimate the true incidence of complications in the surgical community at large. Recently, a national survey of 77 604 cases of laparoscopic cholecystectomy performed in 4292 hospitals was reported.[53] A total of 33 deaths occurred, 18 of which were related to operative injuries. Intestinal and vascular injuries occurred in 0.14% and 0.25% of cases, respectively, and were the most lethal types of complications encountered. Complications that required laparotomy occurred in 1.2% of patients, and the rate of bile duct injury was 0.6%. As has been suggested by several groups, physician training and experience appear to be among the most important determinants on the incidence of laparoscopic complications.[49,54–56]

The principal types of complications associated with laparoscopic surgery can be classified as shown in Table 4–3. Insertion of the Veress needle and trocars may result in injury to the major vessels, the gastrointestinal tract, and the bladder. The incidence of trocar-related

TABLE 4–3. LAPAROSCOPIC COMPLICATIONS

Insertion Related	Post Insertional Complications	Pneumoperitoneum Related
Major vascular injury	Gastrointestinal perforation acute or delayed	CO_2 embolism
Gastrointestinal injury	Laceration/bleeding from solid organs	Hypercarbia
Bladder injury	liver, spleen, kidney	Respiratory acidosis
CO_2 embolism	Hernias of abdominal wall	Subcutaneous emphysema
Abdominal wall hemorrhage		Pneumothorax
		Pneumomediastinum

complications ranges from 1:500 to 1:2000 cases.[54] Trocar injuries may occur with either a closed or open insertion technique, although the risk is greater with the closed method, especially during blind insertion of the first trocar.[57] Excessive use of force is often a factor in such injuries, particularly those that involve retroperitoneal structures. The retractable guards found on most disposable trocars may provide an added margin of safety, but they will not prevent serious injuries from occurring.

Most insertion-related vascular complications involve the aorta, inferior vena cava, iliac artery and vein, or mesenteric vessels. Injuries incurred with the Veress needle sometimes can be managed conservatively if the patient is stable and the site of injury is inspected carefully after laparoscopic access to the peritoneal cavity has been gained. Trocar injuries to major intra-abdominal vessels always must be treated by open laparotomy. Exclusion of such injuries should be the first priority of the laparoscopist following insertion of the initial trocar and video telescope. Major vascular injury always should be suspected in any patient who experiences sudden hemodynamic collapse during a laparoscopic procedure,[58] especially if the decompensation is related temporally to insertion of a trocar. In such cases, one should discontinue gas insufflation immediately and quickly lower CO_2 pressure to 8 mm Hg, because of the possibility of a CO_2 embolism. The endoscope should *not* be removed, but a rapid scan of the abdomen and retroperitoneum should be carried out with the video telescope to search for hemorrhage.[59] If retroperitoneal blood or a retroperitoneal hematoma is present, an exploratory laparotomy should be performed immediately and the bleeding site compressed until the patient has been stabilized. Delay in performing laparotomy on the patient with a major vascular injury only increases the risk of exsanguination and death. Sudden hemodynamic collapse of the patient undergoing laparoscopy may also result from CO_2 embolism, tension pneumothorax, or cardiac dysrhythmias. If laparoscopic inspection of the peritoneal cavity reveals no evidence of

vascular injury, a CO_2 embolism should be suspected and managed as described above.

Injuries to the gastrointestinal tract may be incurred at any point during the laparoscopic surgical procedure. The management of intestinal injuries from laparoscopy depends on the extent of the injury. Suspected injuries due to the Veress needle first should be inspected carefully with a laparoscope after gaining access at an alternative site; treatment may consist of either observation or laparoscopic suturing of the injury. If intestinal laceration occurs with the trocar, the trocar should be left in place while an open laparotomy is performed. Management of trocar injuries to the bowel with laparoscopic techniques may be possible in carefully selected cases.[60] Gastrointestinal injuries also may occur from electrocautery and laser burns, or from lacerations by laparoscopic instruments. If unrecognized, such injuries may result in delayed perforation with peritonitis, sepsis, and death.[52,61]

The risk of bladder injury during trocar insertion should be minimal if the bladder has been decompressed with a Foley catheter. Lacerations to solid organs (liver, spleen) may occur from laparoscopic instruments or when an upper abdominal alternative insertion site is used. Abdominal wall complications that may occur owing to trocar injuries include bleeding, hematomas, and hernias. Injury to abdominal wall vessels (eg, inferior epigastric artery) usually can be avoided by transilluminating the abdominal wall with a laparoscope before placing the trocar. Inspection of all trocar sites at the completion of the laparoscopic procedure should be performed routinely to avoid unrecognized bleeding from these sites. Hernias that develop postoperatively through a laparoscopic port site have a high incidence of incarceration and Richter hernia formation because of the small size of the fascial defect.[62–64] Closure of the fascia at all port sites 10 mm or greater in diameter is recommended to avoid this complication.

A number of complications may develop as a result of CO_2 pneumoperitoneum. These include CO_2 embolism, hypercarbia, subcutaneous emphysema, and, rarely, pneumomediastinum and pneumothorax. Improper placement of the Veress needle also may result in insufflation of the preperitoneal space or CO_2 emphysema involving the omentum, intestinal mesentery, and retroperitoneum. Hypercarbia and the accompanying acidosis usually can be managed by increasing minute ventilation and lowering the CO_2 insufflation pressure. Subcutaneous emphysema may exacerbate the degree of hypercarbia, but it is otherwise of no consequence clinically and usually resolves within 24 to 48 hours of surgery. Cardiac complications of pneumoperitoneum include transient dysrhythmias and bradycardia from increased vagal stimulation.

■ DIAGNOSTIC LAPAROSCOPY

Laparoscopy was first used clinically as a diagnostic tool to evaluate abdominal pathology. Ascites of unknown origin and liver disorders were the most common conditions for which diagnostic laparoscopy originally was utilized. Diagnostic laparoscopy has been employed increasingly in recent years for a wide variety of conditions that include patients with acute and chronic abdominal pain, intra-abdominal malignancies, and abdominal trauma.

Diagnostic laparoscopy usually is carried out with a 5-mm or 10-mm trocar placed at the umbilicus. A second 5-mm trocar is placed in the upper or lower abdomen to allow manipulation or biopsy of intra-abdominal structures. Diagnostic laparoscopic evaluation of the peritoneal cavity should be performed in an orderly sequence, just as with open laparotomy. In the lower abdomen, the right colon, appendix, sigmoid colon, bladder, and inguinal floor should be visualized. Examination of the uterus, fallopian tubes, and ovaries in women may be facilitated by a cervical tenaculum placed transvaginally for manipulation of the uterus. In the upper abdomen, the liver, gallbladder, stomach, spleen, and diaphragm are examined. The small intestine may be examined from the ligament of Treitz to the ileocecal valve, although this usually requires two accessory ports and appropriate atraumatic instruments for grasping and "running" the bowel.

EVALUATION OF ABDOMINAL PAIN

Laparoscopy has been a useful means for evaluating patients with unexplained abdominal pain. In the setting of acute abdominal pain, laparoscopy may establish or exclude the diagnosis of appendicitis and other conditions that require therapeutic surgical intervention. The negative laparotomy rate for acute appendicitis may be reduced by 20% to 40% if diagnostic laparoscopy is carried out prior to laparotomy.[65–67] In one series of 70 patients with a variety of causes of acute abdominal pain, the etiology of the pain was correctly identified by laparoscopy in 69 patients.[68] The majority of patients in this series had either appendicitis or gynecologic pathology. Patients with chronic abdominal pain present a more difficult diagnostic dilemma. Laparoscopy should be considered in such patients if physical examination and conventional diagnostic tests are unrevealing. Easter and associates[69] performed diagnostic laparoscopy in 70 patients with chronic abdominal complaints. Positive findings were present in 47% of patients, and laparoscopy resulted in subsequent therapeutic interventions with positive clinical outcomes in 27 (39%) patients. The most common finding in these patients was intra-abdominal adhesions. Laparoscopy also may play a valuable role in treating the critically ill patient with suspected intra-abdominal sepsis.[70] The advantage of laparoscopy in this group of patients is that it can be performed in the intensive care unit under local anesthesia. Additionally, a negative laparoscopic exam potentially would avoid the morbidity of unnecessary laparotomy in this group of seriously ill patients.

EVALUATION OF ABDOMINAL MALIGNANCIES

Dedicated laparoscopists have used laparoscopy to diagnose and stage intra-abdominal malignancies for many years. The value of laparoscopy in this setting is to be able to eliminate unnecessary laparotomies in patients with unresectable tumors or who need a biopsy and tissue diagnosis. Laparoscopic guidance may be used to obtain directed percutaneous needle biopsies or to biopsy a tumor directly, using instruments with cautery capability. Ascites, if present, should be aspirated and sent for cytologic examination. Diagnostic laparoscopy has been used for patients with liver tumors, retroperitoneal tumors, lymphomas, pancreatic tumors, and for patients with malignant ascites.[71,72] The accuracy of laparoscopic liver biopsy has been estimated to be 90%.[73] Laparoscopy successfully identified malignant abdominal neoplasms in 17 (68%) of 25 patients in one series with no false negative results.[69] Retroperitoneal tumors were diagnosed accurately by laparoscopic examination in 16 (84%) of 19 patients in one recent report, with adequate tissue-cell typing obtained in all patients with lymphomas.[68]

Conventional preoperative imaging techniques in patients with gastrointestinal tract malignancies frequently fail to detect small hepatic and peritoneal metastases.[74–76] Laparoscopy is highly successful in detecting those surface tumor implants that preclude curative surgical resection. Warshaw and associates[77] performed laparoscopy in 72 patients with pancreatic carcinoma who subsequently underwent exploratory laparotomy. Peritoneal metastases were accurately detected in 22 (96%) of 23 cases. Most implants were small (1 to 3 mm) and not detected by computerized tomographic (CT) or magnetic resonance imaging (MRI) scans. Furthermore, none of 24 patients with negative laparoscopy were found to have tumor implants at laparotomy. The overall incidence of peritoneal metastases in patients with a negative CT scan in this series was 36%. Therefore, the use of laparoscopy in conjunction with preoperative radiologic imaging techniques, potentially could eliminate unnecessary laparotomies in a substantial number of patients.

Laparoscopy also has been used to detect peritoneal implants in patients with gastric carcinoma.[78–80] The clinical impact of laparoscopy in this setting is less clear, however, since most of these patients undergo resection even if metastases are present. Other potential staging applications for laparoscopy include carcinomas of the distal esophagus and cardia,[81–82] second-look laparoscopy for ovarian carcinoma,[76] and pelvic lymph node staging for prostate carcinoma.[83] In the future, the diagnostic accuracy of laparoscopy in these patients may be enhanced further by use of laparoscopic ultrasound and radionuclide probes that detect tumors currently inaccessible to the laparoscope.[84,85]

ABDOMINAL TRAUMA

Laparoscopy now is being used in some centers to evaluate patients with abdominal trauma.[86,87] The appropriate indications for diagnostic laparoscopy in trauma patients have not been defined clearly, but many include patients with blunt trauma, penetrating stab wounds, and tangential gunshot wounds.[88,89] Laparoscopy should not delay laparotomy in patients with clear indications for operation. Suspected diaphragmatic injury is a relative contraindication to laparoscopy because of the risk of tension pneumothorax from the CO_2 pneumoperitoneum. Patients with injuries to major blood vessels also may be at increased risk of developing a CO_2 embolism.

Laparoscopy in trauma patients has been performed in emergency rooms under local anesthesia or in the operating room under general anesthesia.[86,87] If the procedure is to be done under local anesthesia, a small 4- or 5-mm laparoscope should be inserted initially at the umbilicus. CO_2 insufflation pressures should be kept at 8 mm to 10 mm Hg to prevent undue patient discomfort and to minimize the risk of pneumoperitoneum-related complications. A second 5-mm port usually is placed in the upper abdomen. A suction/irrigation cannula is inserted through this port to remove blood from the field and to manipulate organs. Both lateral gutters and the pelvis should be aspirated of blood, and the patient should be observed for ongoing bleeding. Individual organs also may be examined, although detection of bowel injuries from penetrating trauma may be difficult. The presence of a large amount of blood in the peritoneal cavity should be an indication for immediate laparotomy.

Berci and associates[86] recently evaluated the role of diagnostic laparoscopy in 150 patients with abdominal trauma. In 84 (56%) patients no hemoperitoneum was found, and none of these patients required exploratory laparotomy. Laparoscopy was positive in 66 patients. Thirty-eight (25%) patients had minor injuries and were observed. One of these patients subsequently required laparotomy for a missed sigmoid colon perforation. Significant hemoperitoneum, requiring immediate laparotomy, was present in the remaining 28 (19%) patients, and all but one patient in this group had a definable injury that required open surgical repair. Fabian and associates[87] reported similar results in 182 patients undergoing diagnostic laparoscopy.

■ LAPAROSCOPIC CHOLECYSTECTOMY

Laparoscopic cholecystectomy has become widely accepted as the procedure of choice for patients with symptomatic cholelithiasis.[4] Laparoscopic cholecystectomy clearly has been shown to be associated with decreased pain, shorter hospitalization, a reduced period of postoperative disability[2,3,16] and decreased hospital costs.[90] The majority (>90%) of patients with gallstones are candidates for this procedure, and it has been estimated that 85% of all cholecystectomies performed in the United States in 1993 will be done laparoscopically.[91] The technique for laparoscopic cholecystectomy and a detailed analysis of the results are presented in Chapter 67.

A summary of the results of several large series of laparoscopic cholecystectomy are shown in Table 4–4.[4,49,51,52,92,93] The rate of conversion to open cholecystectomy has ranged from 1.8% to 4.7%. This conversion rate is generally higher early in the surgeon's experience. Factors that increase the likelihood of conversion to open cholecystectomy include increasing age, male sex, multiple severe attacks of biliary colic, and acute cholecystitis.[94] Deaths have been rare and most have been due to associated medical conditions. However, deaths due to technical complications, such as bile duct and intestinal injuries, have been reported.[52] The incidence of common bile duct injury in these combined series has been ≤0.5%, which is only slightly higher than the incidence reported for open cholecystectomy.[95–97]

Despite the favorable outcomes in specialized centers, the rapid introduction of laparoscopic cholecystectomy into the surgical community has been associated with an increase in the number of bile duct injuries that have been referred to tertiary care centers.[98–100] Following the implementation of laparoscopic cholecystectomy in New York State, an increased number of complications was also reported, and the rate of bile duct injury was estimated to be seven to eight times that associated with open cholecystectomy.[101,102] Many of these injuries undoubtedly occurred during the learning curve of the surgeon's experience,[49] and fewer technical complications of laparoscopic cholecystectomy can be expected as additional experience accrues. In addition to the experience of the surgeon, other risk factors for bile duct injury during laparoscopic cholecystectomy include chronic scarring in Calot's triangle, acute cholecystitis, and obesity.[103] Recently, a National Institutes of Health Consensus Conference on *Gallstones and Laparoscopic Cholecystectomy* concluded that the outcome of laparoscopic cholecystectomy is influenced to a large extent by the training, experience, skill, and judgement of the surgeon performing the procedure.[104] The panel also recommended that laparo-

TABLE 4–4. RESULTS OF LAPAROSCOPIC CHOLECYSTECTOMY

Author, Year	Number of Patients	% Converted[a]	% Mortality	% Major Complications	% Common Bile Duct Injury
Larson et al, 1992[92]	1963	4.5	0.1	2.0	0.3
Southern Surgeons, 1991[49]	1518	4.7	0.07	1.5	0.5
Cuschieri et al, 1991[51]	1236	3.6	0	1.6	0.3
Soper et al, 1992[4]	618	2.9	0	1.6	0.2
Lillemoe et al, 1992[93]	400	1.8	0	5.0	0.5
Wolfe et al, 1991[52]	381	3.0	0.8	3.4	0

[a]Converted to open operation

scopic cholecystectomy should be converted promptly to open cholecystectomy if there was uncertainty about the anatomy, if excessive bleeding occurred, or if other problems arose. Conversion to open cholecystectomy under these circumstances should not be viewed as a complication or failure of laparoscopic cholecystectomy, but rather as a reflection of sound surgical judgement. Because of the increased numbers of complications associated with introducing laparoscopic cholecystectomy into surgical practice, the panel also recommended that strict guidelines be developed for training in laparoscopic surgery, for determination of competence, and for monitoring of quality.

LAPAROSCOPIC COMMON BILE DUCT EXPLORATION

The ideal current approach to the treatment of choledocholithiasis is unclear. Endoscopic retrograde cholangiopancreatography (ERCP) may be used to evaluate patients with suspected common bile duct stones preoperatively and to perform endoscopic sphincterotomy and stone removal if necessary. However, 3% to 5% of patients undergoing cholecystectomy will have unsuspected common bile duct stones found on intraoperative cholangiography.[105,106] These patients may be approached in one of several ways: (1) postoperative ERCP with or without endoscopic sphincterotomy and stone extraction, (2) conversion to open cholecystectomy and common bile duct exploration, or (3) laparoscopic common bile duct exploration. Laparoscopic exploration of the bile duct usually is performed using a transcystic duct approach as described in Chapter 69. The limitations of this approach are that (1) it is difficult to examine the common hepatic duct proximal to the cystic duct and (2) larger stones (>8 mm) cannot be removed through the cystic duct. Alternatively, a laparoscopic choledochotomy may be performed which allows removal of larger stones and provides freer access to the proximal bile duct. However, this approach is technically demanding, since it requires placement of a

T tube and drain and the bile duct must be sutured over the T tube laparoscopically.

In experienced hands, laparoscopic common bile duct exploration has been successful in clearing the bile duct of stones in >90% of cases.[107–109] The recovery time for patients undergoing transcystic duct–common bile duct exploration is similar to that for laparoscopic cholecystectomy; the recovery time has been longer in patients undergoing laparoscopic choledochotomy. The advantages of a laparoscopic approach to choledocholithiasis, therefore, is that the risks and costs of the second procedure (ERCP and sphincterotomy) are avoided. However, there is a lack of controlled trials comparing the laparoscopic and endoscopic approaches. Currently, the optimal method for managing choledocholithiasis is determined by the expertise of the individual surgeon and endoscopist who are performing these procedures.

■ LAPAROSCOPIC APPENDECTOMY

Laparoscopic appendectomy for acute appendicitis was initially reported by Schreiber in 1987,[110] 4 years after Semm[11] had first performed an incidental appendectomy through the laparoscope. Since that time, the safety and efficacy of this procedure have been documented in several centers.[38,111–113] The largest experience to date is from Pier and associates,[112] who, in 1991, reported results in 639 attempted cases. Laparoscopic appendectomy was performed for acute appendicitis in 70% of cases and only 2% of patients required conversion to an open procedure. Major complications occurred in 1% of patients and included postoperative abscess (3 cases), appendiceal stump leak (1 case), and bleeding requiring conversion to open appendectomy (3 cases). Similar rates of technical complications and conversion to open appendectomy have been demonstrated in other reports as well.[38,111,113–115]

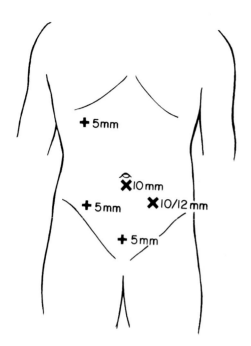

Figure 4–16. Port sites for laparoscopic appendectomy. Primary port sites are indicated by *X.* Sites for placement of an additional 3rd or 4th port are indicated by +. The umbilical and left lower quadrant ports are generally 10 to 12 mm in diameter.

Laparoscopic appendectomy usually is performed using three or four laparoscopic ports as shown in Fig 4–16. The precise number, size, and site for port placement vary according to surgeon preference and skill, the difficulty of the procedure and the anatomic findings. Generally, a 10-mm port is inserted at the umbilicus for placement of the laparoscope. A 10-mm to 12-mm port is placed in the left lower midabdomen; this port is used for the dissecting instruments, clip applier, and if necessary, an endoscopic linear stapler. A third 5-mm port may be placed at any of the other locations shown and for the more difficult cases, a fourth port may be required as well. The procedure should begin with a diagnostic evaluation of the peritoneal cavity. If the appendix is normal, a standard algorithm should be followed for examining the abdominal cavity and determining whether an appendectomy is indicated. If pathology is localized to the appendix, then a method for providing traction on the appendix and mesoappendix should be employed. This can be done with an atraumatic grasper, an endoscopic Babcock clamp, or a suture loop tied around the appendix. However, the appendix itself should be handled as little as possible to avoid perforation and fragmentation. The mesoappendix may be divided with a combination of cautery and clips or with a linear stapler. Ligation of the base of the appendix is accomplished either with a pre-tied suture loop (Endoloop, Ethicon Endosurgery, Inc., Cincinnatti, OH) or with an endoscopic linear stapler. The lin-

ear stapler provides the most secure closure of the appendiceal stump, but adds significantly to the cost of the procedure. Double ligation of the appendiceal stump proximally with Endoloops has been shown to be a safe and suitable method for most appendectomies.[113–115] Inversion of the stump is not necessary and is difficult technically. Use of the endoscopic linear stapler is recommended for patients in whom there is involvement of the base of the appendix by the inflammatory process. One should avoid using cautery or laser to divide the appendix itself because of the risk of delayed necrosis of the stump. Once the appendix is free, it may be removed by retracting the specimen into the shaft of a 10- to 12-mm cannula or by placing it into an entrapment sac. Whichever method is chosen, the goal is to remove the appendix without contacting the abdominal incision, thus minimizing the risk of wound contamination.

The potential benefits of laparoscopic versus open appendectomy include improved diagnostic capabilities, reduced morbidity owing to fewer wound infections and other complications, and reduced postoperative disability. However, open appendectomy for nonperforated appendicitis already is associated with a low complication rate and a short hospital stay. Consequently, the margin of benefit provided by a laparoscopic approach may not prove as dramatic as with laparoscopic cholecystectomy. Perhaps the most important advantage provided by laparoscopic appendectomy is an improved ability to diagnose other intra-abdominal disease processes. Historically, the incidence of negative laparotomy for acute appendicitis has ranged from 10% to 40%,[116–117] with the highest rates occurring in women of child-bearing age.[118] The accuracy of laparoscopy to diagnose acute appendicitis has been demonstrated already[65,119] and, in the view of most laparoscopists, the diagnostic capabilities of laparoscopy are far superior to that which can be obtained via a conventional appendectomy (gridiron or McBurney) incision. In women, the pelvic organs and most of the gastrointestinal tract are visualized readily, whereas the view through a small right lower quadrant incision is limited. Whether these improved diagnostic capabilities of laparoscopy will translate into significantly better patient outcomes is unclear. Laparoscopy also may allow more precise placement of an incision in the right lower quadrant, if an open approach is ultimately required.

Recently, the benefits of laparoscopic versus open appendectomy have been analyzed by several groups. Nowzaradan and associates[38] retrospectively compared 100 consecutive patients undergoing laparoscopic appendectomy versus 100 unselected patients treated by open appendectomy. The patients who underwent the laparoscopic procedure were discharged from the hospital earlier and had a more rapid return to full physical activity than the patients treated by open appendectomy. Wound infections occurred in 17.1% of all patients undergoing open appendectomy versus 1.3% of patients treated laparoscopically. In a similar type of uncontrolled comparison, Schirmer and associates[113] reported laparoscopic results that were comparable to, but not better than, the open procedure. Three small trials that prospectively randomized patients with suspected appendicitis to either approach were recently reported.[114,120,121] In two of the series, patients treated laparoscopically had shorter hospital stays, fewer postoperative complications, and an earlier return to full activity than the patients who underwent the open procedure. In the third trial, there were no differences in postoperative outcome parameters between the two groups.[121] Operating times were slightly longer in the laparoscopic groups in all trials. Laparoscopic appendectomy also appears to be more expensive than the open procedure.[115] These increased costs may offset any potential savings realized from earlier discharge of the patient from the hospital.

■ LAPAROSCOPIC ANTIREFLUX PROCEDURES

The surgical approach to the treatment of gastroesophageal reflux has been altered recently by the development of laparoscopic antireflux operations.[122,123] Most patients with symptomatic gastroesophageal reflux can be managed by changes in diet and lifestyle and by antisecretory medications. However, for patients with complicated gastroesophageal reflux disease, surgical therapy with the Nissen fundoplication has been shown to be more effective than medical treatment, with H-2 blockers in controlling the symptoms and signs of esophagitis.[124] Despite the successful impact of surgical therapy on gastroesophageal reflux disease, few patients have been referred for surgery in recent years because of the pain and morbidity associated with the large upper midline abdominal incision through which the Nissen procedure is performed. Laparoscopic antireflux operations have the potential for diminishing pain and morbidity associated with the open procedure while providing a definitive and perhaps superior alternative to long-term medical therapy.

Antireflux operations that have been performed laparoscopically are the Nissen fundoplication (360° wrap) and the Toupet procedure (200° to 270° wrap). In many respects, these procedures are ideally suited to a laparoscopic approach because no tissue is removed from the patient and the operation being performed should be identical to its open counterpart.[125–127] The indications for laparoscopic antireflux operations include the failure of medical therapy with persistence of symptoms and/or signs of esophagitis, the develop-

TABLE 4–5. CONTRAINDICATIONS TO LAPAROSCOPIC ANTIREFLUX OPERATIONS

Absolute	Relative
Previous vagotomy or partial gastrectomy	Morbid obesity
Shortened esophagus	Previous failed antireflux surgery
	Esophageal motility disorder
	Delayed gastric emptying

ment of complications such as stricture or ulceration, and the presence of Barrett's esophagitis.[128] Laparoscopic Nissen fundoplication also has been performed in infants and children with significant gastroesophageal reflux.[129] Contraindications to the laparoscopic antireflux procedure are listed in Table 4–5. Careful preoperative evaluation is essential to select the appropriate patients for operation. Diagnostic studies should include an upper gastrointestinal (GI) endoscopy with biopsy, esophageal manometry, and pH testing. Manometry and pH testing are especially important to demonstrate hypotonicity of the lower esophageal sphincter and to exclude the presence of either a primary motor disorder of the esophagus or alkaline reflux esophagitis.[130]

For laparoscopic Nissen fundoplication, the patient is placed in a modified lithotomy position as shown in Fig 4–17. This allows the surgeon to stand between the patient's legs and to operate facing straight forward. The sites we have used for laparoscopic port placement are shown in Fig 4–18. Ports should be placed cephalad so that the instruments will easily reach the esophageal hiatus. Special instruments facilitating this procedure include an angled (30°) laparoscope, endoscopic Babcock graspers, cautery scissors, curved instruments for dissecting around the esophagus, and an atraumatic retractor for the liver. The procedure is performed in a manner similar to the open Nissen fundoplication (see Chapter 39) as shown sequentially in Figs 4–19 and 4–20. The left lobe of the liver is elevated with a retractor, but the left triangular ligament should not be divided as this makes retraction of the liver more difficult. The stomach and epiphrenic fat pad are retracted inferiorly with an endoscopic Babcock clamp to place tension on the esophageal hiatus. The dissection at the esophageal hiatus should be carried out to identify the esophagus, both vagal nerve trunks, and the right and left crura of the diaphragm. The gastrophrenic peritoneum, between the left crus and the superior pole of the spleen, must be divided so that the esophagus can be encircled. Short gastric vessels usually need to be divided with endoclips to mobilize the gastric fundus sufficiently to allow a loose wrap. If the esophageal hiatus is significantly enlarged, the crura are reapproximated posterior to the esophagus.

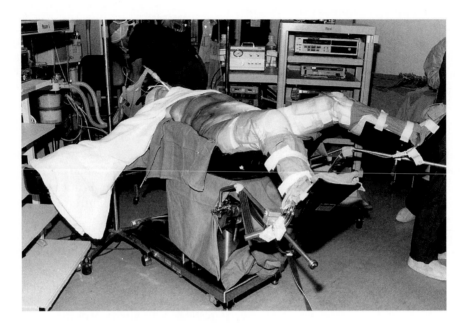

Figure 4–17. Patient position for laparoscopic Nissen fundoplication. The patient is in a modified lithotomy position using Lloyd Davies stirrups. The bean bag cushion is beneath the patient to prevent movement during tilting of the operating room table.

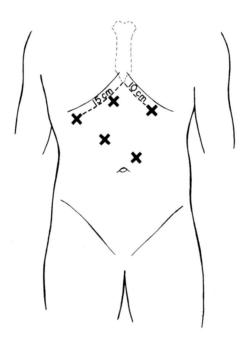

Figure 4–18. Port sites for laparoscopic Nissen fundoplication. All ports are 10 to 12 mm in diameter. The initial port is placed superior and to the left of the umbilicus; the right and left subcostal ports are inserted 15 cm and 10 cm from the xiphoid, respectively. These distances are measured with the abdomen distended by the pneumoperitoneum.

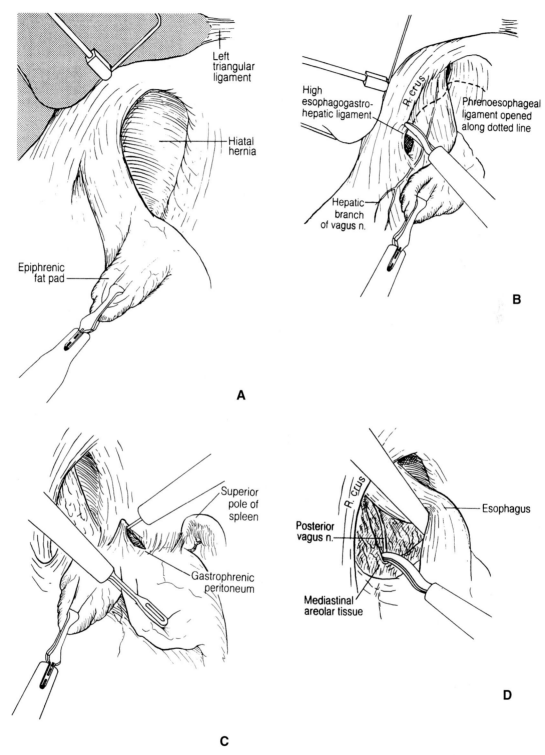

Figure 4–19, Mobilization of the esophagus and stomach for Nissen fundoplication. **A**. Initial exposure. The left lobe of the liver is lifted cephalad. An endoscopic grasper (Babcock clamp) placed on the epiphrenic fat pad reduces the hiatal hernia and provides traction on the distal esophagus. **B**. Dissection begins to the right of the esophagus with cautery scissors. The phrenoesophageal membrane is incised and the right crus of the diaphragm and anterior wall of the esophagus are identified. **C**. The gastrophrenic ligament is divided to the left of the esophagus. This step is facilitated by rolling over the fundus of the stomach. Short gastric branches may need to be divided to adequately mobilize the fundus. **D**. Dissection is continued behind the esophagus where the posterior vagus nerve is identified. The dissection should stay close to both crura to avoid entering the pleura. A window then is created between the left crus of the diaphragm and the posterior esophageal wall. *Continued*

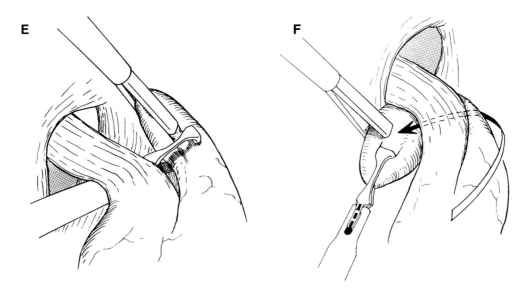

Figure 4–19, cont'd. E and **F**. The fundus is elevated anteriorly and a Babcock clamp is passed behind the esophagus. The stomach is placed into the jaws of the clamp and is then pulled behind the esophagus to the right side. (From Cuschieri AE. Hiatal hernia and reflux esophagitis. In: Hunter JG, Sackier JM (eds), *Minimally Invasive Surgery*. New York, NY: McGraw-Hill; 1993:100–103)

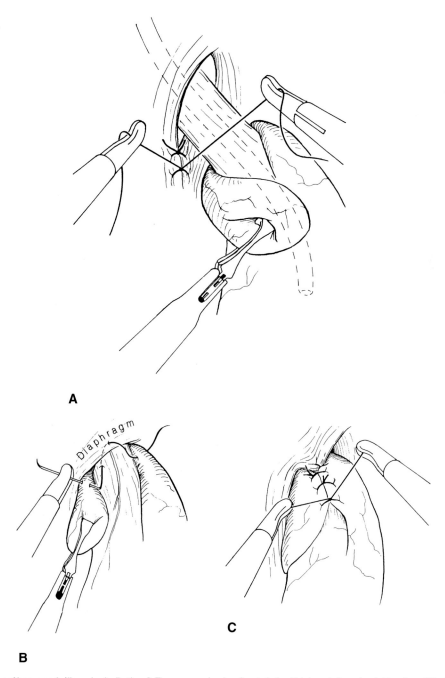

A

B

C

Figure 4–20. Completion of laparoscopic Nissen fundoplication. **A**. The crura may be closed posteriorly with interrupted nonabsorbable sutures if the hiatus is dilated. **B**. and **C**. Interrupted sutures are placed on the 360° wrap. The fundus should be anchored to the esophagus with at least one suture to prevent the Nissen from "slipping." Anchoring the wrap to the diaphragm as shown is optional. (From Cuschieri AE. Hiatal hernia and reflux esophagitis. In: Hunter JG, Sackier JM (eds), *Minimally Invasive Surgery*. New York, NY: McGraw-Hill; 1993:104)

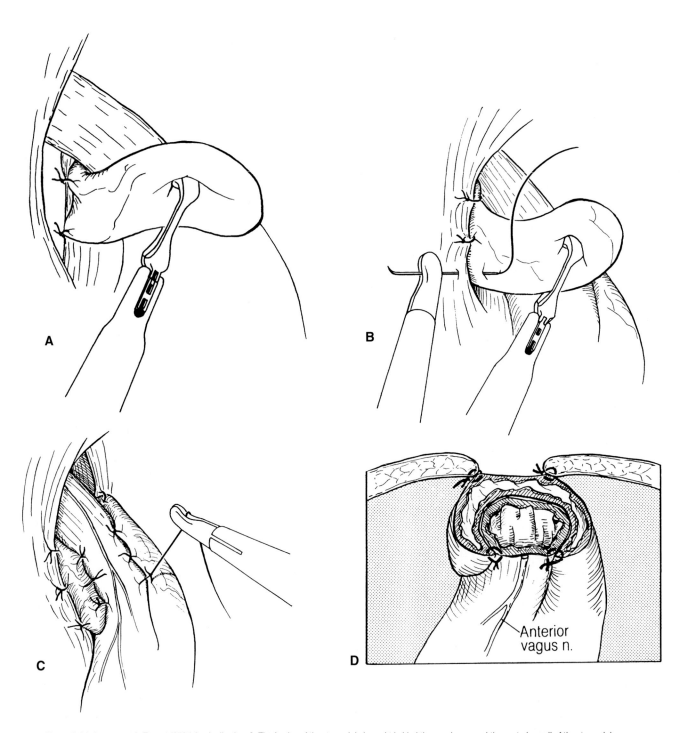

Figure 4–21. Laparoscopic Toupet (270°) fundoplication. **A**. The fundus of the stomach is brought behind the esophagus and the posterior wall of the stomach is anchored to the left crus of the diaphragm with two or three interrupted sutures. **B**. The fundus is next anchored to the right crus of the diaphragm in a similar manner. **C**. The wrap is completed by suturing it to the anterior surface of the esophagus on either side of the anterior vagus nerve. **D**. Cross sectional view showing a 270° wrap with four-point fixation. (From Cushieri AE. Hiatal hernia and reflux esophagitis. In: Hunter JG, Sackier JM (eds), *Minimally Invasive Surgery*. New York, NY: Mc-Graw-Hill; 1993:107)

The gastric wrap should be done over an esophageal dilator to prevent excessive tightening that may result in postoperative dysphagia and the gas bloat syndrome. A bougie, 60 Fr in size or equivalent (38 to 42 Fr with an 18-Fr nasogastric tube), is used for this purpose.[128] A 1 to 2-cm wrap consisting of two or three interrupted nonabsorbable sutures is carried out. The esophageal wall should be incorporated in at least one of these sutures to prevent the Nissen from slipping. It is relatively easy to tie the sutures using extracorporeal knots and a knot-pushing device. In the Toupet partial fundoplication, the gastric fundus is passed beyond the esophagus and anchored posteriorly to the right and left crura of the diaphragm (Fig 4–21). Anteriorly the fundus is anchored to the esophagus on either side of the anterior vagus nerve to achieve a 270° wrap.

To date, the results of the laparoscopic Nissen fundoplication have been excellent. Repairs of simple type I sliding hiatal hernias or combined type I and type II and paraesophageal hernias have been reported.[131–133] The length of hospitalization has averaged 2 to 4 days; complete relief of symptoms has occurred in >90% of patients.[123,131,134] The incidence of postoperative dysphagia and gas bloat syndrome has been comparable to that for the open Nissen procedure. Pneumothorax occasionally has occurred as a result of the violation of the pleura during dissection of the lower esophagus in the setting of CO_2 pneumoperitoneum,[135] but usually resolves without intervention. Current follow-up of the laparoscopic Nissen fundoplication has been relatively short in most series, but if the early positive results can be sustained, it is possible that many antireflux operations will be performed laparoscopically in the future.

■ LAPAROSCOPIC OPERATIONS FOR PEPTIC ULCER DISEASE

Surgery for peptic ulcer disease has declined in frequency in recent years because of the effectiveness of medical therapy and the morbidity associated with most antiulcer operations. However, with the development of minimal access surgery, there has been a renewed interest in the surgical treatment of peptic ulcer disease. For patients with uncomplicated peptic ulcer disease, highly selective (proximal gastric) vagotomy has emerged, in recent years, as the surgical procedure of choice. Highly selective vagotomy denervates the parietal cells of the proximal stomach while maintaining innervation of the antrum and pylorus; therefore acid secretion is effectively suppressed, but complications of diarrhea, dumping, and delayed gastric emptying associated with truncal vagotomy and drainage or resection are

much less common.[136,137] Several laparoscopic methods for duplicating the physiologic outcome of highly selective vagotomy have been reported clinically: (1) complete anterior and posterior highly selective vagotomy,[138–140] (2) posterior truncal vagotomy with anterior highly selective vagotomy,[141] and (3) posterior truncal vagotomy with anterior gastric seromyotomy.[142] The technical aspects to performing these procedures have been described in detail by several groups.[143,144]

Laparoscopic anterior and posterior highly selective vagotomy represents a direct adaptation of the standard open highly selective vagotomy procedure. In this operation, complete division of all branches of the anterior and posterior nerves of Latarjet, from the distal esophagus and gastroesophageal junction to the crow's foot of the antrum, is carried out. Preliminary results of this technique have been reported in two small series of patients[139,140] who have undergone surgery for chronic duodenal ulcers. No complications were reported in either of these studies, and acid secretion was reduced in patients who are studied postoperatively. Recurrent ulceration has not been observed, but the follow-up interval has been short.[139]

The technical difficulty of performing bilateral highly selective vagotomy and the risk of incomplete denervation of the parietal cells have led some investigators to simplify the operation by combining posterior truncal vagotomy with anterior highly selective vagotomy (Fig 4–22)[145] or anterior gastric seromyotomy.[146] Since posterior truncal vagotomy is performed more reliably than complete posterior highly selective vagotomy, there is less risk of technical failure of the operation. By preservation of the anterior vagal fibers to the gastric antrum and pylorus, gastric emptying should be maintained adequately.[147] Bailey and Zucker[144] have reported early results in 30 consecutive patients undergoing this procedure. In a 2 year follow-up, recurrent ulceration had occurred in two patients, both of whom had prepyloric ulcers.

Posterior truncal vagotomy with anterior gastric seromyotomy (Taylor procedure) was first performed by Katkhouda in 1989.[142] The rationale for anterior gastric seromyotomy, as originally reported by Taylor,[146] was the anatomic observation that the anterior vagus nerve branches course obliquely through the seromuscular layers of the stomach 1 to 2 cm from the lesser curvature, before they reach the parietal cells. By dividing this seromuscular layer from the gastroesophageal junction to within 6 cm of the pylorus, the parietal cells being supplied by branches of the anterior vagus should be completely denervated (Fig 4–23). Anterior gastric seromyotomy has been reported to be easier to perform than anterior highly selective vagotomy,[148] but a comparison of the efficacy of the two approaches in terms of control of acid secretion has not been done. Katkhouda

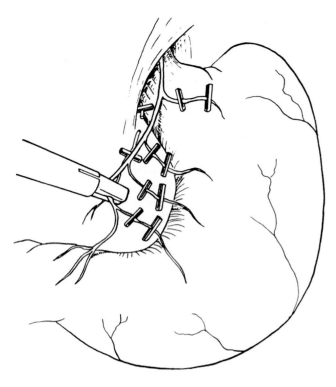

Figure 4–22. Laparoscopic posterior truncal vagotomy and anterior highly selective vagotomy. (From Katkhouda N, Mouiel J. Laparoscopic treatment of peptic ulcer disease. In: Hunter JG, Sackier JM (eds), *Minimally Invasive Surgery.* New York, NY: Mc-Graw-Hill; 1993:128)

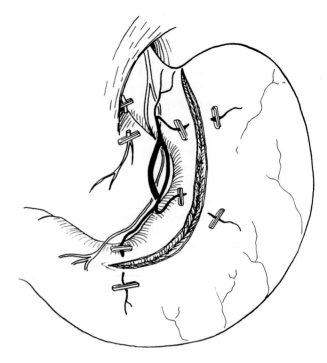

Figure 4–23. Posterior truncal vagotomy and anterior lesser curve seromyotomy. (From Katkhouda N, Mouiel J. Laparoscopic treatment of peptic ulcer disease. In: Hunter JG, Sackier JM (eds), *Minimally Invasive Surgery.* New York, NY: McGraw-Hill; 1993:126)

and Mouiel[143] have reported 60 patients (mean age of 33 years) with duodenal ulcers refractory to medical therapy treated with the laparoscopic Taylor procedure. An 80% reduction in acid production was observed at 1 month postoperatively and, 6 months after surgery; complete healing of the ulcers was documented in 58 (96.7%) patients. In the remaining two patients, scarring at the site of previous ulceration was seen without active disease; however, recurrent ulceration developed in one patient 2 years postoperatively. Operative and postoperative complications of the procedure have included pneumothorax (1 patient), gastroesophageal reflux (1 patient) and gastric bezoars (3 patients). Gastric perforation as a result of the seromyotomy has been reported in experimental studies,[148] but it was not observed in this large clinical series. Closure of the seromyotomy with two overlapping layers of suture is recommended to prevent this complication and to achieve hemostasis.

Laparoscopic bilateral truncal vagotomy has been reported in combination with either pyloric dilatation or pyloromyotomy. Pyloric dilatation is performed under direct laparoscopic control using a balloon dilator. Approximately 20% of patients develop some degree of pyloric stenosis; repeat dilatations often are required.[143] Side effects of the procedure include diarrhea and

dumping. Laparoscopic pyloromyotomy is an experimental technique that uses a specialized stapling device to excise the anterior pyloric muscle and reanastomose the anterior stomach to the duodenum.[149] The safety and efficacy of this procedure and its clinical role are under investigation. Thoracoscopic truncal vagotomy has been reported in patients with recurrent peptic ulceration who have previously had a gastric drainage procedure.[150] The thoracoscopic approach may be particularly suitable for patients with an incomplete vagotomy after prior vagotomy and pyloroplasty or antrectomy. Preliminary clinical reports[151] have indicated that laparoscopic hemigastrectomy and Billroth II gastrojejunostomy is feasible technically in selected patients. Whether this approach will be safe, appropriate, and advantageous for patients with peptic ulcer disease will be the subject of further study.

Laparoscopic treatment of perforated duodenal ulcer has been reported in several centers.[37,143,152,153] The most common approach has been to combine simple closure of the perforation with an omental patch and copious irrigation of the abdominal cavity. Some patients who have undergone operation within a few hours of the onset of symptoms also have been treated with simultaneous laparoscopic highly selective vagotomy. Vereecken[37] reported 30 patients with perforated ulcers who were treated laparoscopically. Two patients were converted to open operation and one patient died from multiorgan system failure. On average, oral intake was resumed on postoperative day 4 and patients were discharged on the 9th postoperative day. No patients required surgical reintervention or developed recurrent ulceration at a mean follow-up interval of 5 months postoperatively.

■ LAPAROSCOPIC FEEDING TUBE INSERTION

Percutaneous endoscopic gastrostomy (PEG) has become the preferred method for providing enteral access in patients who require long-term nutritional support. Contraindications that require a surgical approach rather than PEG insertion include esophageal obstruc-

tion from malignancies, inability to transilluminate the abdominal wall with the gastroscope, and the presence of ascites. Furthermore, in many patients, a jejunostomy feeding tube is preferable to a PEG, especially if there is a history of gastroesophageal reflux, previous gastric surgery, or delayed gastric emptying. However, an endoscopic approach to jejunostomy tube placement has been unsatisfactory because of problems in maintaining the tip of the tube beyond the pylorus.[154] Open surgical placement of feeding tubes can be performed under local anesthesia but has been associated with postoperative ileus, pain, wound healing problems, and infection. Recently, techniques have been developed for laparoscopic insertion of jejunostomy[155] and gastrostomy[156] feeding tubes.

The procedure usually is performed under general anesthesia, although local anesthesia has been used in

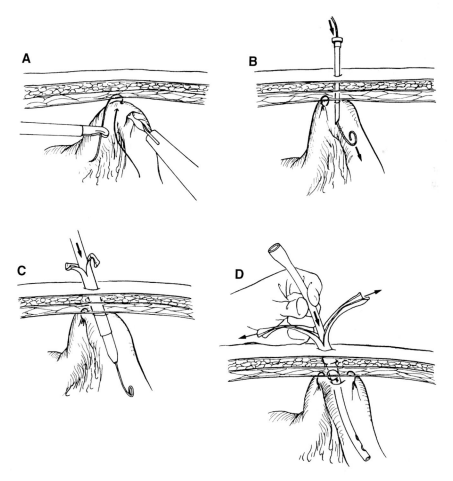

Figure 4–24. Laparoscopic feeding tube insertion. **A.** The bowel is secured to the abdominal wall with a single interrupted suture. This suture may be placed laparoscopically or by combined percutaneous and laparoscopic methods (see text). **B.** The jejunostomy tube is placed in three steps using a modified Seldinger technique. A needle is passed transcutaneously into the bowel and a soft guidewire is inserted through the needle. **C.** The needle is removed and a 10-Fr peel-away catheter and dilator are passed over the guidewire into the bowel. **D.** The dilator is removed and an 8-Fr feeding catheter is inserted through the peel-away sheath which then is removed. Additional sutures may be placed to anchor the jejunum to the posterior abdominal wall. (From Sangster W, Hunter JG. Laparoscopic access for enteral nutrition. In: Hunter JG, Sackier JM (eds), *Minimally Invasive Surgery.* New York, NY: McGraw-Hill; 1993:118)

selected cases. Three laparoscopic ports are inserted at the umbilicus (10 mm), right lower quadrant (10 mm) and upper midline (5 mm). The videotelescope usually is placed through the right lower quadrant port. The jejunum is identified at the ligament of Treitz and an appropriate site for placement of the tube is selected 25 to 40 cm distally. The subsequent steps in the procedure are demonstrated in Fig 4–24. The jejunum first must be anchored to the posterior abdominal wall. This usually is accomplished by percutaneously passing a suture on a straight needle into the abdomen where it is then passed through the seromuscular layer of the jejunum and back through the abdominal wall. A total of three sutures are necessary to adequately stabilize the jejunum. These sutures then can be tied externally. Alternatively, the jejunum may be secured with fasteners inserted via percutaneous needles[157] or by intracorporeal suturing of the jejunum to the posterior abdominal wall.[158] The jejunostomy tube is inserted using the Seldinger technique and employing a standard introducer and peel-away sheath kit. The basic steps are described below (Fig 4–24B through 24D). A needle is inserted percutaneously into the jejunum. A guidewire then is passed through the needle, the needle is removed, and the tract is dilated over the guidewire with a 12-Fr dilator and sheath. The dilator is removed and a 10-Fr catheter is inserted through the sheath. The sheath then is peeled away leaving the feeding tube in the jejunum. The position is confirmed by injecting the tube with saline, and the catheter is sutured externally to the skin. Tube feedings may be started immediately postoperatively. The technique for gastrostomy tube insertion is essentially identical except that a larger (18 Fr) balloon-tipped catheter is used. Stamm gastrostomy[159] and Janeway gastrostomy[160] also have been reported using laparoscopic techniques.

Sangster and Swanstrom[155] reported successful laparoscopic jejunostomy tube insertion in 23 consecutive patients. In most cases, operating time was less than 45 minutes. All patients were receiving full nutritional support within 48 hours of tube placement. The only complications were a superficial abscess in one patient and minor skin breakdown in two patients.

■ LAPAROSCOPIC COLON RESECTION

Colon resection is one of the most common major abdominal surgical procedures performed with approximately 200 000 cases done in the United States each year.[161] Therefore, it is not surprising that minimally invasive approaches to the treatment of colon and rectal disorders would be attempted. Colon resection for benign and malignant disease, colostomy formation and colostomy closure, and operations for rectal prolapse

now have been performed laparoscopically. Laparoscopic colon resections are technically demanding procedures because of the need to mobilize a segment of bowel, divide the mesenteric blood supply to that bowel, and create a water-tight anastomosis. Successful completion of each of these components of the operation depends on advanced laparoscopic skills that include the ability to operate from multiple viewpoints, familiarity with complex laparoscopic surgical instrumentation, and dexterity in laparoscopic suturing.

Intestinal resections may be performed using laparoscopic techniques exclusively or, as is more commonly done, in a laparoscopically assisted fashion in which a portion of the operation is performed extracorporeally through a small abdominal incision. Laparoscopic intestinal resections using totally intracorporeal methods have been reported both experimentally[162,163] and clinically.[164] The principal technical features that currently limit this approach are difficulties in reanastomosis of the bowel and removal of large specimens through small incisions. Recent advances in stapling technology already have overcome some of the barriers to laparoscopic intestinal resection and reanastomosis. However, specimen removal remains problematic because of the need for histologic evaluation of the intact bowel segment to stage colonic neoplasms.

In laparoscopic-assisted colectomy, the initial portion of the operation is done laparoscopically, including mobilization of the bowel segment and division of its mesenteric blood supply. A small incision (3 to 7 cm) then is made over the site of the mobilized bowel, which is exteriorized through the incision. Transection at anastomosis is performed in an open fashion using standard anastomotic techniques. The anastomosis itself can be performed rapidly and with the same integrity as in conventional open surgery. This approach also provides an uncomplicated means for removing the specimen from the abdomen. Theoretically at least, the smaller abdominal incision and reduced manipulation of the intra-abdominal viscera required of laparoscopic-assisted colectomy versus standard open colectomy should preserve many of the traditional benefits of a minimally invasive approach.

Patients in whom laparoscopic colectomy is contraindicated include those with large bowel obstruction or colonic perforation. Malignant neoplasms account for the majority of procedures in most published reports, but the appropriateness of laparoscopic treatment of colon cancer has been debated. Areas of concern include the possibility of inadequate staging, the adequacy of lymph node sampling and mesenteric resection, and the potential for implantation of tumor cells in the abdominal cavity. Tumor seeding of wound tracts of patients undergoing laparoscopic resection for colon cancer already has been observed[165] and is a major cause for

cock clamps. The lateral peritoneal attachments then are divided with cautery scissors. The ureters should be identified during right or left colectomy. The peritoneum of the bowel mesentery is incised and the mesenteric vessels are ligated with sutures, endoscopic clips, or a vascular stapler. Transillumination of the mesentery with a second light source may facilitate identification of mesenteric vessels. If the anastomosis is to be performed extracorporeally, the bowel should be exteriorized prior to transecting it. Following completion of the anastomosis, the mesenteric defect is closed and the bowel is returned to the abdominal cavity.

When the site of the planned anastomosis is at or below the level of the peritoneal reflection, it may be possible to use a totally intracorporeal approach by using a circular stapler passed transanally to create the anastomosis. The resected bowel segment may be removed either transanally or through a small abdominal incision. The stapling anvil for the proximal segment of colon may be placed in one of two methods: the proximal colon may be brought out through a small incision to allow the anvil and purse-string suture to be placed under direct vision and then dropped back into the abdominal cavity or alternatively, the anvil is passed transanally into the proximal bowel and the purse-string suture is placed with laparoscopic techniques. The distal rectal stump either is stapled closed or secured with a second purse-string suture. With either approach, the anvil in the proximal bowel then is manipulated down to the rectum laparoscopically and is attached to the stapler. As in open surgery, the anastomosis then should be tested with a proctoscope and air to ensure its integrity. Advances in stapling technology undoubtedly will lead to increased use of totally intracorporeal methods for performing bowel resections.

In addition to several small reports,[166–168] a few large uncontrolled trials[164,169–172] of laparoscopic colon resection have been reported and are summarized in Table 4–6. The operations performed have included right hemicolectomy, left hemicolectomy, low-anterior resection, abdominoperineal resection and subtotal colectomy. Phillips and associates[164] used totally intracorporeal methods in 40 (78%) of 51 patients, but most other reports have employed primarily laparoscopically assisted techniques. Polyps and colon cancer were the most common indications for operation. The number of lymph nodes examined per specimen was deemed to be adequate and consistent with pathology data from historical controls. Conversion to open colectomy was required in 8% to 41% of patients in these reports. Complications occurred in 8% to 28% of patients. When compared to conventional open colectomy, reduced pain medication requirements and earlier hospital discharge were demonstrated, but the degree of benefit was not as striking as for laparoscopic cholecys-

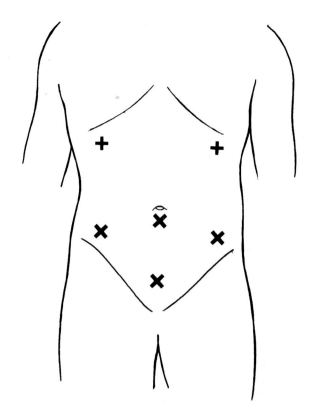

Figure 4–25. Port sites for laparoscopic colectomy. All ports should be 10 to 12 mm in diameter. The principal port sites are indicated by *X*. Supplemental ports should be placed opposite the side of the planned colectomy (ie, in the right upper quadrant for left colectomy and in the left upper quadrant for right colectomy).

concern. These observations suggest the need for controlled clinical trials to assess not only the cost effectiveness and safety of laparoscopic colon resection but to address the oncologic validity of the technique. The potential benefits of laparoscopic colectomy, in terms of postoperative pain and recovery, certainly cannot justify the operation unless the well-established principles of oncologic surgery can be followed.

Laparoscopic colon resections usually are performed via four or five 10-mm laparoscopic ports as shown in Fig 4–25. The fifth port, which is optional in some cases, is placed opposite the side of the planned colectomy in either upper quadrant. In patients with tumors, the adjacent bowel may be tattooed colonoscopically with India ink prior to the planned laparoscopic procedure so that the lesion is easily identifiable at laparoscopy. The patient should be placed in the modified lithotomy position. This allows the surgeon or assistant to stand between the patient's legs and also provides access to the rectum for distal resections. A bean-bag mattress is helpful in securing the patient to the operating table and allowing one to tilt the table. After inserting the laparoscopic ports, the bowel segment to be resected is grasped and retracted with atraumatic endoscopic Bab-

TABLE 4–6. RESULTS OF MAJOR SERIES OF LAPAROSCOPIC COLECTOMY

	Welton[169]	Phillips[164]	Falk[170]	Monson[171]	Zucker[172]
Number of Patients	87	51	66	40	65
Operative Time: Mean (range)	195 min (35–590 min)	138 min (75–390 min)	—	Right: 210 min (120–310 min) Left: 240 min (150–330 min)	142 min (110–217 min)
Conversion to Open Colectomy	8 (9%)	4 (8%)[a]	27 (41%)	7 (18%)	2 (3.1%)
Discharge Day	5	4.6 (1–30)	4–5	8 (5–14)[b]	4.1 (3–8)
Complications	24 (28%)	4 (8%)	16 (24%)	6 (15%)	4 (6.2%)
Deaths	0	1 (2%)	0	1 (2.5%)	0

[a]An additional seven patients were converted to laparoscopically assisted colectomy.
[b]The average length of hospitalization after open colectomy was 14 days.

tectomy. The average length of hospitalization in these reports ranged from 3.9 to 8 days.

Two groups have compared outcomes in patients undergoing the laparoscopic approach to outcomes in traditional open colon resections. Falk and associates[170] divided patients into three groups: (1) successful laparoscopic colectomy, (2) attempted laparoscopic colectomy converted to open colectomy, and (3) standard open colectomy. Patients who underwent successful laparoscopic colectomy were discharged from the hospital earlier, but overall costs were similar owing to the longer operating times and increased instrumentation expense of the laparoscopic approach. Wexner and colleagues[173] recently reported preliminary results in a small prospective randomized trial of 10 patients undergoing laparoscopic versus open total abdominal colectomy for benign disease. Patients treated by laparoscopic total abdominal colectomy had a longer duration of postoperative ileus and longer length of hospitalization than the open group. Operating time was also 35% longer in the laparoscopically treated patients.

OTHER COLON PROCEDURES

Laparoscopy is an ideal method for performing colostomy in patients who require fecal diversion and have nondilated bowel.[174] The technique is applicable to the creation of either loop or end colostomies. One of the laparoscopic ports should be inserted through the site at which the colostomy is to be placed. The extent of the dissection is minimal, since only the lateral peritoneal attachments of the left colon need to be mobilized. The apex of the sigmoid loop then is brought out through an enlarged port incision, where it is either matured as a loop colostomy or is divided with a stapler and matured as an end colostomy.

Laparoscopic closure of a left-sided colostomy after Hartmann's procedure also has been reported.[169] The stoma is mobilized externally and the anvil from a circular stapler then is inserted into it. A purse-string suture is placed and then tied around the anvil post. Some degree of adhesiolysis usually can be performed under direct vision through the stoma site and makes placement of the other laparoscopic ports easier. The fascia at the stoma opening is closed around a laparoscopic port and pneumoperitoneum is established. Further adhesiolysis and mobilization of the rectal stump is carried out laparoscopically through three or four additional ports. Mobilization of the splenic flexure of the colon may be necessary to achieve a tension-free anastomosis. The anastomosis can be completed using a circular stapler passed transanally.

Laparoscopic rectopexy for rectal prolapse has been reported by several groups.[175–177] Early results have been satisfactory in terms of resumption of normal bowel function, and recurrences have not been observed.

■ LAPAROSCOPIC HEPATIC AND PANCREATIC PROCEDURES

The application of laparoscopic techniques to the treatment of a variety of hepatobiliary and pancreatic diseases other than cholelithiasis is currently under evaluation. Partial hepatectomy in patients with liver tumors has been performed using ultrasonic dissection and high voltage electrocautery.[178] Laparoscopic treatment of hepatic cysts by unroofing the cyst and packing the cyst cavity with omentum has been reported by several groups.[179–181] Laparoscopic ultrasound may be useful to delineate the extent of the cyst and its relationship to the underlying hepatic anatomy.[181]

Palliative procedures for bypass of patients with unresectable pancreatic cancer have been performed laparoscopically, including cholecystojejunostomy[182] and gastrojejunostomy.[183] Whether these procedures achieve better or more cost-effective palliation than the currently available endoscopic and radiologic techniques will need to be evaluated. Laparoscopic pancreatic resections have been accomplished experimentally[184] and clinically. Gagner and associates have performed laparoscopic pancreaticoduodenectomy (Whipple procedure) in three patients and distal pancreatectomy for benign pancreatic tumors (2 insulinomas, 1 cystadenoma) in three patients.[183a]

■ LAPAROSCOPIC SPLENECTOMY

Splenectomy has been performed laparoscopically in carefully selected patients by a number of groups.[185–187] Patients should have a near normal–size spleen and good clinical performance status. Contraindications to the laparoscopic approach include marked splenomegaly and an uncontrollable bleeding diathesis. Consideration should be given to preoperative splenic artery embolization during the learning curve of the surgeon's experience and also in obese patients.[188]

The sequential steps in performing laparoscopic splenectomy have been described by Phillips.[188] The patient is positioned with the left arm extended and the left side elevated 20° with a flank roll. Five laparoscopic ports are used, as shown in Fig 4–26. The first step in the procedure should be ligation of the splenic artery, which is accomplished by entering the lesser sac via the gastrocolic omentum. The splenic artery is isolated along the superior border of the pancreas and is ligated with endoscopic clips. The splenic flexure of the colon then is mobilized; the inferior pole branches to the spleen are isolated and divided. Vessel ligation may be accomplished with clips or sutures tied extracorporeally. Endoloops also may be used for larger vessels, but their application first requires that the vessel be divided, after achieving preliminary control, with clips or a grasping instrument. The spleen is retracted medially and the splenorenal attachments are divided with the cautery. The spleen then is lifted anteriorly with an atraumatic fan retractor and the hilar vessels are dissected, ligated, and divided. This allows better access to the short gastric vessels that are divided between endoscopic clips. The remaining splenophrenic attachments are divided with the cautery. The spleen then is placed in an impermeable nylon entrapment sac and removed at the umbilical port site. If histologic evaluation of the spleen is unimportant, the specimen may be morcel-

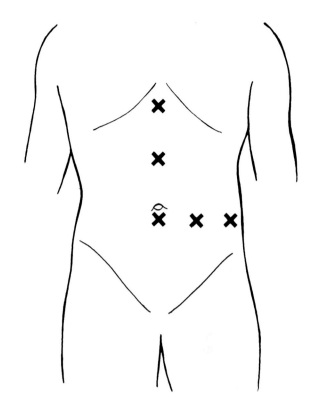

Figure 4–26. Port sites for laparoscopic splenectomy. (From Phillips EH. Laparoscopic splenectomy. In: Hunter JG, Sackier JM (eds), *Minimally Invasive Surgery*. New York, NY: McGraw-Hill; 1993:309–313. Reprinted with permission).

lated within the bag and removed through the port incision. For removal of the intact spleen, the umbilical incision is extended inferiorly.

Phillips and associates[189] have attempted laparoscopic splenectomy in 10 patients. The clinical diagnoses in these individuals were immune thrombocytopenia purpura (6 patients), Hodgkin's lymphoma (1 patient) and hemolytic anemia (3 patients). Four patients were converted to open splenectomy; the mean operating time was 155 minutes and blood loss averaged 350 mL. Two patients required blood transfusions postoperatively. There were no complications and patients were discharged an average of 3.3 days postoperatively.

Recently, a transabdominal lateral flank approach has been utilized successfully in performing laparoscopic splenectomy.[190] The patient is placed in the right lateral decubitus position (left side up) and four 10 to 11-mm trocars are inserted in the lateral abdominal and flank region. The sequential steps in the dissection are (1) mobilization of the splenic flexure of the colon, (2) division of the splenorenal ligament, (3) isolation and division of the splenic hilar vessels, and (4) division of the short gastric vessels. Placement of the spleen in an entrapment sac is faciliated by leaving the spleen suspended from its ligamentous attachments to the diaphragm while the spleen is maneuvered into the bag. The principal advantage of the lateral approach is that exposure is simplified owing to gravity retraction of the liver, spleen, and stomach medially and the intestines inferiorly. Consequently, operative times and blood loss may be reduced when compared to the anterior transabdominal approach.[190]

While these data indicate that laparoscopic splenectomy can be successfully performed by experienced laparoscopists, this is a technique that requires advanced skills and is associated with potentially hazardous bleeding. The benefits and risks of laparoscopic splenectomy should be investigated in a larger number of patients before this approach can be widely recommended.

■ LAPAROSCOPIC HERNIA REPAIR

Inguinal hernia repair is one of the most commonly performed surgical procedures, with approximately 500 000 patients undergoing operation in the United States each year.[191–193] Conventional herniorrhaphy consists of ligation or reduction of the hernia sac and suture reconstruction of the inguinal floor. The operation is simple to perform and in most cases, can be carried out under local anesthesia as an outpatient procedure. However, the traditional types of groin hernia repairs (Bassini repair and McVay repair) have been associated with recurrence rates of 5% to 10% for primary hernias and 10% to 30% for recurrent hernias.[194–196] Other types of open hernia repair, including the Shouldice repair[197] and the Lichtenstein tension-free hernia repair[198] with mesh, have been associated with low recurrence rates, but they are not widely employed by most practicing surgeons. Moreover, open hernia repair often is associated with considerable postoperative pain and a delayed return to unrestricted physical activity and employment (4 weeks or more). Complications of ilioinguinal nerve injury, spermatic cord injury, orchitis, and epididymitis may delay the recovery process further. These "imperfections" in conventional herniorrhaphy, along with the success of laparoscopic cholecystectomy, have provided incentive for the development of laparoscopic hernia repair.

Several different techniques for laparoscopic hernia repair have, to date, been utilized in humans. Some of these initial approaches have included ligation of the hernia sac and staple closure of the internal inguinal ring,[199] insertion of a mesh plug to fill the hernia defect,[200–201] iliopubic tract repair,[201] and various types of preperitoneal patch repair.[203–205] The preperitoneal patch repair is the most generally accepted method for laparoscopic hernia repair and entails placement of a large prosthetic patch to cover the hernia defect and inguinal floor. This operation is analagous to the open

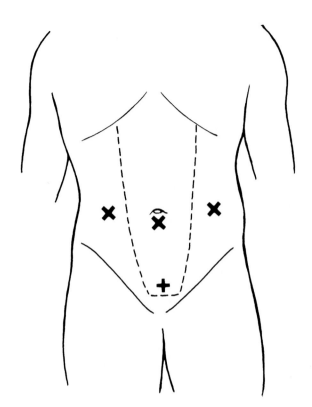

Figure 4–27. Port sites for laparoscopic hernia repair. The three primary ports (*X*) are 10 to 12 mm in size to allow insertion of the hernia stapler. In some cases, a fourth port (5 mm), in the suprapubic region, may be useful in providing additional retraction.

preperitoneal approach advocated by Stoppa,[206] who used a large tension-free patch to cover the entire inguinal myopectineal orifice. A hernia recurrence rate of only 1.4% has been reported with the Stoppa repair.[207]

Laparoscopic inguinal hernia repair usually is performed under general anesthesia. Three 10 to 12-mm laparoscopic ports are placed transabdominally into the peritoneal cavity: one at the umbilicus and one each in the right and left midabdomen at about the level of the umbilicus (Fig 4–27). Inspection of the inguinal floor is carried out bilaterally. Prior to any dissection, the surgical landmarks identifiable laparoscopically include the internal inguinal ring, vas deferens, spermatic vessels, inferior epigastric vessels, and the iliac artery and vein (Fig 4–28). One can distinguish readily between indirect, direct, and femoral hernias. The peritoneum overlying the inguinal floor is incised and, along with the hernia sac, is dissected off the underlying structures. In cases in which the indirect sac is large, the distal sac simply may be disconnected and left in situ. The dissection is complete once the sac has been reduced and the peritoneum has been elevated such that Cooper's ligament, the pubic tubercle, and iliopubic tract are clearly defined.[208] A large sheath (3 inches by 5 inches) of prosthetic mesh then is placed over the entire myopectineal

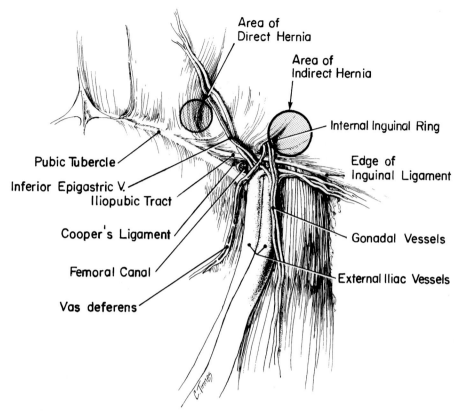

Figure 4–28. Anatomic landmarks for laparoscopic hernia repair. A preperitoneal view of the anatomy of the inguinal floor on the right side is shown here. (v = vessels). (From Geis P, et al. *Surgery* 1993;114:767)

orifice and secured in place with a stapling device or with sutures (Fig 4–29). The peritoneum then is closed over the mesh with staples or sutures in order to reduce the frequency of postoperative adhesions. Direct intraperitoneal placement of the mesh, which was carried out in some early studies,[209] has been discontinued, mostly because of the risk of adhesion formation. Recently, extraperitoneal laparoscopic hernia repair has been carried out by confining CO_2 insufflation and laparoscopic port placement to the preperitoneal space.[204] Expansion of the preperitoneal space with balloon dilation has greatly improved access and has facilitated dissection of the preperitoneal space at the level of the inguinal floor. The advantages of this extraperitoneal approach are that it avoids the potential risks to intra-abdominal organs associated with transperitoneal laparoscopy.

Preliminary data from two large uncontrolled multiinstitutional trials have analyzed the safety and efficacy of the laparoscopic approach to hernia repair. McFadyen and colleagues[203] tabulated data from 16 surgeons who performed 847 laparoscopic hernia repairs in 752 patients (Table 4–7). Preperitoneal placement of a large prosthesis over the inguinal floor was associated with the lowest incidence of recurrent hernia. The vari-

ous plug techniques have been associated with high rates of hernia recurrence and have been abandoned.[91] The complication rate ranged from 4.4% to 19.8%, but most complications were minor and consisted of small local hematomas, groin pain, and transient postoperative urinary dysfunction. Bladder injury, reported in four patients, was the most common serious complication. Fitzgibbons and associates[205] reported 597 patients who underwent 736 hernia repairs using the prosthetic patch procedure. The types of hernias treated were: indirect inguinal (362), direct inguinal (302), femoral (20), and combined (52). Bilateral hernias were repaired in 139 (23.3%) patients and 117 (19.6%) patients had recurrent hernias. There have been 16 (2.2%) definite hernia recurrences and 9 (1.2%) possible recurrences during an average follow-up period of 6 months. There was one postoperative death due to myocardial infarction. Perioperative complications have included local hematomas (7.5%), urinary dysfunction (3.7%), thigh pain or numbness (3.9%), groin pain (12.9%), orchitis (2%), and testicular or spermatic cord swelling (5%). Persistent thigh pain or numbness was seen in three patients (0.5%). These symptoms have occurred most commonly in the distribution of either the femoral branch of the genitofemoral nerve or the lat-

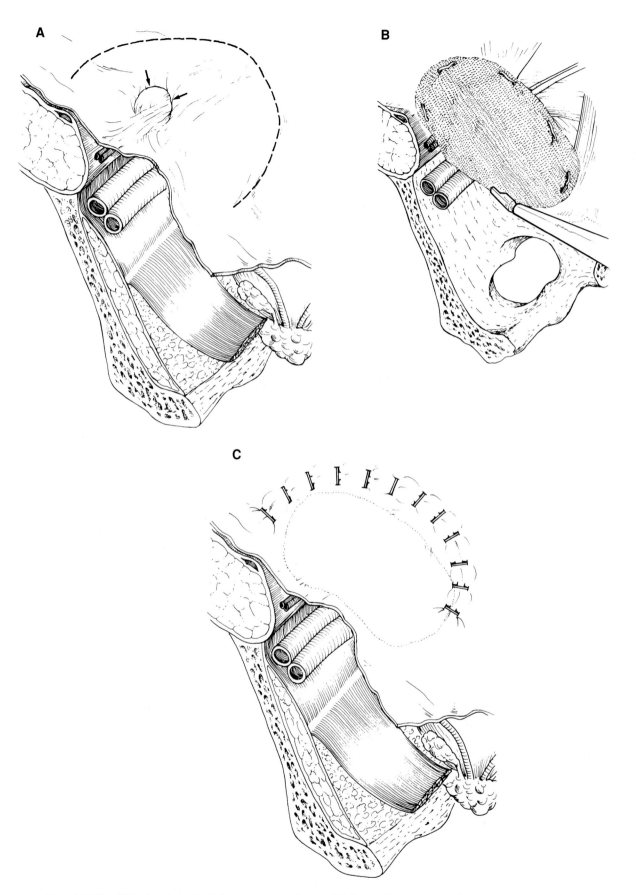

Figure 4–29. View of the left inguinal region during laparoscopic hernia repair. **A**. Indirect hernia (*arrow*) showing location of incision (*dotted line*) of peritoneum. **B**. Placement and staple fixation of the mesh. **C**. Closure of the peritoneum over the mesh with staples. (Modified from Soper NJ, et al. *N Engl J Med* 1994 (330;409-419)

TABLE 4–7. EARLY RESULTS OF LAPAROSCOPIC INGUINAL HERNIA REPAIR

Method of Repair	Patients	Number of Hernias	Recurrences (%)	Follow-up	Incidence Complications[a]
Sac Ligation and Internal Ring Closure	87	98	2 (2.0%)	24 mo.	4.4%
Plug and Patch	74	84	6 (7.1%)	8 mo.	13.5%
Iliopubic Tract Suture	28	30	2 (6.6%)	<6 mo.	19.8%
Prosthetic patch across inguinal floor	563	635	9 (1.4%)	5.6 mo.	9.0%

[a]Most complications were minor and consisted of transient postoperative urinary dysfunction, groin pain or small local hematomas.
(From MacFadyen BV, Arregui ME, Corbitt JD, et al. Complications of laparoscopic herniorrhaphy. *Surg Endosc* 1993;7:155–158)

eral cutaneous nerve of the thigh.[210] This complication, as well as more serious injuries in the femoral nerve, can be prevented by avoiding placement of staples posterior to the iliopubic tract or more than 1.5 cm lateral to the internal ring.[211]

Despite a significant rate (2% to 4%) of early recurrence following laparoscopic hernia repair, the operation has been viewed favorably by many groups because it does appear to result in reduced postoperative pain and an earlier return to full physical activity compared to conventional herniorrhaphy.[199,201,203–205,212,213] In a study of 163 patients, Schultz[213] reported minimal use of analgesics and found that patients were able to resume the normal activities of daily living an average of 2.4 days postoperatively and returned to work an average of 4.5 days after surgery. However, reduced postoperative pain and early physical rehabilitation also have been characteristic of open tension-free hernioplasties in which a mesh prosthesis is used to bridge the hernia defect.[214]

Therefore, the potential advantages of laparoscopic hernia repair must be weighed against several controversial aspects of the procedure.[91,215] Most other laparoscopic procedures performed to date have attempted to duplicate their open counterparts, whereas laparoscopic hernia repair represents a departure from conventional herniorrhaphy technique. The favorable results reported with the open Stoppa technique[206] may not be reproduced using current laparoscopic techniques. Many hernia recurrences develop 5 years or more after the original operation,[194] whereas average follow-up has been short (≤ 6 months) in all trials of laparoscopic herniorrhaphy. Thus, the potential exists for an excessively high recurrence rate to appear in the future for a procedure that has been widely implemented without adequate evaluation in controlled clinical trials. Also, early reports have originated from centers with special interest and expertise in this technique and may not reflect those results obtainable by the average general surgeon who is well trained in open hernia repair.

Several other factors also should be considered in determining the advisability of laparoscopic hernia repair.[91] Laparoscopic hernia repair requires a general anesthetic. There is a small risk of serious injury to intra-abdominal structures that does not exist with an extra-abdominal inguinal hernia repair. Complications, including infection and adhesion formation, may occur from prosthetic mesh placement. Finally, laparoscopic hernia repair may be more expensive. In contrast to laparoscopic cholecystectomy, these costs are not offset by decreased in-patient hospital costs. A recent comparison of conventional open hernia repair versus laparoscopic repair indicated an average increase in cost of 135% with the laparoscopic approach.[216] These various aspects of laparoscopic hernia repair should be investigated in controlled clinical trials with long-term follow-up before the procedure is used more widely.

■ LAPAROSCOPIC ADRENALECTOMY

In many respects, the adrenal glands are ideally suited to laparoscopic excision, since most adrenal tumors are small and pathologically benign. However, laparoscopic access to the adrenals is complicated by their cephalad location in the retroperitoneum superior to the kidneys and deep to other intra-abdominal viscera. Recently, a variety of minimally invasive approaches have been utilized for performing adrenalectomy.[217–220] These approaches have been patterned after the standard open operative techniques for performing adrenalectomy: anterior transabdominal approach, lateral flank approach, and posterior retroperitoneal approach.

The advantage of the transabdominal approach is that the endoscopic view is the same as for other laparoscopic procedures. However, this method is technically difficult because of the need to mobilize and retract overlying intra-abdominal organs and has been associated with prolonged operating times.[220–222] Laparoscopic adrenalectomy that uses the transabdominal

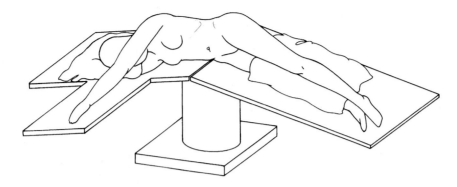

Figure 4–30. Patient position for laparoscopic left adrenalectomy. The patient is in a lateral decubitus position with the left side up. For right adrenalectomy, the right side is up. Pressure points (axilla, hips) should be padded well. (From Brunt LM, Soper NJ. Laparoscopic adrenalectomy. In: Arregui ME, Fitzgibbons RF, Katkhouda N, et al. (eds), *Principles of Laparoscopic Surgery: Basic and Advanced Techniques.* New York, NY: Springer-Verlag; 1995, pp 366–378)

lateral flank approach has been the most successful technique utilized to date and is discussed in detail below. A posterior retroperitoneal approach to laparoscopic adrenalectomy is theoretically attractive because of the directness of this approach and because this method eliminates the need to retract intra-abdominal organs. Retroperitoneal endoscopic adrenalectomy first was developed experimentally, using direct retroperitoneoscopy with CO_2 insufflation of the retroperitoneal space.[217] However, clinical application of this technique is, at this time, uncertain because of limitations imposed by the small confines of the retroperitoneal working space and the large amount of retroperitoneal fat encountered in most patients.

The most successful method for performing adrenalectomy laparoscopically has been the transabdominal lateral flank approach.[223] For this approach, the patient is placed in the lateral decubitus position with the side that harbors the adrenal lesion facing up (Fig 4–30). Flexion of the operating room table may be helpful in expanding access to the flank area. Pressure points (axilla, hips) should be padded well to avoid nerve compression injuries. A total of four laparoscopic ports are placed as shown in Fig 4–31. All ports should be 10 mm in diameter to allow complete flexibility in placing the videotelescope and dissecting instruments. Mobilization of the splenic flexure of the colon on the left, and hepatic flexure of the colon and right lobe of the liver on the right, are necessary to allow placement of the more dorsal fourth port in the posterior axillary line. Cautery scissors are used to dissect out the adrenal gland, and endoscopic clips are used to ligate discrete arterial branches and the adrenal vein. Particular caution should be exercised in dissecting out the right adrenal vein, which is short, broad (1 cm in diameter), and empties directly into the inferior vena cava. Adherence to established principles of open adrenal surgery

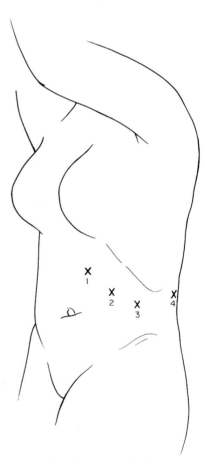

Figure 4–31. Port sites for laparoscopic left adrenalectomy. The initial port is inserted in the midsubcostal region. Additional ports are placed in the anterior axillary, midaxillary and posterior axillary lines. For right adrenalectomy, the ports are placed in a similar location in the right flank. (From Brunt LM, Soper NJ. Laparoscopic adrenalectomy. In: Arregui ME, Fitzgibbons RF, Katkhouda N, et al (eds), *Principles of Laparoscopic Surgery: Basic and Advanced Techniques.* Springer-Verlag. 1995, pp 366–378)

with meticulous hemostasis and extracapsular dissection of the adrenal is critical to avoid bleeding complications and to prevent implantation of adrenal tissue or tumor in the retroperitoneum. Once the adrenal gland has been dissected free, it is placed in an impermeable entrapment sac and removed at the mid-subcostal port site.

Laparoscopic adrenalectomy using the lateral flank approach was attempted by Gagner in 18 patients with a variety of adrenal neoplasms.[223] Conversion to open adrenalectomy was necessary in only one patient who had a 15-cm angiomyolipoma of the right adrenal gland. Bilateral adrenalectomy for adrenal hyperplasia from Cushing's disease was performed laparoscopically in three patients. The average operative time per adrenal gland removed was 2.3 hours and was slightly longer for right (2.7 hours) than for left (1.8 hours) adrenalectomy. Patients were discharged from the hospital an average of 4 days postoperatively (range of 2 to 19 days), and postoperative transfusions were necessary in two patients. Our group has recently obtained similar success in seven patients treated with laparoscopic adrenalectomy using this approach.[224]

These preliminary results suggest that, in carefully selected patients, laparoscopic adrenalectomy may be considered as an alternative to an open surgical approach. Large adrenal tumors (>6 cm) with a suspicion of malignancy should, at this time, contraindicate the laparoscopic approach. Patients with pheochromocytomas may be considered candidates for laparoscopic adrenalectomy provided the lesion has been clearly localized, the patient is medically stable, and has been prepared pharmacologically for surgery.[225] Laparoscopic adrenalectomy should not alter current guidelines for the management of asymptomatic adrenal masses.

■ CREDENTIALING AND TRAINING

Prior to 1989, most surgical training programs did not provide for residency experience in laparoscopic surgical techniques. The rapid development of laparoscopic cholecystectomy and market-driven public demand for this new procedure presented the surgical community with an unprecedented need for retraining an entire generation of surgeons. The academic medical centers were unprepared to meet the private sector demand, and this void was filled primarily by free-standing and industry-sponsored short (2 to 3 day) courses consisting of didactic sessions and a variable degree of hands-on laboratory experience.[226] This variability in training and the inevitable learning curve associated with laparoscopic cholecystectomy have been factors in the increased incidence of biliary complications and common bile duct injuries reported with this procedure.[98–100] In New York State, where hospitals are required to report adverse events to the Department of Health, an alarming increase in serious complications and even deaths from laparoscopic cholecystectomy was reported.[101] The subsequent investigation in New York led the Department of Health to issue a memorandum establishing statewide guidelines for privileging and credentialing in laparoscopic surgery. These New York guidelines have served as a "wake-up call"[227] for hospitals and practicing surgeons alike that laparoscopic surgery requires specific skills that differ from traditional open surgical methods and necessitates separate privileging mechanisms. Although some surgical organizations have published guidelines for privileges and credentialing in laparoscopic surgery,[228] ultimately the responsibility must lie at the local level, in hospitals and in surgery departments. The increasing implementation of advanced laparoscopic surgical procedures and the introduction of new operative approaches will continue to require careful monitoring and strict privileging guidelines to ensure issues of safety, efficacy, and quality control.

Laparoscopic surgery also has unquestionably added a new dimension to surgical residency education and training.[4,229] More advanced laparoscopic procedures, especially those performed infrequently, may present a special challenge to resident training. As minimally invasive techniques advance, it is likely that traditional surgical education will need to be supplemented by increased use of hands-on laboratory courses. The development of computer-driven video technologies and virtual-reality techniques may expand the possibilities for surgical training. Undoubtedly, many of the challenges of residency training in laparoscopic surgery will diminish as the next video generation of students enters our surgical training programs.

REFERENCES

1. Spaw AT, Reddick EJ, Olsen DO. Laparoscopic laser cholecystectomy: analysis of 500 procedures. *Surg Laparosc Endosc* 1991;1:2–7
2. Soper NJ, Barteau JA, Clayman RV, et al. Comparison of early postoperative results for laparoscopic vs standard open cholecystectomy. *Surg Gynecol Obstet* 1992;174:114–118
3. Barkun JS, Barkun AN, Sampalis JS, et al. Randomized controlled trial of laparoscopic vs minicholecystectomy. *Lancet* 1992;340:1116–1119
4. Soper NJ, Stockman PT, Dunnegan DL, Ashley SW. Laparoscopic cholecystectomy: the new "gold standard"? *Arch Surg* 1992;127:917–921
5. Rosin D. History. In: Rosin D (ed), *Minimal Access Medicine and Surgery: Principles and Techniques.* Oxford, England: Radcliffe Medical Press; 1993:1–9

6. Kelling G. Zur colioskopie. *Arch Klin Chir* 1923;126:226–229

7. Jacobeus HC. Kurze ubersicht uber meine erfahrungen mit der laparoskopie. *Munch Med Woechenschr* 1911;58:2017–2019

8. Kalk H. Erfahrungen mit der laparoskopie. *Z Klin Med* 1929;111:303–348

9. Veress J. Neues instrument zur ausfuhrung von brust oder bauchpunktionen. *Dtsch Med Wochenshr* 1938;41:1480–1481

10. Semm K. History. In: Sanfilippo JS, Levine RL (eds), *Operative Gynecologic Endoscopy*. New York, NY: Springer-Verlag; 1989

11. Semm K. Endoscopic appendectomy. *Endoscopy* 1983;15:59–64

12. Berci G, Cuschieri A. *Practical Laparoscopy*. East Sussex, England: Ballière Tindall; 1986

13. Cuschieri A, Hall AW, Clark J. Value of laparoscopy in diagnosis and management of pancreatic carcinoma. *Gut* 1978;19:672–677

14. DuBois F, Icard P, Berthelot G, et al. Coelioscopic cholecystectomy: preliminary report of 36 cases. *Ann Surg* 1990;211:60–62

15. Filipi CJ, Fitzgibbons RJ, Salerno GM. Historical review: diagnostic laparoscopy to laparoscopic cholecystectomy and beyond. In: Zucker KA (ed), *Surgical Laparoscopy*. St. Louis, MO: Quality Medical; 1991:3–21

16. Reddick EJ, Olsen DO. Laparoscopic laser cholecystectomy: a comparison with mini-lap cholecystectomy. *Surg Endosc* 1989;3:131–133

17. Reddick EJ, Olsen D, Daniell J, et al. Laparoscopic laser cholecystectomy. *Laser Med Surg News Adv* February 1989:38–40

18. A tiny TV camera is fast transforming gallbladder surgery. *The Wall Street Journal* December 10, 1990

19. Talamini MA, Gadacz TR. Laparoscopic equipment and instrumentation. In: Zucker KA (ed), *Surgical Laparoscopy*. St. Louis, MO: Quality Medical, 1991:23–55

20. Duppler DW. Laparoscopic instrumentation, videoimaging, and equipment disinfection and sterilization. *Surg Clin N Amer* 1992;72:1021–1032

21. Satava RM, Poc W, Joyce G. Current generation video endoscopes: a critical evaluation. *Am Surg* 1988;54:73–77

22. Hasnain JU, Matjasko MJ. Practical anesthesia for laparoscopic procedures. In: Zucker KA (ed). *Surgical Laparoscopy*. St. Louis, MO: Quality Medical; 1991:77–86

23. Versichelen L, Serreyn R, Rolly G, Vanderkerckhove D. Physiopathologic changes during anesthesia administration for gynecologic laparoscopy. *J Reprod Med* 1984;29:697–700

24. Soper NJ, Hunter JG. Suturing and knot tying in laparoscopy. *Surg Clin N Amer* 1992;2:1139–1152

25. Clayman RV, Kavoussi LR, McDougall EM, et al. Laparoscopic nephrectomy: a review of 16 cases. *Surg Laparosc Endosc* 1992;1:29–34

26. Absten GT. Lasers and cautery in laparoscopy. In: Graber JN, Schultz LS, Pietrafitla JJ, Hickok DF, et al (eds). *Laparoscopic Abdominal Surgery*. New York, NY: McGraw-Hill; 1993:41–56

27. Hunter JG. Laser physics and tissue interaction. In:

Hunter JG, Sackier JM (eds). *Minimally Invasive Surgery*. New York, NY: McGraw-Hill; 1993:23–31

28. Odell RC. Laparoscopic electrosurgery. In: Hunter JG, Sackier JM (eds). *Minimally Invasive Surgery*. New York, NY: McGraw-Hill; 1993:33–41

29. Voyles CR. The laparoscopic buck stops here! *Am J Surg* 1993;165:472–473

30. Soderstrom RM, Levy BS. Bowel injuries during laparoscopy: causes and medicolegal questions. *Contemp Ob Gyn* 1985;27:41–45

31. Bordelon BM, Hobday KA, Hunter JG. Laser vs electrosurgery in laparoscopic cholecystectomy: a prospective randomized trial. *Arch Surg* 1993;128:233–236

32. Mintz M. Risks and prophylaxis in laparoscopy: a survey of 100,000 cases. *J Reprod Med* 1977;18:269–272

33. Peterson HB, Greenspan JR, Ory HW. Death following puncture of the aorta during laparoscopic sterilization. *Obstet Gynecol* 1981;59:133–134

34. Johannsen G, Andersen M, Juhl B. The effect of general anaesthesia on the haemodynamic events during laparoscopy with CO_2-insufflation. *Acta Anaesthesiol Scand* 1989;33:132–136

35. Hanley ES. Anesthesia for laparoscopic surgery. *Surg Clin N Amer* 1992;72:1013–1019

36. Gomar C, Fernandez C, Villalonga A, Nalda MA. Carbon dioxide embolism during laparoscopy and hysteroscopy. *Ann Fr Anesth Reanim* 1985;4:380–382

37. Vereecken L. Laparoscopic treatment of perforated gastroduodenal ulcer. *Surg Endosc* 1993;7:123

38. Nowzaradan Y, Barnes JP Jr, Westmoreland J, Hojabri M. Laparoscopic appendectomy: treatment of choice for suspected appendicitis. *Surg Laparosc Endosc* 1993;3:411–416

39. Drouard F, Delamarre J, Caprin J-P. Cutaneous seeding of gallbladder cancer after laparoscopic cholecystectomy. *N Engl J Med* 1991;325:316

40. Soper NJ, Hunter JG, Petrie RH. Laparoscopic cholecystectomy during pregnancy. *Surg Endosc* 1992;6:115–117

41. Morrell DG, Mullins JR, Harrison PB. Laparoscopic cholecystectomy during pregnancy in symptomatic patients. *Surgery* 1992;112:856–859

42. Miles RH, Carballo RE, Prinz RA, et al. Laparoscopy: the preferred method of cholecystectomy in the morbidly obese. *Surgery* 1992;112:818–823

43. Schirmer BD, Dix J, Edge SB, et al. Laparoscopic cholecystectomy in the obese patient. *Ann Surg* 1992;216:146–152

44. Unger SW, Scott JS, Unger HM, Edelman DS. Laparoscopic approach to gallstones in the morbidly obese patient. *Surg Endosc* 1991;5:116–117

45. Schauer PR, Luna J, Ghiatas AA, et al. Pulmonary function after laparoscopic cholecystectomy. *Surgery* 1993;114:389–399

46. Peters JH, Ortega A, Lehnerd SL, et al. The physiology of laparoscopic surgery: pulmonary function after laparoscopic cholecystectomy. *Surg Laparosc Endosc* 1993;3:370–374

47. Ponsky JL. Complications of laparoscopic cholecystectomy. *Am J Surg* 1991;161:393–395

48. Lightdale C. Indications, contraindications and compli-

cations of laparoscopy. In: Sivak M (ed). *Gastroenterologic Endoscopy.* Philadelphia, PA: WB Saunders; 1987: 1039–1044

49. Southern Surgeon's Club. A prospective analysis of 1518 laparoscopic cholecystectomies. *N Engl J Med* 1991;324: 1073–1078

50. Dubois F, Berthelot G, Levard H. Laparoscopic cholecystectomy: historic perspective and personal experience. *Surg Endosc* 1991;1:52–57

51. Cuschieri A, Dubois F, Mouiel J, et al. The European experience with laparoscopic cholecystectomy. *Am J Surg* 1991;161:385–387

52. Wolfe BM, Gardiner BN, Leary BF. Endoscopic cholecystectomy: an analysis of complications. *Arch Surg* 1991;126: 1192–1198

53. Deziel DJ, Millikan KW, Economou SG, et al. Complications of laparoscopic cholecystectomy: a national survey of 4,292 hospitals and an analysis of 77,604 cases. *Am J Surg* 1993;165:9–14

54. Bailey RW. Complications of laparoscopic general surgery. In: Zucker KA (ed). *Surgical Laparoscopy.* St. Louis, MO: Quality Medical Publishing; 1991;311–342

55. Beadle, EM. Complications of laparoscopy. In: Graber JN, Schultz LS, Pietrafitla JJ, Hickok DF, et al. (eds). *Laparoscopic Abdominal Surgery.* New York, NY: McGraw Hill; 1993:75–82

56. Orlando R, Russell JC, Lynch J, Mattie A. Laparoscopic cholecystectomy: a statewide experience. *Arch Surg* 1993; 128:494–499

57. Sigman HH, Fried GM, Garzon J, et al. Risks of blind versus open approach to celiotomy for laparoscopic surgery. *Surg Laparosc Endosc* 1993;4:296–299

58. Cuschieri A, Berci G. Laparoscopic biliary surgery: Instruments and basic operative techniques for laparoscopic surgery. London, England: Blackwell Scientific; 1990:15–37

59. Semm K. *Operative Manual for Endoscopic Abdominal Surgery.* Chicago, IL: Year Book; 1987:130–213

60. Reich H. Laparoscopic bowel injury. *Surg Laparosc Endosc* 1992;2:74–78

61. Peters JH, Gibbons GD, Innes JT, et al. Complications of laparoscopic cholecystectomy. *Surgery* 1991;110:769–778

62. Mealy K, Hylar J. Small bowel obstruction following laparoscopic cholecystectomy. *Eur J Surg* 1991;157:675–676

63. Kiilholma P, Makinen J. Incarcerated Richter's hernia after laparoscopy. *Eur J Obstet Gynecol Reprod Biol* 1988;28: 75–77

64. Radcliffe AG. Richter's herniation of the small bowel through the trocar site following laparoscopic surgery. *J Laparoendosc Surg* 1993;3:520–522

65. Leape LL, Ramenofsky ML. Laparoscopy for questionable appendicitis: can it reduce the negative appendectomy rate? *Ann Surg* 1980;191:410–413

66. Deutsch AA, Zelikovsky A, Reiss R. Laparoscopy in the prevention of unnecessary appendicectomies: a prospective study. *Br J Surg* 1982;69:336–337

67. Paterson-Brown S. Laparoscopy as an adjunct to decision making in the 'acute abdomen'. *Br J Surg* 1986;73: 1022–1024

68. Salky B. Diagnostic laparoscopy. *Surg Laparosc Endosc* 1993;3:132–134

69. Easter DW, Cuschieri A, Nathanson LK, Lavelle-Jones M. The utility of diagnostic laparoscopy for abdominal disorders: audit of 120 patients. *Arch Surg* 1992;127:379–383

70. Bender JS, Talamini MA. Diagnostic laparoscopy in critically ill intensive care unit patients. *Surg Endosc* 1992; 6:302–304

71. Warshaw AL, Castillo CF. Laparoscopy in preoperative diagnosis and staging for gastrointestinal cancers. In: Zucker KA (ed). *Surgical Laparoscopy.* St. Louis, MO: Quality Medical; 1991:101–113

72. Greene FL. Laparoscopy in malignant disease. *Surg Clin N Amer* 1992;72:1125–1137

73. Jeffers L, Spiegelman G, Reddy KR, et al. Laparoscopically directed fine needle aspiration for the diagnosis of hepatocellular carcinoma: a safe and accurate technique. *Gastrointest Endosc* 1988;34:235–237

74. Lightdale CL. Clinical applications of laparoscopy in patients with malignant neoplasms. *Gastrointest Endosc* 1982;28:99–102

75. Cuschieri A. Laparoscopy for pancreatic cancer: does it benefit the patient? *Eur J Surg Oncol* 1988;14:41–44

76. Spinelli P, Difelice G. Laparoscopy and abdominal malignancies. *Prob Gen Surg* 1991;8:329–347

77. Warshaw AL, Zhuo-Yun G, Wittenberg J, et al. Preoperative staging and assessment of resectability of pancreatic carcinoma. *Arch Surg* 1990;125:230–233

78. Possik RA, Franco EL, Pires DR, et al. Sensitivity, specificity, and predictive value of laparoscopy for the staging of gastric cancer and for the detection of liver metastases. *Cancer* 1986;58:1–6

79. Shandall A and Johnson C. Laparoscopy or scanning in oesophageal and gastric carcinoma? *Br J Surg* 1985;72: 449–451

80. Gross E, Bancewicz J, Ingram G. Assessment of gastric cancer by laparoscopy. *Br Med J* 1984;288:1577

81. Dagnini G, Caldironi W, Martin G, et al. Laparoscopy in abdominal staging of esophageal carcinoma. *Gastrointest Endosc* 1986;43:400–402

82. Watt I, Stewart I, Anderson D, et al. Laparoscopy, ultrasound and computed tomography in cancer of the oesophagus and gastric cardia: a prospective comparison for detecting intra-abdominal metastases. *Br J Surg* 1989;76: 1036–1043

83. Kerbl K, Clayman RV, Petros JA, et al. Staging pelvic lymphadenectomy for prostate cancer: a comparison of laparoscopic and open techniques. *J Urol* 1993;150:396–399

84. Okita K, Kodma T, Oda M, et al. Laparoscopic ultrasonography: diagnosis of liver and pancreatic cancer. *Scand J Gastroenterol* (suppl) 1984;19 (suppl 94):91–100

85. Fornari F, Civardi G, Cavanna L, et al. Laparoscopic ultrasonography in the study of liver diseases. Preliminary results. *Surg Endosc* 1989;3:33–36

86. Berci G, Sackier JM, Paz-Partlow M. Emergency laparoscopy. *Am J Surg* 1991;161:332–335

87. Fabian TC, Croce MA, Stewart RM, et al. A prospective analysis of diagnostic laparoscopy in trauma. *Ann Surg* 1993;217:557–565

88. Berci G. Emergent and urgent laparoscopy. In: Hunter JG, Sackier JM (eds). *Minimally Invasive Surgery.* New York, NY: McGraw Hill; 1993:291–295

89. Sosa JL, Sims D, Martin L, Zeppa R. Laparoscopic evaluation of tangential abdominal gunshot wounds. *Arch Surg* 1992;127:109–110

90. Bass EB, Pitt HA, Lillemoe KD. Cost-effectiveness of laparoscopic cholecystectomy vs. open cholecystectomy. *Am J Surg* 1993;165:466–471

91. Soper NJ, Brunt LM, Kerbl K. Laparoscopic general surgery. *N Engl J Med* 1994;330:409–419.

92. Larson GM, Vitalie GC, Casey J, et al. Multi-practice analysis of laparoscopic cholecystectomy in 1,983 patients. *Am J Surg* 1992;163:221–226

93. Lillemoe KD, Yeo CJ, Talamini MA, et al. Selective cholangiography: Current role in laparoscopic cholecystectomy. *Ann Surg* 1992;215:669–674

94. Sanabria JR, Gallinger S, Croxford R, Strasberg SM. Risk factors in laparoscopic cholecystectomy for conversion to open cholecystectomy, *J Amer Coll Surg* 1994;179:696–704.

95. Gilliland TM, Traverso LW. Modern standards for comparison of cholecystectomy with alternative treatments for symptomatic gallstones with emphasis on long-term relief of symptoms. *Surg Gynecol Obstet* 1990;170:39–44

96. McSherry CK. Cholecystectomy: the gold standard. *Am J Surg* 1989;158:174–178

97. Roslyn JJ, Binns GS, Hughes EF, et al. Open cholecystectomy: a contemporary analysis of 42 474 patients. *Ann Surg* 1993;218:129–137

98. Davidoff AM, Pappas TN, Murray EA, et al. Mechanisms of major biliary injury during laparoscopic cholecystectomy. *Ann Surg* 1992;215:196–202

99. Moossa AR, Easter DW, Van Sonnenberg E, et al. Laparoscopic injuries to the bile duct: a cause for concern. *Ann Surg* 1992;215:203–208

100. Soper NJ, Flye MW, Brunt LM, et al. Diagnosis and management of biliary complications of laparoscopic cholecystectomy. *Am J Surg* 1993;165:522–526

101. *Laparoscopic Surgery.* New York State Department of Health Memorandum; Series 92–201: June 12, 1992.

102. Bernard H, Hartman TW. Complications after laparoscopic cholecystectomy. *Am J Surg* 1993;165:533–535

103. Rossi RL, Schirmer WJ, Braasch JW, et al. Laparoscopic bile duct injuries: risk factors, recognition, and repair. *Arch Surg* 1992;127:596–602

104. NIH Consensus Conference. Gallstones and laparoscopic cholecystectomy. *JAMA* 1993;269:1018–1024

105. Hunter JG, Soper NJ. Laparoscopic management of bile duct stones. *Surg Clin N Amer* 1992;72:1077–1097

106. Tompkins RK, Pitt HA. Surgical management of benign lesions of the bile ducts. *Curr Prob Surg* 1982;19:327–398

107. Petelin JB. Laparoscopic approach to common duct pathology. *Surg Laparosc Endosc* 1991;1:33–41

108. Petelin JB. Laparoscopic management of common bile duct pathology. *Soc Min Inv Therap* 1992;1(suppl):40

109. Phillips EH, Carroll BJ, Pearlstein AR, et al. Laparoscopic choledochoscopy and extraction of common bile duct stones. *World J Surg* 1993;17:22–28

110. Schrieber J. Early experience with laparoscopic appendectomy in women. *Surg Endosc* 1986;1:211–216

111. Gangal MT, Gangal MH. Laparoscopic appendectomy. *Endoscopy* 1987;19:127–129

112. Pier A, Gotz F, Bacher C. Laparoscopic appendectomy in 625 cases: from innovation to routine. *Surg Laparosc Endosc* 1991;1:8–13

113. Schirmer BD, Schmieg RE Jr, Dix J, et al. Laparoscopic versus traditional appendectomy for suspected appendicitis. *Am J Surg* 1993;165:670–675

114. Attwood SEA, Hill ADK, Murphy PG, et al. A prospective randomized trial of laparoscopic versus open appendectomy. *Surgery* 1992;112:497–501

115. Fritts LL, Orlando R. Laparoscopic appendectomy: a safety and cost analysis. *Arch Surg* 1993;128:521–525

116. Adiss DG, Shaffer N, Fowler BS, et al. The epidemiology of appendicitis and appendectomy in the United States. *Am J Epidemiol* 1990;132:910–925

117. Bongard F, Landers DV, Lewis F. Differential diagnosis of appendicitis and pelvic inflammatory disease. *Am J Surg* 1985;150:90–96

118. Reiertsen O, Rosseland AR, Hoivik B, Solheim K. Laparoscopy in patients admitted for acute abdominal pain. *Acta Chir Scand* 1985:151:521–524

119. Whitworth CM, Whitworth PW, Sanfillipo J, Polk HC. Value of diagnostic laparoscopy in young women with possible appendicitis. *Surg Gynecol Obstet* 1988;167:187–190

120. McAnena OJ, Austin O, O'Connell PR, et al. Laparoscopic versus open appendicectomy: a prospective evaluation. *Br J Surg* 1992;79:818–820

121. Tate JJT, Dawson JW, Chung SCS, et al. Laparoscopic versus open appendicectomy: prospective randomised trial. *Lancet* 1993;342:633–637

122. Dallemagne B, Weerts JM, Jehaes C. et al. Laparoscopic Nissen fundoplication: preliminary report. *Surg Laparosc Endosc* 1991;1:138–143

123. Hinder RA, Filipi CJ. The technique of laparoscopic Nissen fundoplication. *Surg Laparosc Endosc* 1992;2:265–272

124. Spechler SJ and The Department of Veteran's Affairs Gastroesophageal Reflux Disease Study Group. Comparison of medical and surgical therapy for complicated gastroesophageal reflux disease in veterans. *N Engl J Med* 1992;326:786–792

125. Nissen R. Gastropexy and "fundoplication" in surgical treatment of hiatus hernia. *Am J Dig Dis* 1961;6:954–961

126. DeMeester TR, Johnson LF, Kent AH. Evaluation of current operations for the prevention of gastroesophageal reflux. *Ann Surg* 1974;180:511–525

127. Thor KBA, Silander T. A long-term randomized prospective trial of the Nissen procedure vs. a modified Toupet technique. *Ann Surg* 1989;210:719–724

128. McKernan JB, Wolfe BM, MacFadyen BV Jr. Laparoscopic repair of duodenal ulcer and gastroesophageal reflux. *Surg Clin N Amer* 1992;72:1153–1167

129. Lobe TE, Schropp KP, Lunsford K. Laparoscopic Nissen fundoplication in childhood. *J Ped Surg* 1993;28:358–361

130. Wiener GJ, Richter JE, Cooper JB, et al. The symptom index: a clinically important parameter of ambulatory 24-hour esophageal pH monitoring. *Am J Gastroenterol* 1988;83:358–361

131. Cuschieri AE, Schimi S, Nathanson LK. Laparoscopic reduction, crural repair, and fundoplication of large hiatal hernia. *Am J Surg* 1992;163:425–430

132. Congreve DP. Laparoscopic paraesophageal hernia repair. *J Laparoendosc Surg* 1992;2:45–48

133. Kuster GGR, Gilroy S. Laparoscopic repair of paraesophageal hiatal hernias. *Surg Endosc* 1993;7:362–363

134. Weerts JM, Dallemagne B, Hamoir E, et al. Laparoscopic Nissen fundoplication: detailed analysis of 132 patients. *Surg Laparosc Endosc* 1993;3:359–364

135. Cuschieri AE. Hiatal hernia and reflux esophagitis. In: Hunter JG, Sackier JM (eds), *Minimally Invasive Surgery.* New York, NY: McGraw-Hill; 1993:87–111

136. Johnston D. Operative mortality and post-operative morbidity of highly selective vagotomy. *Br Med J* 1974; 4:545–547

137. Hoffman J, Olesen A, Jensen HE. Prospective 14 to 18 year follow-up study after parietal cell vagotomy. *Br J Surg* 1987;74:1056–1059

138. Frantzides CT, Ludwig KA, Quebbeman EJ, Burhop J. Laparoscopic highly selective vagotomy: technique and case report. *Surg Laparosc Endosc* 1992;2:348–352

139. Helms B, Czarnetzki D. Laparoscopic proximal selective vagotomy. *Minim Invasive Ther* 1992;1(suppl 1):118

140. Legrand M, Detroz B, Honore P, Jacquet N. Laparoscopic highly selective vagotomy. Minim Invasive Ther 1992;1(suppl 1):90.

141. Bailey RW, Flowers JL, Graham SM, Zucker KA. Combined laparoscopic cholecystectomy and selective vagotomy. *Surg Laparosc Endosc* 1991;1:45–49

142. Katkhouda N, Mouiel J. A new technique of surgical treatment of chronic duodenal ulcer without laparotomy by videocoelioscopy. *Am J Surg* 1991;161: 361–364

143. Katkhouda N, Mouiel J. Laparoscopic treatment of peptic ulcer disease. In: Hunter JG, Sackier JM (eds), *Minimally Invasive Surgery.* New York, NY: McGraw Hill; 1993:123–130

144. Bailey RW, Zucker KA. Laparoscopic management of peptic ulcer disease. In: Zucker KA (ed), *Surgical Laparoscopy Update.* St. Louis, MO: Quality Medical Publishing; 1993:241–286

145. Hill GL, Barker CJ. Anterior highly selective vagotomy with posterior truncal vagotomy: a simple technique for denervating the parietal cell mass. *Br J Surg* 1978;65: 702–705

146. Taylor TV. Lesser curve superficial seromyotomy—an operation for chronic duodenal ulcer. *Br J Surg* 1979;66: 733–737

147. Taylor TV, Holt S, Heading RC. Gastric emptying after anterior lesser curve seromyotomy and posterior truncal vagotomy. *Br J Surg* 1985;72:620–622

148. Shapiro S, Gordon L, Dayhkovsky L, et al. Development of laparoscopic anterior seromyotomy and right posterior truncal vagotomy for ulcer prophylaxis. *J Laparoendosc Surg* 1991;1:279–286

149. Pietrafitta JJ, Schultz LS, Graber JN, Hickok DF. Experimental transperitoneal laparoscopic pyloroplasty. *Surg Laparosc Endosc* 1992;2:104–110

150. Laws HL, Naughton MJ, McKernan JB. Thoracoscopic vagectomy for recurrent peptic ulcer disease. *Surg Laparosc Endosc* 1991;2:24–28

151. Goh P, Tekant Y, Issac J, et al. The technique of laparoscopic Billroth II gastrectomy. *Surg Laparosc Endosc* 1992;2:258–260

152. Mouret P, Francois Y, Vignal J, et al. Laparoscopic treatment of perforated peptic ulcer. *Br J Surg* 1990;77:1006.

153. Swanstrom L. Laparoscopic repair of perforated ulcer: treatment algorithm and follow-up. *Surg Endosc* 1993; 7:122

154. Ponsky JL, Aszod A. Percutaneous endoscopic jejunostomy. *Am J Gastroenterol* 1984;79:113–116

155. Sangster W, Swanstrom L. Laparoscopic-guided feeding jejunostomy. *Surg Endosc* 1993;7:308–310

156. Duh QY, Way LW. Laparoscopic gastrostomy using T-fasteners as retractors and anchors. *Surg Endosc* 1993;7: 60–63

157. Duh QY, Way LW. Laparoscopic jejunostomy using T-fasteners as retractors and anchors. *Arch Surg* 1993;128: 105–108

158. Sangster W, Hunter JG. Laparoscopic access for enteral nutrition. In: Hunter JG, Sackier JM (eds), *Minimally Invasive Surgery.* New York, NY: McGraw Hill; 1993:113–121

159. Reiner DS, Leitman IM, Ward RJ. Laparoscopic Stamm gastrostomy with gastropexy. *Surg Laparosc Endosc* 1991; 1:189–192

160. Lathrop JC, Felix EJ, Lauber D. Laparoscopic Janeway gastrostomy utilizing an endoscopic stapling device. *J Laparoendosc Surg* 1991;1:335–339

161. Pappas TN. Laparoscopic colectomy—the innovation continues. *Ann Surg* 1992;216:701–702

162. Soper NJ, Brunt LM, Fleshman JW, et al. Laparoscopic small bowel resection and anastomosis. *Surg Laparosc Endosc* 1993;3:6–12

163. Fleshman JW, Brunt LM, Fry RD, et al. Laparoscopic anterior resection of the rectum using a triple stapled intracorporeal anastomosis in the pig. *Surg Laparosc Endosc* 1993;3:119–126

164. Phillips EH, Franklin M, Carroll BJ, et al. Laparoscopic colectomy. *Ann Surg* 1992;216:703–707

165. Fusco MA, Paluzzi MLO. Abdominal wall recurrence after laparoscopic-assisted colectomy for adenocarcinoma of the colon: report of a case. *Dis Colon Rectum* 1993;36:858–861

166. Cooperman AM, Katz V, Zimmon D, Botero G. Laparoscopic colon resection: a case report. *J Laparoendosc Surg* 1991;1:221–224

167. Jacobs M, Verdeja JC, Goldstein HS. Minimally invasive colon resection (Laparoscopic colectomy). *Surg Laparosc Endosc* 1991;3:144–150

168. Fowler DL, White SA. Laparoscopy-assisted sigmoid resection. *Surg Laparosc Endosc* 1991;1:183–188

169. Welton M, Peters W, Fleshman J, et al. Laparoscopic colorectal surgery: early results. [Abstract] *Am Society of Colorectal Surgery* 1993

170. Falk PM, Beart RW Jr, Wexner SD, et al. Laparoscopic colectomy: a critical appraisal. *Dis Colon Rectum* 1993; 36:28–34

171. Monson JRT, Darzi A, Carey PD, Guillou PJ. Prospective evaluation of laparoscopic-assisted colectomy in an unselected group of patients. *Lancet* 1992;340:831–833

172. Zucker KA, Martin D, Pitcher D, Ford S. Laparoscopic assisted colon resection. *Surg Endosc* 1993;7:121

173. Wexner SD, Johansen OB, Nogueras JJ, Jagelman DG. Laparoscopic total abdominal colectomy: a prospective trial. *Dis Colon Rectum* 1992;35:651–655

174. Lange V, Meyer G, Schardey HM, Schildberg FW. Laparoscopic creation of a loop colostomy. *J Laparoendosc Surg* 1991;1:307–312

175. Berman IR. Sutureless laparoscopic rectopexy for procidentia: technique and implications. *Dis Colon Rectum* 1992;35:689–693

176. Cuschieri A, Shimi S, Banting S, Velpen GV. Laparoscopic repair of total rectal prolapse. *Surg Endosc* 1993; 7:125

177. Darzi A, Henry MM, Guillun PJ, Monson JRT. Stapled laparoscopic rectopexy for rectal prolapse. Surg Endosc 1995;9:301–303

178. Gagner M, Rheault M, Dubuc J. Laparoscopic partial hepatectomy for liver tumor. *Surg Endosc* 1992;6:99

179. Way LW and Wetter A. Laparoscopic treatment of liver cysts. *Surg Endosc* 1992;6:89

180. Fabiani P, Katkhouda N, Iovine L, Mouiel J. Laparoscopic fenestration of biliary cysts. *Surg Laparosc Endosc* 1991;1:162–165

181. Mårvik R, Myrvold HE, Johnsen G, Røysland P. Laparoscopic ultrasonography and treatment of hepatic cysts. *Surg Laparosc Endosc* 1992;3:172–174

182. Fletcher DR, Jones RM. Laparoscopic cholecystojejunostomy as palliation for obstructive jaundice in inoperable carcinoma of pancreas. *Surg Endosc* 1992;6:147–149

183. Mouiel J, Katkhouda N, White S, Dumas R. Endolaparoscopic palliation of pancreatic cancer. *Surg Laparosc Endosc* 1992;3:241–243

183a. Gagner M. Personal communication

184. Soper NJ, Brunt LM, Dunnegan DL, Meininger TA. Laparoscopic distal pancreatectomy in the porcine model. *Surg Endosc* 1993;7:120

185. Carroll BJ, Phillips EH, Semel CJ, Fallas M, Morgenstern L. Laparoscopic splenectomy. *Surg Endosc* 1992;6:183–185

186. Delaitre B, Maignien B. Laparoscopic splenectomy—technical aspects. *Surg Endosc* 1992;6:305–308

187. Thibault C, Mamazza J, Létourneau R, Poulin E. Laparoscopic splenectomy: operative technique and preliminary report. *Surg Laparosc Endosc* 1992;2:248–253

188. Phillips EH. Laparoscopic splenectomy. In: Hunter JG, Sackier JM (eds), *Minimally Invasive Surgery.* New York, NY: McGraw-Hill; 1993:309–313

189. Phillips EH, Carroll BJ, Fallas MJ. Laparoscopic splenectomy. *Surg Endosc* 1993;7:121

190. Park A, Gragner M. The lateral approach to laparoscopic splenectomy. *Surg Endosc* 1994;8:239

191. Selected data on hospitals and use of services. Section C. In: Polister P and Cunico E (eds). *Socioeconomic Factbook for Surgery.* Chicago, IL: American College of Surgeons; 1989:25–42

192. Vayda E, Mindell WR, Rutkow IM. A decade of surgery in Canada, England, and the United States. *Arch Surg* 1982;117:846

193. Goldsmith MF. Some new twists to one of the most common procedures in US general surgery. *JAMA* 1989; 262:3248–3249

194. Lichtenstein IL, Shore JM. Exploding the myths of hernia repair. *Am J Surg* 1976;132:307–310

195. Peters JH, Ortega AE. Laparoscopic inguinal hernia repair. In: Hunter JG, Sackier JM (eds), *Minimally Invasive Surgery.* New York, NY: McGraw Hill; 1993:297–308

196. Condon RE, Nyhus LM. Complications of groin hernias. In: Nyhus LM, Condon RE (eds), *Hernia* 3rd ed. Philadelphia, PA: JB Lippincott; 1989:253–269

197. Wantz GE. The Canadian repair of inguinal hernia. In: Nyhus LM, Condon RE (eds), *Hernia* 3rd ed. Philadelphia, PA: JB Lippincott; 1989:236–252

198. Lichtenstein IL, Shulman AG, Amid PK, Montllor MM. The tension-free hernioplasty. *Am J Surg* 1987;157:188–193

199. Ger R, Monroe K, Duvivier R, Mishrick A. Management of indirect inguinal hernias by laparoscopic closure of the neck of the sac. *Am J Surg* 1990;159:370–373

200. Schultz L, Graber J, Pietrafitta J, Hickok D. Laser laparoscopic herniorrhaphy: a clinical trial preliminary results. *J Laparoendosc Surg* 1990;1:41–45

201. Corbitt JD. Laparoscopic herniorrhaphy. *Surg Laparosc Endosc* 1991;1:23–25

202. Gazayerli MM. Anatomical laparoscopic hernia repair of direct or indirect inguinal hernias using the transversalis fascia and iliopubic tract. *Surg Laparosc Endosc* 1992;2:49–52

203. MacFadyen BV, Arregui ME, Corbitt JD, et al. Complications of laparoscopic herniorrhaphy. *Surg Endosc* 1993;7:155–158

204. McKernan JB, Laws HL. Laparoscopic repair of inguinal hernias using a totally extraperitoneal prosthetic approach. *Surg Endosc* 1993;7:26–28

205. Fitzgibbons R, Annibali R, Litke B, et al. A multicentered clinical trial on laparoscopic inguinal hernia repair: preliminary results. *Surg Endosc* 1993;7:115

206. Stoppa RE, Rives JL, Warlaumont CR, et al. The use of dacron in the repair of hernias of the groin. *Surg Clin N Amer* 1984;64:269–285

207. Stoppa RE, Warlaumont CR. The preperitoneal approach and prosthetic repair of groin hernia. In: Nyhus LM, Condon RE (eds), *Hernia* 3rd ed. Philadelphia, PA: JB Lippincott; 1989:199–221

208. Spaw AT, Ennis BW, Spaw LP. Laparoscopic hernia repair: the anatomic basis. *J Laparoendosc Surg* 1991;1:269–277

209. Salerno GM, Fitzgibbons RJ, Filipi CJ. Laparoscopic inguinal hernia repair. In: Zucker KA (ed), *Surgical Laparoscopy.* St. Louis, MO: Quality Medical; 1991:281–293

210. Kraus M. Laparoscopic identification of preperitoneal nerve anatomy in the inguinal area. *Surg Endosc* 1993; 7:114

211. Eubanks S, Newman L, Goehring L, et al. Meralgia paresthetica: a complication of laparoscopic herniorrhaphy. *Surg Laparosc Endosc* 1993;3:381–385

212. Geis WP, Crafton WB, Novak MJ, Malago M. Laparoscopic herniorrhaphy: results and technical aspects in 450 consecutive procedures. *Surgery* 1993;114:765–774

213. Schultz LS. Laparoscopic inguinal herniorrhaphy. In: Graber JN, Schultz LS, Pietrafitta JJ, Hickok DR (eds), *Laparoscopic Abdominal Surgery.* New York, NY: McGraw-Hill; 1993:255–270

214. Amid PK, Shulman AG, Lichtenstein IL. Critical scrutiny of the open "tension-free" hernioplasty. *Am J Surg* 1993; 165:369–371

215. Rutkow IM. Laparoscopic hernia repair: the socioeconomic tyranny of surgical technology. *Arch Surg* 1992;127:1271

216. Gill BD, Traverso LW. Continuous quality inventory: open versus laparoscopic groin hernia repair. *Surg Endosc* 1993;7:120

217. Brunt LM, Molmenti EP, Kerbl J, et al. Retroperitoneal endoscopic adrenalectomy: an experimental study. *Surg Laparosc Endosc* 1993;3:300–306

218. Gagner M, Lacroix A, Bolte E. Laparoscopic adrenalectomy in Cushing's syndrome and pheochromocytoma. *N Engl J Med* 1992;327:1033

219. Sardi A, McKinnon W. Laparoscopic adrenalectomy for primary aldosteronism. *JAMA* 1993;269:989–990

220. Matsuda T, Terachi T, Mikami O, et al. Laparoscopic adrenalectomy: initial results of 15 cases. *Minim Invasive Ther* 1993;2(suppl):52

221. Go H, Takeda M, Nishiyama T, et al. Laparoscopic adrenalectomy. *J Urol* 1993;149:450A

222. Higashihara E, Tanaka Y, Horie S, et al. Laparoscopic adrenalectomy: the initial 3 cases. *J Urol* 1993;149: 973–976

223. Gagner M, Lacroix A, Bolte E, Pomp A. Laparoscopic adrenalectomy. The importance of a flank approach in the lateral decubitus position. *Surg Endosc* (in press).

224. Brunt LM, Norton JA, Quasebarth M, Soper NJ. Laparoscopic adrenalectomy. *Minim Invasive Ther* 1993; 2(suppl):53

225. Brunt LM, Soper NJ. Laparoscopic adrenalectomy. In: Arregui ME, Fitzgibbons RF, Katkhouda N, et al (eds), *Principles of Laparoscopic Surgery: Basic and Advanced Techniques.* New York, NY: Springer-Verlag; (in press)

226. Forde KA. Endosurgical training methods: is it surgical training that is out of control? *Surg Endosc* 1993; 7:71–72

227. Greene FL. New York State Health Department ruling— a "wake-up call" for all. *Surg Endosc* 1992;6:271

228. Society for American Gastrointestinal Surgery. Granting of privileges for laparoscopic general surgery. *Am J Surg* 1991;161:324–325

229. Schirmer BD, Edge SB, Dix J, Miller AD. Incorporation of laparoscopy into a surgical endoscopy training program. *Am J Surg* 1992;163:46–52

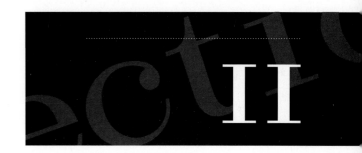

EVALUATION OF GASTROINTESTINAL DISORDERS

5

Gastrointestinal Bleeding

Bruce E. Stabile ▪ *Michael J. Stamos*

▪ HISTORY

The earliest reports of gastrointestinal (GI) bleeding are as ancient as the first known medical writings. Clinical descriptions date to beyond 5000 years ago, and the Ebers papyrus reported acute hemorrhage as a complication of peptic ulceration.[1] With no understanding of the pathophysiology of hemorrhagic shock, early therapeutic recommendations, including those of Hippocrates, were counterproductive. Various forms of therapeutic bloodletting, including phlebotomy and the application of leeches, were commonly recommended even through the last century. Successful resuscitation from hemorrhagic shock became possible with a greater understanding of the physiology of the circulatory system and the introduction of intravenous infusion therapy and blood banking techniques. Barium contrast radiography and general anesthesia were important contributions that enabled the surgeon to manage patients with gastrointestinal (GI) bleeding effectively. Recently introduced techniques, such as fiberoptic endoscopy and visceral arteriography, have expanded the diagnostic and therapeutic capabilities of the clinician.

Despite the proliferation of sophisticated diagnostic and therapeutic techniques, the overall mortality of GI bleeding has remained unchanged at 8% to 10%.[2] The constancy of the mortality rate probably reflects the overall improved care of an aged, less fit patient population. Virtually all studies indicate advanced age as a predictor of mortality; death among patients younger than 50 years has become a rarity. In addition to age, a number of other risk factors for morbidity and mortality from GI bleeding have been identified (Table 5–1).

It is estimated that 1% to 2% of all acute medical and surgical hospital admissions are for GI bleeding.[3] The diversity of etiology and lesion location makes GI bleeding a diagnostic and therapeutic problem that affects all ages, nationalities, ethnic groups, and socioeconomic strata. Although the majority of cases of acute bleeding subside spontaneously, recurrence is common. The morbidity and mortality of the condition derives from the consequences of hypovolemic shock on the myocardium and central nervous system. Since the preponderance of GI bleeding occurs in middle-aged to elderly adults who require intensive medical and surgical care, the social and economic consequences of GI bleeding are considerable. It is imperative that a rapid, cost-effective, and efficient evaluation and treatment plan be executed in all cases. This, in turn, requires a detailed understanding of the various etiologies of upper and lower GI hemorrhage. Preliminary to any diagnostic efforts, however, it is an accurate assessment of the rate and volume of blood loss and its consequences upon the patient's hemodynamic condition.

▪ CLINICAL PRESENTATION

Upper GI tract hemorrhage is defined as that emanating from a bleeding site proximal to the ligament of Treitz. Hematemesis or grossly bloody emesis correlates

TABLE 5–1. RISK FACTORS FOR MORBIDITY AND MORTALITY IN GASTROINTESTINAL HEMORRHAGE

Age >60 years
Shock at presentation
Hematemesis
Hematochezia
Transfusion requirement of 6 or more units
Coronary artery disease
Chronic pulmonary disease
Acute pulmonary failure
Chronic renal failure
Cirrhosis
Acute hepatic failure
Sepsis
Multiple organ failure syndrome
Coagulopathy
Recent cerebrovascular accident
Multiple trauma
Major burn
Malignancy
Immunosuppression
Postoperative status

highly with massive upper GI tract hemorrhage. Thin, dark, granular, or so-called "coffee-ground" emesis also suggests active or recently subsided upper GI hemorrhage, but of a less severe degree. Melena or liquid black, foul-smelling stool typically accompanies upper GI hemorrhage and represents the degradation of blood that has traversed the small and large intestine. However, melena can arise from the small intestine at a site distal to the ligament of Treitz; therefore, it also can be a symptom of lower GI hemorrhage. Hematochezia, or the passage of bright red- or maroon-colored blood and clots from the rectum, is typical of lower GI hemorrhage emanating from the distal small bowel or large bowel. Hematochezia may occasionally accompany massive upper GI bleeding, resulting from the rapid transit induced by the cathartic effects of blood in the intestinal tract. This clinical scenario is virtually always accompanied by significant hemodynamic instability. Blood streaking on the formed stool generally signifies minor bleeding from a lesion distal to the sigmoid colon. Chemical, or guaiac, testing of the stool for the presence of occult blood loss may be positive as a result of minor bleeding from any site within the GI tract.

■ EVALUATION OF GASTROINTESTINAL BLEEDING

Several elements are important in the evaluation of GI hemorrhage. The first is the severity of the presenting hemorrhage. This assessment is based on the patient's history and physical examination, the degree of initial hemodynamic compromise, and the patient's early re-

sponse to resuscitative efforts. The second element is the anatomic level and nature of the bleeding lesion. This can be assessed by endoscopy, angiography, or by radionuclide scanning techniques. Although successful therapeutic intervention is not necessarily predicated on an exact knowledge of all elements of evaluation, the quality of patient care is enhanced by such knowledge.

INITIAL EVALUATION AND RESUSCITATION

Assessment of Hemodynamic Status

Once the diagnosis of acute GI hemorrhage is suspected, the first priority is a rapid assessment of the patient's hemodynamic status. The early symptoms and signs of hemorrhagic shock occur with acute blood volume losses of 15% to 20% and include weakness, pallor, diaphoresis, and skin that is cool to palpation.[4] These findings derive from the adrenergic stimulation and vasoconstriction consequent to rapid intravascular volume loss. Acute losses of 20% to 40% of blood volume result in moderate hemorrhagic shock manifested by tachycardia, hypotension, mental confusion, or agitation, and oliguria. With volume losses >40%, profound shock ensues with prostration, a depressed level of consciousness, a thready pulse, and severe oliguria or anuria. Myocardial ischemia, manifested by angina pectoris, dysrhythmias or ischemic changes on electrocardiogram (EKG), may occur, particularly in patients of advanced age or with coronary artery disease. Such profound shock leads to irreversible vital organ injury and death if not rapidly treated.

In all patients with acute GI hemorrhage, resuscitative measures take precedence over the diagnostic pursuit. Two large-bore intravenous catheters should be inserted and an immediate blood sample obtained for determination of hematocrit, coagulation parameters, and for typing and cross-matching of blood products. It is important to note that a normal hematocrit in no way negates the diagnosis of acute GI hemorrhage, since anemia develops only when sufficient time elapses for hemodilution to occur. A low initial hematocrit suggests bleeding ongoing for a number of hours or days and/or the presence of chronic anemia from chronic blood loss or some other cause. Along with establishment of intravenous access, an important initial measure is to supply oxygen to the patient by nasal cannulae or mask. Volume resuscitation with an isotonic crystalloid solution is instituted and appropriate clinical monitoring begun, including serial vital signs, mental status and hematocrit determinations, urinary output, and continuous EKG and pulse oximetry. Additional laboratory evaluation should be obtained, consisting of complete blood count, platelet count, prothrombin time, partial thromboplastin time, electrolytes, blood urea nitrogen, creatinine, and liver function tests.

During the initial resuscitative phase either normal saline or lactated Ringer's solution is infused rapidly until 1 to 2 L have been delivered. Additional fluid therapy is dictated by the patient's clinical response. A central venous catheter or pulmonary artery catheter may be indicated to guide the resuscitative efforts in patients with preexisting cardiac or pulmonary disease. If pulse, blood pressure, and other parameters of organ perfusion quickly return to normal, the intravenous infusion can be decreased to maintenance rates. If the patient shows no response to the rapid infusion of 2 L of crystalloid solution, then massive blood loss usually has occurred, and early transfusion of blood products may be required. This is particularly true if the initial hematocrit value is 30% or less. In all circumstances, the blood bank should have 6 units of packed, cross-matched red blood cells available for immediate use and should be instructed to maintain this level of availability as units are used.

While the early resuscitative efforts are in progress, a rapid history and physical examination should be performed. History-taking should emphasize the current episode and clinical presentation, GI diseases with known bleeding potential, and diseases and drugs that affect coagulation, particularly the use of alcohol, tobacco, and nonsteroidal anti-inflammatory agents. The physical examination should focus on the vital organ systems and the stigmata of chronic liver disease. The abdominal examination is particularly important with reference to possible GI tract malignancy or chronic liver disease, manifested by hepatosplenomegaly, ascites and the cutaneous signs of portal hypertension. The rectal exam is critical regarding the color and character of the stool and the presence of anorectal masses.

UPPER VERSUS LOWER GASTROINTESTINAL BLEEDING

A nasogastric tube should be placed in any patient with suspected or known upper GI hemorrhage. If the patient has vomited a large quantity of blood, or if blood or coffee-ground material is aspirated, the diagnosis of upper GI tract hemorrhage is largely proven (Table 5–2). Because of the intermittent nature of the bleeding and the infrequency of duodenogastric reflux in some patients, a negative nasogastric aspirate result may be imprecise.[5] To assure that duodenal contents are being sampled, bile staining of the aspirated fluid should be in evidence. If the gastric aspirate is completely colorless, elicitation of the gag reflex in the patient commonly results in reflux of duodenal contents into the stomach. This may help to identify the occasional patient with active or recent duodenal hemorrhage with minimal or no spontaneous reflux into the stomach.

Whenever the level of GI bleeding is unclear on initial assessment, gastric lavage using room temperature

TABLE 5–2. RELATIONSHIP BETWEEN THE MANIFESTATION OF GASTROINTESTINAL BLEEDING AND THE LIKELIHOOD OF AN UPPER VERSUS A LOWER GI BLEEDING SOURCE

Bleeding Manifestation	Likelihood of Upper GI Source	Likelihood of Lower GI Source
Hematemesis	Assured	Ruled out
Melena	Probable	Possible
Hematochezia	Unlikely	Highly probable
Blood streaked stool	Ruled out	Assured
Occult blood in stool	Possible	Possible

normal saline should be performed to sample the gastric contents and evacuate clots or old blood. Gastric lavage is most effective when room temperature solution is used, since cold solutions interfere with the highly temperature-sensitive coagulation enzymes.[6] Removal of clots from the stomach also promotes contraction of the stomach and enhances vasoconstriction. Most importantly, it prepares the stomach for upper endoscopy evaluation.

Whenever the nasogastric aspirate is negative for blood and the clinical presentation suggests a lower GI source, the first specific diagnostic maneuver should be rigid proctosigmoidoscopy. This, like nasogastric intubation, can be done in the emergency room or at the bedside, since it requires no specialized equipment or support. Although most major lower GI hemorrhages are found to be emanating from >25 cm above the anal verge, proctosigmoidoscopy allows excellent evaluation for the presence of bleeding internal hemorrhoids, rectal tumors or polyps, or diffuse hemorrhagic mucosal disorders. The rigid scope is particularly useful, since it allows the endoscopist to irrigate and evacuate the rectum and rectosigmoid colon as the instrument is passed proximally, obviating the need for preparation of the bowel prior to examination.

■ DIAGNOSIS OF UPPER GASTROINTESTINAL BLEEDING

UPPER GASTROINTESTINAL ENDOSCOPY

Whenever GI hemorrhage is thought to derive from a source proximal to the ligament of Treitz, or whenever the issue is in doubt, the first invasive diagnostic maneuver should be upper GI flexible endoscopy. This technique has a diagnostic accuracy of approximately 95% and an overall complication rate of less than 1%.[7] The diagnostic accuracy of the test is great, if performed within the first 12 hours of bleeding; thus, the examination should be accomplished as soon as possible after initial resuscitation and stabilization of the patient.[8] Upper endoscopy can identify bleeding lesions, such as diffuse mucosal erosions, Mallory-Weiss mucosal tears, and vascular malformations, that are typically overlooked by other modalities. Endoscopy also allows a qualitative assessment of bleeding rate, provides prognostic information regarding rebleeding potential, and offers numerous therapeutic interventions for specific lesions.[9]

ANGIOGRAPHY

Angiography is rarely used or indicated for upper GI hemorrhage. In the rare instance where upper endoscopy is unavailable or nonrevealing and the bleeding site still is thought to be proximal to the ligament of Treitz, celiac axis arteriography may be indicated. If bleeding is <0.5 mL/min, extravasated contrast is unlikely to be seen.[10] Likewise, if bleeding is intermittent or venous in nature, the study is insensitive. On the other hand, angiodysplastic lesions, particularly arteriovenous malformations, often can be seen in the absence of active bleeding, by virtue of the abnormal vascular architecture and premature venous filling that are characteristic. When positive, upper GI angiography has the potential for therapeutic intervention by embolization of the feeding vessel.[11]

UPPER GASTROINTESTINAL BARIUM RADIOGRAPHY

Barium contrast radiography is no longer pertinent to the diagnosis of acute hemorrhage. The test is diagnostic in only approximately three-fourths of cases and offers no therapeutic potential.[12] Furthermore, the presence of barium in the GI tract obviates the possibility of angiographic examination. For these reasons, upper GI contrast studies should be reserved for those patients with chronic or intermittent bleeding that probably is due to an ulcer or mass lesion.

■ CAUSES AND TREATMENT OF UPPER GASTROINTESTINAL BLEEDING

The keys to successful management of upper GI bleeding are adequate early resuscitation, including blood transfusion as indicated, and early accurate diagnosis of the source of bleeding. In most circumstances, upper endoscopy provides not only the exact source of bleeding but also an accurate assessment of the bleeding rate. Because all sources of upper GI bleeding involve a disruption of the mucosa, pharmacologic inhibition of gastric acid secretion is provided empirically.[13] Whenever active bleeding is seen endoscopically, a nasogastric tube is replaced and maintained to constant low suction to provide an ongoing monitor of bleeding activity.

PEPTIC ULCER DISEASE

Despite a decline in the frequency of peptic ulcer disease during the past three decades, it remains the most common cause of upper GI bleeding. In a recent literature review encompassing more than 10 000 patients with upper GI hemorrhage, peptic ulcer disease accounted for 27% to 46% of all cases.[14] While duodenal ulcer remains slightly more prevalent than gastric ulcer, recent data suggest that gastric and duodenal ulcers bleed with roughly equal frequencies.[7]

For duodenal ulcer, there is a distinct association between hemorrhage and ulcer location.[15] Most bleeding duodenal ulcers are located in the posterior wall of the duodenal bulb just beyond the pylorus (Fig 5–1). These ulcers penetrate through the full thickness of the duo-

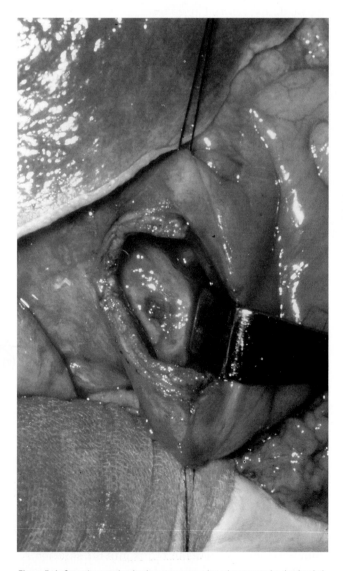

Figure 5–1. Operative anterior duodenostomy exposing a large posterior duodenal ulcer crater with a visible vessel in its center.

denal wall and into the gastroduodenal artery, with resultant hemorrhage.[16] Since the majority of gastric ulcers are situated along the lesser curve of the stomach, deep penetration of these ulcers can result in erosion and hemorrhage from branches of the left gastric artery. Because the vascularity of the stomach wall is uniformly great, gastric ulcers in any location are at risk for major hemorrhage. This is particularly true for giant gastric ulcers of >3 cm.[17]

Patients with chronic ulcer disease have an approximate 20% chance of experiencing a major bleeding episode. Hemorrhage is the most important cause of mortality from the disease and accounts for >40% of all ulcer-associated deaths.[18] Bleeding from gastric ulcer tends to be more severe and more lethal than bleeding from duodenal ulcer; however, this merely may reflect the older population in which gastric ulcer is found.

Most bleeding episodes resulting from gastroduodenal ulceration have an acute onset and are intermittent in nature. Approximately three-fourths of all such bleeding events subside spontaneously without therapeutic intervention.[15] While the onset of bleeding often is preceded by exacerbation of typical dyspeptic ulcer pain, this is by no means inevitable, and the pain almost always subsides immediately after the onset of hemorrhage. Because of a significant association between rebleeding and mortality, predictors of rebleeding are an important issue in the management of patients with ulcer hemorrhage.[19] Numerous factors have been found to have predictive value for rebleeding. Age >60 years, admission hemoglobin <8 g/dL, shock at the time of admission, coagulopathy, an ulcer diameter of >1 cm, active pulsatile bleeding, and a visible vessel or adherent red clot on endoscopy all have been associated with an increased risk of rebleeding.[20–22] Since the major morbidity and mortality attending ulcer hemorrhage derives from the repeated episodes of hypotension and the associated myocardial ischemia, early endoscopic or operative intervention is indicated whenever rebleeding is predicted or occurs.

Nonoperative Management

Despite a large experience with pharmacologic therapy, there has been little proven success in stopping active ulcer bleeding. Antacids, H_2-receptor antagonists, omeprazole, prostaglandins, vasopressin, as well as somatostatin and its analog have all been evaluated and found to be ineffective.[23] The same is true for use of these agents to prevent early rebleeding from peptic ulcer disease.

The major advances that have occurred in recent years in the treatment of ulcer hemorrhage have derived from various hemostatic methodologies applied through the flexible endoscope. In 1989, a National Institutes of Health consensus conference concluded that endoscopic hemostatic therapy was useful and should be applied in patients at high risk for persistent or recurrent ulcer hemorrhage.[24] Specifically, patients with an initial large blood volume loss, endoscopic evidence of active bleeding, or a visible vessel should be subjected to initial endoscopic therapy, if available. While laser, electrocautery, heater probe, and injection therapy all have been shown to have efficacy in ameliorating ulcer bleeding, there are no significant differences among the four treatment modalities with respect to effectiveness. However, because of the expense, technical requirements, and potential for transmural perforation, laser therapy is the least desirable alternative. While individual trials have shown no significant survival advantage to endoscopic therapy, recent meta-analyses strongly suggest significant improvement in mortality as well as in control of bleeding.[25,26] Thus, it is prudent to apply endoscopic hemostatic techniques at the time of initial diagnostic endoscopy when peptic ulcer is found to be the cause of significant hemorrhage.[27] Since the techniques are generally safe and inexpensive, even the temporary cessation or attenuation of massive ulcer hemorrhage is of value in providing adequate time for mobilization of the operating room team for emergency surgery.[28]

Transcatheter angiographic embolization of the bleeding artery has been used with success in ulcer bleeding. Various embolic agents, such as gelfoam, wire coils and detachable balloons, all can be effective but in general, angiographic therapy is unavailable or unsuccessful in patients who are poor candidates for emergency surgical intervention.[11] Angiographic embolization typically has been successful in >50% of cases, whereas intra-arterial infusion of vasopressin has been less effective and has the additional disadvantage of adverse cardiovascular effects.[23] Thus, if angiographic intervention is used, embolization is preferred since ischemic complications in the upper GI tract are rare.

Operative Treatment

Indications for operation in bleeding peptic ulcer include (1) severe hemorrhage unresponsive to resuscitative efforts, (2) prolonged bleeding with loss of one-half or more of the estimated blood volume, (3) recurrence of hemorrhage after initial control with nonoperative measures, (4) repeated hospitalization for bleeding, and (5) a coexisting additional indication for operation.[15,16] The choice of operation depends on the age and condition of the patient and the size, location, and bleeding rate of the ulcer.

The mainstays of successful therapy for bleeding duodenal ulcer are suture ligation of the bleeding artery and vagotomy. Truncal vagotomy and pyloroplasty is the most appropriate procedure for elderly patients, those with severe concurrent illness, and those suffering shock from exsanguinating hemorrhage.[16] The operation is quick, easy and frequently life-saving.

However, this operation has an early rebleeding rate that may exceed 10% and may lead to mortality.[29] Therefore, in the younger patient without other risk factors, truncal vagotomy combined with antrectomy should be considered. Whenever possible, reconstruction of GI continuity is done by gastroduodenostomy. If a large, deep, posterior ulcer crater precludes safe mobilization of the duodenum for anastomosis, the duodenum is closed with the ulcer in situ and a gastrojejunostomy is performed. This technique has the theoretical advantage of removing a high-risk ulcer from the acid stream, with consequent reduction of postoperative rebleeding. The combined operation, when applied to selected patients, has an excellent record for minimizing postoperative rebleeding and is attended by a mortality rate of <5%.[30]

Since 1977, proximal gastric vagotomy has been used in select patients with bleeding duodenal ulcer.[31] The operation consists of duodenotomy or pyloroduodenotomy for exposure and suture control of the bleeding ulcer. A proximal gastric vagotomy then is performed. The duodenal incision is closed longitudinally rather than vertically, as in a pyloroplasty, thus preserving antropyloric function and normal gastric emptying. Experience with this approach has been relatively limited, with <350 cases reported.[32,33] The combined postoperative mortality has been 4.8% and the early rebleeding rate has been 2.6%. Recurrent ulcer has developed in 5.6% of patients with a mean follow-up of 3.5 years. Proximal gastric vagotomy has a legitimate role for acute bleeding duodenal ulcer, but it should be used only in younger, low-risk patients without exsanguinating hemorrhage.[32]

For bleeding gastric ulcer, distal gastrectomy to include the ulcer is the operation of choice.[34] Since most bleeding gastric ulcers are situated in the antrum of the stomach, the distal resection includes only one-third to one-half of the stomach. For ulcers situated higher on the lesser curve, the gastrectomy can be tailored with extension of the resection proximally along the lesser curve. Gastric ulcers located in the pyloric channel or in the prepyloric area require the addition of a vagotomy to the gastric resection, since they are characterized by a hypersecretory pathophysiology similar to that found in duodenal ulcer patients.[34] Gastric ulcers located in the proximal stomach exclusive of the lesser curvature can be treated by generous wedge excision of the ulcer combined with a vagotomy. Because this approach has rebleeding rates that are higher than those attending antrectomy, it should not be used for ulcers amenable to a limited distal gastric resection. In all instances of antrectomy without vagotomy, the reconstruction should be a gastroduodenostomy, since gastrojejunostomy is complicated by a higher incidence of marginal ulceration.[35]

In the rare circumstance in which gastrinoma is known to be the cause of a bleeding peptic ulcer, standard ulcer operations should be abandoned and a total gastrectomy should be performed. In the vast majority of such instances, the reason for bleeding is patient noncompliance with the medical regimen. Since curative resection of gastrinoma is unreliable over the long term, total gastrectomy may be justified.

Bleeding from a postoperative recurrent peptic ulcer following an acid-reducing procedure always represents a failure of the operation, and a more suggestive surgical approach is mandated. In the majority of such instances, the cause for ulcer recurrence is an inadequate vagotomy.[35] Because revagotomy is an unreliable solution, antrectomy should be performed.

Gastritis—Mucosal Erosions

Gastric hemorrhage from diffuse mucosal inflammation and superficial erosions is rarely severe or life threatening.[36] Most patients presenting with bleeding gastritis have ingested some substance that is toxic to the gastric mucosa or impairs its intrinsic defense mechanisms against acid-peptic injury. Alcohol, salicylates and other nonsteroidal anti-inflammatory drugs are the most commonly ingested substances that lead to acute hemorrhagic gastritis. Bleeding in such cases is due to a superficial mucosal injury with erosions and capillary oozing. In most instances, bleeding is not massive and is accompanied by mild to moderate pain. It usually is self-limited and stops spontaneously in 90% of cases with simple withdrawal of the offending substance.[37] In a study of more than 100 patients with alcohol-induced gastric mucosal bleeding, 84% of patients required <6 units of blood transfusion and >90% responded to nonoperative treatment.[38] Alcoholic patients with cirrhosis and portal hypertension are prone to refractory bleeding from the gastric mucosa owing to a combination of coagulopathy, mucosal congestion, and relative ischemia with impaired mucosal regeneration.[39] Bleeding in such patients can be brisk and refractory to therapeutic maneuvers other than those that decrease portal venous pressure.

Hemorrhagic erosive gastroduodenitis from the stress syndrome is the equivalent of an organ failure lesion. It occurs almost exclusively in seriously ill patients suffering from multiple trauma, shock, sepsis, major burn, or central nervous system trauma. It is often a component of the multiple organ failure syndrome.[40] Because it is considered to be mediated by complex neurohumoral mechanisms, the common final pathway may be mucosal ischemia, resulting in critical impairment of intrinsic mucosal defenses. The lesion is characterized by multiple superficial mucosal erosions that are typically located in the proximal stomach. However, the entire stomach and duodenum may be involved in one-third of cases.

Prophylaxis

Because of improvements in the supportive care of critically ill patients, the stress ulcer syndrome is encountered less frequently. Prophylactic measures also have served to decrease the incidence of stress bleeding. Patients without intensive supportive care and stress ulcer prophylaxis develop shallow erosions in the gastric mucosa within 72 hours of major trauma, sepsis, or prolonged hypotension. Only about 20% of patients clinically manifest the gastric erosions, most by overt bleeding. A recent multicenter prospective study has identified respiratory failure and coagulopathy as the most important risk factors for stress ulcer bleeding.[41] Prophylaxis is directed at suppression or neutralization of gastric secretion. Specific regimens designed to enhance gastroduodenal mucosal resistance or promote epithelial renewal also may be efficacious. Once fully developed, the stress ulcer syndrome is attended by a 50% or greater mortality rate.[41,42] Although death is more often the result of the underlying original insult, the presence of upper GI hemorrhage adds significantly to mortality rates of such patients, as compared to similarly ill patients without hemorrhage.

Treatment

Intervention for bleeding gastritis rarely is required. Endoscopic means, such as electrocoagulation or heater probe application, can be effective for multiple punctate bleeding sites, but they are ineffective for diffuse mucosal hemorrhage. In such cases, selective intra-arterial infusion of vasopressin has been reported to stop the bleeding in 75% to 80% of patients.[43] Surgical therapy seldom is required for bleeding gastritis and only total gastrectomy is effective when hemorrhage is severe. Both gastric devascularization and vagotomy, combined with a drainage procedure and suture ligation of major bleeding points, have been effective, in anecdotal reports.[14] Total and subtotal gastrectomy have the advantage of ablation of all or most of the bleeding sites, but these procedures are attended by significant morbidity and mortality rates. In general, every effort should be made to avoid operation. The patient should be managed with cardiovascular, pulmonary, and coagulation mechanism support and by treatment of sepsis, when present. Enteral nutritional support also has been shown to be necessary for epithelial maintenance and renewal. Surgical mortality ranges from 40% to 55%.[23]

BLEEDING ESOPHAGOGASTRIC VARICES

Approximately one-third of patients with portal hypertension experience upper GI hemorrhage, and bleeding correlates with moderate- to large-sized gastroesophageal varices (Fig 5–2).[23] Bleeding presumably results from variceal rupture when the overlying atten-

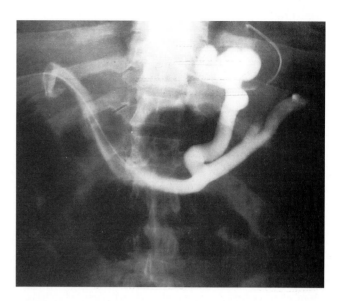

Figure 5–2. Percutaneous transhepatic portogram showing large gastric varices and left gastric (coronary) vein.

uated mucosa is eroded or traumatized. Hemorrhage is usually massive, but intermittency is the rule, with 75% stopping at least temporarily.[44] The intermittent nature of the bleeding is probably due to decompression of the bleeding varix with clot formation at the rupture site, followed by clot lysis and rebleeding. Patients with severe coagulopathy associated with chronic liver disease characteristically have little or no ability to form clots, and their bleeding tends to be unrelenting. The mortality attending the initial variceal hemorrhage may be 50% in untreated patients, with more than half of the deaths resulting from exsanguination.[44] Most of the remainder are due to hepatic failure or sepsis. Of those patients surviving the initial bleeding episode, approximately one-third rebleed within 6 weeks, and more than two-thirds will rebleed within 1 year of the initial bleed.[44,45] Exclusive of the acute hemorrhage, longevity is determined by the functional hepatic reserve and the progression of the underlying hepatic disease.

Medical Management

Management of the patient with variceal hemorrhage requires attention to considerations not usually needed in nonvariceal hemorrhage. Most important is the correction of reversible coagulopathy with replacement of clotting factors through the use of vitamin K, fresh frozen plasma, and platelet transfusions. Although widely practiced, pharmacologic therapy with intravenous vasopressin is unproven as a means of controlling variceal hemorrhage. Previous studies have suggested a benefit with respect to bleeding, but no difference in survival has been noted.[46] A more recent placebo-controlled trial demonstrated no efficacy of intravenous infusion of vasopressin with respect to control of bleeding or mortality.[47] Concomitant use of nitroglycerine with vasopressin infusion has been demonstrated to reverse the deleterious cardiovascular effects of vasopressin without diminishing its putative therapeutic efficacy.[48] Intra-arterial vasopressin has not been shown to be superior to intravenous infusion.[49] Thus, while the efficacy of vasopressin in controlling variceal hemorrhage may be limited, it should be administered only intravenously and with concomitant nitroglycerine.

The naturally occurring peptide, somatostatin, and its long acting synthetic analog, octreotide, also have been administered intravenously as a means of decreasing splanchnic blood flow and portal venous pressure. Somatostatin is at least as effective as vasopressin in controlling acute variceal hemorrhage and has fewer complications.[50] Placebo-controlled trials have not demonstrated efficacy convincingly, with regard to hemostasis.[51,52] However, it is clear that no survival benefit, thus far, has been demonstrated with the use of somatostatin. A single study has suggested that intravenous metoclopramide may have a role in controlling hemorrhage from esophageal varices.[53] The putative mechanism of action is the reduction of intravariceal venous pressure by constriction of the lower esophageal sphincter.

Direct tamponade of bleeding varices through the use of a variety of balloon tamponade tubes has been available for more than 50 years. The most commonly used tube is the Sengstaken-Blakemore (Rusch, Inc. Duluth, GA), which is equipped with both a gastric and an esophageal balloon as well as a gastric aspiration port. The Minnesota tube is similar but has a separate port for aspiration of the esophagus. With balloon inflation and direct compression of the bleeding varices, initial hemostasis is obtained in 85% to 89% of cases.[23] With deflation of the balloons and release of the tamponade, rebleeding occurs in up to 60% of cases.[54] There has been no survival benefit demonstrated by this temporizing measure. Use of such tables requires considerable expertise and bedside vigilance. Major complications, such as aspiration, airway obstruction, and esophageal necrosis and rupture, have been reported in up to 20% of cases.[55] In general, balloon tamponade is used as a stop-gap measure in patients with exsanguinating hemorrhage from gastroesophageal varices when other less dangerous control methods are unavailable or have failed.

Endoscopic Therapy

Emergency upper endoscopy is indicated in all patients with suspected variceal hemorrhage. Since other potential bleeding lesions are particularly common in patients with portal hypertension, endoscopic evaluation is essential in establishing the true identity of the offending lesion. Variceal injection sclerotherapy has emerged in recent years as the emergency intervention

of choice and now is applied almost universally at the time of initial diagnostic endoscopic examination. A variety of sclerosant agents can be injected via the endoscope through a small-gauge long needle directly into and/or around the bleeding varices. Injection sclerotherapy accomplishes immediate control of variceal bleeding in 70% of cases. With repeated sclerotherapy sessions, definitive control can be obtained in up to 95% of patients.[56] Unfortunately, up to 50% of patients rebleed during the initial hospitalization and some additional treatment program must be undertaken. Numerous randomized prospective trials comparing sclerotherapy and standard medical management have demonstrated a significant benefit from chronic endoscopic therapy.[23] Improved rebleeding rates, as well as mortality rates, have been achieved. Thus, the therapeutic efficacy of endoscopic sclerotherapy appears to be well established compared to other medical means of managing bleeding esohageal varices. However, no efficacy has been shown by the use of schlerotherapy as a prophylactic means of preventing initial hemorrhage in patients with known portal hypertension and asymptomatic varices.[45] The principal drawbacks of sclerotherapy include the need for multiple sessions in order to ablate the variceal complex, as well as the development of esophageal ulcerations and strictures.[23] Sclerotherapy-induced ulcers may bleed and occasionally perforate, in which case mortality is excessive. Despite these and other complications, sclerotherapy is currently the initial treatment of choice for bleeding esophageal varices.

Endoscopic esophageal variceal ligation is a recently introduced technique that represents an extension of the widely used rubber band ligation of anorectal hemorrhoids. The goals of variceal ligation are the same as those of endoscopic sclerotherapy. Strangulation and necrosis lead to eventual fibrosis and obliteration of the mucosal and submucosal portal venous collaterals, effectively precluding subsequent variceal hemorrhage. Thus far, endoscopic ligation of varices has been shown to be at least as effective as sclerotherapy and has been attended by a lower complication rate.[57] Specifically, the incidence of esophageal ulceration and stricture has been reduced. With additional experience, endoscopic variceal ligation may replace sclerotherapy as the preferred initial intervention.

Operative Treatment

Surgery for bleeding esophagogastric varices remains the definitive method for stopping acute hemorrhage and preventing its recurrence. Two general types of operations are applicable; these include esophagogastric devascularization procedures and surgical decompression of the portal venous system. Surgical procedures are used most often for the prevention of recurrent hemorrhage rather than for treatment of unremitting bleeding. In many centers, emergency surgery for variceal bleeding is reserved for patients who have failed at least two sessions of sclerotherapy and who have reasonable hepatic function (Child-Pugh class A and B patients). Patients with poor function (Child-Pugh class C patients) are usually continued on some form of nonsurgical management, since the mortality rate attending emergency operation in such patients is prohibitive.[58]

Nonshunt or devascularization procedures span the gamut from simple esophageal transaction and reanastomosis using a circular stapling device, to the extensive thoracoabdominal gastroesophageal devascularization procedure of Sugiura.[59] The latter operation involves devascularization of the thoracic and abdominal esophagus, proximal stomach, esophageal transaction and reanastomosis, splenectomy and pyloroplasty via a thoracoabdominal incision. The operation is a major undertaking but has the theoretical advantage of maintaining portal venous hepatic perfusion. Excellent results have been reported from Japan with a rebleeding rate of 1.5% and a 10 year actuarial survival rate of 72% when performed electively, and 55% when performed urgently.[60] Unfortunately, such results have not been forthcoming from other countries. In the United States, simple esophageal transaction and reanastomosis has been the more frequently performed nonshunt procedure. This operation has been used in decompensated patients with active bleeding, with disappointing results.[61]

The standard operative procedure for bleeding varices is still portosystemic vascular anastomosis to decompress the hypertensive portal venous system and varices. The end-to-side portacaval shunt has been practiced the most widely, since it is the easiest and most reliable operation to stop bleeding.[23] The shunt totally diverts portal venous flow into the vena cava and decompresses the entire splanchnic venous bed. Operative mortality varies widely, depending on the patient's Child-Pugh class, and on whether the procedure is performed urgently or electively. The side-to-side portacaval shunt was developed in an attempt to preserve a portion of hepatopetal portal venous flow while still adequately decompressing the varices. Unfortunately, the large gradient between portal and systemic venous pressures usually dictates that the total shunting of portal flow into the vena cava occurs. The only demonstrated advantage of the side-to-side or central shunt is improved control of postoperative ascites.[62] The interposition portacaval shunt and the mesocaval shunt use prosthetic grafts to create side-to-side shunts, again to preserve some portion of hepatopetal flow.[45] Small-diameter grafts have been used to control the amount of flow diverted to the systemic venous system, but graft thrombosis remains a problem.[63] The proximal splenorenal shunt involves splenectomy and end-to-side

anastomosis of the splenic vein to the left renal vein and represents another form of functional side-to-side or central shunt.

Selective shunting, as represented by the distal splenorenal (Warren) shunt, is designed to decompress the variceal channels while maintaining high pressure and hepatopetal flow in the remainder of the portal venous system.[64] It involves isolation of the esophagogastric variceal bed from the remainder of the splanchnic system by division of the coronary vein and all other venous drainage routes, except the short gastric veins. The splenic vein is divided at its confluence with the superior mesenteric vein and then anastomosed to the left renal vein. Thus, the esophagogastric varices are decompressed via the short gastric veins and the splenic vein into the systemic venous circulation. Hepatopetal portal venous inflow from the superior mesenteric vein is preserved. When compared with portacaval shunts in six randomized prospective trials, the distal splenorenal shunt showed no benefits with regard to rebleeding or survival.[23,45] In some comparisons, however, the selective shunt has been associated with significantly reduced hepatic encephalopathy, particularly in nonalcoholic cirrhotic patients. Because of greater technical difficulty, a slightly higher thrombosis rate and lack of decompression of the splanchnic bed or liver, the distal splenorenal shunt is not recommended for patients with acute bleeding or significant ascites.

The newest intervention for bleeding gastroesophageal varices is the transjugular intrahepatic portocaval shunt (TIPS).[65] This procedure is performed in the angiography suite under local anesthesia and involves introduction of a needle into the internal jugular vein. The needle then is advanced via the vena cava into a hepatic vein, through the hepatic parenchyma and into a portal vein. A guidewire then is threaded through the needle and an angioplasty balloon is used to expand the hepatic parenchymal tract between the hepatic and portal veins. An expandable stent then is placed in the parenchymal tract to establish a shunt between the two veins. Although introduction of the TIPS procedure has been met with considerable enthusiasm, concerns regarding the durability of the shunt remain. TIPS has been shown to be effective in approximately 80% of bleeding patients, yet stenosis of the intrahepatic shunt has occurred in up to 25% of patients in follow-up of <1 year.[66] Repeat dilatations and placement of additional stents are required to ensure long-term patency in most patients. TIPS has been used very successfully as a temporizing measure for patients awaiting liver transplantation.[67] Its efficacy as a durable substitute for a surgical portosystemic shunt remains to be demonstrated. It does represent an additional relatively nonmorbid method for controlling unrelenting variceal hemorrhage in high-risk patients.

Orthotopic liver transplantation is the most aggressive and definitive approach to variceal hemorrhage from portal hypertension. Transplantation is reserved for patients with advanced hepatocellular liver disease complicated by variceal bleeding rather than for variceal bleeding per se.[68] Patients with good hepatocellular reserve should not be considered transplant candidates, since shunt procedures are reliable methods of controlling variceal bleeding. Patients who are considered transplant candidates initially are treated endoscopically or with TIPS. If a surgical shunt is required in a transplant candidate, a mesocaval or splenorenal shunt is preferred so as not to violate the portal vein or vena cava prior to transplantation.

Isolated-bleeding gastric varices associated with splenic vein thrombosis are readily treated by splenectomy.[69] Since gastric varices are more often a sequelae of generalized portal hypertension, it is important to document the splenic vein thrombosis prior to undertaking this operation. Nonoperative methods for controlling varices in the gastric fundus are difficult technically and usually ineffective. Even though splenectomy is a proven therapy for sinistral portal hypertension, angiographic transcatheter splenic artery embolization also has been suggested for poor operative-risk patients. However, splenic abscess may follow splenic infarction.[23]

ESOPHAGEAL EROSIONS AND ULCERS

Less than 3% of all upper GI bleeding is the result of severe gastroesophageal acid reflux disease.[36] Bleeding derives from either severe erosive esophagitis or from a single, deeply penetrating esophageal ulcer. Esophageal ulcers are relatively uncommon and most are found in the presence of Barrett's epithelium. The ulcer typically is located at the junction of normal squamous epithelium and the proximal extent of the metaplastic columnar epithelium. Whether due to erosive esophagitis or to a true ulcer, hemorrhage associated with reflux esophagitis rarely is massive and almost always self-limited.

When hemorrhage from esophagitis or esophageal erosions is unremitting, endoscopy should be undertaken to obtain hemostasis.[23] Because the majority of inflammatory bleeding lesions in the esophagus are superficial, the success rate of endoscopic hemostatic therapy is high. Following cessation of bleeding, aggressive medical therapy, such as histamine H_2 antagonists or omerprazole, should be instituted. In most instances, effective control of acid reflux is sufficient to prevent recurrent hemorrhage.

In most instances, bleeding from deep esophageal ulcers also can be treated endoscopically.[23] Assessment of the likelihood of malignancy is an important issue in such cases, particularly in the presence of Barrett's ep-

ithelium. Bleeding from esophageal ulcers unresponsive to endoscopic control is rare. However, in such cases, emergency operation may be required. If the suspicion of malignancy is great, or there is severe dysplasia in Barrett's epithelium, resection by esophagogastrectomy may be indicated. If malignancy is not an issue, esophagotomy and oversewing of the bleeding ulcer can be performed. This should be accompanied by an antireflux procedure, such as a Nissen fundoplication, in which the closed esophagotomy is covered by the gastric wrap.

MALLORY-WEISS SYNDROME

An uncommon cause of upper GI bleeding is a mucosal tear that results from rapid and forceful dilation of the gastroesophageal junction. Mallory-Weiss tears account for approximately 15% of acute upper GI bleeds, with more than 80% related to antecedent episodes of forceful vomiting, retching, coughing or straining.[70] Most occur in alcoholic patients and may be complicated by the presence of portal hypertension. More then 80% of the mucosal tears are located on the lesser curvature of the gastroesophageal junction. The lesion is typically 1 to 4 cm in length and approximately three-fourths are located entirely in gastric mucosa; the remaining one-fourth extend into the squamous epithelium of the distal esophagus.[70] Multiple tears are present in a minority of patients. Although once thought to be associated with rather massive hemorrhage, it now is recognized that most mucosal tears result in mild to moderate bleeding with spontaneous cessation in >90% of patients. In the remaining minority, either brisk arterial bleeding or massive venous bleeding owing to preexisting portal hypertension result in prolonged, potentially exsanguinating hemorrhage. Such cases account for the overall 3% to 4% mortality associated with the lesion.[14]

In most instances of hemorrhage from Mallory-Weiss tears, only supportive therapy is required. Particular attention should be directed at correcting coagulopathy in affected patients. Brisk or persistent bleeding is managed best by endoscopic electrocoagulation or heater-probe techniques.[23] Angiographic therapy with intra-arterial infusion of vasopressin or transcatheter embolization of the left gastric artery or one of its branches also can be effective.[43] Operative intervention is required only rarely. Emergency operation consists of an anterior gastrotomy near the cardia, with direct oversewing of the mucosal tear. Rebleeding from Mallory-Weiss tears, whether treated operatively or nonoperatively, is distinctly uncommon.

TUMORS OF THE UPPER GASTROINTESTINAL TRACT

Neoplastic lesions arising from the esophagus, stomach, or duodenum almost invariably cause occult upper GI tract bleeding. Thus, while anemia is common, overt bleeding is unusual and when present, is not typically massive. This is particularly true for esophageal neoplasms, and duodenal tumors. Gastric neoplasms are occasionally complicated by exigent hemorrhage. Gastric adenocarcinoma and to a lesser extent, lymphoma, may present as ulcerative lesions with persistent hemorrhage from central tumor necrosis and bleeding. These complications result from tumor vessels incapable of vasospasm.[71] Adenomatous polyps, which are benign lesions, only rarely bleed overtly. Leiomyomas, on the other hand, are notorious for presenting with brisk hemorrhage from their central ulcerations. Moreover, their malignant counterpart, leiomyosarcomas, behave similarly, but they may attain very large sizes and may be complicated by profuse bleeding.

The treatment for upper GI hemorrhage due to tumors is almost exclusively surgical. Endoscopy and angiography have limited therapeutic roles in bleeding from neoplasms, but they may be attempted in cases of advanced unresectable primary malignancies of the stomach or duodenum.[23] Metastic lesions may be approached similarly; however, these therapies are usually ineffective except as very short-term temporizing measures. Thus, in the vast majority of patients, a direct surgical approach is required. The specific operation is tailored to the type and extent of tumor found. For small lesions such as suspected or proven leiomyomas, simple wedge excision constitutes adequate therapy. Any previously unbiopsied tumor should be submitted for immediate frozen-section pathologic examination to rule out malignancy. If malignancy is found, a standard cancer operation should be performed, if the patient's condition allows it. Known malignant lesions of the stomach, such as adenocarcinoma, lymphoma, and leiomyosarcoma, should be treated by subtotal or total gastrectomy. Malignant tumors of the duodenum usually may be excised locally or resected by antrectomy that includes the duodenal bulb. Benign tumors of the third and fourth portions of the duodenum may be resected locally or treated by distal duodenectomy without pancreatectomy.

VASCULAR MALFORMATIONS

Vascular malformations are a relatively uncommon but important cause of upper GI bleeding, and they represent a group of pathologic entities of incompletely understood etiologies. Vascular malformations account for approximately 2% to 4% of upper GI bleeding and typically are found in elderly patients, although some, such as hereditary hemorrhagic telangiectasia, are clearly congenital.[14,72] Acquired lesions often are associated with chronic renal failure and dialysis or aortic valvular disease.[23,73] The typical angiodysplastic lesion is

<1 cm in diameter, flat or only slightly raised above the normal mucosal contour, and stellate in appearance, with obviously dilated and tortuous vascular elements. The lesions are multiple in approximately two-thirds of patients.[14,73] Bleeding presumably occurs when the lesions are abraided by food in transit and usually is not exsanguinating, although recurrent bleeding is the rule. Between episodes of overt bleeding, occult blood loss often is present.

In most cases, vascular malformations are amenable to endoscopic ablation.[23] This is true particularly when lesions are small and bleeding is slow. Large vascular lesions are far less responsive to endoscopic coagulation as are those diffusely involving the mucosa. In such cases, surgical resection is the appropriate treatment. An operation also should be considered for patients with multiple episodes of rebleeding that follow attempts at endoscopic control. Patients with Osler-Weber-Rendu syndrome may benefit from a trial of estrogen-progesterone therapy, if surgical resection is not feasible.[74]

DEULAFOY'S LESION

Deulafoy's lesion is an abnormally large submucosal artery in the stomach that is prone to acute upper GI hemorrhage when erosion of the overlying mucosa and vascular wall necrosis occur. Approximately 80% of these lesions are found within 6 cm of the gastroesophageal junction on the lesser curvature of the stomach.[75] The bleeding that emanates from the large and abnormally located artery is typically intermittent and brisk. The etiology of the lesion is unknown.

Since bleeding from Deulafoy's lesion often is life threatening, therapeutic intervention should be immediate and aggressive. While endoscopic means have met with occasional success, the safest course is surgical wedge resection of the offending lesion.[76] Simple gastrotomy and oversewing of the large submucosal artery also may be an effective, though perhaps less reliable, alternative. Overall mortality is 23%.[76]

AORTOENTERIC FISTULA

The most common form of aortoenteric fistula is found between the proximal anastomotic suture line of an aortic prosthetic graft and the distal duodenum.[77] In some cases the fistula appears to be the result of a primary graft infection, with pseudoaneurysm formation and subsequent fistulization through the adjacent duodenal wall.[78] In other cases, evidence for preexisting graft infection is lacking and it is presumed that there is direct-pressure necrosis of the adherent duodenal wall from the pulsatile motion of the aortic-graft anastomosis. Thus, transmural pressure necrosis of the duodenum exposes the vascular suture line to infection, which results in dehiscence and bleeding into the duodenum. Although much less common, primary aortoduodenal fistula can also occur in the unoperated patient with an abdominal aortic aneurysm that erodes and ruptures into the lumen of the overlying adherent duodenum.[79]

In all its varieties, hemorrhage caused by aortoduodenal fistula is classically massive, but often is presaged by a smaller, brief, sentinel hemorrhage.[78] This may represent the stage of evolution of the fistula during which the duodenal mucosa is undergoing pressure necrosis, just prior to overt fistulization. Once the fistula is actually established, bleeding is truly massive and exsanguination is inevitable, unless surgical intervention occurs.

The important initial step with suspected aortoduodenal fistula is upper endoscopy for visualization of the distal duodenum.[23] If overt bleeding or mucosal erosion or hematoma is evident in the distal duodenum of a patient with known aortic graft or aneurysm, the diagnosis should be assumed and no further investigation is required. If endoscopic diagnosis is not possible, an abdominal computed tomography scan, magnetic resonance imaging, or abdominal aortogram may be helpful in demonstrating a pseudoaneurysm at the aortic-graft anastomosis.

Whenever the diagnosis of aortoduodenal fistula is seriously entertained, emergency laparotomy should be performed.[79] Since infection is an important factor in the pathogenesis of the fistula, operative management should include removal of the prosthetic graft, closure of the duodenal fistula, and extraanatomic bypass to revascularize the lower limbs. In the more controlled setting, an axillobifemoral bypass graft first is constructed and is followed immediately by laparotomy, removal of the aortic graft, oversewing of the infrarenal aortic stump, and closure of the duodenal defect.[77] In the presence of active hemorrhage, laparotomy should be performed first, followed immediately by extraanatomic bypass.

HEMOBILIA

Hemobilia is a rare cause of upper GI bleeding that most often results from blunt or penetrating hepatic injury, with fistula formation within the liver between a vascular structure and the biliary ductal system.[80] Bleeding is usually mild to moderate and is accompanied by right upper quadrant pain. Jaundice from acute extrahepatic biliary obstruction owing to blood clot formation in the common bile duct also is evident. Nontraumatic causes of hemobilia include hepatic abscesses and occasionally, choledocholithiasis or oriental cholangiohepatitis.

The diagnosis of hemobilia is typically made on upper endoscopy, with findings of bleeding from the ampulla of Vater.[23] When bleeding is active, visceral angiography usually demonstrates the vascular-biliary fistula within the liver. In the majority of cases, angiographic embolization of the artery feeding the fistula is curative.[81] In patients with massive hemobilia or in those unresponsive to angiographic embolization, laparotomy and ligation of the right or left hepatic artery may be required. Hepatic resection rarely is required, usually in cases of neoplasm or calculus disease that are not amenable to more conservative therapy.[80]

HEMOSUCCUS PANCREATICUS, PANCREATIC PSEUDOCYSTS AND PSEUDOANEURYSMS

Upper GI hemorrhage may derive from a variety of mechanisms that are consequent to chronic pancreatitis. The autodigestive inflammatory process imparted by pancreatitis can lead to weakening of the arterial wall and pseudoaneurysm formation in any of the arteries supplying or adjacent to the pancreas (Fig 5–3). The most commonly involved arteries are the splenic, gastroduodenal, pancreaticoduodenal, and left gastric artery.[82] Gastrointestinal hemorrhage results when these pseudoaneurysms rupture and decompress either directly into the stomach or duodenum or, less com-

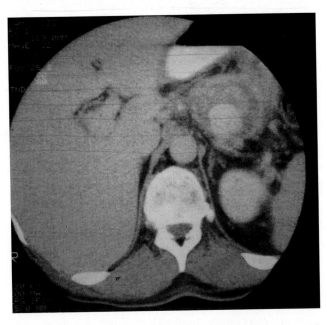

Figure 5–3. Abdominal computed tomography scan showing large retrogastric pseudoaneurysm caused by pancreatitis. Unclotted, flowing arterial blood in the center of the pseudoaneurysm is surrounded by a thick layer of freshly clotted blood.

monly, into the pancreatic duct. In the latter situation, bleeding into the duodenum via the ampulla of Vater also occurs. Such bleeding is termed *hemosuccus pancreaticus*.[83] GI hemorrhage deriving from all of these mechanisms is typically moderate to massive in magnitude. Although it may be initially intermittent, bleeding inevitably recurs; the outcome is usually fatal if intervention is not initiated.

The diagnosis of upper GI hemorrhage related to pancreatic disease is dependent upon an index of suspicion based on known history of pancreatitis. The initial diagnostic maneuver is upper endoscopy that may reveal a bleeding site anywhere in the stomach or duodenum without typical signs of chronic ulcer disease, neoplasm, or other mucosal abnormalities. If bleeding is from the ampulla of Vater, in the absence of jaundice or biliary colic but in the presence of pancreatic disease or trauma, hemosuccus pancreaticus should be

suspected. Whenever this occurs, or when bleeding into the upper GI tract from a pancreatic pseudoaneurysm or pseudocyst is suspected, visceral arteriography of the celiac axis and its branches should be undertaken immediately. Arterial embolization should be performed both proximal and distal to the bleeding site because of the rich collateral flow through the pancreas (Fig 5–4).[82] If bleeding is successfully controlled, pseudocysts >5 cm should be treated specifically. If angiographic control is unsuccessful, emergency laparotomy for arterial ligation proximal and distal to the bleeding pseudoaneurysm should be undertaken. In cases of large pseudocysts, intracystic suture ligation of the vessel may be accomplished. Occasionally, pancreatic resection is the only means of obtaining secure vascular control. Pancreatic resection usually is required in cases of hemosuccus pancreaticus, since the bleeding site is typically within the pancreatic parenchyma.

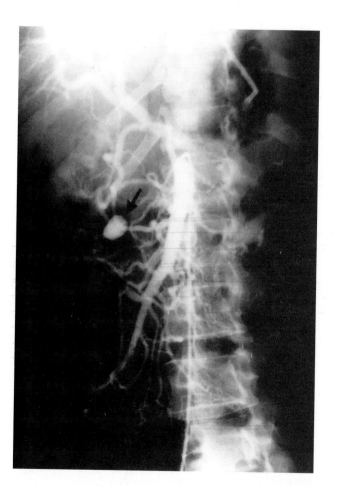

A

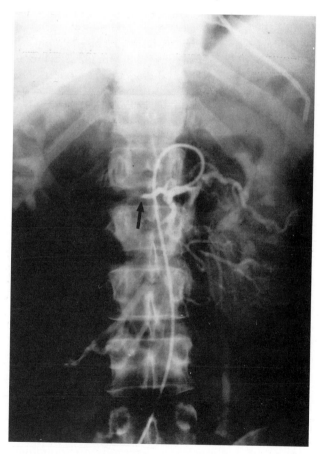

B

Figure 5–4. A. Superior mesenteric arteriogram demonstrating pseudoaneurysm of inferior pancreaticoduodenal artery (*arrow*) in the head of the pancreas. **B.** Repeat arteriogram immediately following selective transcatheter embolization of the inferior pancreaticoduodenal artery showing cessation of flow and nonfilling of the pseudoaneurysm (*arrow*).

■ DIAGNOSIS OF LOWER GASTROINTESTINAL BLEEDING

In the past, there has been unnecessary confusion in the diagnosis of lower GI bleeding. Such confusion has resulted from difficulties in diagnosis prior to the advent of modern endoscopic techniques and a tendency to group all cases of lower GI hemorrhage together, regardless of the quality or quantity of blood loss. Factors that have contributed to the diagnostic difficulty include the often intermittent nature of the bleeding; the anatomic configuration and expanse of the colon and small intestine; the absence of mucosal lesions, in many cases; and the forward egress of shed blood, which obscures endoscopic visualization. For purposes of clarity and clinical applicability, it is appropriate to categorize and evaluate lower GI bleeding on the basis of the severity and activity of the hemorrhage. There are three separate categories: (1) minor self-limited bleeding, (2) major, but self-limited, bleeding, and (3) major or massive ongoing bleeding. Since a given lesion may present as any one of these categories, classification distinctly influences patient management. In addition, the presenting symptoms and severity of the acute episode often can give clues to the diagnosis, thus aiding in the selection of appropriate diagnostic and therapeutic maneuvers.

PATTERNS OF LOWER GASTROINTESTINAL BLEEDING

Massive Ongoing Bleeding

The management of patients with massive lower GI bleeding remains controversial. A lack of randomized prospective trials comparing the efficacies of the various available treatment modalities has contributed to such controversy. In addition, many studies purporting to evaluate the management of such patients include those with acute major self-limited lower GI bleeding as well. Patients with unremitting massive lower GI hemorrhage are clearly a minority, constituting only 10% to 20% of patients presenting with hemodynamically significant lower GI bleeding. The remaining 80% to 90% of patients can be expected to stop bleeding spontaneously. Inclusion of such patients complicates any study designed to assess diagnostic or therapeutic efficacy.

There are four initial management choices for patients with continuing major lower GI bleeding: (1) urgent colonoscopy, (2) nuclear scintigraphy, (3) angiography, and (4) urgent surgery (Fig 5–5). Of these options, all but nuclear scintigraphy are potentially therapeutic as well as diagnostic.

Major Self-Limited Bleeding

Patients who present with hemodynamic compromise and a history of recent or ongoing hematochezia usually

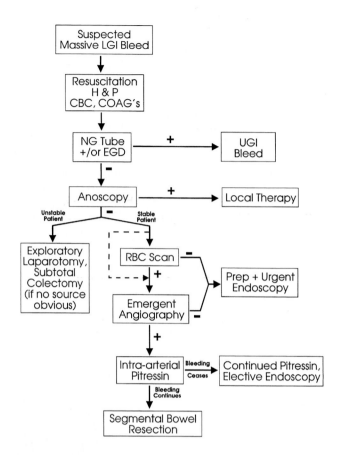

Figure 5–5. An algorithm for the management of patients with suspected major ongoing lower gastrointestinal bleeding.

respond to initial resuscitation with crystalloids. The majority (>75%) cease bleeding spontaneously. The continued passage of shed blood, for as long as 24 hours following cessation of bleeding, particularly with a small bowel or proximal colonic source, complicates differentiation of such patients from those with continued bleeding. The potential dire consequences of ongoing massive bleeding dictate an aggressive initial diagnostic and therapeutic approach. Following initial resuscitation, appropriate monitoring measures should be instituted, upper GI source should be excluded, and a decision regarding further diagnostic and/or therapeutic measures should be made. The usual options include nuclear scintigraphy, angiography and colonoscopy. Continued observation and supportive therapy is yet another option.

Minor Self-Limited Bleeding

Patients with minor, hemodynamically insignificant lower GI bleeding can be subcategorized further based on factors such as patient age, preexisting medical conditions, and the nature of the bleeding episode or episodes. Most often the presenting minor hemorrhage is attributed appropriately to hemorrhoidal disease, but it may be due to a variety of other causes. In fact, the majority of neoplasms that present with bleeding are associated with only minimal visible blood loss.

Further evaluation and treatment of a patient with a recent minor hemorrhage should be dictated by the nature of the bleeding episode, as well as the clinical suspicion. Rigid proctoscopy or flexible sigmoidoscopy is mandatory in the evaluation of such patients. In young patients with a clinical history and proctoscopic findings consistent with hemorrhoidal bleeding, therapy should be directed at controlling hemorrhoids, who have close follow-up and further evaluation, as dictated by the subsequent course. In older patients with significant risk factors or a suspicious clinical history, flexible sigmoidoscopy or colonoscopy should be performed prior to attributing the bleeding to hemorrhoidal disease.

NUCLEAR SCINTIGRAPHY

Bleeding scans incorporating technetium sulfur colloid or technetium 99m–labeled (^{99m}Tc) red blood cells utilize external gamma counters to detect intraluminal extravasation of blood. The scans are noninvasiveness and potentially sensitive in detecting bleeding as slow as 0.1 mL/min. With the use of tagged red blood cells, these scans can detect intermittent bleeding.[84,85] Sulfur colloid scans are very sensitive in detecting active bleeding and can be completed in >1 hour. However, significant hepatic and splenic uptake may obscure bleeding sites in the upper abdomen. Additionally, rapid intravascular clearance of the radiolabel requires that active bleeding be present at the time of scanning. ^{99m}Tc-labeled red blood cell scans require more time because of the labeling process, but allow repeated scanning for up to 24 hours after injection. The scans also provide better localization by demonstrating the anatomic contours of the egress path of the labeled red blood cells on sequential images (Fig 5–6). The disadvantages of these scans include a relative lack of specificity, especially for small bowel lesions, absence of any therapeutic potential, and the possibility for an attendant delay in therapy. The results reported in the literature for nuclear scintigraphy have been extremely variable, with sensitivities and specificities ranging from 40% to 92%.[84-90] This fluctuation is most likely the result of the variability in patient selection, timing of the examination, and operator expertise. However, when used urgently to study selected hemodynamically stable patients with significant bleeding, the test has excellent sensitivity in predicting continued hemorrhage. Thus, its use is encouraged as a screening test prior to angiography and limits the application of an invasive procedure with potential nephrotoxicity. Additionally, the angiographic approach can be directed to the appropriate mesenteric vessel and thereby can minimize the volume of contrast injection and the time spent in the angiography suite.

Nuclear scintigraphy is perhaps ideal for patients

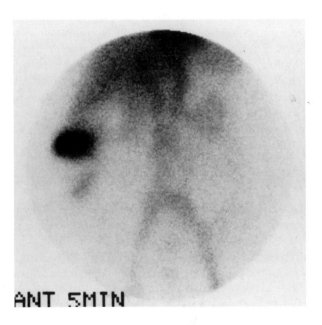

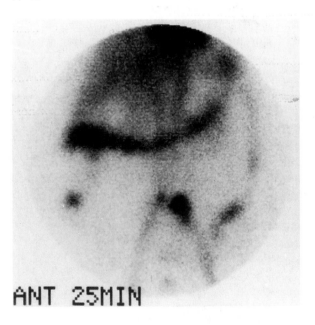

A   B

Figure 5–6. A. Technetium-99m labelled red blood cell scan showing concentration of the radionuclide in the right upper quadrant of the abdomen. **B**. Delayed view showing advancement of the radionuclide into the transverse colon providing specific localization of the bleeding site to the hepatic flexure of the colon. (Courtesy of Dr. Carol Marcus)

who present with significant bleeding, but who respond rapidly to resuscitative measures. The difficulties often encountered in clinically determining the presence or absence of ongoing bleeding and the risk of early rebleeding make the tagged red blood cell scan particularly useful in this setting. With a negative predictive value of 92%, the information derived is often useful in determining the acuity of a hemorrhage.[88] Around-the-clock availability of nuclear scintigraphy scanning is absolutely essential, since timing of the scans is correlated directly with success in localizing the bleeding site.

ANGIOGRAPHY

Visceral angiography involves selective catheterization of the mesenteric vessels and injection of contrast with inspection for extravasation and pooling of media within the intestinal lumen (Fig 5–7). The technique allows detection of bleeding rates as low as 0.5 mL/min.[91] Owing to the often intermittent nature of lower GI bleeding, angiographic examination should be performed on actively bleeding patients without unnecessary delays.[92] To improve both the efficacy and safety of the examination, adequate intravascular volume replenishment is essential prior to injection of the nephrotoxic contrast media. In the setting of prior localization of the bleeding site by nuclear scintigraphy or endoscopic examination, direct selective catheterization of the appropriate vessel can be performed initially. However, in the absence of preangiographic localization, initial superior mesenteric artery catheterization and visualization should be carried out. If this is unsuccessful in visualizing the bleeding site, catheterization of the inferior mesenteric artery and, if necessary, the

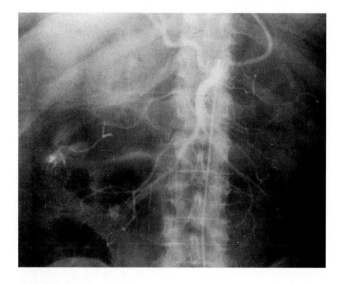

Figure 5–7. Superior mesenteric arteriogram demonstrating extravasation of contrast medium from the right colic artery.

celiac artery, are performed. Although mid-rectal and low-rectal lesions may require hypogastric injection, most, if not all such lesions should be easily localized by preangiographic rigid proctoscopy.

Upon successful angiographic visualization of the site of hemorrhage, the catheter is advanced superselectively, closer to the site of bleeding, for intra-arterial infusion of vasopressin. Vasopressin causes very effective arterial and venous vasoconstriction, as well as bowel contraction. These effects act in concert to significantly reduce local blood flow and to promote thrombosis at the bleeding site. Infusion at a rate of 0.2 units/min initially is begun. This can be increased safely to 0.4 units/min as necessary.[93,94] Cessation of bleeding is confirmed by repeat angiography 15 to 30 minutes after infusion is begun. If effective, infusion should be continued at the effective dose for 24 to 48 hours and then slowly tapered.[92,94] Because of first pass metabolism of vasopressin in the liver, intra-arterial infusion is extremely safe. However, reported complications include cardiac, visceral, and peripheral ischemia.[93–96] If vasopressin is effective in stopping the bleeding, the chance of rebleeding from the offending lesion may still be as high as 50%.[92] Most patients who rebleed do so within the first 12 hours after discontinuation of vasopressin infusion. Thus, the selective catheter should be left in position, with a slow infusion of nonheparinized saline, for an additional 24 hours. This enables rapid reinstitution of vasopressin should bleeding recur. If transcatheter intra-arterial vasopressin fails to control the bleeding, the patient should be readied urgently for segmental bowel resection. An alternative approach for patients considered to be prohibitive operative risks is transcatheter embolization using gel foam, wire coils, or autologous blood clot. However, a significant incidence of postembolic bowel infarction of the colon has limited the application of this technique.[97] Additional benefits of angiographic examination include visualization of nonbleeding vascular malformations, neoplasms, or other lesions that may be responsible for bleeding.

COLONOSCOPY

Although colonoscopy has proven useful in evaluating patients with occult chronic GI bleeding and those who have stopped bleeding after an acute self-limited hemorrhage, the use of the procedure in patients with truly massive ongoing lower GI bleeding remains controversial.[98] Many of the studies that have reported an advantage of endoscopic evaluation and therapy of acutely bleeding patients have excluded unstable patients. Technical difficulties with emergency colonoscopy include a significant absorption of light by blood and a drastic impairment of visualization due to clot in the colonic lumen. Actual visualization of ongoing bleeding is relatively uncommon and indirect, and potentially misleading indicators of bleeding sites, such as mucosal erosions, adherent clots, or blood filling a diverticulum, often are relied upon.[99,100] In the event of localization of a bleeding site (usually an arteriovenous malformation or a diverticulum), a variety of therapeutic modalities are of potential benefit, including bicap electrocautery, heater-probe coagulation, injection sclerotherapy, and laser photocoagulation. The risk of colonic perforation in the urgent setting is significantly higher than in elective colonoscopy. Thus, the procedure should be attempted only by the experienced endoscopist. Furthermore, because of the notorious inability of endoscopy to identify anatomic sites accurately within the colon, exclusive of the cecum and rectum, tattooing of the bleeding site with submucosal injection of an agent, such as methylene-blue or India ink, should be performed. This allows accurate intraoperative localization of the site should the patient continue to bleed or rebleed and require emergency surgery.

Colonoscopic examination of the patient with a major, but self-limited, hemorrhage is the test of choice after a negative bleeding scan and/or arteriogram.[101] The colonoscopy should be performed semiemergently, since sensitivity and specificity are related to visualization of the actual bleeding site.[102] Although the source of lower GI bleeding is grossly obvious at endoscopy in a minority of patients, in the majority the etiology is a superficial mucosal lesion (diverticulum, vascular malformation). Thus, any evidence of recent bleeding may be rather subtle and relatively obscured by rapid healing.

BARIUM ENEMA RADIOGRAPHY

Although once considered the diagnostic standard in acute lower GI bleeding, barium enema radiography no longer has a role in the care of patients with active hemorrhage. The deletion of the procedure from the armamentarium of the clinician was brought about by recognition of its extremely poor sensitivity and the emergence of more effective diagnostic and therapeutic modalities, such as angiography and endoscopy. Since most of the lesions that cause acute lower GI bleeding are superficial, barium contrast studies fail to detect them. Additionally, because of retention of barium within the lumen of the GI tract, the examination obscures the findings of other more specific tests, such as angiography and endoscopy.

■ OPERATIVE INTERVENTION FOR LOWER GASTROINTESTINAL BLEEDING

Despite attempts at less invasive methods for controlling acute massive lower GI hemorrhage, a subset of patients require urgent operative intervention. A formal exploratory laparotomy is mandatory in these patients, with thorough examination of the entire GI tract. The initial step should be to determine visually the location of blood within the GI tract. Although this may be misleading, it may provide some clue as to the location of the bleeding source. If blood is present only distal to a competent ileocecal valve in a patient with hemodynamically significant ongoing bleeding, the source is almost certainly colonic in origin.

The next maneuver should be careful inspection and gentle palpation of the entire GI tract, starting proximally to rule out sources such as small bowel tumors and Meckel's diverticulum. In the absence of an obvious source or localization of the bleeding, intraoperative upper endoscopy should be considered in those patients who have not had the study preoperatively. With the advantage of a preoperative localizing test, and after a brief operative exploration, a segmental bowel resection that includes the offending lesion may be performed. With the security of localization and the benefit of the cathartic effect of intraluminal bleeding, it is usually safe to perform a primary anastomosis. In the setting of severe hemodynamic instability of preexisting malnutrition, an end stoma and mucous fistula should be considered. Without preoperative or intraoperative localization of the bleeding source, a "blind" subtotal colectomy is the accepted standard of treatment. A primary ileorectal anastomosis can be performed safely, in most cases. This procedure has an acceptable operative mortality of <10%, a rebleeding rate of <10%, and gives acceptable postoperative bowel function to virtually all patients with adequate sphincter control.[103] Blind segmental colectomies, either right or left, have no place in the treatment of lower GI hemorrhage. Such procedures have operative mortalities comparable to that of total abdominal colectomy, and rebleeding rates of 20% to 50%.[104] An additional maneuver to consider when performing a total colectomy is placement of a bowel clamp at the planned site of distal resection (rectosigmoid junction), followed by irrigation of the rectal segment and repeat proctoscopy to definitely rule out a rectal source of bleeding.

A final option is emergency laparotomy with on-table colonic lavage and intraoperative colonoscopy to identify the bleeding site, followed by segmental colectomy.[104,105] This approach can be effective when performed by an experienced surgeon and a skilled endoscopist, but caution should be exercised in the unstable patient. Attempts at intraoperative endoscopic localization of colonic bleeding sites are best reserved for relatively stable patients who are projected to have poor bowel function after a total abdominal colectomy.

■ CAUSES AND TREATMENT OF LOWER GASTROINTESTINAL BLEEDING

DIVERTICULAR DISEASE

In Western society, diverticulosis of the colon is present in over 50% of the population over the age of 60 years.[106] The vast majority of colonic diverticula are pulsion-type pseudodiverticula that derive from high intraluminal pressure and segmentation of the bowel. Thus, the common variety are not true diverticula but rather are outpouchings of the mucosa and submucosa through the muscular layer at sites of penetration of the vasa recta (Fig 5–8). Most of these lesions are located between the mesenteric and antimesenteric taenia coli. Enlargement of a colonic diverticulum leads to stretching and splaying of the small vasa recta over the dome of the lesion. Hemorrhage results from weakening and erosion of the vessel with decompression into the bowel lumen. The exact pathogenesis of the hemorrhage is unknown, but histopathologic observations have confirmed changes in the intima and media of the vasa recta, thereby suggesting that the primary lesion resides within the vessel rather than the mucosa.[91]

The exact risk of bleeding in a patient with known diverticular disease is not well defined, but has been estimated to be between 4% and 17%.[91] The hemorrhage tends to be rather massive and probably is attributable to the arterial source.[107] Patients with diverticular bleeding typically have minimal accompanying abdominal symptoms, although the cathartic effect of the blood may cause some intestinal cramping. In the majority of cases, bleeding ceases spontaneously, but in a distinct minority (10% to 20%), it continues unabated in the absence of intervention.[106] The risk of rebleeding following a self-limited hemorrhage is approximately 25%, but increases to 50% among patients who have suffered two prior episodes of diverticular bleeding.[104] Right-sided colonic diverticula, while much less common than left-sided or sigmoid diverticula, are considered by some experts to be responsible for a disproportionally higher incidence of diverticular hemorrhage. However, this finding is not well confirmed, and there is often difficulty in distinguishing between bleeding from arteriovenous malformations and bleeding from diverticula, in the absence of detailed angiographic or endoscopic evidence. The overall high prevalence of diverticulosis in the population at risk for lower GI bleeding makes the exact diagnosis of many bleeding episodes problematic. Thus, the diagnosis of diverticular bleeding often is made from indirect evidence and in many cases, it is essentially a diagnosis of exclusion.[108] Nevertheless, in most series, diverticular disease is a major cause of significant lower GI hemorrhage and accounts for >50% of cases.[23]

ARTERIOVENOUS MALFORMATIONS

Acquired arteriovenous malformations (AVMs) are lesions that occur primarily in the cecum and ascending colon of elderly patients.[109] They are found less commonly in the ileum and even less frequently in the descending and sigmoid colon.[110,111] AVMs are often referred to as angiodysplasia and have been appreciated as a lesion of the lower GI tract for more than 50 years. Angiography and colonoscopy have dramatically increased the recognition of AVMs, but have contributed little to the explanation of their pathogenesis (Fig 5–9). The angiographic criteria for identification of an AVM include (1) early and prolonged filling of the draining vein, (2) clusters of small arteries, and (3) visualization of a vascular tuft. Submucosal venous hypertension due to colonic muscular contractions has been implicated as an etiology.[109,110] Also, it has been suggested that anatomic characteristics of the cecum predispose to AVM formation. The contribution of AVMs to the spectrum of lower GI bleeding remains debatable, with some investigators attributing only a small minority of bleeding episodes to them, while others regard AVMs as the most frequent cause of lower GI bleeding in the elderly population.

The pattern of bleeding of an AVM is typically one of recurrent episodes. Although a given episode may be hemodynamically significant, continued massive bleeding is distinctly uncommon. Fatigue, or even angina or syncope, are common accompanying symptoms that reflect the chronic blood loss from AVMs. The intermit-

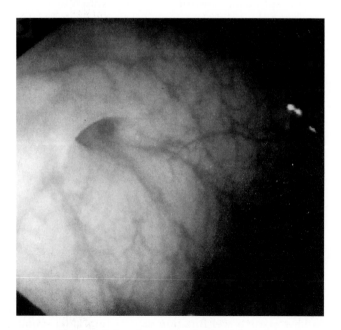

Figure 5–8. Endoscopic appearance of a sigmoid diverticulum.

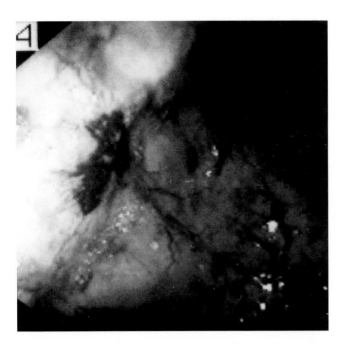

Figure 5–9. Endoscopic visualization of a nonbleeding colonic arteriovenous malformation.

tent nature of the bleeding frequently foils attempts at definitive diagnosis if they are not performed during the bleeding episode.

INFLAMMATORY BOWEL DISEASE

Ulcerative colitis and, to a lesser extent, Crohn's colitis, occasionally present with major or even massive lower GI hemorrhage. Although other colitides can present with bleeding, these are rarely massive in quantity.[112] When relatively minor and hemodynamically insignificant, bleeding from ulcerative or Crohn's colitis often responds to conservative measures directed at the inflammatory disease itself. When hemodynamically significant, surgical intervention usually is required. It is the diffuse nature of the bleeding that typically precludes successful nonoperative intervention in the majority of such cases. In patients with a prior history of inflammatory bowel disease, there is little diagnostic dilemma. However, among patients with hemorrhage as the presenting symptom, rigid proctoscopy readily demonstrates the mucosal inflammation, in most instances.

Following initial resuscitation, a decision regarding a trial of conservative therapy must be made. If operative intervention is indicated, the patient is explored through a midline incision, and a total abdominal colectomy, end ileostomy, and formation of a Hartmann's pouch is performed. There is essentially no place for proctocolectomy in this setting, since hemodynamically significant bleeding rarely, if ever, emanates from the distal segment. However, proctoscopic examination of this segment should be done in the operating room. The Hartmann's pouch should be formed above the peritoneal reflection to minimize difficulties with later restoration of continuity by ileorectostomy or, more commonly, by an ileal pouch–anal anastomosis.

TUMORS OF THE COLON AND RECTUM

Overall, colonic and rectal neoplasms account for approximately 5% to 10% of all hospital admissions for lower GI bleeding.[97,113] Symptomatic bleeding from a benign colonic or rectal polyp is distinctly unusual, with the possible exception of juvenile polyps. The vast majority of symptomatic bleeding episodes owing to tumors of the colon and rectum result from malignant neoplasms. Proximal colonic tumors have a high propensity for occult bleeding that manifests as weakness due to anemia. Perhaps the most important factor in the delayed presentation of patients with proximal colonic tumors is the lack of recognition of even moderate bleeding owing to the mixing of blood with stool.

On clinical history, neoplasms arising in the rectosigmoid segment can be confused easily with hemorrhoidal bleeding. The treatment of hemorrhoids as the presumptive site of bleeding should be preceded by flexible sigmoidoscopy in all patients beyond the age of 40 or 50 years. In younger patients, treatment of the hemorrhoids without further investigation is appropriate if there are no identifiable risk factors, a consistent clinical history, and anoscopic evidence of acute internal hemorrhoidal disease. Failure to respond to directed therapy should be followed, without delay, by additional diagnostic investigation.

MECKEL'S AND OTHER SMALL INTESTINAL DIVERTICULA

Meckel's diverticulum is a congenital true (full-thickness) diverticulum of the ileum. Occurring on the antimesenteric border of the distal ileum, it represents an embryologic remnant of the vitelline duct.[91] The diverticulum usually contains normal ileal mucosa, but in up to 50% of cases it harbors gastric, pancreatic or other ectopic tissue. Although a Meckel's diverticulum is present in approximately 2% of the normal population, symptoms attributable to the diverticulum are rare.[114] Bleeding, when it occurs, is usually associated with the presence of ectopic gastric mucosa. Bleeding usually is seen in infants and children, and occasionally in young adults. In patients beyond adolescence, the diagnosis often is delayed because it is not considered early in the clinical course, and because of difficulty in localizing the bleeding site. ^{99m}Tc and Meckel's diverticulum scans detect ectopic gastric mucosa with up to 80% accuracy but give only indirect evidence regarding bleeding, and false-positive scans are a potential pitfall (Fig 5–10).[104,115] Excision

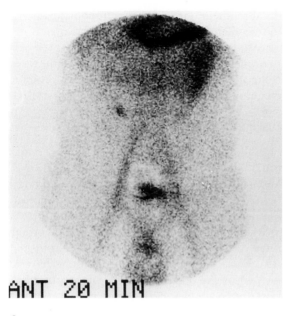

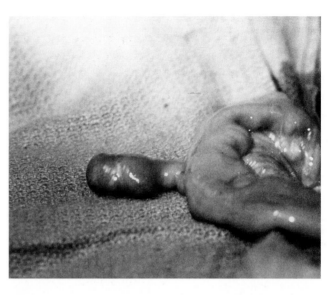

Figure 5–10. A. Meckel's scan showing concentration of radionuclide in the right side of abdomen (Courtesy of Dr. Carol Marcus). **B**. Confirmatory operative finding of a Meckel's diverticulum containing ectopic gastric mucosa.

of a Meckel's diverticulum for bleeding always should include a segment of ileum (sleeve resection) to assure inclusion of the adjacent ulceration. Simple diverticulectomy is inadequate for bleeding.

Non-Meckel's diverticula of the small intestine are acquired pulsion pseudodiverticula caused by intestinal dyskinesia.[116] They are located most commonly on the mesenteric border of the jejunum and can be difficult to visualize at operation owing to concealment by mesenteric fat (Fig 5–11). When these diverticula bleed, specific preoperative diagnosis and localization are rare. More commonly, the lesions are seen on barium contrast radiographic studies performed after cessation of bleeding of obscure origin. When discovered in this manner, targeted therapy usually is not indicated, since they often are found in coexistence with colonic diver-

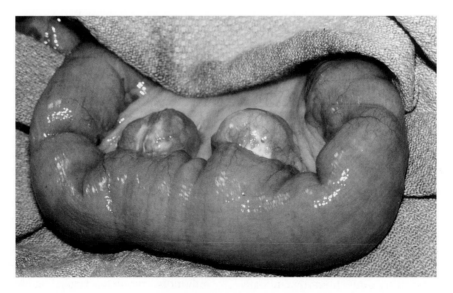

Figure 5–11. Jejunal diverticula located on the mesentric surface within the leaves of the mesentery.

ticula and other potential bleeding lesions.[117] Identification of jejunal or ileal diverticula in the patient with active lower GI bleeding should lead to visceral arteriography, since nuclear scintigraphy has poor specificity for small intestinal hemorrhage. Definition of the bleeding site by arteriography also allows selective placement of an indwelling mesenteric arterial catheter that facilitates intraoperative localization of the bleeding bowel segment. Alternatively, intraoperative enteroscopy (endoscopy of the small intestine) may be used to localize the bleeding site. If all of the small bowel diverticula present can be removed without an extensive enterectomy, this is advisable. When generalized diverticulosis is present, a more limited resection, guided by bleeding-site localization, is required.

■ OBSCURE GASTROINTESTINAL BLEEDING

For practical purposes, obscure GI bleeding is defined herein as intermittent GI bleeding for which no source has been determined, despite rigorous endoscopic and radiologic investigation. Obscure GI bleeding may constitute up to 5% of all patients who present with GI bleeding.[118] The typical presentation is one of intermittent acute bleeds accompanied by a resultant chronic anemia. The acute bleeding episodes frequently require transfusion.

Crucial to the accurate diagnosis and localization of the bleeding site to educate the patient to alert the treating physician at the earliest sign of acute bleeding. Owing to the frequency of a proximal site of bleeding in the colon or small intestine, and the intermittent nature of the bleeding, the urgent use of diagnostic procedures such as endoscopy and nuclear scintigraphy should be triggered by even subtle signs of acute exacerbation. Arteriography, if not already performed, should be pursued with special attention to evidence of angiodysplasia, particularly of the small intestine.

Enteroclysis radiographic examination of the small intestine is performed by infusing barium and air directly into the duodenum via a tube. It is able to detect small bowel tumors, but has poor discriminatory ability for superficial mucosal lesions. Enteroscopy is an additional diagnostic technique that utilizes a specially designed scope that allows inspection of a variable amount of the jejunum, although it requires a very experienced endoscopist. Alternatively, a pediatric colonscope can be used to visualize the entire duodenum and proximal jejunum.

Various provocative tests, most of which utilize arteriography and heparin or thrombolytics to precipitate or exacerbate acute bleeding, also have been described and may be considered.[104,119] However, caution should be exercised and surgical standby is mandatory when at-

tempting such potentially dangerous maneuvers. Additionally, a method to specifically localize the site of observed bleeding and to assist in the planned operative intervention is required. In most circumstances, this involves superselective catheterization of the bleeding mesenteric vessel.

In spite of all attempts at nonoperative diagnosis and localization, operative exploration is required in a significant percentage of patients with obscure GI bleeding.[120,121] Exploratory laparotomy is first conducted with meticulous examination of the entire intestinal tract, from the gastroesophageal junction to the intraperitoneal rectum. Transillumination of the bowel wall with a fiberoptic light source, in a darkened operating room, may define otherwise occult vascular lesions. Failure to localize a probable bleeding site should prompt intraoperative endoscopy. A pediatric colonoscope may be inserted orally and passed, with assistance, through a lengthy portion of the small intestine. Endoscopic and surgical coordination is important and any possible bleeding site should be identified carefully with serosal sutures or clips. When appropriate, the patient should be positioned in the lithotomy position to allow colonoscopic examination with retrograde cannulation of the ileocecal valve and inspection of the remaining distal small intestine not visualized by the upper enteroscopy. Endoscopic transillumination of the intestine with the room darkened may detect submocosal angiodysplasia not visible on the mucosal surface. Lastly, vigorous hydration of the patient may be helpful by accentuating the thin-walled veins that constitute the bulk of angiodysplastic lesions.[110] In the vast majority of cases of obscure GI bleeding, resection of the segment of small intestine or colon containing the offending lesion is curative.[118]

COLONIC AND ANORECTAL VARICES

Portosystemic collaterals exist between the colon and the retroperitoneum naturally.[122] Furthermore, collaterals between the superior rectal and the middle and inferior rectal venous circuits are constant and dependable portosystemic communications. In the presence of portal hypertension, these naturally occurring collateral pathways may become clinically important in the context of lower GI bleeding. Although anal varices often are present in patients with cirrhosis and portal hypertension, they only infrequently cause significant blood loss. However, when anal varices are found to be the source of bleeding, excision by hemorrhoidectomy is potentially treacherous, and simple oversewing of the offending varix with a locking suture usually is curative.[104]

Colonic varices and rectal varices proximal to the sphincter complex are more problematic. Usually diag-

TABLE 5–3. UNCOMMON MEDICAL CONDITIONS ASSOCIATED WITH GASTROINTESTINAL BLEEDING

Medical Condition	Frequency of GI Bleeding (%)
Chronic renal failure	very common
Disseminated intravascular coagulation	40–60
Thrombocytopenia	1–50
Amyloidosis	10–45
Hereditary hemorrhagic telangiectasia	13–30
Hemophilia A and B	8–25
Pseudoxanthoma elasticum	11–15
Ehlers-Danlos Syndrome	6–12
Anticoagulation therapy	3–12

nosed by endoscopy or angiography, they are best treated by nonselective portosystemic shunting. TIPS, as a temporizing measure prior to liver transplantation, is a viable option in patients with limited hepatic reserve. Colon resection should be reserved for selected patients, since it is associated with an almost prohibitive mortality.[122]

■ UNCOMMON CAUSES OF GASTROINTESTINAL BLEEDING

There are a number of uncommon medical conditions that are associated with GI bleeding (Table 5–3). The actual lesions are highly variable, but they are located more often in the stomach and duodenum than in other sites. The frequency of chronic minimal blood loss is undoubtedly high in these conditions, although acute massive hemorrhage is relatively unusual.

REFERENCES

1. Allan RN. History, epidemiology, mortality. In: Dykes PW, Keighley MRB (eds), *Gastrointestinal Hemorrhage*. Boston, MA: Wright PSG; 1981
2. Bogoch A. Hematemesis and melena. part I: etiology and medical aspects. In: Bockus HL (ed), *Gastroenterology*, vol 1, Philadelphia, PA: WB Saunders; 1974
3. Palmer ED. Upper gastrointestinal hemorrhage. *JAMA* 1975;231:853
4. Gann DS, Amaral JF. Pathophysiology of trauma and shock. In: Zuidema GD, Rutherford RD, Ballinger WF (eds). *The Management of Trauma*. Philadelphia, PA: WB Saunders; 1985
5. Cellar RE, Gavaler JS, Alexander JA, et al. Gastrointestinal hemorrhage: the value of a nasogastric aspirate. *Arch Intern Med* 1990;150:1381
6. Leather RA, Sullivan SN. Iced saline lavage: a tradition without foundation. *Can Med Assoc J* 1987;136:1245
7. Sugawa C, Steffes, CP, Nakamaura R, et al. Upper GI bleeding in an urban hospital. *Ann Surg* 1990;212:521
8. Foster DN, Miloszewski KJA, Losowsky MS. Stigmata of recent hemorrhage in diagnosis and prognosis of upper gastrointestinal bleeding. *Br Med J* 1978;1:1173
9. Fleischer D. Endoscopic therapy of upper gastrointestinal bleeding in humans. *Gastroenterology* 1986;90:217
10. Baum S. Angiography and the gastrointestinal bleeder. *Radiology* 1982;143:569
11. Walker TG, Waltman AC. Angiographic diagnosis and therapy of upper gastrointestinal hemorrhage. In: Bennet JR, Hunt RH (eds), *Therapeutic Endoscopy and Radiology of the Gut*. Baltimore, MD: Williams & Wilkins; 1990: 167–177
12. Steer ML, Silen W. Diagnostic procedures in gastrointestinal hemorrhage. *N Engl J Med* 1983;309:646
13. Collins R, Langman M. Treatment with histamine H_2 antagonists in acute upper GI hemorrhage. *N Engl J Med* 1985;313:660
14. Steffes C, Fromm D. The current diagnosis and management of upper gastrointestinal bleeding. *Adv Surg* 1992; 25:31
15. Stabile BE, Passaro E Jr. Duodenal ulcer: a disease in evolution. *Curr Prob Surg* 1984;21:1
16. Stabile BE. Current surgical management of duodenal ulcers. *Surg Clin N Am* 1992;72:335
17. Chua CL, Jevara PR, Low CH. Relative risks of complications in giant and nongiant gastric ulcers. *Am J Surg* 1992;164:94
18. Jones SC, Axon ATR. Bleeding peptic ulcer—endoscopic and pharmacologic management. *Postgrad Med J* 1991; 67:606
19. Stabile BE, Passaro E Jr. Surgery for duodenal and gastric ulcer disease. *Adv Surg* 1993;26:275
20. MacLeod IA, Mills PR. Factors identifying the probability of further hemorrhage after acute upper gastrointestinal hemorrhage. *Br J Surg* 1982;69:256
21. Branichi FJ, Boey J, Fok PJ, et al. Bleeding duodenal ulcer: a prospective evaluation of risk factors for rebleeding and death. *Ann Surg* 1990;211:411
22. Wara P. Endoscopic prediction of major rebleeding—a prospective study of stigmata of hemorrhage in bleeding ulcer. *Gastroenterology* 1985;88:1209
23. Peterson WL, Laine L. Gastrointestinal bleeding. In: Sleisenger MH, Fordtran JS (eds), *Gastrointestinal Disease*. Philadelphia, PA: WB Saunders; 1993
24. NIH Consensus Conference. Therapeutic endoscopy and bleeding ulcers. *JAMA* 1989;262:1269
25. Cook DJ, Guyatt GH, Salena BJ, et al. Endoscopic therapy for acute nonvariceal upper gastrointestinal hemorrhage—a meta-analysis. *Gastroenterology* 1992;102:139
26. Sacks HS, Chalmers TC, Blum AL, et al. Endoscopic hemostasis: an effective therapy for bleeding peptic ulcers. *JAMA* 1990;264:494
27. Ralph-Edwards A, Himal HS. Bleeding gastric and duodenal ulcers: endoscopic versus surgery. *Can J Surg* 1992; 35:177
28. Sugawa C, Joseph AL. Endoscopic interventional management of bleeding duodenal and gastric ulcers. *Surg Clin N Am* 1992;72:317

29. McConnell DB, Baba GC, Deveney CW. Changes in surgical treatment of peptic ulcer within a Veterans Hospital in the 1970s and the 1980s. *Arch Surg* 1989;124:1164

30. Palumbo LT, Sharpe WS. Active bleeding duodenal ulcer—management during ten-year period. *Surg Clin N Am* 1967;47:239

31. Johnston D. Division and repair of sphincteric mechanism at the gastric outlet in emergency operation for bleeding peptic ulcer: a new technique for use in combination with suture ligation of the bleeding point and highly selective vagotomy. *Ann Surg* 1977;186:723

32. Stabile BE. Surgical treatment of peptic ulceration. *Curr Opin Gen Surg* 1993;1:206

33. Brancatisano R, Falk GL, Hollinshead JW, et al. Bleeding duodenal ulceration: the results of emergency treatment with highly selective vagotomy. *Aust N Z J Surg* 1992; 62:725

34. Jordan PH Jr. Surgery for peptic ulcer disease. *Curr Prob Surg* 1991;28:265

35. Stabile BE, Passaro EJ. Recurrent peptic ulcer. *Gastroenterology* 1976;70:124

36. Laine L. Upper gastrointestinal hemorrhage. *West J Med* 1991;155:272

37. Larson DE, Farnell MB. Upper gastrointestinal hemorrhage. *Mayo Clinic Proc* 1983;58:371

38. Elerding SC, Moore EE, Wolz JR, et al. Outcome of operations for upper gastrointestinal tract bleeding. *Arch Surg* 1980;115:1473

39. Sarin SK, Sreenivas DV, Lahoti D, et al. Factors influencing development of portal hypertensive gastropathy in patients with portal hypertension. *Gastroenterology* 1992; 102:994

40. Laine L, Weinstein WM. Subepithelia hemorrhages and erosions of human stomach. *Dig Dis Sci* 1988;33:490

41. Cook DJ, Fuller HD, Guyatt GH, et al. Risk factors for gastrointestinal bleeding in critically ill patients. *N Engl J Med* 1994;330:377

42. Zuckerman GR, Shuman R. Therapeutic goals and treatment options for prevention of stress ulcer syndrome. *Am J Med* 1987;83(suppl 6A):29

43. Johnson WC, Widrich WC. Efficacy of selective splanchnic arteriography and vasopressin perfusion in diagnosis and treatment of gastrointestinal hemorrhage. *Am J Surg* 1976;131:481

44. Graham DY, Smith JL. The course of patients after variceal hemorrhage. *Gastroenterology* 1981;80:800

45. Henderson JM. Portal hypertension and shunt surgery. *Adv Surg* 1993;26:233

46. Merigan TC Jr, Platkin JR, Davidson CS. Effect of intravenously administered posterior pituitary extract on hemorrhage from bleeding esophageal varices: a controlled evaluation. *N Engl J Med* 1962;266:134

47. Fogel MR, Knauer M, Andres LL, et al. Continuous intravenous vasopressin in active upper gastrointestinal bleeding: a placebo-controlled trial. *Ann Intern Med* 1982;96:565

48. Gimson AES, Westaby D, Hegarty J, et al. A randomized trial of vasopressin and vasopressin plus nitroglycerin in the control of acute variceal hemorrhage. *Hepatology* 1986;6:410

49. Chojkier M, Groszmann RJ, Atterbury CE, et al. A controlled comparison of continuous intra-arterial and intravenous infusions of vasopressin in hemorrhage from esophageal varices. *Gastroenterology* 1979;77:540

50. Jenkins SA, Baxter JN, Corbett W, et al. A prospective randomized controlled clinical trial comparing somatostatin and vasopressin in controlling acute variceal hemorrhage. *Br Med J* 1985;290:275

51. Burroughs AK, McCormick PA, Dughes MD, et al. Randomized, double-blind, placebo-controlled trial of somatostatin for variceal bleeding: emergency control and prevention of variceal rebleeding. *Gastroenterology* 1990;9:1388

52. Valenzuela JE, Schubert T, Fogel MR, et al. A multicenter randomized, double-blind trial of somatostatin in the management of acute hemorrhage from esophageal varices. *Hepatology* 1989;10:958

53. Hosking SW, Doss W, El-Zeing H, et al. Pharmacologic constriction of the lower aesophageal sphincter: a simple method of arresting variceal hemorrhage. *Gut* 1988; 29:1098

54. Haddock G, Garden OJ, McKee RF. Esophageal tamponade in the management of acute variceal hemorrhage. *Dig Dis Sci* 1989;34:913

55. Novis GH, Duys GO, Barbezat O, et al. Fiberoptic endoscopy and the use of the Sengstaken tube in acute gastrointestinal hemorrhage with portal hypertension and varices. *Gut* 1976;17:258

56. Terblanche J, Yakoob HI, Bomman PC, et al. Acute bleeding varices—a five year prospective evaluation of tamponade and sclerotherapy. *Ann Surg* 1981;194:521

57. Stiegmann G, Goff JS, Michaletz-Onody PA, et al.: Endoscopic sclerotherapy as compared with endoscopic ligation for bleeding esophageal varices. *N Engl J Med* 1992;326:1527

58. Hasan F, Levine BA. The role of endoscopic scleropathy in the management of esophageal varices. *Dig Dis Sci* 1992;10(suppl 1):38

59. Johansen K, Helton WS. Portal hypertension and bleeding esophageal varices. *Ann Vasc Surg* 1992;6:553

60. Sugiura M, Futagawa S. Esophageal transection with paraesophageal devascularizations (the Sugiura Procedure) in the treatment of esophageal varices. *World J Surg* 1984;8:673

61. Langer BF, Greig PD, Taylor BR. Emergency surgical treatment of variceal hemorrhage. *Surg Clin N Am* 1990; 70:307

62. Resnick RH, Iber FL, Ishihara AM, et al. A controlled study of the therapeutic portacaval shunt. *Gastroenterology* 1974;67:843

63. Sarfeh IJ, Rypins EB, Mason GR. A systematic appraisal of portacaval H-graft diameters: clinical and hemodynamic perspectives. *Ann Surg* 1986;204:356

64. Warren WD, Millikan WJ, Henderson JM, et al. Splenopancreatic disconnection: Improved selectivity of distal splenorenal shunt. *Ann Surg* 1986;204:346

65. Zemel G, Katzen BT, Becker GJ, et al. Percutaneous transjugular portosystemic shunt. *JAMA* 1991;266:390

66. Brewer TG. Treatment of acute gastroesophageal variceal hemorrhage. *Med Clin N Am* 1993;77:993

67. Woodle ES, Darcy M, White HM, et al. Intrahepatic portosystemic vascular stents: a bridge to hepatic transplantation. *Surgery* 1993;113:344

68. Wood RP, Shaw BW Jr, Rikkers LF. Liver transplantation for variceal hemorrhage. *Surg Clin N Am* 1990;70:449

69. Thavanathan J, Heughan C, Cummings TM. Splenic vein thrombosis as a cause of variceal hemorrhage. *Can J Surg* 1992;35:649

70. Sugawa C, Benishek D, Walt AJ. Mallory-Weiss Syndrome—a study of 224 patients. *Am J Surg* 1983; 145:30

71. Allum WH, Brearley S, Wheatley KE, et al. Acute hemorrhage from gastric malignancy. *Br J Surg* 1990;77:19

72. Vase P, Grove O. Gastrointestinal lesions in hereditary hemorrhage telangectasia. *Gastroenterology* 1986;91: 1079

73. Gilmore PR. Angiodysplasia of the upper gastrointestinal tract. *J Clin Gastroenterol* 1988;10:386

74. Van Cutsem E, Rutgeerts P, Vantrappen G. Treatment of bleeding gastrointestinal vascular malformations with oestrogen-progesterone. *Lancet* 1990;335:953

75. Veldhuyzen Van Zanten SJO, Bartelsman JFWM, Schipper MEI, et al. Recurrent massive hematemesis from Dieulafoy vascular malformations—a review of 101 cases. *Gut* 1986;27:213

76. Bech-Knudsen F, Toftgaard C. Exulceratio simplex Dieulafoy. *Surg Gynecol Obstet* 1993;176:139

77. Peck JJ, Eidemiller LR. Aortoenteric fistulas. *Arch Surg* 1992;127:1191

78. Wilson SE, Van Wagenen P, Passaro E Jr. Arterial infection. *Curr Prob Surg* 1978;15:1

79. Wheeler WE, Hanks J, Raman VK. Primary aortoenteric fistulas. *Ann Surg* 1992;58:53

80. Goodnight JE, Blaisdell FW. Hemobilia. *Surg Clin N Am* 1981;61:973

81. Rosch J. Peterson BD, Hall LD, et al. Interventional treatment of hepatic arterial and venous pathology: a commentary. *Cardiovasc Intervent Radiol* 1990;13:183

82. Stabile BE, Wilson SE, Debas HT. Reduced mortality from bleeding pseudocysts and pseudoaneurysms caused by pancreatitis. *Arch Surg* 1983;118:45

83. Grisendi A, Lonardo A, Della Casa G, et al. Hemoductal pancreatitis secondary to gastroduodenal artery-ruptured pseudoaneurysm: a rare cause of hematemesis. *Am J Gastroenterol* 1991;86:1654

84. Alavi A, Ring EJ. Localization of gastrointestinal bleeding: Superiority of ^{99m}Tc sulfur colloid compared with angiography. *Am J Radiol* 1981:137:741

85. Hunter JM, Pezim ME: Limited value of technetium 99m-labeled red cell scintigraphy in localization of lower gastrointestinal bleeding. *Am J Surg* 1990;159:504

86. Bentley DE, Richardson JD. The role of tagged red blood cell imaging in the localization of gastrointestinal bleeding. *Arch Surg* 1991;126:821

87. Markisz JA, Front D, Royal HD, et al. An evaluation of ^{99m}Tc-labeled red blood cell scintigraphy for the detection and localization of gastrointestinal bleeding sites. *Gastroenterology* 1982;83:394

88. Nicholson ML, Neoptolemos JP, Sharp JF, et al. Localiza tion of lower gastrointestinal bleeding using in vivo tech netium-99m-labelled red blood cell scintigraphy. *Br J Surg* 1989;76:358

89. Orecchia PM, Hensley EK, McDonald PT, et al. Localization of lower gastrointestinal hemorrhage: experience with red blood cells labeled in vitro with technetium [99m]Tc. *Arch Surg* 1985;120:621

90. Winzelberg GG, Froelich JW, McKusick KA, et al. Radionuclide localization of lower gastrointestinal hemorrhage. *Radiology* 1981;139:465

91. Ure T, Vernava AM, Longo WE. Diverticular Bleeding. *Sem Col Rect Surg* 1994;5:32

92. Browder W, Cerise EJ, Litwin MS. Impact of emergency angiography in massive lower gastrointestinal bleeding. *Ann Surg* 1986;204:530

93. Rahn NH, Tishler JM, Han SY, et al. Diagnostic and interventional angiography in acute gastrointestinal hemorrhage. *Radiology* 1982;143:361

94. Baum S, Rosch J, Dotter CT, et al. Selective mesenteric arterial infusions in the management of massive diverticular hemorrhage. *N Engl J Med* 1973;288:1269

95. Athanasoulis CA, Baum S, Rosch J, et al. Mesenteric arterial infusions of vasopressin for hemorrhage from colonic diverticulosis. *Am J Surg* 1975;129:212

96. Renert WA, Button KF, Fuld SL, et al. Mesenteric venous thrombosis and small bowel infarction following infusion of vasopressin into the superior mesenteric artery. *Radiology* 1972;102:292

97. Leitman IM, Paull DE, Shires GT. Evaluation and management of massive lower gastrointestinal hemorrhage. *Ann Surg* 1989;209:175

98. Forde KA: Colonoscopy in acute rectal bleeding. *Gastrointest Endosc* 1981;27:219

99. Jensen DM, Machicado GA. Diagnosis and treatment of severe hematochezia. The role of urgent colonoscopy after purge. *Gastroenterology* 1988;95:1569

100. Treate MR, Forde KA. Colonoscopy, technetium scanning, and angiography in acute rectal bleeding: an algorithm for their combined use. *Surg Gastroenterol* 1983;2:135

101. Brandt LJ, Boley SJ. The role of colonoscopy in the diagnosis and management of lower intestinal bleeding. *Scan J Gastroenterol* 1984;19(suppl 102):61

102. Gostout CJ: Acute gastrointestinal bleeding—a common problem revisited. *Mayo Clin Proc* 1988;63:596

103. Drapanas T, Pennington DG, Kappelman M, et al. Emergency subtotal colectomy: preferred approach to management of massively bleeding diverticular disease. *Ann Surg* 1973;177:519

104. Finne CO III. The aggressive management of serious lower gastrointestinal bleeding. *Prob Gen Surg* 1992; 9:597

105. Berry R, Campbell B, Kettlewell MGW. Management of major colonic haemorrhage. *Br J Surg* 1988;75:637

106. McGuire HW, Haynes BW. Massive hemorrhage from diverticular disease of the colon: guidelines for therapy based on bleeding pattern in fifty cases. *Ann Surg* 1972; 175:847

107. Behringer GE, Albright NL. Diverticular disease of the colon: a frequent cause of massive rectal bleeding. *Am J Surg* 1973;125:419

108. Parsa F, Gordon HE, Wilson SE. Bleeding diverticulosis of the colon: a review of 83 cases. *Dis Col Rect* 1975;18:37

109. Church JM. Angiodysplasia. *Sem Col Rect Surg* 1994;5:43

110. Richardson JD. Vascular lesions of the intestines. *Am J Surg* 1991;161:284

111. Vu H, Adams CZ, Hoover EL. Jejunal angiodysplasia presenting as acute lower gastrointestinal bleeding. *Am Surg* 1990;5:302

112. Escudero-Fabre A, Cummings O, Kirklin JK, et al. Cytomegalovirus colitis presenting as hematochezia and requiring resection. *Arch Surg* 1992;127:102

113. Jensen DM, Machicado GA. Endoscopic diagnosis and treatment of bleeding colonic angiomas and radiation telangiectasia. *Perspect Col Rect Surg* 1989;2:99

114. Soltero MJ, Bill AH. The natural history of Meckel's diverticulum and its relation to incidental removal: a study of 202 cases of diseased Meckel's diverticulm found in King County, Washington, over a fifteen-year period. *Am J Surg* 1968;132:168

115. Ludtke FE, Mende V, Kohler H, et al. Incidence and frequency of complications and management of Meckel's diverticulum. *Surg Gynecol Obstet* 1989;160:537

116. Longo WE, Vernava AM. Clinical implication of jejunoileal diverticular disease. *Dis Col Rect* 1992;35:381

117. Ross CB, Richards WO, Sharp KW, et al. Diverticular disease of the jejunum and its complications. *Am Surg* 1990;56:319

118. Szold A, Katz LB, Lewis BS. Surgical approach to occult gastrointestinal bleeding. *Am J Surg* 1992;163:90

119. Rosch J, Kozak BE, Keller FS. Interventional diagnostic angiography in acute lower gastrointestinal bleeding. *Sem Intervent Radiol* 1988;5:10

120. Desa LA, Ohri SK, Hutton KAR, et al. Role of intraoperative enteroscopy in obscure gastrointestinal bleeding of small bowel origin. *Br J Surg* 1991;78:192

121. Ress AM, Benacci JC, Sarr MG. Efficacy of intraoperative enteroscopy in diagnosis and prevention of recurrent, occult gastrointestinal bleeding. *Am J Surg* 1992;163:94

122. Strong SA. Colonic, anorectal and peristomal varices. *Sem Col Rect Surg* 1994;5:50

6

Jaundice

Kim U. Kahng ▪ *Joel J. Roslyn*

The diagnosis and management of patients with jaundice can be one of the more perplexing and challenging problems confronting physicians and surgeons. The diagnosis may be elusive, and the treatment less than straightforward. During the last decade, our evolving ability to image the biliary tract and facilitate the diagnostic evaluation of these patients has led to the development of logical algorithms for clinical management. Innovative techniques for access to the biliary tract have resulted in new and creative means of management, prompting reevaluation of existing treatment principles for patients with biliary obstruction. In addition, an improved understanding of the pathophysiology of hyperbilirubinemia has influenced therapeutic regimens and has contributed to more rational approaches for patient care.

Jaundice is a generic term for the yellow pigmentation of the skin, mucus membranes, or sclera that is caused by a heterogeneous group of disorders. The predilection for scleral icterus is due to the abundance of scleral elastin, which has a high affinity for bilirubin. The clinical manifestations of jaundice are the direct result of increased serum levels of bilirubin, a normal metabolite of hemoglobin. Normal serum bilirubin concentration ranges from 0.2 to 1.0 mg/dL. Jaundice is clinically apparent when the serum bilirubin level exceeds 2.5 mg/dL. Kernicterus is a specific clinical entity seen in early infancy in which very high levels of unconjugated bilirubin result in deposition and consequent neural destruction in the basal ganglia of the brain.

The disorders that cause jaundice have been classified in a variety of ways (Table 6–1). The basis for each system has focused on the ultimate medical or surgical treatment, the derangement in bilirubin metabolism, unconjugated or conjugated hyperbilirubinemia (Table 6–2), or the nature of the disorder, hepatocellular or obstructive. It is helpful to divide the causes of obstructive jaundice into two categories, cholestasis from parenchymal liver disease or mechanical obstruction from a blockage of either the intrahepatic or extrahepatic biliary tract. A number of benign and malignant processes can cause mechanical obstruction to the flow of bile.

Medical jaundice is an imprecise term that does little to clarify etiology, pathophysiology, or clinical sequelae of the disorder. It encompasses a broad range of problems having little in common other than that they do not require surgical intervention. Disorders included in medical jaundice are infections or chemical hemolytic anemias or other noxious agents and drugs; defects in transport, storage, or excretion of bilirubin; and diseases that cause hepatocellular damage. *Surgical jaundice* can be distinguished from medical jaundice by a thorough history, complete physical exam, and simple laboratory tests.

A rational approach to the evaluation and management of both medical and surgical jaundice can be greatly facilitated by understanding the essentials of bilirubin metabolism.

TABLE 6–1. CLASSIFICATION OF JAUNDICE

Medical
 Hepatocellular Disease
 Unconjugated Hyperbilirubinemia

Surgical
 Biliary Obstruction
 Conjugated Hyperbilirubinemia

■ METABOLISM OF BILIRUBIN

SOURCES OF BILIRUBIN

Bilirubin is a yellowish-red pigment and organic ion with the chemical structure ($C_{33}H_{36}O_6N_4$), as shown in Fig 6–1. The total amount of bilirubin produced under normal circumstances is 300 mg/day.[1,2] Fifteen to twenty percent of the total daily bilirubin production is derived from nonerythropoietic sources, primarily the hepatic metabolism of heme-containing proteins and enzymes. The destruction of maturing erythroid cells in the bone marrow as a consequence of ineffective erythropoiesis accounts for a small fraction of nonerythropoietic bilirubin production. The term *early labeled fraction* is also used to refer to nonerythropoietic bilirubin production. When radiolabeled glycine is administered to human subjects, it is incorporated into bilirubin. The 15% to 20% of the isotope that appears in the stool within several days constitutes the early labeled fraction from nonerythropoietic sources. The remainder of the isotope is not detected until 120 days later. This late fraction represents the major source of daily bilirubin production, which is the catabolism of red blood cells (Fig 6–2). These circulating cells, whose life span is approximately 100 to 120 days, are destroyed by mononuclear phagocytes in the reticuloendothelial system. Catabolism of the senescent red blood cell includes hydrolysis of globin with release of amino acids by proteolytic enzymes, oxidation of the iron fraction to ferritin, and breakdown of the heme group by a microsomal oxidizing system. The porphyrin ring of the heme group is catalyzed by microsomal membrane-bound heme oxygenase to bile pigments with release of carbon monoxide. Biliverdin is then converted by biliverdin reductase to bilirubin. Unconjugated bilirubin is a lipid-soluble, nonpolar pigment released from the reticuloendothelial system.

BILIRUBIN TRANSPORT

Unconjugated bilirubin has a high affinity for albumin to which it binds in a reversible, noncovalent manner. Bilirubin is transported by albumin in the plasma, which serves to protect tissues from its potentially toxic effects.

Bilirubin may be displaced from albumin by certain organic anions. In addition, transport of unconjugated bilirubin is influenced by plasma pH and specific physicochemical factors. The bilirubin-albumin complex enters the sinusoidal circulation of the liver via the portal or hepatic arterial systems.

METABOLISM OF BILIRUBIN

The metabolism of bilirubin is a complicated, multistage procedure that involves the liver, intestine and kidney (Fig 6–3). The hepatic metabolism of bilirubin occurs in three phases: uptake, conjugation, and excretion. Unconjugated bilirubin disassociates from albumin at the plasma membrane of the hepatocyte. This process, along with the entry of bilirubin into the hepatocyte, presumably is regulated by a carrier-mediated transport system, although the exact mechanism remains unclear. Once in the hepatocyte, bilirubin binds to specific cytoplasmic anionic proteins, designated as acceptor proteins Y and Z and more recently, ligandin. These proteins may be pivotal in the overall transport process by minimizing the efflux of bilirubin back into the plasma.

TABLE 6–2. CLASSIFICATION OF JAUNDICE BASED ON TYPE OF HYPERBILIRUBINEMIA

Unconjugated
 Overproduction
  Hemolysis
  Ineffective erythropoiesis
 Decreased hepatic uptake
  Drugs
  Prolonged fasting
  Sepsis
 Decreased glucuronyl transferase activity
  Gilbert's syndrome
  Crigler-Najjar
  Neonatal jaundice
  Acquired
   Drugs
   Hepatocellular disease[a]

Conjugated
 Impaired hepatic excretion
  Familial/hereditary
   Dubin-Johnson syndrome
   Rotor syndrome
   Cholestatic jaundice of pregnancy
  Acquired
   Hepatocellular disease[a]
   Drugs
   Sepsis
 Extrahepatic biliary obstruction

[a]In hepatocellular disease, uptake, conjugation, and excretion of bilirubin are all impaired. Since excretion which is the rate-limiting step is impaired to the greatest extent, conjugated bilirubinemia predominates in hepatocellular disease.

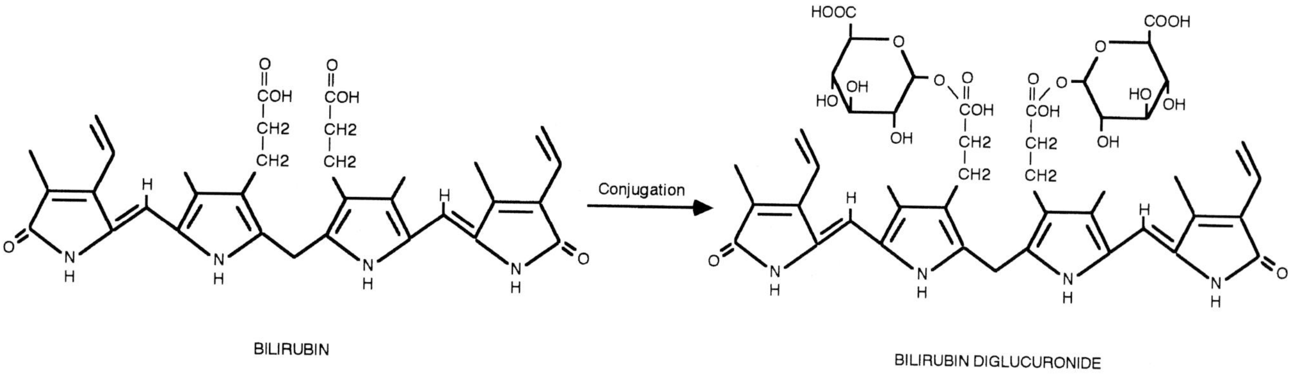

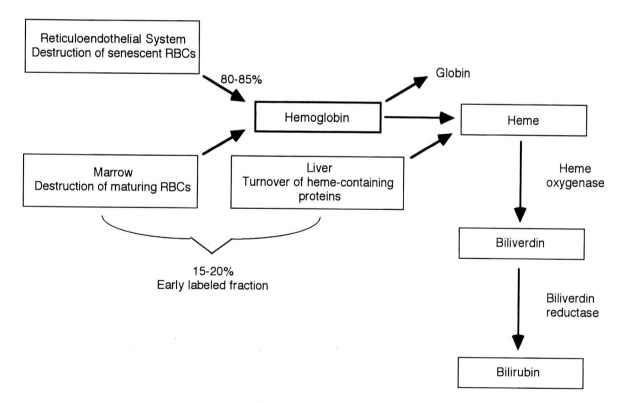

Figure 6–1. Structure of bilirubin and conjugated bilirubin.

Figure 6–2. Sources of bilirubin.

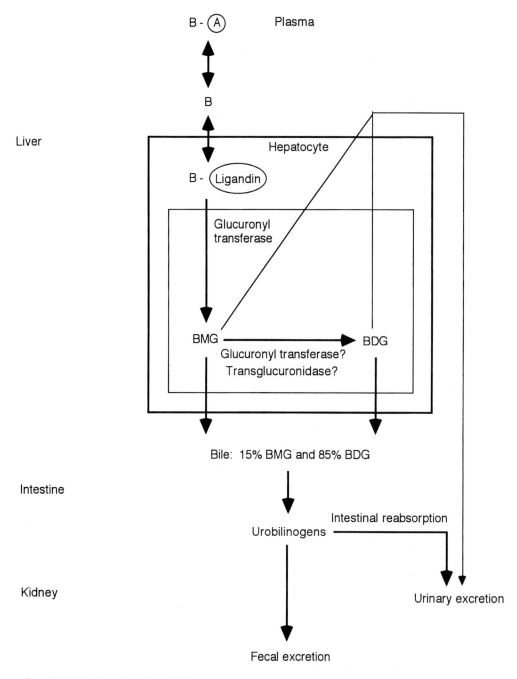

Figure 6–3. Metabolism and excretion of bilirubin. **A.** albumin. **B.** bilirubin. BMG: bilirubin monoglucuronide; BDG: bilirubin diglucuronide.

In the cell, unconjugated bilirubin bound to the ligandin is carried to the smooth endoplasmic reticulum, where it is converted to a water-soluble moiety. Glucuronyl transferase catalyzes the initial conjugation of bilirubin with uridine diphophate glucuronic acid, a derivative of glucose, to form bilirubin monoglucuronide (BMG). Further conjugation of BMG to bilirubin diglucuronide (BDG) may be catalyzed by the same enzyme; however, some authors have postulated a role for a plasma membrane transglucuronidase. Both BMG and BDG are transferred into the bile canaliculus and excreted in bile, which is 85% BDG and 15% BMG. Thus, bilirubin, in a conjugated and water soluble form, enters the biliary tract and drains into the duodenum.

An important phase in the metabolism of bilirubin, particularly from the perspective of the clinician, occurs in the small intestine. Bacteria present in the distal small bowel convert conjugated bilirubin to a series of compounds that are collectively termed urobilinogen. The intermediary products are mesobilirubinogen and stercobilinogen. These colorless compounds are further reduced into urobilin, also known as stercobilin, which gives stool its characteristic brown color. A small percentage of urobilinogen is reabsorbed in the terminal ileum and colon and excreted by the kidney. Its absence in urine may indicate complete biliary obstruction, while its presence in elevated amounts may result from increased production of bilirubin, as in hemolysis. Acholic stool occurs when bilirubin substrate is unavailable for conversion to urobilinogen and stercobilin.

Since unconjugated bilirubin is tightly bound to albumin, it is not excreted by the kidney. In contrast, conjugated bilirubin is water soluble and nonprotein bound. Therefore, it is filtered by the renal glomeruli and excreted in the urine. As the plasma level of conjugated bilirubin rises, renal excretion increases to a maximum of approximately 220 mg/day. This rate of excretion approaches the rate of hepatic production, which is approximately 250 mg/day. At this point, plasma bilirubin no longer increases beyond a plateau of 25 to 30 mg/dL. Higher plasma bilirubin levels suggest the presence of acute renal failure.

■ APPROACH TO THE PATIENT WITH JAUNDICE

PERSPECTIVE

An orderly approach to the diagnosis of jaundice is essential for instituting the appropriate therapy in a timely manner. The variety of diagnostic tests and therapeutic options that now exists makes it imperative that the management of patients with obstructive jaundice be conducted in a rational way. A number of studies have attempted to identify the most efficacious and cost-effective manner of patient evaluation. As this era of cost-containment continues to evolve, it will become increasingly important that we develop specific algorithms for the care of the jaundiced patient, who most likely will be evaluated by a primary care physician, a gastroenterologist, and a surgeon. The interdependence of these physicians mandates that they have a close working relationship and a general understanding of all disorders that can result in jaundice.

HISTORY

Significant information leading to a focused differential diagnosis can be gleaned from a carefully performed history. Many patients with clinical jaundice seek medical attention only after a family member notices a change in the color of their skin or eyes. Scleral icterus is the most common presenting symptom and typically is present when the serum bilirubin level exceeds 2.5 mg/dL.

The first issue that must be resolved is whether the patient does have evidence of jaundice. Other maladies can be confused with jaundice, and several key points and questions can be helpful in focusing the attention of the clinician in one direction or another. Consumption of large quantities of certain foods or drugs may lead to discoloration of the skin, mimicking jaundice. Yellowish appearance of the skin can develop when large amounts of carrots or tomatoes are eaten. The pigmentation that is characteristic of patients with Addison's disease can also simulate jaundice. These conditions should be easily distinguishable based on clinical presentation, even without the benefits of laboratory examination.

When obtaining a history from a jaundiced patient, it is helpful to distinguish among causes that are congenital or hereditary, infectious, neoplastic, hematologic, or related to exposure or consumption of drugs or alcohol. Age of presentation, gender, travel history, diet and social history, associated constitutional symptoms, presence of pruritus, and pain are important factors that should be considered in developing an appropriate differential diagnosis. The reported color of urine and stool will help to classify the problem as unconjugated or conjugated hyperbilirubinemia. Onset of jaundice at a young age or its presence for a long period of time is consistent with a hereditary or congenital disorder affecting hepatic metabolism of bilirubin. Constitutional symptoms, such as anorexia, weight loss, or easy fatiguability, suggest a chronic or subacute process affecting parenchymal function. These may be the only symptoms in a patient with a pyogenic liver abscess. Abdominal pain usually indicates an inflammatory or acute obstructive process such as acute hepatitis or acute extrahepatic biliary obstruction. The insidious development of deep jaundice in the absence of acute pain is characteristic of neoplastic obstruction, particularly when associated with weight loss. Pruritus is very common in patients with obstructive jaundice and generally is not present in individuals with hemolytic anemias. Dark urine suggests conjugated hyperbilirubinemia and acholic stools point to complete biliary obstruction.

PHYSICAL EXAM

Patients presenting with jaundice require a complete physical examination with emphasis on specific areas. The first site where hyperbilirubinemia can be detected is the sclera, as a result of the affinity of elastin for bilirubin. Scleral icterus generally will appear when the serum bilirubin level approaches 2.5 mg/dL. Yellowing of the skin or mucous membranes does not become readily apparent until the serum bilirubin level exceeds 6.0 mg/dL.

Physical findings that suggest chronic liver disease include hepatosplenomegaly, spider angiomata, gynecomastia, cutaneous xanthomas, and ascites. The liver should be carefully palpated and assessed for size as well as degree of tenderness. A large, tender liver with a rounded edge or surface is characteristic of acute congestion or inflammation and often is present in patients with congestive heart failure or acute hepatitis. A large, nodular liver is typical of patients with carcinomatous involvement (primary or metastatic) or an infiltrative process such as lymphoma, Hodgkin's disease, or amyloidosis. A bruit heard over the liver is suggestive of hepatocellular carcinoma. Spider angiomata are telangiectatic vascular malformations that often are noted on the upper trunk and back in patients with cirrhosis. Gynecomastia in males often is found in the presence of chronic liver disease. Both spider angiomata and gynecomastia are the result of disordered estrogen metabolism. Palmar erythema and Dupuytren's contracture also are suggestive of chronic liver disease.

Patients with malignant obstruction of the distal common bile duct will often have a large, distended, easily palpable gallbladder, or Courvoisier's gallbladder. The lack of tenderness, despite the degree of gallbladder distention, reflects the slow, insidious development of biliary obstruction. The presence of occult blood in the stool of a jaundiced patient is suggestive of a malignancy.

LABORATORY EXAMINATION

Based on the history and physical examination, the astute clinician can construct a differential diagnosis. This is refined by considering specific data in the context of the clinical presentation. A key early step in the laboratory evaluation of the jaundiced patient is to characterize the nature of the hyperbilirubinemia.

The standard test for bilirubin is the van den Bergh reaction. The basis for this colorimetric test is the differing solubility of conjugated and unconjugated bilirubin. The so-called direct reaction occurs when a color change is noted in an aqueous medium. This is used to measure conjugated bilirubin, which is water soluble. The total amount of bilirubin, both conjugated and unconjugated, is measured when the reaction is carried out in alcohol or methanol. The amounts of total and conjugated bilirubin is calculated (indirect fraction) as the difference between total and conjugated (direct reaction) bilirubin. A more precise means of measuring bilirubin levels is high-performance liquid chromatography (HPLC), although this rarely is done in clinical situations.

Total bilirubin levels rise secondary to overproduction or impaired uptake of bilirubin, impaired gluicuronide conjugation, decreased excretion of bilirubin by the liver, and extrahepatic biliary obstruction. Other than conveying the degree of hyperbilirubinemia, the total serum bilirubin concentration does not distinguish among these possible etiologies. The presence of predominantly unconjugated hyperbilirubinemia is associated with hemolysis, ineffective erythropoiesis, drugs, prolonged fasting, sepsis, and genetic derangements such as Gilbert's syndrome and Crigler-Jajar syndrome. Hepatocellular disease impairs excretory function to a greater degree than the ability to conjugate bilirubin and therefore, the hyperbilirubinemia in this setting is predominantly of the conjugated type. It is very difficult to distinguish between hepatocellular disease and extrahepatic biliary obstruction solely on the basis of conjugated hyperbilirubinemia. The presence of bilirubin in the urine is evidence of conjugated bilirubin, since the unconjugated fraction is not filtered by the kidney. Bilirubin can be detected in the urine by dipstick, Ictotest tablets, or by shaking the urine and looking for the characteristic yellow foam. The combination of conjugated hyperbilirubinemia, bilirubinuria, and clay-colored stool is very suggestive of extrahepatic biliary obstruction; further studies should be pursued as appropriate. In the context of extrahepatic biliary obstruction, neoplastic obstruction tends to produce higher total bilirubin values than benign problems such as choledocholithiasis.

Liver function tests can provide critical information in the early assessment of the jaundiced patient. Marked elevation of aminotransferases generally is seen with hepatocellular injury, although abnormalities may be seen in obstructive diseases as well. Aspartate aminotransferase (AST, SGOT) and alanine aminotransferse (ALT, SGPT) catalyze the transfer of amino groups from aspartate and alanine to the keto groups of ketoglutarate leading to the formation of oxaloacetate and pyruvate. Since AST is present in a number of tissues other than the liver, it is a less specific indicator of hepatocellular injury than ALT. AST and ALT may be increased in virtually any hepatic disorder, but they are most elevated in the presence of extensive hepatic necrosis. Extrahepatic biliary obstruction, in the absence of cholangitis, is characterized by only mild elevations of AST and ALT. The most sensitive indicator of extrahepatic biliary obstruction, regardless of etiology or location, is serum alkaline phosphatase. Elevation of this enzyme, however, may be caused by any of several isoenzymes derived from liver, intestine, bone, and placenta. Electrophoresis and other sophisticated methodologies can be used to identify these isoenzymes, although the source of the elevated alkaline phosphatase usually can be identified on the basis of clinical findings. Hepatobiliary alkaline phosphatase is secreted by the biliary ductular endothelium. The increased serum levels found in acute biliary obstruction result from back diffusion or leak from the ducts. The serum alkaline phosphatase level is often only minimally elevated in parenchymal liver disorders, whereas it is severely deranged in obstructive jaundice. An important caveat is that serum alkaline phosphatase may remain significantly elevated long after biliary obstruction has been relieved (Fig 6–4). In situations where the source of an elevated alkaline phosphatase is elusive, the determination of serum 5′-nucleotidase may be useful. This enzyme is present in a number of tissues, but significant elevations are usually indicative of biliary obstruction. Other enzymes, including leucine aminopeptidase and glutamyltranspeptidase (GGT), are nonspecific and may be associated with a number of organ-specific and systemic disorders unrelated to the liver.

Measurements of proteins that are exclusively synthesized by the liver can be helpful in confirming extensive hepatic injury; however, they provide little information about specific etiologies. Serum albumin is recognized widely as an indicator of hepatic synthetic function, but its long half-life limits its role in diagnosing acute hepatic injury. The prothrombin time is one of the more useful tests for hepatic function. It is dependent on normal hepatic synthesis of clotting factors and sufficient uptake of vitamin K. A prolonged prothrombin time often indicates significant hepatic injury. The inability to normalize the prothrombin time despite the parenteral administration of vitamin K is a grave prognostic sign.

The surgeon most often is involved in the diagnostic evaluation and treatment of patients with presumed extrahepatic biliary obstruction. In this setting, the typical laboratory profile includes conjugated hyperbilirubinemia, bilirubinuria, marked elevation of alkaline phosphatase, normal or minimally elevated aminotranspeptidases, and normal hepatic synthetic function. While

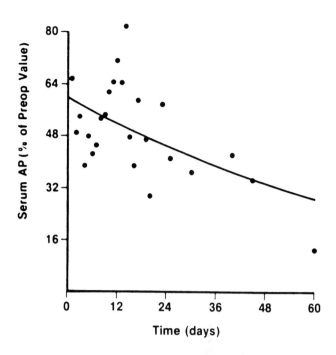

Figure 6–4. Serum alkaline phosphatase after relief of obstructive jaundice in 98 patients. The slow rate of decline results in persistently elevated levels long after biliary obstruction has been relieved. (From Pellegrini CA. Pathophysiology of biliary obstruction. In: Way LW, Pellegrini CA (eds), *Surgery of the Gallbladder and Bile Ducts.* Philadelphia, PA: WB Saunders; 1987:112)

characteristic of biliary obstruction, appropriate therapy and intervention requires anatomic definition of the site of obstruction.

■ RADIOLOGIC EVALUATION OF EXTRAHEPATIC BILIARY OBSTRUCTION

Although critical, the differentiation of jaundice from hepatocellular disease owing to extrahepatic biliary obstruction may be impossible on the basis of laboratory evaluation alone. The combination of clinical assessment and radiologic examination provides an accurate diagnosis in 98% of patients.[3] Documentation of intrahepatic or extrahepatic biliary dilatation is an essential step in the evaluation and treatment of the jaundiced patient.

PLAIN ABDOMINAL RADIOGRAPHS

Abdominal radiographs may be useful in the evaluation of a patient with an acute surgical abdomen, but generally they contribute little to the assessment of those presenting with jaundice. Duct dilatation will not be revealed on plain films. Cholelithiasis may be documented in 20% to 30% of patients who have calcified stones. Speckled calcification in the region of the head of the pancreas may be suggestive of chronic pancreatitis.

ABDOMINAL ULTRASONOGRAPHY

Biliary obstruction generally is characterized ultrasonographically by biliary dilatation (Fig 6–5), although this may be conspicuously absent in up to 15% of patients.[4] The absence of dilated ducts in the presence of jaundice may suggest secondary biliary cirrhosis or hepatic parenchymal pathology. Ultrasonography is often the initial study performed to determine the presence and level of intrahepatic and extrahepatic biliary dilatation, particularly since recent technologic advances have led to accuracy rates similar to those of computed tomography (CT).[5] Prospective evaluation of ultrasonography suggests that the level of obstruction can be defined in over 90% of patients with biliary obstruction.[6,7] In the presence of distal obstruction, dilatation of the extrahepatic ducts occurs prior to any change in the intrahepatic ducts. The extent to which the ductal system is dilated may not correlate with the degree of hyperbilirubinemia. Duct dilation may not be apparent in the presence of acute biliary obstruction. The reservoir function of the gallbladder may serve to decompress the biliary tract so that a time lag exists between the onset of obstruction and the ultrasonographic demonstration of biliary duct dilatation.[8] Ductal architecture can be assessed sonographically, and diagnostic findings of intrahepatic biliary dilatation include parallel intrahepatic channels (Fig 6–6).[9] Color-flow Doppler sonography may assist in distinguishing dilated ducts from portal venous and hepatic arterial branches.[10]

Sonography can provide useful information regarding the nature and etiology of the biliary obstruction. The sonographic signs of cholelithiasis and choledocholithiasis have been well described. Mass lesions may be visualized, although the reliability with which benign diseases can be distinguished from malignant processes remains unclear. The absence of stones or a mass may be suggestive of a small cholangiocarcinoma. Persistent intraluminal echoes without shadowing, irregularly defined shadows arising from a mass, echogenic bands crossing a bile duct, and biliary dilatation in the presence of a collapsed gallbladder are all sonographic findings that are consistent with the diagnosis of cholangiocarcinoma.[11,12]

ENDOSCOPIC ULTRASONOGRAPHY

During the last 15 years, endoscopic ultrasonography has evolved as a useful clinical tool in the assessment of patients with benign and malignant gastrointestinal diseases.[13,14] A recent prospective study of 60 patients with periampullary masses or obstructive jaundice suggests that endoscopic ultrasonography may be more accurate than combined ERCP and CT scan in defining the nature and extent of the cause of biliary obstruction.[15] The ability to evaluate and integrate information about mucosal, vascular, ductal, and parenchymal abnormalities in a single examination makes endoscopic ultrasonography particularly valuable. In this era of cost-containment, it is essential that we more fully evaluate the role of this technique in the overall evaluation and management of the patient with obstructive jaundice.

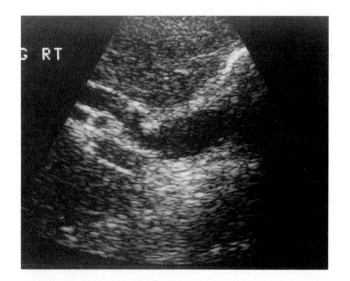

Figure 6–5. Sagittal right anterior oblique scan that demonstrates a dilated common bile duct, measuring 2 cm in diameter, anterior to the portal vein. (From Friedman AC, Dachman AH (eds), *Radiology of the Liver, Biliary Tract, and Pancreas.* St. Louis, MO: Mosby Year-Book; 1994)

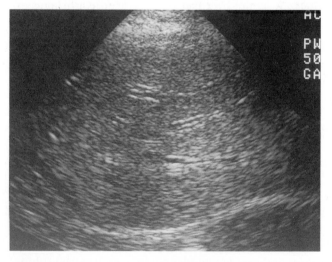

Figure 6–6. Transverse scan of the right lobe of the liver showing multiple parallel channels indicative of intrahepatic ductal dilatation. (From Friedman AC, Dachman AH (eds), *Radiology of the Liver, Biliary Tract, and Pancreas.* St. Louis, MO: Mosby Year-Book; 1994)

COMPUTERIZED TOMOGRAPHY

Although CT offers little advantage over ultrasonography in the detection of biliary dilatation, CT scans trace the course of the bile duct, visualize adjacent structures more accurately and define the cause of biliary obstruction. The use of intravenous contrast, especially when delivered as a rapid bolus, assists in distinguishing bile ducts from portal vessels. In addition, small 1 to 2 cm masses in the liver parenchyma can be visualized. Oral contrast identifies the duodenum and small bowel, which is helpful in discerning portions of the biliary tract and pancreas (Fig 6–7). For these reasons, CT frequently is performed as the first imaging study for the jaundiced patient. It is less operator-dependent than ultrasonography and more likely to demonstrate both the level and cause of biliary obstruction.[16] The CT diagnosis of biliary obstruction is based on the demonstration of dilated intrahepatic or extrahepatic ducts, seen as linear branching or circular structures. Dilatation of the common bile duct does not always denote pathology. Abrupt termination of a dilated duct is suggestive of a neoplasm, but the possibility of a non-calcified gallstone also must be considered.[17] In general, ultrasonography is more sensitive than CT for detecting cholelithiasis in the gallbladder; however, CT is better for documenting ductal stones.[18–20] The pattern of duct dilatation noted on CT is useful in identifying specific conditions that may cause segmental or diffuse obstruction, such as sclerosing cholangitis or Caroli's disease.

MAGNETIC RESONANCE IMAGING

The role of magnetic resonance imaging (MRI) in the evaluation of the biliary tract remains unclear.[21] Conventional biliary imaging currently includes ERCP and percutaneous transhepatic cholangiography (PTC). While both techniques provide excellent visualization of the biliary tract, they are invasive tests with well-recognized morbidity. Early experience with new and more sophisticated MRI techniques suggests that MRI cholangiography ultimately may prove quite useful in the evaluation and characterization of biliary tract pathology.[22,23]

BILIARY SCINTIGRAPHY

Historically, isotopic scanning was the optimal means of imaging the biliary tract. Despite limited resolution, the dynamic nature of scintigraphy offers a theoretical advantage over the static images of the newer noninvasive imaging techniques. Scintigraphic studies use radioisotope-labeled compounds that are excreted in the bile. The most commonly employed agents for biliary excretory scintigraphy are technetium 99m (^{99m}TC)-labeled iminodiacetic acid (IDA) derivatives. Serial gamma–camera images of the right upper quadrant are obtained following intravenous administration of the radiolabeled agent. The images are influenced by hepatic blood flow, reticuloendothelial function, and biliary excretion. Focal hepatic abnormalities appear as photopenic areas. Normal hepatic uptake without evidence

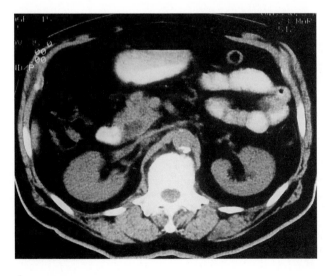

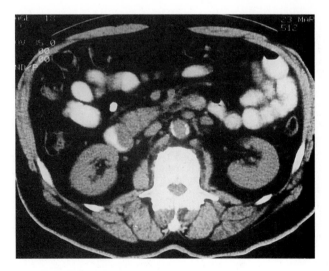

A   **B**

Figure 6–7. Computed tomography of ampullary carcinoma. **A**. Dilated common bile duct and pancreatic duct within the head of the pancreas. **B**. The next caudal image showing a soft tissue mass protruding into the barium within the duodenum. (From Friedman AC, Dachman AH (eds), *Radiology of the Liver, Biliary Tract, and Pancreas.* St. Louis, MO: Mosby Year-Book; 1994)

of activity within the gut is suggestive of biliary obstruction. False positives, however, are not uncommon. Even though biliary scintigraphy is a test with high specificity and sensitivity for acute cholecystitis, its role in the evaluation of the jaundiced patient is quite limited.

TRANSHEPATIC CHOLANGIOGRAPHY

Visualization of the biliary tract is best accomplished by instillation of contrast material directly into a bile duct. The techniques of PTC and ERCP have rendered intravenous cholangiography obsolete. PTC was first introduced more than 50 years ago, although the technique has been significantly modified during the past years.

Since PTC is an invasive procedure, the decision to proceed with it must be considered carefully. Relative contraindications include significant coagulopathy or the presence of ascites. Assessment of the coagulation profile is particularly important in the presence of jaundice. An elevated prothrombin time requires correction with Vitamin K administration prior to PTC. In the presence of biliary obstruction, we recommend periprocedural administration of antibiotics. Coverage should focus on gram negative organisms, avoiding nephrotoxic antibiotics when possible. PTC is performed using local anesthesia, although intravenous sedation and occasionally, general anesthesia, may be required. A 22-gauge flexible Chiba needle is directed through the abdominal wall and into the liver. Entry into a bile duct is confirmed by aspiration of bile or injection of contrast material. In most patients, the intrahepatic and extrahepatic ducts can be visualized with great clarity (Fig 6–8A). This test is an important diagnostic tool for delineating malignant and benign strictures of the bile duct. At the time PTC is performed, an indwelling catheter can be placed to provide either external or internal biliary drainage (Fig 6–8B). Thus, PTC can be both diagnostic and therapeutic. In our experience, it is particularly useful when dealing with proximal or hilar pathology.

The successful performance of PTC is dependent on a number of factors, including the expertise of the in-

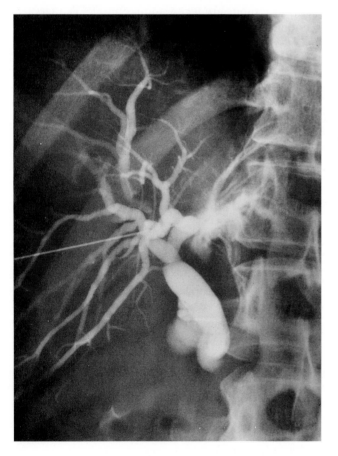

A

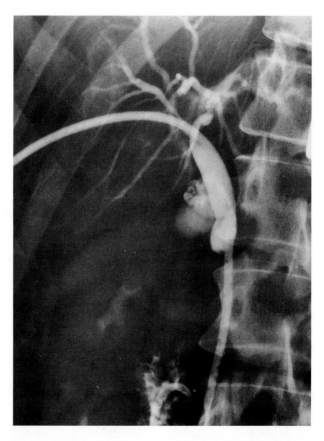

B

Figure 6–8. Percutaneous transhepatic cholangiography and drainage for pancreatic carcinoma. **A.** Percutaneous cholangiogram demonstrating distal common bile duct obstruction. **B.** Subsequent placement of a 10-Fr Cope indwelling catheter through the obstruction into the duodenum. (From Friedman AC, Dachman AH (eds), *Radiology of the Liver, Biliary Tract, and Pancreas.* St. Louis, MO: Mosby Year-Book; 1994)

terventional radiologist and the degree of biliary dilatation. With sufficient experience, virtually all systems with significant biliary dilatation can be intubated and opacified.[24] Even in the absence of dilated ducts, a success rate of 50% to 60% can be expected, although multiple passes of the Chiba needle may be required.[25,26] This procedure is not without risk and the morbidity rate is reported to be 2% to 4%. Complications include bleeding, hemobilia, bile leaks, and sepsis.[27] While PTC provides accurate information about the level of obstruction, caution must be exercised in establishing a diagnosis based on cholangiographic criteria alone.

ENDOSCOPIC RETROGRADE CHOLANGIOPANCREATOGRAPHY

The management of patients with obstructive jaundice was revolutionized by the introduction of ERCP more than 25 years ago.[28] Since that early report, the technology and instrumentation of this procedure has been refined and the use of ERCP has become standard. ERCP is a combined endoscopic and radiologic procedure that allows inspection of the duodenum and ampullary region as well as direct intubation and radiographic visualization of the bile duct and pancreatic duct. It is indicated for diagnostic purposes and for definition of biliary and/or pancreatic anatomy. In addition, ERCP can be a therapeutic modality, since access to the bile duct and the pancreatic duct is provided. Procedures that can be performed include sphincterotomy, stone removal, dilation of a stricture, and stent placement (Fig 6–9). In patients with normal gastroduodenal anatomy, the success rate for duct intubation approaches 98%. Even in patients who have had gastric resection and gastroenterostomy, there is a reported 65% to 85% success rate in identifying and cannulating the papilla.[29] Success rates are, of course, operator dependent. Complications of ERCP include pancreatitis, cholangitis, and pancreatic sepsis. Advantages of ERCP over PTC include the ability to visualize the stomach, duodenum, ampullary region, and the opportunity to assess the pancreatic duct. Additional capabilities include manometry, biopsy, and the collection of bile for cytology and other purposes.

DIAGNOSING OBSTRUCTIVE JAUNDICE: A UNIFIED APPROACH (FIG 6–10)

Great controversy exists regarding the optimal approach to the patient whose history, examination and laboratory profile suggest the possibility of obstructive jaundice. Computer programs have been introduced as a possible aid to clinicians, but their true role remains unclear.[30] The role of ultrasonography and CT scan is also unclear.[31–33] Additionally, the information obtained from ultrasonography and CT scan is different from either PTC or ERCP. These latter procedures serve to define biliary anatomy and may offer therapeutic ac-

cess to the bile duct. ERCP is a more sensitive imaging test for detecting biliary obstruction than ultrasonography or CT scan.[34] PTC is particularly useful when proximal pathology is suspected, based on prior screening studies, or when endoscopic expertise is not available. Other considerations in the selection of PTC versus ERCP include the need for therapeutic options.

■ PATHOPHYSIOLOGY OF JAUNDICE

MORPHOLOGIC CHANGES

The systemic sequelae of hyperbilirubinemia and obstructive jaundice have become well recognized in recent years. Long standing biliary obstruction can result in alteration of both hepatic and systemic function. Regardless of the etiology of bile duct obstruction, common bile duct dilatation is a frequent sequelae, with the degree and extent determined by the nature of the obstruction, duration of the process, and local factors. Dilatation is most marked in patients with neoplastic obstruction, since the process is indolent and the native duct is otherwise normal. In contrast, patients with obstruction owing to an inflammatory process or choledocholithiasis typically will have dilatation that is less impressive. This occurs in part because the obstruction is usually incomplete and the walls of the duct are thickened as a result of inflammation. Regardless of the etiology, longstanding biliary obstruction is associated with bile plugging within the canaliculi, centrilobular bile stasis, and periductular extravasation of bile with reactive edema and infiltration of polymorphonuclear leukocytes. Bile duct proliferation can occur with periportal and intralobular fibrosis, leading to biliary cirrhosis.

RENAL FAILURE

Clinical Syndrome
The clinical relationship between obstructive jaundice and renal failure was recognized more than 50 years ago.[35,36] The incidence of renal failure in patients undergoing surgical procedures for relief of obstructive jaundice is approximately 10%.[37] The mortality rate in this subset of patients is extremely high (32% to 100%).[38,39] The level of hyperbilirubinemia correlates with the postoperative decrease in creatinine clearance.[40,41] The etiology of acute renal failure in the presence of obstructive jaundice is multifactorial and includes renal ischemia, prostaglandin mediated alterations in renal microcirculation, myocardial depression, reduction of intravascular volume, and sepsis.

Etiology
Early investigators reported that hemodynamic instability and hypotension might be, in part, responsible for renal

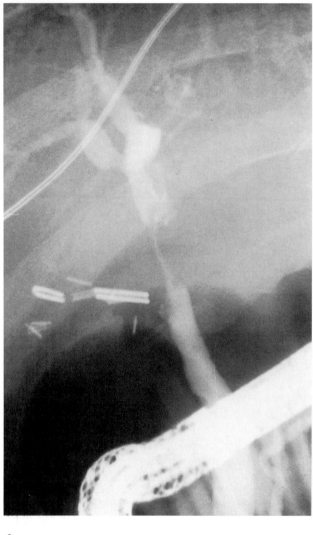

A

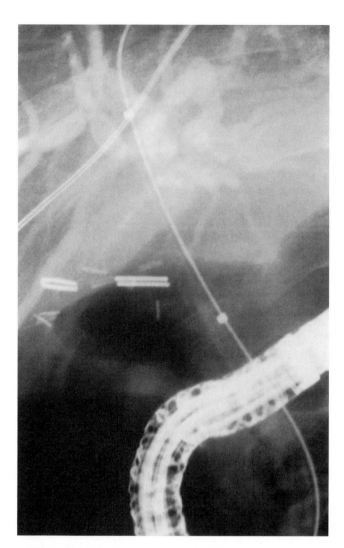

B

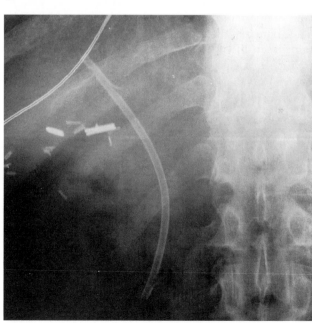

C

Figure 6–9. Endoscopic diagnosis and therapy of a biliary stricture. **A.** Endoscopic cholangiogram showing a stricture of the proximal common bile duct after open cholecystectomy. **B.** Balloon dilatation of the stricture. The radiopaque markers show the proximal and distal ends of the balloon. **C.** Subsequent stent placement. (From Friedman AC, Dachman AH (eds), *Radiology of the Liver, Biliary Tract, and Pancreas.* St. Louis, MO: Mosby Year-Book; 1994)

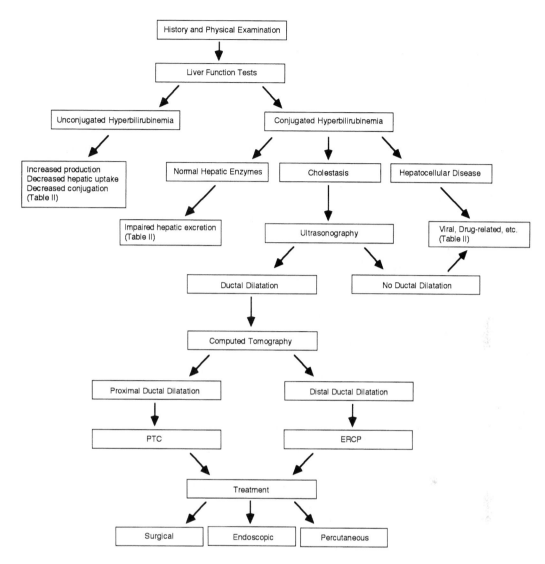

Figure 6–10. Flow diagram showing the approach to the jaundiced patient.

failure occurring in patients requiring surgery for obstructive jaundice.[42] Hemorrhage in jaundiced dogs is associated with a higher mortality rate than in control animals. Moreover, bile duct–ligated dogs are more prone to hypotension with severe hemorrhage than are controls.[43] This apparent alteration in the hemodynamic response to volume depletion in jaundiced subjects is accompanied by changes in baseline hemodynamic and circulatory function. Chronic bile duct ligation is associated with decreased systemic arterial pressure,[44] decreased peripheral vascular resistance,[45] and decreased responsiveness to norepinephrine.[46] More recent studies demonstrating increased levels of atrial natriuretic peptide in experimentally induced obstructive jaundice suggest a possible mechanism for the observed derangements in sodium and water metabolism.[47] Measurement of body water compartments in patients with obstructive

jaundice suggests that reduction of the interstitial volume and a marginally reduced plasma volume may be determinant factors in the pathogenesis of the renal and hemodynamic disturbances observed in patients with biliary tract obstruction.[48] Considerable evidence suggests that bile duct ligation results in significant alterations in renal blood flow, with redistribution within the kidney itself, and that these changes probably are mediated by prostaglandin.[49–51] Whether bile, bile acids, or bilirubin have a direct toxic effect on the kidney remains unclear.

Endotoxin absorbed from the gastrointestinal tract into the protal circulation is normally cleared by the reticuloendothelial system (RES) of the liver. The RES is suppressed in patients with biliary obstruction, and this decrease in clearance of endotoxins results in spillover into the systemic circulation with endotoxemia.[52] The importance of this factor to the development of renal failure in patients with obstructive jaundice is underscored by a recent report suggesting that the prevention of endotoxemia in this setting preserves renal function.[53]

Treatment

Prevention would appear to be essential in the clinical management of postoperative renal failure in patients with obstructive jaundice. Recognizing that the jaundiced patient may be volume depleted and that sympathetic tone of the vasculature may be blunted, hydration must be adequate prior to the induction of general anesthesia. Urine output often is not a reliable indicator of volume status, since bile salts stimulate increased water excretion and renal mechanisms may be impaired. Invasive monitoring often is indicated in the jaundiced patient, particularly if other co-morbid conditions are present. In addition to volume replenishment, a number of treatments have been advocated for the management of acute renal failure in the jaundiced patient. Although early experimental studies suggested that the administration of mannitol preserves renal blood flow and function and reduces mortality in the perioperative period,[40] more recent human studies have provided conflicting data.[54] Whether prevention of systemic endotoxemia protects renal function remains unclear.[55] The risk of developing postoperative renal failure correlates with the degree of hyperbilirubinemia; thus, the concept of reducing jaundice by biliary drainage has some scientific rationale. However, the effect of preoperative biliary drainage on renal function has not been specifically addressed.

SEPSIS

Clinical Syndrome

Sepsis associated with obstructive jaundice is manifested by two distinct syndromes: cholangitis and alterations in the host defense mechanism. More than 100 years ago, Charcot described the clinical triad of fever, right upper quadrant pain, and jaundice that characterizes cholangitis. Typically, cholangitis occurs in the presence of infected bile and obstruction. Although cholangitis most frequently is associated with choledocholithiasis,[56] it is being reported with increasing frequency in patients with benign and malignant bile duct strictures.[57] Cholangitis has been reported to occur following T tube cholangiography, percutaneous liver biopsy, THC, ERCP, and removal of common bile duct stones.[58]

Etiology

Although bactibilia is a factor in septic complications observed in jaundiced patients undergoing surgery, considerable evidence indicates that there are specific alterations in host-defense mechanisms that are responsible for the jaundice-associated sepsis syndrome.

In the setting of biliary obstruction, it has been proposed that the absence of bile from the gut initiates a cascade of events that lead to altered phagocytic function and changes in the reticuloendothelial system. Specifically, the absence of bile is associated with an increase in the bacterial count in the gut and a loss of structural integrity of the small bowel mucosa. These changes facilitate bacterial translocation with an increase in lipopolysaccharides (LPS) transported to the liver. LPS induces release of cytokines and cellular mediators. Circulating tumor necrosis factor (TNF) is increased in animals with biliary obstruction.[59] Treatment with specific anti-TNF agents reduces circulating TNF levels, but has a variable effect on associated mortality in an animal model of jaundice.[60] The role of TNF and other cytokines in the sepsis syndrome of jaundice remains unclear, but their actions may be responsible for the observed inhibition and reduction of phagocytic function and clearance of LPS.[61–63] Kuppfer cell activity decreases with biliary obstruction with an inverse correlation with systemic endotoxemia. These changes in the host defense system and the inability to clear LPS results in tissue damage and ultimately, organ failure.

Treatment

The initial treatment of postoperative patients with presumed cholangitis should be aimed toward stabilization and correction of any technical factors that might be contributing to sepsis. Specific strategies recommended for the management of patients with cholangitis will be discussed in greater detail in Chapter 58. Our increasing understanding of the pathogenesis of sepsis syndrome in biliary obstruction has provided some interesting and innovative approaches to the management of this disorder. Preoperative administration of bile salts to jaundiced patients appears to prevent systemic and portal endotoxemia, and it also prevents postoperative renal dysfunction.[64] Several studies suggest that lactulose inactivates endotoxin, prevents septic related complications in jaundiced animals, and reduces mortality rates.[64,65] Lactulose-induced inhibition of TNF production by monocytes in response to endotoxin may help explain the beneficial effect of this agent.[66] The hypothesis that absence of bile salts from the gut may predispose to sepsis in the setting of obstructive jaundice has prompted the evaluation of preoperative administration of bile salts as a therapeutic modality. Data suggests that preoperative administration of sodium deoxycholate to jaundiced patients prevents systemic and portal endotoxemia and also prevents postoperative renal dysfunction,[67] perhaps by a TNF-mediated mechanism.[68] Although polymyxin B has been shown to bind endotoxin[69] and improve survival in an animal model,[70] human studies have failed to reveal any beneficial effect of its use in the prevention of sepsis.[71]

BLEEDING

Clinical Syndrome

In the jaundiced patient, the anatomic and physiologic relationship of the biliary tract to the liver and the portal circulation makes bleeding an important consideration undergoing surgery. Bleeding can occur (1) from inadequate local hemostasis or injury to a major vessel, (2) following instrumentation through the liver with intrahepatic vascular injury and hemobilia, (3) as a consequence of portal hypertension, or (4) secondary to a coagulopathy. Clinical experience indicates that excessive bleeding due to coagulopathy is not uncommon in jaundiced patients undergoing biliary tract surgery.

Etiology

Jaundice-associated coagulopathy may result from hepatocellular dysfunction and vitamin K deficiency. Normal hepatic function is essential for the synthesis of specific coagulation factors II, VII, IX, X and prothrombin. Severe liver dysfunction leads to reduced synthesis of these factors and results in hypoprothrombinemia. Vitamin K is the fat soluble vitamin that is a critical cofactor in the synthesis of coagulation proteins by the liver. In the setting of biliary obstruction, reduction in intestinal bile salt concentration decreases vitamin K absorption and may further impair the clotting mechanism in patients with compromised hepatic function on the basis of cholestasis and/or sepsis.

Treatment

The coagulopathy caused by vitamin K deficiency that occurs with biliary obstruction can be reversed, at least partially, by the administration of exogenous vitamin K. This should be given preoperatively and can be expected to facilitate normal production of prothrombin complex proteins within 8 to 10 hours. Additional doses can be given postoperatively, as necessary. This is in contrast to the situation which chronic liver disease in which vitamin K administration theoretically would have no beneficial effect on the abnormal clotting mechanism. Transfusion of fresh frozen plasma may be life saving and should correct the coagulopathy of obstructive jaundice.

■ TREATMENT OF OBSTRUCTIVE JAUNDICE

IMPACT OF JAUNDICE ON CLINICAL OUTCOME

Clinicians are concerned with the systemic manifestation of hyperbilirubinemia. The risk of operation in patients with jaundice and biliary obstruction has now been well defined. A series of reports suggested that the perioperative morbidity and mortality for surgery in patients with obstructive jaundice approached 50% and 25%, respectively. A number of specific factors, includ-

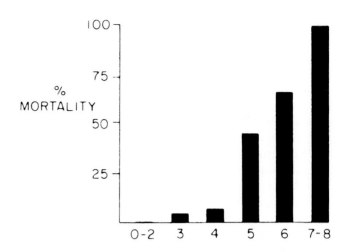

Figure 6–11. Correlation of risk factors with mortality in biliary tract surgery. The risk factors used were malignant obstruction, age > 60 years, serum albumin < 3.0 g/dL, hematocrit < 30%, white blood cell count > 100 IU, and serum creatinine > 1.3 mg/dL. (From Pitt HA, Cameron JL, Postier RG, et al. Factors affecting mortality in biliary tract surgery. *Am J Surg* 1981;141:66)

ing age, underlying disease process, presence of biliary sepsis, degree of malnutrition, and the status of renal and hepatic function, have been proposed as predictive of an adverse outcome.[72–74] In one series, the mortality rate was directly correlated with the number of risk factors present (Fig 6–11).[35] Death is often the result of sepsis, renal failure, gastrointestinal hemorrhage, or multiorgan failure. Recognition of the relationship between hyperbilirubinemia and surgical outcome has led to the hypothesis that alleviation of the obstruction or reduction of the degree of hyperbilirubinemia would influence outcome and reduce morbidity and mortality.

THERAPEUTIC GOALS AND STRATEGY

The management of patients with jaundice should focus on diagnosis, amelioration of symptoms, and relief of biliary obstruction. A rational approach for diagnostic evaluation has been previously described. In addition to jaundice, the most bothersome symptom associated with uncomplicated biliary obstruction is pruritus. Although the mechanism of generalized pruritus remains unclear, cholestyramine, a bile salt–sequestering resin, may be helpful in decreasing the pruritus associated with partial bile duct obstruction.[75] In the absence of bile acids in the intestine, as with complete biliary obstruction, cholestyramine has little role in treatment of pruritus. Antihistamines have not proven very helpful, and the best treatment is relief of the obstruction. Biliary decompression also should help reverse the adverse effects of jaundice on renal, cardiovascular, and immune function. Restoration of uninterrupted bile flow, by either surgical, endoscopic or radiologic means, remains the cornerstone of management in the patient with biliary obstruction and jaundice.

Relief of biliary obstruction leads to a prompt choleresis. However, the rate of return of serum bilirubin levels to normal is unpredictable. There is no correlation between duration of obstruction and rate of return of serum bilirubin or alkaline phosphatase levels to normal. Indeed, human studies suggest that as the preoperative serum bilirubin levels become higher, the chances of postoperative return to normal become diminished. After biliary drainage or decompression, serum bilirubin levels fall at an average rate of 8% per day, so that values are approximately 25% of the preoperative value by day 10 and are about 10% of the preoperative value weeks after operation.

ROLE OF PREOPERATIVE PERCUTANEOUS BILIARY DRAINAGE

In the late 1970s, a number of authors began to recommend preoperative biliary drainage (PBD) for patients with obstructive jaundice. These early retrospective and uncontrolled reports were enthusiastic about the efficacy of this new modality.[76-78] Although considerable data suggested that the degree of hyperbilirubinemia could be markedly reduced by preoperative drainage, there was a growing concern that many patients would sustain early and late complications related to the biliary drainage procedure, and thereby limit the benefit of this intervention. Subsequently, three randomized, controlled prospective studies performed in South Africa,[79] England,[80] and the United States,[81] all failed to demonstrate any significant benefit from the routine use of preoperative biliary drainage in patients with obstructive jaundice. Data suggest that the length of hospital stay and hospital-based charges actually are increased in patients undergoing preoperative biliary drainage as opposed to surgery alone (Fig 6–12). A fourth prospective study suggested that PBD does, in fact, reduce the surgically related complications but that this effect is offset by drainage-related complications.[82] Although routine preoperative PBD cannot be recommended, it may play a very important role in select patients who are malnourished or in whom definitive management needs to be delayed. In addition, the preoperative placement of a transhepatic catheter may be very helpful to the surgeon, facilitating the intraoperative identification of the bile duct.

TECHNIQUES FOR BILIARY DRAINAGE

The primary goal in the management of patients with obstructive jaundice is achieving biliary drainage. The ideal situation is to be able to provide internal drainage of bile flow and avoidance of an external biliary fistula. Currently available therapeutic options include surgery, percutaneous management using radiologic guidance, and endoscopic intubation.

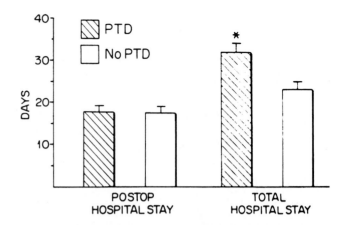

Figure 6–12. Mean postoperative and total hospital stay for 75 patients with obstructive jaundice treated by either surgery alone (no PTD), or surgery following preoperative biliary drainage (PTD). In the PTD group, surgery was delayed until total serum bilirubin was < 10 mg/dL or the estimated mortality risk was < 10%. While no difference in postoperative hospital stay was seen, total hospital stay was significantly longer (*p < 0.005) in the PTD group. (From Pitt HA, Gomes AS, Lois JF, et al. Does preoperative percutaneous biliary drainage reduce operative risk or increase hospital cost? *Ann Surg* 1985;201:545)

Technologic developments have greatly facilitated the radiologic and endoscopic approach to biliary drainage. A number of factors should be considered in the selection of which technique to use: nature of the underlying problem or lesion, biliary and GI anatomy, desired goal, and local expertise. The role of each modality in the management of specific disorders are discussed in the appropriate chapters. Surgery, percutaneous biliary drainage, and endoscopy should not be viewed as competitive techniques, but rather as complementary approaches. Patients often are managed best by a multidisciplinary approach that incorporates surgical, radiologic or percutaneous, and endoscopic techniques. The specific indications for the various options that exist, technical aspects of their performance, and potential complications will be discussed in great detail elsewhere in this text.

Surgery

When surgery is indicated for the jaundiced patient, the surgeon must decide what would be the most appropriate procedure. The surgical management of common duct stone disease may include choledochotomy with stone removal, transduodenal sphincteroplasty, choledochoduodenostomy, or other biliary enteric bypass.[83] Specific indications for these procedures, technical details, and potential complications will be discussed elsewhere in this text. Although a number of alternatives exist for the management of patients with benign bile duct strictures, most of these individuals will require some form of surgical repair, either choledochojejunostomy or Roux-en-Y hepaticojejunostomy.[84] The role of postoperative stents in this setting continues to be contro-

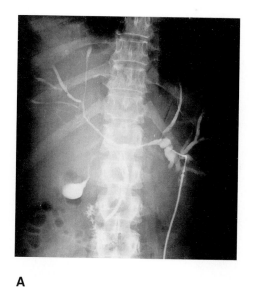

A

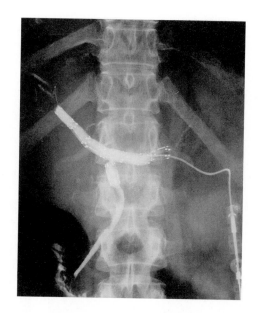

B

Figure 6–13. Biliary drainage of obstructed left and right ductal systems owing to a bulky liver metastasis from ovarian carcinoma. **A.** Cholangiogram by injection into the left ductal system revealing compression and displacement of the right and left hepatic ducts by the centrally located metastasis. **B.** Bile ducts are patent after placement of Gianturco Z stents. (From Friedman AC, Dachman AH (eds), *Radiology of the Liver, Biliary Tract, and Pancreas.* St. Louis, MO: Mosby Year-Book; 1994)

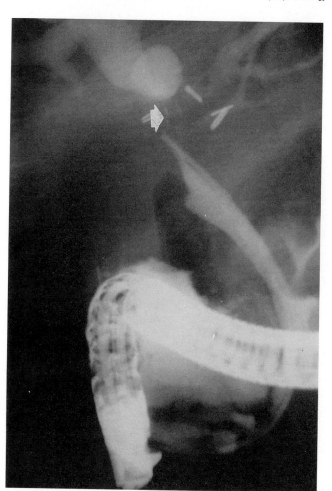

A

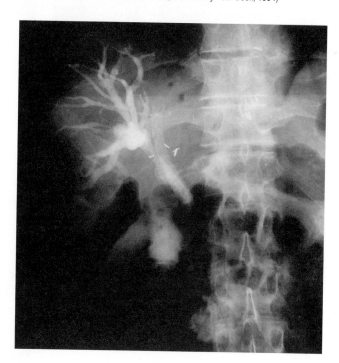

B

Figure 6–14. Internal biliary drainage for cholangiocarcinoma. **A.** ERCP shows narrowing at the confluence and obstruction of both right and left ductal systems. **B.** Placement of two Wallstents established internal drainage of both ductal systems. (From Friedman AC, Dachman AH (eds), *Radiology of the Liver, Biliary Tract, and Pancreas.* St. Louis, MO: Mosby Year-Book; 1994)

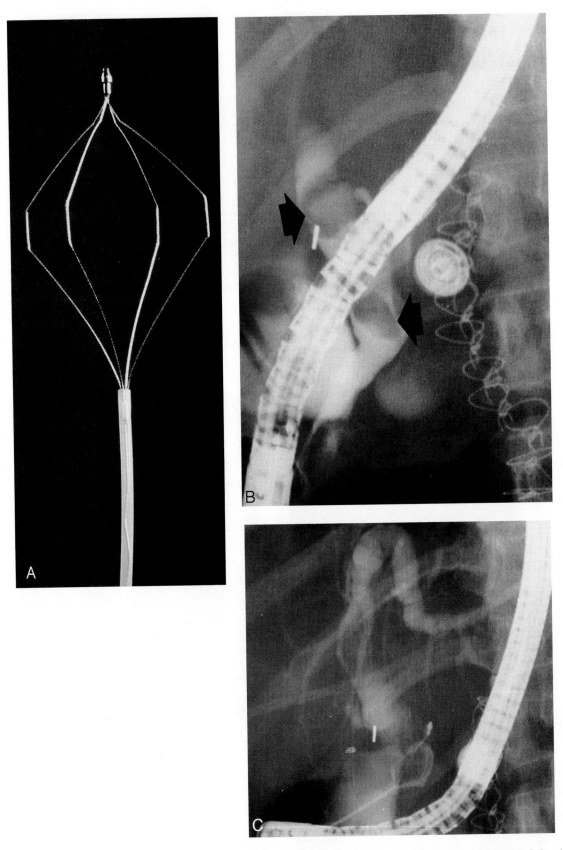

Figure 6–15. Endoscopic approach to common bile duct stones. **A.** Retrieval basket. **B.** Demonstration by ERCP of two stones in the common bile duct. **C.** One of the stones is extracted using the retrieval basket (the other stone has already been removed). (From Friedman AC (ed), *Radiology of the Liver, Biliary Tract, Pancreas, and Spleen.* Baltimore, MD: Williams & Wilkins; 1987)

versial.[85,86] Although patients with extrahepatic biliary tract carcinomas may have multiple symptoms, the vast majority present with jaundice. Surgery, whether for cure or palliation, continues to be the mainstay of therapy for patients with bile duct cancers.[87,88] Controversy exists concerning the ability of unilateral drainage to provide adequate biliary decompression with tumors that have occluded the communication between the right and left hepatic ductal systems.[89,90] Comparison of patients with unresectable malignant hilar strictures managed surgically suggests that unilateral drainage produces similar results to bilateral drainage and that complete hilar obstruction may not be a contraindication to unilateral operative biliary decompression.[91]

Radiologic and Percutaneous Drainage Techniques

Interventional biliary radiology has become a mainstay in the treatment of patients with obstructive jaundice. PTC is an invasive procedure and patient assessment and preparation should be similar to that used for individuals undergoing a formal surgical procedure. Prophylactic administration of antibiotics is recommended when PTC is performed in the setting of biliary obstruction and should be continued for 24 to 48 hours. After the cholangiogram has been obtained, a guidewire can be passed across the obstruction and in most cases, a Cope loop-type self-retaining catheter, made of a soft pliable material, can be inserted to provide internal drainage (Fig 6–8). The most significant complications with this procedure are hemobilia and biliary sepsis.[92] This technology provides for tumor biopsy, balloon dilatation, and placement of biliary endoprostheses. The two most widely used types of endoprostheses are the self-expandable Gianturco Z or Wallstent stents (Figs 6–13 and 6–14) and the balloon-expandable Palmaz stent. These prostheses are particularly helpful in the management of patients with malignant strictures.[93] Compared to surgical palliation, the impact of these stents on the quality of life for patients with malignant biliary strictures remains unclear.[94]

Endoscopic Techniques

Numerous advances have occurred in therapeutic biliary endoscopy since sphincterotomy was first introduced in 1973. In addition to its role in the management of chronic pancreatitis, endoscopic sphincterotomy, with or without stent placement, may be the procedure of choice in patients with retained or recurrent common bile duct stones (Fig 6–15), choledocholithiasis and acute pancreatitis, and benign or malignant biliary strictures (Fig 6–9). Endoscopic stents and drains may be inserted at the time of diagnostic ERCP and sphincterotomy to provide immediate relief from suppurative cholangitis. Nasobiliary drains have proven quite useful as a temporizing maneuver for short-term drainage. The indications, compli-

cations, and results with endoscopic biliary drainage are similar to those of the percutaneous techniques described above. Specific indications and results will be discussed in the chapters dealing with common duct stones, biliary strictures, and pancreatic and biliary tumors.

REFERENCES

1. Wolkoff A. Bilirubin metabolism and hyperbilirubinemia. *Semin Liver Dis* 1983;3:1
2. Isselbacher KJ. Jaundice and hepatomegaly. In: Wilson JD, Braunwald E, Isselbacher KJ, et al (eds), *Harrison's Principles of Internal Medicine*, 12th ed. New York, NY: McGraw-Hill; 1991:264–268
3. O'Connor KW, Snodgrass PJ, Swonder JE, et al. A blinded prospective study comparing four current noninvasive approaches in the differential diagnosis of medical versus surgical jaundice. *Gastroenterology* 1983;84:1498
4. Beinart C, Efremedis S, Cohen B, Mitty HA. Obstruction without dilatation. Importance in evaluating jaundice. *JAMA* 1981;245:353
5. Laing FC, Jeffrey RB, Wing VW, Nyberg DA. Biliary dilatation: defining the level and cause by real-time US. *Radiology* 1986;160:39
6. Eyre-Brook IA, Ross B, Johnson AG. Should surgeons operate on the evidence of ultrasound alone in jaundiced patients? *Br J Surg* 1983;70:587
7. Gibson RN, Yeung E, Thompson JN, et al. Bile duct obstruction: radiologic evaluation of level, cause and tumor resectability. *Radiology* 1986;160:43
8. Scheske GA, Cooperberg PL, Cohen MM, Burhenne HJ. Dynamic changes in the caliber of the major bile ducts, related to obstruction. *Radiology* 1980;135:215
9. Conrad MR, Laday MJ, Janes JO. Sonographic "parallel" channel sign of biliary tree enlargement in mild to moderate obstructive jaundice. *AJR Am J Roentgenol* 1978;130:279
10. Ralls PW, Mayekawa DS, Lee KP, et al. The use of color Doppler sonography to distinguish dilated intrahepatic ducts from vascular structures. *AJR Am J Roentgenol* 1989;152:291
11. Levine E, Maklad NF, Wright CH, Lee KR. Computed tomographic and ultrasonic appearances of primary carcinoma of the common bile duct. *Gastrointest Radiol* 1979;4:147
12. Machan L, Muller NL, Cooperberg PL. Sonographic diagnosis of Klatskin tumors. *AJR Am J Roentgenol* 1986;147:509
13. DiMagno EP, Buxton JL, Regan PT, et al. Ultrasonic endoscope. *Lancet* 1980;1:629
14. Sivak MV, Kaufman AR. Endoscopic ultrasonography in the differential diagnosis of pancreatic disease: a preliminary report. *Scand J Gastroenterol* 1986;21(suppl):130
15. Snady H, Cooperman A, Siegel J. Endoscopic ultrasonography compared with computed tomography with ERCP in patients with obstructive jaundice or small peripancreatic mass. *Gastrointest Endosc* 1992;38:27
16. Baron RL, Stanley RJ, Lee JKT, et al: Prospective comparison of the evaluation of biliary obstruction using com-

puted tomography and ultrasonography. *Radiology* 1982; 145:91

17. Jeffrey RB, Federle MP, Laing FC, et al. CT of choledocholithiasis. *AJR Am J Roentgenol* 1983;140:1179

18. Mitchell SE, Clark RA. A comparison of CT and sonography in choledocholithiasis. *AJR Am J Roentgenol* 1984; 142:729

19. Barron RC. Common bile duct stones: reassessment of criteria for CT diagnosis. *Radiology* 1987;162:419

20. Cronan JJ. Ultrasound diagnosis of choledocholithiasis: reappraisal. *Radiology* 1986;161:133

21. Leander P, Golman K, Klaveness J, et al. MRI contrast media for the liver: efficacy in conditions of acute biliary obstruction. *Invest Radiolog* 1990;25:1130

22. Semelka RC, Shoenut JP, Kroeker MA, et al. Bile duct disease: prospective comparison of ERCP, CT, and fat suppression MRI. *Gastrointest Radiol* 1992;—:347

23. Morimoto K, Shimoi M, Shirakawa T, et al. Biliary obstruction: evaluation with three-dimensional MR cholangiography. *Radiology* 1992;183:578

24. Jain S, Long RG, Scott J, et al. Percutaneous transhepatic cholangiography using the "Chiba" needle - 80 cases. *Br J Radiol* 1977;50:175

25. Harbin WP, Mueller PR, Ferrucci JT. Transhepatic cholangiography: complications and use patterns of the fine-needle technique. A multi-institution survey. *Radiology* 1980;135:15

26. Mueller PR, Harbin WP, Ferrucci JT, et al. Fine needle cholangiography: Reflections after 450 cases. *AJR Am J Roentgenol* 1980;136:85

27. Sarr MG, Kaufmann SL, Zuidema GD, Cameron JL. Management of hemobilia associated with transhepatic biliary drainage catheters. *Surgery* 1984;95:603

28. McCune WS, Shorb PE, Moscowitz H. Endoscopic cannulation of the ampulla of Vater: a preliminary report. *Ann Surg* 1968;167:752

29. Osnes M, Myren J. Endoscopic retrograde cholangiopancreatography (ERCP) in patients with Billroth II partial gastrectomies. *Endoscopy* 1975;7:225

30. Camma C, Garofalo G, Almasio P, et al. A performance evaluation of the expert system "jaundice" in comparison with that of three hepatologists. *J Hepatol* 1991;13:279

31. Baron RL, Stanley RJ, Lee JKT. Prospective comparison of the evaluation of biliary obstruction using computed tomography and ultrasonography. *Radiology* 1982;145:91

32. Borsch G, Wegener M, Wedmann B, et al. Clinical evaluation, ultrasound, cholescintigraphy, and endoscopic retrograde cholangiography in cholestasis: a prospective study. *J Clin Gastroenterol* 1988;10:185

33. O'Connor K, Snodgrass PJ, Swonder JE, et al. A blinded prospective study comparing four current noninvasive approaches in the differential diagnosis of medical versus surgical jaundice. *Gastroenterology* 1983;84:1498

34. Pasanen PA, Partanen K, Pikkarainen P, et al. Diagnostic accuracy of ultrasound, computed tomography, and endoscopic retrograde cholangiopancreatography in the detection of obstructive jaundice. *Scand J Gastroenterol* 1991;26:1157

35. Heyd CG. "Liver deaths" in surgery of the gallbladder. *JAMA* 1931;97:1847

36. Helwig FC, Schutz CB. A liver kidney syndrome. Clinical pathological and experimental studies. *Surg Gynecol Obstet* 1930;55:570

37. Wait RB, Kahng KU. Renal failure complicating obstructive jaundice. *Am J Surg* 1989;157:256–263

38. Dawson JL. The incidence of postoperative renal failure in obstructive jaundice. *Br J Surg* 1965;52:663

39. Bouillot J-L, Ledorner G, Alexandre J-HL. Facteurs de risque de la chirurgie des icteres obstructifs: etude retrospective a propos de 176 patients. *Gastroenterol Clin Biol* 1985;9:238

40. Dawson JL. Post-operative renal function in obstructive jaundice: effect of mannitol diuresis. *Brit Med J* 1965;1:82

41. Evans HJR, Torrealba V, Hudd C, et al. The effect of preoperative bile salt administration on postoperative renal function in patients with obstructive jaundice. *Brit J Surg* 1982;69:706

42. Williams RD, Elliott DW, Zollinger RM. The effect of hypotension in obstructive jaundice. *Arch Surg* 1960;81:182

43. Cattell WR, Birnstingl MA. Blood volume and hypotension in obstructive jaundice. *Brit J Surg* 1967;54:272

44. Shasha SM, Better OS, Chaimovitz C, et al. Hemodynamic studies in dogs with chronic bile-duct ligation. *Clin Sci* 1978;55:109

45. Alon U, Berant M, Mordechovvitz D, et al. Effect of isolated cholemica on systemic hemodynamics and kidney function in conscious dogs. *Clin Sci* 1982;63:59

46. Bomzon A, Gali D, Better OS, et al. Reversible suppression of the vascular contractile response in rats with obstructive jaundice. *J Lab Clin Med* 1985;105:568

47. Oms L, Martinez-Rodenas F, Valverde J, et al. Reduced water and sodium intakes associated with high levels of natriuretic factor following common bile duct ligation in the rabbit. *Br J Surg* 1990;77:752

48. Sitges-Serra A, Carulla X, Piera C, et al. Body water compartments in patients with obstructive jaundice. *Br J Surg* 1992;79:553

49. Levy M, Wexler MJ, Fechner C. Renal perfusion in dogs with experimental hepatic cirrhosis: role of prostaglandins. *Am J Physiol* 1983;245:F521

50. Zambraski EJ, Dunn MJ. Importance of renal prostaglandins in control of renal function after chronic ligation of the common bile duct in dogs. *J Lab Clin Med* 1984;103:549

51. Kahng KU, Monaco DO, Schnabel FR, Wait RB. Renal vascular reactivity in the bile duct ligated rat. *Surgery* 1988; 104:250

52. Katz S, Grosfeld JL, Gross K, et al. Impaired bacterial clearance and trapping in obstructive jaundice. *Ann Surg* 1984;199:14

53. Pain JA, Cahill CJ, Gilbert JM, et al. Prevention of postoperative renal dysfunction in patients with obstructive jaundice: a multicentre study of bile salts and lactulose. *Br J Surg* 1991;78:467

54. Gubern JM, Sancho JJ, Simo J, Sitges-Serra A. A randomized trial on the effect of mannitol on postoperative renal function in patients with obstructive jaundice. *Surgery* 1988;103:39

55. Pain JA, Cahill CJ, Gilbert JM, et al. Prevention of postoperative renal dysfunction in patients with obstructive jaun-

dice: a multicentre study of bile salts and lactulose. *Br J Surg* 1991;78:467

56. Pitt HA, Zuidema GD. Factors influencing mortality in the treatment of pyogenic hepatic abscess. *Surg Gynecol Obstet* 1975;140:228

57. Thompson JE Jr, Tompkins RK, Longmire WP Jr. Factors in the management of acute cholangitis. *Ann Surg* 1982; 195:137

58. Bilbao MK, Dotter CT, Lee TG, Katon RM. Complications of endoscopic retrograde cholangiopancreatography (ERCP): a study of 10,000 cases. *Gastroenterology* 1976;70:314

59. Bemelmans MHA, Greve JW, Gouma DJ, Buurman WA. Cytokines, tumor necrosis factor and interleukin-6 in experimental biliary obstruction in mice. *Hepatology* 1992; 15:1132

60. Bemelmans MHA, Gouma DJ, Greve JW, Buurman WA. Effect of antitumour necrosis factor treatment on circulating tumour necrosis factor levels and mortality after surgery in jaundiced mice. *Br J Surg* 1993;80:1055

61. Holman JM Jr, Rikkers LF. Biliary obstruction and host defense failure. *J Surg Res* 1982;32:208

62. Tanaka N, Ryden S, Berqvist L, et al. Reticulo-endothelial function in rats with obstructive jaundice. *Br J Surg* 1985; 72:946

63. Greve JW, Gouma DJ, Soeters PB, Buurman WA. Suppression of cellular immunity in obstructive jaundice is caused by endotoxins: A study with germ-free rats. *Gastroenterology* 1990;98:478

64. Cahill CJ. Prevention of postoperative renal failure in patients with obstructive jaundice—the role of bile salts. *Br J Surg* 1983;70:590

65. Pain JA, Bailey ME. Experimental and clinical study of lactulose in obstructive jaundice. *Br J Surg* 1986;63:774

66. Greve JW, Gouma DJ, van Leeuwen PAM, Buurman WA. Lactulose inhibits endotoxin induced tumor necrosis factor production by monocytes: an in vitro study. *Hepatology* 1989;10:454

67. Cahill CJ, Pain JA, Bailey ME. Bile salts, endotoxin and renal function in obstructive jaundice. *Surg Gynecol Obstet* 1987;165:165(b):519–22

68. Greve JW, Gouma DJ, Buurman WA. Bile acids inhibit endotoxin induced tumours necrosis factor production by monocytes: an in vitro study. *Gut* 1990;31:198

69. Corrigan JJ, Keirnat JF. Effect of polymyxin B on endotoxin activity in gram negative septicaemia model. *Ped Res* 1979;13:48–51

70. Ingoldby CJH. The value of polymyxin B in endotoxemia due to experimental obstructive jaundice and mesenteric ischemia. *Br J Surg* 1980;67:565

71. Ingoldby CJ, McPherson GAD, Blumgart LH. Endotoxemia in human obstructive jaundice. effect of polymyxin B. *Am J Surg* 1984;147:766

72. Pitt HA, Cameron JL, Postier RG, Gadacz TR. Factors affecting mortality in biliary tract surgery. *Am J Surg* 1981; 141:66

73. Blamey SL, Fearon KGH, Gilmour WH, et al. Predictors of risk in biliary surgery. *Br J Surg* 1983;70:535

74. Dixon JM, Armstrong CP, Duffy SW, Davies GC. Factors affecting morbidity and mortality after surgery for obstructive jaundice: a review of 373 patients. *Gut* 1983;24:845

75. Carey JB, Williams G. Relief of the pruritus of jaundice with a bile-acid sequestering resin. *JAMA* 1961;176:432

76. Nakayama T, Ikeda A, Okuda K. Percutaneous transhepatic drainage of the biliary tract. *Gastroenterology* 1978; 74:554

77. Hansson JA, Hoevels, J, Simert G, et al. Clinical aspects of nonsurgical percutaneous transhepatic drainage in obstructive lesions of the extrahepatic bile ducts. *Ann Surg* 1979;189:58

78. Ferrucci JT, Mueller PR, Harbin WP. Percutaneous transhepatic biliary drainage: technique, results and applications. *Radiology* 1980;135:1

79. Hatfield ARW, Tobias R, Terblanche J, et al. Preoperative external biliary drainage in obstructive jaundice: a prospective controlled clinical trial. *Lancet* 1982;2(8304):896–9

80. McPherson GAD, Benjamin IS, Hodgson HJF, et al. Preoperative percutaneous transhepatic biliary drainage: the results of a controlled trial. *Br J Surg* 1984;71:371

81. Pitt HA, Gomes AS, Lois JF, et al. Does preoperative percutaneous biliary drainage reduce operative risk or increase hospital cost? *Ann Surg* 1981;201:545

82. Smith RC, Pooley M, George CRP, Faithful GR. Preoperative percutaneous transhepatic internal drainage in obstructive jaundice: a randomized, controlled trial examining renal function. *Surgery* 1985;97:641

83. Tompkins RK. Surgical management of bile duct stones. *Surg Clin North Am* 1990;70:1329

84. Millis JM, Tompkins RK, Zinner MJ, et al. Management of bile duct strictures: an evolving strategy. *Arch Surg* 1992; 127:1077

85. Innes JT, Ferrara JJ, Carey LC. Biliary reconstruction without transanastomotic stent. *Ann Surg* 1988;54:27

86. Lillemoe KD, Pitt HA, Cameron JL. Postoperative bile duct strictures. *Surg Clin North Am* 1990;70:1355

87. Tompkins RK, Saunders K, Roslyn JJ, Longmire WP Jr. Changing patterns in diagnosis and management of bile duct cancer. *Ann Surg* 1990;211:614

88. Lai ECS, Chu KM, et al. Choice of palliation for malignant hilar biliary obstruction. *Am J Surg* 1992;163:208

89. Hall RI, Denyer ME, Chapman AH. Percutaneous-endoscopic placement of endoprostheses for relief of jaundice caused by inoperable bile duct stricutres. *Surgery* 1990;107:224

90. Deviere J, Baize M, de Touef J, Cremer M. Long-term follow-up of patients with hilar malignant stricture treated by endoscopic internal biliary drainage. *Gastrointest Endosc* 1988;34:95

91. Baer HU, Rhyner M, Stain SC, et al. The effect of communications between the right and left liver on the outcome of surgical drainage for jaundice due to malignant obstruction at the hilus of the liver. *Hepatobil Surgery* 1994;9:7

92. Gunther RW, Schild H, Thelen M. Percutaneous transhepatic biliary drainage: experience with 311 procedures. *Intervent Radiol* 1988;11:65

93. McLean GK, Burke DR. Role of endoprostheses in the management of malignant biliary obstruction. *Radiology* 1989;170:961

94. Lai ECS, Tompkins RK, Mann LL, Roslyn JJ. Proximal bile duct cancer: quality of survival. *Ann Surg* 1987; 205:111

7

Diarrhea and Constipation

Rolando H. Rolandelli

When healthy, the human digestive tract absorbs most ingested nutrients, leaving only resistant fibers, bacteria, mucus and cellular debris for elimination in feces. A certain amount of water is retained in feces to allow defecation without pain or effort. As fiber in the diet increases, stool volume, water, and frequency also increase.[1] Men produce softer and larger volumes of stool than women. During the luteal phase of the menstrual cycle, stool becomes harder and has a slower transit time.

Diarrhea results from an increase in stool volume with an associated decrease in consistency. However, since stool volume is difficult to quantify, even in the hospitalized patient, the most widely accepted criteria for defining diarrhea are consistency and frequency. More than three semiliquid stools per day is considered diarrhea. Constipation is defined as a decrease in the frequency of stools, regardless of volume and consistency, to less than one stool every 3 days or to less than two stools per week. The prevalence of constipation in the United States is 2%, with 4 million people seeking medical consultation every year.[2] More than $369 million per year is spent for cathartics and laxatives dispensed by drugstores and hospitals in the United States.[3]

The causes of diarrhea and constipation, as well as the diagnostic and therapeutic approaches, are quite different in ambulatory patients as compared to hospitalized patients. In the outpatient setting, diarrhea and constipation usually are symptoms of the primary disease. However, in the hospitalized patient, diarrhea and constipation are often epiphenomena of other diseases. This chapter reviews the different types of diarrhea and constipation, in both ambulatory and hospitalized patients, with respect to pathophysiology, clinical presentation, diagnosis, and treatment.

■ COLONIC PHYSIOLOGY

The healthy colon is the most efficient absorptive organ of the gastrointestinal tract. It absorbs more than 95% of the sodium, chloride, and water entering the cecum.[4] This absorptive efficiency allows the colon to compensate for sudden changes in ileal effluent. In experimental conditions, the cecum can be perfused with volumes of up to 4.5 L/24 hours before an increase in fecal output is noted.[5] The absorption of sodium and water by the colonic mucosa is an active process that depends upon the availability of an energy source for epithelial cells. The colonic epithelium can utilize various fuels; however, n-butyrate is oxidized in preference to glutamine, glucose, or ketone bodies.[6] Since n-butyrate cannot be produced by mammalian cells, the colonic epithelium relies on luminal bacteria to produce it by fermenting dietary fiber. The lack of n-butyrate, such as that resulting from inhibition of fermentation by broad-spectrum antibiotics, leads to less sodium and water absorption and thus, to diarrhea.[7] Conversely, the perfusion of the colonic lumen with n-butyrate stimulates sodium and water absorption.[8] N-butyrate, acetate, and propionate are short-chain fatty acids (SCFA) produced by bacterial fermentation; these constitute the main anions in stool.[9] Other physiological effects of SCFA on the colon include stimulation of blood flow, mucosal cell renewal, and regulation of intraluminal pH with homeostasis of the bacterial flora.

While dietary fiber is the main substrate for bacterial fermentation in the normal colon,[10] not all dietary fibers are equally fermented[11]: lignin is not fermented and produces bulk, celluloses are only partially fermented, and pectins are completely fermented. Colonic transit time and stool bulk depend upon the fermentability of the various fibers ingested. Poorly fermented fibers increase luminal bulk and accelerate transit time; highly fermentable fibers provide minimal bulk and slow transit time. Consequently, the type of fiber source has an impact on both the etiology and the treatment of colonic diseases. As a result, in populations with a high intake of roughage, i.e, water insoluble fibers[12] constipation, diverticulosis, and colon cancer are all uncommon. Water insoluble fibers are therapeutic for constipation (creating bulk), and water soluble fibers are therapeutic for diarrhea (generating SCFA).

Fermentation in the colon is made possible by its distinctive morphology.[13] The colon can be divided into three anatomical segments: the right colon, the left colon, and the rectum. The right colon is the fermentation chamber of the human gastrointestinal tract; in both the cecum and ascending colon, bacteria are metabolically active. The left colon is a site of storage and desiccation of stool. The rectum is the reservoir through which defecation can be deferred until a more convenient time.

Transit through the colon is controlled by the autonomic nervous system. Parasympathetic nervous fibers supply the colon via the vagi and the pelvic nerves. Nerve fibers reaching the colon are arranged in several plexuses: the subserous, myenteric (Auerbach), submucous (Meissner), and mucous plexuses. The neurons of the myenteric plexus are concentrated along the tenia and are sparse between the tenia, where the longitudinal muscle layer is thin. Sympathetic nerve fibers originate in the superior and inferior mesenteric ganglia and reach the colon by way of perivascular plexuses.

The motility pattern is different in the three anatomic segments. In the right colon, *antiperistalsic* waves generate retrograde flow of colonic contents back to the cecum.[14] In the left colon, contents are propelled caudad by *tonic contractions*, separating them into a series of globular masses. A third type of contraction, called *mass peristalsis*, is interspersed with the propulsive and retropulsive contractions and occurs at varying intervals, more frequently after meals. Each mass peristalsis contraction is able to advance a column of colonic contents through one-third of the colonic length. Finally, the rectum will undergo receptive relaxation to accommodate stool until defecation takes place.

Hormones also play a role in regulating colonic motility. Thyroid hormone, gastrin, vasoactive intestinal polypeptide (VIP), and cholecystokinin increase colonic motility, while glucagon and somatostatin decrease it. Serotonin indirectly increase colonic motility by increasing intestinal secretions.

Multiple drugs influence colonic motility. Opiates significantly decrease transit time through the right colon and inhibit defecation. Opiate antagonists, such as naloxone, stimulate colonic motility. Various other drugs decrease intestinal motility, including α adrenergic agonists, prostaglandin synthetase inhibitors, calcium channel blockers, lithium, chlorpromazine, and trifluoperazine.

■ DIARRHEA IN THE AMBULATORY PATIENT

An excessive fecal output (>500 cc or gm/day) may result from either malabsorption of nutrients or from mucosal secretion. Malabsorbed nutrients produce a high osmotic load in the stool, whereas mucosal secretion is usually watery and hyposmolar. Malabsorption usually is a chronic condition, while secretory diarrhea in most cases is an acute event. Stools from malabsorptive diarrhea, or steatorrhea, are greasy and yellowish with a rancid odor, and typically float in water. Stools from secretory diarrhea are clear and watery, and they are often stained with blood. A third form of diarrhea may have components of both steatorrhea and secretory diarrhea as well as an inflammatory exudate that includes blood. This form is called exudative diarrhea and is characteristic of inflammatory bowel diseases (Table 7–2).

MALABSORPTIVE DIARRHEA (STEATORRHEA)

Fat is the first nutrient to be lost in feces whenever nutrient absorption is adversely affected by a pathological condition. Fat absorption requires enzymatic degradation, emulsification, uptake by specific sites of the intestinal mucosa (tip of the villi), reesterification by the intestinal mucosa and lymphatic transport. Carbohydrates and proteins are degraded more easily and can be absorbed anywhere in the intestinal mucosa. Moreover, the colon can compensate for carbohydrate or protein malabsorption by transforming their carbon skeletons into SCFA. Malabsorbed fat adds to stool volume (steatorrhea) and produces colonic secretion leading to further loss of nutrients, water, and electrolytes. The consequence of fat malabsorption is a loss of ab-

TABLE 7–1. CLASSIFICATION OF DIARRHEA

Malabsorptive diarrhea
  Luminal disorders
    Hepatobiliary disease
    Pancreatic insufficiency
    Bacterial overgrowth
      Jejunal diverticulosis
      Scleroderma
  Mucosal abnormalities
    Crohn's disease
    Ulcerative colitis
    Celiac disease
    Tropical sprue
    Radiation enteritis
  Lymphatic disease
    Whipple's disease
    Lymphangiectasia
    Lymphomas

Secretory diarrhea
  "Food Poisoning"
    Salmonella
    Shigella
    Staphylococcus
    Clostridium Welchi
  "Travellers diarrhea"
  Infections in immunocompromised patients
    Cytomegalovirus
    Yersinia
  Endocrine tumors
    Zollinger-Ellson syndrome
    VIPoma

sorbed calories with progressive weight loss and malnutrition. Fat soluble vitamins K, A, D, and E also can be malabsorbed in steatorrhea, leading to their respective vitamin deficiency syndromes.

The most common cause of malabsorptive diarrhea is chronic alcoholism, which causes cirrhosis and pancreatic insufficiency. The lack of both bile salts and pancreatic enzymes creates suboptimal conditions for digestion and absorption. The second most common cause of malabsorptive diarrhea is mucosal inflammation from Crohn's disease or radiation enteritis. In both of these illnesses there may be a combination of factors leading to malabsorption, including bacterial overgrowth and previous intestinal resection. Relatively uncommon causes

TABLE 7–2. DIARRHEA CHARACTERISTICS

	Malabsorptive	Secretory	Exudative
Presentation	Chronic	Acute	Subacute
Stool Consistency	Greasy	Watery	Bloody
Osmolar Gap	Positive	Negative	Either
Blood	absent	rare	common

of malabsorptive diarrhea include lymphatic diseases, scleroderma, celiac sprue disease, and Whipple disease.

SECRETORY DIARRHEA

The most common cause of secretory diarrhea is the ingestion of foods contaminated with enteropathogens or enterotoxins (Table 7–1). Immunosuppression resulting from the Acquired Immune Deficiency Syndrome (AIDS) or from immunosuppresant drugs given to patients after transplantation is commonly associated with diarrhea. Five to ten percent of all patients with AIDS will develop cytomegalovirus (CMV) ileocolitis,[15] and disseminated CMV has been identified in 90% of AIDS patients at autopsy.[16] Chronic diarrhea due to CMV is a common cause of malnutrition in AIDS patients. In addition, CMV colitis may lead to bleeding or perforation and may require emergency surgery. CMV infection is, in fact, the most common indication for surgery in AIDS patients, with a mortality after surgery for CMV colitis of 86% at 6 months, usually from sepsis and pneumonia.[17]

Patients afflicted with secretory diarrhea may become depleted of water and electrolytes; children and the elderly are particularly susceptible to dehydration. When severe, infections producing secretory diarrhea may damage the mucosal barrier of the intestine and produce translocation of bacteria and endotoxins.

Hormone-secreting tumors may present with watery diarrhea. In the Zollinger-Ellison syndrome, at least half of the patients develop secretory diarrhea. The Verner-Morrison, or watery-diarrhea-hypokalemia-alkalosis syndrome, is caused by excessive production of vasoactive intestinal polypeptide (VIP), pancreatic polypeptide and prostaglandin E1 and E2. Secretory diarrhea is also a typical feature of the carcinoid syndrome produced by carcinoid tumors in the gastrointestinal tract or lungs. These tumors typically secrete serotonin or substance P.

EXUDATIVE DIARRHEA

Exudative diarrhea is the most common manifestation of ulcerative colitis. Patients with active ulcerative colitis have frequent stools containing blood and mucus. When the disease involves the rectum, urgency, tenesmus, and incontinence are also common. Patients with granulomatous colitis (Crohn's disease of the colon) may also have exudative diarrhea.

DIAGNOSTIC WORKUP IN DIARRHEAL STATES

As previously mentioned, quantification of stool output can be very difficult in both the ambulatory and hospital settings. In some elderly individuals incontinence can be confused for diarrhea. A normal volume of stool can produce frequent soiling in an incontinent patient; whenever possible, stool volume should be measured in

TABLE 7–3. SPECIFIC ANTIBIOTIC THERAPY FOR ACUTE INFECTIOUS DIARRHEA

Enteropathogen	Antibiotic
Amebiasis	Metronidazole 750 mg po tid × 10 days
Campylobacter	Erythromycin 250 mg po qid × 5 days
Giardia	Metronidazole 250 mg po tid × 7 days
Salmonella (sepsis)	Ampicillin 1 g IV q 4 h × 10 days
Shigella	Trimethoprim-sulfamethoxazole 2 DS po bid × 10 days
Vibrio cholerae	Tetracycline 500 mg po qid × 2 days
Yersinia enterocolitica	Tetracycline 250 mg po qid × 7 days

order to diagnose diarrhea. Rectal tubes and adult diapers can be used in the elderly population to provide an objective assessment of stool output. A volume >300 cc of stool or more than three large, liquid stools per day is indicative of diarrhea.

Recent conditions at or near the time of development of the diarrhea provide useful diagnostic clues. Sudden onset of watery stools after the ingestion of suspicious foods, recent ravel, or recent antibiotic therapy will suggest the diagnosis of secretory diarrhea. Association with other symptoms is also important, such as aggressive peptic ulcer disease in individuals with the Zollinger-Ellison syndrome. A history of alcohol abuse points to pancreatic insufficiency and malabsorptive diarrhea. Recurrent episodes of exudative diarrhea, in association with constitutional symptoms (fever, weight loss, growth retardation), indicate inflammatory bowel disease.

STOOL ANALYSIS

For all patients with diarrhea, a stool sample should be taken for isolation of enteropathogens and assay of *Clostridium difficile* toxin. Prior antibiotic therapy is not essential to the development of *Clostridium difficile* colitis. In equivocal cases, the differentiation between malabsorptive and secretory diarrhea can be made by the measurement of electrolytes and osmolality in stool. The stool osmotic gap is calculated by subtracting 2 X (Na + K) from the measured osmolality.[18] A negative osmotic gap is indicative of secretory diarrhea, whereas a positive osmotic gap indicates malabsorptive diarrhea. The diagnosis of malabsorptive diarrhea can be investigated further by measuring fecal fat. The Van de Kamer test requires stool collection for 72 hours while the patient ingests 100 gm/day of fat. An excretion of more than 7 grams/day of fat is diagnostic for steatorrhea. When stool collection is impossible (e.g., in incontinent patients) Sudan staining of a spot sample of stool can reveal fat malabsorption. In addition, urine analysis for laxatives (bisacodyl, phenolphthalein, and danthron)

may unmask surreptitious laxative abuse. Blood assays for gastrin, VIP, and other enterohormones should be obtained when the history and stool analysis suggests secretory diarrhea of endocrine origin.

Endoscopic examination of the colon by sigmoidoscopy or colonoscopy may reveal mucosal changes associated with inflammatory bowel disease or pseudomembranes associated with *Clostridium difficile* colitis. Small bowel biopsy is the only recourse to establish the diagnosis of celiac disease, Whipple's disease, lymphangiectasia, amyloidosis, and other rare conditions. Some diarrheal conditions, such as jejunal diverticulosis and scleroderma, are associated with small bowel bacterial overgrowth. Bacteria residing in diseased small bowel can ferment carbohydrates and amino acids as do normal colonic flora. Since hydrogen is produced only by bacteria in the body and is excreted mostly in exhaled air, small bowel fermentation can be investigated by a breath hydrogen test. Exhaled hydrogen is measured under basal conditions and after the administration of lactulose. A high baseline level (>40 ppm) or an early rise after lactulose administration (<3 hours) is indicative of small bowel bacterial overgrowth.

THERAPY

The most effective treatment for diarrhea is outright elimination of the specific disease that increases stool output. For instance, diarrhea as a result of a VIPoma will cease with the complete excision of the tumor. Unfortunately, complete elimination of disease is not possible in most cases of diarrhea, and treatment is limited to reducing stool output with antidiarrheal medications.

The various drugs used for the treatment of diarrhea are listed in Table 7–4. Binders and bacterial flora promoters are the first line of treatment, in most cases. In the United States, opiates are probably the drugs most frequently used for diarrhea. Although very effective, they may cause such side effects as depressed mental status; in infectious diarrhea, they may cause additional bacterial overgrowth. In order to avoid chemical dependency on diphenoxylate, atropine is added to produce unpleasant side effects at large doses. The secretion inhibitor, octreotide, has gained wide popularity in recent years. It is effective in the secretory diarrheas of AIDS and of endocrine origin. One disadvantage to octreotide use is the pain associated with subcutaneous injection. For patients who may require octreotide for a prolonged period of time, a pump for continuous subcubtaneous infusion is tolerated better than intermittent injections.

In patients with steatorrhea, dietary counseling and enzyme replacement are the mainstays of treatment. The diet should be low in long-chain triglycerides and

TABLE 7–4. ANTIDIARRHEAL MEDICATIONS

Binders
  Bile salts
    Cholestyramine
  Enterotoxins
    Kaolin
    Charcoal

Bacterial flora promoters
  Bacterial inocula
    Lactobacillus acidophilus
  Fermentable fibers
    Pectin

Motility agents
  Opiates
    Diphenoxylate/atropine
    Loperamide
    Codeine

Secretion inhibitors
  Alpha-adrenergic agents
    Clonidine
    Lidamidine
  Calcium channel blockers
    Verapamil
  Glucocorticoids
    Prednisone
  Prostaglandin synthetase inhibitors
    Indomethacin
    Salicylates
  Chlorpromazine derivatives
    Trifluoperazine
  Somatostatin analogue
    Octreotide

Miscellaneous
  Lithium carbonate

supplemented with medium-chain triglycerides, which are absorbed more easily.

Patients with exudative diarrhea that is caused by ulcerative colitis can be treated with a variety of medications, including sulfasalazine and other derivatives of the 5-aminosalicylic acid. When the disease becomes resistant to medical therapy or after 10 years, a restorative proctocolectomy is the treatment of choice. Patients with Crohn's disease limited to the colon also may benefit from a colectomy, although the disease usually recurs in the small bowel.

■ DIARRHEA IN THE HOSPITALIZED PATIENT

Diarrhea is common in surgical patients and ranges from a simple inconvenience to a life-threatening condition. Disruption of bacterial homeostasis is the most common disturbance of colonic physiology that results in diarrhea. The colon harbors the most luxurious bac-

terial flora of the body. Bacterial species and growth are controlled closely by several factors, including motility, availability of fermentation substrates (dietary fiber), bacterial activity and their metabolic products (SCFA). These factors are affected by the diagnostic and therapeutic measures received by surgical patients. Colonic motility is affected by surgical procedures that lead to postoperative ileus. The use of opiates and other drugs also slows colonic transit. In preparation for surgery, the colon is cleansed of bacteria by mechanical agents, cathartics and enemas, and bacterial counts are reduced with intestinal antibiotics. After surgery, oral diets are modified (bland, mechanical, low residue) to reduce the work load of the gastrointestinal tract. These modifications eliminate fiber from the diet and deprive colonic bacteria of a fermentation substrate. Bacterial fermentation also is impaired by the administration of systemic antibiotics. Decreased availability of SCFA[19] to the colonic mucosa impairs absorption of water and sodium and raises the colonic pH (Table 7–5).

These physiologic disturbances to the colon are sufficient to produce diarrhea, even in the absence of infectious microorganisms. This explains many cases of antibiotic-associated diarrhea in which no other cause can be identified. In a small number of surgical patients, *Clostridium difficile* toxin is found in diarrheal stools.

CLOSTRIDIUM DIFFICILE COLITIS

The pathogenesis of *Clostridium difficile* colitis is still a matter of debate. *Clostridium difficile* is found as part of the colonic flora of infants and in nearly 10% of adults.[20] Adults rarely develop colitis unless hospitalized. In hospitals, outbursts of *Clostridium difficile* diarrhea have been noted in certain geographical areas, leading to the theory of a transmissible disease.[21] A few

TABLE 7–5. CAUSES OF DIARRHEA IN THE HOSPITALIZED PATIENT

Drug induced
  Antibiotic agents
    Pseudomembranous colitis
  Antimetabolites, colchicine

Tube feedings
  Nutrient composition
    High fat
    Low fiber
  Faulty technique
    Boluses into the small bowel
    Boluses with hyperosmolar medication

Postresectional
  Gastrectomy
  Enterectomy
  Colectomy

cases of *Clostridium difficile* colitis without prior antibiotic therapy have been reported.[22,23] All of these intriguing phenomena can be explained on the basis of the pH sensitivity of the *Clostridium difficile*. This bacterium grows and produces its toxins in an alkaline environment.[24] In healthy adults, the acidity of the stomach destroys *Clostridium difficile*. This gastric barrier is eliminated with the administration of antacids and other agents that block acid secretion; this explains the outbreaks in hospitals, particularly in intensive care units where prophylaxis for upper gastrointestinal bleeding is common. If the *Clostridium difficile* survives the gastric environment, it normally will be eliminated by acidity in the colon. However, administration of antibiotics decreases the production of SCFAs[19] and consequently, increases colonic pH, allowing the *Clostridium difficile* to grow and produce toxin. Colonic stasis, such as that caused by surgery, allows further growth of *Clostridium difficile*, which explains the high incidence of pseudomembranous colitis in the postoperative period.[25]

Toxins secreted by the *Clostridium difficile* produce an exudate firmly adherent to the mucosa; thus, this disease is named pseudomembranous colitis. The severity of *Clostridium difficile* colitis is highly variable and may range from a few loose stools to fulminant toxic megacolon. The diagnosis of this illness is made by the presence of *Clostridium difficile* toxin in stool or the presence of pseudomembranes in the colon. The treatment for pseudomembranous colitis is discontinuation of the antibiotics that caused it, and the use of binders such as cholestyramine or Kaolin/pectin. If the patient remains symptomatic, the use of oral metronidazole or vancomycin is recommended.

In some patients *Clostridium difficile* invades the colonic wall, and the cytotoxins reach systemic circulation.[26] These patients become septic and the clinical condition rapidly deteriorates. The resolution of diarrhea in patients with pseudomembranous colitis associated with toxic megacolon is an ominous sign.[27] These patients require an emergency colectomy to remove the septic focus, along with the creation of an ileostomy.[28,29]

TUBE-FEEDING RELATED DIARRHEA

Other surgical patients who develop diarrhea do so while receiving tube feedings. The incidence of diarrhea related to tube feedings ranges from 2.3%[30] to 50%,[31] depending on the severity of the underlying illness. Some factors associated with tube-feeding diarrhea are hypoalbuminemia, administration of H2 antagonists, and antibiotics. All other causes of diarrhea should be ruled out before discontinuing the tube feedings.

A common practice in hospitals is to administer medications via the feeding tube. Most medications available in a liquid form, suspension or elixir, are made palatable by the addition of a monosaccharide (eg, sorbitol) which makes them hyperosmolar. Other medications are hyperosmolar regardless of the vehicle used in the preparation, eg, potassium chloride. These medications can produce diarrhea, particularly when they are infused into the jejunum.[32] Faulty technique in the administration of tube feedings, such as boluses into the jejunum, also produce diarrhea.

Defined formula diets used for tube feedings can produce diarrhea owing to hyperosmolarity (elemental diets) and high fat content.[33] We also have found that fiber-free liquid formulas produce diarrhea in normal subjects.[34] The administration of a fiber-free liquid formula results in lower production of SCFA and less absorption of water and electrolytes. These changes reverse with the addition of pectin to the diet.[34] We found that a fiber-supplemented diet produced less diarrhea than a fiber-free formula in acutely ill patients.[35]

POSTRESECTIONAL DIARRHEA

Patients undergoing resections of the gastrointestinal tract often develop diarrhea in the postoperative period. Gastric resection can lead to diarrhea owing to rapid emptying of hyperosmolar foods into the jejunum (dumping syndrome) or because of concomitant vagotomy. Small bowel resection may result in diarrhea, depending on the extent and site of resection. Up to 50% of the small bowel length can be excised without malabsorptive diarrhea; however, resection of more than 80% of the small bowel will inexorably lead to malabsorption and dependency on parenteral nutrition.[36] Resection of large segments of ileum is more likely to result in diarrhea than resection of an equivalent length of jejunum, mainly from the interruption of the enterohepatic circulation of bile salts. Resection of the right colon and ileocecal valve accelerates intestinal transit and may produce diarrhea until adaptation occurs.

Postgastrectomy syndromes can be improved with dietary modifications and medications that reduce intestinal transit. Dumping symptoms can be attenuated by apportioning meals in small amounts, avoiding concentrated sweets, and frequently diluting the osmolar load with water. Water soluble fibers, such as pectin and guar gum, are effective in reducing gastric emptying and in slowing small bowel transit.[37] Octreotide, a somatostatin analogue, has been used successfully to treat dumping syndrome because of its inhibitory properties on gastrointestinal motility and secretion.

Short bowel syndrome is characterized by malabsorptive diarrhea requiring parenteral nutrition in order to maintain fluid and nutrient balances. Some patients may develop sufficient hyperplasia and hypertrophy of the remaining bowel to compensate for lost bowel. All of these patients develop gastric hypersecretion that can contribute to malabsorption and diarrhea, in addition to exposing the patient to the risk of peptic ulcer disease. Agents that block gastric secretion (H2 antagonists) have become routine in the management of patients with short bowel syndrome. Some patients will benefit from the administration of cholestyramine, a bile salt binder; however, the diarrhea will worsen in others. Pectin has a variety of helpful effects, including delayed gastric emptying, bile salt binding, slowing of intestinal transit, stimulation of mucosal cell proliferation, and rescue of malabsorbed calories in the form of SCFA.

Segmental resections of the colon usually are well tolerated without the development of diarrhea. Regardless of the segment and length of intestine resected, many patients develop diarrhea when oral feedings resume. A common cause of early diarrhea is the use of full liquids which contain hyperosmolar liquids and lactose.

■ CONSTIPATION IN THE HOSPITALIZED PATIENT

The significance of constipation is perceived differently by individuals, depending upon their preconceived notions of normality for frequency of bowel movements. Some patients are deeply concerned if they do not evacuate daily, while others are not even aware of how frequently they have bowel movements. Aside from the paucity of bowel movements, patients with chronic constipation may complain of various symptoms. In a survey of patients with constipation, 50% perceived constipation as the low frequency of bowel movements; 20% perceived it as the necessity to strain, stool hardness, and occurrence of pain; and 30% perceived it as a combination of both.[38] Frequency of bowel movements varies according to the volume of stools, which in turn, depends on the fiber content of the diet. Populations in North America and Western Europe eliminate between 80 and 120 gm/day of stool while populations in Third World countries eliminate 300 to 500 gm/day of stool.[39] Populations that consume a Western diet have a frequency of stools ranging from three movements per day to three movements per week in 98% of subjects.[40] Criteria proposed by Devroede for the diagnosis of constipation are (1) stool weight less than 35 gm/day, (2) weekly stool frequency less than three for women and five for men while consuming more than 30 gm of dietary fiber daily, and (3) more than 3 days without a bowel movement.[41]

ETIOLOGY

There are many causes of chronic constipation (see Table 7–6). Luminal obstructions of the colon are the most worrisome because of the possibility of obstructing

TABLE 7–6. CONSTIPATION AS EPIPHENOMENA OF OTHER DISEASES

Luminal obstruction
  Neoplasm, volvulus, intussusception, diverticular disease, Endometriosis, ischemic colitis, anastomotic stricture

Outlet obstruction
  Anal stenosis, anal fissure, rectal procidentia, rectocele, pubis rectalis syndrome, descending perineum syndrome

Visceral neuropathy
  Congenital aganglionosis (Hirshsprung's disease)
  Acquired aganglionosis (Chagas' disease)

Visceral myopathy
  Colonic inertia
  Megacolon, Megarectum

Central neuropathy
  Cerebral neoplasms, Parkinson's disease,
  Spinal cord disease (trauma, multiple sclerosis)

Psychiatric disorders
  Psychoses, depression, anorexia nervosa

Endocrine and metabolic disorders
  Hypothyroidism, hypopituitarism, diabetes mellitus
  Mucoviscidosis, porphyria, lead poisoning

colon cancer. Elderly individuals who experience a change in bowel habits always should be screened with a barium enema or colonoscopy for colon cancer. Colonic volvulus and diverticular disease are more common in the elderly than in younger patients. In young females, the colon may become involved with endometriosis and create obstruction. In patients with vascular disease in other territories (cerebral, cardiac, aortoiliac), ischemic colitis should be suspected, especially in those who have had aortic reconstruction without reimplantation of the inferior mesenteric artery. Patients with previous colonic surgery are at risk for developing anastomotic stricture, particularly those with prior low anterior resections of the rectum and stapled anastomoses.

Anorectal pathology is another common cause of chronic constipation. Patients with external hemorrhoids or anal fissure may involuntarily defer bowel movements because of the pain associated with defecation. Rectal procidentia and rectocele may physically obstruct the passage of stool through the anal canal. During defecation the anorectal angle normally increases from a resting value of 90° to approximately 135°. This angle widens with relaxation of the pubis rectalis muscle. In some individuals there is no relaxation of the pubis rectalis or there may even be a paradoxical contraction, with inability to defecate. This syndrome, called paradoxical pelvic floor contraction, spastic pelvic floor syndrome, anismus, or dyschezia can produce chronic constipation.

The innervation of the colon can be affected locally, as in Hirschsprung's and Chagas' disease, or systemically, as in spinal cord disease. Although Hirschsprung's disease is usually diagnosed in the newborn or during infancy, a few individuals are able to evacuate with the help of laxatives and enemas and do not seek medical care until adulthood. These are typically men in their twenties presenting with acute colonic complications such as obstruction, hemorrhage, or perforation. Chagas' disease is produced by the *Trypanosoma cruzi* parasite which generates a neurotoxin that selectively damages the autonomic nervous system of the colon, the esophagus, and the cardiac conduction system. This disease is endemic to South America, although some cases have been reported in Texas.[42] Constipation and neurogenic bladder may arise as sequelae of spinal cord injuries.

The largest group of patients with chronic constipation suffers from idiopathic visceral myopathy. These patients have a slow transit through the colon and, in severe instances, colonic inertia. Depending on the level of the defect, the colon may dilate proximally, leading to a megacolon with or without megarectum. Constipation owing to idiopathic megacolon often is treated with laxaties, further impairing colonic motility. Idiopathic slow transit constipation, also known as Arbuthnot Lane's disease, is almost entirely limited to women, and is commonly associated with gynecological problems (ovarian cysts, infertility and galactorrhea), epilepsy, Raynaud's phenomenon and psychiatric disorders.

The lack of symptom specificity, the wide range of potential causes, and frequent coexistence of those causes of constipation make the diagnostic process crucial. The best approach to the diagnosis and treatment of chronic constipation involves a multidisciplinary team that includes a surgeon, gastroenterologist, nutritionist, and psychologist.

DIAGNOSTIC WORK-UP OF CHRONIC CONSTIPATION

In patients with chronic constipation, several pathologies may coexist which independently can perpetuate constipation. For example, a patient may develop constipation from obstructed defecation caused by rectal intussusception and then develop a slow transit time. Therapeutic measures directed at accelerating transit (colectomy) will not help this patient unless the rectal intussusception is corrected. Consequently, patients with chronic constipation require an integrated approach to assess all potential factors affecting colonic motility and defecation.

HISTORY

A detailed history will assist in determining whether additional investigation should be made. Many patients with irritable bowel syndrome feel a compelling need to evacuate daily and often complain of bloating and abdominal discomfort if more than 24 hours have elapsed without a bowel movement. Upon further questioning, many also are found to have periods of diarrhea alternating with constipation. This association should alert the surgeon to the diagnosis of irritable bowel syndrome. It is not uncommon for these patients to seek surgical intervention for relief of symptoms, but even if incidental abnormalities can be corrected (eg, rectocele) symptoms will persist, or even worsen, after surgery.

When the history confirms the diagnosis of chronic constipation (a consistent pattern of fewer than two bowel movements per week) a full investigation is warranted. Identification of events prior to the onset of symptoms may help determine the cause of constipation. For example, in the presence of rectal intussusception or prolapse, hysterectomy or posterior colporrhaphy tend to aggravate obstructed defecation. Exercise or lifting may precipitate a failure of the pelvic floor, particularly in multiparous women.

Clinical signs of obstructed defecation include straining, rectal fullness, an urgency to defecate, and a sense of incomplete evacuation. Some patients develop elaborate methods of rectal emptying, such as rectal intubation and irrigation. Others require direct manual disimpaction of the rectum or through the vagina when stool is impacted in a rectocele. Patients with procidentia can feel the rectum slide through the anal canal and often have to reduce it manually. Urinary stress incontinence due to cystocele is very common in patients with procidentia or rectocele.

PHYSICAL EXAMINATION

Abdominal examination is usually unrewarding in chronic constipation. Rectal examination, however, can provide important information. The anus should be inspected for hemorrhoids and fissures that may cause painful defecation. Elderly individuals with chronic constipation often develop a descending perineum syndrome. The anus normally lies above a line connecting the coccyx and the symphysis pubis. In descending perineum syndrome, the anus will lie several centimeters below the ischial tuberosities; it is drawn lower upon straining. Partial or full thickness rectal prolapse in these patients also may be present. Partial thickness prolapse presents with radial folds, whereas full thickness prolapse presents with circular folds. Digital assessment of sphincter tone and sensory thresholds may reveal anal stricture, anal sphincter weakness (long-standing prolapse), and decreased sensation (neuropathies). Women with symptoms of obstructed defecation should be given a complete pelvic exam to rule out contributing gynecological problems, such as cystocele, enterocele, or uterine prolapse. Rectoceles can be demonstrated by assessing the thickness of the rectovaginal septum during a combined rectal and vaginal exam.

The dynamics of the rectal wall can be visualized through a rigid proctosigmoidoscope by asking the patient to perform a Valsalva maneuver. In cases of intussusception ("hidden" prolapse) the folding of the rectal wall can be seen. If the sigmoidoscope is introduced beyond the rectum, it will descend through the anus when the patient performs a Valsalva maneuver. Proctosigmoidoscopy may also reveal mucosal pathology such as a solitary rectal ulcer or colitis cystica profunda (often associated with rectal intussusception). A stool sample should always be obtained for occult blood testing. The presence of blood in stool, overt or occult, should alert the physician to the possibility of luminal pathology.

SPECIALIZED RADIOGRAPHY

All patients with possible luminal pathology should undergo a double contrast barium enema and a colonic transit-time measurement. In patients with obstructed defecation, a defecography and anorectal manometry should also be obtained. A double contrast barium enema may demonstrate a luminal narrowing causing obstruction, a mass leading to intussusception, and dilatation of the colon.

A colonic transit time is mandatory for a definitive confirmation of the diagnosis of constipation; it also assesses severity and locates segmental defects versus a global defect in colonic transit. The study is performed 48 hours after discontinuation of laxatives. According to the original method, described by Hinton, Lennard-Jones and Young,[43] 20 radiopaque barium-impregnated markers are ingested before breakfast. Plain films of the abdomen are obtained on days 4 and 6. The number of markers and their distribution along the colon are recorded. A normal colonic transit should carry the markers throughout the colon in 5 days. A slow transit is demonstrated by a persistence of markers in the colon beyond day 6.

Defecography involves instilling contrast media into the rectum and recording the act of defecation with static radiographs and videofluoroscopy videotape.[44,45] The static radiographs allow measurement of the anorectal angle and the relationship between the anus and the coccyx/pubis plane under resting conditions and upon straining. The videotape is used to detect "hidden" prolapse or rectal intussusception, which can be missed in static radiographs, especially if only part of the rectal circumference is involved. Videofluoroscopy also demonstrates the coordinated function of the muscles involved in defecation.

ANORECTAL LABORATORY

Functional studies of the defecation physiology are essential in deciding whether surgery is indicated in a patient with chronic constipation.[46,47] These studies include anorectal manometry, electromyography, sensory thresholds measurement, and colonic myoelectric activity.

Anorectal manometry most commonly is performed through open-tipped multilumen catheters perfused with fluid. These catheters are connected to a transducer and register the internal and external sphincter pressures and the presence of the anorectal inhibitory reflex.[48] In patients with Hirschsprung's disease, the anorectal inhibitory reflex is abolished.[49] The results of anorectal manometry are less consistent in patients with idiopathic constipation. In these patients, some authors have reported elevated resting anal pressures,[50] while others have found reduced resting pressures.[51] Through endoscopically placed colonic mucosal electrodes electromyography records the action potential derived from the muscles of defecation.[52] In patients with paradoxical pelvic floor contraction, the pubis rectalis muscle remains contracted during defecation. In patients with long-standing constipation, the nerves supplying the external sphincter and the puborectalis muscles can be damaged as a result of perineal descent.[53] The pattern of myoelectrical activity in response to medications can differentiate between neurogenic and myogenic disorders and can indicate the appropriate therapy. Sensory threshold measurements may disclose a high rectal threshold (insensitivity) in patients with idiopathic constipation and the extent of denervation or myopathy in the colonic wall.

A rectal biopsy should be obtained in all patients with suspected aganglionosis.[54] The histological specimens are examined for ganglion cells.[55] Since acetylcholinesterase is increased significantly in Hirschsprung's disease, a more reliable method for diagnosis of this disease is the staining of biopsy specimens for acetylcholinesterase.[56] This method has a 99% accuracy rate in differentiating Hirschsprung's disease from idiopathic constipation. Routine hematoxylin/eosin staining fails to demonstrate ganglion cells in 39% of patients without Hirschsprung's disease.

TREATMENT FOR CHRONIC CONSTIPATION

Better understanding of the role of dietary fiber in colonic physiology has dramatically changed the management of chronic constipation. Dennis Burkitt is credited with the pioneering work on dietary fiber, colonic transit time, and the epidemiology of colonic diseases.[12] More recent studies demonstrate a wide variety of components in dietary fiber with diverse effects on colonic physiology.[57] Structural plant fibers, such as the celluloses and hemicelluloses present in bran, are fermented only partially by bacteria; thus, they hold water, produce bulk, and thereby accelerate transit time.[58] The use of fiber as a bulking agent is more "physiologic" and is preferred over the laxatives and cathartics used in the "prefiber era." Laxatives and cathartics stimulate elicit stools by increasing colonic secretion and motility. When used chronically in combination with a low fiber intake, they result in an inert colon.

Constipation caused by luminal obstruction requires immediate treatment, usually surgical. Often pathologies producing luminal obstruction coexist, such as synchronous diverticulosis and cancer, or intussusception and cancer. Another cause of luminal obstruction is anastomotic stricture. Because most surgeons reserve the use of staplers for low anterior resection of the rectum, these anastomotic strictures usually are found in close proximity to the anal verge. Transabdominal resection of the stricture and recreation of a coloproctostomy can be technically impossible. When possible, resection of a strictured anastomosis in the low rectum can risk the function of the sphincter complex.

Constipation as a result of outlet obstruction can be caused by anal or rectal abnormalities. Anal fissure is best treated by lateral subcutaneous internal sphincterotomy.[59] Anal stenosis can be a sequela of a hemorrhoidectomy or Crohn's disease. The treatment of anal stenosis ranges from simple dilatation to anoplasty, depending on its cause and severity. In patients with chronic constipation caused by rectal pathologies, colonic transit studies play a major role for the surgeon when deciding what operation to perform. A patient with rectal prolapse and a normal colonic transit can be treated by rectopexy. However, rectal prolapse with a slow colonic transit and a redundant sigmoid colon is treated best by sigmoidectomy with tacking of the distal rectum to the presacral fascia.

When performing a rectopexy for obstructed defecation, a posterior rectopexy is the preferred procedure, rather than an anterior sling.[60] In an anterior rectopexy, the rectum becomes constrained, either by the sacrum or the sling itself, and fecal impaction may ensue, particularly when the constipation is combined with a slow transit time. Placing the sling posteriorly, first on the sacrum and then on the sides of the rectum, leaves the anterior wall of the rectum free to expand during defecation. Postoperative hemorrhage and urogenital dysfunction is less common with the posterior approach because it avoids the presacral venous plexus and sacral nerves. In the posterior rectopexy, the sling first is sutured to the midline of the sacrum, which is free of vessels and nerves, and then to the sides of the rectum.[61] In an anterior rectopexy, the sling is laid over the anterior and lateral aspects of the rectum and then sutured to

the sides of the sacrum where nerves exit the spine and veins join to form the presacral plexus. In addition, the triangular shape of the sarcum forces the creation of a cone, with the sling narrower at the caudad aspect. However, the posterior approach creates a line of sutures that allows the sling to wrap around the rectum in a cylindrical shape.

Which synthetic material is best to use to create a sling is still a matter of debate. In Europe, an Avalon sponge has been used successfully.[62] This material promotes intense fibrosis that firmly attaches the rectum to the side walls of the pelvis. However, Avalon has been implicated in the development of sarcomas in experimental animals and is not approved for use in the United States. Teflon and dacron can be used, provided the procedure does not involve entering the intestinal lumen. Polypropelene mesh has gained a greater acceptance in the United States, since it creates a strong sling that becomes included in autogenous tissues.

The presence of a rectocele, in association with rectal intussusception or prolapse, requires a surgical approach through both the perineum and the abdomen. The rectum is dissected from the vagina via either a transvaginal or a transrectal approach[63] prior to the rectopexy. Once the rectum has been reduced out of the sacral hollow via traction from above, the rectovaginal septum is reinforced with sutures (colporrhaphy), and the redundant vaginal wall is excised. Patients with a previous hysterectomy may have an unsupported vaginal cuff, rendering a weak pelvic floor that may cause other organs to prolapse. In such cases, the vaginal cuff should be sutured to the sacrum and the excess of peritoneum in the Douglas pouch should be excised. Pelvic floor disorders present in various combinations and may be diagnosed first by a gynecologist, a coloproctologist or a urologist. The surgical treatment requires an integrated approach designed to address all of the pelvic floor abnormalities at once.

Visceral neuropathies affecting the colon are the anganglionoses, congenital or acquired. The acquired form (Chagas' disease) is caused by neurotoxins produced by *Trypanosoma cruzi*. Patients with Chagas' disease develop constipation and megacolon during the course of several years. Most of these patients can be treated conservatively with laxatives and enemas, although some require urgent surgery for perforation or volvulus. The definitive treatment for Chagasic megacolon is subtotal colectomy and ileorectal anastomosis.[64]

Congenital megacolon usually becomes symptomatic soon after birth, although some patients with milder forms of Hirschsprung's disease (short segment, late onset) do not seek medical attention until adulthood. Congenital megacolon always requires surgical treatment. In newborns, a temporary colostomy is created as a temporizing measure until a body weight of 20 lbs is reached. The definitive treatment for early-onset Hirschsprung's disease is segmental resection of the diseased colon and endoanal or coloanal anastomosis. In late-onset Hirschsprung's disease anorectal myomectomy is the operation of choice.[65] This operation is essentially an extended internal sphincterotomy that includes the muscularis of the aganglionic segment, usually 8 to 10 cm from the dentate line. With longer aganglionic segments, or after failed anorectal myomectomy, a low anterior resection of the rectum with coloanal anastomosis is recommended.[66]

Most patients with chronic constipation suffer from an idiopathic visceral myopathy. The objective signs of constipation are usually found in association with additional complaints not solely attributable to constipation.[67] In fact, many of these patients meet the criteria that define irritable bowel syndrome. As mentioned above, appropriate therapy is best determined by a multidisciplinary team. In those patients selected for surgery, the procedure is planned based on the extent and severity of the myopathy, as determined by colonic transit studies. When the rectum is spared by the myopathy, a subtotal colectomy with ileorectal anastomosis is the preferred procedure, although some surgeons prefer a cecoproctostomy in order to reduce diarrhea.[68] With rectal involvement, a restorative proctocolectomy with ileal pouch anal anastomosis is now the treatment of choice.[69]

In treating chronic constipation caused by central neuropathies such as Parkinson's disease, multiple sclerosis, amyotrophic lateral sclerosis, or spinal cord injury, a combination of bulking agents and enemas can establish a pattern of regular bowel movements. However, for some paraplegic patients who also suffer from incontinence and nonhealing decubitus ulcers, a colostomy can provide greater relief and simplify their care. To prevent fecal impaction, a transverse colostomy is preferred to sigmoid colostomy.

Constipation related to psychiatric, metabolic, and endocrine disorders is managed conservatively. These conditions must be ruled out prior to performing surgery for visceral myopathy.

FACTORS CAUSING CONSTIPATION

Constipation is highly prevalent in hospitalized patients (Table 7–7). One of the causes of constipation is the lack of sufficient fiber in the diet, consumed orally or received via tube feeding. Immobilization in bed, pain, and analgesic use are other factors causing constipation. In the critically ill patient, dehydration, electrolyte imbalance, and uremia contribute to a slower colonic transit time. A common cause of constipation and fecal impaction in the hospital is the barium used for contrast radiographs of the gastrointestinal tract.

TABLE 7–7. CAUSES OF CONSTIPATION IN THE HOSPITALIZED PATIENT

Bowel rest
Low fiber tube feedings
Immobilization
Dehydration, hypokalemia, uremia
Narcotics, anticholinergics, antidepressant, iron, barium
Acute intestinal pseudo-obstruction (Ogilvie syndrome)

COLONIC PSEUDO-OBSTRUCTION

A serious form of constipation seen in surgical patients is acute intestinal pseudo-obstruction or Ogilvie's syndrome.[70] This syndrome is characterized by acute dilatation of the cecum and ascending colon. The pathogenesis of this syndrome is not fully understood; one hypothesis suggests a massive sympathetic stimulation to the spinal segments S2 to S4, creating segmental paralysis of the descending and sigmoid colon. Patients affected with Ogilvie's syndrome are usually in their sixth decade, and have suffered trauma or surgery involving the pelvis. In addition to constipation, these patients develop nausea, vomiting, abdominal pain, and fever. Occasionally, they may have diarrhea instead of constipation. Typically, the cecum is distended without a clear point of distal obstruction. When the diameter of the cecum exceeds 13 cm the chances of ischemia or perforation are high (23%). The treatment of choice is transanal decompression with colonoscopy. Surgical decompression is required when transanal decompression is not effective. This can be accomplished with a cecostomy or colostomy. In cases of ischemia, a formal resection is indicated.

■ SUMMARY AND CONCLUSIONS

Diarrhea and constipation are multifactorial phenomena of diverse etiology. Patients seeking attention for diarrhea may have malabsorptive, secretory, or exudative diarrhea. Malabsorption is common in chronic alcoholism and with mucosal abnormalities such as Crohn's disease and radiation enteritis. Secretory diarrhea is caused by infectious agents (CMV in AIDS) or endocrine tumors (VIPoma). Hospitalized patients are susceptible to developing diarrhea due to *Clostridium difficile* colitis, tube feeding intolerance and resections of segments of the GI tract. Diagnostic measures for diarrhea include stool osmolality, culture, and fat content. Diarrhea usually is treated symptomatically with binders, bacterial flora promoters, motility agents, and secretion inhibitors.

Chronic constipation can be caused by luminal or outlet obstruction, visceral neuropathy or myopathy, central neuropathy, psychiatric, and endocrine or metabolic disorders. History, physical exam, and physiological studies are essential in planning the appropriate therapy. Physiological studies include colonic transit time, defecography, anorectal manometry, electromyography, sensory thresholds and myoelectrical activity. The most common form of chronic constipation is idiopathic visceral myopathy. When surgery is required, the most common procedures performed are subtotal colectomy with ileorectal anastomosis or restorative proctocolectomy, depending on rectal involvement. In the hospital setting, patients are particularly at risk for developing acute colonic pseudo-obstruction (Ogilvie's syndrome). Disturbances of bowel transit in hospitalized patients can be reduced by the use of fiber supplements in oral diets and tube feedings, the avoidance of broad spectrum antibiotics and opiates, and adequate hydration and electrolyte homeostasis.

REFERENCES

1. Davies GJ, Crowder M, Reid B, Dickerson JWT. Bowel function measurements of individuals with different eating patterns. *Gut* 1986;27:164–169
2. Sonnenberg A, Koch TR. Epidemiology in the United States. *Dis Colon Rectum* 1989;32:1–8
3. Schouten WR, Gordon PH. Constipation. In: Gordon PH, Nivatvongs S (eds), *Principles and Practice of Surgery for the Colon, Rectum, and Anus.* St. Louis, MO: Quality Medical; 1992:907–956
4. Phillips SF, Giller J. The contribution of the colon to electrolyte and water conservation in man. *J Lab Clin Med* 1973;81:733–746
5. Devroede GJ, Phillips SF. Conservation of sodium, chloride, and water by the human colon. *Gastroenterology* 1969; 56:101–109
6. Roediger WEW. Utilization of nutrients by isolated epithelial cells of the rat colon. *Gastroenterology* 1982;83:424–429
7. Roediger WEW, Moore A. Effect of short chain fatty acids on sodium absorption in isolated human colon perfused through the vascular bed. *Dig Dis Sci* 1981;26:100–106
8. Roediger WEW, Rae DA. Trophic effects of short chain fatty acids on mucosal handling of ions by the defunctionalized colon. *Br J Surg* 1982;69:23–25
9. Roediger WEW. Role of anaerobic bacteria in the metabolic welfare of the clonic mucosa in man. *Gut* 1980;21:793–798
10. Miller TL, Wolin MJ. Fermentations by saccharolytic intestinal bacteria. *Am J Clin Nutr* 1976;32:164–172
11. Nyman M, Asp NG. Fermentation of dietary fiber components of rat intestinal tract. *Br J Nutr* 1982;47:357–366
12. Burkitt DP, Walker ARP, Painter NS. Effect of dietary fibers on stools and transit times and its role in the causation of disease. *Cancer* 1972;2:1408
13. Cumming JH, Branch WJ. Fermentation and the production of short ion and the production of short the human

14. Ritchie JA, Truelove SC, Ardran GM, Tuckey MS. Propulsion and retropulsion of normal colonic contents. *Dig Dis Sci* 1971;8:697–703
15. Drew WL, Buhles W, Erlich KS. Herpes virus infections (cytomegaiovirus, herpes simplex virus, varicella-zoster virus): how to use gangcyclovir (DHPG) and acyclovir. *Inf Dis Clin N Am* 1988;2:495
16. Wexner SD. Sexually transmitted diseases of the colon, rectum and anus. *Dis Colon Rectum* 1990;33:1048
17. Wexner SD, Smithy WB, Trillo C, et al. Emergency colectomy for cytomegaiovirus ileocolitis in patients with the acquired immune deficiency syndrome. *Dis Colon Rectum* 1988;31:755
18. Shiau YF, Feldman GM, Resnick MA, Coff PM. Stool electrolyte and osmolality measurements in the evaluation of diarrheas disorders. *Ann Int Med* 1985;102:773–775
19. Hoverstad T, Carlstedt-Duke B, Lingaas E, et al. Influence of ampicillin, clindamycin, and metronidazole on faecal excretion of short-chain fatty acids in healthy subjects. *Scand J Gastroenterol* 1986;21:621–626
20. Stark PL, Lee A, Parsonage BD. Colonization of the large bowel by *Clostridium difficile* in healthy infants: quantitative study. *Infect Immunol* 1982;35:895–899
21. McFarland LV, Mulligan ME, Kwork RYY, Stamm WE. Nosocomial acquisition of *Clostridium difficule* infection. *N Eng J Med* 1989;320:204–210
22. Peiken SR, Galdibini J, Bartlett JG. Rote of *Clostridium difficile* in a case of nonantibiotic-associated pseudomembranous colitis. *Gastroenterology* 1980;79:948–951
23. Gurian L, Ward TT, Katon RM. Possible food-borne transmission in a case of pseudomembranous colitis due to *Clostridium difficile.* Influence of gastrointestinal secretions on *Clostridium difficile* infection. *Gastroenterology* 1982;83:465–469
24. Rolfe RD. Role of volatile fatty acids in colonization resistance to *Clostridium difficule. Inf Immunol* 1984;45:185–191
25. Church JM, Fazio VW: A role for clonic stasis in the pathogenesis of disease related to *Clostridium difficile. Dis Colon Rectum* 1986;29:804–809
26. Qualman SJ, Petric M, Kermali MA, et al. *Clostridium difficile* invasion and toxin circulation in fatal pediatric pseudomembranous colitis. *Am J Clin Pathol* 1990;94:410–416
27. Burke GW, Wilson ME. Mehrez IO. Absence of diarrhea in toxic megacolon complicating *Clostridium difficile* pseudomembranous colitis. *Am J Gastroenterol* 1988;83:304–307
28. Bradley SJ, Weaver DW, Maxwell NPT, Bouwrnan DL. Surgical management of pseudomembranous colitis. *Ann Surg* 1988;54:329–332
29. Morris JB, Zollinger RM, Stellato TA. Role of surgery in antibiotic-induced pseudomembranous colitis. *Ann J Surg* 1990;160:535–539
30. Cataldi-Betcher EL, Seltzer MH, Slocum BA. Complications occurring during enteral nutrition support. *JPEN* 1983;7:546–552
31. Kelly TWJ, Patrick MR, Hillman KN. Study of diarrhea in critically ill patients. *Cell Care Med* 1983;11:7–9

32. Hill DB, Henderson LM, McClain CJ. Osmotic diarrhea induced by sugar-free theophylline solution in critically ill patients. JPEN 1991;15:332–336

33. Gottschlich MM, Warden GD, Michel MA. Diarrhea in tube-fed burn patients: incidence, etiology, nutritional impact, and prevention JPEN 1988;12:338–345

34. Zimmaro DM, Rolandelli REI, Koruda MJ, Settle RG, Rombeau JL: Isotonic tube feeding formula induces liquid stool in normal subjects: reversal by pectin. JPEN 1989;13:117–123

35. Guenter PA, Settle RG, Perlmutter S, Marino PL, DeSimone GA, Rolandelli RH: Tube feeding-related diarrhea in acutely ill patients JPEN 1991;15:277–280

36. Rombeau JL, Rolandelli RH. Enteral and parenteral nutrition in patients with enteric fistulas and short bowel syndrome. Surg Clin NA 1987;67:551–571

37. Lawetz O, Blackburn AM, Bloom SR. Effect of pectin on gastric emptying and gut hormone release in dumping syndrome. Scand J Gastroenterol 1983;18:327–336

38. Moore-Guillon V. Constipation: What does it mean? J R Soc Med 1984;77:108–110

39. Burkitt DP. Fibre as protective against gastrointestinal disease. Am J Gastroenterology 984;29:249–252

40. Connell AM, Hilton C, Irvine C, et al. Variation of bowel habit in two population samples. Br Med J 1965;2:1095–1099

41. Devroede GJ. Constipation mechanisms and management. In: Sleisenger MH, Fordtran JS (eds), Gastrointestinal Disease, 3rd ed. Philadelphia, PA: WB Saunders; 1983

42. Monroe LS. Gastrointestinal parasites. In: Berk JE (ed), Bockus Gastroenterology, 4th ed. Philadelphia, PA: WB Saunders; 1985

43. Hinton JM, Lennard-Jones JE, Young AC. A new method for studying gut transit time using radioopaque markers. Gut 1969;10:842–847

44. Mahieu P, Pringot J, Bodart P. Defecography I. Description of a new procedure and results in normal patients. Gastrointest Radiol 1984;9:247–251

45. Mahieu P, Pringot J, Bodart P. Defecography II. Contribution to the diagnosis of defecation disorders. Gastrointest Radiol 1984;9:253–261

46. Fleshman OW, Fry RD, Kodner IJ. The surgical management of constipation. Baillieres Clin Gastroenterol 1992;6:145–162

47. Bassotti G, Betti C, Pelli MA, Morelli A. Extensive investigation on clonic motility with pharmacological testing is useful for selecting surgical options in patients with inertia colica. Am J Gastroenterology 1992;87:143–147

48. Coller JA. Clinical application of anorectal manometry. Gastroenterol Clin N A 1987;16:17–33

49. Lawson JON, Nixon HH. Anal canal pressures in the diagnosis of Hirschsprung's disease. J Pediatr Surg 1967;2:544–552

50. Taylor I, Hammond P, Darby C. An assessment of anorectal motility in the management of adult megacolon. Br J Surg 1980;67:754–756

51. Read NW, Timms JM, Barfield LJ, et al. Impairment of defecation in young women with severe constipation. Gastroenterology 1986;90:53–60

52. Snooks SJ, Swash M. Electromyography and nerve latency studies. In: Gooszen HG, Hoedemaker HC, Wetermand IT, Keighley MRB (eds), Disordered Defecation. Dordrecht, The Netherlands: Nijhoff;1987

53. Snooks SJ, Bames PRH, Swash M, Henry MM. Damage to the inervation of the pelvic floor musculature in chronic constipation. Gastroenterology 1985;89:977–981

54. Aldridge RT, Campbell PE. Ganglion cell distribution in the normal rectum and anal canal: a basis for the diagnosis of Hirschsprung's disease by anorectal biopsy. J Pediatr Surg 1968;3:475–490

55. Weinberg AG. The anorectal myenteric plexus: its relation to hypoganglionosis of the colon. Am J Clin Pathol 1970;54:637–642

56. Causse E, Vaysse P, Fabre J, et al. The diagnostic value of acetylcholinesterase butyl-cholinesterase ration in Hirschsprung's disease. Am J Clin Path 1987;88:477–480

57. Kirway KO, Smith AN, McConnell AA, et al. Action of different bran preparations on colonic function. Br Med J 1974;4:187–189

58. Stephen AM, Cummings JH. Water-holding by dietary fiber in vitro and its relationship to fecal output in man. Gut 1979;10:722–729

59. Notaras MJ. The treatment of anal fissure by lateral subcutaneous internal sphincterotomy—a technique and results. Br J Surg 1971;58:96–100

60. Ripstein CB. Definitive corrective surgery. Dis Colon Rectum 1972;15:334–346

61. Yoshioka K, Heyen F, Keighley MRB. Functional results after abdominal rectopexy for rectal prolapse. Dis Colon Rectum 1989;32:835–838

62. Wells C: New operation for rectal prolapse. Proc R Soc Med 1959;52:602–603

63. Sehapakayak S. Transrectal repair of rectocele: an extended armamentarium of colorectal surgeons: a report of 355 cases. Dis Colon Rectum 1985;18:237–243

64. Cutait DE, Cutait R. Surgery of Chagasic megacolon. World J Surg 1991;15:188

65. Bentley JFR. Some new observations on megacolon in infancy and childhood with special reference to the management of megasigmoid and megarectum. Dis Colon Rectum 1964;7:462–470

66. McCready RA, Beart RW Jr. Adult Hirschsprung's disease: results of surgical treatment at the Mayo Clinic. Dis Colon Rectum 1980;23:401

67. Kamm MA, Hawley PR, Lennard-Jones JE. Outcome of colectomy for severe idiopathic constipation. Gut 1988;29:969

68. Preston DM, Hawley PR, Lennard-Jones JE, Todd IP. Results of colectomy for severe idiopathic constipation in women (Arbuthnot Lane's disease). Br J Surg 1984;71:547

69. Nicholls RJ, Kamm MA. Proctocolectomy with restorative ileoanal reservoir for severe idiopathic constipation: report of two cases. Dis Colon Rectum 1988;31:968

70. Vanek VW, Al-Salti M. Acute pseudo-obstruction of the colon (Ogilvie's syndrome): an analysis of 400 cases. Dis Colon Rectum 1986;29:203–210

8

Abdominal Pain

David W. McFadden

Nearly everyone has experienced abdominal pain. Whether self-limited, as with gastroenteritis, or imminently life-threatening, as in perforated peptic ulcer or colon cancer, the physical and psychosocial impacts may be overwhelming. Recent studies have demonstrated a 25% prevalence of severe gastrointestinal symptoms in the elderly, with chronic constipation and abdominal pain predominating.[1,2] Acute and chronic forms of digestive diseases account for approximately 10% of the cost of health care in the United States and more than 200 000 deaths per year.[3] Approximately 250 000 people miss work each day because of digestive or abdominal problems. Abdominal pain accounts for more hospital admissions in the United States than any other disease category.[4]

The physician and patient usually differ in their perspectives on the complaints of the patient. This disparity in perception is sometimes an aid, but may be an impediment, especially when the physician's orientation to disease categories results in a perceived dehumanization of the patient. In evaluating abdominal pain, it is important to consider the patient as well as any underlying disease.

Symptoms are the subjective manifestations of a disturbance in function and represent pathophysiologic states rather than specific diseases.[5] In the gastrointestinal tract, numerous alterations in physiologic function can be implicated that affect secretion, absorption, motility, synthesis, digestion, and transport. The resultant symptoms include abdominal (or extraabdominal) pain, dysphagia or odynophagia, anorexia, weight loss,

nausea and vomiting, bloating or distention, constipation, flatulence, and diarrhea.[6] Signs of disease are the objective demonstrations of a pathologic process. These include tenderness, rigidity, masses, altered bowel sounds, bleeding, malnutrition, jaundice, and stigmata of hepatic dysfunction.[5,7]

The case history remains one of the most useful tools in the diagnosis of digestive diseases.[3] The surgical consultant should review thoroughly every detail of the illness with the patient. The art of physical examination is also of great importance in the diagnosis of abdominal pain. Combining the elicited symptoms from a complete history and the signs from a comprehensive physical examination allows the surgeon to establish a differential diagnosis. It is important to formulate a thorough, but cost-effective diagnostic evaluation, which may require blood tests, radiographs, and histologic confirmation.[8]

■ PAIN

Pain, from the Latin *poena* meaning punishment, penalty, or torment, is the singular sensory experience that humans use to identify disease within themselves. It is one of the greatest motivational drives known to man.[5] Most diseases of the abdominal viscera are associated with pain sometime during their course (Fig 8–1). A brief review of abdominal embryology and pain physiology will assist the clinician in evaluating the patient with acute or chronic abdominal pain.

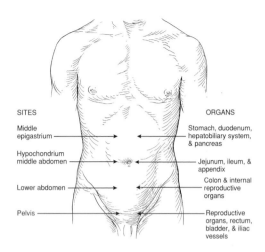

Figure 8–1. Pain map of the abdomen.

The gastrointestinal tract comprises a foregut, midgut, and hindgut. Each segment has its own blood supply and innervation and retains these relationships throughout development and into adulthood. The foregut extends from the oropharynx to the duodenum at the level of the entrance of the common bile duct, and includes the pancreas, liver, biliary tree, and spleen. The midgut is composed of the distal duodenum, jejunum, ileum, appendix, ascending colon, and proximal two-thirds of the transverse colon. The hindgut consists of the remainder of the colon and rectum down to the cloacal bulge, which constitutes the interface between the surface ectoderm and endoderm of the cloaca, corresponding to the dentate line.[5,8]

The peritoneum is a continuous visceral and parietal layer. Although both layers are mesodermally derived, they develop separately. Importantly, and for diagnostic reasons, the nerve supply to each layer is separate. The visceral layer, ie, the layer surrounding all intraabdominal organs, is supplied by autonomic nerves (sympathetic and parasympathetic), and the parietal peritoneum is supplied by somatic innervation (spinal nerves).[4] The pathways relaying the sensation of pain differ for each layer and differ in quality as well. Visceral pain is characteristically dull, crampy, or aching; parietal pain is sharp, severe, and persistent.[8]

Normal embryologic development of the abdominal viscera proceeds with bilateral midline autonomic innervation that results in visceral pain, usually perceived as arising from the midline. The position of pain in the midline is determined by the embryologic origin of the involved viscus. Epigastric pain is typical of foregut origin. Periumbilical pain signifies pain emanating from the midgut. Hypogastric or lower abdominal midline pain indicates a hindgut origin. Pelvic pain is more typical of disease originating in structures derived from the cloaca.[5]

For abdominal pain to be recognized by the patient, nociceptors, or pain receptors, must be noxiously stimulated. Two types of neuronal fibers are involved. A-δ fibers are rapid transmitters and give rise to sharp, well-localized pain sensations. These fibers are distributed to muscle and skin and are involved with the somatic pain transmission through spinal nerves. C fibers are slow transmitters and generate the sensation of dull, poorly localized pain that is more gradual in its onset and of longer duration.[8] These fibers are located intramurally in hollow viscera and in the capsule of solid organs. They are found in muscle, periosteum, and the parietal peritoneum. These fibers are involved in visceral pain transmission through the autonomic nervous system.[5]

Different neural pathways are responsible for pain mediation, depending on whether the source of the pain is the parietal peritoneum or the visceral peritoneum. The anterior and lateral abdominal walls are supplied by nerves arising from spinal segments T7 to L1. The posterior abdominal wall is innervated from spinal segments L2 to L5. Pain arising from the abdominal wall is relayed to the spinal cord through the spinal nerves. Because these pain fibers enter the spinal cord ipsilaterally, pain is perceived as originating from that side. Also, such pain localizes to the area of the abdomen from which it originates. In contrast, pain arising from intraabdominal viscera is perceived to arise in the midline because sensory input from such viscera enters the spinal cord on both sides.[4,5]

Abdominal pain can be divided into three categories: visceral, somatic, and referred. The aforementioned intramural sensory receptors of the abdominal organs are responsible for visceral pain. A diverse group of destructive stimuli to the abdominal viscera are painless. For example, almost all abdominal organs are insensitive to pinching, burning, stabbing, cutting, and electrical and thermal stimulation. The same is true for the application of acid and alkali to normal mucosa.[8]

There are four general classes of visceral stimulation that result in abdominal pain. These include (1) stretching and contraction, (2) traction, compression, and torsion, (3) stretch, and (4) certain chemicals. The mediating receptors for these responses are located intramurally in hollow organs, on serosal structures such as the visceral peritoneum and capsule of solid organs, intramesenteric (especially associated with large mesenteric vessels and ligaments), and within the mucosa. These receptors are polymodal, or responsive to both mechanical and chemical stimuli. Mucosal receptors respond primarily to chemical stimulation.[8] The major forces that evoke visceral pain arise from geometric forces, such as stretching and distention, that result in increased wall tension. Other factors held responsible for visceral pain include ischemia and inflammation.[4] Visceral pain almost always heralds in-

TABLE 8–1. POSSIBLE ORIGINS FOR REFERRED PAIN

Right Shoulder
  Diaphragm
  Gallbladder
  Liver capsule
  Right-sided pneumoperitoneum

Left Shoulder
  Diaphragm
  Spleen
  Tail of pancreas
  Stomach
  Splenic flexure
  (Colon)
  Left-sided pneumo-peritoneum

Right Scapula
  Gallbladder
  Biliary tree

Left Scapula
  Spleen
  Tail of pancreas

Groin/Genitalia
  Kidney
  Ureter
  Aorta/Iliac artery

Back-Midline
  Pancreas
  Duodenum
  Aorta

traabdominal disease, but may not indicate the need for surgical therapy. When visceral pain becomes superceded by somatic pain, the need for surgical intervention becomes likely.[9]

Somatic or visceral pain arises from irritation of the parietal peritoneum. Mediated mainly by spinal nerve fibers that supply the abdominal wall, somatic pain is localized and is perceived as arising from one of the four quadrants of the abdominal wall. In contrast to visceral pain where geometric changes are responsible for the stimulation of nerve endings, somatic pain arises as a response to acute changes in pH or temperature, as seen in bacterial or chemical inflammation.[5,8] In addition, somatic pain is felt in response to sudden increases in pressure, as with a surgical incision. Somatic pain is perceived as sharp and pricking and is usually constant. In many clinical situations, it is probable that the perception of pain results from multiple stimuli. The pain of pancreatic cancer probably arises from the combination of serosal stretch, vascular and mesenteric compression, and direct neural infiltration. The sensitivity of visceral receptors also are affected by circumstances. Pressure or chemical application to normal gastric mucosa is usually painless, but if the mucosa is inflamed, these same stimuli are quite painful.[8]

Referred pain is felt in an area of the body other than the site of its origin, and is one of the characteristic qualities of abdominal pain. Referred pain usually arises from a deep structure, is superficial at its distant presenting location, and frequently is sharp, localized, and persistent at the distant site. It occurs secondary to the existence of shared central pathways for afferent neurons arising from different sites.[9] Two associated features of referred pain are skin hyperalgesia and increased muscle tone of the abdominal wall. A classic example is the ruptured spleen that results in irritation of the left hemidiaphragm, which is innervated by the same cervical nerves. In this setting, referred pain is perceived as arising in the left shoulder (Kehr's sign), also supplied by those nerve roots. A knowledge of referred pain and its patterns may be of diagnostic assistance when other evidence of disease is lacking or absent (Table 8–1).

■ ACUTE ABDOMINAL PAIN

Acute abdominal pain is loosely defined as pain that is present for less than eight hours. The key to the management of the patient with acute abdominal pain is early diagnosis. No aspect of diagnosis is more important than a careful and thorough history. If possible, it is best to allow the patient to give his or her entire current history before asking specific questions. This should include a past medical history and information concerning associated illnesses. A history of prior similar symptoms also should be sought, as well as the presence of any prodromal symptoms.[9]

The character and onset of the pain are important. Colicky pain usually indicates some type of obstructive process, as in bowel obstruction, passing a ureteral calculus, or acute cholecystitis. Colic represents hyperperistalsis of the smooth muscle in an attempt to move fluid or an object past the obstruction. Between attacks, the pain lessens or disappears. During attacks, the pain is persistent and unrelenting. The pain seen with infectious processes such as appendicitis or diverticulitis is sustained and gradually worsens over time. Clues to the underlying cause of pain may be deduced by the type of onset. Pancreatitis is usually gradual in onset and commonly follows an episode of alcohol abuse. In contrast, a perforated hollow viscus produces a sudden onset of pain that the patient may be able to time precisely. The location of the pain is very helpful in establishing the diagnosis. This is especially true with somatic pain that results from an irritation of the parietal peritoneum (Fig 8–1).

Other factors must also be considered in the evaluation of the patient with abdominal pain. These include any previous history of intraabdominal disease, previous abdominal surgery, and current medications. Familial or concomitant diseases in family members also should be sought. A woman's precise menstrual history should be obtained because this may be the sole clue to the presence of gynecologic pathology.[10]

The first and most important step in the physical examination of the patient with an acute abdomen is a careful observation of the body habitus and facial expression of the patient. An unwillingness to change body position suggests an underlying peritonitis. Hip flexion with the knees drawn up to maintain comfort suggests tension on the abdominal wall and possible peritoneal irritation.[9] Restriction of diaphragmatic excursion with respiration, as noted by shallow breathing and the use of accessory respiratory muscles, is also consistent with peritoneal irritation. In contrast, the presence of colicky pain frequently is manifested by intense movement in an effort to alleviate pain followed by restful intervals between colicky periods. Inspection of the abdomen for hernial bulges, masses, distention, or areas of inflammation should follow. Careful auscultation of the abdominal cavity for the presence or absence and quality of bowel sounds is performed. The presence and location of bruits should be noted. A careful auscultation of the chest, particularly in the diaphragmatic area, should be undertaken to document diaphragmatic movement and to search for the possibility of basilar pneumonia that may simulate an acute abdominal condition. Gentle palpation of all quadrants of the abdomen should be performed last. Gentle, rather superficial, palpation of the abdomen should be performed initially, proceeding from the quadrant with the least symptomatology to the most painful area. Peritoneal signs or masses, suggested by the superficial exam, then may be confirmed by a deeper, but still gentle, palpation. Classic rebound tenderness is frought with examiner error, and a percussion test is kinder and more specific.[5] Having the patient cough, laugh, or maximally distend the abdomen may localize the disease, especially in children.[11] Patients in pain who have been examined by previous unskilled examiners are often quite sensitized to the manipulations that are used to elicit rebound. Therefore, a skilled examiner must use other diversions to confirm peritonitis. Other techniques, such as using a stethoscope to depress and release the abdomen, the so-called stethoscope test, is useful. Similarly, shaking the pelvis from side to side may elicit true rebound tenderness. Uncommonly, hyperesthesia is present, but is defined as exquisitely sensitive skin to gentle touch. Hyperesthesia exists because the dermatome corresponding to that supplied by the same nerve roots as an area of parietal peritoneum is being irritated by an intraabdominal inflammatory process.

Many laboratory tests may offer useful information in the evaluation of the patient with an acute abdominal condition. Minimally, a complete blood count, urine analysis, serum amylase, and, for women with lower abdominal pain, a beta human chorionic gonadotropin, or pregnancy test, should be requested. A set of serum electrolytes, blood urea nitrogen, creatinine, and glucose are useful in determining the hydration status, renal function, and basic metabolic state of the patient. Liver chemistries are helpful in the patient with upper abdominal pain or stigmata of liver disease. In general, laboratory tests should not be performed unless their results could alter the need for additional tests or therapy.[12] Frequently, at the time of venipuncture, an intravenous cannula can be inserted and used for hydration and/or administration of medication.

Four radiologic views of the chest and abdomen are essential in the patient without an obvious diagnosis.[13] The physician must be aware of the time, and the stress a trip to the radiology suite creates for the patient, and assure the stability of the hemodynamic status of the patient prior to this endeavor. An upright and supine film of the abdomen and an upright and lateral radiograph of the chest then are performed. Although only 10% of patients with an acute abdomen have abnormalities on screening roentgenography, it is still suggested to obtain them unless a clear-cut diagnosis is established.[14] Pneumoperitoneum, gas-fluid levels, fecaliths, gallstones, ascites, and obliteration of the psoas shadows are all helpful diagnostic findings that can be seen on the four screening films.[15] Contrast gastrointestinal studies, ultrasonography, computed axial tomographic scans, and arteriography may all be suggested or required given the findings and clinical suspicions of the evaluating physician.[16,17]

No laboratory or radiologic maneuver should be performed unless its result will alter the need for additional tests or treatment. If the patient clinically has appendicitis, of what benefit is an abdominal series to look for a fecalith? Also, test results should not duplicate previous tests. Gallstones delineated by ultrasound do not require additional radiologic examinations. A balance should be sought and should include cost, yield, morbidity, and accuracy. Finally, avoid the "Mount Everest" syndrome,[18] wherein a test is performed because the facilities exist for its performance.

Numerous surgical causes exist for the patient presenting with acute abdominal pain, and these are covered in those chapters dealing with the specifics of organ systems. A recent review of nearly 1200 patients presenting to the emergency ward with abdominal pain affords some interesting findings.[19] The most common diagnosis was nonspecific abdominal pain, occurring in 35% of patients. Appendicitis (17%), intestinal obstruction (15%), urologic causes (6%), and gallstones (5%) were the leading surgical causes. The largest number of admissions occurred in the age groups 10 to 29 years old (31%) and 60 to 79 years old (29%). Surgical procedures were required in 47% of patients. The increased proportion of elderly patients in this recent study mirrors the rise in the elderly population. Large series of elderly patients presenting with acute abdominal pain have found the leading diagnoses to be cholelithiasis, nonspecific pain, malignancy, incarcerated hernia, ileus, and gastroduodenal ulcer.[5] The presence of comorbid processes, especially cardiovascular disease, stresses the need for rapid diagnosis and timely operative surgery, if needed.[2]

■ GYNECOLOGIC CAUSES OF THE ACUTE ABDOMEN

Organ systems other than those classically associated within the realm of the alimentary tract also must be considered. Gynecologic causes of acute abdominal pain include pelvic inflammatory disease, ectopic pregnancy, tubo-ovarian cysts, torsion, hemorrhage or abscess, and Mittelschmerz disease.[10] Pelvic inflammatory disease (PID) must be considered in virtually every woman of reproductive age with lower abdominal pain. It can be divided into tubo-ovarian abscess with or without rupture. Whereas PID is usually appreciated bilaterally, the abscess is unilateral in over 70% of cases. Acute pain is reported by 90% of patients, fever/chills by 50%, fever in 60%, and leukocytosis in 68%.[10] Pelvic examination usually reveals extreme pelvic tenderness and increased pain on cervical motion.[20] Peritoneal signs in the upper abdomen suggest leakage or rupture, usually requiring surgical intervention. Differentiation of pelvic inflammatory disease from acute appendicitis is particularly difficult, especially in women of childbearing age, and the rate of false positive explorations approaches 40%. Table 8–2 outlines a few of the salient differences.

Ectopic pregnancies occur in 1 of 200 pregnancies, leading to 50 000 cases per year in the United State. Risk factors include prior slapingitis, tubal ligation, prior tubal repair, presence of an intrauterine device, and prior ectopic pregnancy. Pain and abnormal uterine bleeding are seen in 97% and 86% of patients, respectively.[21] Chorionic gonadotropin testing and culdocentesis are essential for diagnosis.

Hemorrhage from functional ovarian cysts also can simulate an acute surgical abdomen. Symptoms typically begin at or near the time of ovulation. Pain is classically severe, abrupt in onset, and frequently bilateral. Serum pregnancy testing should distinguish this process from ectopic pregnancy. Operation may not be required in the former process. Adnexal torsion presents with lower abdominal, lateralized pain that may be colicky. As with other pelvic conditions, ultrasonography and laparoscopy are helpful tools in diagnosis and management.[12]

TABLE 8–2. APPENDICITIS VS PELVIC INFLAMMATORY DISEASE

Finding	Appendicitis	PID
Nausea, Vomiting	+++	+
Menstrual cycle	No Preference	60% in first 14 days
History of venereal disease	+	+++
Duration of symptoms	32 hours	65 hours
Cervical motion of adnexal tenderness	+	+++
Guarding, tenderness	Right lower quadrant	Bilateral

■ UROLOGIC CAUSES OF THE ACUTE ABDOMEN

Urologic conditions that may simulate an acute surgical abdominal condition include renal, perirenal or bladder infections, obstructions of the ureter, renal pelvis or bladder, and acute intrascrotal events. Uncomplicated pyelonephritis is rarely a diagnostic problem and uncommonly presents as an acute abdominal event. In contrast, renal and perirenal abscesses may present acutely, and may mimic appendicitis, diverticulitis, or cholecystitis. An intravenous pyelogram (IVP) is abnormal in most cases, as is the urinalysis. Acute ureteral or renal pelvic obstruction is the most common condition to be confused with nonurologic causes of the acute abdomen. Urinalysis, plain abdominal radiography, and IVP are usually confirmatory.[22]

Acute testicular torsion and other intrascrotal events present with prominent abdominal pain in 25% to 50% of cases. A careful examination of the scrotum usually will reveal an elevated testicle on the affected side, along with profound tenderness.[22]

■ THE ACUTE ABDOMEN IN SPECIFIC CONDITIONS

Nonsurgical simulators of the acute abdomen include pulmonary, cardiac, neurologic, metabolic, toxic, infectious, and hematologic conditions (Table 8–3).

Acute abdominal pain in the pediatric patient is covered in Chapters 77 and 78, but Table 8–4 outlines the differential diagnoses. In the first few years of life, congenital abnormalities are the most common source of abdominal symptoms of surgical importance.[23] Histories are difficult to obtain, and physical examination in the newborn or infant can be extremely misleading in that no discernible tenderness may be present. Plain abdominal films should be used more liberally in the pediatric population. In older children, the history and physical findings are elicited more easily, and diagnosis is easier. Certain features in children should be mentioned. Anorexia is frequently absent in children with

TABLE 8–3. NONSURGICAL CAUSES OF THE ACUTE ABDOMEN

Metabolic
  Diabetic ketoacidosis
  Porphyria
  Adrenal insufficiency
  Uremia
  Hypercalcemia

Neurogenic
  Herpes Zoster
  Abdominal epilepsy
  Spinal cord tumor, infection
  Nerve root compression

Cardiopulmonary
  Pneumonia
  Myocardial infarction
  Myocarditis
  Empyema
  Costochondritis

Toxic
  Insect bites
  Venoms (scorpion, snake)
  Lead poisoning
  Drugs

Miscellaneous
  Hemolytic crises
  Rectus sheath hematoma

appendicitis or other intraabdominal inflammatory conditions.[11] The sigmoid colon is often redundant in children. If adjacent to an inflamed appendix, diarrheal symptoms may predominate, leading to a false diagnosis of gastroenteritis. In children, microscopic hematuria and pyuria are seen more commonly with appendicitis, whereas leukocytosis is seen less commonly.[23]

Acute abdominal conditions after cardiac surgery occur in only 1% of patients. Abdominal complications are responsible for 7% to 10% of the total mortality after cardiac surgery because of their associated 25% to 60% mortality. Gastrointestinal bleeding, acute cholecystitis, mesenteric ischemia, pancreatitis, and acute colitis are the most commonly reported diagnoses.[24]

The immunocompromised host comprises a heterogenous group that includes patients receiving allografts, chemotherapy, immunosuppressive drugs for autoimmune disorders, and the patient with the acquired immunodeficiency syndrome (AIDS).[25–28] Each of these groups have specific abdominal complications that must be appreciated and suspected by the evaluating physician (Table 8–5).

Acute, nonspecific abdominal pain is a frequent final diagnosis, accounting for up to 43% of patients with abdominal pain presenting to emergency wards.[29] One retrospective British study found this to be the 6th and 10th most common cause of hospital admission for women and men, respectively.[19] One long-term study found that 77% of these patients remain healthy and free of symptoms at five years follow-up, 7% had been readmitted (one-third of whom had acute appendicitis), and the rest had diagnosed recurrences of acute nonspecific abdominal pain. Malignancy was found in only one of 230 patients, or 4% of patients more than 50 years of age.[29]

Abdominal wall pain is an alternate diagnosis to be considered in patients with acute abdominal pain. Causes to be evaluated include iatrogenic peripheral nerve injuries, hernia, myofascial pain syndromes, the rib tip syndrome, abdominal pain of spinal origin, and spontaneous rectus sheath hematomas.[30]

Each year nearly 10 000 new spinal cord–injury patients are added to the approximately 200 000 paraplegics residing in the United States. Acute abdominal conditions are common, yet difficult to diagnose, in these patients. One excellent review of 21 patients found that the interval between the spinal cord injury and the hospitalization for the acute abdominal complaint averaged 15 years. The average patient was 43 years old. Diseases most commonly seen were acute cholecystitis (36%), perforated peptic ulcer (14%), and renal disease (9%). Physical examination was frequently not helpful. Leukocytosis was seen in 57%, and radiologic studies (plain radiographs, computed tomography (CT) scans, oral cholecystograms, sonograms, and barium studies) led to the correct diagnosis in 77% of cases.

TABLE 8–4. PEDIATRIC ACUTE ABDOMEN

Infants	Children	Adolescents
Viral enteritis	Meckel's diverticulitis	Pelvic inflammatory disease
Intussusception	Cystitis	
Pyelonephritis	Viral enteritis	Appendicitis
Gastroesophageal reflux	Appendicitis	Mittelschmerz
Bacterial enterocolitis	Crohn's Disease	Crohn's Disease
Pneumonitis	Bacterial enterocolitis	Pancreatitis
Appendicitis	Pneumonitis	Pneumonia
Pyloric stenosis	Pancreatitis	Hematocolpos
Testicular torsion	Ruptured tumors	Bacterial entercolitis
Mesenteric cysts	Poisoning	Viral enteritis
Ruptured tumors	Pyelonephritis	Peptic Ulcer
Pancreatitis	Trauma (child abuse)	Poisoning
Meckel's diverticulitis		Trauma
Hirschsprung's disease		Ectopic pregnancy
Strangulated hernia		Pregnancy
Poisoning		Appendicitis
Trauma (child abuse)		Cholelithiasis
		Psychosomatic

TABLE 8–5. ACUTE ABDOMEN IN THE IMMUNOCOMPROMISED PATIENT

Cytomegalovirus Infection
  Interstitial pneumonitis
  Mononucleosis
  Pancreatitis
  Hepatitis
  Cholecystitis
  Gastrointestinal ulceration

Pancreatitis
  Steroid
  Azothiaprine
  Cytomegalovirus
  Pentamidine

Hepatitis
  A, B, C.
  Cytomegalovirus
  Ebstein-Barr virus

Cholecystitis
  Cytomegalovirus
  Acalculous
  Campylobacter

Hepatosplenic Abscess
  Fungal
  Mycobacterial
  Protozoal
  Splenic rupture

Bowel Perforation
  Lymphoma, leukemia (especially after chemotherapy)
  Cytomegalovirus
  Colon ulcers
  Kaposi's sarcoma
  Pseudomembranous colitis
  Mycobacterial
  Iatrogenic

Acute Graft vs Host Disease

Pseudoacute Abdomen

Fecal Impaction

Standard Abdominal Processes
  Appendicitis
  Cholecystitis
  Diverticulitis
  Bowel obstruction
  Ulcer disease
  Pelvic inflammation disease
  Urinary tract infection
  Perirectal abscess
  Lymphadenitis

Neutropenic Enterocolitis

dence of nausea and vomiting. Fever was seen in 29% of patients and decreased bowel sounds in 76% of patients. The most common diagnosis was intramural hematoma of the bowel (86% of all patients). The jejunum was the most frequent site for hematoma (67%), with the ileum (28%) the second most common site. Other diagnoses reported were bowel infarction in 6% of patients, volvulus in 4% of patients, and miscellaneous causes in 6% of patients. Overall patient mortality was 14%. The challenge for the surgeon is to differentiate those patients with intramural hematoma from the minority of patients who will require surgery. Laparotomy is recommended for those patients who fail to improve or who worsen over a 24 to 36 hour observation period.

■ CHRONIC ABDOMINAL PAIN

The patient with chronic abdominal pain remains a common medical and surgical problem. The diagnosis often is elusive, despite a variety of investigations. As Hutchinson stated 70 years ago: "In the treatment of the chronic abdomen the most important thing is to catch the patient early. If she (sic) has once set her feet on the slipper slope which leads to successive operations she is undone."[30]

The pain pattern in patients with chronic abdominal pain can provide important diagnostic clues. Bouts of pain with entirely normal interregnums usually is explained by a discrete intermittent disorder of physiology. Examples include acute intermittent porphyria, internal hernias, endometriosis and occasionally, choledocholithiasis.[8] Chronic abdominal pain that is present most or all of the time is usually the result of a clear pathophysiologic abnormality,[33] such as chronic pancreatitis, or pancreatic or colonic malignancy. Other cases of chronic abdominal pain may have no specific pathophysiologic abnormality. Nonulcer dyspepsia and irritable bowel syndrome are frequently applied diagnoses; however, in reality, these are diagnoses of exclusion.[34]

Circumstances that elicit the abdominal pain also may provide diagnostic clues. Monthly intervals of pain suggest endometriosis. Pain following drug ingestion is suggestive of acute intermittent prophyria (barbiturates) or pancreatitis (steroids, thiazides, tetracyclines). Pain after eating should stimulate the work-up of mesenteric ischemia, chronic pancreatitis, or pancreatic cancer.[8]

The reason for chronic abdominal pain that has been present for most of the time for several months usually is obvious. Weight loss suggests depression, malignancy, or chronic pancreatitis. Fevers are present with intraabdominal abscesses, autoimmune disorders, and malignancy.

Overall mortality was 10%, and there was a 38% operative morbidity rate.[31]

Acute abdominal pain in the patient on oral anticoagulation is another difficult clinical situation. In a recent review of 51 cases from the literature,[32] all patients were found to have pain, and there was a 78% inci-

Physical examination may disclose jaundice, mass, ascites, or neurologic asymmetries.[8]

Two other sources of chronic abdominal pain should be mentioned. Pain arising from the abdominal wall is misdiagnosed frequently. Specific diagnoses include iatrogenic peripheral nerve injuries, hernias, myofascial pain syndromes, the rib tip syndrome, abdominal pain of spinal origin, and spontaneous rectus sheath hematoma.[30] In 1926, Carnett developed a simple test that, when positive, localizes the origin of symptoms to the parietes rather than the viscera. Carnett's test is performed by palpating the abdomen of the supine patient in the usual way. With the palpating fingers located over the tender spot, the patient is asked to contract the abdominal muscles by raising his head from the bed. Once the muscles are tensed, pressure is reapplied and the patient is asked if the pain is changed. If the cause of the symptoms is intraabdominal, the tensed muscles should shield the viscera and result in diminished tenderness. On the other hand, if the source resides in the abdominal wall the pain will be worse or no better.

Numerous psychiatric disorders also are associated with chronic abdominal pain.[35] Diagnoses include primary affective disorders, somatization disorders, psychogenic (conversion) pain, hypochondriasis, anxiety states, substance abuse disorders, schizophrenia, chronic factitious disorder with physical symptoms (Munchausen syndrome), and malingering.

The control of intractable abdominal pain, when associated with diseases that cannot be satisfactorily treated, is one of the most challenging and frustrating problems that the clinician has to face.[8] Examples include unresectable pancreatic carcinoma and chronic pancreatitis. Pharmacologic management, along with behavioral and psychological therapies, are frequently applied with some success. Neurosurgical and/or chemical ablation techniques may be required in select cases.

REFERENCES

1. Fenyo G. Acute abdominal disease in the elderly. *Am J Surg* 1982;143:751
2. Shamburek RD, Farrar JT. Disorders of the digestive system in the elderly. *N Engl J Med* 1990;322:438
3. Spiro HM. Gastrointestinal consultation. In: Moody FG, et al (eds), *Surgical Treatment of Digestive Diseases.* 2nd ed. Chicago, IL: Year Book; 1990:3–10
4. McFadden DW, Zinner MJ. Approach to the patient with acute abdomen and fever of abdominal origin. In: Yamada T, et al (eds), *Textbook of Gastroenterology.* Philadelphia, PA: JB Lippincott; 1991:692–707
5. McFadden DW, Zinner MJ. Gastroduodenal disease in the elderly. *Surg Clin North Am* 1994;74:113
6. Hyatt JR. Management of the acute abdomen: a test of judgment. *Postgrad Med* 1990;87:38
7. Eastwood GL, and Avanduk C (eds), *Manual of Gastroenterology: Diagnosis and Therapy.* Boston, MA: Little Brown; 1989:121–124
8. Klein KB, Mellinkoff SM. Approach to the patient with abdominal pain. In: Yamada T, et al (eds), *Textbook of Gastroenterology.* Philadelphia, PA: JB Lippincott; 1991: 660–679
9. Cutler BS, Dodson TF, Silva WE, Vander Salm TJ (eds), *Manual of Clinical Problems in Surgery.* Boston, MA: Little Brown; 1984:57–61
10. Burnett LS. Gynecologic causes of the acute abdomen. *Surg Clin North Am* 1988;68:385
11. Nesblett WW, Pietsch JB, et al. Acute abdominal conditions in children and adolescents. *Surg Clin North Am* 1988;68:415
12. Paterson-Brown S, Vipond MN. Modern aids to clinical decision-making in the acute abdomen. *Br J Surg* 1990;77:93
13. Levine MS. Plain film diagnosis of the acute abdomen. *Emerg Med Clin North Am* 1985;3:541
14. Eisenberg RL, Heineken P, et al. Evaluation of plain abdominal radiographs in the diagnosis of abdominal pain. *Ann Surg* 1983;197:464
15. Roh JJ, Thompson JS, et al. Value of pneumoperitoneum in the diagnosis of visceral perforation. *Am J Surg* 1983;146:830
16. Schaff MI, Tarr RW, et al. Computed tomography and magnetic resonance imaging of the acute abdomen. *Surg Clin North Am* 1988;68:233
17. Balthazar EJ, Chako AC. Computerized tomography in acute gastrointestinal disorders. *Am J Gastroenterol* 1990; 85:1445
18. Pickleman J. Abdominal Pain. In: Davis JH (ed), *Clinical Surgery.* St Louis, MO: CV Mosby; 1987:537
19. Irvin TT. Abdominal pain: a surgical audit of 1190 emergency admissions. *Br J Surg* 1989;76:1121
20. Sweet RL, Gibbs RS. *Infectious Diseases of the Female Reproductive Tract,* 2nd ed. Baltimore, MD: Williams and Wilkins; 1990
21. Weckstein LN. Current perspective on ectopic pregnancy. *Obstet Gynecol Surg* 1985;40:259
22. Koch MO, McDougall WS. Urologic causes of the acute abdomen. *Surg Clin North Am* 1988;68:399
23. Hatch EI. The acute abdomen in children. *Ped Clin North Am* 1985;32:1151
24. Rosemurgy AS, McAllister E, Karl RC. The acute surgical abdomen after cardiac surgery involving extracorporeal circulation. *Ann Surg* 1988;207:323
25. Glenn J, Funkhouser WK, et al. Acute illnesses necessitating urgent abdominal surgery in neutropenic cancer patients. *Surgery* 1989;105:778
26. Stellato TA, Shek RR. Gastrointestinal emergencies in the oncology patient. *Semin Onc* 1989;16:521
27. Villar HG, Warneke JA, et al. Role of surgical treatment in the management of complications of the gastrointestinal

tract in patients with leukemia. *Surg Gynecol Obstet* 1987;165:217

28. Wade DS, Nava HR, et al. Neutropenic colitis. *Cancer* 1992;69:17
29. Jess P, Bjerregaard B, Brynitz S, et al. Prognosis of acute nonspecific abdominal pain. *Am J Surg* 1982;144:338
30. Gallegos NC, Hobsley M. Abdominal wall pain: an alternative diagnosis. *Br J Surg* 1990;77:1167
31. Neumayer LA, Bull DA, Mohr JD, et al. The acutely affected abdomen in paraplegic spinal cord patients. *Ann Surg* 1990;212:561

32. Euhus DM, Hiatt JR. Management of the acute abdomen complicating oral anticoagulation therapy. *Ann Surg* 1990;56:581
33. Alpers DH. Functional gastrointestinal disorders. *Hosp Pract* 1983;37:139
34. Weddington WW. Psychiatric aspects of chronic abdominal pain. *Drug Ther* 1982;17:45
35. McFadden DW, Zinner MJ. Manifestations of gastrointestinal disease. In: Schwartz S (ed), *Principles of Surgery*, 6th ed. New York, NY: McGraw-Hill; 1994:1015–1042

9

Functional Gastrointestinal Syndromes

Howard R. Mertz ▪ *Emeran A. Mayer*

In general the term *functional* is used to describe a disorder in which patient symptoms are unexplained by any detectable anatomic, biochemical, or physiological abnormality. Since most functional gastrointestinal symptoms include abdominal discomfort or pain, this discussion will be limited to those conditions in which pain or discomfort is a principal symptom. Gastrointestinal functional disorders encompass several organ-specific syndromes: noncardiac chest pain in the esophagus, nonulcer dyspepsia (NUD) in the stomach, sphincter of Oddi dysfunction (SOD) in the biliary tract, and the irritable bowel syndrome (IBS) in the small and large intestine. There are several other disorders that often are considered functional in origin. Chronic abdominal pain syndromes without correlation to physiologic events in the gastrointestinal tract may be considered functional; however, since they are unlikely to be related to function or dysfunction of the gut, they should not necessarily be considered gastrointestinal in origin. Other functional syndromes include constipation, painless diarrhea, nausea, and idiopathic vomiting. Given the similar natural history, epidemiology and possibly, pathophysiology, NUD and IBS will be discussed together. SOD is somewhat distinct and will be discussed separately.

▪ DEFINITIONS OF IBS AND NUD

Since there are no specific diagnostic tests for IBS and NUD, definitions are critical for diagnosis. Inconsis-

tency in inclusion criteria have seriously hampered many studies of these syndromes.[1]

Manning was the first to describe several symptoms highly predictive of IBS: looser bowel movements associated with discomfort, more frequent bowel movements associated with discomfort, relief of discomfort with defecation, bloating sensation with visible abdominal distention, increased mucus in the stool and a sense of incomplete rectal emptying after defecation. The more symptoms that are present, the greater the likelihood of the diagnosis. The criteria are less predictive in the elderly (Table 9–1).[2] A panel of experts at the 1986 International Congress of Gastroenterology in Rome proposed a modification of the Manning criteria to better describe IBS: abdominal pain relieved by defecation together with an alteration in the frequency or consistency of bowel movements or disturbed defecation.[3] The advantage of the new system is the requirement that patients have discomfort in addition to some alteration in bowel movements.

NUD is a syndrome of chronic intermittent upper abdominal discomfort that the patient or physician believes is related to the upper digestive tract, and in which an ulcer has been ruled out. There are a number of specific entities that fulfill these criteria, some of which are organic in origin. Biliary colic, gastroparesis, gastroesophageal reflux disease, chronic pancreatitis, postgastrectomy syndromes, and intestinal angina are organic causes of NUD symptoms that must be excluded by history, physical examination, and appropriate studies.

TABLE 9–1. MANNING CRITERIA FOR IBS

Abdominal discomfort associated with more frequent bowel movements
Abdominal discomfort associated with loose bowel movements
Relief of discomfort with defecation
Increased mucus per rectum
Sense of incomplete rectal evacuation
Abdominal bloating sensation with visible distention

Allied Symptomatology

    Alternating constipation and diarrhea
    Chronic fluctuating course
    Stress-exacerbation of symptoms
    Absence of nocturnal awakening due to symptoms

Management of these disorders is often challenging and requires an accurate diagnosis. However, based on an appropriate history and an absence of physical or laboratory findings, the experienced practitioner is able to make a confident diagnosis. Surgical therapy is not indicated for these disorders, and may, in fact, worsen symptoms.[4,5,6] Avoidance of overmedication and repeated diagnostic adventures for changes in symptomatology is important because the natural history is benign, minor changes in symptomatology are common, and patients frequently press for additional tests and treatment. In functional disorders, it is vital to assess the person as well as the patient to understand why they are presenting at any given point in time, why symptoms may have flared up, and what personal issues have made coping with chronic symptoms more difficult.

■ HISTORY

For decades IBS had been considered psychosomatic or primarily the result of emotional problems and neuroses. However, in 1947, Almy showed the profound influence emotions have on the motility of the colon in health and even more so in IBS.[7] In 1961, Chaudhary and Truelove found a subset of IBS patients with frequent high-amplitude sigmoid colon contractions associated with their typical discomfort and coined the term *spastic colon*.[8] In 1977, Snape reported abnormal myoelectric patterns in IBS.[9] However, subsequent carefully designed studies have failed to confirm any consistent abnormal myoelectric pattern specific for IBS. Thus, there is currently no convincing evidence for a primary motility abnormality in the etiology of IBS.[1]

Sensory abnormalities in IBS were first reported in 1973 by Ritchie, who found hypersensitivity to balloon distention of the sigmoid colon.[10] Using a barostat de-

vice to administer isobaric distentions, Malagelada later showed hypersensitivity to gastric distention in NUD.[11] To evaluate IBS subjects who complained of excessive gas, Lasser and Levitt used an argon washout technique. They found no quantitative or qualitative difference in intraluminal gas, but they did find an increased sensitivity to the gas perfusion in these subjects.[12] Hypersensitivity has been found repeatedly in IBS and NUD, and it is thought to be a key element in symptom generation.[13]

Although psychoneuroses have long been appreciated in patients with IBS and NUD, an understanding of this aspect of the syndromes has been recently advanced. Whitehead[14] and Drossman[15] each found that neurosis is very common in the IBS patient seeking medical care, but not in the person with functional complaints of similar intensity who does not present for medical treatment. This suggests that IBS is not a psychologic disorder, but that psychologic disorders represent a comorbid condition, exacerbating and compounding the symptoms, and impelling the patient to present for medical care. Drossman also found a higher prevalence of past and present physical and sexual abuse in female IBS patients. It is not known whether these experiences incite IBS or whether they cause emotional problems that lead to inadequate coping and increased utilization of the health care system. A higher rate of surgeries also was found in the female IBS patients.[16] An understanding of gastrointestinal functional disorders is still developing and the integration of the observed disturbances in gastrointestinal motor events, sensory function, and central nervous system abnormalities is the goal of current investigation.[17]

■ EPIDEMIOLOGY

Mail surveys have shown that in Western populations, symptoms consistent with IBS are found in approximately 15% of persons, yet a small fraction present their complaint to a physician.[18] In the Western population seeking medical attention there is a 3:1 preponderance of female patients, but in India this ratio is reversed, and the prevalence in Western countries based on telephone interviews does not show an increase in female sufferers. The usual age of onset is the 3rd or 4th decade, with onset after age 65 distinctly unusual. A careful history usually reveals symptoms of gastrointestinal distress dating back to childhood or early adulthood, defined by the patient as a "sensitive" or "nervous" stomach, for example. The epidemiology of NUD is similar, with a preponderance of middle-aged female patients.

■ ANATOMY

MUSCLE AND SEROSA

The muscle wall of the gastrointestinal tract, from the stomach to the rectum, comprises two layers of smooth muscle. There is a circular layer beneath the submucosa and a longitudinally-oriented layer beneath the circular layer. The longitudinal muscle is wrapped by serosa, forming the visceral peritoneum. The organ is held loosely in its position by the mesentery that carries the blood supply and innervation.

INNERVATION

There are four components to the innervation of the gastrointestinal tract: the extrinsic afferent system (sensory information carried from the gut), the efferent system (effector information carried to the gut), the intrinsic nervous system, and the higher centers (including the spinal cord, brainstem, and cortex).

Afferent innervation to the gut is supplied by the vagus nerve, spinal nerves, and sacral parasympathetics. The vagus nerve is composed of predominantly (>80%) afferent fibers and supplies the stomach, pancreaticobiliary tract, the small intestine, and the colon, with the exception of the rectum.[19] The sacral afferent fibers run with the efferent parasympathetics in the pelvis to innervate the colon, rectum and anal canal. *Vagal and sacral afferents* (parasympathetic) predominantly innervate the mucosa and muscular layers of the gut. The mucosal afferents are especially sensitive to stroking (eg, passing a probe over the mucosa).[19] The afferents in the muscular layers function as tension receptors, since they are activated by distention or contraction of the viscus.[20]

Nerve endings of *spinal (splanchnic) afferents*, in contrast to the vagal and sacral afferents, are predominantly located in the mesentery. These fibers course along the blood vessels in the mesentery and respond to torsion or distortion of the mesentery.[21,22] (Table 9–2)

Efferent innervation to the gut is carried by these same nerves. In general, the parasympathetic efferents are stimulatory and the sympathetic efferents are inhibitory. There are a number of reflex loops in which information arising from the gut is carried to ganglia (prevertebral, inferior mesenteric, superior mesenteric, celiac), which in turn triggers efferent signals to alter gut secretion and motor events. An example is the inhibition of motor activity in one part of the colon in response to distention in another part.[23] In addition, spinal and supraspinal reflex loops modulate efferent outflow. For example, relaxation of the internal anal sphincter with rectal distention is a spinal reflex, and gastric fundic relaxation with esophageal distention is a supraspinal reflex mediated by the vagus nerve.

TABLE 9–2. AFFERENT INNERVATION OF THE GUT

Anatomic Area	Sensation	Pathway
Mucosa	Chemosensitivity Stroking	Parasympathetic (vagal, sacral)
Muscularis	Distention	Parasympathetic (vagal, sacral)
Serosa	Torsion	Sympathetic (thoracolumbar spinal nerves)

The *intrinsic nervous system* is a complex and autonomous network of interconnecting neurons that control local activity. These functions are the ones that continue after extrinsic denervation. Such functions include intestinal secretion, peristalsis and initiation, and propagation of the migrating motor complex.

Central centers from the spinal cord to the brainstem to the cortex process and interpret sensory information and initiate efferent messages to the gut. Sensory information is modulated at the spinal level by central descending inputs exerted from the reticular activating system in the medulla. Generally, this input is inhibitory and in the normal subject, it prevents the vast number of afferent stimuli that arise from the gastrointestinal tract from reaching consciousness or causing pain (Fig 9–1).

■ PATHOPHYSIOLOGY

Various motor, sensory, secretory, psychological, and behavioral abnormalities all have been reported in the functional disorders of the gastrointestinal tract. Recently, several hypotheses have been proposed to provide a unifying framework for many of the observed abnormalities.[1,17] The major abnormalities that have been identified will be discussed.

MOTOR ABNORMALITIES

An exaggerated colonic motor response to stress has been reported in IBS.[24] However, in response to stress, such as criticism or inappropriate delay in a medical setting, IBS patients also have a greater emotional stress response.[25] An increase of 3 cycles/min colonic myoelectric activity is seen,[9] but has also been found in psychoneurotics without IBS.[26] Perhaps least controversial is the observation of increased small bowel clustered contractions in IBS patients and their association with the subjects' typical pain.[27,28] Both discrete clustered contractions (DCCs) and prolonged propagated contractions (PPCs) are more frequent in IBS, particularly dur-

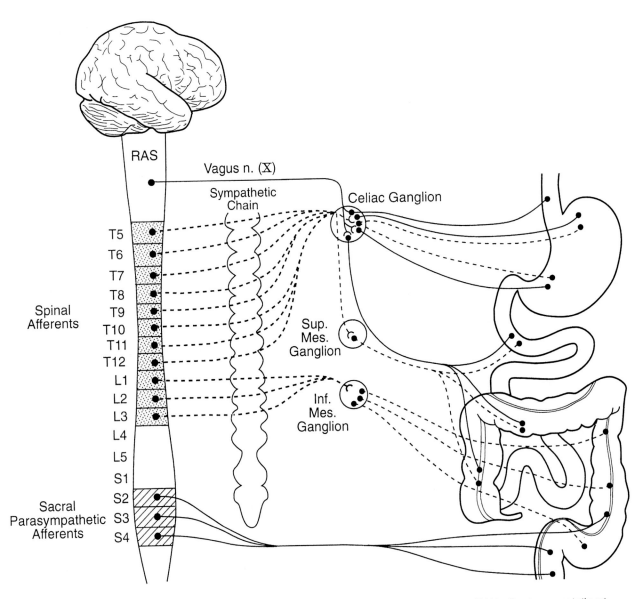

Figure 9–1. Central centers from the spinal cord to the brainstem to the cortex process and interpret sensory information and initiate efferent messages to the gut.

ing stress. However, PPCs and DCCs also are seen in normal controls when testing is more unpleasant (larger diameter tubes, tubes passed into the cecum from above and inpatient recording), and can be associated with discomfort as well.[29,27] Again, the motor responses may be primary or secondary to an increased stress response of the IBS patient to the "unpleasantness" of a medical setting and/or upper intestinal intubation.

Motor abnormalities also have been described in NUD. Gastric compliance is not different from normals,[11] but antral hypomotility and delayed emptying is seen in about 50% of NUD.[30] Correction of the delayed emptying with prokinetic agents, however, does not generally improve subjective symptoms, which suggests

that this delay in transit is not responsible for symptoms.[31] Because of great variability in methods and IBS inclusion criteria in the motility literature, many studies are questionable and others are not comparable.[1] As a result, it is difficult to implicate dysmotility as a primary abnormality in gastrointestinal functional disorders.

SECRETORY ABNORMALITIES

The ileal mucosa of subjects with diarrhea-predominant IBS has been shown to secrete sodium and chloride with saline perfusion and to increase secretion in response to perfusion with low concentrations of bile acids. In contrast, normal subjects absorb sodium and chloride with

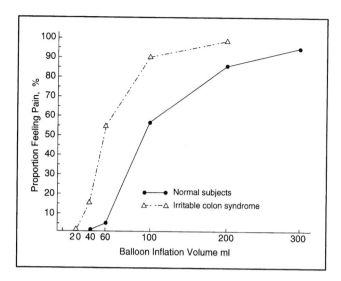

Figure 9–2. Onset of pain at different volumes of balloon inflation (From Ritchie J. *Gut* 1973;14:125–132)

saline perfusion and, at the same low concentrations of bile acids, absorb sodium and chloride. The normal ileum also will secrete sodium and chloride at supraphysiologic bile-acid concentrations.[32] Analogous to motor events in the gut, this physiologic abnormality may be the manifestation of the hyperactive sensory (afferent) portion of an afferent-efferent reflex arc. Altered intestinal secretion may play an etiologic role in the diarrhea of IBS. It also may explain the improvement of symptoms in IBS patients treated with soluble fiber, which absorbs bile acids in addition to its other properties. Altered secretion in the colon may cause the increased mucus production seen in some individuals with IBS.

VISCERAL HYPERSENSITIVITY

Visceral hypersensitivity, principally to painful distention, has been described in a variety of organs in functional disorders. Rectosigmoid colon hypersensitivity to balloon distention,[10] small intestinal hypersensitivity to gas perfusion,[12] and gastric hypersensitivity to balloon distention[11,33,34] are all well documented and reproducible abnormalities(Fig 9–2). Hypersensitivity is reported predominantly for noxious sensation (discomfort and pain) rather than for normal sensations (fullness, gas) and can, therefore, be referred to as hyperalgesia.[35] It appears that the hypersensitivity is limited to visceral organs in these subjects, since cutaneous thresholds for painful stimuli are not lower in IBS.[36] An additional sensory abnormality that is well characterized in IBS and NUD is aberrant cutaneous referral of visceral sensations to locations remote from the stimulus[33,37] (Fig 9–3). The combination of aberrant referral and hyperalgesia suggests altered processing of afferent information at the spinal level.[13] An increase in the excitability of certain dorsal horn neurons (central sensitization) can result from neuroplastic changes in response to nerve injury or tissue irritation.

Supraspinal centers play an important role in modulating sensory input from the periphery. Animal studies demonstrate that descending inhibition from the brainstem reticular activating system (RAS) to the dorsal horn neurons in the spinal cord plays an important principal role in modulating pain thresholds.[38] When the spinal cord is cooled above the level studied, an increased excitability and a lower threshold for depolarization is seen, which indicates a descending inhibitory pathway that exerts a tonic influence, under normal conditions. Conditioning or learning may effect this de-

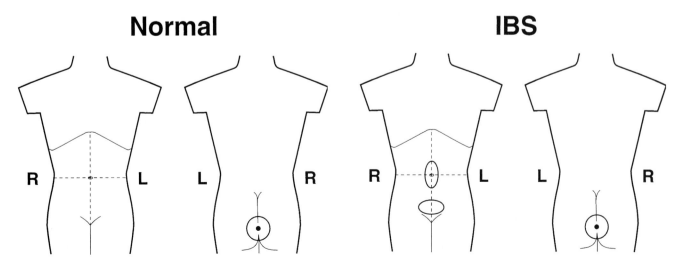

Figure 9–3. Aberrant cutaneous referral of visceral sensations to locations remote from the stimulus is a sensory abnormality well-characterized in IBS and NUD.

scending control. When monkeys are conditioned to expect a cutaneous noxious stimulus after an auditory cue, dorsal horn neuronal deplorization is detected after the auditory cue, but before the stimulus. This demonstrates that central descending control to the dorsal horn can be very specific and focal.[39] Genetics influence the descending inhibitory pathway, as well. Mice with high pain thresholds can be bred with a corresponding increase in opiate receptors in the RAS.[40] Individual differences in the amount of descending inhibition would be expected in a population, with some individuals relatively resistant to pain and others more sensitive to it. In humans, a reduction in descending inhibition could lead to the hyperalgesia and altered vicerosomatic referral areas observed in IBS and NUD.

SLEEP

Sleep abnormalities are common in IBS and NUD, with at least 30% of subjects reporting subjective difficulty with sleep.[41,42] An increased proportion of rapid eye motion (REM) phase sleep and an increased prevalence of sleep apnea have been documented in IBS by sleep electroencephalograms (EEGs).[43]

Fibromyalgia and IBS are syndromes that overlap. In IBS, 61% of patients in one survey complained of chronic musculoskeletal pain, and 63% complained of constant tiredness, both features of fibromyalgia.[41] Another survey showed that 34% of fibromyalgia patients also have IBS.[44]

Normal subjects can develop musculoskeletal pains after sleep deprivation.[45] In fibromyalgia, sleep disruption is common, and low-dose amitriptyline has been shown to improve patients' musculoskeletal symptoms and revert sleep EEGs to normal.[46] If fibromyalgia and functional gastrointestinal syndromes are analogous, correction of sleep abnormalities may explain the benefit of tricyclic antidepressents in IBS.[47,48]

PSYCHOLOGICAL ISSUES

Psychological abnormalities are seen in 70% to 80% of IBS patients who present to major centers for evaluation, whereas nonpatients who do not seek medical care for their IBS symptoms have no more psychopathology than control subjects.[14,15] Anxiety and depression are the common mood disorders seen. Somatization, hostility, phobic behavior, obsessive/compulsive traits and interpersonal sensitivity are all increased in IBS patient populations.[14] Current evidence suggests that the neuropsychologic abnormalities do not correlate with measures of luminal sensitivity or to disease severity, but rather seem to be independent comorbid conditions that may separate the IBS patient from the non-IBS patient.[14,35] This concept is corroborated by similar findings in subjects with lactase deficiency, where neuroticism is strongly increased among those who present for medical evaluation.[49] Treatment of psychologic abnormalities has been shown to lessen abdominal symptoms, whether treatment is with antidepressants or psychotherapy.[47,50] Whether it is a primary cause of symptoms or a comorbid condition leading to health-care utilization, identification and treatment of psychologic issues is critical to management of functional disorders.

Stress is commonly associated with exacerbation or onset of symptoms, particularly with severe emotional trauma such as the loss of a parent.[51,52] The presence of past or present physical and sexual abuse is increased in IBS and is a stressor that seems to provoke symptoms. As noted above, mental stress can evoke alterations in gastrointestinal motility (DCCs) associated with symptoms.[28] Additionally, stress reduction through relaxation training can raise sensory thresholds to painful rectal distention in IBS.[28a] Corticotropin releasing factor (CRF), a central mediator of the stress response, causes sensory thresholds to noxious rectal distention to fall when administered intravenously to normal volunteers.[53] It is possible that CRF mediates hyperalgesia and symptoms in IBS patients with anxiety and other psychological states. The exact mechanism for stress-induced exacerbation of IBS symptoms is not known, but could relate to changes in motility, changes in intestinal sensitivity, or exacerbation of psychologic dysfunction.

Behavioral issues also play a role in the presentation of the functional patient to the doctor. IBS patients report three times as many nongastrointestinal symptoms as healthy controls and 1.5 times as many symptoms as non-IBS patients.[54] IBS patients make twice as many visits to their physicians for these complaints as compared to controls and IBS nonpatients. Illness behavior in IBS patients may result from early-life conditioning; IBS patients are more likely to have been rewarded with toys and candy when they were sick as children.[35,52] Recurrent abdominal pain can be a mechanism for obtaining emotional support, attention, avoidance of unwanted activities, or disability. The request for emotional support in the traditional medical setting may be expressed as: "Doctor, my abdominal pain is worse." What the patient may mean to say is, "I am having a lot of problems now and need the interest and support of a strong and caring person." Patients often feel grateful if further testing and treatment is undertaken, interpreting it as an indication that the physician takes the complaints seriously and is interested in helping. Ongoing investigations and therapeutic trials can be complicated by false-positive findings and placebo responses to medications, both of which are common. The sick role can have consequences for these patients; female IBS patients are four times as likely to have a hysterectomy as compared to controls, and more likely to have other surgery, as well.[55]

Other behaviors, such as nervous air swallowing, can lead to NUD and IBS symptoms. Volunteers asked to swallow air every few seconds for an hour can develop bloating and visible distention.[56] Anxious functional patients commonly swallow air, which leads to symptoms such as belching and fullness. Behavior contributions also include lifestyles that generate stress, absence of stress outlets, sleep deprivation, and poor diet.

DIET

In NUD, questionnaire data has not found any specific food, alcohol, coffee, or tea consumption to be linked to symptoms.[57] Although patients often note sensitivity to fat intake, a double-blind challenge was unable to confirm this.[58]

Literature evaluating the role of dietary triggers of IBS and NUD symptoms are very limited; however, patients frequently emphasize the importance of diet in symptom generation. Based on exclusion diets and questionnaires, wheat, corn, dairy products, coffee, tea, and citrus fruits all have been implicated in IBS.[59] Many patients also report sensitivity to dietary fats, spicy foods, uncooked vegetables, and fruits. True food allergies have not been proven to be related to IBS when double-blind testing is performed; therefore, these "trigger foods" are more likely mediators of changes in motility, sensation, or secretion in the irritable intestine.

Lactase deficiency or sorbitol ingestion certainly can mimic IBS, and should be ruled out early in the patient evaluation. Complex carbohydrates that may arrive undigested into the colon are fermented by colonic bacteria into carbon dioxide, methane, and hydrogen gas. For patients with visceral hypersensitivity, the distention caused by this gas production may provoke abdominal symptoms. Avoidance of beans, cauliflower, broccoli, cabbages, and uncooked legumes is reasonable as a trial for patients who complain of gaseous distention or flatulence.

In summary, although the pathophysiology of gastrointestinal functional disorders is unclear, several consistent abnormalities have been found. It is likely that visceral hypersensitivity causes symptoms of discomfort in response to normal or altered gastrointestinal motor activity. Stress and diet may play a role in the motor and/or sensory dysfunction, while psychological and behavioral factors probably influence the decision of the patient to seek medical care (Fig 9–4).

■ NATURAL HISTORY

Functional gastrointestinal disorders present in the 3rd or 4th decade of life, but also can present in childhood and in the elderly. A careful history in the late-onset functional patient usually reveals either severe emotional precipitating factors or a longer history of less severe abdominal symptoms. The syndromes are generally lifelong, with a course punctuated by remissions and exacerbations. Intercurrent illness can be a trigger for

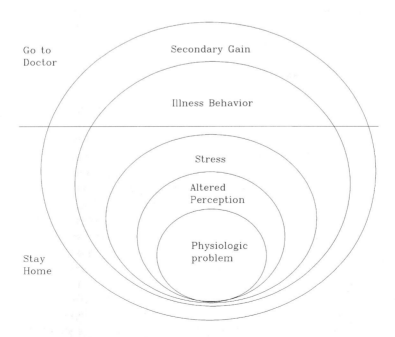

Figure 9–4. A patient's decision to seek medical care is based on a number of factors.

IBS. Patients may suffer IBS symptoms for up to 6 months after acute gastroenteritis.[60] It is likely that other acute or chronic gastrointestinal diseases can lead to functional symptoms. Other triggers include stress, illness, surgery, medication, and dietary factors. Although morbidity can be significant, mortality is not increased.

■ DIAGNOSIS

There are no pathognomonic signs or symptoms that establish the diagnosis of NUD or IBS. Therefore, diagnosis is based on compatible symptomatology and the exclusion of other organic disorders.

IBS must be separated from other gastrointestinal diseases that present with lower (periumbilical and below) abdominal pain (Table 9–1). The Manning criteria are useful to distinguish IBS from organic disorders by symptoms. When two symptoms are present, sensitivity for IBS is 53% and when three symptoms are present, sensitivity is 93%. When patients with organic gastrointestinal disease are questioned, 42% have two Manning criteria and 26% have three or more.[61] IBS is suspected when a patient complains of abnormal bowel habits and lower abdominal discomfort. The initial evaluation is a complete history and physical exam. A history of acute onset of symptoms, onset in a person more than 50 years old, significant weight loss, progressive symptoms, or symptoms awakening the patient from sleep all make the diagnosis of IBS less likely and dictate more aggressive evaluation. Fever, blood or melena per rectum, or dehydration point to an organic etiology as well. Conversely, chronic fluctuating symptoms, stress exacerbation, prominent postprandial symptoms and a family history of IBS make the diagnosis more likely (Fig 9–5).

On physical exam, tenderness may be present in IBS, particularly a palpable tender sigmoid loop, but the tenderness usually is not severe. Severe abdominal tenderness that persists with distraction suggests an alternate diagnosis. Occult blood in the stool cannot be at-

TABLE 9–3. DIFFERENTIAL DIAGNOSIS IN IBS

Obstructive luminal lesion (especially colon carcinoma)
Inflammatory bowel disease
Collagenous colitis
Pseudoobstruction
Constipation
Mesenteric ischemia
Infectious colitis (*C. difficile,* Amoebic, *Campylobacter* jejuni)
Gynecologic disorders (endometriosis, ovarian carcinoma)
Drug-induced diarrhea or constipation
Lactase deficiency

tributed to IBS. All female patients should have a careful pelvic exam to evaluate for endometriosis, ovarian carcinoma, and other gynecologic disorders. Synchronization of lower abdominal pain with menstrual periods can be seen in endometriosis and in IBS.[55]

The laboratory evaluation of periumbilical and lower abdominal discomfort includes a CBC, erythrocyte sedimentation rate, amylase, and complete chemistries. In IBS, these are all normal.

If the history is compatible with IBS, the physical is essentially normal, and the basic laboratory evaluation is normal, further evaluation is based on bowel habits. For the patient with alternating diarrhea and constipation, a flexible sigmoidoscopy effectively excludes an obstructing lesion or colitis. If sigmoidoscopy is negative, the diagnosis of IBS can be made. For patients with diarrhea, stool samples for ova and parasites, for *Clostridium difficile* (if antibiotics have been taken in the last few months), for fecal leukocytes, and fat should be obtained. If negative, a flexible sigmoidoscopy with random biopsies to rule out collagenous or microscopic colitis is performed prior to making the diagnosis of IBS. For the patient with constipation-predominant symptoms, empiric treatment with fiber and stool softeners (and, if necessary, judicious laxatives) is utilized. If constipation remains a problem, a flexible sigmoidoscopy or barium enema should be performed to exclude anatomic causes of obstruction. If negative, a sitzmark transit study of the colon is very helpful. When markers are retained throughout the colon, the diagnosis is colonic inertia. If markers pool in the pelvic colon and rectum, paradoxic pelvic floor contraction syndrome (the anal sphincter and levators contract inappropriately during defecation efforts) may be present. If the transit study is normal, complaints of constipation are most likely the result of the sensation of incomplete evacuation (with no stool in the rectum), to alterations in stool form (hard), or to straining or to bloating abdominal distention. All of these symptoms are part of either the Manning or the Rome criteria for IBS.

NUD can be diagnosed when there is chronic upper abdominal discomfort, particularly with meals. There are a number of disorders that can produce upper abdominal discomfort that must be ruled out prior to making the diagnosis of NUD (Table 9–4). The history is generally adequate to rule out biliary colic, which tends to last longer, radiate to the scapula or back, and be sharper and more abrupt in onset than functional dyspepsia. Chronic pancreatitis also presents differently, with prolonged pain that typically radiates to the back and is exacerbated by alcohol with a delay of many hours, and the accompaniment of steatorrhea, weight loss, and often diabetes.

Symptoms of heartburn are specific for gastroesophageal reflux disease; however, atypical reflux can be

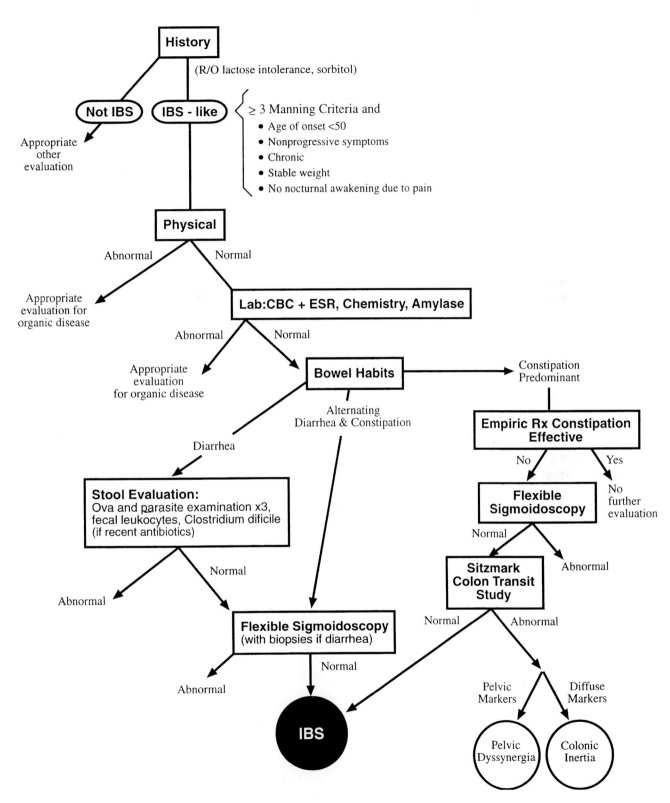

Figure 9–5. Evaluation of chronic lower abdominal pain, (periumbilical and below).

TABLE 9–4. DIFFERENTIAL DIAGNOSIS IN NONULCER DYSPEPSIA

Gastroesophageal reflux
Peptic ulcer
Crohn's disease
Biliary colic
Chronic pancreatitis
Irritable bowel syndrome
Abdominal wall syndrome
Mesenteric ischemia
Giardia lamblia
Abdominal mass lesion
Anorexia nervosa variant

more difficult to differentiate from functional dyspepsia. Atypical reflux can present with hoarseness, cough, asthma, and epigastric pain, without classic heartburn symptoms. When the presentation is epigastric discomfort, clues to reflux include exacerbations by meals, caffeine, alcohol, onions, spicy foods, peppermint, chocolate, or recumbency. The diagnosis of gastroesophageal reflux disease can be established by endoscopy, histologic evaluation of the distal esophagus if gross esophagitis is not seen, the Bernstein acid perfusion test, and the "gold standard" 24 hour pH study.

Gastric cancer can present with insidious symptoms, no physical findings and can even respond to acid inhibition with healing of the associated gastric ulceration. Cancer must be suspected in persons with onset at more than 40 years of age, progressive symptoms, weight loss, occult blood loss, and in persons from high risk areas such as Japan, parts of China, and Russia.

Peptic ulcer classically presents with sharp or burning epigastric pain relieved by meals, exacerbated by hunger, and with nocturnal symptoms. Ulcer risk factors include smoking, aspirin, and the use of nonsteroidal anti-inflammatory drugs (NSAIDs). By definition, NUD implies a similarity to peptic ulcer symptoms. The question is when to investigate patients with ulcer-like complaints. The American College of Physicians recommended endoscopy only after a 6 to 8 week trial of acid-suppression fails to resolve symptoms.[62] This strategy assumes that 6 to 8 weeks of acid inhibition will heal peptic ulcers and that, during this period, behaviors that may cause ulcers or reflux could have changed.

The evaluation of a patient with dyspepsia should take into account age, severity of symptoms, duration of symptoms, and the presence of weight loss. For instance, the yield of endoscopy in patients more than 40 years old is 30%, and increases to 60% in patients more than 65 years old.[63] Early endoscopy generally is recommended for patients more than 40 years of age, those with a long history of symptoms and no prior evaluation, those with significant weight loss, and those with pro-

gressive symptoms.[64] When relief of symptoms after 6 to 8 weeks of empiric acid inhibition and behavioral changes is incomplete, or relapse occurs, then endoscopy (esophagogastroduodenoscopy) should be performed. There is a role for 24 hour esophageal pH monitoring to diagnose gastroesophageal reflux disease when endoscopy is negative. For patients with severe symptoms, symptoms that are partially relieved by acid suppression, or those that require either high-dose H2 blockers or proton pump inhibitors for relief should be evaluated for reflux before long-term medication is prescribed (Fig 9–6).

Recently, rectal balloon distention has been used to diagnose IBS, with a sensitivity of >60% and a specificity of 95% (vs normal controls).[65,66] In NUD, gastric balloon distention can prospectively separate functional disease from organic disease, with a sensitivity of 70% and a specificity of 95%.[67] However, all functional disorders are diagnoses of exclusion, particularly since they can coexist with organic disease.

■ MANAGEMENT

There is no cure for the underlying pathology that generates symptoms in IBS, NUD and the other functional gastrointestinal syndromes. However, it is possible to treat the exacerbating factors and to aid the patient in self-management.

It is important to diagnose functional disorders, thereby ruling out organic disease to the satisfaction of the patient and physician with an expeditious and complete evaluation. This approach relieves patient anxiety that can exacerbate the symptoms and prevents patients from "doctor-shopping" in the hopes of diagnosing an organic ailment. The diagnosis of functional disorders should be made in a positive way, such as in the following manner: "Your symptoms and course of illness are classic for the irritable bowel syndrome and the negative tests confirm this." If the diagnosis is made solely by exclusion (eg, "The tests show nothing, so this must be a functional illness."), the patient will wonder if the physician is unsure or if the right test was performed (Table 9–5).

PSYCHOLOGICAL TREATMENT IN IBS AND NUD

Addressing the psychological and behavioral issues that are so common in these patients has been proven to reduce gastrointestinal symptoms as well as improving the underlying psychologic disorder.[50] For patients with more severe symptoms or possible psychopathology, a multidisciplinary approach utilizing gastroenterologic and psychologic expertise is advisable. The psychologic assessment and treatment (if necessary) needs to be in-

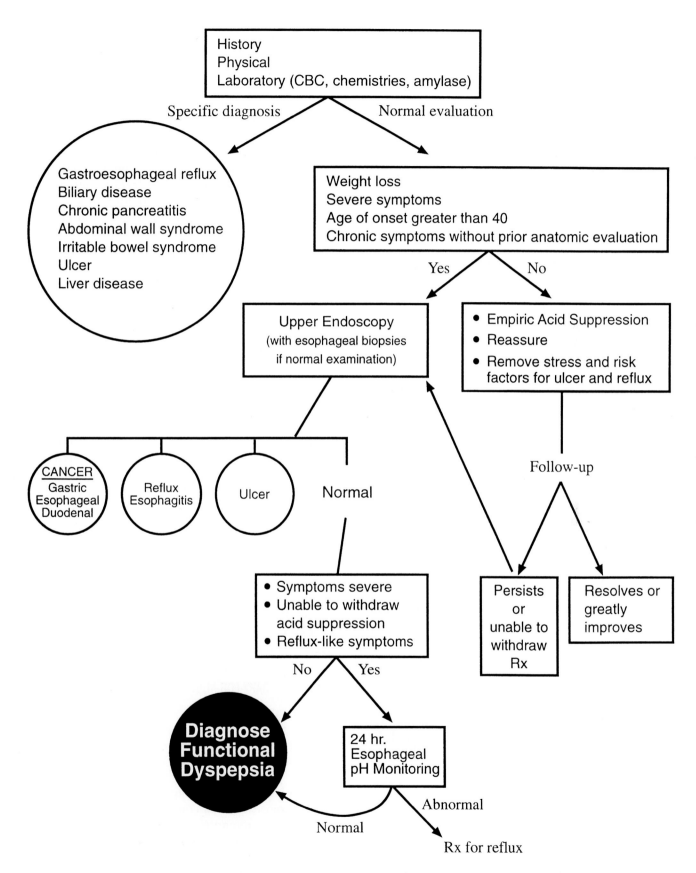

Figure 9–6. Evaluation of chronic upper abdominal discomfort and nausea.

TABLE 9–5. TREATMENT OF FUNCTIONAL DISORDERS

Make a Diagnosis
  Exclude appropriate organic diseases
  Make a positive diagnosis (not purely by exclusion)
  Reassurance through a firm diagnosis

Address Psychopathology
  Psychological evaluation
  Counselling if appropriate
  Stress management if appropriate
  Pharmacotherapy if appropriate (depression, panic)

Behavioral Changes
  Relaxation techniques
  Biofeedback
  Self-management of illness
  Lifestyle changes if appropriate

Fiber and Dietary Modifications

Medications
  Low-dose tricyclic antidepressants
  Antidiarrheal agents if appropriate
  Antispasmodics (occasionally useful)

troduced early as a useful device to improve symptoms, to manage stresses that clearly cause symptoms and to aid in the selection of medications. To minimize resistance of patients, it should be made clear that the psychological evaluation and treatment is part of the medical evaluation process and in no way replaces medical therapy, but supplements it. The patient needs to understand the role of psychological factors in exacerbating real symptoms and the benefits of a combined psychological and medical approach. The patient should not be made to feel that the doctor considers the symptoms purely psychological, wishes to dismiss the patient as "crazy," and is transferring care to a psychologist.

Psychological therapies that have proven useful include traditional psychotherapy[50] and meditation with hypnosis and guided imagery.[68] Judicious use of anxiolytics and antidepressants may be helpful. Stress management using education, biofeedback, and other relaxation techniques can prevent or reduce symptoms. The use of diaries to correlate symptoms with stresses, foods, bowel habits, menses, as well as other factors, are useful to understand the triggers for symptoms and also to help the patient toward self-management. Behavior modification plays an important role in management; lifestyle changes and training in self-management are valuable and ideally should be addressed before any medications are used.

MEDICAL THERAPY FOR IBS

No consistent effectiveness has been shown for any drug therapy in IBS.[69] Placebo response rates up to 60%

make drug evaluation more difficult and point out the strong psychological factors in symptom generation.

For IBS, medical therapy almost always should include a fiber supplement to help regularize bowel function, whether the patient complains of alternating bowel habits, constipation, or diarrhea-predominant symptoms. For diarrhea-predominant symptoms or fecal urgency, antidiarrheal agents such as loperamide can dramatically improve symptoms. When constipation exacerbates symptoms, a stool softener should supplement fiber. If symptoms are more difficult to control, osmotically active laxatives that do not lead to gas production (milk of magnesia, mineral oil, and low-dose polyethylene glycol solution) are helpful and should not lead to "cathartic colon." If constipation is severe or refractory to empiric therapy, evaluation with a sitzmark transit study may detect colonic inertia or pelvic dyssynergia. These entities have specific treatments (higher-dose laxatives, low-residue diet, prokinetic drugs, possibly colectomy for inertia, and biofeedback therapy for pelvic dyssynergia).

Dietary triggers vary between patients, but trials of withdrawal of lactose, spicy foods, fatty foods, and uncooked vegetables and fruits is reasonable. Use of food diaries helps to identify dietary triggers and to establish patient cooperation and autonomy.

Pharmacotherapy with low-dose tricyclic antidepressants has yielded some benefits in controlled trials.[47,48] These trials excluded patients with depression and used doses lower than the standard doses for depression, so the benefit is unlikely to be the result of treatment of depression. The benefits pharmocotherapy may relate to improved sleep or to alterations in neurochemistry, which is the postulated mechanism of action of amitriptyline in diabetic neuropathic pain.[70] Antispasmodic drugs (anticholinergics such as dicyclomine and probanthene) may offer temporary relief for cramping pain or diarrhea. The relief generally is not pronounced or long lasting and primarily may offer the patient a sense of control over the symptoms.

MEDICAL THERAPY FOR NUD

It is difficult to make general recommendations for the medical treatment of NUD, since it is a heterogeneous disorder. Trials of various types of therapy, with careful documentation of response, is probably the best approach.

There are mixed data supporting the use of H2 inhibitors for NUD when compared to placebo.[71–73] It is reasonable to administer antacids or H2 blockers as a trial. Dietary counseling with trials of avoidance of spicy foods, fatty foods, alcohol, caffeine, and milk products may be beneficial. For subjects with predominantly postprandial symptoms of bloating and early satiety, smaller and more frequent meals should be consumed. Currently, there is no evidence to support eradication of H pylori, since H pylori gastritis is equally common in dyspeptic and normal patients and suppression or eradication of the bacterium has not led to consistent improvement in symptoms.[74] There is evidence that prokinetic agents improve symptoms in a subset of patients with NUD. Cisapride has been shown superior to placebo for dyspeptic symptoms in some studies[75,76] but not in others.[31,77] When benefit was noted, symptom relief often was superior at night. Since symptoms at night may be reflux-related, and none of the studies excluded reflux with Bernstein or 24 hour esophageal pH tests, it is possible that the cisapride benefit is related to inhibition of gastroesophageal reflux.

If long-term prokinetic drugs or acid antisecretory drugs are contemplated, a 24 hour pH test is probably cost-effective, since it may lead to improved compliance with antireflux measures, appropriate use of proton pump inhibitors (omeprasole), and surgical fundoplication.

SURGERY IN FUNCTIONAL GASTROINTESTINAL DISEASE

Surgery has no role in the treatment of functional gastrointestinal disease. Therefore, surgery should be avoided unless there are clear indications. Functional patients often search persistently for treatments for their symptoms, which likely explains the higher rates of hysterectomies and other abdominal surgeries in IBS patients.

Outcome after surgery may be worse in patients with functional disease. Among patients who inadvertently have gastric surgery for NUD, symptoms generally worsen and there is a much higher likelihood of postgastrectomy syndromes than in those with true ulcer.[4] When patients have prominent psychiatric histories and/or no evidence of ulcer at operation, results can be very disappointing. This led one group to name this postoperative problem The Albatross Syndrome.[5]

Symptoms of IBS developed de novo in 10% of women after hysterectomy, in one prospective study.[6] In a retrospective study, women who had had a hysterectomy were more likely than controls to experience the IBS symptoms of constipation, straining, bloating, and a sense of incomplete rectal evacuation. They did not present for medical evaluation for these symptoms more than the controls, however, implying that they did not present initially for hysterectomy because of health care–seeking behavior.[78] It may be that the IBS symptoms developed subsequent to the operations. In this same study, women, after a cholecystectomy, were more likely to have incomplete rectal evacuation and fecal urgency than controls with asymptomatic gallstones.[78] These studies imply either that surgery can provoke IBS or that IBS patients are more likely to have surgery. Either interpretation offers a caution to operating when the symptoms of patients are compatible with functional disease.

Many patients with functional illnesses may doctor-shop, looking for a miracle cure, particularly one which is rapid, complete, and requires no physiologic exploration (ie, surgery). It is prudent to seek symptoms of functional illness and pursue appropriate nonsurgical management when indications for surgery are predominantly for pain and organic pathophysiology does not explain the symptoms well.

■ SPHINCTER OF ODDI DYSFUNCTION

The term sphincter of Oddi dysfunction (SOD) is applied to a heterogeneous group of disorders with actual or presumed dysfunction of the sphincter of Oddi. SOD is defined as a benign, acalculous obstruction to the flow of bile and/or pancreatic fluid through the sphincter of Oddi, which can result in pain, cholestasis, or pancreatitis. These disorders are manifested clinically as functional biliary-type pain, with or without evidence of biliary obstruction, postcholecystectomy syndrome, recurrent idiopathic pancreatitis, and papillary stenosis.

The concept of disordered sphincter of Oddi function is relatively new, having been introduced by Nardi in 1966.[79] Geenen and associates firmly established the existence of the syndrome in 1989 when a double-blind randomized study treated presumed SOD with endoscopic sphincterotomy or sham sphincterotomy and found significant improvement in pain in the sphincterotomy group. Elevated resting pressure in the sphincter of Oddi was the strongest predictor of improvement via sphincterotomy.[80] SOD is probably part of a continuum comprising pancreaticobiliary obstruction by papillary stenosis (owing to stricture), sphincter muscle dysfunction causing intermittent pancreaticobiliary obstruction, and pure functional disease in which pancreaticobiliary-type pain may or may not be related to abnormalities of sphincter function.

ANATOMY AND PHYSIOLOGY

The sphincter of Oddi is located at the confluence of the pancreatic duct, common bile duct and duodenum. There are three components to the sphincteric smooth muscle: sphincter ampullae, sphincter choledochus, and sphincter pancreaticus. The innervation is thought to be vagal.

The function of the sphincter of Oddi is not entirely clear, since patients rarely experience physiologic perturbation after sphincterotomy. The most likely function is to form a mechanical barrier preventing bacteria and parasites from gaining access to the liver, gallbladder, and pancreas. The sphincter also maintains a tonic pressure in the biliary tree so that bile flow between meals fills the gallbladder. The sphincter relaxes with meals, under the influence of cholecystokinin which coordinates contraction of the gallbladder to induce bile flow into the duodenum.

Measurement of sphincter pressure is feasible now in certain biliary endoscopy centers. Endoscopic water-perfused manometry reveals consistent findings in healthy subjects and subjects with sphincter dysfunction.[81,82] Normal resting sphincter tone is approximately 20 mm Hg punctuated by intermittent phasic contractions of amplitude up to several 100 mm Hg.[83,84] The majority of these contractions are propagated anterograde. Cholecystokinin causes a reduction in sphincter pressure in normal subjects.[85]

EPIDEMIOLOGY

SOD is a disorder predominantly seen in females. Most series show a female to male ratio of >9:1.[80,85,86] The bulk of recognized cases is in young to middle-aged postcholecystectomy patients. Psychological comorbidity and concurrent functional bowel disorders have not been studied in any systematic way.

PATHOPHYSIOLOGY

Geenen and associates[80] classify SOD into three categories. Type I patients have biliary-type pain, abnormal liver enzymes, a dilated common bile duct, and delayed biliary drainage. Type II patients have biliary-type pain and one or two of the other three findings. Type III patients, the largest subgroup, are those with pain and none of the abnormalities indicative of biliary obstruction (Table 9–6). Although each subset can have clinical improvement after surgical or endoscopic sphincterotomy, the proportion of patients who improve is greatest in type I and least in type III. Based on the response to sphincterotomy and the high prevalence of abnormal sphincter of Oddi manometry, some of these patients have unequivocal evidence for disease caused by SOD, particularly in type I. Others, especially type III patients and type II patients with normal manometric findings, do not improve after sphincterotomy and may have a different pathophysiology (hypersensitive biliary tree, nonulcer dyspepsia, gastroesophageal reflux, peptic ulcer, or abdominal wall pain syndrome). Based on the abnormal viscerosomatic referral patterns seen and the absence of clear biliary pathology, NUD is the most common diagnosis in type III patients.

Patients with postcholecystectomy syndrome frequently have impaired biliary flow at the level of the ampulla. Dynamic hepatobiliary isotopic scanning shows a high prevalence of delayed bile duct emptying without fixed obstruction or anatomic abnormality.[87] Elevated sphincter of Oddi pressures and abnormal responses to neural and hormonal signals are also very common in this patient group and are the most likely explanation for delayed drainage.[82,85] There is no convincing evidence that cholecystectomy alone causes SOD. It is more likely that the observed sphincter abnormalities are present preoperatively, as well, and account for much of the symptomatology that leads to the cholecystectomy.

Recurrent idiopathic pancreatitis and recurrent pancreatic-type pain also may be the result of dysfunction of the pancreatic portion of the sphincter of Oddi.[88] A high prevalence of hypertensive sphincter pancreaticus has been found in individuals with these disorders, just as it has in the biliary syndromes.[82]

The presumed etiology of symptoms and disease relates to pancreaticobiliary obstruction. Originally the Nardi test was used to document intermittent obstruction from papillitis. A positive test required pain and elevation of liver enzymes after morphine and neostigmine injection. The Geenen classification system includes indicators of biliary obstruction: common bile duct dilatation, delayed dye emptying, and intermittent elevations of liver enzymes. Bile duct pressures above the sphincter are elevated in type II SOD, presumably owing to obstructed outflow.[83] Although pain in this syndrome presumably is the result of increased pressures in the pancreaticobiliary tree, this has not been well studied. Whether some patients, particularly those who do not benefit from sphincterotomy, have hypersensitivity to distention of the pancreaticobiliary tree has not been examined.

For those patients who do not have measurable sphincter abnormalities or evidence for obstruction to explain their biliary-type pain, there is a good possibil-

TABLE 9–6. CLASSIFICATION OF SPHINCTER OF ODDI DYSFUNCTION

Type I
1. Unexplained biliary-type pain lasting for more than 6 months after cholecystectomy
2. Common bile duct dilatation greater than 12 mm by ERCP
3. Delayed common bile duct drainage by ERCP (>45 min)
4. Abnormal liver enzymes on 2 occasions

Type II
1. Unexplained biliary-type pain lasting for more than 6 months after cholecystectomy
2. One or two of the other three criteria (2, 3, 4 above)

Type III
1. Unexplained biliary-type pain lasting for more than 6 months after cholecystectomy
2. None of the other three criteria (2, 3, 4 above)

From Geenen JE, et al. *N Eng J Med* 1989;320:82–87

ity that nonulcer dyspepsia or irritable bowel syndrome is the cause of these symptoms. It is known that balloon distention in abdominal organs, ranging from the esophagus to the sigmoid colon, can reproduce biliary pain in postcholecystectomy syndrome.[89] This may occur as a result of aberrant referral, or from diffuse gut hypersensitivity with summation of afferent inputs from various locations, causing pressures in the biliary tree to reach threshold levels for discomfort.

DIAGNOSIS

The diagnosis of SOD currently is based on the clinical criteria used by Geenen and associates (Table 9–6). This system is accepted and leads to reproducible treatment results when utilized by different groups.[90,91] Geenen's group advocates sphincter of Oddi manometry as well, since it predicted response to sphincterotomy in type II patients. Others have found manometry less useful[90,91] and are concerned by the rate of normal manometry in type I patients (14% to 35%).[82,92] The Nardi test is too insensitive (approximately 30% positive predictive value) in predicting abnormal sphincter manometry and response to sphincterotomy.[80,86]

There are numerous etiologies of pancreaticobiliary-type pain that must be ruled out before a diagnosis of SOD is made. These include biliary and pancreatic organic disease and nonpancreaticobiliary disease. Nonulcer dyspepsia and IBS should be considered also (Table 9–7).

MANAGEMENT

SOD type I patients uniformly respond well to endoscopic sphincterotomy,[92,93] which has an acceptable risk-to-benefit ratio, although the chance of complications is higher in SOD than in other disorders.[94]

SOD type II has a high (55%) prevalence of measurable sphincter abnormalities.[80,82] Elevated sphincter pressure could be used as a criteria for performing endoscopic sphincterotomy, since the patients with elevated basal pressure have better pain improvement after sphincterotomy. Type II patients with normal sphincter pressures were no more likely to improve after sphincterotomy than after sham sphincterotomy.[80]

Type III patients have a low prevalence (28%) of abnormal sphincter motility and do not respond well to endoscopic sphincterotomy. Whether sphincter manometry can separate a group of responders is not known. Particularly in this group, a search for other gastrointestinal and extraintestinal disorders should be sought. NUD and IBS are commonly occurring disorders that could mimic symptoms from the pancreaticobiliary tree.[89] Evaluation of suspected type III SOD patients should include a psychosocial evaluation similar to IBS and NUD.

TABLE 9–7. DIAGNOSES TO EXCLUDE IN POSSIBLE SPHINCTER OF ODDI DYSFUNCTION

Biliary Tract Disease
Occult calculous disease
Microlithiasis
Biliary cyst
Biliary stricture (includes chronic pancreatitis)
Biliary neoplasia

Pancreatic Disease
Chronic pancreatitis
Pancreas divisum
Pancreatic stone or stricture
Recurrent acute pancreatitis

Other Disease
Gastroesophageal reflux disease
Nonulcer dyspepsia
Irritable bowel syndrome
Musculoskeletal pain
Peptic ulcer
Adhesions

Patients with recurrent idiopathic pancreatitis should be considered for pancreatic sphincter of Oddi manometry, if this is available.

Drug therapy for SOD also may be beneficial. Two randomized, placebo-controlled trials using nifedipine in type II patients have demonstrated improvement in the majority of the treated patients.[95,96] Transcutaneous nerve stimulation (TENS) also has been reported to increase serum-vasoactive peptide levels and reduce sphincter of Oddi pressures.[97] These measures do not offer the potential of permanent improvement like sphincterotomy, but are safer and suggest there is potential for future medical therapies for this condition.

■ SUMMARY

Functional gastrointestinal disorders include a variety of syndromes. These syndromes have variable presentations and may be groups of disorders with different pathophysiology but with similar symptomatic presentations. In general the functional disorders of the gut do not lead to increased mortality and are not associated with other organic diseases. There are often psychological factors influencing symptom flare-ups and health care–seeking, which must be addressed. Therapy is conservative, with treatment to reduce symptoms rather than to cure the underlying condition. In sphincter of Oddi dysfunction, a subset of patients are cured by sphincterotomy. Clinical skill must be utilized to differentiate organic from functional disease and to avoid excessive evaluation and treatment. A good doctor-patient relationship is critical to the ongoing management.

REFERENCES

1. McKee DP, Quigley EMM. Intestinal motility in irritable bowel syndrome: is IBS a motility disorder? part II. *Dig Dis Sci* 1993;38:1773–1782

2. Manning AP, Thompson WD, Heaton KW. Towards positive diagnosis in the irritable bowel syndrome. *Br Med J* 1978;2:653–654

3. Thompson WG, Creed F, Drossman DA, et al. Functional bowel disease and functional abdominal pain. *Gastroenterology Intl* 1992;5:75–91

4. Amdrup E. Variations in food tolerance after partial gastrectomy. The relationship between pathological findings at operation and type and intensity of postgastrectomy symptoms. *Acta Chir Scand* 1961;120:410–421

5. Johnstone FR, Holubitsky IB, Debas HT. Postgastrectomy problems in patients with personality defects: The "Albatross" syndrome. *Can Med Assoc J* 1967;96:1559–1564

6. Prior A, Stanley KM, Smith ARB, Read NW. Relation between hysterectomy and the irritable bowel: a prospective study. *Gut* 1992;33:814–817

7. Almy TP, Kern F, Tulin M. Alterations in colonic function in man under stress: experimental production of sigmoid spasm in healthy persons. *Gastroenterology* 1947;8:616–626

8. Chaudhary NA, Truelove SC. Human colonic motility: a comparative study of normal subjects, patients with ulcerative colitis and patients with irritable colon syndrome, I. resting patterns of motility. *Gastroenterology* 1961;40:1–17

9. Snape WJ Jr, Carlson GM, Matarazzo SA, Cohen S. Evidence that abnormal myoelectrical activity produces colonic motor dysfunction in the irritable bowel syndrome. *Gastroenterolgy* 1977;72:383–387

10. Ritchie J. Pain from distension of the pelvic colon by inflating a balloon in the irritable colon syndrome. *Gut* 1973;14:125–132

11. Mearin F, Cucala M, Azpiroz F, Malagelada J-R. The origin of symptoms on the brain-gut axis in functional dyspepsia. *Gastroenterology* 1991;101:999–1006

12. Lasser RB, Bond JH, Levitt MD. The role of intestinal gas in functional abdominal pain. *N Engl J Med* 1975;293:524–526

13. Mayer EA, Raybould HE. Role of visceral afferent mechanisms in functional bowel disorders. *Gastroenterology* 1990;99:1688–1704

14. Whitehead WE, Bosmajian L, Zonderman AB, Costa PT Jr, Schuster MM. Symptoms of psychological distress associated with irritable bowel syndrome. *Gastroenterology* 1988;95:709–714

15. Drossman DA, McKee DC, Sandler RS, et al. Psychosocial factors in the irritable bowel syndrome. A multivariate study of patients and nonpatients with irritable bowel syndrome. *Gastroenterology* 1988;95:701–708

16. Drossman DA, Leserman J, Nachman G, et al. Sexual and physical abuse in women with functional or organic gastrointestinal disorders. *Ann Intern Med* 1990;113(11):828–833

17. Mayer EA, Gebhart GF. Functional bowel disorders and the visceral hyperalgesia hypothesis. In: Mayer EA, Raybould HE (eds), *Basic and Clinical Aspects of Chronic Abdominal Pain.* New York, NY: Elsevier; 1993;3–28

18. Talley NJ, Zinsmeister AR, Van Dyke C, Melton LJ. Epidemiology of colonic symptoms and irritable bowel syndrome. *Gastroenterology* 1991;101(4):927–934

19. Grundy D, Scratcherd T. Sensory afferents from the gastrointestinal tract. In: Schultz SG, Wood JD, Rauner BB (eds): *Handbook of Physiology.* vol 1. (sect 6) New York, NY: Oxford University Press; 1989;593–620

20. Iggo A. Afferent C-fibers and visceral sensation. In: Cervero F, Morrison JFB (eds), *Progress in Brain Research.* vol 67. New York, NY: Elsevier; 1986;29–38

21. Jaenig W, Morrison JFB. Functional properties of spinal visceral afferents supplying abdominal and pelvic organs, with special emphasis on visceral nociception. *Progr Brain Res* 1986;67:87

22. Morrison JFB. Splanchnic slowly adapting mechanoreceptors with punctate receptive fields in the mesentery and gastrointestinal tract of the cat. *J Physiol* 1977;233:349–362

23. Szurszewski JH, King BF. Physiology of prevertebral ganglia in mammals with special reference to inferior mesenteric ganglion. In: Schultz SG, Wood JD, Rauner BB (eds), *Handbook of Physiology.* vol 1 (sect 6) New York, NY: Oxford University Press, 1989;519–592

24. Narducci F, Snape WJ, Battle WM, et al. Increased colonic motility during exposure to a stressful situation. *Dig Dis Sci* 1985;30(1):40–44

25. Welgan P, Meshkinpour H, Beeler M. The effect of anger on colon motor and myoelectric activity in irritable bowel syndrome. *Gastroenterology* 1988;94:1150–1156

26. Latimer P, Sarna S, Campbell D, et al. Colonic motor and myoelectric activity: a comparative study of normal subjects, psychoneurotic patients, and patients with irritable bowel syndrome. *Gastroenterology* 1981;80:893–901

27. Kellow JE, Gill RC, Wingate DL. Prolonged ambulant recordings of small bowel motility demonstrate abnormalities in the irritable bowel syndrome. *Gastroenterology* 1990;98(suppl 5, pt 1):1208–1218

28. Kumar D, Wingate DL. The irritable bowel syndrome: a paroxysmal motor disorder. *Lancet* 1985;2:973–977

28a. Monnikes H. Personal communication.

29. Kellow JE, Phillips SF. Altered small bowel motility in irritable bowel syndrome is correlated with symptoms. *Gastroenterology* 1987;92:1885–1893

30. Malagelada JR, Stanghellini V. Manometric evaluation of functional upper gut symptoms. *Gastroenterology* 1985;88:1223–1231

31. Jian R, Ducrot F, Ruskone A, et al. Symptomatic, radionuclide and therapeutic assessment of chronic idiopathic dyspepsia. A double-blind placebo-controlled evaluation of cisapride. *Dig Dis Sci* 1989;34:657–664

32. Oddsson E, Rask-Madsen J, Krag E. A secretory epithelium of the small intestine with increased sensitivity to bile acids in irritable bowel syndrome associated with diarrhea. *Scand J Gastroenterol* 1978;13:409–416

33. Mertz H, Sytnik B, Galen S, Mayer EA. Evidence for altered spinal processing of gastric afferent information in nonulcer dyspepsia. *Gastroenterology* 1993;104:A551

34. Lemann M, Dederding JP, Flourie B, et al. Abnormal perception of visceral pain in response to gastric distension in chronic idiopathic dyspepsia. The irritable stomach syndrome. *Dig Dis Sci* 1991;36:1249–1254

35. Whitehead WE, Engel BT, Schuster MM. Irritable bowel syndrome. Physiological and psychological differences between diarrhea-predominant and constipation-predominant patients. *Dig Dis Sci* 1980;25:404–413

36. Cook IJ, Van Eeden A, Collins SM. Patients with irritable bowel syndrome have greater pain tolerance than normal subjects. *Gastroenterology* 1987;93:727–733

37. Moriaty KJ, Dawson AM. Functional abdominal pain: further evidence that whole gut is affected. *Br Med J* 1982; 284:1670–1672

38. Lumb MB. Brainstem control of visceral afferent pathways in the spinal chord. In: Cervero F, Morrison JFB (eds), *Visceral Sensation, Progress in Brain Research*, vol 67. New York, NY: Elsevier; 1986;279–293

39. Dubner R, Hoffman DS, Hayes RL. Neuronal activity in medullary dorsal horn of awake monkeys trained in a thermal discrimination task, III. task-related responses and their funcational role. *J Neurophysiol* 1981;46:444–464

40. Marek P, Yirmiya R, Liebeskind JC. Genetic influences on brain stimulation-produced analgesia in mice: II. Correlation with brain opiate receptor concentration. *Brain Res* 1990;507:155–157

41. Whorwell PJ, McCallum M, Creed FH, Roberts CT. Noncolonic features of irritable bowel syndrome. *Gut* 1986; 27:37–40

42. Fefer L, Mertz H, Kodner A, Mayer EA. 24 hr ambulatory gastroduodenal manometry in normals (N) and patients with nonulcer dyspepsia (NUD). *Gastroenterology* 1992; 102:A447

43. Kumar D, Thompson PD, Wingate DL, et al. Abnormal REM sleep in the irritable bowel syndrome. *Gastroenterology* 1992;103:12–17

44. Yunus M, Masi AT, Calabro JJ, et al. Primary fibromyalgia (fibrositis): clinical study of 50 patients with matched normal controls. *Semin Arthritis Rheum* 1981;11:151–171

45. Moldofsky H, Scarisbrick PS. Induction of neurasthenic musculoskeletal pain syndrome by selective sleep stage deprivation. *Psychosom Med* 1976;38:35–44

46. Watson R, Leibman KD, Jenson J. Alpha-delta sleep. EEG characteristics, incidence, treatment, psychophysiological correlates and personality. *Sleep Res* 1985;14:226

47. Greenbaum DS, Mayle JE, Vanegran LE. Effects of desipramine on irritable bowel syndrome compared with atropine and placebo. *Dig Dis Sci* 1987;32:257–266

48. Myren J, Lovland B, Larssen S-E, Larsen S. A double-blind study of the effect of trimipramine in patients with the irritable bowel syndrome. *Scand J Gastroenterol* 1984;19: 835–843

49. Whitehead WE, Enck P, Schuster MM. Psychopathology in patients with irritable bowel syndrome. In: *Nerves and the Gastrointestinal Tract*. New York, NY: Academic Press; 1989;465–476

50. Guthrie E, Creed F, Dawson D, Tomenson B. A controlled trial of psychological treatment for the irritable bowel syndrome. *Gastroenterology* 1991;100:450–457

51. Hill OW, Blendis L. Physical and psychological evaluation of nonorganic abdominal pain. *Gut* 1967;8:221–229

52. Lowman BC, Drossman DA, Cramer EM. Recollection of childhood events in adults with irritable bowel syndrome. *J Clin Gastroenterol* 1987;9:324–330

53. Lembo T, Plourde V, Moennikes H, et al. Corticotropin-releasing factor (CRF) produces rectal hyperalgesia in humans. *Gastroenterology* 1993;104:A541

54. Sandler RS, Drossman DA, Nathan HP, McKee DC. Symptom complaints and health care seeking behavior in subjects with bowel dysfunction. *Gastroenterology* 1984;87: 314–318

55. Whitehead WE, Cheskin LJ, Heller BR, et al. Evidence for exacerbation of irritable bowel syndrome during menses. *Gastroenterology* 1990;98(6):1485–1489

56. Gierczak S, Chami T, Schuster MM, Whitehead WE. Gastrointestinal symptoms produced by air swallowing. *Gastroenterology* 1993;104:A512.(Abstract)

57. Talley NJ, McNeil D, Piper DW. Environmental factors and chronic unexplained dyspepsia. Association with acetaminophen but not other analgesics, alcohol, coffee, tea, or smoking. *Dig Dis Sci* 1988;33(6):641–648

58. Taggart D, Billington BP. Fatty foods and dyspepsia. *Lancet* 1966; August 27:464–466

59. Jones VA, McLaughlan P, Shorthouse M, et al. Food intolerance: a major factor in the pathogenesis of the irritable bowel syndrome. *Lancet* 1982;ii:1115–1117

60. Chaudhary NA, Truelove SC. The irritable bowel syndrome. *Quart J Med* 1962;31:307–322

61. Talley NJ, Phillips SF, Melton LJ, et al. Diagnostic value of the Manning criteria in irritable bowel syndrome. *Gut* 1990;31:77–81

62. Health and Public Policy Committee American College of Physicians. Endoscopy in the evaluation of dyspepsia. *Ann Intern Med* 1985;102:266–269

63. Fjosne U, Kleveland PM, Waldum H, et al. The clinical benefit of routine upper gastrointestinal endoscopy. *Scand J Gastroenterol* 1986;21:433–440

64. Talley NJ, Phillips SF. Nonulcer dyspepsia: potential causes and pathophysiology. *Ann Intern Med* 1988;108: 865–879

65. Prior A, Sorial E, Sun W-M, Read NW. Irritable bowel syndrome: differences between patients who show rectal sensitivity and those who do not. *Eur J Gastroenterol Hepatol* 1993;5:343–349

66. Mertz H, Mayer EA. Evidence for the alteration of splanchnic afferent pathways in IBS patients. *Gastroenterology* 1995;109:40–52

67. Mertz H, Kodner A, Niazi N, Mayer E. Are rectal sensory thresholds a biological marker of IBS disease activity? *Gastroenterology* 1995;109:40–52.

68. Whorwell PJ, Prior A, Faragher EB. Controlled trial of hypnotherapy in the treatment of severe refractory irritable bowel syndrome. *Lancet* 1984;2:1232–1234

69. Klein KB. Controlled treatment trials in the irritable bowel syndrome: a critique. *Gastroenterology* 1988;95:232–241

70. Max MB, Culnane M, Schafer SC, et al. Amitryptiline relieves diabetic neuropathy pain in patients with normal or depressed mood. *Neurology* 1987;37:589–596

71. Gotthard R, Bodemar G, Brodin U, Jonsson KA. Treatment with cimetidine, antacid, or placebo in patients with dyspepsia of unknown origin. *Scand J Gastroenterol* 1988; 23:7–18

72. Saunders JH, Oliver RJ, Higson DL: Dyspepsia: incidence of nonulcer disease in a controlled trial of ranitidine in general practice. *Br Med J* 1986;292:665–668

73. Nyren O, Adami H, Bates S, et al. Absence of therapeutic benefit from antacids or cimetidine in nonulcer dyspepsia. *N Engl J Med* 1986;314:339–343

74. Marshall BJ, Valenzuela JE, McCallum RW, et al. Bismuth subsalicylate suppression of helicobacter pylori in nonulcer dyspepsia: a double-blind placebo-controlled trial. *Dig Dis Sci* 1993;38(9):1674–1680

75. Rosch W. Cisapride in non-ulcer dyspepsia. *Scand J Gastroenterol* 1987;22:161–164

76. Van Outryve M, De Nutte N, Van Eeghem P, Gooris JP. Efficacy of cisapride in functional dyspepsia resistant to domperidone or metoclopramide: a double-blind, placebo-controlled study. *Scand J Gastroenterol* 1993; 28(suppl 195):47–53

77. Corinaldesi R, Stanghellini V, Raiti C, et al. Effect of chronic administration of cisapride on gastric emptying of a solid meal and on dyspeptic symptoms in patients with idiopathic gastroparesis. *Gut* 1987;28:300–305

78. Heaton KW, Parker D, Cripps H. Bowel function and irritable bowel symptoms after hysterectomy and cholecystectomy—a population based study. *Gut* 1993;34: 1108–1111

79. Nardi GL, Acosta JM. Papillitis as a cause of pancreatitis and abdominal pain: role of evocative test, operative pancreatography and histologic evaluation. *Ann Surg* 1966; 164:611–618

80. Geenen JE, Hogan WJ, Dodds WJ, et al. The efficacy of endoscopic sphincterotomy after cholecystectomy in patients with sphincter-of-Oddi dysfunction. *N Eng J Med* 1989;320(2):82–87

81. Guelrud M, Mendoza S, Rossiter G, Villegas M: Sphincter of Oddi manometry in healthy volunteers. *Dig Dis Sci* 1990;35(1):38–46

82. Sherman S, Troiano FP, Hawes RH, et al. Frequency of abnormal sphincter of Oddi manometry compared with the clinical suspicion of sphincter of Oddi dysfunction. *Am J Gastroenterol* 1991;86(5):586–590

83. Meshkinpour H, Mollot M, Eckerling GB, Bookman L. Bile duct dyskinesia; clinical and manometric study. *Gastroenterology* 1984;87:759–762

84. Bar-meir S, Geenen JE, Hogan WJ, et al. Biliary and pancreatic duct pressures measured by ERCP manometry in patients with suspected papillary stenosis. *Dig Dis Sci* 1979;24:209–215

85. Rolny P, Arleback A, Funch-Jensen P, et al. Paradoxical response of sphincter of Oddi to intravenous injection of cholecystokinin or ceruletide. Manometric findings and results of treatment in biliary dyskinesia. *Gut* 1986; 27:1507–1511

86. Tanaka M, Ikeda S, Matsumoto S, Yoshimoto H, Nakayama F: Manometric diagnosis of sphincter of Oddi spasm as a cause of postcholecystectomy pain and the treatment by endoscopic sphincterotomy. *Ann Surg* 1985; 202(6):712–719

87. Grimon G, Buffet C, Andre L, et al. Biliary pain in postcholecystectomy patients without biliary obstruction. *Dig Dis Sci* 1991;36(3):317–320

88. Venu RP, Geenen JE, Hogan W, et al. Idiopathic recurrent pancreatitis: an approach to diagnosis and treatment. *Dig Dis Sci* 1989;34:56–60

89. Kingham JGC, Dawson AM. Origin of chronic right upper quadrant pain. *Gut* 1985;26:783–788

90. Thatcher BS, Sivak MV, Tedesco FJ, et al. Endoscopic sphincterotomy for suspected dysfunction of the sphincter of Oddi. *Gastrointest Endosc* 1987;33(2):91–95

91. Roberts-Thomson IC, Toouli J. Is endoscopic sphincterotomy for disabling biliary-type pain after cholecystectomy effective? *Gastrointest Endosc* 1985;31(6):370–373

92. Rolny P, Geenen JE, Hogan WJ, Venu RP. Clinical features, manometric findings and endoscopic therapy results in group I patients with sphincter of Oddi dysfunction. *Gastroenterology* 1991;37:252 (Abstract)

93. Neoptolemos JP, Bailey IS, Carr-Locke DL. Sphincter of Oddi dysfunction: results of treatment by endoscopic sphincterotomy. *Br J Surg* 1988;75:454–459

94. Sherman S, Ruffolo TA, Hawes RH, Lehman GA: Complications of endoscopic sphincterotomy: a prospective series with emphasis on the increased risk associated with sphincter of Oddi dysfunction and nondilated bile ducts. *Gastroenterology* 1991;101:1068–1075

95. Sand J, Nordback I, Koskinen M, et al. Nifedipine for suspected type II sphincter of Oddi dyskinesia. *Am J Gastroenterol* 1993;88(4):530–535

96. Khuroo MS, Alizargar S, Yattoo GN. Efficacy of nifedipine therapy in patients with sphincter of Oddi dysfunction: a prospective, double-blind, randomized, placebo-controlled, cross over trial. *J Clin Pharmacol* 1992;33:477–485

97. Guelrud M, Rossiter A, Souney PF, et al. The effect of transcutaneous nerve stimulation on sphincter of Oddi pressure in patients with biliary dyskinesia. *Am J Gastroenterol* 1991;86(5):581–585

10

Nausea and Vomiting

Edward E. Whang ▪ *Stanley W. Ashley* ▪ *Edward H. Livingston*

Nausea is an unpleasant sensation, referred to the pharynx and upper abdomen and associated with the feeling that vomiting is imminent. *Vomiting,* or *emesis,* refers to the forceful oral expulsion of gastric contents. *Retching* is the rhythmic respiratory activity associated with emesis; it may occur in isolation, if the stomach is empty.

Nausea and vomiting are clues to the existence of pathology and, in the surgical patient, to the need for therapy. Acute symptoms can be indicative of intra-abdominal catastrophes; chronic symptoms suggest functional or long-standing mechanical disorders. However, these symptoms also accompany a broad spectrum of medical diseases and are complications of a variety of therapeutic interventions. Therefore, knowledge of the diverse etiologies of nausea and vomiting, as well as an understanding of pathophysiologic mechanisms, is essential for the surgeon treating patients with abdominal disorders.

▪ HISTORY

Herodutus described the ancient Egyptian practice of monthly emesis.[1] They believed that, "All diseases to which men were subject proceed from the food itself." Hippocrates also advocated monthly vomiting.[2] Systematic physiologic studies of the mechanisms resulting in vomiting were first described in the 17th century. Chirac concluded that emesis results from compression of a flaccid stomach by the abdominal muscles and diaphragm.[3] This observation was confirmed by Hunter in

1840.[4] The contemporary model for the neural control of emesis was first proposed by Borison and Wang in 1952.[5] They demonstrated the existence of two distinct sites in the brainstem critical for mediating emesis.

The relationships among nausea, vomiting, surgery, and anesthesia were described in 1848 by John Snow.[6] He hypothesized that movement, shortly after awakening from anesthesia, produced the symptoms, and he recommended wine and opium for treatment. One of the great advances in surgery was the introduction of gastric suction.[7] In 1932, Wangensteen demonstrated a substantial reduction in morbidity and mortality with the use of nasogastric suction in the management of nausea and vomiting due to ileus or bowel obstruction.[8] That this technique remains the mainstay of treatment for postoperative nausea and vomiting is a testament to the significance of his observations. Few recent advances in the therapy of postoperative nausea and vomiting have had a comparable impact.

▪ PHYSIOLOGY

Nausea, retching, and vomiting represent characteristic, precisely coordinated responses of the somatic muscles and viscera. Three distinct sequential phases have been described.[9]:

1. **Preejection.** The subjective sensation of nausea develops during this prodromal phase. Autonomic hyperactivity is highlighted by cold sweat-

ing, cutaneous vasoconstriction, papillary dilation, hypersalivation, tachycardia, and reduced gastric secretion. The proximal stomach relaxes, while tone in the proximal small intestine increases.

2. **Ejection.** During retching, the mouth is closed and there is rhythmic, synchronous contraction of the diaphragm, abdominal muscles, and external intercostal muscles against a closed glottis. Intrathoracic pressure falls while intra-abdominal pressure rises. As a result, gastric contents traverse the lower esophageal sphincter and oscillate between the stomach and esophagus. During vomiting, the diaphragmatic hiatus relaxes, permitting transfer of intraabdominal pressure to the thorax. The upper esophageal sphincter relaxes, and the forceful ejection of gastric contents through an open glottis and mouth results.

3. **Postejection.** The period following emesis is characterized by muscular weakness and lethargy.

NEURAL CONTROL OF VOMITING

The *emetic center,* located in the lateral reticular formation of the medulla oblongata, coordinates the neural circuits that mediate the emesis response (Fig 10–1). The *chemore-ceptor trigger zone (CTZ)*[10], located in the area postrema on the floor of the fourth ventricle, contains receptors that are activated by toxins in the blood and cerebrospinal fluid (CSF). Activation of the chemoreceptor trigger zone results in the stimulation of the emetic center through neural pathways between the two centers. The overall effect is emesis in response to circulating toxins.

Visceral afferent nerve fibers transmit emetic signals from the gut to the emetic center.[11] Mechanoreceptors, located in the intestinal submucosal plexus and muscular wall, are activated by contraction as well as distention of the bowel, and mucosal chemoreceptors are activated by intraluminal irritants.[12] In turn, they activate visceral afferent nerves that ultimately stimulate the emesis center. This mechanism is responsible for vomiting induced by bowel obstruction, peritoneal inflammation, intestinal ischemia, and chemical irritation.

The vestibular labyrinthine system is essential for induction of emesis by motion stimuli. Electrical stimulation of the cerebral cortex, hypothalamus, and thalamus can evoke emesis. Psychologic stimuli, acting through **higher centers,** descend through cerebral pathways and also may induce vomiting. Nausea and vomiting also can be evoked by mechanical stimulation of pharyngeal afferents projecting to the brainstem via the glossopharyngeal nerves. A brainstem pressure detector

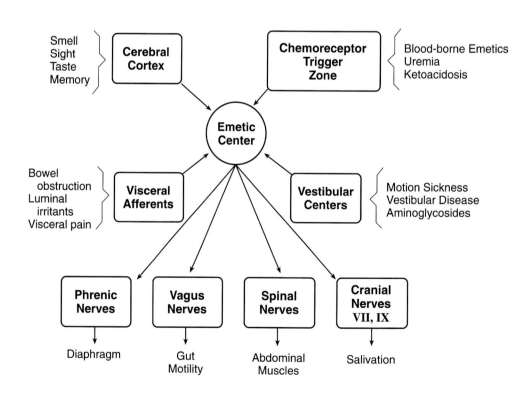

Figure 10–1. The neural control of vomiting. The neural pathways mediating the emesis response.

tector has been implicated in the nausea and vomiting caused by increased intracranial pressure.

The afferent and efferent arcs of the vomiting response are mediated through a variety of neurotransmitters, both in the Central Nervous System and in the periphery.[13] Of these, the evidence for a physiologic role for dopamine, histamine, opiates, and serotonin is most convincing.

HORMONAL INFLUENCES

Hormonal control of nausea and vomiting is not understood as well as neural control. Peptide YY (PYY) is the most potent hormone associated with vomiting and has been proposed as an endogenous circulating emetogen.[14] Elevated β-hCG and progesterone levels might contribute to the nausea and vomiting that occurs during pregnancy.[15] Elevated levels of serum Adrenal Cortico-Trophin Hormone vasopressin, and norepinephrine have been found in the syndrome of recurrent paroxysmal vomiting.[16] However, controlled radioimmunoassay studies have failed to demonstrate a clear correlation between symptom onset or severity and plasma level of any hormone.[17]

■ ETIOLOGY

GASTROINTESTINAL OBSTRUCTION

Regurgitation, rather than true vomiting, occurs with *esophageal obstruction,* which can be the result of neoplasms, strictures, or rings.

Gastric outlet obstruction causes chronic nausea and vomiting. Patients with this disorder may vomit undigested food particles for up to 12 hours after a meal. Peptic ulcer disease (PUD) is the most common etiology. In a review of 738 patients with PUD, gastric outlet obstruction was found to be a complication in 12%.[18] The majority of these patients have chronic disease, with marked structural deformities of the antrum and duodenal bulb. However, symptoms also can be transient or recurrent with pyloric channel ulcers, which can induce local edema and pylorospasm. Other etiologies for mechanical gastric outlet obstruction include gastric carcinoma, Crohn's disease, pancreatitis, pancreatic pseudocyst, and pancreatic cancer.

Mechanical *small bowel obstruction* results in nausea and vomiting accompanied by crampy abdominal pain, distention, and obstipation. The most common etiologies for small bowel obstruction are postoperative adhesions (75%), malignancies (8%), hernias (8%), volvulus (3%), and inflammatory bowel disease (1%).[19] Proximal obstruction tends to present early (1 day), with pain and vomiting predominating within the symptom complex. Distal small bowel obstruction occurs

later (2 to 3 days), with abdominal pain, distention, and obstipation preceding vomiting.

Although obstipation, abdominal pain, and distention are more prominent symptoms in patients with **colonic obstruction,** nausea and vomiting may occur as well. The most common causes of large bowel obstruction are carcinoma (65%), volvulus (15%), and diverticular disease (10%).[20] Other etiologies include hernias, peritoneal carcinomatosis, fecal impaction, intussusception, postradiation and ischemic strictures, foreign bodies, and inflammatory bowel disease.

POSTGASTRECTOMY SYNDROMES

Nausea and vomiting are characteristic of several postgastrectomy syndromes. Bilious vomiting is a consistent finding in **alkaline reflux gastritis.** This complication occurs most frequently following Bilroth II (BII) reconstruction, but it also is seen after Bilroth I (BI) reconstruction and after pyloroplasty. *Postsurgical gastroparesis syndrome* occurs after vagotomy and antrectomy with BI or BII reconstruction, vagotomy with drainage, or Roux-en-Y reconstruction done for relief of alkaline reflux gastritis. The syndrome is characterized by nausea, vomiting, and pain, with gastric stasis in the absence of mechanical obstruction. The physiological basis for this syndrome is unclear, but may be related to decreased gastric reservoir capacity, alteration of the pyloric sphincter mechanism, and vagotomy.[21]

Intermittent mechanical obstruction of the afferent limb of a BII reconstruction leads to the *afferent loop syndrome.* It is characterized by postprandial midepigastric pain that is relieved by emesis of large volumes of bilious vomitus. In contrast to *efferent loop obstruction,* the vomitus of afferent obstruction is devoid of food particles. Other mechanical etiologies of postgastric-surgery vomiting include anastomotic obstruction, jejunal intussusception, internal herniation, adhesions, and recurrent ulcer.

FUNCTIONAL DISORDERS OF THE GASTROINTESTINAL TRACT

Gastroparesis refers to a gastric motility disorder in which the transit of intraluminal contents into the duodenum is impaired without mechanical obstruction.[22] Nausea and vomiting are accompanied by bloating, early satiety, and recurrent bezoar formation. Vomiting of large volumes of solid food several hours after a meal is typical. Defects of antral function and resultant delayed emptying of solids are most pronounced. Patients with gastroparesis often have normal gastric transit of liquids, indicating that the factors that regulate fundic tone are normal. The severity of symptoms do not correlate well with objective findings are radionuclide-emptying studies.

Gastroparesis is most frequently idiopathic; however, predisposing factors, especially reversible conditions, should be sought. Gastroparesis can be induced by drugs, particularly narcotics, aluminum-containing antacids, anticholinergics, β-adrenergic agents, tricyclic antidepressants, and diphenhydramine. Gastroparesis is also a component of systemic disorders such as diabetes mellitus and scleroderma. Gastroparesis diabeticorum usually is associated with long-term insulin dependence and manifestations of peripheral neuropathy, and is probably secondary to a vagal neuropathy. Recordings of intragastric contractile activity indicate a loss of phase 3 of the migating myoelectric complex (MMC), the powerful contractions that sweep along the GI tract and serve to push chyme forward.[22] MMC phase 3 activity also is lost in patients who have undergone surgical vagotomy.

Nonulcer dyspepsia is a term used to describe a disorder characterized by persistent epigastric distress associated with nausea, early satiety, belching, and bloating, in the absence of objective gastric pathology.[23] Delayed gastric emptying and duodenogastric bile reflux are found in some of these patients, but the pathophysiology and diagnostic criteria are poorly defined. Evaluation is directed at ruling out diseases that can cause similar symptoms, including peptic ulcer disease, gastric carcinoma, gastroesophageal reflux, biliary tract disease, chronic pancreatitis, and irritable bowel syndrome.

Intestinal pseudo-obstruction represents a group of syndromes characterized by the signs and symptoms consistent with small intestinal or colonic obstruction, in the absence of intrinsic or extrinsic occlusion of the gut lumen.[24] Impaired intestinal motility is the primary defect and can be the result of derangements in intestinal musculature or neural control, systemic diseases, or medications.

Acute pseudo-obstruction most commonly occurs as an isolated colonic disorder (Ogilvie's syndrome).[25] It generally occurs in elderly patients as a complication of other illnesses, including cardiac disease, major surgery, infection, and trauma. Nausea and vomiting is rare; in fact, worrisome symptoms usually are absent, and the physical examination is unimpressive except for the marked abdominal distention.[24] Patients with this syndrome typically continue to pass flatus and have diarrhea while the abdominal distention is progressing. Abdominal x-ray films reveal a massively dilated colon with well-preserved haustral markings and a minimum of small bowel air. Differentiation from mechanical colonic obstruction is generally dependent upon water soluble contrast enema or sigmoidoscopic examinations.

The clinical course of chronic intestinal pseudo-obstruction is more variable. The motility disturbances in this disorder can affect every part of the gastrointestinal tract, and the regions involved determine the clinical presentation. Esophageal involvement produces dysphagia and heartburn; gastric and intestinal involvement result in nausea, vomiting, bloating, and abdominal discomfort; colonic involvement leads to distention and constipation. Etiologies for this syndrome are divided into the myopathic disorders, such as scleroderma, amyloidosis, and hollow visceral myopathy, and the neuropathic disorders, including the idiopathic variant, which is believed to result from a derangement of the myenteric plexus. Neuropathic and myopathic forms of this disorder sometimes can be distinguished on the basis of distinctive manometric profiles, but a full-thickness biopsy of the affected segment often is required to establish a diagnosis.

INFECTION AND IMMUNITY

Nausea and vomiting, associated with diarrhea, abdominal cramps, headache, and myalgia that occurs during a 24 to 48 hour period, are almost diagnostic of viral gastroenteritis. Two parvoviruslike agents, the Norwalk agent and the Hawaii agent, are most frequently implicated in acute, self-limited cases.[26] Nausea and vomiting may occur in immunosuppressed patients in association with cytomegalovirus and herpes simplex infections of the gastrointestinal tract.

Diarrhea is usually a more prominent symptom than vomiting in bacterial gastroenteritis, except in cases caused by nontyphoid *Salmonella*, in which vomiting can be severe. Food poisoning with bacterial toxins is a common cause of acute nausea and vomiting. Toxins of *Staphylococcus aureus*, *Clostridium perfringens*, or *Bacillus cereus* cause illness within 24 hours after exposure. Acute infectious hepatitis may produce nausea and vomiting before right upper quadrant tenderness or icterus become apparent. These symptoms usually abate as the jaundice becomes more pronounced.

A variety of systemic infections or infections with foci distant from the gastrointestinal tract may induce nausea and vomiting, particularly in children. Graft-versus-host disease after allogeneic bone marrow transplantation also leads to nausea and vomiting.

PREGNANCY

Nausea occurs in 50% to 90% of all pregnancies. Vomiting occurs in 25% to 55% of pregnancies.[15] The incidence of symptoms is higher in younger women, obese women, women from Western cultures, and women who experience nausea and vomiting while taking oral contraceptives. Symptoms begin shortly after the first missed menstrual period, peak in the third month, and usually disappear by the fourth month. Symptom severity is not correlated with a higher risk for fetal abnormalities, death, or low birth weight.

Hyperemesis gravidarum is diagnosed in pregnant women who develop fluid and electrolyte disturbances or nutritional deficiency from intractable vomiting. The incidence is 3.5 per 1000 deliveries.[27] There is no association with toxemia of pregnancy or fetal abnormalities. Vomiting begins after the first missed menstrual period and usually disappears during the third month. There is a higher incidence in women with multiple gestation or molar pregnancies. Severe metabolic disturbances in untreated patients may result in death. Treatment is directed at fluid and electrolyte replacement and supportive psychotherapy.

MEDICATIONS

Nausea and vomiting are frequently reported drug side-effects.[28,29] Drugs and their metabolites can induce nausea and vomiting by activating receptors in the chemoreceptor trigger zone, gastrointestinal tract, or both. They may also inhibit enzymes responsible for degrading emetogenic neurotransmitters.

A list of drugs causing nausea and vomiting is shown in Table 10–1.

CHEMOTHERAPY

The toxicities most universally recognized as being associated with chemotherapy are nausea and vomiting.[30–32] These symptoms are frequently the limiting toxicity, requiring chemotherapeutic regimens to be altered. Antitumor efficacy is often sacrificed by using lower dosages or less potent agents in an effort to reduce nausea and vomiting. Up to 20% of patients have been reported to withdraw from some treatments because of nausea and vomiting.

Chemotherapy-induced nausea and vomiting occurs in three well-characterized syndromes.[33] The acute syndrome, which has the greatest prevalence, begins 1 to 2 hours after drug administration, peaks within 4 to 10 hours, and subsides within 12 to 24 hours. Delayed nausea and vomiting occurs 1 to 5 days after treatment, with a peak frequency between 48 and 72 hours. Symptoms are generally less severe than in the acute form, but may be of greater duration. Anticipatory nausea and vomiting is a conditioned reflex associated with poor control of emesis during prior treatments. Symptoms occur before the treatment actually is administered.

Chemotherapeutic agents exhibit a broad range of emetogenicity, as shown in Table 10–2. Cisplatin is the agent acknowledged to be the most emetogenic. Reducing peak plasma concentrations of the agents through the use of continuous infusion schedules, in contrast to bolus infusions, has been shown to reduce the severity of symptoms.[34] In combination chemotherapy, the degree of nausea and vomiting is additive.

Patient characteristics correlated with reduced symptom severity include male sex, age, and a history of heavy alcohol use.[35] There appears to be a significant psychological component, since severity increases in patients suffering from depression or anxiety disorders. A roommate suffering from nausea and vomiting also may increase symptom severity.

It is important to remember that the etiologies of nausea and vomiting in patients receiving chemotherapy for malignancies also include structural manifestations of tumor growth (brain metastasis or bowel obstruction), metabolic complications (hypercalcemia), as well as factors unrelated to the cancer or its therapy.

RADIOTHERAPY

Nearly 50% of patients treated with a radiation dose of at least 230 cGy experience vomiting.[36] Epigastric radiation causes earlier and more severe symptoms than does radiation directed at other parts of the body. Neutron radiotherapy is more emetogenic than gamma radiotherapy.[37]

The mechanism causing these effects is unknown, but inflammatory mediators and other humoral factors released during radiation-induced tissue damage may stimulate receptors in the Chemoreceptor Trigger Zone.[37] Following cranial or whole body radiation, cerebral edema with concomitant increases in intracranial pressure may lead to vomiting.

Up to 15% of patients develop late complications of radiation to the gastrointestinal tract, including mu-

TABLE 10–1. DRUGS CAUSING NAUSEA AND VOMITING

Drug Class	Mechanism/Site of Action
Aminoglycosides	Vestibular damage
Bromocriptine	Area postrema
Cholinomimetics	Area postrema
Levodopa	Area postrema
Opiates	Area postrema
Theophylline	Area postrema
Ipecac	Gastric afferent nerves
Ergot alkaloids	Area postrema
Cardiac glycosides	Area postrema

TABLE 10–2. EMETOGENIC POTENTIAL OF CHEMOTHERAPEUTIC AGENTS

High Emetogenic	Moderately Emetogenic	Mildly Emetogenic
Actinomycin-D	Asparaginase	Bleomycin
Cisplatin	Azacitidine	Etoposide
Carmustine	Carboplatin	Fluorouracil
Dacarbazine	Cyclophosphamide	Methotrexate
Nitrogen mustard	Doxorubicin	Vincristine
Streptozocin	Mitomycin	

Adapted from Strum SB, McDermed JE, Pileggi J, Riech LP, Whitaker H. Intravenous metoclopramide: prevention of chemotherapy-induced nausea and vomiting: a preliminary evaluation. *Cancer* 1984;53:1432–1439

cosal ulceration, intestinal obstruction and fistulia, malabsorption, and arteritis with gradual vascular occlusion.[38] All of these changes can produce nausea and vomiting months to years after radiation therapy.

MISCELLANEOUS ETIOLOGIES

Nausea and vomiting due to seasickness, carsickness, spectacle sickness, wide-screen movies sickness, flight simulator sickness, and vestibular end-organ disease require intact vestibular afferent pathways. A unifying pathophysiologic concept explains each of these disorders as examples of a single sensory conflict syndrome. The conflict develops between information given by one set of sensations and that given by another set (intermodality conflict) or between actual and anticipated signals (neural mismatch).[39] It is apparent that endogenously produced motion, such as running and jumping, rarely cause symptoms, and that actual physical motion is not even necessary for motion sickness to develop.

Increased intracranial pressure, whether caused by intracerebral tumors, pseudotumor cerebri, or CNS infections, produce vomiting that is often, but not necessarily, projectile. Symptoms tend to be more pronounced in the morning.

Metabolic causes of nausea and vomiting include diabetic ketoacidosis, uremia, adrenal insufficiency (particularly during adrenal crisis), and electrolyte imbalances.

Vomiting is a component of anorexia nervosa and bulimia. Patients suffering from anorexia nervosa attempt to lose weight primarily through reduced intake, but they may use vomiting as an adjunctive measure. Delayed gastric emptying has been described in these patients, although its relevance is not clear.[40] Bulimia, on the other hand, is characterized by episodes of binge eating followed by vomiting and may be associated with laxative and diuretic abuse. The magnitude of vomiting in these disorders is sometimes great enough to induce fatal metabolic complications.

■ VOMITING IN THE PEDIATRIC PATIENT

An infant who begins vomiting in the first days of life should be evaluated for the presence of gastrointestinal obstruction caused by necrotizing enterocolitis, intestinal atresia, malrotation, meconium ileus, Hirschsprung's disease, imperforate anus, or gastric torsion.[41] Intestinal obstruction should be suspected in any infant who (1) exhibits >20 cc of fluid on gastric aspirate, especially if it is bile-stained, (2) vomits and has abdominal distention during the first 24 to 36 hours of life, and/or (3) does not pass meconium stool by 48 hours.[42] Vomiting accompanied by bloody diarrhea suggests is-

chemic or dead bowel. Other causes of vomiting in the first few days of life include infections, such as meningitis, sepsis, necrotizing enterocolitis, and pyelonephritis. In infants, these infections can be present in the absence of fever. Metabolic acidosis or hyperammonemia, owing to inborn errors of amino acid metabolism, renal insufficiency, obstructive uropathy, or increased intracranial pressure that is due to hydrocephalus, subdural hematoma, and cerebral edema, are additional etiologies in the newborn.

The differential diagnosis of vomiting in the older infant (4 weeks to 2 years) include gastrointestinal obstruction resulting from hypertrophic pyloric stenosis, enteric duplications, malrotation with volvulus, intussusception, incarcerated hernia, complications of Meckel's diverticulum, and Hirschsprung's disease. The characteristically projectile, nonbilious vomiting of pyloric stenosis begins when the infant is 2 to 6 weeks old. Intussusception is the most common cause of obstruction between 3 months and 6 years. In infants under the age of 4 months, vomiting may be the sole presenting symptom.[43] Nonobstructive etiologies include gastroenteritis and gastroesophageal reflux. Pediatric patients particularly are prone to vomiting during the course of a variety of infections, including pneumonia, pertussis, otitis media, streptococcal pharyngitis, cervical adenitis, urinary tract infection, and viral hepatitis.

In the older child (>2 years), gastroenteritis is the most common cause of vomiting, but appendicitis, peptic ulcer, and posttraumatic injuries also should be considered. Accidental ingestion of drugs or chemical agents always should be considered in vomiting of acute onset.

Cyclic vomiting occurs in children between 2 and 5 years of age and is characterized by recurrent attacks of vomiting, fever, headaches, and abdominal pain. Frequency of vomiting ranges from once a month to several times a day. The etiology is unknown, although a seizure disorder and psychosocial stress have been proposed.

Reye's syndrome should be considered in a child with vomiting and altered mental status. It typically follows a viral infection (influenza or varicella, most commonly) and has been associated with aspirin use. Encephalopathy and hepatomegaly with fatty degeneration of the viscera occur. Laboratory confirmation is based on a three-fold or greater elevation of serum ammonia and transaminase levels.

■ EVALUATION OF THE PATIENT

EVALUATION OF SYMPTOMS

The precise nature of the symptoms should be delineated. Nausea should be differentiated from anorexia and early satiety, which have different diagnostic and therapeutic implications. Likewise, vomiting should be differentiated from regurgitation and rumination. *Regurgitation,* indicative of esophageal disease, consists of the return of gastric or esophageal contents to the pharynx in the absence of active muscular contractions that occur with vomiting. *Rumination* refers to repeated cycles of regurgitation followed by swallowing of the regurgitated material. The act is usually involuntary, effortless, and is not associated with abdominal discomfort or nausea.

Duration of Symptoms

Acute nausea and vomiting accompany intraabdominal crises. In the absence of marked abdominal pain, acute symptoms usually are associated with an infectious, toxic, or drug etiology. The etiologies of chronic nausea and vomiting are more varied and the diagnosis more difficult.

Timing

Nausea and vomiting early in the morning, and prior to meals, is typical during pregnancy and is seen in patients with uremia, alcoholism, and increased intracranial pressure.

Relation to Meals

Vomiting due to viral gastroenteritis or active gastric ulcer occurs in the immediate postprandial period. Symptoms that occur with gastric outlet obstruction or delayed gastric emptying often occur several hours after eating.

Content of Vomitus

Undigested food suggests regurgitation and esophageal disease. Partially digested food suggests gastric outlet obstruction, high small–bowel obstruction or gastroparesis. The presence of bile indicates gastroduodenal patency and is, therefore, rare in gastric outlet obstruction. A feculent odor suggests ischemic injury to the gut, gastrocolic fistula, or long-standing obstruction of ileus with bacterial overgrowth. Blood and coffee grounds–appearing emesis indicate mucosal injury.

Associated Symptoms

Pain is often the chief complaint in abdominal emergencies. Vomiting often relieves pain due to peptic ulcer disease, but not that caused by pancreatitis or biliary tract disease. Weight loss, anorexia, and early satiety are typical of patients with malignant etiologies of gastric outlet obstruction. In contrast, patients with benign causes of gastric outlet obstruction retain a normal appetite. Fever and myalgia suggest a viral infection. Headache, neck stiffness, disturbed vision, and mental status changes suggest CNS lesions. Inappropriate attitudes to symptoms, especially in young women, should suggest an eating disorder.

HISTORICAL FACTORS

A thorough drug ingestion history, as well as a history of systemic illnesses predisposing to impaired GI motility, such as diabetes, should be sought. Infection or bacterial toxin-induced illness is suggested by a history of family or friends acquiring similar symptoms, particularly if the same food was ingested by affected individuals.

PHYSICAL FINDINGS

The abdomen should be examined for the presence of distention, tenderness, masses, scars, a succussion splash, and the quality of bowel sounds. A hernia should be sought and the stool examined for occult blood. Evidence of weight loss, dehydration, and hypovolemia is elicited by determining the presence of postural hypotension. Fundoscopic examination can reveal increased intracranial pressure. Detailed neurologic examination is indicated when a generalized gastrointestinal motility disorder is suspected. Cranial nerve palsies, extrapyramidal signs, peripheral neuropathy, signs of autonomic neuropathy (such as orthostatic hypotension, absence of sweating, abnormal pulse and blood pressure responses to a Valsalva maneuver) should be sought. These signs might suggest a neural basis for impaired GI motility.

LABORATORY TESTS

Pregnancy should be excluded in women of childbearing age prior to radiographic studies. Serum chemistries may reveal electrolyte and metabolic disturbances that may cause vomiting. Hypochloremic, hypokalemic metabolic alkalosis is a consequence of vomiting and indicates the need for replacement therapy. Determination of serum drug levels (digoxin, for example) may be indicated based on the history.

RADIOLOGICAL AND ENDOSCOPIC TESTS

Abdominal series and contrast studies may reveal lesions producing symptoms, or they may offer indirect evidence of mechanical obstruction or motility disturbances, such as gastric dilation, retained food and secretions, delayed emptying of contrast, and intestinal dilation with slow transit. Abdominal computed tomographic (CT) scanning is indicated when pancreatic disease is suspected or when extrinsic compression is seen during contrast studies.

Since delayed clearance of contrast can limit further studies, a contrast enema should be performed prior to an upper gastrointestinal series, if distal obstruction is considered. Likewise, residual contrast can obscure CT scan interpretation. If leakage from the gastrointestinal tract is a concern, Gastrograffin is the contrast agent of choice. However, Gastrograffin may stimulate motility in ileus, but it also may exacerbate symptoms in cases of mechanical bowel obstruction.

Endoscopy is more sensitive and specific than radiological studies in the diagnosis of foregut mucosal lesions, but is less likely to provide information on motor function. Findings may be normal even with severe gastrointestinal motility disorders.

GASTRIC EMPTYING STUDY

Gastric emptying may be evaluated after mechanical obstruction has been eliminated as the basis for symptoms. Dual isotope gamma scintigraphy is used to quantitate gastric emptying of meals labeled with radioactive isotopes. Technetium 99m (^{99m}Tc)-DTPA and indium 113 m (^{113m}In)-DTPA are used to label liquids, and ^{99m}Tc-sulfur colloid incorporated into chicken liver is the most commonly employed solid marker.[44] Although these studies can establish the presence of delayed gastric emptying, they do not distinguish among the various causes of gastroparesis. Positive results can be found even in patients with anorexia nervosa.[40]

MANOMETRY

Manometry of the stomach and small intestine has seen limited clinical application, despite the fact that it is well established in the evaluation of foregut motility. Gastrointestinal manometry may play a greater role in the future, as comprehensive databases of motility patterns in health and disease are established.[45] Manometry might be particularly useful in distinguishing pseudo-obstruction from mechanical obstruction. A disorganized pattern of infrequent, low-amplitude contractions is typical of pseudo-obstruction, whereas clustered contractions separated by periods of quiescence are characteristic of mechanical obstruction.[46]

ANCILLIARY STUDIES

Labyrinthine function tests can reveal vestibular disease, while CT or magnetic resonance imaging (MRI) examinations of the head can disclose intracranial lesions. Autonomic function tests, such as the sweat test and recordings of the cardiac response to vagal stimulation, may indicate generalized disorders of autonomic regulation. Psychogenic vomiting should be considered and psychiatric consultation requested. It should be remembered that psychogenic vomiting is a diagnosis of exclusion and that psychiatric symptoms may be a consequence of chronic nausea and vomiting.

DIAGNOSTIC LAPAROTOMY

Indications for laparotomy include obstruction, perforation, and peritonitis. Other reasons for laparotomy in cases of long-standing nausea and vomiting are less compelling. When a complete evaluation yields no diagnosis, laparotomy or laparoscopy occasionally may be indicated, if symptoms are intractable and responsible for significant disability and a compromised nutritional state. At laparotomy, if no structural lesion is found, full-thickness intestinal biopsies are taken and examined for the presence of smooth muscle and neural pathology (Fig 10–2).

■ COMPLICATIONS OF VOMITING

The mechanical stress induced by protracted retching and vomiting may result in gastroesophageal mucosal tears (Mallory-Weiss syndrome) or free perforation of the esophagus (Boerhaave syndrome). These syndromes are also associated with hiatal hernia. The high intraabdominal pressure associated with retching is transmitted to the herniated segment located in the thorax. Rapid gastric and esophageal distention results in tears in the region of the gastroesophageal junction. High intra-abdominal pressures are transmitted through the venous system, resulting in cutaneous capillary rupture manifested as petechiae. Postoperatively, the dramatic fluctuations in intraabdominal and intrathoracic pressure may result in wound dehiscence or bleeding.

Aspiration pneumonia is one of the most significant causes of postoperative morbidity. Frequently, this complication results from postoperative emesis. Normally, the glottis is closed during vomiting, but this protective mechanism may be lost with anesthetics, alcohol intoxication, or brainstem damage, increasing the risk of postemesis aspiration pneumonia.

Metabolic consequences of protracted emesis include malnutrition, dehydration, hyponatremia, hypokalemia, and metabolic acidosis or alkalosis. Hypochloremic, hypokalemic metabolic alkalosis is produced by the loss of hydrogen, potassium, and chloride ions in the vomitus, contraction of the extracellular fluid space without a commensurate loss of bicarbonate from this compartment, and a hypokalemia-induced shift of hydrogen ions into the intracellular compartment. Hypokalemia also results from urinary potassium losses. The alkalosis is associated with the delivery of sodium bicarbonate to the kidneys at a rate that exceeds the maximum renal tubular capacity for bicarbonate reabsorption. In the distal tubule, sodium-potassium countertransport leads to potassium excretion. This mechanism is stimulated by increased levels of aldosterone

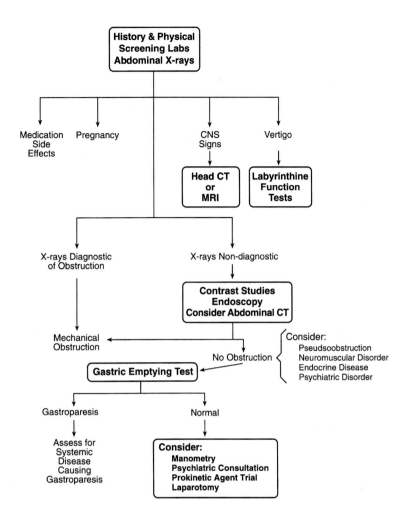

Figure 10-2. The diagnostic algorithm for chronic/recurrent nausea and vomiting.

associated with volume contraction. As the potassium is depleted, a paradoxic aciduria results, since hydrogen ions can substitute for potassium on the countertransporter. Hyponatremia results from the loss of sodium in the vomitus and from renal losses in association with bicarbonate excretion. Increased urinary excretion of sodium paradoxically occurs in the face of systemic sodium depletion. Antidiuretic hormone (ADH) levels are elevated with volume contraction and contribute to the hyponatremia.

■ **TREATMENT**

The therapy for specific gastrointestinal disorders is described in subsequent chapters. Here the pharmacology of antiemetics and their clinical uses are outlined (Fig 10–3).

ANTIDOPAMINERGIC AGENTS

These agents induce antiemetic effects by acting as dopamine receptor antagonists, primarily at the chemoreceptor trigger zone, but also in the periphery. Their most important side-effects are the result of dopamine inhibition, and include extrapyramidal reactions, galactorrhea, and gynecomastia.

Phenothiazines

These were the first group of drugs demonstrated to have substantial antiemetic activity.[47] Prochlorperazine (Compazine) and chlorpromazine (Thorazine) are the phenothiazines most used frequently for nausea and vomiting. These agents display antihistaminic and anticholinergic activity and therefore are effective against motion sickness. Prochlorperazine has been shown to have an effect significantly greater than placebo, but

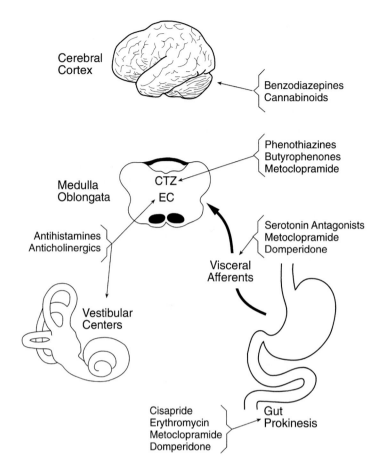

Figure 10–3. Site of action of antiemetic agents.

less than that of tetrahydrocannabinol or high-dose metoclopramide in cytotoxic chemotherapy-induced emesis.[48]

Butyrophenones
These include haloperidol (Haldol) and droperidol. The antiemetic use of Haloperidol is primarily limited to the treatment of terminally ill patients. Droperidol, because of its more prolonged duration of action, is used in the management of postoperative nausea and vomiting.

Substituted Benzamides
The prototype is metoclopramide (Reglan). These were originally developed as prokinetic agents for the treatment of diabetic gastroparesis and for use during radiological procedures. Metoclopramide increases lower esophageal sphincter pressure and relaxes the pyloric sphincter mechanism. Gastric emptying is accelerated in patients who are diabetic or who have undergone vagotomy.[49] Small intestinal transit also is accelerated. At standard doses, metoclopramide is ineffective as an

antiemetic agent but, at high doses (2 mg/kg intravenously every 2 hours), it has potent antiemetic activity against chemotherapy-induced symptoms. Both antidopaminergic and antiseritonergic actions are observed at these high doses, with the antiseritonergic action actually more relevant to its antiemetic effect.[50]

Domperidone
This is an imidazole agent that penetrates the blood-brain barrier poorly and therefore is less likely to produce extrapyramidal reactions than the other dopamine receptor antagonists. Its role in the treatment of chemotherapy-induced emesis has been limited because of case reports in which large doses of intravenous domperidone have led to cardiac arrest.[51] The intravenous form of domperidone subsequently was withdrawn, although cardiac arrests had not occurred with recommended doses. Because of the relatively minor side-effect profile, oral formulations of domperidone are gaining popularity as antiemetics for pediatric patients undergoing chemotherapy.[52]

CORTICOSTEROIDS

Dexamethasone, methyprednisolone, and prednisone are mildly effective antiemetic agents. The mechanism of their antiemetic actions is unknown, but may be related to their antiinflammatory properties[53] or their ability to alter cellular permeability.[54] They are used primarily in combination with other antiemetic agents in the management of symptoms in patients undergoing chemotherapy.

CANNABINOIDS

Dronabinol (delta-9-tetrahydrocannabinal or THC) and nabilone have been found to be superior to placebo, and equivalent or superior to oral prochloperazine, in the management of chemotherapy-induced nausea and vomiting.[55] Side effects consisting of dysphoria, hallucination, sedation, vertigo, dry mouth, and disorientation (particularly in older patients) limit their use. They are seldom used as first-line therapy but are employed in patients unable to tolerate other antiemetic regimens.

BENZODIAZEPINES

Lorazepam and alprazolam are used in the management of anticipatory vomiting and anxiety related to chemotherapy administrations. Their antiemetic potency is low, and their anxioloytic, sedative, and amnesic properties may account for their beneficial effects.[56]

ANTICHOLINERGIC AGENTS

Hyoscine hydrobromide (scopolamine hydrobromide) is administered as a transdermal preparation, since it is rapidly metabolized by the liver and has a short duration of action in oral and parenteral forms. It acts as an antagonist at muscarinic receptors and is useful for treating motion sickness and postoperative nausea and vomiting. It is ineffective in treating chemotherapy-induced emesis. In palliative care settings, a subcutaneous infusion of scopolamine and morphine has been used to control the retching, nausea, vomiting, and pain induced by intestinal obstruction.[57]

ANTIHISTAMINES

Diphenhydramine, cyclizine, and promethazine block H1 receptors at the level of the vestibular afferents and within the brain stem. They are commonly used in the treatment of motion sickness and postoperative nausea and vomiting.

ANTISEROTONERGIC AGENTS

Odansetron (Zofran) is the first member of the newest family of antiemetic drugs.[58] They are specific antagonists at the serotonin $5HT_3$ receptor. Comparative trials have demonstrated odansetron to be superior to metoclopramide in the treatment of chemotherapy-induced nausea and vomiting.[59] Side effects, all of which are mild and transient, include headache, lightheadedness, diarrhea, rash, and increases in serum aminotransferase levels. Extrapyramidal reactions are not seen with these agents. These agents were developed specifically to treat chemotherapy-induced symptoms. It has not yet been determined how useful odansetron will be in treating other forms of nausea and vomiting.

PROKINETIC AGENTS

These agents enhance the transit of materials through the gastrointestinal tract. They have been used in the treatment of gastroesophageal reflux, gastroparesis, nonulcer dyspepsia, postoperative ileus, chronic intestinal pseudoobstruction, and colonic motor disorders.[49] Cisapride is related structurally to metoclopramide but has no antidopaminergic activity and therefore, induces no extrapyramidal side-effects. By stimulating the release of acetylcholine from enteric neurons, it stimulates gastrointestinal motility.[49] Its only side-effect is increased stool frequency. Macrolides, such as erythromycin, stimulate the onset of migrating motor complexes even at dosages that are less than required for antibiotic potency.[60] Motilin, a 22 amino–acid gut hormone, plays a physiologic role in initiating MMCs. It appears that erythromycin may act as an agonist at the motilin receptor.[49]

■ APPROACH TO THE PATIENT WITH POSTOPERATIVE NAUSEA AND VOMITING

Postoperative nausea and vomiting and postoperative ileus are well-recognized syndromes that lead to significant morbidity and prolong hospitalization. The incidence of nausea and vomiting after abdominal operations is reported to be 23% to 41% for nausea alone, and 16% for nausea with vomiting.[61] The incidence is greater in female patients and is correlated inversely with age.[62,63] Diabetes, obesity, pregnancy, gastroesophageal reflux, dehydration, and electrolyte imbalances, such as occurs with prolonged fasting and bowel preparations, increase the incidence.

The incidence of symptoms varies with the nature of the procedure, with intraabdominal procedures resulting in the highest rates. Emergency operations in which the stomach has not been adequately decompressed are particularly likely to produce this syndrome. The incidence is correlated directly with the duration of surgery and anesthesia. Although recent series would suggest a reduction in the incidence of ileus with laparoscopy, nausea or vomiting develop in 92% of patients following procedures in which the peritoneal cavity is insufflated.[64] Postoperatively, motion, hypotension, hypoglycemia, and pain exacerbate symptoms.

Nausea and vomiting can accompany visceral pain from a variety of causes, including biliary tract disease, pancreatitis, peritonitis, nephrolithiasis, and myocardial infarction.

Individual intravenous and inhalational anesthetic agents have varying emetogenic potential.[65] Balanced anesthesia techniques that employ opiate analgesics produce a two- to five-fold higher incidence of postoperative symptoms than standard methods. After local and spinal anesthesia, symptoms occur in 9%[66] and 15% to 35%[67] of patients, respectively.

Management of patients with nausea and vomiting in the immediate postoperative period consists of intravenous hydration, analgesia, and bedrest. If oxygen is administered, tight-fitting face masks should be avoided, as they can heighten claustrophobic sensations in nauseated patients. Antiemetic agents traditionally used during the postoperative period include droperidol, metoclopramide, and prochlorperazine. Of these agents, intravenous droperidol has been shown to have the greatest efficacy.[68] The role of odansetron in the treatment of postoperative nausea and vomiting is being investigated.[69] Routine use of prophylactic antiemetics after surgery is unwarranted. They induce undesirable side effects, including sedation, dysphoria, and extrapyramidal symptoms, and they carry a theoretical risk of masking symptoms of postoperative bowel obstruction. However, judicious use of these agents might be indicated in patients with a predisposition to developing severe symptoms or after procedures where vomiting would be particularly detrimental.

Nausea and vomiting accompanied by abdominal pain and distention, particularly if they occur beyond the third postoperative day, are increasingly ominous and indicate the need for reevaluation. A major challenge in the management of postoperative nausea and vomiting is the prompt recognition of bowel obstruction, since a delay in diagnosis may result in intestinal strangulation.

Bowel obstruction occurring in the early postoperative period (within 1 month after operation or during the same hospitalization) constitutes 5% to 29% of all cases of bowel obstruction.[70] It is a complication in 2.2% of all surgical procedures.[71] Surgery of the colon, rectum, or appendix, and surgery for trauma and other emergency conditions are risk factors for the development of early postoperative small bowel obstruction. This predisposition may be related to the degree of contamination or infection resulting from emergency procedures involving the colon.

Abdominal radiographs are often diagnostic of me-

chanical obstruction. Contrast studies are less reliable and may offer a false sense of security. In one series, 38% of patients in whom orally administered contrast material passed into the colon still required operation.[72] The value of contrast studies lies in their ability to differentiate partial from complete small bowel obstruction. This distinction is largely irrelevant in the postoperative period, because a diagnosis of partial obstruction or ileus beyond the third postoperative day should be investigated as urgently as a diagnosis of mechanical bowel obstruction. Uncomplicated ileus occurring after surgery only lasts transiently in the small bowel, 24 to 48 hours in the stomach, and 48 to 72 hours in the colon.[73] Occasionally, inhibition of bowel function is prolonged, lasting days to weeks, and is termed postoperative paralytic ileus. Paralytic ileus persisting beyond the third postoperative day may be the result of an underlying abscess, anastomotic leak, occult wound infection or bowel incarcerated in a fascial dehiscence, or misdiagnosed mechanical bowel obstruction.

An initial trial of nasogastric decompression is warranted, and fluid and electrolyte imbalances should be corrected. Frequent clinical examinations are imperative. Deterioration in the clinical course or an absence of improvement by 48 hours is an indication for contrast studies of the gastrointesinal tract, or laparotomy. This approach is used for all patients whose symptoms are compatible with early postoperative bowel obstruction, regardless of the likelihood that the underlying cause may be ileus.[70]

REFERENCES

1. Garrison F, *An Introduction to the History of Medicine.* Philadelphia, PA: WB Saunders; 1929
2. Nasser M, A prescription of vomiting: historical footnotes. *Int J Eating Dis* 1993;13:129–131
3. Mayo H, *Outlines of Human Physiology,* 2nd ed. London, England: Burgess and Hill; 1829
4. Hunter J, *Observations on Certain Parts of the Animal Oeconomy.* Philadelphia, PA: Haswell, Barrington, and Haswell; 1840
5. Wang SC, Borison HL, A new concept of the organization of the central emetic mechanism: recent studies on the site of action of apomorphine, copper sulfate, and cardiac glycosides. *Gastroenterology* 1952;22:1–12
6. Snow J, *On Narcotism by the Inhalation of Vapours.* 1848, London, England: Royal Society of Medicine Services; 1848 (Facsimile ed, 1991)
7. Kussmaul CA, Meilung von ileus durch magenausspulung. *Berl Klin Wochenschr* 1884;21:669–685
8. Wangensteen OH, The early diagnosis of acute intestinal obstruction with comments on pathology and treatment: with a report on successful decompression of three cases of mechanical small bowel obstruction by nasal siphonage. *West J Surg Obstet and Gynecol* 1932;40:1–17

9. Andrews PL, Hawthorn J, The neurophysiology of vomiting. *Baillieres Clin Gastroenterol* 1988;2:141–168

10. Borison HL, Borison R, McCarthy LE, Role of the area postrema in vomiting and related functions. *Fed Proc* 1984;43:2955–2958

11. Andrews PLR, et al. The abdominal visceral innervation and the emetic reflex: pathways, pharmacology, and plasticity. *Can J Physiol Pharmacol* 1990;68:325–345

12. Andrews PLR. Vagal afferent innervation of the gastrointestinal tract. In: Cervero F, Morrison JFB (eds), *Brain Research*. London, England: Elsevier Science; 1986:65–86

13. Leslie RA, et al. The neuropharmacology of emesis: the role of receptors in neuromodulation of nausea and vomiting. *Can J Physiol Pharmacol* 1990;68:279–288

14. Harding RK, McDonald TJ. Identification of PYY as an emetic peptide in the dog. *Peptides* 1989;10:21–24

15. Baron TH, Ramirez B, Richter JE. Gastrointestinal motility disorders during pregnancy. *Ann Intern Med* 1993; 118:366–375

16. Sato T, et al. Recurrent attacks of vomiting and psychotic depression: a syndrome of periodic catecholamine and prostaglandin discharge. *Acta Endocrinol* 1988;117:189–197

17. Kucharczyk J, Harding RK, Regulatory peptides and the onset of nausea and vomiting. *Can J Physiol Pharmacol* 1990;68:289–293

18. Weiland D, et al. Gastric outlet obstruction in peptic ulcer disease: an indication for surgery. *Am J Surg* 1982;143:90–93

19. Lipsett PA. Small bowel obstruction. In: Cameron JL (ed), *Current Surgical Therapy*. St Louis, MO: Mosby Year Book; 1992:98–101

20. Stanislav GV, Michelassi F. Obstruction of the large bowel. In: Cameron JL (ed), *Current Surgical Therapy*. St Louis, MO: Mosby Year Book; 1992:165–168

21. Herrington JL. Remedial operations for postgastrectomy and postvagotomy syndromes. In: Cameron JL (ed), *Current Surgical Therapy*. St Louis, MO: Mosby Year Book; 1992:86–97

22. Read NW, Houghton LA. Physiology of gastric emptying and pathophysiology of gastroparesis. *Gastroenterol Clin North Am* 1989;18:359–373

23. Talley NJ, Phillips SF. Nonulcer dyspepsia: potential causes and pathophysiology. *Ann Intern Med* 1988;108: 865–879

24. Camilleri M, Phillips SF. Acute and chronic intestinal pseudo-obstruction. *Adv Intern Med* 1991;36:287–306

25. Ogilvie H. Large intestine colic due to sympathetic deprivation. *Br Med J,* 1948;2:671–673

26. Ouyang A. Approach to the patient with nausea and vomiting. In: *Textbook of Gastroenterology*. Philadelphia, PA: JB Lippincott; 1991:647–659

27. Feldman M. Nausea and vomiting. In: Sleisenger MH, Fordtran JS (eds), *Gastrointestinal Disease: Pathophysiology, Diagnosis, Management*. Philadelphia, PA: WB Saunders; 1989:222–238

28. Mitchelson F. Pharmacological agents affecting emesis: a review I. drugs. 1992;43:295–315

29. Mitchelson F. Pharmacological agents affecting emesis: a review II. drugs. 1992;43:443–463

30. O'Brien BJ, et al. Impact of chemotherapy-associated nausea and vomiting on patients' functional status and on costs: survey of five Canadian centers. *Can Med Assoc J* 1993;149:296–302

31. Grunberg SM, Hesketh PJ. Control of chemotherapy-induced emesis. *N Engl J Med* 1993;329:1790–1796

32. Lindley CM, Bernard S, Fields SM. Incidence and duration of chemotherapy-induced nausea and vomiting in the outpatient oncology population. *J Clin Oncol* 1989;7: 1142–1149

33. Graves T. Emesis as a complication of cancer chemotherapy: pathophysiology, importance, and treatment. *Pharmacotherapy* 1992;12:337–345

34. Jordan NS, et al. The effect of administration rate on cisplatin-induced emesis. *J Clin Oncol* 1985;3:559–561

35. Pisters KMW, Kris MG. Management of nausea and vomiting caused by anticancer drugs: state of the art. *Oncology* 1992;6(suppl 2):99–104

36. Stewart DJ. Cancer therapy, vomiting, and antiemetics. *Can J Physiol Pharmacol* 1990;68:304–313

37. Young RW. Mechanisms and treatment of radiation-induced nausea and vomiting. In: Davis CJ, Lake-Bakaar GV, Grahama-Smith DG (eds), *Nausea and Vomiting: Mechanisms and Treatment*. Berlin, Germany: Springer-Verlag; 1986:94–109

38. Kokal WA. The impact of antitumor therapy on nutrition. *Cancer* 1985;55:273–278

39. Oman CM. Motion sickness: a synthesis and evaluation of the sensory conflict theory. *Can J Physiol Pharmacol* 1990; 68:294–303

40. McCallum RW, Grill BB, Lange R. Definition of a gastric emptying abnormality in patients with anorexia nervosa. *Clin Res* 1981;29:667A

41. Fuchs S, Jaffe D. Vomiting. *Pediatr Emerg Care* 1990;6: 164–170

42. Talbert JL, Felman AH, DeBusk FL, Gastrointestinal surgical emergencies in the newborn infant. *Pediatrics* 1970; 76:783–797

43. Newman J, Schuh S, Intussusception in babies under four months of age. *Can Med Assoc J* 1987;136:266–269

44. Brown ML, Malagelada JR. Gastric emptying tests. In: Wahner HW (ed), *Nuclear Medicine: Quantitative Procedures*. Boston, MA: Little, Brown; 1983:171–181

45. Malagelada JR, Camilleri M. Unexplained vomiting: a diagnostic challenge. *Ann Intern Med* 1984;101:211–218

46. Richards W, Parish K, Williams LF. The usefulness of small-bowel manometry in the diagnosis of gastrointestinal motility disorders. *Am Surgeon* 1989;56:238–244

47. Moertel CG, Reitemeier RJ, Gage RP. A controlled clinical evaluation of antiemetic drugs. *JAMA* 1963;186:116–118

48. Gralla RJ, et al. Antiemetic efficacy of high-dose metoclopramide: randomized trials with placebo and prochlorperazine in patients with chemotherapy-induced nausea and vomiting. *N Engl J Med* 1981;305:905–909

49. Reynolds JC, Putnam PE. Prokinetic agents. *Gastroenterol Clin North Am* 1992;21:567–595

50. Fozard JR, Mobarok Ali AT. Blockade of neuronal tryptamine receptors by metoclopramide. *Eur J Pharmacol* 1978; 49:109–112

51. Joss RA, et al. Sudden death in cancer patients on high dose domperidone. *Lancet* 1982;1:1019

52. Allan SG. Antiemetics *Gastroenterol Clin North Am* 1992;21: 597–611

53. Rich WM. Abdulhayoglu G, Di Saia PJ. Methylprednisolone as an antiemetic during cancer chemotherapy—a pilot study. *Gynecol Oncol* 1980;9:193–198

54. Livrea P, et al. Acute changes in blood-CSF barrier permselectivity to serum proteins after intrathecal methotrexate and CNS irradiation. *J Neurol* 1985;231:336–339

55. Sallan SE, et al. Antiemetics in patients receiving chemotherapy for cancer: a randomized comparison of delta-9-tetrahydrocannabinol and prochlorperazine. *N Engl J Med* 1980;302:135–138

56. Bowcock SJ, et al. Antiemetic prophylaxis with high-dose metoclopramide or lorazepam in vomiting induced by chemotherapy. *Br Med J* 1984;288:1879

57. Baines M, Carter RL, Oliver DJ. Medical management of intestinal obstruction in patients with advanced malignant disease: a clinical and pathological study. *Lancet* 1985;990–993

58. Hasketh PJ, Gandara DR. Serotonin antagonists: a new class of antiemetic agents. *J Natl Cancer Inst* 1991;83: 613–620

59. Marty M, et al. Comparison of the 5-hydroxytryptamine (serotonin) antagonist ondansetron (GR38032F) with high-dose metoclopramide in the control of cisplatin-induced emesis. *N Engl J Med* 1990;322:816–821

60. Otterson MF, Sarna SK. Gastrointestinal motor effects of erythromycin. *Am J Physiol* 1990;269:G355–363

61. Benson JM, et al. Nausea and vomiting after abdominal surgery. *Clin Pharmacol* 1992;11:965–967

62. Lerman J. Surgical and patient factors involved in postoperative nausea and vomiting. *Br J Anesth* 1992;69(suppl 1):24S–32S

63. Camu F, Lauwers MH, Verbessem D. Incidence and aetiology of postoperative nausea and vomiting. *Eur J Anesth,* 1992;9(suppl 6):25–31

64. Bodner M, White PF. Antiemetic efficacy of ondansetron after outpatient laparoscopy. *Anesthesiology* 1991;73:250–254

65. Rabey PG, Smith G. Anaesthetic factors contributing to postoperative nausea and vomiting. *Br J Anaesth* 1992; 69(suppl 1):40S–45S

66. Ratra CK, Badola RP, Bhargava KP. A study of factors concerned in emesis during spinal anaesthesia. *Br J Anaesth* 1972;44:1208–1211

67. Spelina KR, Gerber HR, Pagels IL. Nausea and vomiting during spinal anaesthesia. Effect of metoclopramide and domperidone: a double blind trial. *Anaesth,* 1984;39: 132–137

68. Rowbotham DJ. Current management of postoperative nausea and vomiting. *Br J Anesthesiology* 1992;69(suppl 1):46S–59S

69. Baber N, et al. Clinical pharmacology of ondansetron in postoperative nausea and vomiting. *Eur J Anaesth* 1992;9(suppl 6):11–18

70. Frykberg ER, Phillips JW. Obstruction of the small bowel in the early postoperative period. *South Med J* 1989;82: 169–173

71. Quan SHQ, Stearns MW. Early postoperative intestinal obstruction and postoperative intestinal ileus. *Dis Colon Rectum* 1961;4:307–318

72. Dunn JT, Halls JM, Berne TV. Roentgenographic contrast studies in acute small-bowel obstruction. *Arch Surg* 1984;119:1305–1308

73. Livingston EH, Passaro EP Jr. Postoperative ileus. *Dig Dis Sci* 1990;35:121–132

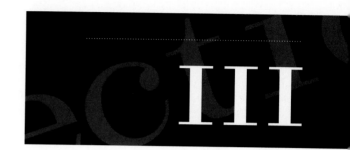

III

ABDOMINAL WALLS

11

Incisions, Closures, and Management of the Wound

Harold Ellis

■ INCISIONS AND CLOSURES OF THE WOUND

It is probably no exaggeration to state that, in abdominal surgery, wisely chosen incisions and correct methods of making and closing such wounds are factors of great importance. Any mistake, such as a badly placed incision, inept methods of suturing, or ill-judged selection of suture materials, may result in serious complications such as hematoma formation, infection, stitch abscess, an ugly scar, an incisional hernia, or, worst of all, complete disruption of the wound.

It should be the aim of the surgeon to employ the type of incision considered to be the most suitable for the particular operation about to be performed. In doing so, three essentials should be achieved:

1. Accessibility
2. Extensibility
3. Security

The incision must give ready and direct access to the anatomy to be investigated and also must provide sufficient room for the required procedure to be performed. A satisfactory operative field is obtained not only by means of a well-made and adequate incision, but also by means of the apt use of retractors and packs, the correct posture of the patient on the operating table, and efficient illumination.

The incision should be extensible in a direction that will allow for any probable enlargement of the scope of the operation, but it should interfere as little as possible with the functions of the abdominal wall.

The closure of the wound must be reliable and ideally, should leave the abdominal wall as strong after the operation as it was before.

TYPES OF INCISIONS

The incisions most often used for exploring the abdominal cavity may be classified as follows:

- **Vertical.** These incisions may be midline or paramedian and supraumbilical or infraumbilical. They may be extended well below or well above the umbilicus; for example, in resections of the colon or in the exposure of an aortic aneurysm.
- **Transverse and oblique.** The best examples are the McBurney gridiron incision for appendectomy, the Kocher subcostal incision for displaying the gallbladder and bile ducts, the Pfannenstiel infraumbilical incision, commonly employed for gynecologic surgery, and the transverse or oblique lateral incision for exposure of the colon.
- **Abdominothoracic.** This incision is used particularly for extensive exposure of the liver and of the esophagogastric junction.

CHOICE OF INCISION

The choice of the incision depends on many factors. These include the organ to be investigated, the type of surgery to be performed, whether speed is an essential consideration, the build of the patient, the degree of obesity, and the presence of previous abdominal incisions. There is no hard and fast rule; often the paramount consideration is the individual preference of the surgeon.

Most surgeons, for example, prefer a vertical, upper abdominal midline or paramedian approach to the stomach and duodenum. In cases of extreme emergency—a ruptured aortic aneurysm or a serious closed abdominal injury—there is no doubt that the midline incision gives the most rapid access and can, if necessary, be extended rapidly to the whole length of the abdomen. If the patient is thin and has a narrow subcostal angle, a transverse incision has little advantage, whereas if the patient is obese with a wide subcostal angle, a subcostal oblique incision gives excellent access to the biliary system and the spleen.

The McBurney muscle-split right iliac fossa incision is ideal for appendectomy and can be enlarged readily, either medially or laterally, should the need arise.

If a colostomy or ileostomy is likely to be fashioned, this must be taken into consideration in planning the incision. Thus, an abdominoperineal excision of the rectum is performed best through a lower midline or right paramedian incision, allowing the maximum distance from the siting of the left iliac fossa colostomy. Similarly, a long, left paramedian incision is useful in total colectomy when the ileostomy stoma is to be sited on the right lower abdominal wall.

If possible, reentry into the abdomen should be performed through the previous incision, especially if the incision is weak or is the site of an incisional hernia, since the hernia can be repaired at the same time. There is a distinct risk that a second incision placed alongside the previous wound, especially if heavily undercut, would cut off the blood supply of the skin between the two incisions, resulting in necrosis of the skin bridge.

Many surgeons have advocated oblique and transverse incisions on the grounds that these are stronger and less liable to disrupt and herniate. These virtues are put forward to mitigate the undoubted fact that these incisions are more tedious to perform than the midline approach. The same argument has been used for the paramedian incision.

Many of the studies reported in the past (and the clinical impressions of many experienced surgeons) made no allowance for the fact that midline incisions often are carried out in cases of great urgency, such as hemorrhage, trauma, and sepsis, or in reopening previous laparotomy wounds, perhaps already the site of an incisional hernia. The other, more sophisticated incisions, tend to be used in selected and elective cases. One would hardly wonder that more complications were found in the former than the latter!

Obviously, only carefully conducted prospective controlled trials can compare one incision with another. We have carried out controlled trials in which those patients in whom the vertical incision was desirable were randomly assigned to have either median and paramedian incisions performed, and those in whom an oblique or transverse incision could be performed randomly received this approach or a paramedian incision.[1] All incisions were closed by the same mass nylon technique. The results are demonstrated in Table 11–1 and show that, in our experience, no virtue could be demonstrated between these three incisions with regard to dehiscence and herniation. (This subject is discussed further in Chapter 14).

DESCRIPTION OF INDIVIDUAL INCISIONS

Midline Epigastric Incision

Most operations on the stomach, duodenum, gallbladder, pancreas, spleen, and hiatus can be performed through a midline epigastric incision, which has a number of advantages. It is almost bloodless, no muscle fibers are divided, and no nerves are injured. It affords good access to the upper abdominal viscera, and is very quick to make as well as to close; it is unsurpassed when speed is essential. A midline epigastric incision also can be extended the full length of the abdomen by curving around the umbilical scar or, with perfect safety, by incising straight through the umbilicus.

The incision is placed exactly in the midline and extends from the tip of the xiphisternum, usually to about 1 cm above the umbilicus. The skin, subcutaneous fat, linea alba, extraperitoneal fat, and peritoneum are divided seriatim. The extraperitoneal fat is abundant and vasculinar in the upper half of the incision, and small vessels here need to be coagulated with diathermy. The

TABLE 11–1. CONTROLLED RANDOMIZED TRIAL OF MEDIAN/PARAMEDIAN/TRANSVERSE INCISIONS FOR MAJOR LAPAROTOMIES (1-YEAR FOLLOW-UP)

Group A: Paramedian vs Transverse
46 paramedian—8 incisional hernias (17%)
50 transverse—7 incisional hernias (14%)
(Not significant; $P > .05$)

Group B: Paramedian vs Median
40 paramedian—7 incisional hernias (18%)
39 median—9 incisional hernias (23%)
(Not significant; $P > .05$)

(From Ellis H, Coleridge-Smith PD, et al: *Postgrad Med J* 1984;60:27)

falciform ligament of the liver is best avoided by opening the peritoneal cavity well to the left or preferably, to the right of the midline under the belly of the rectus muscle, as shown in Fig 11–1.

If the falciform ligament interferes with the exposure of the stomach or duodenum, or if it cramps the movements of the surgeon in any way, it should be clamped in two places, divided, and ligated.

Midline Subumbilical Incision

The midline subumbilical incision is similar to, and may extend to, the epigastric midline incision. Below the umbilicus, the linea alba is narrow and not infrequently, the rectus sheath on one or the other side is opened inadvertently. However, this is of little consequence.

As a general rule, in any vertical incision placed in the epigastrum to avoid the falciform ligament, the peritoneum should be opened at the bottom end of the incision, whereas in subumbilical vertical incisions, the peritoneum should be incised in the upper part to avoid injury to the bladder. The peritoneum always should be opened with the greatest care. A safe method is to pick up a fold of peritoneum with dissecting forceps, shake it to ensure that no other structure has been caught up with it, clip it with two artery forceps placed slightly apart, and then divided this raised fold with the utmost care, using a knife with its blade held almost horizontally. This small opening then is enlarged to admit two

fingers that then are used to protect the underlying viscera while the peritoneum is being divided throughout the whole length of the wound. Special care is required when operating on the patient with intestinal obstruction because of the loops of distended bowel immediately below the incision. Special care is also required when reopening the abdomen following previous surgery; the surgeon must assume that there will be underlying adhesions. Under such circumstances, the initial incision into the peritoneal cavity, must be performed with infinite precautions since a loop of intestine could be immediately under the scalpel edge. If the surgeon suspects that this is so, it is wise to try another area of peritoneum, preferably at one or the other end of the incision and away from the immediate mass of adhesions. Once the peritoneum has been entered, the edges of the peritoneum are held up with forceps so that the line of attachment of the adhesions can be seen and divided under direct vision.

Upper Paramedian Incision

An upper paramedian incision can be made on either the right or left side of the midline. The incision is vertical, starting at the costal margin, finishing about 2 to 8 cm below the umbilicus, and placed 2.5 to 5 cm from the midline. Extra access can be obtained by sloping the upper extremity of the incision upward to the xiphoid (Fig 11–2).

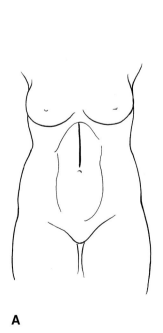

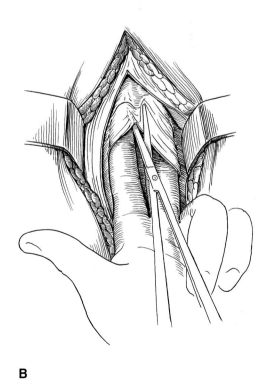

A   **B**

Figure 11–1. Epigastric midline incision. **A.** Surface markings. **B.** The linea alba and peritoneum are divided. The falciform ligament is avoided by opening the peritoneal cavity to the left or right of the midline.

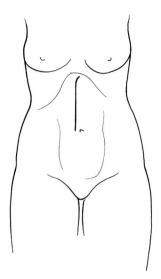

Figure 11–2. Upper paramedian incision, surface markings; extra access can be obtained by sloping the upper extension of the incision upward toward the xiphoid.

After the anterior sheath of the rectus muscle has been exposed, it is incised for the whole length of the wound; then the inner portion of the rectus sheath is dissected from the rectus muscle with particular care being taken at the fibrous intersections of the rectus sheath, which are situated at the level of the umbilicus, below the xiphoid, and halfway between the two. At these three points, segmental vessels invariably are encountered and require diathermy coagulation. Once the muscle is free, the rectus can be drawn laterally (Fig 11–3), since the posterior rectus sheath is free from the muscle. The posterior sheath and the peritoneum then are incised vertically, again for the whole length of, and in a line with, the skin incision.

Lower Paramedian Incision

The lower paramedian incision is similar to the above and, indeed, can be continuous with it to enable exposure of the abdomen from the costal margin to the pubis. It differs only in that the inferior epigastric vessels are encountered and need to be divided and tied. The posterior layer of the rectus sheath is absent below the semilunar fold of Douglas in the lower half of the incision (Fig 11–4).

Lateral Paramedian Incision

A modification of the standard paramedian incision has been described by Guillou and his associates.[2] This comprises a vertical incision placed at the junction of the middle and outer one-third of the width of the rectus sheath (the anterior rectus sheath at this point consists of two layers). The anterior sheath is dissected from the rectus muscle, which is slid laterally in the

usual fashion. The posterior sheath or peritoneum, or both, are divided in the same sagittal plane as the anterior sheath. Theoretically, the wide-shutter mechanism provided by such a lateral incision in the sheath should diminish the risk of wound dehiscence and incisional hernia, since the wound is splinted by the rectus muscle.

If necessary, the upper or lower extremity of the incision can be angled inward, toward the xiphoid (Fig 11–5A) or the pubic symphysis. The lines of section of

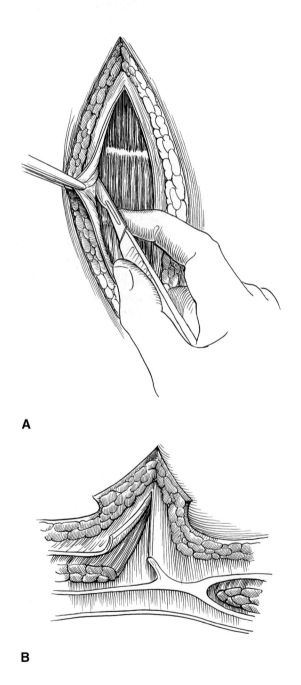

A

B

Figure 11–3. A. Dissection of the rectus muscle from the anterior rectus sheath. **B.** Paramedian incision in transverse section.

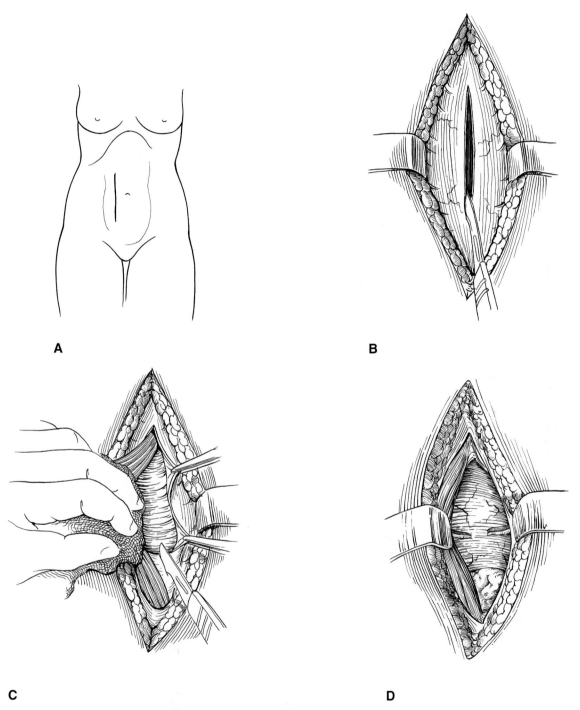

Figure 11–4. Lower paramedian incision. **A**. Surface markings. **B**. Incision of the anterior rectus sheath. **C**. Retraction of rectus abdominis. **D**. Location of the branches of the inferior epigastric vessels that run across the lower part of the incision. *Continued*

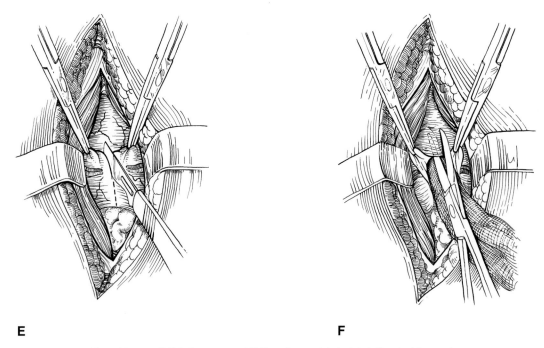

Figure 11–4, cont'd. E. Peritoneum opened. **F**. The peritoneum is incised the full length of the wound.

the conventional and lateral paramedian incisions are shown in Fig 11–5B.

Guillou and his associates advocated closure of the incision in two layers, the peritoneum and posterior rectus sheath being closed with catgut, and the anterior sheath with continuous Prolene. However, we carried out a prospective, randomized trial in which the peritoneum was closed in 77 cases as compared to 75 cases in which it was left open.[3] Patients were followed up for between 1 and 2 years. There were no cases of burst abdomen; no incisional hernias developed in patients in whom the lateral paramedian incision was performed and the peritoneum closed; and only one incisional hernia developed in the group in whom the peritoneum was left open (Fig 11–5C).

Excellent results have been claimed by the Leeds group. Together with Alan Pollock of Scarborough, we have carried out a prospective trial, comparing this technique with the conventional midline incision.[4] At follow-up at 1 year, of 159 midline incisions, 20 had developed an incisional hernia (12.6%) compared with only two incisional hernias noted in 170 patients (1.2%) with the lateral paramedian incision ($P<.001$).

The disadvantages of this incision are the length of time required for its performance and the virtual impossibility of performing the incision when a previous laparotomy scar is being reopened.

Vertical Muscle-Splitting Incision

The vertical muscle-splitting incision is carried out in exactly the same way as the conventional paramedian in-

cision, but the rectus muscle is split longitudinally in its medial one-third or preferably, in its medial one-sixth, after which the posterior sheath of the rectus muscle and the peritoneum are opened in the same line. This incision can be made and closed quickly, and it affords good access. It is popular in many clinics and is particularly valuable in reopening the scar of a previous paramedian incision. In such circumstances, it is very difficult, or indeed impossible, to dissect the rectus muscle away from the scar tissue of the rectus sheath, and only a muscle split is possible under these circumstances.

Kocher Subcostal Incision

A right subcostal incision is used frequently in surgery of the gallbladder and biliary passages and is of particular value in unduly obese patients and muscular patients. Less often, a left-sided subcostal incision is employed, particularly in elective splenectomy.

The subcostal incision commences exactly at the midline about 2.5 to 5 cm below the xiphisternum and extends downward and outward about 2.5 cm or so below the costal margin for a length of about 12 cm. After the rectus sheath is divided, the rectus muscle is divided along the length of the wound, using diathermy to control branches of the superior epigastric artery. The lateral abdominal muscles are cut in an outward direction for a short distance. Although the small eighth thoracic nerve will almost invariably be divided, the large ninth nerve must be seen and preserved to prevent weakening of the abdominal musculature. The incision then is deepened to open the peritoneum (Fig 11–6).

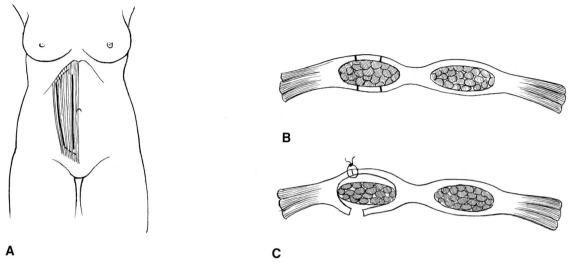

Figure 11–5. A. Lateral paramedian incision compared with conventional paramedian incision. Note that the upper or lower extension may be angled medially (*dotted line*) for greater access. **B.** Lateral paramedian and conventional paramedian incisions compared in transverse section. **C.** Closure of the incision; it is sufficient to suture the anterior rectus sheath, leaving the posterior sheath open.

The incision may be continued across the midline into a double Kocher incision, which provides excellent access to the upper abdomen. This is useful in carrying out total abdominal gastrectomy in an obese patient, in extensive hepatic resections, or in providing anterior access to both suprarenal glands.

It should be noted that the rectus muscle can be cut transversely and, provided its anterior and posterior sheaths are closed, no serious weakening of the abdominal muscle results because the incision passes between adjacent nerves without injuring them. The rectus muscle has a segmental nerve supply, so there is no risk of a transverse incision depriving the distal part of the muscle of its innervation. Healing of the scar, in effect, simply results in the formation of a man-made additional fibrous intersection in the muscle.

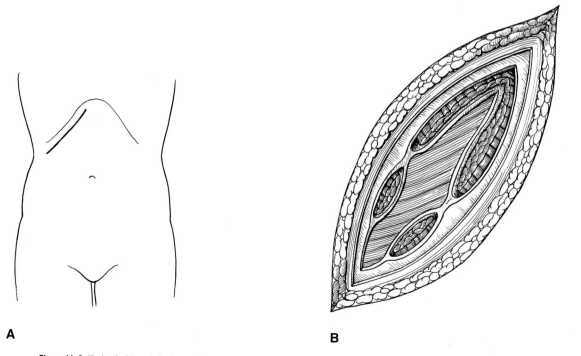

Figure 11–6. Kocher incision. **A.** Surface markings. **B.** Division of rectus and medial portions of the lateral abdominal muscles.

McBurney Gridiron or Muscle-Split Incision

This is the incision of choice in most cases of acute appendicitis and was described by Charles McBurney in 1894.[5] The level and length of the incision will vary according to the thickness of the abdominal wall and the suspected position of the appendix. Often, careful palpation of the abdomen when the patient is fully anesthetised will reveal a mass, thus facilitating placement of the incision directly over the diseased organ. If nothing can be felt, the incision is centered at McBurney's point, in other words, the junction of the middle and outer one-third of the line that joins the umbilicus to the anterior superior ilac spine. Usually, the incision is placed transversely in the line of the skin creases, which gives excellent results in terms of cosmetics. If the patient is obese or if it is anticipated that it may be necessary to extend the incision, then the incision should be placed obliquely, which enables it to be extended laterally as a muscle-cutting incision (Fig 11–7).

After the skin and subcutaneous tissues are divided, the external oblique aponeurosis is divided in the direction of its fibers, exposing the underlying internal oblique muscle. A small incision then is made in this muscle, adjacent to the outer border of the rectus sheath. The opening is enlarged with the points of the scissors to permit the introduction of two index fingers between the muscle fibers so that the internal oblique and transversus can be retracted with a minimal amount of damage (Fig 11–8).

A fold of peritoneum then is picked up and nicked with a knife, after which the peritoneal incision is stretched with the index fingers. This procedure tends to produce a circular hole in the peritoneum that, at

completion of the operation, is easy to close with a purse-string suture.

If further access is required, the wound can be easily enlarged by dividing the anterior sheath of the rectus muscle in line with the incision, after which the belly of the rectus muscle is retracted medially. As already mentioned, wide lateral extension of the incision can be achieved by a combination of division and splitting of the oblique muscles laterally.

Oblique Muscle-Cutting Incisions

This extension of the McBurney incision by division of the oblique muscles laterally and the rectus sheath medially provides good access to the iliac fossa and can be used for a right- or left-sided colonic resection, cecostomy, or sigmoid colostomy. It bears the eponym of the Rutherford-Morison incision.

Pfannenstiel Incision

This is a popular incision for gynecologic operations and also gives access to the retropubic space in the male for extraperitoneal retropubic prostatectomy.

The Pfannenstiel incision is usually about 12 cm long and is placed in the curving interspinous crease, its central point being approximately 5 cm above the symphysis pubis (Fig 11–9). Both anterior rectus sheaths are exposed and divided for the whole length of the wound. Artery forceps are clipped to the upper and lower edges of the sheath, which then is widely separated above and below from the underlying rectus muscles. It is necessary to separate the aponeurosis in an upward direction, almost to the umbilicus and downward to the pubis. The rectus muscles then are retracted laterally and the peritoneum opened vertically in the midline, with care being taken not to injure the bladder at the lower end of the wound.

The exposure afforded with this incision is somewhat limited and should not be used when a procedure outside the pelvis might be necessary. An advantage of using it is that it leaves an almost imperceptible scar because it is placed in the skin crease and, in any case, is hidden by the pubic hair.

Thoracoabdominal Incision

The thoracoabdominal incision, either right or left, converts the pleural and peritoneal cavities into one common cavity and thereby gives excellent exposure. The right incision may be particularly useful in elective and emergency hepatic resections. The left incision may be used effectively in resection of the lower end of the esophagus and proximal portion of the stomach.

The patient is placed in the "cork-screw" position. The abdomen is tilted about 45° from the horizontal by means of sand bags, and the thorax is twisted into the fully lateral position (Fig 11–10). This position allows

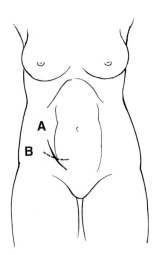

Figure 11–7. Surface markings of the right iliac fossa appendicectomy incision. **A.** The classic McBurney incision is obliquely placed. **B.** Most surgeons today use a more transverse skin-crease incision.

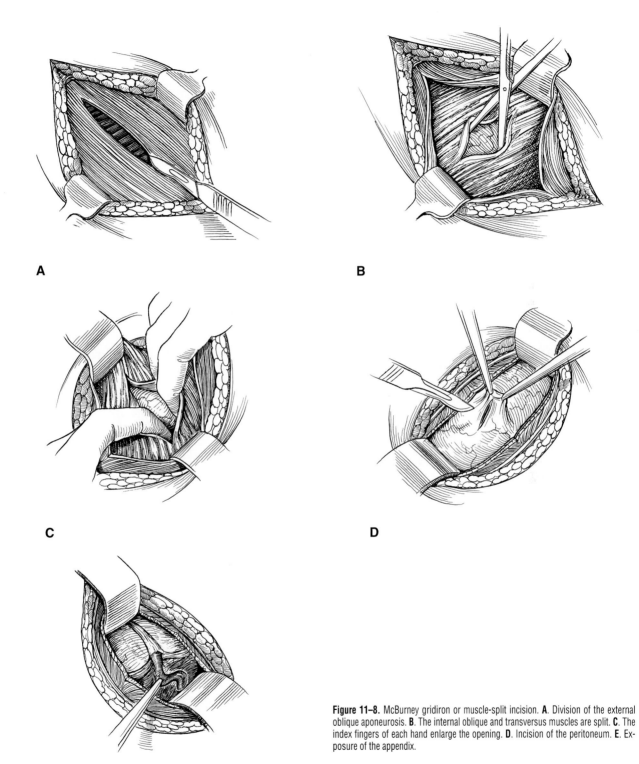

A

B

C

D

E

Figure 11–8. McBurney gridiron or muscle-split incision. **A**. Division of the external oblique aponeurosis. **B**. The internal oblique and transversus muscles are split. **C**. The index fingers of each hand enlarge the opening. **D**. Incision of the peritoneum. **E**. Exposure of the appendix.

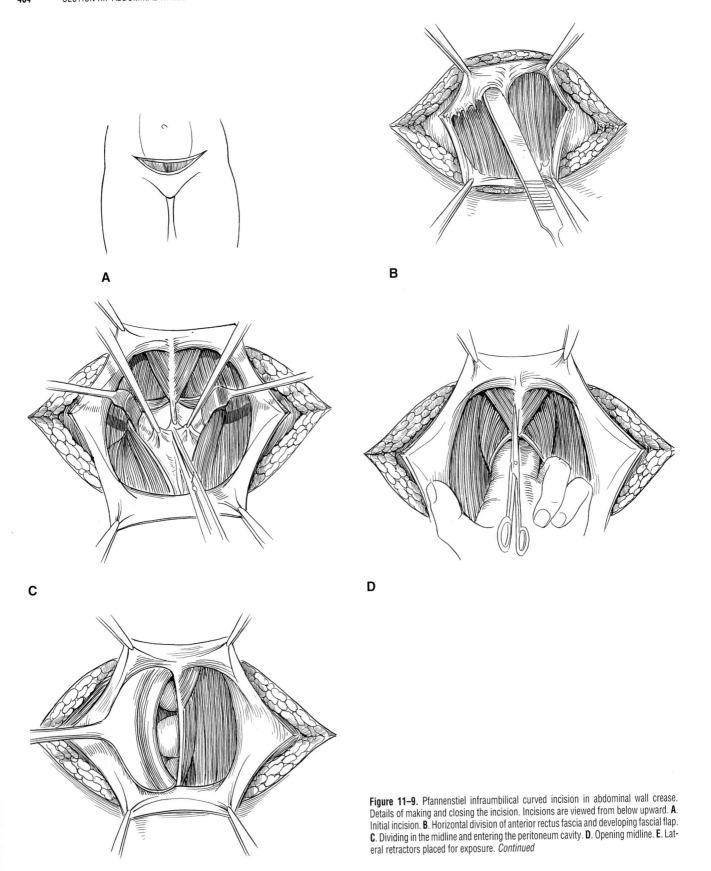

A

B

C

D

E

Figure 11–9. Pfannenstiel infraumbilical curved incision in abdominal wall crease. Details of making and closing the incision. Incisions are viewed from below upward. **A**. Initial incision. **B**. Horizontal division of anterior rectus fascia and developing fascial flap. **C**. Dividing in the midline and entering the peritoneum cavity. **D**. Opening midline. **E**. Lateral retractors placed for exposure. *Continued*

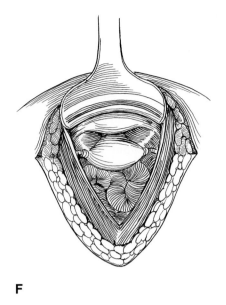

F

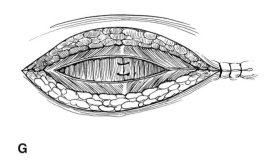

G

Figure 11–9, cont'd. F. Inferior retractors placed for exposure. **G**. Closure midline and inferior rectus.

maximal access to both the abdomen and the thoracic cavity.

The abdominal part of the incision may comprise a midline or left upper paramedian incision, which allows preliminary exploration of the abdomen. To this is then added an obliquely placed limb that continues along the line of the eighth interspace. The eighth interspace is identified easily, since it lies immediately caudad to the inferior pole of the scapula (Fig 11–10). Alternatively, an oblique upper abdominal incision is used, which continues directly into the thoracic part of the incision.

After the abdomen is opened, the chest incision is deepened through the latissimus dorsi and serratus anterior, and the obliquus externus and its aponeurosis. The intercostal muscles of the eighth space are divided to open the pleural cavity. The incision is continued across the costal margin, which is divided with a solid scalpel. It is useful at this stage to resect a short segment of costal cartilage; this allows easier closure of the chest wall. A Finochietto self-retaining chest retractor is inserted and slowly opened; this allows wide retraction of the intercostal space, and it is not usually necessary to resect a rib. The diaphragm is split radially, picking up and tying the branches of the phrenic vessels before their division.

Closure of this extensive incision is carried out by suturing the diaphragm using two layers of thread, inserting an underwater tube drain into the pleural cavity through a separate stab incision, closing the chest muscles in layers using catgut or Dexon, and then closing the abdominal part of the incision by the mass suture technique.

CLOSURE OF THE ABDOMINAL INCISION

The ideal method of abdominal wound closure has not been discovered. It should be technically so simple that the results are as good in the hands of a trainee as in those of the master surgeon; it should be free from the complications of burst abdomen, incisional hernia, and persistent sinuses; it should be comfortable to the patient and should leave a reasonably aesthetic scar.

My preferred technique of mass closure of the laparotomy incision using nylon is described below. (The controversies concerning techniques of closure and the suture materials employed are discussed at length elsewhere in this chapter). Until recently, layered closure of

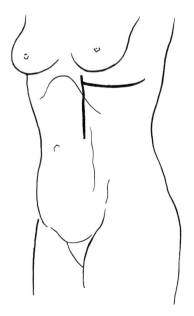

Figure 11–10. Surface markings of the thoracoabdominal incision.

the abdominal wall was considered sacrosanct, with great emphasis placed on closure of the peritoneal layer. It is now fully realized, both from clinical observations and laboratory animal studies, that healing of the incision takes place by formation of a dense fibrous scar that unites the opposing faces of the laparotomy wound en masse. The purpose of the sutures is to coapt the wound edges and to act as a splint while this dense fibrous scar deposits and matures. Wide bites must be taken (Fig 11–11), a minimum of 1 cm from the wound edge, and placed at intervals of 1 cm or less. The suture length should measure at least four times the wound length to ensure an adequate reserve of suture length in the wound when the suture is placed on tension, as may occur during abdominal distention.[6]

To take wide bites of the full thickness of the abdominal wall, this author employs the large Moynihan 5/8 needle to which is swagged a double loop of nylon 75 cm long (150 cm nylon in total) (Fig 11–12). By passing the needle through the loop, the end of the suture line can be anchored firmly. One loop is used at the up-

per extremity and one at the lower extremity of the incision, so that only one nylon knot needs to be tied at the middle of the incision (Fig 11–13). Some surgeons prefer to use a single length of nylon, and others favor interrupted nylon sutures.

For the midline incision, all layers of the abdominal wall, apart from skin and subcutaneous fat, are incorporated and the skin then is closed with interrupted nylon sutures. A similar technique is used for the paramedian incision by picking up the anterior and posterior rectus sheaths. The transrectus incision will incorporate the medial sliver of rectus muscle in the suture loops (Fig 11–14). Transverse and subcostal Kocher incisions[7] also can be safely closed with this technique. If the peritoneum cannot be included in the suture or if, in a grossly distended abdomen or in a thin elderly person, the peritoneum tears, this is of no consequence, as was demonstrated in a controlled trial comparing closures of laparotomy wounds with and without peritoneal suture.[3]

Mass closure is impossible only with the wide para-

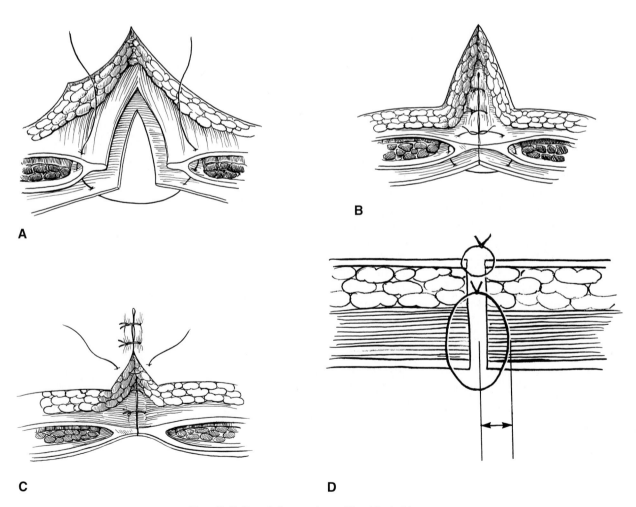

Figure 11–11. Stages in the mass closure of the midline incision.

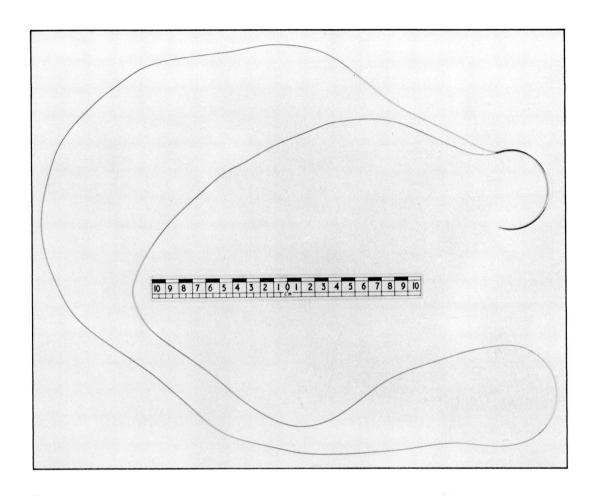

A

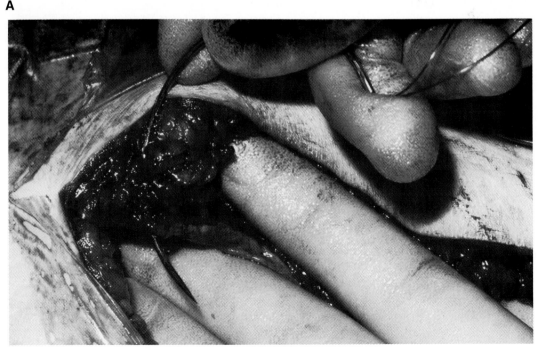

B

Figure 11–12. Moynihan 5/8 hand needle swaged to a double loop of nylon.

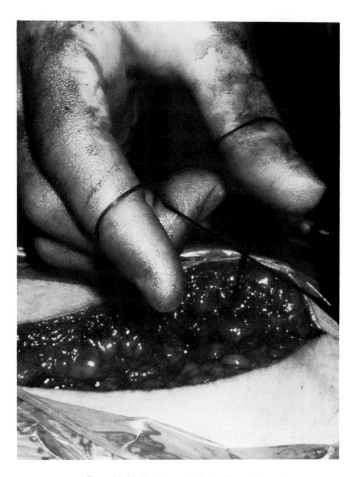

Figure 11–13. Technique of anchoring the nylon loop.

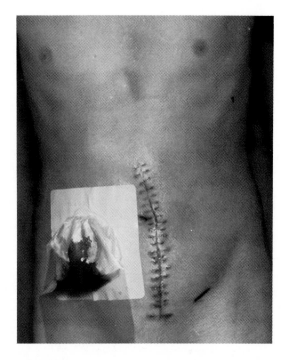

Figure 11–15. Emergency total colectomy for ulcerative colitis. The scar of the separate left iliac fossa stab drain can be seen, and the ileostomy has been brought out through a separate incision. Drains and stomas through the main incision are always to be avoided.

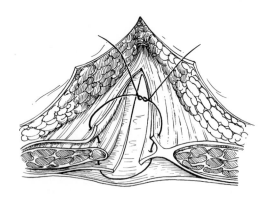

Figure 11–14. Mass closure of the paramedian incision.

median incision. For this incision, the posterior rectus sheath, together with the peritoneum and the anterior rectus sheath, are closed separately.

Drains and ostomy stomas invariably should be brought out through a separate stab wound in order to prevent weakening of the main laparotomy incision (Fig 11–15).

The use of tension sutures is not mentioned here because this author never employs them in the primary closure of laparotomy incisions but reserves them entirely for resuture of a burst abdomen. Tension sutures are painful and leave an ugly scar. No published evidence of controlled studies which demonstrate that they reduce the risk of evisceration or of incisional herniation can be found, and they have been abandoned by most surgeons.

■ MANAGEMENT OF THE WOUND

CLEAN WOUNDS

Postoperative management of the laparotomy wound is usually a straightforward affair (which will be discussed later). One then must consider the care of wound drains and finally, deal with the complications of abdominal wound healing.

Most surgeons like to apply a dressing to the abdominal wound and keep it thus covered until the sutures have been removed and healing has taken place. This is certainly the practice of most surgeons in the United Kingdom, and it is employed in most hospitals in many parts of the world. For a clean uncomplicated abdominal incision, this dressing is probably an unnecessary ritual, yet it is one that is expected by the nursing staff, by most physicians, and by the majority of patients. A piece of sterile gauze kept in place by strips of nonreactive adhesive certainly does no harm.

However, there are two circumstances in which dressings may be a disservice to the patient. The first is when the gauze is completely covered by an occlusive nonporous strip of adhesive; this will prevent evaporation of sweat from the skin and exudate from the wound and will encourage the growth of bacteria in the moist microatmosphere beneath the occlusive dressing. There inevitably will be an increase in the incidence of superficial wound infections and stitch abscesses under such circumstances. Some years ago we carried out a series of experiments in which one-half of the abdominal incision was dressed with conventional gauze and the other half covered with a completely waterproof occlusive dressing. The experiment was abandoned rapidly when the high frequently of stitch abscesses in the occluded portion of the wound was noted. The second hazard is the high incidence of skin reactions to some of the adhesive tapes currently in use; this complication can pro-

duce considerable discomfort to the patient and can be avoided by the use of nonreactive tapes.

Under normal circumstances the dressing applied in the operating theatre need not be disturbed until the time comes to remove the sutures. Earlier inspection and change of the dressing are called for if the dressing becomes displaced, if it becomes soaked with blood or serum, or if pyrexia and local pain raise the suspicion of wound infection. However trivial, wound infections occur in a series of clean abdominal wounds always should be a matter of concern to the surgeon. There should be a complete review of the methods adopted by the surgical and nursing team both in the operating room and in the postoperative period, in an attempt to pinpoint the reason for this complication and the possibility of some flaw in the technique employed by the surgeon.

But is this dressing ritual of clean, sutured abdominal wounds really necessary? In an interesting report published of a study, all dressings from clean wounds were removed on postoperative day 2 and, if all appeared well, the wound was exposed.[8] Drains, if used, were dressed separately. This technique was accompanied by no evidence of an increased incidence of wound sepsis. To quote these authors:

> What then is the explanation of our observations that postoperative dressings may be removed from a wound healing *per primam* after the second day, without increasing the incidence of infection? The answer must lie in the fact that wound edges, carefully approximated, are sufficiently sealed by coagulum and overlying epithelial regrowth to resist contamination. Of additional importance, it would seem, is the fact that an exposed wound is a dry wound, and few bacteria retain their vitality on a dry surface. These studies have shown that clean, surgically closed wounds, managed by a technique of early exposure, do not have an increased incidence of infection. Our infection rates of 1.4 percent in clean wounds and 5 percent in contaminated wounds are comparable to the incidence of infection in clean wounds of from 1 to 5 percent generally reported.
>
> Thus the major potential disadvantage of this type of wound care, namely increased risk of infection, has not materialized.
>
> The advantages to early wound exposure appear to outweigh the possible disadvantages. These advantages are: the healing wound remains clean and dry with less surface moisture or evidence of minor inflammation than the wound dressed with occlusive bandages; daily inspection or palpation of the wound is possible; and the patient does not have the annoyance of tape and bandages to contend with. We have been most gratified by the acceptance by patients of this technique of wound care.
>
> It should be emphasized that this technique of early wound exposure is being reported on wounds that are clean and are surgically closed. It is not being used on grossly infected wounds or on granulating wounds.[8]

If wound dressings are omitted from the majority of surgical patients, there is, naturally, a striking savings of nursing time, labor, and expensive dressing materials. The patient is relieved of the discomforts of wound dressings, and the surgeon can observe the wound easily and informally.

Many units employ this exposure technique with complete satisfaction and this author has often used it without any problems.

A randomized trial of 170 consecutive patients undergoing either inguinal hernia repair or high saphenous ligation with one of three surgical options (1) a dry dressing of gauze, (2) a polyurethane film dressing (Opsite), and (3) immediate exposure was reported.[9] There was no difference in dressing comfort or dressing preference between the different groups, and the quality of the final scar was also no different. There was 1 wound infection in the 53 exposed wounds, 3 infections in the 59 treated with gauze dressing, and no less than 5 infections in the 54 with an occlusive dressing. The higher infection rate in the polyurethane-dressed group, although not reaching statistical significance, probably was due to the moist environment beneath the dressing.

CLOSURE OF THE SKIN INCISION

The suturing of the skin incision often is left to the house surgeon, and frequently it does not receive the meticulous attention it deserves. It is important that accurate coaptation of the lips of the wounds be obtained; if bits of fat are allowed to protrude between the edges because of slack and inaccurate suturing, or if the edges are strangulated by sutures that are tied too tightly, then uncomplicated healing can hardly be expected. Braided sutures of silk or thread should be avoided, since braided material undoubtedly potentiates superficial stitch abscesses. Unbraided nylon should be employed wherever possible; admittedly, it is a little more difficult to tie than braided material, but the reward of clean healing is well worth the additional effort. Another perfectly satisfactory technique in clean wounds is to use subcuticular continuous Dexon. Its use is particularly advantageous in children, since it avoids the pain and discomfort of suture removal. Closure with microporous tape is also a satisfactory method, particularly when no tension on the wound is anticipated, but this technique is unsatisfactory when profuse drainage from the wound is expected.

Nylon skin sutures usually are removed between postoperative days 7 and 10. If Dexon is used as a subcuticular stitch, it can be left, of course, to absorb completely. Quite often, however, the exposed ends of the suture above and below the wound need to be snipped away.

This author never uses deep tension sutures except for closure of a burst abdomen (vide infra), but if they have been employed, they are left in place for 14 days.

Drains

No hard and fast rules regarding the time for removal of drainage tubes can be laid down, because the length of time will, of necessity, vary with the purpose for which they have been inserted. Generally, however, drains that have been introduced to give vent to oozing of blood or serum should be withdrawn at the end of 24 to 48 hours. Again, in cases of general peritonitis or when there is gross contamination of the abdominal cavity during operation, the drains that have been inserted should not be allowed to remain in situ for more than 3 days; however, where a localized abscess (eg, appendix abscess) has been drained, the tube or tubes will have to remain in position for a longer period. After a few days they should be rotated and shortened, until eventually they are replaced by tubes of smaller caliber. In cases of cholecystectomy with exploration of the common bile duct, a drain usually is inserted in the region of the gallbladder fossa to allow for the escape of serum or possibly bile. When there is little or no discharge from such tubes, it is best to remove them on or about postoperative day 3; however, if there is a discharge of bile, it would be unwise to remove these tubes until the discharge has ceased or is minimal. There is one useful general rule: whenever possible, abdominal drains should be passed through separate stab wounds. This avoids contamination of the main abdominal incision.

When dealing with the various operations in which drainage is called for, we will attempt to indicate where the drains should be placed and how long they should remain in position.

INCISIONS WITH COMPLICATIONS

Stitch Abscesses

Stitch abscesses are usually seen about postoperative day 10 but may occur earlier, before any of the skin stitches have been removed or even some days or weeks after the wound apparently has healed. Stitch abscesses may be superficial or deep. When deep, they may be felt as rounded, indurated masses in the depths of the wound, and they are painful to the touch. When superficial, they may appear as brown or mauve-colored fluctuating circumscribed blisters more or less in line with the incision. They produce a certain amount of uneasiness and pain in the wound, and although some of the more deeply situated abscesses may become absorbed and disappear, the superficial ones are evacuated best by incising the blistered area and expressing the contents, which very often include a knot of catgut or silk with some blood-stained pus. Cultures then should be taken, with the responsible organisms being identified and appropriate tests for sensitivity carried out, although antibiotic treatment rarely will be necessary. Such sinuses heal rapidly as soon as the offending stitch is removed, leaving only a slight scar.

Cellulitis

In cases of cellulitis of the wound, the appearances are usually quite typical. As a result of the surrounding inflammatory edema, the stitches appear to be buried deep in the skin. The edges of the wound are covered here and there with inspissated pus or blood; there may be some oozing of serum between the sutures, and a faint red blush will be discernible in the region of the line of incision or stitch holes, extending outward for a variable distance.

The hemolytic streptococcus or *Staphylococcus aureus* may be responsible but, after abdominal surgery, the bowel organisms (*Escherichia coli*, *Streptococcus faecalis*, *Bacteroides*, etc) are the most common offenders.

The condition becomes evident a few days after operation and generally is associated with raised temperature and constitutional symptoms such as headache, anorexia, and malaise. By removal of a few skin stitches to relieve tension, by application of heat to the affected area, and by wise use of antibiotics, these wounds often can be induced to heal without further complications.

The effective use of antibiotics depends on (1) knowledge of the organisms involved, (2) their sensitivities to the various antibiotic agents available, and (3) maintenance of an adequate concentration of drug.

At times, a localized abscess may form or suppuration may be extensive and may involve some of the deeper layers of the abdominal wall. In such an instance, drainage often can be effected by judicious use of a sinus forceps in the wound; if that fails, an incision should be made over the abscess and the contents evacuated, after which a small tube should be inserted to afford drainage. If there is extensive associated cellulitis, administration of the selected antibiotics is indicated until the acute phase has subsided. It must be stressed, however, that pus requires drainage; there is no antibiotic that substitutes for this fundamental surgical principle.

When there is a large collection of blood or pus under the skin or when there is much fat in the abdominal wall that has become infected during the process of operation (eg, appendectomy for perforated gangrenous appendicitis), infection with *E. coli* and *Bacteroides* is prone to occur, causing the formation of an extensive abscess. Such wounds have a dusky, mottled appearance, are boggy and tender, with tenderness rendering it impossible at times to elicit the signs of fluctuation; the appearance should guide the surgeon to remove a stitch or two and to probe the depths of the wound for deep-seated pus, which, when located, is often found to be brown, oily, and foul smelling and, being under great pressure, will gush from the depths of the wound with considerable force and will flood the surrounding area rapidly. In such cases, it is best to open the wound in part, irrigate it with hydrogen peroxide followed by warm normal saline solution, and provide adequate drainage.

Gas Gangrene Infection of Abdominal Wounds

When one considers how often abdominal wounds become contaminated with septic peritoneal fluid, and even with colonic contents, it is surprising that gas gangrene infection of abdominal wounds is so rare.

Analysis of the reported cases of gas gangrene infection following gastrointestinal surgery has revealed that a perforated gangrenous appendix, operations on the bowel for closed-loop obstruction such as volvulus of the sigmoid colon, and cecostomy or colostomy for large gut obstruction have commonly been featured. In addition, cases have been reported following gunshot injuries and wounds of the abdominal wall and viscera associated with lacerations or crushing of muscles. Interestingly enough, due no doubt to rapid and efficient treatment, gas gangrene is now remarkably unusual in wartime injuries. One report[10] recorded only four examples of gas gangrene, with no deaths, among 4900 battle casualties in the Korean War,[10] and another reported that gas gangrene was a rare occurrence in the Vietnam campaign.[11] In the Yom Kippur war of 1973, it has been noted that no case of gas gangrene occurred among 624 consecutive battle casualties evacuated to three base hospitals in Israel.[12] In a personal communication, General Robert Scott, RAMC, told this author that there has not been a single case of clostridial infection among the wounded troops in Northern Ireland nor among the British casualties in the Falklands.

A rare but interesting group consists of those patients in whom gas gangrene complicated cholecystectomy. This complication may take various forms:

1. There may be a primary gas gangrene infection of the acutely inflamed gallbladder, usually in a desperately ill patient presenting with the features of fulminating peritonitis. The diagnosis may be made preoperatively by detection of gas in the gallbladder on plain x-rays of the abdomen.
2. The clostridial infection may follow cholecystectomy and may involve the abdominal wall, the liver and gallbladder bed, or the peritoneal cavity.

In a personal case,[13] a 35-year-old male was submitted to a routine cholecystectomy for chronic cholecystitis and cholelithiasis. The ducts were normal. The immediate postoperative course was satisfactory but, after 24 hours, the pulse rate began to rise and the patient looked pale and ill. Three hours later his pulse rate had risen to 160 beats per minute, and his blood pressure had dropped to 90/50 mm Hg; he was toxic, restless, anxious, and disoriented. There was slight pyrexia (99°F). His abdomen was tender in the region of the wound, but there were no other abnormal physical signs. Thirty hours after the initial operation the wound was reopened, with the patient under general anesthesia. Immediately, the musty smell of gas gangrene could be detected, and there was thin yellow pus with bubbles of gas both in the abdominal wall and within the peritoneal cavity. The liver was swollen and bright red. An immediate swab of the pus strongly suggested clostridial infection on microscopy, and subsequent cultures grew *Clostridium welchii* and a penicillin-sensitive *S. aureus*. Histologic examination of a small piece of muscle taken from the abdominal wall revealed coagulation necrosis, with separation of the muscle fibers from their sarcolemmal sheaths; clostridia could be seen in the interstitial tissue. The wound was swabbed out with hydrogen peroxide and closed with drainage. The patient was treated with intramuscular penicillin and streptomycin and also was given polyvalent antigas gangrene serum (the latter two drugs would be omitted today); he made an entirely smooth recovery.

Gas gangrene infection following abdominal surgery may result either from inoculation of a necrotic nidus in the wound from the air, instruments, dressings in the operating room or, much more commonly, from liberation of clostridia contained within the alimentary tract or biliary system. Clostridia can almost invariably be recovered from normal stools, and they may be found, although much less often, when bile, gallbladder wall, or even gallstones are cultured anaerobically. Indeed, as a general rule, it can be stated that clostridial infection following surgical procedures in modern operating rooms results from organisms derived from the patient's own bowel.

Clinical Manifestations.

Gas gangrene infections are ushered in by severe pain in the wound, usually 12 to 72 hours after operation; the pain is often, but not invariably, associated with a high temperature (39° to 41° C [103° to 106°F]), rapid pulse rate (120 to 140 beats per minute), severe shock, and a feeling of apprehension. The patient is gravely ill from the start; the usual malar flush associated with pyogenic infection is replaced by a greyish pallor, weakness, and profuse sweating; the mental state is often one of apathy and indifference.

When such wounds are examined in the early stages, the edges are found to be edematous, red, and acutely inflamed; later they become dusky, dark brown, and finally black from putrefaction. In some cases the reddened area around the skin incision takes on the yellowish brown or bronze tint that is so characteristic of this infection. The wound is crepitant and discharges pus containing gas bubbles and an irritating brownish, watery fluid that has a peculiar foul odour. To an experienced observer with a keenly discriminating sense of smell, there is a characteristic acrid or "mousy" odour. Difficulty often is experienced in differentiating infection produced by clostridia in secondary mixed infection in abdominal wounds. It should be remembered that crepitation may result from nonclostridial organisms, especially in diabetics. Demonstration on x-ray films of gas in the soft tissues may permit an earlier diagnosis than one rendered by clinical findings alone. Because there are not satisfactory laboratory tests for early bacteriologic diagnosis of gas gangrene, it is practical to explore surgically, and without delay, any wound suspected of being infected. Valuable information can, of course, be obtained from immediate microscopic examination of the exudate.

Treatment.

As soon as the condition is recognized, the following treatment should be carried out:

1. Debridement of wounds and any surrounding areas of cellulitis is the most important single therapeutic factor. When gas gangrene is suspected in the immediate postoperative phase after an elective abdominal operation, the patient must be taken to the operating room and given a general anesthetic, after which the incision should be opened widely and deeply into the muscular layers, with all necrotic tissue being removed. Necrotic tissue is, of course, nonviable, noncontracting, and nonbleeding, and it requires ablation.

2. The wound should be thoroughly cleaned with hydrogen peroxide (20 volumes); there is no doubt that this irrigation of the wound at the time of debridement, and subsequently, is of distinct value.

3. The antibiotic of choice is penicillin; 1 million units should be given intramuscularly at once, and treatment should be continued at a dosage of 500 000 units every 8 hours. If the patient is sensitive to penicillin, a member of the tetracycline group or erythromycin may be used. There is no firm evidence that antigas gangrene serum has any value, and because of its high risk of allergic reactions, most authorities now have abandoned its use.

4. Although there have been no controlled clinical trials, there is strong evidence that hyperbaric oxygen is of considerable value in treating clostridial infection. Its use owes much to the enthusiasm of Boerema in Holland.[14] The high

PO$_2$ within the chamber, at a pressure of 3 atm, immediately stops clostridial organisms from multiplying and inactivates the toxin, while maintaining the viability of damaged tissue. There is much to be said for transferring the patient, if at all possible, to such a unit for expert care. An important report has been published on 88 patients treated over a 10 year period at a hyperbaric center. Interestingly, the most common cause was amputation for ischemic gangrene (32 cases); however, 10 of their cases followed intestinal surgery.

Postoperative Acute Dermal Gangrene

Spreading gangrene of the superficial tissues following surgery, trauma, drug injections, or sepsis is fortunately a rare occurrence. Because of this rarity, few surgeons encounter more than two or three of these alarming cases during their clinical experience, with the result that there has been much confusion over the nomenclature, the bacteriology, and the treatment of this condition. Excellent reviews on this subject have been published.[16–19]

Ledingham and Tehrani[20] divided acute dermal gangrene into two categories: *(1) necrotizing fasciitis* is a progressive and usually rapid necrotizing process affecting the subcutaneous fat, the superficial fascia, and the superior surface of the deep fascia. Initially, the skin is intact, but it becomes gangrenous secondary to interruption of its deep blood supply, and *(2) progressive bacterial gangrene* is a slowly progressive lesion that affects the total thickness of the skin, but does not involve the deep fascia. Pus formation is variable. In both types, most lesions follow wounds or sepsis of the abdominal wall or perineum; however, occasionally they may be seen peripherally.

Necrotising Fasciitis The disease was described by Meleney in 1924,[21] but the name *necrotising fasciitis* was introduced by Wilson in 1952.[22] It may present with nonspecific redness, swelling, and edema around the primary wound or area of sepsis but, in other cases, there may be the appearance of cellulitis in an area some distance from the primarily affected region, which retains a normal appearance. If the condition is untreated there is rapid progression, in a matter of days, to frank gangrene of the skin, beneath which the underlying fascia is grey, ragged, and stringy. This fascial involvement is much more extensive than that of the overlying skin. In addition to these local features, there are severe systemic disturbances, including toxemia, dehydration, and mental apathy. The condition is distinguished readily from gas gangrene because of the absence of crepitus, the absence of muscle involvement, and the failure to isolate clostridia from tissues or exudate.

Necrotising fasciitis can occur postoperatively, particularly after abdominal or perineal operations; it can follow trauma and has been reported after illicit drug injections, as well as after dental extraction. Occasionally, no preceding history can be elicited, but there might be some easily forgotten trauma, such as a minor laceration or an insect bite. For example, one report describes two cases, one following stretching of an anal fissure and another resulting from intertrigo, both in diabetic subjects.[23]

In many cases, the patient has some underlying condition that may reduce resistance to infection, and of these diabetes is clearly the most common. It must be kept in mind, however, that necrotising fasciitis also may occur in previously healthy subjects. In a report on 124 patients with necrotising infection encountered during more than 20 years, 61 were diabetic, 33 were in renal failure, 21 had advanced liver disease, and 17 were malnourished. The mortality rate was 25%. In a review of 27 patients with necrotising fasciitis, no fewer than 21 had associated chronic disease; 13 were diabetic, 8 had arteriosclerosis, 5 were obese, 4 were alcoholic, 3 had metastatic cancer, and 2 were in chronic renal failure.[25] From the point of view of etiology, 9 followed abdominal operations, 9 had perineal disease, 7 resulted from chronic skin ulcers, 1 had a colonic perforation, and 2 were of unknown etiology. The severity of this condition is shown by the fact that 20 of these 27 patients died, including 9 of the 11 diabetics. In another review of 28 patients with necrotising fasciitis of the perineum, no fewer than 11 were diabetic.[26] Of the diabetic patients, 8 died, whereas there were only two deaths in the 17 nondiabetic patients. These authors consider that the high mortality of this condition in the perineal region is the result of the difficulty of carrying out complete debridement in this anatomic situation. Yet another report[27] notes that all five patients with necrotizing fasciitis with secondary involvement of the retroperitoneal tissues died, presumably owing to the impossibility of radical excision of all the involved tissues.[27]

Although in Meleney's original series, hemolytic streptococci were isolated exclusively,[21] no single microbe pathognomonic for necrotising fasciitis has been found. Modern bacteriologic techniques usually reveal mixed cultures. Indeed, in one series, the number of organisms cultured varied from 1 isolate in 4 of their patients to as many as 11 bacterial types.[25] In this study, the predominant organisms were *Bacteroides, E. coli,* enterococci, and clostridia. Probably the most common combination is the nongroup A streptococci with *Bacteriodes fragilis.* It may be that early use of modern antibiotics may have eliminated the hemolytic streptococci, which might possibly have been an important initiating factor in the disease process. The dangers of streptococcal infection, even in the antibiotic era, are stressed in a report that presents nine patients with life- or limb-threatening streptococcal infection and in three of whom no source of infection was found; in the others, the precipitating injuries were only minor abrasions or contusions. All but two of these patients, however, had serious preexisting medical problems; diabetes in four, cachexia or recent weight loss in three, arterial vascular disease in three, obesity in three, long-term steroid use in two, and cirrhosis in one. Death occurred in five of these patients (56%) with multiple organ failure and serious coagulation disorders.

Progressive Bacterial Gangrene. This condition also was described by Meleney,[29] and some of the confusion in distinguishing this entity from necrotising fasciitis stems from the fact that both conditions often bear his name.

Progressive bacterial gangrene usually presents with nonspecific cellulitis around the wound or near the site of sepsis and very slowly extends during the next few days. The central area becomes purple and then develops all the features of gangrene. Dead, leathery, liquefying sloughs of skin that are black or mud brown and are bathed in thin watery pus undergo a slow but steady disintegration; on separating, they leave a comparatively healthy base covered with pale-pink, waterlogged granulation tissues. Surrounding this area of gangrene is an advancing, often serpiginous, purplish zone that is here and there slightly undermined, although undermining is not a prominent feature. It then fades off into a peripheral erythematous margin that eventually flattens to the level of the healthy skin. When this condition affects the scrotum, it is known as Fournier gangrene.[30]

In the past, this lesion frequently was called postoperative progressive synergistic gangrene because it was believed to be caused by two organisms that were more active in combination than alone. Meleney[29] originally incriminated a nonhemolytic microaerophilic streptococcus and *S. aureus,* but several synergistic pairs have been subsequently demonstrated, including *Proteus* and *Staphylococcus albus.* In one report, it was found that the most common organisms isolated in eight patients were coliforms, with a wide variety of associated bacteria, and the authors concluded that synergism between some of these groups may exist, but presumably not more so than in many other wounds similarly infected.

Fortunately both of these forms of acute dermal gangrene are relatively rare in modern surgical practice. Presumably, antibiotics have helped to reduce the incidence of the condition, and many of the cases reported in recent years, as we have noted, have been in patients in whom ischemia and reduced host defense mechanisms have been present; many have been diabetics or have been on steroids. Whereas earlier reports describing these conditions stressed the importance and apparent specificity of the invading organisms, nowadays

the main problems are the vicious cycle of infection, local ischemia, and reduced host defense mechanisms.

Treatment. The local treatment of both these conditions includes radical excision of the necrotic tissue. In necrotising fasciitis, total debridement of all necrotic tissue must be performed until the skin and subcutaneous tissue can no longer be separated from the deep fascia. In progressive bacterial gangrene, the skin must be excised until healthy bleeding tissue is encountered. The wound is loosely dressed with gauze and is inspected at least daily; any evidence of extension of the gangrenous tissue is an indication for further debridement. Parenteral antibiotic therapy is instituted immediately; metronidazole and a cephalosporin are a useful combination, but therapy will be modified according to subsequent bacteriologic findings. The general condition of the patient is of major importance and includes any associated factors, particularly diabetes and renal or hepatic failure. Once the necrotising process is arrested and systemic toxicity alleviated, the denuded areas will require split-skin grafting.

Hematoma

The incidence of hematoma occurring in clean operative wounds is about 2%. The risk is increased in patients with a bleeding diathesis, the most common cause of which is iatrogenic (ie, the use of anticoagulants). Hematomas are, of course, caused by faulty hemostasis of the layers of the abdominal wall, but they are not serious unless they become infected. They usually give rise to an aching pain in the wound that is accompanied by a slight rise in temperature. Small hematomas may be difficult to detect, but on careful palpation they may be felt as small, hard, rounded areas, usually underneath the line of the skin incision. Sometimes they may be more deeply placed between the layers of the abdominal wall. When they are near the surface, they may produce a brown or mauve blister that is tender, soft, and fluctuating. Since these small hematomas usually resolve, they may be left alone. If large, and particularly if soft, they should be aspirated with a wide-bore needle, or the edges of the wound that overlies them should be separated with a probe or a sharp-pointed scalpel, and the contents evacuated. A small drain then should be inserted into the cavity to prevent reaccumulation of serum and to facilitate the process of healing.

If there is considerable extravasation of blood giving rise to a fluctuating mass, it is best to return the patient to the operating room and open the wound, evacuate the clot, and ligate or coagulate with diathermy any bleeding vessels that are visible, after which the wound should be closed, with drainage being provided.

If cultures taken from the wound during operation do not yield a growth of microorganisms, no postoperative antibiotic treatment is indicated; if infection with associated cellulitis occurs, then appropriate antibiotic therapy should be prescribed.

Keloid Scars

There is no doubt that some persons have a greater tendency to form keloid scars than others. Crockett[31] discussed susceptibility in 12 different areas of the body, according to the severity and consistency of keloid formation: (1) keloid seen consistently: presternal region and upper back, (2) keloid may be severe or may occur in susceptible people: bearded area, ear, deltoid and preaxial region of upper limb, anterior chest wall excluding the midline, and scalp and forehead, (3) keloid change is rarely severe: lower back, abdomen, lower limb, postaxial region of upper limb, central area of face, and genitalia. Keloid scars are much more common among black people, in whom they tend to occur in more florid form than in other races. Women are affected more frequently than men, and young adults are affected more frequently than other age groups, but no one is exempt.

The cause of keloid is unknown. It occurs in human but not in animal scar tissue and is essentially an excessive accumulation of collagen in response to trauma, which may be (1) surgical, (2) thermal, (3) accidental, (4) infectious, or (5) minimal. Keloid scars may grow progressively, and they are always unsightly and discolored.

The appearance of a keloid scar is unmistakable. It is shiny pink or red; it is raised above the level of the surrounding skin and is firm and hard, with a surface that may be smooth, rough, or grooved. It has irregular feelers projecting laterally from the parent stem. The various marks made by the needle while the skin is being sutured are likewise keloid in appearance; they are red, shotty, and angry looking. Although the margins of the keloid may appear sharply defined, they are not actually so, and on palpation the hardened knotty scar tissue can be felt spreading downward from the surface into the subcutaneous tissues and in some cases, even the deep fascia and muscles. A keloid scar has the microscopic appearance of a soft fibroma, and it never becomes malignant.

In the past, many authorities made a distinction between a hypertrophic scar and keloid formation. The scar that showed moderate hypertrophic tendencies and then either regressed or remained stable was called a hypertrophic scar, whereas the scar in which deposits of collagen continued to enlarge beyond the original size and shape of the wound was labeled keloid. However, modern investigations have indicated that the only difference between these types of scar formation is the quantity (not the quality) of collagen deposited in the abnormal scar.

In an interesting scanning electron microscopic study of hypertrophic scar and keloid scar, no significant difference was found between the two.[32] In both there was greatly increased density of collagen. The bundle arrangement was less obvious than in a normal scar, and the confluence of collagen gave a homogeneous appearance. Fiber diameter was about one-half to three-quarters of that in normal skin, and cross-stranding was frequent. Capillaries were absent, and some whorled nodules were observed. A steroid-treated hypertrophic scar showed a dense homogeneous arrangement of collagen with small fiber size that differed from that of active hypertrophic scar only in a relative increase in interstitial space. A hypertrophic scar treated by compression showed some parallelism of small fiber bundles and some return of waviness.

Another fascinating study involved 10 consecutive patients with keloid formation who volunteered for an experiment.[33] In each patient, the keloid was excised and the wound meticulously sutured. At the time of the excision, an autotransplant of the keloid was made into a small full-thickness defect on the anterior abdominal wall. In nine patients the keloid recurred after excision, but the time of recurrence varied from 1 month to 8.5 months. In many patients, the recurring keloid strikingly followed the outline of the original lesion. In four patients, skin grafts had been used to close the defects, with the skin being taken from the proposed recipient site on the anterior abdominal wall; keloid occurred beneath and around these grafts. However, only 1 of the 10 keloid grafts developed new keloid at the site of transplantation. In all the others, no keloid occurred, and over the course of 3 years all became softer, paler, and flatter. Some regressed so completely that they became difficult to see. These experiments seem to exclude the possibility of any general systemic influence; they point very strongly to a local factor.

Treatment. Prophylaxis is important. This comprises the prompt application of pressure to a scar which is likely to become hypertrophic, for example, in a burn scar or in a patient who has developed a keloid elsewhere. This requires the use of a specially fitted elastic pressure garment, sleeve or legging, which must be worn continuously for many months.

For the established keloid, the surgeon should avoid, if at all possible, further surgery. Straightforward excision and suture is followed almost inevitably by an even larger and uglier scar. Radiation has been used before or after excision or skin grafting in an attempt to prevent exuberant scar formation, but its effect is doubtful, and the use of irradiation in young people in a nonmalignant condition, with its risks of late malignant change, is not recommended.

The injection of triamcinolone into the keloid is well

worth trying and can be repeated after 6 weeks if improvement is noted. The treatment is painful and, in children, may require a general anesthetic.

A keloid may grow to such a size that an attempt at removal becomes almost inevitable. The patient must be warned that recurrence is likely. The most effective technique is to shave the scar down to its base followed by application of a split-skin graft. This is followed by prolonged use of an appropriate pressure garment.

Calcification and Ossification in Abdominal Scars

Calcium salts may be deposited in any dead or degenerate tissue; this deposition is termed *dystrophic calcification.* Common examples of this occur in hematoma, atheroma, degenerate long-standing colloid goiters, and benign and malignant tumors (eg, uterine fibroids, meningioma, and breast cancer), as well as in gaseous material and in the fibrous tissue of scars.

The composition of the calcium salts deposited in this process is the same as that of normal bone, but the exact mechanism of this calcification is not understood.

Wherever there is dystrophic calcification, ossification also may occur, and bone marrow, as well as bone lamellae, may form at the sites of pathologic ossification. When this occurs in abdominal wounds, it may be that osteoblasts are liberated from the xiphoid, which is so often nicked in carrying out a high midline incision. One study reports that 3 of 15 patients undergoing resection of the xiphoid at laparotomy developed bone in the scar.[34] However, many examples of ectopic ossification in wounds may be found in which this could not possibly have taken place. Under these circumstances, it is believed that tissue fibroblasts differentiate into osteoblasts. Transitional epithelium in the urogenital tract has a remarkable propensity for stimulating ossification in the adjacent stroma, and ossification along the fistulous tract after cystotomy is well known.

Another interesting review is of six patients with heterotopic bone formation in abdominal scars together with reports of 44 other examples.[35] Of these 50 cases, 41 were in males; the age ranged from 25 to 81 years. Of particular interest is the fact that all patients had been subjected to a vertical abdominal incision. In general, the bone formation occurred within a few months, mostly within 1 year, of operation. In all cases, the abdominal wound had healed by primary intention, and none of the patients had any known endocrine, metabolic, or biochemical disorders. No specific suture material or closure technique could be held responsible.

Quite often, careful palpation of an abdominal scar many months or years after surgery will reveal hard, calcified, or ossified tissue; in the latter case, an x-ray film of the abdomen will reveal the bony tissue (Fig 11–16). If the patient notices this mass in the scar, reassurance is usually all that is necessary, and this author has not

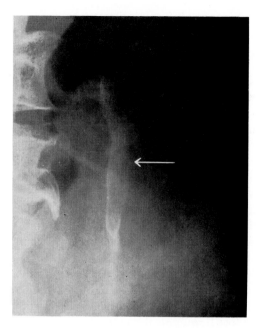

Figure 11–16. Ossification (*arrow*) in an old upper paramedian incision scar.

personally been asked by a patient to remove the ossified plaque. However, it is not uncommon to encounter this bony tissue on reopening an abdominal scar to carry out a further laparotomy. It is then an easy enough matter to excise the bony tissue; sound healing of the laparotomy wound will take place after routine wound closure.

Abdominal Wound Disruption and Evisceration

Disruption of abdominal wounds has been discussed under various names such as separation of abdominal wounds, broken-down abdominal incisions, postoperative dehiscence of abdominal wounds, postoperative eventration, and burst abdomen. The name adopted here would appear to be the one most generally accepted.

Disruption of an abdominal wound may be partial or complete. It is partial when one or more layers have separated but either the skin or the peritoneum remains intact, with rapid development of an often massive full-length incisional hernia. When it is complete, all the layers of the abdominal wall have burst apart, and this may or may not be associated with protrusion of a viscus evisceration.

Wound disruption is a grave and tragic complication that may follow any abdominal operation in either sex at any age, and when it occurs, it presents many serious problems in management of the case.

Incidence. Estimates of the incidence vary between 0% and 3%.[36] Most surgeons would regard an incidence of

3% as being unduly high and would consider a fair estimate for all cases to be in the region of 0.5% to 1%. Nevertheless, careful study of the publications dealing with this subject does reveal some discouragingly high figures. For example, one such report recorded a 3.5% incidence of burst abdomen in 370 abdomens closed with polydioxanone.[37] In reading these reports and in evaluating the percentage figures given for wound breakdown, it is important to look critically at the material studied. Some reports have considered all laparotomies (including appendectomies performed through right iliac fossa) as muscle-splitting incisions. Although dehiscence and herniation of such incisions may occur, they are certainly unusual. A number of studies have included only elective operations and have excluded reopened abdominal wounds and emergency cases, which, as will be discussed later, account for a considerable proportion of wound failures. Retrospective studies are less reliable than careful prospective trials; one can never be sure that perusal of notes reveals every example of wound disruption. A terminal case with gaping skin edges just kept together by a few skin sutures, but with gut exposed in its deeper recesses, may not find its way into the hospital statistics.

In recent years, there has been a considerable drop in the incidence of burst abdomens in many reports, a result of the spread in popularity of the mass closure technique, usually combined with the use of nonabsorbable suture material and with closely placed, wide bites of the abdominal wall. In our own experience, between 1975 and 1977, 341 major abdominal wounds were closed by the layered technique with a 3.8% incidence of dehiscence that fell to 0.8% in 788 patients when the mass closure technique was introduced.[38]

Later in this chapter the incidence of burst abdomen among patients treated by mass abdominal closure, as well as the incidence of this complication in various prospective clinical trials of different methods of wound closure—trials that have exploded many of our preconceived ideas about this controversial subject—will be discussed.

Mortality. The death rate in reported series varies considerably and may be as high as 44%, although the average operative mortality in a collective review is 18.1% (range 9.4% to 43.8%).[39] Much depends on the group of patients under study. In a series of nearly 3000 operations for duodenal ulcer performed in Veterans Administration hospitals in the United States, 67 instances of burst abdomen (2.2%), with 11.9% mortality were reported. Because burst abdomens occurred particularly among elderly patients who had wound infection, pneumonia, obstruction or who were undergoing emergency operation for hematemesis, this mortality well might have been expected on the basis of these other factors.

In studying any series of cases, it can be seen that many patients eventually would have died from the primary disease for which the operation was performed; the disruption merely precipitated the fatal outcome.

Etiology. No single cause can account for all wound disruptions; as a rule, a combination of factors is responsible. Basically, the abdominal wound may disrupt either completely or partially (with a resultant incisional hernia) because of one or more of the following reasons (Fig 11–17):

1. The knot may break or undo, a technical error that should be avoided but that is still seen from time to time.
2. The suture material may rupture, either because it is too weak for the tensions placed upon it or because it is destroyed rapidly in the tissues. This factor should be avoidable by correct selection of the suture material.
3. The sutures cut through the tissues, either because the sutures are placed too close to the wound edge or because of excessive weakening of the tissues from such factors as jaundice, uremia, protein depletion, or, most importantly, sepsis. This will be compounded if the tension placed on the healing wound is increased by abdominal distention, coughing, or straining.

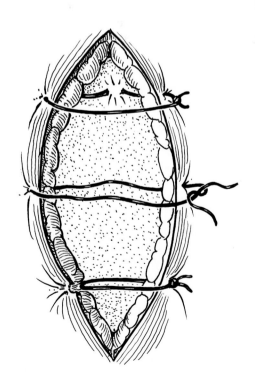

Figure 11–17. The three causes of wound disruption: upper suture has broken, middle suture knot has become undone, and lower suture has pulled through tissue.

The clinical study of wound healing is complicated considerably by the fact that it is uncommon for any one factor to exist in isolation, and it may be difficult, indeed, to determine which factor is of greatest importance in a particular case. Consider, for example, the patient who undergoes laparotomy for carcinoma of the pancreas. The patient may be elderly, intensely jaundiced, anemic, and protein depleted and, of course, is suffering from what is often advanced malignant disease. Immediately after operation, the patient may develop uremia, thus putting additional stress on the wound by going into postoperative ileus as well as developing severe pulmonary collapse. Perhaps the patient may be on cytotoxic drugs. Which factor or factors are blamed if the abdominal wound bursts apart? What role, if any, does the choice of the incision, the suture material, or the technique of closure play in this disaster?

Age and Sex. Disruption of abdominal wounds is more common in patients over 60 years of age than in younger patients.

The sex incidence shows a predominance for males, the ratio being about 4:1.

Type of Anesthesia. It would seem obvious that the type of aesthesia employed for the operation plays an insignificant role, since it has been established beyond dispute that disruption occurs with equal frequency after local, spinal, and inhalation anesthesia.

Nevertheless, it is true that a badly administered inhalation anesthetic associated with straining and struggling of the patient and entailing, as it does, hasty, forcible, and perhaps inaccurate suture of the abdominal wall under great tension, can be a contributing factor, especially when the suturing is performed by inept hands.

Factors in Technique. Although it is generally accepted that faulty methods of closure, increased intra-abdominal pressure, and other mechanical factors in the immediate postoperative period, such as operations for malignant disease in patients more than 60 years of age and in poor-risk patients, and diseases associated with malnutrition, hypoproteinemia, anemia, and vitamin deficiencies leading to poor and ineffectual healing are the primary preoperative causes of wound dehiscence, a number of cases are attributable directly to certain factors in the operative technique itself.

It should be noted that, until recently, many aspects of the relationship between surgical technique and wound disruption were based on clinical impression. Valuable though this may be, it cannot be compared with the results of carefully planned prospective clinical trials. As a result of such trials, many long-held beliefs have not been seriously questioned or disproved.

Incisions. At one time, many authorities preached that midline incisions, particularly in the upper abdomen, were more prone to disruption than paramedian incisions. These statements were based on collected statistics, but they failed to take into account the fact that midline incisions were often employed to gain rapid access to the abdomen in desperate emergency situations. In studies from my unit, we have shown that if other factors also are taken into consideration, there is no significant difference between median and paramedian wounds.[41,42] It is true that the incidence of dehiscence with the McBurney muscle-splitting appendix incision is extremely low, although incisional hernias may follow this incision, especially in the presence of infection or obesity, in elderly subjects, and when a tube drain is employed for a considerable period of time. Transverse abdominal incisions have a low incidence of breakdown, but these tend to be used in elective procedures and not in emergency situations. The Kocher subcostal gallbladder incision is certainly not free from the risk of disruption and herniation.

We have studied a group of 96 patients who received either vertical and transverse incisions randomly. There was one total wound disruption of a paramedian incision, but no statistical difference between the incidence of incisional hernia at 1 year between the two groups.[43]

It should be noted that a report from Leeds claimed exceptionally good results from the use of the lateral paramedian incision.[44] Thus, in a series of 850 cases, there was not a single burst abdomen, and follow-up at 1 year showed only three incisional hernias, a rate of 0.37%. In a randomized study, 207 laparotomies with either midline, medial paramedian, or lateral paramedian incisions were performed.[2] There was only one burst abdomen in the median group. Fourteen incisional hernias developed, but none of these occurred in the lateral paramedian group; there was no significant difference between the incidence of incisional hernias in the midline and medial paramedian incisions. It should be noted that two important groups of patients are excluded from this series; these are patients undergoing emergency laparotomy for severe hemorrhage, and patients who previously have been submitted to laparotomy, so that further surgery was performed through the same incision.

The placing of a colostomy or ileostomy stoma in the incision definitely increases the risk of disruption of the wound and the risk of formation of a ventral hernia. Wherever possible, the stoma should be fashioned through a separate small incision. To a rather lesser extent, the same advice applies to the placing of abdominal drainage tubes.

Suture Material Employed. Catgut is still used extensively by many surgeons throughout the world for closure of abdominal laparotomy wounds. The usual practice is to employ a continuous suture of 0 to 1 chromic catgut for the posterior rectus sheath and peritoneum, and either continuous or interrupted sutures of 1 chromic catgut for the anterior sheath of linea alba. However, controlled studies have shown a disastrously high failure rate when catgut alone is employed.[45–47]

Most surgeons, impressed by these results, use nonabsorbable sutures in the anterior sheath or linea alba. Steel wire gives excellent results, but it is undoubtedly difficult to use; therefore, like many surgeons, this author uses monofilament nylon.

Many surgeons are anxious about employing nonabsorbable suture material in closing abdominal wounds after dealing with frankly infected and heavily contaminated cases. However, it has been shown that monofilament nylon is extremely unreactive, and healing often will take place even when there is gross suppuration and when the superficial layers of the wound have broken down, actually exposing the nylon in the anterior sheath.[48] In some of these cases, it is true—a persistent sinus may form, especially over the knot at the end of the continuous suture. However, it is a simple matter to remove the knot from the depths of the sinus without having to clear the entire length of the nylon and after removal, the sinus rapidly dries.

Many surgeons now employ biodegradable synthetic polyester sutures. Since the aponeurosis of the abdominal incision is slow to heal, and since braided sutures, if infected, show a high tendency to produce a persistent sinus, a slowly absorbable monofilament polyester should be employed. Examples of this are polydioxanone (PDS) and polyglyconate (Maxon).

Technique of Laparotomy Closure. Most surgeons believe that the peritoneum must be sutured during closure of an abdominal incision. Yet is is known from clinical observations and from animal studies that raw peritoneal defects heal rapidly, that in obese, straining patients with poor tissues, the peritoneal stitches often tear through as fast as they are inserted with no obvious later deleterious effects, and that some surgeons heretically fail to observe the rule and leave the peritoneum unsutured without apparent disaster. Undoubtedly, the question is of some importance. If leaving the peritoneum open makes no difference in abdominal wound healing, then an unnecessary routine can be abandoned, and the occasional considerable difficulty in obtaining peritoneal closure can be avoided. However, if it should be shown that there is a higher incidence of wound failure when the peritoneum is not sutured, then obviously this procedure must retain its currently emphasized role in laparotomy closure. In a 1976 study no differences were found in the bursting strengths of abdominal incisions in dogs, regardless of whether the peritoneal layer had been sutured.[49]

In a randomized prospective study comparing 77 patients undergoing laparotomy through a lateral paramedian incision in whom the peritoneum was closed with 1 chromic catgut to 75 patients in whom the peritoneum was left open, it was reported that in both groups the anterior sheath was closed with monofilament nylon, using a mass closure technique.[33] At follow-up of between 1 and 2 years there had been no cases of burst abdomen. No incisional hernias had developed in patients in whom the peritoneum was closed, and only a single incisional hernia occurred in the group in whom the peritoneum was left open. The difference between these two groups was not statistically significant.

Almost since the beginning of abdominal surgery the masters of technique have preached the importance of meticulous layer-by-layer closure of the abdominal wall, and, indeed, this certainly has strong esthetic appeal.

In 1941, Jones and associates[50] reported a burst abdomen rate of 11% when incisions were sutured with two layers of catgut, and 7% when sutured with catgut for peritoneum and interrupted steel wire for the anterior rectus sheath. However, only one burst abdomen occurred in 81 operations after steel-wire closure with interrupted mass far-and-near sutures incorporating all layers of the abdominal wall apart from the skin. It is interesting that the "far-near" stitch was first used in 1900 by Smead, a resident to Finney in Baltimore. During the course of a complicated operative procedure, Smead suggested that the operation be finished with a closure that was safe and rapid. Finney agreed, and Smead performed what is believed to be the first far-near mass closure of the abdomen, a technique often referred to in the United States as the Smead-Jones method.

Theoretical arguments have been supporting the value of a closure employing nonabsorbable sutures that include all layers of the abdominal wall, apart from skin, and that also incorporate wide bites of tissue on either side of the line of incision.[6,51] When put to the practical test, this technique was not found wanting. In paramedian elective laparotomies, one trial reported one burst abdomen and no hernias among 108 cases using all-coats interrupted wire sutures;[52] another reported no wound disruptions in 186 laparotomies closed with continuous all-coats nylon.[53] Yet another group closed 280 midline wounds with all-coats continuous nylon, again without a single wound dehiscence;[54] a similar finding was reported in 120 laparotomies subjected to mass closure using steel wire,[46] and a most remarkable achievement of only one dehiscence in a series of 1505 closures using all-coats nylon was also reported.[6]

Because of the extremely encouraging results reported in these trials, this author has switched over to the use of a nylon continuous suture to close the full thickness of the abdominal incision apart from the skin, which is sutured separately with interrupted fine nylon. Bites are taken at least 1 cm from the edge of the wound and are placed close together (a maximum of 1 cm apart). The introduction of this technique produced a quite dramatic improvement in results. From 1975 to 1977, 341 layered closures were performed, and there were 13 burst abdomens (3.8%). From 1977 to 1980 the mass closure technique was used in 788 patients, with 6 burst abdomens, an incidence of 0.8%.[37] In closing the lateral paramedian incision, only the anterior sheath of the rectus need be closed by this method.

Factors Responsible for Poor Healing of the Tissues.

General State of the Patients. Surgeons with any degree of experience recognize that wound healing is not often a problem in a healthy young patient undergoing routine abdominal surgery. However, the surgeon soon comes to learn that problems will be encountered when the patient is obese, emaciated, elderly, cachectic, toxemic, jaundiced, diabetic, anemic, uremic, alcoholic, protein-depleted, scorbutic, or is suffering from any diseased state associated with prolonged steroid medication. It goes without saying that these depressing conditions are rarely encountered in isolation.

Vitamin C is essential for collagen synthesis. In man, the half-life of the vitamin is 16 to 20 days, and it takes 90 to 120 days to deplete the 2- to 3-gm body pool and produce degrees of vitamin C deficiency, which may be found in patients with peptic ulcer (who usually avoid fresh fruit and vegetables), in those with severe dysphagia (eg, from carcinoma of the esophagus), and in recluses (eg, those who exist on a diet of tea, bread, margarine, and jam). It has been demonstrated that there is a fall in the vitamin C level in the blood of patients after operation that returns to normal in about a week.[55] However, those patients who have received blood during the operation have persistently low vitamin C blood levels. The white cells are responsible for both the storage and the transportation of ascorbic acid in man. Hemorrhage depletes this reserve, and it is not replaced by stored blood. The leukocyte ascorbic acid level falls to a deficiency level after 7 days of storage. It was suggested that this deficiency may account for the increased incidence of abdominal wound dehiscence, as well as anastomotic leakage, that has been noted in patients undergoing emergency surgery for bleeding peptic ulcer.

Any experienced surgeon will have the clinical impression that uremia inhibits wound healing, and certainly this was our observation in the early days of renal dialysis and kidney transplantation, before modern technology enabled us to maintain our patients postoperatively at a relatively low level of blood urea. Surprisingly, very few reports dealing with wound healing and abdominal dehiscence even mention the incidence of

uremia. A 1965 research study produced uremia in dogs with uranyl nitrate and showed that abdominal wound breakdown occurred in these uremic animals that could be prevented by adequate renal dialysis.[56] In a series of experiments carried out in rats rendered uremic by unilateral nephrectomy with contralateral heminephrectomy, researchers demonstrated significant diminution in the bursting strength of laparotomy wounds and of small bowel anastomoses.[57] Using fibroblasts in culture, these researchers also demonstrated marked inhibition of fibroblast growth in uremic serum. Regrettably, there is little clinical observation on wound healing in uremic patients. Several series reported the following: (1) of 12 patients with acute postoperative uremia following renal surgery, seven of them had complete wound dehiscence of their muscle-splitting lumbar incisions,[58] and (2) of 19 operations performed in patients undergoing long-term peritoneal dialysis, eleven were elective and included two hernia repairs, whereas the remaining eight were emergency operations.[59] Of these 19 patients, four developed fascial dehiscence, and one had a superficial wound breakdown. The authors of these reports were unable to find any other reports of surgery in patients on chronic renal dialysis. The subject of wound healing in uremic patients merits much greater attention on the part of the surgeon.

Obstructive jaundice in the rat was shown to decrease the strength of abdominal incisions and to delay fibroplasia and angiogenesis in the healing wound.[60] In a clinical study of healing of laparotomy wound in 326 consecutive patients, 21 patients were jaundiced during or after surgery.[61] Of these patients, three suffered complete disruption of the abdominal wound, and an additional four patients subsequently developed incisional hernia: a total wound failure of 33%. This compared with 6 disruptions and 10 further incisional hernias at the time of review of the 305 nonjaundiced patients, giving a total wound failure rate of 5%. This difference was highly significant statistically. Interestingly, this risk of dehiscence was negated when the switch to the mass closure technique was made.[62]

Because of the multifactorial situation in seriously ill patients which has already been emphasized, many other individual factors are suggested rather than definitely proved as causes of wound breakdown. These include malignant disease, severe systemic sepsis (for example pancreatitis), wound infection and obesity. Increased abdominal pressure may impose stress on the freshly sutured abdominal wound sufficient to produce disruption. This may be brought about as a result of postoperative vomiting, explosive coughing, hiccup, and gross abdominal distention.

To sum up, the prevention of wound disruption depends on the anesthetist, the surgical technique employed, the nature of the disease, and the patient's diet.

The anesthetist, with skill, can diminish coughing and vomiting and can give the surgeon that relaxation of the abdominal wall that favours gentle handling and ease in suturing the wound. The surgeon must neglect no point of technique that will contribute to firm and secure approximation of the edges of the wound, and must remember the vitamin C requirements and nutritional demands of the patient.

Clinical Picture of Wound Disruption. There are many clinical types of wound disruption. For example, the progress of the patient appears to be satisfactory, although the temperature may be slightly raised and meteorism may be troublesome; then, when the stitches are removed on day 7 or 8, the wound will literally fall apart, or a day or two after removal of the sutures, the dressings and sometimes even the binder and bedclothes may be drenched with a pink serosanguineous discharge. This pink discharge is almost pathognomonic of dehiscence; when it occurs early, that is, before day 7, the wound should be examined. With a stitch or two removed, the edges of the wound are gently separated with a probe, and the deeper layers are inspected to determine if union is satisfactory. Sometimes this pink discharge is associated with a large subcutaneous hematoma or a soft and tympanitic boggy swelling that distends the wound. Both these findings should be investigated in the operating room, and if a large hematoma has formed, it should be evacuated, with the depths of the wound examined to see if any separation has occurred. The soft tympanitic swelling generally indicates that a knuckle of gut has burst through all the layers of the abdominal wall and lies under the skin incision; although the skin incision may remain intact, the condition is, in itself, an indication that immediate repair is imperative.

Another type of disruption is one in which the wound appears to be soundly healed. There may or may not be the pink discharge previously described, but the patient, following some excessive strain, may feel a sudden "give" in the wound which, when examined, will be found to be torn asunder with the gut eviscerated. It is surprising how painless this condition may be and how little, if any, shock results; shock, in fact, is rarely seen in cases of dehiscence of the wound except when evisceration is extensive. In cases in which the edges of the skin incision have separated, the surgeon, after having inspected and probed the depths of the wound, often may believe that what is seen is actually rectus sheath or muscle fibers coated with fibrinous clot. More often than not, however, it is the omentum, the transverse colon, or a portion of the small intestine that is protruding into the depths of the wound, and the best way of ascertaining the truth is to explore the wound in the operating room.

In another type of disruption the immediate postoperative course is very stormy. There is usually consider-able postoperative vomiting and marked distention; hiccup may be troublesome, respiratory complications are frequent, and suppuration of the wound is common.

When postoperative rupture occurs in a wound that is frankly suppurating, the onset is nearly always gradual. An abscess forms, which is usually drained; in the discharge, portions of the sloughing aponeurotic sheath of fibers of muscle are carried away, followed by separation of the deeper layers; the matted omentum and intestine are often adherent to the necrotic muscle.

Disruption generally follows removal of the sutures between days 7 and 10, but it may occur later (on day 14) when supporting or stay sutures have been used, or even later than this after the wound appears to be soundly healed, especially in cases of ascites or when suppuration is a late complication.

Prognosis. As previously stated, the mortality rate with this condition has been computed by different authorities as being between 9% and 44% with an average of 18%.

The earlier the accident is recognized and treated, the better will be the prognosis, especially in clean cases in which the dehiscence is partial or, if complete, is not associated with prolapse of the intestine. When there is extensive suppuration of the wound or general peritonitis, the prognosis is very grave. The primary condition for which the patient was operated on causes death more often than does the rupture itself or the measures required in its treatment.

Treatment. There are three methods of treatment in common use today:

1. Packing the wound, followed by strapping with adhesive plaster
2. Temporary packing and strapping, followed by secondary suture
3. Immediate resuture

Packing and strapping of the wound are indicated (1) when the condition of the patient is such that any secondary operative procedure would be too hazardous; that is, when the patient is in a critical state and is suffering from shock, (2) when the disrupted wound is foul and freely suppurating, and (3) when there is no gross prolapse of the viscera.

Therefore, in the severe, critical case, strapping is to be preferred to resuturing. In the desperate case, the problem is to get the patient safely through the immediate crisis with the least possible interference. As soon as the patient has recovered from the early effects of the wound disruption and the treatment by strapping, and provided there is no evidence of gross infection, secondary suture (when indicated) may then be carried out with much less risk.

It is true that postoperative ventral hernia is an invariable sequel to this method of treatment, but it can be repaired at a later date which comparative safety and success.

When strapping is indicated, the patient is given an appropriate intramuscular injection of morphine or pethidine (meperidine). The wound is gently cleansed with warm normal saline, and any minor degree of visceral protrusion is replaced carefully. It should be noted that this technique is impractical when there is excessive prolapse of the bowel; in this situation a relaxant anesthetic is essential to reduce the viscera within the abdominal cavity with ease and safety. The wound edges are sprayed with Polybactrin, a bulky dry gauze dressing is applied, and the wound is held together with generous strips of elastoplast placed transversely across the abdomen. Alternatively, a Velcro abdominal belt can be used for this purpose. If all goes well, the dressings can be changed in a few days, and the process can be repeated at intervals until healing takes place. In some cases, a secondary suture of the skin can be carried out at this stage, but in other instances, one may elect to allow the wound to heal entirely by granulations.

Resuture of the disrupted wound is recommended for the majority of cases and especially for those in which the edges of the wound, although they may be frayed and torn, are relatively clean. It also may be recommended for those cases in which shock is absent or, if present, is responding readily to treatment, in which sepsis is controllable, and in which the accident has occurred early in the postoperative phase and is recognized promptly.

As soon as the condition is recognized, an intramuscular injection of morphine and atrophine premedication should be given, and the wound and protruding viscera should be freely bathed with warm normal saline solution and covered with large sterile towels wrung out in the same solution, over which a many-tailed bandage of Velcro abdominal support is lightly applied. The patient should be cautioned against coughing or straining.

When the patient has been moved to the operating room, a nasogastric tube is passed, and the gastric contents are aspirated. The patient is then anesthetized. After the binder and the dressings have been removed, the surrounding skin and prolapse viscera are again washed with saline solution. The edges of the abdominal wall are then lifted upward, and the prolapsed gut is replaced below the level of the peritoneal edges. At this stage the wound is mopped dry and painted with Cetrimide or chlorhexidine (Hibitane). Disintegrated fragments of suture material are extracted, and the wound edges are freshened by snipping away necrotic tissue and edematous skin tags. It will be noted in many cases that the edges of the wound are swollen and boggy and that the peritoneum and posterior sheath of the rectus muscle are glued together and retracted outward, a state of affairs that immediately suggests that any thought of suturing layer by layer is quite out of the question. Were this attempted, the surgeon would, in any case, at once realize that the tissues are too friable and cheesy to permit it. If only a very small area of the wound has been disrupted, this portion alone should be sutured. However, if more than half of the wound has been disrupted, the correct procedure is to open the remaining part and suture the whole wound afresh.

Resuture is performed as follows: hook retractors are placed at each extremity of the wound, and these are handed to an assistant whose sole duty it is to exert firm, upward traction, not only during the introduction of the sutures but until the last through-and-through suture has been tied, at which stage the retractors are removed. The sutures will consist of strong monofilament nylon and are inserted 2.5 cm from the margin of the wound and about 2.5 cm apart and are made to transfix all the layers of the abdominal wall on both margins of the wound (Fig 11–18). As they are introduced, the free ends are clipped with hemostats. The sutures are threaded though 5 cm rubber tubing and firmly tied. For the reapproximation of the skin edges, interrupted nylon sutures are placed between the through-and-through sutures (Fig 11–19).

The skin sutures are removed on postoperative day 10; the through-and-through sutures are left in for 3

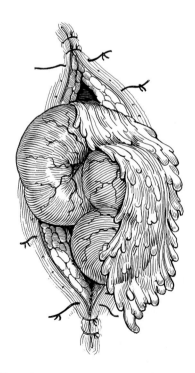

Figure 11–18. Wound disruption. Prolapse of small intestine and omentum with little evidence of healing in wound margins.

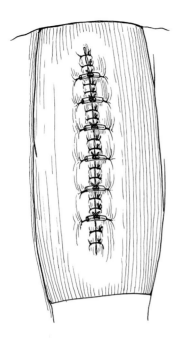

Figure 11–19. Retension sutures tied and held in position and supported by rubber tubing.

weeks. Active measures should be taken to combat peritonitis, including gastric suction and decompression, intensive antibiotic therapy, and intravenous fluid replacement.

Incisional Hernia

An incisional hernia is one that develops in the scar of a surgical incision. It may be a small, even insignificant, bulge through the wound, revealed only when the patient is asked to lift the legs off the examination couch, to sit up, or to cough, and may often not even have been noticed by the patient. However, it may also be a large, unsightly and uncomfortable affair (Fig 11–20). Only those hernias with a narrow neck and large sac are at risk of strangulation; those with a wide neck are a nuisance but not usually a danger. Rarely, a particularly thin-walled large incisional hernia may actually ulcerate at its fundus so that omentum protrudes or there is even the development of an intestinal fistula.

Incidence. Many surgeons consider incisional hernias a rarity. In some instances this is owing to the excellent technique of the surgical team, for example, Donaldson and colleagues at St. James' Hospital, Leeds, using the lateral paramedian incision, found only a single incisional hernia in 231 laparotomies.[44] However, while admiring these excellent figures, the rarity of incisional hernias claimed by others may be because patient follow-up is not meticulously, carefully, and specifically examined for the presence of a hernia. A patient lying flat on the bed may appear to have a beautifully healed scar,

but in searching for herniation we accept any bulge at all in the wound when the legs are lifted, with sitting up, or with coughing. In our study of 1129 major laparotomy wounds in adults assessed at regular intervals for 12 months after operation, we detected 84 incisional hernias (7.4%).[37] Others have reported similar figures in carefully studied series: 961 patients 6 months after laparotomy with 96 incisional hernias (10%)[63]; 213 laparotomies at 6 months and 29 hernias (13%)[64]; a 4.7% incidence of herniation at 6 months in a consecutive series of 200 laparotomies, dehiscence having occurred in 1% of the patients.[65]

Most studies of the incidence of incisional hernia give results at 6, or, at the most, 12, months after surgery. Between 2.5 and 5.5 years after operation, we studied 363 patients known not to have had incisional hernia at 1 year after operation.[66] Twenty-one patients (5.8%) were found to have developed incisional hernias. Interestingly, none of the causal factors, which will be discussed, were found to be associated with the development of these late hernias. In addition, six of the patients were unaware of the presence of the hernia, and none of the patients were inconvenienced by it or requested surgical repair or a supporting corset. We can give no explanation of how mature collagen can stretch to form an incisional hernia a year or more after sound healing has occurred. Perhaps scar tissue is a more dynamic tissue than has previously been thought, so that metabolic stresses on the patient might result in some disturbance on the dynamic equilibrium of the new collagen. It is interesting to note another of the late development of incisional hernia in studies carried out at 3 and 5 years after laparotomy.[67]

The time of the development of incisional hernia was

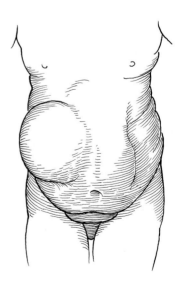

Figure 11–20. Massive incisional hernia.

documented in a series of 500 incisional hernia repairs performed at the Shouldice Clinic in Toronto.[68] The time of occurrence was reported as follows:

Within 2 weeks	5.6%
Within 6 months	52.2%
Within 1 year	67.8%
Within 2 years	78.6%
Within 3 years	88.4%
Within 4 years	93.2%
Within 5 years	97.0%

A further 1.4% occurred between years 5 and 30, and there were inadequate histories in the remaining 1.6%.

Etiology. Many factors have been implicated in the development of incisional hernia but prospective trials have replaced conjecture by solid information. In our own study, of 1129 major laparotomies in which there were 19 burst abdomens and 84 incisional hernias, we found that wound herniation was more common at a statistically significant level in the elderly, in men, in the obese, in patients undergoing bowel surgery, and in patients with incisions >18 cm.[37] There was no significant difference related to the type of incision used (midline, paramedian, or transverse), nor was there any difference between the complication rate in wounds closed by a consultant or a registrar; however, the incidence was higher in the hands of senior registrars. Postoperative complications, particularly chest infection, abdominal distention, and wound infection were the most significant factors associated with herniation, and these factors tended to occur in combination. The study included 104 patients whose wounds were closed with absorbable polyglycolic acid, and among these patients there were 12 hernias (11.5%), a significantly higher proportion than in those in whom the mass closure technique with nylon was used (Table 11–2).

The part played by wound sepsis appeared to be the most important; 48% of the 179 patients who developed a wound infection went on to develop an incisional hernia (Table 11–3).

TABLE 11–2. COMPARISON OF NYLON AND DEXON SUTURES FOR MASS CLOSURE: INCIDENCE OF WOUND DEHISCENCE, HERNIATION, AND SINUS FORMATION

Factor	Total (%)	Nylon (%)	Dexon (%)
Number of cases	210	106	104
Dehiscence	2 (0.95)	1 (0.94)	1 (0.96)
Wound herniation	16 (7.6)	4 (3.8)	12 (11.5[a])
Sinus formation	22 (10.5)	10 (9.4)	12 (11.5)

[a]P <.05.
(From Bucknall TE, Ellis H, 1981.)

TABLE 11–3. INCIDENCE OF WOUND HERNIATION RELATED TO SOME SUGGESTED CAUSAL FACTORS[a]

Factor	All Patients (n = 1129)	Patients Who Developed Hernias (n = 84)	X[a] Test
Patients			
Mean age (years)	46.1	58.2	P <.001
Men	510	62	P <.0001
Obesity	200	30	P <.0001
Taking steroids	20	1	NS
Jaundiced	45	3	NS
Incision			
Midline	544	48	NS
Paramedian	558	35	NS
Transverse	27	1	NS
Length >18 cm[b]	155/419	31/36	P <.001
Suture			
Mass (nylon)	684	49	NS
Mass (polyglycolic acid)	104	12	P <.05
Two layer (catgut and nylon)	177	9	NS
One layer (nylon)	164	14	NS
Surgeon			
Consultant	424	18	P <.005
Senior registrar	471	47	P <.005
Registrar	207	19	NS
Operation			
Local antiseptic	867	63	NS
Drain	548	44	NS
Bowel surgery	378	43	P <.01
Malignancy	258	13	NS
Emergency	184	14	NS
Postoperative complications			
Chest infection	195	32	P <.0001
Abdominal distention	148	24	P <.0005
Wound infection	179	41	P <.00001

[a]Values are numbers of patients.
[b]Measuring commenced 1978; 419 patients included.
NS, Not significant
(From Bucknall TE, Cox PJ, et al: *Br Med J* 1982;284:931)

A prospective study in which 98 incisional hernias occurred in 961 patients undergoing laparotomy (10%) showed that the most important determinants were chest complications, male sex, age over 65, and wound infection.[63]

It has been pointed out that a burst abdomen is an important predisposing factor to incisional herniation,[69] and that more than one-quarter of resutured burst abdomens went on to develop this complication.

During the period 1979 to 1984, our unit at Westminster studied 877 patients who had undergone elective or emergency major laparotomies and who had been followed for a minimum of 6 months.[70] Midline, conventional paramedian, and transverse incisions were used during this time period, but all had a common method of wound closure to the rectus sheath by the continuous nylon mass closure technique. The incidence of incisional hernia was 6% in the 699 fresh incisions. It rose to 12% in the 142 patients in whom the incision was carried out by reopening a previous wound (P <.05) and rose to no less than 44% in the 36 patients in whom the laparotomy was carried out through a previous incisional hernia (P <.01). With the exception of jaundice, none of the other commonly accepted risk factors for incisional herniation were increased significantly in those patients with reopened wounds who subsequently developed a hernia, when compared with patients who did not develop a hernia. Thus, there is a considerably increased risk of incisional herniation when laparotomy is performed through a previous abdominal incision.

Repair of Incisional Hernias. Repair of incisional hernias is considered fully in Chapter 14.

REFERENCES

1. Ellis H, Coleridge-Smith PD, et al. Abdominal incisions—vertical or transverse? *Postgrad Med J* 1984;60:27
2. Guillou PJ, Hall TJ, et al. Vertical abdominal incisions—a choice? *Br J Surg* 1980;67:395
3. Gilbert JM, Ellis H. Peritoneal closure after lateral paramedian incision. *Br J Surg* 1987;74:113
4. Cox PJ, Ausobsky JR, Ellis H. Towards no incisional hernias: lateral paramedian versus midline incisions. *J R Soc Med* 1986;79:711
5. McBurney C. The incision made in the abdominal wall in cases of appendicitis, with a description of a new method of operating. *Ann Surg* 1894;20:38
6. Jenkins TPN. The burst abdominal wound: a mechanical approach. *Br J Surg* 1976;63:873
7. Kocher T. *Textbook of Operative Surgery,* 2nd ed. London, England: Black; 1903
8. Hermann RE. Early exposure in the management of the postoperative wound. *Surg Gynecol Obstet* 1965;120:503
9. Law NW, Ellis H. Exposure of the wound—a safe economy in the NHS. *Postgrad Med J* 1987;63:27
10. Howard JM, Invi FK. Clostridial myositis—gas gangrene: observations of battle casualties in Korea. *Surgery* 1954; 36:1115
11. Whelan TJ, Burkhalter WE, et al. Mangement of war wounds. In: Welch CE (ed), *Advances in Surgery,* 3rd ed. Chicago, IL: Year Book; 1968:227
12. Klein RS, Berger SA, et al. Wound infections during the Yom Kippur War: observations concerning antibiotic prophylaxis and therapy. *Ann Surg* 1975;182:15
13. Elliot-Smith A, Ellis H. *Clostridium welchii* infection following cholecystectomy. *Lancet* 1957;2:723
14. Boerema I, Groeneveld PHA. *Proceedings of the 4th International Congress on Hyperbaric Medicine.* London, England: Bailliere, Tindall and Cassell; 1970
15. Darke SG, King AM, et al. Gas gangrene and related infection: classification, clinical features and aetiology, management and mortality. A report of 88 cases. *Br J Surg* 1977;64:104
16. Gozal D, Ziser A, et al. Necrotising fasciitis. *Arch Surg* 1986;121:233
17. Janevicius RV, Hann SE, et al. Necrotizing fasciitis. *Surg Gynecol Obstet* 1982;154:97
18. Kingston D, Seal DV. Current hypotheses on synergistic microbial gangrene. *Br J Surg* 1990;77:260
19. Pessa ME, Howard RJ. Necrotising fasciitis. *Surg Gynecol Obstet* 1985;161:357
20. Ledingham Inca, Tehrani MA. Diagnosis, clinical course, and treatment of acute dermal gangrene. *Br J Surg* 1975; 62:364
21. Meleney FL. Hemolytic streptococcus gangrene. *Arch Surg* 1924;9:317
22. Wilson R. Necrotizing fasciitis. *Ann Surg* 1952;18:416
23. Percival R, Hargreaves AW. Necrotizing fasciitis: an alternative approach. *Postgrad Med J* 1982;58:756
24. Stone HH, Fabian TC, et al. Management of acute full-thickness losses of the abdominal wall. *Ann Surg* 1981;193: 612
25. Rouse TM, Malamgoni MA, et al. Necrotizing fasciitis: a preventable disaster. *Surgery* 1982;92:765
26. Oh C, Lee C, et al. Necrotizing fasciitis of perineum. *Surgery* 1982;91:49
27. Woodburn KR, Ramsay G, et al. Retroperitoneal necrotizing fasciitis. *Br J Surg* 1992;79:342
28. Aitken DR, Mackett MCT, et al. The changing pattern of hemolytic streptococcal gangrene. *Arch Surg* 1982;117:561
29. Meleney FL. A differential diagnosis between certain types of infectious gangrene of the skin. *Surg Gynecol Obstet* 1933;56:847
30. Hirn M, Niinikoski J. Management of perineal necrotiang fasciitis. *Ann Chir Gynecol* 1989;78:277
31. Crockett DJ. Regional keloid susceptibility. *Br J Plast Surg* 1964;17:245
32. Harvey-Kemble JV. Scanning electron microscopy of hypertrophic and keloid scar. *Postgrad Med J* 1976;52:219
33. Calnan JS, Copenhagen HJ. Autotransplantation of keloid in man. *Br J Surg* 1967;54:330
34. Watkins GL. Bone formation scars after xiphoidectomy. *Arch Surg* 1964;89:731
35. Apostolidis NS, Legakis NC, et al. Heterotopic bone formation in abdominal operation scars. *Am J Surg* 1981; 142:555
36. Chevrel JP. *Surgery of the Abdominal Wall.* Berlin, Germany: Springer-Verlag; 1987:106
37. Wissing J, Vroonhoven TJ, et al. Fascia closure after midline laparotomy: results of a randomized trial. *Br J Surg* 1987;74:738
38. Bucknall TE, Cox PJ, et al. Burst abdomen and incisional hernia: a prospective study of 1129 major laparotomies. *Br Med J* 1982;284:931
39. Poole GV. Mechanical factors in abdominal wound closure: the prevention of fascial dehiscence. *Surgery* 1985; 97:631
40. Mendoza CB, Postlethwait RW, et al. Incidence of wound disruption following operation. *Arch Surg* 1970;101:396

41. Bucknall TE. Factors influencing wound complications: a clinical and experimental study. *Ann R Coll Surg Engl* 1983;65:71

42. Bucknall TF and Ellis H. Abdominal wound closure—a comparison of monofilament nylon and polyglycolic acid. *Surgery* 1981;89:672

43. Ellis H, Coleridge-Smith PD, et al. Abdominal incisions—vertical or transverse? *Postgrad Med J* 1984;60:407

44. Donaldson DR, Hegarty JH, et al. The lateral paramedian incision-experience with 850 cases. *Br J Surg* 1982;69:630

45. Goligher JC, Irvin TT, et al. A controlled clinical trial of three methods of closure of laparotomy wounds. *Br J Surg* 1975;62:823

46. Leaper DJ, Pollock AV, et al. Abdominal wound closure: a trial of nylon, polyglycolicacid and steel sutures. *Br J Surg* 1977;64:603

47. Tagart REB. The suturing of abdominal incisions: a comparison of monofilament nylon and catgut. *Br J Surg* 1967; 54:952

48. Bucknall TE, Teare L, et al. The choice of a suture to close abdominal incisions. *Eur Surg Res* 1983;15:59

49. Karipineni RC, Wilk PJ, et al. The role of the peritoneum in the healing of abdominal incisions. *Surg Gynecol Obstet* 1976;142:729

50. Jones TE, Newell ET, et al. The use of alloy steel wire in the closure of abdominal wounds. *Surg Gynecol Obstet* 1941; 72:1056

51. Dudley HAF. Layered and mass closure of the abdominal wall. *Br J Surg* 1970;57:664

52. Goligher JC. Visceral and varietal sutures in abdominal surgery. *Am J Surg* 1976;131:130

53. Kirk RM. Effect of method of opening and closing the abdomen on incidence of wound bursting. *Cancer* 1972; 2:352

54. Martyak SN, Curtis LE. Abdominal incision and closure: a systems approach. *Am J Surg* 1976;131:476

55. McGinn FP, Hamilton JC. Ascorbic acid levels in stored blood in patients undergoing surgery after blood transfusion. *Br J Surg* 1976;63:505

56. Nayman J, McDermott FT. Wound dehiscence in acute renal failure: clinical and experimental studies. *Med Res* 1965;1:180

57. Colin JF, Elliot P, et al. The effects of uremia upon wound healing: an experimental study. *Br J Surg* 1979;66:793

58. Androulakakis PA. Uraemia and wound healing. *Br J Surg* 1980;67:380

59. Moffat FL, Deitel M, et al. Abdominal surgery in patients undergoing long-term peritoneal dialysis. *Surgery* 1982; 92:598

60. Bayer I, Ellis H. Jaundice and wound healing: an experimental study. *Br J Surg* 1976;63:392

61. Ellis H, Heddle R. Does the peritoneum need to be closed at laparotomy? *Br J Surg* 1977;64:733

62. Taube M, Ellis H. Mass closure of abdominal wounds following major laparotomy in jaundiced patients. *Ann R Coll Surg Engl* 1987;69:276

63. Pollock AV. Laparotomy. *J R Soc Med* 1981;74:480

64. Johnson CD, Bernhardt LW, et al. Incisional hernia after mass closure of abdominal incisions with Dexon and Prolene. *Br J Surg* 1982;69:55

65. Irvin TT, Stoddard CJ, et al. Abdominal wound healing: a prospective clinical study. *Br Med J* 1977;2:351

66. Ellis H, Gajra H, et al. Incisional hernias: when do they occur? *Br J Surg* 1983;70:290

67. Harding KG, Mudge M, et al. Late development of incisional hernia: an unrecognized problem. *Br Med J* 1983; 286:519

68. Akman PC. A study of five hundred incisional hernias. *J Int Coll Surg* 1962;37:125

69. Grace RH, Cox S. Incidence of incisional hernia after dehiscence of the abdominal wound. *Am J Surg* 1976;131:210

70. Lamont PM, Ellis H. Incisional hernia in reopened abdominal incisions—an overlooked risk factor. *Br J Surg* 1988;75:374

12

Intestinal Stomas

Ira J. Kodner

An intestinal stoma is an opening of the intestinal or urinary tract onto the abdominal wall, constructed surgically or appearing inadvertently. A colostomy is a connection of the colon to the skin of the abdominal wall. An ileostomy involves exteriorization of the ileum on the abdominal skin. In rare instances, the proximal small bowel may be exteriorized as a jejunostomy. A urinary conduit involves a stoma on the abdominal wall that serves to convey urine to an appliance placed on the skin. The conduit may consist of an intestinal segment or, in some cases, a direct implantation of the ureter, or even the bladder, on the abdominal wall.

Information about the types and numbers of stomas constructed, complications of stomas, and resultant impairment of an individual's life has been limited because the diseases for which stomas are constructed are not mandated as reportable in the United States. Therefore the United Ostomy Association (UOA), a voluntary group of 40000 members with stomas of various types, undertook the mission of collecting data from patients in the United States and Canada who have an intestinal stoma. A review of 15000 such entries shows the peak incidence for ileostomy construction owing to ulcerative colitis to occur in persons between 20 and 40 years of age, with a lower peak but in the same age range, for patients with Crohn's disease. The second largest peak represents colostomies constructed because of colorectal cancer, and this peak is in patients 60 to 80 years of age. When complications were analyzed according to original indication for surgery, we found that many patients knew they had complications but were not aware

of the exact nature of the complication. Postoperative intestinal obstruction occurred in all categories of disease, as did retraction of the stoma and abscess formation. There was a preponderance of hernia formation in patients who had surgery for colorectal cancer, whereas abscess, fistula, and stricture formation were the major complications in the patients with Crohn's disease. As new surgical procedures are devised, a justification for their utilization is often the reduction of the level of handicap that exists among patients who have had construction of a conventional ostomy. The UOA survey revealed that patients resumed household activities 90% of the time, vocational activities 73% of the time, social activities 92% of the time, and sexual activities 70% of the time. It is taken into account that patients who have proctectomy for cancer frequently lose their sexual function because of autonomic denervation and not because of the presence of a stoma.

Changes that have improved the quality of life of the patient with a stoma include the development and availability of improved stoma equipment. Specialized surgical techniques, some of which are described in this chapter, have been developed that facilitate the subsequent maintenance of an ostomy. In addition, specialized nursing techniques applied both preoperatively and postoperatively have enhanced the care of the patient with a stoma.

The overall incidence of stoma construction appears to be decreasing and will probably continue to do so. There are now fewer abdominoperineal resections for cancer because of the advent of new surgical techniques, especially the use of stapling devices, as well as an increased use of local treatment for selected rectal tumors. The incidence of permanent ileostomies is decreasing because of the popularization of sphincter-saving procedures for patients with ulcerative colitis and familial polyposis. The surgical procedures that eliminate permanent stomas, however, have resulted in an increasing use of temporary loop ileostomies, which are usually more difficult stomas to manage.

■ COMMON COMPLICATIONS OF STOMAS

Each type of stoma is associated with a particular spectrum of complications, but some problems are common to all intestinal stomas. The specific ones are dealt with under each category of stoma. A common complication, regardless of the stoma type, is destruction of the peristomal skin, which is usually caused by poor location or construction of the stoma. In addition to the acute maceration and inflammation of the skin, pseudoepitheliomatous hyperplasia may arise at the mucocutaneous border of stomas subjected to chronic malfitting appliances. Appearance of a fistula adjacent to a stoma usually indicates recurrence of Crohn's disease. One of the difficult complications to handle, especially in an obese patient, is improper location of the stoma, which prohibits maintenance of the seal of an appliance. A special problem arises in the patient who has portal hypertension because the construction of a stoma results in the creation of a portosystemic shunt, and varices can form in the peristomal skin.

Other common problems include the need for precautions with medications, especially time-released enteric medications, which may pass through a shortened intestinal tract unabsorbed. Laxatives also can be devastating to the patients with no colon or with a proximal colostomy. The ostomy patient, in some cases, has chronic difficulty maintaining proper fluid and electrolyte balance, and diuretics in these patients can be especially difficult to manage. The usual intestinal preparations prior to diagnostic testing should be altered for the patient with an intestinal stoma.

The data from the UOA registry indicate that patients have regained a good quality of life following construction of an intestinal stoma. Conventional ileostomy and sigmoid colostomy account for 73% of the patients in the UOA data registry. Colorectal cancer, chronic ulcerative colitis, and Crohn's disease account for 88% of the patient diagnoses. Ileostomy revisions are most commonly performed for Crohn's disease. Parastomal hernia occurred in 9.5% of patients with sigmoid colostomy, of which 26% required surgical treatment. The incidence of surgery to correct stoma complications was 10.5% for patients with a conventional ileostomy and 7.5% for patients with a sigmoid colostomy.

The data from the UOA registry suggest that emphasis should be placed on proper construction of standard stomas. The stoma location should be chosen and marked preoperatively, even if there is only a remote possibility of need for an intestinal stoma during the operative procedure.

■ COLOSTOMY

The most common indication for fashioning a colostomy is cancer of the rectum. Since a colostomy is an opening of the large intestine with no sphincteric controls, its location would obviously be better on the abdominal wall than in the perineum where an appliance cannot be maintained. A distal colorectal anastomosis in an elderly patient with a poorly functioning anal sphincter may result in what is essentially a "perineal colostomy." In these cases, it often behooves the surgeon to construct a good colostomy rather than to preserve an incompetent anus. Colostomies are also constructed as treatment for obstructing lesions of the distal large intestine and for actual or potential perforations.

TYPE BY ANATOMIC LOCATION

Traditionally, the type of colostomy has been categorized by the part of the colon used in its construction. The most common type has been called an "end-sigmoid" colostomy. However, if the inferior mesenteric artery is transected during an operation for cancer of the rectum, the blood supply to the sigmoid colon is no longer dependable, and it should not be used for stoma construction. Therefore, an "end-descending" colostomy is usually preferable to an end-sigmoid colostomy. Other types of colonic stomas include the transverse colostomy and cecostomy. The physiology of the colon should be taken into account when considering stoma construction. The right side of the colon absorbs water and has irregular peristaltic contractions. Stomas made from the proximal half of the colon usually expel a liquid content. The left colon serves as a conduit and reservoir and has a few mass peristaltic motions per day. The content is more solid, and in many cases the stoma output can be regulated by irrigation.

TYPE BY FUNCTION

More important than the anatomy of the colon is the function that the colostomy is intended to perform. There are two considerations: (1) to provide decompression of the large intestine, and (2) to provide diversion of the feces.

Decompressing Colostomy

A decompressing stoma does not necessarily provide diversion of feces. These colostomies are constructed most often for treatment of obstructing cancer of the rectum or sigmoid colon. They are frequently done on an emergency basis, with no opportunity for preparation of the intestine. Recently, there has been interest in cleansing of the colon and total abdominal colectomy with ileorectal anastomosis rather than construction of a temporary decompressing stoma. Nevertheless, decompressing stomas are still useful and safe. Their use provides opportunity for a subsequent definitive cancer operation without compromise of the principles of cancer surgery. The major disadvantage of a decompressing stoma is that it does not necessarily provide complete fecal diversion. This carries the risk of potentially fatal sepsis if there is disruption of intestinal continuity distal to the stoma.

Types of Decompressing Stomas. There are three types of decompressing stomas: (1) the so-called "blow-hole" decompressing stoma constructed in the cecum or transverse colon, (2) a tube type of cecostomy, and (3) a loop-transverse colostomy.

Cecostomy and "Blow-Hole" Stoma. A cecostomy should be constructed only rarely because it is difficult to manage postoperatively. It should be reserved for the severely, acutely ill patient with massive distention and impending perforation of the colon. This is seen most often with distal obstructing cancer or in some of the pseudoobstruction syndromes seen in elderly or immunocompromised patients. Because these operations are done on an urgent basis and the abdomen is usually distorted by intestinal dilatation, the choice of site for an incision is over the dilated cecum. The location of this incision or of an intended decompressing transverse colostomy is selected by placing a marker on the umbilicus when an abdominal film is obtained.

A disadvantage of a cecostomy or loop colostomy done through a small incision is that one cannot evaluate other parts of the colon for potential ischemic necrosis due to massive dilatation. The construction of a blow-hole cecostomy or transverse colostomy (Fig 12–1) is carried out by making a 4- to 6-cm transverse incision over the most dilated part of intestine and then placing a series of interrupted, seromuscular, absorbable sutures between the peritoneum and the seromuscular layer of the bowel to be decompressed. This should be done through an incision sufficient to allow subsequent incision of the intestine and suturing of the intestine to the skin. The bowel wall will be very thin, and it is not unusual to have leakage of gas as the sutures are being placed. It may be helpful to irrigate with a di-

lute solution of kanamycin throughout this procedure to prevent infection of the abdominal wall.

Once the first layer of sutures has been placed and the intestine is sealed from the remainder of the abdominal cavity, needle decompression of the gas-distended viscus is performed to reduce the tension on the intestinal wall. When this procedure is completed, a second layer of absorbable sutures is placed between the seromuscular layer of the intestine and the fascia of the abdominal wall. Subsequently, the colon is incised, usually with release of a large amount of liquid and gas. The full thickness of intestine then is sutured to the full thickness of skin, again with absorbable sutures, and an appliance is placed over the stoma. Postoperatively, it is not unusual for there to be significant inflammation in the abdominal wall around such a stoma, and after a period of weeks, significant prolapse may occur. Therefore these stomas should be used for short periods of time, with definitive resection performed as soon as possible.

A tube cecostomy (Fig 12–2) is constructed by making a similar incision or by approaching the cecum through a laparotomy incision. A purse-string suture is placed in the cecal wall, and a large mushroom-tipped or Malecot catheter is placed in the cecum. The purse-string suture secures the catheter. Usually a second purse-string suture is placed, and the tube is brought through a right lower quadrant incision. The cecum then is sutured to the peritoneum of the abdominal wall. The advantage of this stoma is that there is less chance of prolapse. The major disadvantage is that the tubes usually become blocked with feces, drain poorly, and sometimes leak stool adjacent to the drain.

Loop-Transverse Colostomy. This is a decompressing stoma as well, although when properly constructed (Fig 12–3), it will serve as a diverting stoma for approximately 6 weeks or until the posterior wall recesses far enough below the wall of the abdomen that stool can enter the distal loop. These stomas are constructed for reasons similar to those described for the blow-hole type stoma and to provide temporary diversion for protection of complicated distal anastomoses. The other advantage is that, when properly constructed, a loop-transverse colostomy can serve as a long-term stoma. The incidence of prolapse is not prohibitive. Parastomal hernias can occur if the fascia is not closed tightly enough, and these stomas usually cannot be regulated by irrigation techniques.

The site can be chosen for this stoma in an emergency situation as previously described, or it can be marked electively on the abdominal wall in preparation for potential construction in patients who are to have low colorectal anastomoses or in those in whom it is anticipated that inflammatory reaction will be encoun-

Text continued on page 433

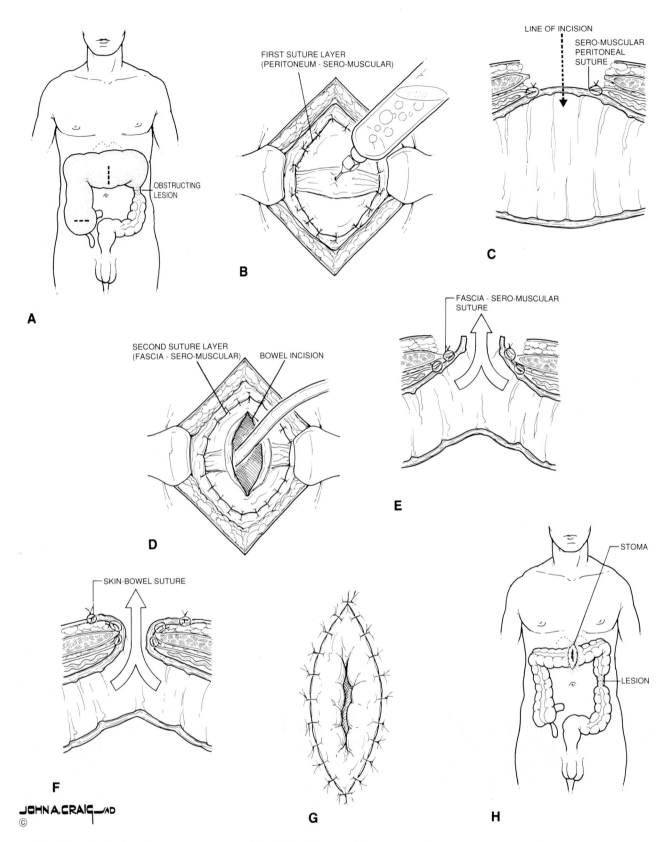

Figure 12–1. Construction of blow-hole cecostomy or colostomy. **A.** The incision is located over the most dilated aspect of the intestine. **B.** After the peritoneum is quarantined, gas is allowed to escape, decompressing the bowel. **C.** Placement of the quarantine sutures. **D.** The colon is opened, and more adequate aspiration is effected. **E.** Details of the second level of quarantine sutures between fascia and seromuscular layer of colonic wall (should be completed before the bowel is opened). **F, G.** The stoma is completed by placement of sutures between skin and colonic wall. **H.** Completed blow-hole stoma.

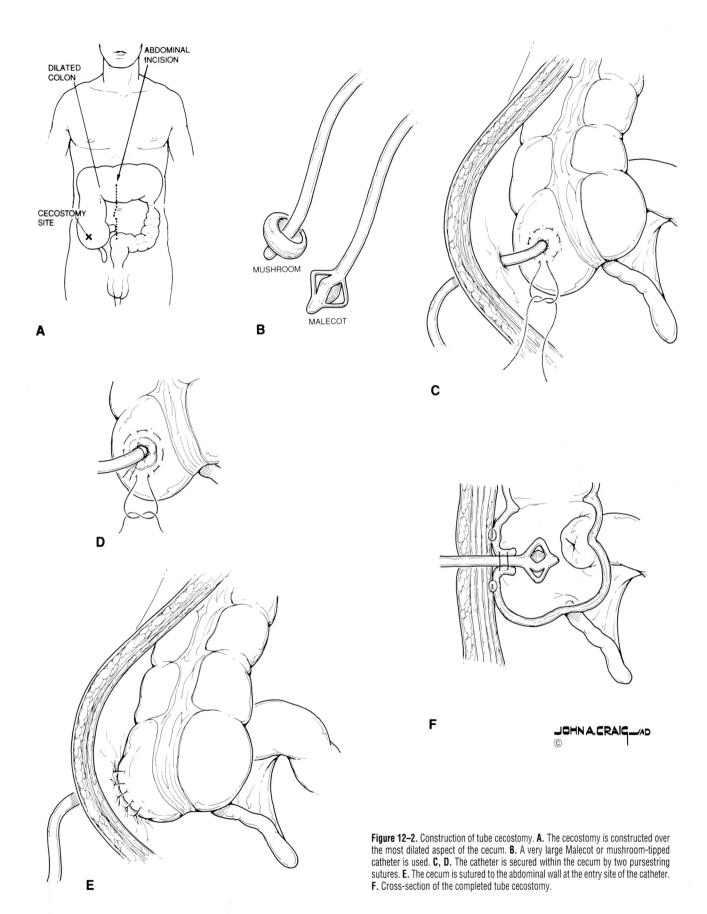

A. DILATED COLON — ABDOMINAL INCISION — CECOSTOMY SITE

B. MUSHROOM — MALECOT

C.

D.

E.

F.

JOHN A. CRAIG _AD
©

Figure 12–2. Construction of tube cecostomy. **A.** The cecostomy is constructed over the most dilated aspect of the cecum. **B.** A very large Malecot or mushroom-tipped catheter is used. **C, D.** The catheter is secured within the cecum by two pursestring sutures. **E.** The cecum is sutured to the abdominal wall at the entry site of the catheter. **F.** Cross-section of the completed tube cecostomy.

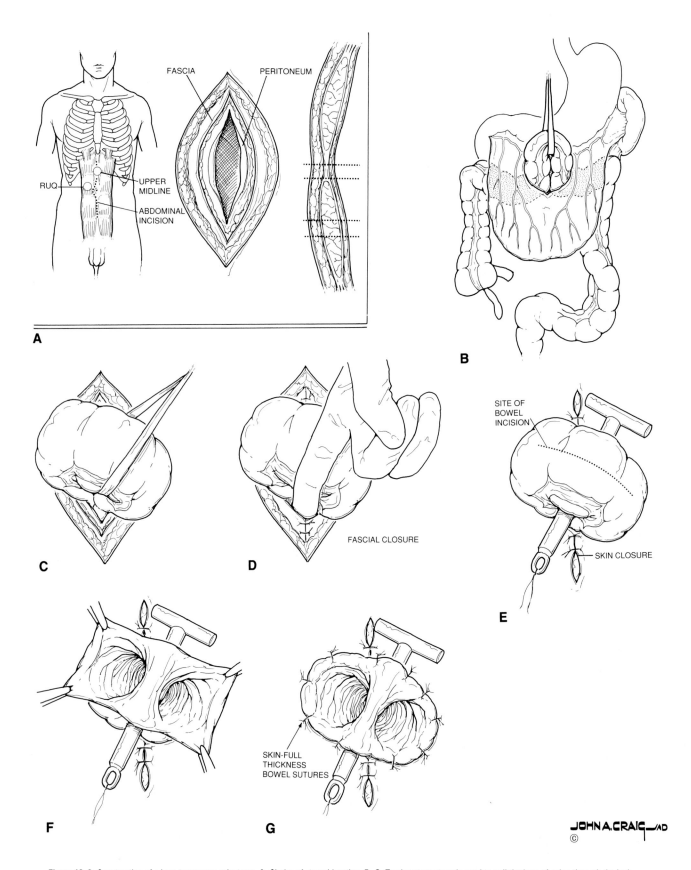

Figure 12–3. Construction of a loop-transverse colostomy. **A.** Choice of stomal location. **B, C.** Tracheostomy tape is used to pull the loop of colon through the incision. **D.** The fascia is closed tightly around the loop of intestine. **E, F, G.** The loop of colon is opened over a supporting rod and is sutured to the skin of the abdominal wall.

tered and require temporary diversion of intestinal content as a safeguard against contamination from a leaking anastomosis. This occurs occasionally in patients with severe diverticulitis. In an elective situation, the stoma can be placed through the rectus muscle either on the right or left side, depending on later intentions of closing or resecting the colostomy site in continuity with a cancer operation, or it can be brought through the midline (Fig 12–3A). The midline location allows tight closure of the fascia of the linea alba around the stoma, thus reducing the incidence of hernia and prolapse, and it makes dissection easier at the time of closure because the midline incision may be opened to allow proper mobilization of the colon for closure.

Construction of the loop colostomy requires the colon to be mobile enough to be brought to the level of the abdominal wall (Fig 12–3B). If this cannot be done or if the colon is so massively dilated that loop colostomy is not safe, one should resort to the use of a blow-hole colostomy as previously described, in which only one wall of the intestine is utilized and tension on the mesentery is avoided. The loop-transverse colostomy is constructed by placing a tracheostomy tape around the colon at the site chosen for the colostomy. The transverse colon at this site is usually dissected free of the overlying omentum in the embryonic peritoneal fusion planes. The tracheostomy tape and colon are brought through an avascular window in the omentum to allow better sealing between the colon and the abdominal wall (Fig 12–3B, C). The fascia is then closed on either side of the loop of colon tightly enough to allow snug passage of one fingertip. This usually seems frighteningly tight but is necessary to prevent postoperative hernia and prolapse.

The skin then is closed, also snugly, on either side of the loop of colon. The tracheostomy tape then is replaced by a T-shaped plastic rod that frequently has a suture through each end of it so that it can be easily repositioned should it be displaced (Fig 12–3E). The wound is protected, and attention is directed to the protruding loop of colon, which is incised either longitudinally or transversely to allow the best separation of the edges of the colon (Fig 12–3F). Full thickness of intestine is then sutured to full thickness of skin with absorbable suture material (Fig 12–3F). If this stoma is properly constructed, the posterior wall will bulge upward, providing the desired diversion as well as decompression. An appliance then is applied either over the rod or beneath the rod, depending on the tension of the stoma.

In the postoperative period, the appliance is emptied or changed as necessary, and the wound is kept clean. The rod is usually left in place for 1 week and then is easily removed. The colostomy appliance is fashioned as necessary as the contour of the stoma and skin opening change. Patients with this type of stoma usually are not taught to irrigate, because irrigation is infrequently successful. After the immediate postoperative period, the patient usually is instructed to empty the appliance as necessary and to change the entire appliance every 1 or 2 days, depending on the condition of the skin and the ability to maintain an adequate seal of the appliance to the skin.

CLOSURE OF A TEMPORARY COLOSTOMY. The most important consideration in dealing with closure of a temporary colostomy is deciding when it is safe to restore intestinal continuity. Distal integrity and adequacy of sphincter muscle function must be carefully evaluated before closure of the stoma is undertaken. The reason for constructing the stoma initially must be taken into account, and contrast studies and endoscopy should demonstrate clearly that the original reason no longer exists.

Adequate function of the anal sphincter must be demonstrated before the temporary colostomy is closed. This can be done by formal manometric and electromyographic studies or by giving the patient a 500 mL enema and asking him to hold it until he can comfortably walk to a toilet and expel the enema. If the sphincter does not work and cannot be repaired, the patient will be better off with a properly constructed end colostomy than with attempts to preserve a nonfunctional sphincter. Once it is decided that it is safe to close the colostomy, the procedure should be undertaken with the same skill and precaution as required for a colon anastomosis (Fig 12–4). The literature reflects a high complication rate for colostomy closure, and this rate is used to rationalize not constructing such colostomies. Although this type stoma is used infrequently, not to use it can result in disaster; and if the same surgical skill is used in closure as in constructing an anastomosis, the complication rate of closure should approach zero.

The closure is begun by making a circumferential incision around the stoma, including a small rim of skin (Fig 12–4A). If the stoma has been placed in the midline, the midline incision may be opened on either side of it to allow adequate mobilization. The circumferential incision is deepened until the peritoneal cavity is entered and the colon and surrounding omentum can be separated from the abdominal wall. The colon then is brought through the incision, and the serosal surface is clearly defined circumferentially (Fig 12–4B, C). This involves resecting omentum and fibrofatty tissue from the serosal surface. Once this step is completed, the stoma is ready for closure, which can be accomplished by a linear stapling device (Fig 12–4D, E), by a hand-sutured closure (Fig 12–4F, G), or if the bowel has been compromised in any way, by complete transection of the colon and construction of a formal end-to-end anastomosis. Caution must be taken to ensure that no small in-

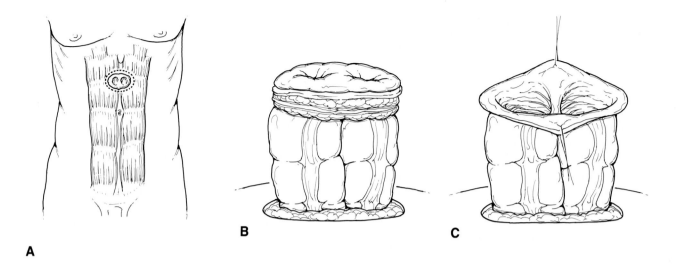

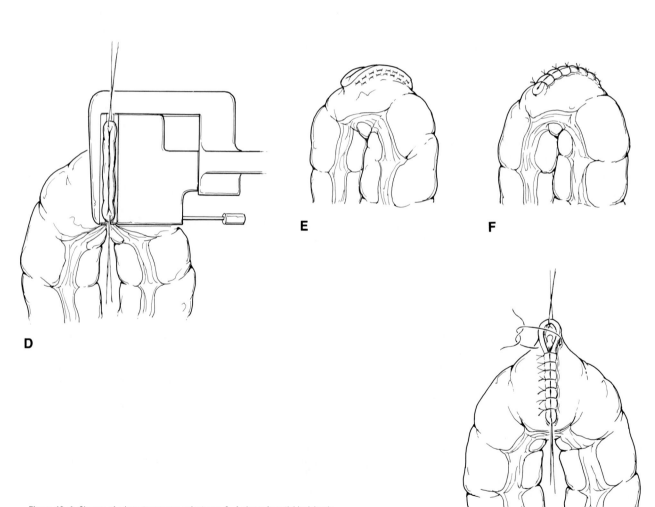

Figure 12–4. Closure of a loop-transverse colostomy. **A.** A circumferential incision is made around the stoma, with reopening of the midline incision if needed. **B, C.** The colon is mobilized adequately. **D, E.** Staple closure of the colostomy. **F, G.** Suture closure of the colostomy.

JOHN A. CRAIG AD
©

testine has been injured and that no significant bleeding has been left unattended. Once this has been accomplished, the colon is returned to the abdominal cavity, and the abdomen is closed. Usually the skin itself is left open for delayed primary closure.

Diverting Colostomy

A diverting colostomy is constructed to provide complete diversion of intestinal content. It must be done when there is breech of distal bowel continuity such as occurs with traumatic injury, diverticulitis, perforated unresectable cancer, or a leaked or threatened anastomosis. The end colostomy can be constructed to allow external radiation of an unresectable rectal cancer, subsequently to be followed by an attempt at a definitive cancer operation and possibly a takedown of the colostomy. In this situation, a sling of polyglycolic acid mesh may be used to keep the small intestine out of the field of radiation. An end, totally diverting colostomy is also constructed when there is destruction of the distal rectum or anus as a result of trauma, Crohn's disease, hidradenitis, or multiple sphincter injuries. It is most commonly constructed when it is necessary to remove the rectum either because of cancer or, rarely, because of inflammatory bowel disease limited to the rectum or anus.

Choices for Construction.
A completely diverting colostomy can be constructed only by complete transection of the colon. When this is done, the proximal component is brought up as an end colostomy, and the distal component is either brought up as a mucous fistula or is left closed within the abdominal cavity (as in a Hartmann resection). The technique of stoma construction is the same as that which is described for the end colostomy after proctectomy. A mucous fistula is constructed in the inferior aspect of the incision by using similar techniques or by bringing the distal bowel out through a separate small incision. It is necessary to construct a formal mucous fistula only if there is risk of distal obstruction from either the disease process or a tight anal sphincter, or if there is severe inflammatory destructive change in the rectum. If the distal component is closed and left within the abdominal cavity, it should be fixed to the fascia in the inferior aspect of the incision so that easy access exists should the closed end have to be converted to a formal mucous fistula. The old operation of so-called double-barreled Divine colostomy should be abandoned because the closely adjacent stomas make application of an appliance very difficult. Short-term diversion also can be achieved by a properly constructed loop-transverse colostomy. Adequate diversion can be expected in most cases, for 6 weeks, and this is a satisfactory middle ground, except for those cases in which there is actual disruption distally. For them, complete separation of the colon is compulsory.

Construction of an End Colostomy (Fig 12–5).
An end, completely diverting, colostomy usually is located in the left lower quadrant, where the site is chosen preoperatively by placing a vertical line through the umbilicus and another line transversely through the inferior margin of the umbilicus and by affixing a disk the size of a stoma faceplate to designate the stoma opening through the rectus muscle and on the summit of the infraumbilical fat fold (Fig 12–5A). An alternative location is through the midline fascia, not necessarily at the umbilicus. Although this site seems initially esthetically unappealing, it allows construction of a stoma with a lesser incidence symptomatic of hernia formation because of the ability to tightly close the linea alba around the stoma.

Once a site is chosen, the patient should be evaluated in multiple body configurations to verify the adequacy of the stoma site. A most common mistake is to choose the site with the patient supine and then find when the patient rises to a standing or sitting position that the chosen site is completely obscured by fat folds, scar tissue, or a protruding skeletal structure. The location should be adjusted up or down, even considering the use of upper quadrants of the abdomen, if necessary, to allow proper fixation of an appliance and easy access by the patient. The site usually is marked with ink in the patient's room and then is scratched into the skin with a needle in the operating room after induction of anesthesia. This is totally painless for the patient and does not leave a permanent tattoo should colostomy not be needed.

An end colostomy most often is constructed after removal of the rectum for low-lying malignancy (see Chapter 49). The operation is performed through a midline incision. The entire left colon is mobilized on its mesentery, including at least partial mobilization of the splenic flexure (Fig 12–5B). The inferior mesenteric artery is transected at its origin, and the mesentery is incised to the junction of the descending and sigmoid colon. Because of the transection of the inferior mesenteric artery and the possibility of preoperative radiation, the entire sigmoid colon must be removed, necessitating construction of the colostomy using the well-vascularized descending colon.

If the colostomy is to be brought through the left lower quadrant, an opening in the abdominal wall is made at the previously marked site by excising a 3-cm disk of skin. The undesirable oval configuration of a stoma is avoided by placing traction clamps in the dermis, the fascia, and the peritoneum. These clamps are held in alignment when the opening is made through the abdominal wall. This duplicates the configuration of the abdominal wall when the abdomen is closed and should allow construction of a desirable circular stoma.

The fat, fascia, muscle, and posterior peritoneum are then incised longitudinally (Fig 12–5A). No fat is excised. The opening then is dilated to allow passage of

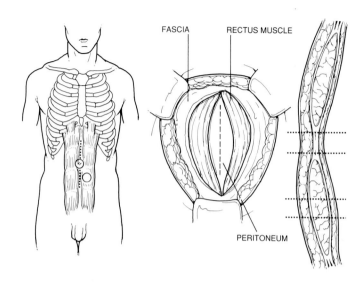

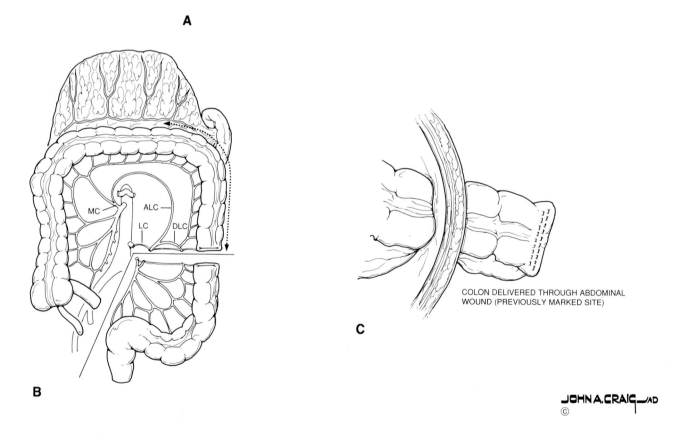

Figure 12–5. Construction of an end (diverting) colostomy. **A.** Selection of stoma location and technique of incision of the abdominal wall at the colostomy site. **B.** Technique of colonic mobilization and provision of adequate blood supply for the colostomy.

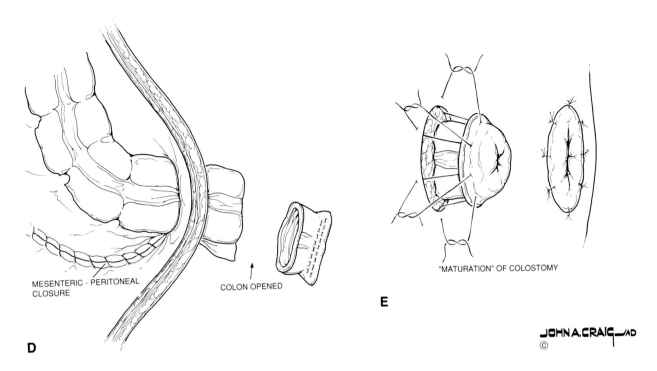

MESENTERIC - PERITONEAL CLOSURE

COLON OPENED

"MATURATION" OF COLOSTOMY

E

D

JOHN A. CRAIG—AD
©

Figure 12–5, cont'd. C, D, E. Final stages of constructing a "mature" end colostomy. IMA - inferior mesenteric artery; MCA - middle colic artery; ALC - ascending left colic artery; DLC - descending left colic artery

two fingers, and the closed end of the colon is pulled through the abdominal wall (Fig 12–5C). The mesentery of the colon then is sutured to the lateral abdominal wall with a running, nonabsorbable suture to avoid potential herniation of the small intestine between the colon and the abdominal wall. After the wound is closed and protected, attention is directed to completing the colostomy (Fig 12–5C to E). The stoma is completed by excising the staple or suture line and by placing chromic catgut sutures between the full thickness of colon and skin. If the stoma is constructed because of inflammatory bowel disease or radiated bowel, a spigot configuration is utilized by applying principles similar to those for ileostomy construction. This facilitates a good appliance seal for anticipated high volume, liquid effluents.

If the colostomy will be brought through the midline, no fixation of the mesentery is necessary. The intended midline colostomy is brought through the abdominal incision, and the entire incision is closed, with the sutures adjacent to the colostomy being tied last. At least a few interrupted sutures are placed on either side of the colostomy even if a running closure of the abdominal wall is used. As the last sutures are tied, the colon is pulled through the abdominal wall, and the surgeon's finger is placed adjacent to the stoma as a spacer to avoid compromise of the blood supply to the stoma. The skin

is closed and the wound is protected as attention is directed to the colostomy, where either the staple line is excised or the clamp is removed, and full thickness of colon is sutured to full thickness of skin with interrupted absorbable sutures. Because of the mobilization of the mesentery and the midline position of the colostomy, the small bowel falls beneath it, and nothing need be done with the mesentery of the colon itself.

Once the stoma construction is complete, an appliance is applied in the operating room. The simplest is a one piece appliance with a skin barrier that can be cut to the appropriate size of the stoma. This same appliance can be used for colostomy and ileostomy. The pouch is allowed to fall to the patient's side because, in the postoperative period, the patient will be supine rather than upright the majority of time. The appliance, which need not be sterile, is held in place with the skin adhesive of the appliance and is secured with strips of nonallergenic tape placed in "picture-frame" fashion. The remaining wound dressing is applied. Tincture of benzoin should never be used to maintain adhesion of an appliance to the skin because it has a high risk of initiating contact dermatitis. If colostomy function does not begin within 4 or 5 days, the stoma is irrigated with small volumes (250 mL) of normal saline to initiate stoma function. The enterostomal therapy nurses are involved early in the care of the stoma and in teaching the patient and family to provide long-term care of the colostomy. In most cases, the patient is taught the technique of stoma irrigation, and then each individual decides in the more distant postoperative course if he wishes to irrigate the stoma or not.

LONG-TERM COLOSTOMY MANAGEMENT

The patient with a properly constructed, well-functioning colostomy may elect to irrigate once a day or every other day and to wear only a minimal appliance in the intervening period, although the patient should be instructed always to carry an appliance should episodes of diarrhea occur. Simple appliances exist to allow absorption of mucus and deodorized passage of gas during the period between irrigations, if the patient elects to irrigate.

Irrigation

The advantages of irrigating the colostomy include the absence of need for wearing an appliance at all times, the provision of a more regulated life-style, the reduced passage of uncontrolled gas, less leakage of stool between irrigations, and the general feeling of comfort that some people experience after irrigating the colostomy. The disadvantages are that it is a time-consuming ritual and that some people feel discomfort when the bowel is distended during irrigation. Irrigation carries a minimal risk of perforation. Absorption of water during the irrigation process can be significant, and the patient with an irritable bowel syndrome will usually not achieve adequate control by irrigation and may be frustrated by attempting to do so. The principle of irrigation is based on the fact that the distal colon displays a few mass peristaltic motions each day and that these can be stimulated by distention of the intestine. It has been shown that 80% of people who irrigate daily can depend on the discharge from the colostomy being one or two movements per day. Poor results from irrigation can be anticipated if the patient has an irritable bowel syndrome, a peristomal hernia, irradiated bowel, inflammatory bowel disease, poor eyesight, reduced manual dexterity, or simply fear of dealing with the intestine at the abdominal wall. A preoperative history of irritable bowel syndrome is most important because these patients must never be promised regular function of their colostomies.

The technique of irrigation, usually performed in the morning, uses a cone tip that fits into the stoma only enough to provide a seal and to allow the instillation of 500 to 1000 mL of water. It is not necessary to dilate the stoma, and a finger is inserted only periodically to determine the direction for placement of the cone tip. Once the water has been instilled, a drainage bag is applied, and the individual can proceed with morning chores while the colostomy empties in response to the stimula-

tion. Between irrigations the patient usually wears a security pouch, which permits passage of gas through a charcoal filter and provides a small pad to absorb any mucus normally secreted by the colonic mucosa.

Ischemia or infection causing partial loss of the intestinal wall or separation of the stoma from the skin also can result in stricture of the colostomy. A tight stricture makes irrigation impossible and frequently causes the patient significant discomfort because of the resulting partial obstruction. Because the stricture is always at skin level, it's correction is simple and no patient should suffer because of a colostomy stricture.

COLOSTOMY COMPLICATIONS

General Considerations

A common problem experienced by the patient with a colostomy is irregularity of function, which most often is related to irritable bowel syndrome or radiation of the intestine. Many problems are related to improper location of the stoma, which allows seepage of mucus and maceration of the skin because an appliance seal cannot be adequately maintained. Parastomal hernia formation is common, and prolapse less so. Patients experience episodes of diarrhea and constipation depending on their underlying disease, dietary habits, and episodic infections. Patients with colostomies are troubled with gas and odor problems because there is no sphincter around the stoma and gas can be passed uncontrollably. This problem is usually regulated by diet and, in some cases, by administering mild antidiarrheal agents when social activity dictates. Minimal bleeding around a stoma is common because the mucosa is exposed to environmental trauma. Of course, prolonged bleeding should be evaluated to be sure that there is not a recurrence of the primary disease process. The same is true of cramps and diarrhea. These can be acceptable occasionally, but anything of a prolonged or severe nature must be evaluated.

Evaluation of the UOA data registry shows that hernia formation is the most common complication of end colostomy, with obstruction, abscess, and fistula presenting less frequently. Of all of the complications that occur, few require surgical correction. Fecal impaction does occur with a colostomy and can be managed by a combination of oil and detergent given as a retention irrigation in the hospital or by the simple combination of salad oil, warm water, and mild liquid detergent at home.

Stoma Stricture

The problem of stoma stricture is eliminated by suturing the full thickness of the colon to the skin of the abdominal wall at the time of initial construction. Stricture of stomas resulted from formation of a serositis in previous times when it was believed unsafe to open the colon initially, and it was opened in a delayed fashion.

Even for the transverse-loop colostomy, the colonic wall should be sutured primarily to the skin of the abdominal wall. The process has come to be called "maturation" of the colostomy.

Paracolostomy Hernia

Paracolostomy hernia frequently occurs because the stoma is located lateral to the rectus muscle, although it can occur when all is done according to acceptable surgical principles. Once a parastomal hernia becomes symptomatic, usually when located in the left lower quadrant, the best treatment is to move the colostomy to the midline and to use tight closure of the linea alba. No highly successful operations have been devised for primary repair of paracolostomy hernias. These hernias are interesting in that they usually do not result from a weakness in the abdominal wall but instead from pouch formation within the rectus sheath. This may be why the incidence is lessened by construction in the midline. It is often possible to relocate the colostomy without formal laparotomy by dissecting circumferentially at the site of the colostomy and then passing the closed end of colon to the midline where a circular opening is fashioned for the new stoma. This, of course, cannot be done in the presence of dense and excessive adhesions.

Colostomy Prolapse

Prolapse of the colostomy is seen most often with the transverse-loop colostomy. It probably results from operating when the colon is dilated. The opening becomes excessive once the colon decompresses. The surgical treatment of this complication is difficult, and the best treatment is to rid the patient of the primary disease and restore intestinal continuity. If this is not possible, the loop colostomy should be converted to an end colostomy with a mucous fistula.

Colostomy Perforation

Perforation of the colon just proximal to the stoma most often occurs during careless irrigation with a catheter, or during contrast x-ray studies when a catheter is placed in the colostomy and a balloon is inflated. This occurrence represents a surgical emergency and must be dealt with by laparotomy and reconstruction of the colostomy with adequate drainage, if there is significant fecal or barium contamination. Cases of mild inflammation with extravasation of air only can be managed with antibiotics and localized drainage, and surgery can be avoided.

■ ILEOSTOMY

An ileostomy is an opening constructed between the small intestine and the abdominal wall, usually by using distal ileum but sometimes more proximal small intes-

tine. The stoma is constructed on a permanent basis for patients who require removal of the entire colon, and usually the rectum, for inflammatory bowel disease, either Crohn's disease or ulcerative colitis. The use of a loop ileostomy is becoming more frequent because of the complex sphincter-preserving operations being performed for ulcerative colitis and familial polyposis. For these operations, (restorative proctocolectomy) it is necessary to have complete diversion of intestinal flow while the pouches are allowed to heal and adapt. The loop ileostomy is also useful in cases where multiple and complex anastomoses must be performed distally, usually for Crohn's disease. As the sphincter-preserving operations are used more, diminishing numbers of permanent ileostomies will be constructed, but similar principles and techniques will be utilized in constructing the temporary loop ileostomies. The same principles used in constructing an ileostomy can be applied to the construction of a urinary conduit, especially the use of a loop stoma for the obese patient.

The surgical construction of an ileostomy must be more precise than that for a colostomy because the content is liquid, high volume, and corrosive to the peristomal skin. Therefore, the stoma must be accurately located preoperatively, and it must have a spigot configuration to allow an appliance to seal effectively and precisely around the stoma.

Various types of ileostomies can be constructed. The most common has been the end ileostomy, using a technique popularized by Brooke and Turnbull. The loop ileostomy is used, as described, to protect diseased areas or surgical procedures distally. The loop—end ileostomy is a stoma that uses the principles of a loop ileostomy but is constructed as a permanent stoma when the mesentery and its blood supply need special protection. The continent ileostomy, a technique devised by the Swedish surgeon Nils Kock, is an internal pouch that does not require the wearing of an external appliance. The urinary conduit is a stoma constructed of small intestine to provide a conduit to the outside for the urinary tract.

DETERMINATION OF ILEOSTOMY LOCATION

The location of the ileostomy must be carefully chosen before surgery (Fig 12–6). It should avoid any deep folds of fat, scars, and bony prominences of the abdominal wall. The site is chosen by drawing a vertical line through the umbilicus and a transverse line through the inferior margin of the umbilicus and applying a disk the size of a stoma faceplate (approximately 8 cm in diameter) to determine the location. The disk is allowed to abut on both of the lines in the right lower quadrant, and the site is marked with ink. The patient then is brought to an exaggerated sitting position and allowed

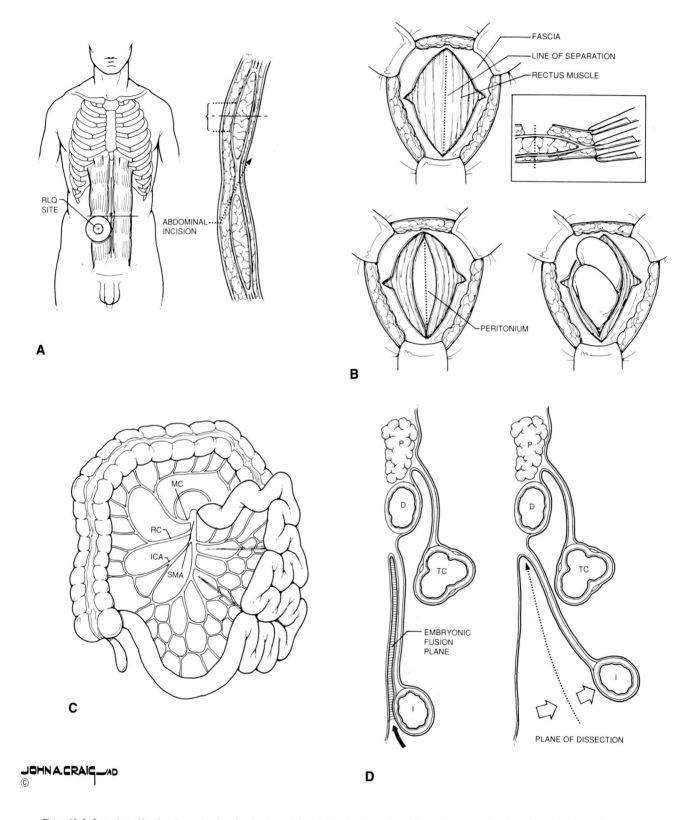

A

B

FASCIA

LINE OF SEPARATION

RECTUS MUSCLE

PERITONIUM

C

MC

RC

ICA

SMA

D

P

D

TC

I

EMBRYONIC FUSION PLANE

P

D

TC

I

PLANE OF DISSECTION

RLQ SITE

ABDOMINAL INCISION

JOHN A. CRAIG—AD
©

Figure 12–6. General considerations in construction of an ileostomy. **A.** Locating the ileostomy site and the use of a paramedian skin incision that slants to the midline fascia, allowing preservation of the peristomal skin. **B.** Technique for making the abdominal wall opening. **C.** Vascular supply of the distal ileum, which must be used to maintain viability of the ileostomy (MC = middle colic artery, RC = right colic artery, ICA - ileocolic artery, SMA = superior mesenteric artery). **D.** Plane of mobilization of the distal ileum to allow construction of an ileostomy without tension (P = pancreas, D = duodenum, TC = transverse colon, I = ileum).

to turn in various directions to be sure the site is adequate in all positions. If not, the location should be adjusted to bring the stoma to the summit of the infraumbilical fat fold to be sure that there is clearance for fitting of an appliance. When the patient is in the operating room and anesthesia has been administered, the chosen site is scratched with a fine needle before preparation of the abdominal skin is carried out. The majority of complications arising from ileostomies can be avoided by taking these precautions in marking the site for the stoma preoperatively. Even in cases in which the use of a stoma seems remote, the precaution of marking the site preoperatively should be taken. In addition, whenever possible, patients should be seen by an enterostomal therapist and an ostomy visitor so that they can be given information about the stoma and its care. The visit from an ostomate (someone who has done well with a similar stoma) is helpful because it allows the patient to know that the surgery can be survived and that life can be carried on productively and normally with the presence of a stoma. The discussion should avoid excessive details about types of equipment and types of stoma problems during the postoperative period.

When an ileostomy is anticipated, the choice of abdominal incision is a left paramedian skin incision, slanting the incision to midline fascia (Fig 12–6A). This gives the advantage of opening the fascia through the midline to provide a simple, effective closure and at the same time preserve all the right lower quadrant peristomal skin for maintenance of the appliance seal.

End Ileostomy

The construction of the ileostomy begins early in the operative procedure. When the colon is mobilized for colectomy, as is the usual case when an ileostomy is to be constructed, full mobilization of the mesentery of the distal ileum should be carried out (Fig 12–6D). This is an important and often neglected part of the procedure. There is an embryonic fusion plane of the mesentery of the small intestine to the right posterior abdominal wall. The ileum can be elevated on this mesentery up to the duodenum, allowing extreme mobility of the terminal ileum. The ileocolic artery then is transected as part of the colectomy, and the remaining blood supply to the small intestine is preserved (Fig 12–6C). It is important to preserve the most distal arcade of vessels and mesenteric tissue on the ileum at the segment of the intended ileostomy. This blood supply is prepared early in the operative procedure so that if there is any question about the vascularity of the distal ileum, it will be known long before the abdomen is closed. The preservation of this distal bit of mesentery and fat on the ileum sometimes appears to cause excess bulk around the ileostomy, but this fat soon atrophies, allowing a well-vascularized stoma of appropriate size. The intestine is transected with a linear-cutting type of stapling instrument so that the end of the ileum can be easily pulled through the abdominal wall without increased risk of contamination. This can, of course, be accomplished as well by suturing the end of the ileum.

When the colectomy has been completed, an opening is prepared in the right lower quadrant of the abdominal wall at the previously marked site (Fig 12–6B). This is accomplished by placing traction clamps on the dermis, fascia, and peritoneum so that the round configuration of the stoma will be maintained. A 3-cm disk of skin is excised, the fat is preserved, and a longitudinal incision approximately 3 to 4 cm long is made through all layers, with each layer being retracted with three small retractors as the incision is deepened. The operating surgeon pushes upward on the abdominal wall from the inside as the incision is deepened. The fascia is incised longitudinally as well, and frequently a small lateral notch is placed on each side. The muscle is separated, and any vessels are coagulated. The posterior fascia and peritoneum then are incised, and the surgeon inserts two fingers through the opening to be sure that it will accommodate the intestine. The ileum is brought through the abdominal wall to the intended length, usually about 6 cm (Fig 12–7B). The serosa of the ileum is protected with a moist pad, and the mesentery of the distal ileum is sutured to the right lateral abdominal wall with a continuous suture (Fig 12–7C). This prevents torsion of the intestine and herniation of the small bowel around the post of the ileostomy and perhaps reduces the incidence of stoma retraction and prolapse. The superior end point of this running suture becomes obscure and often involves suturing to the falciform ligament. Whatever tissue is necessary is used to close the gap completely.

The abdomen then is closed. The incision is protected, and attention is directed to the ileostomy where the staple line or suture line is excised, verifying the adequacy of blood supply (Fig 12–7D). If the blood supply of the stoma is questioned, more of the ileum should be resected.

The next objective is to make a protruding, everting stoma. This is accomplished by placing 3–0 chromic catgut sutures through the full thickness of intestine, the seromuscular area of the ileum at the base of the stoma, and the dermis (Fig 12–7E). Sutures through the skin should be avoided, because any stellate scarring will prevent the maintenance of the required seal of the application. Eight of these sutures should be placed, one in and one between each quadrant, and as traction is applied after they are all placed, the stoma should evert nicely.

After the stoma is completed, an ileostomy appliance is applied. A simple appliance in which the skin barrier can be cut to the size of the stoma is best. The pouch is

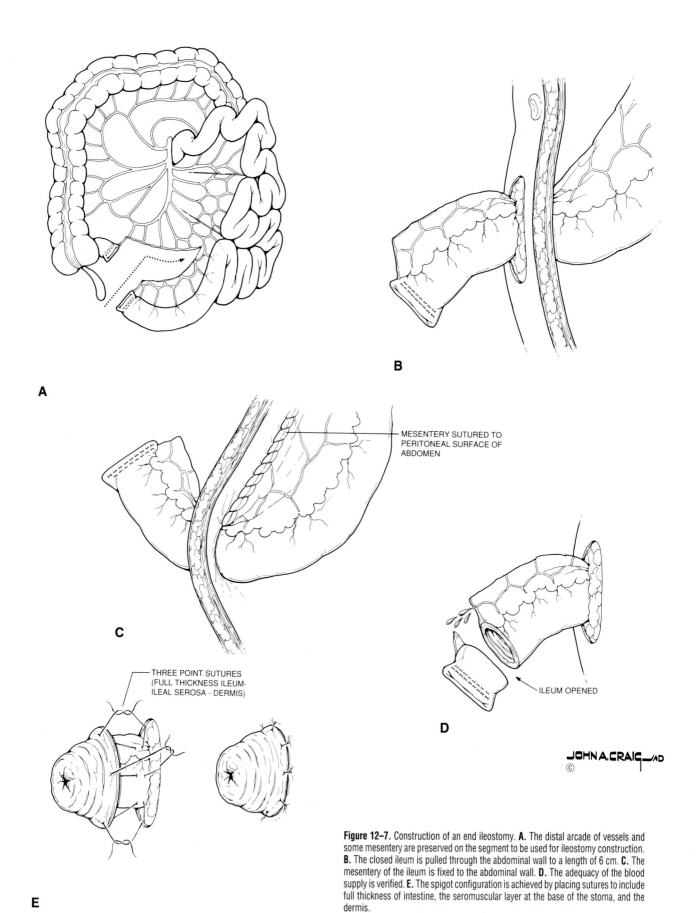

A

B

MESENTERY SUTURED TO
PERITONEAL SURFACE OF
ABDOMEN

C

ILEUM OPENED

D

THREE POINT SUTURES
(FULL THICKNESS ILEUM-
ILEAL SEROSA - DERMIS)

E

JOHN A. CRAIG ᴀᴅ
©

Figure 12–7. Construction of an end ileostomy. **A.** The distal arcade of vessels and
some mesentery are preserved on the segment to be used for ileostomy construction.
B. The closed ileum is pulled through the abdominal wall to a length of 6 cm. **C.** The
mesentery of the ileum is fixed to the abdominal wall. **D.** The adequacy of the blood
supply is verified. **E.** The spigot configuration is achieved by placing sutures to include
full thickness of intestine, the seromuscular layer at the base of the stoma, and the
dermis.

allowed to hang to the side, and a stoma skin adhesive, not benzoin, is applied to the appliance if needed. The pouch is taped in position using a picture-frame configuration of nonallergenic tape. In the immediate postoperative period, if there is any question about leakage around the appliance or malfitting of the appliance, it should be changed and the skin cleaned immediately. It is important to preserve the integrity of the peristomal skin, and all the nursing staff should be attuned to this importance. The leaking appliance should not be left for changing by the next shift or for the enterostomal therapist the next morning, because the skin can be damaged during this waiting period.

Loop Ileostomy

The loop ileostomy stoma is constructed when both diversion of the intestinal flow and decompression of the distal intestine are required. The location is chosen exactly as one would choose the site for an end ileostomy. The construction can then follow one of two techniques. The technique popularized by Turnbull at the Cleveland Clinic involves choosing the site in the intestine for the intended loop ileostomy and then placing orienting sutures proximally and distally (Fig 12–8A). A loose suture with one knot can be placed proximally and one with two groups of knots distally. It is important to maintain this orientation as the stoma is constructed.

The opening in the abdominal wall is made the same as for an end ileostomy (Fig 12–6B), but the loop of intestine is drawn through this abdominal opening by a tracheostomy tape placed through the mesentery and around the intestine (Fig 12–8B). As the intestine is drawn through the abdominal wall, care is taken to orient the proximal functioning loop in the inferior position. This involves placing a partial twist on the loop of intestine. In massively obese patients with a shortened mesentery, it is necessary to make a conical configuration of the opening in the abdominal wall, with the internal opening being much larger than the external opening at the skin. If this maneuver is used, it is best to place a row of tacking sutures between the peritoneum and the loop of intestine to maintain position and orientation. Once the loop is drawn through the abdominal wall, the abdomen is closed, maintaining the orientation of the loop. It is usually not necessary to fix the mesentery of the ileum to the abdominal wall when constructing a loop ileostomy. The wound is then protected, and attention is directed to the stoma.

The tracheostomy tape is replaced by a small plastic rod, which is commercially available (Fig 12–8C). It is not sutured to the peristomal skin, but it often has a heavy suture tied around each side so that should the rod dislodge, it can be drawn back through the mesentery rather than being pushed through, with risk of injuring the mesentery. The loop of intestine is opened by

making a four-fifths circumferential incision at the superior aspect of the loop, allowing 1 cm of ileum above the skin level in the superior aspect (Fig 12–8D). The recessive limb thus is formed superiorly, and sutures are placed between the full thickness of ileum and dermis at this level. As the inferior aspect of the stoma is constructed, sutures are placed as previously described between the full thickness of ileum, the seromuscular area at the base of the stoma, and the dermis. As these sutures are tied, the stoma should assume a spigot configuration supported by the rod, with the intestine closed tightly on either side of the rod. If their use is indicated, a few small pieces of Penrose drain can be placed in the subcutaneous tissue as the sutures are tied. These provide short-term drainage of the parastoma tissue and should be removed after 24 hours. The ileostomy appliance may be placed beneath the rod or over the rod, depending on the tension of the mesentery. The rod is left in place for 1 week, and the same ileostomy care is provided as previously described.

Another technique for constructing a protecting and completely diverting ileostomy is that popularized by Abcarian and Prasad that more recently has been used to protect the anastomosis for restorative proctocolectomy (Fig 12–9). This technique involves transecting the ileum with a linear-cutting stapling instrument. No compromise of the mesentery is involved. The opening in the abdominal wall is made in identical fashion to that previously described; but when the intestine is pulled through, the proximal component is excised, and the stoma is constructed as previously described for an end ileostomy. The recessive limb at the base of the stoma has one corner of the staple line excised, and the full thickness of ileum is sutured to the dermis at the superior aspect of the stoma. This allows a small recessive limb that serves to decompress the distal intestine.

Closure of Loop Ileostomy. When endoscopic procedures and contrast studies have shown that the pouch is intact or that the distal anastomoses have healed securely, consideration can be given to closing the loop ileostomy. If the primary procedure has involved the anal sphincter mechanism, careful physical examination and manometric studies should verify the adequacy of sphincter function before intestinal continuity is restored.

For closure of the loop ileostomy (Fig 12–10), a circumferential dissection is carried out, with a minimal rim of skin included, until the peritoneal cavity is entered and clean peritoneal surface of abdominal wall can be palpated circumferentially. Once this is accomplished, the loop of intestine can usually be brought easily through the circular incision in the abdominal wall. Closure then is completed by excising the rim of fibrous tissue, with care being taken to preserve all of the intestine (Fig 12–10B, C). The choice of closure then varies

Text continued on page 448

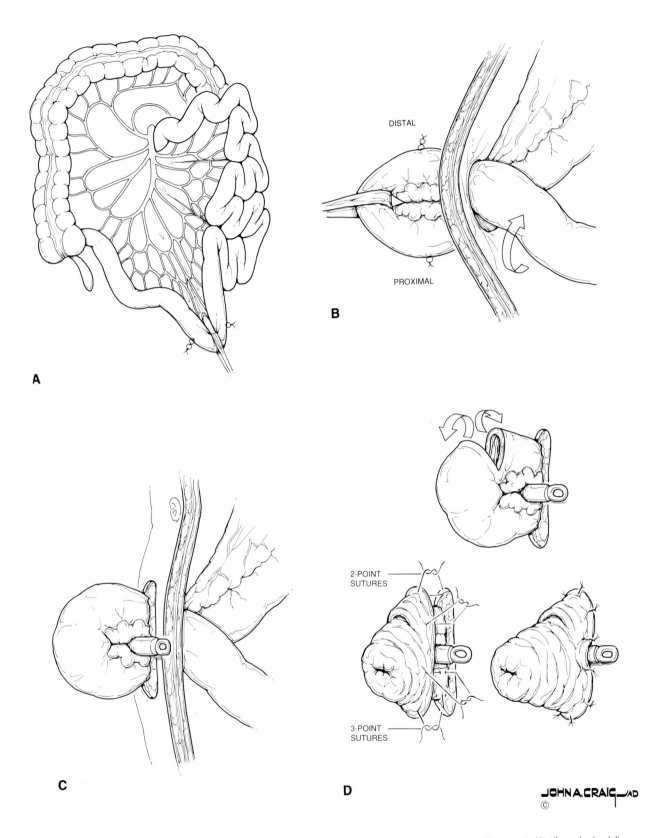

Figure 12–8. Construction of a loop ileostomy. **A.** A tracheostomy tape is placed at the segment for the intended ileostomy with sutures to identify proximal and distal limbs. **B.** The loop is pulled through the abdominal wall while its proper orientation is maintained. **C.** The tape is replaced by a plastic rod. **D.** The spigot configuration is completed.

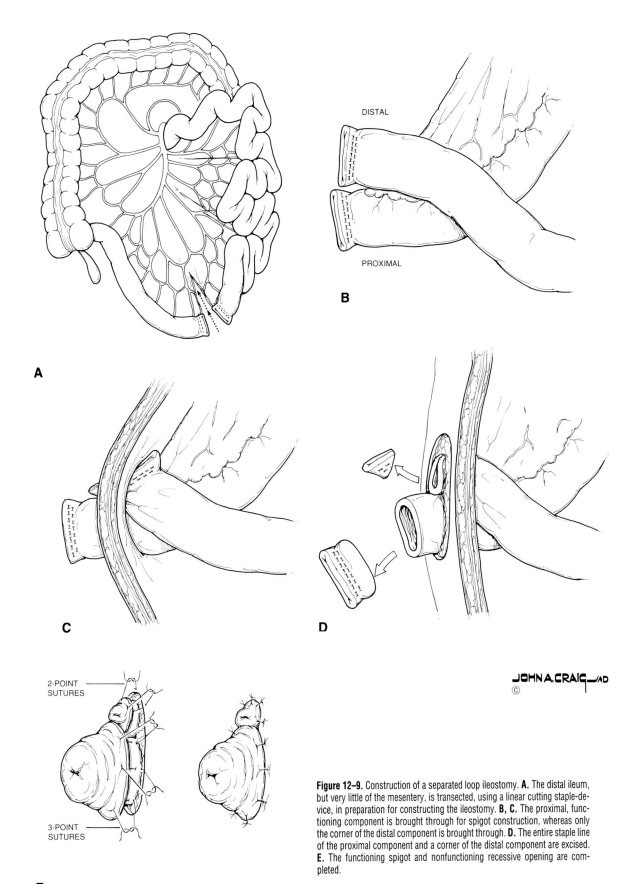

A

B

DISTAL

PROXIMAL

C

D

JOHN A. CRAIG_—AD
©

E

2-POINT
SUTURES

3-POINT
SUTURES

Figure 12–9. Construction of a separated loop ileostomy. **A.** The distal ileum, but very little of the mesentery, is transected, using a linear cutting staple-device, in preparation for constructing the ileostomy. **B, C.** The proximal, functioning component is brought through for spigot construction, whereas only the corner of the distal component is brought through. **D.** The entire staple line of the proximal component and a corner of the distal component are excised. **E.** The functioning spigot and nonfunctioning recessive opening are completed.

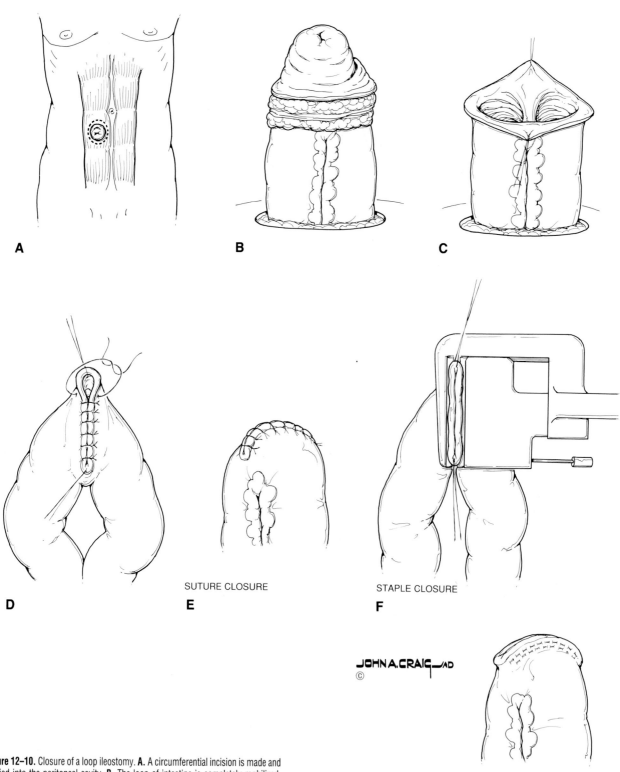

A

B

C

D

E
SUTURE CLOSURE

F
STAPLE CLOSURE

JOHN A. CRAIG AD
©

G

Figure 12–10. Closure of a loop ileostomy. **A.** A circumferential incision is made and carried into the peritoneal cavity. **B.** The loop of intestine is completely mobilized. **C.** The fibrofatty tissue is completely excised, preserving all the intestine. **D, E.** A suture closure can be performed, or a transverse stapled closure (**F, G**) can be affected.

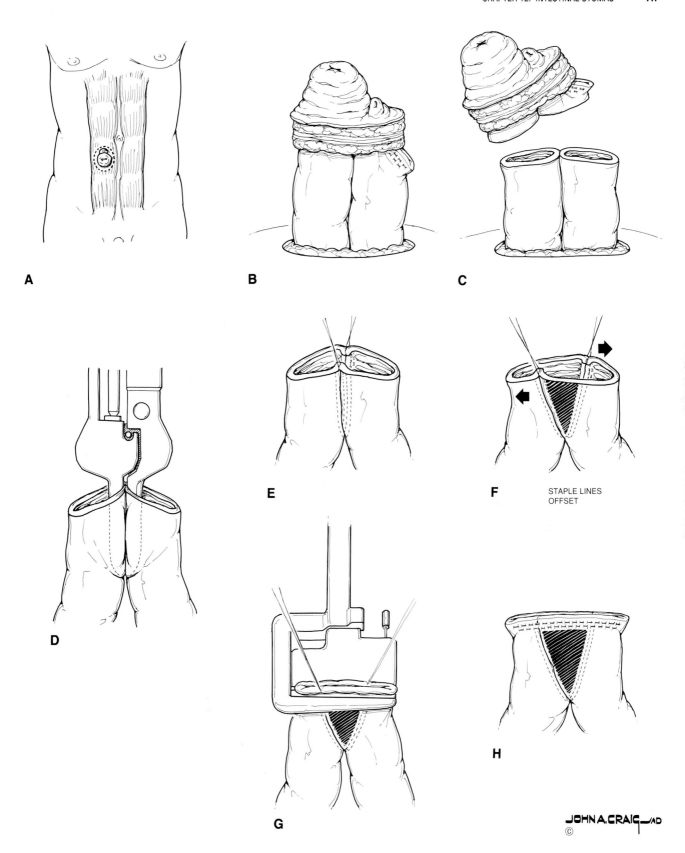

Figure 12–11. Closure of a separated loop ileostomy. **A.** A circumferential incision is made and carried into the peritoneal cavity. **B, C.** The stoma site and residual staples are excised. **D.** A linear-cutting stapler is applied to the antimesenteric side of the intestine. **E, F.** The components of the staple line are offset. **G, H.** The functional end-to-end closure is completed with a linear stapling instrument.

between hand-sutured transverse closure (Fig 12–10D, E), stapled transverse closure (Fig 12–10F, G), or formal construction of an anastomosis.

For closure of the separated-loop ileostomy (Fig 12–11), the mobilization is carried out in similar fashion, and a functional end-to-end closure is performed. A linear-cutting stapler is applied and removed, and the enterotomy is closed transversely. The intestine should be rotated so that antimesenteric surfaces are used for the staple line. If this type of closure is utilized, it is important to offset the staple lines so that there is no possibility of their healing together and causing an obstruction. After intestinal continuity is restored, the abdominal wall is closed, and the skin is left open for delayed primary closure.

Loop-end Ileostomy

A loop-end ileostomy should be constructed in the rare circumstances in which it is unsafe to resect the mesentery of the distal ileum or when there is tension created on the mesentery as the ileum is brought to the abdominal wall for construction of the ileostomy. This occurs in the patient with a thickened mesentery or a very obese abdominal wall or in a patient who has had multiple surgical procedures that altered the mesentery. These conditions preclude dealing with the usually pliable, mobile tissue. This technique is especially useful in the obese patient who requires construction of a urinary conduit after cystectomy and radiation. The technique is especially helpful because a supporting rod can be placed beneath the stoma for 1 week to help avoid retraction through a thick abdominal wall (Fig 12–12).

Constructing a loop-end ileostomy involves transecting the ileum as previously described, but the closed end will remain closed (Fig 12–12A). The staple line is inverted with seromuscular sutures, or if it is to be used for a urinary conduit, only absorbable sutures are used to close the end of the ileum, because stone formation has been reported around staples (Fig 12–12B). The orienting sutures are then placed as described for construction of a loop ileostomy, and a tracheostomy tape is placed so that when the loop of ileum is pulled through the abdominal wall, the closed recessive end will be superior and just within the abdominal cavity (Fig 12–12C). The construction of the loop-end stoma then proceeds exactly as that described for the loop ileostomy (Fig 12–12D to F). However, in this case in which the stoma will be permanent, the mesentery of the distal ileum is fixed to the abdominal wall (Fig 12–12D). If the stoma will be used as a urinary conduit, the loop of the conduit should be brought through the abdominal wall before the ureteral anastomoses have been carried out. It is a disconcerting problem to have the ureters fixed and then find there is an inadequate length of ileum to bring through the abdominal wall. It

is also easier to place the ureteral stents when the construction is done in this fashion.

A special problem has been found in patients with the loop-end ileostomy in that there continues to be mucous secretion from the recessive limb, and after a period of several months, this secretion may interfere with perfect seal of the ileostomy appliance. If interference does occur, it may become necessary to resect the distal limb and convert the stoma to a proper end ileostomy. This is a small price to pay, however, because it is an easy operation to remove the recessive limb, and it can be done without opening the abdominal cavity. Of more importance is the fact that the loop configuration during the initial procedure has allowed maintenance of blood supply and a protruding configuration under circumstances in which this otherwise may have been impossible, and that would have resulted in major complications.

Postoperative Care and Complications

The components of an ileostomy appliance are a skin barrier, some type of adhesive disk, a faceplate, and a drainable pouch. In fact, most ileostomy appliances are now commercially available as one-piece or semidisposable two-piece units. The one in common use has a skin barrier with a fixed plastic ring so that the stoma opening can be cut precisely, the skin barrier applied, and the pouch snapped directly onto the plastic ring, thus allowing easy drainage and disposal of the pouch part of the appliance. The skin barrier component should need changing only every 4 to 5 days in a patient with a properly protruding and located stoma. A well-constructed ileostomy should allow the patient to display normal physical vigor, to eat a well-balanced, palatable diet, and to engage in normal recreational and sexual activity. There should be no prolapse or retraction, the skin should remain normal, and the appliance should not leak. Between 500 and 800 mL of thick liquid content should be passed per day.

Before the concept of stoma eversion was conceived, in approximately 1960, the majority of patients who underwent construction of an ileostomy had serious postoperative complications, usually related to the serositis, which caused a partial obstruction at the stoma itself. These patients suffered massive fluid and electrolyte imbalance and often death, which was related to the enormous sequestration of fluid secondary to the small bowel obstruction. This condition was called "ileostomy dysfunction" and was anticipated after the construction of each stoma. This devastating problem essentially has been eliminated, since stomas have been everted and serositis has been prevented as the result of using the Turnbull and Brooke technique. The output from an ileostomy should not be excessive, even in the immediate postoperative period.

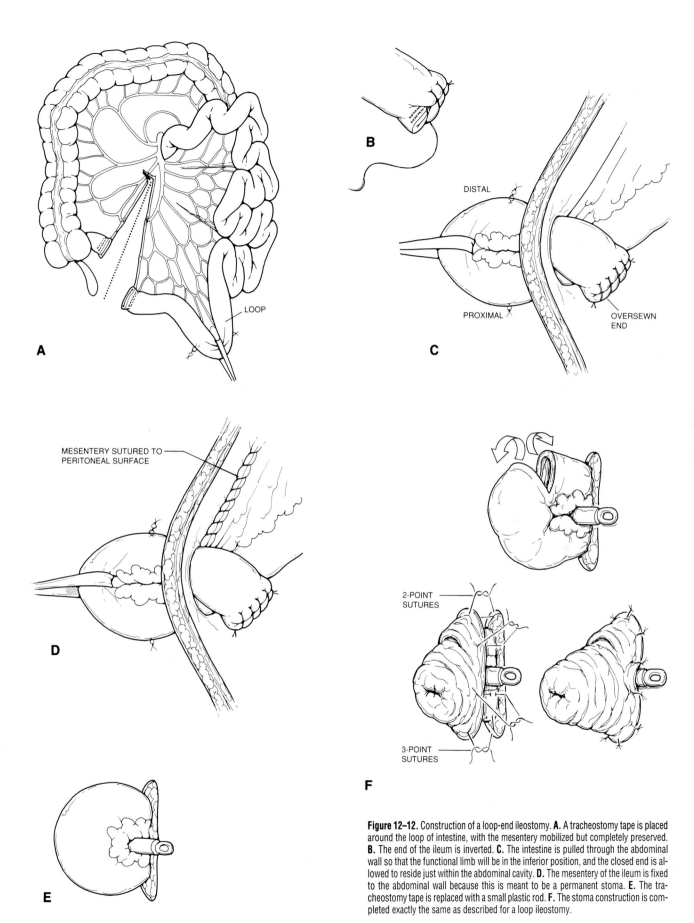

A

B

C

DISTAL

PROXIMAL

OVERSEWN
END

D

MESENTERY SUTURED TO
PERITONEAL SURFACE

LOOP

E

2-POINT
SUTURES

3-POINT
SUTURES

F

Figure 12–12. Construction of a loop-end ileostomy. **A.** A tracheostomy tape is placed around the loop of intestine, with the mesentery mobilized but completely preserved. **B.** The end of the ileum is inverted. **C.** The intestine is pulled through the abdominal wall so that the functional limb will be in the inferior position, and the closed end is allowed to reside just within the abdominal cavity. **D.** The mesentery of the ileum is fixed to the abdominal wall because this is meant to be a permanent stoma. **E.** The tracheostomy tape is replaced with a small plastic rod. **F.** The stoma construction is completed exactly the same as described for a loop ileostomy.

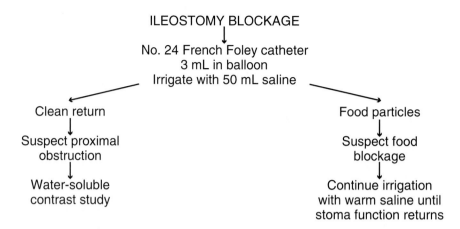

Figure 12–13. Ileostomy blockage algorithm (From Kodner IJ. Stoma complications. In: Fazio VW (ed), *Current Therapy in Colon and Rectal Surgery.* Philadelphia, PA: BC Decker; 1990:420–425

Patients with ileostomies do have problems, most often related to maintenance of the seal of the appliance because of poor location or defective configuration of the stoma. In some cases, it is necessary either to revise the stoma locally to bring it into a spigot configuration or to relocate it so an appliance can be securely applied. The more common problems experienced by ileostomy patients involve odor and gas control, because there is no sphincter in the ileostomy. The patients usually can manage these problems by paying attention to foods and medications ingested, by using various deodorant products, and by maintaining meticulous personal hygiene.

The only unusual long-term risk to the ileostomy patient is that of dehydration, which occurs especially in hot weather and during strenuous physical activity. The individuals should be instructed to maintain adequate intake of fluids and electrolytes. They should routinely have medications on hand for simple diarrhea so that control can be achieved before dehydration occurs. Many patients with ileostomies will at times present with acute blockage of the stoma, which is usually related to food indiscretion. It is hazardous to perform digital exam of an ileostomy, and this should *never* be done. Patients will have ingested some fibrous food with a high residual component and will present with cramping abdominal pain, dehydration, and vomiting. These patients should be admitted to the hospital and started on intravenous fluid replacement, and the stomal problem should be dealt with as follows. A 24 Fr Foley catheter is placed in the stoma, and the balloon is inflated with 3 to 5 mL of saline just beneath the fascia. The stoma is then irrigated with 50 mL of saline. There will be either a clear return or return of food particles. If the return is clear, it suggests more proximal obstruction, and a wa-

ter soluble contrast study should be done for evaluation. If the problem is a food blockage, the instillation of the contrast material often will prove therapeutic. If it is due to a more proximal blockage, it must be dealt with as a small intestinal obstruction. If food particles are returned from the initial irrigation, the irrigation must be continued with warm saline until stoma function returns and the blockage is eliminated. This procedure often requires 12 to 24 hours and intravenous fluid supplementation.

Some patients develop a high ileostomy output because of dietary indiscretion, infectious disease, short bowel syndromes, or recurrence of inflammatory bowel disease. The cause must be determined and each problem dealt with individually. It is important to maintain fluid and electrolyte balance as these problems are being resolved. Special care must be provided for the patient with the short bowel syndrome to maintain electrolyte balance and to compensate for the vitamin B_{12}, calcium, and fat malabsorption that occurs with absence of the distal ileum.

Another special problem that may occur with an ileostomy is the formation of a paraileostomy fistula. This usually represents recurrence of Crohn's disease and should be dealt with based on the extent of the Crohn's disease. While evaluation and treatment are being carried out, the appliance should be modified so that the fistula is allowed to drain into the appliance, and no attempt should be made to cover the fistula opening. This usually is achieved by modification of the configuration of the skin barrier component of the appliance.

Patients and those individuals aiding in the care of the ileostomy should be in the habit of observing the ileostomy for injury. There are no pain fibers in the ileum, and it is not unusual for a patient to lacerate the stoma with a malfitting appliance without noticing the injury, especially on the inferior aspect of the stoma.

Destruction of the peristomal skin can be so severe as to require split-thickness skin graft for definitive management. In these cases and in others in which the skin is injured around the stoma, a special ileostomy appliance may be utilized. It is based on maintenance of the seal to the mucosa of the ileum rather than to the peristomal skin. This appliance is used infrequently, when it is the only solution to complicated peristomal skin problems. Its use requires wearing supportive belts to maintain the appliance in place, but the skin can be treated with medicated pads during this period.

Review of the UOA data registry overall shows a low incidence of complications from ileostomy and an even lower incidence of need for corrective surgery. A study by McCleod showed that 72% of the patients with conventional ileostomy lead normal lives and that only 9% had a restricted life-style because of the stoma. Ninety percent of the patients spent <1 hour a day dealing with their stomas.

■ CONTINENT ILEOSTOMY

The continent ileostomy, or Kock pouch, has been used as an alternative to a conventional ileostomy for selected patients with ulcerative colitis or familial polyposis. It involves construction of an internal pouch with a continent nipple valve. The continent ileostomy allows placement of the stoma in an inconspicuous location and avoids the need for wearing an appliance permanently. It does require multiple intubations of the pouch daily to allow emptying. The complication rate for construction of this continent ileostomy has been high because of the difficulty in maintaining continence of the nipple valve and position of the pouch so that intubation can be easily accomplished. This operation should probably be done only in centers where it is performed frequently and where the complications are managed by an experienced team. The continent ileostomy can be constructed as a primary procedure for patients with ulcerative colitis. It may also be considered for patients who have an existing ileostomy that malfunctions, is poorly located, or causes severe injury to the peristomal skin because of allergic reaction to the ostomy equipment. However, the pouch has been used infrequently as primary treatment for patients with familial polyposis and ulcerative colitis since the advent of the ileal-anal pull-through or "restorative proctocolectomy." Most surgeons agree that the continent ileostomy is contraindicated for patients with Crohn's disease because of the significant risk of recurrent disease. It is also not to be recommended for patients who have a well-functioning end ileostomy.

The advantages of a continent ileostomy are that a patient need not wear an appliance, the patient is continent between intubations, there are no stoma complications, and he may experience a better quality of life. The disadvantages are that not all patients are continent, it does require multiple intubations during the day, there can be difficulty in intubation, and the surgery is prolonged and carries an increased risk of complications. If the procedure fails, the individual will lose a significant amount of small intestine. Also, psychologic factors may have been involved in the original motivation for choosing the internal ileostomy that are not alleviated by the more complicated surgical procedure.

CONSTRUCTION OF CONTINENT ILEOSTOMY

The construction of an intestinal reservoir for feces was first described in 1967 by Nils Kock. His original description of a U-shaped pouch was based on the theory that interruption of coordinated peristalsis would enhance capacity. Since then, J- and S-shaped pouches have been used with similar results. An S-shaped pouch is described here.

The construction of a continent ileostomy, or Kock pouch, can be broken into four components: (1) the creation of a pouch, (2) the creation of a nipple valve, which provides continence, (3) the suspension of the pouch from the abdominal wall in such a way as to prevent slippage of the nipple valve, and (4) the creation of a stoma.

The terminal ileum should be transected as close to the cecum as possible (Fig 12–14A). The S-shaped reservoir is fashioned from a 30- to 45-cm segment of distal ileum, starting 15 cm from the cut end (Fig 12–14B). The last 15 cm is used for the outlet (5 cm) and nipple valve (10 cm). The intestine is tacked in place in the shape of an S, using interrupted seromuscular sutures of 2-0 polyglycolic acid placed at the edge of the mesentery. Each limb of the S should be 10 to 15 cm long. The intestine is opened along the entire portion of the S, with the surgeon taking care to incise close to the mesenteric border on the outer limbs of the S and exactly at the antimesenteric surface of the central limb. A single-layer continuous suture line of 2-0 synthetic absorbable suture is first placed between the two walls of the central limb and the inner walls of the two outer limbs (Fig 12–14C). The sutures that begin on the posterior wall continue onto the anterior wall as the suture line reaches the outer wall of each of the two outer limbs of the S. The anterior wall is completed by continuing the suture from each direction, using an inverting full-thickness technique (either "baseball" or Connell) until the sutures meet in the middle. Before the pouch is closed, the nipple valve must be constructed.

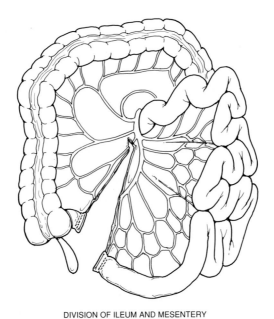

DIVISION OF ILEUM AND MESENTERY

A

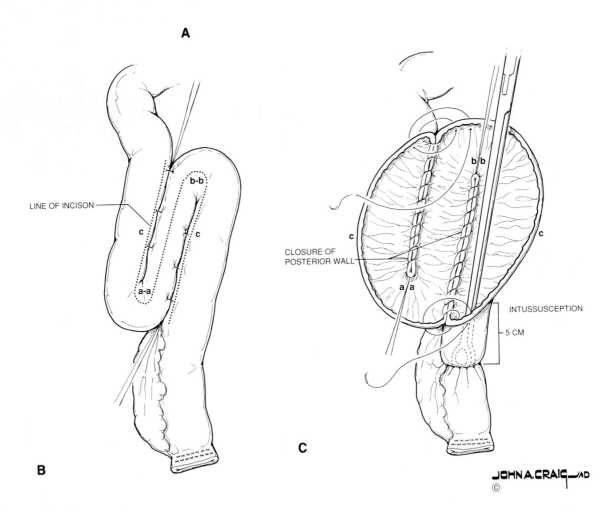

LINE OF INCISON

CLOSURE OF
POSTERIOR WALL

INTUSSUSCEPTION

5 CM

B

C

JOHN A. CRAIG AD
©

Figure 12–14. Construction of a continent ileostomy. **A.** The colectomy should be completed with as much distal ileum preserved as possible. **B.** Alignment of the components of the S-shaped pouch and nipple valve and the line of incision to open pouch. **C.** The pouch construction is begun with continuous 2-0 synthetic absorbable suture material. *Continued*

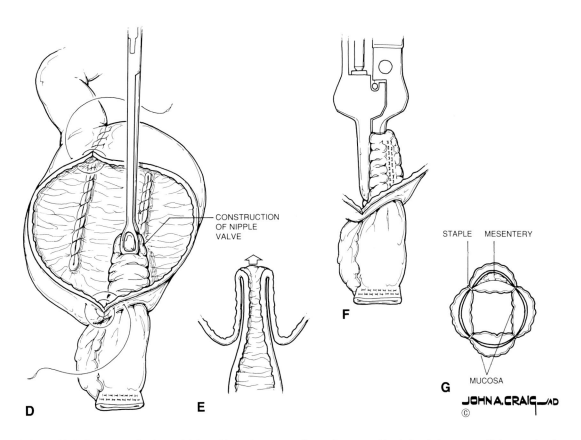

Figure 12–14, cont'd. D. The anterior wall of the pouch is formed by continuous suture from each corner, and the nipple valve is constructed before complete closure of the pouch. **E.** The ileum is intussuscepted to form the 5 cm long nipple valve. **F, G.** The intussusception is maintained by placement of multiple lines of staples adjacent to the mesentery and on the antimesenteric borders.

The 15 cm of ileum distal to the pouch will become the nipple valve and stoma. Prior to completion of the anterior wall suture, with the pouch mostly open, the nipple valve is made by intussuscepting the ileum into the pouch (Fig 12–14D, E). A Babcock clamp is passed into the distal ileum from within the pouch and is closed onto the full thickness of the bowel at a point 5 cm from the pouch. The clamp is drawn into the pouch, intussuscepting the bowel on itself to form the nipple valve. The valve is maintained in this position by placing a line of GIA staples on either side of the mesentery and a third row of staples on the antimesenteric aspect (Fig 12–14F). Occasionally it is possible to place four staple lines equidistant around the circumference of the nipple valve (Fig 12–14G). A linear-cutting staple instrument with the cutting blade removed is used to place the staple lines. One arm of the instrument is inserted into the lumen of the nipple from within the pouch before closing and firing the instrument. These staple lines make a serosa-to-serosa fixation of the nipple valve and prevent its unfolding. The anterior wall of the pouch is then completed as previously described (Fig 12–15A). A 5-cm outlet of distal ileum remains that will

pass through the abdominal wall and allow construction of a flush stoma.

The right lower quadrant stoma site is created as described earlier in this chapter, with the opening placed below the belt line and within the rectus muscle. Before the outlet is passed through the abdominal wall opening, a sling of soft synthetic mesh (1 cm × 10 cm) is passed through a window made in the mesentery of both the pouch and nipple valve under the major vessels as they fold into the nipple valve mesentery (Fig 12–15B, C). The strip of mesh maintains the nipple configuration and helps secure the pouch to the abdominal wall. Seromuscular absorbable sutures are used to fix the mesh to the base of the outlet (Fig 12–15D). The two ends of the sling are left long because they are sutured together at the antimesenteric surface of the outlet. This facilitates delivery of the outlet through the stoma site and allows a securing suture of nonabsorbable material to be placed through the sling into the anterior fascia. As the outlet is readied to be drawn through the abdominal wall, a row of three untied seromuscular sutures is placed on the shoulders of the pouch medial and lateral to the outlet (Fig 12–15E). These sutures, in-

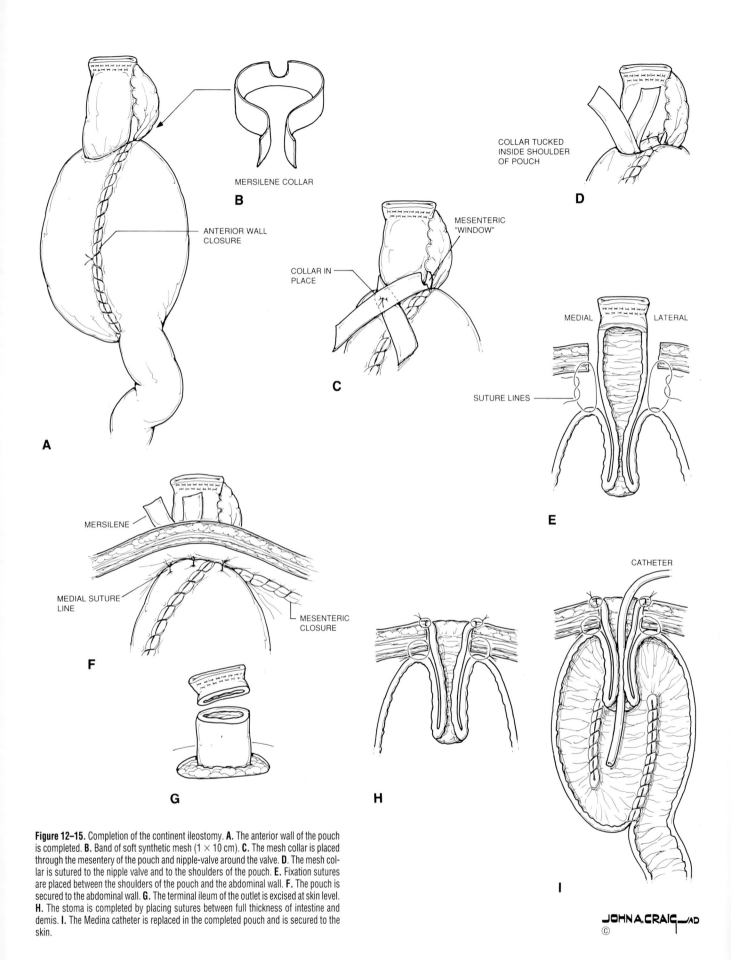

B MERSILENE COLLAR

ANTERIOR WALL CLOSURE

A

COLLAR TUCKED INSIDE SHOULDER OF POUCH

D

MESENTERIC "WINDOW"

COLLAR IN PLACE

C

MEDIAL   LATERAL

SUTURE LINES

E

MERSILENE

MEDIAL SUTURE LINE

MESENTERIC CLOSURE

F

G

H

CATHETER

I

Figure 12–15. Completion of the continent ileostomy. **A.** The anterior wall of the pouch is completed. **B.** Band of soft synthetic mesh (1 × 10 cm). **C.** The mesh collar is placed through the mesentery of the pouch and nipple-valve around the valve. **D.** The mesh collar is sutured to the nipple valve and to the shoulders of the pouch. **E.** Fixation sutures are placed between the shoulders of the pouch and the abdominal wall. **F.** The pouch is secured to the abdominal wall. **G.** The terminal ileum of the outlet is excised at skin level. **H.** The stoma is completed by placing sutures between full thickness of intestine and demis. **I.** The Medina catheter is replaced in the completed pouch and is secured to the skin.

corporating the posterior fascia and peritoneum, are used to fix the pouch to the anterior abdominal wall. The outlet is delivered through the stoma site and the pouch drawn toward the abdominal wall. The sutures then are tied, first laterally and then medially (Fig 12–15F). A permanent securing suture is placed through the tails of the sling and the anterior fascia, and the ends of the mesh are trimmed.

If possible, the cut edge of the small intestine's mesentery is sutured to the anterior abdominal wall (Fig 12–15F). A continuous suture is placed from the outlet of the pouch to the falciform ligament. The pouch in its final position should rest at the right pelvic brim, with the antimesenteric surface (anterior wall) of the pouch directed inferiorly.

The terminal ileum at the outlet should be excised at skin level (Fig 12–15G). The stoma is finally completed by placing absorbable sutures between the subcuticular layer of the skin and the full thickness of the intestinal wall (Fig 12–15H). A Medina catheter is passed through the stoma into the pouch and is secured to the skin to prevent slippage of the tube into or out of the pouch (Fig 12–15I). There should be minimal resistance and no deviation from a straight passage. The pouch should be drained in this manner for 2 weeks before intermittent clamping is begun during the third week. Finally, the pouch should be extubated and reintubated every 4 hours until the intervals gradually increase to 6 or 8 hours.

The nipple valve provides increasing continence as pressure rises in the pouch. Should the nipple valve lose its configuration and prolapse or should it slip through the mesenteric aspect of the pouch (the weakest point), either incontinence or obstruction will result. These two problems, along with "pouchitis," are the most common complications following the continent ileostomy procedure. As a result, many variations of pouch construction have been used in attempts to prevent or correct these problems.

If a fistula should form from the nipple valve or if the nipple valve should slip, it may be possible to preserve the pouch and construct a new nipple valve (Fig 12–16). The technique involves resecting the pouch outlet, including the nipple valve, after fully mobilizing the pouch from the abdominal wall and pelvis (Fig 12–16B). The terminal ileum is transected 15 cm proximal to the pouch (Fig 12–16C). The pouch then is rotated 180 degrees on its mesentery (Fig 12–16D). A new nipple valve is created as previously described by intussuscepting the new outlet on itself and placing staple lines along the valve to secure the fold (Fig 12–16E to G). The opening in the pouch wall created when the old outlet was resected serves as the entry to the pouch to perform this maneuver. The proximal ileum's cut edge is then anastomosed to the pouch through a second enterotomy in a position that allows the pouch to lie comfort-

ably in the right lower quadrant as before (Fig 12–16D). If at all possible, the existing stoma site should be preserved and reused. The pouch then is resuspended by using a mesh sling as described, and the stoma is constructed (Fig 12–16H, I). The pouch should be protected by constant drainage through an indwelling Medina catheter for at least 1 week. Because the pouch will not require expansion and the patient will not need education, the prolonged period of progressive clamping should not be necessary.

■ URINARY CONDUIT

The urinary conduit is constructed of a segment of intestine with well-maintained vascularity so that it can be connected to the urinary tract to allow egress of urine through the abdominal wall via a stoma constructed exactly like an ileostomy. It is not intended to have any type of reservoir capacity but merely to provide an open conduit. This urinary conduit is constructed most often after removal of the urinary bladder for invasive cancer. It is also used for management of severe obstructive uropathy, the congenital abnormalities of spina bifida, meningomyelocele, or bladder exstrophy, and for trauma to the spinal cord resulting in a severely neurogenic bladder. The incidence of this surgery for congenital and traumatic disorders is decreasing as other means of emptying the bladder are devised. The cystectomy, construction of the urinary conduit, and ureterointestinal anastomosis are most often carried out by urologists, but the construction of the stoma, as well as restoration of intestinal continuity, may be done by a surgeon more experienced in intestinal and stoma surgery.

The basic principles of construction of the conduit and stoma involve isolation of a segment of intestine, with maintenance of the mesenteric blood supply and enough mobility to allow the distal end to be used as a stoma and the proximal end to serve as the site for ureteral implantation. It is most important to maintain the isoperistaltic direction of the intestine, especially if the conduit is constructed of sigmoid colon. The conduit must not be made of radiated bowel, even if this requires using either colonic or proximal small intestinal conduits. If the stoma is improperly constructed, there may be stasis of urine, resulting in reflux and damage to the proximal tract.

The surgical technique consists of choosing a long enough segment of small intestine to allow the stoma to be constructed at the level of the abdominal wall and still allow the proximal end to reach close enough to the retroperitoneum to preclude tension on the ureterointestinal anastomoses (Fig 12–17). Usually, 18 to 20 cm of intestine is enough, but this must be modified if there is a shortened mesentery or a massively obese abdominal wall. It is in these latter situations that the loop-end

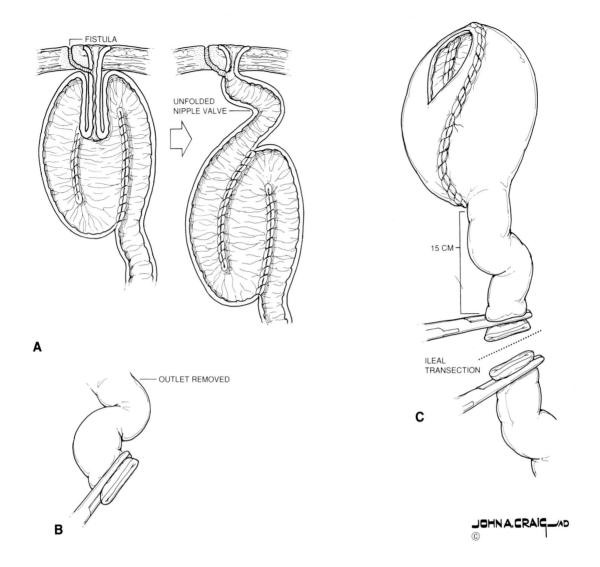

Figure 12–16. Preservation of the continent ileostomy after fistula formation or loss of the nipple configuration. **A.** Fistula between skin and nipple valve (*left*) and slipped nipple valve (*right*). **B.** The faulty nipple valve and outlet are excised. **C.** The distal ileum is transected 15 cm proximal to pouch, leaving enough intestine to reconstruct the valve and stoma. *Continued*

stoma, supported over a small rod, can be advantageous. After the segment of intestine is chosen, the mesentery at the distal point is incised to allow enough mobility for reaching the abdominal wall. The mesentery at the proximal site of transection is incised only in a limited fashion, and care must be taken to preserve a generous blood supply (Fig 12–17A). Intestinal continuity is restored, with the intended conduit positioned posterior to the restored intestine (Fig 12–17B). The ileoileal anastomosis may be completed in any fashion that uses sutures or staples. The conduit is then cleaned of intestinal content, and the proximal end is closed. Closure must be done with absorbable sutures, because staples can lead to stone formation. It then is preferable

to make the opening in the abdominal wall and to construct the stoma as previously described for an ileostomy (Fig 12–17C, D). This procedure ensures that the ureteral anastomosis will be completed with the conduit in its final position and without the need for applying tension to bring the intestine through the abdominal wall. The ureteral anastomoses are performed, and stents are placed (Fig 12–17E). All aspects of the stoma construction are the same as for an ileostomy except that the appliance must contain a valve to allow constant drainage since the volume of urine is high and its weight would tend to pull the appliance off if constant drainage were not maintained. In the distant postoperative period, this problem is solved by the patient's emptying the appli-

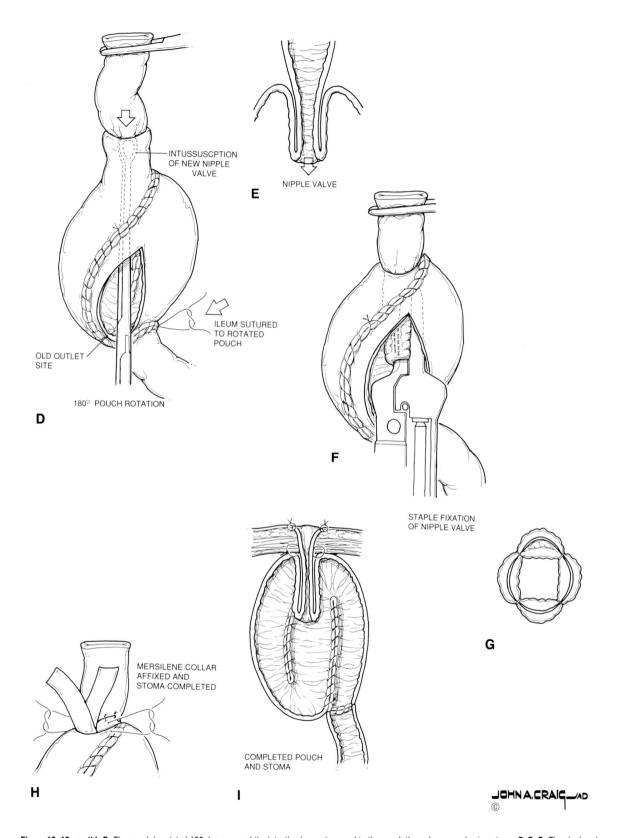

INTUSSUSCPTION
OF NEW NIPPLE
VALVE

NIPPLE VALVE

E

ILEUM SUTURED
TO ROTATED
POUCH

OLD OUTLET
SITE

180° POUCH ROTATION

D

F

STAPLE FIXATION
OF NIPPLE VALVE

G

MERSILENE COLLAR
AFFIXED AND
STOMA COMPLETED

COMPLETED POUCH
AND STOMA

H   I

JOHN A. CRAIG AD
©

Figure 12–16, cont'd. D. The pouch is rotated 180 degrees, and the intestine is anastomosed to the pouch through a second enterostomy. **E, F, G.** The nipple valve is reconstructed as before through the enterotomy made by resecting the old valve. **H, I.** The pouch is fixed to the abdominal wall, and the stoma is completed.

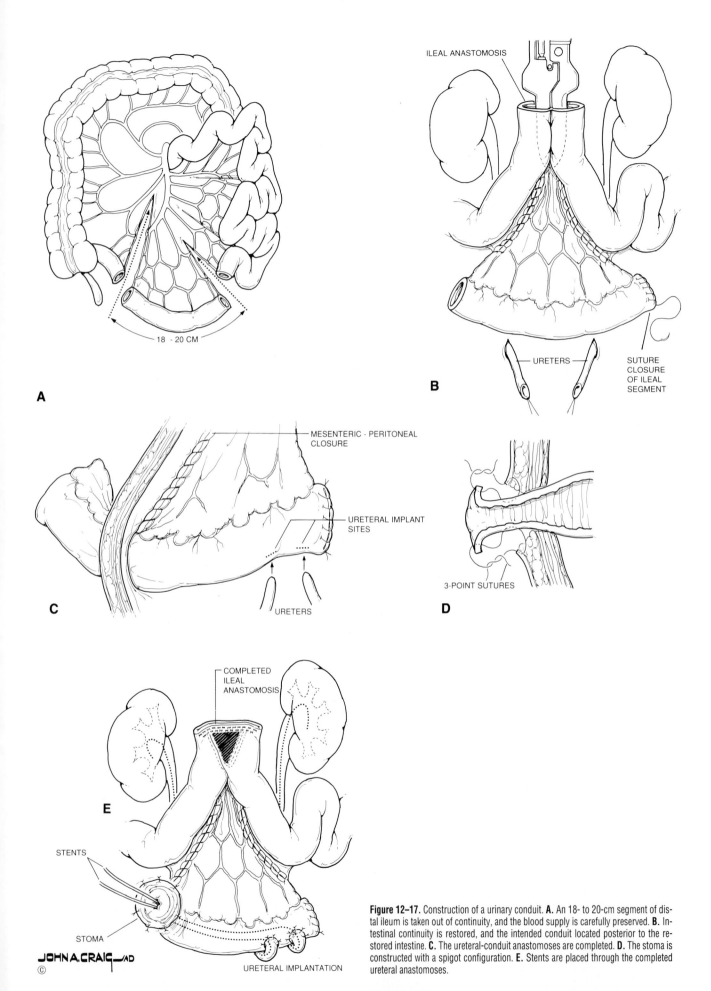

A

18 - 20 CM

B

ILEAL ANASTOMOSIS

URETERS

SUTURE
CLOSURE
OF ILEAL
SEGMENT

C

MESENTERIC - PERITONEAL
CLOSURE

URETERAL IMPLANT
SITES

URETERS

D

3-POINT SUTURES

E

COMPLETED
ILEAL
ANASTOMOSIS

STENTS

STOMA

URETERAL IMPLANTATION

JOHN A. CRAIG AD
©

Figure 12–17. Construction of a urinary conduit. **A.** An 18- to 20-cm segment of distal ileum is taken out of continuity, and the blood supply is carefully preserved. **B.** Intestinal continuity is restored, and the intended conduit located posterior to the restored intestine. **C.** The ureteral-conduit anastomoses are completed. **D.** The stoma is constructed with a spigot configuration. **E.** Stents are placed through the completed ureteral anastomoses.

ance frequently and by sleeping attached to a night drainage system.

COMPLICATIONS OF URINARY CONDUIT

The most common complication of a urinary conduit is a leaking appliance because of improper placement or construction of a flush rather than a protruding stoma. Although some urologists believe that a flush stoma is less susceptible to injury, most surgeons disagree with this concept and believe that a spigot configuration is best. Not infrequently, sutures are placed in the skin rather than in the dermis during stoma construction. This leads to a circumferential series of radial scars that preclude maintenance of the seal of the appliance. Because the stoma effluent is thin liquid, the appliance seal must be precise to avoid injury to the peristomal skin. If there is stasis in the conduit and poor seal of an appliance, an odor will develop and become the cause of great concern to the patient. It is not unusual to have to revise and sometimes relocate flush urinary conduit stomas. If this is done, care must be taken to ensure that the length of the conduit is adequate. If it is not, it is possible to add a segment of small intestine so that a proper stoma can be constructed without having to revise the ureterointestinal anastomoses.

The patient who does not maintain adequate personal hygiene and acidification of the urine may develop stone formation, with crystal formation around the stoma itself. This development can be alleviated by acidifying the urine or by placing a small amount of vinegar in the appliance. If the stoma has been constructed within the field of radiation, the radiation can break down the skin around the stoma. This requires relocation of the stoma to a nonradiated location on the abdominal wall. Relocation should be done even if the upper quadrants need to be used. Recent advances have employed the principles of Kock pouch construction, previously described, to allow construction of a continent urinary diversion.

■ INTESTINAL FISTULA

The formation of an intestinal fistula is not planned by the surgeon. Therefore it must be dealt with as it occurs. Applying modern principles of stoma care to maintain the integrity of the peristomal skin until definitive treatment of the fistula can be carried out should obviate the need for the damage to the skin from primitive means of preventing severe destruction of the skin and abdominal wall. These stomal care techniques, coupled with intravenous nutritional supplementation, should alleviate forever uncontrolled intestinal drainage from abdominal wounds.

SELECTED READINGS

Birnbaum EH, Fleshman JW. Anal Manometry. In: Kuijpers HC (ed), *Colorectal Physiology: Fecal Incontinence.* Boca Raton, FL: CRC Press; 1993:111–118

Birnbaum EH, Myerson RJ, et al. Chronic effects of pelvic radiation therapy on anorectal function. *Dis Colon Rectum,* 1994;37:909–915

Bricker EM. Bladder substitution after pelvic avisceration. *Surg Clin North Am* 1950;30:1511

Burch JM, Martin RR, et al. Evolution of the treatment of the injured colon in the 1980s. *Arch Surg* 1991;126:979–984

Butcher HR, Jr., Sugg WL, et al. Ileal conduit method of ureteral urinary diversion. *Ann Surg* 1962;156:682

Byers JM, Steinberg JB, et al. Repair of parastomal hernias using polypropylene mesh. *Arch Surg* 1992;127:1246

Chappuis CW, Frey DJ, et al. Management of penetrating colon injuries: a prospective randomized trial. *Ann Surg* 1991;213:492

Chechile G, Klein EA, et al. Functional equivalence of end and loop ileal conduit stomas. *J Urol* 1992;147:582

Corman JM, Odenheimer DB. Securing the loop—historic review of the methods used for creating a loop colostomy. *Dis Colon Rectum* 1991;34:1014

Corman ML. Colon and Rectal Surgery (3rd ed). Philadelphia, PA: JB Lippincott; 1993

Crile G Jr, Turnbull RB Jr. Mechanism and prevention of ileostomy dysfunction. *Ann Surg* 1954;140:459

Dinnick T. The origins and evolution of colostomy. *Br J Surg* 1934;22:142

Doughty D. Role of the enterostomal therapy nurse in ostomy patient rehabilitation. *Cancer* 1992;70(suppl):1390

Fallon WF Jr. The present role of colostomy in the management of trauma. *Dis Colon Rectum* 1992;35:1094

Feinberg SM, McLeod RS, et al. Complications of loop ileostomy. *Am J Surg* 1987;153:102

Fleshman JW. Loop ileostomy. *Surgical Rounds* 1992;Feb:129

Fleshman JW, Cohen Z, et al. The ileal reservoir and ileoanal anastomosis procedure: factors affecting technical and functional outcome. *Dis Colon Rectum* 1988;31:10

Fleshman JW, Kodner IJ, et al. Anal incontinence. In: Zuidema G (ed), *Shackelford's Surgery of the Alimentary Tract.* Philadelphia, PA: WB Saunders; 1993

Fleshman JW, Soper NJ. Medical management of benign anal disease. In: Quigley EMM, Sorrell MF (eds), *Medical Care of the Gastrointestinal Surgical Patient.* Baltimore, MD: Williams & Wilkins; 1994

Fry RD, Kodner IJ. Anorectal diseases. In: Levine BA, Copeland EM, Howard RJ, et al (eds), *Current Practice of Surgery.* New York, NY: Churchill-Livingstone; 1993

Fry RD, Shemesh EI, et al. Perforation of the rectum and sigmoid colon during barium-enema examination: management and prevention. *Dis Colon Rectum* 1989;32:759

Fucini C, Wolff BG, et al. Bleeding from peristomal varices: perspectives on prevention and treatment. *Dis Colon Rectum* 1991;34:1073

Garcia D, Hita G, et al. Colonic motility: electric and manometric description of mass movement. *Dis Colon Rectum* 1991;34:577

Geraghty JM, Talbot IC. Diversion colitis: histological features in the colon and rectum after defunctioning colostomy. *Gut* 1991;32:1020

Gordon PH, Nivatvongs S. *Principles and Practice of Surgery for the Colon, Rectum, and Anus.* St. Louis, MO: Quality Medical;1992

Gottlieb LM, Handelsman JC. Treatment of outflow tract problems associated with continent ileostomy (Kock pouch): report of six cases. *Dis Colon Rectum* 1991;34:936

Grundfest-Broniatowski S, Fazio V. Conservative treatment of bleeding stomal varices. *Arch Surg* 1983;118:981

Jeter KF. These Special Children. A book for parents of children with colostomies, ileostomies, & urostomies Palo Alto, CA: Bull; 1982

Jeter KF. Perioperative teaching and counseling. *Cancer* 1992; 70(suppl):1346

Kaveggia FF, Thompson JS, et al. Placement of an ileal loop urinary diversion back in continuity with the intestinal tract. *Surgery* 1991;110:557

Kodner IJ. Colostomy and ileostomy. *Clin Symp* 1978;30:1

Kodner IJ. Stoma complications. In: Fazio VW (ed), *Current Therapy in Colon and Rectal Surgery.* BC Decker; 1989:420

Kodner IJ: Colostomy. Indications, techniques for construction, and management of complications. *Semin Colon Rectal Surg* 1991;2:73

Kodner IJ, Fleshman JW, et al. Intestinal stomas. In: Schwartz SI (ed), *Maingot's Abdominal Operations,* vol 9. Stamford, CT: Appleton & Lange; 1989:1143

Kodner IJ, Fry RD, et al. Intestinal stomas: their management. In: Veidenheimer MC (ed), *Seminars in Colon & Rectal Surgery.* Philadelphia, PA: WB Saunders; 1991:65

Kodner IJ, Fry RD, et al. Current options in the management of rectal cancer. *Adv Surg* 1991;24:1

Kodner IJ, Fry RD, et al. Intestinal stomas: their management Philadelphia, PA: WB Saunders; 1991:65

Kodner IJ, Fry RD, et al. Colon, rectum, and anus. In: Schwartz SI (ed), *Principles of Surgery,* vol 6. New York, NY: McGraw-Hill; 1993:1191

Köhler LW, Pemberton JH, et al. Quality of life after proctocolectomy: a comparison of Brooke ileostomy, Kock pouch, and ileal pouch-anal anastomosis. *Gastroenterology* 1991; 101:679

MacKeigan JM, Cataldo PA. *Intestinal Stomas: Principles, Techniques, and Management.* St. Louis, MO: Quality Medical;1993

MacLeod JH. Colostomy irrigation—a transatlantic controversy. *Dis Colon Rectum* 1972;15:357

Mazor A, Lacey D, et al. Angiogenesis, type IV collagen, and PCNA do not predict metastasis in localized colorectal cancer. *Society of Surgical Oncology Symposium* 46:1993 (Abstract)

McLeod RS, Fazio VW. Quality of life with the continent ileostomy. *World J Surg* 1984;8:90

McLeod RS, Lavery IC, et al. Patient evaluation of the conventional ileostomy. *Dis Colon Rectum* 1985;28:152

Moran BJ, Jackson AA. Function of the human colon. *Br J Surg* 1992;79:1132

Myerson RJ, Michalski JM, et al. Adjuvant radiation therapy for rectal carcinoma: predictors of outcome. *Radiology* 1993; 189:214 (Abstract)

Myerson RJ, Shapiro SJ, et al. Carcinoma of the anal canal. *Am J Clin Oncol* 1994;18(1):32–39

Nightingale JMD, Lennard-Jones JE, et al. Oral salt supplements to compensate for jejunostomy losses: comparison of sodium chloride capsules, glucose electrolyte solution, and glucose polymer electrolyte solution. *Gut* 1992;33:759

Orsay CP, Kim DO, et al. Diversion colitis in patients scheduled for colostomy closure. *Dis Colon Rectum* 1993;36:366

Parks SE, Hastings PR: Complications of colostomy closure. *Am J Surg* 1985;149:672

Pearl RK, Prasad ML, et al. End-loop stomas: the new generation of intestinal stomas. *Contemp Surg* 1985;27:270

Pearl RK, Prasad ML, et al. Early local complications from intestinal stomas. *Arch Surg* 1985;120:1145

Pemberton JH, Phillips SF, et al. Quality of life after Brooke ileostomy and ileal pouch-anal anastomosis: comparison of performance status. *Ann Surg* 1989;209:620 (discussion)

Prasad ML, Pearl RK, et al. End-loop colostomy. *Surg Gynecol Obstet* 1984;158:380

Prasad ML, Pearl RK, et al. Rodless ileostomy. A modified loop ileostomy. *Dis Colon Rectum* 1984;27:270

Rolstad BS, Wilson G, et al. Sexual concerns in the patient with an ileostomy. *Dis Colon Rectum* 1983;26:170

Rombeau JL, Wilk PJ, et al: Total fecal diversion by the temporary skin-level loop transverse colostomy. *Dis Colon Rectum* 1978;21:223

Shemesh EI, Kodner IJ, et al. Statistics from the ostomy registry. *Ostomy Quart* 1987;24:70

Shirley F, Kodner IJ, et al. Loop ileostomy: techniques and indications. *Dis Colon Rectum* 1984;27:382

Soliani P, Carbognani P, et al. Colostomy plug devices: a possible new approach to the problem of incontinence. *Dis Colon Rectum* 1992;35:969

Starke J, Rodriguez-Bigas M, et al. Primary adenocarcinoma arising in an ileostomy. *Surgery* 1993;114:125

Svaninger G, Nordgren S, et al. Sodium and potassium excretion in patients with ileostomies. *Eur J Surg* 1991;157:601

Thompson JS, Williams SM. Technique for revision of continent ileostomy. *Dis Colon Rectum* 1992;35:87

Trelford JD, Goodnight J, et al. Total exenteration, two or one ostomy. *Surg Gynecol Obstet* 1992;175:126

Turnbull RB Jr, Weakley F (eds), *Atlas of Intestinal Stomas.* St. Louis, MO:CV Mosby; 1967

Unti JA, Abcarian H, et al. Rodless end-loop stomas: seven-year experience. *Dis Colon Rectum* 1991;34:999

Wexner SD, Taranow DA, et al. Loop ileostomy is a safe option for fecal diversion. *Dis Colon Rectum* 1993;36:349

Wiesner RH, LaRusso NF, et al. Peristomal varices after proctocolectomy in patients with primary sclerosing cholangitis. *Gastroenterology* 1986;90:316

Winslet MC, Drolc Z, et al. Assessment of the defunctioning efficiency of the loop ileostomy. *Dis Colon Rectum* 1991;34:699

Winslet MC, Poxon V, et al. A pathophysiologic study of diversion proctitis. *Surg Gynecol Obstet* 1993;177:57

13

Preoperative and Postoperative Management

Carson D. Liu ▪ *David W. McFadden*

The successful outcome of surgery depends on a comprehensive preoperative evaluation, patient preparation, skilled surgical technique, and meticulous postoperative care. Patient management techniques have advanced and enabled healthcare providers to evaluate and monitor patient treatment and progress more effectively. A better understanding of the natural history of diseases allows for improved preoperative and postoperative management.

▪ PREOPERATIVE MANAGEMENT

The care of the patient in the preoperative period comprises a diagnostic work-up, interpretation of the results, a decision regarding the necessity of surgery, and preparation for surgery. The surgeon acquires the necessary data through a history and physical examination, preoperative screening tests, and medical speciality consultations. Using this information, the main decision of the surgeon at this stage is whether surgery is warranted in lieu of the potential risks.

HISTORY AND PHYSICAL EXAMINATION

The physician-patient relationship is established at the onset of history-taking. During the initial encounter, communication is established between physician, pa-

tient, and the patient's family. The surgeon should use this time to minimize the psychological stresses of surgery by informing the patient of the probable outcome and specific situations the patient will find himself in after the procedure. Also, the surgeon should discuss any issues that may involve family members. For example, donation of designated blood by relatives should be discussed well before the proposed surgery.

The initial evaluation of surgical patients must include a complete history and physical examination. Preparation of the patient for the physiological stress of surgery requires an accurate diagnosis. The history provides focal points to help tailor the physical examination and the ordering of preoperative tests. A precise history enables the physician to make the correct diagnosis in 70% to 80% of cases. A systematic approach in history-taking will initiate a comprehensive discussion between patient and physician. An organ system approach (neurological, psychological, pulmonary, cardiac, gastrointestinal, hepatic, renal, endocrine, vascular, nutrition) is one such method. This sort of methodical approach enables the physician to assess preoperative risks accurately. Information regarding past medical problems will help to determine suspected risk factors, and a list of medications and allergies will assist treatment plans postoperatively.

The social history is of importance in preoperative preparation and postoperative management. A quantitation of tobacco usage, alcohol ingestion, recreational drug usage, and caffeine intake should be assessed. Tobacco usage is discouraged preoperatively for those patients undergoing general anesthesia. Chronic alcohol ingestion is associated with malnutrition, hepatic dysfunction, and central nervous system disorders. Chronic caffeine ingestion has been implicated as the most common cause of postoperative headaches. Abuse of intravenous drugs is associated with a higher incidence of hepatitis B, hepatitis C, human immunodeficiency virus, and subacute bacterial endocarditis. Risks should be discussed with the patient when patients refuse to cease usage of the above drugs, and these discussions should be documented in the patient's chart.

CARDIAC PREOPERATIVE EVALUATION

The morbidity and mortality of a procedure can be assessed by the tolerance of the patient to the stress of surgery. Cardiac risk factors are a major concern during the preoperative assessment. The preoperative evaluation often is performed by a team of physicians that includes the surgeon, anesthesiologist, internist, and cardiologist. History, physical examination, chest radiographs, and electrocardiogram are used to determine if there is preexisting cardiac pathology. An electrocardiogram and chest radiograph are required for patients with a known history of cardiac problems, men older than 40 years of age, and women older than 55 years of age.

Patients older than 65 years of age with a known cardiac history should be considered as candidates for placement of a pulmonary artery catheter, preoperatively, to assess hemodynamic parameters. The Swan-Ganz catheter will determine cardiac index, stroke index, ventricular stroke work, and oxygen transport measurements. Preoperative medical treatment is focused at maximizing hemodynamic parameters. Younger patients with cardiac symptoms initially may be screened with two-dimensional echocardiograms to rule out anatomical defects. Other tests, such as multiple-gated acquisition (MUGA) scans and dipyridamole-thallium 201 scans provide important data on the extent of coronary artery disease. Determination of whether coronary angiography or coronary artery bypass is needed should be decided preoperatively before elective abdominal surgery.

Various categories stratifying the risks of patients for preoperative cardiac complications have been described.

Cardiac Risk Factors

Patients are classified by the degree of their illnesses in the American Society of Anesthesiologists (ASA) Physical Status Scale (Table 13–1). Each patient is grouped into a specific ASA scale. This scale is the best predictor of noncardiac deaths and is easy to use.

TABLE 13–1. AMERICAN SOCIETY OF ANESTHESIOLOGISTS (ASA) SCALE

Class I	Normal healthy individual
Class II	Patient with mild systemic disease
Class III	Patient with severe systemic disease that is not incapacitating
Class IV	Patient with incapacitating systemic disease that is a constant threat to life.
Class V	Moribund patient who is not expected to survive 24 hours with or without surgery
E	Added for emergency procedures

ASA classification for prediction of noncardiac deaths. Class I patients have a mortality rate of 1% to 6%, class II patients have a mortality rate of 4% to 11%, and class III patients are estimated to have a mortality rate of 22% to 27%. Class IV patients are always at risk of death due to organ failure, and their mortality rates are dependent on stability of organ function. Class V patients have a mortality rate near 100% within 24 hours, and surgery is the last resort.

Goldman's Criteria

Surgical patients undergoing general anesthesia can be categorized by their risk of experiencing an untoward cardiac event. Nine factors were identified by Goldman to predict cardiac outcome.[1] The cardiac risk index has an excellent predictive value for postoperative cardiac complications (Table 13–2).

Of the total 53 points allowable, 28 points are possible to manipulate by maximizing the medical condition of the patient or by waiting 6 months after a myocardial infarction before undertaking surgery. The total point value summed up will classify each patient into a Gold-

TABLE 13–2. GOLDMAN'S CARDIAC RISK SCALE

Criteria	Points
History	
Age >70 years old	5
Myocardial infarction within 6 months	10
Physical Exam	
S3 gallop or jugular venous distention	11
Significant aortic valvular stenosis	3
Electrocardiogram	
Rhythm other than sinus or PAC on previous EKG	7
>5 PVC/min	7
General	
pO_2 <60, or pCO_2 >50, K <3.0 or HCO_3 <20, BUN <50, Cr >3.0 mg/dL, abnormal SGOT, signs of chronic liver disease.	3
Operation	
Intraperitoneal, intrathoracic, or aortic operation	3
Emergency Surgery	4
Total Possible Score	53

man class of I-IV, with an associated risk of complications (Table 13–3).

The use of Goldman's criteria are superior in estimating *cardiac* risk factors as compared to the ASA scale. The risk of cardiac death is similar in both class II and class III patients, but the incidence of life-threatening complications is much higher in class III patients.

The Acute Physiology and Chronic Health Evaluation (APACHE II)

The APACHE II score is used to assess degrees of physiological derangement. The scoring system comprises temperature, respiratory rate, arterial pH, serum potassium, hematocrit, heart rate, oxygenation, serum sodium, serum creatinine, white blood cell count, Glasgow coma score, and advancing age. The weighting system is based on a scale of 0 to 4, with higher scores representing larger degrees of deviation from normal values. Additional points are given for advancing age and chronic illnesses (history of cardiovascular, respiratory, hepatic, renal or immune disorders). The sum of all of these factors is used as the APACHE II score. Healthy individuals will have a score of 0 to 5. Scores higher than 35 are associated with >80% chance of death.

The APACHE II scoring system is not as accurate in postoperative cardiac surgery patients who receive coronary bypass. These patients have unusually high scores but low mortality rates.

Respiratory Evaluation

Respiratory problems are important factors in the morbidity and mortality of surgical patients after general anesthesia. A pulmonary evaluation is used to identify and reduce risk factors related to surgery. A minimal knowledge of respiratory physiology is necessary for understanding the various respiratory pathologies that may prohibit general anesthesia.[2] Respiratory parameters of interest to the surgeon are tidal volume (TV), functional residual capacity (FRC), and vital capacity (VC) (Fig 13–1). Tidal volume is the amount of air exchanged during a normal resting respiratory cycle. Nor-

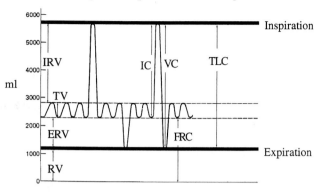

Figure 13–1. Static lung volumes measured by spirometry. IRV: inspiratory reserve volume; TV: tidal volume; ERV: expiratory reserve volume; RV: residual volume; IC: inspiratory capacity; VC: vital capacity; FRC: functional reserve capacity; TLC: total lung capacity. (Adapted from Guyton AC. *Textbook of Medical Physiology.* 7th ed. Philadelphia, PA: WB Saunders; 1986

mal tidal volume averages 7 to 8 cc/kg. An average of 10 cc/kg is used as an estimate of tidal volume when setting the ventilator after endotracheal intubation.

FRC is the volume remaining in the lungs after exhalation of the tidal volume. Normal FRC is approximately 15 to 30 cc/kg. FRC decreases with age, prolonged bed rest, thoracic surgery, and general anesthesia. VC is the amount of air exhaled after a maximal inhalation. Normal VC is 30 to 70 cc/kg.

A theoretical value, the critical closing volume (CCV), is used to describe the volume remaining in the lungs when microatelectasis begins (Fig 13–2). In normal individuals, the CCV is between the FRC and residual volume (RV). CCV increases with age, while FRC decreases with general anesthesia. When CCV exceeds FRC, the patient experiences spontaneous atelectasis as well as closure of small airways. Fig 13–3 and Table 13–4 describe the conditions that decrease FRC and confirm how age and smoking are major causes of increase in CCV. When FRC decreases to the point where it is less than CCV, obligatory atelectasis occurs.

TABLE 13–3. CARDIAC RISK INDEX

Class	Total Points	% Life Threatening Complication	% Cardiac Death
I	0–5	0.7	0.2
II	6–12	5.0	2.0
III	13–25	11.0	2.0
IV	≥ 26	22.0	56.0

Predicted risks utilizing the total scores from Goldman's scoring system. (Adapted from Goldman L, Caldera DL, Nussbaum SR, et al. Multifactorial index of cardiac index in noncardiac surgical procedures. *N Engl J Med* 1977;297:845–850)

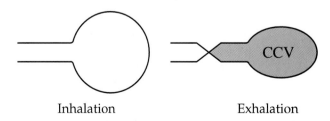

Figure 13–2. Critical Closing Volume of Alveoli. Schematic representation of the CCV (ie, the volume remaining in the alveoli when small airways collapse).

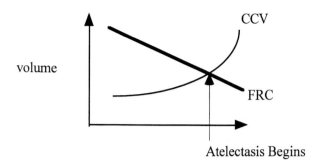

Figure 13-3. Relationship of FRC and CCV. Atelectasis will occur as CCV. increases with age, smoking history, or pulmonary and FRC decreases from surgery.

Static lung volumes change after surgery, especially after upper abdominal and thoracic surgery.[3] There is a decrease in VC of 50% to 60% and a compensatory increase in respiratory rate to maintain minute ventilation. FRC decreases for the first 4 days after surgery until a nadir is reached. Many of these deficits last for up to 2 weeks after surgery, but some can persist for up to 4 months.

Location of the surgical incision also affects postoperative respiratory patterns. It is well known that incisions in the chest or upper abdomen significantly decrease sighing and coughing reflexes. Postoperative pain and narcotics also blunt the sighing and coughing reflexes. Sighing is important, since it is a normal mechanism used to preserve lung volume in the awake individual. This mechanism expands the distal alveoli and is an efficient way of reducing alveolar collapse that occurs naturally during sleep and long periods of recumbency. Sighing is markedly decreased in postoperative patients, and its need must be considered during patient management.

Breathing mechanisms shift from a predominantly diaphragmatic-driven to a rib cage–driven breathing pattern in postoperative patients. This postoperative diaphragmatic dysfunction is a reflex phenomenon rather than an actual paralysis, and its etiology is unclear. Voluntary diaphragmatic contradiction is preserved in the postoperative patient. Postoperative incentive spirometry and early ambulation help to minimize postoperative atelectasis.

Pulmonary Risk Factors

Several preoperative pulmonary risk factors have been identified (Table 13–5). Obesity, smoking, asthma, chronic obstructive pulmonary disease, and age are among the most important.

A major risk factor for pulmonary complications is obesity. An increased body mass will increase the total cellular oxygen consumption as well as increase carbon dioxide production. Obese patients work harder to maintain respiration because of an inefficient or stiff chest wall that mimics a restrictive ventilatory pattern. These patients also are thought to be at higher risk for pulmonary infections postoperatively, with a noticeably increased rate of atelectasis. Patients with morbid obesity should have baseline arterial blood gas and pulmonary function tests preoperatively, if major upper abdominal or chest surgery is planned. A transverse rather than a vertical incision should be considered. Postoperatively, the head of the bed should be elevated to reduce diaphragmatic elevation and the work of breathing.

Smoking is another significant contributor to postoperative complications. Tobacco usage of 20 pack-years or more is a recognized risk factor for patients undergoing major surgery. Patients who quite smoking at least eight weeks before surgery can reduce their risks of postoperative complications. Smoking cessation allows the small airways to become more normal, as well as allowing the regeneration of functional cilia that clear respiratory mucus. Studies of postoperative respira-tory secretion clearance have utilized mucus made radiopaque with tantalum powder. Factors found to worsen mucous transport are smoking, narcotic analgesia, prolonged bedrest, and presence of an endotracheal tube. If the patient is unable to quit smoking, or time is a constraint, the use of preoperative bronchodilators, chest physiotherapy, and a short course of antibiotics may be beneficial.

Age has been cited as a relative risk factor for the development of pulmonary complications, although age alone is not associated with an increased risk for surgery. The duration of anesthesia is associated with a

TABLE 13–4. CAUSES OF FRC AND CCV CHANGES

FRC Decreases	CCV Increases
Supine Position	Age
General Anesthesia	Smoking
Obesity	Pulmonary Edema
Abdominal Pain	Emphysema
Pregnancy	

TABLE 13–5. SUMMARY OF PULMONARY RISK FACTORS

Age greater than 65 years
Obesity
Tobacco usage history
Prolonged hospitalization
Upper abdominal surgery or thoracic surgery
COPD or asthma history

greater incidence of pulmonary complications. Anesthesia of 3.5 hours or longer is associated with an increased incidence of pulmonary complications.[4] The type of anesthesia used also alters the risk of pulmonary complications. Although no difference exists between general and spinal anesthesia, the use of regional anesthesia is associated with less pulmonary complications.

Patients with asthma have been identified as having a higher complication rate, postoperatively. Patients requiring steroids for control of their asthma will have poor wound healing and may develop adrenal insufficiency. Halothane has been recommended as the best inhalation anesthetic agent for patients with asthma because of its rapid induction, increased pulmonary compliance, and decreased salivation. Certain anesthetics (D-tubocurarine, cyclopropane, and thiopental) have been associated with increased incidence of postoperative wheezing.

Patients undergoing laparoscopic procedures wherein CO_2 is used any experience acidosis secondary to hypercarbia. Arterial blood gases may need to be assayed intraoperatively, especially in patients with previous cardiac problems.

RENAL ASSESSMENT

Renal function should be evaluated preoperatively to prevent further deterioration from nephrotoxic agents or massive fluid administration during surgery. The history will reveal whether a patient has chronic renal failure, and laboratory screening tests will detect evidence of acute or chronic renal failure.

The extent of renal failure is determined preoperatively by clinical manifestations and routine laboratory evaluations, such as serum creatinine and blood urea nitrogen (BUN). BUN alone is not accurate at portraying renal function. The glomerular filtration rate (GFR) can be roughly estimated clinically by measuring the serum BUN and creatinine. A 24 hour creatinine clearance is more accurate for determining GFR. The serum creatinine level is affected by GFR, renal tubular secretion, and rate of production. After 20 years of age, creatinine production decreases by 5% every 10 years.[5] Normal values of creatinine clearance for men are from 90 to 130 mL/min and normal values for women range from 80 to 125 mL/min. Creatinine (Cr) clearance is determined by the following equation:

$$\text{Clearance Cr} = (\text{Volume} \times \text{Urine Cr})/\text{Plasma Cr}$$

Creatinine is preferentially secreted by the renal tubules during acute renal failure, causing the 24 hour creatinine clearance to overestimate GFR by as much as 50%.[6]

It is useful in acute renal failure to discriminate the type of inciting event (prerenal, renal, postrenal). Prerenal failure is caused by decreased perfusion of the kidneys and is easily reversed with volume repletion, correction of cardiac failure, or reversal of systemic hypotension. Urine osmolality is high and a urinary sodium concentration of less than 10 mEq/L is indicative of a prerenal mechanism of failure. If the etiology remains equivocal, the fractional excretion of sodium (FE_{Na}) will help to clarify the prerenal status.

$$FE_{Na} = \frac{U_{Na}/P_{Na}}{U_{Cr}/P_{Cr}} \times 100$$

U_{Na} is the urine sodium concentration; P_{Na} is the plasma sodium concentration; U_{Cr} is the urine creatinine; and P_{Cr} is the plasma creatinine concentration. If the fractional excretion of sodium is <1, then a prerenal etiology needs to be determined (Table 13–6). If the FE_{Na} is >1, then other etiologies should be investigated (Table 13–7). Prerenal failure should be corrected immediately to prevent permanent ischemic renal injury. Swan-Ganz monitoring of wedge pressure, systemic vascular resistance, and cardiac output have proven to be effective in diagnosing and correcting the etiologies of prerenal failure.

Etiologic factors of postrenal failure often entail an obstructive component involving the ureters, bladder, or the urethra. Tumors, renal stones, and benign prostatic hypertrophy are common causes of postrenal obstruction. Mechanical decompression can be achieved easily by inserting Foley catheters, stents, or nephrostomy tubes to relieve the mechanical obstruction.

NUTRITIONAL ASSESSMENT

Nutritional status of each patient needs to be assessed preoperatively to ensure a normal healing response to operative trauma (Table 13–8). Abnormal nutritional

TABLE 13–6. ETIOLOGIES OF PRERENAL FAILURE

Hypovolemia
  Hemorrhage
  Burns
  Third-space losses (peritonitis, intestinal ileus)
  Gastrointestinal losses
  Iatrogenic (diuretic use)
  Sweating

Decreased intravascular volume
  Congestive heart failure
  Myocardial infarction
  Cirrhosis, hepatorenal syndrome, ascites
  Nephrotic syndrome

Catabolic states
  Sepsis
  Postoperative phase
  Steroids
  Starvation with stress

TABLE 13–7. ETIOLOGIES OF INTRARENAL AND POSTRENAL FAILURE

Toxins
  Radiographic contrasts
  Antibiotics (aminoglycosides, amphotericin B, sulfonamides, penicillins, cephalosporins, tetracycline, rifampin, polymyxin)
  Other drugs (captopril, nonsteroidal anti-inflammatory agents, furosemide, methoxyflurane, phenytoin)
  Rhabdomyolysis

Vascular Disease
  Renal artery thrombi, stenosis, or embolus
  Renal vein thrombosis
  Dissecting aortic aneurysm with or without involvement of renal arteries

Glomerular or autoimmune disorders
  Goodpasture's syndrome
  Systemic lupus erythematosis
  Scleroderma
  Polyarteritis nodosa
  Henoch-Schonlein purpura
  Wegener's granulomatosis
  Serum sickness
  Poststreptococcal glomerulonephritis
  Hemolytic-uremic syndrome
  Thrombotic thrombocytopenic purpura
  Preeclampsia
  Abruptio placentae
  Postpartum renal failure

Postrenal
  Obstruction of urethra, bladder, or ureters
  Injury to ureter or bladder during surgery

status also is associated with an impaired immune system. Weight loss of 20% or more not only increases the surgical mortality rate, but also increases the infection rate by more than 300%. A dietary history may be helpful to determine if nutritional deficiencies exist. Serum albumin <3 grams/dL or a serum transferin level of <150 mg/dL are accepted indicators of malnutrition. Anthropometric studies also are advocated to determine nutritional status. Immune competence can be estimated by total lymphocyte counts >1000/μL of blood or by measuring cell-mediated immunity. The degree of delayed hypersensitivity is estimated with subcutaneous injections of *Candida,* mumps, and *Trichophyton.* Cell-mediated immunity can be judged as impaired when a normal response of 5 mm in duration is not seen by 72 hours.

A common cause of malnutrition in the preoperative patient is inadequate protein intake.[7] Studies of hospitalized patients have revealed that 30% to 50% of patients have moderate to severe malnutrition caused by their primary disease, such as malignancy or gastrointestinal loss. Thus, a vicious cycle begins with malnutrition, causing impaired wound healing and decreased resistance against infections. Sepsis and worsening malnutrition may ensue with associated hypermetabolic

states. Interruption of this cycle is essential for survival of the patient.

The body is composed of approximately 20% fat, 14% protein, and a small amount of glycogen stored in the liver and muscle. The rest of body composition is water. Even smaller amounts of glucose, amino acids, fatty acids, and triglycerides are present in the extracellular fluid for energy resources. Existing glycogen can provide approximately 800 to 1200 kcal of energy, consumed within the first 8 to 24 hours of fasting. The skeletal muscle mass is protein storehouse, but all protein serves a structural or functional purpose. The most efficient energy storehouse is fat, which serves a relatively minor function as insulation. An average person who performs a moderate amount of work requires approximately 3000 kcal per day. The starving person requires less because of adaptation. The response of the body to starvation is directed towards supplying glucose to the brain, which requires 144 grams per day. Adaptation is facilitated by decreasing the catabolism of protein during gluconeogenesis and increasing fat utilization. Altered levels of insulin and glucagon also help to prevent further protein catabolism during prolonged starvation.

Traditional surgical therapy used to prevent protein breakdown during early starvation is administration of a small amount of carbohydrate, such as dextrose, in the intravenous fluid. A minimum of 100 gm/day of dextrose will decrease protein consumption. If the patient is malnourished upon admission, enteral feeding or intravenous parenteral nutrition must be considered because the protein-sparing effects of intravenous fluid will not address the ongoing deficits.

Preoperative nutritional support may be required in patients with inflammatory bowel disease or certain ma-

TABLE 13–8. COMMON CAUSES OF PREOPERATIVE MALNUTRITION

Alcoholism

Inability to Absorb Nutrients
  Short-bowel syndrome
  Gastrointestinal fistulas
  Malabsorption (inborn)
  Diarrhea or vomiting for prolonged period

Increased Metabolic Demands
  Sepsis
  Malignancy
  Burns
  Trauma
  Chronic Illness

Iatrogenic
  Hemodialysis
  Steroids
  Immunosuppression
  Chemotherapy

lignancies. Nutritional support may require placement of a jejunostomy or gastric tube perioperatively to allow enteral nutrition after surgery. Judgement as to the mode of therapy should be directed at convenience, invasiveness of support, and the more physiologic manner of obtaining nutrition.

Whenever possible, enteral nutrition should be used. Enteral nutrition is preferred, since it may prevent bacterial translocation across the intestinal epithelium in the fasted patient. When the enteric method is not used, intestinal epithelial breakdown occurs, and bacteria traverse into the lymphatics and bloodstream. Early postoperative enteral nutrition has been shown to increase both wound and colonic anastomotic strength.[8] Enteral nutrition is contraindicated in several conditions, primarily in certain gastrointestinal or neurological deficiencies (Table 13–9).

The purpose of nutritional support is to meet the body's demands without exceeding them. The delivery of excess nutrients may be harmful. Excess glucose or protein intake can cause hypertonic dehydration, liver dysfunction, and carbon dioxide retention.[9,10] Both enteral nutrition and total parenteral nutrition have risks associated with administration (Tables 13–10, 13–11).

After evaluation of the nutritional status of the patient, a decision is made to administer maintenance caloric supplement or an anabolic caloric level of replacement. The calculation of the maintenance calorie needs can be calculated by the Harris-Benedict formula.

$$\text{Male: Basal Energy Expenditure (BEE)} = 13.7 \times \text{wt(kg)} + 5 \times \text{Ht (cm)} - 6.8 \times \text{age (yr)}$$

$$\text{Female: BEE} = 655 + 9.6 \times \text{wt(kg)} + 1.7 \times \text{ht(cm)} - 4.7 \times \text{age(yr)}$$

$$\text{Oral Maintenance} = \text{BEE} \times 1.2$$

$$\text{Oral Anabolic} = \text{BEE} \times 1.6$$

A simpler way of estimating caloric needs is 35 kcal/kg/day for maintenance and 45 kcal/kg/day for anabolic calorie supplementation.

PREOPERATIVE LABORATORY TESTS

Awareness of cost containment has made preoperative testing more streamlined in elective cases. A cost savings of 35% to 50% can be achieved by obtaining preoperative tests on an outpatient basis. Certain radiographs and blood tests can be useful in identifying preoperative risk factors.

Screening tests have been drastically reduced over the past years to contain rising medical costs. Routine screening tests are strikingly inefficient when used as primary tools during the risk assessment phase. Routine

TABLE 13–9. RELATIVE CONTRAINDICATIONS TO ENTERAL FEEDING

Laryngeal incompetence
Gastric outlet obstruction
Intestinal obstruction
Ileus
Severe acute pancreatitis
Gastrointestinal fistula
Toxic megacolon
Severe diarrhea
Severe gastroesophageal reflux
Tracheoesophageal fistula
Necrotizing enterocolitis
Shock
Coma

screening tests are diagnostically useful in only 5% of all patients. Overall, patient management is altered in only 0.22% of elective surgical cases with their use.[11] Therefore, before embarking upon extensive preoperative evaluation, the history and physical should be used as a guide.

Urinalysis

One of the most common preoperative tests performed is the routine urinalysis. Specimens need to be examined quickly after collection to avoid misleading changes within the specimen over time (ie, bacterial overgrowth or degradation of protein casts). The routine urinalysis should test for protein, ketones, glucose, specific gravity, and a microscopic examination including cell differentiation.

Proteinuria is a marker for glomerular disease and may signify such conditions as intrinsic kidney diseases or congestive heart failure. Urinary ketones may represent starvation or the diabetic state. Diabetic ketosis can be confirmed by the detection of serum acetone. The presence of urinary glucose is suggestive of diabetes. Urinary specific gravity can give an estimate of the patient's free water status in certain disease states, but may be falsely high in a patient with osmotic diuresis from diabetes or proteinuria. The presence of red blood cells can signify various renal pathologies, except when

TABLE 13–10. POSSIBLE COMPLICATIONS OF ENTERAL NUTRITION

Diarrhea, cramping, or bloating
Aspiration
Hyperglycemia
Osmotic diuresis
Fluid and electrolyte imbalance
Tube malfunction/leak
Erosion of nares
Otitis media

TABLE 13–11. POSSIBLE COMPLICATIONS OF TOTAL PARENTERAL NUTRITION

Line sepsis
Pneumothorax
Hemothorax
Subclavian artery injury
Air embolus
Catheter tip erosion through superior vena cava
Venous thrombosis
Hyperglycemia
Hyperosmolar diuresis
Carbon dioxide retention
Encephalopathy
Electrolyte alterations
Liver dysfunction

catheterization is used to obtain the specimen. Microscopic hematuria may signify renal calculi, urinary tract infections, renal tuberculosis, renal vein thrombosis, malignant nephrosclerosis, and subacute bacterial endocarditis. When the urine sample is centrifuged and examined under the microscope, a few leukocytes may be normally present in female patients. The number of epithelial cells is important to distinguish the possibility of a poorly collected specimen. An increased number of leukocytes in the urine usually signifies an infection of the urinary tract. Over 50% of leukocytes are lysed rapidly in hypotonic alkaline urine at room temperature, further supporting the necessity to process specimens rapidly. Casts are formed in renal tubules and usually are derived from gelled protein precipitation. Occasional hyaline casts are seen after high fevers, exercise, secondary heart failure, or postural proteinuria.

Complete Blood Count

A complete blood count (CBC) comprises a hemoglobin, hematocrit, white blood cell count (WBC), automated differential, and a platelet count. A CBC is more useful in female patients to determine the hemoglobin level preoperatively, with an estimated 6% to 13% probability of abnormal results. The occurrence of an abnormal CBC in all hospital admissions is minimal. Less than 0.5% of asymptomatic patients will have an abnormal leukocyte count, and a differential WBC count is useful in only 2.8% of all patients. A differential count should be ordered during emergency cases, suspected infection, or in patients with previously abnormal white blood cell counts. Most hospitals will perform a manual differential count when a high white blood cell count is noted.

Electrolytes, Blood Urea Nitrogen, Creatinine and Glucose

Automated machines have made many blood tests inexpensive and efficient. The electrolytes, blood urea nitrogen (BUN), creatinine, and glucose usually are or-

dered and reported as a sequential multiple analysis-7 (SMA-7). When an SMA-7 is ordered routinely, an unexpected abnormality rate of only 0.2% is seen.[11] Some hospitals charge the same whether an SMA-7 is ordered or whether 2 to 3 individual serum tests are ordered. The most important electrolyte to check is the serum potassium, which needs to be maintained between 3.5 to 5.0 mEq/L to decrease the risk of perioperative cardiac arrhythmias.[12]

Prothrombin Time and Partial Thromboplastin Time

The measurement of routine prothrombin times (PT) and partial thromboplastin times (PTT) during the preoperative evaluation has a probability of .008% of diagnosing an unknown bleeding tendency. In the absence of clinical history, trauma, or liver dysfunction, the probability of discovering an abnormal PT or PTT is extremely low. Risk factors during history-taking that require measurement of PT or PTT include a history of previous excessive bleeding during surgery or dental work, a family history of bleeding, or the use of medications that may interfere with clotting mechanisms. In addition, patients using nonsteroidal antiinflammatory agents may need to have a bleeding test performed to assess platelet adherence. A patient undergoing major cardiac or vascular surgery should have a PT and PTT prior to surgery.

Chest Radiographs

Chest roentgenograms are performed as a routine screening test nearly 60% of the time. The abnormalities seen on chest x-ray rarely alter patient management; the most common abnormality is chronic respiratory disease. The following are indications for a preoperative chest x-ray in asymptomatic patients.

- Known pulmonary or cardiac disease history
- Anticipated chest surgery
- Age >40 years
- High risk for postoperative pulmonary complications
- Positive tuberculin test or high risk for unsuspected pulmonary infection

Electrocardiogram

Routine electrocardiography (EKG) should be obtained in men older than 40 years of age and women older than 55 years of age. A history of cardiac disease or a family history of cardiac disease also may justify preoperative EKGs. The electrocardiogram will have a high incidence of nonspecific ST and T wave changes in all age groups, which may not be helpful in most preoperative evaluations. Data obtained from the EKG need to be correlated with the history of the patient and the family history for cardiac diseases.

FLUIDS AND ELECTROLYTES

Management of fluid and electrolyte metabolism remains challenging in the perioperative care of surgical patients. Adequate preoperative hydration is essential in severely ill patients undergoing general anesthesia, since surgical procedures produce changes in the distribution of fluids and electrolytes. Bodily fluids are primarily water. As a person ages, the lean body mass decreases with water-free fat replacing body mass. Water contributes approximately 50% of the body weight in females and 60% in males. The body is divided into two functional compartments; the intracellular and extracellular fluid compartments. With the use of isotopic dilution techniques, the body compartments have been accurately measured. Forty percent of total body weight is intracellular. The extracellular fluid constitutes 20% of the total body weight. Only 5% of the total body weight is within the intravascular system (Fig 13–4). The primary electrolytes in the extracellular compartment are sodium and chloride; the primary electrolytes in the intracellular compartment are potassium, magnesium, and phosphate. Proteins in the plasma also are found in relatively high concentrations. The ionic difference between the intracellular and extracellular compartments is maintained by the cell membrane. The dissolved proteins in the plasma selectively pass through the semipermeable cell membrane, and are the primary components in creating an effective osmotic pressure. In the extracellular fluid compartment, various layers of cells are joined by tight junctions to help maintain homeostasis of the different ions. The increased effective plasma osmotic pressure from proteins causes a lower inorganic anion concentration in plasma as compared to the interstitium (Fig 13–5). When there is a loss of plasma protein or red blood cells during hemorrhage, intravenous replacement of hypotonic fluids will affect the interstitial free-fluid and electrolyte levels. Initial therapy with isotonic solutions or hypertonic solutions are more beneficial at maintaining intravascular volume.

Approach To Fluid and Electrolyte Therapy

The surgeon must observe and match the fluid and electrolyte losses during the preoperative and postoperative periods. Replacement of electrolytes and fluid account for normal maintenance requirements, abnormal losses secondary to the disease or surgery, and correction of preexisting abnormalities.

In a normal individual, insensible water gains result from oxidation of carbohydrates, creating approximately 250 cc/day (range: 125 to 800 cc/day). Insensible water losses include evaporation through skin and lungs, averaging 600 cc/day (range: 600 to 1,500 cc/day). Sensible water losses include urinary losses of 800 to 1500 cc/day and intestinal losses of 250 cc/day during bowel movements.

Maintenance fluid requirements in a normal adult are approximately 35 cc/kg per 24 hours. In children, a

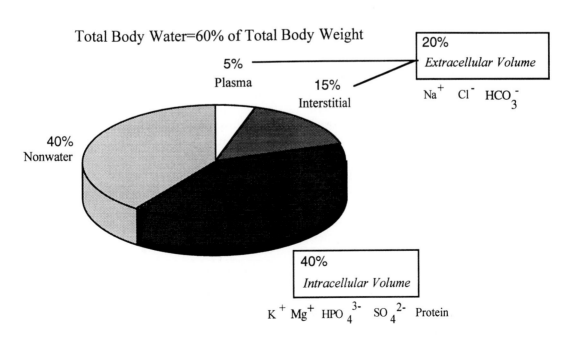

Figure 13–4. Percentages of various compartments and their predominant electrolytes.

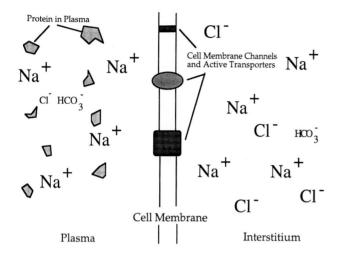

Figure 13–5. The semipermeable cell membrane contain various channels and co-transporters which allow proteins to remain in the plasma, and a larger concentration of chloride to be maintained in the interstitium to balance the effective osmotic pressure.

useful guideline in calculating maintenance fluid requirements is as follows:

- First 10 kg - 1000 cc/24 hrs.
- Second 10 kg - 500 cc/24 hrs.
- For every kg >20 kg - add 25 cc/kg per 24 hrs.

For example, a 25 kg child would require 1000 + 500 + 125 = 1625 cc/24 hrs or approximately 68 cc/hrs. It is important to remember that the above estimate of maintenance fluid requirements is for a normal individual and the ultimate goal of hydration is to obtain a minimum urine output of 0.5 cc/kg per hour.

Extracellular fluid volume deficits are the most common disorders in surgical patients. Losses in fluid volume include obligatory electrolyte losses at variable concentrations. Some common causes of fluid losses include emesis, nasogastric tube suctioning, diarrhea, fistula drainage, hemorrhaging, fluid sequestration in injured or inflamed tissues, or burns. Severe volume depletion causes shifts in fluid and electrolytes from the intracellular compartment to the extracellular compartment. When a significant loss of fluid occurs, all organ system functions become depressed. The normal febrile response is blunted, the immune system is suppressed, and central nervous system function is diminished. A patient with protracted peritonitis may not manifest expected clinical findings and present with a normal WBC, euthermia, and little complaints of abdominal pain.

When a sufficient volume of fluid is lost, renal hypoperfusion occurs and oliguria may be found. The fractional excretional of sodium and the presence of urinary sediment are useful in monitoring urinary function.

Several laboratory tests may indirectly reflect changes

in the extracellular fluid (ECF) volume. The blood urea nitrogen usually rises during deficiencies in ECF. Serum creatinine may not always increase proportionately in young adults, but in the elderly, blood urea nitrogen and creatinine parallel one another during ECF deficiencies. The concentration of red blood cells, white blood cells, and platelets are slightly elevated during ECF volume deficits. Serum sodium does not parallel changes of other blood components, being the major extracellular cation. The body has a remarkable ability to maintain sodium concentrations despite thirst, antidiuretic hormone, or aldosterone. The body can usually maintain the serum sodium between 135 to 145 mEq/L. A low sodium level represents an excess of total body water or a deficiency of total body sodium. In contrast, a high sodium level represents a deficiency in water or an excess of total body sodium. The serum sodium concentration can be multiplied by 2 and added to 10. A normal extracellular osmolality can be assumed if the value is within 5% of a normal serum osmolality of 290 mOsm/L.

Various compositions of intravenous fluid may be used for preoperative maintenance and replacement therapy (Table 13–12). Lactated Ringer's solution has been a popular choice to replace extracellular fluid losses because of its approximation to physiologic ionic concentrations. Isotonic sodium chloride is useful to replace hyponatremia and hypochloremia during initial intravenous fluid replacement. Normal serum has approximately 103 mEq/L of chloride while normal saline, or 0.9% NaCl, contains 154 mEq/L of chloride. If the amount of chloride administered exceeds the excretory ability of the kidneys, a dilutional acidosis may develop as a result of decreasing bicarbonate concentrations relative to carbonic acid levels. Another popular choice by surgeons is 5% dextrose in 0.45% NaCl with 20 mEq/L of KCl. This choice of maintenance fluid is an excellent replacement to match free-water insensible losses. It also provides dextrose to prevent protein wasting during the fasting state.

In the postoperative period, proper replacement of fluids may be difficult depending on the amount of blood loss, the length of surgery, and the adequacy of preoperative hydration. If the patient is monitored with a right-sided (CVP) heart catheter, replacement of flu-

TABLE 13–12. CONCENTRATIONS OF ELECTROLYTES IN INTRAVENOUS FLUID AS COMPARED TO EXTRACELLULAR FLUID

Solution	Na	K	Ca	Mg	Cl	HCO$_3^-$
Extracellular fluid	142	4	5	3	103	27
Lactated Ringer's	130	4	2.7	—	109	28
0.9% sodium chloride	154	—	—	—	154	—
D$_5$ 0.45% sodium chloride	77	—	—	—	77	—

ids can be much easier in the immediate postoperative period. If there is less cardiovascular monitoring, frequent assessments may need to be performed to replace fluid and electrolyte losses.

Surgeons tend to underestimate intraoperative blood losses by nearly 40%. Immediately after surgery, sequestration of fluid will continue to enter third-space compartments for the first 12 to 24 hours. The recommended fluid for replacement of acute fluid sequestration is a hypertonic solution such as 5% dextrose in lactated Ringer's solution. Hypertonic solutions have traditionally been used to maintain intravascular volume, rather than hypotonic solutions. Once adequate perfusion is achieved, as evidenced by reduction of tachycardia, a minimum urine output of 30 to 40 cc/hr, and warm and well perfused extremities, a maintenance fluid rate can be established with a hypotonic solution (D5-½ NS with 20 mEq/L of KCl).

Approach to Electrolyte Replacement

A normal adult ingests 75 to 120 mEq of sodium per day. A child ingests approximately 3 mEq/kg/per day. Abnormalities in sodium are very rare in elective surgical patients. In hospitalized patients, common causes of sodium imbalances are listed in Tables 13–13 and 13–14.

TABLE 13–13. HYPERNATREMIA (Na+ >145 mEq/L)

Pure Water Loss
Impaired thirst drive (hypothalamic injury or tumor)
Inability to obtain water (infants, dementia, coma)
Increased insensible water loss (mechanical ventilation)

Excessive Na+ Intake:
Iatrogenic (excessive intravenous replacement)
Accidental (drowning in seawater)
Glucocorticoid/mineralocorticoid excess (Cushing's syndrome, primary aldosteronism, ectopic ACTH hormone production)

Loss of Water in Excess of Na+ Losses:
Gastrointestinal loss (vomiting, diarrhea, intestinal fistula)
Renal loss secondary to central cause (central diabetes insipidus: head trauma, posthypophysectomy, tumor, sarcoidoisis, tuberculosis, Wegener's granulomatosis, syphyllis, histiocytosis, CNS infection, congenital)
Renal loss secondary to impaired concentrating ability by kidneys (osmotic diuresis: diabetic ketosis, chronic renal failure from polycystic kidneys, interstitial disease, medullary cystic disease, postobstructive diuresis secondary to partial urinary obstruction, diuresis phase of arf, mannitol, tube feeds, infant formula)
Excessive diuretic use, hypokalemia, hypercalcemia, decreased protein uptake, prolonged, excessive H2O intake, sickle cell disease/trait, multiple myeloma, amyloidosis, SJogren's syndrome, nephrogenic diabetes insipidus).

Pharmacologic Causes
alcohol, phenytoin, amphotericin B, lithium, demeclocycline, propoxyphene, colchicine, vinblastine, sulfonylurea hypoglycemic agents

Skin Loss (massive burns)

TABLE 13–14. HYPONATREMIA (Na+ <130 mEq/L)

Pseudohyponatremia with normal serum osmolality (hyperglycemia, hyperlipidemia, hyperproteinemia, infusion of mannitol)
Renal loss (diuretic use, renal salt wasting in renal tubular acidosis or advanced chronic renal disease, osmotic diuresis, mineralocorticoid deficiency)
Third space loss (burns, sweating, hemorrhagic pancreatitis)
Associated with decreased extracellular fluid volume (vomiting, diarrhea)
Associated with increased extracellular fluid volume (congestive heart failure, cirrhosis, ascites, nephrotic syndrome, renal failure)
Associated with normal extracellular fluid volume (syndrome of inappropriate antidiuretic hormone, CNS diseases including cerebrovascular accident, delirium tremens, multiple sclerosis, pulmonary diseases including pneumonia, lung abscess, tuberculosis, carcinoma, pain, acute psychosis, hypothyroidism, positive pressure ventilation, porphyria)
Pharmacologic causes (antidiuretic hormone, nicotine, morphine, barbiturates, isoproterenol, nonsteroidal antiinflammatory drugs, acetaminophen, amitriptyline, colchicine, cyclophosphamide)
Psychogenic polydypsia
Excessive beer drinking

Symptoms and signs caused by hypernatremia include restlessness, weakness, delirium, maniacal behavior, tachycardia, decreased saliva and tears, dry and sticky mucous membranes, red swollen tongue, flushed skin, fever, and oliguria. A change in sodium concentration always will affect the extracellular fluid volume concomitantly, whereas the opposite does not always occur. Treatment requires rehydration with a hypotonic salt solution during a 24 hour period. Rapid correction should be avoided to prevent cerebral edema.

Signs and symptoms of hyponatremia include muscle twitching, hyperactive tendon reflexes, increased intracaranial pressure with concomitant changes in blood pressure and pulse, increased salivation and lacrimation, watery diarrhea, oliguria, or anuria. Treatment is dependent on the cause of hypervolemia, and will require either water restriction, if water intoxication is involved, or sodium replacement, if a true sodium depletion is present.

Normal intake of potassium, in an adult, is 40 to 60 mEq/24 hrs and 2 mEq/kg per 24 hours, in a child. There is a minimum daily K+ loss of 30 to 45 mEq in urinary losses independent of the serum level of potassium. Hyperkalemia will cause EKG changes and eventually impede cardiac conduction. Initial symptoms may be weakness, irritability, or confusion. Loss of deep tendon reflexes may be an early diagnostic clue. When hyperkalemia is noticed, an EKG should be performed. If there are EKG changes manifested by peaked T waves, decreased R waves, deepened S waves, depressed ST segments, or prolonged QRS waves, urgent measures should be taken. Treatment should include calcium gluconate (10 cc of 10% intravenously during 2 minutes), one ampule of sodium bicarbonate intravenously, and 60cc of 50% dextrose with 10 units of regular insulin, intravenously. Monitoring of blood glucose should be performed for several hours after administration. Diuresis with furosemide may be used with hydration in less urgent situations. If the above measures are insufficient, hemodialysis should be considered, if the potassium level remains above 7.5 mEq/L or cardiac irritability is noted.

ANTIBIOTICS

Perioperative antibiotic usage certainly has reduced infection rates. Preoperative prophylactic antibiotics have reduced morbidity rates in elective clean-contaminated cases where body organs or cavities containing bacteria are opened. During abdominal surgery, transection of any portion of the gastrointesinal tract can implant bacteria into the peritoneal cavity or wound.

Wound infections occur in 1.7% of clean surgical cases, 8.8% in clean-contaminated wounds, 17.5% for contaminated wounds, and 41.6% for dirty wounds (Table 13–15).[13] The use of prophylactic antibiotics, such as a first generation cephalosporin, has been shown to reduce abscess formation and wound infections in most clean-contaminated and contaminated cases. Additional coverage for gram negative bacteria or anaerobic coverage is warranted in special cases, such as colon surgery or biliary obstruction, or contaminated or dirty cases.

Penetrating abdominal trauma victims do not have the luxury of undergoing bowel preparation prior to surgery. Antibiotic therapy coverage must account for the bacterial contamination present prior to their administration. Therapy is broadened to cover most enteric and skin organisms until culture results are available. At that time, the surgeon may narrow the spectrum of antibiotics. The most consistent risk factor predisposing patients to intraabdominal infection after trauma is colon injury.[14]

An increased incidence of abdominal infections is seen in blunt trauma patients who were restrained with seatbelts during automobile accidents. In trauma patients, a higher incidence of abdominal infections occur from the existence of multiple risk factors. Penetrating objects are not sterile and seed bacteria upon entry into a body cavity. Bacterial contamination is augmented with multiple vascular catheter insertions during minimal sterile techniques in a rushed emergency room. Furthermore, the pathophysiology of shock, with its associated immunosuppression and hypoperfusion of visceral organs, predisposes these patients to infections.

Studies on laboratory animals have shown the optimal timing of prophylactic antibiotics to be within 3 hours of bacterial inoculation. Tissue seeding of bacteria was decreased if antibiotics were administered within this time frame. Human studies have revealed that preoperative prophylactic antibiotics were associated with a 7% infection rate, whereas an infection rate of 33% was noted in patients who received antibiotics intraoperatively only, and an infection rate of 30% existed in patients who received antibiotics postoperatively.[15] A tabulation of recommended prophylactic antibiotics are listed in Table 13–16.

Many medical conditions are associated with increased wound infections (Table 13–17). A heightened awareness, perioperatively, will enable early diagnosis of wound infections in high-risk patients.

SKIN PREPARATION

Preparation of the patient's skin for surgery begins the night before surgery. Preoperative baths or showers with antiseptics will reduce the probability of a *Staphylococcus aureus* wound infection. Chlorhexidine baths or showers have been shown to reduce wound infection rates when given the night before surgery.[16] The hair in the operative field should not be removed unless it inhibits accurate closure of wounds. If removal of hair is needed, clippers should be used rather than shaving.[17] Shaving, either the night before or immediately before surgery, has been shown to increase wound infection rates.[18]

At the time of surgery, the patient's skin can be prepared with a povidone-iodine solution or gel in either 10% or 1% concentrations. Other solutions, such as hexachlorophene compounds or triclosan compounds, are as effective as povidone-iodine solutions. The mechanical cleansing of the skin with these agents will significantly reduce the number of bacteria, especially at intertriginous folds and the umbilicus. Drying of the painted povidone-iodine material must occur to reduce bacterial floral. After draping the operative site, any pooled iodine at the edges of the operative site must be removed to prevent skin irritation. Chlorhexidine should be used with caution around the face, since deafness has been reported.[19]

BOWEL PREPARATION

The distal ileum and colon contain enormous amounts of bacteria. The highest concentration of pathogenic bacteria exists in the right colon. During surgery, tran-

TABLE 13–15. WOUND CLASSIFICATION AND ASSOCIATED INFECTION RATE

Class	Wound	Infection Rate (%)
I	Clean	1.7
II	Clean contaminated	8.8
III	Contaminated	17.5
IV	Dirty	41.6

TABLE 13–16. PROPHYLACTIC ANTIBIOTICS RECOMMENDED FOR SURGICAL PROCEDURES

	Antibiotic	Dose
Aerobic gram positive & gram negative organisms	Cefazolin	1 gm IV
Gram negative aerobes & anaerobes	Metronidazole & Gentamicin	500 mg IV 1.5 mg/kg IV
Single-agent coverage of gram negative aerobes and anaerobes	Cefoxitin or Doxycycline	1 gm IV 200 mg IV

Adapted from Scientific American Medicine. Care of the Surgical Patient. Ch. VI, sect. 3, pp 4. 1994, Scientific American, Inc., New York

section across this mucosa will expose the peritoneal cavity to a large bacterial load. Mechanical cleansing is used to decrease wound infections and peritonitis during elective colonic surgery. Oral nonabsorbable antibiotics also are used to reduce the bacterial load within the lumen of the bowel. The numbers of aerobic bacteria, such as *Escherichia coli*, and anaerobic bacteria, such as *Bacteroides fragilis*, are reduced with oral antibiotics.

Mechanical cleansing of the bowel traditionally has involved a liquid diet, cathartics, and enemas. Elderly patients may not tolerate the metabolic disturbances associated with a prolonged regimen. Whole-gut lavage now is performed with balanced electrolyte solutions that usually contain polyethylene glycol. Patients are placed on a liquid diet 2 days prior to surgery, when the mechanical cleansing is begun. On the day prior to surgery, patients ingest the lavage preparation at a rate of 1L for 2 to 4 hours.

Oral antibiotics, usually consisting of 1 gm each of neomycin base and erythromycin base, are given on the day before surgery, at 1 PM, 2 PM, and 11 PM for a planned surgery at 8 AM the next day. These antibiotics are directed towards the aerobic and anaerobic flora present in the colon. The timing of administration of these oral agents is critical for its efficacy. If the surgery is planned for later in the day, the timing of oral antibiotics should be adjusted to cover the 19 hours prior to surgery. No more than three doses of the neomycin-erythromycin regimen should be given, otherwise resistant flora will emerge. The substitution of metronidazole for neomycin may be as effective. The goal is to reduce the bacterial load within the lumen and not to sterilize the gut. An additional dose of antibiotic, usually a cephalosporin, is given intravenously 1 hour before surgery.

In emergency situations, where bowel preparations are not feasible, intraoperative lavage can be performed. Some investigators use 8 to 10 L of normal saline irrigated through the distal ileum, which may allow for a primary anastomosis after colon resection. Other surgeons have had good results using topical ampicillin powder applied to subfascial spaces.

Bowel preparations are advocated for noncolonic abdominal surgery to facilitate operative manipulation of the colon. The reduction of colonic bacterial flora may help to decrease translocation of bacteria postoperatively.

MANAGEMENT OF DIABETES MELLITUS

Patients with a history of diabetes should have their medical regimen re-evaluated prior to surgery. The home glucose monitoring of the patient will delineate the efficacy of their selfcare. The urinalysis and serum glucose also will verify the history. A hemoglogin A_{1c} concentration of <6% is the best way of diagnosing well-controlled diabetes mellitus. If the patient is well controlled, preoperative management entails a reasonable caloric intake with 50% carbohydrates. Ingestion of smaller meals with snacks will minimize postprandial hyperglycemia. Patients who take oral hypoglycemic agents should have their medication discontinued on the day of operation. The half-life of chlorpropamide extends beyond 36 hours and should not be resumed until after surgery. On the morning of surgery, insulin at 0.1 units/kg/L is added to intravenous fluids containing 5% dextrose. Patients on subcutaneous injections of insulin preoperatively will require their dosage of insulin at a reduced level on the morning of surgery. Patients who have blood glucose level less than 250 mg/dL can have one-half of their dose of NPH and regular insulin on the morning of surgery. They should also receive intravenous solutions containing 5% dextrose to simulate their usual morning carbohydrate load. If the preoperative glucose levels can have one-half of their dose of NPH and regular insulin on the morning of surgery. They should also receive intravenous solutions containing 5% dextrose to simulate their usual morning carbohydrate load. If the preoperative glucose level is <250 mg/dL, two-thirds of the usual amount of NPH and regular insulin is administered on the morning of surgery.

TABLE 13–17. RISK FACTORS ASSOCIATED WITH WOUND INFECTION

Diabetes Mellitus
Uremia
Poor blood supply or severe undermining of skin
Wound closed under tension
Malnutrition
Liver failure
Anemia
Sepsis
Hypoxia
Age
Obesity
Steroids and immunosuppressants
Chemotherapy
Previous local radiation treatments

Postoperatively, patients are monitored routinely before meals and at bedtime, or every 6 hours, if fasting. Regular insulin can be given subcutaneously in the postoperative care of diabetic patients. We prefer to give it intramuscularly since blood flow and therefore, absorption, is more consistent with this technique. If the blood glucose levels remain uncontrolled with increased dosages of insulin, the patient needs to be placed in a closely monitored area with continuous intravenous administration of insulin.

The stress of trauma or surgery may cause a diabetic patient to suffer from diabetic ketoacidosis. Symptoms of polydypsia, polyuria, weakness, malaise, nausea, vomiting, and abdominal pain are not reliable immediately after operation. The patient may show signs of dehydration from the hyperosmolar diuresis induced by hyperglycemia. Kussmaul's respirations and ketotic breath are seen with severe acidosis. Blood serum levels of glucose are usually >350 mg/dL ketones >5 mmol/L, and bicarbonate levels are reduced. Electrolyte imbalances occur in diabetic ketoacidosis with pseudohyperkalemia and variable sodium levels, depending on the amount of free water lost. If time permits, correction of fluid and electrolytes with continuous infusion of insulin is the treatment of choice in postoperative patients. If urgent surgical intervention is needed in the preoperative ketoacidotic patient, a blood pH of >7.3 and a bicarbonate level >20 mEq/L are desired. A higher level of insulin can be infused with large fluid replacements, as long as blood sugars are followed closely. If the pH <7.1, bicarbonate administration should be given. Ideally, 48 hours of stable blood glucose levels should be obtained before elective surgery is performed.

Diabetic patients should be examined for possible infectious sites, especially in the lower extremities. Closer attention needs to be placed on the chronic conditions seen in chronic diabetics (ie, vascular insufficiency, nephropathy, neuropathy, and silent cardiac ischemia).

■ POSTOPERATIVE MANAGEMENT

PAIN MANAGEMENT

All surgical procedures will produce postoperative pain of variable intensity. Severe pain impairs respiratory excursion and may worsen atelectasis. Postoperative pain also is implicated in prolonging gastrointestinal ileus, urinary retention, and the increasing bedrest that may worsen the risk of deep vein thrombosis. The increased levels of catecholamines increases myocardial oxygen consumption and work.

Postoperative pain management has improved with patient-controlled analgesic (PCA) devices that alleviate pain upon request of the patient. The increased usage of epidural catheters also has improved postoperative pulmonary toilet after major abdominal surgery. Postoperative pain is less intense and shorter in duration in patients who receive epidural narcotics, as compared to patients who receive intravenous narcotics. Normalization of pulmonary VC and peak expiratory flow is achieved with postoperative epidural anesthesia. The introduction of intramuscular nonsteroidal anti-inflammatory agents also have decreased the use of narcotics. Nonsteroidal anti-inflammatory agents have proven useful in patients who are tolerant to opiates and in the elderly. Many hospitals have specialized anesthesia consultant teams to aid in prescribing a variety of analgesics in difficult cases. Most physicians inadequately prescribe narcotics, and nurses tend to give less than the prescribed amounts to prevent the feared side effects of respiratory depression or narcotic addiction. Studies have shown that narcotic addiction does not develop in the postoperative patient unless a routine dosage of narcotics is given for >2 weeks.

POSTOPERATIVE FEVERS

Low-grade temperatures >38°C occur in nearly 40% of postoperative patients.[20] Fevers in the early postoperative period usually are not related to infections. Infections tend to cause fevers approximately 3 days after surgery, although this is not an absolute rule and preexisting occult infections may flourish in the early postoperative phase. The approach to postoperative fevers requires a physical examination to determine if confirmatory tests are needed. Ordering a battery of tests, the "shotgun" approach, in postoperative patients with fevers is cost inefficient. Frequent examinations of the patient, including auscultation of the lungs and examination of the surgical wounds, will narrow the choice of laboratory tests. Most early postoperative fevers develop from mechanical ventilation during general anesthesia. Postoperatively, a poor cough reflex, in addition to preexisting pulmonary disease or upper abdominal incisions will increase pulmonary atelectasis. Prolonged atelectasis may lead to the development of pneumonia. Prevention of atelectasis, and the associated fevers, requires early ambulation by the patient, deep breathing, and incentive spirometry.

Urinary tract infections are common in older male patients with benign prostatic hypertrophy, or in patients with indwelling catheters. Wound infections are seen later in the postoperative course unless clostridium or streptococcus are the causative bacteria. If cellulitis or wound drainage is noted, the wound should be promptly opened and drained to prevent erosion though fascial layers. Physical examination of the patient may suggest the need for diagnostic tests, including chest x-rays, blood cultures, complete blood count, sputum culture, urinalysis, and urine cultures.

HYPOTHERMIA

Hypothermia may occur in patients undergoing operations in which the abdominal cavity is opened for a prolonged period. Convection of heat occurs via the intestinal blood supply and evaporation of fluids at the peritoneal and visceral surfaces. Postoperatively, severe hypothermia may be detrimental to coagulation by prolonging the clotting time. Careful monitoring of core temperatures in the operating room, or in the recovery unit, can be achieved easily via a Swan-Ganz catheter with a temperature probe, or a rectal thermometer. Reversal of hypothermia can be achieved by warming intravenous fluids or blood products in the operating room. In the recovery room, warming blankets, using circulating warm water or air, are effective.

MANAGEMENT OF DRAINS AND TUBES

Patients may return from the operating room with a host of tubes and drains placed during surgery. Nurses and physicians need to be aware that each of these tubes have special requirements. An operative sketch of tubes and their placements in the operative note will reduce possible confusion.

Nasogastric Tubes

Nasogastric tubes are used to empty the stomach and duodenum of secretions and swallowed air. Theoretically, this decreases downstream fluid transport, which allows the gut to rest and remain undistended, and to protect anastomoses. Numerous studies have shown that routine use of nasogastric tubes are unnecessary in a variety of gastrointestinal surgeries.

Sump nasogastric tubes frequently are misused when the sump port is plugged to prevent reflux of bilious material. Patency of the sump tubing must be maintained with continuous suction through the gastric port. An increased rate of aspiration is associated with a nonfunctioning nasogastric tube. The Levin tube has the advantage of patient comfort, but patency is more difficult to maintain. Levin nasogastric tubes need to be placed on intermittent suction in order to prevent self-collapse of the tubing or continuous suctioning against the stomach wall. Often the first complaint of patients is pain in the posterior pharynx secondary to the nasogastric tube. Topical sprays and lozenges may help to alleviate some of the discomfort.

Long Intestinal Tubes

Long intestinal tubes (Cantor or Miller-Abbott) are used occasionally in patients with recurrent, chronic, or early postoperative partial small bowel obstructions. A latex bag filled with mercury is at the end of a tube equipped with multiple side ports. The patient is repositioned at various times to allow the progression to the site of partial obstruction. The goal is to have peristalsis propel the tube distally to decompress the bowel. In theory, bowel-wall edema exists proximal to the partially obstructed site, making the partial obstruction worse. Once decompression of the edematous proximal bowel is achieved, resolution of the obstruction may occur. Removal of the tube is performed by pulling the tube out one to two feet every hour. It should be noted that many partial small bowel obstructions will need surgical relief.

Gastric tonometry

Gastric tonometry (pHi), a new monitoring tool, is used in the intensive care unit to estimate visceral blood flow. If consists of a modified nasogastric tube with a latex balloon at the tip of the tube. The balloon is intermittently filled with normal saline and left in the stomach for a prescribed time. Hydrogen ions diffuse freely through the latex balloon and into the normal saline, which is removed and analyzed for H^+ concentration. Using the Henderson-Hasselbach equation, the amount of hydrogen ions retrieved intraluminally compared to arterial pH represents gastric perfusion, which correlates with oxygen delivery to the visceral organs. It is debatable whether the gastric pHi can replace the right-sided heart catheter. Studies on the predictive value of gastric tonometry have shown it to be helpful in determining whether a patient can be weaned from the mechanical ventilator.

$$pHi = 6.1 + \log HCO3/(gastric\ pCO2 \times 0.0307)$$

In one study, patients with a reduced pHi (gastric pHi of 7.09 to 7.36) during weaning could not be weaned from the ventilator. Patients who had no change in the gastric pHi were weaned successfully from the ventilator.[21] Other studies have shown gastric tonometry to be an early predictor of death in multisystem organ failure, as compared to calculating oxygen delivery and oxygen consumption.[22] Further studies will determine the role of gastric tonometry in the intensive care patient.

Closed-Suction Drains

Closed-suction catheters are used routinely and are associated with a reduced incidence of drain-related infection and complication. The care of closed-suction drains is simple and patients can be taught to change a bandage around the exit site of the drain and to measure drain output on a daily basis. Patients often are sent home with closed-suction drains and instructed to return to clinic for removal when a certain minimal output is achieved.

Penrose Drains

The Penrose drain is one of the oldest types of drain and usually is brought through the skin via a separate skin incision. Management of this drain entails frequent changing of the gauze covering the drain. The drain is gradually removed when drainage from the site is diminished. The slow withdrawal of the Penrose tube breaks the newly formed fibrin around the drain and allows continued drainage of the deep cavity. Once the drain is removed completely, a bandage is placed over the exit site and secondary wound healing is allowed to take place.

Foley Catheters

Bladder catheters are routinely left in place after general anesthesia to monitor urine output in the immediate postoperative period. The most common complication of Foley catheters is urinary tract infections. The distal urethra is colonized with bacteria, causing ascending urinary tract infections in approximately 10% to 25% of patients. Urinary tract infections tend to develop within 3 to 4 days after catheterization, in 95% of patients. *Escherichia coli* is the most common pathogen of urinary tract infections, followed by *Enterobacter,* staphylococcus, streptococcus, and enterococcus species. The usual presentation of urinary tract infection is postoperative fever or sepsis which may be confirmed by urine microscopy and culture. Methods such as a strict closed-catheter system have reduced the infection rate. Urinary tract infections are easily preventable by removing catheters as soon as possible. Once diagnosed, antibiotics such as sulfomethaxosole-trimethoprim, ampicillin, or ciprofloxacin are used routinely.

POSTOPERATIVE COMPLICATIONS

Cardiovascular complications often occur in the elderly patient undergoing general or spinal anesthesia. Optimization of the cardiac status of the patient should be performed preoperatively. Careful volume management during and after the surgery must be managed by the physician. Patients with previous cardiac disease should be aware of the risks of general surgery and be informed of possible postoperative angina or arrhythmias. Hypertension in the postoperative period is exacerbated by pain or hypoxia. Adequate pain management and supplemental oxygen should be administered before any antihypertensive medication. Most postoperative hypertension can be managed with sublingual nifedipine until the patient is able to resume preoperative oral medications.

Respiratory Complications

Respiratory complications are common in postoperative patients. Atelectasis occurs in all patients within five to ten minutes of induction of general anesthesia. Up to 40% of postoperative patients will have radiographic changes consistent with atelectasis. Lower abdominal incisions and transverse abdominal incisions may lower the incidence of atelectasis and pneumonias. Preoperative education, incentive spirometry, and pulmonary toilet may help to reduce atelectasis in the early postoperative period. Incentive spirometry has been shown to be of less value in the late postoperative period. Preoperative antibiotics for active bronchitis should be continued after the operation to prevent pneumonias. The use of bronchodilators is helpful in patients with reactive airway disease and chronic obstructive pulmonary disease. A lack of efficacy in studies with aerosolized bronchodilators and intermittent positive-pressure bronchodilation has virtually eliminated their use. Hand-held nebulizers are just as effective. The best treatment to prevent complication is early ambulation.

Wound Infection

The incidence of wound infection correlates with the wound classification at the time of surgery. Wounds are classified into four different groups that correlate with infection rates.

The majority of class I and II wounds will heal by primary intention without complications, whereas primary closure of class IV wounds will have a 50% wound-infection rate.[23] Careful scrutiny of the wound is needed by the surgeon, if contaminated wounds are closed. Some surgeons advocate closure of severely contaminated wounds with closed suction drains. If the wound is left open, antiseptic agents, such as povidone-iodine solutions or Dakin's solution, have been shown to inhibit fibroblastic activity during wound healing,[24] and should not be used except in extremely dirty wounds. The traditional manner of using wet-to-dry wound packings, using normal saline for gentle debridement of open wounds, usually will keep a wound clean. Once the bacterial count is $<10^5/gm$, the wound can be closed as a delayed primary closure 4 to 5 days after surgery.

A wound needs to be opened upon recognition of infection to prevent abscess formation and erosion through fascial layers. The role of antibiotics is questionable if no signs of cellulitis are present. Staphylococcal infections with their associated cellulitis will benefit from a short course of intravenous antibiotic therapy. Anaerobic wound infections often are characterized by local pain and palpable crepitus. Wound infections with streptococcus or clostridium species will manifest with fevers immediately in the postoperative course. A particular synergistic wound infection, Meleney's infection, is observed with *Staphylococcus aureus* and microaerophilic nonhemolytic *Streptococcus*. Examination of the wound may reveal the presence of subcutaneous air. Aggressive debridement of all necrotic tissue and high-dose broad spectrum antibiotic administration is instituted immediately. Some of the predisposing factors for wound infections are listed in Table 13–17.

Thromboembolism

Pulmonary embolism occurs in 500 000 to 600 000 patients annually with approximately 67 000 patients dying within the first hour of diagnosis and another one-third eventually dying. Deep venous thrombosis (DVT) is the third most common cause of death in the United States. Patients presenting with the acute onset of dyspnea in the postoperative period should always be suspected of having a pulmonary embolus. If the diagnosis is made early, only 8% to 10% die after initiation of early treatment. Recognition of risk factors which predispose patients to thromboembolism is critical to early diagnosis (Table 13–18). The majority of pulmonary emboli form in the deep venous systems of the lower extremities, while a small percentage develop in the deep pelvic venous system. The sudden onset of dyspnea is the most common presenting symptom of pulmonary embolism. Half of all affected patients will have rales at the involved side. Only 28% of patients will have the classic symptoms of pleuritic chest pain, dyspnea, and hemoptysis, making the clinical diagnosis difficult.[25]

Prevention of thromboembolism begins with placement of pulsatile lower-extremity stockings prior to the onset of general anesthesia. If pelvic surgery is involved, subcutaneous injections of heparin or low-dose coumadin therapy also should be considered. Patients with hypercoagulable states by history should have a hematology consultation considered before operation, to determine adequate therapy during surgery.

Once a suspicion of pulmonary embolus is entertained, treatment with heparin should be initiated. Confirmation of the diagnosis is difficult. Ventilation-perfusion (V/Q) scans are a useful noninvasive technique. Unfortunately, a majority of V/Q scans are inde-

terminate. Pulmonary angiography is the gold standard to diagnose embolus to the lung, but the stability of the patient and renal function make the test impractical to use in many clinical settings. Duplex scanning of the lower extremities or plethysmography is helpful if DVT are visualized, but the absence of DVT in the lower extremities does not rule out embolism.

Patients who have DVT diagnosed without pulmonary embolization occurring may undergo placement of an inferior vena cava filter or receive anticoagulation therapy. Placement of a caval filter is useful in patients who may continue to have further embolizations.

Heparin accelerates the action of antithrombin III by binding to factor XIIa, XIa, IXa, Xa, and thrombin, decreasing thrombus formation. A standard preoperative prophylactic regimen consists of 5000 units administered subcutaneously followed by another 5000 units 8 to 12 hours postoperatively. The prophylactic dose is much lower than a therapeutic dose for the treatment of pulmonary embolization. Low-dose prophylactic heparin can decrease the incidence of DVT by 68% and pulmonary embolism by 49%.[26]

Dextran given intravenously has been used as a prophylactic agent for DVT formation. Dextran, initially used as a volume expander, is available as Dextran 40 or Dextran 70. Dextran is a glucose polymer that decreases viscosity and platelet interactions within damaged endothelium. Dextran also increases clot fibrinolysis.[27] Dextran is administered in a volume of 500 mL during 6 hours before surgery and then every day for 2 to 5 days after surgery. The problems with dextran include volume overload, lack of efficacy, and high cost.

Oral therapy with warfarin is the standard therapy for long-term treatment of venous thromboembolism. Warfarin inhibits the vitamin K–dependent coagulation factors, II, VII, IX and X, and protein C. An aim to prolong prothrombin times to 1.5 to 2 times control values can prevent recurrence of thromboembolism. Patients are admitted to the hospital for discontinuation of warfarin and initiation of heparin prior to surgery.

Antiplatelet therapy with aspirin has been appealing because of the simplicity and low cost. Unfortunately, the results from clinical trials have been conflicting. At this time, aspirin can not be recommended as prophylaxis for deep venous thrombosis.

Graduated compression stockings and intermittent pneumatic leg compression boots are effective at preventing DVT in the low-risk patient. The physical compression of the lower extremities eliminate stasis in the proximal veins and increases the fibrinolytic activity. Compression stockings need to be used until patients are able to ambulate after surgery. Compression stockings used in conjunction with heparin may be even more efficacious than either one used alone.

TABLE 13–18. RISK FACTORS PREDISPOSING TO THROMBOEMBOLISM

Cancer
Advancing age
Pelvic surgery
Stroke
Inflammatory bowel disease
Obesity
Prior history of thromboembolism
Prolonged immobilization
Sepsis
Estrogen therapy
Pregnancy
Congestive heart failure
Lupus anticoagulant
Nephrotic syndrome
Inherited (protein C or S deficiencies, antithrombin III deficiency)

Modified from Consensus Conference. Prevention of venous thrombosis and pulmonary embolism. *JAMA* 1986;256:744–757

Upper Gastrointestinal Hemorrhage

The incidence of life-threatening upper gastrointestinal bleeding has been decreased with routine administration of antiulcer medications. Histamine, or H2, receptor antagonists have been less effective than antacids in preventing massive upper gastrointestinal bleeding. Administration of 30 cc of antacids every 1 to 2 hours to maintain the gastric pH above 4.0 is considered adequate prophylaxis. Recently, continuous infusions of H2 receptor antagonists rather than intermittent dosing have been shown to be more efficacious in preventing gastric stress ulcerations. Antacids and H2 blockers cause bacterial overgrowth and increase the risk of aspiration pneumonia. The use of sucralfate does not alter gastric pH and may, therefore, prevent bacterial overgrowth. Further prevention of upper gastrointestinal hemorrhage is directed towards maintaining the protective enteral barrier. The gastrointestinal mucosal barrier can be maintained with enteral nutrition.

REFERENCES

1. Goldman L, Caldera DL, Nussbaum SR, et al. Multifactorial index of cardiac index in noncardiac surgical procedures. *N Engl J Med* 1977;297:845–850
2. Jackson MCV. Preoperative pulmonary evaluation. *Arch Intern Med* 1988;148:2120–2127
3. Lawrence VA, Page CP, Harris GD. Preoperative spirometry before abdominal operations. A critical appraisal of its predictive value. *Arch Intern Med* 1989;149:280–285
4. Latimer RG, Dickman M, Day WC, et al. Ventilatory patterns and pulmonary complications after upper abdominal surgery determined by preoperative and postoperative computerized spirometry and blood gas analysis. *Am J Surg* 1971;122:622–632
5. Rowe JW. Clinical research on aging: strategies and directions. *N Engl J Med* 1977;297:1332
6. Carrie BJ, Golbetz HV, Michaels AS, et al. Creatinine: an inadequate filtration marker in glomerular diseases. *Am J Med* 1980;69:177
7. Bistrian BR, Blackburn GI, Hallowell E, et al. Protein status of general surgical patients. *JAMA* 1974;230:858–860
8. Moss G, Greenstein A, Levy S, et al. Maintenance of GI function after bowel surgery and immediate enteral full nutrition, I. doubling of canine colorectal anastomotic bursting pressure and intestinal wound mature collagen content. *JPEN* 1980;4:535
9. Gault MH, Dixon ME, Doyle M, et al. Hypernatremia,azotemia and dehydration due to high protein tube feeding. Ann Intern Med 1968;68:778–791
10. Askanazi J, Elwyn DH, Silverberg PA, et al. Respiratory distress secondary to a high carbohydrate load: a case report. *Surgery* 1980;87:596–598
11. Kaplan EB, Shiner LB, Beckman AJ, et al. The usefulness of preoperative laboratory screening. *JAMA* 1985;253:3576
12. Corr PB, Burton BE. Biochemical and metabolic factors contributing to malignant ventricular arrhythmias. In: Josephson ME, (ed), *Ventricular Tachycardia: Mechanisms and Management.* Mt. Kisco, NY: Futura; 1982:97
13. Daly JM, Copeland EM, Dudrick SJ. Preparation of the Patient. In: Nyhus LM, Baker RJ, (ed), *Mastery of Surgery.* Boston, MA: Little, Brown; 1984:3–18
14. Feliciano DV, Spjut-Patrinely. Preoperative, intraoperative, and postoperative antibiotics. *Surg Clin North Am* 1990;6:698–701
15. Fullen WD, Hunt J, Altemeier WA. Prophylactic antibiotics in penetrating wounds of the abdomen. *J Trauma* 1972;12:282
16. Hayek LJ, Emerson JM, Gardner AMN. A placebo-controlled trial of the effect of two preoperative baths or showers with chlorhexidine detergent on postoperative wound infection rates. *J Hosp Infect* 1987;10:165
17. Masterson TM, Rodeheaver GT, Morgan RF, et al. Bacteriologic evaluation of electric clippers for surgical hair removal. *Am J Surg* 1984;148:L301
18. Hamilton HW, Hamilton KR, Lone FJ. Preoperative hair removal. *Can J Surg* 1977;20:269
19. Bicknell PG. Sensorineural deafness following myringoplasty operations. *J Laryngol Otol* 1971;85:957
20. Kenan S, Lievergall M, Simchen E, et al. Fever following orthopedic operations in children. *J Pediatr Orthop* 1986;6:139
21. Mohsenifar Z, Hay A, Hay J, et al. Gastric intramural pH as a predictor of success or failure in weaning patients from mechanical ventilation. *Ann Intern Med* 1993;119:794–798
22. Marik PE. Gastric intramucosal pH. A better predictor of multiorgan dysfunction syndrome and death than oxygen-derived variables in patients with sepsis. *Chest* 1993;104:225–229
23. Cruse PJE, Foord R. The epidemiology of wound infection: a 10 year prospective study of 62 939 wounds. *Surg Clin North Am* 1980;60:27
24. Lineaweaver W, Howard R, Soucy D, et al. Topical antimicrobial toxicity. *Arch Surg* 1985;120:267
25. Killewick LA, Martin R, Cramer M, et al. Pathophysiiology of venous claudication. *J Vasc Surg* 1984;1:507–511
26. Consensus Conference. Prevention of venous thrombosis and pulmonary embolism. *JAMA* 1986;256:744–757
27. Hull RD, Raskob GE, Hirsch J. Prophylaxis of venous thromboembolism: an overview. *Chest* 1986;89:374S–383S

14

Hernias

Jack Abrahamson

A hernia may be defined generally as a protrusion of abdominal viscera outside the abdominal cavity through a natural or acquired defect. However, this definition does not include internal hernias in which abdominal viscera, usually the small bowel, enter preformed intraperitoneal sacs commonly found around the duodenum, cecum, and sigmoid colon.

■ INGUINAL HERNIA

HISTORY

The earliest record of inguinal hernia dates back to approximately 1500 BC. The ancient Greeks were well aware of inguinal hernias, and the term derives from the Greek word meaning an offshoot, a budding, or bulge. The Latin word *hernia* means a rupture or tear. Trusses and bandages generally were used to control the herniation. In the earlier part of the first century AD, Celsus described the operation in vogue at that time in the Greco-Roman area.[1] Through an incision in the neck of the scrotum, the hernial sac was dissected off the spermatic cord and transected at the external inguinal ring. The testis usually was excised as well. The incision was generally left open. Later, a mass ligature of the sac and cord at the external ring was recommended, with excision of the sac, cord, and testis distal to the ligature, as described by Paul of Aegina in 700 AD.

Guy de Chauliac, in 1363, differentiated between inguinal and femoral hernia and described the technique of reduction for strangulation.[2] In 1556, Franco illustrated the use of a grooved director to cut the strangulating neck of the hernia while avoiding the bowel.[3] Casper Stromayr, in 1559, published a comprehensive textbook on hernia in which he distinguished direct from indirect hernia and advised that the testicle need not be removed during an operation for the former.[4]

Little information was added to the literature until the beginning of the 18th century. From this time until the early 19th century the anatomy of the inguinal region was described and accurately defined. The dawn of modern surgery began in 1865 when Joseph Lister introduced his method of antisepsis by carbolic spray. By the beginning of the 20th century, Koch had developed methods of asepsis, which was followed by modern dry and wet heat sterilization.

Tissue Repairs

Marcy, an American surgeon and a pupil of Lister, was the first to introduce antiseptic techniques in the repair of hernia. He was also the first to recognize the importance of the transversalis fascia and of closing the internal ring. In 1871, he published his report of two patients operated on in the previous year in whom he used carbolized catgut to suture the ring.[5] A French pupil of Lister, Lucas-Championniere, brought antisepsis to France.[6] In 1881 he reported that the first case in which the aponeurosis of the external oblique muscle was slit to reveal the canal, which allowed dissection and ligation of the sac at the internal ring under direct vision. The depressing fact at this time was that the best surgical centers in both Europe and North America were reporting mortality rates of up to 7% for hernia operations. The recurrence rate after 1 year was 30% to 40%, and almost all hernias had recurred by the end of 4 years.

The greatest contribution to hernia surgery was that of the Italian surgeon Edoardo Bassini.[7–12] His clear insight into the anatomy and physiology of the inguinal region enabled him to dissect and reconstruct the inguinal canal to preserve the functional anatomy. He laid the inguinal canal open widely by splitting the aponeurosis of the external oblique. He next opened the transversalis fascia from the pubic tubercle to beyond the internal ring. In this way he was able to dissect and ligate the sac high in the retroperitoneal space. He realized the importance of repairing the transversalis fascia and of reinforcing the posterior wall of the canal: using interrupted sutures of silk, he sutured the internal oblique and transversus abdominis muscles, as well as the upper leaf of the transversalis fascia in one layer to the lower leaf of the transversalis fascia and the inguinal ligament. The rectus sheath was incorporated into the medial end of the repair. The aponeurosis of the external oblique muscle was resutured in front of the spermatic cord.

Bassini first performed this operation in 1884 and reported it in 1887. He published his results in 1887, 1888, 1889, 1890, and finally, in 1894.[7–12] He reported 206 operations with no operative mortality. The patients varied from young children to elderly men. His series included cases operated on for strangulation; bilateral repairs were done, and associated cryptorchidism was dealt with at the same operation. Bassini reported an almost 100% follow-up of his patients for 5 years, with 11 wound infections and only eight recurrences. These phenomenal results earned him the title of "Father of Modern Herniorrhaphy."

During the next 100 years, most inguinal hernias were repaired by the Bassini method or variations of it. Some of the variations were unsuccessful because of the lack of understanding of the functional anatomy of the area and others were improvements and reduced the incidence of recurrent hernia.

Notable among the improvements is the multilayered repair described by Shouldice in 1953.[13] This method has become popular in the past 20 years and is probably the most successful of the "pure tissue" methods, suturing only the local tissues without the addition of any prosthetic material. The recurrence rate in primary hernia repair, as reported from the Shouldice Hospital in Toronto, is <1%. Others, such as Myers and Shearburn, have confirmed these results.[14] However, this method is rather complicated and, in some cases, calls for extensive dissection and suturing under tension. Modern pioneers in the field of tissue repairs, such as Berliner and Lichtenstein, have developed simpler but equally successful methods.[15,16]

In 1898, George Lotheissen first reported the technique of suturing the musculoaponeurotic arch (conjoined tendon) to the pectineal (Cooper's) ligament, as opposed to the inguinal (Poupart's) ligament popularized by Bassini.[17] The Lotheissen method had the added advantage of repairing the femoral ring as well as the inguinal defects and was popular in Europe for repair of both of these types of hernia. It was especially recommended for a strangulated femoral hernia. This repair was popularized in the United States around 1940 by McVay who showed, by anatomical dissections, that the transversus abdominis muscle and its fascia are normally inserted onto the pectineal ligament.[18] He stressed the importance of preserving this anatomical plane. McVay stated that, since the fascia transversalis was not attached to the inguinal ligament and since they were in two different planes, there was no anatomic reason for suturing them together. Rutledge has used this technique extensively and in 1988 published his 25 year experience, with a success rate equal to that of the leading hernia centers that use a variety of other techniques.[19] In 1993 he described the method in detail and brought his experience to date.[20]

Critics of the Cooper ligament repair are of the opinion that, since this ligament is lower down and further posterior to the inguinal ligament, a great deal more tension is brought about by bringing the conjoined tendon down to Cooper's ligament and that this tension is not adequately relieved by the so-called relaxing incision. The anatomical fact that the transversalis fascia inserts onto Cooper's ligament does not oblige the surgeon to attempt to reattach the attenuated and torn fascia to its original anatomical site. Furthermore, since the normal anatomy is either rearranged or destroyed when doing a tissue repair of an inguinal hernia, there is no special anatomic logic for bringing down the conjoined tendon with extra tension to Cooper's ligament to preserve the original plane. These critics also state that the Bassini principle of suturing the conjoined tendon to the inguinal ligament has proved itself in many hundreds of thousands of cases. The Cooper's ligament operation is a more difficult one, involving much wider dissection and tedious suturing and is not popular. In good hands, it undoubtedly does give excellent results. The technique is most valuable when repairing a recurrent inguinal hernia when the inguinal ligament is destroyed. Lotheissen originally used his operation in this setting.

In spite of superb results in special centers or by surgeons particularly interested in the subject, the overall results of hernia repair today are far from satisfactory, with recurrence rates varying from 10% to 30%.[21] The basic cause of this unacceptable situation is faulty technique on the part of the operating surgeon owing mainly to ignorance of the functional anatomy and physiology of the abdominal wall. This leads to incomplete dissection and often, to repair under tension. Other factors include the use of wrong suture materials and infection. These factors are especially common in early recurrence.

A hernia repair done with undue tension is doomed to failure. This failure is not usually the result of some inherent weakness of the tissues, but is an ischemic necrosis of the tissues caused by pressure of sutures under tension. The problem is that most inguinal hernia repairs are based on the Bassini principle of suturing the so-called conjoined tendon to the inguinal ligament. The ease with which this can be done depends on the individual anatomy of the patient. In some cases, the musculoaponeurotic arch of the conjoined tendon is low and close to the inguinal ligament, but in others it is high, with a wide gap between it and the inguinal ligament. In this situation, the only way the two sutures can be approximated is with great tension, by a determined surgeon. Some surgeons compromise by using "relaxing" incisions or "slides" to lessen the tension, but the contribution of this maneuver in reducing the incidence of recurrence is questionable. A further anatomic variation is the index of aponeurosis to muscle in the musculoaponeurotic arch of the conjoined tendon, which has a wide range of variation. When much aponeurotic tissue is present, the sutures will hold to a greater degree, but the fleshy muscular arch will cut through more easily, especially if sutured under tension.

Darn Repairs

To overcome these problems, operators have sought the ideal tensionless or tension-free repair. There has always been general agreement that the first step, after dealing with the sac, is to repair the weakened or torn posterior wall of the inguinal canal, the transversalis fascia, and to tighten the stretched internal inguinal ring around the cord. This means doing a Marcy-type of repair.[5] Some surgeons have been satisfied with this procedure alone, but others have sought a means of reinforcing the posterior wall with either natural tissue or biologic or synthetic material in the form of a tension-free darn between the conjoined tendon and the inguinal ligament.

The earliest of these darners was McArthur, who, in 1901, reported using pedicled strips of the external oblique aponeurosis woven between the conjoined tendon and the inguinal ligament.[22] He was followed in 1910 by Kirschner, who used fascial grafts from the thigh.[23] In 1918 Handley introduced the "darn and stay-lace" procedure, using silk.[24] Gallie and LeMesurier, in 1921, published the use of fascia lata strips used as sutures woven into the muscles, the inguinal ligament, and the tissues of the posterior wall of the inguinal canal

"much as one would darn a sock."[25] Others, such as Mair, used strips of skin cut off the edges of the incision and denuded of dermis.[26]

These living tissues were difficult to harvest and tended to be absorbed. They also caused complications inherent in the tissue used. The recurrence rate was still significant.

In the search for a suitable substitute, in 1937 Ogilvie introduced his "silk lattice repair," using nonabsorbable silk sutures;[27] he was followed by Maingot in 1940, 1941, and 1979, who advocated floss silk for his darn.[28-30] McLeod also reported using silk for the posterior lattice repair.[31] Silk, being a biologic substance, lost most of its strength within a few months and also caused major problems in infected wounds. The twisted or braided threads allowed organisms to settle within the suture material. The silk was deep in the infected wounds and perpetuated chronic sinuses and was also incorporated in the infected granulomatous scar tissue and thus was difficult to remove. This was especially true for the floss silk.

Soon after nylon became available, Nichols and Diack, and Aries, explored its use in surgery in experimental animals.[32,33] In 1942, Melick first reported the use of braided, multifilament nylon for the repair of inguinal hernia.[34] There were also a number of reported animal experiments with this synthetic material.[35-37] Following his animal experiments, Haxton, in 1945, stated that he had used monofilament nylon in 300 operations to suture various tissues, including skin.[37] While not specifically stated, it is assumed that he used the material for repair of hernias.

Moloney introduced the forerunner of the modern nylon darn technique in 1948.[38] He advocated first a Bassini-type suture of continuous monofilament nylon to bring down the conjoined tendon to the inguinal ligament, but with no attempt to approximate these two structures forcefully if the suture were too tight. This suture then was followed by a second continuous suture passing laterally from the pubic tubercle between good strong tissue in the rectus sheath and the tendinous portion of the internal oblique muscle above to the inguinal ligament below and ending beyond the internal ring. His recurrence rate was less than 1%.[39,40] These results have been confirmed by others.[41-49] For the sake of accuracy, it should be noted that not all of the surgeons in these reports were using a strict tensionless darn. Some were, in fact, doing a Bassini-type repair, with a continuous suture repeated once or twice. This author reported a series of more than 1000 cases of inguinal hernia repaired by his modification of the nylon darn, with a recurrence rate in primary repairs of 0.8%.[47,49] There was one recurrence in the last 300 cases of primary repair, a rate of 0.33%.

This is a tensionless technique in which, after dealing with the sac, the posterior wall of the canal is repaired by approximating the rectus sheath and conjoined tendon to the inguinal ligament with a continuous monofilament nylon suture. When these structures cannot be brought together easily, the gap between them is narrowed as far as possible, without creating tension. A tensionless darn is now applied using a continuous nylon thread in three runs, between the rectus sheath and conjoined tendon above and the inguinal ligament below. Each run of nylon slopes in a different direction so that the threads interweave to form a strong permanent latticework that reinforces the repair or the gap between the conjoined tendon and the inguinal ligament. This technique has become popular because of its simplicity, general applicability, and very low recurrence rate. In a recent survey of consultant surgeons in the United Kingdom, it was found that 35% used a nylon darn as their sole method of repair (ie, more than by any other method).[50] The Shouldice repair alone or combined with other methods was used by only 20% of the consultants. In the United States, Mansberger reported his series of darn repairs done according to the Moloney technique.[51]

Patch Graft Repairs

While the darners were darning, the patchers were seeking the ideal patch in the form of a sheet of natural tissues, biological materials, metals, or synthetic sheets or weaves to fill in the gap in the weakened posterior wall of the canal. The earliest reports, from 1900 to 1909, were those of Witzel and Goepel, in Germany; Bartlett, in the United States, and McGavin, in Britain.[52-55] They used silver-wire filigree sheets shaped to fit the size and contours of the gap in the tissues and sutured to the borders of the defect. In most cases, however, the wire corroded and fragmented and was rejected through chronic sinuses, and the hernia recurred.

Tantalum metal sheets were introduced by Burke in 1940,[56] and tantalum gauze by Throckmorton in 1948.[57] They were further reported on separately by Lam, Koontz, and Jefferson,[58-60] in 1948. However, metal fatigue caused fragmentation of this material, followed by recurrence of the hernia. Later reports noted skin sinuses due to these fragments and even erosion through the peritoneum and into small bowel, causing bowel fistulae.[61-63] Thus, the method was abandoned. Instead, surgeons sought sheets of natural tissues. Flaps of fascia from the thigh were hinged on the region of the inguinal ligament and swung up to be sutured to the anterior abdominal wall. Conversely, flaps of aponeuroses of the external or internal oblique muscle or of the anterior rectus sheath were turned down and sutured to the inguinal ligament. Others brought sheets of fascia as free grafts from the thigh, fascia lata, or abdominal wall and even sheets of skin, as reported by Mair in 1945,[26] to be sutured to the edges of the posterior wall of the inguinal

canal. These methods proved uniformly disappointing, and no real progress was made until the development of modern synthetic polymer plastics in the form of sheets of woven or knitted mesh of polyamide and the newer polypropylene. These were popularized by Usher in 1958.[64] The material is cheap and universally available, is easily cut to the required shape, is flexible and pleasant to handle, and is practically indestructible in human tissues. The threads are monofilament, extremely smooth, and inert and thus elicit little tissue reaction. Consequently, they are not rejected, even in the presence of infection. Collagen tissue can be laid down through the interstices of the weave so that the material is incorporated into healthy new tissue.

Sheets of woven or knitted synthetic polyester threads are used extensively in Europe, especially by French surgeons, but are not popular in the United States because of the fear of chronic infection perpetuated by the multifilament threads used to manufacture these prostheses.

Another synthetic material in the polymer series is polytetrafluoroethylene (PTFE), originally introduced as a mesh woven from monofilament threads. Animal experiments were reported by Harrison in 1957[65]; however, its use in humans was disappointing[66], and it is no longer used in this form. It has reappeared in a new expanded form that is microporous and has been extensively used for vascular prostheses. It is now available in sheets of varying thicknesses. It causes little tissue reaction, is partly invaded by connective tissue and collagen, is not easily infected, and is extremely strong. Because of these characteristics it has been used for the repair of hernias.[67-70] However, because of its high price and poor incorporation into the tissues, it is not popular.

In recent years, sheets of woven monofilament polyamide or knitted monofilament polypropylene have been used extensively.[16,71-73] This synthetic mesh usually is used to strengthen the repair of the transversalis fascia and is sutured either deep to or superficial to the transversalis fascia to create a strong and tensionless repair. It also is used as a simple inlay or onlay graft, sutured to the abdominal wall and inguinal ligament without the need to repair the fascia transversalis. Modern herniologists such as Lichtenstein and Gilbert have simply laid a swatch of the synthetic mesh, without sutures, deep to or in front of the repaired fascia transversalis.[16,73] They also have reported using a rolled-up strip or folded piece of the mesh to plug a wide internal ring, femoral hernias, or recurrent inguinal hernias. In this way, modern herniorrhaphy is rapidly becoming a simple, "tensionless and sutureless" operation.[73-78]

Preperitoneal Repairs

A history of inguinal hernia repair would be incomplete without a mention of the abdominal or preperitoneal approach. This approach was recorded by the ancient Hindus for cases of strangulated hernia. It was described in Europe in the Middle Ages and in the 16th century and was recommended toward the end of the 19th century. All these procedures were performed transperitoneally. Even as late as 1919, LaRoque described a gridiron transperitoneal incision for hernia repair.[79] The modern era of transabdominal, but extraperitoneal, repair of hernia was introduced by Cheatle in 1920.[80] He first used a midline incision, but later changed to a low transverse or Pfannenstiel incision. He peeled the peritoneum off the abdominal wall and bladder and was able to transect the sac and repair the internal ring from above. Various modifications and different incisions were described in reports from 1936 to 1954 that stressed the ease of exposure of the anatomy when approached from above and the facility of repair of inguinal and femoral hernias.[81–84] This approach was strongly recommended by Nyhus in 1960 and popularized by his group and by Read, in 1968 and 1979.[85–87] Read recommended this route for the use of prosthetic material, which also was endorsed by Nyhus, McVay, and Wantz.[18,88–92]

The approach from above has not been popularly adopted for routine hernia repair. Undoubtedly, the foremost proponent today of the preperitoneal approach is Stoppa, who recommends it especially for problematic cases in which repeated repairs of multiple recurrent hernia have been done and in which the tissues have become scarred and weakened and the normal anatomy destroyed. For these cases, he developed an operation he calls the great prosthesis for reinforcement of the visceral sac (GPRVS) in which, through a midline abdominal incision, a large sheet of prosthetic mesh is placed between the peritoneum and the abdominal wall to close off all hernial openings. He reported his technique and results in 1984, 1987 and 1989 and brought his experience up-to-date in 1992.[72,93–97]

The surgeon today can choose between four basic techniques for hernia repair as classified by Gilbert in 1987[73]; pure tissue repair, combined tissue and prosthetic repair, pure prosthetic repair, and nylon darn. He can use the method with which he is most comfortable, but must keep in mind that only a recurrence rate well below 1%, with a long and diligent follow-up, is acceptable.

Laparoscopic Repair for Inguinal Hernia

The tidal wave of minimal access surgery has inevitably swept hernia repair along in its surge. Laparoscopic transperitoneal closure of the internal orifice of groin hernias by a series of metal clips was introduced by Ger in 1977.[98] Since then several methods have evolved, but routine clinical application of the technique began only in 1990. The most popular method today is the introduction of the laparoscope and instruments through several ports in the abdominal wall after induction of pneumoperitoneum under general anesthesia. The pelvic peritoneum is opened in the region of the hernia and the sac is transected, after which a patch of synthetic mesh is placed over the hernial opening and fixed in place with metal clips. The peritoneum is replaced to cover the mesh and to isolate it from the intestines. Several extraperitoneal approaches are evolving in an attempt to avoid the risks and complications of opening the peritoneal cavity.[99,100] In the pediatric age group laparoscopic repair of inguinal hernia has been reported by Easter.[101]

The advantages of laparoscopic herniorrhaphy are that, in experienced hands, the method is quick and relatively atraumatic, bilateral repairs can be done at the same operation, clinically unsuspected contralateral hernias can be identified and repaired, and some of the complications of traditional hernia surgery, such as orchitis, epididymitis, wound infection and neuralgia, can be largely avoided. Only small openings are made in the abdominal wall; thus postoperative recovery and return to normal activities is rapid and practically painless.

On the other hand, the disadvantages include the need for a general anesthetic and violation of the abdominal cavity, with the future risk of adhesions as well as new hernias at the sites of introduction of the ports. The method has not been perfected, definitive instrumentation has not yet been developed, there is at yet no ideal synthetic material for intraperitoneal placement. The complications recorded include small and large bowel perforation, bladder laceration, adhesions, bowel obstruction, mesh erosion into the bladder, transient testicular pain, palpable mesh, mesh migration into the scrotum, scrotal hydrocele, and pelvic osteitis, the pros and cons of which have been discussed by many authors.[99,100,102–112]

The early results of laparoscopic herniorrhaphy are promising but the follow-up period is short and the number of cases is limited. The success of this new method must be measured against the gold standard of conventional hernia repair, which, in most of the cases, are done on an ambulatory basis without the need for admission to a hospital or general anesthesia.

INCIDENCE

The true incidence of inguinal hernia is not known, although fairly accurate estimates are available, based on different surveys.

Inguinal hernias in children are found in 10 to 20 per 1000 live births. The male to female ratio is 4:1. Almost all are indirect, with <1% presenting as direct hernias. Premature infants have a much higher incidence of inguinal hernias approximately 7% to 10%. The smaller the premature baby, the higher the incidence of hernias.

The overall incidence of inguinal hernias in adults in the Western hemisphere varies between 10% and 15%. The male to female ratio is 12:1. The incidence varies between 5% and 8% in patients 25 to 40 years of age. Hernias are present in ≥45% of males at 75 years of age and older. In 1993, Lichtenstein reported that over 700 000 groin hernia operations are performed annually in the United States.[113]

ANATOMY

The inguinal (Poupart) ligament is actually not a ligament but the curved inward free lower edge of the external oblique muscle between its origin on the iliac crest and its insertion at the pubis. It stretches from the anterior superior iliac spine to the pubic tubercle. The external oblique muscle is entirely aponeurotic in the inguinal region. Its fibers pass forward and downward to fuse with and to form the anterior rectus sheath and to fuse with the aponeurotic fibers of the external oblique muscle on the opposite side at the midline. Its lower free edge, the inguinal ligament, curves posteriorly and superiorly to form the shelf-like floor of the inguinal canal. At its insertion at the pubic tubercle, the fibers of the inguinal ligament flare out in a fan-like fashion to fuse with the anterior rectus sheath above (the reflected part of the inguinal ligament). These fibers also fuse with fibers from the opposite inguinal ligament along the upper border of the pubic bone (the superior pubic ligament), across the top and front of the pubic bones, fusing with the periosteum of the pubis, and downward to the superior pubic ramus to form the lacunar (Gimbernat) ligament. It continues on the superior pubic ramus along the pectineal line to form the pectineal (Cooper) ligament. The aponeurosis of the external oblique muscle forms the anterior wall of the inguinal canal and splits in a triangular fashion over the pubic bone (the external ring) through which the spermatic cord or round ligament emerges. The apex of the split is strengthened by intercrural fibers.

The next two layers, the internal oblique and the transversus abdominis muscles, arch over the spermatic cord in a lateromedial direction from their origin on the iliac crest and lateral part of the inguinal ligament to their insertion in the anterior rectus sheath and medial one-third of the inguinal ligament. In this way, they form the anterior wall of the inguinal canal in its lateral third, the roof of the canal in the middle third, and part of the posterior wall of the canal in its medial third. The lower edge of the internal oblique muscle is usually fleshy as it arches over the canal but is aponeurotic higher up. The lower edge of the transversus abdominis muscle is usually aponeurotic. Fibers of the internal oblique muscle pass down to envelop the cord and to constitute the cremaster muscle. The musculoaponeu-

rotic arch formed by these two muscles is called the conjoined tendon, even though the two muscles usually only fuse close to the anterior rectus sheath.

Deep to the transversus abdominis lies the endoabdominal fascia. The part of this fascia that lies in contact with the transversus abdominis muscle is called the transversalis fascia. It passes downward to emerge from behind the lower free edge of the transversus abdominis muscle and forms the posterior wall of the inguinal canal. The fascia is inserted along the pectineal line and contributes the anterior wall of the femoral sheath. After passing the inguinal ligament, a variable condensation of the transversalis fascia is named the iliopubic tract. The spermatic cord or round ligament emerges from the retroperitoneal space through the internal inguinal ring, which is bounded medially and inferiorly by a condensation of the transversalis fascia and superiorly and laterally by the aponeurotic lower edge of the transversus abdominis. The inferior epigastric artery passes upwards, close to the medial edge of the internal ring. That part of the transversalis fascia medial to the inferior epigastric vessels is known as Hesselbach's triangle, which is bounded by the vessels laterally, the conjoined tendon and rectus sheath superiorly, and the inguinal ligament inferiorly. Indirect inguinal hernias pass through the internal ring lateral to the inferior epigastric vessels, and direct hernias bulge forward medial to the vessels, through Hesselbach's triangle, pushing the attenuated transversalis fascia ahead of them or emerging through a tear in the fascia.

Between the fascia transversalis and the peritoneum is a loose layer of areolar tissue and fat.

ETIOLOGY

Much controversy surrounds the question of the cause of inguinal hernias. It is assumed that three factors are involved: the presence of a preformed sac, repeated elevations in the intra-abdominal pressure, and weakening of the body muscles and tissues with time. A patent processus vaginalis is held to be the prime cause of indirect inguinal hernia in infants and children, and probably in adults as well; yet almost all other mammals have a permanently patent processus vaginalis and only very rarely suffer from inguinal hernia. On the other hand, simple closure of the sac at the internal ring (herniotomy) cures indirect hernia in children. Jan found, at postmortem examination, that at least 20% of adults have a patent processus vaginalis, yet they did not have a hernia during life.[114] Surana reported this figure to be as high as 20% to 30%.[115,116]

Enormously high intra-abdominal pressures are generated when an individual coughs or strains, yet the abdominal wall usually maintains its integrity in spite of preformed weak areas, notably the transversalis fascia and the internal inguinal ring. This is generally explained on the basis of a "shutter mechanism." The muscles of the abdominal wall must contract to raise the intra-abdominal pressure. As the external oblique muscle contracts, it becomes tense and presses on the weak posterior wall of the inguinal canal and so reinforces it and also tends to pull the inguinal ligament upward (ie, convex cranially). At the same time, the muscular arch passing over the cord also sharply contracts, and as its fibers shorten, the arch is straightened out and comes to lie on, or close to, the raised inguinal ligament and so protects the weak posterior wall of the canal. As this "shutter" comes down, it passes in front of the internal ring and so counteracts the pressure on the ring from inside the abdomen. The very act of contraction of the abdominal muscles in coughing or straining, which tends to blow out the internal ring and the transversalis fascia, automatically, and at the exact same time, brings into play mechanisms that prevent the occurrence of this damage.

Raised intra-abdominal pressure such that which occurs during pregnancy can make a hernia appear for the first time, as can other causes of raised intra-abdominal pressure such as ascites or in cases of continuous ambulatory peritoneal dialysis or ventriculoperitoneal shunt.

The third factor involved in the etiology of inguinal hernia is the weakening of the muscles and fascias of the abdominal wall with advancing age, lack of physical exercise, adiposity, multiple pregnancies, and loss of weight and body fitness, as may occur after illness or operation. It has been suggested that abnormalities in the structure of collagen, such as a reduction in polymerized collagen and a decreased concentration of hydroxyproline, will lead to a loss of binding between the collagen fibers.[117] This mechanism is important in some cases, especially in cases of repeated recurrent hernia and perhaps, in cases of a familial tendency to hernia.

Animals that walk on all four limbs have a body structure similar to that of man, yet they rarely suffer from inguinal hernia. It is, therefore, often stated that the change to the upright posture and two-legged propulsion has brought about alterations in the functional anatomy of man, such as a reduction in the mechanical efficiency of the shutter mechanism, that lead to a greater propensity to develop inguinal hernias.

The cause of hernia is probably multifactorial. In the case of indirect hernia, a preformed sac of processus vaginalis is probably present, but bowel is prevented from entering by efficient muscular action. A sudden and unusually high increase in intra-abdominal pressure may be sufficient to overcome this protective mechanism, and a hernia may quite suddenly appear. This may be seen in the case of fit young men who perform a strenuous physical act that they are not accustomed to doing. In men weakened by age, adiposity, illness, chronic cough, constipation, and urinary obstruction, the protecting mechanisms deteriorate until they are no longer able to prevent the bowel from entering the preformed sac.

In direct hernia, there is no preformed sac; in fact, there is no real peritoneal sac at all. Because of the factors mentioned previously, the protective mechanisms fail. The weakened transversalis fascia, on its own, cannot withstand the repeatedly raised intra-abdominal pressure and stretches, ballooning out in front of the advancing bowel, or simply tears and allows the peritoneum-covered bowel to pass through it.

The reason that inguinal hernias are more common in the elderly may be linked to the findings of Rodrigues who, in 1990, reported a decrease in oxytalan fibers and an increase in the amorphous substance of the elastic fibers as a function of age, which may be responsible for alterations in the resistance of the transversalis fascia.[118]

CLASSIFICATION

To compare different methods for repair of hernia, it is important that the same type, grade, or stage of hernia is discussed for any meaningful assessment of results. Also, for those surgeons who believe that graded or more extensive repairs are indicated for different stages of severity of hernia, an anatomic and functional classification is necessary to describe and evaluate these repairs. In 1967 Casten published a three-staged classification of inguinal and femoral hernia and a method for repair of each stage.[119] In 1970 Halverson described four groups of groin hernia and the repair he recommended for each group.[120] In 1987 and 1988 Gilbert discussed his simple classification of five types of inguinal hernia in which he elegantly combines the anatomic and functional aspects and the operation he uses for each type.[48,121] This was expanded by Robbins, who added two more types.[78] Nyhus proposed a new classification in 1993,[90] and in the same year, Rutkow described and discussed the classification developed by Bendavid of the Shouldice Hospital.[122] This is a most comprehensive and all-embracing system based on the type, stage, and dimension of the hernia (TSD) and certainly is the most thorough of all hernia classifications proposed to date. However, complexity of the Bendavid classification will somewhat reduce its clinical usefulness. On the other hand, Gilbert's "pocket" classification is sufficiently comprehensive and applicable to modern hernia surgery and yet is simple enough to memorize and use clinically. It will be described in the section on repair of inguinal hernias.

CLINICAL MANIFESTATIONS

History

A complete inguinal hernia may be present at birth or may appear shortly afterward but, in adults, the development is usually more insidious. The exception to this is the rapid onset, even within hours or a day or two, of an "acute" inguinal hernia, usually indirect, following sudden unexpected and unusual exertion and accompanied by pain and even occasionally, by ecchymosis in the inguinal region. Such an occurrence at work may lead to claims for industrial compensation. In the usual case, the patient may feel some discomfort in the groin and notice a small bulge above the inguinal crease when coughing or straining that immediately subsides. As the hernia develops, it appears when the patient stands and reduces when he lies down. As it grows larger, it may not reduce spontaneously when he is lying down, and the patient learns to reduce it manually. In the early stages, when the hernia is stretching and tearing the tissues of the abdominal wall as it grows, the patient may complain of much discomfort and even pain in the region, especially when walking or straining. Later, when the hernia is established, the complaints usually are concerned with the presence of an unesthetic bulge of the groin and scrotum that interferes with walking and other activities and causes a heavy dragging sensation. Patients often complain of an unpleasant sickening feeling in the pit of their stomachs when they are straining. This may be the result of tension on the mesenteries as the bowel is forced down into the hernia. The hernia may be incarcerated or irreducible because of adhesions between the sac and the contents or because of adhesions between the loops of bowel and omentum, especially in long-standing hernias in which the matted mass of contents cannot pass back through the relatively narrow hernial orifice. Bowel and omentum may be caught by pressure on the edge of the hernial orifice, leading to interference with its blood supply and to strangulation of the hernial contents, in which case an obvious emergency manifests itself with extreme pain and signs of intestinal obstruction and later signs of gangrenous bowel.

Examination

In infants and children, there is usually no problem with the diagnosis. The child presents with an obvious bulge in the groin that may go down into the scrotum. The swelling disappears when the child lies down, or may be reduced easily. When the parents describe a typical hernia but it cannot be seen when examining the child, it will usually appear when the child coughs or strains. In the case of infants, pressure on the lower abdomen may cause the hernia to appear, especially if the child cries or pushes against the examiner's hand. The cord may be rolled on the pubis by the examiner's finger, looking for a thickened cord or for the "silk" sign attributed to the sac rolling on itself, but these signs are not reliable.

In adults, clinical examination will reveal a bulge that increases in size and turgor with coughing and that usually can be reduced (a gurgling sound will be produced) when the patient is supine. Smaller hernias only may become visible as a bulge when the patient coughs. When the patient stands, a cough impulse can be felt at the tip of the finger after introducing it into the inguinal canal through the external ring by invaginating the scrotum.

An *indirect hernia* is sausage- or pear-shaped and lies parallel to the inguinal ligament. After reduction it reappears more laterally and runs down above the inguinal ligament towards the scrotum. A *direct hernia* is more rounded, more medial, bulges forward, and tends not to go down into the scrotum. After reduction, it reappears in a forward direction. When an indirect hernia is present, a finger inserted through the external ring into the inguinal canal will pass laterally and upwards of the internal ring. In the case of a direct hernia, the finger will pass directly backward into the abdomen through the opening in the transversalis fascia. When the hernia is reduced and the examiner applies manual pressure over the internal ring and requests the patient to stand and to cough, an indirect hernia will not reappear, whereas a direct hernia will immediately bulge forward. These signs are not always clear-cut. A long-standing, large indirect hernia will stretch the internal ring until it occupies most of the transversalis fascia; its appearance is no different from a direct hernia. A small direct hernia protruding through a narrow tear of the transversalis fascia will appear clinically like an indirect hernia. The differentiation is of academic interest only. The true nature of the hernia is revealed at operation and is handled accordingly.

An incarcerated hernia is soft and nontender, but irreducible. A strangulated hernia is tense, swollen, tender, and irreducible and becomes red, edematous, and inflamed.

DIFFERENTIAL DIAGNOSIS

In infants and children, a hernia must be differentiated from a hydrocele of the tunica vaginalis, which usually clears up by 6 months of age and does not require any treatment. It also must be differentiated from an encysted hydrocele of the cord or canal of Nuck, in the female, which also usually disappears spontaneously but occasionally needs to be cured surgically. However, a communicating hydrocele is a hernia containing fluid, with a narrow passage from the peritoneal cavity into which the bowel has not yet entered, and should be treated as for a hernia.

The diagnosis of inguinal hernia in the adult is usually not difficult, but occasionally it may have to be differentiated from femoral hernia or from enlarged inguinal lymph nodes owing to lymphogranuloma venereum, syphilis, tuberculosis, plague, cat scratch fever, or involvement with primary malignant disease such as lymphoma or with secondary carcinomatous deposits. A saphenous varix also may mimic inguinal hernia, as may a subcutaneous lipoma and a tuberculous psoas abscess may point in the groin and be confused with hernia.

Herniography and Scintigraphy

Since the 1960s, herniography has been recommended for the diagnosis of inguinal hernia in a number of reports.[123–128] Radiopaque contrast material is injected intraperitoneally, and the patient is maneuvered through various positions in an attempt to introduce the material into an actual or potential hernial sac that can then be demonstrated radiographically. This technique undoubtedly does reveal true or potential hernial sacs, but it has failed to gain popularity because of the ease with which most hernias can be diagnosed by simple clinical means. It may, however, be of some use in specially selected cases, for instance, to confirm or exclude the presence of an inguinal hernia in sportsmen and others complaining of unexplained groin pain.[129]

There is no real indication for herniography in infants and children, however small the risk may be. The diagnosis of hernia is usually obvious and if not, there is no harm in waiting until it is. Herniography may reveal a contralateral patent processus vaginalis in a child with an inguinal hernia, but this is not a real indication for operation.

As mentioned previously, children and adults on continuous ambulatory peritoneal dialysis have a greater tendency than usual to develop inguinal as well as other hernias. It also has been suggested that a suspected hernia or patent processus vaginalis can be simply and elegantly diagnosed in these patients by adding radionuclide to the dialysis fluid and scanning for this with the patient standing so that the radiomaterial will collect in the hernia or processus vaginalis.[114,130] If present, a herniorrhaphy should be done at the start of the dialysis.

A fairly rapid onset of a hernia should alert the surgeon to the possibility of its being secondary to raised intra-abdominal pressure resulting from cirrhotic or malignant ascites or chronic incomplete intestinal obstruction caused by a carcinoma of the colon. Indeed, inguinal hernia is such a common finding in the older age groups that one must be wary of arbitrarily attributing abdominal complaints to the hernia. In case of doubt, intra-abdominal pathology, and especially malignant disease, should be sought by the appropriate investigations. Occasionally, on opening the hernial sac there is a gush of excess intraperitoneal fluid. This ascites should be aspirated and sent for cytologic examination. It or one or more small white nodules on the inner surface of the hernial sac may be the first indication of intraperitoneal miliary spread of carcinomatosis and should be histologically examined.[131]

TREATMENT

Indications for Operation

All inguinal hernias in children should be repaired without delay because of the risk of complications of incarceration and strangulation, which include gangrene of the bowel, testis, and ovary, and because of the increased wound infection and recurrence rate following these operations. It has been estimated that the complication rate when operating urgently for a strangulated hernia in a child is 20 times that of a planned procedure. An elective pediatric hernia repair should be a pleasant and minor ambulatory procedure with practically no complications and no mortality.

In adults, the risk of a hernia operation is negligible, and the recurrence rate, when a good repair has been done, is so small that there is hardly any reason for not operating on all hernias as soon as they are diagnosed. This is especially so when one considers the morbidity and mortality and the high recurrence rate when the operation is for a neglected strangulated hernia, especially in the elderly with their associated medical problems. The elderly patient should be operated on electively because of the associated medical problems rather than citing these problems as causes for not operating.

Rorbaek-Madsen reported a series of patients of median age 84 years, operated electively and as emergencies for groin hernias.[132] In those operated electively there was a 5% complication rate whereas in those who underwent an emergency operation, the complication rate was 57%, and the mortality rate was 14%. He concludes that elective hernia repair can be carried out safely even in the presence of serious coexisting disease, whereas emergency hernia repair carries a high risk of complications even in the absence of coexisting disease. Gavrilenko reported a series of 260 elderly and senile patients operated on electively for groin hernia with a 1.2% complication rate and no mortality and concluded that it is safe to perform elective hernia repair in the elderly and senile even in the presence of concomitant diseases.[133] Gardner, in his series of patients more than 80 years of age operated for inguinal hernia both electively and as emergencies, showed that deaths were the result of complications of the primary hernia disease rather than the associated diseases, indicating that one should treat hernias in the elderly early, before complications develop.[134]

The small, wide-necked direct inguinal hernias in elderly patients that pop out and back on coughing can be left alone unless they show signs of growing. Some hernias can be controlled by suitably fitted trusses. However, these are uncomfortable and difficult to keep in place. They often slide off the hernial opening and allow the hernia to slip out alongside the cushion of the truss; they do not always prevent strangulation. They can never cure the hernia and, on the contrary, cause ischemia and wasting of the tissues around the hernia because of constant pressure. Additionally, they make future repairs more difficult and less certain. It has been reported that most of the 40 000 trusses sold in the United Kingdom annually are a wasted expense since the mortality from elective hernia repair is now almost zero.[135] Virtually no patient need be refused on medical grounds. A truss should not be supplied before a reliable surgical opinion is obtained.

Preoperative Assessment and Preparation

As is true for any other operation, the general condition of the patient should be assessed by appropriate clinical examinations and laboratory tests. A history and simple clinical examination is all that is required for the usual healthy child. Some anesthetists still request a hemoglobin measurement and a urine test, although most have dispensed with this. In the adult, cardiovascular, pulmonary, renal, and other conditions such as diabetes mellitus should be looked for and controlled. It is especially important that elderly patients be brought to an optimal physical state before the operation. Smokers should be urged to stop the habit or at least suspend it for some weeks prior to operation. Grossly overweight patients should be advised to reduce before the operation. Some hernia centers, such as the Shouldice Hospital in Toronto, refuse to operate on obese candidates. However, most surgeons resign themselves to the fact that obese patients will not lose much weight and so operate on them without delay.

Anesthesia

Infants and Children. Small infants and babies are traditionally given a general anesthetic including intubation for hernia repairs, but this practice is now in a state of flux. Small premature babies have a strong tendency to develop apnea and bradycardia after general anesthesia and surgery and may die unexpectedly. It is now suggested that small babies weighing approximately 1000 gm or less should be operated on with local anesthesia. Babies who are premature at birth retain this risk of postoperative apnea and bradycardia for even a year or more and even after they have gained normal weights. In order to overcome this problem, there is a strong movement to keep the babies conscious during the operation by using regional anesthesia in the form of continuous caudal anesthesia given through an epidural catheter. In this way, the level and duration of anesthesia can be accurately titrated and the incidence of postanesthetic apnea reduced. Single-dose caudal epidural and subarachnoid anesthetics also could be used but their duration of action may be insufficient for some operations. The frequency of significant episodes of ap-

nea in these babies after general anesthesia for inguinal herniotomy is estimated to be between 15% and 31%, and these usually occur during the first 12 hours after the operation. This method has proved to be safe and free of complications, so much so that some anesthetists advocate discharging the baby from the hospital with or without an apnea monitor several hours after the operation. Most, however, prefer to hospitalize the baby for at least 24 hours for more definitive monitoring. This technique is discussed both by Henderson and Peutrell who both point out the importance of the subject when one considers that approximately one-third of babies with birth weights under 1000 gm will need inguinal herniotomy, the majority of them during their first year of life.[136,137]

Young children and teenagers are difficult to manage with regional or local infiltration anesthesia and are usually given a general anesthetic.

Adults. In adults, local infiltration anesthesia is commonly used for the repair of inguinal hernia. The patient is awake and can cooperate during the operation by coughing or raising his trunk to test the repair, avoiding the postoperative discomforts of a general anesthetic such as coughing and vomiting. The local infiltration method is most suited to ambulatory surgery in which the patient leaves the hospital on the same day; it also decreases costs.[138] Many thousands of inguinal hernias are repaired annually under local anesthesia.[78,139–141]

Spinal or epidural anesthesia is also excellent. Epidural anesthesia is rapidly gaining in popularity. It has been demonstrated that there was no statistically significant difference between cardiac output, mean arterial pressure, total peripheral resistance, and heartrate in patients receiving either a general anesthetic or a regional field block.[142] There is, however, a cost benefit to local anesthesia by avoiding the costs of a general anesthetic and the recovery room. Nausea and vomiting are less common after regional anesthesia than after a general anesthetic. The heart, lungs, and brain are relatively unaffected and epidural anesthesia is titratable if a catheter is used.

Regional anesthesia does have another advantage over general anesthesia in that there is less postoperative pain which has been explained on the basis of the "wind-up phenomenon."[78,143] There is intense stimulation of the pain pathways at the spinal cord level at the time of the operation that sensitizes or "winds up" the nervous or neuronal connections involved and so facilitates the transmission of painful impulses for a time afterwards. Good local or regional anesthesia spares the central nervous system from the barrage of impulses through a blockade of the pain fibers so that there is less postoperative pain. The neural blockade suppresses the formation of the sustained hyperexcitable state in the central nervous system that is responsible for the postoperative pain; following cessation of the operation, there is a gradual diminution of this sensory blockade, giving a prolonged postoperative pain-free period.

A further advantage of regional anesthesia is that, since there is less motor involvement in epidural anesthesia, the patients can be discharged a few hours after the operation. General anesthesia is still widely used, often on an ambulatory basis as well. Both surgeon and anesthetist should be flexible with regard to the type of anesthesia to be used, suiting it to the general condition and preference of the patient. The type of anesthesia used has no influence on the recurrence rate.[138,144–146]

Skin Preparation. Shaving the skin before the operation is controversial since it damages the skin in the form of minor cuts and scratches. If the shaving is done on the preoperative day, these minor wounds have sufficient time to become infected, thus increasing the incidence of infected hernia wounds. An alternative is to use an electric shaver, but it too may cause skin damage. Some surgeons avoid this problem by using a depilatory cream. Other surgeons will not allow any form of hair removal. Operating in an unshaven pubic area is unpleasant and is also a nuisance and the problem can be reasonably overcome by shaving the area shortly before the operation. There are a variety of ways of cleansing the skin in the operating room. This author prefers having the area of the lower abdomen and upper thigh scrubbed for 5 minutes with a povidone-iodine scrub, which is then dried and the skin painted with a povidone-iodine solution.

OPERATIONS FOR INGUINAL HERNIA REPAIR

Herniotomy In Infants and Children

Premature infants, full-term infants, children, teenagers and young adults who have a simple indirect inguinal hernia do not need a complicated repair. Their basic defect is failure of the processes vaginalis to close. Neither the anatomy nor function of the inguinal mechanism or any of its constituent parts—the muscles, ligaments, fascia, and nerves—is in any way defective. The surgeon must correct the basic defect in as simple a manner as possible, taking care not to damage the surrounding inguinal structures. Wide surgical dissection of the inguinal region and the mechanical rearrangement of the structures in different types of herniorrhaphies destroys the shutter mechanism. Also, the more dissection and manipulations in the region, the greater the likelihood of damaging delicate important structures. Injuries to the vas deferens and the vascular supply to the testis may lead to problems of fertility and sterility in later life.[147–151] The urinary bladder, femoral

vein, and nerves in this region also may be damaged. All that is needed to repair an indirect inguinal hernia in this group is to close the patent processus vaginalis, the hernial sac, at its neck, in other words, at its connection with the general peritoneal cavity. There are, however, certain exceptions to this rule. Children at high risk for recurrent hernias should probably have a formal herniorrhaphy performed. These include those with ascites, children with a ventriculoperitoneal shunt, those on continuous ambulatory peritoneal dialysis,[152] children suffering from malnutrition and growth failure, and those with connective tissue disorders such as the Ehlers-Danlos, Hunter-Hurler and Marfan syndromes.

Once the diagnosis has been established, the operation should be carried out without delay because of the risk of strangulation, especially in infants under 6 months of age. More than one-half of the cases of strangulation occur during this time. Approximately one-third of all strangulated inguinal hernias occur during the first year of life. Also, the smaller the child, the greater the risk of gangrene of the ovary or testis from compression and obstruction of their blood supply in the strangulating ring. Hernias in premature infants can be observed but should be repaired a few days before the baby is discharged from the hospital, for the simple reason that it is easier to operate on a somewhat bigger baby. Boley reported recently that an irreducible ovary palpated in an inguinal hernia of a child is at a significant risk of torsion developing into gangrene.[153] In his series of 386 girls with inguinal hernias, 15 (4%) had irreducible ovaries at the time of the operation and four of these 15 (27%) were found to be twisted and infarcted. Other series report 2% to 33% of strangulated ovaries. Because of this, an asymptomatic irreducible ovary should be considered as an incarcerated hernia and operated on as an emergency.

In newborn infants, the external and internal rings overlie each other. There is no real inguinal canal. When the newborn has a hernia, the spermatic cord and the hernial sac pass almost straight out from the abdominal cavity, through the internal and external rings. As the infant grows, the internal ring moves laterally away from the external ring and the inguinal canal begins to form. At 1½ years of age the edges of the rings still overlap so that the spermatic cord and the hernial sac still pass almost directly out of the abdomen. By about 2 years of age, the rings have separated and the proper inguinal canal can be identified between them. It is clear, therefore, that up to two years of age, the neck of the sac easily can be approached directly through the external and internal rings and ligated and transected flush with the peritoneum—a simple herniotomy.

The technique described by this author in 1973 consists of making a small transverse incision through the skin directly over the external ring, remembering that the pubic symphysis in an infant is higher than would appear initially.[154] Scarpa's fascia is elevated between two toothed dissecting forceps and incised. The cord, with its coverings, is isolated in the region of the pubis by bluntly dissecting and separating the fat around it and the external ring is exposed. The cord is elevated and its covering layers of external spermatic fascia, the cremaster and the internal spermatic fascia are gently teased open just distal to the external ring to reveal the hernial sac anteromedial to the cord structures. The sac is separated from the other constituentes of the cord by dissection in the correct plane between it and other cord structures. After approximately 1.5 cm of the sac has been freed and any contents milked back into the peritoneal cavity, the sac is cross-clamped with an artery forceps and transected distal to the clamp. Nothing more need be done about the distal part of the sac except to ensure that its cut-across end is open and has not stuck together to seal off the sac. There is no need to dissect out or remove the distal stump of the sac; doing so will cause bleeding, hematoma, and unnecessary damage and complications.

Using the artery forceps as a grip and with the assistant holding the distal cord tense, the proximal stump of the sac is freed up through the internal ring to the level of the extraperitoneal fat. A small area of peritoneum around the neck of the sac also can be cleared, if desired. By rotating the clamp several times, the sac is twisted tightly, thus ensuring that it is empty. While the clamp is pulled up fairly strongly, the sac is transfixed and ligated just distal to the most proximal twist and the excess stump excised. With this high ligation, the stump should now retract and disappear. The cord structures are returned and the opening in the coverings of the cord repaired with a few interrupted fine sutures. By pulling on the testis, the cord will retract into the depths of the wound. A long-acting anesthetic such as bupivacaine can be injected or simply inserted into the wound to reduce postoperative pain. Scarpa's fascia may be approximated with one suture of synthetic absorbable material and the skin closed with a fine 5-0 continuous subcuticular synthetic absorbable suture.

In the child more than 2 years of age, the external and internal rings become progressively more widely separated so that direct dissection through them is no longer possible. In this case, a short transverse skincrease incision is made over the region of the internal ring, more laterally and higher than that for the infants (Fig 14–1A). The lateral part of the incision may even cross the groin. The incision is carried down to the aponeurosis of the external oblique muscle where it forms the anterior wall of the inguinal canal in front of the internal ring. The aponeurosis is now split in the line of its fibers, opposite the internal ring, taking care to stop short of the external ring (Fig 14–1B). This maneuver opens the inguinal canal and exposes the cord in the region of the internal ring. Here the cremasteric fascia and the internal spermatic fascia are seen to pass down from the conjoined tendon onto the cord. These coverings are separated gently to reveal the sac and the cord structures (Fig 14–1C). Care must be taken not to split the coverings at too high a level since this would damage the conjoined tendon—a structure most important for the integrity of the inguinal shutter mecha-

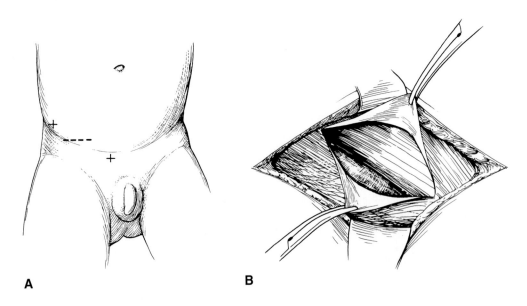

A   **B**

Figure 14–1. Herniotomy. **A.** Short transverse incision over the region of the internal ring. **B.** Aponeurosis of external oblique has been slit open to expose the contents of the inguinal canal. The cord covered by the cremaster muscle is seen filling the canal. *Continued*

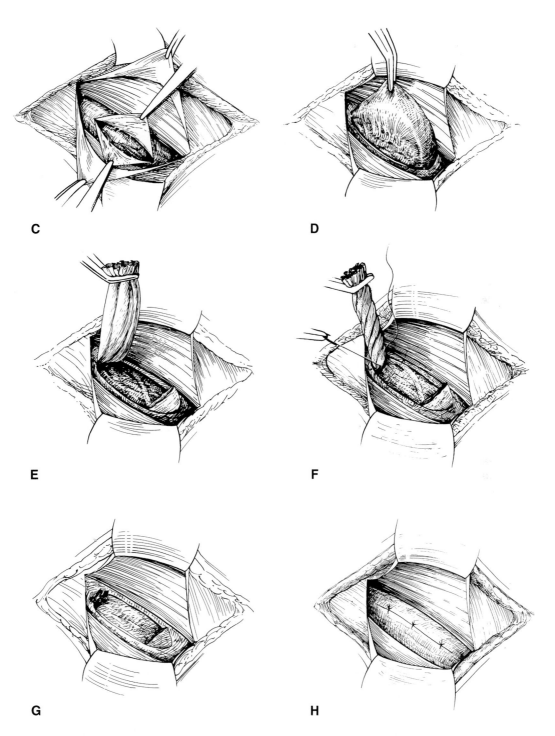

Figure 14–1, cont'd. C. The cremaster muscle has been split open to expose the elements of the spermatic cord. **D.** The hernial sac just distal to the neck is being dissected free of the cord structures. **E.** The sac has been clamped and transected. **F.** The proximal end of the sac has been dissected free to beyond the neck, twisted empty, strongly retracted, and transfixed. **G.** The excess of the proximal end of the sac has been excised, and the distal part of the sac is left undisturbed. **H.** The cremaster has been repaired. *Continued*

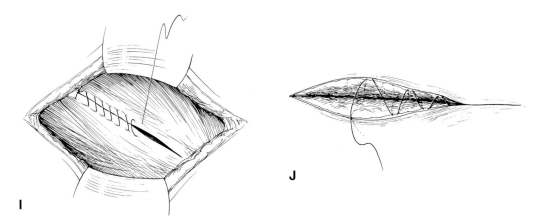

Figure 14–1, cont'd. I. The slit in the aponeurosis has been closed. **J.** The skin is closed with a fine intradermal suture. After Rejovitzky, MD.

nism. A high split through the conjoined tendon also will make finding the sac difficult. The hernial sac just distal to the neck is dissected free of the other cord structures (Fig 14–1D), milked empty, clamped across and transected distal to the clamp (Fig 14–1E). As in the infant, the distal part of the sac is left in place after ensuring that its cut end is open. As before, the proximal stump of the sac is dissected clean up to the neck and a little beyond, while the assistant keeps the other cord structures tense. The sac is twisted empty, strongly retracted, transfixed, ligated, and the excess excised (Fig 14–1F, G). The coverings of the cord are repaired with a few fine interrupted sutures (Fig 14–1H). At this stage, a long-acting local anesthetic such as bupivacaine can be injected into the wound as well as in the iliohypogastric and the ilioinguinal nerves or simply instilled into the wound to reduce postoperative pain. The slit-open aponeurosis of the external oblique is closed with a continuous synthetic monofilament nonabsorbable suture (Fig 14–1I). Scarpa's fascia and the skin are closed as for the babies (Fig 14–1J). This procedure of herniotomy is suitable for all ages, from 2 years to even young adults.

Herniotomy in females is essentially the same as in males but easier, since the sac is not intimately associated with cord structures and the round ligament can be ligated together with the sac, if necessary. However, the ovary may be present in the hernial sac and must be returned to the abdomen before the sac is clamped and transected. Care is needed to avoid damage to the fallopian tube and ovary in the occasional sliding hernia in which these structures form part of the wall of the sac.

Herniotomy in the child is usually a simple outpatient procedure. The child is brought to the hospital in a fasting state just before the scheduled time for operation. Preoperative medication usually is not given. The parents remain with the child in the operating room until he is asleep and are with him when he awakes. The child may be discharged about 2 to 3 hours later, once he is awake and taking some fluids. Complications are extremely rare and minor, there is no mortality and recurrence is rare, but may occur when a large hernia has left a wide internal ring or when the posterior wall of the inguinal canal is damaged at operation or the sac was missed.

Recurrent hernia in infants and children, after repair of a primary inguinal hernia by herniotomy only, varies between 0.8% and 3.8%, although the true figure is probably higher. Fifty percent are evident by 6 months after the operation and approximately 80% by the end of 2 years. The rest appear sporadically even into early adulthood.[155]

Bilateral Repair and Contralateral Exploration in Pediatric Hernias

Herniotomy in the child is simple and quick, so that both sides can be repaired at the same session when bilateral inguinal hernias are present. Routine exploration is controversial. A patent tunica vaginalis on the opposite side does not necessarily constitute a true hernia nor is it an indication that an operation will be needed in the future. A recently closed processus vaginalis can be easily reopened at operation. A hernial sac also can be artificially produced. Jan reported a postmortem study where he demonstrated an open processus vaginalis in 20% of groins in adults without a clinically apparent inguinal hernia.[114] In a series in which all infants had a contralateral exploration, 100% of infants up to 1 week of age were found to have a patent processus vaginalis on the contralateral side.[115] This percentage dropped steadily as the child got older, so that in children of 2 years of age, they found only 25% with contralateral patent processus vaginalis. In another series, only 10.3% of children operated upon for unilateral inguinal hernia with no contralateral exploration developed a contralateral hernia after years of follow-up.[115] The high number of unnecessary contralateral explorations increases anesthetic time and the risks of complications. In a follow-up series of 116 children operated on one side for inguinal hernia, a diminished size of the testis on the side of the operation in six patients, complete testicular atrophy in one patient and iatrogenic cryptorchism in three patients were found.[116] Their conclusion and my belief is that, since a true hernia on the opposite side will develop in only 10% or perhaps even 15% of cases, it does not seem reasonable to subject the other 85% to 90% of children to an unnecessary procedure. For the same reason, this author objects to procedures to look for a patent processus vaginalis on the side opposite the clinically obvious hernia, such as preoperative herniography, preoperative and intraoperative laparoscopy, intraoperative blind probing from within the abdominal cavity through the opened sac of the hernia, and injection of air into the peritoneal cavity at operation. Chatterjee recently discussed papers from Japan, Indonesia and Pakistan reporting 5.8%, 3.7%, and 2%, respectively, of children who developed a contralateral hernia after having been operated on one side for inguinal hernia. In view of this, he comes to the same conclusions.[156]

Herniorrhaphy

In most adults, simple herniotomy is not sufficient to prevent recurrence of the hernia. The natural barriers to herniation, the muscles and fascias of the region, have failed, and their function must be replaced by a mechanical barrier of either natural tissues in the area or synthetic materials.

The Incision. Since inguinal hernias are almost exclusively repaired by the anterior or groin approach, this technique will be described in detail. The preferred incision is a transverse one centered over the internal ring (Fig 14–2A). Depending on the build of the patient, the line of the incision may cross the inguinal crease, but this is of no consequence as long as the incision follows Langer lines. In obese people, there is a convenient, slightly curved skin fold that can be followed (Fig 14–2B). The incision should be a long one, stretching from the line of the anterior superior iliac spine laterally but avoiding damage to the superficial external pudendal vessels to reduce postoperative edema of the penis and scrotum, almost to the midline medially. This gives good exposure of the rectus sheath at the important medial end of the repair and to the region lateral to the internal ring and also avoids strong retraction which increases the incidence of wound infection. A well-placed and well-closed incision heals cleanly with a delicate scar, and it is of no importance whether it is a few centimeters longer or shorter, whereas good exposure is vital to a good operation.

The Dissection. The skin and fat and the condensed layer of the superficial fascia of the abdominal wall are incised down to the aponeurosis of the external oblique muscle. Dissection throughout the operation must be meticulous, and careful hemostasis must be observed to avoid hematomas and infection. There is no need to dissect the fat off the aponeurosis. The external ring is identified and the external oblique aponeurosis is slit at the level of the apex of the external ring by making a small incision with the scalpel in the aponeurosis in the line of the fibers, at about the midpoint of the proposed line of incision. Each side is grasped with an artery forceps. The slightly opened tip of a pair of scissors is inserted in the incision, and the scissors are pushed to split the aponeurosis laterally past the internal ring and medially into the external ring (Fig 14–2C). This maneuver parts the fibers and avoids cutting them. The inguinal canal then is exposed (Fig 14–2D). The cord and it coverings are cleared off the inner aspect of the inguinal ligament up to the pubic tubercle by blunt dissection with gauze-tipped artery forceps. The superior leaf of the aponeurosis of the external oblique is mobilized, especially cranially and medially. It is peeled by blunt gauze dissection off the aponeurosis of the internal oblique muscle and the anterior rectus sheath to expose the anterior surface and edge of the rectus sheath and the fibers of the aponeurosis of the internal oblique muscle. It is important that a wide area be exposed to obtain strong healthy aponeurotic tissue well away from the canal for the repair.

The spermatic cord and its covering are mobilized. A plane is opened medially between the cord and the pubis, and this is developed laterally toward the internal ring. Fibers of the conjoined tendon passing over the cord are swept cranially by blunt dissection to rejoin the conjoined tendon. It is convenient to encircle the cord with a rubber tape for retraction. At this stage the iliohypogastric nerve, ilioinguinal nerve, and the genital branch of the genitofemoral nerve are visible and should be preserved, if possible. It is also now clear whether an indirect or direct hernia or both are present. The cord is "skeletonized" by removing its coverings, as well as any preperitoneal fat adherent to it in the form of a so-called "lipoma." Only the essential constituents remain, leaving a thin cord to facilitate snug closure of the internal ring and reconstruction of the inguinal canal (Fig 14–2E). A bulky fat cord may be compressed and strangulated in the new canal. The skeletonization includes removal of all of the cremaster muscle from the edges of the internal ring to the pubic tubercle. This is an essential maneuver because it exposes and allows good inspection of the internal ring and the transversalis fascia, as well as the musculoaponeurotic arch of the internal oblique and transversus abdominis muscles—the conjoined tendon.

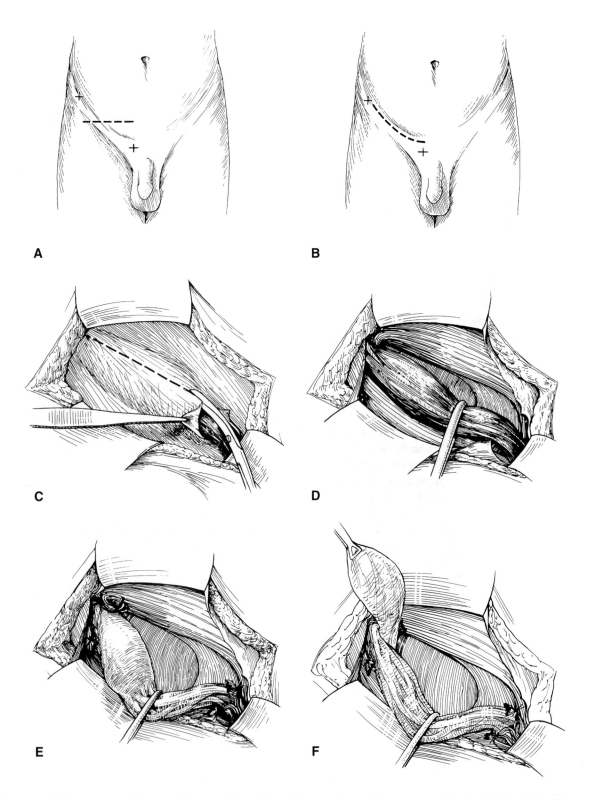

Figure 14–2. Adult hernia incision and dissection. **A.** Transverse incision. **B.** Curved skin crease incision. **C.** The aponeurosis of the external oblique is being slit open. **D.** The inguinal canal is exposed and the spermatic cord mobilized. **E.** The spermatic cord has been skeletonized, and the internal ring and posterior wall of the canal have been defined. **F.** A medium-sized sac has been dissected free of the cord elements. *Continued*

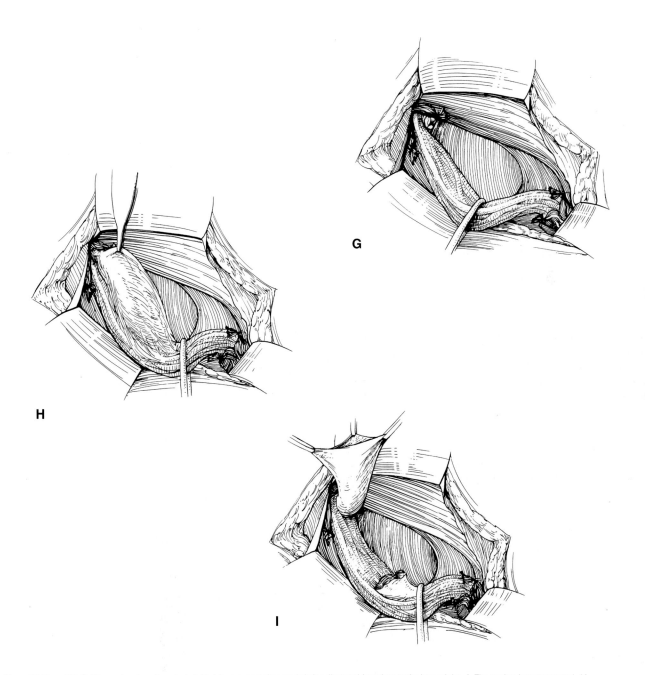

Figure 14–2, cont'd. G. The sac has been invaginated. **H.** A long or complete sac is being dissected free close to the internal ring. **I.** The sac has been transected. After Rejovitzky, MD.

Tons reported a series of hernias repaired by the Shouldice technique comparing removal of the cremaster with nonremoval and found a higher recurrence rate when it was not removed.[157]

The Sac. For many centuries the sac was considered the most important element in the repair of inguinal hernia, and even today, in many descriptions of the operation, one is urged to ligate it as high as possible in the retroperitoneum. Several maneuvers were described to retract the stump of the sac cranially and fix it high up behind the muscles of the abdominal wall. Complicated techniques were used for transfixing and ligating or suturing the upper end of the sac. These were considered vital for the prevention of recurrence of the hernia. Today far less importance is attached to the method of disposal of the sac. The critical means of avoiding recurrence is to do a good repair. An indirect sac should be dissected up into the retroperitoneum beyond the internal ring. The purpose of this is to clear the edges and outer and inner surfaces around the internal ring so as to be able to suture them safely and securely. When dealing with a large indirect hernia with a widely stretched internal ring or with a large direct hernia, one must take care when freeing the sac not to damage the urinary bladder. It may be hidden in preperitoneal and perivesical fat, rendering it more vulnerable. If the bladder has been inadvertently opened, it should be closed immediately in two layers with continuous fine absorbable material, suturing the mucosa and the muscle layers separately, and a catheter should be inserted.

An indirect sac of medium length can be freed off the cord in a convenient plane up to the retroperitoneum and simply invaginated (Fig 14–2G). A larger sac or a complete sac can be lifted off the cord at a convenient site close to the internal ring (Fig 14–2H). After ensuring that none of the constituents of the cord, such as the vas deferens, is adherent to it and that the sac is empty, it may be cut across (Fig 14–2I). The distal section may be left undisturbed. Attempts at removing it are unnecessary and may lead to bleeding, hematoma, or damage to the vas deferens or testicular vessels. One must simply ensure that the cut-across end is open and not bleeding. The open end of the proximal part of the sac may be elevated by some artery forceps, freed up to the level of the retroperitoneum, and simply inverted into the abdominal cavity. There is no special advantage to ligating or suturing this end of the sac, as far as the security of the hernia repair is concerned. In wide hernias with a dilated internal ring, there may be some advantage to closing the sac in that it helps to prevent prolapsed bowel that interfere with suturing of the internal ring. Leaving a peritoneal defect in the region of the internal ring is of no consequence. It has been shown that peritoneal defects close rapidly, within hours or days.[158–162] In 1971 it was re-

ported that sutured peritoneum was rendered ischemic which, in turn, caused adhesions in an attempt to secure an alternative blood supply.[163] It is common practice in many surgical centers throughout the world to leave the peritoneum unsutured when closing abdominal incisions.[164] In a report of hernia repairs in which the sac was not ligated, there were no complications or recurrence attributable to this.[165] In a series of indirect hernias in which one group of patients in whom the sac was simply amputated and the defect in the peritoneum allowed to retract into the abdomen was compared with a second similar group in whom the sac was ligated, there was no difference in the recurrence rate after several years of follow-up.[166] However, the incidence of severe pain was greater in the ligated group. This was attributed to the fact that the peritoneum has a rich nerve supply and is consequently a very sensitive membrane. Suturing and ligating the peritoneum causes ischemia and necrosis, which probably cause the increased pain. This author's routine practice is simply to invert short sacs and to transect and invert longer ones without suture or ligation.

In women, an indirect sac usually is resected together with the round ligament, and the internal ring is closed as part of the repair of the posterior wall of the inguinal canal.

With direct hernias, no true sac is present. The bowel, covered by peritoneum, some preperitoneal fat, and remaining fibers of the transversalis fascia, is replaced into the abdominal cavity when the posterior wall of the canal is repaired.

Sliding hernias are no longer a problem once one accepts the principle that high ligation of the sac is of no importance. With an indirect hernia the sac is freed up into the retroperitoneum to clear the internal ring and is inverted into the peritoneal cavity. A longer sac may be transected just below the sliding bowel, and the sac and contents inverted into the peritoneal cavity. A sliding direct hernia is inverted when repairing the posterior wall of the canal.

When a double or "pantaloon" hernia is present, both the indirect and direct peritoneal sacs are freed up to the retroperitoneal space. The medial wall of the indirect sac is put on tension, and this maneuver slides the direct sac laterally behind the inferior epigastric vessels. The resultant combined sac is dealt with as is done in an indirect hernia repair.

The Suture Material. The process of healing takes approximately 1 year. After the first 6 months, the wound has gained about 80% of its final strength. Therefore, it is apparent that any suture material that will not hold the tissues for at least 6 months will be unsuitable for hernia repair. Catgut and the newer synthetic absorbable sutures lose 50% of their strength within 14 days, disintegrate within 6 weeks and are unsuitable for hernia repair.

Biologic materials such as silk, cotton, or linen lose 40% of their strength within 6 weeks and begin to disintegrate by 3 months. They cause much tissue response, perpetuate infection by organisms lurking within the twist or braid, and behave as foreign bodies, causing chronic sinuses when the wounds are infected. They have no place in hernia repair and should be abandoned. Even the more modern polyesters and nylons may perpetuate sepsis when twisted or braided.

Monofilament nonabsorbable synthetic sutures of the nylon type, if sufficiently thick, are practically indestructible in human tissues.[167,168] They are strong, smooth, inert, and excite little tissue reaction. They do not cause a foreign body reaction in infected wounds and, when exposed in a purulent wound, become covered with granulation tissue. These monofilament synthetic nonabsorbable sutures are the most suitable available for hernia repair. Polyamide and polypropylene, in sizes 00, 0 or 1, are most commonly used. They are pliable and comfortable to handle, but attention must be paid to knot security. They are also commercially available in the form of ready-made loops swaged onto atraumatic needles so that they need not be tied or knotted at one end. A further advantage of the smoothness and pliability of the threads is that when used as a continuous stitch, the suture can slide in the tissues and adjust itself to the varying strains.

Monofilament stainless steel wire also has excellent properties. It is inert and causes little tissue reaction. It remains intact and retains its strength almost indefinitely. However, it is difficult to handle, rather springy, and tends to form kinks. For these reasons, most surgeons avoid using it. However, the Shouldice Hospital has used 34- or 32-gauge steel wire most successfully for many years for many thousands of hernias and continues to do so.

Pure Tissue Repairs

The Shouldice Operation. This repair is probably the most popular of those using only local tissues, and has been well summarized.[169–171] It is basically a multilayered Bassini operation. The Shouldice Hospital uses only 34- or 32-gauge stainless steel wire continuous sutures, although outside that institution most surgeons find it more convenient to use a synthetic monofilament nonabsorbable suture. Almost all of the operations are done under local anesthesia. The principles of the repair include meticulous dissection and hemostasis, clear demonstration of the internal ring from which the spermatic cord is freed, and complete excision of the cremaster muscle. A concomitant femoral hernia is sought from below by incising the cribriform fascia in the thigh and later from above after slitting open the transversalis fascia and exposing the retroperitoneal space.

Repair of the transversalis fascia and tightening of the internal ring is the basis of the tissue type of repair. After suitable exposure of the transversalis fascia and the internal ring and freeing of the spermatic cord from its edges, the indirect hernial sac is dissected and dealt with as previously discussed. The medial pillar of the internal ring is caught by two artery forceps and is lifted off the preperitoneal fat. The tip of a pair of scissors is passed behind the medial pillar medially to the pubic tubercle, separating the transversalis fascia from the preperitoneal fat and from the inferior epigastric vessels, which are preserved. An index finger then is passed along this tract to examine the state of the transversalis fascia and the femoral canal. Next, the transversalis fascia is slit open with scissors from the medial pillar of the internal ring between the two artery forceps up to the pubic tubercle (Fig 14–3A). The upper flap is grasped by artery forceps and is lifted to allow a wide dissection between it and the preperitoneal fat (Fig 14–3B). The lower flap is similarly freed off the underlying fat and past the free edge of the inguinal ligament after dividing the cremasteric vessels to expose the condensation in the iliopubic tract. The first layer of the repair is now begun (Fig 14–3C) by suturing the free edge of the lower flap high behind the upper flap to the posterior aspect of the transversalis fascia as well as to the posterior aspect of the rectus sheath and of the aponeurosis of the transversus abdominis. The 34-gauge continuous stainless steel suture is passed through the strong fascia lateral to the pubic tubercle and tied. Big bites of tissue are taken when suturing, on the "mass closure" principle. Sutures should be 2 to 4 mm apart and the bites placed alternately more or less forward or backward to spread the tension. All the tension of the repair should not be placed on the same line of a few fibers. The suture is continued laterally up to and including the opened internal ring. By suturing the lateral corner of the lower flap high and laterally, as well as the stump of the cremaster, the transversalis fascia is tightened around the emerging cord. The wire suture is not tied at this stage but continues for the next layer. It begins at the lateral end of the repair, suturing the free edge of the upper flap of transversalis fascia to the base of the lower edge and the iliopubic tract and to the inguinal ligament up to the pubic tubercle where the steel suture is tied to its original tail (Fig 14–3D). This double layer of overlapped transversalis fascia and muscles forms a new strong posterior wall of the canal, constitutes a new, tight internal ring around the cord, and holds back a direct hernia, the stump of an indirect sac, as well as the preperitoneal fat.

This posterior wall is further strengthened by another double layer that sutures the conjoined tendon to the inguinal ligament and lower flap of the external oblique aponeurosis. A second length of wire is passed

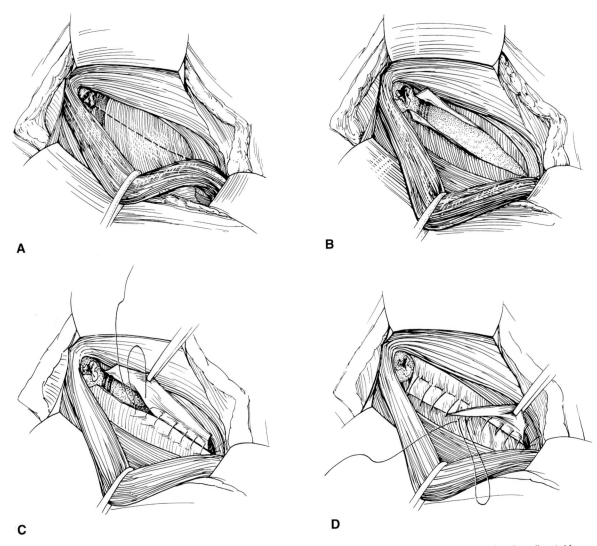

A

B

C

D

Figure 14–3. The Shouldice operation. **A.** The transversalis fascia is being incised. **B.** The upper and lower flaps of the transversalis fascia have been dissected free and elevated to expose the extraperitoneal fat and the inferior epigastric vessels. **C.** The first layer of the Shouldice operation. **D.** The second layer. *Continued*

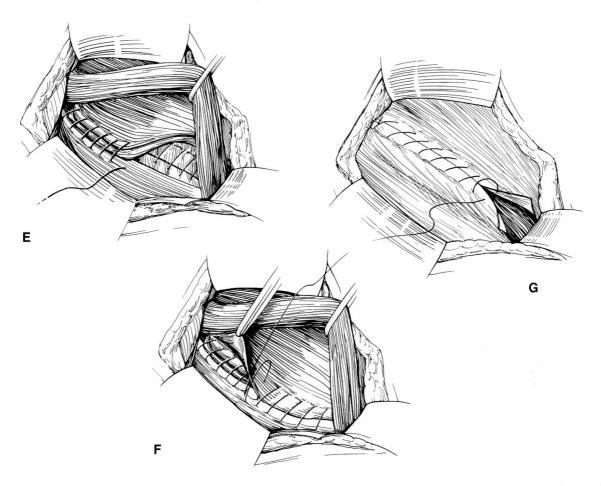

Figure 14–3, cont'd. E. The third layer. **F.** The fourth layer. **G.** The external oblique aponeurosis has been repaired in front of the spermatic cord. After Rejovitzky, MD.

through the inguinal ligament at the medial edge of the new internal ring and then takes a bite of the posterior surface of the aponeurotic tendon of the transversus abdominis and is tied. This suture is continued medially up to the pubic tubercle (Fig 14–3E) and returns again laterally to suture the anterior rectus sheath and the lower aspect of the conjoined tendon from the front to the inner surface of the lower flap of the external oblique aponeurosis (Fig 14–3F). This line is continued back to the internal ring, further reinforcing the ring around the emergent cord, and the suture is tied to its original tail. The cord is now laid on this four-layered buttress, and the external oblique aponeurosis is closed in front of the cord in a single or double layer, once more with a continuous steel suture (Fig 14–3G). The first line of a double closure begins at the medial end and sutures the lower flap to the posterior aspect of the upper flap until the lateral end is reached and then returns to suture the edge of the upper flap to the anterior surface of the lower flap back to the medial end, where it is tied, leaving the cord to emerge through a reconstituted external ring. The subcutaneous layers are closed with a continuous absorbable suture to eliminate the dead space, and the skin edges are approximated with clips.

The recurrence rate for primary hernia repairs is <1%. One cannot argue with the superb results of the Shouldice Hospital in Toronto, which have been produced by a highly specialized group of surgeons dedicated to the repair of these hernias. One is, however, disturbed by the fact that they reject certain patients such as the obese, as well as all incarcerated or strangulated hernias and this may be a factor in their good results. The method is complicated and requires a great deal of dissection. Although descriptions of the method stress that the posterior wall of the canal is repaired by suturing transversalis fascia, this is, in fact, often not possible because of this fascia's being a weak and ragged structure, especially in the elderly with large direct hernias and in patients with recurrent hernias. Although the flaps of transversalis fascia are undoubtedly included in the sutures, the bites also include elements of the conjoined tendon above and the iliopubic tract and inguinal ligament below, so that what is actually being done in many cases is a Bassini-type repair four times over. The nature of the repair is such that many are done under tension, even though the Shouldice Hospital contends that the tension is spread by the continuous suture.

The Berliner Approach. In 1984, Berliner described his disappointing results using the classical Bassini and Cooper ligament repairs, which led him to change to the Shouldice operation.[15] However, it soon became apparent to him that four layers were not necessary to but-

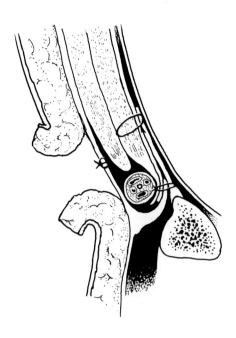

Figure 14–4. The Berliner approach. The diagram shows the two-layered overlap repair of the posterior wall of the inguinal canal and the external oblique aponeurosis sutured in front of the cord. After Rejovitzky, MD.

tress the posterior wall, and he reduced this to three layers. After several years with results comparable to those of the Shouldice Hospital, he dispensed with the third layer as well. He now does only the two-layer overlap repair of the transversalis fascia and transversus abdominis aponeurosis to the inguinal ligament with an equally low recurrence rate. The steps include dissection and slitting open of the transversalis fascia as is performed for the Shouldice operation (see Fig 14–3A and B); then a first continuous suture approximates the undersurface of the transversalis fascia and transversus abdominis aponeurosis superiorly to the inferior incised margin of transversalis fascia (Fig 14–3C). The second continuous suture approximates the superior margin of transversalis fascia and transversus abdominis aponeurosis to transversalis fascia, where it forms the anterior femoral sheath, and to the inguinal ligament (Fig 14–3D). To quote Berliner: "The operation is less complex, anatomically correct, and physiologically sound" (Fig 14–4).[15]

The Lichtenstein Repair. In the second edition of his book, published in 1986, Lichtenstein describes his "classical" pure tissue repair.[16] After the posterior wall of the canal is exposed and the internal ring prepared, the cord is skeletonized, and the sac is dealt with. Next, the lower edge of the transversus abdominis aponeurosis, with the transversalis fascia attached to it, is brought down and sutured to the inguinal ligament

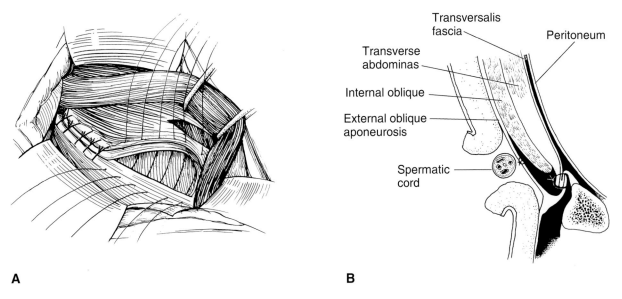

A

B

Figure 14–5. The Lichtenstein repair. **A.** The single-layer repair of the posterior wall of the inguinal canal and the relaxing incision. **B.** The single-layer repair of the posterior wall of the inguinal canal and the external oblique sutured behind the cord. After Rejovitzky, MD.

with a series of staggered, interrupted nonabsorbable synthetic sutures. The tension on this line of sutures is relieved by a relaxing incision in the anterior rectus sheath (Fig 14–5A). This is another variant of the Bassini technique but takes into account the fact that the lower edge of the internal oblique muscle is fleshy, does not hold sutures, and therefore is not included in the repair. The external oblique aponeurosis usually is sutured behind the cord (Fig 14–5B). Lichtenstein reports an overall recurrence rate of 0.7% for almost 6000 consecutive herniorrhaphies—results as good as those of the Shouldice Hospital but with even less dissection and fewer lines of suture than Berliner's modified and simplified Shouldice procedure.[16]

The Wilkinson Technique. This is a pure tissue technique that combines the Bassini repair with a local tissue-flap reinforcement of the posterior wall of the canal, as well as increasing the indirect course of the spermatic cord. After the preparatory dissection has been completed and the sac dealt with, without slitting open the transversalis fascia, the lower edge of the aponeurosis of the transversus abdominis and the internal oblique muscle are sutured down to the shelving margin of the inguinal ligament with a continuous suture (Fig 14–6A). Next, the inferior leaf of the aponeurosis of the external oblique muscle is passed upward behind the cord and is sutured to the external surface of the internal oblique muscle (Fig 14–6B). This flap reinforces the posterior wall of the canal. The superior leaf of the external oblique muscle then is sutured over the inferior leaf, but in front of the cord, with two continuous suture

lines (Fig 14–6C). This achieves an overlap of two layers of external oblique aponeurosis to strengthen the posterior wall of the canal, with the cord taking an S course between the layers (Fig 14–6D and E). In 1988, Wilkinson reported a recurrence rate of 1.2% in 1455 primary hernia repairs.[172]

The Cooper Ligament Repair. Rutledge has used general anesthesia routinely for his large series of cases, since wide dissection and deep suturing must be done.[19] Perioperative antibiotic coverage is given and a catheter is placed in the bladder. The standard anterior approach is used. The posterior wall of the inguinal canal is split open widely and the preperitoneal plane is freed. The hernia sacs are dealt with, and the Cooper's ligament is cleared. The femoral artery and vein are cleared and all fat and glands in the femoral canal are removed. The anterior femoral fascia is mobilized and carefully preserved. The lower edge of the aponeurosis of the transversus abdominis muscle is exposed and trimmed clean, together with the lower edge of the internal oblique. A long relaxing incision is made in the anterior rectus sheath just medial to its lateral edge for about 10 to 12 cm, starting from the pubic tubercle. The preperitoneal tissues are inverted with a continuous absorbable suture to keep them off the region for repair.

Rutledge uses interrupted silk sutures for the actual repair, although a monofilament synthetic nonabsorbable suture is more commonly used today. Beginning at the pubic tubercle, a series of sutures is placed between the lower edge of the aponeurosis of the transversus abdominis and Cooper's ligament up to the medial wall of

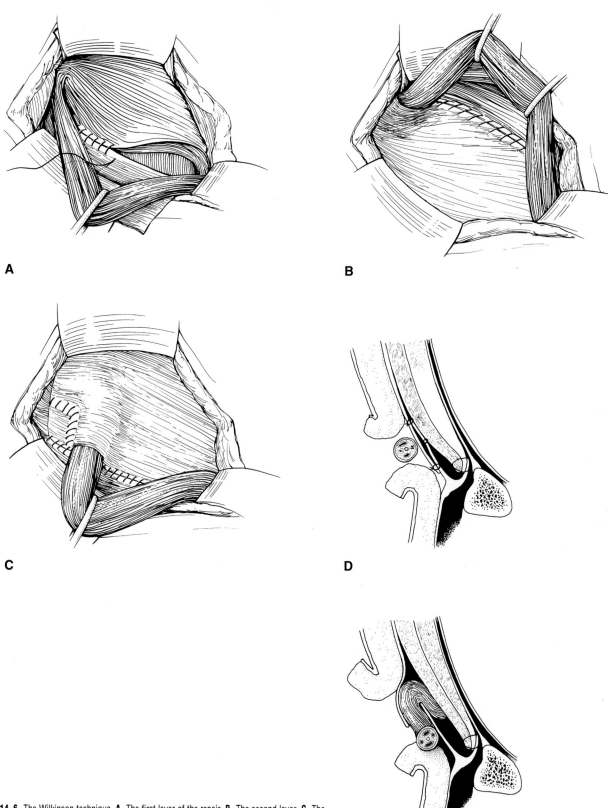

A

B

C

D

E

Figure 14–6. The Wilkinson technique. **A.** The first layer of the repair. **B.** The second layer. **C.** The third layer. **D.** Diagram of the repair. **E.** Diagram showing S course of cord. After Rejovitzky, MD.

the femoral vein. If the internal oblique is aponeurotic in this area, it is included in the sutures. Additional sutures between Cooper's ligament and the anterior femoral fascia ensure the closure of the femoral canal. The repair is continued laterally by a series of sutures between the musculoaponeurotic arch above and the anterior femoral fascia going beyond the internal ring so that the cord is displaced obliquely and laterally. The sutures then are tied from medial to lateral. Since there have been reported cases of herniation through the relaxing incision, Rutledge recommends placing an inlay patch of polypropylene mesh into the defect and suturing it to the edges of the incised anterior rectus sheath with a continuous polypropylene suture.[20] Occasionally a sheet of polypropylene mesh is placed on the whole repair as well as on the mesh patch of the relaxing incision, as an onlay graft, and sewn down around its edges. The cord is replaced onto the repair and the external oblique aponeurosis closed in front of the cord to reconstitute the inguinal canal. Rutledge uses the Cooper's ligament repair on all groin hernias in adults, primary or recurrent, regardless of the presenting type, with excellent results reported in more than 1500 cases. Whether or not the relaxing incision is efficacious is a subject of much discussion.[172,173,174]

Darn Repairs

The Abrahamson Nylon Darn Repair. A good hernia repair should last the patient for the rest of his life, no matter what his age at the time of the operation. The surgeon must bear in mind this responsibility. A 1982 report showed that almost 6% of recurrences occurred during the first postoperative month, 39% during the first year after primary repair, and 24% occurred later than 10 years after the operation.[175] The Shouldice Hospital has reported that late recurrence is not uncommon in cases followed for 10 to 40 years. As the causes of early recurrence after hernia repair were eliminated (faulty technique, ignorance of the functional anatomy and physiology of the abdominal wall, repair with tension, the use of incorrect suture material, and infections), it became apparent that even with the finest technique and materials and the best intentions, a percentage of hernias will recur over the years because of factors beyond the control of the surgeon. These are mainly the natural weakening of the tissues and deterioration of body fitness with time and aging, increased adiposity, raised intra-abdominal pressure owing to chronic cough, constipation, and obstructive disease of the urinary bladder. It was realized that some form of reinforcement was needed to overcome the problems of aging scar tissue and of muscles and tendons approximated by sutures, especially in direct hernia repair.

A variety of natural and foreign materials were used for this reinforcement, but with little success, until the

advent of strong, smooth, resistant, and pliable monofilament nylon. The principle of the nylon darn operation for the repair of inguinal hernia is to reinforce the weakened or torn posterior wall of the inguinal canal with the muscles of the musculoaponeurotic arch, as well as with a simple lattice work of monofilament nylon suture under no tension, on which is laid a buttress of fibrous tissue, without the normal tissues being torn or necrosed. The nylon sutures are anchored into strong, healthy tissues far from the area of herniation. The nylon darn solves the problem of early recurrence since the nylon lattice will hold the area intact for the first year, until the natural connective tissue collagen scar matures to its full strength. However, the muscle and scar tissue is not able to withstand the constant wear and tear of repeated stress over many years. As they fail, the nylon, which is practically indestructible in human tissues, will once more come into its own and will maintain the integrity of the repair for many years, until the end of the patient's life.

The technical details of the operation were described in 1987 and 1988.[47,49,176] The incision and meticulous dissection and preparation of the tissues are as described previously. No special dissection of a direct sac is needed, although occasionally it is convenient to reduce a sac prolapsing through a punched-out hole in the transversalis fascia and to suture the opening. A large sliding hernia with much preperitoneal fat may occasionally be conveniently reduced and the edges of the tear in the transversalis fascia closed with a continuous suture to render the repair more manageable. The transversalis fascia is not split open. The repair is begun by suturing the medial edge of the rectus sheath and the musculoaponeurotic arch (conjoined tendon) to the posterior portion of the inguinal ligament and to the iliopubic tract with a continuous 2-0 polyamide or polypropylene suture (Fig 14–7A). The suture is begun at the medial end of the repair by catching fascia on the pubis, passing through the medial end of the inguinal ligament and the remains of the fascia transversalis and then taking a good bite through the lowest portion of the medial edge of the rectus sheath and tendon and tied. The suture continues laterally in a simple over-and-over fashion including, along the lower edge, some fibers of the inguinal ligament, the iliopubic tract, and the lower part of the transversalis fascia. Along the upper edge, the medial edge of the rectus sheath is sutured as far laterally as possible, after which the suture takes in part of the transversalis fascia as well as the lower edge of the aponeurosis of the transversus abdominis and also the aponeurotic part of the internal oblique. The fleshy part of the internal oblique is not included in the suture. Fairly large bites of tissue are taken along the upper edge. Suture bites on the inguinal ligament are staggered, some more forward and others further behind so

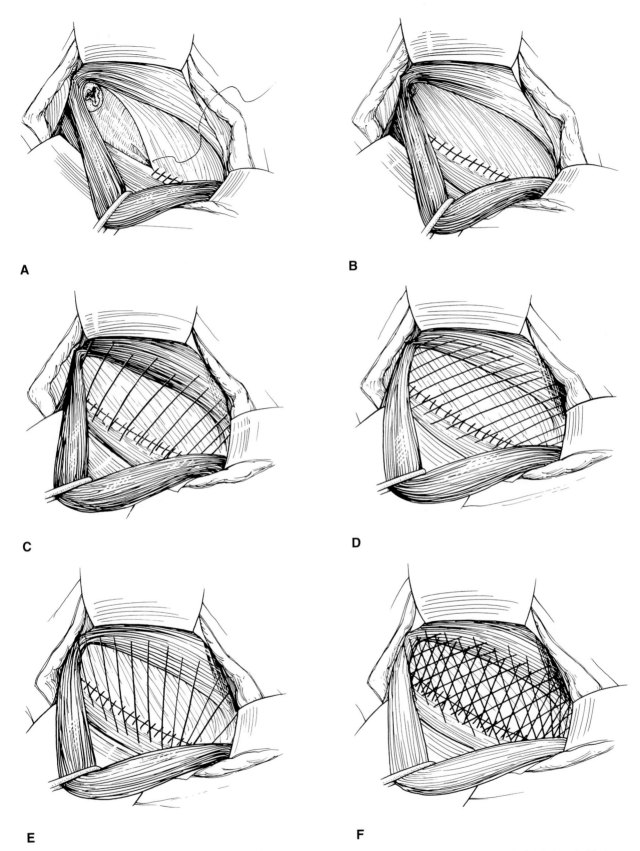

A

B

C

D

E

F

Figure 14–7. The Abrahamson nylon darn repair. **A.** Suture of the musculoaponeurotic arch to the inguinal ligament. **B.** Completed repair of posterior wall of the inguinal canal and snug closure of the internal ring. **C.** The first run of the nylon darn. **D.** The second run. **E.** The third run. **F.** The completed darn. *Continued*

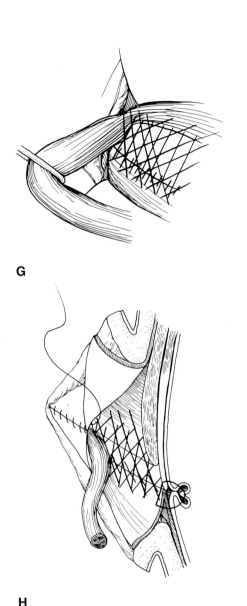

G

H

Figure 14–7, cont'd. G. The internal ring reinforced anteriorly, superiorly, and inferiorly. **H.** Diagram of the repair. After Rejovitzky, MD.

arch, in order to reinforce the ring against an indirect recurrence. At this point the suture is tied (Fig 14–7B).

Up to this stage, the procedure constitutes a tissue repair and its strength depends on that of the tissues used. If no more is done, some cases will develop early recurrence and others late recurrence. This repair has the advantage of closing the rent in the transversalis fascia and of tightening the internal ring and providing a thick musculoaponeurotic barrier for the posterior wall of the canal. It also provides a smooth, flat bed on which to lay the darn.

The darn is done with 0 monofilament nylon thread (polyamide 6), 1.5 m long and doubled to form a loop 75 cm long, with the free ends swaged onto an atraumatic curved 40 mm round-bodied needle. Starting at the medial end (Fig 14–7C) a bite is taken of the most medial fibers of the inguinal ligament where they sweep over the pubic tubercle. The point of the needle then is pushed under the lateral edge of the rectus muscle and sheath just above where they are inserted into the pubis, and a deep, wide bite is taken of the muscle and sheath so that the needle appears on the anterior surface of the sheath and is extracted. The needle is then simply passed through the tail end of the loop, and tightened, eliminating the inconvenience of a knot. The suture is continued laterally, taking bites of the inguinal ligament below and deep wide bites of the rectus muscle and its sheath to ensure a good darn in the critical medial angle of the repair where recurrences tend to occur. When the rectus sheath can no longer be used, the sutures pass onto the conjoined tendon. Each stitch is laid in a vertical fashion. The stitches on the inguinal ligament are staggered to spread the tension between the fibers. At the upper end the suture passes over the muscular lower part of the internal oblique and transversus abdominis but takes a deep and wide bite of the white aponeurotic part of the conjoined tendon. The stitches are held slightly tight—just enough to straighten the thread, and are not placed under tension. This vertical line of sutures is continued laterally, in front of, and even slightly beyond, the internal ring, displacing the cord laterally. The same suture changes direction and returns medially as the second layer of the darn (Fig 14–7D). It passes in front of the covered internal ring. The stitches are now laid in a sloping fashion, passing upwards and medially from the inguinal ligament to the conjoined tendon and later the rectus sheath, crossing the stitches of the first run at an angle. The bites on the inguinal ligament also are staggered and a bit anterior to those of the first run, in order to spread the tension. Large bites are taken, as before, of the aponeurotic fibers of the conjoined tendon, and placed this time more cranially than the first row. No tension is placed on the sutures. At the medial end, a bite is taken on the inguinal ligament at the pubic tubercle and of the lower end of the rectus sheath and tied.

that all of the repair will not be secured to only a few fibers of the inguinal ligament. The aim is to approximate the rectus sheath and conjoined tendon to the inguinal ligament. This is easily done without tension, or under minimal tension, in most cases. When this is not possible, we do not force the approximation under tension but leave a gap, usually only a narrow one, between the upper elements of the repair and the inguinal ligament. At the lateral end, the edges of the internal ring are picked up and included in the sutures to achieve a fairly tight and snug closure of the ring around the cord. This line of sutures is carried laterally beyond the internal ring for 1 to 2 cm, with the object of covering the internal ring with the musculoaponeurotic tissue of the

The third line of sutures is the same as the second except that the stitches slope cranially and laterally from the inguinal ligament (Fig 14–7E). The suture is passed through the medial end of the inguinal ligament and the rectus sheath, then through the loop, and tightened. At the medial end, the suture takes up all of the inguinal ligament where it forms the lower edge of the external ring and it then passes onto the inguinal ligament more laterally. At this stage, the original repair line, as well as the first two runs of the darn, occupy most of the inguinal ligament and there may no longer be any room left on the inguinal ligament for a third line, which may get "pushed" forward onto the aponeurosis of the external oblique muscle (which of course is the continuation of the inguinal ligament). This gives an added advantage of wrapping the inguinal ligament and lower flap of the aponeurosis of the external oblique around the inferior edge and anterior wall of the repair. The upper end of the sutures of the third run should be placed at a higher level than the second run. Big bites are taken of the tissues and the needle is brought out as high as possible.

When the space between this line and the inguinal ligament below is narrow, there is not enough room left above for the third run. In these cases, the emerging needle hooks up some of the external oblique aponeurosis along its line of fusion with the internal oblique. In these cases, at the completion of the repair, when the anterior wall of the canal has been closed by suturing the cut edges of the external oblique aponeurosis, the blue sutures of the polyamide can be seen as a series of parallel lines on the surface of the upper part of the external oblique aponeurosis. The third run of the darn should be continued laterally beyond the internal ring and tied. The stitches of each run should be sufficiently close to form a close darn (Fig 14–7F). There should not be large gaps through which a hernia could recur. Gaps should be filled while doing any of the three runs. It is of no importance if some of the stitches are placed in different directions and at different angles. Because of the slope of the sutures, the second and third runs reinforce the repair below and above the internal ring (Fig 14–7G).

The cord is laid on the darn, and the anterior wall of the inguinal canal is reconstituted in front of the cord (Fig 14–7H) by suturing together the cut edges of the aponeurosis of the external oblique with a continuous suture of 2-0 monofilament nylon. Scarpa fascia and the subcutaneous fat are not sutured. The skin is closed, preferably with a continuous intradermal (subcuticular) suture of 5-0 synthetic absorbable thread, but alternatively Michel clips may be used. Clips are removed on the second postoperative morning, less than 48 hours after the operation.

This author reported more than 1000 repairs of primary and recurrent hernia using this technique. In a fol-

low-up of maximum of 15 years, the recurrence rate for primary repairs was 0.8% and was 0.33%, in the last 300 cases.

The nylon darn repair for inguinal hernia resembles the mass closure technique for abdominal incisions. The monofilament nylon thread must be thick enough not to cut through the tissues but not so thick as to be unpliable and difficult to handle. Large mass bites of full-thickness tissue must be taken to hold the sutures. The stitches should not be so close as to cause ischemia of the tissues between them, but not so far apart as to allow extrusion of abdominal contents. The sutures in the conjoined tendon must be carefully placed in good, healthy tissue at a distance from the stretched and attenuated muscles around the hernia. The smooth nylon can slide in the tissues and adjust the tension on individual sutures during relaxation and exercise.

Mixed Tissue/Prosthetic Repairs

With the realization that pure tissue repairs may develop recurrences years after the operation, surgeons developed techniques for reinforcing the repair with sheets of synthetic mesh laid either deep to the tissue repair as an "underlay" graft or in front of the repair as an "overlay" graft. Polypropylene mesh usually is used.

The Lichtenstein Plastic Screen Reinforcement

A knitted polypropylene mesh is recommended and has been used since 1969 as a simple means of reinforcement for all direct and recurrent hernias. A 3 × 8 cm sheet of the mesh screen is laid onto the new posterior wall (Fig 14–8) and is secured by interrupted nonabsorbable sutures to the lacunar ligament, inguinal ligament, and the transversus aponeurosis. The screen is split at the internal ring, and the two tails are brought around the cord and tacked down with one suture. In 1986 Lichtenstein stated that "the porous mesh permits

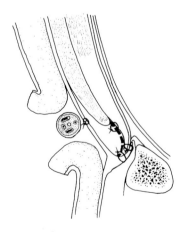

Figure 14–8. Lichtenstein plastic screen reinforcement. After Rejovitzky, MD.

the penetration and deposition of a thick layer of reactive fibrous tissue that permanently buttresses the posterior canal wall repair."[16]

The Gilbert Classification and Tissue/Prosthetic Repair. In 1987 Gilbert described his anatomic/functional classification for the diagnosis and treatment of inguinal hernia. It is probably the best example today of the logical application of mixed tissue/prosthetic repair in which the type of repair is adapted to the type of hernia.[121]

Gilbert Type I. The Gilbert type I hernia has a snug internal ring through which a peritoneal sac of any size passes (Fig 14–9A). Once this sac has been surgically reduced, it will be contained by the existent internal ring. The canal floor is intact. After the sac has been mobilized, it is invaginated within the abdominal cavity. When local anesthesia is used, the patient may cough and strain, but the sac does not reappear. To reinforce the canal floor against future direct herniation, a polypropylene mesh overlay graft is fashioned in the approximate shape of the Hesselbach triangle and is placed over the transversalis fascia (Fig 14–9B). This graft is held in place without direct suturing, by approximating the aponeurotic arch of the transversus abdominis to the inguinal ligament in two layers in front of the mesh, using a continuous 3-0 polypropylene monofilament suture (Fig 14–9C). The external oblique aponeurosis is repaired in front of the cord.

Gilbert Type II. The type II hernia has a moderately enlarged internal ring. It admits one finger but is smaller than two fingerbreadths. After reduction of the indirect peritoneal sac, it will protrude when the patient coughs or strains (Fig 14–10A). The canal floor is otherwise intact. To avoid the wide dissection, transection, and multiple-layer resuture of the Shouldice technique, a simple and equally effective method has been devised by Gilbert. A cylindrical plug, fashioned from a rolled-up strip of polypropylene mesh is passed completely through the internal ring (Fig 14–10B). It expands by partially unwinding and blocks the anatomically and functionally defective internal ring. The plug remains in place without sutures and is incorporated into the

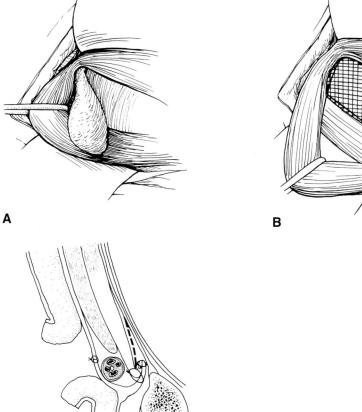

A

B

C

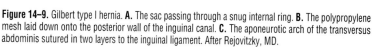

Figure 14–9. Gilbert type I hernia. **A.** The sac passing through a snug internal ring. **B.** The polypropylene mesh laid down onto the posterior wall of the inguinal canal. **C.** The aponeurotic arch of the transversus abdominis sutured in two layers to the inguinal ligament. After Rejovitzky, MD.

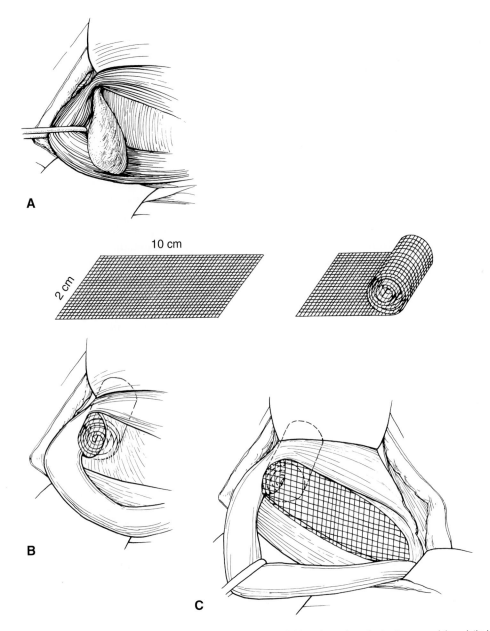

Figure 14–10. Gilbert type II hernia. **A.** The sac passing through a moderately enlarged internal ring. **B.** The polypropylene plug has been passed through the internal ring. **C.** The polypropylene mesh laid down onto the posterior wall of the inguinal canal. After Rejovitzky, MD.

collagen and scar tissue that forms around it. To ensure against future herniation, an overlay graft is placed over the posterior wall of the canal (Fig 14–10C) and is held in place as the floor is reinforced in two layers in front of the mesh, the same as for type I. The external oblique aponeurosis is re-sutured in front of the cord.

In 1987 Gilbert reported a series of 101 cases of type I and II hernias repaired by a revolutionary but ingeniously simple new sutureless and tension-free method.[73,121] After the sac has been dealt with, an "umbrella plug" fashioned from a square of polypropylene mesh is passed through the internal ring to behind the transversalis fas-

cia where it opens to hold back the sac and the extraperitoneal fat (Fig 14–11A and B). The plug is held in place by the shutter mechanism of the internal ring. To ensure against the later development of a direct hernia, a swatch of polypropylene mesh is laid onto the posterior wall of the canal, and the lateral end is slit to encompass the emerging cord (Fig 14–11C). The anterior wall of the canal is resutured in front of the cord. Both pieces of mesh are held in place by the body's internal hydrostatic forces and eventually will be incorporated into the tissues and prevent recurrence of an indirect or direct hernia. By means of this sutureless technique,

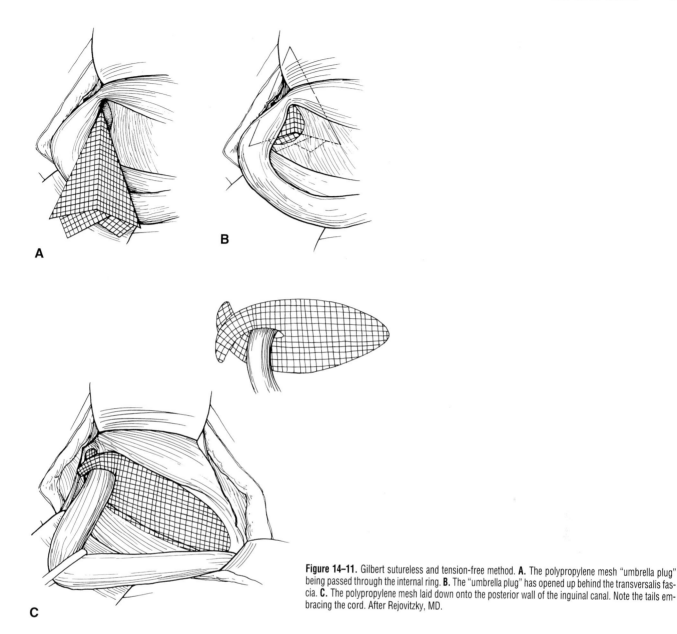

Figure 14–11. Gilbert sutureless and tension-free method. **A.** The polypropylene mesh "umbrella plug" being passed through the internal ring. **B.** The "umbrella plug" has opened up behind the transversalis fascia. **C.** The polypropylene mesh laid down onto the posterior wall of the inguinal canal. Note the tails embracing the cord. After Rejovitzky, MD.

there is a minimum of disturbance of the tissues, the shutter mechanism is left intact, and the musculoaponeurotic arch is not destroyed by sutures. There is also a minimum of postoperative discomfort. Since the Gilbert type I and II hernias constitute about 75% of all indirect hernias, this method, if proved successful, will contribute greatly to the ease and shortening of the time for repair of these hernias, as well as patient comfort. In 1992 Gilbert reported a series of 482 cases repaired by this sutureless technique with only one recurrence, owing to omission of the onlay swatch.[74]

Gilbert Type III. The type III hernia has a large internal ring, two fingerbreadths or more, as is often seen with large scrotal and sliding hernias. The reduced indirect

peritoneal sac will prolapse out immediately without any effort on the part of the patient (Fig 14–12A). This situation calls for a complete reconstruction of the internal ring and of the posterior wall of the canal. The transversalis fascia is slit completely open, and the upper and lower flaps are lifted and freed from the underlying preperitoneal fat (Fig 14–12B). An underlay polypropylene mesh graft is laid on the preperitoneal fat (Fig 14–12C). The transversalis fascia and the musculoaponeurotic arch of the transversus abdominis are approximated in two overlapping layers to the inguinal ligament, and, at the same time, a new snug internal ring is constructed (Fig 14–12D). The slit-open anterior wall of the canal, the external oblique aponeurosis, is reconstituted in front of the cord.

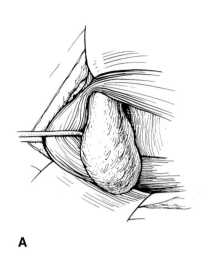

A

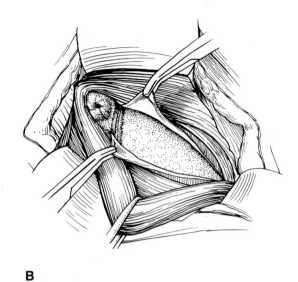

B

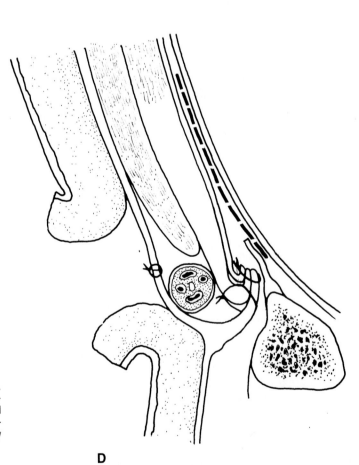

C

D

Figure 14–12. Gilbert type III hernia. **A.** The sac passing through a large internal ring. **B.** The transversalis fascia has been slit open and freed from the underlying preperitoneal fat. The sac is invaginated. **C.** The polypropylene mesh laid on the preperitoneal fat. **D.** The transversalis fascia and musculoaponeurotic arch of the transversus abdominis sutured in two layers to the inguinal ligament in front of the underlay polypropylene mesh graft. After Rejovitzky, MD.

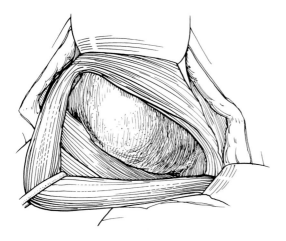

Figure 14–13. Gilbert type IV hernia. After Rejovitzky, MD.

Gilbert Type IV. The type IV hernia is a typical direct hernia characterized by a large or full blow-out of the posterior wall of the canal (Fig 14–13). The internal ring is intact. This hernia is dealt with in the same manner as a type III hernia with an underlay graft and complete two-layer overlap repair of the posterior wall (Fig 14–12C and D).

Gilbert Type V. The type V hernia is a direct hernia protruding through a punched-out hole in the transversalis fascia. The internal ring is intact (Fig 14–14A). This hernia is similar to a punched-out recurrent hernia through the posterior wall of the canal, and both are dealt with similarly. The herniation is invaginated after freeing it from the edges of the defect and a polypropylene rolled-up plug is passed completely through the defect where it expands somewhat and remains in place (Fig 14–14B, C, and D). If it is technically possible, a polypropylene mesh onlay graft is placed on the posterior wall and is covered by suturing the transversalis fascia and transversus abdominis aponeurosis to the inguinal ligament (Fig 14–14E). If the posterior wall is strong, only the plug is inserted and held in place by the Lichtenstein four- or five-stitch technique. The external oblique aponeurosis is resutured in front of the cord.

In 1987, Gilbert reported that he had used his classification and types of repair for the past 5 years and had not yet had a single recurrence in primary or recurrent hernias.[73,121]

The Rutkow Mesh-Plug Hernioplasty. In 1989, Rutkow and associates went further than Gilbert's limitation of using the plug and mesh repair for only types I and II hernias by extending its use to the Gilbert type III hernias as well.[177] As their confidence in the method increased, they used it for types IV and V, as well, and also for double or pantallon hernias, which they designated as type

VI, and for femoral hernias, designated type VII. In 1993, Robbins and Rutkow reported their results of 1563 "mesh-plug" hernioplasties on types I through VII hernias, primary as well as recurrent, with the remarkably low recurrence rate of 0.1%.[122] They also use a flat piece of polypropylene mesh, as does Gilbert, but they roll it into a cone instead of folding it into Gilbert's umbrella. The size of the plug is adjusted according to the size of the internal ring or the hernial defect and the pointed narrow end of the cone is inserted first. In type III hernias, the shutter mechanism has usually been destroyed so, to ensure that the plug will not be ejected, it is sutured around its wide base to the edges of the crura with a few interrupted polyglactin absorbable sutures. This is also found to be advisable in some type II hernias. The same technique of suturing the base of the cone to the edges of the defect is used in types IV through VIII as well, no matter how large the defect and whether primary or recurrent. An overlay graft of flat polypropylene mesh then is placed with the sutureless technique on the anterior surface of the posterior wall of the inguinal canal. This is cut to fit the size and shape of the inguinal canal. Its lateral portion is split to embrace the cord. The external oblique is repaired in front of the cord. Epidural anesthesia is used as the method of choice and all patients are discharged several hours after completion of their operation. Postoperative pain is significantly decreased owing to the minimal dissection and the absence of tension, as well as to the epidural anesthetic. They do not use any perioperative prophylactic antibiotics and have had virtually no problems with infection or rejection of the mesh grafts.

Pure Prosthetic Repairs

The Lichtenstein Tension-Free Repair. In the second edition of his book on hernia repair, Lichtenstein describes a preliminary report of more than 300 cases of direct and indirect hernia treated by a new concept.[16] At that stage the maximum follow-up was only 2 years, but no recurrence was noted. In 1993, Lichtenstein reported that, since 1984, all primary direct and indirect hernias in adult men had been treated by the tension-free technique without closure of the defect.[113] In more than 3000 cases there were only four recurrences that occurred early in their experience. There were no failures in the last five years. The procedure is performed under local anesthesia in an outpatient facility. The skin and subcutaneous tissues are incised and the external oblique aponeurosis is slit open to reveal the inguinal canal. The cord is elevated from the posterior wall of the canal. An indirect sac is dissected free and invaginated into the abdomen. If there is a large direct hernia, the sac may be invaginated by an absorbable imbricating suture to allow positioning of the screen on a flat surface.

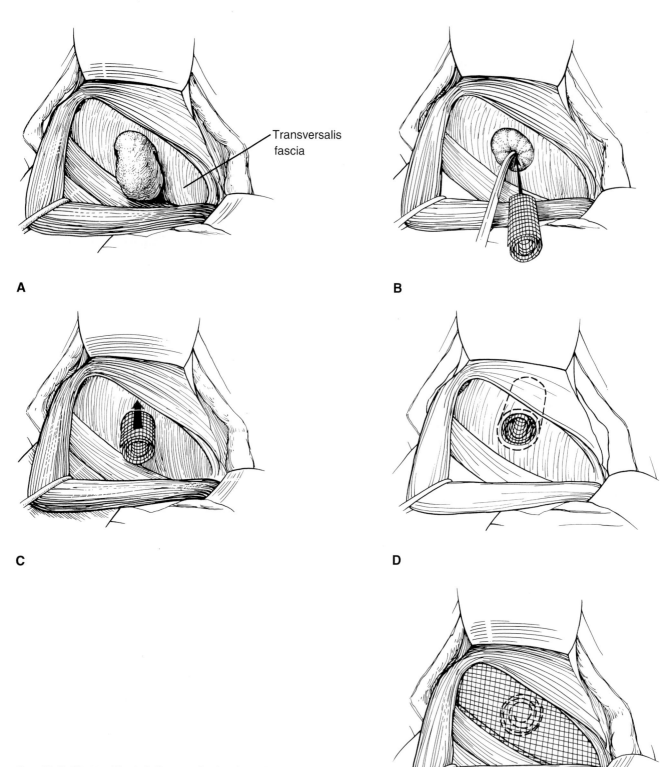

Transversalis
fascia

A

B

C

D

Figure 14–14. Gilbert type V hernia. **A.** The sac passing through a punched-out defect of the posterior wall of the canal. **B.** The sac is being invaginated. **C.** The "plug" of polypropylene mesh is passed through the punched-out defect. **D.** The "plug" has expanded. **E.** The polypropylene mesh onlay graft placed onto the posterior wall of the inguinal canal. After Rejovitzky, MD.

E

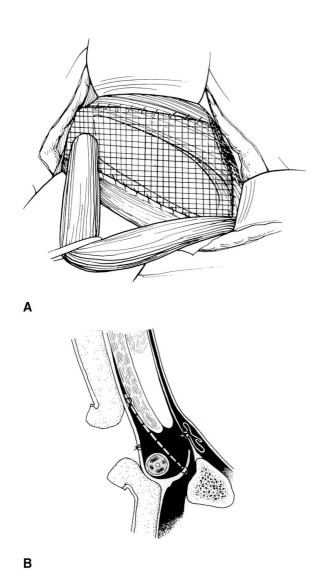

A

B

Figure 14–15. The Lichtenstein tension-free repair. **A.** The sheet of polypropylene mesh attached to the abdominal wall. **B.** The inverted sac of the hernia and the points of attachment of the polypropylene mesh. After Rejovitzky, MD.

A sheet of polypropylene mesh measuring approximately 8 × 6 cm is trimmed to fit the area exposed and used to reconstruct the entire floor of the inguinal canal without any attempt to close the defect by suture. The mesh is sutured along its lower edge to the pubic tubercle, the lacunar ligament, and the inguinal ligament to beyond the internal ring with a continuous suture of the monofilament 3-0 polypropylene. The medial edge is sutured to the rectus sheath, also with a continuous suture of 3-0 polypropylene. The superior edge is tacked down to the aponeurosis or muscle of the internal oblique with a few interrupted sutures. The lateral edge of the mesh is slit and the two tails passed around to embrace the cord at the internal ring; they then are crossed over each other and tacked down to the inguinal ligament with one

polypropylene suture (Fig 14–15, A and B). This creates a new internal ring and shutter mechanism. The external oblique aponeurosis then is resutured in front of the cord. This is a completely tensionless repair and requires no formal reconstruction of the canal floor; it is a revolutionary departure from the tissue repairs used for the past 100 years since Bassini.

The Rives Prosthetic Mesh Repair. In contrast to Lichtenstein's tension-free repair, Rives recommends placing the sheet of polypropylene mesh in a deeper plane (ie, deep to the transversalis fascia between it and the peritoneum).[178] This procedure necessitates slitting the transversalis fascia and freeing it widely. A larger sheet of mesh is used. The lower margin is folded over in a hem and is fixed by a series of interrupted sutures of 2-0 monofilament polypropylene along the pectineal (Cooper) ligament and the fascia iliaca (Fig 14–16A). The mesh then is slipped behind the cord and is passed upward behind the transversus abdominis aponeurosis, transversalis fascia, and rectus sheath and is fixed by interrupted sutures to the full, combined thickness of the internal oblique and transversus muscles and the outer edge of the rectus muscle and sheath (Fig 14–16B and C). The superior border or superolateral edge is split to accommodate the cord and the ends of the tail also are fixed to the full thickness of the two deeper muscles. The advantage of this method is that it uses healthy strong tissues far from the hernial defect to anchor the prosthesis, which also is kept in place by the intra-abdominal pressure forcing it up against the posterior aspect of the anterior abdominal wall. The prosthesis is further fixed by being incorporated into a layer of scar tissue. The mesh is covered by suturing the musculoaponeurotic arch of the transversus abdominis and internal oblique muscle, and transversalis fascia above to the transversalis fascia and inguinal ligament below. The external oblique muscle is closed in front of the cord. This method is intended for very large hernias or for recurrent inguinal hernias with large defects of the abdominal wall. A similar technique of giant prosthetic reinforcement of the visceral sac performed through an anterior groin incision has also been described.[92,179]

Rives also uses a midline subumbilical abdominal approach with preperitoneal dissection to place a large sheet of mesh over the inner surface of the anterior, inferior, and posterior abdominal wall in the inguinal region, between the peritoneum and the abdominal wall on the side of the hernia (Fig 14–17). He recommends this approach especially for difficult recurrent hernias in which the pectineal (Cooper) ligament has been destroyed and the anatomy of the inguinal region has been scarred and distorted.[178]

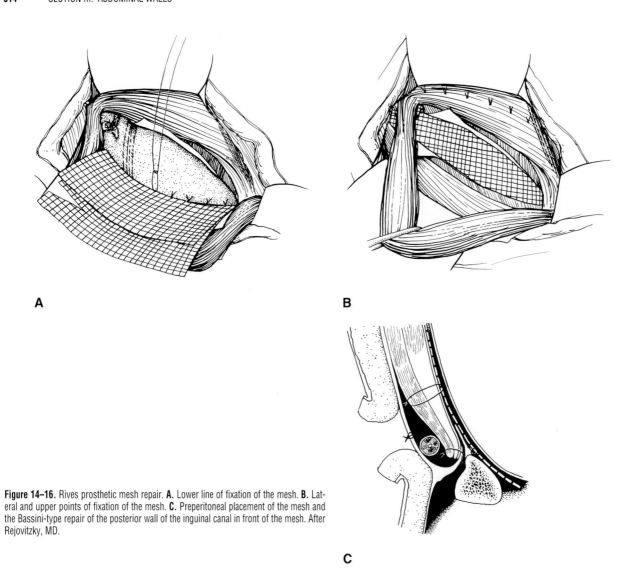

Figure 14–16. Rives prosthetic mesh repair. **A.** Lower line of fixation of the mesh. **B.** Lateral and upper points of fixation of the mesh. **C.** Preperitoneal placement of the mesh and the Bassini-type repair of the posterior wall of the inguinal canal in front of the mesh. After Rejovitzky, MD.

A   B

Figure 14–17. Rives abdominal approach showing the points of attachment of the mesh in the preperitoneal plane. After Rejovitzky, MD.

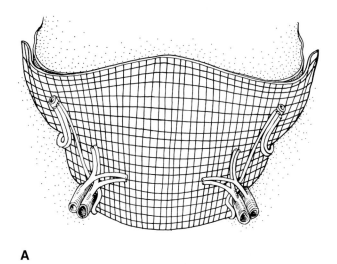

A

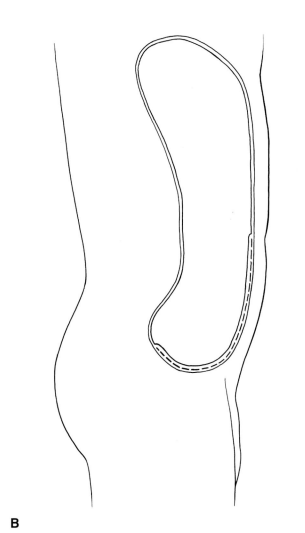

B

Figure 14–18. Stoppa great prosthesis for reinforcement of the visceral sac (GPRVS). **A.** The mesh spread around the peritoneum of the lower abdomen. **B.** The mesh in the preperitoneal plane, stretching from the level of the umbilicus and across the floor of the pelvis, covering all actual and potential hernial orifices. After Rejovitzky, MD.

The Stoppa Great Prosthesis for Reinforcement of the Visceral Sac. This pure prosthetic type of repair is unique and quite revolutionary in concept and requires a complete mental turnabout in one's approach to hernia surgery, which has always been concerned with, or perhaps even obsessed by, methods for the repair of the defect of the weakened, stretched, or torn abdominal wall breached by hernias. Stoppa's method is not primarily concerned with these openings in the abdominal wall parietes and practically ignores them. The principle of the method, as described by Stoppa, is "extensive prosthetic reinforcement of the peritoneum" by a large sheet of knitted polyester fiber (dacron, mersilene) placed between the peritoneum and the anterior, inferior, and posterior, and lateral abdominal walls through a midline lower abdominal incision.[72,180] The mesh stretches around the lower abdomen and pelvis from one side to the other like a bucket, enveloping the lower half of the parietal peritoneum with which it becomes incorporated by collagen and scar tissue. This acts as a large prosthetic buttress of the peritoneal envelope and renders it quite inextensible and no longer able to herniate through any of the actual or potential hernial orifices (Fig 14–18A and B).

When correctly placed, the large prosthesis does not require any anchoring sutures. It is kept in place by Pascal's principle of hydrostatic pressure: "the intraabdominal pressure acting via the peritoneal envelope holds the prosthesis solidly against the abdominal wall. In this way the prosthesis is immediately fixed in position, then reinforced by the cicatricial investment of the dacron mesh." The method does not cause any further damage to the abdominal wall in the region of the groin.

Stoppa has used this technique since 1968 and summarized his experience in 1987.[187] This important addition to the armamentarium of the hernia surgeon will no doubt be used extensively in the future. Stoppa stresses the ease and speed with which this procedure is performed and recommends it especially in cases of complicated hernial lesions or multiple recurrence in which the inguinal anatomy has been largely scarred and distorted or destroyed. It is particularly useful in elderly patients with large bilateral hernias. Most surgeons will no doubt continue to repair inguinal hernias by the more conventional methods, as does Stoppa and his group. However, this group has engendered such confidence in the method that they now recommend it for routine use in patients more than 60 years of age even with a unilateral hernia, and at the slightest doubt in the patients under 60 years of age, such as those with bilaterial hernias, with a weak abdominal wall, or whose work demands heavy physical labor. They summarized their indications for GPRVS as "those hernias that present a high risk of recurrence such as recurring hernias, bilateral groin hernias, groin hernias associated with low incisional hernias, simultaneous direct and indirect hernias, large hernias, recurring hernias when Poupart's and/or Cooper's ligaments are destroyed, and prevascular hernias."[96,97] To this list he added those hernias related to collagen diseases such as Ehlers-Danlos and Marfan syndromes and patients in whom surgery is a risky proposition because of old age, obesity or cirrhosis. This is indeed a long list of patients who make up 30% to 40% of groin hernias in Stoppa's practice. He reports a series of 2000 cases of GPRVS followed from 1 to 12 years with recurrence rates of 0.56% for primary groin hernias and 1.1% for recurrent groin hernias—a truly remarkable success story when one considers that the "best" cases were operated on by conventional inguinal methods, whereas the "worst" cases were repaired by GPRVS.

Postoperative Recovery

Patients whose hernias have been repaired under local anesthesia usually leave the hospital on the same day. Those who have had a general, spinal, or epidural anesthetic may also be discharged on the same day but are often kept overnight. Postoperative pain can be reduced to a minimum in those cases not treated by a local anesthetic, by injecting a long-acting local anesthetic such as bupivacaine into the tissues of the groin region and into the iliohypogastric and ilioinguinal nerves. Alternatively, the local anesthetic agent can be simply instilled into the wound to flood the area before closing the external oblique aponeurosis. These methods of producing postoperative analgesia are efficient.[181]

When necessary, simple nonopiate analgesia can be given orally.

In 1925, Herzfeld, working in an overcrowded hospital in a socioeconomically depressed area, introduced ambulatory daycare hernia surgery in infants and children and showed that there was no relationship between early discharge and postoperative complications or recurrences.[182,183] Once it became accepted that there is no relationship between early mobilization and the risk of recurrence of the hernia, postoperative hospitalization became superfluous for most patients. There was no specific service that the institution could contribute to their postoperative comfort which was not available to them at home. However, the socioeconomic and medical status of a patient may make him unsuitable for same-day discharge. This was confirmed in the Lancet in 1985[144]; it was found that in practice, about one-third of patients were discharged on the day of operation, about one-third were kept in overnight and discharged less than 24 hours after the operation, and the remaining one-third was discharged only after four to five days because of age, medical and socioeconomic reasons.[184–190]

In the private hernia centers in the United States, the patients are usually of a higher socioeconomic status, making for a certain amount of selection of patients. The result is that practically all of the patients are discharged on the same day of the operation. This applies to many thousands of patients from such centers as Lichtenstein's in California, Gilbert's in Florida and Rutkow's in New Jersey. Yet at the Shouldice Hospital, the patients are kept in for three days postoperatively and for five days if bilateral repairs are done. In the United States, Bellis recently reported his personal series of 27 267 cases of inguinal herniorrhaphy done under local anesthesia and with the use of mesh, all discharged on the same day.[191] In my department, about half of the patients are operated under local anesthesia and are discharged on the same day. The rest are given spinal or general anesthesia and are discharged the next morning, usually less than 24 hours postoperatively. A very few may stay on for an extra day or two because of medical or socioeconomic reasons. All patients are encouraged to ambulate on the day of the operation and to be as active as possible thereafter.

The modern tendency to close the skin with an intradermal continuous absorbable suture has simplified wound care. Good alternatives are closing the skin with adhesive bands, or Michel clips. These methods avoid having a foreign body, the suture, pass through the skin to the subcutaneous layers and thus possibly introduce infection along the suture track. All dressings are removed on the first postoperative morning. The wound should be clean and dry and sealed by this time. Patients may shower or bathe as they wish. Clips are removed on the second postoperative morning, that is, less than 48 hours after the operation.

No restrictions are placed on physical activities. Patients are encouraged to return to a normal active lifestyle as soon as possible, within the initial limitations of postoperative discomfort. The repair immediately after the operation is as strong as it will ever be if strong monofilament nylon or a synthetic nonabsorbable mesh was used and was anchored into healthy tissues. The darn or the prosthetic material is indestructible from the practical point of view and will hold the repair indefinitely. The collagen scar tissue contributes no strength to the repair for the first few months and little strength thereafter. There is therefore no advantage in limiting postoperative activities. This has been substantiated by a series of thousands of cases. During the past 45 years, it has been shown repeatedly that there is no evidence that lengthy rest reduces the chance of recurrence and that the opposite is usually the case. For almost 50 years, patients at the Shouldice Hospital have traditionally walked from the operating room table to their bed and yet this center has a remarkably low recurrence rate. Patients who return to work and resume heavy lifting have the same recurrence rate as those who return to nonstrenuous work. Indeed, several series have shown that persons with sedentary occupations have double the risk for recurrences as opposed to those who return to heavy manual labor. Barwell showed that the recurrence rate depends less on the activity of the patient and more on the technique used for repair and the ability of the surgeon.[192] However, even though we allow patients to return to normal activities, that does not mean that they do so. Motivation on the part of the patient is the most important factor influencing the time of return to work. In my own practice, I find that highly motivated, self-employed professionals are back in their offices within a few days of the operation. Less motivated, salaried employees with generous sick leave and pay benefits may quickly return to their private activities but are in no hurry to return to work, especially if their family doctor easily provides sick leave certificates. In these cases, they may return to work only after three to eight weeks or more, depending on the degree of physical effort entailed in their work. This represents a great loss to the national work force and income. Although there is no fixed rule, 10 days to 2 weeks leave postoperatively is considered sufficient for a sedentary worker and 3 weeks for a manual laborer.[194–196]

GIANT INGUINAL HERNIA

A giant inguinal hernia is defined as one that reaches below the midlevel of the thigh when the patient stands. The truly large ones reach to below the knees or even almost to the ankles and may contain most of the small and large bowel and the stomach as well. The hernia usually grows over years and with time, the skin of the huge scrotum becomes grossly thickened, edematous and leathery. The inguinal canal is overstretched and the layers of the abdominal wall in the region are thinned out. The internal and external rings are wide open and displaced and come to lie opposite each other so that the normal oblique line of the inguinal canal disappears. The musculoaponeurotic arch is also greatly stretched and attenuated and may be at a relatively great distance from the inguinal or pectineal (Cooper's) ligaments. Patients suffer great discomfort from the weight and size of the enormous hernia and will walk with great difficulty or may be practically immobilized. Furthermore, the weight of the hernia drags down the skin of the abdomen over the penis which gets buried deep down at the end of a long tunnel and cannot be reached so that the patient loses control of his urinary stream, causing the skin of the lower abdomen, scrotum and thighs to be constantly excoriated and infected.

The management of a truly giant inguinal hernia may be a major surgical challenge. The repair can be done from below through a standard groin approach and the defect can usually be closed satisfactorily by any of the standard repairs such as the Shouldice, or the author's nylon darn or the Cooper's ligament techniques. In more problematic cases, a prosthetic mesh can be inserted through the groin approach. Stoppa advises repairing them through a midline abdominal approach using his great prosthesis for the reinforcement of the visceral sac (GPRVS).[96] The spermatic cord on the side of the hernia is usually very elongated and twisted and the testis grossly edematous and enlarged. In most reported cases, preservation of the testis was impossible because of technical reasons, and orchidectomy was done. Two difficult problems arise: returning the many loops of bowel, stomach and omentum to the abdominal cavity, and dealing with the enormous, edematous and superfluous scrotum. The bowel can usually be coaxed back into the abdominal cavity though some pressure may be needed. The resultant pressure and upward displacement of the diaphragm may make respiratory assistance mandatory for even a few days postoperatively. Preoperative stretching of the abdominal wall by pneumoperitoneum is not successful since the inflated air escapes into the huge hernial sac. Other methods that have been suggested include bowel resection such as subtotal colectomy and a relaxing midline epigastric incision. The scrotum is dealt with by amputation followed by plastic reconstruction of a neoscrotum and skin coverage for the penis by local skin flaps.[193] This can be done at the time of the hernia repair or postponed for later as a second stage procedure. The problems are compounded when the patient presents with strangulation of the hernia. After suitable resuscitation, the hernia is explored and if the patient's general condition and the condition of the strangulated bowel allow for return of the hernial content to the abdomen and repair of the hernia, this should be done. If this is not possible, the strangulating neck of the hernia may be incised or even the inguinal ligament partly or wholly cut across and bowel resection done where necessary. The wound is closed and after a few weeks when the patient has recovered and the swollen and edematous bowel has returned to normal, the hernia repair can be done. There is a very high mortality associated with strangulation of these giant hernias.[197,198]

SPORTS HERNIA

This is a vexing and somewhat confusing subject much written about in the sports medicine literature. Some of the reports, such as Taylor's in 1991,[199] describe series of cases of frank inguinal hernias treated successfully in patients who happen to be sportsmen, a situation which apparently does not warrant a special grouping. Others report cases of athletes complaining of chronic undiagnosed groin pain who undergo surgical exploration of the groin. In some cases, a shorter or longer patent processus vaginalis is found but it is not clear whether this is a true hernia. It is reported that most of these athletes return to their normal activities after repair of this hernia with a marked improvement in the level of pain. In other reports, series of similar cases are reported of sportsmen complaining of chronic undiagnosed groin pain who were operated on for exploration of the groin.[200,201] It is claimed that, in the majority of them, distention of the posterior inguinal wall or even a "significant bulge" is present, representing an early direct inguinal hernia, and that the majority are cured of their pain after repair of the posterior inguinal wall. However, in about 20% of cases, no pathology is found, or else it is a pathology that does not require surgical treatment such as "avulsion of fibers of the internal oblique muscle from the pubic tubercle." These patients have undergone an unnecessary operation. Herniography is advised in an attempt at more accurate preoperative diagnosis to confirm the presence of distention of the posterior inguinal wall, to avoid unnecessary operations on normal subjects. Van den Berg published his series of herniography done for unexplained groin pain or anterior abdominal wall pain with no false-positive results and no complications, and advises the use of this examination in these cases.[129] It is not clear whether athletes who complain of chronic undiagnosed groin pain and in whom no obvious groin hernia is present should be advised to undergo an operative exploration of the groin.

COMPLICATIONS OF INGUINAL HERNIA REPAIR

Hernia repair is safe, but, like all operations, it may be attended by general or specific complications.

General Complications

The general complications include pulmonary atelectasis, pulmonary embolism, pneumonia, thrombophlebitis, and urinary retention. Most can be avoided by good preoperative preparation and by early and active ambulation. Postoperative urinary retention should be a rare phenomenon. Prostatic patients with symptoms severe enough to need prostatectomy may conveniently have this procedure combined with simultaneous herniorrhaphy. Alternatively, the prostate should be dealt with first and the hernia repaired some weeks later. If the prostatic complaints are borderline and there is no clear indication for prostatectomy, or if the patient refuses the operation but requests repair of his hernia, the problem can be overcome by the introduction into the bladder via the urethra of a fine #5 or #8 neonatal teflon feeding tube immediately after the induction of anesthesia. The catheter is removed 24 hours postoperatively. Urinary retention may be treated by temporary

catheterization with a fine neonatal feeding tube as above, and with phenoxybenzamine (Dibenzyline). Persistent cases may need prostatectomy. The most potent cause of postoperative urinary retention is probably distention atony brought about by overfilling of the bladder owing to over-enthusiastic infusion of fluids during and after the operation, especially when general, spinal, or epidural anesthesia is used. Herniorrhaphy causes only minor surgical trauma and there is no need for large volumes of intravenous fluids. The infusion may be removed within an hour of cessation of the operation and oral fluids can be taken a few hours later.

Local Complications

Hemorrhage. Ecchymosis of the skin around the incision is common. Occasionally, mild ooze of blood may seep into the skin of the penis and scrotum. The discoloration may appear alarming, but the blood absorbs and disappears within a matter of days. Scrotal hematomas may reach large proportions but usually absorb with time. Sometimes they may need to be aspirated or evacuated surgically, although this is often not possible because of the blood having oozed into the scrotal tissues. Rarely, these hematomas become infected, and the resulting abscess must be drained.

Serious hemorrhage may occur during the operation. It usually is the result of injury to the inferior epigastric vessels during suturing and is handled by ligating these vessels. More serious is a tear in the external iliac vessels, which may necessitate formal exposure and repair of the arterial or venous wall.

Bladder Injury. The urinary bladder may be opened inadvertently when dissecting the sac of a direct or large indirect hernia. This usually can be avoided if direct sacs are not dissected but simply inverted when the posterior wall of the canal is repaired. It is also less likely to happen if indirect sacs are invaginated and not ligated high. The opening in the bladder is sutured in two layers and a urethral catheter is placed in the bladder for 8 days.

Testicular Complications. Testicular swelling, orchitis, and testicular atrophy are the result of interference with the blood supply and probably the lymphatic drainage of the testis. They are rarely the result of tearing and ligation of the testicular artery but may be the result of tying off the veins in the spermatic cord when the cremaster muscle is resected, and when the distal part of the sac has been dissected unnecessarily.

Another cause of testicular swelling or atrophy may be congestion owing to closing the internal ring too snugly around the cord. The testicular swelling may take some weeks to subside and occasionally leads to testicular atrophy. In the case of planned or accidental transection of the cord, apparently no damage is done in about one-third of the cases, if the testis has a good collateral blood supply and the cremaster has not been excised below the level of the pubic tubercle. In the other two-thirds, some degree of testicular swelling, pain, tenderness, and fever ensue, and one-half of these cases go on to atrophy of the testis. In the others, some degree of permanent damage to the testis ensues. Rarely, acute necrosis and gangrene of the testis occur and often are complicated further by infection and abscess formation. This is best treated by antibiotics, early reoperation, and excision of the necrotic testis and cord. The wound is left open.

In children and young adults, testicular damage will have serious consequences owing to reduced fertility. It has been reported that 6.65% or 8500 patients with infertility had had inguinal hernioplasty with or without subsequent atrophy of the testis, and semen quality was reduced markedly owing to ischemic orchitis or immunological reactions.[148] Kald found a 2.7% rate of testicular atrophy in patients years after hernia repair,[202] and Fong and Wantz urged minimal cord dissection, leaving intact all significant distal hernial sacs and no dissection beyond the pubic tubercle.[203] They recommend the properitoneal approach for all recurrent hernias to avoid difficult dissection of the cord.

Vas Deferens Injuries.
Transection of the vas deferens is an unusual accident. In the young adult, it is best treated by immediate anastomosis. In older men, the torn ends are simply ligated. It must be stressed that, besides obvious tearing or cutting of the vas deferens, it may also be damaged, especially in children, by undue pressure, traction, kinking, and especially by squeezing between the ends of a dissecting forceps. These traumas lead to damage to the wall and mucosa of the vas, with consequent fibrosis and obstruction. The problem of transection or obstruction of the vas deferens is not just the failure of the sperm to reach the seminal vesicles, nor just the pressure atrophy leading to degeneration of the spermatic tubercles, but also the production of serum antisperm antibodies. Vasilev reported eight cases of sterility following iatrogenic obstruction of the vas after repair of inguinal hernias.[147] Reanastomosis was done in six by microsurgery with marked improvement in the spermatological indices in three. Sandhu discusses the problem of oligospermia after vas deferens injury at hernia operations.[149] Matsuda points out that in his series, the incidence of unilateral vas deferens obstruction was 26.7% for subfertile patients with a history of inguinal hernia repair during childhood.[150,151] He also states that the true incidence of vasal disruption caused by inguinal hernia operations in infancy is unknown but is probably greater than his series indicates. A significant percentage of patients with vasal obstruc-

tion caused by infant inguinal herniorrhaphy have serum antisperm antibodies despite the absence of sperm granulomas.

Bowel Injuries.
Small bowel may be injured if caught in the transfixion suture when the sac is ligated. Cecum or sigmoid colon may be opened or devascularized when they form part of the wall of a sliding hernia. These complications are avoided if the sac is invaginated and not suture ligated. They are serious injuries and require experience and judgment for correct and successful management.

Nerve Injury.
The nerves in the region often are injured during inguinal hernia operations. The main nerves are the iliohypogastric, ilioinguinal, and the genital branch of the genitofemoral. In theory, they should be preserved but, in practice, this is not always possible. The iliohypogastric nerve is often transected when the upper leaf of the external oblique aponeurosis is elevated. The ilioinguinal nerve may be torn when the cord is mobilized, and the genital branch of the genitofemoral nerve is usually resected when the cremaster muscle is excised. These injuries cause varying degrees of anesthesia or paresthesia in the region of the sensory distribution of the nerves, which pass after some weeks or months. Fortunately, extensive crossing and overlapping between these nerves limit the area of discomfort. Sometimes nerves are caught in sutures and cause severe burning pain on movement. This too usually passes spontaneously but occasionally may require injection for nerve blocking or even exploration for release of the entrapped nerve. Rarely, the femoral nerve may be caught in a suture during a Cooper's ligament repair or a large prosthetic repair, causing paresis or paralysis of the muscles supplied by the nerve and requiring exploration and release of the entrapped nerve. These so-called postherniorrhaphy neuralgias often are compounded by personality and behavior problems as well as by hopes of financial compensation.

Wound Infection.
Wound infection is a potent cause of recurrence of hernias. In specialized ambulatory surgery units the incidence of postoperative wound infections is around 1% or less. In general hospitals, the incidence may be as high as 5%. Furthermore, these figures may not reflect the true incidence of wound infection since they are published by the surgical units who do the operations, and several recent surveys show that 50% to 75% of the true incidence of hernia wound infections occur after the patients have left the hospital and are unknown to the surgeon so that the overall incidence may be even four or five times that usually reported.[204–208]

Wound infection varies in degree from the mildest and insignificant to the castastrophic. There may be only some minor redness of the skin edges, a discharge of some clear serous fluid, or a small stitch abscess. These do not influence the recurrence rate and do not need any specific treatment. More serious is frank cellulitis in and around the wound that may progress to fasciitis and necrosis of the tissues on each side and in the depths of the incision, or to abscess formation and purulent discharge from the wound. Careful preoperative skin preparation, strict sterility discipline, atraumatic dissection, and gentle tissue handling will reduce wound infection to an absolute minimum. Antibiotic therapy should be initiated as soon as cellulitis is observed. This treatment may be sufficient to abort the problem. Once wound infection is established, the wound should be widely opened to allow free drainage. If monofilament nylon sutures were used, the wound will heal even if the sutures are exposed, and the hernia usually will not recur. Even where a prosthetic mesh was inserted, the wound usually heals. The mesh need rarely be removed. Postoperative suction drainage significantly reduces the incidence of wound hematoma, seroma, and infection following repair of large hernias, recurrent hernias, difficult hernias requiring much dissection, and otherwise complicated hernias.[209]

There is no general consensus about the use of prophylactic antibiotics in hernia surgery.[15,20,78,102,198,199,204,206,209–217] A routine inguinal hernia repair should not need antibiotic coverage. Ronaboldo, in 1993, reports that 72% of wound infections occur after discharge from hospital and incur high costs to the patient and the medical services. Thus, prophylactic antibiotics should be considered for clean cases of hernia since they are easy to use and cost-effective if given orally. There is no clear evidence to show that the postoperative infection rate is lower when antibiotics are used. Detailed attention to gentle operating techniques is probably more important. An antibiotic "umbrella" cannot cover up for bad surgery. Some surgeons irrigate the operation site at intervals with an antibiotic or bactericidal solution, but there is no evidence to show that this influences the rate of infection.[15,102,198,199,211,216]

When dealing with very large hernias, or recurrent hernias or hernias with infected granulomas from previous operations, or with incisional hernias, antibiotic coverage is commonly used because bacteria may remain present in wounds for prolonged periods of time. A wound once considered infected should always be considered so.[218] It has been recommended that perioperative antibiotics should be used when reoperating a recurrent hernia.[218,219] Houch found that repair of incisional hernia has a significantly higher infection rate than other clean operations, ten times that for clean laparotomies and 20 times that for inguinal herniorrhaphy, and especially so if the original incision was infected.[219] The high rate of infection is significantly reduced if perioperative antibiotics are used.[219] Repair of an incisional hernia or a recurrent hernia should not be classified as a clean surgical procedure but should be regarded as a contaminated operation requiring perioperative antibiotics.[219]

Postherniorrhaphy Paravesical Suture Granulomas. Several publications have recently reported the finding of a palpable mass close to the urinary bladder, caused by a foreign body reaction to sutures used in the repair of an inguinal or femoral hernia. The mass may be found some months after the hernia operation or even up to 11 years as in one reported case. Lynch reported 11 cases.[220] Some of the cases had urinary symptoms, probably not linked to the presence of the mass that was found abutting on the bladder. In these cases, a malignant tumor was suspected clinically. Neulander reported a case of a patient with carcinoma of the urinary bladder where the palpable mass was thought to be a pelvic metastasis.[221] The treatment for postherniorrhaphy paravesical granuloma is excision.

HERNIA REPAIR COMBINED WITH OTHER OPERATIONS

Bilateral Hernia Repair

Bilateral hernias in children are usually repaired at the same operation. In adults, the subject has been controversial. There are certain distinct advantages to simultaneous bilateral inguinal herniorrhaphy. At the cost of little extra operating time, the patient is saved double admissions to hospital, two separate anesthetics, extra total operating time and twice the convalescent time. The financial benefit to the patient and to the health-providing authorities is obvious. If it can be shown that all this can be achieved at no extra risk to the patient of postoperative complications or an increase in the recurrence rate, then the method should be recommended. This has, in fact, been shown to be so.[19,139,141,145,222–226] These patients were operated under local, regional, or general anesthesia and most were discharged within 24 hours. At the Shouldice Hospital, the two operations are performed 48 hours apart when local anesthesia is used, to avoid toxic doses.[227,228] However, when general anesthesia is used for an unrelated reason, both operations are done at the same time.

It is difficult to find a dissenting opinion. The confidence in the safety of bilateral simultaneous herniorrhaphy is enhanced by reports that it can be safely combined with other procedures such as transurethral or open suprapubic or retropubic prostatectomy. Bilateral simultaneous inguinal herniorrhaphy therefore can be recommended as both safe and economical. It does not increase the recurrence rate.[174] However, it is safer to defer the second side if the first is difficult or prolonged, or involves more dissection than usual.

Incidental Appendectomy. Although in some cases it is possible to remove the appendix when repairing an inguinal hernia, the temptation to do so is best resisted. There is no reason to remove a normal appendix. The exposure is not always safe, and since the bowel lumen must be opened, an element of risk of infection is introduced. An infected herniorrhaphy is not worth the negligible and theoretical benefit of removing a healthy appendix.

Other Operations. A patient scheduled to undergo an operation under general anesthesia may request to take advantage of the same anesthesia to repair his inguinal hernia as well. Generally speaking, there is no real contraindication to this request, provided that the patient's general condition allows a longer procedure and that proper standards of sterility are maintained. In this author's department, we have combined inguinal herniorrhaphy with prostate, thyroid, breast, biliary, gynecological as well as with other hernia operations such as umbilical or epigastric. We believe that the concern about wound infection, recurrence, and extra anesthetic time are exaggerated.

Simultaneous Prostatectomy and Herniorrhaphy. Combined prostatectomy and inguinal herniorrhaphy by either the conventional inguinal route or properitoneal approach was reported.[229,230] In 1988 this author summarized a series of 76 patients with this combined operation.[231] Inguinal herniorrhaphy and prostatectomy are the most frequently performed surgical procedures in the older male population. Not infrequently, inguinal hernia and hypertrophy of the prostate occur together in the same patient. Julke found that 60% of all men more than 50 years of age had pathological voiding function with either residual urine or pathological flow rates or both.[232] While this may not necessarily be a risk factor for the development of inguinal hernia, it certainly occurs in the same age group in which inguinal hernia is most common in males. Besides their anatomic proximity, a close interrelationship may exist between the two entities. Herniorrhaphy, in the presence of untreated but compensated prostatic hypertrophy, may be complicated by urinary retention. The increased intra-abdominal pressure associated with straining in prostatic hypertrophy may be a factor in the development of an inguinal hernia. These considerations, together with the obvious advantage to the patient of having one operation to cure two pathologies, as well as the economic benefit, encouraged the development of a combined but simple approach to both problems.

The series of cases reported began in 1980 and was comprised of patients 51 to 93 years of age with benign prostatic hypertrophy and unilateral or bilateral inguinal hernia.[231] Both procedures were done through the same transverse (Pfannenstiel) incision extended slightly to the side of the hernia. The prostatectomy was either transvesical or retropubic. Bilateral hernias were repaired at the same operation. Four of the unilateral hernias were recurrent after one or more previous repairs. The hernia repair extended the surgery time by 20 to 30 minutes without increasing the morbidity rate. There was one mild wound infection, which cleared up after open drainage, without recurrence of the hernia. So far there has been only one recurrence; that was in a case early in the series in which one side of a simultaneous bilateral hernia repair recurred 2 years after the operation.[174]

Gonzalez compared three groups of men: the first group had inguinal hernia repair combined with transurethal resection of the prostate; the second was a group of men having inguinal hernia repair only; and the third group had transurethral resection of the prostate alone.[233] The first group had the highest incidence of preoperative risk factors because of age and associated medical problems, yet there was no significant difference in operative or postoperative complications. After a 4-year follow-up period, there were no recurrences in the first group. The length of hospitalization was the same in the three groups. There were no deaths. He concludes that combined repair of inguinal hernia and transurethral resection of the prostate is practical, safe, and effective. Furthermore, only one anesthetic, one operation, one hospitalization, and one convalescence is required; all of this with morbidity and mortality comparable to inguinal hernia repair or prostatectomy alone. There have been several reports of simultaneous unilateral or bilateral herniorrhaphy by the standard groin approach combined with transurethral as well as open prostatectomy in hundreds of cases,[234] many of which were poor risk patients. There are also reports of preperitoneal herniorrhaphies done simultaneously with radical retropubic prostatectomies and radical cystoprostatectomies with no complications attributable to the hernia repair and with no increase in the morbidity or recurrence rate.

RECURRENT HERNIA

Etiology

The success of a hernia operation depends almost entirely on the skill, knowledge, understanding, and experience of the surgeon. The best results are achieved in specialized units by dedicated surgeons who confine their practice to hernia surgery. The need for specialized units has recently been discussed.[50,122,235–237] It follows, therefore, that most failed herniorrhaphies, especially the early recurrences, are the result of failure on the part of the surgeon. Late recurrences are usually owing to tissue failure, but here, too, the surgeon is partly to blame in that he failed to take the necessary preventive measures at the original operation. The causes of failure have been discussed earlier in this chapter and are dealt with in greater detail in a 1994 report by Abrahamson.[174] Recurrent hernias are more often direct than indirect, indicating that when repairing an indirect hernia, surgeons do not pay enough attention to the state of the posterior wall of the canal and fail to reinforce it to prevent later failure in the form of a direct hernia.

Tension is a cardinal factor, if not the most important one, in the failure of a hernia repair, and has been discussed earlier in the chapter. Tissues sutured under tension will tend to pull apart but are prevented from doing so by the sutures. However, the tissues pulling on the sutures create an area of ischemic pressure necrosis where the suture meets the tissue. This process of ischemic pressure necrosis will progress until there is no longer any tension, which usually occurs when the tissues have returned to their previous unsutured position and the hernia will recur through the resultant gap. A second mechanism is the cutting out of the sutures from the tissues when the suture tension becomes greater than the strength or holding capacity of the tissues. This depends on several factors but in normal, healthy tissues, it mainly depends on the distance of the suture passing through the tissues from the cut edge and the angle that the suture makes with the line of the fibers of the tissue, as well as the type of tissue. The greater the mass of tissue enclosed in the suture, the more the suture is at right angles to the fibers, and the more aponeurotic the tissue, the less likely is the suture to cut out. The highly successful newer techniques of hernia repair—the tensionless repair of Lichtenstein, the sutureless technique of Gilbert, and the mesh-plug hernioplasty of Rutkow—are all based on the absolute absence of tension.

Infection also will lead to the breakdown of hernia repairs. It has been estimated that approximately 50% of recurrent hernias are the result of infection. Recurrences were four times greater in infected than noninfected repairs in the Shouldice Hospital series. Berliner reported that four out of ten infected wounds in his series developed recurrences.[216] These figures are typical for most published series. The mechanisms by which infected wounds break down are not entirely clear. When there is a frank cellulitis and tissue necrosis, it is obvious why there is complete breakdown of the repair. In less severe reactions, where absorbable or nonabsorbable biological sutures such as silk have been used, the breakdown products of the inflammatory process may hasten the disintegration of the sutures before the wound is strong enough to hold together on its own, so that the wound, unsupported by the sutures, will fall apart.

The inflammation and edema lead to softening and weakening of the tissues, rendering them unable to hold the suture against the strains to which the wound is subjected, so that the tissues will tear and allow the suture to cut out. The infection, with the ensuing inflammation and edema, will cause the tissues to swell, but the mass of tissue enclosed in each suture will attempt to swell against the unyielding ring of the thread, causing pressure necrosis of these tissues and loosening of the suture.

At this stage, even though the wound may heal and the sinuses close, the sutures no longer give the vital support to the tissues. The repair will heal with scar tissue that will eventually give way under the stresses and strains to which it is subjected and the hernia will recur.

The suture material must be nonabsorbable and monofilament, either stainless steel wire or synthetic sutures of the nylon type. There is no logical reason for the use of absorbable sutures nor of biological sutures. Twisted or braided mutifilament sutures also should be avoided. The incidence of recurrence is higher with these sutures. A smooth monofilament nylon, a continuous suture with big bites of tissue spreads the tension evenly throughout the suture line and has more "give" under stress.

The size of the hernia has a negative influence on the outcome of a hernia repair. The larger the hernia, the greater the incidence of recurrence. The tissues have been stretched and attenuated by longstanding pressure, and the large defect is more difficult to close by any method. Previous operative trauma, as reflected by the number of recurrences and repairs the hernia has undergone, will increase the chances of a further recurrence.

An emergency operation on a strangulated hernia in an infant or a child increases the recurrence rate. The tissues are swollen, edematous, and soft and the detailed anatomy is blurred, leading to intraoperative trauma such as overstretching of the internal ring, tearing of the musculoaponeurotic arch of the conjoined tendon, tearing of the posterior wall of the canal, and to later recurrence of the hernia. In the adult, however, there is no clear evidence that an emergency operation at the time of strangulation increases the recurrence rate. Inadequate dissection of the sac of an indirect hernia will leave a preformed passage for a recurrent hernia.

A missed or overlooked hernia may occasionally be the cause of a recurrent hernia. When an obvious direct hernia is found at operation, failure to explore the cord for the presence of an indirect hernia as well, or at least for the presence of a patent processus vaginalis, will lead to the development of an indirect recurrence. Other often overlooked causes are one or more small herniations of extraperitoneal fat through the transversalis fascia or even higher up through the internal oblique and transversus abdominis muscles. Attempts should be made to reduce them and to suture each opening; the posterior wall of the canal and the conjoined musculoaponeurotic arch then should be reinforced with a nylon darn or prosthetic patch.

It is commonly but incorrectly held that orchiectomy will enhance the chances for a better repair and avoid recurrence of a hernia; there is no evidence for this. An undescended testis associated with a hernia in the adult should be removed. The testes also may be removed when repairing hernias in males with carcinoma of the prostate. Rarely, the cord may be torn when repairing a multiple recurrent hernia, and the testis left with very few attachments to provide collateral circulation. In this situation, it is best removed.

The type of operation done for the repair of an inguinal hernia does not influence the recurrence rate. All the recognized techniques have a more or less 1% recurrence rate or even less when done by an experienced hernia surgeon who is familiar with the method and applies it to a suitable patient. On the other hand, even the best method can be botched by an inexperienced and/ or ignorant surgeon.

The general conditions that may lead to recurrence of a repaired hernia are listed and discussed in the section on postoperative ventral abdominal hernias and are also dealt with in greater detail in a report by this author.[174] Contrary to the commonly held belief, obesity has not been shown to be a factor in the occurrence or recurrence of inguinal hernia. In fact, it has been found that obesity even has a certain protective influence in inguinal hernia development.[238] Others have found that a larger proportion of patients with recurrent inguinal hernia were near or below ideal body weight. It seems, however, from most reports, that the percentage of ideal body weight of a patient has no apparent effect on the recurrence rate. The situation is quite the opposite when dealing with postoperative ventral abdominal (incisional) hernias where overweight plays a major role in the production of and in the failure of the operative repair of the hernia.

In 1981, Cannon reported on the profound influence that tobacco smoking has on the production of inguinal hernia and recurrence after repair.[239] The concept has been developed further by others and, in 1991, Read summarized the subject and quoted numerous references.[240] It appears that circulating proteases are released by the lungs leading to free, active, and unbound neutrophil elastase in the plasma of cigarette smokers and that the systemic protease-antiprotease imbalance is a response to cigarette smoking. The uninhibited proteolysis leads to emphysema, hernia, abdominal aortic aneurysm, and skin degeneration.

Inguinal hernia often develops in patients with ascites and there is a high recurrence rate after repair of the hernias in these patients. The mechanism appears to be the opening of a latent processus vaginalis by the increased intra-abdominal hydrostatic pressure. The same effect applies in children and adults with ascites from other causes as well as those with ventriculoperitoneal shunts for hydrocephalus, and those on peritoneal dialysis, especially children on continuous ambulatory peritoneal dialysis (CAPD).[114,152,241,242] In children, there is a high incidence of recurrence of the inguinal hernia if only high ligation of the sac (herniotomy) is done. Children should be carefully evaluated for hernia when they become candidates for peritoneal dialysis and hernias should be promptly repaired as an elective inpatient procedure, with a formal herniorrhaphy performed. In males under two years of age, a bilateral repair should be done even if only a single hernia is present. Once a peritoneal dialysis catheter has been placed, radionuclide substances can be introduced with the dialysis fluid and actual or potential hernias can be demonstrated on groin scans.[114,130] Inguinal herniorrhaphy can be performed safely on patients on peritoneal dialysis, with the dialysis restarted immediately after the operation. In patients with liver cirrhosis and refractory ascites, there is a high recurrence rate of repaired hernias, and the treatment of the ascites is a major determinant of the success of the hernia repair. If the ascites cannot be controlled by medical means, then a peritoneovenous shunt should be inserted separately or concomitantly with the herniorrhaphy. Patients with ascites owing to intra-abdominal malignant disease also tend to develop hernia. This may be the first manifestation of their disease.

Multiple recurrences of repeated repairs of a hernia may, in some cases, be the result of disorders of collagen production, maintenance, and absorption.[239,243–245] In 1987, Peacock recommended a procedure to repair a recurrent direct inguinal hernia based on the hypothesis that recurrence is the result of a localized disorder of collagen metabolism. Stimulation of net collagen synthesis and deposition to restore the balance between collagen synthesis and collagenolysis is achieved by the inductor qualities found in normal human perifascial tissue. The hernial defect is corrected by grafting tissues rich in inductor substances.[244]

Incidence

The incidence of recurrent hernia after primary repair varies widely, from less than 1% in special interest centers to 30% in general surveys. The longer and more complete the follow-up, the higher the recurrence rate. Recurrence after more than one repair is higher and increases with the number of repairs. In a series of 350 recurrent hernia repairs by nylon darn that this author reported in 1988 and had followed-up for 2 to 15 years, the recurrence rate was 2.8 percent.[176]

Operations for Repair of Recurrent Hernia

The findings at operation will vary between two extremes. On one hand there are fairly well preserved tissues and on the other extreme and especially after multiple repairs, the tissues are largely destroyed, distorted, and scarred. The usual structures used to anchor repairs such as the inguinal and pectineal ligaments have also disappeared. The hernia bulges through a large defect between the thigh and the abdominal wall. These have been called inguino-femoral hernias or hernias through Fruchaud's space or the myopectineal orifice.

When small defects are present and the repair is otherwise satisfactory, especially in the elderly, a limited repair of only the defect need be done after the sac has been freed and invaginated. The edges of the defect may be approximated by a continuous monofilament nylon suture and reinforced by a small onlay darn of the same suture. In 1986 Lichtenstein reported his new concept for a simplified tension-free repair for this type of recurrence.[16] After the sac has been dealt with, a plug fashioned from a rolled-up 2 × 20 cm strip of polypropylene mesh is inserted to fill the hole and is sutured to the edges (Fig 14–19).

In the majority of cases of indirect or direct recurrence, what is left of the previous repair must be taken apart and the normal anatomy restored by meticulous dissection of the anatomic layers. Every bit of usable tissue must be preserved. After suitable preparation, there is usually sufficient tissue of good strength to allow for performance of one of the standard hernia repairs. It is sometimes useful to place a vacuum drain in the wound of repaired recurrent hernias.[209] This reduces the incidence of hematoma and infection.

Surgeons at the Shouldice Hospital use their multilayered operation also for recurrent hernia. They have been

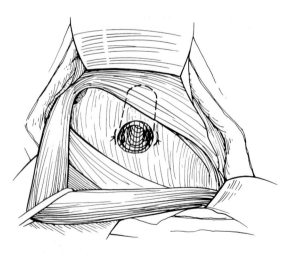

Figure 14–19. Lichtenstein "simplified tension-free repair" showing the polypropylene plug and the suture tacking technique. After Rejovitzky, MD.

running a trial of prosthetic mesh repair for this type of recurrence.[246] They found that mesh was needed in recurrent indirect inguinal hernia in 0.95%, and in recurrent direct inguinal hernia, in 4.7% of cases. Similarly, Berliner reported that, in his series, biomaterial was required to effect a tension-free repair in only four of 350 recurrent inguinal hernias.[247] On the other hand, surgeons such as Gilbert, Lichtenstein, and Rutkow believe that all recurrences should be repaired with prosthetic mesh by one of their standard tensionless procedures.[74,76,78] Lichtenstein reported a series of 1500 recurrent inguinal hernias treated by his tension-free method and followed up for 3 to 20 years with only a 1.6% recurrence rate.[113] In the past 5 years there have been only two failures in 390 cases, a recurrence rate of less than 1%.

When much tissue has been destroyed by one or more previous attempts at repair, it is usually not possible to approximate the edges of the defect without tension, and there is no alternative to the use of a prosthetic mesh. It may be applied by the Lichtenstein onlay graft[16] or the Rutkow mesh-plug hernioplasty technique,[78] but larger defects are best repaired by the Rives method[71] of placing a large prosthetic mesh between the peritoneum and abdominal wall by the inguinal approach (see Fig 14–16) or the abdominal extraperitoneal approach (see Fig 14–17). These methods have been elegantly described and illustrated by Wantz.[90–92]

Stoppa strongly advises using his great prosthesis for reinforcement of the visceral sac (GPRVS) for large multiple recurrent hernia and especially bilateral cases.[95] This avoids the difficult and tedious dissection of scarred and distorted tissues demanded by the inguinal approach and the efforts to approximate the edges of firm and fixed defects of the abdominal wall. All these difficulties are simply ignored by the abdominal lower midline extraperitoneal approach and by wrapping the peritoneum of the lower abdomen in the envelope of prosthetic nylon mesh.

When a recurrent hernia is repaired by the inguinal approach, the spermatic cord must be meticulously dissected free from the scar tissue around it, and the testis usually can be preserved. However, orchidectomy should be considered when the cord has been damaged or in a complicated recurrent hernia. Signed informed consent should be obtained before the operation in cases in which this likelihood may arise. An advantage of the Stoppa GPRVS is that there is no need to dissect the cord or to endanger the testis.

STRANGULATED HERNIA

Strangulation is the most serious complication of hernia. As previously mentioned, the incidence is highest in the first few months of life and the younger the patient, the greater the tendency to irreducibility. Approximately 90% of strangulated hernias in infants can be manually reduced, but complications can still develop after reduction so it is best to admit these babies after reduction for observation and to operate on the hernia two days later.

In adults, Gallegos estimated the cumulative probability of strangulation for inguinal hernia as 2.8% after three months, rising to 4.5% at the end of 2 years.[248] Thus, the greatest rate is in the first 3 months after appearance of the hernia. Thus, patients with a short history of inguinal hernia should be operated earlier than those with longer histories who have been on the waiting list for some time. Strangulation occurs more frequently with incarcerated hernias, with advanced age, and in large hernias with relatively small openings. The initiating cause of strangulation is not clear. Whatever the cause, for some reason the bowel becomes relatively too wide for the opening through which it passes, leading to compression of the mesenteric veins. The increased venous pressure causes edema of the bowel wall and further compression and obstruction of the veins, going on to venous infarction and gangrene of the loops of bowel and omentum in the hernia. This process takes only a few hours, making strangulation an urgent situation. The local findings are extreme pain and tenderness, swelling of the hernia, edema, redness of the skin, and irreducibility. The systemic manifestations are those of bowel obstruction and gangrenous bowel, leading to serious fluid and electrolyte imbalance.

The mortality rate is related directly to the length of time of strangulation and the age of the patient. Manual reduction of the hernia should be attempted, with the patient sedated, if necessary. In the majority of cases, manual reduction is successful and allows a delay of a few days while the edema and systemic symptoms return to normal. The hernia then can be operated on electively. This delay is important since hernias operated on when strangulated are associated with higher mortality, morbidity, infection, and recurrence rates, especially in elderly patients. A fair amount of sustained pressure may be used in the attempt at reduction. When strangulation is advanced or if gangrene has set in, it is practically impossible to reduce the hernia. Reduction en masse, in which the hernial sac itself, together with its strangulated contents, is pushed through the hernial defect in the abdominal wall and comes to lie in the extraperitoneal space where the process of strangulation continues, is a rare complication of strenuous attempts at reduction. In this case, relief of symptoms is not immediate, as occurs with successful reduction, and urgent operation is indicated. Irreducibility also indicates the need for urgent operation to relieve a strangulated hernia. The systemic effects of strangulation, as well as other incidental conditions such as diabetes mellitus, arrhythmias, and cardiac failure, are treated as intensively as possible in the

short time available while the operating room is prepared. Operation must not be delayed for prolonged preoperative assessment or treatment. A nasogastric tube is passed, and an indwelling catheter is placed in the bladder. Perioperative antibiotics are given.

The operation is usually done with the patient under general anesthesia, although spinal or epidural anesthesia is also suitable. Local anesthesia usually is not used for a strangulated hernia. The usual standard transverse incision is made, and the subcutaneous fat is dissected off the hernial sac. The sac is opened and the contents examined before the inguinal canal is opened or the tissues are dissected. It is vital to know the state of the bowel and omentum in the sac before they are allowed to escape into the abdominal cavity. Loops of bowel proximal and distal to the obstruction are extracted and examined, especially the bands of pressure at the hernial neck. If the bowels are satisfactory in color and peristalsis, they are returned to the abdomen, and repair of the hernia proceeds as usual. If necessary, the neck of the hernia may be dilated with a finger to extract or return the bowel. Rarely, the tight neck may need to be incised over a grooved probe. If the color of the bowel is questionable, it is worth covering it with a warm moist pad for some 10 minutes. If the normal pink color and peristalsis return and the paraintestinal vessels can be seen or felt to pulsate, the bowel is returned to the abdominal cavity.

Omentum in a questionable state is simply resected. If the bowel is frankly gangrenous or there are questionable areas that do not recover, resection and end-to-end anastomosis should be done. If the hernial opening is sufficiently wide and the bowel mesenteries long enough, they can be done via the hernia, but if the bowel cannot be sufficiently exteriorized, it is far safer to make an abdominal incision higher up and do the resection comfortably and safely. A good approach is to do a lower transverse transrectus incision on the right side. It is quite adequate for a small bowel resection. However, if large bowel is gangrenous, a midline incision is preferable for adequate exposure.

In strangulated hernias, especially if bowel resection is done, the incidence of wound infection rises, so prosthetic implants are best avoided when the hernia is repaired. The wound should be drained for 24 hours by vacuum through a nylon catheter to avoid collections of fluid, hematoma, and wound infection.

■ FEMORAL AND RELATED HERNIAS

There are several weaknesses and potential canals in the area between the inguinal ligament and the superior pubic ramus through which hernias may occur. The most common hernia in this region is the femoral hernia.

FEMORAL HERNIA

Incidence

Although it is the second most common of the naturally occurring abdominal wall hernias, femoral hernia constitutes only 5% of them. In clinical practice, one encounters about one femoral hernia for every 10 inguinal hernias. They are more common in females, the female to male ratio being 4:1. It is not unusual for males who develop femoral hernia to have had a previous repair of an inguinal hernia. It is not clear in these cases whether both hernias occurred because of the weakness of the abdominal wall in the area. The femoral hernia may have been present at the time of the first operation but missed, or may have developed later, also on the basis of the same etiology. Alternatively, it is postulated that repair of the inguinal hernia causes tension on the transversalis fascia and pulls up the inguinal ligament, leading to weakening of the tissues of the femoral canal and to herniation. Femoral hernia constitute about 2% of abdominal wall hernias in men, but about one-third in women, in whom they are almost as frequent as inguinal hernias. Femoral hernia is twice as common on the right as on the left side and may be bilateral in about 1 out of 15 cases. Femoral hernia is very prone to strangulation. Gallegos found that the cumulative probability of strangulation for femoral hernia in adults was 22% in the first 3 months and 45% at 21 months.[248] This is 10 times the rate for inguinal hernia. It is estimated that about one-third of femoral hernias will strangulate. This high percentage accounts for the fact that almost half the strangulated groin hernias encountered clinically are femoral hernias, even though inguinal hernia is much more common than femoral hernia.

Etiology

In contrast to inguinal hernia, femoral hernia is rare in infancy and childhood, so the etiology is probably not congenital. There is no evidence of a preformed sac. Chapman reported a series of 1134 cases of groin hernias in childhood of which only six were femoral hernias, an incidence of 0.5%.[249] The correct diagnosis was made in only two cases preoperatively. These two had undergone inguinal hernia repair a few months previously and the groin mass reappeared shortly after the operation, leading him to conclude that the femoral hernias were missed. Asai reported a case of femoral hernia in a 9 year–old boy.[250] He could find only 25 cases in the Japanese literature of femoral hernia in childhood ranging in age from 1 month to 9 years. The female to male ratio was 3:2, five cases were bilateral and 48% of the cases were incarcerated when first seen. Luque reported 11 cases of femoral hernia in childhood, of which six were diagnosed preoperatively.[251] The hernia usually appears after middle age, suggesting

that natural weakening of the tissues and loss of elasticity is the basic cause. It is more common in multiparous women.

Anatomy

The transversalis fascia emerges above from behind the musculoaponeurotic arch of the internal oblique and the transversus abdominis muscles and passes down to attach to the pectineal ridge. In this way it closes off the area between the inguinal ligament and the superior pubic ramus and separates the abdomen from the thigh (Fig 14–20A and B). This area is mainly filled by the iliopsoas and pectineus muscles and the femoral artery, vein, and nerve passing from the abdomen to the thigh. At its most medial end, there exists a potential canal, the femoral canal, through which the common type of femoral her-

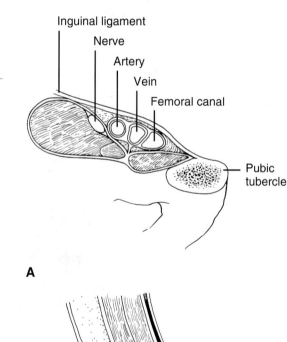

A

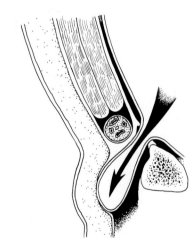

B

Figure 14–20. Femoral hernia. **A.** The structures posterior to the inguinal ligament. **B.** The femoral hernia passing through the femoral canal and bulging in the groin below the inguinal ligament. After Rejovitzky, MD.

nia emerges. It is bounded anteriorly by the inguinal ligament, medially by the lacunar part of the inguinal ligament (Gimbernat), posteriorly by the pubic ramus and the pectineal ligament, and medially by the femoral vein and sheath. The canal is filled by loose areolar tissue and femoral lymph nodes. With weakening and giving way of the transversalis fascia closing the canal, the peritoneal sac of the femoral hernia transverses the narrow confines of the rigid canal and passes into the loose subcutaneous area of the thigh. Here it is able to expand and pass forward to bulge below the inguinal ligament. It may even pass upwards to cross the inguinal ligament. The sac is covered with extraperitoneal fat and contains either small bowel, omentum, or both. The sac is relatively large compared to the narrow neck, which has no room to expand so that strangulation is common.

Clinical Manifestations

The patient may notice a small reducible lump in the medial aspect of the groin. The lump is often permanent because of incarceration of the hernia. Commonly, especially in elderly females, the patient is unaware of the presence of a femoral hernia, and the first indication of its existence is when she appears with strangulation of the hernia. It is thus mandatory to inspect the femoral orifices in all elderly patients, especially females, who present with intestinal obstruction. Aspects of the diagnosis of femoral hernia are discussed in a series of 98 cases in which the referral diagnosis was correct in 36 cases.[252] The correct preoperative diagnosis was made in 85 of the cases. There were four deaths in this series, all of which were urgent admissions with incarcerated bowel and all were not diagnosed before admission. Of the cases with strangulated small bowel at operation, 70% with an incorrect initial diagnosis required resection whereas only 20% with a correct initial diagnosis required resection. He concludes that femoral hernias are frequently incorrectly diagnosed and that this situation is associated with a worsened outcome in urgent cases. Chamary also stresses the high morbidity and mortality associated with emergency surgery and intestinal obstruction in femoral hernia.[217] The differential diagnosis is usually not difficult. Enlargement of femoral lymph nodes is about the only condition that may mimic a femoral hernia.

Treatment

All femoral hernias, with few exceptions, should be operated on and repaired as soon as possible after diagnosis. Even the elderly and sick can withstand a simple repair done under local anesthesia. The frequency and the high morbidity and mortality rate of strangulated femoral hernia, especially in the old and frail, is a mandatory indication to operate on these patients electively, despite their brittle condition. An attempt should always be made to reduce a strangulated femoral hernia, although this procedure is much less frequently successful than with inguinal hernia. A confusing clinical picture can present in cases of a Richter-type hernia, in which only part of the wall of small bowel is strangulated in the hernia but the rest of the lumen is open so that intestinal obstruction is not present. An irreducible strangulated femoral hernia is an urgent emergency. While the operating room is prepared, an intravenous infusion is set up, a nasogastric tube and a urinary catheter are passed, and measures are taken to correct the fluid and electrolyte imbalance and any medical condition that may be present.

Operation

The usual approach for elective repair of a femoral hernia is through a small transverse thigh incision below the inguinal ligament. There is no real indication in these cases for the higher and more complicated Lotheissen approach through the inguinal canal, and even less indication for the transabdominal preperitoneal route. The incision is located in the medial aspect of the thigh, below the inguinal ligament, and is centered over the femoral canal. In strangulated hernia, the incision is placed over the swelling. The subcutaneous fat is split to reveal the mass of extra peritoneal fat enveloping the sac. This mass is freed by blunt finger dissection and is dislocated forward. The inguinal ligament and pectineal fascia and the neck of the hernia are exposed by gauze dissection. The exposure is practically bloodless. The mass of extraperitoneal fat is split to reveal the sac which is dissected up to and beyond its narrow neck, then opened to inspect its contents. Adhesions between bowel and omentum and the sac wall should be freed. The bowel and omentum are returned to the abdominal cavity. It may be necessary, especially with a strangulated hernia, to digitally dilate the neck from within the sac in order to return the bowel. Rarely, the lacunar part of the inguinal ligament, or even part of the inguinal ligament itself, must be incised to free the neck of the hernia. In these cases, care must be taken not to damage an abnormal obturator artery. The sac may now be transfixed and ligated at the neck or simply snipped off and the stump returned to the abdominal cavity. The extraperitoneal fat is excised. The margins of the femoral canal now have been cleared and are exposed for closure of the defect.

The repair is done with monofilament polypropylene or polyamide 2-0. Ideally, the inguinal ligament should be sutured to the pectineal (Cooper's) ligament with a few interrupted stitches. However, except for large hernial openings, this procedure is usually technically difficult because of the natural rotation of the pelvis and the depth of the pectineal ligament. The simplest alternative is the purse-string repair (Fig

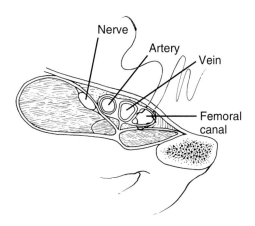

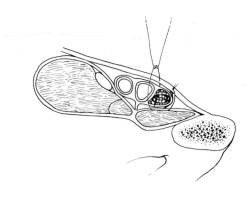

Figure 14–21. Femoral hernia. The Ellis purse-string closure of the femoral canal. After Rejovitzky, MD.

Figure 14–22. Lichtenstein polypropylene plug for repair of a femoral hernia. After Rejovitzky, MD.

14–21).[253] A thick bite is taken through the inguinal ligament, then alternately through the lacunar ligament, the pectineal fascia, the fascia over the medial aspect of the femoral vein, and finally, once more through the inguinal ligament close to the initial entry of the stitch. The purse-string is closed and tied. A figure-eight closure was described by Devlin,[254] and Lichtenstein described his simple technique in which, after the sac is dealt with, a plug made from a rolled-up strip of polypropylene mesh is fitted snugly into the femoral canal and held there by a few polypropylene tacking sutures (Fig 14–22).[16,255] This tension-free repair should ensure against recurrences, which tend to occur more often after femoral hernia repairs than they do after repair of inguinal hernias. The subcutaneous fat and fascia are approximated by a few absorbable sutures and the skin closed with an absorbable synthetic 5-0 continuous intradermal suture.

When dealing with a strangulated hernia from which gangrenous bowel must be resected, it is usually difficult and unsafe to perform the resection through the hernial opening. It is advisable to resect comfortably through a second small laparotomy incision.

Another popular method to deal with the hernia as well as with the bowel resection is the Lotheissen approach through the posterior wall of the inguinal canal. The Henry preperitoneal approach through a lower midline abdominal incision is also popular, especially for incarcerated or strangulated femoral hernias. It is claimed that the hernial opening is better seen and more easily repaired from above and that incarcerated or strangulated bowel can be more easily and safely released and resected. Berliner reported a series of 44 cases of incarcerated or strangulated femoral hernias on which he operated using the Henry approach, which he found to be effective and safe.[256] An added bonus

was the finding of an unsuspected contralateral femoral hernia in 16% of the cases.

Bendavid has published several papers on the subject of femoral hernia in which he stresses the high recurrence rate following femoral hernia repair and the even higher rate following repair of recurrences.[257–260] He suggests that all femoral hernias should probably be repaired with a prosthetic mesh and that it is mandatory to do so when dealing with recurrences. For this purpose he has designed an "umbrella" of polypropylene mesh and also a relaxing incision for femoral herniorrhaphy.

FEMORAL-RELATED HERNIAS

Hernias below the inguinal ligament, apart from the common femoral hernia, are rare. The least uncommon of them is the prevascular hernia that appears in the groin between the inguinal ligament and the femoral vessels. It may be a primary hernia or may develop as a recurrent hernia following repair of an inguinal hernia. These hernias are difficult, if not impossible, to repair by the conventional inguinal methods since the posterior border is composed of the femoral vessels, which cannot be used for anchoring the sutures. Furthermore, when a prevascular hernia develops after repair of an inguinal hernia the inguinal ligament itself may be torn, as well as the transversalis fascia, the iliopubic tract, and the anterior femoral sheath. These hernias are therefore best repaired with a prosthetic nylon mesh by the transabdominal preperitoneal route, either by the Rives unilateral repair (see Fig 14–17) or the Stoppa (GPRVS) bilateral repair (see Fig 14–18).

An external femoral hernia passes from the abdomen under the inguinal ligament lateral to the femoral artery. Similar hernias may develop more laterally in the region of the iliopsoas muscle. These lateral hernias may be repaired by suturing the inguinal ligament to the pectineal ligament or the fascia of the iliopsoas. Where this is not possible, the Rives or Stoppa transabdominal preperitoneal prosthetic mesh repairs should be done.

Rare hernias may pass behind the femoral vessels, under the pectineal fascia, and through the lacunar ligament of Gimbernat and may even be associated with an ectopic testis that has passed through the femoral canal.

OMPHALOCELE AND GASTROSCHISIS

History

Ambrose Pare, in the 16th century, first described omphalocele and gastroschisis. Successful primary repair of these conditions was reported by Hamilton at the beginning of the 19th century, although he succeeded only with small defects. In the 19th century, nonoperative treatment was introduced but apparently fell out of favor until Grob revived its use in 1963. The concept of mobilizing flaps of abdominal wall skin to cover unopened omphaloceles, where the abdominal wall defect was too large to be closed primarily, was reported by Olshausen at the end of the 19th century, and later by Williams. Gross established this method on a sound footing in 1948. Ruptured omphaloceles were almost universally fatal, even though Reid reported the successful management of some cases in 1913.

Gastroschisis was recognized as distinct from omphalocele in 1953 by Moore and Stokes who pointed out the main differences: there was no sac in gastroschisis and the umbilical cord was normally inserted into the abdominal wall.[261] The bowel prolapsed through what appeared to be a defect lateral to the insertion of the umbilicus. Some successful operations for gastroschisis were probably done before this date.

Embryology

The abdominal wall begins to form during the fourth week of gestation by the infolding of the head and tail folds and the two lateral folds. These four folds are destined to meet in the middle of the midline at the site of the future umbilicus. Meanwhile the midgut grows longer until the abdominal cavity can no longer accommodate it, so that it prolapses in the form of a loop through the still open umbilicus. During the tenth gestational week, the prolapsed midgut returns to the now enlarged abdominal cavity, rotating anticlockwise as it goes in. Failure of the four folds to meet at their destined point at the umbilicus will result in a herniation of the intestines into the umbilical cord through the defect in the abdominal wall, resulting in an omphalocele. The defect is round and in the midline. The prolapsed bowel is covered by a partially translucent membrane in continuity with the covering of the umbilical cord, which itself is inserted near the apex of the bulge. If the migration of the four folds is halted at an earlier stage, more complicated defects may occur involving thoracic and pelvic organs. An omphalocele may rupture before, during, or after birth.

Gastroschisis appears to be caused by a different mechanism, apparently linked to the as yet not clearly understood disappearance of the right umbilical vein, which may result in an abdominal wall defect to the right of the umbilical vein or what appears to be the right hand edge of the umbilicus. Gastroschisis is almost always on the right side, with a normal umbilical cord normally attached to the abdominal wall at the umbilicus and to the left of the gastroschisis defect. There is no sac. The prolapsed loops of bowel lie on the abdominal wall, exposed to the amniotic fluid.

Etiology and Incidence

The incidence of omphalocele and gastroschisis is one in 3000 to 5000 births. About half of the infants are stillborn. The cause of these defects is unknown. There is no evidence for a hereditary basis. The incidence is greater in babies with trisomy syndromes. About one-third of the babies have other associated anomalies that may be serious and even life-threatening. These are mainly cardiovascular, genitourinary, and craniofacial. Bowel atresia also may be present and is considered to be the result of pressure ischemia by the edge of the abdominal wall defect.

Clinical Manifestations

Small omphaloceles may have an umbilical ring defect of 1 to 2 cm in diameter and contain only a loop or two of small bowel, but the defect may be 10 cm or more in diameter and the sac may contain small bowel, colon, stomach, and liver. A small defect with a narrow sac may contain only one loop of small bowel and may not be diagnosed at birth. In these cases, there is a distinct danger of clamping the sac and the bowel and excising a piece of the bowel when tying the umbilical cord. If an omphalocele is left untreated, the coverings will dry within a few days and cracks will appear. At this stage, infection creeps in under the dry and crusted peel. Eventually the coverings fall apart and the bowel will prolapse.

In the case of gastroschisis, the unprotected prolapsed loops of bowel have been exposed to the irritating effect of the amniotic fluid from an early stage of gestation. The bowel is dilated and grossly thickened, edematous, and granular. The loops are matted together and also partly covered by thick, tough fibrous material. The total length of bowel appears to be shorter than normal though it is not clear whether the bowel is actually anatomically shorter or whether it is only functionally so owing to the length having been taken up by the dilated bowel. Areas of ischemia or even frank atresia may be seen where the bowel is pressed up against the edge of the abdominal wall defect. The inflammatory changes brought about in the bowel by the chemical irritation of the amniotic fluids lead to a state of paralytic ileus.

Treatment

Immediately after birth, as soon as the diagnosis is established, the area of the omphalocele or exposed bowel must be covered with a sterile gauze pack soaked with saline. A nasogastric tube must be placed in the stomach and attached to a low-grade vacuum to aspirate swallowed air. An intravenous infusion must be set up. It must be recognized that these are major neonatal problems requiring highly specialized management in a pediatric intensive care unit.

After suitable preparation, these infants are operated under general anesthesia with intubation and relaxation. Omphaloceles with a defect of up to 5 to 6 cm usually can be closed with a one-stage procedure. An unopened sac, or the remains of a ruptured sac, is excised and the bowels examined to exclude nonrotation, atresia, or other problems that may need to be dealt with. The abdominal wall is forcefully stretched by inserting fingers of each hand and pushing out hard from the inside in all directions. A determined surgeon usually can achieve sufficient space to replace the bowel easily. The defect of the abdominal wall then can be closed by a full-thickness mass closure with a continuous monofilament nylon thread, or interrupted sutures may be used. The skin is closed with a running intradermal 5-0 absorbable synthetic suture.

The same method is used when dealing with gastroschisis, although the problem is less the width of the defect, which is often quite narrow, but rather the difficulty of returning the mass of swollen and matted loops of bowel into the abdomen. This is the preferred treatment when it can be achieved, even if some pressure is needed on the loops of bowel to coax them.

There are two options for dealing with larger omphaloceles or gastroschisis. One is simply to ignore the wide defect and defer its closure for a later date but to cover the omphalocele or the prolapsed bowel with skin of the abdominal wall which has been mobilized laterally almost to the midline of the back, superiorly up onto the chest wall, inferiorly down to the pubis and sutured in the midline. If the child survives, the large ventral abdominal hernia is repaired at the age of 1 year or later.

The second option and the one more popularly used, is to manually stretch the abdominal wall as above and then to construct a silo of silastic sheeting to enclose the bowels. This is a reinforced sheet of silicon with an extremely smooth surface and strong enough to hold sutures even under tension. The technique is to clear the

skin off the edge of the defect and to suture the one edge of the piece of silastic all around to the full thickness of the defect but not to the skin. The two lateral edges of the silastic are then sutured together where they meet to construct a cylinder enclosing the prolapsed bowel. The walls of the cylinder are then sutured across close to the bowel to create a pouch with the bowel inside. The excess of the silicon is trimmed and the silicon suspended from the top of the incubator. This slight traction draws up the abdominal walls and stretches them slowly. The silicon is twisted every 1 or 2 days to force some of its contents into the abdomen, or squeezed and sutured across at a lower level. In this fashion, after 5 to 7 days, the bowel should be totally in the abdomen and the infant is returned to the operating room where, under general anesthesia, the pouch is removed and the abdominal defect closed and covered with the skin. The process must be completed before 7 to 9 days because of the danger of infection, with sepsis of the pouch and its contents. During this time, the infant receives total parenteral nutrition and antibiotics and the silon pouch is kept sterile with povidone iodine.

The reason for this seemingly complicated maneuver is that the infant will not survive forceful replacement of the bowel and closure of the abdomen under great tension. The greatly increased volume of the abdominal contents under tension will force up the diaphragms and practically immobilize them. The pressure of the intra-abdominal contents on the inferior vena cava will obstruct it and reduce or even stop the venous return to the heart. Furthermore, the pressure on the mesenteric venous system and on the bowel walls will obstruct and thrombose the veins leading to ischemic necrosis of the intestines. These factors will cause the infant to expire within minutes or hours of completion of the operation.

Another method not often used now is to treat unruptured omphaloceles by the open method. The sac was either painted daily with dessicating agents to keep it dry and sterile, hoping to form a hard eschar under which epithelialization slowly took place until the eschar peeled off or the sac was kept moist by constantly wetting it with antiseptic solutions while epithelium slowly crept in from the edges and covered the sac. However, some of the substances used on the sac turned out to be toxic and sepsis with peritonitis often set in. Nonetheless, a fair number of infants survived and had their residual abdominal hernia repaired at a later date. This method is occasionally used today, mainly in infants with severe associated anomalies who are too sick to stand a general anesthetic.

The postoperative management involves long-term respiratory support, correction of acidosis and blood gas and acid-base monitoring. A prolonged period of total parenteral nutrition may be needed until the bowels recover normal function, especially in cases of gastroschisis. Approximately two-thirds of these babies survive. The mortality is not necessary the result of the abdominal wall defect, which may have been successfully treated, but may be owing to severe associated anomalies, especially in the omphalocele babies where these are more common.

■ UMBILICAL HERNIA

When the umbilical scar in infants does not close completely or if it fails and stretches in later years, the abdominal contents protrude through the opening and constitute an umbilical hernia. Midline hernias abutting on the umbilicus superiorly and inferiorly are called paraumbilical hernias and are usually included in this group.

HISTORY

Umbilical hernias have been known to occur since biblical times and are still the source of much superstition and ignorance. Celsus mentioned the repair of an umbilical hernia in the first century AD,[1] and William Cheselden reported the repair of one in 1740.[262] In 1901, William J. Mayo described a series of 19 instances of his classic transverse overlapping operation using nonabsorbable sutures.[263]

INCIDENCE

Estimates of the incidence of umbilical hernia at birth vary greatly. In Caucasian infants, they range between 10% to 30%. In children of African descent, it may be several times greater. Premature infants commonly have umbilical hernias, even 70% or more. Down, Beckwith-Wiedman, and other syndromes have umbilical hernias as one of the components. Children with raised intra-abdominal pressure owing to ascites, CAPD, or ventriculoperitoneal shunt, also tend to develop an umbilical hernia.[114,152,241,242] The majority of congenital umbilical hernias close spontaneously during the first few years of life. By 5 to 6 years of age, only about 10% are still present. However, some may continue to constrict and close through 10 years of age.

The incidence of umbilical hernia in the adult is unknown. It is more common in the female, with a female to male ratio of 3:1, and it is more common in people of African origin.

ETIOLOGY AND ANATOMY

The embryo develops a head, tail, and two lateral folds that grow towards each other to form the abdominal cavity. At about the sixth week of gestation, the rapidly growing intestinal tract cannot be contained by the abdominal cavity and prolapses out through the future umbilical ring. By the tenth week, the midgut rotates and enters the abdominal cavity and the four folds meet to form a narrow umbilical ring which, at birth, is only wide enough to allow the passage of the umbilical arteries and vein. When the cord is ligated, the arteries and vein thrombose, the umbilical ring continues to contract and to close by scar tissue. If this process is halted before complete closure of the umbilical ring, an umbilical hernia will be produced. The cord will separate normally and the granulation tissue covering the umbilicus will be epithelialized. If bowel or omentum prolapse through the incompletely closed umbilicus before or after birth, an umbilical hernia is formed. The hernial opening varies between a few millimeters in diameter to up to 4 cm.

The cause of umbilical hernia in adults is unknown, as is its possible relationship to the presence of an umbilical hernia in childhood. It is said that 10% of adults with umbilical hernias have a history of umbilical hernia in childhood. It occurs more frequently in middle-aged women and is often associated with fair to gross adiposity and with multiple pregnancies. It also may develop in cases of gross ascites owing to liver cirrhosis, congestive cardiac failure, nephrosis, peritoneal dialysis, and malignant disease. The cause is probably multifactorial, with raised intra-abdominal pressure acting on the weakened and stretched scar tissue of the umbilicus.

The defect in the abdominal wall is usually 2 to 5 cm in diameter, but large openings (up to 10 cm in diameter) are also common. Larger rings, even up to 20 cm in diameter, are occasionally seen. The opening is often relatively narrow compared to the size of the sac, which may be large, long, and multiloculated, protruding forwards and downwards even to overhang the pubis. The hernia also may spread in all directions, burrowing into the subcutaneous fat. Smaller hernias usually contain only some omentum, but transverse colon, loops of small bowel, and even stomach enter as the hernia grows. These hernias frequently become incarcerated and irreducible because of adhesions between the loops of bowel, the omentum, and the sac.

CLINICAL MANIFESTATIONS

The diagnosis is not difficult. In infants, when the baby cries or strains, the swelling appears at the umbilicus and bulges forwards. The sac may contain a loop of small bowel, but if the diameter of the opening is <7 mm, the hernia is either empty or only some omentum is present or enters with straining. Strangulation is extremely rare.[264] Since most umbilical hernias in childhood tend to close spontaneously, there is no immediate hurry to operate on them. The operation can be postponed until the age of 4 to 6 years, unless the hernia is symptomatic or parenteral pressure cannot be resisted. Hernial openings >2 cm in diameter and those with thin sharp edges, tend not to close. Most with openings <2 cm in diameter and with thick rounded edges, do close. It is advisable to operate on children before they enter school.

The situation in adults is quite the opposite. Most umbilical hernias are symptomatic and there is no tendency for spontaneous closure. Adult patients with small umbilical hernias often complain of quite severe pain in the region, especially when coughing or straining. Larger hernias are usually painless but uncomfortable because of their weight dragging on the abdomen. The skin over the hernia is stretched and often very thin and may even be ulcerated by pressure necrosis. Other skin lesions such as intertrigo in the inferior fold between the hernia and the abdominal wall are common, especially in obese women, since the combination of sweaty moisture, warmth, and friction causes large areas of ulceration and weeping dermatitis, with accumulation of decomposing and foul-smelling discharges. Many patients seek surgery for esthetic reasons and for relief of the discomfort, but the real danger is the risk of the commonly occurring strangulation of the hernial contents. The use of girdles, corsets, trusses, and other means of applying pressure to the hernia should be discouraged. They are uncomfortable and usually do not fulfill the function for which they are designed.

Incarcerated umbilical hernias and those that have undergone episodes of irreducibility and strangulation should be repaired surgically, whatever the general condition of the patient, after suitable assessment and preparation. It is less risky to operate electively on a treated and stabilized patient than to do an emergency procedure on a sick, unprepared, and uncontrolled fat, elderly patient with gangrenous bowel. Associated medical conditions should be an indication for elective operation rather than a reason for rejecting the patient.

Flat hernias with wide openings and no real sac need not be repaired unless they show signs of growing.

Patients with umbilical hernia owing to ascites from cirrhosis and portal hypertension need special consideration. The operation is associated with a high morbidity and mortality rate, with leakage of the ascitic fluid through the wound, progressive encephalopathy, and hemorrhage from ruptured esophageal varices. Recurrence of the hernia is also common because of pressure from the ascites. One should be selective with these patients and probably only operate on symptomatic hernias. Intensive medical treatment and even peritoneovenous shunting to control the ascites should be instituted before the operation and, in most cases, a prosthetic mesh repair should be done.

TREATMENT

In childhood, the operation for the repair of an umbilical hernia is performed under general anesthesia and usually can be done conveniently as an outpatient procedure, just as is done for inguinal hernias. A curved, concave up "smile" incision is made in a skin crease below the umbilicus and encircling it from 3 o'clock to 9 o'clock. The skin flap is raised, using fine skin hooks and a small blade. The subcutaneous fat is dissected off the aponeurosis of the external oblique to clear the opening of the hernia and to demonstrate the sac that is cleared of fat on its inferior and lateral aspects. A fine artery forceps is passed around the superior aspect of the sac and used as a retractor to clear the rest of the sac and the aponeurosis around the hernial opening. The distal end of the sac is freed from the skin of the umbilicus by sharp dissection. The sac now can be inverted into the abdominal cavity through the hernial defect or alternatively, it can be opened to inspect and return any contents to the abdominal cavity. The sac is then simply snipped off at its base. The hernial opening is closed transversely with a few interrupted sutures, or a continuous suture, of 3-0 nonabsorbable monofilament nylon passing through the full thickness of the abdominal wall at the edge of the defect. Hemostasis is assured and the skin of the umbilicus is tacked down to the aponeurosis with two synthetic absorbable 4-0 sutures. The skin is closed with a continuous 5-0 synthetic absorbable suture. There is no need to excise excess skin that will contract down to form a normal-looking umbilicus. A gauze ball is pressed into the umbilical concavity, covered with gauze, and held down by strips of plaster. The dressing is removed after a few days. Postoperative complications such as skin necrosis, wound infection, seroma or hematoma are unusual and require no special active treatment. Recurrence of the hernia is extremely rare.

A thin adult patient with a small umbilical hernia does not need any special preparation, and the operation can be done with local anesthesia. More commonly, the patient is an obese female, often presenting with hypertension, cardiovascular and renal disease, diabetes, and chronic lung disease. If the operation can be delayed, the patient should be urged to lose weight. The associated medical conditions must be treated and respiratory exercises begun so that the patient is in an optimal state for the operation. The skin around the hernia may need special preoperative care in cases with dermatitis and moist intertrigo, especially when dealing with large hernias. The author prefers to wash the skin of the abdominal wall, including the affected areas, several times daily for a few days preoperatively with povidone-iodine scrub, followed by painting with povidone-iodine solution, which is allowed to dry. The moist areas are kept exposed to warm air to facilitate drying and healing.

The operation is best done with the patient under general anesthesia.

Traditionally, the Mayo overlap repair has been used (Fig 14–23A). An elliptic transverse incision is made to excise the skin, umbilical scar, fat, and the hernial sac (Fig 14–23B and C). The ring then was enlarged by incising the abdominal wall laterally on each side (Fig 14–23D). The hernial contents were returned to the peritoneal cavity, and the defect was closed by overlapping the upper flap of abdominal wall over the lower by using two rows of staggered interrupted full-thickness silk sutures (Fig 14–23E and F). It was believed that a wide area of contact between the upper and lower fascial sheets would promote strong adhesion between them and ensure a good repair. However, it has been shown experimentally that opposing sheets of fascia tend not to adhere to each other and that, on the contrary, two cut edges of fascia opposed to each other and in contact promote the development of strong collagen tissue and a lasting bond. Consequently, other techniques are more commonly used today.

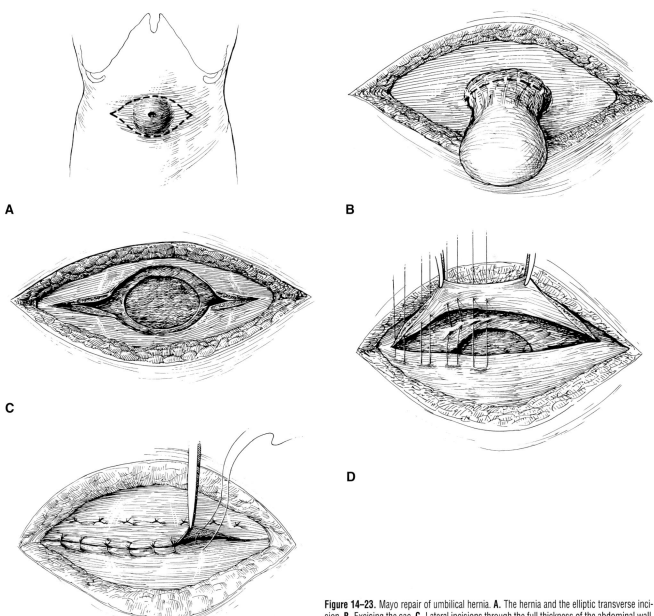

A

B

C

D

Figure 14–23. Mayo repair of umbilical hernia. **A.** The hernia and the elliptic transverse incision. **B.** Excising the sac. **C.** Lateral incisions through the full thickness of the abdominal wall. **D.** First row of sutures. **E.** Second row of sutures. After Rejovitzky, MD.

E

Small Umbilical Hernias

Small umbilical hernias in adults are dealt with as in children. The umbilical cicatrix need not be excised. A curved "smile" incision, concave cranially, is made around the inferior aspect of the hernia in the skin crease between the hernia and the abdominal wall. The skin flap with umbilical cicatrix is raised by incising the subcutaneous fat (Fig 14–24A). The fascial edge of the hernial opening and the neck of the sac are exposed. A wide area of anterior rectus sheath around the opening is cleared of fat. The neck of the sac is circumcised along the edge of the hernial opening so that it may be lifted away from the abdominal wall (Fig 14–24B). The contents of the hernia are extracted, and adhesions between them and the sac are freed. The bowel is returned to the peritoneal cavity. The omentum and the sac are excised.

The opening is closed transversely with a series of interrupted monofilament polypropylene or polyamide sutures. It is more convenient to place all the sutures in position before tying them individually (Fig 14–24C). Alternatively, a continuous suture may be used. Good full-thickness bites are taken of the abdominal wall along the upper and lower margins of the hernial opening at least 1.5 cm from the edge. These sutures are at a right angle to the line of the fascial fibers so that there is less of a tendency for them to cut out. Coughing and straining postoperatively tend to close the line of repair rather than strain it outwards, since the fibers pull in a transverse direction rather than craniocaudally. After careful hemostasis, the deep surface of the skin of the umbilical cicatrix is tacked down to the fascia in the region of the repair by a few fine absorbable sutures to preserve the natural appearance of the umbilicus. The skin is closed with a 5-0 synthetic absorbable intradermal suture or with clips.

MEDIUM-SIZED UMBILICAL HERNIA

The larger hernias, up to about 10 cm in diameter, can still be closed transversely, but an onlay nylon darn of the anterior rectus sheaths should be added. A transverse elliptic incision is used to excise the umbilicus and excess skin and fat. The neck of the sac is isolated at the edge of the hernial opening (Fig 14–25A). The anterior rectus sheaths are cleared of subcutaneous fat for a wide area around the margins of the hernia to expose enough surface for the onlay darn. The neck of the sac is carefully circumcised along the hernial margin (Fig 14–25B). Fingers may now be inserted into the sac to guide the scissors used to slit the sac radially (Fig 14–25C). The loops of bowel and omentum are carefully freed from all the loculations of the sac and are returned to the abdominal cavity. The upper and lower edges of the hernial opening are approximated by a

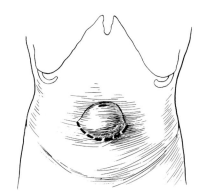

A

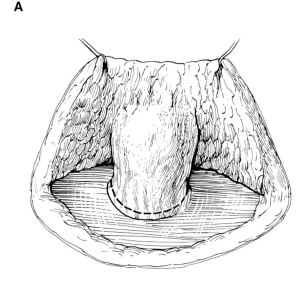

B

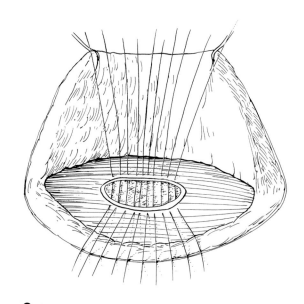

C

Figure 14–24. Small umbilical hernia. **A.** The "smile" incision; raising the flap of skin and cicatrix. **B.** Incising the hernia sac. **C.** The sutures in place. After Rejovitzky, MD.

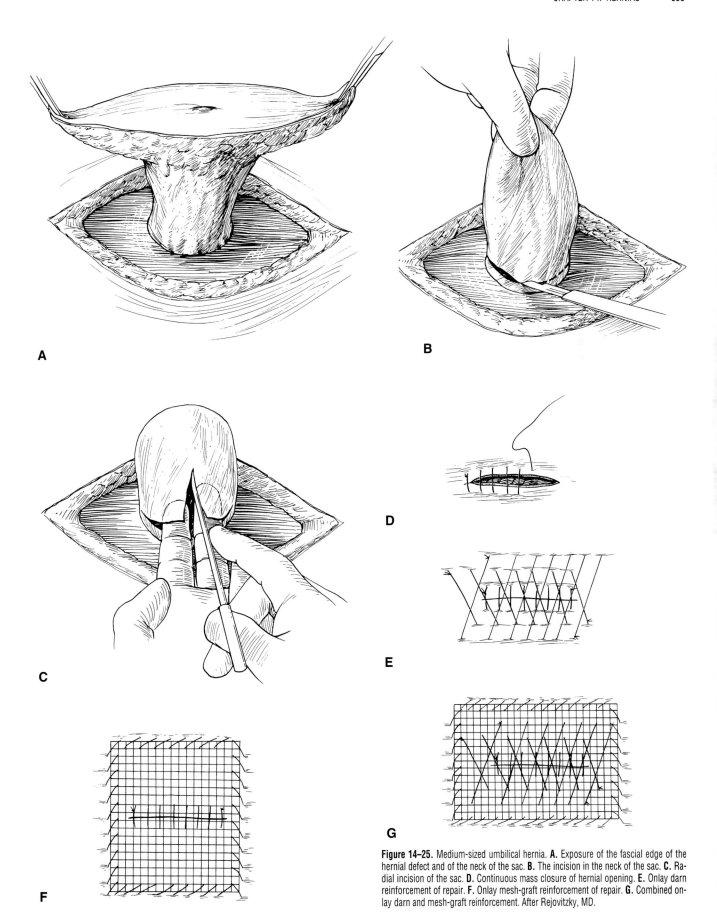

Figure 14–25. Medium-sized umbilical hernia. **A.** Exposure of the fascial edge of the hernial defect and of the neck of the sac. **B.** The incision in the neck of the sac. **C.** Radial incision of the sac. **D.** Continuous mass closure of hernial opening. **E.** Onlay darn reinforcement of repair. **F.** Onlay mesh-graft reinforcement of repair. **G.** Combined onlay darn and mesh-graft reinforcement. After Rejovitzky, MD.

continuous mass closure technique using heavy monofilament polyamide or polypropylene suture and taking large bites of the full thickness of the abdominal wall well away from the hernial margin (Fig 14–25D). Two lines of oblique sutures are used for the darn (Fig 14–25E). The first line should go beyond, both above and below, the original transverse suture line. The second line of the darn should be placed even further beyond the first. Strong bites are taken of the rectus sheath. One or two vacuum drains are inserted through separate stab wounds to evacuate secretions. Absorbable subcutaneous sutures may be used and the skin closed. Some surgeons prefer suturing an onlay prosthetic nonabsorbable mesh graft instead of the onlay darn (Fig 14–25F). Others use both the darn and a mesh sutured over it (Fig 14–25G).

Large Umbilical Hernias

The larger umbilical hernial openings are difficult to repair and cannot be simply sutured transversely without undue tension, which would cause tissue necrosis, cutting out of the sutures, and early recurrence. These large defects may be closed by one of two methods: prosthetic mesh or shoelace repair.

Prosthetic Mesh Repair. A sheet of polypropylene mesh or expanded polytetrafluoroethylene (PTFE) is trimmed to the shape of the hernial opening, with an extra edge of at least 4 cm beyond it and is placed between the abdominal contents and the peritoneum. The edges of the mesh are fixed by interrupted polyamide or polypropylene mattress sutures passing through the entire thickness of the abdominal wall about 4 cm from the edge of the defect (Fig 14–26A and B). It is convenient to pass all the sutures through the mesh first and then to place

the mesh in its intra-abdominal position, passing the ends of the sutures through the abdominal wall and finally tying each end to its fellow. The dead space is drained by one or two vacuum drains and the skin closed. Because of complications that may occur when the bowel is in direct contact with the synthetic mesh, care must be taken to place omentum between the bowel and the prosthesis. Alternatively, the mesh may be placed in the plane between the rectus muscles and the posterior rectus sheath, as is described in the section on incisional hernias.

Shoelace Repair. This is the method which the author prefers for the repair of large umbilical hernias, as described for the repair of large postoperative ventral abdominal hernias (see Fig 14–38).[265] In this case a long vertical, elliptic incision is used, excising the umbilicus and the excess skin and fat. The rectus sheaths are cleared from around the hernial opening and for a distance above and below the defect. Each rectus sheath is slit about 1 to 1.5 cm from the edge of the defect to expose the rectus muscle. Each slit is continued upward and downward beyond the defect to meet at the midline but to end about 1 to 1.5 cm lateral to it. The two ribbons of anterior rectus sheath along the midline are sutured together by a continuous suture of O monofilament polyamide in the form of a commercially available loop on a round-bodied curved needle, to form a new midline. At the same time, the unopened sac and the hernial contents are returned to the abdominal cavity. Care must be taken to invert the sac and to empty its contents into the abdominal cavity to avoid a type of reduction en masse. If necessary, the sac is opened. The lateral cut edges of the rectus sheaths then are brought closer together and parallel

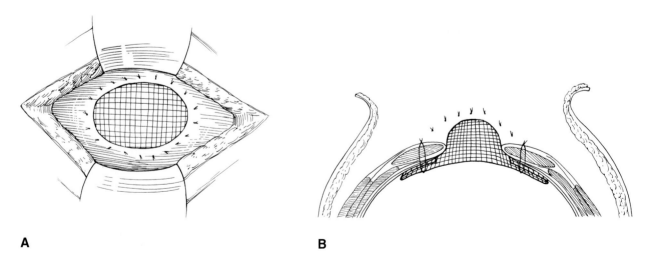

A   **B**

Figure 14–26. Prosthetic mesh repair of large umbilical hernia. **A.** Completed repair. **B.** Intraperitoneal mesh graft and method of fixation to full thickness of abdominal wall. After Rejovitzky, MD.

to each other by a to-and-fro polyamide loop 1 shoelace suture, which substitutes functionally for the missing rectus sheath. The dead space is drained by vacuum drains and the skin closed.

POSTOPERATIVE COMPLICATIONS

Postoperative complications of umbilical hernia repair include mainly local hematoma formation and wound infection, both of which increase the likelihood of recurrence of the hernia. With proper care, both complications should be rare. The overall recurrence rate should be less than 5%.

STRANGULATED UMBILICAL HERNIA

When dealing with strangulated hernias, the general condition of the patient should be intensively treated in as short a time as possible while the operating room is being prepared. Nasogastric intubation and suction must be instituted. Perioperative antibiotics should be given. The hernia repair is the same as for elective cases. Gangrenous bowel should be resected and reanastomosed through the hernial opening. Because of the higher risk of wound infection, prosthetic mesh grafts are best avoided when gangrenous bowel has been resected. Repairs done with monofilament nylon will heal, even if the wound is left open or if it is opened later in the postoperative period because of infection.

■ EPIGASTRIC HERNIA

Epigastric hernias are protrusions of abdominal contents through the interstices between the decussating fibers of the aponeuroses of the sheet muscles of the abdominal wall in the midline (the linea alba), between the umbilicus and the xiphoid process of the sternum. A paraumbilical hernia is really an epigastric hernia abutting on the umbilicus.

HISTORY

Epigastric hernias were first described in 1285, although the term was introduced by Leveille in 1812. This hernia was regarded as reflecting serious intra-abdominal disease, but it is now known to be a local condition only, with no other intra-abdominal associations.

INCIDENCE

The frequency of epigastric hernia in the general population is estimated to be about 5%. It is occasionally found in newborns and children, but is more common in early adulthood and middle age. This hernia is three times more common in men than in women. Up to 20% of epigastric hernias may be multiple, but usually only one is dominant.

ETIOLOGY

The cause of epigastric hernia is unknown, but since it occurs even in newborn children, it is assumed to be the result of a structural congenital weakness of the linea alba between the xiphoid process of the sternum and the umbilicus. It is possibly owing to a lack of fibers at the midline decussation, which allows preperitoneal fat to herniate between the gaps. The fact that it is common between 20 and 50 years of age probably reflects a balance between a congenital defect and a rise of intra-abdominal pressure, adiposity, and weakening of the muscles in adults. It is more frequent in people with a wide linea alba (diastasis of the recti muscles).

ANATOMY

The midline opening in the fascia is usually elliptic, with the long axis lying transversely, or diamond shaped (Fig 14–27A and B). The size is usually only a few millimeters, but openings several centimeters in diameter are not unusual. Wider defects rarely are seen. Usually only a small amount of preperitoneal fat protrudes through the defect, although a small empty sac may be present as well (Fig 14–27C). Larger sacs usually contain some omentum, but small bowel, transverse colon, or even part of the stomach wall also may be present.

CLINICAL MANIFESTATIONS

The usual epigastric hernia is symptomless and is a chance finding by the patient or his doctor. Occasionally, especially once the hernia has been discovered, the patient may complain of mild or even severe pain in the mass and of exquisite tenderness to touch. The pain of epigastric hernia is exacerbated by exertion and relieved by rest in the supine position. The smaller hernias may become painful because of strangulation of the preperitoneal fat nipped by the sharp fascial edges of the opening. Omentum in the sac may strangulate, in which case the hernia may become swollen, painful, and tender, and the overlying skin may redden. Larger hernias containing bowel may also strangulate, but this is rare.

The real danger of epigastric hernia is to attribute to it symptoms caused by more serious intra-abdominal disease. For this reason, when it is not absolutely clear that the hernia is the source of the complaints, intra-abdominal pathology such as hiatus hernia, peptic ulcer, or cholelithiasis or malignant disease of the gastrointestinal tract should be ruled out.

The diagnosis is not usually difficult, although in obese people the typical smooth, rounded, slightly tender lump may be lost in the depths of the subcutaneous fat.

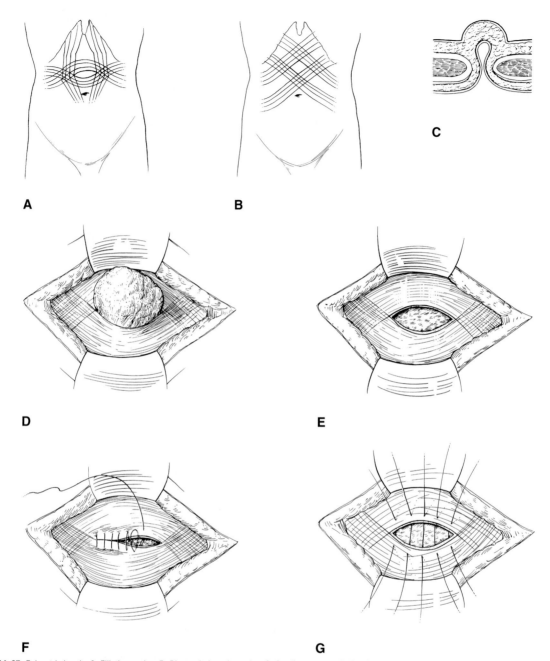

Figure 14–27. Epigastric hernia. **A.** Elliptic opening. **B.** Diamond-shaped opening. **C.** Small empty sac. **D.** herniated fat exposed. **E.** Herniated fat and sac have been excised. **F.** Repair by continuous suture. **G.** Repair by interrupted sutures. After Rejovitzky, MD.

TREATMENT

Small, symptomless epigastric hernias may safely be left untreated. The larger ones and those causing discomfort should be repaired.

Simple Closure

The operation can be done under local anesthesia, although with children or adults with larger hernias, especially in obese patients, a general anesthetic is preferable.

The herniated fat is exposed through a small transverse incision and is excised (Fig 14–27D). The fascial opening in the linea alba and some centimeters of fascia around it are cleared of fat. A small sac, if present and empty, is simply returned to the peritoneal cavity. If the sac is not empty and the contents cannot be easily reduced, it is best opened. Omentum adherent to the inside of the sac can be excised together with the sac (Fig 14–27E). Formal closure of the sac or peritoneum is unnecessary. The opening in the fascia is closed transversely with a continuous suture or a few interrupted sutures of fine monofilament polypropylene or polyamide, taking generous bites of the edges (Fig 14–27F through I). The subcutaneous fat may be closed with synthetic absorbable suture material and the skin edges approximated with a 5-0 synthetic absorbable continuous intradermal suture. Recurrence of the hernia is most unusual.

If, with time, one or more new epigastric hernias appear, they can be repaired in a similar fashion. There is little reason for doing a major repair of all of the linea alba from the sternum to the umbilicus through a long vertical incision when repairing a single small epigastric hernia. Most patients do not develop more than one epigastric hernia and do not need the major procedure. Repair of the usual small epigastric hernia is a minor ambulatory operation and can be repeated easily.

Reconstruction of Linea Alba

The rare case that develops more hernias probably reflects a generalized weakness of the midline fascia and is often associated with marked diastasis of the recti muscles. In this case, complete reconstruction of the linea alba from the umbilicus to the sternum is indicated and is done with the patient under general anesthesia. Several methods are advocated for this reconstruction. This author prefers the simple extraperitoneal procedure, using a modification of the shoelace technique, which is described in the discussion on the repair of postoperative ventral hernia. In this way, a strong new linea alba is constructed, the rectus muscles are approximated in the midline, and the diastasis is eliminated by suturing together the lateral cut edges of the rectus sheaths and fixing them in the midline to the new linea alba (Fig 14–28A).

Other methods are the vertical mass closure with bites that include not only the linea alba but also part of the anterior and posterior rectus sheath (Fig 14–28B) and the vertical overlap technique done by making a vertical incision along the anterior rectus sheath to create a medial flap, which is then doubled-breasted (Fig 14–28C).

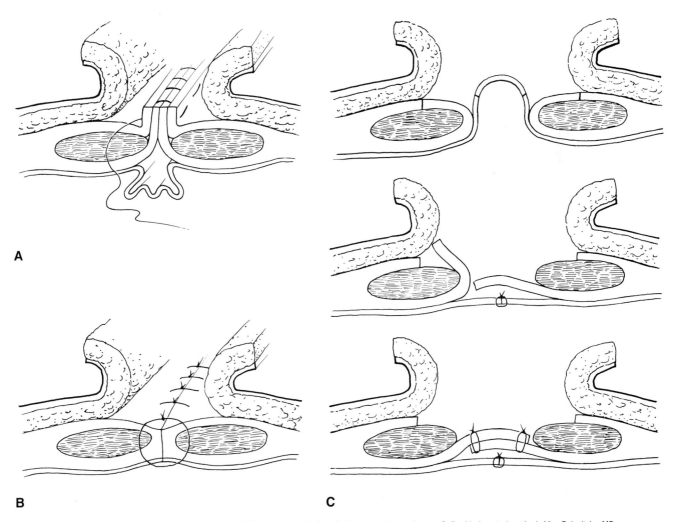

A

B

C

Figure 14–28. Reconstruction of linea alba. **A.** Modified shoelace technique. **B.** Interrupted mass closure. **C.** Double-breasted method. After Rejovitzky, MD.

Not surprisingly, Stoppa uses a prosthetic buttressing repair regardless of the diameter of the defect, as he described in 1981.[93] The linea alba is opened through a midline incision. A 6 × 12 cm strip of mesh is inserted into the retromuscular prefascial space or between the omentum and the peritoneum and is fixed in place by biologic adhesive. The edges of the linea alba are then reapproximated by simple over-and-over suturing or by an overlapping suture if diastasis of the recti muscles is present.

REPAIR OF LARGER HERNIAS

The rare, large epigastric hernia also can be repaired transversely, as was described for moderately sized umbilical hernia, and is best done with general anesthesia (see Fig 14–25). The anterior rectus sheaths are cleared of fat around the edge of the hernial defect. The sac is excised, and the upper and lower edges of the fascial opening are approximated by a continuous mass closure technique using a heavy monofilament nylon loop and taking large bites of the full thickness of the abdominal wall. The repair is reinforced by an onlay nylon darn.

The rare, still larger epigastric hernias should be treated as large postoperative ventral hernias by the shoelace method (see Fig 14–38) or should be closed with a sheet of prosthetic mesh (see Fig 14–26).[265]

■ OBTURATOR HERNIA

An obturator hernia is one of the rarest forms of hernia. Most surgeons will see no more than one, or perhaps two, in an entire career.

INCIDENCE

Since many cases are probably not reported, it is difficult to know what the true incidence of this condition is. The largest series, consisting of 20 cases, was reported from Thailand in 1974,[266] and an updated report on obturator hernia published in 1978.[267] Approximately 0.5% of mechanical intestinal obstructions are the result of strangulated obturator hernia. The hernia is more common in females, with a female-to-male ratio of 6:1. Reasons cited for this one-sided distribution include the broader female pelvis, a wide obturator canal, and pregnancy. The age of patients in reported cases varies from 12 to 93 years, but most cases occur in patients during their seventh and eighth decades. Aging, loss of body weight, and chronic lung disease are associated with obturator hernia. Overall, the hernia is found more frequently on the right side than on the left. In women, it appears more often on the right side, and in men, it appears more often on the left side. Bilateral obturator hernias occur in about 6% of cases, and other associated groin hernias are not uncommon.

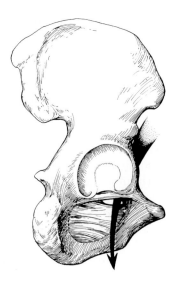

Figure 14–29. Direction of obturator hernia through the obturator canal. After Rejovitzky, MD.

ANATOMY

The hernia passes through the obturator canal, which is bounded above by the superior pubic ramus and below by the sharp, free upper edge of the obturator membrane (Fig 14–29). The canal is about 3 cm long and runs obliquely forward, downward, and medially. The obturator vessels and nerve pass through this canal from the abdomen to the medial aspect of the thigh. The nerve and vessels usually lie posterolateral to the hernial sac and must be avoided if the hernial orifice needs to be incised to be widened. The sac is long and narrow as it passes through the firm canal and balloons out in the thigh, deep to the pectineus muscle. Shorter sacs may end in the canal. While the hernia may contain a loop of small bowel, in a small hernia only part of the bowel wall may be in the sac, thus forming a Richter hernia. Unusual cases have been reported of the appendix, Meckel's diverticulum, omentum, bladder, and even ovary and fallopian tube being caught in the hernia.

CLINICAL MANIFESTATIONS

There are four cardinal features of obturator hernia, although they appear together in less than 5% of these patients. Intestinal obstruction is the most common sign and occurs in 88% of patients. It is usually in the form of acute obstruction with strangulation. The second most common feature is the Howship-Romberg sign, which is found in almost 50% of patients who characteristically complain of pain down the inner surface of the thigh, in the knee joint, and often in the hip joint as well. This is referred pain from the cutaneous branch of the anterior division of the obturator nerve and is owing to compression of the nerve in the narrow and unyielding canal. In the elderly, this pain is often misinterpreted as arthritic in origin. The nerve also contains motor fibers, and compression may lead to weakness and wasting of the adductors and to loss of the adductor reflex in the thigh. The third most common point, elicited in about 30% of patients, is a history of repeated attacks of intestinal obstruction that pass spontaneously and are probably the result of intermittent compression of the small bowel in the hernia, followed by remissions. The fourth sign is a palpable mass high in the medial aspect of the thigh at the origins of the adductor muscles. It is present in only 20 percent of cases. The mass is best felt with the thigh flexed, adducted, and rotated outwards. Patients rarely complain of a lump in the groin, because large obturator hernias are unusual and many of the patients are too elderly to notice it. Also, since obturator hernia is not always thought of in cases of intestinal obstruction, the attending physician does not examine for a lump in this unusual situation.

Two further signs may point to the diagnosis in cases with strangulation of an obturator hernia. One is the presence of ecchymosis in the medial part of the groin below the inguinal ligament due to seeping of blood-stained effusions from the infarcted hernia and bowel. The second is the presence of a tender mass in the obturator area felt laterally on vaginal examination. Cases of strangulated obturator hernia in elderly women presenting late with an abscess in the thigh following bowel necrosis have been reported.[268]

TREATMENT

All obturator hernias should be operated on soon after diagnosis, since the risk of strangulation is extremely high. There is no place for conservative treatment, nor is it technically possible considering the high incidence of potentially lethal complications of obturator hernia and the danger of not recognizing the condition.[269] In a series of 13 cases with 14 hernias, only five were diagnosed preoperatively. All presented with small bowel obstruction and half required a bowel resection. All were emaciated and elderly with a high morbidity and mortality rate; 15.4% of these patients died.

In the unusual case of diagnosis of an obturator hernia that is not strangulated, the operation for repair can be done electively with no special preparations besides the usual preoperative assessments. The usual case, however, presents as acute intestinal obstruction with strangulation of unknown cause, since, in most cases, the hernia is not thought of or found. The preoperative preparations will include placement of a nasogastric tube and intravenous correction of fluid and electrolytes.

There are three operative approaches for the repair of obturator hernia: the lower abdominal midline transperitoneal approach, the lower abdominal midline extraperitoneal approach, and the exposure in the thigh. Tsubona stressed the high incidence of bilateral obturator hernia and suggests that the added advantage of the retropubic extraperitoneal approach is that a contralateral hernia can be looked for and simultaneously repaired.[270]

Thigh Operation

Theoretically, the thigh operation should be the ideal approach, since it is both extra-abdominal and directly aimed at the obturator foramen. However, it is seldom used as the primary approach for elective surgery or in cases of strangulation, because access is narrow and deep between the muscles, inspection and reduction of the hernial contents is not safe in cases of strangulation, and repair of the hernial defect is difficult. Occasionally, however, it is necessary as a counter incision when faced with problems in reducing an obturator hernia through one of the abdominal approaches. A vertical incision is made in the upper and medial point of the thigh along the adductor longus muscle, which is displaced medially (Fig 14–30). The pectineus muscle is either split or cut across to expose the sac, which is opened. The contents are inspected and reduced, the sac is excised, and the hernial opening is closed with a continuous monofilament polypropylene or polyamide suture. If the bowel in the hernia is strangulated and not viable, a laparotomy incision must be done for safe resection and anastomosis.

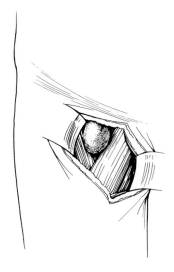

Figure 14–30. Thigh approach for repair of obturator hernia. After Rejovitzky, MD.

Abdominal Midline Extraperitoneal Approach

The midline extraperitoneal approach is the best method for dealing with an obturator hernia when the diagnosis has been made preoperatively. It allows good exposure of the internal opening of the obturator canal without interfering with the abdominal contents. An incision is made from the umbilicus to the pubis in the midline, without breaching the peritoneum, which is peeled off the bladder in the midline, and also laterally to expose the superior pubic ramus and the obturator internus muscle. The sac will be seen as a projection of peritoneum passing into the obturator canal and is incised at its base. The contents are reduced into the peritoneal cavity, the sac is transected at the neck, and the peritoneal defect is closed. The sac may now be extracted from the canal by traction, or an artery forceps may be passed down into the sac to grasp the distal end and to extract the sac by inversion. The internal opening of the obturator canal is closed with a continuous monofilament nylon suture, taking bites of the tissues around it, such as the periosteum of the superior pubic ramus and the fascia on the internal obturator muscle. Care must be exercised not to injure the obturator nerve and vessels. Alternatively, a sheet of prosthetic mesh may be laid down to cover the area and tacked down around its edges. The peritoneum is allowed to return to the pelvic wall, and the abdominal incision is closed. Other extraperitoneal approaches have been described but are seldom used. They are mainly muscle-cutting or muscle-splitting techniques through a skin incision above and parallel to the inguinal canal.

Abdominal Midline Transperitoneal Approach

The midline transperitoneal approach is the most common method for repair of obturator hernia, since most cases are unexpectedly encountered during laparotomy for intestinal obstruction of unknown cause. The collapsed small bowel is followed until it disappears into the anterolateral pelvic wall at the internal opening of the obturator canal, at which point the obstructed and dilated proximal loop of small bowel is also found. A careful attempt at reduction by gentle traction on the loops of bowel is often successful. This attempt may be augmented by pressure on the hernial sac over the medial aspect of the thigh. In two of the three cases that this author has treated, these maneuvers were not successful, but a short, sharp strike with the fist in the upper inner aspect of the thigh over the area of the sac ejected the loop of strangulated bowel out of the obturator canal. The third case was a Richter type of lateral strangulation of the small bowel wall that was easily extracted. The internal opening of the obturator canal is very rigid and cannot be digitally dilated. Extraction of the bowel can be made easier by carefully incising the sharp edge of the obturator membrane, using a grooved

probe to avoid damage to the bowel. Care must be taken to identify and avoid injury to the obturator nerve. If these maneuvers fail, a counter incision must be made in the thigh (Fig 14–30). The sac is excised, and the canal opening is closed as described above. Nonviable bowel is resected and the abdomen is closed in the usual manner.

Results

The mortality rate has been reduced to approximately 10% in spite of the advanced age and poor general condition of most of these patients, mainly because of better care of the fluid and electrolyte balance preoperatively and because of the cardiovascular and pulmonary support postoperatively. Recent reports quote a recurrence rate of less than 5%.

■ PERINEAL HERNIAS

Perineal hernias are protrusions of the abdominal contents through the muscles and the fascia that form the floor of the pelvis. They are also called pelvic hernias, ischiorectal hernias, pudendal hernias, posterior labial hernias, subpubic hernias, hernias of the pouch of Douglas, and vaginal hernias. This type of hernia should not be confused with a rectocele, a cystocele, or a colpocele, which are related to a relaxation of the pelvic floor usually caused by childbirth.

Scarpa, in 1821, first reported a case, but de Garengeot is supposed to have seen one in 1731.[271] The condition is extremely rare, and fewer than 100 cases have been reported—mainly in single case reports.

Perineal hernias are primary, spontaneously occurring hernias. A secondary or postoperative type may occur following abdominoperineal resection of the rectum and related procedures.

PRIMARY PERINEAL HERNIAS

Etiology
Primary perineal hernias usually occur between the fifth and seventh decades of life and are five times more common in women than in men, perhaps because of childbirth and the broader female pelvis. A deep, elongated pouch of Douglas is thought to be a congenital predisposing factor in perineal hernias. Other factors include obesity, ascites, pelvic infections, and obstetric trauma.

Anatomy
The pelvic floor is formed by the levator ani and the iliococcygeus muscles and their fascia (Fig 14–31). The circumference of the pelvic outlet is bounded anteriorly by the pubic symphysis and the subpubic ligament, laterally by the pubic rami and ischial tuberosities, and

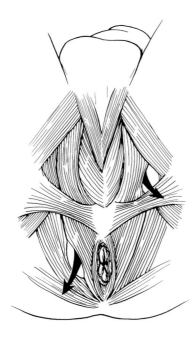

Figure 14–31. Anatomy of perineal hernias. After Rejovitzky, MD.

posteriorly by the sacrotuberous ligaments and the coccyx. The transversus perinei muscles divide the space into the urogenital triangle anteriorly and the ischiorectal fossae posteriorly. Two types of perineal hernia are described, anterior and posterior, depending on their relationship to the transversus perinei muscles.

The anterior perineal hernia occurs almost exclusively in women. It enters in front of the broad ligament and lateral to the bladder, passes through the paravesical fossa of Waldeyer, and emerges anterior to the transversus perinei muscle. These hernias may enter the labium majus and become known as labial or pudendal hernias.

Posterior perineal hernias occur in both men and women but are more frequent in women. In men, the hernia enters between the bladder and the rectum and appears in the ischiorectal fossa or perineum, posterior to the transversus perinei muscle and lateral to the median raphe. In women, the hernia enters between the rectum and the uterus and passes posterior to the broad ligament and lateral to the uterosacral ligament. It may pass through the levator ani muscle or between it and the iliococcygeus muscle, or even directly through the iliococcygeus muscle. It may remain in the midline and pass forward to press into the vaginal wall or backward into the rectum. It may also lie in the ischiorectal fossa below the lower margin of the gluteus maximus muscle and may be confused with a sciatic hernia.

A lateral pelvic hernia, through the hiatus of Schwalbe, also has been described. In this case, the peritoneal sac passes through a gap in the line of origin of the levator ani muscle from the fascia of the internal obturator muscle. It passes anteriorly into the labium majus and posteriorly into the ischiorectal fossa.

Anterior perineal hernias contain intestine or bladder. Posterior perineal hernias may contain omentum, small bowel, or rectum. The hernias have a wide neck and usually soft borders with no rigid fibrous ring, so that incarceration or strangulation are rare.

Clinical Manifestations

The patient may complain of a soft protruberance that is easily reduced when the recumbent position is assumed. Symptoms are usually mild. In cases of anterior hernia, minor urinary discomfort may have been noted. In cases of posterior hernias in which the mass may assume a large size and even protrude below the lower edge of the gluteus maximus muscle, sitting may be difficult or impossible. A dragging sensation may be felt on standing or straining. Rarely, constipation may be attributed to the hernia. A posterior hernia protruding into the posterior wall of the vagina may interfere with labor.

Physical examination will reveal a soft and easily reducible mass with a cough impulse. The direction in which it reduces will indicate the anatomic nature of the hernia. Strangulation is rare since the hernial defect is usually large and bounded by soft and often atrophied muscle. If it occurs, local pain, swelling, and signs of inflammation will develop, together with the signs and symptoms of intestinal obstruction. The hernia will become tender and irreducible. Bimanual, rectal, and vaginal examinations will help to differentiate perineal hernia from cystoceles and rectoceles. Perineal abscess, lipoma, fibroma, and polyps could possibly be confused with perineal hernia. Rectal prolapse must sometimes be differentiated from a perineal hernia. The two may coexist, with the perineal hernia appearing anterior to the prolapsed rectum. Lubat has reported the elegant demonstration by CT of two cases of posterior perineal hernia showing the contents and the anatomical relations.[272]

Treatment

Three options are available for surgical repair: the abdominal, the perineal, or the combined approach. The abdominal approach is preferable since it allows better exposure of the anatomy of the defect and a more secure repair. With the patient under general anesthesia, the abdomen is opened through a midline subumbilical incision. The bowel will disappear through a defect in the pelvic floor and usually can be reduced easily. Occasionally, mild traction or even outside pressure on the hernia may be needed. The empty sac is everted and excised. Small defects can be closed by interrupted sutures of monofilament polyamide or polypropylene. Since atrophied muscle tissue is used for the repair, the recurrence rate is high. Recurrence can be avoided by using a sheet of prosthetic non-absorbable mesh to reinforce the repair. It is laid on the pelvic floor of the region to cover the repair and is tacked down by nonabsorbable monofilament sutures. When the defect is large and the edges are thin and friable, they cannot be approximated. In these cases, a synthetic nonabsorbable mesh prosthesis is sutured to cover the defect. The rectovesical pouch then may be eliminated by a series of sutures.

The perineal route is a more direct approach to the hernial sac and avoids a laparotomy, but exposure and repair of the defect is more difficult. The method is not suitable for dealing with a strangulated hernia or with bowel of questionable viability. A transverse or longitudinal incision is made in the skin over the hernia. The sac is freed from the surrounding muscles and is excised. The hernial contents are reduced into the pelvic cavity and the defect is repaired with interrupted monofilament nonabsorbable synthetic sutures.

In extreme cases in which a large strangulated hernia cannot be reduced by the abdominal approach alone, a combined abdominal and perineal route may be necessary.

INCISIONAL PERINEAL HERNIA

Etiology
An incisional perineal hernia may follow abdominoperineal resection of the rectum or pelvic exenteration. It occurs as a result of the excision of the levator ani muscles and the pelvic fascia with incomplete repair of the pelvic floor. The addition of excision of the coccyx is thought to be an aggravating factor. Women are more frequently affected than men. The hernia is rare since many of the patients do not survive very long after the original operation. Another reason is that there are relatively fewer abdominoperineal resections of the rectum since more and lower anterior resections of the rectum are being done.

Treatment
Minor degrees of pelvic herniation, as manifested by bulging of the perineum after abdominoperineal resection, are quite common and do not require treatment. Although operation is not indicated when there is evidence of recurrence of malignant disease, large uncomfortable hernias hanging between the thighs and those with skin ulceration should be repaired. The operation is a major procedure and should not be lightly undertaken. Although the abdominal or perineal route may be used, the former is preferable since it allows better exposure of the anatomy of the defect, especially for freeing the loops of bowel that often have firmly adhered to the sac. Since there is no pelvic floor to repair, the large defect must be closed with a sheet of nonabsorbable synthetic mesh prosthesis.

■ SPIGELIAN HERNIA

Adriaan van der Spieghel (1578–1625), a Flemish anatomist, was a pupil of Fabricius of Padua. He became professor of anatomy and surgery in that city and was the first to describe accurately the semilunar line, as well as the caudate lobe of the liver to which his name was given. Spigelius, as he was known in Italy, never described a hernia. He described the fascia through which this hernia occurs. The Spigelian fascia is the aponeurotic part of the transversus abdominis muscle between the medial border of its muscular part and the insertion of the aponeurosis into the posterior rectus sheath.

INCIDENCE

Almost 1000 cases have been described in the literature. In one review of the subject, in 1984, the mean age was 50 years, and the ratio of women to men was 1.4:1.[273] The ratio of hernias on the right side to hernias on the left side was 1.6:1. The hernia was bilateral in 24 of 744 patients. In 10 cases there were more than one hernia on the same side. Most of the hernias were located below the level of the umbilicus; only 28 were above this level. The youngest recorded patient was 6 days old, and the oldest was 94 years of age.[274,275] Incarceration at the time of the operation occurred in 69 of 325 patients (21.2%). The hernial sac was situated subcutaneously in only 15 cases, while in most cases the hernia was located between the musculoaponeurotic layers of the anterior abdominal wall.

ANATOMY

The semilunar line that marks the lateral border of the rectus sheath stretches from the tip of the ninth rib cartilage to the pubic tubercle. The Spigelian fascia, which is really a strip of aponeurosis, runs parallel and lateral to the outer border of the rectus sheath, where its fibers fuse with those of the internal and external oblique muscle aponeuroses to form the rectus sheath. The Spigelian fascia varies in width. At its upper end, it hardly exists since the muscular part of the transversus abdominis usually reaches up to the semilunar line. It gets wider as it passes down to the level of the umbilicus and is widest in that part between the level of the umbilicus and where it meets the arcuate fold of Douglas. Several reports describe the insertion of the transversus abdominis and internal oblique muscles into the rectus sheath as a series of microbundles of muscle and microtendons in a parallel arrangement, with gaps between them that are filled by fibrofatty septae.[276,277] The usual protective gridiron arrangement of the abdominal wall musculature does not exist here so that factors such as aging of the tissues, obesity, increased abdominal pressure due to coughing, constipation, prostatism, sudden lifting of a heavy weight,

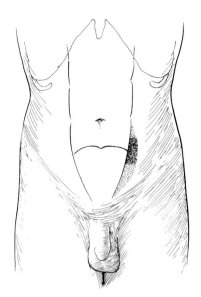

Figure 14–32. Spigelian hernia. Sites of most common occurrence. After Rejovitzky, MD.

and pregnancies may force the preperitoneal fat through the fibrofatty septae and thus cause a Spigelian hernia.

Most of the hernias occur in the area between the level of the umbilicus and the level of the arcuate line, or fold of Douglas, where the Spigelian fascia is widest and presumably weakest (Fig 14–32). The hernias occur particularly at the point where the semilunar and arcuate lines meet, since it is at this point that all the fibers of the transversus abdominis muscle pass in front of the rectus muscle. There is no posterior rectus sheath below this point. The rearrangement of the fibers at this point is believed to cause an area of functional weakness where the hernias can more easily occur. Hernias at the upper reaches of the semilunar line are not usually true Spigelian hernias since there is rarely any Spigelian fascia there. These hernias usually pass through the posterior rectus sheath along the medial side of the semilunar line and expand in the rectus sheath and are called intravaginal hernias.

Hernias below the level of the arcuate line of Douglas pass through the conjoined tendon of the transversus abdominis and internal oblique muscles and are called "low" Spigelian hernias. At the lowest levels they may behave like direct inguinal hernias. Other hernias, such as umbilical, epigastric, or inguinal, may be associated with Spigelian hernia.

As the hernia develops, preperitoneal fat pushes its way through the slit-like defects of the Spigelian fascia and the aponeurosis of the internal oblique muscle, dragging a protrusion of peritoneum with it (Fig 14–33A). The hernia meets resistance from the aponeurosis of the external oblique muscle but is able to mush-

room in the loose areolar tissue between the internal oblique and external oblique muscles (Fig 14–33B). Because of anatomic variations, a small number of hernias pass through the aponeurosis of the transversus abdominis muscle only and lie between that muscle and the internal oblique muscle (Fig 14–33C). In this way, almost all Spigelian hernias are interstitial (interparietal). Rarely, the hernia may pierce the aponeurosis of the external oblique muscle and lie in the subcutaneous tissues of the abdominal wall (Fig 14–33D). The hernia

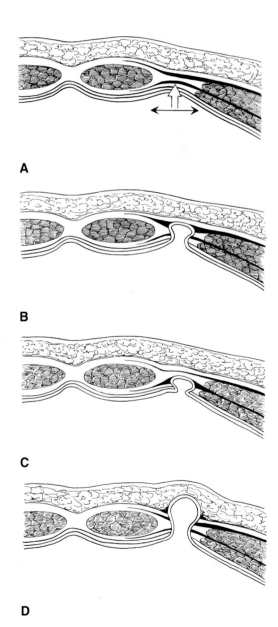

A

B

C

D

Figure 14–33. Spigelian hernia. **A.** Breaching the Spigelian fascia. **B.** The most common type has passed through the transversus abdominis and the internal oblique aponeuroses and is spreading out in the interstitial layer deep to the external oblique aponeurosis. **C.** The less common type in the interstitial layer between the transversus abdominis aponeurosis and the internal oblique muscle. **D.** The least common subcutaneous type. After Rejovitzky, MD.

is unable to spread medially because of the resistance of the rectus sheath, but it can develop laterally and inferiorly and may come to lie alongside the anterior superior iliac spine or even in the inguinal region.

Spigelian hernias are usually <2 cm in diameter but, occasionally, larger hernias, even up to 11 cm in diameter, are seen. The smaller peritoneal sacs are usually empty, but the larger ones may contain omentum, small or large bowel, or even part of the stomach wall.

CLINICAL MANIFESTATIONS

Patients complain of pain or a lump or both at the site of herniation. The pain is sharp and constant or intermittent, or there is a dragging, uncomfortable feeling. If strangulation of the hernial contents is present, the pain will be severe and constant and associated with symptoms and signs of complete or partial (Richter) intestinal obstruction, going on to gangrene and peritonitis. Localized perforation into the sac may cause an abdominal wall abscess and even fistula.

When a mass is present along the semilunar line, especially in the region below the umbilicus, the diagnosis becomes easier. The mass may be reducible, after which the hernial defect in the fascia may be felt. There is usually tenderness present in the region of the defect. The palpable mass of a Spigelian hernia, whether it be subcutaneous or interstitial, usually persists during abdominal contraction. When the hernia is incarcerated and irreducible, it may be confused with lipoma, desmoid tumor, hematoma of the rectus sheath, or even an appendix abscess.

Roentgenologic investigations by plain x-ray films or with contrast media, especially tangential views, may be helpful in confirming the diagnosis by showing bowel outside the abdominal cavity at the site of pain, tenderness, or mass. However, ultrasound examination is the best, easiest, and most reliable test available for diagnosing Spigelian hernia. Testa showed that ultrasound diagnosis is accurate in 86% of the cases.[278] Hodgson believes that the greatest degree of diagnostic accuracy can be achieved by a combination of ultrasound and tangential radiographs.[279] If the hernia is reduced and no mass is palpable, ultrasound scanning will show a break in the echogenic shadow of the semilunar line corresponding to the fascial defect. Whether or not the hernia is palpable, if it is not reduced, the hernial sac and contents will be demonstrated passing through the defect in the Spigelian fascia and lying in an interstitial or subcutaneous plane. Scanning by thin-section CT will also confirm the presence of a Spigelian hernia, but CT is more expensive and not universally available. Spigelian hernia may be an elusive diagnosis and may mimic other intra-abdominal conditions. For this reason it should be kept

in mind and, if necessary, sought through these special examinations. As they become more available, the diagnosis of Spigelian hernia will probably become more common.

TREATMENT

Since at least 20% of Spigelian hernias present with strangulation, the proper treatment is operative repair, which is more conveniently done with the patient under general anesthesia, although local or regional methods can be used. A transverse or oblique skin incision is made over the lump or over the fascial defect. A subcutaneous hernia will immediately reveal itself, but more commonly the hernia is interstitial, and the external oblique muscle must be split in the line of its fibers to demonstrate the sac. It is freed from the surrounding tissues down to the neck. The sac is opened and the contents reduced back into the peritoneal cavity. Some adhesions between the contents and the sac wall may have to be freed. The sac may now be excised or inverted. It is not necessary to tie or suture it. The defect in the fascia of the transversus abdominis and the internal oblique muscle is closed with a continuous suture of monofilament polyamide or polypropylene. The slit in the external oblique muscle is similarly repaired and the skin closed. The repair heals well and few recurrences have been reported.

■ LUMBAR HERNIA

ANATOMY

The lumbar region is the area between the twelfth rib above, the iliac crest below, the erector spinae muscles behind, and a vertical line from the tip of the twelfth rib to the iliac crest anteriorly. Hernias in this region are extremely rare and tend to occur mainly through the inferior lumbar triangle (of Petit), which is bounded below by the iliac crest, in front by the posterior edge of the external oblique muscle, and behind by the anterior border of the latissimus dorsi muscle (Fig 14–34). The floor is covered by lumbar fascia, deep to which are the internal oblique and transversus muscles. The triangle is absent when the free border of the latissimus dorsi overlaps the external oblique fibers.

The superior lumbar triangle may also be the site of these rare hernias. It is bounded by the twelfth rib and the lower border of the serratus posterior inferior muscle, by the posterior border of the internal oblique muscle, and, behind, by the quadratus lumborum and erector spinae muscles. The floor is formed by the transversalis aponeurosis, and the space is covered by the latissimus dorsi.

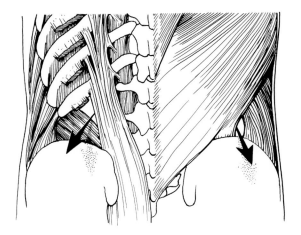

Figure 14–34. Lumbar hernia showing the superior and inferior lumbar triangles. After Rejovitzky, MD.

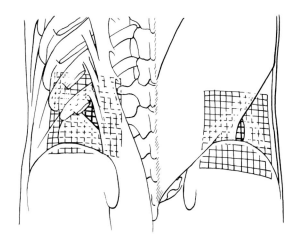

Figure 14–35. Prosthetic mesh repair of lumbar hernia. After Rejovitzky, MD.

Clinical Manifestation

Congenital lumbar hernias have been reported in newborns and children, but are rare. Mehta reported a case in a newborn male and collected 30 pediatric cases from the literature.[280] They occur in otherwise normal babies but may be associated with the lumbo-costo-vertebral deficiency syndrome and other congenital lesions. However, they usually occur in persons between 50 and 70 years of age. Two-thirds of the cases are reported in men, and hernias on the left side are more common. They also may be bilateral. Acquired lumbar hernias may follow trauma, poliomyelitis, loin incision, and the use of iliac crest as a donor site for bone grafting.

Lumbar hernias rarely strangulate. They tend to grow and may assume large proportions, overhanging the iliac crest. Patients complain of a dragging discomfort in the hernia. Examination will reveal a soft swelling that is easily reducible. A cough impulse is usually present, and the hernia increases in size on straining.

TREATMENT

Operative repair should be done with the patient under general anesthesia and lying on his/her side. An oblique skin crease incision or a vertical incision is made over the area of the hernia, and the sac is dissected down to its neck. The sac is opened and the contents reduced. The empty sac can be simply inverted or excised. Numerous complicated procedures have been described for repair of the hernia, involving muscle slides and muscle or fascial flaps and grafts. They should be abandoned in favor of simpler repairs. When good tissue is present and the defect is small, it can be closed by a continuous monofilament polyamide or polypropylene suture. When the defect is large and the tissues are poor, the hernia is best repaired with a large sheet of prosthetic nonabsorbable mesh of polypropylene, or PTFE laid between the peritoneum and the abdominal wall muscles and fixed around its periphery by a series of monofilament synthetic nonabsorbable sutures passed through the full thickness of the abdominal wall (Fig 14–35).

■ SCIATIC HERNIA

ANATOMY

Sciatic hernia is a protrusion from the pelvis of a peritoneal sac through the greater sciatic notch, above or below the piriformis muscle, or through the lesser sciatic notch (Fig 14–36). It passes backward and downward to the buttock where it lies deep to the gluteus maximus muscle. The hernia usually contains small bowel, but colon, omentum, bladder, fallopian tube, ovary, Meckel's diverticulum, and even ureter has been reported. The condition is rare. Most surgeons will not see any cases during their entire career. Cases have been reported in children younger than 1 year of age, but most were found in adults between the ages of 20 and 60 years.[281–283]

CLINICAL MANIFESTATIONS

The patient may complain of pain in the buttock that radiates down the sciatic nerve, or a mass, or both. The pain may be confused with intermittent claudication. On examination, a reducible mass may be felt deep to the gluteus maximus. Most cases were not diagnosed preoperatively but were found only at laparotomy for intestinal obstruction.

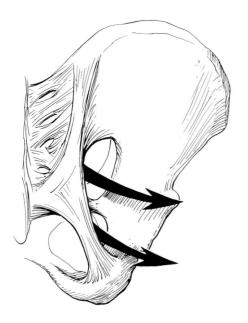

Figure 14–36. The superior and inferior sciatic foramina and the direction of the sciatic hernias. After Rejovitzky, MD.

TREATMENT

The hernia usually is approached through a lower midline abdominal incision. In the female the bowel will be seen entering the hernia behind the broad ligament. Even when intestinal obstruction is present, the bowel usually can be reduced with light traction. Where needed, the opening can be dilated with a finger or else the piriformis muscle may be partially incised, taking great care to avoid the many nerves and vessels in the region. The sac then is everted and excised and the opening repaired by suture of the edges with monofilament polyamide or polypropylene. When this repair is not possible, the opening can be plugged with a rolled-up strip of polypropylene mesh held in place with a few stitches (see Fig 14–19).[16] Larger defects should be covered with a sheet of polypropylene mesh.

The posterior or transgluteal method may be used for uncomplicated and reducible sciatic hernias diagnosed preoperatively. The gluteus maximus muscle is approached through a gluteal incision and is detached at its origin to expose the hernia. The sac is dissected free and opened. The contents are reduced and the sac is dealt with. The defect is sutured closed using local tissues or polypropylene mesh.

■ POSTOPERATIVE VENTRAL ABDOMINAL HERNIA

A postoperative ventral abdominal, or incisional, hernia is the result of failure of the lines of closure of the abdominal wall following laparotomy. The approximated

tissues separate, and abdominal organs, mainly bowel, bulge through the gap, which is covered from inside outwards with peritoneum, scar tissue, and skin (Fig 14–37). These hernias may grow to reach enormous proportions, and the truly giant hernias may contain most of the abdominal contents.

HISTORY

Major abdominal surgery developed rapidly during the latter part of the last century and with it rose the incidence of postoperative hernias. For more than 100 years, attempts have been made to develop successful methods for repairing them, but most attempts were followed by a high incidence of complications and a high recurrence rate.

Repair of this hernia is one of the few instances in surgery in which implants of foreign material were used

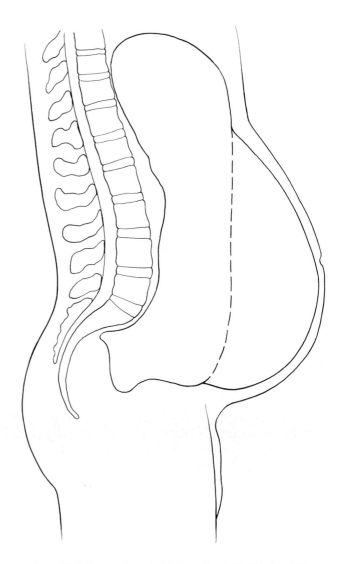

Figure 14–37. Postoperative ventral abdominal hernia. After Rejovitzky, MD.

to bridge gaps, before the use of natural tissues. Witzel in 1900, Goepel also in 1900, Bartlett in 1903, and McGavin in 1909 advocated the use of a silver-wire filigree.[52–55] Koontz and Throckmorton, each in 1948, used tantalum gauze.[57,59] Sheets of stainless steel and tantalum also were used. These metals fragmented within a short time, and the hernia recurred in many cases. Furthermore, the fragments of metal caused skin sinuses and even perforation of the bowel.

Fascia lata grafts used in the form of strips or sheets have been reported.[22–24, 284–287] The use of skin in sheets or strips has also been advocated.[26] These tissues tended to be absorbed and were associated with a high recurrence rate. Harvesting the grafts was often a problem, as were complications such as sinus formation, dermoid cysts, and even malignant change.

Shortly after the advent of synthetic plastic material, pliable plastic sheets and the polyvinyl alcohol sponge were used.[288,289] The modern era of prosthetic hernia repair began in 1958 when Usher reported his experience with polyamide mesh.[64] Later, braided polyester mesh, polypropylene mesh and expanded polytetrafluoroethylene (PTFE) were introduced. These latter three materials have revolutionized the surgery for postoperative hernia so that historic methods should now be abandoned.

Darn techniques of repair of postoperative hernia were introduced early in the century. A variety of sutures were used, including strips of fascia lata or skin and even animal tendon. Biologic threads of silk, cotton and linen were also tried. In 1949 Gosset revived the use of full-thickness strips of auto graft skin in the form of a reinforcing darn repair.[290] The darn technique is an excellent method for repair of these hernias, but it was not universally accepted because of the lack of a suitable suture material. However, in 1948 Abel reported his initial experiences with closing abdominal incisions and repairing hernias with monofilament stainless steel wire.[291] His later reports summarized his technique.[292,293] Hunter reported his experience using monofilament nylon and suturing only the anterior rectus sheaths.[294] He avoided approximating the rectus sheaths under tension. This author further modified and developed this nylon darn technique and, since 1973, has been using the "shoelace" method for the repair of ventral postoperative hernias. Results were reported in 1984, 1985, and 1987, and the operative technique is detailed in a paper published in 1988.[265,295–297] The advantages of this method include its relative simplicity and the fact that the abdominal cavity is not opened. The recurrence rate is low.

INCIDENCE

In the best centers, the incidence of postoperative hernia has been at least 10% as shown by long-term follow-up studies.[298–301] Where less emphasis is placed on the niceties of abdominal wound closure, the incidence is much higher. Earlier short-term studies have the erroneous impression that most postoperative hernias appear within the first year after the operation and that 80% appear within the first 2 years. Recent studies, however, show that about two-thirds appear within the first 5 years and that at least another third appear 5 to 10 years after the operation. As longer and more accurate follow-up studies are done, it will probably be shown that with aging and weakening of the tissues, postoperative hernias may appear even more than 10 years after the original operation. With the all-around improvement in surgical management and the constant perfecting of better methods for abdominal closure, the incidence of postoperative ventral hernia can be expected to drop. In a recent publication, Hesselink reported on 417 patients who underwent incisional hernia repair.[302] With a mean follow-up period of 34.9 months, the overall recurrence rate was 36%. Of these recurrences, 45% appeared in the first year, 64% in the second year, and 78% within the first three years. The cumulative recurrence rate after 5 years was 41%. After the second, third, and fourth attempts at repair, the recurrence rate was 56%, 48%, and 47%, respectively. Factors such as obesity, diabetes mellitus, lower abdominal incision, and wound infection had a higher rate of incisional hernia and recurrence after repair but were not statistically significant. The most important factor was the size of the hernia. Hernias <4 cm wide had a recurrence rate of 25% while those >4 cm recurred in 41%. The author stresses the importance of the technique of wound closure and hernia repair.

ETIOLOGY

Many factors, singly or in various combinations, may cause failure of the wound to heal satisfactorily and may lead to the development of a postoperative hernia.[174] The two main causes are poor surgical technique and sepsis. The situation is similar to that found after repair of inguinal hernias in that there are two types of postoperative ventral hernias, early and late.

Early Hernias

The early-occurring type, which appears soon after the original laparotomy closure, often involves the whole length of the wound, grows rapidly, and becomes large. This early failure usually is the result of technical failure on the part of the surgeon.

Poor Surgical Technique

Nonanatomic Incisions. Nonanatomic incisions are typified by the vertical pararectus incision along the outside of the lateral border of the rectus sheath, which destroys the nerve and vascular supply to the tissues medial to the incision, causing them to atrophy. The more lateral the incision, the greater the damage. Generally speaking, the best and simplest access to the abdominal cavity is through the midline or transverse incisions. The lateral paramedian incision may prove to have a low incidence of postoperative hernia.[303]

It is commonly believed that incisional hernias and recurrent incisional hernias are more common in vertical (ie, midline or paramedian) incisions and less common in transverse or oblique incisions. However, carefully controlled trials have shown that, when all wounds are closed by the mass technique, there is no difference in the incidence of burst abdomen, eventration, postoperative hernia, or recurrent postoperative hernia. The important factors are the type of closure and the type of suture material used.[174,304–309]

Layered Closures. Layered closures are followed by a greater incidence of postoperative hernias than are wounds closed by the single-layer mass closure technique. This may be owing to the fact that many more sutures are used, which are closely placed, and because insufficiently sized bites of each thin layer are taken.

Inappropriate Suture Material. The process of wound healing, collagen formation, and maturation, the laying down of the collagen fibers in parallel lines according to the lines of stress, and the healed wound gaining its maximum strength takes about 1 year. Approximately 80% of the final wound strength is reached after 6 months. It follows, therefore, that the wound must be supported for at least this time. The sutures are entirely responsible for the integrity of the wound for the first 6 months, so any material that does not survive and maintain most of its strength for this time is not suitable for wound closure. Reliable trials have shown that wounds closed with nonabsorbable suture material are followed by a far lower incidence of postoperative hernias than wounds closed with absorbable material. Thus, catgut and the synthetic absorbable sutures should not be used for closure of laparotomy wounds. Biologic sutures such as silk, cotton, and linen disintegrate after 2 months and also should not be used. Furthermore, these sutures, especially silk, perpetuate wound infection and sinuses.

The ideal suture material for abdominal closure, especially of midline incisions, is monofilament stainless steel wire (SW gauge 28) used in the form of interrupted mass closure, taking large bites of the musculoaponeurotic layers of the abdominal wall. This is the method preferred by the author. The peritoneum is not sutured as a separate layer, nor is it included in the mass suture, if it can be avoided. There is no advantage to suturing the peritoneum, and there are certain disadvantages.[164,310–312] Monofilament stainless steel wire sutures were introduced by Abel in 1948.[291] In 1975 Goligher re-

ported a less than 1% early postoperative hernia rate when using stainless steel wire mass closure and no late postoperative hernias.[313] This author has been using this method almost exclusively for 30 years, and personal experience confirms the above findings. The technique of passing and tying the steel sutures is simple and easily mastered, with some practice. Interrupted heavy monofilament polypropylene or polyamide sutures may be used but are also not convenient to knot. A good alternative is mass closure with a continuous heavy (1 or metric 4) monofilament polyamide or polypropylene as a single thread or, preferably, in the form of a commercially available loop.[314]

Suturing Technique. It is still widely but erroneously believed that when an abdominal incision is closed, a great number of small sutures closely placed and tightly tied, with each taking a small bite of tissue, are neater and better than fewer, widely spaced, loosely tied sutures that take a large mass bite of the tissues. However, small sutures take only a small amount of tissue close to the cut edge of the incision. In vertical abdominal incisions at, or near, the midline, these sutures pull in the line of fibers of the aponeurotic muscles and, since they are so close to the incision, easily cut out of the tissues. A small, tightly tied suture causes ischemia and necrosis of the tissues it contains and also of an area on each side of the suture. When these small, tightly tied sutures are placed close to each other, their ischemic areas merge and thus, cause necrosis of a strip of tissue all along the edge of the incision, which separates, together with the sutures, from the rest of the abdominal wall, leading to failure of the wound.

Tension. Closing wounds with tension is bad surgery. The lateral pull of the abdominal wall muscles against the suture, which tends to pull them in the opposite direction, creates an area of pressure necrosis where the suture meets the tissue. This pressure necrosis is a primary cause of wound dehiscence.[315] The problems of tension have been discussed further in the section on inguinal hernias.

Maingot succinctly summarized these failures on the part of the surgeon as "inept methods of suture."[29]

Sepsis. Sepsis, the second major cause of early wound failure, is a contributing factor, if not the most important one, in more than 50% of postoperative hernias that develop in year 1 after operation. It may range from frank acute cellulitis, with fasciitis and necrosis of the tissues on each side of the incision, to low-grade chronic sepsis around sutures such as braided or twisted silk. The latter case is very difficult to overcome, since the infecting organisms lurk in the spaces between the fibers of the suture thread and constantly reinfect the tissues. The infection causes inflammation and edema of the tissues, which become soft and weakened so that the sutures tear the tissues and pull out under the strain of the intra-abdominal pressure (see also the section on inguinal hernias).

Drainage Tubes. Drainage tubes brought out through the operation wound are a potent cause of postoperative hernias.[316] Since the tissue planes along the track of the drain are not sutured, an open and weak passage is present through all the layers of the wound through which a hernia may develop. Furthermore, after the first 24 hours, there is a rapid rise in the wound infection rate, since the drain allows for two-way traffic of secretions outwards and organisms inwards to the wound and abdominal cavity. Also, the irritation caused by the drain causes edema or softening and tearing of the tissues and cutting out of the sutures.

Obesity. Obesity is associated with a high percentage of postoperative hernias, as well as with recurrences following repair of these hernias. Ellis' group found that obesity was associated with a three-fold increase in herniation and recurrence.[317] Read and Manninen confirmed that obesity plays a major role in the production of these hernias as well as in recurrence following their repair.[309,318] It is difficult to pinpoint the actual reasons for this or the technical factors involved. Cutting through large masses of fat and the increased retraction needed may raise the infection rate in these patients and lead to recurrence. Tissues infiltrated with fat may not be able to hold the sutures, especially since the excess of intra- and extra-abdominal accumulations of many kilograms of fat may add enormous tension on the sutures, causing the tissues to tear under the strain and to bring about a defect in the abdominal wall. Furthermore, obese patients tend to develop postoperative complications such as paralytic ileus, atelectasis, pneumonia, and deep venous thrombosis that may increase the incidence of incisional hernia. Some surgical centers will refuse to operate for repair of a postoperative hernia on an obese patient until he or she loses the excess fat.

General Condition

The general condition of the patient influences the rate of postoperative ventral hernia. The factors include age, generalized wasting, malnutrition and starvation, hypoproteinemia (especially hypoalbuminemia), avitaminosis (especially Vitamin C), malignant disease, anemia, jaundice, diabetes mellitus, chronic renal failure, liver failure, ascites, prolonged steroid therapy, immunosuppressive therapy, and alcoholism.

Postoperative Complications

Postoperative complications increase the incidence of postoperative hernias. They especially include prolonged postoperative paralytic ileus and intestinal obstruction with abdominal distention, which places enormous vertical tension on the wound by increasing its length and, at the same time, raising the lateral pull on the sutures by increased girth of the abdomen. Chest complications such as chronic obstructive lung disease, pulmonary collapse, bronchopneumonia, emphysema, and asthma are also factors. The pulmonary complications are more frequent and more severe in patients who smoke.

Type of Operation

Certain types of operations have a tendency to be followed by hernia. These include laparotomy for generalized or localized peritonitis in patients with perforated peptic ulcer, appendicitis, diverticulitis, and acute pancreatitis. Also included are operations for intra-abdominal malignant disease, chronic inflammatory bowel disease, and reoperation through the original wound, especially within the first 6 months after the initial procedure.[319] The cause of the wound failure is not in the operation itself but in the presence of many of the factors previously mentioned.

Postoperative Wound Dehiscence

Postoperative wound dehiscence or "burst abdomen," whether covered by skin or with frank evisceration, is often followed by postoperative hernia whether resutured or treated by the open method. This is not surprising, since practically all the conditions mentioned previously are also the causal factors in burst abdomen.[320]

Late Hernias

Tissue Failure. The etiology of the late-occurring hernia is not clear. The hernia develops in what apparently is a perfectly healed wound that has functioned satisfactorily for 5, 10, or even more years after the operation. The incidence is not related to the method used for closing the original incision and is presumably the result of the failure of the collagen in the scar, although there seems to be no obvious reason why mature collagen that has served well for a number of years should change its structure. Rodrigues has recently shown a decrease in oxytalan fibers and an increase in the amorphous substance of the elastic fibers as a function of age.[118] This may be the factor responsible for alterations in the resistance of the transversalis fascia and abdominal wall scar tissue. The aging and weakening of the tissues and the raised intra-abdominal pressure associated with chronic cough, constipation, and prostatism are cited as factors.

Collagen Abnormalities. Abnormal collagen production and maintenance have been shown to be associated with recurrent hernias in certain patients.[243,244,321] There is a deficiency of collagen and abnormalities in its physico-chemical structure, manifesting in reduced hydroxy-proline production and in changes in the diameter of the collagen fibers. These changes have been demonstrated in these patients in other sites such as skin, lung, and pericardium, and may be associated with the imbalance between proteolytic enzymes and their inhibitors and the other enzyme abnormalities found in patients with emphysema and those who smoke. In 1970 Read observed that the rectus sheath in patients with direct inguinal hernias was lighter for a given area than that of normal controls.[322] This observation led to further investigations, and in 1978 he postulated that inguinal hernia is part of a widespread connective tissue disorder associated with emphysema and smoking[277] and in 1981, together with his associate Cannon, he called this syndrome "metastatic emphysema."[239] Read summarized his findings as related to the cause of inguinal hernia and recurrences.[240,245] These collagen mechanisms may play a part in the development of late postoperative hernias. Electrical stimulation has been shown experimentally in animals and in clinical use in humans to have a positive effect on the speed and strength of wound healing.[323,324]

ANATOMY

A hernia may develop in any abdominal incision, but most are found in midline or paramedian incisions. They are also commonly seen in wounds for appendectomy, subcostal incisions for cholecystectomy, or scars following closure of colostomy. In recent years high epigastric hernia following sternal splitting incisions for cardiac operations and lower abdominal hernias through incisions for dialysis catheters have become more common. More recently hernias are being reported in the incisions for the ports used to gain access to the abdominal cavity in laparoscopic surgery.

The hernial opening may vary in size since the original incision may have been a short one or all or only part of a long incision may have failed to heal. Several defects may exist along one incision, making for multiple hernias in one scar. In the early appearing hernias, all of a long incision may have parted, leaving a long and wide defect. The sac of the hernia is often quite large and long and multiloculated, even with small hernial defects. It protrudes forward, downward, and to the sides, burrowing into the subcutaneous fat, and may even overhang the pubis and thighs. These hernias may reach enormous proportions and constitute a serious surgical challenge. The hernia may contain omentum, transverse colon, loops of small bowel, and even stomach. Adhesions between the contents and the sac wall are common and may be responsible for the hernia being incarcerated and irreducible.

CLINICAL MANIFESTATIONS

The patients complain of an unsightly bulge in the operation scar as well as of pain and discomfort. They often suffer from a heavy, sickening, dragging sensation aggravated by coughing and straining. In large dependent hernias, areas of skin may undergo pressure ischemic necrosis and may ulcerate, and rarely, the hernia may rupture. If the hernia strangulates, the symptoms of intestinal obstruction and ischemic bowel will supervene. There is often a history of repeated mild attacks of incomplete obstruction manifesting as colicky pains and vomiting. Intertrigo may develop in the deep crease between the hernia and the abdominal wall, and the skin may become moist, infected, and odorous. Obese patients with large, pendulous hernias are practically immobilized and find life almost unbearable.

INDICATIONS FOR OPERATION

Not all postoperative ventral hernias need to be repaired. One frequently finds a low, wide bulge down the length of the old incision. When it does not bother the patient and shows no signs of growing, there is no indication for reoperating. For most other types, repair should be undertaken. The patient may request operation for esthetic reasons for a large and unsightly hernia. Pain and discomfort are indications. Large hernias with small openings have a high risk of strangulation and should be repaired. A history of recurrent attacks of subacute obstruction, incarceration and irreducibility, and strangulation are definitive indications.

PREOPERATIVE MANAGEMENT

Repair of a large postoperative ventral hernia is a major undertaking and requires careful preoperative assessment and preparation of the patient. The repair should be delayed for at least 1 year after the operation that caused the hernia or after a previous attempt at repair. This is the time it takes for collagen to mature and for the tissues to reach their final "dry" state. One should also wait for at least 1 year after all infection and sinuses have healed. This is an arbitrary period in view of the work of Davis and Houck, both of whom show that bacteria may remain alive in old infected wounds, even many years after the wounds have apparently healed, and can reinfect later repairs of incisional hernias where the original closure was infected.[218,219] One may, however, be forced to operate earlier because of threatened or actual strangulation or in cases in which, in spite of treatment and waiting, persistent sinuses remain. Some cases with chronic purulent discharge, especially if associated with retained foreign bodies such as fragments of metal sheet, wire mesh, or synthetic mesh, may have to be staged. With the patient under general anesthesia, the wound is first cleared of the foreign bodies and infected sutures, and sinuses, and pockets are widely opened. The wound is left open to heal by granulation. Later, after 1 year, if possible, the actual repair may be done.

Most repairs are done as single elective operations, but they also may be combined with other planned or emergency intra-abdominal procedures.

Obesity and smoking are associated with a higher recurrence rate after hernia repair. Thus, obese patients must be urged to reduce weight before the operation, although they often seem unable to do so, and smokers should be urged to stop the habit, preferably some months before the operation.

Associated cardiovascular, respiratory, and renal conditions, diabetes, hypertension, and other general illnesses must be diagnosed, assessed, and treated. The operation is usually elective and must be delayed until the patient is in an optimal state. Respiratory exercises are begun a few weeks prior to the operation.

Intertrigo and infected and moist dermatitis are cleansed with povidone-iodine scrub several times daily, are painted with povidone-iodine solution, and are exposed to warm, dry air until healed.

The patient is investigated for coexisting abdominal pathology so that it can be dealt with at the same operation. This will avoid the embarrassing pitfall of further surgery for missed pathology soon after a major repair of a large abdominal hernia.

Preoperative pneumoperitoneum therapy is used in some centers to stretch the abdominal cavity so that it will more easily accommodate the hernial contents.[325] The aim is to prevent respiratory and cardiac embarrassment that may be caused by forceful reduction of the hernial contents raising and limiting the movements of the diaphragm, interfering with the venous return to the heart, and reducing the respiratory volume. This author does not use this method, finding it tedious and time consuming and unpleasant for the patient. The problem of returning even the largest hernial contents to the abdominal cavity is eliminated when using the ingenious technique described by Dixon in 1929 for reconstructing the linea alba.[326] Most patients cope well with this procedure, but the elderly and especially fat and short patients with large hernias and those with chronic lung disease may need respiratory assistance for some hours or even days postoperatively until they stabilize.

The abdomen is scrubbed and painted with povidone-iodine several times in the 24 hours preceding the operation, with special attention to the umbilicus, the groin, and the crease between the hernia and the abdominal wall. Prophylactic subcutaneous heparin usually is given. Perioperative antibiotics are used. However, in view of the reports of Davis and Houck mentioned above, and comments by Read, it appears that antibiotics should be used more liberally when repairing postoperative hernias, since a high proportion of them follow previous infected wounds and the procedure should, in fact, be considered a contaminated operation.[218,219,327] The arguments for antibiotics become even stronger when a foreign body such as a prosthetic mesh will be used for the repair. General anesthesia with good relaxation is the rule, although small hernias in thin subjects can be repaired using local or general anesthesia.

OPERATIVE METHODS FOR REPAIR

With the development of modern synthetic nonabsorbable suture material, three basic methods have emerged for repair of these distressing hernias: resuture, shoelace darn repair, or synthetic nonabsorbable mesh closure. The method chosen depends largely on the size of the hernial defect.

The size of the hernia itself can be best and most dramatically assessed with the patient standing and coughing, but more important is the size of the defect and its behavior, which should be examined with the patient supine. The surgeon's hand, with fingers straightened, is inserted into the defect, and the patient is requested to raise his head and shoulders forwards without the aid of his hands. If necessary, he is asked to raise his straightened legs at the same time. The test should be done both with the hernia out and with the hernia and its contents reduced back into the abdominal cavity and held there by the surgeon's hand. A small defect is one in which the musculoaponeurotic edges come together or almost do so and which is suitable for closure by resuture. Attempts at resuturing wider hernias will result in tension and, almost inevitably, in recurrence of the hernia. This author, however, prefers to repair these narrow hernias not by resuture, but by the shoelace technique. This is a quick, easy, extraperitoneal method that simply returns the unopened hernial sac and its contents to the abdominal cavity and thus avoids the tedious and perhaps risky dissection of the adherent loops of bowel on the inner surface of the sac and abdomen. Since the defect is narrow, the lateral cut edges of the rectus sheaths (see below) come together in the midline and are anchored to the new linea alba.

Hernias with a wider defect also can be conveniently repaired by the shoelace darn technique.[265] This method is preferred even for the giant hernias for the same reason as detailed in the previous paragraph. Thomas reported on a new method of fascial partition/release for repair of incisional hernias. He reported good results but the method has the disadvantage of cutting across and sliding muscle planes.[328]

The third method for repair of these hernias involves the use of sheets of woven or knitted mesh of synthetic nonabsorbable materials such as polypropylene, polyester, or sheets of expanded polytetrafluoroethylene (PTFE) placed across the defect and stitched to the abdominal wall. The most common and most favored material today is knitted polypropylene. This method of repair of large postoperative ventral abdominal hernias is a good one and has undoubtedly become popular. However, it may involve the resection of the hernial sac and the dissection of the adherent loops of bowel, with the risk of fistula formation. A large foreign body is used, and the whole procedure is often time consuming and requires prolonged anesthesia, whereas the shoelace technique is simple and quick and entirely extraperitoneal. This author does not use the synthetic mesh technique as a routine repair, preferring to reserve it for hernia cases with large defects of the anterior abdominal wall following postoperative infections with fasciitis and sloughing, for trauma, or for cases in which repeated attempts at repair of the hernia have led to destruction of part of the abdominal wall. Some surgeons advise the use of prosthetic mesh in every case of incisional hernia repair, irrespective of the size.

Repair by Resuture

The operation is best done with the patient under general anesthesia with good relaxation. The old scar is excised in an elliptic fashion and is carefully separated from the hernial sac. The skin on each side of the incision then is further freed to expose the complete sac down to the musculoaponeurotic borders of the hernial defect and part of the abdominal wall beyond it. The sac is opened, and all adherent omentum and loops of bowel are dissected off its inner surface and also off the inner surface of the abdominal wall for a few centimeters on each side of the defect, remembering that it is better to leave bits of sac wall or peritoneum adherent to the wall of the freed bowel rather than to leave bits of the bowel wall stuck to the sac or peritoneum. The sac and its peritoneal lining, scar tissue, and old suture material are excised up to the edge of the hernial defect to expose the normal tissues of the linea alba.

The abdomen then is closed with interrupted mass sutures of monofilament stainless steel wire of SW gauge 28, passing through the abdominal wall at least 3 cm from the edge of the defect. They should not be tightly tied and should be spaced 2 cm apart. A heavy monofilament nylon thread may be used instead of the steel wire. Alternatively, a continuous heavy monofilament nylon loop (#1) mass closure can be used, taking large bites, as with the interrupted closure. The length of the nylon used for the continuous mass closure should be at least four times the length of the incision. The excess skin is excised, and the wound is closed over the repair with automatic staples or with continuous fine monofilament nylon sutures.

Hernias through paramedian incisions are repaired in the same manner. In this case the medial edge of the defect will be the intact linea alba and what remains of the rectus sheath alongside it. The lateral edge will be composed of anterior and posterior rectus sheath and the rectus muscle between them, with all three layers fused by scar tissue along the edge. The mass sutures are passed through these two sides.

The Shoelace Darn Repair

This method is based on the understanding of the functional anatomy of the abdominal wall, which it reconstructs as close to normal as possible in order to restore the normal function of its separate parts and as a whole.

The flat muscles of the abdominal wall are normally in a state of tonic contraction, which tends to shorten them. However, since the muscles of one side are fixed to those of the other side along the midline of the linea alba, they are not able to shorten; instead, they pull against each other in a balanced fashion so that they act as a dynamic girdle, flattening the abdominal wall and holding back the contents of the abdomen (Fig 14–38A). With the vertical splitting of the midline at operation and failure of the wound to heal postoperatively, the two halves separate as the hernia develops. The flat muscles have lost their midline anchor and therefore can no longer pull against each other in their normal balanced fashion. Instead, their tonic contraction now causes them to shorten so that the gap between the recti muscles widens (Fig 14–38B). Each rectus abdominis muscle is pulled laterally and becomes curved with the concave side medially (Fig 14–38C). There is no loss of tissue in the usual case nor is there a defect of the muscles and fasciae of the abdominal wall, apart from the linea alba along the edges of the hernial opening, which was largely destroyed when the original sutures tore out and is not suitable for use in repairs.

To restore the normal anatomy and function, the operation reconstructs a strong new linea alba midline anchor, allows the rectus muscles to straighten and return to lie alongside each other at the midline, and also reconstructs the anterior rectus sheaths and fixes them to the new linea alba.

A further anatomic consideration is the fact that the external oblique muscle at its upper and lower parts, which arise from the thoracic cage and from the pelvis, is relatively short and more difficult to elongate. Since this muscle comprises most of the anterior rectus sheath, it is relatively difficult to return the anterior rectus sheath to the midline, especially in the epigastrium. On the other hand, the posterior rectus sheath is made up of the internal oblique and transversus abdominis muscles, which have their origin in the lumbar region and are, therefore, relatively longer and more easily stretched, thus allowing easier sliding of the posterior rectus sheath back to the midline. This makes it possible to cover even enormous defects in the abdominal wall with the strong aponeurotic layer of the posterior rectus sheath when reconstituting the linea alba.

The first of the two basic steps in the repair is to reconstitute the strong new midline anchor for the flat muscles by reconstructing a new linea alba, by suturing together a strip of fascia from the medial edge of each anterior rectus sheath.[326] The second-step is to restore the recti muscles to their normal position and to draw the flat muscles back to their former length by drawing closer together the lateral cut edges of the anterior rectus sheaths where the medial strips were split off. This step is accomplished with a continuous suture of heavy monofilament nylon that passes to and fro between the cut edges and that also substitutes functionally and anatomically for the missing anterior rectus sheaths.

A vertical elliptic incision is used, excising the old scar. In obese patients with a large apron of fat hanging below the pubis, panniculectomy and abdominoplasty are combined with repair of the hernia. In this case a long transverse incision is used at the level of the suprapubic crease and is extended almost to the back, curving up at its lateral ends. The skin and fat of the apron and of the abdominal wall are freed upward off the musculoaponeurotic layer to well up onto the anterior chest wall. After repair of the hernia the apron and the excess skin and fat of the lower abdominal wall, usually up to the level of the umbilicus, are excised. Should it become necessary, an inverted midline V of the remaining skin and fat is excised to create a tucked in waistline (Fig 14–38D).

In the usual case, the skin and fat are dissected off the sac of the hernia, as well as off the rectus sheath on each side (Fig 14–38E). The anterior rectus sheaths should be exposed sufficiently to allow for splitting off of the medial ribbon, as well as for suturing the second, the shoelace, layer. Time need not be wasted on accurate delineation of the medial edge of the rectus sheaths or on leaving an absolutely clean surface on the hernial sac. With the first continuous suture for construction of the new midline, the sac, together with the adherent bits of scar tissue, and even old sutures that cannot be easily removed, are returned to the abdominal cavity. The new linea alba is now constructed, using a vertical strip 1 to 1.5 cm wide split off the medial edge of each anterior rectus sheath as follows: (1) the abdominal wall around the hernial opening is defined, (2) an incision is made in each anterior rectus sheath about 1 cm or more from its medial edge to confirm the presence of rectus muscle, (3) the incision is extended up and down the entire length of the hernial opening and for about 2 cm beyond, keeping the ends of the incision away from and parallel to the midline, above and below the hernia (Fig 14–38F and G), and (4) the two strips are sewn together from above downward by a continuous over-and-over suture of O (metric 3.5) monofilament polyamide loop, starting at the top corners of the incision and incorporating the whole width of each strip. This not only creates the new linea alba but also returns the unopened sac and its contents to the abdominal cavity (Fig 14–38H). The sac remains unopened throughout the operation. If it is opened inadvertently, it is closed with a synthetic absorbable suture. There is no need to open the sac and become involved in the tedious dissection for freeing the masses of adherent bowel from the sac walls and from each other unless dealing with an emergency case of strangulation and bowel obstruction or with a patient with a recent history of bowel obstruction. There appears to be no reported case of mechanical obstruction following simple inversion of the sac. We have repaired more than 500 ventral hernias by this technique during the past 20 years and have not yet encountered a mechanical complication. It would appear that its occurrence is more theoretical than real.

In this way the posterior rectus sheaths and the rectus muscles have been approximated at the midline. The rectus muscles have been stretched wide and thinned, with their fibers running in many different directions. A sometimes alarming gap remains between the lateral cut edges of the rectus sheaths (Fig 14–38I). This gap is closed by the second suture, for which a 6-m 0 or 1 length of heavy monofilament polyamide is used, doubled to form a loop 3 m long. Alternatively, two commercially available 1 (metric 4) loops of monofilament can be used, each starting at one end of the incisions in the rectus sheaths and meeting in the middle of the line of the repair, where they are tied one to the other. The polyamide loops are available in monofilament threads 2 m long, doubled to make a loop 1 m long. On special order a 3-m long thread, doubled to form a 1.5-m loop, can be obtained.

The usual suture begins at the top end of the incision in the rectus sheaths from inside the sheath and passes out on that side, returning inside through the opposite corner and slipping through the loop. The flat muscles are now restored to their former lengths, and the recti muscles are restored to their normal thickness and position by the continuous heavy monofilament nylon suture passing to and fro in front of the rectus abdominis muscles, between the cut edges of the anterior rectus sheaths, and through the strong new midline anchor for the whole length of the hernia, in the manner of a shoelace tightening a boot (Fig 14–38J). Each bite on the rectus sheath passes vertically from above down, from outside in, and from inside out at least 2 cm from the edge, so that it crosses and pulls on the fibers of the rectus sheath at a right angle, thereby preventing the sutures from cutting out (Fig 14–38K).

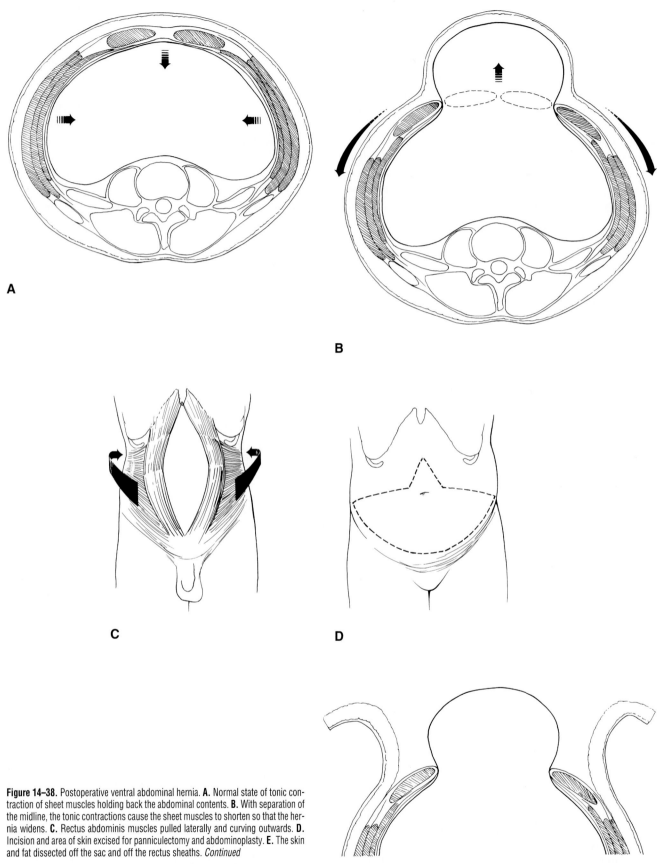

Figure 14–38. Postoperative ventral abdominal hernia. **A.** Normal state of tonic contraction of sheet muscles holding back the abdominal contents. **B.** With separation of the midline, the tonic contractions cause the sheet muscles to shorten so that the hernia widens. **C.** Rectus abdominis muscles pulled laterally and curving outwards. **D.** Incision and area of skin excised for panniculectomy and abdominoplasty. **E.** The skin and fat dissected off the sac and off the rectus sheaths. *Continued*

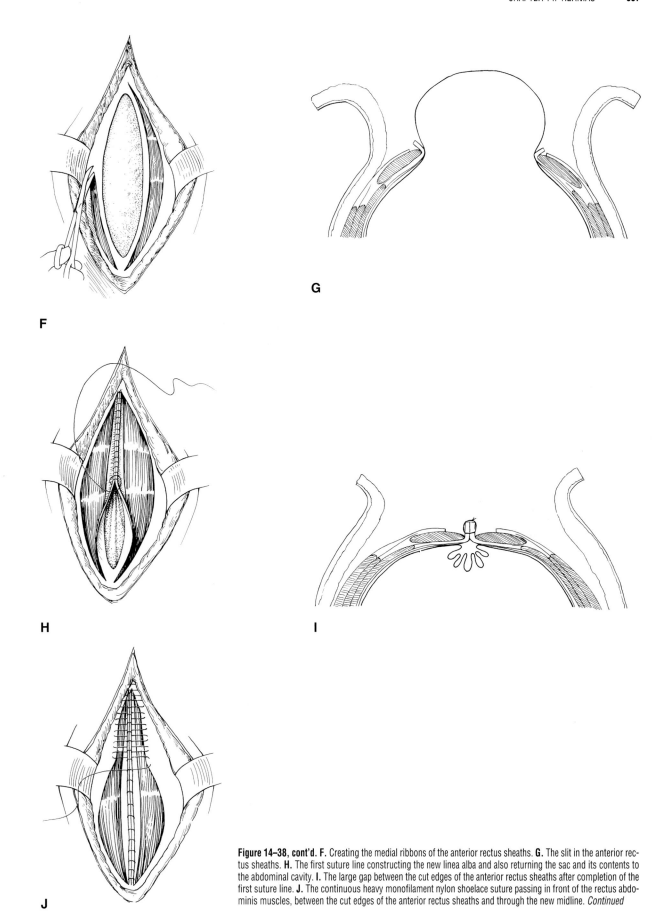

Figure 14–38, cont'd. F. Creating the medial ribbons of the anterior rectus sheaths. **G.** The slit in the anterior rectus sheaths. **H.** The first suture line constructing the new linea alba and also returning the sac and its contents to the abdominal cavity. **I.** The large gap between the cut edges of the anterior rectus sheaths after completion of the first suture line. **J.** The continuous heavy monofilament nylon shoelace suture passing in front of the rectus abdominis muscles, between the cut edges of the anterior rectus sheaths and through the new midline. *Continued*

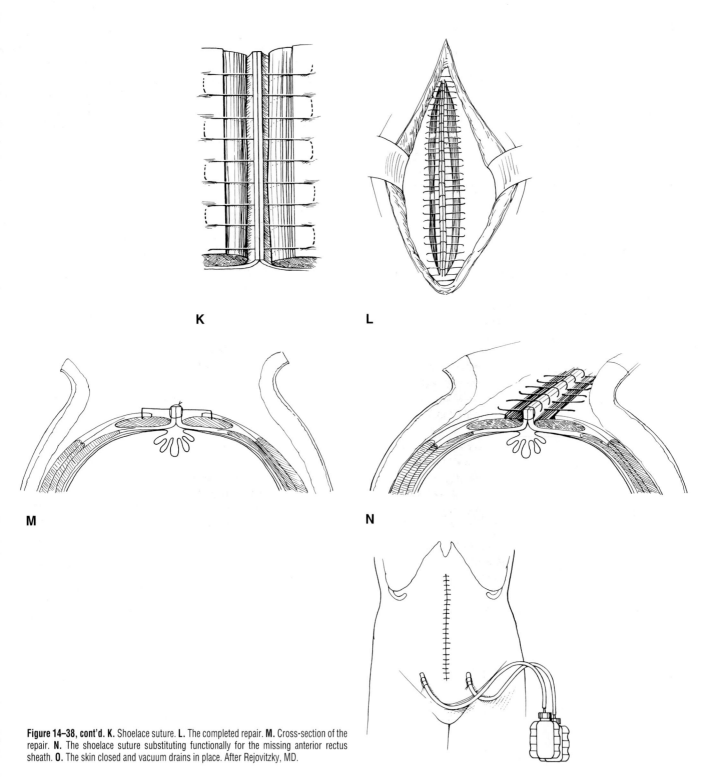

Figure 14–38, cont'd. K. Shoelace suture. **L.** The completed repair. **M.** Cross-section of the repair. **N.** The shoelace suture substituting functionally for the missing anterior rectus sheath. **O.** The skin closed and vacuum drains in place. After Rejovitzky, MD.

The sutures should be approximately 0.5 cm apart and fairly tense to narrow the gap considerably between the cut edges of the rectus sheaths. Good anesthesia with relaxation is important at this stage. Each suture is fixed at its midpoint by passing through the new midline, thus preventing bow-stringing and reherniation between the sutures. At the bottom end of the repair, the nylon is tied with a loop-in-the-loop (Aberdeen) knot. The cut edges of the rectus sheaths have been brought parallel to each other (Fig 11–38L), and the rectus muscles are narrowed and thicker and at the midline in their normal anatomic positions, with their fibers running parallel to each other. With narrow or moderately wide hernias the edges of the anterior rectus sheaths may be approximated by this suture line. In the usual case of a large hernia, a gap of at least a few centimeters remains, with the continuous pliable to-and-fro shoelace suture adjusting itself to the differing widths and tension across the fascial defect and thus functionally substituting for the missing anterior rectus sheaths (Fig 14–38M and N).

The excess skin and fat are excised. A vacuum drain is placed on either side, and each is brought out through a separate stab. The incision is closed with automatic staples or a continuous suture of fine monofilament polyamide thread (Fig 14–38O).

In cases in which only part of the original incision has herniated and the remainder is still intact, the complete incision should be included in the repair to spread the tension evenly along the greater length.

Hernias through paramedian or more lateral vertical incisions are repaired in a similar manner. In the usual paramedian incision, the rectus sheath on one side of the hernia is intact and can be used as in the ordinary midline case. On the other side, the anterior and posterior rectus sheaths and the rectus muscle between them have fused with scar tissue along the edge of the defect. The ribbon of anterior rectus sheath can be split off and sutured as though the incision were in the midline. In the more lateral incision, this applies to both edges.

When other incisions with hernias exist on either or both sides of the main hernia, as after colostomy closures or appendectomies, these are dealt with when the second, or shoelace, layer of heavy monofilament nylon is placed. Each suture is passed through the cut edge of the rectus sheath and is then continued outward to take strong bites of each edge of the secondary hernial defect and then back again across the main repair. In this way, the abdominal wall is laced, with the sutures stretching across the main and secondary hernial defects (Fig 14–39).

The operation is entirely extraperitoneal and involves

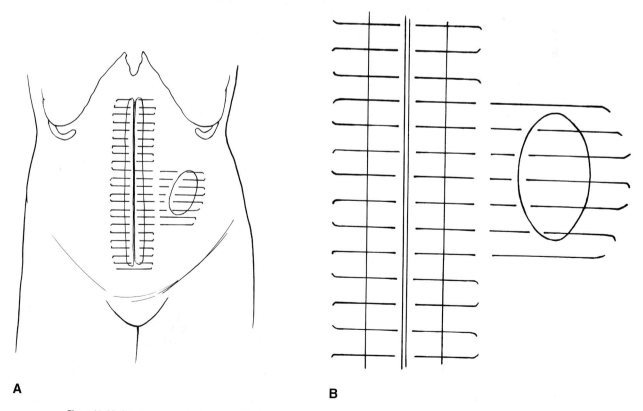

Figure 14–39. Simultaneous repair of accompanying hernias. **A.** Postcolostomy hernia. **B.** Diagram of technique. After Rejovitzky, MD.

only two simple suture lines placed in normal healthy tissue. Consequently, the postoperative recovery is smooth and rapid. As soon as the patient is fully awake, the nasogastric tube is removed, and the patient may start to drink. Ambulation is begun the evening of the operation. The intravenous infusion is removed that evening or the next morning, and the patient is encouraged to walk, eat, and drink normally. When dealing with the elderly, with very obese patients, with heavy smokers, with patients with chronic lung disease, and particularly with patients who had excessively large hernias, we prefer to preempt postoperative respiratory difficulties by maintaining the patient on a ventilator for 12 to 24 hours or even longer. Since this is a routine postoperative procedure in this type of patient, we do not hesitate to apply it to the repair of large hernias as well.

Complications are few and usually minor. The most serious local complication is infection, which is a potent cause of recurrence of the hernia. Strict precautions must be taken with regard to sterility. The dissection must be clean and atraumatic. Meticulous hemostasis is important throughout the operation, since any collections may lead to infection. The vacuum drains usually function for 24 to 48 hours, by which time there is no more discharge, and they are then removed.

In this author's series of 500 cases, there were no deaths and only a 2% recurrence rate. Since the operation is entirely extraperitoneal and technically simple and quick, it is eminently suitable for elderly patients with other general medical problems.[329]

Hernias in the epigastrium and those in the lower abdomen may abut on the costal arch or on the pubis, respectively, where there may be a gap with the base of the hernia fixed to the skeleton so that the rectus muscles cannot be brought together in the midline. The defect can be dealt with by making the medial ribbon of the anterior rectus sheath wider in this area and elongating the slit in the rectus sheath well up onto the chest wall or down onto the pubis. This procedure allows good aponeurotic cover for the gap, which is reinforced by the shoelace suture substituting for the missing muscles and anterior rectus sheath. If the upper or lower gap does not appear sufficiently reinforced, further layers of nylon can be added in different oblique directions in the form of a darn.

It is inevitable that one would consider the fate of the repair should any of these patients need further surgery. One patient in my series underwent a negative laparotomy for abdominal pains in another hospital 1 year after the repair of her hernia. This author has reoperated on two other patients, 2 years and 5 years after the repair, both for carcinoma of the colon. A standard midline incision was used in the three cases. The smooth nylon was easily extracted. There was no bare rectus muscle alongside the midline. The defect in the ante-

rior rectus sheath had apparently been filled by collagenous connective or scar tissue. No evidence of the large inverted sac was found. The first case was closed with a continuous monofilament nylon mass closure, and the other two by mass closure with interrupted monofilament stainless steel sutures. These women showed no evidence of recurrence of the hernia more than 10 years following their last operation.

Prosthetic Mesh Repair

The use of sheets of nonabsorbable synthetic mesh prostheses placed across the defect and stitched to the abdominal wall has revolutionized the repair of abdominal wall defects and has rendered obsolete most of the older types of operations.[29,326,330–335] It is an excellent method for repair of large postoperative ventral abdominal hernias and is universally used. This author, however, does not use it as routine repair, preferring to reserve it for hernia cases with large defects of the anterior abdominal wall, following postoperative infections with fasciitis and sloughing of the tissues of the abdominal wall, for cases involving trauma or excision of sections of the abdominal wall for tumors, or after multiple attempts at repair of a postoperative hernia with destruction of tissues. The reason for this choice is that the method involves the resection of the hernial sac and the tedious freeing of adherent loops of bowel, with the risk of fistula formation. It is often a time-consuming procedure, requiring prolonged anesthesia, whereas the shoelace technique is simple, quick, entirely extraperitoneal, restores the normal anatomy, and is quite adequate for most cases.

Choice of Material. The ideal mesh is one that is cheap and universally available, is easily cut to the required shape, is flexible, slightly elastic and pleasant to handle. Additionally, it should be practically indestructible and capable of being rapidly fixed and incorporated by human tissues. It must be inert and elicit little tissue reaction and consequently, not rejected, even in the presence of infection. It must be sterilizable and noncarcinogenic.

Polypropylene mesh (Prolene, Marlex) meets the requirements of the ideal prosthesis and is today the most commonly used material for repair of all types of hernia. It consists of a monofilament thread of polypropylene, knitted in a fairly loose manner. It stimulates almost no biological response from the tissues or significant rejection and is rapidly incorporated by fibroblasts and granulation tissue that pass through and fill the interstices between the knit. There are no crevices and the surface of the thread is extremely smooth so that it is hardly colonizable by bacteria and thus withstands infection exceptionally well. Even when exposed in an infected wound, it will be covered rapidly and incorporated by the granulation tissue. Polypropylene mesh can be cut to any shape, it does not unravel, and holds sutures exceptionally well without tearing. If a sheet is not large enough, it can be joined to other sheets by simple continuous suture with a monofilament polypropylene thread. It remains pliable in the tissues and can be easily incised, if a new laparotomy becomes necessary. This can be followed by any conventional form of resuture of the abdominal wall. Lichtenstein carried out a series of laboratory and clinical investigations, comparing various prosthetic materials and, in 1991, reported that monofilament polypropylene stimulates a strong fibroblastic response throughout the interstices and also has a marked resistance to infection.[102] For all these reasons, polypropylene knitted mesh has become the standard by which all other prosthetic meshes must be measured.

The next most popular prosthesis is also a knitted mesh but has a multifilament polyester fiber thread (dacron, mersilene). This is an excellent material, cheap and freely available and is very popular in French surgical centers. It is also recommended by some English and American surgeons. Its main advantage is that it is light and extremely supple, has a pleasant, soft feel, and is strong and elastic. Because of its softness, it easily conforms to all shapes and surfaces without any tendency to recoil. Its surface is slightly granular and excites a greater tissue inflammatory response than polypropylene. While some surgeons see the latter two as negative qualities, those that use this material consider these characteristics advantageous. They believe that the granular surface creates friction between the mesh and the tissues, especially the peritoneum, thus preventing slippage of the mesh. The more extreme inflammatory response causes a rapid invasion of the mesh by fibroblasts and granulation tissue, quickly and strongly fixing the mesh in the tissues. For these reasons, the knitted polyester mesh is particularly suitable for the Stoppa GPRVS procedure when no sutures are used to fix the mesh, but friction and rapid incorporation is relied on while the intra-abdominal pressure holds the mesh in place. The two main disadvantages of this material is that it tends to tear easily if sutured under tension, especially with interrupted sutures, and the mutifibered braided thread makes this mesh less resistant to infection. The crevices and spaces between the filaments making up the thread are 10 microns or less in size, and consequently, bacteria that are approximately 1 micron in size can safely colonize these spaces, since leukocytes are too large to squeeze into 10 microns. These colonies will continually reinfect the tissues and perpetuate the infection, leading to failure of the repair and recurrence. Wantz, who very strongly recommends this mesh for the GPRVS procedure, reported in 1991 that, in the presence of infection, the mesh does not always need to be removed.[141] Wide exposure of the mesh, local irrigation, and systemic an-

tibiotics, may permit the ingrowth of granulation tissue and reintegration of the prosthesis.

Another synthetic material available, although less commonly used, is expanded polytetrafluoroethylene (ePTFE, Teflon, Gore-Tex). This material has been extensively and successfully used for vascular prostheses and is available in microporous sheets of varying thicknesses. It is extremely strong, yet very pliable, soft, smooth, and slippery to the touch. The material is biologically inert and causes little, if any, tissue reaction, with no tendency to be rejected. Theoretically, its porous microstructure should provide a lattice for the invasion of fibroblasts and granulation tissue. However, this is not as efficient as are knitted meshes with wide spaces that are more easily invaded.[177] The Lichtenstein group claims that penetration of fibroblasts from the host tissue into the depth of ePTFE is only approximately 10% after three years, and that this is further decreased in the presence of infection.[336] This poor penetration leads to defective fixation and slippage of the prosthesis and recurrence of the hernia. A further disadvantage is that ePTFE is made up of spaces between the synthetic material and that many of these spaces can be shown to be <10 microns in size. ePTFE sheets can be cut to any shape and do not unravel. They hold sutures very well without tearing and sheets can be joined together by simple suture. The material retains its pliability in the tissues. The biological inertness of ePTFE, while being a disadvantage as far as incorporation is concerned, may be of some advantage in certain situations where the material is used to bridge large gaps of the abdominal wall, where the unprotected bowel comes into contact with the prosthesis. ePTFE may produce fewer adhesions, even in the presence of infection, and perhaps may reduce the risk of bowel adhesions, obstruction, enterocutaneous fistula and sinus formation, with extrusion of the prosthesis and recurrence of the hernia, although this is disputed. Although there may be certain advantages of ePTFE, its high cost limits its availability since knitted polypropylene mesh is much cheaper and, on the whole, probably better.

Absorbable synthetic meshes are available (polyglactin, polyglycolic acid) but have been proved to be unsuccessful for the repair of incisional and other hernias. It was hoped that these absorbable materials would provide a lattice for the laying down of new collagen tissue and then become absorbed, leaving the new buttress of scar tissue to cure the hernia. However, this new tissue is not able to withstand natural stresses and strains, leading to an unacceptably high rate of recurrence. It has been suggested that these absorbable synthetic meshes be used in infected areas to bridge hernia defects, in situations where one would hesitate to insert a nonabsorbable foreign body mesh, with the hope that the hernia will be closed and the mesh absorbed, leaving only scar tissue. The recurrence rate is very high, but whatever recurrences develop could be repaired at a later date with nonabsorbable mesh. Greene reported using a knitted mesh of polyglycolic acid in 59 critically ill patients to successfully bridge abdominal wall defects and to prevent evisceration after celiotomy.[337] Postoperative ventral hernias were common 4 to 6 months later. Those patients who survived would probably not have done so, had this method not been used, and Greene recommends the technique for quickly achieving a secure tension-free closure of abdominal wounds in situations such as in generalized intra-abdominal sepsis or posttrauma. ePTFE is unsuitable for the reconstruction of contaminated abdominal wall defects and polypropylene mesh may be more suitable, although it has a high risk of complications such as visceral adhesions, and erosion of the intestine and skin.[338]

Certain complications are common to all mesh materials, nonabsorbable and absorbable, that come into contact with the bowels and other intra-abdominal organs, whether the prosthesis is placed intraperitoneally, as an underlay graft, or as in inlay or onlay graft where the defect in the abdominal wall has not been closed with host tissue. These include adhesions, bowel obstruction, erosion into bowel with enterocutaneous fistula formation, and erosion of the mesh into the urinary bladder. Recently, in animal experiments, the phenomenon was demonstrated whereby translocation of enteric bacteria takes place from the bowel to biomaterials in the peritoneal cavity within hours or days, even though the bowel remains normal.[339] These complications are not common but have been recorded from several sources so that it is clear that intraperitoneal placement of prosthetic mesh or other contact of the mesh with the bowels should be avoided, if possible. If this is unavoidable, care should be taken to place omentum between the bowels and the graft. These complications do not occur when the mesh is placed in the preperitoneal space away from the abdominal contents.[102,103,106–108]

It was believed that synthetic absorbable mesh had little tendency to form adhesions or enteral fistulas when in contact with the bowel, and it was therefore recommended and used as a screen or double patch together with a nonabsorbable mesh to close incisional hernias where no tissues are available to place between the bowel and the nonabsorbable mesh. It was hoped that the absorbable screen would shield the bowel from the nonabsorbable mesh until a neoperitoneum could be formed on the under surface of the permanent mesh, by which time the temporary mesh would be absorbed and would disappear.[141,340] However, it now appears that the absorbable mesh does not have any special characteristics as far as fewer adhesions and fistulae are concerned.[336,340,341] Prosthetic mesh placed superficially and covered only by skin, may erode through the

skin and become exposed through the resultant ulcer. It has always been advised that the mesh be fixed with only synthetic nonabsorbable monofilament sutures, preferably of the same material as itself. Polypropylene, polyamide, and PTFE sutures are available. Biologic suture material such as silk, cotton, or linen must not be used. However, some authors have recently reported using interrupted sutures of synthetic absorbable material (polyglactin, polyglycolic acid) for fixing the prosthesis, and claim that, since the mesh is rapidly invaded by fibroblasts and granulation tissue and is firmly incorporated into the tissues, the sutures used to hold it in place are only temporarily useful until this process of incorporation has taken place. These superfluous sutures may then be absorbed and will disappear.

Types of Operations. Many variations and combinations of mesh repair have been described (Fig 14–40). A piece of mesh cut to the shape of the defect, but slightly larger, may be sutured in place, deep to the peritoneum or between the peritoneum and the abdominal wall. A piece of mesh the size and shape of the defect may be sutured as an inlay graft to the edges of the defect. A larger piece may be used as an onlay graft on the abdominal wall. Large sheets of mesh may be sutured to almost the whole of the inner surface of the abdominal wall, deep to the peritoneum, or to the outer surface of the musculoaponeurotic abdominal wall as an onlay

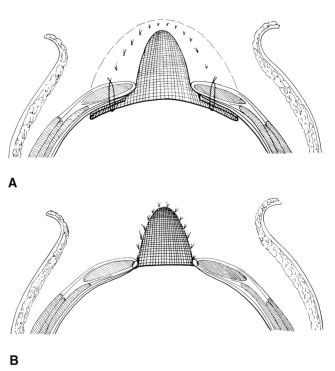

A

B

Figure 14–40. Variations of prosthetic mesh repair. **A.** Underlay graft. **B.** Inlay graft. *Continued*

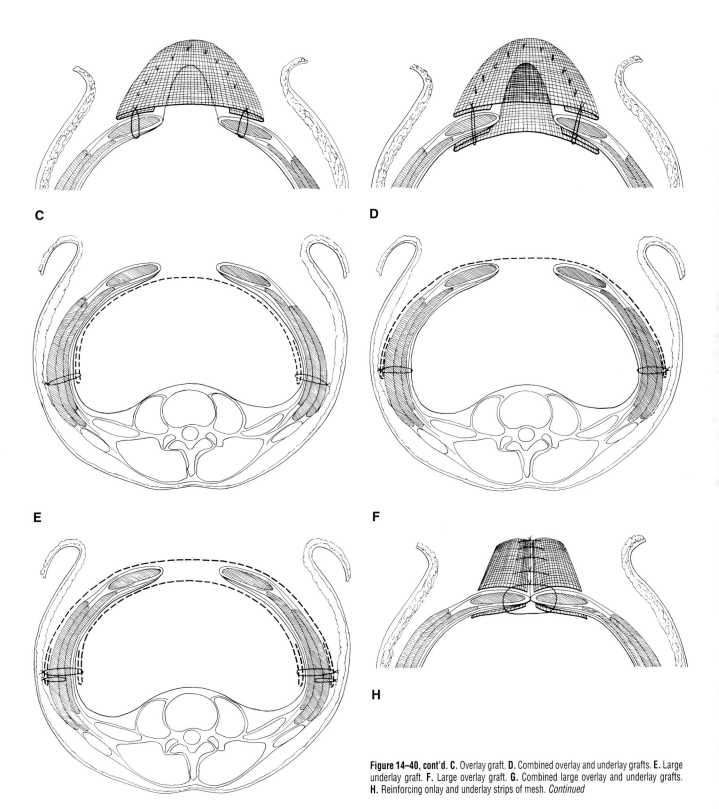

Figure 14–40, cont'd. C. Overlay graft. **D.** Combined overlay and underlay grafts. **E.** Large underlay graft. **F.** Large overlay graft. **G.** Combined large overlay and underlay grafts. **H.** Reinforcing onlay and underlay strips of mesh. *Continued*

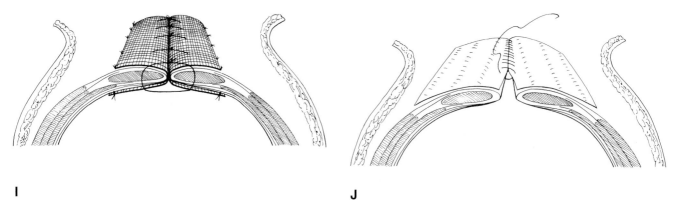

I   J

Figure 14–40, cont'd. I. Wrap-around mesh reinforcement of wound edges. **J.** Two sheets of mesh sutured to abdominal wall, then sutured to each other to draw together the edges of the wound. After Rejovitzky, MD.

graft between the abdominal wall and subcutaneous fat. Reinforcing strips of mesh may be used to hold sutures more securely, or sheets of mesh may be wrapped around the edges of the hernial opening to avoid sutures cutting out. Another interesting variation is the use of two equal pieces of mesh sutured to a large area of the abdominal wall on each side of the defect by several vertical rows of sutures. Their opposing medial edges are then approximated and sutured together under some tension, bringing the two sides of the abdominal wall defect closer together. An excellent method which has been popular in France for some years now, is the Rives-Stoppa technique of placing the sheet of prosthetic mesh in the plane between the posterior rectus sheath and the rectus muscles,[95,178] and has been popularized in the United States, as well.[90,141] This has distinct advantages over the underlay intraperitoneal, inlay or overlay methods.

Operative Technique. As previously mentioned, prosthetic mesh repair is a major procedure, and attention must be paid to good preoperative assessment and preparation of the patient, as well as to local preparation of the skin. The operation is done under general anesthesia. The originally popular method this author now seldom uses is as follows: (1) the old scar is excised by a vertical elliptic incision and carefully separated from the hernial sac, (2) the skin flaps on each side are dissected off the sac to well beyond the edge of the hernial defect, clearing the fat off the rectus sheath and the aponeurosis and muscle of the external oblique, (3) the sac is opened vertically along the middle, and its inner surface, as well as the peritoneal surface of the anterior abdominal wall, is cleared of all adherent omentum and bowel, and (4) a piece of polypropylene mesh then may be prepared and sutured to the inner aspect of the abdominal wall, as was described for the larger umbilical hernias (see Fig 14–26).

However, this author prefers to spread the tension on the repair and use a full-sized sheet of mesh (23 × 35 cm) that is spread out on the inner aspect of the abdominal wall (the inner surface of the peritoneum). This is sutured with interrupted U stitches of monofilament polypropylene or polyamide (metric 4) sutures to the full thickness of the abdominal wall so that the knots lie on the outer surface of the external oblique muscle. All the sutures are passed through the edges of mesh without a needle and clipped with artery forceps (Fig 14–41A). Each suture runs parallel to the edge of the graft. The ends of the sutures of one side are threaded onto a large needle and passed through the abdominal wall, or an Albaran or Reverdin needle may be used. Each end is tied to its fellow in a mattress fashion, pulling the mesh into position (Fig 14–41B). This is then repeated with the lower border, the upper border and finally, the remaining lateral border. In this way, all the bowel and omentum are returned to the abdominal cavity and retained there by the sheet of mesh (Fig 14–41C and D). The sutures must be placed well lateral through the abdominal wall to bring the mesh under some tension. Excess loose mesh should be avoided. Where possible, the omentum should be spread and interposed between the bowel and the mesh. Cases have been reported of erosion and fistula in a loop of bowel in contact with the mesh. Omentum will presumably help to avoid this.

The two halves of the hernial sac are then sutured to each other with a continuous simple over-and-over suture of synthetic absorbable material. This does not add strength to the repair but serves to cover and isolate the polypropylene mesh. A second full-sized sheet of mesh may be used as an onlay graft laid on the outer surface of the external oblique muscles and sewn down along its edge with a continuous over-and-over suture of 1 (metric 4) monofilament nylon in the form of a loop (Fig

14–41E and F). Again, big bites are taken of the abdominal wall and of the edge of the mesh. Two vacuum drains are inserted through stab wounds. The excess skin and fat are excised, and the wound is closed with automatic staples or a continuous fine monofilament nonabsorbable thread.

Ideally, each thread passed through the inner mesh and the abdominal wall also should be passed through the outer mesh and only then should it be tied. The reinforcement afforded by the graft then will lessen the chance of the sutures' cutting out from the abdominal wall. Furthermore, less suturing will be required, since the same set of sutures will serve both mesh grafts. However, it is rather awkward coping with two grafts and the bowel at the same time, as well as ensuring the correct tension of the grafts.

In obese patients with pendulous abdomens, a transverse suprapubic incision is used, and panniculectomy with abdominoplasty is added, as was described in the section on shoelace repair.

The postoperative management is the same as that for the shoelace repair. The patients are mobilized the same evening of the operation and are encouraged to return to their normal activities as soon as possible. However, they are advised to avoid unusually excessive physical effort for some months, until the mesh graft has been firmly incorporated.

Postoperative complications are similar to those of the shoelace repair. If infection supervenes and does not respond to antibiotic treatment, the wound may have to be laid open to allow free drainage. Removal of the exposed graft is usually not necessary. The area should be washed regularly with saline solution to remove discharges and loose debris. With time, the graft will be covered with healthy granulation tissue. Healing may be accelerated at this stage by covering the area with a split-skin mesh graft, or the wound may be left to close on its own.

Rives-Stoppa Technique. In 1987 Rives published his account of his prosthetic mesh technique for repair of incisional hernias where the mesh is placed in the plane behind the rectus muscles and laid onto the anterior aspect of the posterior rectus sheaths.[178] This was later elaborated upon by Stoppa.[95] The technique was popularized in the United States by Wantz in his paper of 1991 and his book of the same year.[90,141] The essential steps are as follows: (1) under general anesthesia, the old scar is excised and the hernia sac dissected free down to the myoaponeurotic edges of the hernial opening, (2) the sac is then opened and its contents inspected, (3) all adherent loops of bowel are freed and returned to the peritoneal cavity, (4) the excess sac is excised and the peritoneum and sac are closed with a running absorbable synthetic suture; where there is insuffi-

cient peritoneum to close the sac, Rives advises to suture the omentum to the edges of the residual defect or else to close it with a sheet of absorbable mesh of polyglactin, so that the prosthetic nonabsorbable mesh for the actual repair will not come in contact with bowel for fear of adhesions, sepsis, and fistula, (5) the bed for the permanent prosthesis is prepared by slitting open the medial edge of each rectus sheath along the hernial defect and for 8 to 10 cm above and below it, and (6) the rectus muscles are separated from the posterior rectus sheaths up to the whole length of the lateral edge of the sheath. Rives, Stoppa, and Wantz advise using a sheet of knitted, braided polyester fiber (mersilene, dacron) cut longer than the length of the defect and wide enough to stretch from one lateral edge of the rectus sheath to the other. This sheet then is fixed under slight tension with a few nonabsorbable monofilament synthetic sutures.[90,95,141,178] Thus, it will lie on the closed peritoneum and posterior rectus sheaths and will stretch above and below the defect and also from one lateral edge of the rectus sheath to the other, and in the plane behind the rectus muscles. The sutures are passed through the edge of the mesh and then along the line of the lateral edges of the rectus sheath (linear semilunaris), from inside the sheath, through the whole thickness of the abdominal wall and out through stab holes in the skin, using an Albaran or Reverdin needle (Fig 14–41G). The sutures are tied so that the knots come to lie on the outer surface of the external oblique muscle and each stab wound is closed with a suture or staple. The upper and lower edges of the mesh are sutured in a similar fashion. When the hernial defect reaches the upper part of the abdominal wall, the upper edge of the mesh is passed down to lie under the diaphragm. In the lower abdomen, below the arcuate line of Douglas, the graft comes to lie in the preperitoneal plane and should be long enough to hang into the pelvis in the retropubic space of Retzius and in the spaces of Bogros. In this case, it should be fixed with a few sutures to the back of the pubis and along the pectineal lines. Two vacuum drains are laid on the graft and brought out through separate stab wounds. The two anterior rectus sheaths then are sutured together along their cut medial edges with a continuous synthetic absorbable or nonabsorbable monofilament suture. The excess skin is excised and the wound is closed. The method is described and beautifully illustrated by Wantz, in both his paper and book.[90,141] This is an excellent repair that incorporates several important principles. The mesh graft does not come into contact with the bowel. The graft lies at a deep plane, covered by muscle and aponeurotic sheath, thereby lessening the risk of infection as well as the risk of erosion through the skin. The graft has wide margins beyond the edges of the hernia defect so that there is a wide area for strong incorporation of the graft. This

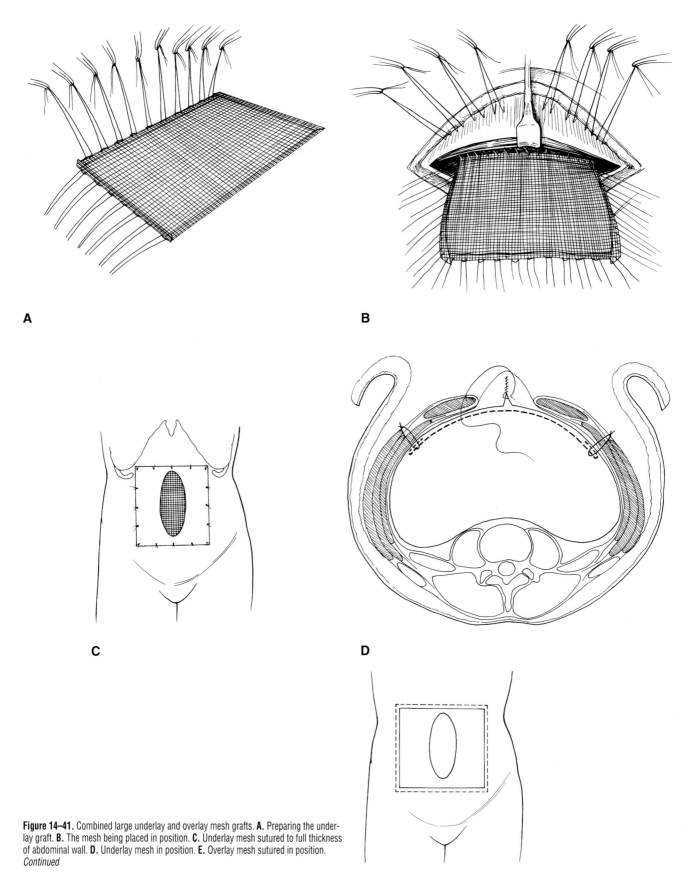

Figure 14–41. Combined large underlay and overlay mesh grafts. **A.** Preparing the underlay graft. **B.** The mesh being placed in position. **C.** Underlay mesh sutured to full thickness of abdominal wall. **D.** Underlay mesh in position. **E.** Overlay mesh sutured in position. *Continued*

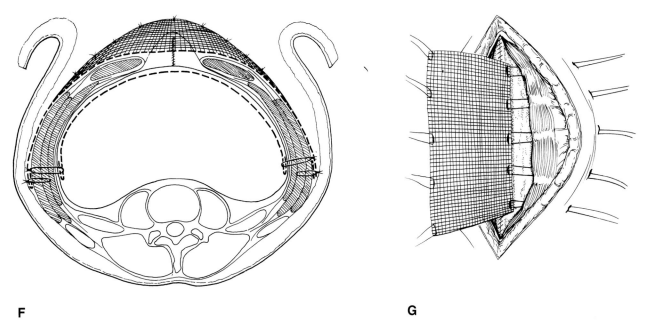

F   **G**

Figure 14–41, cont'd. F. Completed combined repair before placing vacuum drains and closing skin. **G.** Rives-Stoppa technique. Mesh passing behind rectus abdominis muscle. After Rejovitzky, MD.

avoids slippage and recurrent hernia between the graft and the edge of the defect. The graft lies in a plane between the abdominal cavity and the abdominal wall so that it is compressed and held in place by the natural forces of the intra-abdominal pressure against the abdominal wall. The wider the margins of the graft beyond the defect, the stronger will be the forces over a larger area holding the graft in place.

This author has used this method with much satisfaction in quite a large series of cases. However, knitted polypropylene mesh was used, which is made of a monofilament thread instead of the multifilament polyester fiber. Furthermore, we do not open the sac of the hernia, so as not to get involved in the tedious dissection of adherent loops of bowel and the risks of opening the bowel, such as fistula formation or wound sepsis. Instead, the bed is prepared for the graft as is done in the first stage of the shoelace operation, by separating a ribbon of aponeurosis off the medial edge of each rectus sheath and suturing them together with a continuous monofilament polyamide thread to construct a strong new midline linea alba and, at the same time, invert the hernial sac into the peritoneal cavity. This maneuver has the advantages of bringing the rectus sheaths closer together so that a narrower prosthesis can be used and also of making for a smooth bed of posterior rectus sheath on which to lay the graft well separated from the bowels.

The method of fixation of the mesh has evolved through several stages. The synthetic nonabsorbable

mesh should be fixed in place with synthetic monofilament nonabsorbable suture that will hold it in place until it is fully incorporated into the host tissue. When the mesh is placed on the anterior surface of the posterior rectus sheath, it is conveniently fixed in place by interrupted U sutures passing through the full thickness of the abdominal wall from in front of the external oblique, through to the mesh and back again with the knot tied on the surface of the external oblique muscle. Far fewer sutures are used than was previously considered necessary, even with large sheets of mesh. Stoppa has shown that each edge of the mesh needs an anchoring suture at each corner and usually not more than three further sutures in between. Inserting many sutures is time-consuming and does not affect the recurrence rate. Originally, in order to place these sutures far out from the edge of the hernia, it was necessary to expose a very wide area of the external oblique muscle by dissecting off and lifting a large flap of the skin and fat of the abdominal wall. This leads to extensive dead spaces where fluids could accumulate postoperatively and possibly lead to seromas, hematomas, and infection. However, Rives and Stoppa devised the ingenious method of passing the suture through the thickness of the abdominal wall with an Albaran- or a Reverdin-type needle and through a series of stab wounds in the skin and fat around the periphery of the abdominal wall (Fig 14–41G). Thus, there is no longer a need to raise flaps of skin and fat, yet the knots are still tied on the surface of the external oblique muscle and far from the edge of the hernial defect. It is most important not to place the suture close to the edge of the hernial defect where the tissues are thin, scarred and fibrotic, ischemic and weak. Sutures close to the edge tend to tear out so that the prosthesis will slide away from the edge of the defect, leaving a gap through which a recurrent hernia will emerge. The sutures must be placed far from the defect through thick healthy abdominal wall.

The surgeons of the Lichtenstein group have developed a simple and elegant method of stapling the mesh when it is placed on the anterior surface of the posterior rectus sheath, using an articulating stapler.[342] They place a line of staples along the edge of the mesh into the rectus sheath. This rapid and simple technique holds the mesh in place and prevents it from rolling over itself until incorporation is complete. They believe that the line of staples is not a tension-bearing line, so that deep firm sutures through the abdominal wall are not necessary to hold the mesh in place. They do, however, make sure to cover the mesh so that it is held in place by the physical principle of Pascal. In 1991, Costalat reported a series of 70 cases of incisional hernia repaired by the Rives-Stoppa method where the sheet of mesh was fixed circumferentially, quickly and easily, with a fascia stapler, and even under tension.[343] The clips were placed in the "lateral linea alba" (ie, the semilunar line). Their follow-up was 3 months, and the maximum was 5 years. One case recurred, due to a technical error.

It is interesting to note a report of the use of percutaneous sutures through small incisions in the skin similar to the Rives-Stoppa technique, but with a straight needle from outside the abdomen in, and from inside out, for placement and fixation of synthetic mesh in the groin, when repairing inguinal hernias laparoscopically.[344]

Marlex-Peritoneal Sandwich. A new method has been developed for the repair of incisional hernia whereby the prosthetic sheet of polypropylene mesh is implanted between two layers of host tissues like a sandwich.[345] This is done by slitting open the hernial sac and scar tissue vertically in the midline, and freeing all adherent bowel and omentum from the inner surface. The cut edge of one flap then is sutured to the medial edge of the opposite rectus sheath to close the abdominal cavity. The sheet of mesh is laid down on the anterior surface of this flap and each edge is sutured to the medial edge of the rectus sheath on its ipsilateral side. The mesh then is covered by the second half of the sac, the cut edge of which is sutured to the medial edge of the opposite rectus sheath, thus completing the sandwich with the mesh in the middle. This is an easy and attractive method but has the disadvantage of having to open the peritoneal cavity and separate all the adherent bowel from the sac. This maneuver is time-consuming and has certain po-

tential complications. A further disadvantage is that the method does not reconstruct the normal anatomy and function of the elements of the abdominal wall as is achieved in the shoelace or the Rives-Stoppa methods. The advantage of the method is its relative simplicity and the fact that the prosthesis is separated from the bowel and from the subcutaneous fat and skin.

■ POSTOPERATIVE HERNIAS THROUGH NONVERTICAL INCISIONS

Postoperative incisional hernias may follow a variety of procedures in which a vertical midline or paramedian incision usually is not used. They include hernias following appendectomy, closure of colostomy, or subcostal incisions for cholecystectomy or splenectomy, hernias through suture holes or drain wounds, laparoscopic port wounds and hernias in lumbar incisions following nephrectomy or other urologic procedures and lumbar sympathectomy. Parastomal hernia may be included in this category.

APPENDECTOMY

Hernia following appendectomy through a gridiron muscle-splitting incision is usually the result of infection of the wound in advanced appendicitis, with or without perforation, and is associated with local purulent peritonitis. Other common causes are placing a drain through the incision and tying sutures too tightly in the fleshy internal oblique and transversus abdominis muscles, leading to necrosis of the muscle.

Two types of hernia occur. In the more common type, there is an obvious reducible bulge with a cough impulse, with the hernia passing through all the layers of the abdominal wall. Less common is the interstitial or interparietal type in which the hernia passes through a defect in the transversus abdominis and internal oblique muscles, but not through the intact aponeurosis of the external oblique. The hernia mushrooms out in the plane between the external oblique and internal oblique muscles and may be missed easily. In this case, when the patient complains of pain in the region, a vague mass may be present in the abdominal wall, and a cough impulse may be felt by a hand placed flat on the scar. In patients suspected of this condition, the diagnosis should be confirmed by ultrasound scanning or CT to avoid an unnecessary explorative operation. These investigations also should be done in patients who continue to complain of pain in what clinically appears to be a well-healed scar.

Operative repair is done by excising the old scar, freeing the sac from the parietal layers of the abdominal wall, and reducing the inverted sac back into the abdominal cavity. The transversus abdominis and internal oblique muscles are usually well preserved, and the defect in both layers may be simply closed by approximating the edges with a loosely sutured and loosely tied continuous mass closure suture of heavy monofilament nonabsorbable material. This closure should begin and end a few centimeters away from the defect. The aponeurosis of the external oblique muscle is sutured as a separate layer with a continuous monofilament nonabsorbable suture. When the tissues are thin and atrophic, an overlap type of repair may be used for the two inner muscles, but these cases are best treated with a sheet of polypropylene mesh, with a margin measuring at least 6 to 8 cm beyond the periphery of the defect, placed between the peritoneum and the transversus abdominis muscle and sutured around its borders with interrupted polypropylene sutures to the full thickness of the abdominal wall.

CLOSURE OF COLOSTOMY

Wounds following closure of colostomy are, for practical purposes, always infected by colonic organisms. These wounds are best closed by a single layer of mass closure sutures of stainless steel wire through all three muscular layers, with the skin left open to heal by secondary intention. Hernias following closure of colostomy are usually the result of incorrect closure as well as infection. An attempt at repair should be delayed for at least 1 year after the wound has healed and sinuses have closed, by which time the tissues and scar have matured and occult organisms hopefully have disappeared. The scar then is excised and the peritoneal sac is freed from the muscle layers, inverted, and reduced. The muscle layers are best repaired in one layer of mass closure interrupted stainless steel sutures, and the skin then is closed. When the edges cannot be approximated without tension, a prosthetic polypropylene mesh graft should be placed extraperitoneally, as described for postappendectomy hernias.

SUBCOSTAL INCISIONS

Hernias in subcostal incisions may be owing to placement of the incision too close to the subcostal margin, poor suturing technique, and infection. However, the most common cause is probably bringing a drain out through the incision.[316] Usually the whole length of the incision has herniated and the old scar must be excised. The peritoneum is freed and the sac excised after adherent bowel and omentum are released. The anterior rectus sheath and external oblique aponeurosis are separated from the posterior rectus sheath and the transversus and internal oblique muscles. The posterior rectus sheath, peritoneum, and the two inner muscles are sutured as one layer, using the continuous mass closure

technique with a loop of O (metric 3.5) monofilament polyamide, starting at the medial end. The anterior rectus sheath and aponeurosis of the external oblique are sutured with a continuous loop of the same suture material, and the skin is closed. Rarely, an intraperitoneal polypropylene mesh prosthetic reinforcement is needed and is sutured to the full thickness of the abdominal wall, and often to the costal margin as well. Special aspects of this repair have been discussed by this author in another report.[346]

SUTURE HOLES, DRAIN WOUND AND PORT WOUND HERNIAS

Hernias coming through suture holes, drain wounds, and laparoscopic port wounds may be quite large, but the hernial defect is usually small. The hernial sac is dissected free and is inverted into the abdominal cavity. The defect is closed in one layer with a few interrupted monofilament nonabsorbable mass sutures.

LUMBAR INCISIONS

The common incision used in the lumbar region may be quite destructive because it cuts across muscles and neurovascular bundles and usually is followed by herniation. The hernia usually manifests as a generalized bulge with no well-defined sac or neck, and repair of these hernias may be problematic. The layers are dissected free, but it is usually unnecessary to open the peritoneum. Attempts at excising the sac may only complicate matters further, since the small and large bowel and especially the blood supply to the colon may all be firmly adherent to its inner aspect. When good muscle is present, it may be repaired in layers with continuous monofilament nonabsorbable suture. When the muscles are thin and atrophied, an overlap technique may appear feasible, but usually a prosthetic repair is indicated. A large sheet of polypropylene mesh is inserted in the plane between the peritoneum and muscles and is spread from the paraspinal muscles posteriorly to the rectus sheath anteriorly and from above the twelfth rib superiorly to below the iliac crest inferiorly. The mesh is fixed around its periphery with interrupted polypropylene sutures passing through the full thickness of all the musculoaponeurotic layers of the abdominal wall (see Fig 14–35).

PARASTOMAL HERNIA

Parastomal hernia is a postoperative hernia through the incision made for the bowel, ileum or colon, to pass from the abdomen to the skin. It may be a difficult problem to manage. The incidence is 5% to 10% of cases of ileostomy or colostomy. It is lowest when the stoma is brought through the rectus muscle. Devlin described four types of parastomal hernias as follows:[347]

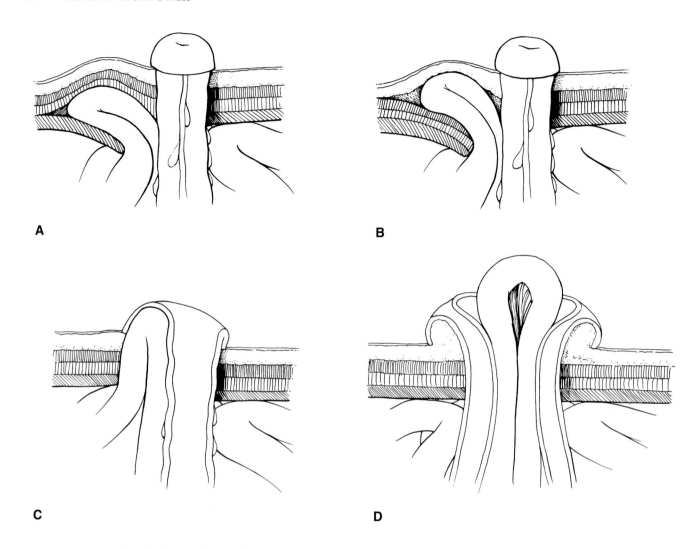

Figure 14–42. Types of parastomal hernia. **A.** Interstitial. **B.** Subcutaneous. **C.** Intrastomal. **D.** Perstomal. After Rejovitzky, MD.

Interstitial (Fig 14–42A), in which the herniated bowel extrudes alongside the bowel for the stoma, then burrows into one of the intermuscular planes

Subcutaneous (Fig 14–42B), in which the herniated bowel extrudes from the abdomen alongside the bowel for the stoma and bulges into the subcutaneous fat alongside the stoma (the most common type)

Intrastomal (Fig 14–42C), which is found in the spout type of stoma, usually ileostomies, and in which the herniated bowel extrudes from the abdomen alongside the bowel for the stoma and enters the plane between the emerging and the everted part of the bowel

Perstomal (Fig 14–42D), in which there is prolapse of the stomal bowel, with loops of bowel entering the hernial space produced between the layers of the prolapsed bowel.

Strangulation of these hernias is not common but has been reported. The hernias develop either because of technical errors in the placement or construction of the stoma, or because of factors associated with the patient such as obesity, malnutrition, advanced malignancy, or old age.

Indications for Operation

Not all parastomal hernias need repair. Most are small and do not bother the patient. Others can be controlled by special colostomy fittings. Operative repair is indicated when the hernia is large and interferes with stomal management such as bag fitting or enemas, or when the stoma is displaced by the hernia to the point where it cannot be seen by the patient. A large hernia with a small neck is at risk for strangulation and is an indication for repair, as is strangulation or a history of recurrent obstruction. Some patients demand operation for esthetic reasons. Patients must be assessed preoper-

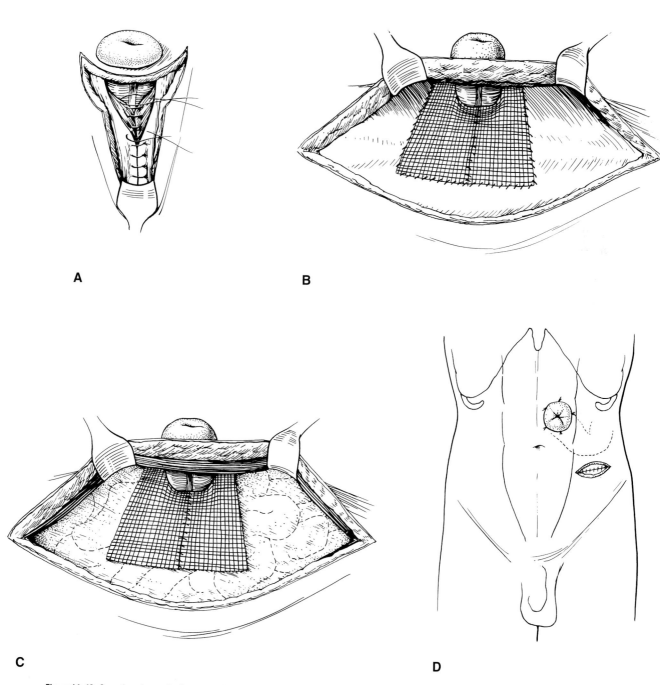

Figure 14–43. Operations for repair of parastomal hernia. **A.** Local repair. **B.** Subcutaneous prosthetic mesh repair. **C.** Extraperitoneal prosthetic mesh repair. **D.** Relocation of stoma and repair of original colostomy wound. After Rejovitzky, MD.

atively. Those with recurrent or inoperable carcinoma should not be operated on. Patients with inflammatory bowel disease may need further resection.

Operations

Three types of operations for parastomal hernia are available: local repair, prosthetic repair, and subcutaneous repair. *Local repair* (Fig 14–43A), which involves dissection around the stoma and efforts to suture the defect in the muscle layers, results in an unacceptably high incidence of recurrence and is not recommended. *Prosthetic repair* may be either subcutaneous, extraperitoneal, or intermuscular. In 1981, Leslie described a *subcutaneous repair* that involves reducing the hernia, repairing the defect in the muscles, and reinforcing the abdominal wall in the area with a sheet of polypropylene mesh as an onlay graft.[348] The mesh is partly slit so that it can be passed around the bowel of the stoma, around which it is wrapped like a sleeve. The edges of the mesh are sutured to the external oblique muscle and aponeurosis (Fig 14–43B). This procedure has been associated with much infection and sinus formation. A similar procedure has recently been described by de Ruiter[349] who designed a sheet of polypropylene mesh with a polypropylene ring fused in the middle. The device is sutured to the external surface of the external oblique muscle and the colon is brought out through the ring.

The *extraperitoneal prosthetic repair* is a more extensive procedure but gives better results. The previous laparotomy incision is reopened, and the extraperitoneal plane is opened to and around the bowel to the stoma. A wide sheet of polypropylene mesh is slit to its center point, where a circle of material slightly smaller than the circumference of the emerging bowel is excised. The mesh is slipped around the bowel, which passes along the slit until it fits into the hole in the middle of the mesh. The slit in the mesh is then resutured so that the mesh fits snugly around the bowel and onto it for a short distance. The corners of the mesh are tacked down to the peritoneum to hold it from slipping until it is incorporated into the tissues (Fig 14–43C). Byers reported a similar intraperitoneal procedure done through the original laparotomy incision.[350] A strip of polypropylene mesh 3 cm wide is sutured on each side of the colon where it passes through the abdominal wall. Each suture passes through both strips as well as through both edges of the hernia defect, thereby repairing the defect and reinforcing it at the same time.

Relocation of Stoma

The stoma must be relocated if the parastomal hernia cannot be repaired as described above, if the stomal site is unsatisfactory, or if the stoma itself is problematic. This is usually done with a localized approach through the old colostomy incision or with a regular laparotomy through the previous operative scar. The stoma is freed and is relocated to a more satisfactory site, and the old stomal wound is closed (Fig 14–43D). This is the best method for dealing with troublesome parastomal hernias, but it is not necessarily indicated in every case. In 1993, Alexandre described a procedure which combines relocation of the stoma together with prosthetic mesh reinforcement of the new opening, and of the previous opening which is closed with sutures, and of the surrounding area by placing a large mesh in the plane between the transversus abdominis muscle and the oblique muscles.[351] A round hole is cut in the mesh to allow the passage of the bowel.

REFERENCES

1. Celsus AC. *Of Medicine.* Translated by James Grieve, London; England; 1756:419
2. de Chauliac G. *La grande chirurgie composee en 1363. Revue avec des notes, une introduction sur le moyenage. Sur la vie et les oeuvres de Guy de Chauliac par E.* Nicaise. Paris, France: Felix Alcan; 1890:522
3. Franco P. *Traite des Hernies Contenant une Ample Declaration de Toutes Leurs Especes et autres Excellentes Parties de la Chirurgie, Assauoir de la Pierre, des Cataractes des Yeux, et autres Maladies, Desquelles comme le Cure Est Perilleuse, aussi Est Elle de Peu d'Hommes Bien Exercee.* Lyon, France: Thibauld Payan; 1556.
4. Stromayr C. *Die Handschrift des Schnitt und Augenarztes.* Berlin, Germany: Caspar Stromayer, Idra-Verlagsanshalt; 1925.
5. Marcy HO. A new use of carbolised cat gut ligatures. *Boston Med Surg J* 1871;83:315
6. Lucas-Championniere J. *Chirurgie Operatoire: Cure Radicale des Hernies; avec une Etude Statistique de Deux Cents Soixante-quinze Operations et cinquante Figures Intercalees dans le Texte.* Paris, France: Rueff et Cie; 1892
7. Bassini E. Nuovo metodo per la cura radicale dell'ernia inguinale. *Atti Congr Associ Med Ital* 1887;2:179
8. Bassini E. Sulla cura radicale dell'ernia inguinale. *Arch Soc Ital Chir* 1887;4:380
9. Bassini E. Sopra 100 casi di cura radicale dell'ernia inguinale operata col metodo dell'autore. *Arch Ed Atti Soc Ital Chir* 1888;5:315
10. Bassini E. Nuovo Metodo per la Cura Radicale dell'Ernia Inguinale. Padua, Italy: Prosperini; 1889
11. Bassini E. Ueber die Behandlung des Leistenbruches. *Arch Klin Chir* 1890;40:429
12. Bassini E. Neue Operation—Methode zue Radicalbehandlung der Schenkelhernia. *Arch Klin Chir* 1894;47:1
13. Shouldice EE. The treatment of hernia. *Ontario Med Rev* 1953;20:670
14. Myers RN, Shearburn EW. The problem of recurrent inguinal hernia. *Surg Clin North Am* 1973;53:555
15. Berliner SD. An approach to groin hernia. *Surg Clin North Am* 1984;64:197
16. Lichtenstein IL. *Hernia Repair Without Disability,* 2nd ed. St Louis, MO: Ishiyaku Euroamerica; 1986

17. Lotheissen G. Zur radikol Operation der Schlenkelhernien. *Zentralbl Chir* 1898;23:548

18. McVay CB, Halverson K. Preperitoneal hernioplasty. In: Beahrs OH, Beart RW Jr (eds), *General Surgery Therapy.* New York, NY: John Wiley and Sons; 1981:10

19. Rutledge RH. Cooper's ligament repair: a 25-year experience with a single technique for all groin hernias in adults. *Surgery* 1988;103:1

20. Rutledge RH. The Cooper ligament repair. *Surg Clin North Am* 1993;73:471

21. Rand Corp (Santa Monica, California). Conceptualization and measurement of physiological health for adults. *Rand Corp Publ* 1983;15:3

22. McArthur LL. Autoplastic suture in hernia and other diastases: preliminary report. *JAMA* 1901;37:1162

23. Kirschner M. Die praktischen Ergebnisse der freien Fascien-Transplanation. *Arch Klin Chir* 1910;92:888

24. Handley WS. A method for the radical cure of inguinal hernia (darn and stay-lace method). *Practitioner* 1918;100:466

25. Gallie WE, Le Mesurier AB. The use of living sutures in operative surgery. *Can Med Assoc J* 1921;11:504

26. Mair GB. Preliminary report on the use of whole skin-grafts as a substitute for fascial sutures in the treatment of herniae. *Br J Surg* 1945;32:381

27. Ogilvie WH. Hernia, In: Maingot R (ed), *Postgraduate Surgery,* vol 3. East Norwalk, CT: Appleton-Century-Crofts; 1937:367

28. Maingot R. The floss silk lattice posterior repair operation for direct inguinal hernia. *Br Med J* 1941;1:777

29. Maingot R. A further report on the "keel" operation for large diffuse incisional hernias. *Med Press* 1958;240:989

30. Maingot R. The floss-silk lattice repair for inguinal hernias. *Br J Clin Pract* 1979;3:97

31. McLeod C. The treatment of indirect inguinal hernia: a critical review of a small personal series. *Lancet* 1955;2:106

32. Nichols HM, Diack AW. Animal experiments with nylon sutures. *West J Surg Obstet Gynec* 1940;48:42

33. Aries LJ. Experimental studies with synthetic fiber (nylon) as a buried suture. *Surgery* 1941;9:51

34. Melick DW. Nylon suture. *Ann Surg* 1942;115:475

35. Stonham FV. New nylon suture material. *Ind Med Gaz* 1942;77:283

36. Localio SA, Casale W, Hinton JW. Wound healing—experimental and statistical study. III. experimental observations. *Surg Gynec Obstet* 1943;77:243

37. Haxton H. Nylon for buried sutures. *Br Med J* 1945;1:12

38. Moloney GE, Gill WG, Barclay RC. Operations for hernia: technique of nylon darn. *Lancet* 1948;2:45

39. Moloney GE. Results of nylon darn repairs of herniae. Lancet 1958;1:273

40. Moloney GE. Darning inguinal hernias. *Arch Surg* 1972;104:129

41. Shuttleworth KED, Davies WH. Treatment of inguinal herniae. *Lancet* 1960;1:126

42. Leacock AG, Rowley RK. Results of nylon repairs in inguinal hernias. *Lancet* 1962;1:20

43. Ellis H. Inguinal hernia. *Br J Hosp Med* 1970;4:9

44. Callum KG, Doig RL, Kinmonth JB. The results of nylon darn repair for inguinal hernia. *Arch Surg* 1974;108:25

45. Lifschutz H, Juler GL. The inguinal darn. *Arch Surg* 1986;121:717

46. Morris GE, Jarrett PEM. Recurrence rates following local anaesthetic day case inguinal hernia repair by junior surgeons in a district general hospital. *Ann R Coll Surg (Engl)* 1987;69:97

47. Abrahamson J, Eldar S. Primary and recurrent inguinal hernias—repair with nylon darn. *Theor Surg* 1987;2:91

48. Abrahamson J, Berliner SD, Gilbert AI, Obney N. Inguinal hernia—100 years since Padua. *Contemp Surg* 1988;32:95

49. Abrahamson J, Eldar S. The nylon darn repair for primary and recurrent inguinal hernias. *Contemp Surg* 1988;32:33

50. Morgan M, Swan AV, Reynolds A, Beech R, Devlin HB. Are current techniques of inguinal hernia repair optimal? A survey in the United Kingdom. *Ann R Coll Surg (Engl)* 1991;73:341

51. Mansberger JA, Rogers DA, Jennings WD, Leroy J. A comparison of a new two-layer anatomic repair to the traditional Shouldice herniorrhaphy. *Am Surg* 1992;58:211

52. Witzel O. Ueber den Verschluss von Bauchwunden und Bruchpforten durch versenkte Silberdrahtnetze. (Einheilung von Filigranpelotten). *Zentralbl Chir* 1900;27:257

53. Goepel R. Ueber die Verschliessung von Bruchpforten durch Einheilung geflochtener, fertiger Silberdrahtnetze (Silberdrahtpelotten). *Verh Dtsch Ges Chir* 1900;29:174

54. Bartlett W. An improved filigree for the repair of large defects in abdominal wall. *Ann Surg* 1903;38:47

55. McGavin L. The double filigree operation for the radical cure of inguinal hernia. *Br Med J* 1909;2:357

56. Burke GL. The corrosion of metals in the tissues; and an introduction to tantalum. *Can Med Assoc J* 1940;43:125

57. Throckmorton TD. Tantalum gauze in the repair of hernias complicated by tissue deficiency. *Surgery* 1948;23:32

58. Lam CR, Szilagyi DE, Puppendahl M. Tantalum gauze in the repair of large postoperative ventral hernias. *Arch Surg* 1948;57:234

59. Koontz AR. Preliminary report on the use of tantalum mesh in the repair of ventral hernias. *Ann Surg* 1948;127:1079

60. Jefferson NC, Dailey UG. Incisional hernia repaired with tantalum gauze: preliminary report. *Am J Surg* 1948;75:575

61. Adler RH. An evaluation of surgical mesh in the repair of hernias and tissue defects. *Arch Surg* 1962;85:836

62. Thorbjarnarson B, Goulian D. Complications from use of surgical mesh in repair of hernias. *NY State J Med* 1967;(May):1189

63. Bothra R. Late onset small bowel fistula due to tantalum mesh. *Am J Surg* 1973;125:649

64. Usher FC, Ochsner J, Tuttle LLD Jr. Use of marlex mesh in the repair of incisional hernias. *Am Surg* 1958;24:969

65. Harrison JH. A Teflon weave for replacing tissue defects. *Surg Gynecol Obstet* 1957;104:584

66. Gibson LD, Stafford CE. Synthetic mesh repair of abdominal wall defects: follow up and reappraisal. *Am Surg* 1964;30:481

67. Sher W, Pollack D, et al. Repair of abdominal wall defects—Goretex vs Marlex grafts. *Am Surg* 1980;46:618

68. Jenkins SD, Kramer TW, et al. A comparison of prosthetic

materials used to repair abdominal wall defects. *Surgery* 1983;94:392

69. Hamer-Hodges DW, Scott NB. Replacement of an abdominal wall defect using expanded PTFE sheet (Gore-Tex). *J R Coll Surg (Edinb)* 1985;30:65

70. Bauer JJ, Salky BA, et al. Repair of large abdominal wall defects with expanded polytetrafluoroethylene (PTFE). *Ann Surg* 1987;206:765

71. Rives J. Surgical treatment of the inguinal hernia with dacron patch: principles, indications, technic and results. *Int Surg* 1967;47:360

72. Stoppa RE, Rives JL, et al. The use of dacron in the repair of hernias of the groin. *Surg Clin North Am* 1984;64:269

73. Gilbert AI. Prosthetic adjuncts to groin hernia repair. Paper presented at Seminar "Advances and Improvements in Hernia Surgery," Miami, FL, March 12–14, 1987.

74. Gilbert AI. Sutureless repair of inguinal hernia. *Am J Surg* 1992;163:331

75. Shulman AG, Amid PK, Lichtenstein IL. Prosthetic mesh plug repair of femoral and recurrent inguinal hernias: the American experience. *Ann R Coll Surg (Engl)* 1992;74:97

76. Shulman AG, Amid PK, Lichtenstein IL. The safety of mesh repair for primary inguinal hernias: results of 3019 operations from five diverse surgical sources. *Am Surg* 1992;58:255

77. Amid PK, Shulman AB, Lichtenstein IL. Critical scrutiny of the open "tension-free" hernioplasty. *Am J Surg* 1993; 165:369

78. Robbins AW, Rutkow IM. The mesh-plug hernioplasty. *Surg Clin North Am* 1993;73:501

79. LaRoque GP. The permanent cure of inguinal and femoral hernia; a modification of the standard operative procedures. *Surg Gynec Obstet* 1919;29:507

80. Cheatle GL. An operation for the radical cure of inguinal and femoral hernia. *Br Med J* 1920;2:68

81. Henry AK. Operation for femoral hernia by a midline extraperitoneal approach: with a preliminary note on the use of this route for reducible inguinal hernia. *Lancet* 1936;1:531

82. Musgrove JE, McCready FJ. The Henry approach to femoral hernia. *Surgery* 1949;26:608

83. McEvedy PG. Femoral hernia. *Ann R Coll Surg (Engl)* 7;484: 1950

84. Mikkelsen WP, Berne CJ. Femoral hernioplasty: Suprapubic extraperitoneal (Cheatle-Henry) approach. *Surgery* 1954;35:743

85. Nyhus LM, Condon RE, Harkins HN. Clinical experiences with preperitoneal hernial repair for all types of hernia of the groin. *Am J Surg* 1960;100:234

86. Read RC. Preperitoneal exposure of inguinal herniation. *Am J Surg* 1968;116:653

87. Read RC. Bilaterality and the prosthetic repair of large recurrent inguinal hernias. *Am J Surg* 1979;138:788

88. Nyhus LM, Condon RE (eds), *Hernia,* 2nd ed. Philadelphia, PA: JB Lippincott; 1978:212

89. Nyhus LM. Iliopubic tract repair of inguinal and femoral hernia. The posterior (preperitoneal) approach. *Surg Clin North Am* 1993;73:487

90. Wantz GE. *Atlas of Hernia Surgery.* New York, NY: Raven; 1991:101

91. Wantz GE. Giant prosthetic reinforcement of the visceral sac for repair of a re-recurrent inguinal hernia. *Postgrad Gen Surg* 1992;4:109

92. Wantz GE. The technique of giant prosthetic reinforcement of the visceral sac performed through an anterior groin incision. *Surg Gynecol Obstet* 1993;176:497

93. Stoppa R, Henry X, et al. Prostheses de paroi abdominale. *Forum Chir* 1981;21:28

94. Stoppa R. Hernia of the abdominal wall. In: Chevrel JP (ed), *Surgery of the Abdominal Wall.* Berlin, Germany: Springer-Verlag; 1987:155

95. Stoppa R. The treatment of complicated groin and incisional hernias. *World J Surg* 1989;13:545

96. Stoppa RE. In: Wantz GE (ed), Giant prosthetic reinforcement of the visceral sac for repair of a re-recurrent inguinal hernia. *Postgrad Gen Surg* 1992;4:109

97. Stoppa R, Moungar F. Hernia surgery today [editorial] (La chirurgie herniaire, aujourd'hui). *G Chir* 1992; 13:517

98. Ger R, Mishrick A, Hurwitz J, Romero C, Oddsen R. Management of groin hernias by laparoscopy. *World J Surg* 1993;17:46

99. Ferzli G, Massaad A, Albert P, Worth MH, Jr. Endoscopic extraperitoneal herniorrhaphy versus conventional hernia repair: a comparative study. *Curr Surg* 1993;50:291

100. McKernan JB, Laws HL. Laparoscopic repair of inguinal hernias using a totally extraperitoneal prosthetic approach. *Surg Endosc* 7:26, 1993.

101. Easter DW. Inguinal hernia in pediatrics: initial experience with laparoscopic inguinal exploration of the asymptomatic contralateral side. *J Laparoendosc Surg* 1992;2:361

102. Lichtenstein IL, Shulman AG, and Amid PK. Laparoscopic hernioplasty. *Arch Surg* 1991;126:1449

103. Filipi CJ, Fitzgibbons RJ, Jr., Salerno GM, Hart RO. Laparoscopic herniorrhaphy. *Surg Clin North Am* 1992; 72:1109

104. Rutkow IM. Laparoscopic hernia repair: the socioeconomic tyranny of surgical technology. *Arch Surg* 1992; 127:1271

105. Macintyre IM. Laparoscopic herniorrhaphy [Editorial]. *Br J Surg* 1992;79:1123

106. Toy FK, Smoot RT, Jr. Laparoscopic hernioplasty update. *J Laparoendosc Surg* 1992;2:197

107. Arregui ME, Nauarrete J, Davis CJ, Castro D. Laparoscopic inguinal herniorrhaphy: techniques and controversies. *Surg Clin North Am* 1993;73:513

108. Layman TS, Burns RP, Chandler KE, et al. Laparoscopic inguinal herniorrhaphy in a swine model. *Am Surg* 1993;59:13

109. Sailors DM, Layman TS, Burns RP, et al. Laparoscopic hernia repair: a preliminary report. *Am Surg* 1993;59:85

110. Talamini MA. Laparoscopic appendectomy and herniorrhaphy. *Adv Surg* 1993;26:387

111. MacLean LD. The repair of inguinal hernias. [Editorial] *Ann Surg* 1995;221:1

112. Fitzgibbons RJ Jr, Camps J, Cornet DA, Nguyen NX, et al. Laparoscopic inguinal herniorrhaphy: results of a multicenter trial. *Ann Surg* 1995;221:3

113. Lichtenstein IL, Shulman AG, Amid PK. The cause, prevention, and treatment of recurrent groin hernia. *Surg Clin North Am* 1993;73:529

114. Jan TC, Wu CC, Yang CC, Lee YM. Detection of open processus vaginalis by radionuclide scintigraphy. *Kao Hsiung I Hsueh Ko Hsueh Tsa Chih* 1992;8:54

115. Surana R, Puri P. Is contralateral exploration necessary in infants with unilateral inguinal hernia? *J Pediatr Surg* 1993;28:1026

116. Surana R, Puri P. Fate of patent processus vaginalis: a case against routine contralateral exploration for unilateral inguinal hernia in children. *Pediatr Surg Int* 1993; 8:412

117. Peacock EE Jr. Biology of hernia. In: Nyhus LM, Condon RE (eds), *Hernia*, 2nd ed. Philadelphia, PA: JB Lippincott; 1978:79

118. Rodrigues-Junior AJ, de-Tolosa EM, de Carualho CA. Electron microscopic study on the elastic and elastic related fibres in the human fascia transversalis at different ages. *Gegenbaurs Morphol Jahrb* 1990;136:645

119. Casten DF. Functional anatomy of the groin area as related to the classification and treatment of groin hernias. *Am J Surg* 1967;114:984

120. Halverson K, McVay B. Inguinal and femoral hernioplasty: a 22 year study of the author's methods. *Arch Surg* 1970;101:127

121. Gilbert AI: Overnight hernia repair: updated considerations. *South Med J* 1987;80:191

122. Rutkow IM, Robbins AW. Demographic, classificatory, and socioeconomic aspects of hernia repair in the United States. *Surg Clin North Am* 1993;73:413

123. Ducharme JC, Bertrand R, Chacar R. Is it possible to diagnose inguinal hernia by x-ray? *J Can Assoc Radiol* 1967; 18:448

124. Lunderquist A, Rafstedt S. Roentgenologic diagnosis of cryptorchism. *J Urol* 1967;98:219

125. White JJ, Haller JA, Dorst JP. Congenital inguinal hernia and inguinal herniography. *Surg Clin North Am* 1970; 50:823

126. Swischuk LE, Stacy T. Herniography: radiologic investigation of inguinal hernia. *Radiology* 1971;101:139

127. Thompson W, Longerbeam JK, Reeves C. Herniograms. An aid to the diagnosis and treatment of groin hernias in infants and children. *Arch Surg* 1972;105:71

128. Gullmo A, Broome A, Smedberg S. Herniography. *Surg Clin North Am* 1984;64:229

129. Van den Berg JC, Strijk SP. Groin hernias: role of herniography. *Radiology* 1992;184:191

130. Suga K, Kaneko T, Nishigauchi K, et al. Demonstration of inguinal hernia by means of peritoneal 99mTc-MAA scintigraphy with a load produced by standing in a patient treated by continuous ambulatory peritoneal dialysis. *Ann Nucl Med* 1992;6:203

131. Nicholson CP, Donohue JH, Thompson GB, Lewis JE. A study of metastatic cancer found during inguinal hernia repair. *Cancer* 1992;69:3008

132. Rorbaek-Madsen M. Herniorrhaphy in patients aged 80 years or more: a prospective analysis of morbidity and mortality. *Eur J Surg* 1992;158:591

133. Gavrilenko BG, Bannyi AV, Pagava AZ, Melinik BS. Surgical treatment of inguinal hernias in elderly and very old patients. *Klin Khir* 1992;2:29

134. Gardner B, Palasti S. A comparison of hospital costs and morbidity between octogenarians and other patients undergoing general surgical operations. *Surg Gynecol Obstet* 1990;171:299

135. Law NW, Trapnell JE. Does a truss benefit a patient with inguinal hernia. *BMJ* 1992;304:1092

136. Henderson K, Sethna NF, Berde CB. Continuous caudal anesthesia for inguinal hernia repair in former preterm infants. *J Clin Anesth* 1993;5:129

137. Peutrell JM, Hughes DG. Epidural anaesthesia through caudal catheters for inguinal herniotomies in awake expremature babies. *Anesthesia* 1993;48:128

138. Gilbert AI. Technique may save $1000 per hernia repair. *Med Trib.* Oct 24, 1979.

139. Lichtenstein IL. Herniorrhaphy. A personal experience with 6,321 cases. *Am J Surg* 1987;153:553

140. Gilbert AI. Inguinal hernia repair: biomaterials and sutureless repair. *Perspec Gen Surg* 1991;2:113

141. Wantz GE. Incisional hernioplasty with mersilene. *Surg Gynec Obstet* 1991;172:129

142. Behnia R, Hashemi F, Stryker SJ, Ujiki GT, Poticha SM. A comparison of general versus local anesthesia during inguinal herniorrhaphy. *Surg Gynecol Obstet* 1992;174:277

143. Amado WJ. Anesthesia for hernia surgery. *Surg Clin North Am* 1993;73:427

144. Lancet. British hernias. *Lancet* 1985;1:1080

145. Ris H-B, Aebersold P, Kupfer K, et al. 10 Jahre Erfahrung mit einer modifizierten Operationstechnik nach Shouldice fur Inguinalhernien bei Erwachsenen. II. Welche Faktoren beeinflussen die Rezidivgenese von Inguinalhernien? *Chirurgie* 1987;58:100

146. De Wilt JHW, Ijzermans JNM, Hop WCJ, Jeekel J. De behandeling van recidief van hernia inguinalis. *Ned Tijdschr Geneeskd* 1990;134:531

147. Vasilev VI. Herniotomy as a cause of male infertility. *Khirurgiia Mosk* 1990;8:70

148. Yavetz H, Harash B, Yogev L, et al. Fertility of men following inguinal hernia repair. *Andrologia* 1991;23:443

149. Sandhu DP, Osborn DE, Munson KW. Relationship of azoospermia to inguinal surgery. *Int J Androl* 1992;1:504

150. Matsuda T, Horii Y, Yoshida O. Unilateral obstruction of the vas deferens caused by childhood inguinal herniorrhaphy in male infertility patients. *Fertil Steril* 1992; 58:609

151. Matsuda T, Muguruma K, Horii Y, et al. Serum antisperm antibodies in men with vas deferens obstruction caused by childhood inguinal herniorrhaphy. *Fertil Steril* 1993;59:1095

152. Khoury AE, Charendoff J, Balfe JW, et al. Hernias associated with CAPD in children. *Adv Perit Dial* 1991;7:279

153. Boley SJ, Cahn D, Lauer T, et al. The irreducible ovary: a true emergency. *J Pediatr Surg* 1991;26:1035

154. Abrahamson J. Repair of inguinal hernias in infants and children: the approaches of a pediatric surgeon. *Clin Pediatr* 1973;12:617

155. Vibits H, Pahle E. Recurrences after inguinal herniotomy in children: long time follow-up. *Ann Chir Gynecol* 1992;81:300

156. Chatterjee SK. Inguinal hernia. [Editorial comment]. *Pediatr Surg Int* 1993;8:453

157. Tons C, Klinge U, Kupczyk-Joeris D, et al. Controlled study of cremaster resection in Shouldice repair of primary inguinal hernia. *Zentralbl Chir* 1991;116:737

158. Robbins GF, Brunschweig A, Foote FW. Deperitonealization: clinical and experimental observations. *Ann Surg* 1949;130:466

159. Trimpi HD, Bacon HE. Clinical and experimental study of denuded surfaces in extensive surgery of the colon and rectum. *Am J Surg* 1952;84:596

160. Eskeland G. Regeneration of parietal peritoneum. *Acta Path Microbiol Scand* 1964;62:459

161. Ellis H, Harrison W, Hugh TB. The healing of peritoneum under normal and pathological conditions. *Br J Surg* 1965;52:471

162. Raftery AT. Regeneration of parietal and visceral peritoneum. A light microscopical study. *Br J Surg* 1973; 60:293

163. Ellis H. The cause and prevention of postoperative intraperitoneal adhesions. *Surg Gynecol Obstet* 1971;133:497

164. Ellis H, Heddle R. Does the peritoneum need to be closed at laparotomy? *Br J Surg* 1977;64:733

165. Ferguson DJ. Closure of the hernial sac—pro and con. In: Nyhus LM, Condon RE (eds), *Hernia*, 2nd ed, Philadelphia, PA: JB Lippincott; 1978:152

166. Smedberg SGG, Broome AEA, Gullmo A. Ligation of the hernial sac? *Surg Clin North Am* 1984;64:299

167. Douglas DM. Tensile strength of sutures: B.P.C. method of test; loss when implanted in living tissue. *Lancet* 1949;2:497

168. Moloney GE. The effect of human tissues on the tensile strength of implanted nylon sutures. *Br J Surg* 1961; 48:528

169. Welsh DRJ, Alexander MAJ. The Shouldice repair. *Surg Clin North Am* 1993;73:451

170. Panos RG, Beck DE, Maresh JE, Harford FJ. Preliminary results of a prospective randomised study of Cooper's ligament versus Shouldice herniorrhaphy techniques. *Surg Gynecol Obstet* 1992;175:315

171. Tanner WA, Ng CY. Shouldice hernia repair—a five year audit. *Ir J Med Sci* 1993;162:13

172. Wilkinson LH, Floyd VT, et al. Inguinal hernia—a different technique. *Contemp Surg* 1988;32:47

173. Lichtenstein IL, Amid PK, Shulman AG. The iliopubic tract: the key to inguinal herniorrhaphy? *Int Surg* 1990; 75:244

174. Abrahamson J. Factors and mechanisms leading to recurrence of hernias. In: Bendavid R (ed), *Prostheses in Abdominal Wall Hernia*, 1st ed. Georgetown, Texas: RG Landes; 1994

175. Warlaumont C. Les hernies de l'aine. Place des protheses an tulle de Dacron dans leur traitement (a propos de 1236 hernies operees). *These Med Amiens* 1982.

176. Abrahamson J, Eldar S. The nylon darn repair for recurrent inguinal hernias. Paper presented at Collegium Internationale Chirurgiae Digestivae (CICD)) 10th World Congress, Copenhagen; Sept 1988.

177. Rutkow IM. *Socioeconomics of Surgery*. St. Louis, MO: CV Mosby; 1989

178. Rives J. Major incisional hernias. In: Chevrel JP (ed), *Surgery of the Abdominal Wall.* New York, NY: Springer-Verlag, 1987:116

179. Wantz GE. Giant prosthetic reinforcement of the visceral sac. *Surg Gynecol Obstet* 1989;169:408

180. Stoppa R. Hernia of the abdominal wall. In: Chevrel JP (ed), *Surgery of the Abdominal Wall.* Berlin, Germany: Springer-Verlag; 1987:155

181. Spittal MJ, Hunter SJ. A comparison of bupivacaine instillation and inguinal field block for control of pain after herniorrhaphy. *Ann R Coll Surg (Engl)* 1992;74:85

182. Hertzfeld. The radical cure of hernia in infants and young children. *Edinb Med J* 1925;32:281

183. Hertzfeld G. Hernia in infancy. *Am J Surg* 1938;39:422

184. Black N. Day case surgery. *Lancet* 1992;339:61

185. Collopy BT. Improving appropriate use of surgical services. *Qual Assur Health Care* 1991;3:221

186. Farquharson EL. Early ambulation with special reference to herniorrhaphy as an outpatient procedure. *Lancet* 2:517, 1955.

187. Glassow F. Short stay surgery (Shouldice technique) for repair of inguinal hernia. *Ann R Coll Surg (Engl)* 1976; 58:133

188. Grotzinger U. Ambulatory hernia surgery. *Ther Umsch* 1992;49:478

189. Mamie C, Forster A. Ambulatory surgery. Attitude of patients. *Presse Med* 1992;21:657

190. Millat B, Gignoux M, Hay JM. Surgical treatment of inguinal hernia in short-term hospitalization: prospective survey of 500 consecutive unselected cases. Associations Francaises de Recherche en Chirurgie. *Presse Med* 1992; 21:1796

191. Bellis CJ. Immediate return to unrestricted work after inguinal herniorrhaphy: personal experiences with 27,267 cases, local anesthesia and mesh. *Int Surg* 1992;77:167

192. Barwell NJ. Recurrence and early activity after groin hernia repair. *Lancet* 1981;2:985

193. Hodgkinson DJ, McGrath DC. Scrotal reconstruction for giant inguinal hernias. *Surg Clin North Am* 1984;64:307

194. Rider MA, Baker DM, Locker A, Fawcett AN. Return to work after inguinal hernia repair. *Br J Surg* 1993;80:745

195. Robertson GSM, Burton PR, Haynes IG. How long do patients convalesce after inguinal herniorrhaphy? Current principles and practice. *Ann R Coll Surg (Engl)* 1993;75:30

196. Christensen T, Kehlet H. Postoperative fatigue. *World J Surg* 1993;17:220

197. Leibovitch I, Gutman M, Skornick Y, Rozin RR. Giant inguinoscrotal hernia with ensuing fatal complications. *Isr J Med Sci* 1990;26:408

198. Fadiran OA, Lawal OO, Jeje J, et al. Giant inguino-scrotal hernia: a case report. *Cent Afr J Med* 1992;38:127

199. Taylor DC, Meyers WC, Moylan JA, et al. Abdominal musculature abnormalities as a cause of groin pain in athletes. Inguinal hernia and pubalgia. *Am J Sports Med* 1991; 19:239

200. Malycha P, Lovell G. Inguinal surgery in athletes with chronic groin pain: the "sportsman's" hernia. *Aust NZ J Surg* 1992;62:123

201. Hackney RG. The sports hernia: a cause of chronic groin pain. *Br J Sports Med* 1993;27:58

202. Kald A, Nilsson E. Quality assessment in hernia surgery. *Qual Assur Health Care* 1991;3:205

203. Fong Y, Wantz GE. Prevention of ischemic orchitis during inguinal hernioplasty. *Surg Gynecol Obstet* 1992; 174:399

204. Ranaboldo CJ, Karran SE, Bailey IS, Karran SJ. Antimicrobeal prophylaxis in "clean" surgery: hernia repair. *J Antimicrob Chemother* 1993;31(suppl B):35

205. Simchen E, Wax Y, Galai N, Israeli A. Discharge from hospital and its effects on surgical wound infections. The Israeli Study of Surgical Infections (ISSI). *J Clin Epidemiol* 1992;45:1155

206. Karran SJ, Karran SE, Toyn K, Brough P. Antibiotic prophylaxis in clean surgical cases and the role of community surveillance. *Eur J Surg Suppl* 1992;31–32

207. Michaels JA, Reece-Smith H, Faber RG. Case-control study of patient satisfaction with day-case and inpatient inguinal hernia repair. *J R Coll Surg (Edinb)* 1992;37:99

208. Bailey IS, Karran SE, Toyn K, Brough P, Ranaboldo C, Karran SJ. Community surveillance of complications after hernia surgery. *BMJ* 1992;304:469 (See erratum *BMJ* Mar 21, 1992;304:739)

209. Beacon J, Hoile RW, Ellis H. A trial of suction drainage in inguinal hernia repair. *Br J Surg* 1980;67:554

210. Bohnen JM. Antimicrobial prophylaxis in general surgery. *Can J Surg* 1991;34:548

211. Chassin JL. *Operative Strategy in General Surgery, an Expositive Atlas*, vol 2. New York, NY: Springer-Verlag; 1984

212. Hopkins CC. Antibiotic prophylaxis in clean surgery: peripheral vascular surgery, noncardiovascular thoracic surgery, herniorrhaphy, and mastectomy. *Rev Infect Dis*, 1991:13(suppl 10):S869

213. Lazorthes F, Chiotasso P, Massip P, et al. Local antibiotic prophylaxis in inguinal hernia repair. *Surg Gynecol Obstet* 1992;175:569

214. Platt R, Zucker JR, Zaleznik DF, et al. Prophylaxis against wound infection following herniorrhaphy or breast surgery. *J Infect Dis* 1992;166:556

215. Read RC, Barone GW, Hauer-Jensen M, Yoder G. Preperitoneal prosthetic placement through the groin. The anterior (Mahorner-Goss, Rives-Stoppa) approach. *Surg Clin North Am* 1993;73:545

216. Berliner SD. Biomaterials in hernia repair, In: Nyhus LM, Condon RE (eds), *Hernia*, 3rd ed. Philadelphia, PA: JB Lippincott; 1989:541

217. Chamary VL. Femoral hernia: intestinal obstruction is an unrecognized source of morbidity and mortality. *Br J Surg* 1993;80:230

218. Davis JM, Wolff B, Cunningham TF. Delayed wound infection: an 11 year survey. *Arch Surg* 1982;117:113

219. Houck JP, Rypins EB, Sarfeh IJ, et al. Repair of incisional hernia. *Surg Gynecol Obstet* 1989;169:397

220. Lynch TH, Waymont B, Beacock CJ, Wallace DMA. Paravesical suture granuloma: a problem following herniorrhaphy. *J Urol* 1992;147:460

221. Neulander E, Kaneti J, Lissmer L, et al. Post-herniorrhapy paravesical granuloma simulating pelvic metastasis in a patient with bladder cancer. *Int Urol Nephrol* 1992;24:273

222. Palumbo LT, Sharpe WS. Primary inguinal hernioplasty in the adult. *Surg Clin North Am* 1971;51:1293

223. Stott MA, Sutton R, Royle GT. Bilateral inguinal hernias: simultaneous or sequential repair? *Postgrad Med J* 1988; 64:375

224. Serpell JW, Johnson CD, Jarrett PE. A prospective study of bilateral inguinal hernia repair. *Ann R Coll Surg (Engl)* 1990;72:299

225. Wantz GE. The Canadian repair. Personal observations. *World J Surg* 1989;13:516

226. Miller AR, Van Heerden JA, Naessens JM, O'Brian PC. Simultaneous bilateral hernia repair: a case against conventional wisdom. *Ann Surg* 1991;213:272

227. Obney N. Shouldice technique for the repair of inguinal hernias: results and complications. Paper presented at seminar "Advances and Improvements in Hernia Surgery," Miami, March 12–14, 1987.

228. Obney N. Inguinal Hernia—100 years since Padua. *Contemp Surg* 1988;32:95

229. McDonald DF, Huggins C. Simultaneous prostatectomy and inguinal herniorrhaphy. *Surg Gynecol Obstet* 89:621, 1949.

230. Jasper WS Sr. Combined open prostatectomy and herniorrhaphy. *J Urol* 1974;111:370

231. Abrahamson J, Issaq E. Combined operation for prostatic hypertrophy and inguinal hernia. Paper presented at International College of Surgeons 26th World Congress, Milan, Italy, July 1988.

232. Julke M, Schmid R, Thalmann C, et al. Inguinal hernia as a sequela of disordered bladder emptying. *Helv Chir Acta* 1992;59:331

233. Gonzalez-Ojeda A, Marquina M, Calva J, et al. Combined inguinal herniorrhaphy and transurethral prostatectomy. *Br J Surg* 1991;78:1443

234. Issaq E, Abrahamson J, Elder S, Kedar SS. Economic and other advantages in combined prostatectomy and hernia repair. *Theor Surg* 1987;2:78

235. Kingsnorth AN, Gray MR, Nott DM. Prospective randomised trial comparing the Shouldice technique and plication darn for inguinal hernia. *Br J Surg* 1992; 79:1068

236. Wyatt JP. Prospective randomized trial comparing the Shouldice technique and plication darn for inguinal hernia. *Br J Surg* 1993;80:403

237. Kingsnorth AN, Gray MR, Nott DM. Prospective randomised trial comparing the Shouldice technique and plication darn for inguinal hernia [letter]. *Br J Surg* 1993;80:403

238. Abramson JH, Gofin J, Hopp C, et al. The epidemiology of inguinal hernia: a survey in Western Jerusalem. *J Epidemiol Community Health* 1978;32:59

239. Cannon DJ, Read RC. Metastatic emphysema, a mechanism for acquiring inguinal herniation. *Ann Surg* 1981;194:270

240. Read RC. A review: the role of protease-antiprotease imbalance in the pathogenesis of herniation and abdominal aortic aneurysm in certain smokers. *Postgrad Gen Surg* 1992;4:161

241. Hurst RD, Butler BN, Soybel DI, Wright HK. Management of groin hernias in patients with ascites. *Ann Surg* 1992;216:696

242. Pauls DG, Basinger BB, Shield CF, III. Inguinal hernior-

rhaphy in the continuous ambulatory peritoneal dialysis patient. *Am J Kidney Dis* 1992;20:497

243. Peacock EE, Jr. Biology of hernia. In: Nyhus LM, Condon RE (eds), *Hernia,* 2nd ed. Philadelphia, PA: JB Lippincott; 1978:79

244. Peacock EE Jr. Biological aspects of inguinal hernia. Paper presented at seminar "Advances and Improvements in Hernia Surgery," Miami, March 12–14, 1987

245. Read RC. The development of inguinal herniorrhaphy. *Surg Clin North Am* 1984;64:185

246. Bendavid R. The rational use of mesh in hernias. A perspective. *Int Surg* 1992;77:229

247. Berliner SD. Clinical experience with inlay expanded polytetrafluoroethylene soft tissue patch as an adjunct in inguinal hernia repair. *Surg Gynecol Obstet* 1993;176;323

248. Gallegos NC, Dawson J, Jarvis M, Hobsley M. Risk of strangulation in groin hernias. *Br J Surg* 1991;78:1171

249. Chapman WH, Barcia PJ. Femoral hernia in children: an infrequent problem revisited. *Mil Med* 1991;156:631

250. Asai A, Takehara H, Okada A, et al. A case of femoral hernia in a child. *Tokushima J Exp Med* 1992;39:145

251. Luque-Mialdea R, deTomas-Palacios E, Cerda-Berrocal J, et al. Femoral hernia in children (Hernia femoral en el niño). *An Esp Pediatr* 1993;38:135

252. Corder AP. The diagnosis of femoral hernia. *Postgrad Med J* 1992;68:26

253. Ellis H. Strangulated external hernia, In: Ellis H (ed), *Intestinal Obstruction*. New York, NY: Appleton-Century-Crofts; 1982:175

254. Devlin HB. Femoral hernia, In: Devlin HB (ed), *Management of Abdominal Hernias*. London, England: Butterworths; 1988:121

255. Lichtenstein IL, Shore JM. Simplified repair of femoral and recurrent inguinal hernia by a "plug" technic. *Am J Surg* 1974;128:439

256. Berliner SD. The Henry operation for incarcerated and strangulated femoral hernias. *Arch Surg* 1992;127:314

257. Bendavid R. A femoral "umbrella" for femoral hernia repair. *Surg Gynecol Obstet* 1987;165:153

258. Bendavid R. Femoral hernias: primary versus recurrence. *Int Surg* 1989;74:99

259. Bendavid R. Recurrent femoral hernia treated by the insertion of a marlex umbrella. *Postgrad Gen Surg* 1992; 4:117

260. Bendavid R. Surgical workshop: a relaxing incision for femoral herniorrhaphy. Postgrad Gen Surg 1992;4:174

261. Moore TC, Stokes GE. Gastroschisis: report of two cases treated by a modification of Gross' operation for omphalocele. *Surgery* 1953;33:112

262. Cheselden W. The anatomy of the human body. London, England: Livingstone, Dodsley, Cadell, Baldwin and Lowndes; 1740

263. Mayo WJ. An operation for the radical cure of umbilical hernia. *Ann Surg* 1901;31:276

264. Rudran V, Jones R. Strangulated umbilical hernia in a child. *Br J Gen Pract* 1992;42:440

265. Abrahamson J, Elder S. "Shoelace" repair of large postoperative ventral abdominal hernias: a simple extraperitoneal technique. *Contemp Surg* 1988;32:24

266. Martin MC, Welch TP. Obturator hernia. *Br J Surg* 1974; 61:547

267. Gray SW, Skandalakis JE: Strangulated obturator hernia. In: Nyhus LM, Condon RE (eds), *Hernia,* 2nd ed. Philadelphia, PA: JB Lippincott; 1978:427

268. Hannington-Kiff JG. Obturator hernia: an elusive diagnosis. *J R Soc Med* 1992;85:508

269. Yip AWC, Ahchong AK, Lam KH. Obturator hernia: a continuing diagnostic challenge. *Surgery* 1993;113:266

270. Tsubono T, Fukuda M, Muto T. A case of bilateral obturator hernias: image diagnosis and description of a retropubic operative approach. *Surg Today* 23:159, 1993.

271. de Garengeot RJC. *Traite des Operations de Chirurgie,* 2 ed Paris, France: Huart; 1731:369

272. Lubat E, Gordon RB, Birnbaum BA, Megibow AJ. CT diagnosis of posterior perineal hernia. *AJR Am J Roentigenol* 1990;154:761

273. Spangen L. Spigelian hernia. *Surg Clin North Am* 64:351, 1984.

274. Azuma T, Nakamura S, Hatakeyama G, Nagahara N, et al. A Spigelian hernia in an infant. *Osaka City Med J* 1992;38:155

275. Ondo-N'Dong F, Lorofi R. Comes G, et al. Spigelian hernia: apropos of a series of 31 cases. *J Chir (Paris)* 1992; 129:210

276. Zimmerman LM, Anson BJ, et al. Ventral hernia due to normal banding of the abdominal muscles. *Surg Gynecol Obstet* 1944;78:535

277. Read RC: Spigelian hernia. In: Nyhus LM, Condon RE (eds), *Hernia,* 2nd ed. Philadelphia, PA: JB Lippincott; 1978:375

278. Testa T, Fallo E, Celoria G, et al. Spigelian hernia: its echotomographic diagnosis and surgical treatment. *G Chir* 1992;13:29

279. Hodgson TJ, Collins MC. Anterior abdominal wall hernias: diagnosis by ultrasound and tangential radiographs. *Clin Radiol* 1991;44:185

280. Mehta MH, Patel RV, Mehta SG: Congenital lumbar hernia. *J Pediatr Surg* 1992;27:1258

281. Attah M, Jibril JA, Yakubu A, et al. Congenital sciatic hernia. *J Pediatr Surg* 1992;27:1603

282. Gaffney LB, Schanno J. Sciatic hernia: a case for congenital occurrence. *Am J Surg* 1958;95:974

283. Black S. Sciatic hernia. In: Nyhus LM, Condon RE (eds), *Hernia,* 2nd ed. Philadelphia, PA: JB Lippincott; 1978:443

284. Gallie WE, Le Mesurier AB. Living sutures in the treatment of hernia. *Can Med Assoc J* 1923;13:468

285. Gallie WE, Le Mesurier AB. The transplantation of the fibrous tissues in the repair of anatomical defects. *Br J Surg* 1924;12:289

286. Gallie WE. Closing very large hernial openings. *Ann Surg* 1932;96:551

287. Hamilton JE. The repair of large or difficult hernias with mattressed outlay grafts of fascia lata: a 21 year experience. *Ann Surg* 1968;167:85

288. Thompson W. Radical cure of inguinal hernia with a plastic insert. *Lancet* 1948;2:182

289. Schofield TL. Polyvinyl alcohol sponge: an inert plastic

for use as a prosthesis in the repair of large hernias. *Br J Surg* 1955;42:618

290. Gosset J. Bandes de peau totale comme materiel de suture autoplastique en chirurgie. *Chirurgie* 1949;75:277

291. Abel AL, Hunt AH. Stainless steel wire for closing abdominal incisions and for repair of herniae. *Br Med J* 1948;2:379

292. Abel AL, Clain A. The surgical treatment of large incisional herniae using stainless steel wire. *Br J Surg* 1960; 48:42

293. Abel AL, Clain A. Incisional hernia. Considerations in the surgical treatment of large incisional hernias using stainless steel wire. In: Nyhus LM, Harkins HN (eds), *Hernia*. Philadelphia, PA: JB Lippincott; 1964:390

294. Hunter RR. Anatomical repair of midline incisional hernia. *Br J Surg* 1971;58:888

295. Abrahamson J, Eldar S. A new method of repair of large postoperative ventral abdominal hernias. *Dig Surg* 1984; 1:117

296. Abrahamson J, Eldar S. A new method of repair of large postoperative ventral abdominal hernias. Paper presented at American College of Surgeons 71st Annual Clinical Congress, Chicago, Oct 1985.

297. Abrahamson J, Eldar S. Extraperitoneal repair of large postoperative ventral abdominal hernias—shoelace technique. *Theor Surg* 1987;2:70

298. Bucknall TE, Ellis H. Abdominal wound closure: a comparison of monofilament nylon and polyglycolic acid. *Surgery* 1981;89:672

299. Ellis H, Gajraj H, George CD. Incisional hernias, when do they occur? *Br J Surg* 1983;70:290

300. Harding KG, Mudge M, et al. Late development of incisional hernia: an unrecognised problem. *Br Med J* 1983; 286:519

301. Mudge M, Hughes LE. Incisional hernia: a 10 year prospective study of incidence and attitudes. *Br J Surg* 1985;72:70

302. Hesselink VJ, Luijendijk RW, De Wilt JHW, et al. An evaluation of risk factors in incisional hernia recurrence. *Surg Gynecol Obstet* 1993;3:228

303. Donaldson DR, Hegarty JH, et al. The lateral paramedian incision—an experience with 850 cases. *Br J Surg* 1982;69:630

304. Pollock AV. Laparotomy. *J R Soc Med* 1981;74:480

305. Richards PC, Balch CM, Aldrete JS. Abdominal wound closure: a randomized prospective study of 571 patients comparing continuous versus interrupted suture techniques. *Ann Surg* 1983;197:238

306. Ellis H, Coleridge-Smith PD, Joyce AD. Abdominal incisions: vertical or transverse? *Postgrad Med J* 1984;60:407

307. Chevrel JP. Postoperative complications. In: Chevrel JP (ed), *Surgery of the Abdominal Wall*. Berlin, Germany: Springer-Verlag; 1987:83

308. Abrahamson J. Epigastric, umbilical and ventral hernia. In: Cameron JL (ed), *Current Surgical Therapy—3*, Toronto, Canada: BC Decker; 1989:417

309. Manninen MJ, Lavonius M, Perhoniemi VJ. Results of incisional hernia repair: a retrospective study of 172 unselected hernioplasties. *Eur J Surg* 1991;157:29

310. Ellis H. Internal overhealing: the problem of intraperitoneal adhesions. *World J Surg* 1980;4:303

311. Elkins TE, Stovall TG, Warren J, et al. A histologic evaluation of peritoneal injury and repair: implications for adhesion formation. *Obstet Gynecol* 1987;70:225

312. Stark M. Suturing of peritoneum. *World J Surg* 1993; 17:419

313. Goligher JC, Irvin TT, et al. A controlled clinical trial of three methods of closure of laparotomy wounds. *Br J Surg* 1975;62:823

314. Rubio PA. Closure of abdominal wounds with continuous nonabsorbable sutures: experience in 1697 cases. *Int Surg* 1991;76:159

315. Bartlett LC. Pressure necrosis is the primary cause of wound dehiscence. *Can J Surg* 1985;28:27

316. Ponka JL. *Hernias of the Abdominal Wall*. Philadelphia, PA: WB Saunders; 1981

317. Bucknall TE, Cox PJ, Ellis H. Burst abdomen and incisional hernia: a prospective study of 1129 major laparotomies. *Br Med J* 1982;284:931

318. Read RC, Yoder G. Recent trends in the management of incisional herniation. *Arch Surg* 1989;124:485

319. Lamont PM, Ellis H. Incisional hernia in re-opened abdominal incisions: an overlooked risk factor. *Br J Surg* 1988;75:374

320. Efron G. Abdominal wound disruption. *Lancet* 1965;1: 1287

321. Peacock EE Jr. Subcutaneous extraperitoneal repair of ventral hernias: a biological basis for fascial transplantation. *Ann Surg* 1975;181:722

322. Read RC. Attenuation of the rectus sheath in inguinal herniation. *Am J Surg* 1970;120:610

323. Franke A, Tessmann D, Busch H, et al. Bipolar impulses or direct current as an adjuvant treatment of incisional hernia? Comparative experimental animal study. *Z Exp Chir Transplant Kunstliche Organe* 1990; 23:55

324. Pekarsky VV, Shpilevoy PK, Deruchina MS, Gluschuk SP. Inplantable electric stimulator-alloprosthesis in repair of postoperative hernias. *PACE* 1991;14:135

325. Moreno IG. Chronic eventrations and large hernias: preoperative treatment by progressive pneumoperitoneum. *Surgery* 1947;22:945

326. Dixon CF. Repair of incisional hernia. *Surg Gynecol Obstet* 1929;48:700

327. Read RC. [Editorial comment]. *Curr Surg* 1990;47:278

328. Thomas WO III, Parry SW, Rodning CB. Ventral/incisional abdominal herniorrhaphy by fascial partition/release. *Plast Reconstr Surg* 1993;91:1080

329. Abrahamson J, Eldar S. Abdominal incisions. *Lancet* 1989;1:847

330. Judd ES. The prevention and treatment of ventral hernia. *Surg Gynecol Obstet* 1912;14:175

331. Gibson CL. Operation for cure of large ventral hernia. *Ann Surg* 1920;72:214

332. Nuttal HCW. Rectus transplantation for midline incisional herniae. *Br J Surg* 1937;25:344

333. Watson LF. *Hernia: Anatomy, Etiology, Symptoms, Diagnosis, Differential Diagnosis, Prognosis, and the Operative and Injec-*

tion Treatment, 2nd ed. London, England: Henry Kimpton; 1938

334. Wells CA. Hernia—incisional and umbilical. *Ann R Coll Surg (Engl)* 1956;19:316

335. Madden JL. *Atlas of Technics in Surgery,* 2nd ed. New York, NY: Appleton-Century-Croft; 1964

336. Amid PK, Shulman AG, Lichtenstein IL. Selecting synthetic mesh for the repair of groin hernia. *Postgrad Gen Surg* 1992;4:150

337. Greene MA, Mullins RJ, Malangoni MA, et al. Laparotomy wound closure with absorbable polyglycolic acid mesh. *Surg Gynecol Obstet* 1993;176:213

338. Bleichrodt RP, Simmermacher RKJ, Van der Lei B, Schakenraad JM. Expanded polytetrafluoroethylene patch versus polypropylene mesh for the repair of contaminated defects of the abdominal wall. *Surg Gynecol Obstet* 1993;176:18

339. Mora EM, Cardona MA, Simmons RL. Enteric bacteria and ingested inert particles translocate to intraperitoneal prosthetic materials. *Arch Surg* 1991;126:157

340. Flament JB, Palot JP. Use of two prostheses in the surgical repair of recurrent hernias. (Trivellini G, Danelli PG, eds), *Postgrad Gen Surg* 1992;4:135

341. Amid PK, Shulman AG, Lichtenstein IL. An experimental evaluation of a new composite mesh with the selective property of incorporation to the abdominal wall without adhering to the intestines. *J Biomed Mater Res* 1994;28:373

342. Amid PK, Shulman AG, Lichtenstein IL. A simple stapling technique for prosthetic repair of massive incisional hernias. *Am Surg* 1994;60:934

343. Costalat G, Noel P, Vernhet J. Method for the correction of ventral hernia using a parietal prosthesis held by a metal stapler: a propos of seventy cases. *Ann Chir* 1991; 45:882

344. Rosenthal D, Franklin ME Jr. Use of percutaneous stitches in laparoscopic mesh hernioplasty. *Surg Gynecol Obstet* 1993;176:491

345. Matapurkar BG, Gupta AK, Agarwal AK. A new technique of "Marlex-peritoneal sandwich" in the repair of large incisional hernias. *World J Surg* 1991;15:768

346. Abrahamson J. Treatment of a giant abdominal incisional hernia by intraperitoneal Teflon mesh implant. (Druart ML, Limbosch JM, eds). *Postgrad Gen Surg* 1992; 4:121

347. Devlin HB. Peristomal hernia. In: Dudley H (ed), *Operative Surgery Alimentary Tract and Abdominal Wall,* vol 1, 4th ed. London, England: Butterworths; 1983:441

348. Leslie DR. The parastomal hernia. *Aust NZ J Surg* 1981; 51:485

349. De Ruiter P, Bijnen AB. Successful local repair of paracolostomy hernia with a newly developed prosthetic device. *Int J Colorectal Dis* 1992;7:132

350. Byers JM, Steinberg JB, Postier RG. Repair of parastomal hernias using polypropylene mesh. *Arch Surg* 1992; 127:1246

351. Alexandre JH, Bouillot JL. Paracolostomal hernia: repair with use of a Dacron prosthesis. *World J Surg* 1993;17:680

15

Biliary and Gastrointestinal Fistulas

Scott M. Berry ▪ *Josef E. Fischer*

▪ BILIARY FISTULAS

A fistula is an abnormal transmural communication between two epithelialized surfaces. Biliary fistulas, like other fistulas, can be external or internal, spontaneous or postoperative. Biliary fistulas have been reported to arise from the gallbladder, cystic duct remnant, common bile duct, and hepatic ducts.[1–17] Internal fistula tracts usually terminate in the duodenum, colon, stomach, common bile duct, or lung.[4,7,9–15,17] External fistulas usually exit the body through drains, drain tracts, incisions, or the skin of the right upper quadrant, right flank, or umbilicus.[6,8,16,18–35] In developed countries, biliary fistulas most commonly occur after hepatobiliary or pancreatic surgery. Neoplasia, such as pancreatic adenocarcinoma or cholangiocarcinoma, and inflammation, such as occurs with echinococcal cysts, amebic abscesses, or untreated cholelithiasis, are more common etiologic agents of biliary fistulas in developing nations. The clinical presentation of biliary fistulas is variable and depends on their anatomic course and the underlying disease process. Appropriate nonoperative and/or operative management also depends on the underlying anatomy and pathology.

HISTORY

Thilesus is credited with the first report of spontaneous external biliary fistulas in 1670.[1,36] In 1890, Courvoisier described 499 cases of perforated gallbladder, of which 169 resulted in spontaneous external biliary fistulas.[36,37]

Modern biliary tract surgery has made spontaneous external biliary fistulas very rare, even though biliary tract stone disease is exceedingly common. Since the advent of cholecystectomy by Langenbuch in 1882,[38] there have been less than 75 cases of spontaneous external biliary fistulas reported.[1]

Spontaneous internal biliary fistula are more common and usually result from gallstone-associated acute or chronic cholecystitis. Fistulous communication between the biliary passages and other viscera have been regarded as pathologic curiosities because of their variety and unusual nature.[39] In 1854, Courvoisier published the first report of gallstone passage through a cholecystoduodenal fistula causing a small bowel obstruction at the terminal ileum, a phenomena generally termed *gallstone ileus*.[40] In 1872, Roth reported an 8% incidence of internal biliary fistulas in patients dying from biliary tract stone disease.[4] In 1890, Courvoisier reported internal biliary fistula in 4.8% of patients dying of biliary tract stone disease, and in 2.6% of patients with gallstones who died of other causes.[4,37]

The first case of choledochoduodenal fistula is reported in the London Medical Gazette in 1940. Since that time, approximately 150 cases of choledochoduodenal fistulas have been reported.[41] In the past, 80% of these fistulas were the result of peptic ulcer disease.[41–43] However, choledochoduodenal fistula has become a well-described complication of endoscopic sphincterotomy. Whether the widespread use of this procedure has now made it the most common cause of choledochoduodenal fistulas is unknown.[42,43]

Cholecystobiliary fistula (Mirizzi syndrome) was first described in 1948.[12] Since that time, sporadic reports have appeared in the literature. In 1989, Csendes and associates[44] reported the incidence of the Mirizzi syndrome in 17 395 patients undergoing surgery for biliary tract stone disease to be 1.3%, and suggested dividing the syndrome into four types, depending upon the percent circumference of the common bile duct involved. Type I lesions exhibit external compression of the common bile duct and represent 11% of Mirizzi syndrome cases. Type II lesions involve less than one-third of the common bile duct circumference and represent 41% of cases. Type III lesions involve up to two-thirds of the common bile duct diameter and include 44% of cases. In type IV lesions, the common bile duct is completely destroyed. Fortunately, only 4% of Mirizzi syndrome cases are of this type.

Postoperative external biliary fistulas followed the development of biliary tract surgery. Initial surgical management of gallstones evolved from allowing cutaneous perforation of the gallbladder, prior to the 1600s, to incision of subcutaneous biliary abscesses with percutaneous removal of stones. A cholecystostomy, carried out by Bobbs in 1876, is the first report of a persistent postoperative external biliary fistula, albeit intentional. Incision of the gallbladder with suture to the anterior abdominal wall was performed by both Simms and Kocher in 1878. Langenbuch performed the first cholecystectomy in 1882. With improvements in perioperative, anesthesia, and intraoperative technique, the incidence of biliary fistula after open cholecystectomy is now 0.02% to 0.2%.[45] Although the exact incidence of biliary fistula after laparoscopic cholecystectomy is unknown, it is probably higher than for open cholecystectomy.[46–54]

Cystic-duct remnant fistulas are rare. The most commonly involved viscus is the duodenum (57%), followed by the colon (29%), and the stomach (14%).[55]

Biliary fistula after pancreatoduodenectomy was reported not long after descriptions of the operation appeared in 1935,[56] and are currently the second most common complication following pancreatoduodenectomy.[23,57] The first large series of hepatic resections, reported by Keen in 1899, heralded the birth of biliary fistulas following hepatic resection.[58] Currently, biliary fistulas complicate 1% to 3% of liver resections, except in cirrhotic livers or when left trisegmentectomies are performed. Biliary fistulas complicate 30% of these particular cases.[59] After liver transplantation, biliary fistulas occur in 10% to 15% of patients.[60,61]

EPIDEMIOLOGY AND ETIOLOGY

Spontaneous causes of biliary fistulas have become rare, with early intervention for biliary tract stone disease, bile duct cancer, and hepatic abscess.[36] In underdeveloped countries, untreated biliary tract stone disease, amebic abscesses, and echinococcal cysts are the most common causes of cholecystoenteric and hepatodochoenteric or cutaneous fistulas, and the epidemiology reflects the incidence of these diseases. Spontaneous internal biliary fistulas are usually cholecystoduodenal (77%), cholecystocolic (15%), cholecystogastric (6%), or cholecystocholedochal (2%).[7] In >90% of cases, biliary-enteric fistulas arise from biliary calculi with associated acute and chronic cholecystitis.[4,5] Other causes include peptic ulcer disease, endoscopic sphincterotomy, pancreatobiliary malignancy, tuberculosis, mucormycosis, polyarteritis nodosa, and *Salmonella typhi*.[1,36] An inflammatory or neoplastic process that causes gallbladder, common bile duct, or liver adherence and eventual erosion into surrounding structures is the common basis for internal fistula formation (Table 15–1). Spontaneous external fistulas are now exceedingly rare. Their pathophysiology is the same as for internal spontaneous fistulas, cholelithiasis, cholangiocarcinoma, echinococcosis, and amebiasis as common causes.[1,36,62,63]

Because the most common cause of spontaneous biliary fistulas in advanced countries is biliary tract stone disease, the incidence of this complication mirrors the inci-

TABLE 15–1. BILIARY FISTULAS

	Etiology and Occurrence (%)	Anatomic Characteristics
Spontaneous	Cholelithiasis: 2–8	Cholecystoduodenal Cholecystocolic Cholecystogastric Cholecystocholedochal
	Echinococcus: 2–22	Hepatodochopleural Hepatodochobronchial Hepatodochocutaneous
	Amebic abscess: <1	Hepatodochobronchial Hepatodochocutaneous
	Malignancy: <1	Cholecystocutaneous Hepatodochocutaneous
	Peptic ulcer: <1	Choledochoduodenal

Postoperative	Cholecystectomy:
	  Open 0.02–0.2
	  Laparoscopic 0.2–3
	Choledochotomy: 1.3
	Liver resection: 1–3
	  left trisegmentectomy 30
	  cirrhotic liver 30
		Cystic duct-cutaneous
		Hepatodochocutaneous
		Choledochocutaneous
		Choledochocutaneous
		Hepatodochocutaneous

	Liver transplant: 10–15	Choledochocutaneous Hepatodochocutaneous
	Pancreaticoduo- denectomy: 5–30	Choledochocutaneous
Traumatic	Penetrating: 2–4	Biliary tree to adjacent injured organs
	Blunt: <1	Hepatodochocutaneous Hepatodochobronchial

dence of gallstone disease. Cholecystoenteric fistulas are seen chiefly in females 50 to 70 years of age, and the female to male ratio is approximately 3:1. Over 90% of spontaneous fistulas are associated with biliary tract stone disease. In addition, spontaneous biliary fistulas are common in certain groups of stoic native Americans, such as the Pima Indians.[64] Choledochoduodenal fistulas are the only internal biliary fistula not commonly caused by cholelithiasis. Eighty percent of these are the result of posterior-penetrating duodenal ulcers. The epidemiology follows that of peptic ulcer disease, affecting males between the ages of 20 and 50, with a peak incidence at 40 years of age. The female to male ratio is 1:2 to 4. Endoscopic sphincterotomy has become a more prevalent cause of choledochoduodenal fistulas, and may now be the primary etiologic agent in this type of fistula.

Because hepatobiliary and pancreatic malignancy are more common in males, spontaneous biliary fistulas from these causes are more common in males; the female to male ratio is 1:4.

Hepatic infection by echinococcus or amoeba and the surgical treatment of these infectious processes can lead to biliary tract fistulas. In contrast, pyogenic liver abscesses and their surgical treatment are not commonly known to lead to biliary fistulas.[65-70] The most common fistulas occurring in association with echinococcus are hepatodochobronchial or hepatodochopleural and these complicate 2% to 22% of echinococcus cases.[71] In addition, hepatodochocutaneous fistulas following amebic or echinococcal disease have also been reported.[36]

Echinococcus granulosus is a common cause of spontaneous biliary fistulas worldwide.[72] Sheep are the main intermediate host and dogs are the principal host. These infections occur mainly in the sheep-raising areas of the Mediterranean, Middle East, eastern Africa, Australia, New Zealand, and Latin America, although cases in Alaska and Canada have been reported. *Echinococcus multilocularis* causes a similar disease in humans, but occurs in the Northern Hemisphere, Europe, north-central United States, Canada, and Alaska. Rodents are the intermediate host and foxes are the definitive hosts. Man is infected with both species of echinococcus by ingestion of larvae or cysts from infected animals. While echinococcal cysts can occur in any organ, the primary sites are the right lobe of the liver (65%) and the lung (20%).[73] The hepatic cysts calcify or suppurate and erode into adjacent structures; the diaphragm and lung parenchyma in 2% to 22%, the pleural cavity in 1%, or the gastrointestinal tract or skin in less than 0.5%.[73] When daughter cysts are found in the sputum, they are almost always of hepatic, rather than pulmonary origin.[73]

Entamoeba histolytica is another common cause of spontaneous biliary fistulas found worldwide.[74] Although the exact incidence is unknown, amebic infections can, and have, reached epidemic proportions in

developing countries. By contrast, <1% of the United States population is infected with amebiasis and, therefore, biliary fistulas from this cause are not common in the United States. Transmission is by the fecal-oral route and by sexual contact. The disease is much more common in males, with a male-to-female ratio of 7:1. Most infected people are asymptomatic or present with colitis; the most common extraintestinal manifestation is right-sided liver abscess, which, like echinococcal cysts, suppurate through the diaphragm into the lung, or through the abdominal wall.

The majority of external biliary fistulas in developed countries are now postoperative and occur after percutaneous drainage of bile leak after cholecystectomy, hepatic resection, or pancreatic resection.[6,8,55] An emerging major cause of bile duct injury is laparoscopic cholecystectomy. In a recent review of 42 474 patients who underwent open cholecystectomy, only 9 (0.02%) developed postoperative biliary fistulas.[45] In contrast, biliary fistulas complicated 0.2% to 3% of cases after laparoscopic cholecystectomy. The great numbers of cholecystectomies, both open and laparoscopic, performed each year make this the most common antecedent operation of biliary fistula. Because of the prevalence of biliary tract stone disease in females, these fistulas, like spontaneous fistulas, are more common in females. Cystic duct remnants can be found in 30% to 85% of postcholecystectomy patients, and when the cystic duct or common bile duct becomes obstructed, fistulization to the duodenum, stomach, or colon can occur.[55]

Other operations complicated by biliary fistulas include hepatic resection[58,75-77] or transplantation,[78] and pancreatoduodenectomy.[22,23,57] Choledochoduodenostomy results in a 1.3% incidence of external biliary fistulas.[79] The epidemiology is somewhat different for biliary fistulas resulting from hepatic resection or transplantation than for those complicating biliary tract stone disease. Because cirrhosis- or hepatitis-induced hepatoma and metastatic cancer to the liver occur more frequently in males overall, the biliary fistulas associated with these surgical procedures, as well as for the fistulas associated with hepatic transplantation, are more common in males. Biliary fistula is the second most common complication following pancreatoduodenectomy.[23,57]

Blunt and penetrating hepatic trauma results in biliary fistulas in 2% to 4% of cases.[21-25] The great majority (85% to 95%) of these fistulas arise after blunt trauma from motor vehicle accidents. Other causes include falls (4%) and assaults (2%).[24] Most resolve spontaneously after a short period.[80]

ANATOMY

Because the gallbladder is supplied by end arteries, its poorly vascularized fundus is predisposed to pressure ischemia and necrosis when the cystic duct is obstructed.

Intense inflammation causes gallbladder adhesion to surrounding structures such as the first portion of the duodenum, hepatic flexure of the colon, or anterior abdominal wall. Subsequently, perforation can occur into these structures. Spontaneous internal fistulas from the gallbladder usually involve the duodenum (77%), right colon (15%), stomach (6%), or common bile duct (2%). External, spontaneous biliary fistulas involve the right upper quadrant (48%) or umbilicus (27%).[1,4,7,9–15,17]

The cystic duct remnant which remains after cholecystectomy also can be the source of a biliary fistula. The incidence of cystic duct remnant >10 mm in length varies from 63% to 83% after open cholecystectomy. The incidence after laparoscopic cholecystectomy very well may be higher because of reluctance to dissect the cystic duct–common bile duct junction.

The blood supply to the common bile duct is from the coalescence of vascular plexuses that arise from the axial 3-o'clock and 9-o'clock vessels. The blood supply to the axial vessels, and ultimately the common duct vascular network, is from the right hepatic artery above (60%) and the posterior-superior pancreatoduodenal artery below (40%).[81] However, the arterial blood supply to the superior portion of the extrahepatic biliary tree is variable, as is the blood supply to the right lobe of the liver.[82] In up to 17% of cases the common bile duct will be supplied from above by a replaced right hepatic artery.[23,82] Division or ligation of this vessel after extensive distal common bile duct dissection or common bile duct division can lead to complete devascularization of the extrahepatic biliary tree with resultant fistula formation.[23] Because of the anatomic proximity between the common bile duct and the duodenum as it approaches the ampulla of Vater, inflammation of the posterior duodenum by peptic ulceration can lead to adherence and eventual fistulization between these two structures.

PATHOPHYSIOLOGY

Physiology and Pathophysiology

Biliary secretions contain high concentrations of sodium, potassium and bicarbonate (Table 15–2). Since considerable energy is required to produce and secrete this electrolyte-rich fluid, rapid protein, energy, and electrolyte depletion can occur with biliary fistulas. In addition, patients with large bile losses seem to require more daily volume replacement than their measured losses would suggest. The loss of 1 to 2 L of this fluid through a fistula may be very difficult to manage because excessive amounts of sodium are required. This is due, in part, to the high sodium content of these secretions. We have found it useful, on occasion, to use 3% saline for resuscitation.

The 2 to 3 gm bile-acid pool secreted into the bowel

TABLE 15–2. PHYSIOLOGY BILIARY FISTULAS

Volume Output	NPO: 100–1000 mL/day Oral Diet: 1–2 L/day
Electrolytes	Na 130–165 mEq/L K 3–12 mEq/L Cl 90–180 mEq/L HCO 35 mEq/L Trace elements Zn, Cu, Mn
Nutrition	Protein enzyme loss—up to 75 g/day leading to protein malnutrition Enteral fat malabsorption-dermatitis, immune dysfunction because essential fatty acid deficiency
Immune Function	sIgA depleted by complete biliary diversion. Ultimate immune significance unclear but may predispose to translocation
Vitamins	Vitamin K-coagulopathy Vitamin D-osteomalacia, fractures, cardiac arrhythmias

lumen in response to meals circulates 6 to 10 times a day. Reabsorption of the 20 to 30 gm of bile acids presented to the small intestine is extremely efficient, with only 0.5 gm/day entering the colon. Disturbance in the otherwise efficient enterohepatic circulation of bile acids can lead to a number of clinical syndromes, including fat malabsorption, essential fatty–acid deficiency, zinc deficiency, bile-acid diarrhea, oxalosis, vitamin K deficiency with coagulopathy, vitamin D deficiency with osteomalacia, calcium deficiency with pathologic fractures and cardiac arrhythmias.[83,84] Internal biliary fistulas to the duodenum may not alter the enterohepatic circulation to any appreciable extent. However, biliary fistulas to the colon reduce the amount of bile acids available for digestion and, consequently, decrease the concentration of bile acids within the lumen of the small intestine. Impaired solubilization of dietary fat causes increased colonic luminal fat and secretory diarrhea. Diarrhea also can be caused by the presence of increased amounts of bile acids in the colon, leading to colitis. Bile acids also induce colonic mucosal adenylate cyclase, leading to profuse diarrhea.

Gastric mucosal exposure to high concentrations of biliary secretions, such as occurs with cholecystogastric fistulas, can lead to gastric mucosal injury ranging from diffuse gastritis to frank ulceration. Dyspepsia, anorexia, weight loss, and upper gastrointestinal hemorrhage all may occur secondary to the presence of bile acids in the stomach.

External losses of biliary secretions can lead to all of the same syndromes as cholecystocolonic fistulas, with the exception of bile acid–induced diarrhea. Volume depletion, with the resultant volume-contraction alkalosis, can occur rapidly with fistula losses that exceed 200 mL/day. However, more commonly, it occurs insidiously over days and may not be recognized by the clinician. In addition, the high sodium, potassium, and zinc content of biliary secretions can lead to severe deficits of these ions. A tube duodenostomy, which may drain up to 1 L/day, is a controlled biliary fistula and can lead to the same sequelae.

When lipid malabsorption from bile losses is severe, essential fatty acids will be depleted from cell membranes and will result in functional deficits ranging from scaling dermatitis to immunoincompetence. Regardless of whether enteral therapy or parenteral therapy is used, parenteral lipids can be used to supply 3% to 6% of the total caloric provision. This will prevent essential fatty–acid deficiency.

DIAGNOSIS, EVALUATION, AND MANAGEMENT

The signs and symptoms of internal fistulas range from imperceptible to severe. In general, the farther distal biliary fistulas enter into the gastrointestinal tract, the more symptomatic they become. External biliary fistulas usually are apparent and may exit through the right upper quadrant, right flank, or umbilicus. Postoperative fistulas are invariably through a drain, drain tract, or an incision line. The phases of management for biliary fistulas are similar to those for gastrointestinal fistulas, with emphasis on those aspects particularly troublesome when managing biliary fistulas (Table 15–3).

Recognition and Stabilization

Resuscitation. Resuscitating patients with biliary fistulas should proceed by standard life support protocol. After oxygen exchange is ensured, hemodynamic resuscitation should proceed. Volume depletion, with resultant volume-contraction alkalosis, can occur rapidly with fistula losses that exceed 200 mL/day. Normal saline with 30 to 40 mEq/L of potassium added per liter is the most appropriate resuscitation fluid for these patients, who are usually depleted of total body sodium and potassium.

Local Control. Wound care assumes a high priority because, if operation is necessary, it should not be done through a septic, indurated, cellulitic, and denuded abdominal wall.[85] Sump drains usually are not required for biliary fistula control. Simple "bagging" of fistulas may lead to skin closure over the fistula tract, and lead to abscess formation. However, this seems to be less of a problem than it is for gastrointestinal fistulas. Accurate records of fistula output are requisite to daily volume and electrolyte management. Local skin care is crucial and, consequently, many devices have been tried for the local management of fistula drainage.[86–90] Preventing

TABLE 15–3. BILIARY FISTULA TREATMENT GOALS

Resuscitation	Rehydration with normal saline Drainage of sepsis Na, Cl, HCO3, K, Zn, Cu, Mn repletion Local skin care and control of fistula drainage Nutritional management Measures to decrease fistula drainage (somatostatin, sphincter antispasmotics, stents, sphincterotomy)	Within 24–48 hours
Investigation	Definition of anatomy and pathophysiology (nuclear imaging, ERCP, PTCA) CT, MRI, US to localize and drain collections	After 7–10 days
Decision	Assess likelihood of spontaneous closure Plan therapeutic course Decide surgical timing	7–10 days to 4–6 weeks
Definitive Therapy	Operative procedure based on anatomic location and pathophysiology Ensure secure abdominal closure Gastrostomy Jejunostomy	When spontaneous closure is unlikely or after 6–8 weeks
Healing	Continue nutrition support	5–10 days after closure

excoriation or superinfection of the skin surrounding a fistulous tract is paramount. Good control involves integument protection and a mechanism of drainage collection.[86] Preparations useful in preventing skin maceration and breakdown include Karaya powder or seal, ileostomy cement, and glycerine. Ion exchange resins also may be helpful in preventing excoriation. We involve enterostomal therapists very quickly, since they are invaluable in this difficult portion of management. Stoma adhesive or similar products may be very effective; if one can achieve fixation to the skin, these can be left in place, provided that fistula drainage does not leak under the patch. When properly used, the skin underneath is well protected and skin healing can occur.

Somatostatin. Use of somatostatin in biliary fistulas has been advocated, but proof of efficacy is scant. Somatostatin decreases biliary secretions and, when used in biliary fistulas, a 50% reduction in fistula volume has been noted.[75] However, it also was noted that adequate surgical drainage and unobstructed distal bile flow were prerequisites to fistula closure. Thus, we feel that somatostatin may be useful in decreasing biliary fistula output and may accelerate closure but, as is the case for gastrointestinal fistulas, it likely will not affect ultimate closure rates. While it may be a useful adjunct, it does not substitute for the basic principles of adequate drainage and relief of distal obstruction.

Nutritional Management. Biliary juices possess high concentrations of sodium, potassium, and bicarbonate. As stated, patients with large bile losses seem to require more volume than their measured losses would suggest. Repleting the patient nutritionally may be very difficult because of the excessive amounts of sodium required and the energy used to bring plasma sodium concentrations up to that of biliary secretions. Most biliary fistulas can, and should, be cared for with enteral therapy.[91–93] A low-fat diet ostensibly may assist in decreasing fistula drainage. Other dietary restrictions should be dictated by co-morbid conditions, and not the presence of a fistula. Finally, it is occasionally necessary to refeed bile to resupply the enterohepatic circulation, thus increasing the bile-acid pool, among other beneficial effects. The effect has been difficult to quantify, but we believe that it does exist. Consequently, in the presence of large bile fistulas or biliary obstruction, every attempt should be made to refeed bile on a regular basis. Clearly this will require postpyloric nasointestinal tube placement, but we feel that the gains justify feeding-tube placement when a prolonged treatment course seems inevitable. Refeeding will in itself create some problems because of the bacterial contamination. Therefore, bile feeding should be carried out rapidly, without allowing the material to stand for a prolonged period of time. Alternatively, the bile can be refrigerated and warmed immediately prior to infusion into the bowel.

Antibiotics. Unless evidence of cholangitis, cellulitis, or abscess exists, antibiotic use should be reserved. The basic principle of draining purulent collections always should be followed. Antibiotics will not eradicate loculated sepsis without prior drainage. After sphincterotomy, the bile colonization rate approaches 100%. As long as adequate drainage is maintained and the gallbladder has been removed, this colonization poses little threat to the patient. However, the incidence of cholecystitis is 8% to 24% after sphincterotomy when the gallbladder is in situ. Whether antibiotics decrease this complication is unclear. However, in critically ill patients who are not good operative candidates, it seems prudent to attempt bile sterilization. While the presence of a stent may make this goal unobtainable, as long as the stent is not obstructed and bile flows freely, bacterial suppression without complete sterilization may be adequate.

Sphincter of Oddi Spasm. Stenosis at the level of the papilla can cause increased common bile duct pressures. Sphincter of Oddi dysfunction causing persistent biliary fistula is an unproven cause. Most studies of medical interventions that decrease intraductal pressures are targeted at the treatment of biliary dyskinesia. Regardless of the exact mechanism, treatments targeted at decreasing biliary sphincter pressures would seem warranted.

The calcium channel blocking agents nifedipine and nicardipine have both been shown to decrease biliary sphincter pressure because of their ability to relax smooth muscle.[94–96] While studies with nicardipine are lacking, nifedipine has been shown to be effective in relieving the pain associated with biliary dyskinesia. However, studies in biliary fistulas do not exist.[96,97] The action of nifedipine is dose dependent, with little observed change in biliary sphincter pressure at doses <20 mg.[95] Because cardiovascular side effects are common, doses should be titrated to desired response.

Nitrates also relax smooth muscle and can be useful in decreasing biliary sphincter pressure. Glyceryl trinitrate (1.2 mg given sublingual) has been shown to decrease biliary sphincter pressure significantly within 3 minutes of administration.[98] Because of its rapid onset and short duration, patients can dose themselves as needed rather than taking scheduled doses. Because of additive vasodilatory effects, it is probably unwise to use both calcium channel blocking agents and nitrates concurrently. One report of glyceryl trinitrate use in the management of biliary fistulas appears in the literature and suggests a beneficial effect on closure.[99]

Transcutaneous electric nerve stimulation (TENS) has been useful in patients with esophageal spasm, presumably due to vasoactive intestinal peptide (VIP)–releasing properties. TENS decreases biliary sphincter pressures and increases serum VIP levels in patients with biliary dyskinesia. In normal volunteers, TENS increases VIP levels without effect on biliary sphincter pressure.[100] Whether TENS application leads to persistent reduction in biliary tree pressures is unknown.

Prifinium bromide, pinaverium bromide, and hyoscine N-butyl-bromide are antispasmodics that have been shown to decrease sphincter of Oddi pressure.[101,102] Whether these drugs, in addition to the sphincter-altering hormones glucagon,[103,104] secretin,[98] cholecystokinin,[105] and somatostatin,[106] will find clinical utility in the medical treatment of biliary fistulas is still unknown.[107]

Because morphine has been shown to increase common bile duct pressure and biliary sphincter pressure,[108] use of parenteral nonsteroidals (ketorolac), or opiod-like analgesics that do not affect sphincter pressure (buprenophine or tramadol), may be desirable for pain management in patients with biliary fistulas.[109]

Nasobiliary Stents and Sphincterotomy. The morbidity and mortality associated with placement of nasobiliary and internal stents is much lower than the 5% to 8% for percutaneous and surgical decompressive measures.[110] Prior to advances in endoscopic techniques, persistent biliary fistulas all required surgery. When the fistula is not demonstrated by ERCP, sphincterotomy and stenting are unlikely to be successful in promoting fistula closure.[110] The decision to use sphincterotomy alone or to insert an endoprosthesis after sphincterotomy depends on the type of biliary obstruction. Resolution of common bile duct and intrahepatic duct fistulas depends on the etiology and anatomy of the fistula tract. Intrahepatic bile duct fistulas are the most difficult to manage endoscopically. This is mainly owing to the inaccessibility of intrahepatic duct pathology from the retrograde position, in addition to the often complex nature of intrahepatic duct fistulas. Fistulas of the common bile duct or hepatic ducts are usually the result of intraoperative injury, whereas spontaneous rupture of a cystic duct remnant or persistent T tube tract drainage are usually the result of distal obstruction by spasm, stone, tumor, or stricture. Sphincterotomy with placement of endoprosthesis is usually necessary to divert flow away from the fistula tract when common bile duct or hepatic duct injury is present. Sherman and associates[61] reported 18 biliary fistulas following liver transplantation (1.2%), of which 94% were managed successfully by nasobiliary tube (72%), internal stent plus sphincterotomy (17%), or internal stent alone (11%). The average time to closure in this group was 15 days. Conversely, when the intrahepatic ducts are dilated, percutaneous transhepatic drainage may be done with similar results.[27,111] In addition, intrahepatic-duct biliary fistulas occurring after hepatic resection have been treated with percutaneous injection of tetracycline as a sclerosing agent[34] and endoscopic embolization[33] into the well-formed fistula tract. Use of these techniques may avoid technically demanding reoperation.

When distal obstruction is the cause of cystic duct–stump blowout or persistent T tube tract drainage, sphincterotomy and/or removal of the stone without stent placement is all that is usually necessary to promote healing of the fistula tract. Fistulas originating from the gallbladder or cystic duct close rapidly with endoscopic treatment.[111–117] Endoscopic sphincterotomy without stent placement has been successfully used to treat internal cholecystocolonic fistulas,[118,119] bronchobiliary fistulas,[120] and pleurobiliary fistulas[121] with immediate symptomatic relief and closure.

When cystic duct fistula is persistent and not accessible by endoscopic or percutaneous transhepatic decompressive measures, it may be possible to occlude the cystic duct stump via the percutaneously placed drain. This technique involves passing a guidewire through the well-formed tract into the cystic duct stump. An angiographic embolization catheter then is positioned fluoroscopically, and the stump is occluded.[122] The success of this technique is dependent upon prior documentation of an unobstructed distal common bile duct.

Hydatid disease can lead to intrabiliary rupture in 5% to 25% of cases, with resultant biliary-hydatid cyst fistulas. Unless these fistulas are closed at the time of cyst resection, postoperative biliary fistulas will persist in 4% to 7% of patients. In addition, 11% of patients will develop ascending cholangitis.[123] Alper suggests performing choledochoduodenostomy at the time of hydatid cystectomy to obviate these complications, but a decreased incidence of fistula formation has not been documented. In addition, 11% of patients treated with choledochoduodenostomy developed ascending cholangitis.[124] External biliary fistulas following surgery for hydatid disease virtually always close and, therefore, operative intervention should not be considered unless the fistula persists for more than 3 weeks.[125] In the 5% of external biliary fistulas that persist, endoscopic sphincterotomy with or without stent placement will close nearly 100% of fistulas within 4 weeks. The average time to closure after sphincterotomy is 7 days.[125] Endoscopic sphincterotomy obviates the need for reexploration and, therefore, is considered the procedure of choice for these complications.

Investigation

Endoscopic Retrograde Cholangiopancreatography. Biliary fistulas should be investigated by endoscopic retrograde cholangiopancreatography (ERCP). The site of the fistula, the etiology, as well as the status of the distal biliary tree can be ascertained by ERCP in >90% of cases.[118,126,110] Furthermore, ERCP can be performed in the absence of dilated common and intrahepatic ducts. However, if the biliary tree has been ligated or is not in continuity at the level of the common bile duct, ERCP likely will not reveal the fistula. In addition to the direct information that ERCP provides, it also may provide indirect information that influences operative plans. Thus, when ERCP does not demonstrate the fistula, sphincterotomy and stenting are unlikely to be successful and an operation will likely be necessary.[110]

Percutaneous Transhepatic Cholangiography. Percutaneous transhepatic cholangiography (PTCA) provides excellent anatomic detail of the biliary tree and readily can identify the site of most biliary fistulas. In addition, once access is gained into the intrahepatic biliary tree, decompression can also be performed by this route. Access to the biliary tree often is dependent on the size of the intrahepatic ducts. Furthermore, if the distal common duct is obstructed by stone or tumor, interventions to relieve the obstruction will not be possible without endoscopic or surgical intervention. One trial reported spontaneous closure of biliary fistulas in 13 patients managed by the percutaneous technique. However, when the fistula was associated with biliary stricture, half of their patients required surgical intervention for fistula resolution.[111,127] Therefore, PTCA may be useful for anatomic definition and decompression, but it is unlikely that it will be useful for definitive management of a pathologic distal biliary tree.

Nuclear Scans. Nuclear scans may be useful initial tests when postoperative injury of the extrahepatic biliary tree is suspected. Because of their relative ease to perform and their noninvasive nature, they are the procedure of choice in our institution for evaluating the biliary tree in patients suspected of having cystic duct leaks or a biliary tree injury after laparoscopic cholecystectomy. For intrahepatic duct injuries and obvious fistulas, endoscopic or PTCA are necessary for anatomic definition, and nuclear scans can be omitted.

Computed Tomography, Magnetic Resonance Imaging, Ultrasound. These imaging modalities seldom will demonstrate the precise fistula anatomy and, therefore, are not considered primary diagnostic modalities in the evaluation of a biliary fistula. Their utility, as is the case for gastrointestinal fistulas, is the localization of undrained collections, evaluation of the adequacy of collection drainage, and evaluation of tumor recurrence. When symptoms are persistent or sepsis occurs, these studies should be used liberally to localize treatable causes.

Decision

In the absence of distal obstruction, most postoperative biliary fistulas can be managed expectantly with drainage and low-fat diet and will close spontaneously with an average time to closure of 35 days.[25,128,129] If distal obstruction exists, endoscopic sphincterotomy, with or without percutaneous transhepatic or endoscopic transsphincteric stent, will allow decompression while spontaneous closure proceeds, with an average time to closure of 7 days.[26–32] If the fistula persists after these interventions, sclerosis or embolization of the well-formed fistulous tract has been reported.[33,34] If after 6 to 8 weeks of nonoperative management, the fistula persists without signs of closure, an operation may be necessary. This decision should be tempered by the etiology of the fistula, its anatomic location, its physiological and psychological impact on the patient, the medical status of the patient, and the capabilities of the surgeon.

Definitive Therapy

Cholecystic Fistulas. Unless the gallbladder will serve as a decompressive conduit, it should be removed at the time of surgery for cholecystic fistulas. When the fistula is from the cystic duct stump, this should likewise be re-

sected after cholangiography has demonstrated the extent of remaining cystic duct remnant. The secondary fistula defect at the termination of the fistulous tract should be repaired primarily (Fig 15–1). When the termination is in the duodenum, a Heinicke-Mikulicz–type closure of the freshened fistula orifice should be done. When a large duodenal defect results and primary closure is attempted, omental or serosal patch reinforcement, or exclusion and bypass with the tube duodenostomy also should be considered.[34,35] When the stomach is involved, layered primary closure with postoperative gastric decompression is indicated. It is rarely necessary to perform other gastric procedures. Diffuse gastritis and minor ulcerations can be expected to heal after fistula disconnection. When ulceration is severe, gastric wedge resection may be necessary. In addition, if the patient is nutritionally at risk, feeding jejunostomy should be considered.[130–132] When termination is in the colon, primary closure should proceed by established surgical standards. If the colon has been adequately cleared of particulate matter by preoperative bowel preparation, primary closure can proceed. Although rarely necessary, when preparation is suboptimal, consideration can be given to fecal diversion. Finally, it is important to separate the fresh suture lines by interposing healthy tissue after fistula division and repair is complete.

Recently, opinion has moved away from repair of what is still a common cause of internal fistulization, that which occurs with gallstone ileus. The goal of operation should be relief of bowel obstruction. In previous years, repair of the internal fistula was deemed essential; at present, many think this is unnecessary. When there are no symptoms referable to the biliary tract, stomach, or duodenum, the biliary tree should not be approached.

Cholecystocholedochal Fistulas. The treatment of cholecystocholedochal fistulas (Mirizzi Syndrome) depends on the Mirizzi syndrome–type encountered.[12,13,44,133–134] Type I is external compression of the common bile duct, without fistula formation.[44] Consequently, management is similar to that of biliary tract stone disease. Particular attention should be paid to the dissection between the gallbladder and the common bile duct. Chronic inflammation can lead to dense adhesions between these two structures, placing the common bile duct at risk for damage. Mirizzi types II through IV all represent cholecystocholedochal fistulas. The gallbladder should be at least partially removed and the impacted stone extracted. The common bile duct defect then can be managed in three different ways (Fig 15–2). The first involves complete removal of the gallbladder with primary closure of the common bile duct defect after a T tube is inserted through a separate

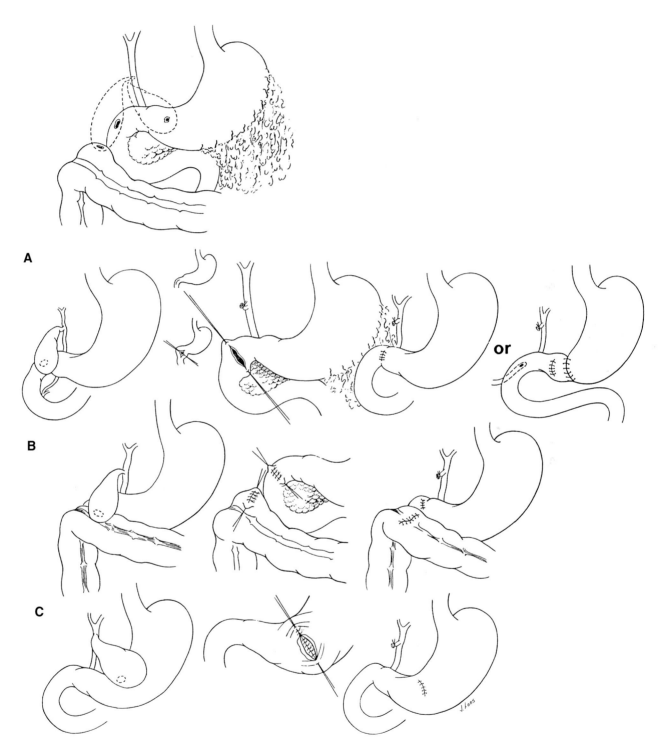

Figure 15–1. Management of cholecystointestinal fistulas. **A.** Cholecystoduodenal fistula management with cholecystectomy and Heinicke-Mickulicz duodenoplasty or cholecystectomy with duodenal exclusion. **B.** Cholecystocolic fistula management with cholecystectomy and layered primary closure of the colonic defect. **C.** Cholecystogastric fistula management with cholecystectomy and layered primary closure of the stomach defect.

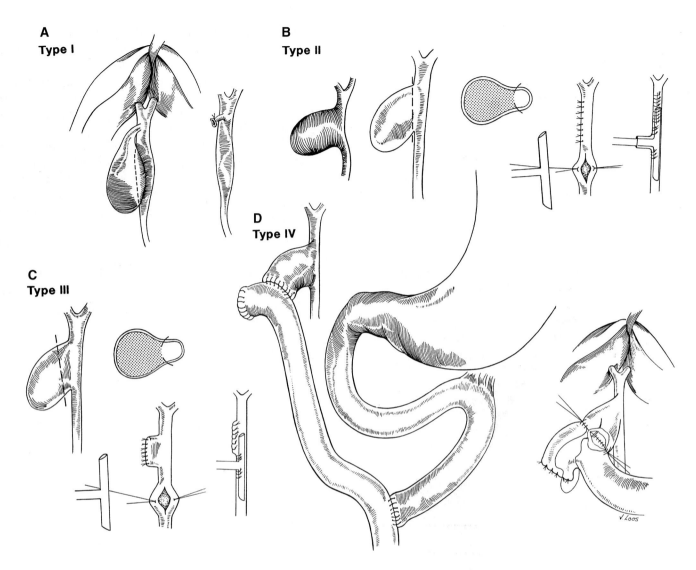

Figure 15–2. Management of the various Mirizzi syndrome types. **A.** Type I lesion is managed by cholecystectomy with particular care when dissecting the plane between the gallbladder and common bile duct. **B.** Type II lesions are managed by cholecystectomy, stone extraction, choledochoplasty, and t tube choledochostomy done through a separate choledochotomy. **C.** Type III lesions are managed by partial cholecystectomy, stone extraction, choledochoplasty using part of the gallbladder wall, and t tube choledochostomy done through a separate choledochotomy. **D.** Type IV lesions are managed by cholecystojejunostomy with stone extraction. Dissection in the fibrotic triangle of Calot should not be attempted.

choledochotomy. This may be appropriate when type II Mirizzi syndrome is present, the duct is well dilated, and the stone and fistula are small.[44,133,134] Narrowing of the common duct is a risk in this type of operation. Alternatively, part of the gall bladder wall can be left intact and used for flap closure over the common duct defect. This may be more appropriate for larger common duct defects, such as with type III lesions. While this type of operation will lessen the risk of narrowing, we nevertheless recommend T tube placement through a separate choledochotomy. Finally, the gallbladder can be partially removed and the remnant anastomosed to the duodenum or to a Roux-en-Y limb of jejunum.[133] This may be the most appropriate treatment for type IV

fistulas because it not only lessens the chance of narrowing, but also obviates the need for extensive dissection in the fibrotic triangle of Calot. In addition, when internal drainage is accomplished through a cholecystojejunostomy or choledochoduodenostomy, T tube placement may be unnecessary.

Choledochoduodenal Fistulas. The exact incidence of choledochoduodenal fistulas is unknown, since many patients will be asymptomatic or have only minor symptoms. Consequently, surgical therapy is reserved for symptomatic patients only. Because the etiology of choledochoduodenal fistulas is peptic ulcer disease in the majority of patients, surgical therapy most often will be directed at the ulcer disease. When ulcer resection is undertaken and a fistulous communication between the common bile duct and duodenum is discovered, the common bile duct should be divided and choledochojejunostomy performed (Fig 15–3). The risk of common duct narrowing or postoperative stricture is great when primary suture repair of the common duct defect is attempted in a nondilated, inflamed common duct. Alternatively, if the common duct is dilated and ulcer surgery preserves the anatomic proximity between the bile duct and duodenum, choledochoduodenostomy can be performed (Fig 15–3). This should be reserved for only the most optimal of situations. If either the bile duct or duodenal stump have questionable blood supply, the anastomosis surely will fail. Finally, cholecystectomy, tube duodenostomy, and T tube drainage of the common bile duct is recommended.

Echinococcal Disease. Biliary fistulas from echinococcal disease occur in 6% of cases and usually are adequately treated at the time the underlying disease process is treated surgically.[136] The cyst is removed and the wall inspected for biliary communications. Small fistulas require no specific treatment, while larger ones should be sutured. The residual cavity then is chemically sterilized.[136] The cyst cavity then can be managed by suture closure, omental or muscle flap obliteration, or closed-suction drainage. Internal drainage and marsupialization are no longer used after hydatid cyst resection. Of those fistulas that persist in the postoperative period, most will close spontaneously, provided the distal common duct is not obstructed by echinococcal debris. Therefore, ERCP and sphincterotomy, with or without nasobiliary stent placement, should be the first step in treating a patient with a postoperative biliary fistula from echinococcal disease.

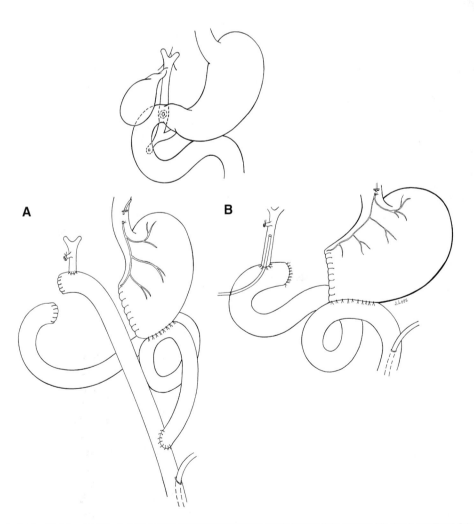

Figure 15–3. Choledochoduodenal fistula management. **A**. Roux-en-Y choledochojejunostomy should be done if the common bile duct is nondilated. Primary repair may lead to narrowing or stricture. **B**. If the common bile duct is dilated, and common duct–duodenal proximity is preserved, side-to-side or end-to-side choledochoduodenostomy can be performed.

Echinococcal disease can also lead to bronchobiliary fistulas. In general, for all types of bronchobiliary communications, it is essential to establish whether an extrahepatic biliary tree communication exists or if common bile duct obstruction is present. Overlooking a communication can lead to therapeutic failure, as will bile duct obstruction. It is also important to identify whether the right pleural cavity is involved, as is the case in over 97% of echinococcal bronchobiliary fistulas.[73] Other important factors to consider when planning an operative approach include the cyst size and the time since rupture.

In most cases, the approach is through a posterolateral right 6th or 7th intercostal space incision. Occasionally, a right thoracoabdominal approach is required. The lower right lobe is freed from the dome of the diaphragm until the fistulous diaphragmatic defect is found. The hepatic cavity is evacuated through this opening and a drain is placed through a separate stab wound. The diaphragmatic defect then is closed. To decrease the chance of postoperative infection, preferably this is done with a monofilament, nonabsorbable suture. If rupture into the lung has been recent, and no pulmonary cavity exists, closure of the bronchial defects with tube thoracostomy drainage of the pleural space is all that is necessary. Finally, a chronic lung abscess with sclerotic walls mandates pulmonary resection.

The transabdominal approach may be useful when the cyst is below the right costal margin, for recent ruptures, or when there are coexistent extrahepatic biliary communications with common bile duct obstruction owing to cysts or debris. Cholecystectomy should be performed at the time of hydatid cyst resection.

Postoperative Fistulas. Management of biliary fistulas occurring after laparoscopic cholecystectomy is dependent upon the injury pattern present. When the fistula arises from the cystic duct stump, expectant management, after documentation of a clear distal common bile duct is the rule. If persistent, endoscopic sphincterotomy should be performed, although stenting is usually unnecessary. Surgery is rarely needed, but should include cholangiography, resection of excessive cystic duct remnant, and secure suture closure of the cystic duct stump. Common duct or major hepatic duct injury is not uncommon after laparoscopic cholecystectomy, occurring in 1% to 2% of cases, compared with a 0.02% to 0.2% incidence after open cholecystectomy.[45–52,54] Regardless of how they occur, these injuries are usually high on the extrahepatic biliary tree, and are seldom amenable to simple repair. Most centers experienced with repair of these injuries agree that Roux-en-Y hepatodochojejunostomy or choledochojejunostomy is usually necessary.[46–50,53,54] The preoperative placement of percutaneous bilateral stents is advocated in a series

of 50 major duct injuries following laparoscopic cholecystectomy in which 10% of patients had unsuspected exclusion of lobar ducts.[46] In addition to making these excluded segments obvious, preoperative stents assist in localization and repair of injured ducts.

Biliary fistulas occur in 1% to 3% of hepatic resection patients. However, in patients undergoing left trisegmentectomies, the occurrence is 30%.[58,137] In a report of 411 patients undergoing hepatic resections there were prolonged biliary leaks in 13 of 411 patients.[58] All closed with expectant management. Another trial reported a 2% biliary fistula rate in 229 patients after hepatic resection for hepatocellular carcinoma.[77] The underlying process that leads to hepatocellular carcinoma seems to be important for predicting postoperative fistula occurrence and the necessity for operative closure. In that study, 77% of resections were for hepatitis-induced carcinoma, and all fistulas were in this group.[77] Forty percent of these patients required operative closure for biliary fistula persisting for >8 weeks. A 6% biliary fistula rate for hepatic resections done for malignancy with vascular occlusion was reported in another study.[76] All of these fistulas healed spontaneously, provided biloma drainage was complete, within 12 to 40 days. Biliary fistulas that persist after hepatic resection can be treated in one of three ways: the involved segment can be resected, the leaking duct can be oversewn, or an anastomosis between the leaking duct and a Roux-en-Y limb of jejunum can be performed.

Carefully performed bilioenteric anastomoses, such as after pancreatoduodenectomy, rarely leak for more than a few days. When they are persistent, suture-line disruption or failure to incorporate a major duct into the anastomosis should be suspected. Alternatively, local factors such as abscess or ischemic necrosis of the bowel or bile duct wall should be considered. The arterial blood supply to the common bile duct must be preserved during pancreatoduodenectomy to avoid ischemic breakdown of the biliary-enteric anastomosis. Biliary fistula is now the second most common complication occurring after pancreatoduodenectomy.[6] In the absence of peritonitis, abscess, cholangitis, or jaundice, expectant management is warranted. Delineation of the defect is necessary to determine operative approach. When the bile duct is in continuity and drains into the bowel, and a single point of extravasation is demonstrated, the fistula can be expected to close gradually. Complete disruption will likely require reoperation. Early operative intervention is chosen for complete ductal disruption or for situations complicated by cholangitis or jaundice. Resection of the distal common duct with a new, more proximal anastomosis to the jejunal limb is indicated. A one-layer anastomosis of fine nonabsorbable suture material is used. An average-sized duct will require approximately 8 sutures. As the anastomosis approaches the common hepatic duct, the chance of success increases. Hepatodochojejunostomy rather than stents may be necessary if common duct viability is questioned. While some surgeons prefer a Roux-en-Y limb of jejunum, others prefer a jejunal loop. There is no clinical or experimental evidence to suggest that one is superior or lessens the chance of cholangitis. One advantage of a simple loop is that barium upper gastrointestinal (GI) examination will allow evaluation of the bilioenteric anastomosis. Whether stents should be placed is unclear. We prefer to use them because they allow for easier fashioning of the anastomosis and provide access to the biliary tree in the postoperative period. When stents are used, we prefer to leave them in place for up to 1 year. Regardless of the method chosen, all agree that an accurate, well-vascularized bilioenteric anastomosis is necessary for success.

Posttraumatic Fistulas. The management of posttraumatic biliary fistulas is dependent upon whether the leak is contained (biloma) or free in the peritoneal cavity. Bilomas are best treated by percutaneous drainage, with operation reserved for persistent fistulas. Free perforation mandates operative repair with postoperative closed-suction drainage.[24] When late biliary fistulas appear, they are most effectively managed without operation, since most close spontaneously within 30 days.[25,129] In patients with persistent fistula, hepatic resection or hepaticojejunostomy to the fistula site may be necessary.[25]

■ GASTROINTESTINAL FISTULAS

In the past most gastrointestinal-cutaneous fistulas were spontaneous. At present, most are acute and iatrogenic, occurring after instrumentation or operation. Presently, a minority are indolent and spontaneous, occurring as a result of neoplasia or inflammation. Internal fistulas are those that communicate with other portions of the gastrointestinal tract or adjacent organs. When short segments of the gastrointestinal tract are bypassed, patients may be relatively asymptomatic and have no significant volume, electrolyte, or nutritional disturbance. If long segments of bowel are bypassed, volume, electrolyte, and nutritional deficits can be profound and the symptomatology prominent as the result of malabsorption from functional short-gut syndrome.

External fistulas make their presence known by drainage of enteric contents onto the skin or out the vagina. Although their presence is usually obvious, their underlying anatomy and pathophysiology may not be. Although the presence of an abnormal external drainage can never truly be considered asymptomatic, external fistulas, particularly distal ones, also can occur without significant volume, electrolyte, and nutritional

disturbance. Because of their diverse etiologies and varying degrees of physiologic significance, gastrointestinal fistulas can have a variety of presentations (Table 15–4).

HISTORY

The earliest record of an enterocutaneous fistula appears in the Old Testament Book of Judges written by Samuel between 1043 BC and 1004 BC. It is the account of Eglon, who sustained an acute posttraumatic enterocutaneous fistula: "And Ehud put forth his hand, and took the dagger and thrust it into his belly . . . And the dirt came out." Celsus described the first reported attempt at surgical repair of a colocutaneous fistula: "It can be sutured, not with any certain assurance, but because this doubtful hope is preferable to certain despair; for occasionally it heals up." In the 18th century, John Hunter advocated a conservative approach to fistulas after he noted that fistulas occasionally close spontaneously: "In such cases nothing is to be done but dressing the wound superficially, and when the contents of the wounded viscus become less, we may hope for cure."

In the early 1900s, enterostomy created in healthy bowel for decompression proximal to an obstruction often would close spontaneously when the obstruction resolved, fostering an unrealistically optimistic attitude toward other gastrointestinal-cutaneous fistulas. After specialized referral centers collected, analyzed, and reported large experiences with fistulas in the 1960s, the true severity of this complication was revealed. Mortality rates approached 60%, which was much higher than had been previously realized.[138] In 1960, Welch and his associates identified sepsis, electrolyte disturbance, and malnutrition as the three major causes of death in patients with fistulas and showed an increasing incidence of these complications as fistula output increased.[138] In addition, they discovered that the greater the fistula output, the greater the morbidity and mortality. Even in

TABLE 15–4. CLASSIFICATION OF GASTROINTESTINAL FISTULAS

Anatomic	Internal/External Anatomic Course	Suggests etiology Prognosticates spontaneous closure Assists planning operative timing and approach
Physiologic	Output (ml/day): Low <200 Moderate 200–500 High >500	Prognosticates mortality Assists physician in anticipating and treating metabolic deficits
Etiologic	Underlying disease process	prognosticates spontaneous closure prognosticates mortality

more contemporary times where parasurgical care is improved, enterocutaneous fistulas still have a 6% to 20% mortality, with malnutrition and sepsis the principal contributing factors.[139] Furthermore, given the ease of monitoring, it is surprising that electrolyte disturbance, defined by abnormal serum electrolyte concentrations for 48 hours or longer, is still quite common. In addition to sepsis, malnutrition and electrolyte disturbance, malignancy contributes to morbidity and mortality, now accounting for 5% to 30% of fistula deaths. This may not be necessarily the result of an increase in the incidence of malignancy, but rather to an increased number of patients with prolonged survival. Now with pro-

longed survival, and aggressive operative therapy, both spontaneous and postoperative fistulas are relatively more common in this population.[128,140,141]

EPIDEMIOLOGY, ETIOLOGY, AND ANATOMY

Knowledge of fistula etiology is crucial for formulation of a successful management plan. This is because the etiology of the fistula, like the site of origin, may provide considerable information regarding spontaneous closure (Table 15–5).

Spontaneous causes account for 15% to 25% of enterocutaneous fistulas. These include radiation, inflam-

TABLE 15–5. GASTROINTESTINAL FISTULAS

Study	Type	Etiology	Malnutrition	Sepsis	Cancer	Mortality
Aguirre[144] (1974)	All intestinal	IBD-20% Surgical-77%	55%	61%	16%	21%
Reber[201] (1978)	All GI	IBD-6% Surgical-94%	—	76%	23%	22%
Soeters[145] (1979)	All GI	IBD-9% Cancer-10% Peptic Ulcer-3% Surgical-72%	87%	55%	36%	43%
Tarazi[180] (1983)	Gastric duodenal	Surgical-98%	71%	63%	21%	30%
Sansoni[276] (1985)	Small intestinal	IBD-56% Cancer-2% Peptic Ulcer-6% Pancreatitis-8% Surgical-25%	—	17%	4%	24%
Gilmartin[200] (1985)	Lateral duodenal	Surgical-92% Trauma-8%	—	15%	8%	15%
Rossi[199] (1986)	Duodenal	Surgical-78% Trauma-10% Peptic Ulcer-6% Cancer-6%	83%	61%	6%	33%
Rose[140] (1986)	All GI	IBD-10% Cancer-6% Peptic Ulcer-3% Pancreatitis-3% Surgical-51%	—	28%	27%	11%
Schein[151] (1991)	Esophageal All intestinal	[a]Surgical-100%	—	26%	—	37%
Prickett[128] (1991)	All GI	—	57%	—	14%	19%
Buechter[152] (1991)	All intestinal	[a]Trauma-100% 2/3 injured bowel 1/2 noninjured bowel	—	47%	0%	13%
Kuvshinoff[139] (1993)	All intestinal	IBD-9% Cancer-4% Pancreatitis-6% Surgical-80%	—	25%	23%	20%

[a]	Includes only postoperative or traumatic fistulas
Surgical	Postoperative fistula
IBD	Inflammatory Bowel Disease (Crohn's and Ulcerative Colitis)
Peptic Ulcer	Gastric and duodenal ulcer disease
All Intestinal	Gastric, duodenal, small and large bowel fistulas
All GI	All intestinal including pancreatic and biliary fistulas

matory bowel disease, diverticular disease, appendicitis, ischemic bowel, indwelling tubes, perforation of duodenal ulcer, pancreatic and gynecologic malignancies, and intestinal actinomycosis or tuberculosis.[159–162] Fistulas that are the result of radiation or recurrent carcinoma are unlikely to close spontaneously.[145] This axiom recently was investigated and still found to be true.[139] Those arising as a result of inflammatory bowel disease often will close and then reopen when enteral feedings are resumed. Therefore, fistulas resulting from radiation, recurrent carcinoma, and inflammatory bowel disease often require surgical closure.[85,163,164] Other than early diagnosis and treatment, there is little a physician can do to prevent occurrence of fistulas from spontaneous causes.

The remaining 75% to 85% of enterocutaneous fistulas are of iatrogenic origin. The operations that antecede the appearance of the fistula are generally of three types: (1) cancer operations, (2) operations for inflammatory bowel disease, and (3) lysis of adhesions that are present as the result of previous surgery. These three types of operations are commonly performed, and numbers alone may make them the most common operations complicated by fistula formation. However, an additional factor that may contribute to postoperative fistula formation is the relative difficulty of these types of operative procedures. Other common operations that precede fistula formation include operations for head and neck, esophageal, pulmonary, pancreatic, gastric, and colonic malignancy; operations for peptic ulcer disease, pancreatitis, and trauma; and operations for diverticulitis.[165–169]

Fistula physiology and etiology provide considerable information about the natural history of each particular fistula. Additional information is obtained from study of the anatomy of the fistula, since the anatomic nature predicts the chance of spontaneous closure[142–147,170,171] and is critical for planning medical management and operative approach. Fistulas occur in every segment of the gastrointestinal tract. Anatomic segments that are outside a body cavity, such as the mouth, pharynx, and rectum, commonly form external fistulas. Those within body cavities may become adherent to surrounding viscera or the abdominal wall when involved by inflammation or neoplasia, thereby resulting in either internal, external, or combined fistulas.

Oral, Pharyngeal and Esophageal Fistulas

The etiology of oropharyngeocutaneous fistulas has shifted from spontaneous fistulas complicating advanced head and neck tumors to fistulas resulting from surgical treatment. Because of tobacco and alcohol use, the patient with head and neck cancer may have poor nutritional status upon presentation. In addition, it may be difficult to maintain oral intake in the presence of painful lesions. Many patients referred for surgical resection also have undergone preoperative radiation therapy. These preoperative factors are additive and, when coupled with the already difficult task of reconstructing the large defects created by radical resections, lead to a 5% to 25% postoperative oropharyngeocutaneous fistula rate.[172] The most common origin of a fistula is where the pharyngeal defect is closed at the base of the tongue. The absence of a serosa, the presence of a segmental blood supply, the necessity for mobilization, and closure performed under tension are intraoperative factors that may contribute to fistulas at this location.

Most esophagocutaneous fistulas are the result of either postoperative leaks at the cervical anastomosis following esophageal resection for cancer, or leaks due to undetected or inadequately repaired cervical esophageal trauma. Their behavior is similar to that of oropharyngeocutaneous fistulas. Esophageal fistulas that occur in the chest are physiologically more significant than cervical esophagocutaneous fistulas. Empyema, mediastinitis, and overwhelming sepsis are common after thoracic esophageal leaks. This has led some to abandon thoracic esophageal anastomoses. Causes of thoracic esophageal leaks include congenital defects, tumor, pulmonary, infections, instrumentation, foreign body and postemetic perforations.[173] When esophageal defects occur in the chest, the usual result is an esophagopleural fistula with empyema and sepsis, an esophagobronchial fistula, or an esophagotracheal fistula. Their presentation is that of severe pneumonia, lung abscess, mediastinitis, or pleural effusion that can proceed very rapidly to overwhelming sepsis and multiple organ failure. Spontaneous thoracic esophagocutaneous fistulas are uncommon. This is probably because overwhelming sepsis, mandating operative intervention, intercedes before spontaneous external drainage can occur. However, thoracic esophagocutaneous fistulas may occur after tube thoracostomy.

Other causes of oropharyngeocutaneous or esophagocutaneous fistulas include trauma, infected congenital neck cysts, anterior cervical fusion, and foreign body perforations.[174–179] Nonoperative treatment usually will result in spontaneous closure. After removal of foreign bodies, drainage of loculated sepsis, and debridement of devitalized tissues, many of these fistulas from less common causes can be closed primarily in layers.

Gastric Fistulas

Gastric fistulas are postoperative in 85% to 90% of cases in most modern series.[180–185] Less common etiologies include inflammation, ischemia, cancer, and radiation. Anastomotic leakage or fistula formation after gastric resection for cancer is an ominous occurrence. Although it happens in only 6% to 8% of cases, it accounts for 50% of deaths following these procedures.[184] Most patients who have gastric leaks develop high fevers, tachycardia, abdominal pain, and abdominal distention in the early postoperative period. Despite cervical esophagostomy, antibiotics, and surgical drainage of the abdomen and thorax, this complication still carries a 50% to 75% mortality.[185–188]

Gastric leak after resections for ulcer disease occurs infrequently. Only 1% to 3% of gastric resection for peptic ulceration will lead to fistula formation. Gastric leak with subsequent fistula formation also can occur after antireflux procedures, usually those done through the chest. The prognosis is much less ominous than gastric fistula occurring after cancer resection, but still carries a considerable mortality.[189–193] A gastric leak will occur in 3% of patients who undergo gastric bariatric operations and most (85%) will present with an intra-abdominal abscess. Percutaneous drainage often will result in a controlled gastrocutaneous fistula. The remaining 15% will present with a gastrocutaneous fistula.[194]

The average time from diagnosis to closure for gastric fistulas is approximately 40 days.[183,189–192,194] The overall mortality is between 15% to 25%. If the fistula output is >200 mL/day, the mortality increases to 40%, and when malnutrition is present the mortality approaches 60%.[182]

Duodenal Fistulas

Fifty to eighty-five percent of duodenocutaneous fistulas are postoperative and occur as the result of complications after gastric resections or operations on the biliary tract, duodenum, pancreas, right colon, aorta, and kidney. The remaining 15% to 50% are the result of trauma, perforated ulcers, and cancer.[34,35,195–197] The overall mortality associated with duodenocutaneous fistulas ranges from 7% to 67%, with an average of 28%.[138,165,198–202] Factors associated with increased mortality include uncontrolled sepsis, age >65, output >500 mL/24 hrs, malnutrition, and multiple operations. Uncontrolled sepsis is by far the most important; when it occurs, mortality is between 70% to 100%.[201,203]

Duodenal fistulas occur in approximately 3% of patients who undergo gastric resections. However, use of catheter duodenostomy may decrease this complication to <1%.[204] Spontaneous duodenocutaneous fistula closure rates from collected series in the literature seem to fall into two distinct groups: those studies that report spontaneous closure rates between 29% to 38%,[144,183,202] and those that report spontaneous closure rates between 83% to 100%.[170,198,205,206] The disparity probably represents differences in the types of fistulas encountered. Edmunds[138] and Malangoni[202] both found that lateral fistulas were less likely to close than end duodenal stump fistulas. Even though closure rates seem disparate, there is agreement that when spontaneous closure does occur, the mean time is 30 to 40 days. In the authors' experience, closure occurs slightly earlier, with a mean time of 21 days.[145]

Small Intestinal Fistulas

Small intestinal fistulas are the most common type of gastrointestinal fistulas encountered. Surgical complications are the dominant etiologic agent in jejunal and ileal fistulas. Most series report 70% to 90% of small intestinal fistulas occur after an operative procedure.[128,139–141,143,145,153] The different complications leading to fistula formation include disruption of an anastomosis, unrecognized injury to the bowel at the time of lysis of adhesions, and inadvertent suture of the bowel at the time of abdominal closure. Roughly half of postoperative fistulas are from disrupted anastomoses and half are from unrecognized bowel injuries. Small bowel fistulas may occur following any intra-abdominal operation, and may occur after operations both with and without intestinal resection. The operations that antecede the appearance of small intestinal fistulas are generally operations for cancer, operations for inflammatory bowel disease, and lysis of adhesions caused by previous surgery. Other operative procedures that may precede fistula formation include those performed for peptic ulcer disease and pancreatitis.[85,142–156,164]

Fistulas may result from anastomoses carried out in less than an adequately prepared bowel, or from a bowel with less than adequate blood supply. Anastomoses also may be jeopardized by hypotension owing to inadequate resuscitation or undue tension placed on the suture line. In addition, when abscesses form adjacent to anastomoses or bowel they may decompress into the bowel lumen. A fistula results when the abscess is drained percutaneously.

Poor nutritional status contributes significantly to anastomotic breakdown and the inadequate response to infection in some patients. When patients are nutritionally depleted, protein synthesis is reduced. Well-vascularized, tension-free anastomoses performed in nutritionally replete patients will decrease postoperative complications in general, and fistula formation in particular.[207] In emergency settings some of these goals are impossible to achieve. In this setting, resection with end ostomies and mucous fistulas, or exteriorization of the fistulized segment, may be necessary.

Spontaneous causes of small bowel fistulas include inflammatory bowel disease, cancer, peptic ulcer disease, and pancreatitis. In Western countries, Crohn's disease is by far the most common cause of spontaneous fistulas.[208–212] The transmural fissures of Crohn's disease cause serosal inflammation which leads to adherence to surrounding structures. When microperforation leads to abscess formation, the abscess discharges into the adherent structure and a fistula results. Twenty to forty percent of patients with Crohn's disease will develop fistulas; roughly half will be external and half will be internal.[208–215] There are two types of external fistulas that occur with Crohn's disease. The first type occurs early in the postoperative period, after resection of a diseased segment, in otherwise healthy bowel. These fistulas behave like non-Crohn's fistulas, have favorable spontaneous closure rates, and should be treated as any other enterocutaneous fistula.[210,213] The other type arises from Crohn's-involved bowel, has a low spontaneous closure rate and should be considered for surgical repair, either early or preferably, when the fistula is closed and the abdominal wall is in reasonable condition.

The remaining spontaneous small bowel fistulas occur as the result of malignancy (2% to 16%), peptic ulcer disease (3% to 6%), and pancreatitis (3% to 8%). Less common causes of external, small intestinal fistulas include actinomycosis, tuberculosis, and lymphoma.

Pouch Fistulas

Total proctocolectomy with permanent ileostomy for ulcerative colitis removes all diseased mucosa and, therefore, is curative.[216–222] However, permanent ileostomy is less than desirable for many of these young, otherwise healthy, patients. In 1947, Ravitch and Sabiston introduced the ileo-anal pull-through procedure. It is not only curative, but also offers the advantage of continence and defecation per anus. However, frequent bowel movements made this procedure less desirable. The addition of various pouches to the ileoanal anastomosis made the ileoanal pull-through the procedure of choice for ulcerative colitis and familial polyposis.[223–234] Construction of the ileal pouch and pouch-anal anastomosis presents technical challenges and, with the introduction of the pouch, led to a new set of complications such as pouchitis, ileoanal strictures, anastomotic separation, pelvic sepsis, pouch leakage, and pouch fistulas.[235–240] Because stool continence, volume, and frequency have reportedly been similar between pouch and primary ileoanal anastomoses, some have resorted to primary ileoproctostomy.[219,235,237] Whether this decreases complications and results in acceptable stool frequency is unknown.

The likely etiology of most pouch fistulas is technical error. Pouch-anal separation may occur because of poor vascular supply to the pouch outlet or tension on the pouch-anal anastomosis when positioning the pouch in the pelvis. Because the ileal segment that forms the pouch-anal anastomosis is furthest from the small bowel mesenteric blood supply, it may be particularly prone to ischemia.

Fistulas may arise from the long continuous suture lines used when forming the pouch, especially when not protected by proximal-diverting ileostomy. These may break down because of poor blood supply or increased intrapouch pressure in the postoperative period when the mucosa continues to secrete mucus and anal sphincter spasm is extreme. A stricture at the pouch-anal anastomosis also may predispose to fistula formation.

It is important that this operation not be attempted for patients with Crohn's colitis. In addition, indeterminate cases of inflammatory bowel disease may actually be Crohn's disease. Because the inflammatory process of Crohn's disease involves the full thickness of bowel wall, mucosal stripping will not eliminate the disease. Patients who have a history of fistula-in-ano or perirectal abscess are suspect of having Crohn's disease.[241] When pouch fistulas occur, pathologic specimens should be reinspected and diagnostic accuracy confirmed.

Fistulas from the pouch may involve the anterior abdominal wall, urinary tract, vulva, vagina, perineum, or adjacent loops of bowel. These fistulas may be recognized by "pouchogram" done prior to ileostomy reversal, necessitating exploration and reestablishment of proximal ileostomy or prolonged periods of nothing by mouth.[238–241] When a pouch fistula develops, operative intervention with repair or reconstruction of the pouch is usually necessary.

Colonic Fistulas

Colocutaneous fistulas are the result of diverticulitis, cancer, inflammatory bowel disease, pancreatitis, appendicitis, radiation therapy, or secondarily from surgical treatment of these diseases. They are generally low output, except for those that have a small bowel communication or component.

Although adjuvant radiotherapy has improved long-term survival of many abdominal and pelvic malignancies, it has led to a 5% to 15% occurrence of radiation-induced gastrointestinal complications.[242–245] Bowel resection with primary anastomosis in irradiated tissues will result in anastomotic breakdown in as many as 31% of cases.[246] In addition, leaks from a colon or rectal anastomosis may not only cause local infective complications and fistula formation, but also spillage of neoplastic cells that subsequently may lead to locally recurrent cancer.[247,248] Techniques such as anastomotic coverage or filling-irradiated dead space with muscle flaps,[249] sigmoid exclusion,[250] or anal pull-through procedures may decrease the incidence of postoperative leaks and fistula formation from irradiated pelvic anastomoses.

The least common type of intestinal fistula is from the appendix.[251,252] Primary appendicocutaneous fistulas are rare and secondary fistulas usually follow simple drainage of an appendiceal abscess.[252–259]

Internal Fistulas

Approximately 20% to 40% of patients with Crohn's disease will develop internal fistulas.[209–215,260–263] Together, Crohn's disease and diverticulitis account for most internal fistulas. The fistulas associated with Crohn's disease are usually enteroenteric, enterovesical, enterocolonic, or colovaginal,[145,263] while those from diverticulitis tend to be colovesical in males and colovaginal in females. Malignancy accounts for the remainder of internal fistulas, although obstruction or perforation owing to malignancy are more common than fistulization. Treatment of internal fistulas is directed at the underlying disorder, with operative intervention reserved for specific complications such as malabsorption, intractable diarrhea, obstruction, recurrent infections, or short bowel syndrome.

The epidemiology of spontaneous fistulas mirrors the epidemiology of the disease processes causing fistula formation. In less developed countries, spontaneous causes, such as appendicitis, diverticulitis, Crohn's disease, neoplasms, and infectious diseases are responsible for most fistulas. The incidence is unknown since most of these patients succumb to their underlying disease process or to the infectious, metabolic or nutritional complications associated with their fistula.

PREVENTION

Postoperative fistulas usually occur in settings of poor patient preparation, such as emergency procedures, or in situations in which the patient has been previously treated with radiation therapy. In the emergency setting, where preoperative preparation is brief, intraoperative techniques to prevent fistula formation assume greater importance. Sound surgical procedure will lessen the chances of fistula formation in the elective setting, and even more so in the emergency setting. Anastomoses should be done in healthy bowel with adequate blood supply. When possible, mechanical bowel preparation should be carried out; most surgeons advocate intraluminal antibiotic preparation, as well. Mechanical bowel preparation to remove particulate fecal matter can decrease colonic bacterial counts from 10^{12-15} to 10^{4-5}. The addition of enteral nonabsorbable antibiotics may decrease these bacterial counts even further, to 10^{2-3}. Systemic antibiotics with activity against enteric organisms should be administered preoperatively, and readministered throughout the procedure.[264–266] Systemic antibiotics, however, do not obviate the need for mechanical preparation or enteral antibiotics. Although it is not clear that enteral antibiotics decrease wound or abdominal infection rates in patients receiving parenteral antibiotics, in the absence of luminal preparation, the incidence of anastomotic breakdown, abscess, and wound infection seems unaffected by systemic antibiotics.[267–270] On-table luminal preparation is advocated by some, but the chances of contamination are great. In clean or clean-contaminated cases, antibiotics may decrease the fre-

quency of anastomotic breakdown as well as prevent abscesses and infections adjacent to the suture line that may cause direct breakdown of an anastomotic suture line.[264] Anastomoses should lay without tension. Meticulous and precise hemostasis should be achieved to prevent unnecessary devascularization and postoperative collections of blood that may become infected and result in abscess formation. The abdominal wall should be closed securely after an anastomosis to prevent exposure of a fresh suture line and to help seal any minor leaks. Fresh anastomoses should not be allowed to come into direct contact with the abdominal closure suture line and should be covered by fat or omentum, when possible. The inflammatory response and intermittent minor leakage that occurs during the healing of an anastomosis usually is sealed off by surrounding healthy tissues, such as peritoneum, adjacent loops of bowel, or omentum. The inflammatory process of two adjacent healing suture lines may predispose to fistula formation. At the end of an abdominal procedure, unless it has been removed, the greater omentum should be placed back in its anatomic position covering the intestines. This will help protect and seal the enteric anastomosis. When this is impossible, some have advocated use of fibrin glue or other connective tissue derivatives to seal the anastomosis.[271]

Dead space should be filled with live tissue or drained with closed suction, especially in previously irradiated areas,[272] and drains should be kept away from the anastomosis. Finally, the patient should be fully hydrated to provide adequate circulatory support and to prevent hypotension that may predispose to fistula formation.

Poor nutritional status may play a major role in anastomotic breakdown and in the inadequate response to infection. If operation can safely be delayed, nutritional preparation may be the most important step in preventing anastomotic breakdown.[205,272,273] Patients with the following nutritional characteristics have been shown to be at increased risk for anastomotic breakdown:

1. Weight loss of 10% to 15% total body weight over a short period (3 to 4 months)
2. Serum albumin concentration <3 gm/dL
3. Serum transferrin concentration <220 mg/dL
4. Anergy to injected recall antigens
5. Inability to perform usual tasks because of weakness or easy fatigability

Oral, Pharyngeal, and Esophageal Fistulas

When flaps are used for reconstruction, vessels should lay as straight and free of tension as possible. This is particularly true for the venous outflow that may become obstructed, leading to flap engorgement and eventual flap loss, suture-line breakdown, and subsequent fistula formation. Creation of false tissue planes during head and neck resections, particularly if the patient was previously irradiated, can devascularize tissue and lead to anastomotic breakdown and fistula formation. Vascularized tissue interposition, such as local muscle flaps, between hollow viscera (esophagus and trachea) will lessen the chances of fistula formation. Reconstruction after thoracic esophageal resections can be reinforced with a pleural patch. This patch may help improve vascularity and seal any minor anastomotic leakage. Whether hand-sewn or stapled anastomoses are superior is debatable, with some authorities maintaining that stapled anastomoses are less prone to breakdown.

Gastric Fistulas

Dividing only the vessels necessary for gastric mobilization while maintaining the gastroepiploic arcade will lessen the chances of gastric necrosis and fistula formation. Adequate duodenal mobilization will ensure tension-free gastroduodenal anastomoses. When mobilization is not possible, use of Billroth II reconstruction may be preferable, as long as duodenal decompression is accomplished. Secure closure of the *angle du mort* when a Hofmeister reconstruction is employed usually can be accomplished by a carefully placed tripartite suture. Postoperative gastric decompression will allow suture lines to seal without increased intraluminal pressure.

Duodenal Fistulas

When either Billroth I or II reconstruction is used, the duodenum should be mobilized adequately to ensure secure closure or anastomosis without necessary dissection. When fistulas involve the duodenum, extensive duodenal mobilization may be necessary to order to resect the affected segments. Duodenal fistulas may be managed appropriately with bypass. Conversely, fistulectomy, freshening of the margins of the fistula site, and Heinicke-Mickulicz closure can be attempted. Resection with end-to-end anastomosis is usually unsafe for duodenal fistulas. Liberal use of tube duodenostomy, in addition to afferent-loop tube placement, will decrease the incidence of postoperative duodenal fistula formation.[34,35,165,195,196,204]

Because the duodenum is in proximity to the right colon, kidney, inferior vena cava, aorta, and pancreas, isolated duodenal trauma is uncommon.[195,196] Associated injuries adversely affect duodenal closure outcome, and therefore, diverticulization at least should be considered during the repair of all duodenal trauma.[166,167] Primary closure, with or without serosal patch, may be adequate only for the least complex of injuries.

Small Intestinal Fistulas

Unless small bowel length is a concern, resection with two layered anastomoses is recommended for small bowel defects. Simple closure of small bowel defects greater than half the bowel circumference may lead to

fistula formation owing to partial obstruction or ischemia, especially when the mesenteric border is involved in the defect. Resection with end-to-end anastomosis should be performed when compromise of the luminal diameter is likely. When closure of multiple defects is necessary and viability is questionable, bypass or proximal diversion should be considered.

Pouch Fistulas

Adequate mobilization of the pouch mesentery is required for tension-free ileoanal anastomoses. Alternatively, when the pouch is positioned in the pelvis, the mesenteric vessels may be compressed as they cross the sacral promontory. Adequate mesenteric mobilization will prevent this from occurring. In addition, particular attention should be paid to the orientation of the pouch. Rotation of the pouch, when positioning it in the pelvis, may impair blood supply, particularly venous drainage. We routinely recommend a diverting ileostomy with all ileoanal pouch procedures.

Colonic Fistulas

Proximal diverting colostomy may allow sufficient time for healing to occur before the suture line is tested by the fecal stream. In addition, some authorities have suggested that rectal tube decompression after Hartman procedure prevents increased pressure in the rectal stump postoperatively and may decrease rectal stump leak and subsequent pelvic sepsis and fistula formation. In addition, pelvic coverage after extensive resections will lessen the chances of fistula formation.[272]

PATHOPHYSIOLOGY

Physiology and Pathophysiology

Fistulas can be classified in physiologic terms by output during a 24 hour period (Table 15–6). Enterocutaneous fistulas result in loss of fluid, electrolytes, trace minerals, and protein; losses may be minimal in distal, low-output fistulas, or extreme in proximal, high-output fistulas. Fistulas are divided into three categories based on output:[143,145,163,170]

1. high-output fistulas, >500 mL per 24 hr
2. moderate-output fistulas, 200 to 500 mL per 24 hr
3. low-output fistulas, <200 mL per 24 hr

Accurate determination of fistula output predicts mortality and assists the physician in preventing and treating metabolic deficits and correcting ongoing losses. There is no correlation between the static measurement of fistula output and spontaneous closure, although it is true that fistula output usually decreases before closure. Anatomic and etiologic factors are much more important for predicting spontaneous closure.

TABLE 15–6. PHYSIOLOGY OF GASTROINTESTINAL FISTULAS

Low Output	Moderate Output	High Output
<200 mL/24h	200–500 mL/24h	>500 mL/24h
Problem electrolytes: K, CL, Mg	Problem electrolytes: Na, K, Cl, HCO$_3$, Zn	Problem electrolytes: Na, K, Cl, HCO$_3$, Mg, Zn, Cu
Feed at 1-1.2x REE	Feed at 1.2–1.3x REE	Feed at 1.2–1.5x REE
Protein: 1–1.5 gm/kg/d	Protein: 1.2–1.8 g/kg/d	Protein: 1.5–2.5 gm/kg/d
RDA: water soluble vitamins	2x RDA: water soluble vitamins	2x RDA: water soluble vitamins
2–5x RDA: vitamin C	5–10x RDA: vitamin C	5–10x RDA: vitamin C
Vitamin K: 10 mg/wk	Vitamin K: 10 mg/wk	Vitamin K: 10 mg/wk

Fluid and Electrolyte Imbalances. Fluid and electrolyte imbalances are defined as abnormalities in serum electrolytes of >48 hours duration, and are primarily associated with high-output fistulas. Such abnormalities occur frequently, given the availability and ease of monitoring acid-base and electrolyte balance. Most commonly, these disturbances involve potassium, sodium, magnesium, phosphate, and zinc. Proximal small intestinal diversion by a fistula may drain up to 4L/day; approximately 2 L arises from swallowed saliva and gastric secretions, and 2 L from pancreatobiliary secretions. The fluid lost is metabolically expensive, since it contains considerable amounts of enzymatic proteins and critical electrolytes. Loss of this fluid can lead to severe volume, electrolyte, and protein depletion.

Malnutrition. Even with safe and effective parenteral therapies, malnutrition remains a major problem in patients with enterocutaneous fistulas.[128,140,141,143,145,151,152,160,180,198–200,275,276] It is most severe and refractory with high-output fistulas. The three main contributing factors are (1) lack of adequate nutrient intake, (2) hypercatabolism associated with sepsis, and (3) the loss of protein-rich, energy-requiring secretions from the fistula. Uncontrolled sepsis is probably the most important factor contributing to the malnutrition associated with enterocutaneous fistulas. Malnutrition does occur without sepsis and usually can be remedied in this circumstance with appropriate nutritional support.[139] However, in the presence of uncontrolled sepsis, it may be impossible to correct nutritional depletion. If uncontrolled sepsis occurs while marked fistula losses continue, metabolic repletion may be impossible.[139] If nutritional stabilization is to proceed, control of sepsis should be an early and singular goal.

Enteral nutrition has been used more frequently to support patients with enterocutaneous fistulas. Use of this modality may be limited by the structural and functional status of the gastrointestinal tract. It is often necessary to provide parenterally at least a portion of nutrition, volume, electrolyte, and vitamin needs of the patient.[207] It is worthwhile to emphasize that a portion of required calories given enterally will increase hepatic protein synthesis and provide some of the beneficial effects associated with enteral nutrition.

Sepsis. Sepsis is the most common complication of enterocutaneous fistulas,[140,141,143,145,151,152,160,180,200,275,276] in addition to being the most common cause of fistula-related death. Computed tomography (CT), magnetic resonance imaging (MRI), or indium scans should be used liberally to localize sepsis, since patients will likely not survive unless all abscesses are drained. If catheter sepsis and other conditions that masquerade as intra-abdominal sepsis are eliminated in a patient dying of sepsis, exploratory laparotomy may be indicated. The entire intestinal tract, from the ligament of Treitz to the rectum should be freed, all abscesses drained, and intestinal continuity restored. The term *refunctionalization* was used for this operation because it was originally intended to restore intestinal continuity for nutrition. Because nutrition can be adequately supplied parenterally, the primary purpose of the procedure now is to drain occult sepsis.

Malignancy. Malignancy is the cause of 3% to 7% of fistulas, is present in 5% to 35% of patients with fistulas, and accounts for 30% to 40% of fistula mortality in most recent reported series.[139–141,143,145,151,152,160,180,200,275,276] Enterocutaneous fistulas that result from malignancy usually signify advanced transmural disease, and consequently carry a poor prognosis. However, with current advancements in oncologic care, these patients often have a reasonable life expectancy. Malignancy should not be considered a contraindication to aggressive nonoperative and operative fistula management. A fistula that is appropriately and aggressively cared for should not alter the natural history of the underlying malignancy to a significant degree. Therefore, a rational treatment plan, based on known tumor biology, should be made. In patients with well-differentiated, slow-growing tumors, an argument for early and aggressive operative management to minimize hospitalization can be made, since operative correction may palliate these patients for many months. In addition, one is reluctant to supply parenteral nutrition to patients with malignancy because parenteral nutrition may enhance tumor growth when given without antineoplastic therapy.

Natural History

There are few other places in surgery where the understanding of the natural history of a disease process is as important as in the management of fistulas. The expected incidence of spontaneous closure, the time it takes for spontaneous closure to occur, and the mortality by anatomic location, pathophysiology, and nutritional status are central to the decision-making process in fistula management (Table 15–7). Indeed, the decisions of whether to operate, when to operate, and what operation to perform are affected most by understanding the natural history of a particular fistula. The highest rate of spontaneous closure has been consistently reported for oropharyngeal, esophageal, duodenal stump, pancreatobiliary, and jejunal fistulas.[85] Fistulas arising from the stomach, ligament of Treitz, or ileum are resistant to spontaneous closure and, therefore, are more likely to require surgical closure.[170] Other characteristics associated with nonhealing fistulas include large adjacent abscesses, intestinal discontinuity, distal obstruction, poor adjacent bowel, fistula tracts <2 cm in length, and enteral defect >1 cm². In addition, fistulas arising from radiation damaged intestine and recurrent carcinoma are not likely to heal. Those that arise from inflammatory bowel disease may close, but will likely reopen as soon as oral intake is resumed.

The average time to closure varies with the anatomic location of the fistula. This knowledge can aid the surgeon in planning a rational time course for nonoperative management. Pharyngeal and esophageal fistulas can be expected to heal in 15 to 25 days, longer if they are in postirradiated tissues. A similar period, or perhaps a slightly longer period, may be expected with duodenal fistulas. Colonic fistulas take longer to heal, approximately 30 to 40 days. Small bowel fistulas,

especially ileal fistulas, may take 40 to 60 days to heal, if at all.[143] In addition, nutritional parameters may be helpful in predicting spontaneous closure of fistulas. Recently published was a 10 year review of 79 patients with 116 fistulas, 80% of which were postoperative, and mortality, mainly owing to sepsis and cancer, was 20.3%.[139] The presence of local sepsis, systemic sepsis, remote sepsis (such as pneumonia or line sepsis), the number of fistulas, fistula output, and the number of blood transfusions were not predictive of spontaneous closure. However, a serum transferrin level >200 mg/dL at the time of presentation, or after 3 weeks of therapy, was an accurate predictor of spontaneous closure. The trend of the serum transferrin, when adequate protein and calories are provided, may be very useful in predicting closure. If serum levels fail to rise after 3 weeks of aggressive nutritional therapy, spontaneous closure is unlikely. Likewise, the authors found that of all the above factors, serum transferrin, retinol binding protein, and prealbumin were predictors of mortality.[139] These measurements tend to identify patients with sepsis or malignancy whose disease is clinically significant.

The mortality associated with a fistula is affected most by the presence of sepsis, the underlying etiology, volume of output, and nutritional status. However, all of these variables are intimately associated with, and affected by, the anatomic location of the fistula. Pharyngeal and cervical esophageal fistulas have a very high spontaneous closure rate and usually represent only minor physiologic stress. Consequently, their fistula-related mortality is low. Duodenal and proximal small bowel fistulas tend to be metabolically significant owing to their high output and, thus, have a 20% to 40% mortality rate.[158,180,199,200] Distal small bowel and colonic fistulas usually have lower outputs. While ileal fistulas tend to remain open, colonic fistulas tend to close, resulting in a fistula-related mortality rate of 20% to 30% for ileal fistulas and 10% to 20% for colonic fistulas.[138–140,144,145,151,162,170,276]

DIAGNOSIS, EVALUATION, AND MANAGEMENT

The ultimate goals in enterocutaneous fistula management are closure of the fistula and reestablishment of intestinal continuity. If 4 to 5 weeks of sepsis-free parenteral nutrition do not result in signs of closure, or if sepsis is present, patients should be taken to the operating room for exploration. Antibiotics and parenteral nutrition are unlikely to be effective in situations where sepsis is persistent. Conservative management and nonoperative management are not necessarily synonymous. Conservative is a term that is relative to the condition and prognosis of the patient, in addition to the etiology, anatomy, and physiology of the fistula. When a patient is resuscitated fully and spontaneous closure of the

TABLE 15–7. NATURAL HISTORY OF GASTROINTESTINAL FISTULAS

	Likely to Close	Unlikely to Close
Anatomic Location	Oro-pharyngeal, esophageal, duodenal stump, pancreaticobiliary, and jejunal	Gastric, lateral duodenal ligament of Treitz, and ileal
Nutritional Status	Well nourished	Malnourished
Sepsis	Absent	Present
Etiology	Appendicitis, diverticulitis, postoperative	Crohn's, cancer, foreign body, radiation
Condition of Bowel	Healthy, adjacent tissue, small leak, quiescent disease, no abscess	Total disruption, abscess, distal obstruction, active disease (Crohn's, tumor)
Miscellaneous	Tract >2 cm in length Defect <1 cm² in size	Epithelialization, foreign body
Transferrin	>200 mg/dL	<200 mg/dL

fistula is unlikely, or when sepsis is unresponsive to percutaneous drainage, prolonged nonoperative management often results in mortality and should be considered radical.

It is helpful to divide management of a patient with an enterocutaneous fistula into various stages. This way the physician can focus on the principal challenges and therapeutic decisions at each stage of management. Fistulas can be tenaciously persistent and resistant to intervention. Having a framework allows the physician and the patient to establish scheduled expectations and it assists in defining realistic goals. The anticipated course of a patient with a fistula can be divided into five sequential, but overlapping, phases: (1) stabilization, (2) investigation, (3) decision, (4) definitive therapy, and (5) healing (Table 15–8).

Recognition and Stabilization

Resuscitation. Postoperative fistulas usually become manifest 5 to 6 days after an operation. A wound abscess appears and is drained, resulting in defervescence; within the next 24 hours, enteric contents appear on the wound dressing. Crystalloid resuscitation, usually 3 to 4 L, to offset intravascular fluid losses sequestered in the

TABLE 15–8. MANAGEMENT PHASES FOR GASTROINTESTINAL FISTULAS

Stabilization	Rehydration Correction of anemia Drainage of sepsis Electrolyte repletion Oncotic pressure restoration Nutrition support institution Control of fistula drainage Institution of local skin care	Within 24–48 hours

Investigation	Fistulogram to define anatomy
	  and pathophysiology
	CT to localize collections and
	  to stage cancer, when present
	EGD or colonoscopy as indicated
		After
		7–10 days

Decision	Assess likelihood of spontaneous closure Plan therapeutic course Decide surgical timing	7–10 days to 4–6 weeks
Definitive Therapy	Plan operative approach Bowel resection with end-to-end anastomosis Ensure secure abdominal closure Gastrostomy Jejunostomy	When spontaneous closure is unlikely or after 4–6 weeks
Healing	Continue nutrition support Transition feedings	5–10 days after closure

bowel and bowel wall is often necessary. Anemia should be corrected to a hematocrit of 35 by transfusion of packed red blood cells. Plasma oncotic pressure should be restored. Organs particularly sensitive to hypoalbuminemia include skin, lungs, and intestines. Several reports have described an association between hypoalbuminemia and impaired gastrointestinal absorption, leading to the conclusion that exogenous albumin administration may promote absorption of intestinal luminal contents.[277–284] We feel that exogenous albumin should be administered until serum albumin reaches 3.0 mg/dL, unless sepsis-induced pulmonary capillary leak is prominent.

Drainage of Abscesses and Local Control. Implantation of enteric bacteria on catheters used for parenteral nutrition does occur, and may be more common with multiple lumen catheters than single lumen catheters.[285] This is particularly true when persistent bacteremia is present. When possible, abscesses should be drained 24 hours prior to line insertion. Prior to operative drainage, when an abscess is evident or is pointing to the abdominal wall, one should inject water soluble dye under fluoroscopy. Information may be gained that otherwise would be unobtainable when fistulas are studied this way.

In the event that an operation should ultimately prove necessary, it should not be done through a septic, indurated, cellulitic, and denuded abdominal wall.[85] Therefore, wound care assumes a high priority with enterocutaneous fistula patients.[86,285–287] Fistula drainage is best controlled by the use of a sump. A latex catheter such as a nephrostomy tube, which is soft at body temperature is preferred because it will not cause further skin or bowel-wall erosion. An air vent to break suction can be made by inserting a 14-gauge IV catheter into the lumen of the drainage tube. This will not only improve local skin care, it also will provide accurate records of fistula output. More recently, high-pressure suction has been advocated with seemingly miraculous results.[90,286,287]

A number of preparations may be used to prevent skin maceration and breakdown. Karaya seal, ileostomy cement, glycerine, or ion exchange resins help keep the skin acidic and prevent activation of pancreatic enzymes. The most effective form of management, in our experience, is Stomadhesive; if one can achieve fixation to the skin, these dressings can be left in place for a week or more. The skin underneath is well protected and skin healing can occur. An enterostomal therapist can be invaluable in this difficult portion of management.

Nutritional Management. The management of enterocutaneous fistulas has evolved significantly over the past three decades and, appropriately, nutritional support has gained a central management role. To optimize nutrient metabolism, circulation and tissue oxygenation must be adequate.[146] However, after initial stabilization, prompt initiation of nutritional support is crucial. The breakdown of lean body mass is relentless and sufficiently rapid so that each day the patient suffers septic starvation, significant deficits are compounded.[85,288–291]

Patients with enterocutaneous fistulas have increased calorie and protein requirements.[289–291] We recommend feeding at a rate that is 1.3 to 1.5 times the basal energy expenditure (BEE). When high-output proximal fistulas are present, needs may be as great as twice the calculated BEE. Although this is likely a high estimate, increased protein is probably more important than calories. Caution should be used in patients who are not septic and whose losses are not excessive to prevent overfeeding.

Weight gain, which is usually reflective of fluid retention more than an increase in body cell mass in an acutely ill patient, should not be a priority. The goal of nutritional therapy in this setting should include nitrogen equilibrium with maintenance or restoration of structural and functional protein synthesis.[146] Generally, healthy individuals require 0.8 to 1.0 gm of protein per kilogram per day. However, external losses and the additional metabolic stress present with enterocutaneous fistulas increases this protein requirement to 1.2 to 2.0 gm of protein per kilogram per day.[143,146,147]

Fluid requirements for maintenance can be estimated from either body weight (30 mL/kg) or body surface area (1500 mL/m^2) and adjusted for existing deficits and ongoing fistula losses. The necessity of keeping accurate records regarding fistula output can not be overstated. With high-output fistulas, the patient may become volume-depleted overnight. Therefore, the fistula losses *must* be added to daily fluid requirements. In addition, patients with fistulas often have a low-grade temperature, which adds 500 to 800 mL/day to their volume requirement for each degree centigrade over 37°. It is rarely necessary to supplement volume or electrolytes in addition to that received via parenteral nutrition except in patients whose fistula outputs are excessive.

We feel that the GI tract should be used, if possible, to provide at least a portion of the nutritional needs of the patient, since this may be sufficient to confer the beneficial effects of enteral nutrition.[292–296] Patients are often intolerant to the osmotic load of glucose-based enteral formulas. Lipid-based enteral formulas present a lower osmotic load than isocaloric carbohydrate-based formulas, and therefore, may be absorbed more efficiently from the GI tract lumen. There must be at least 4 feet of functional bowel, either proximal or distal to the fistula, to be able to use enteral nutrition as a sole nutritional therapy in patients with enterocutaneous fistulas. Respectable rates of fistula closure have been achieved using enteral support, although slightly

less than those achieved with parenteral nutrition.[198,213,286,292–296] Because of mucosal brush-border atrophy and hypoalbuminemia, initially, enteral nutrition may be absorbed poorly, resulting in diarrhea and continued nutritional decay.[297] Because it generally takes 4 to 5 days to attain target caloric provision with enteral therapy, a period of concurrent enteral and parenteral nutrition may be necessary to restore mucosal function.[295,296]

Free amino acids increase the osmolarity of tube feedings and may lead to decreased tolerance. Since dipeptides and tripeptides in the bowel lumen are transported into the mucosal cell and then hydrolyzed to free amino acids, providing protein in the form of free amino acids does not confer any advantage and is probably unnecessary. Oligopeptides from protein hydrolysates are tolerated better and probably are absorbed better than free amino acids and therefore, should be the major protein source of a chemically defined diet.[293,294,296–303]

Patients with high-output enterocutaneous fistulas should receive approximately twice the recommended daily allowance for water soluble vitamins. If the patient has a large, granulating wound where extensive tissue repair will be occurring, vitamin C should be provided at 5 to 10 times the RDA. In addition, patients with fistulas can lose considerable amounts of copper, zinc, and magnesium. We find it useful to monitor serum magnesium levels biweekly and supplement the patient as necessary by adding magnesium directly to the PN solution. While we do not routinely check serum copper or zinc levels, the amount of copper contained in two ampules of commercially prepared vitamin and trace element preparations usually will suffice. Additionally, with high-output fistulas, we routinely add 10 mg/day of elemental zinc to the PN solution.

Antibiotics. Review of large series of patients with fistulas reveal that the average patient receives seven to nine different antibiotics during their hospital course.[128,138–140,145,147,164] To prevent superinfection by resistant organisms, it is important to reserve antibiotics for times when they are needed. Unless a patient is septic, as evidenced by mental-status change, hemodynamic instability, high fever spikes, or the beginning of impaired organ function, antibiotics should be withheld.

The most common organisms causing sepsis in patients with enterocutaneous fistulas are of bowel origin (ie. coliforms, *Bacteroides sp.*, enterococcus). *Staphylococcus sp.* also often plays a role in intra-abdominal sepsis. CT scans should be used liberally if sepsis is suspected. Percutaneous drainage under CT guidance can be very effective in draining suitable abscesses. If sepsis is not controlled by percutaneous drainage and antibiotics, operative therapy is indicated.

Nasogastric Tubes. Unless the intestine is obstructed, there is little evidence that the use of a nasogastric tube is helpful. Several series have been unable to demonstrate improvement of outcome with the use of decompressive tubes.[143,145] Unless the fistula is high in the intestinal tract, the nasogastric tube can be removed, without influencing the amount of fistula drainage.[143] Aside from the patient discomfort from this unproven therapy, the presence of long-term indwelling nasogastric tubes may result in impaired cough, serous otitis media, pharyngitis, alar necrosis, mucosal erosion, and esophageal reflux with late esophageal stricture. If a gastrostomy or tube enterostomy is already present, it can be opened to gravity.

Measures to Decrease Volume of Secretion. Although decreasing fistula output does not improve spontaneous closure rates, it does seem to shorten the time to closure. Orogastric secretions account for 1.5 to 2 L and pancreatobiliary secretions constitute 2 to 2.5 L/day of enteric volume. When added to the 7 to 9 L the small intestine produces each day, it becomes evident that inhibition of these secretions is prudent. Unless a specific contraindication exists, the patient should be placed on therapeutic doses of either a H antagonist or a $H^+ - K^+$ ATPase inhibitor, since stress and prolonged periods of strict NPO may predispose patients to peptic ulceration. Additionally, intestinal intraluminal volume may be decreased by decreasing gastric acid secretion. In addition, diminished gastric acid secretion also may indirectly lessen pancreatobiliary secretion.

Although the efficacy of somatostatin in treatment of pancreatic fistulas is accepted, its role in the treatment of other fistulas is less clear. Somatostatin accelerates gastric emptying but inhibits motility in the remainder of the gastrointestinal tract. A single 50 μg subcutaneous injection of somatostatin increases mouth-to-cecum transit time from 57 to 204 minutes.[304–306] The same dose has been shown to decrease endogenous fluid secretion and increase absorption of water and electrolytes from the small bowel, in patients with diarrhea secondary to neuroendocrine tumors.[148,307–309] Because of these capabilities, the efficacy of somatostatin in enterocutaneous fistulas has been inferred, although never proven. Generalizations about the ability of somatostatin to decrease intraluminal intestinal volume in patients with relatively normal intestinal secretory and absorptive function are tenuous.

The short duration of action of somatostatin necessitated continuous intravenous infusion, in early studies.[310–313] This problem has been resolved by the introduction of the long-acting somatostatin analogue SMS 201-995 (Sandostatin, Sandoz Pharmaceuticals, East Hanover, NJ). Therapeutic equivalence to continuous intravenous infusion can be attained with subcutaneous SMS 201-995, 100-600 μg/day given in two to four divided doses. One series reported the treatment of patients with postoperative enterocutaneous fistulas with parenteral nutrition and SMS 201-995 (100 μg subcutaneously every 8 hours).[313] The mean reduction in fistula output was 55% within 24 hours of instituting SMS 201-995 therapy. This is consistent with our own experience with somatostatin. Spontaneous closure was achieved in 21 (77%) patients after a mean of 5.8 ± 2.7 days. Of the six remaining patients, one died of sepsis, two had distal obstruction and three had total anastomotic disruption. Inability to achieve closure in these six patients is not unexpected. Uncontrolled sepsis, distal obstruction, and total anastomotic disruption should not be expected to be remedied by a subcutaneous injection of SMS 201-995, or any other chemical, for that matter. When compared to parenteral nutrition alone, somatostatin does not seem to improve overall closure rates. Conservative treatment with parenteral nutrition alone succeeds in closing between 60% to 75% of fistulas. In collected series of fistulas treated with parenteral nutrition and somatostatin or SMS 201-995, the closure rate is 60% to 92%, similar to that for parenteral nutrition alone. However, time to closure is decreased from an average of 50 days for parenteral nutrition alone to 5 to 10 days when SMS 201-995 is administered.[148,310–316]

Emotional Support. The external drainage of enteric contents can be a particularly humiliating and demoralizing experience for both the patient and physician. The persistent nature and severe metabolic consequences of many fistulas may necessitate complex and prolonged medical management. This may lead to loss of personal confidence, loss of confidence in the healthcare team, and ultimately to major depression in the patient. Continued involvement and reassurance by the physician, with particular attention to ambulation and physical therapy, will go a long way in minimizing the emotional duress of such an intense medical condition.

Investigation

Radiologic investigations are the single most important entity in defining the anatomy of a fistula. We generally wait 7 to 10 days for the stamina of the patient to improve and the tract to mature sufficiently to be injected with a radiographic contrast media. To provide maximal information, a senior radiologist possessing expertise with equipment and positioning and the senior surgeon responsible for the care of the patient should be present during fluoroscopic evaluation. A water soluble contrast material is injected into the fistula tract through a 5 or 8 pediatric feeding tube. Standard barium gastrointestinal tract examinations, such as an upper GI series, small bowel follow-throughs, and barium enemas, rarely yield information in addition to that obtained from the fistulogram. The ultimate objective of this phase of therapy is to define those characteristics of a fistula which determine whether spontaneous closure is likely (Fig 15–4):

1. Is the bowel in continuity, or has it been completely disrupted?
2. Does the fistula arise from the lateral bowel wall, or is it an end fistula with complete bowel disruption?
3. Is there an associated abscess cavity, how large is it and does the fistula drain into the cavity?
4. What is the condition of the adjacent bowel? Damaged, strictured or inflamed?
5. Is there a distal obstruction?
6. From what part of the gastrointestinal tract does the fistula tract arise?
7. What is etiologic disease process?
8. Is the length of the tract <2 cm?
9. Is the bowel wall defect >1 cm²?

Characteristics associated with nonhealing fistulas include large adjacent abscesses, intestinal discontinuity, distal obstruction, poor adjacent bowel, gastric, ileal, and ligament of Treitz fistulas, fistula tracts <2 cm in length, and enteral defect >1 cm². In addition, fistulas arising from radiation-damaged intestine, inflammatory bowel disease and recurrent carcinoma are not likely to heal.

In general, CT or MRI are not useful in the initial evaluation of a nonseptic patient with an enterocutaneous fistula. If the patient is septic, CT should be used to evaluate the abdomen for undrained abscesses.[317,318] In addition, CT may be useful in evaluation for recurrent tumor, which, if present, may change the entire nature of the therapeutic direction.

Decision

The main goal of therapy in patients with enterocutaneous fistulas is the reestablishment of intestinal integrity. Most favorably, this is achieved by spontaneous closure. However, in unfavorable etiologic, anatomic, and nutritional conditions, this occurs in only one-third of the patients. Even if there are no unfavorable factors present, the ability to predict spontaneous closure in favorable gastrointestinal fistulas is inexact.

Attempts to catalogue characteristics of fistulas that are predictive of spontaneous closure are numerous. The underlying disease, the presence or absence of sepsis, the anatomic location, the condition of the bowel at the fistula site and distally, and the nutritional status of the patient may all carry prognostic significance with regard to the likelihood of spontaneous closure. If at the time of presentation or after 3 weeks of therapy, the serum transferrin level is >200 mg/dL, spontaneous closure is more likely.[139] In addition, when a fistulous tract

is chronic, epithelium may migrate from either end to line the tract, in essence forming an "ostomy". When this occurs, spontaneous closure is highly unlikely and operative therapy usually is required.

If fistula closure has not been achieved spontaneously and no signs of imminent closure are apparent after 4 to 5 weeks of nutritional support in a sepsis-free patient, it is unlikely that the fistula will close, and the patient should be prepared for surgery. If uncontrolled sepsis is present at any time during the clinical course of the patient, urgent drainage of abscesses, or resection of phlegmon with restoration of intestinal continuity, should be carried out. If the condition of the patient is extreme, only drainage of abscesses should be carried out at the initial operation. Diversion of the gastrointestinal tract may be necessary if persistent soiling is likely. Definitive fistula repair carried out at a future time, while disappointing to the patient and surgeon, is preferable to a fatal outcome.

The transplant population may represent the exception to many of the rules accepted when managing fistulas. Because of their ongoing need for immunosuppression, it is probably unwise to subject them to prolonged nonoperative management. Septic complications from fistulas as well as from parenteral nutrition are increased in the immunosuppressed population. In addition, their healing is impaired, as well. Therefore, as soon as there is evidence of short-turnover protein synthesis, early operative correction is recommended. Consideration also should be given to early operative intervention for fistulas arising from malignancy. This is because fistulas complicating malignancy are unlikely to close spontaneously and many, if not most, ultimately require operation. If malignancy is transmural, as is likely, adjunctive therapy will be necessary to optimize recurrence-free interval and survival. As long as the fistula is open, chemotherapy and radiation will not be administered. In addition, current forms of nutritional support are likely to increase tumor growth. Therefore, one should minimize the time of parenteral nutritional support in the absence of surgery or adjunctive treatment.

Definitive Therapy

Alternative Forms of Therapy. Until recently, surgical intervention to close the fistula was the only available option. However, endoscopic injection of congenital tracheoesophageal fistulas has been available since the early 1980s.[318] One report describes endoscopic injections of a fast-hardening amino acid solution into the fistulous tracts of four patients, with successful closure in all four.[319] The fistula tracts included two postoperative esophagopleural fistulas, one bronchobiliary fistula, and one bronchoesophageal fistula. It should be noted that these fistulas were probably not high-output fistu-

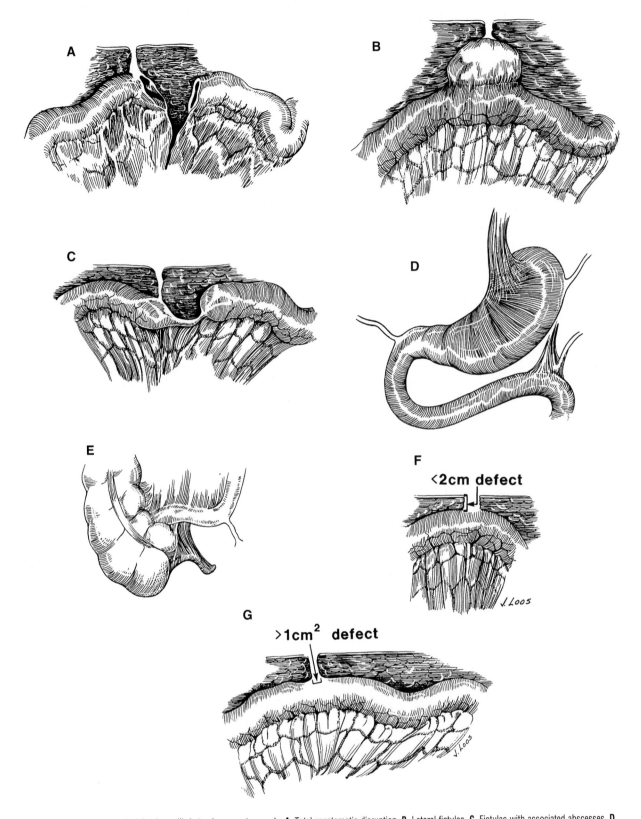

Figure 15–4. Gastrointestinal fistulas unlikely to close spontaneously. **A.** Total anastomotic disruption. **B.** Lateral fistulas. **C.** Fistulas with associated abscesses. **D.** Strictured bowel/distal obstruction. **E.** Gastric, lateral duodenal or ligament or Treitz fistulas. **F.** Ileal fistulas. **G.** Fistulas with tracts <2 cm. **H.** Fistulas with >1 cm² bowel wall defects.

las, and were particularly amenable to this form of therapy. However, between 1988 and 1990 five papers were published, collectively reporting successful results in 30 patients with high-output proximal enterocutaneous fistulas treated by endoscopic injection of fibrin glue.[320–324] Use of this technique in patients with unacceptable operative risk may be warranted. Unfortunately, use is limited by the reach of the endoscope. Additionally, use in colocutaneous fistulas has not been reported, to date.

General Surgical Considerations.

Operation is undertaken in patients whose anatomic features preclude spontaneous closure, and in patients with anatomic features favorable for closure, if 4 to 5 weeks of sepsis-free nutritional support does not lead to closure. If meticulous skin care and control of fistula drainage has been achieved, the operation can be carried out through a healthy abdominal wall, enhancing the chance of secure abdominal closure. Particular attention should be paid to electrolyte and volume status, preoperatively and when there is question, a Swan-Ganz catheter should be placed. Fistula drainage should be cultured and intraluminal antibiotics, as well as targeted intravenous antibiotics, should be administered. If the patient has been receiving enteral nutritional therapy, discontinuation one to two days preoperatively may decrease abdominal distention and aid in attaining a secure abdominal closure. If parenteral nutrition has been used, a full day's order should be submitted the morning of the operation and the rate decreased to 40 mL an hour just prior to operation. This will ensure that the patient does not run out of parenteral nutrition during the procedure, and provides enough volume so that the rate can be re-advanced in the recovery room.

Because many of these patients are hospitalized prior to their operation, their colonizing bacteria may be particularly virulent. The abdomen and operative site should be washed with antibacterial solutions for several days prior to operation. Bowel preparation, and both mechanical and nonabsorbable antibiotic preparation should be carried out. Systemic antibiotics should always be used as these are, by definition, at least clean-contaminated cases. Sufficient time should be allowed for this operation. Extensive dissection is usually necessary, with meticulous technique and hemostasis absolutely essential for the prevention of further fistulization. The operative approach is preferably through a new incision so that the major operative field is relatively clean. Dissection should proceed from the ligament of Treitz to the rectum, with all adhesions freed. The best rates of closure and the lowest incidence of complications are obtained by definitive resection and end-to-end anastomosis.[145,147] Overall, other approaches produce inferior results and should not be attempted unless mitigating

circumstances exist. The anastomosis should be carried out in a clean field away from any previous abscess cavity. The omentum should be placed in its anatomic position with a portion covering the anastomosis. Duodenal fistulas are the exception to the rule of resection with end-to-end anastomosis, partly because of the gravity of the dissection necessary and partly because of very satisfactory outcomes achieved with bypass procedures. Gastrojejunostomy, preferably with vagotomy (but without if the condition of the patient is unstable), gastrostomy, and catheter jejunostomy for feeding will result in closure of most fistulas.

The importance of a secure abdominal wall closure above a fistula cannot be overstated. This may be difficult in patients in whom the abdominal wall has been partially destroyed by sepsis.[88–90] If closure is complicated, a plastic surgery team should be employed to assist in this portion of the operation. In general, prosthetic reconstructions are contraindicated, since they can lead to recurrent fistulas or become infected when used in these contaminated cases. Musculocutaneous flaps should be used if inadequate fascia is available for a tension-free closure. In few other types of cases will deviation from sound surgical principles result in such catastrophic consequences.

A Stamm gastrostomy should be placed at the time of surgery for postoperative gastric decompression. They interfere less with pulmonary toilet and cause less discomfort than nasogastric sump tubes. In addition, they can be used for enteral nutrition supplementation, if necessary. Providing a means of access for postoperative nutritional support is crucial. Feeding jejunostomies should be considered in all patients undergoing enterocutaneous fistula surgery, although one may wish to delay their use in the postoperative period.

Oral, Pharyngeal, and Esophageal Fistulas.

Oropharyngeocutaneous fistulas may often pursue a long subcutaneous course and exit at the lower end of the neck incision. When this occurs, an incision should be made higher in the neck to shorten and control the fistula tract. Not only will this promote healing of the tract, but it will also prevent further tissue loss and possible carotid exposure (Fig 15–5). The patient with an oropharyngeal fistula should be made NPO and a feeding tube should be placed. Antisialogogues usually are not necessary and may result in sialoadenitis, if used. Provided there is no distal obstruction, tumor recurrence, or foreign body to prevent spontaneous closure, expectant management, with particular attention to hydration and nutritional repletion, is indicated. The vast majority of these oropharyngeocutaneous fistulas will heal with nonoperative management, even in irradiated tissues. Because postfistula access is obtained easily and these fistulas tend to be of minor metabolic con-

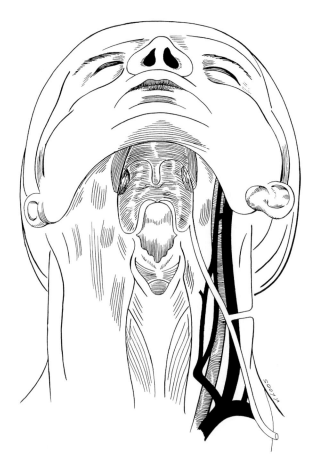

Figure 15–5. Pharyngeocutaneous fistula management. The fistula tract is shortened to provide control and prevent carotid exposure.

enteral nutritional support, a minimum of 250 mL of 10% lipids should be given to the patient by central or peripheral vein every 5 to 7 days to prevent essential fatty–acid deficiency.

Fistulas that persist without signs of closing after 6 to 8 weeks of sepsis-free, nonoperative management should be considered for operative management. Numerous techniques for orocutaneous, pharyngeocutaneous, and cervical esophagocutaneous fistula repair are described in the literature. These include primary closure, skin grafts, local and regional cutaneous flaps, myomucosal flaps, muscle flaps, gastric and colonic interpositions, and free jejunal grafts.[329–341] Appropriate application of these techniques depends on size and location of the fistulous tract.

Gastric Fistulas. Nonoperative care usually involves nasogastric suction, fluid replacement, and aggressive nutritional supplementation. Aggressive drainage of sepsis is paramount if nonoperative treatment is to be attempted, because the mortality doubles when sepsis occurs. With low-output fistulas, it is often possible to feed these patients. Achieving adequate nutrition can be problematic with high-output fistulas. If postfistula access can be obtained, enteral nutrition is preferred. Because as many as 50% of patients with gastrocutaneous fistulas will have malnutrition, parenteral nutrition should be instituted early and continued until the patient can be sustained enterally. Most series report 30% to 50% spontaneous closure of gastrocutaneous fistulas after 4 to 6 weeks of nonoperative management.[180–185] If closure does not occur, fistula resection with layered closure of the stomach is indicated. Decompressive gastrostomy and feeding jejunostomy should be placed. Alternatively, if the gastric remnant is small, nasogastric and nasointestinal tubes can be intraoperatively positioned and secured. If the gastric remnant is not large enough to salvage, completion gastrectomy should be considered.

Duodenal Fistulas. In duodenal fistulas, the same basic rules of nutrition provision pertain as with gastric fistulas.[207,260,292] Simple closure or repair of an established duodenal fistula is associated with a high likelihood of recurrence. Therefore, when primary closure is attempted, omental or serosal patch reinforcement, or exclusion and bypass with tube duodenostomy should also be performed (Fig 15–6).[166,167,205] A preferred approach to duodenal fistulas is to attack the fistula indirectly, by bypassing the fistula and providing a route of gastric drainage, such as gastrojejunostomy. A gastrostomy should be placed as well, thus allowing the bypassed fistula to heal. The use of bypass in duodenal fistulas is in sharp contrast to data that show that treating intestinal fistulas with bypass is not efficacious.[145]

sequence, nonoperative management can be prolonged without undue sequelae. If spontaneous closure has not occurred within 4 to 6 weeks, thyroid function studies should be carried out. Radiation and partial resection of the thyroid during therapy for head and neck cancers may lead to impaired healing from hypothyroidism. In addition, with any nonhealing fistula tract, persistent tumor should be considered and ruled out by biopsy.

Enteral nutritional support with a balanced formulation should be used in patients with oropharyngeocutaneous or esophagocutaneous fistulas when postfistula access can be obtained. The exception may be in the 1% to 2% of neck dissections when the thoracic duct has been injured and has resulted in chylous fistulas.[88] While this is not a true enterocutaneous fistula, nonoperative management is similar to the management of patients with enterocutaneous fistulas. A conservative policy of either parenteral nutrition or enteral nutrition, with medium-chain triglycerides as the major fat source, usually is recommended because, theoretically, both decrease chyle flow.[326–328] Whether giving enteral or par-

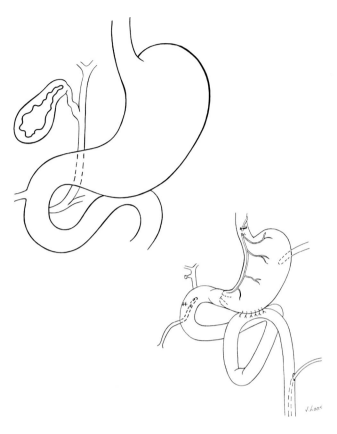

Figure 15–6. Duodenal fistula management. Duodenal fistulas often are managed best by exclusion and bypass. The duodenal repair can be reinforced with omental or jejunal patch. Decompressive-tube duodenostomy and feeding jejunostomy also should be performed.

Small Intestinal Fistulas. Fistulas of the small bowel, with or without a colonic component, are the most common type of fistula encountered by surgeons. Unless they are distal, small bowel fistulas tend to be high-output fistulas. Consequently, volume, electrolyte, and nutritional management are more complicated. Because of the association between fistula output, uncontrolled sepsis, and mortality, the mortality of small bowel fistulas tends to be particularly high, especially as compared with colonic and other fistulas. Factors associated with enterocutaneous fistulas that may raise the average mortality of 20% include age >70 years, a fistula originating in irradiated, ischemic or inflamed bowel, the presence of significant amounts of tumor burden, evisceration, sepsis, output >200 cc per 24 hours, and the presence of malnutrition.[85,86,138–147,153,160,163] Furthermore, the presence of strictured or inflamed bowel, large adjacent abscesses, or distal obstruction all force the surgeon to consider earlier operative repair which would not be considered if these factors were not present. The presence of an abscess and/or undrained sepsis in an unstable patient in whom antibiotics do not obviate the

fever spikes, and/or the beginning of multiple organ system failure, should result in prompt operative intervention, even if an abscess is not present on CT scan. Occasionally, one will find a small, but significant collection. A negative CT scan in a patient with obvious sepsis should prompt renewed efforts to culture an organism from all body fluids. Under these circumstances, *Candida sp* infection of a central line is often the culprit.

In three series from institutions experienced in the care of gastrointestinal cutaneous fistulas, spontaneous closure occurred in only 32% of patients.[139,143,145] The remainder required operative closure. This is particularly true for ileal fistulas in which even the most favorable series reported spontaneous closure rates of only 40%.[169] This tendency for ileal fistulas to stay open recently has been reconfirmed.[139] Smaller ileal diameter, more vigorous ileal motility, the presence of relative obstruction of the ileocecal valve, the increased number of Peyer's patches, and infiltration by lymphocytes may contribute to fistula persistence. Thus, the majority of patients with ileal fistulas will require operation, independent of how favorable the anatomic features appear.

Once surgery has been decided upon, the timing of the operation is the next consideration critical to the outcome of the patient. Under the best of circumstances, the operation often is demanding technically and may lead to further fistula formation, abscess, sepsis, and peritonitis. Unfortunately, the worst time to undertake an operation is within 3 months of the initial operative procedure, since adhesions are likely to be dense and the operation bloody. When possible, 3 to 4 months should pass before attempting reoperation. This will allow adhesions to become more filmy and less adherent. Unfortunately, one usually is required to make a decision about surgery within 6 weeks, so one usually does not have the luxury of allowing the patient to wait 3 months while in the hospital. In one review, it was found that when an operation was carried out within 10 days of fistula formation, the success rate was 67%.[157] When the operation was delayed and carried out between 11 to 42 days, the success rate was 70%, and when the operation was delayed for >42 days, the operative success rate rose to 84%. More impressive, however, was the influence that timing had on mortality. In this study, mortality was 11% to 13% when the operation was done within 10 days, or after 42 days after fistula formation.[157] However, in the intermediate period of between 11 to 42 days after fistula formation, the mortality climbed to 21%. It is our feeling that as long as the patient is gaining metabolically, it is reasonable to pursue a nonoperative management course.

Jejunal fistulas, provided they are not directly at the ligament of Treitz, have a higher likelihood of spontaneous closure than ileal fistulas. After 5 or 6 weeks of medical management in a patient free of significant sepsis, if closure has not occurred, but fistula output is diminishing, serum albumin is rising, and normal bowel function is returning, medical management should continue. Even with complex enterocutaneous fistulas, an additional 10% of fistulas will close after 8 weeks of medical therapy.[156] When the patient is not improving or the anatomy of the fistula is such that spontaneous closure is unlikely, there is little point in delaying the operative procedure, provided it can be done safely.

Once the decision for surgery is made, careful preparation should begin. The abdominal wall should be reevaluated, loculations drained, and cellulitis aggressively treated. If it is clear that a secure abdominal wall closure cannot be obtained through standard incisions, consultation with the plastic surgical service should take place. Rotational flaps or microvascular anastomoses can be performed by plastic surgeons after the intraabdominal portion of the operation is completed. Their contribution of a secure abdominal closure may mean the difference between failure and success.

Prior to surgery, fistula drainage should be carefully cultured so that appropriate antibiotics can be given. If tube feedings are being carried out, these should be slowed so that a respite of 2 to 3 days with antibiotic luminal preparation and cathartics, if appropriate, can be done, as well. Washing of the abdominal wall and surrounding areas with antibacterial solution such as chlorhexidine gluconate (Hibiclens, Stuart Pharmaceuticals, Wilmington, DE) will decrease the bacterial flora. Finally, training of the patient in postoperative pulmonary physiotherapy should begin. In addition to routine preoperative laboratories, particular attention should be paid to the coagulation factors of the patient, since prolonged parenteral nutrition may result in vitamin K deficits. Ample red cell mass, circulating volume, and colloid oncotic preparation should be achieved. Blood, as well as coagulation factor availability, should be ascertained.

The operative approach should take place through a new incision so that the operative field is relatively clean. If this is not possible, the old incision is used, but extended for easier access to the abdomen. In addition, if sepsis still exists in the abdominal wall, the incision should be made remote from this area. Abscess cavities, if present, should be drained through separate stab wounds distant from the primary incision. The operative incision should be planned so that if end-to-end anastomoses will be necessary, which usually is the case, it can be carried out well away from the area of maximal contamination. Fresh anastomoses surrounded by sepsis are likely to fail and will result in high mortality.

After incision, wound protectors or wound towels should be placed to protect the skin and subcutaneous tissues from contamination. Some authorities recommend beginning dissection at the distal ileum and working proximally. In the event that the operation must

then be aborted, internal bypass may be feasible. However, our own finding is that with abdomens having diffuse, dense adhesions, it is best to start working where dissection is easiest. When dissection becomes difficult, laparotomy pads soaked with antibiotic solutions should be applied and dissection continued elsewhere. One can later return to the previous area, which by then will be easier to define. When the fistula-containing loop is identified, the nonoperating hand of the surgeon should remain behind that loop. Dissection then can be directed toward the fistula from all directions. After the fistula tract is identified and separated from the abdominal wall, we temporarily close the bowel wall defect with a suture or an Allis or Babcock clamp. This prevents spillage while the resection margins are cleared of mesentery and the bowel clamps are placed.

Serosal rents created during dissection should be repaired with nonabsorbable Lembert sutures as soon as they are identified. Where full-thickness bowel defects are created, closure should be attempted with two layers of nonabsorbable sutures in Heinicke-Mikulicz fashion. When the mesenteric side of the bowel wall is involved, the blood supply may be compromised. Resection and anastomosis should be considered in this circumstance.

Resection with end-to-end anastomosis is the recommended management of the bowel loop containing the fistula (Fig 15–7). This provides the best chance for permanent resolution. If cancer is present, this may alter the approach. Irradiated bowel is particularly difficult to deal with and, along with duodenal fistulas, may represent an exception to the rule of end-to-end anastomosis. Irradiated bowel is probably best dealt with via stricturoplasty rather than resection and end-to-end anastomosis. Because of the microvascular thrombosis and fibrosis associated with previous radiation therapy, the end artery blood supply to the bowel wall may be inadequate to support a healing anastomosis, making anastomotic failure likely.

When it is unsafe to resect the fistula containing the bowel segment, or if anastomosis would be unwise owing to sepsis, resection with ostomy formation or exteriorization of the two bowel ends can be carried out. Staged closure after sepsis resolves is always superior to attempts at primary anastomosis that are doomed to failure.[180,351,352,353] Bypassing the fistula containing the bowel segment can be done, but it rarely results in closure of the fistula. Because reoperation is usually necessary following the bypass, there is no benefit to using this procedure rather than exteriorization or ostomy formation.[145]

Because the presence of abscess or distal obstruction will cause surgical closure to fail, the bowel should be freed from the ligament of Treitz to the rectum. Once the fistula is resected, the temptation to conclude a fistula operation before this goal is attained may be great.

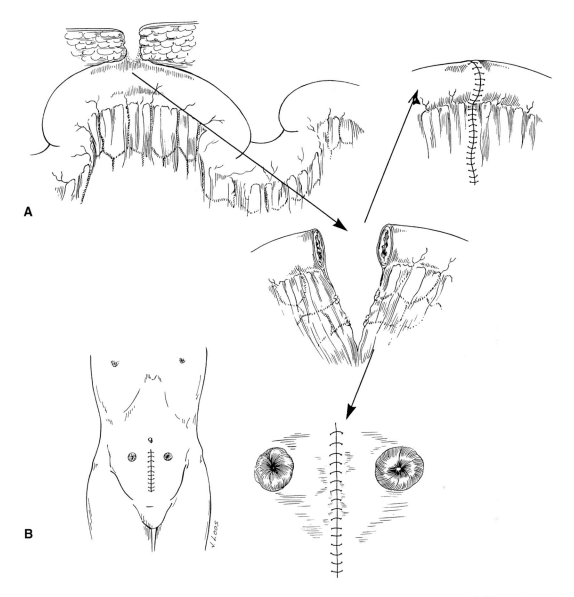

Figure 15–7. Small intestinal fistula management. **A**. Small intestinal fistulas are best managed by resection with end-to-end anastomosis. **B**. When unsafe to perform a primary anastomosis the ends can be exteriorized as end ostomies with anastomosis done when the patient is stable. The proximal effluent should be re-fed into the distal ostomy.

However, if failure supervenes because of this, subsequent reoperation assuredly will be more difficult and the chance of failure greater. One technically superior and complete operation is far better for both patient and surgeon than many inferior and incomplete operations. Therefore, it is advisable to schedule these types of operations to begin early in the day and not to allow other commitments to distract the surgeon for the remainder of the day.

Antibiotic-soaked laparotomy pads should be used throughout the operation. Although many types of antibiotics are used, we prefer kanamycin. The concentration of kanamycin absorbed during the operative proce-

dure is sufficiently low so that renal toxicity is not increased. Irrigation with copius amounts of antibiotic-containing solution should also be done. Final inspection of the entire bowel length and fresh anastomoses should be performed to ensure that inadvertent enterotomies and serosal rents are adequately repaired and that no distal narrowing of the bowel lumen exists. When bowel narrowings are found, stricturoplasties or resection with anastomoses should be performed as necessary.

Decompressive gastrostomy and a feeding jejunostomy should be utilized after every abdominal procedure of this magnitude. The authors do not utilize needle catheter jejunostomies, since a 14 latex nephrostomy tube allows more freedom in the choice of tube feedings in the postoperative period. Finally, a secure abdominal closure is crucial to successful outcome. Prosthetic materials result in recurrence of the fistula.

Some deviation from the standard will be required in pelvic exenteration fistulas, especially when the pelvis has been irradiated.[272] The incidence of recurrence is extraordinarily high, as is the incidence of abscess after a prolonged procedure on irradiated tissue in a denuded pelvis (Fig 15–8). It is absolutely essential to utilize musculocutaneous flaps, preferably gracilis flaps if they are available, to fill the pelvis. This will prevent bowel, especially newly anastomosed bowel, from prolapsing into an infected area with poor blood supply following irradiation. Likewise, the incision in irradiated abdominal wall may be necessarily high and transverse to avoid having to secure closure in an irradiated, indurated abdominal wall.

The presence of recurrent cancer resulting in fistula makes the operative procedure even more difficult. In many situations, significant tumor burden is present, and the chance of operative failure is increased significantly. Resection of the tumor mass should be attempted; however, the primary purpose of the operation is to resect and close the fistula in bowel that is free of tumor. Whenever possible, the bowel, especially the freshly anastomosed bowel, should be walled off from the tumor, even through the use of absorbable mesh such as Vicryl mesh and/or utilization of omentum or an omental flap. The incidence of failure is likely to be highly significant in the presence of cancer. In the final analysis, if the tumor burden is high or there is a massive tumor which cannot be extirpated, bypass may be necessary, with the understanding that the fistula may not be obviated totally, but at least oral nutrition may be resumed and the patient allowed some meaningful time at home.

Finally, there are times when surgery is undertaken in a patient in whom there are multiple extensive abscesses within the abdomen. Under these circumstances, resection and anastomosis of all the fistulas with proximal double-barrel ostomy diversion should be considered. After an appropriate period, contrast studies can be carried out and a limited procedure with closure of the jejunostomy can be performed. When two ostomies are created, feeding of proximal ostomy effluent into the distal limb can be undertaken, when safe. This approach is probably underutilized in critical situations. Mortality may be averted by this maneuver, which is appropriate under desperate circumstances.

Often, there are multiple raw and denuded surfaces that ooze and weep both blood and lymphatic fluid. In addition, there may be areas with large abscesses that will be drained during the course of the procedure. Closed-suction drains should be left in as one would use a closed-suction drain for any abscess, for 5 to 10 days rather than 2 to 3 days. With respect to drainage of areas that are not infected, but merely drain blood and serum, the proximity of these drains to infected and potentially infected areas is such that their use should be looked upon not necessarily as totally prophylactic but as therapeutic. Closed-suction drains, preferably of material that is soft at body temperature and that can be compressed easily so that gentle suction is maintained, are our preference. We do not believe that drain erosion is a problem, but believe that drainage serves a useful purpose by preventing the accumulation of purulence or blood and serum that may turn purulent. Our practice is to remove these drains when they drain <25 cc during a 24 hour period. Occasionally, drainage will decrease and then increase their removal of relatively large amounts of clear serous material. Under those circumstances, it is our belief that the drains are provoking the exudation of fluid. Amylase, cholesterol, and triglyceride levels should be checked to ensure that pancreatic or thoracic duct disruption have not occurred, the drains removed, and their tips cultured.

The nature of nutritional supplementation in gastrointestinal-cutaneous fistulas is evolving. Bowel rest

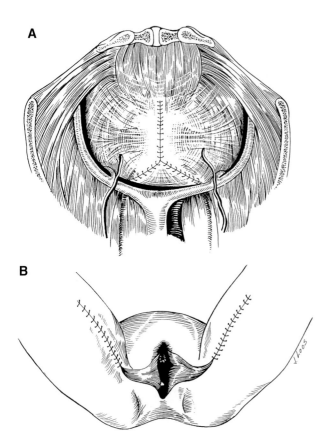

Figure 15–8. Pelvic exenteration management. **A.** The pelvis should be reperitonealized. **B.** When reperitonealization is impossible, advancement flaps of omentum or muscle should be performed.

and the provision of all calories by vein was once thought to be the preferred mode of therapy. However, with the recognition that gut mucosa provides functions other than absorption, the importance of gut feeding is better understood. Provision of gut feeding, even in the presence of sepsis-free parenteral nutrition, has dramatic effects on wound closure and in overall well being. Whether this is the result of increasing gut-mucosal integrity, hepatic protein synthesis, and/or the beneficial immunological effects, is not clear. It is clear that in order to achieve this beneficial effect, one does not have to provide all of the calories by the enteral route. Indeed, it has been estimated that the amount provided is only 20% to 30% of the caloric need.[213] Regardless of whether one can provide the entire caloric need, the provision of some enteral nutrition will yield a better outcome, despite an initial fistula drainage increase.

Recent studies have suggested that alterations in fatty acids supplied to provide the omega-3 polyunsaturated fatty acids, arginine, nucleotides, soluble pectins, and other experimental nutritional supplements gives better results in postoperative patients.[342,343] Only multiple-component formulas are commercially available, and studies on single dietary components are incomplete. Nonetheless, to these authors the evidence is sufficiently compelling so that a decided attempt should be made to provide at least some gut nutrition. When fistulas are very complex, it may be possible to place a feeding tube or jejunostomy and maintain the patient on home enteral nutrition for a prolonged period of time.

Pouch Fistulas. Pouch fistulas may be more difficult to manage than fistulas that occur in otherwise healthy ileum. Most will require preservation or reestablishment of diverting ileostomy for resolution.[344,345]

Treatment with metronidazole, ciprofloxacin, and possibly short-chain fatty-acid enemas for pouchitis should probably be done after diversion is established. In addition, the resected colon should be reinspected to ensure ulcerative colitis and not Crohn's disease was present. Crohn's involvement of the pouch may mandate permanent ileostomy.[346–348]

Many pouch fistulas can be repaired by division and layered closure. In addition, interposed advancement flaps may prevent future fistula formation. Those that can not be salvaged must be resected with either permanent ileostomy or ileostomy with later ileoproctostomy. On occasion, a new pouch can be created with proximal ileostomy for protection. If this is successful, it can be followed by ileostomy closure.[346–348]

Colonic Fistulas. Spontaneous closure in the face of active diverticulitis, cancer, or Crohn's disease is unlikely, but spontaneous closure of postoperative colonic fistulas can be expected to occur in 80% to 90% by 40 to 50 days.[349] Postoperative fistulas tend to be low-output fistulas, and often can be effectively treated with enteral therapy or parenteral nutrition without proximal diverting colostomy.[350]

Most appendicocutaneous fistulas are low-output fistulas and close spontaneously within 3 weeks.[353] If surgical intervention is necessary, excision of the tract with simple closure of the cecum is the treatment of choice.[354] When fistulas occur after an appendectomy is performed in a Crohn's disease–involved cecum, the fistula is virtually always from the terminal ileum and not the appendiceal stump. These fistulas behave as Crohn's disease–related fistulas do; therefore, their management is that of a Crohn's fistula (see below).

Internal Intestinal Fistulas. Symptomatic patients with internal enteroenteral fistulas unresponsive to medical therapy will require operation. Operative intervention for Crohn's disease fistulas is reserved for specific complications such as malabsorption, intractable diarrhea, obstruction, short bowel syndrome, or chronic urinary tract infection. Once diverticulitis has become complicated by abscess or fistula formation, resection of the involved colonic segment is indicated regardless of whether the fistula has closed. Operative indications for malignant internal fistulas are similar to Crohn's disease fistulas. Short life expectancy or prohibitive operative risk will preclude operation for malignant fistulas. In these cases, unless resection will be curative, operation is reserved for specific complications such as malabsorption, intractable diarrhea, obstruction, or short bowel syndrome. Unless specific contraindication exists, such as advanced malignancy, symptomatic enteroenteric or enterocolonic, all colovaginal or colovesical fistulas should be surgically repaired.[214]

Crohn's Disease. Traditionally, Crohn's disease has been treated surgically, in a manner similar to intestinal malignancy. Wide resection with clear margins was offered as the only chance for cure, with severe nutritional and metabolic consequences occurring commonly. However, with the recognition of Crohn's disease as a diffuse abnormality of the gastrointestinal tract, the operative approach has been modified somewhat. Because wide clean margins or microscopic involvement of margins at the time of operation do not alter recurrence rates, conservative resection now is accepted as adequate surgical therapy. In addition, with the understanding that resection will likely not be curative, resection is reserved for symptomatic lesions only.

At operation a large matted mass of bowel may be found in the right lower quadrant of patients with Crohn's ileocolitis. Specific attention should be paid to the length of bowel resected, since postresection short bowel syndrome following repeated resections is common.[355] If resection will place the patient at risk for short bowel syndrome, measures such as stricturoplasty, serosal patching, and intestinal tapering should be considered to preserve intestinal length.[356–358] The margins of resection for Crohn's disease need only be grossly free of disease. The presence of microscopic disease does not increase the likelihood of late recurrence of Crohn's disease as compared to margins completely free of Crohn's disease. In our own practice, the margins are no more than 3 to 4 cm beyond gross fatty overgrowth and mesenteric adenopathy immediately adjacent to the bowel.

En bloc resection of diseased intestine and fistula with end-to-end anastomosis is the preferred treatment for fistulas where both segments of bowel are involved with Crohn's disease. However, when a diseased segment fistulizes to otherwise healthy bowel, the site of the secondary fistula becomes critical in making operative decisions. Repair of the secondary defect should be undertaken (if the stomach, small intestine, right colon, or bladder is involved) by freshening the edges and suturing the defect.[359,360] Intestine containing secondary defects should be resected only if adjacent to diseased bowel that itself requires resection. Sigmoid colon and duodenal defects have a greater tendency to develop fistulas postoperatively,[359,361,362] therefore, if the sigmoid colon is secondarily involved, primary closure can be done safely only if the nutritional status of the patient is good. If the patient manifests poor nutritional status, primary repair with proximal diverting colostomy should be considered.

When the bladder is involved by a Crohn's disease fistula, primary bladder repair with interrupted, layered, absorbable sutures is recommended. A Foley catheter should be left in place for 7 to 10 days. Likewise, colovaginal fistulas can be repaired with layered, absorbable sutures from an abdominal approach, when high on the vaginal wall, and by a perineal approach when midwall or lower.[363] A circumvaginal incision with dissection in the plane of the colovaginal septum usually provides adequate fistula exposure. The fistula tract is excised, and the vaginal wall closed in layers. The vaginal mucosa can be closed from inside the vagina, or as is done in our own practice, extravaginally. The muscular layers of the vagina can be closed externally to interpose layers between the vagina and rectum. In a similar fashion, the bowel wall is closed in two layers externally. Interposition of healthy tissue such as levator or other perineal musculature is useful to prevent fistula redevelopment.

The duodenum usually is not involved with fistulous Crohn's disease,[361] therefore, it can be repaired primarily. However, because postoperative duodenal fistulas carry a high mortality rate, the duodenum should be reinforced by omental or serosal patch, excluded and decompressed by tube duodenostomy, or the duodenal defect diverted into a Roux-en-Y loop.[362]

Diverticulitis. Fistulas associated with diverticulitis have a high spontaneous closure rate. In most patients, resection with end-to-end anastomosis should be carried out after inflammation subsides. End colostomy with oversewing of the rectal stump is preferred, in the acute setting. Although there are reports of successful resection and primary anastomosis in the acute diverticulitis setting, complicated diverticulitis (established abscess or fistula) is probably best handled by Hartman's procedure. Complete resection of diverticula-containing colon is essential to successful treatment. Inadequate sigmoid resection can lead to recurrent diverticulitis. Complications also may occur if diverticula are left at the anastomosis. Primary repair should be undertaken when the bladder is involved by fistula. Foley catheter should be left in place for 10 days for bladder decompression. Likewise, colovaginal fistulas should be repaired with absorbable sutures by an abdominal approach when high on the vaginal wall, and by a perineal approach when midvaginal wall or lower.[363] Interposition of healthy tissue such as levator or other perineal musculature is useful to prevent redevelopment of fistulas.

Malignancy. Fistulas complicating malignancy are unlikely to undergo spontaneous closure. When evaluating a patient for definitive operative therapy there are preliminary questions to be answered:

1. What is the extent of disease?
2. What is the biology of the tumor?
3. What is the life expectancy of the patient?
4. How does the fistula affect the quality of life of the patient?
5. Will operative attempts be palliative or curative?
6. Will chemotherapy or radiation therapy be necessary?
7. What is the operative risk of the patient?

The operative goals for malignant fistulas may be altered by the answers to these questions. When possible, all bowel should be dissected, and resection with end-to-end anastomosis performed. However, freeing the entire bowel length may not be realistic and bypass will be preferred in certain circumstances. In addition, disease-free resection margins may be impossible without massive small bowel resection. The price of profuse diarrhea from short gut syndrome is rarely worth the small gains from such massive resections. Conservative resection is indicated in those cases where cure is unlikely. In addition, abdominal wall resection with extensive reconstruction may be necessary to ensure adequate disease-free margins. We recommend tube gastrostomy in all of these patients.

Healthy, vascularized tissue such as gracilis or rectus femoris muscle flaps should be mobilized to fill the irradiated dead space. This has been shown to decrease the incidence of postoperative fistula formation.[272] If the pelvis has been subjected to prior radiation therapy, segmental resection of the affected bowel may be necessary to ensure adequate healing of the anastomosis.

Healing

It is crucial to continue full nutritional support and antibiotics well into the postoperative period. We believe that antibiotics in this situation are therapeutic and not prophylactic. The postoperative period often is accompanied by a profound hypermetabolic state that places patients at risk for nutritional complications.[288-291] Providing appropriate protein and adequate calories is crucial. Early enteral nutrition can be tried, but it is often impossible to administer all of the nutritional needs of the patient by this route. It is unwise to taper the parenteral nutrition too rapidly. This may leave the patient with inadequate protein and calorie intake to heal what are often tenuous wounds. When starvation occurs in the postoperative period, protein losses may be as high as 70 to 80 gm/day. In the face of such profound protein catabolism, anastomosis, fascia, and wound closure are affected adversely. Parenteral nutrition should be continued to supplement enteral nutrition support until at least 1500 kcal can be taken per day enterally.

Once closure is achieved, either spontaneously or surgically, it may be difficult to persuade these patients to eat. Engaging the assistance of a dietician and the patient's family may be necessary to reestablish oral intake. The traditional dietary advancement from clear liquids through regular diet may not be tolerated by a patient who has not eaten for 4 to 6 weeks. Starting with a soft diet without passing through the preliminary steps may help. In addition, using jejunal tube feedings only at night may decrease satiety. If parenteral nutrition is being used, it may be necessary to wean the rate so anorexia is lessened. Families should bring in the patient's favorite food. Finally, alcohol given prior to a meal may improve appetite.

Even after the fistula is healed, the patient remains at risk for several delayed complications. Short bowel syndrome, after repeated attempts at bowel resection or correction of numerous fistulas, may leave the patient without sufficient absorptive surface. The fistula may recur, especially if the underlying disease process is inflammatory bowel disease or recurrent tumor. Additionally, the fistula site may stricture if an inadequate resection of diseased intestine was performed. Adhesive small bowel obstructions are not infrequent. Although reoperation should be approached cautiously, treatment of these complications should be carried out in accordance with established surgical principles.

Results and Late Complications

Currently, uncontrolled sepsis and malignancy are the leading causes of fistula-related death in most series. Advances in patient monitoring have decreased mortality directly related to electrolyte disturbances, although this complication still occurs in high-output fistulas. Additionally, the exact role that nutritional support has played in decreasing the mortality of enterocutaneous fistulas is debatable. Although it is clear that decreased mortality has been temporally related to advances in nutritional support techniques, causality is difficult to establish. In a 1964 study, it was shown that patients with enterocutaneous fistulas receiving less than 1000 calories/day had a mortality of 58%, while those receiving 1500 to 2000 calories per day had a mortality of 16%.[364] Alternatively, in an extensive 30 year review of enterocutaneous fistulas, it was found that the mortality associated with enterocutaneous fistulas at the Massachusetts General Hospital decreased from 48% to 15%, consistent with current mortality, prior to the institution of parenteral nutrition.[145] Their conclusion was that parenteral nutrition had not decreased the mortality associated with enterocutaneous fistulas. In addition, another group reported their experience with enterocutaneous fistulas: they arbitrarily divided patients into two groups; 1968 to 1971, in which 35% of patients received PN; and 1972 to 1977, in which 71% received PN.[201] The fistula-related mortalities were 10% and 13%, respectively. Their conclusion was that PN had no impact on mortality. Although decreased mortality was not shown, regardless of the fistula site, spontaneous closure rates after 4 to 5 weeks of PN were usually improved. In a recent review from Italy, patients treated between 1981 and 1984 for enterocutaneous fistulas were compared to patients treated between 1985 and 1990. The mortality in the late group was 18% while that of the early, non-PN-treated group was 42%.[365] Although numbers were small, this study compares two groups receiving equivalent modern perioperative and surgical care and, therefore, may be more telling than comparisons between preparenteral and postparenteral nutrition periods. Their findings support the hypothesis that aggressive nutritional support may decrease fistula mortality.

Repeated attempts at resection or correction of numerous fistulas may leave the patient without sufficient absorptive surface. Often, home parenteral support will be necessary while adaptation of the remaining bowel occurs. Additionally, the fistula site may be the source of complications. Stricture with partial obstruction may lead to postprandial crampy abdominal pain and weight loss due to an aversion for enteral nutrition. This is particularly true when the original fistula opening involves a large portion of the diameter of the bowel and repair by other than resection with end-to-end anastomosis is performed. Finally, esophageal stricture may occur after prolonged nasogastric sump decompression. In general, this will become manifest 3 to 4 months after the patient has been discharged from the hospital. Dilation is usually all that is necessary for symptomatic relief, although occasionally resection may be necessary.

We have alluded to the differences in outcome observed between enterally and parenterally nourished patients. In addition, enteral nutrition research has revealed dietary constituents thought to be trophic to the intestinal tract mucosa. Glutamine is an important nitrogen-carrying amino acid and is known to support the small intestinal mucosa. Similarly, SCFAs seem to be the preferred fuel source for the colonocyte.[366–368] Because the metabolic activity of the gastrointestinal tract acts as a regulator of nitrogen flux and protein synthesis, these trophic nutrients may be critical for both local healing and total body nitrogen equilibrium. Therefore, bowel rest may deprive the intestine of the critical metabolic precursors needed to maintain intestinal integrity.

ACKNOWLEDGEMENTS

The authors wish to thank Jean Loos for her excellent artwork.

REFERENCES

1. Birch BRP, Cox SJ. Spontaneous external biliary fistula uncomplicated by gallstones. *Postgrad Med J* 1991;67:391–392
2. Ponsky JL. Complications of laparoscopic cholecystectomy. *Am J Surg* 1991;161:393–395
3. Sedgwick ML, Denyer ME. Treatment of a postoperative cholecystocutaneous fistula by an endoscopic stent. *Br J Surg* 1989;76:159–160
4. Karotkin L. Spontaneous internal biliary fistula. *M Ann Distric of Columbia* 1958;27:623–636
5. Berk JE, Lee RN. Intravenous cholangiography in detection of stone-bearing cystic-duct remnants. *Am J Dig Dis* 1958;3:220–228
6. Jordan GL. Pancreatic resection for pancreatic cancer. In: Howard JM, Jordan GL, Reber HA (eds), *Surgical Diseases of the Pancreas.* Philadelphia, PA: Lea & Febiger; 1987:666–714
7. Glenn F, Reed C, Grafe WR. Biliary enteric fistula. *Surg Gynecol Obstet* 1981;153:527–531
8. Iwatsuki S, Starzl TE. Personal experience with 411 hepatic resections. *Ann Surg* 1988;208:421–434
9. LeBlanc KA, Barr LH, Rush BM. Spontaneous biliary enteric fistulas. *South Med J* 1983;76:1249–1252
10. Lygidakis NJ. Spontaneous internal biliary fistulae: early surgery for prevention, radical surgery for cure; a report of 75 cases. *Med Chir Dig* 1981;10:695–699
11. McSherry CK, Ferstenberg H, Virshup M. The Mirizzi syndrome: suggested classification and surgical therapy. *Surg Gastroenterol* 1982;1:219–225
12. Mirizzi PL. Sindrome del conducto hepatico. *J Int Chir* 1948;8:731–777
13. Piedad OH, Wels PB. Spontaneous internal biliary fistulae, obstructive and non-obstructive types: twenty-year review of 55 cases. *Ann Surg* 1972;175:75–80
14. Rau WS, Matern S, Gerok W, et al. Spontaneous cholecystocolonic fistula: a model situation for bile acid diarrhea and fatty acid diarrhea as a consequence of a disturbed enterohepatic circulation of bile acids. *Hepatogastroenterol* 1980;27:231–237
15. Sane SM, Sieber WK, Girdany BR. Congenital bronchobiliary fistula. *Surgery* 1971;69:599–608
16. Smith EE, Bowley N, Allison DJ, et al. The management of post-traumatic intrahepatic cutaneous biliary fistulas. *Br J Surg* 1982;69:317–318
17. Zwemer FL, Coffin-Kwart VE, Conway MJ. Biliary enteric fistulas: management of 47 cases in native Americans. *Am J Surg* 1979;138:301–304
18. Moosa AR, Easter DW, van Sonnenberg E, et al. Laparoscopic injuries to the bile duct: a cause for concern. *Ann Surg* 1992;215:203–208
19. Hunter JG. Avoidance of bile duct injury during laparoscopic cholecystectomy. *Am J Surg* 1991;162:71–76
20. Phillips EH, Berci G, Carroll B, et al. The importance of intraoperative cholangiography during laparoscopic cholecystectomy. *Am J Surg* 1990;56:798–795
21. Chevallier JM, Jost JL, Menegaux F, et al. Hepatic trauma: experience with 135 consecutive liver injuries (1982–1989) and arguments for conservative surgery. *Langenbeck's Archiv Chirurgie* 1991;376:335–340
22. Schirmer WJ, Rossi RL, Hughes KS, et al. Common operative problems in hepatobiliary surgery. *Surg Clin North Am* 1991;71(6):1363–1389
23. Traverso LW, Freeny PC. Pancreaticoduodenectomy: the importance of preserving hepatic blood flow to prevent biliary fistula. *Am Surg* 1989;55:421–426
24. Bynoe RP, Bell RM, Miles WS, et al. Complications of nonoperative management of blunt hepatic injuries. *J Trauma* 1992;32:308–315
25. Hollands MJ, Little JM. Post-traumatic bile fistulae. *J Trauma* 1991;31:117–120
26. Vaccaro JP, Dorfman GS, Lambiase RE. Treatment of biliary leaks and fistulae by simultaneous percutaneous drainage and diversion. *Cardiovasc Intervent Radiol* 1991;14:109–112
27. Søndenaa K, Skjennald A. Treatment of biliary fistula by percutaneous transhepatic drainage. *Acta Chir Scand* 1989;154:141–143
28. Davids PHP, Rauws EAJ, Tytgat GNJ, et al. Postoperative bile leakage: endoscopic management. *Gut* 1992;33:1118–1122
29. Hoffman BJ, Cunningham JT, Marsh WH. Endoscopic management of biliary fistulas with small caliber stents. *Am J Gastroenterol* 1990;85:705–707
30. Feretis C, Kekis B, Bliouras N, et al. Postoperative external and internal biliary fistulas, unassociated with distal bile duct obstruction: endoscopic treatment. *Endoscopy* 1990;22:211–213
31. Goldin E, Katz E, Wengrower D, et al. Treatment of fistulas of the biliary tract by endoscopic insertion of endoprostheses. *Surg Gynecol Obstet* 1990;170:418–423

32. Liguory C, Vitale GC, Lefebre JF, et al. Endoscopic treatment of postoperative biliary fistulae. *Surgery* 1991;110: 779–784

33. Krige JEJ, Bornman PC, Beningfield SJ, et al. Endoscopic embolization of external biliary fistulae. *Br J Surg* 1990; 77:581–583.

34. Simpson R, Martin R. Use of a controlled duodenal fistula in the management of a major duodenal injury. *Aust NZ J Surg* 1986;56:167–169

35. Eckhauser FE, Strodel WE, Knol JA, et al. Duodenal exclusion for management of lateral duodenal fistulas. *Am Surg* 1988;54:172–177

36. Kuo Y-C, Wu C-S. Spontaneous cutaneous biliary fistula: a rare complication of cholangiocarcinoma. *J Clin Gastroenterol* 1990;12:451–453

37. Reed MWR, Tweedie JH. Spontaneous simultaneous internal and external biliary fistulae. *Br J Surg* 1985;72:538

38. Hardy KJ. Carl Langenbuch and the Lazarus hospital. *Aust NZ J Surg* 1993;63:56–64

39. Judd ES, Burden VG. Internal biliary fistula. *Ann Surg* 1925;81:305–312

40. Courvoisier LG. *Casuistische-Statistische Beitrage Zur Pathologie und Chirurgie der Gallenwege.* Leipzig: FCW Vogel; 1890

41. Naga M, Mogawer MS. Choledochoduodenal fistula. *Endoscopy* 1991;23:307–308

42. Parekh D, Segal I, Ramalho RM. Choledochoduodenal fistula from penetrating duodenal ulcer. *South African Med J* 1992;81:478–479

43. Jorge A, Diaz M, Lorenzo J, et al. Choledochoduodenal fistulas. *Endoscopy* 1991;23:76–78

44. Csendes A, Diaz JC, Burdiles P, et al. Mirizzi syndrome and cholecystobiliary fistula: a unifying classification. *Br J Surg* 1989;75:1139–1143

45. Roslyn JJ, Binns GS, Hughes EFX, et al. Open cholecystectomy: a contemporary analysis of 42 474 patients. *Ann Surg* 1993;218:129–137

46. Branum G, Schmitt C, Baillie J, et al. Management of major biliary complications after laparoscopic cholecystectomy. *Ann Surg* 1993;217:532–541

47. Cates JA, Tompkins RK, Zinner MJ, et al. Biliary complications of laparoscopic cholecystectomy. *Am Surg* 1993; 59:243–247

48. Rossi RL, Schirmer WJ, Braasch JW, et al. Laparoscopic bile duct injuries. *Arch Surg* 1992;127:596–602

49. Cheslyn-Curtis S, Emberton M, Ahmed H, et al. Bile duct injury following laparoscopic cholecystectomy. *Br J Surg* 1992;79:231–232

50. Wootton FT, Hoffman BJ, Marsh WH, et al. Biliary complications following laparoscopic cholecystectomy. *Gastrointest Endosc* 1992;38:183–185

51. Hunter JG. Avoidance of bile duct injury during laparoscopic cholecystectomy. *Am J Surg* 1991;162:71–76

52. Way LW. Bile duct injury during laparoscopic cholecystectomy. *Ann Surg* 1992;215:195

53. Davidoff AM, Pappas TN, Murray EA, et al. Mechanisms of major biliary injury during laparoscopic cholecystectomy. *Ann Surg* 1992;215:196–202

54. Moosa AR, Easter DW, VanSonnenberg E, et al. Laparoscopic injuries to the common bile duct. *Ann Surg* 1992; 215:203–208

55. Woods MS, Farha GJ, Street DE. Cystic duct remnant fistulization to the gastrointestinal tract. *Surgery* 1992;111: 101–104

56. Whipple AO, Parsons WB, Mullins CR. Treatment of carcinoma of the ampulla of Vater. *Ann Surg* 1935;102:763

57. Keck H, Steffen R, Neuhaus P. Protection of pancreatic and biliary anastomosis after partial duodenopancreatectomy by external drainage. *Surg Obstet Gynecol* 1992;174: 329–331

58. Keen WW. Report of a case of resection of the liver for the removal of a neoplasm, with a table of seventy-six cases of resection of the liver for hepatic tumors. *Ann Surg* 1899; 30:267–283

59. Iwatsuki S, Starzl T. Personal experience with 411 hepatic resections. *Ann Surg* 1988;208:421–434

60. Calne R. In: Calne R (ed), *Liver Transplantation: The Cambridge-King's College Hospital Experience.* London, England: Grune and Stratton; 1987

61. Sherman S, Shaked A, Cryer HM, et al. Endoscopic management of biliary fistulas complicating liver transplantation and other hepatobiliary operations. *Ann Surg* 1993; 218:167–175

62. Gibson T, Howat J. Cholecystocutaneous fistula. *Br J Clin Pract* 1987;41:980–982

63. Carragher AM, Jackson PR, Panesar KJS. Case report: subcutaneous herniation of gallbladder with spontaneous cholecystocutaneous fistula. *Clin Radiol* 1990;42:283–284

64. Zwemer FL, Coffin-Kwart VE, Conway MJ. Biliary enteric fistulas. *Am J Surg* 1979;138:301–304

65. Branum GD, Tyson GS, Branum MA, et al. Hepatic abscess. *Ann Surg* 1990;212:655–662

66. Ochsner A, DeBakey M, Murry S. Pyogenic abscess of the liver. *Am J Surg* 1938;40:292–314

67. Lee JF, Block GE. The changing clinical pattern of hepatic abscesses. *Arch Surg* 1972;104:465–470

68. Hill FS, Laws HL. Pyogenis hepatic abscesses. *Am Surg* 1982;48:49–53

69. Altemeier WA, Schowengerdt CG, Whiteley DH: Abscesses of the liver: surgical considerations. *Arch Surg* 1970;101:258–266

70. Bertel CK, van Heerden JA, Sheedy PF. Treatment of pyogenic hepatic abscesses: surgical versus percutaneous drainage. *Arch Surg* 1986;121:554–558

71. Grande D, Ruiz JC, Elizagaray E, et al. Hepatic echinococcosis complicated with transphrenic migration and bronchial fistula: CT demonstration. *Gastrointest Radiol* 1990; 15:115–118

72. Wolfe MS. The cestodes. In: Wyngaarden JB, Smith LH (eds), *Cecil's Textbook of Medicine,* 17th ed. Philadelphia, PA: WB Saunders; 19850

73. Tierris EJ, Avgeropoulos K, Kourtis K, et al. Bronchobiliary fistula due to *Echinococcis* of the liver. *W J Surg* 1977; 1:99–104

74. Krogstadt DJ. Amebiasis and amebic meningoencephalitis. In: Wyngaarden JB, Smith LH (eds), *Cecil's Textbook of Medicine,* 17th ed, Philadelphia, PA: WB Saunders; 1985

75. Railo M. Salmela H, Isoniemi L, et al. Use of somatostatin in biliary fistulas of transplanted livers. *Trans Proc* 1992; 24:391–393

76. Bismuth H, Castaing D, Garden OJ. Major hepatic resec-

tion done under total vascular exclusion. *Ann Surg* 1989; 210:13–19

77. Nagasue N, Kohno H, Chang YC, et al. Liver resection for hepatocellular carcinoma. *Ann Surg* 1993;217;375–384

78. Sherman S, Shaked A, Cryer HM, et al. Endoscopic management of biliary fistulas complicating liver transplantation and other hepatobiliary operations. *Ann Surg* 1993; 218:167–175

79. Parrilla P, Ramirez P, Sanchez-Bueno F, et al. Long-term results of choledochoduodenostomy in the treatment of choledocholithiasis. *Br J Surg* 1991;78:470–472

80. Smith EEJ, Bowley N, Allison DJ, et al. The mangament of post-traumatic intrahepatic cutaneous biliary fistulas. *Br J Surg* 1982;69:317–318

81. Northover JMA, Terblanche J. A new look at the arterial blood supply of the bile duct in man and its surgical implications. *Br J Surg* 1979;66:379–384

82. Michels NA. Blood supply and anatomy of the upper abdominal organs with a descriptive atlas. Philadelphia, PA: JB Lippincott; 1955:139–182

83. Benage D, O'Connor KW. Cholecystocolonic fistula. *J Clin Gastroenterol* 1990;12:192–194

84. Rau WS, Matern S, Gerok W, et al. Spontaneous cholecystocolonic fistula. *Hepatogastroenterol* 1980;27:231–237

85. Fischer JE. Ileal fistula. In: Fischer JE (ed), *Common Problems in Gastrointestinal Surgery*. Chicago, IL: Year Book Medical; 1988:289–297

86. Lange MP, Thebo LM, Tiede SM, et al. Management of multiple enterocutaneous fistulas. *Heart Lung* 1989;18: 386–391

87. Randall HT. Efficacy, feasibility, safety, and cost comparisons of enteral and parenteral elemental nutrition. *Contemp Surg* 1986;28:4–11

88. Blaylock B, Murray M. A jejunal fistula in a granulating wound and jejunal refeeding. *Ostomy/Wound Mgt* 1992; 38(6):8–14

89. Orringer JS, Mendeloff EN, Eckhauser FE. Management of wounds in patients with complex enterocutaneous fistulas. *Surg Gynecol Obstet* 1987;165:79–80

90. Devlin HB, Elcoat C. Alimentary tract fistula: stomatherapy techniques of management. *World J Surg* 1983;7: 489–494

91. Moore FA, Moore EE, Jones TN, et al. TEN versus TPN following major abdominal trauma-reduced septic mortality. *J Trauma* 1989;29:916–923

92. Hamaoui E, Lefkowitz R, Olander L, et al. Enteral nutrition in the early post-operative period: a new semielemental formula versus total parenteral nutrition. *JPEN* 1990;14:501–507

93. Shukla HS, Rao RR, Banu N, et al: Enteral hyperalimentation in malnourished surgical patients. *Indian J Med Res* 1984;80:339–346

94. Fullarton GM, Falconer S, Campbell A, et al. Controlled study of the effect of nicardipine and ceruletide on the sphincter of Oddi. *Gut* 1992;33:550–553

95. Guelrud M, Mendoza S, Rossiter G, et al. Effect of nifedipine on sphincter of Oddi motor activity: studies in healthy volunteers and patients with biliary dyskinesia. *Gastroenterology* 1988;95:1050–1055

96. Khuroo MS, Zagar SA, Yattoo GN. Efficacy of nifedipine therapy in patients with sphincter of Oddi dysfunction; a prospective, double blind, randomized, placebo-controlled, cross over trial. *Brit J Pharmacol* 1992;33:477–485

97. Sand J, Nordback I, Koskinen M, et al. Nifedipine for suspected type II sphincter of Oddi dyskinesia. *Am J Gastroenterol* 1993;88:530–535

98. Carr-Locke DL, Gregg JA, Chey WY. Effects of exogenous secretin on pancreatic and biliary ductal sphincter pressures in man demonstrated by endoscopic manometry and correlation with plasma secretin levels. *Dig Dis Sci* 1985;30:909–917

99. Sharma D, Sunderland GT, Kerr IF. Glyceryl trinitrate in the management of biliary fistulas. *Br J Surg* 1990;77:1029

100. Guelrud M, Rossiter A, Souney PF, et al. The effect of transcutaneous nerve stimulation on sphincter of Oddi pressure in patients with biliary dyskinesia. *Am J Gastroenterol* 1991;86:581–585

101. DiSomma C, Reboa G, Patrone MG, et al. Effects of pinaverium bromide on Oddi's spincter. *Clin Ther* 1986;9:119–122

102. Kobayashi K, Mitani E, Tatsumi S, et al. Studies on papillary function and effects of prifinium bromide and other antispasmodics on motility of the papillary region in humans. *Clin Ther* 1985;7:154–163

103. Rey JF, Greff M, Picazzo J. Glucagon-(1-21)-peptide. study of its action on sphincter of Oddi function by endoscopic manometry. *Dig Dis Sci* 1986;31:355–360

104. Ponce J, Garrigues V, Pertejo V, et al. Effect of intravenous glucagon and glucagon-(1-21)-peptide on motor activity of sphincter of Oddi in humans. *Dig Dis Sci* 1989;34:61–64

105. Rolny P, Arleback A, Funch-Jensen P, et al. Paradoxical response of sphincter of Oddi to intravenous injection of cholecystokinin or ceruletide: manometric findings and results of treatment in biliary dyskinesia. *Gut* 1986;27: 1507–1511

106. Binmoeller KF, Dumas R, Harris AG, et al. Effect of somatostatin analog octreotide on human sphincter of Oddi. *Dig Dis Sci* 1992;5:773–777

107. Sarles JC. Hormonal control of sphincter of Oddi. *Dig Dis Sci* 1986;31:208–212

108. Helm LF, Venu RP, Geenen JE, et al. Effects of morphine on the human sphincter of Oddi. *Gut* 1988;29:1402–1407

109. Staritz M. Pharmacology of the sphincter of Oddi. *Endoscopy* 1988;20:171–174

110. Ponchon T, Gallez JF, Valette PJ, et al. Endoscopic treatment of biliary tract fistulas. *Gastrointest Endosc* 1989;35: 490–498

111. Sedgwick ML, Denyer ME. Treatment of postoperative cholecystocutaneous fistula by an endoscopic stent. *Br J Surg* 1989;76:159–160

112. Goldin E, Katz E, Wengrower D, et al. Treatment of fistulas of the biliary tract by endoscopic insertion of an endoprothesis. *Surg Obstet Gynecol* 1990;170:418–423

113. Feretis C, Kekis B, Bliouras N, et al. Postoperative external and internal biliary fistulas unassociated with distal common bile duct obstruction. *Endoscopy* 1990;22:211–213

114. Hoffman BJ, Cunningham JT, Marsh WH. Endoscopic management of biliary fistulas with small caliber stents. *Am J Gastroenterol* 1990;85:705–707

115. Davids PHP, Rauws EAJ, Tytgat GNJ, et al. Postoperative bile leakage: endoscopic management. *Gut* 1992;33:1118–1122
116. Musher DR, Gouge T. Cutaneous bile fistula treated with ERCP-placed large diameter stent. *Am Surg* 1989;55:653–655
117. Wieman TJ, Corey TS, Shively E. Postoperative percutaneous choledochoscopy. *Am Surg* 1989;55:97–99
118. Marshall T, Kamalvand K, Cairns SR. Endoscopic management of biliary tract disease. *Br Med J* 1990;300:1176
119. Gouldin E, Aharon B, Wengower D, et al. Biliary and colonic cutaneous fistula successfully treated by endoscopic insertion of biliary stents. *J Clin Gastroenterol* 1993;16:58–60
120. Brem H, Gibbons GD, Cobb G, et al. The use of endoscopy to treat bronchobiliary fistula caused by choledocholithiasis. *Gastroenterology* 1990;98:490–492
121. Ramesh GN, Duggal A, Vij JC. Successful management of post-operative pleurobiliary fistula by endoscopic technique. *Gastrointest Endosc* 1991;37:574–576
122. Berger H, Weinzierl M, Neville E, et al. Percutaneous transcatheter occlusion of cystic duct stump in post-cholecystectomy bile leak. *Gastrointest Radiol* 1989;14:334–336
123. Iscan M, Duren M. Endoscopic sphincterotomy in the management of postoperative complications of hepatic hydatid disease. *Endoscopy* 1991;23:282–283
124. Alper A, Arioglu O, Emre A, et al. Choledochoduodenostomy for intrabiliary rupture of hydatid cysts of the liver. *Br J Surg* 1987;74:243–245
125. Vignote ML, Mino G, de la Mata M, et al. Endoscopic sphincterotomy in hepatic hydatid disease open to the biliary tree. *Br J Surg* 1990;77:721
126. Ghazi A, Washington M. Endoscopic retrograde cholangiopancreatology, endoscopic sphincterotomy, and biliary drainage. *Surg Clin North Am* 1989;69:1249–1274
127. Vaccaro JP, Dorfman GS, Lambaise RE. Treatment of biliary leaks and fistulae by simultaneous percutaneous drainage and diversion. *Cardiovas Intervent Radiol* 1991;14:109–112
128. Prickett D, Montgomery R, Cheadle WG. External fistulas arising from the digestive tract. *South Med J* 1991;84:736–739
129. Chevallier JM, Menegaux F, Chigot JP, et al. Hepatic trauma. *Langenbeck's Arch Chir* 1991:335–340
130. Raper S, Maynard N. Feeding the critically ill. *Br J Nurs* 1992;1:273–280
131. Kiver KV, Hats DP, Fortin DF, et al. Pre- and post-pyloric enteral feeding: analysis of safety and complications. *JPEN* 1984;8:95 [abstract]
132. Burtch GD, Shatney CH. Feeding jejunostomy (versus gastrostomy) passes the test of time. *Am Surg* 1987;53:54–57
133. Baer HU, Matthews JB, Schweizer WP, et al. Management of the Mirizzi syndrome and the surgical implications of choledochal fistulas. *Br J Surg* 1990;77:743–745
134. Dewar G, Chung SCS, Li AKC. Management of the Mirizzi syndrome and the implications of cholecystocholedochal fistula. *Br J Surg* 1991;78:378
135. Mishra MC, Vashishtha S, Tandon R. Biliobiliary fistula. *Surgery* 1990;108:835–839
136. Ming-qian X. Diagnosis and management of hepatic hydatidosis complicated with biliary fistula. *Chin Med J* 1992;105:69–72
137. Cole DJ, Ferguson CM. Complications of hepatic resection for colorectal metastasis. *Am Surg* 1992;58:88–91
138. Edmunds LH, Williams GH, Welch CE. External fistulas arising from the gastrointestinal tract. *Ann Surg* 1960;152:445–471
139. Kuvshinoff BW, Brodish RJ, McFadden DW, et al. Serum transferrin as a prognostic indicator of spontaneous closure and mortality in gastrointestinal cutaneous fistulas. *Ann Surg* (in press).
140. Rose D, Yarborough MF, Canizaro PC, et al. One hundred and fourteen fistulas of the gastrointestinal tract treated with total parenteral nutrition. *Surg Gynecol Obstet* 1986;163:345–350
141. Bowlin JW, Hardy JD, Conn JH. External alimentary tract fistulas: analysis of seventy-nine cases, with notes on management. *Am J Surg* 1962;193:6
142. Fischer JE. The management of gastrointestinal cutaneous fistulae. *Contemp Surg* 1986;29:104–108
143. Aguirre A, Fischer JE. Intestinal fistulas. In: Fischer JE (ed), *Total Parenteral Nutrition*. Boston, MA: Little, Brown; 1976:203–218
144. Aguirre A, Fischer JE, Welch CE. The role of surgery and hyperalimentation in therapy of gastrointestinal-cutaneous fistulae. *Ann Surg* 1974;180:393–401
145. Soeters PB, Ebeid AM, Fischer JE. Review of 404 patients with gastrointestinal fistulas: impact of parenteral nutrition. *Ann Surg* 1979;190:189–202
146. Fischer JE. Enterocutaneous fistula. In: Norton LW, Eiseman B (eds.), *Surgical Decision Making*, 2nd ed. Philadelphia, PA: WB Saunders; 1985:146–147
147. Fischer JE. Enterocutaneous fistulas. In: Najarian JS, Delaney JP (eds.), *Progress in Gastrointestinal Surgery*. Chicago, IL: Year Book Medical; 1989:377–387
148. Kingsnorth AN, Moss JG, Small WP. Failure of somatostatin to accelerate closure of enterocutaneous fistulas in patients receiving total parenteral nutrition [letter]. *Lancet* 1986;1:1271
149. Conter RL, Roof L, Roslyn JJ. Delayed reconstructive surgery for complex entero-cutaneous fistulae. *Am Surg* 1988;54:589–593
150. Ayhan A, Tuncer ZS. Radical hysterectomy with lymphadenectomy for treatment of early stage cervical cancer: clinical experience of 278 cases. *J Surg Oncol* 1991;47:175–177
151. Schein M, Decker GAG. Postoperative external alimentary tract fistulas. *Am J Surg* 1991;161:435–438
152. Buechter KJ, Leonovicz D, Hastings PR, et al. Enterocutaneous fistulas following laparotomy for trauma. *Am Surg* 1991;57:354–358
153. Rinsema W, Gouma DJ, von Meyenfeldt MF, et al. Primary conservative management of external small-bowel fistulas: changing composition of fistula series? *Acta Chir Scand* 1990;156:457–462
154. Alvarez RD: Gastrointestinal complications in gynecologic surgery: a review for the general gynecologist. *Obstet Gynecol* 1988;72:533–540
155. Richards WO, Keramati B, Scovill WA. Fate of retained

foreign bodies in the peritoneal cavity. *South Med J* 1986;79:496–498

156. Hugh TB, Coleman MJ, Cohan A. Persistent postoperative enterocutaneous fistula: Pathophysiology and treatment. *Aust NZ J Surg* 1986;56:901–906

157. Fazio VW, Coutsoftides T, Steiger E. Factors influencing the outcome of treatment of small bowel cutaneous fistula. *World J Surg* 1983;7:481–488

158. Nassos TP, Braasch JW. External small bowel fistulas: current treatment and results. *Surg Clin North Am* 1971; 51:687

159. Patrick CH, Goodin J, Fogarty J: Complication of prolonged transpyloric feeding: Formation of an enterocutaneous fistula. *J Pediatr Surg* 1988;23:1023–1024

160. Galland RB, Spencer J. Radiation-induced gastrointestinal fistulae. *Ann Coll Surg Engl* 1986;68:5–7

161. Rubin SC, Benjamin I, Hoskins WJ, et al. Intestinal surgery in gynecologic oncology. *Gynecol Oncol* 1989; 34:30–33

162. Schein M. Free perforation of benign gastrojejunocolic and gastrocolic fistula: report of two cases. *Dis Colon Rectum* 1987;30:705–706

163. Fischer JE. The pathophysiology of enterocutaneous fistulas. *World J Surg* 1983;7:446–450

164. Fischer JE. Enterocutaneous fistula. In: Cameron JL (ed.), *Current Surgical Therapy*. 4th ed. St. Louis, MO: Mosby Year Book; 1992:136–142

165. Feliciano DV, Martin TD, Cruse PA, et al. Management of combined pancreaticoduodenal injuries. *Ann Surg* 1987;205:673–680

166. Simpson R, Martin R. Use of a controlled duodenal fistula in the management of a major duodenal injury. *Aust NZ J Surg* 1986;56:167–169

167. Eckhauser FE, Strodel WE, Knol JA, et al. Duodenal exclusion for management of lateral duodenal fistulas. *Am Surg* 1988;54:172–177

168. Ryan P. Two kinds of diverticular disease. *Ann R Coll Surg Engl* 1991;73:73–79

169. Burch JM, Martin RM, Richardson RJ, et al. Evolution of the treatment of the injured colon in the 1980s. *Arch Surg* 1991;126:979–984

170. MacFayden VB Jr, Dudrick SJ, Ruberg RL. Management of gastrointestinal fistulas with parenteral hyperalimentation. *Surgery* 1973;74:100–105

171. Benson DW, Fischer JE. Fistulas. In: Fischer JE (ed), *Total Parenteral Nutrition*, 2nd ed. Boston, MA: Little, Brown; 1991:253–262

172. Myssiorek D, Becker GD. Extended single transverse neck incision for composite resections: does it work? *J Surg Oncol* 1991;48:101–105

173. Ginsberg RJ, Cooper JD. Esophageal fistula. *World J Surg* 1983;7:455–462

174. Laskin JL. Parotid fistula after the use of external pin fixation: report of a case. *J Oral Surg* 1978;36:621–622

175. Lin JN, Wang KL. Persistent third branchial apparatus. *J Pediatr Surg* 1991;26:663–665

176. Balmaseda MT Jr, Pellioni DJ. Esophagocutaneous fistula in spinal cord injury: a complication of anterior cervical fusion. *Acta Phys Med Rehabil* 1985;66:783–784

177. Rubin JS. Sternocleidomastoid myoplasty for the repair of chronic cervical esophageal fistulae. *Laryngoscope* 1986;96:834–836

178. Fuji T, Kuratsu S, Shirasaki N, et al. Esophagocutaneous fistula after anterior cervical spine surgery and successful treatment using a sternocleidomastoid muscle flap: a case report. *Clin Orthoped Rel Res* 1991;267:8–13

179. Kaplan DK, Thorpe JAC. Use of an omental pedicle graft to repair a large oesophageal defect. *Thorax* 1988;43: 333–334

180. Tarazi R, Coutsoftides T, Steiger E, et al. Gastric and duodenal cutaneous fistulas. *World J Surg* 1983;7:463–473

181. De Villa V, Calvo FA, Bilbao JI, et al. Arteriodigestive fistula: a complication associated with intraoperative and external beam radiotherapy following surgery for gastric cancer. *J Surg Oncol* 1992;49:52–57

182. Kaminsky VM, Dietal M. Nutritional support in the management of external fistulas of the alimentary tract. *Br J Surg* 1975;62:100

183. Halversen RC, Hogle HH, Richards RC. Gastric and small bowel fistulas. *Am J Surg* 1969;118:968

184. Csendes A, Diaz JC, Burdiles P, et al. Classification and treatment of anastomotic leakage after extended total gastrectomy in gastric carcinoma. *Hepatogastroenterol* 1990;37(suppl II):174–177

185. Hölscher AM, Schuler M, Siewert JR. Surgical treatment of adenocarcinomas of the gastroesophageal junction. *Dis Esoph* 1988;1:35–50

186. Troidl H, Kusche J. Vestwela KH. Pouch versus esophagojejunostomy after total gastrectomy: a randomized clinical trial. *World J Surg* 1987;11:699–712

187. Olbe L, Lundell L. Intestinal function after total gastrectomy and possible consequence of gastric replacement. *World J Surg* 1987;11:713–719

188. Escudier B, Belmiba H, Henry-Amar M, et al. Anastomotic fistula complicating total gastrectomy and esophagogastrectomy for cancer of the stomach. *Am J Surg* 1979;138:399–402

189. Hauters P, de Canniere L, Collard JM, et al. Gastrodiaphragmatic fistula after transabdominal Nissen fundoplication. *J Clin Gastroenterol* 1990;12:313–315

190. Gianello P, Baulieux J, Maillet P. Esophageal and gastric fistula after hiatal hernia surgery. *Acta Chir Belg* 1985; 85:169–178

191. Burnett UF, Read RC, Dale Morris W, et al. Management of complications of fundoplication and Barrett's esophagus. *Surgery* 1977;82:521–530

192. Mansour KA, Burton HG, Miles JI, et al. Complications of intrathoracic Nissen fundoplication. *Ann Thorac Surg* 1981;32:173–178

193. Alexandre JH, Fraioli JP, Sage M. Value of water-soluble opaque media in the early detection of fistulae following operation for hiatus hernia. *J Radiol* 1982;63:115–117

194. Buckwalter JA, Herbst CA Jr. Leaks occurring after gastric bariatric operations. *Surgery* 1988;103:156–160

195. Shorr RM, Greaney GC, Donovan AJ. Injuries of the duodenum. *Am J Surg* 1987;154:93–98

196. Pokorny WJ, Brandt ML, Harberg FJ. Major duodenal injuries in children: diagnosis, operative management, and outcome. *J Pediatr Surg* 1986;21:613–616

197. deSa LA, Roddie ME, Williamson RCN. Fata duodeno-

caval fistula resulting from a giant peptic ulcer: case report. *Acta Chir Scand* 1990;156:647–650

198. Garden OJ, Dykes EH, Carter DC. Surgical and nutritional management of postoperative duodenal fistulas. *Dig Dis Sci* 1988;33:30–35

199. Rossi JA, Sollenberger LL, Rege RV, et al. External duodenal fistula: causes, complications, and treatment. *Arch Surg* 1986;121:908–912

200. Gilmartin D, Lane BE. Management of lateral duodenal fistula: a ten-year review. *Irish Med J* 1985;78:311–314

201. Reber HA, Roberts C, Way L, et al. Management of external gastrointestinal fistulas. *Ann Surg* 1978;188:460–467

202. Malangoni MA, Madura JA, Jesseph JE. Management of lateral duodenal fistulas: a study of 14 cases. *Surgery* 1981;90:645–651

203. Smith DW, Lee RM. Nutritional management in duodenal fistula. *Surg Gynecol Obstet* 1956;103:666–672

204. Rodkey GV, Welch CE. Duodenal decompression in gastrectomy. *N Engl J Med* 1960;262:498–501

205. Fischer JE. Enterocutaneous fistula. In: Cameron JL (ed), *Current Surgical Therapy*, 2nd ed. Philadelphia, PA: BC Decker; 1986:81–84

206. Levy E, Cugnenc PH, Frileux P, et al. Postoperative peritonitis due to gastric and duodenal fistulas: operative management by continuous intraluminal infusion and aspiration. Report of 23 cases. *Br J Surg* 1984;71:543–546

207. Meguid MM, Campos AC, Hammond WG. Nutritional support in surgical practice: part II. *Am J Surg* 1990; 159:427–443

208. Lindberg E, Järnerot G, Huitfeldt B. Smoking in Crohn's disease: effect on localisation and clinical course. *Gut* 1992;33:779–782

209. Pettit SH, Irving MH. Does local intestinal ascorbate deficiency predispose to fistula formation in Crohn's disease? *Dis Colon Rectum* 1987;30:552–557

210. Alexander-Williams J, Haynes IG. Conservative operations for Crohn's disease of the small bowel. *World J Surg* 1985;9:945–951

211. Ring KS. Management of abscess and enterocutaneous fistula in a patient with Crohn's disease: case report. *Mt Sinai J Med* 1987;54:450–455

212. Harrison RA, Clark CG. Conservative surgery in Crohn disease. *Surg Annu* 1986;18:29–39

213. Rombeau JL, Rolandelli RH. Enteral and parenteral nutrition in patients with enteric fistulas and short bowel syndrome. *Surg Clin North Am* 1987;67(3):551–571

214. Pettit SH, Irving MH. The operative management of fistulous Crohn's disease. *Surg Gynecol Obstet* 1988;167; 223–228

215. Greenstein AJ, Present DH, Sachar DB, et al. Gastric fistulas in Crohn's disease: report of cases. *Dis Colon Rectum* 1989;32:888–892

216. Winslet MC, Barsoum G, Pringle W, et al. Loop ileostomy after ileal pouch-anal anastomosis: is it necessary? *Dis Colon Rectum* 1991;34:267–270

217. Schoetz DJ, Collier JA, Veidenheimer MC. Can the pouch be saved? *Dis Colon Rectum* 1988;31:671–675

218. Cohen Z, McLeod RS. Stephen W, et al. Continuing evolution of the pelvic pouch procedure. *Ann Surg* 1992; 216:506–512

219. Sugarman HJ, Newsome HH, Decosta G, et al. Stapled ileoanal anastomosis for ulcerative colitis and familial polyposis without a temporary diverting colostomy. *Ann Surg* 1991;213:606–619

220. Schoetz DJ, Coller JA, Veidenheimer MC. Ileoanal reservior for ulcerative colitis and familial polyposis. *Arch Surg* 1986;121:404–409

221. Metcalf AM, Dozois RR, Kelly KA, et al. Ileal "J" pouch-anal anastomosis: clinical outcome. *Ann Surg* 1985;202:735–739

222. Cohen Z, McLeod RS, Stern H, et al. The pelvic pouch and ileoanal anastomosis procedure: surgical technique and initial results. *Am J Surg* 1985;150:601–607

223. Wong WD, Rothenberger DA, Goldberg SM. Ileoanal pouch procedures. *Curr Probl Surg* 1985;22:1–78

224. Nicholls RJ, Pezim ME. Restorative proctocolectomy with ileal reservoir for ulcerative colitis and familial adenomatous polyposis: a comparison of three reservoir designs. *Br J Surg* 1985;72:470–474

225. Nasmyth DG, Williams NS, Johnson D. Comparison of the function of triplicated and duplicated ileal reservoirs after mucosal proctectomy and ileo-anal anastomosis for ulcerative colitis and adenomatous polyposis. *Br J Surg* 1986;73:361–366

226. Pezim ME, Nichols RJ. Quality of life after restorative proctocolectomy with pelvic ileal reservoir. *Br J Surg* 1985;72:31–33

227. Ballantyne GH, Pemberton JH, Beart RW, et al. Ileal J-pouch anal anastomosis: current technique. *Dis Colon Rectum* 1985;28:197–202

228. Fonkalsrud EW. Endorectal ileoanal anastomosis with isoperistaltic reservoir after colectomy and mucosal proctectomy. *Ann Surg* 1984;199:151–157

229. Rothenberger DA, Vermeulen FD, Christenson CE, et al. Restorative proctocolectomy with ileal reservoir and ileoanal anastomosis. *Am J Surg* 1983;145:82–87

230. Keighley MR, Winslet MC, Pringle W, et al. The pouch as an alternative to permanent ileostomy. *Br J Hosp Med* 1987;38:286–293

231. Everett WG. Experience with restorative proctocolectomy with ileal reservoir. *Br J Surg* 1989;76:77–81

232. Metcalf AM, Dozois RR, Beart RW, et al. Temporary ileostomy for ileal pouch-anal anastomosis: function and complications. *Dis Colon Rectum* 1986;29:300–303

233. Parks AG, Nicholls RJ, Belliveau P. Proctocolectomy with ileal reservoir and anal anastomosis. *Br J Surg* 1980;67: 533–538

234. Johnson D, Williams NS, Neal DE, et al. The value of preserving the sphincter in operations for ulcerative colitis and polyposis: a review of 22 mucosal proctectomies. *Br J Surg* 1981;68:874–878

235. Utsunomiya J, Iwama T, Imajo M, et al. Total colectomy, mucosal proctectomy, and ileoanal anastomosis. *Dis Colon Rectum* 1980;23:459–466

236. McHugh SM, Diamant NE, McLeod R, et al. S-pouches versus J-pouches: a comparison of functional outcomes. *Dis Colon Rectum* 1987;30:671–677

237. Taylor BM, Beart RW, Dozois RR, et al. Straight ileoanal anastomosis versus ileal pouch-anal anastomosis after colectomy and mucosal proctectomy. *Arch Surg* 1983; 188:696–701

238. Kusunoki M, Fujita S, Shoji Y, et al. Pouch-vaginal fistulae after ileoanal anastomoses [letter]. *Lancet* 1991;338:315

239. Markham NI, Watson GM, Lock MR. Rectovaginal fistulae after ileoanal pouches [letter]. *Lancet* 1991;337:1295–1296

240. Thoeni RF, Fell SC, Engelstad B, et al. Ileoanal pouches: comparison of CT, scintigraphy and contrast enemas for diagnosing postsurgical complications. *Am J Radiol* 1990;154:73–78

241. Fischer JE, Martin LW, Nussbaum MS, et al. The pull-through procedure: technical factors in influencing outcome, with emphasis on pouchitis. *Surgery* 1993;114: 828–835

242. Mann WJ. Surgical management of radiation enteropathy. *Surg Clin North Am* 1991;71:977–990

243. DeCosse JJ, Rhodes RS, Wentz WB, et al. The natural history of management of radiation induced injury to the gastrointestinal tract. *Ann Surg* 1969;170:369–384

244. Palmer JA, Bush RS. Radiation injuries to the bowel associated with treatment of carcinoma of the cervix. *Surg* 1976;80:458–464

245. Scholfield FF, Holden D, Carr HD, et al: Bowel disease after radiotherapy. *J R Soc Med* 1983;76:463–466

246. Russell JC, Welch JP. Operative management of radiation injuries of the intestinal tract. *Am J Surg* 1979;137: 433–442

247. Galland RB, Spencer J. Surgical management of radiation enteritis. *Surgery* 1986;99:133–138

248. Sauven P, Playforth MJ, Evans M, et al. Early infective complications and late recurrent cancer in stapled colonic anastomoses. *Dis Colon Rectum* 1989;32:33–35

249. Lui RC, Friedman R, Fleischer A. Management of post-irradiation recurrent entero-cutaneous fistula by muscle flaps. *Am Surg* 1989;55:403–407

250. Aitken RJ, Elliot MS: Sigmoid exclusion: a new technique in the management of radiation-induced fistula. *Br J Surg* 1985;72:731–732

251. Welch M, Hoare EM. Late appendicocutaneous fistulae. *J R Coll Surg Edinb* 1991;36:185–186

252. Bergamini C, Bertoncini M, Nanni G. Spontaneous appendicocutaneous fistula: case report and literature review. *Dis Colon Rectum* 1981;24:187–190

253. Rosenberg L, Gordon PH. Tube cecostomy revisited. *Can J Surg* 1986;29:38–40

254. Walker LG, Rhame DW, Smith EB. Enteric and cutaneous appendiceal fistulas. *Arch Surg* 1969;99:585–588

255. Fitz R. Perforating inflammation of the vermiform appendix; with special reference to its early diagnosis and treatment. *Trans Assoc Am Physicians* 1886;1:107–144

256. Shamblin JR, Hudson TL. Recurrent appendicitis after appendectomy. *J Med Assoc Ga* 1965;54:304–305

257. Kelly HA, Herdon E. *The Vermifirm Appendix and Its Diseases.* Philadelphia, PA: WB Saunders; 1905

258. Loennecken W. 20 Ar Gammel AB Dominalfistel Fra Appendix. *Nord Med* 1942;15:2479

259. Hedner J, Jansson R, Lindberg R. Appendicocutaneous fistula: a case report. *Acta Chir Scand* 1978;144:123–124

260. Hill GL, Bourchier RG, Witney GB. Surgical and metabolic management of patients with external fistulas of the small intestine associated with Crohn's disease. *World J Surg* 1988;12:191–197

261. Gilbert JM, Mann CV, Scholefield J, et al. The aetiology and surgery of carcinoma of the anus, rectum and sigmoid colon in Crohn's disease: negative correlation with human papillomavirus type 16 (HPV 16). *Eur J Surg Oncol* 1991;17:507–513

262. Harper PH, Fazio VW, Lavery IC, et al. The long-term outcome in Crohn's disease. *Dis Colon Rectum* 1987;30: 174–179

263. Goldman CD, Kodner IJ, Fry RD, et al. Clinical and operative experience with non-Caucasian patients with Crohn's disease. *Dis Colon Rectum* 1986;29:317–321

264. Stone HN, Haney BB, Kolb LD, et al. Prophylactic and preventive antibiotic therapy: timing, duration, and economics. *Ann Surg* 1978;189:691

265. Meakins JL. Prophylactic antibiotics. In: Wilmore D, Brennan M, Harken A et al (eds.), *Care of the Surgical Patient.* New York, NY: Scientific American; 1989:3. 1–3.9.

266. Burke JF. The effective period of preventive antibiotic action in experimental incisions and dermal lesions. *Surgery* 1961;50:161

267. Coppa GF, Eng K. Factors involved in antibiotic selection in elective colon and rectal surgery. *Surgery* 1988;104:853

268. Kling PA, Dahlgren S. Oral prophylaxis with neomycin and erythromycin in colorectal surgery. *Arch Surg* 1989; 124:705

269. Figueras-Felip J, Basilio-Bonet E, Lara-Eisman F, et al. Oral is superior to systemic antibiotic prophylaxis in operations upon the colon and rectum. *Surg Gynecol Obstet* 1984;158:359

270. Khubchandani IT, Karamchandani MC, Sheets JA, et al. Metronidazole vs erythromycin, neomycin and cefazolin in prophylaxis for colon surgery. *Dis Colon Rectum* 1989; 32:17

271. Marescaux JF, Aprahamian M, Mutter D, et al. Prevention of anastomosis leakage: an artificial connective tissue. *Br J Surg* 1991;78:440–444

272. Jakowatz JG, Porudominsky D, Riihimaki DU, et al. Complications of pelvic exenteration. *Arch Surg* 1985;120: 1261–1265

273. Fischer JE, Sheldon GF, Block GE, et al. Symposium: surgical management of intestinal fistulas. *Contemp Surg* 1978;13:67–85

274. Fischer JE. The management of high-output intestinal fistulas. *Adv Surg* 1975;9:139–176

275. Hollender LF, Meyer C, Avet D, et al. Postoperative fistulas of the small intestine: therapeutic principles. *World J Surg* 1983;7:474–480

276. Sansoni B, Irving M. Small bowel fistulas. *World J Surg* 1985;9:897–903

277. Roediger WEW. Metabolic basis of starvation diarrhoea: implications for treatment. *Lancet* 1986;1:1082

278. Moss G. Malabsorption associated with extreme malnutrition: importance of replacing plasma albumin. *J Am Coll Nutr* 1982;1:89–92

279. Brinson RR, Cyrtis WD, Singh M. Diarrhea in the intensive care unit: the role of hypoalbuminemia and the response to a chemically defined diet. *J Am Coll Nutr* 1987; 6:517–523

280. Brinson RR, Kolts BE. Hypoalbuminemia as an indicator

of diarrheal incidence in critically ill patients. *Crit Care Med* 1987;15:506–509

281. Moss G. Albumin. *Nutr Supp Serv* 1988;8:6–7

282. Schwartz DB, Darrow AK. Hypoalbuminemia-induced diarrhea in the enterally alimented patient. *Nutr Clin Pract* 1988;3:235–237

283. Halvorsen L, Holcroft JW. Albumin: mechanisms of edema formation. *Nutr Clin Pract* 1988;3:222–225

284. Roediger WEW. Metabolic basis of starvation diarrhoea: implications for treatment. *Lancet* 1986;1:1082

285. Ryan JA, Abel RM, Abbott WM, et al. Catheter complications in total parenteral nutrition: a prospective study of 200 consecutive patients. *N Engl J Med* 1974;290:757

286. Medeiros A, Soares CER. Treatment of enterocutaneous fistulas by high-pressure suction with a normal diet. *Am J Surg* 1990;159:411–413

287. Rabinovici R, Reissman P, Eid A, et al. New sump suction appliance for drainage of enterocutaneous fistulae. *Br J Surg* 1988;75:415

288. Reilly JJ, Hull SF, Albert N, et al. Economic impact of malnutrition: a model system for hospitalized patients. *JPEN* 1988;12:371–376

289. Chandra RK. Nutrition, immunity, and infection: present knowledge and future directions. *Lancet* 1983;1:688–691

290. Smythe PM, Schonland M, Brereton-Stiles GG, et al. Thymolymphatic deficiency and depression of cell mediated immunity in protein-calorie malnutrition. *Lancet* 1971; 2:939–943

291. Christou NV, Tellado-Rodriquez J, Chartrand L, et al. Estimating mortality risk in preoperative patients using immunologic, nutritional, and acute-phase response variables. *Ann Surg* 1989;210:69–77

292. Levy E, Frileux P, Cugnenc PH, et al. High-output external fistulae of the small bowel: management with continuous enteral nutrition. *Br J Surg* 1989;76:676–679

293. Deitel M. Elemental diet and enterocutaneous fistula. *World J Surg* 1983;7:451–454

294. Bury KD, Stephens RV, Randall HT. Use of a chemically defined diet for nutritional management of fistulas of the alimentary tract. *Am J Surg* 1971;121:174–183

295. Wolfe BM, Keltner RM, Willmann VL. Intestinal output in regular elemental and intravenous alimentation. *Am J Surg* 1972;124:803–806

296. Voitk AJ, Echave V, Brown RA, et al. Elemental diet in the treatment of fistulae of the alimentary tract. *Surg Gynec Obstet* 1973;137:68–72

297. Adibi SA, Allen ER. Impaired jejunal absorption rates of essential amino acids induced by either dietary caloric or protein-deprivation in man. *Gastroenterology* 1970;59:404

298. Sandler JT. Specific techniques in delivery of liquid diets. In: Deitel M (ed), *Nutrition in Clinical Surgery*. Baltimore, MD: Williams & Wilkins; 1980:43–52

299. Adibi SA. Intestinal transport of dipeptides in man: relative importance of hydrolysis and intact absorption. *J Clin Invest* 1971;50:2266–2275

300. Adibi SA. Intestinal phase of protein assimilation in man. *Am J Clin Nutr* 1976;29:205–215

301. Keohane P, Grimble JK, Brown B, et al. Influence of protein composition and hydrolysis method on intestinal absorption of protein in man. *Gut* 1985;26:907–913

302. Matthews DM. Intestinal absorption of peptides. *Physiol Rev* 1975;55:537–608

303. Matthews DM, Adibi SA. Peptide absorption. *Gastro* 1976;71:151–161

304. Fuessl HS, Carolan G, Williams G, et al. Effect of a long-acting somatostatin analogue (SMS 201-995) on postprandial gastric emptying of ^{99m}Tc-tin colloid and mouth-to-caecum transit time in man. *Digestion* 1987;36: 101–107

305. Moller N, Petrany G, Cassidy D, et al. Effects of the somatostatin analogue SMS 201-995 (sandostatin) on mouth-to-caecum transit time and absorption of fat and carbohydrates in normal man. *Clin Sci* 1988;75:345–350

306. Lembcke B, Cruetzfeldt W, Schleser S, et al. Effect of the somatostatin analogue Sandostatin (SMS 201-995) on gastrointestinal, pancreatic and biliary function and hormone release in normal men. *Digestion* 1987;36:108–124

307. Maton PN, Gardner JD, Jensen RT. Use of long-acting somatostatin analogue SMS 201-995 in patients with pancreatic islet cell tumors. *Dig Dis Sci* 1989;34(suppl 3): 28S–39S

308. Kvols LK, Moertel CG, O'Connell MJ, et al. Treatment of the malignant carcinoid syndrome: evaluation of a long-acting somatostatin analogue. *N Engl J Med* 1986;315: 663–666

309. Edwards CA, Cann PA, Read NW, et al. The effect of somatostatin analogue SMS 201-995 on fluid and electrolyte transport in a patient with secretory diarrhea. *Scand J Gastroenterol* 1986;21(suppl 119):259–261

310. Nubiola-Calonge P, Sancho J, Segura M, et al. Blind evaluation of the effects of octreotide (SMS 201-995), a somatostatin analogue, on small-bowel fistula output. *Lancet* 1987;2(8560):672–674

311. Wallace AM, Newman K. Successful closure of intestinal fistulae in an infant using the somatostatin analogue SMS 201-995. *J Pediatr Surg* 1991;26:1097–1100

312. Chen RJ, Fang JF, Chen MF. Octreotide in the management of postoperative entero-cutaneous fistulas and stress ulcer bleeding. *Am J Gastroenterol* 1992;87:1212–1215

313. Boike GM, Sightler SE, Averette HE. Treatment of small intestinal fistulas with octreotide, a somatostatin analog. *J Surg Oncol* 1992;49:63–65

314. Nubiola P, Badia JM, Martinez-Rodenas F, et al. Treatment of 27 postoperative entero-cutaneous fistulas with the long half-life somatostatin analogue SMS 201-995. *Ann Surg* 1989;210:56–58

315. Borison DI, Bloom AD, Pritchard TJ. Treatment of enterocutaneous and colocutaneous fistulas with early surgery or somatostatin analog. *Dis Colon Rectum* 1992;35: 635–639

316. Julia MV, Parri FJ, Figueras J, et al. Treatment of an enteric fistula with somatostatin in a premature. *Clin Pediatr* 1989;28:149–150

317. Lambiase RE, Deyoe L, Cronan JJ, et al. Percutaneous drainage of 335 consecutive abscesses: results of primary drainage with 1-year follow-up. *Radiology* 1992;184: 167–179

318. Jaques P, Mauro M, Safrit H, et al. CT features of intraabdominal abscesses: prediction of successful percutaneous drainage. *Am J Roentgenol* 1986;146:1041–1045

319. Groitl H, Scheele J. Endoscopic application of fibrin tissue adhesive in the upper gastro-intestinal tract. *Surg Endosc* 1988;2:137

320. Jung M, Manegold BC, Brands W. Endoscopic therapy of gastrointestinal fistulae with fibrin tissue sealant. In: Waclawiczek H-W (ed): *Progress in Fibrin Sealing.* Berlin, Germany: Springer-Verlag; 1989:43–52

321. Marone G, Santoro LM, Torre V. Successful endoscopic treatment of GI-tract fistulas with a fast-hardening amino acid solution. *Endoscopy* 1989;21:47–49

322. Eleftheriadis E, Tzartinoglou E, Kotzampassi K, et al. Early endoscopic fibrin sealing of high-output postoperative enterocutaneous fistulas. *Acta Chir Scand* 1990; 156:625–628

323. Meyer G, Lange V, Wenk H, et al. Endoscopic sealing of gastrointestinal fistulae. *Surg Endosc* 1988;2:116

324. Bianchi A, Solduga C, Ubach M. Percutaneous obliteration of a chronic duodenal fistula. *Br J Surg* 1988;75:572

325. Al-Khayat M, Kenyon GS, Fawcett HV, et al. Nutritional support in patients with low volume chylous fistula following radical neck dissection. *J Laryngol Otol* 1991;105: 1052–1056

326. Bozetti F, Arullani A, Baticci F, et al. Management of lymphatic fistulas by total parenteral nutrition. *J Parenter Enteral Nutr* 1982;6:526–527

327. Hashim SA, Roholt HB, Babayan VK, et al. Treatment of chyluria and chylothorax with medium chain triglycerides. *N Engl J Med* 1964;270:756–761

328. Younus M, Chang RWC. Chyle fistula: treatment with total parenteral nutrition. *J Laryngol Otol* 1988;102:384

329. Myers EN. The management of pharyngocutaneous fistula. *Arch Otolaryngol* 1972;95:10–17

330. Schechter GL. Complications of flaps and grafts in the oral cavity and pharynx. *Laryngoscope* 1983;93:306–309

331. Tsujinaka T, Ogawa M, Kido Y, et al. A giant tracheogastric tube fistula caused by a penetrated peptic ulcer after esophageal replacement. *Am J Gastroenterol* 1988;83: 862–864

332. Chen H, Tang Y, Noordhoff MS. Patch esophagoplasty with musculocutaneous flaps as treatment of complications after esophageal reconstruction. *Ann Plast Surg* 1987;19:448–453

333. Delaere PR, Boeckx WD, Ostyn F, et al. Hypopharyngeal stenosis and fistulas. *Arch Otolaryngol Head Neck Surg* 1988;114:1326–1329

334. Friedman M, Toriumi DM, Strorigl T, et al. The sternocleidomastoid myoperiosteal flap for esophagopharyngeal reconstruction and fistula repair: clinical and experimental study. *Laryngoscope* 1988;98:1084–1091

335. Doberneck RC, Oschwald DL, Orgel MG. Use of a tubed pectoralis major myocutaneous flap for salvage of a failed colonic bypass of the esophagus. *Surg Gynecol Obstet* 1986;162:477–479

336. Jones NF, Eadie PA, Myers EN. Double lumen free jejunal transfer for reconstruction of the entire floor of mouth, pharynx and cervical oesophagus. *Br J Plast Surg* 1991;44:44–48

337. Spiro RH, Shah JP, Strong EW, et al. Gastric transposition in head and neck surgery. *Am J Surg* 1983;146: 483–487

338. Frederickson JM, Wagenfeld JH, Pearson G. Gastric pull-up versus the deltopectoral flap for reconstruction of the cervical esophagus. *Arch Otolaryngol* 1981;107:613–616

339. Guillamondegui OM, Geoffray BG, McKenna RJ. Total reconstruction of the hypo-pharynx and cervical esophagus. *Am J Surg* 1985;159:422–426

340. McConnel FN, Hester TR. Free jejunal grafts for reconstruction of the pharynx and esophagus. *Arch Otolaryngol* 1981;107:476–481

341. Schuller DE. Reconstructive options for pharyngeal and/or cervical esophageal defects. *Arch Otolaryngol* 1985;111:193–197

342. Daly JM, Lieberman MD, Goldfine J, et al. Enteral nutrition with supplemental arginine, RNA, and omega-3 fatty acids in patients after operation: immunologic, metabolic, and clinical outcome. *Surgery* 112:56–67;1992

343. Bower RH, Lavin PT, Licari JJ, et al. A modified enteral formula reduces hospital length of stay in patients in intensive care units. *Crit Care Med* 21:S275;1993 [abstract]

344. Winslet MC, Barsoum G, Pringle W, et al. Loop ileostomy after ileal pouch-anal anastomosis: is it necessary? *Dis Colon Rectum* 1991;34:267–270

345. Schoetz DJ, Collier JA, Veidenheimer MC. Can the pouch be saved? *Dis Colon Rectum* 1988;31:671–675

346. Martin LW, Fischer JE, Sayers HJ, et al. Anal continence following Soave procedure. *Ann Surg* 1986;203:525–530

347. Martin LW, Fischer JE. Preservation of anorectal continence following total colectomy. *Ann Surg* 1982;196: 700–704

348. Fischer JE, Martin LW, Nussbaum MS, et al. The pull-through procedure: technical factors in influencing outcome, with emphasis on pouchitis. *Surgery* 1993;114: 828–835

349. Hagen J, Deitel M, McIntyre JA. Avoidance of a colostomy by nutritional techniques. *Int Surg* 1986;71:32–35

350. Webster MW, Carey LC. Fistulae of the gastrointestinal tract. *Curr Prob Surg* 1976;13:1–50

351. Moreaux J, Vons C. Elective resection for diverticular disease of the sigmoid colon. *Br J Surg* 1990;77:1036–1038

352. Levien DH, Mazier WP, Surrell JA, et al. Safe resection for diverticular disease of the colon. *Dis Colon Rectum* 1989;32:30–32

353. Peer A, Strauss S. Percutaneous drainage of postappendectomy abscesses complicated by enteric communication. *Cardiovasc Intervent Radiol* 1991;14:106–108

354. Law NW, Ellis H. Caecostomy in the management of the sloughed appendix: a report of two cases. *J R Coll Surg Edinb* 1990;35:311

355. Thompson JS. Strategies for preserving intestinal length in the short-bowel syndrome. *Dis Colon Rectum* 1986;30: 208–213

356. Alexander-Williams J, Haynes IG. Conservative operations for Crohn's disease of the small bowel. *World J Surg* 1985;9:945–951

357. Ring KS. Management of abscess and enterocutaneous fistula in a patient with Crohn's disease: case report. *Mt Sinai J Med* 1987;54:450–455

358. Harrison RA, Clark CG. Conservative surgery in Crohn disease. *Surg Annu* 1986;18:29–39

359. Pettit SH, Irving MH. The operative management of fistulous Crohn's disease. *Surg Gynecol Obstet* 1988;167: 223–228

360. Greenstein AJ, Present DH, Sachar DB, et al. Gastric fistulas in Crohn's disease: report of cases. *Dis Colon Rectum* 1989;32:888–892

361. Klein S, Greenstein AJ, Sachar DB. Duodenal fistulas in Crohn's disease. *J Clin Gastroenterol* 1987;9:46–49

362. Ashall G. Closure of upper gastrointestinal fistulas using a Roux-en-Y technique. *J Royal Coll Surg Edinb* 1986;31: 151–155

363. Bauer JL, Sher ME, Jaffin H, et al. Transvaginal approach for repair of rectovaginal fistulae complicating Crohn's disease. *Ann Surg* 1991;213:151–158

364. Chapman R, Foran R, Dunphy JE. Management of intestinal fistulas. *Am J Surg* 1964;108:157–164

365. Sandonato L, Saglimbene F, Sapienza C, et al. Treatment of post-surgery enterocutaneous fistulas: personal experience. *Ann Ital Chir* 1992;63(5):631–634

366. Hagemann RF, Stragand JJ. Fasting and refeeding: cell kinetic response of the jejunum, ileum, and colon. *Cell Tissue Kinetics* 1977;10:3

367. Evans MA, Shronts EP. Intestinal fuels: glutamine, short-chain fatty acids, and dietary fiber. *J Am Diet Assoc* 1992; 92:1239–1249

368. Sakata T, von Engelhardt W. Stimulatory effect of short chain fatty acids on the epithelial cell proliferation in rat large intestine. *Comp Biochen Physiol* 1983;74A:459

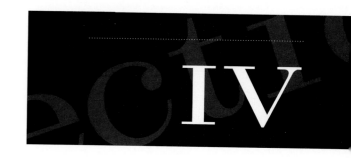

PERITONEUM, RETROPERITONEUM, AND MESENTERY

16

Exploratory Laparotomy

Harold Ellis

In these days of sophisticated preoperative diagnostic techniques, a purely diagnostic laparotomy is performed only rarely. Modern radiology, imaging techniques, and endoscopy generally provide a diagnosis. A diagnostic laparotomy should be considered in patients with fever of unknown origin, cachexia of unknown origin, and rarely, chronic pain, when all tests fail to reveal a cause.

A full exploratory laparotomy, however, must be carried out at the time of elective surgery to exclude, document, or deal with other intra-abdominal pathology. Laparotomy for closed or open abdominal trauma also must involve a careful search of the abdomen since multiple organ involvement is not uncommon.

Laparotomy should be limited in extent only when dealing with an acute abdominal emergency due to perforation, rupture of a viscus, or inflammatory disease. For example, having dealt with a ruptured ectopic pregnancy, a perforated peptic ulcer, an acute cholecystitis, or a ruptured appendix, it would be meddlesome to proceed to further abdominal exploration.

The laparotomy also may be limited when the abdomen is being reexplored and where there are extensive adhesions. Here, discretion must be employed and mobilization of the abdominal viscera limited to what is necessary to carry out the surgical operation and to establish the diagnosis.

■ OPERATIVE TECHNIQUE

The following account is concerned with visual diagnosis in patients undergoing elective surgery for intra-abdominal disease. The organs are investigated in the following order: stomach and duodenum; liver, gallbladder, and bile passages; pancreas and spleen; duodenojejunal flexure and small intestine; appendix and cecum; and colon, omentum, pelvic organs, and retroperitoneum. The diaphragmatic hiatus is examined for evidence of hernia. All these structures can be palpated at laparotomy, but visualization may require division of mesenteric and peritoneal attachments, and the extent of this mobilization will depend on the particular circumstances.

The entire stomach and duodenum are examined methodically. The anterior surface, the greater and lesser curvatures, the omenta with their lymph nodes, and the cardiac and pyloric regions can be palpated and visualized by good retraction. The cardiac portion of the stomach can be inspected and palpated with ease after the left lobe of the liver has been mobilized by division of the left coronary ligament, although this is not performed unless pathology is suspected. Exposure of the posterior surface of the stomach, and the stomach bed itself, can be effected through an incision in the gastrohepatic omentum and also by detaching the gastrocolic ligament from the greater curvature of the stomach (Figs 16–1 and 16–2). This gives an excellent view of

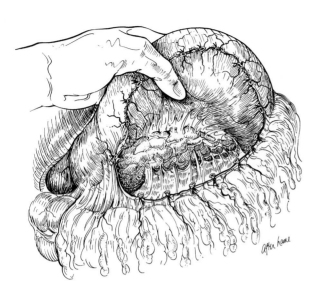

Figure 16–1. Exposure of the pancreas. (Redrawn from Smith R. Operations on the pancreas, In: Rob C, Smith R (eds), *Operative Surgery*, 2nd ed, vol 4. Philadelphia, PA: JB Lippincott; 1969: 304)

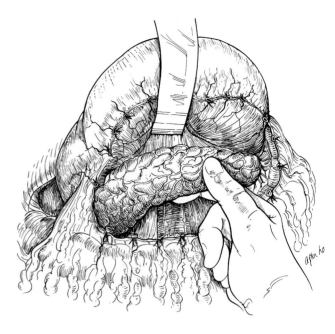

Figure 16–2. Palpation of the body of the pancreas.

the posterior wall of the stomach and a limited view of the posterior wall of the first portion of the duodenum and of the pancreas.

Examination of the duodenum includes testing the patency of the pyloric outlet and searching for the bed of a hidden posterior ulcer. A note is made of any scarring, distortion, or narrowing of the duodenum, and the presence of an ulcer is strongly suggested if gentle rubbing of the duodenal serosa with a gauze swab produces a red speckling appearance, the so-called "red-pepper sign."

If necessary, Kocher's maneuver of mobilizing the duodenum will be necessary so that the sweep of the duodenum and the head of the pancreas can be rotated medially for inspection and palpation (Figs 16–3 and 16–4). Mobilization of the duodenum also exposes the right ureter, the inferior vena cava, and the lower reaches of the common bile duct.

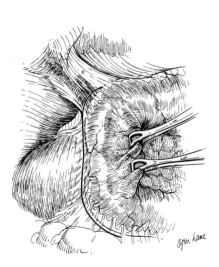

Figure 16–3. Incision for Kocher mobilization of the first three portions of the duodenum. In this illustration, the stump of the cystic duct is visible following previous cholecystectomy.

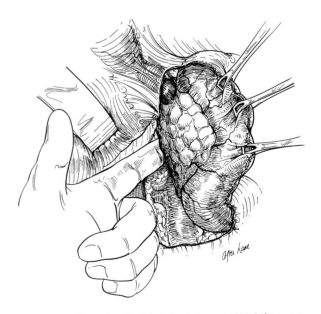

Figure 16–4. Kocher method of mobilizing the duodenum and head of pancreas.

Exposure of the third and fourth portions of the duodenum, the lower half of the head of the pancreas and the root of the superior mesenteric vessels is accomplished by Cattell's method (Fig 16–5). This involves mobilizing the cecum and ascending colon along their right-sided attachment to the posterior abdominal wall and sweeping these structures upward and to the left. The maneuver also gives excellent exposure to the abdominal aorta and is the technique this author prefers when dealing with an abdominal aortic aneurysm, both electively and in the emergency situation.

The liver is explored easily by slipping the hand over its exposed surface. Small angiomas and subserous cysts of the liver are observed frequently at laparotomy and may be mistaken for metastatic deposits. However, neither have the typical umbilicated appearance of secondary nodules, angiomas can be compressed by finger pressure, and both are readily identified visually.

The healthy gallbladder is sea green and can be emptied of its contents by gentle compression with the fingers. Its walls will be thin and elastic. It may be impossible to detect small gallstones in a normal-looking gallbladder, which is tense with bile until the viscus first is milked dry. The signs of chronic cholecystitis are unmistakable; the wall of the gallbladder is thicker and firmer than normal, the sea-green color is toned down by shades of grey, the subserous fatty tissue is augmented, the cystic lymph node feels prominently enlarged and firm; inflammatory adhesions drag up the colon with its omenta; and, usually, calculi are evident.

The common bile duct is examined next. Palpation should be carried out with a finger placed within the foramen of Winslow, while the thumb compresses the structures that lie in the free outer border of the gastrohepatic omentum. The index finger and thumb should be swept upward and downward in the search for stones and enlarged lymph nodes, and an attempt should be made to gauge the caliber of the main ducts. A normal common bile duct is the size of a pencil, approximately 7 mm. The duct is judged to be dilated if it measures 1 cm or more in diameter.

The small intestine, cecum, and appendix then should be examined. The lower small bowel is carefully inspected to exclude the presence of a Meckel's diverticulum, and the mesenteric nodes are felt for the presence of lymphadenitis (simple or tuberculous).

The *colon* should be palpated for a neoplasm polyp, or the presence of diverticula.

Finally, in the female, the pelvic organs are explored systematically.

In many cases of penetrating injury of the abdomen, especially where the wounds of entry or exit are situated in the flanks, the retroperitoneum should be displayed by freely mobilizing the right or the left colon or both, as demonstrated in Figs 16–6, 16–7 and 16–8. These injuries are frequently associated with perforation, laceration, or pulping of the kidney, suprarenal glands, colon, or great vessels. Any of the structures in the retroperitoneal space also may be damaged by blunt trauma. If there is any localized or diffuse swelling caused by blood, urine, bile, or

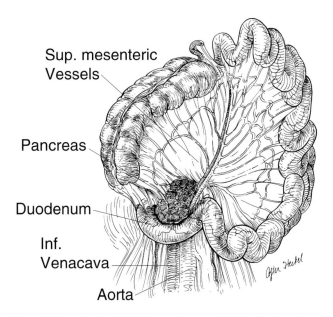

Figure 16–5. Cattell method of obtaining good exposure of third and fourth portions of duodenum, ligament of Treitz, superior mesenteric vessels, and head of pancreas. (Redrawn from Cattell RB, Braasch JW. *Surg Gynecol Obstet* 1960;111:378)

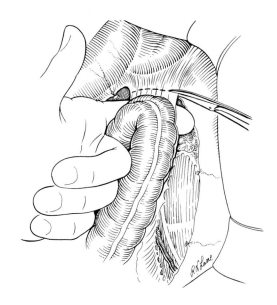

Figure 16–6. Mobilization of the splenic flexure of colon. Division of splenocolic ligament.

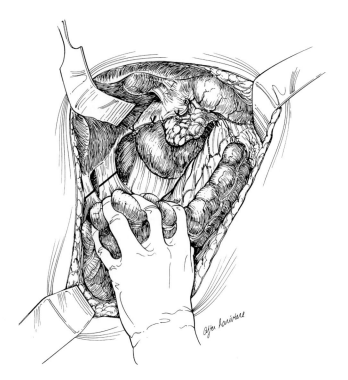

Figure 16–7. Right colon mobilized to obtain good inspection of the retroperitoneal region.

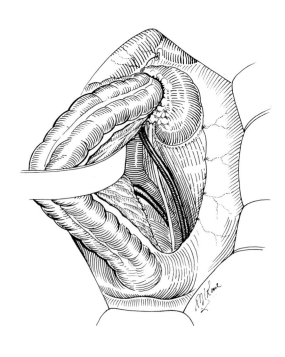

Figure 16–8. Mobilization of the left colon to display the suprarenal gland, kidney, ureter, and blood vessels to the left ovary or testis.

intestinal contents, the retroperitoneal structures should be displayed to determine the extent of the damage. The only exception to this rule is a pelvic hematoma, which is best left undisturbed because of the risk of starting serious hemorrhage from injured pelvic veins.

■ REEXPLORATION OF THE ABDOMEN

The necessity for reexploration of the abdomen is not at all uncommon. When reexploration is performed for a condition involving an entirely different part of the abdomen (eg, a gastrectomy in a patient who has previously been subjected to an appendectomy or hysterectomy), the surgeon obviously will make an entirely fresh incision through an intact portion of the abdominal wall. The only complicating factor in such cases is adhesions resulting from previous surgery. Usually omentum or, less often, loops of bowel will adhere to the serosal aspect of the previous incision, and frequently, local adhesions will be found at the site of the operative intervention. Likewise, omentum or loops of intestine may adhere to the pelvic floor after gynecologic surgery or a previous abdominoperineal excision of the rectum. After cholecystectomy, the duodenum or the hepatic flexure of the colon or omentum may adhere to the gallbladder bed. After gastric surgery, the lesser curve of the stomach usually adheres to the undersurface of the left lobe of the liver, and so on.

In other cases, the surgeon may need to reopen the previous laparotomy wound (eg, revisional gastric surgery, a cholecystectomy performed after vagotomy through an upper midline incision, or a reversal procedure after a previous Hartmann operation). Great care is necessary in opening the abdominal cavity because omentum or bowel is usually adherent to the undersurface of the parietal peritoneum. The liver may adhere to the uppermost extremity of an upper midline incision.

Preferably, the new incision should be extended a little proximal or distal to the old scar, and the peritoneum opened initially through this, it is hoped, unscarred area. If the area has been incised previously, the most delicate approach must be taken in incising the parietal peritoneum. Finger exploration then will reveal the extent of the adhesions. Artery forceps are applied to the peritoneal edges while the assistant applies gentle traction. Under direct vision, the surgeon then must divide the parietal adhesions with scissors or scalpel, keeping rigidly to the avascular line that can be defined where the adhesions attach to the parietal wall. Any attempt to hurry this part of the operation will be met by annoying hemorrhage or, more seriously, by visceral damage. If bowel is densely adherent to the abdominal wall, it is wiser to take a sliver of parietal peritoneum or even subjacent muscle rather than risk opening the gut. I instruct my residents that it is better to have a little parietal wall on the intestine than to have intestinal mucosa on the parietal wall!

17

Peritonitis and Intraperitoneal Abscess

Darryl T. Hiyama ▪ *Robert S. Bennion*

Intra-abdominal infections have been well recognized throughout the history of medicine. Remarkably, however, only within the last century has significant progress been made in the successful treatment of these diseases. Surgical intervention is one of the major reasons for this success and indeed, it may be said that the treatment of intra-abdominal infections remains a classic and defining role of the general or gastrointestinal surgeon. However, the reduction in mortality from 90% at the turn of the century to the estimated 10% to 20% today cannot be ascribed to surgery alone. The armamentarium of improved and effective antibiotics continues to grow along with our understanding of the inflammatory response. The widespread application of computerized tomography has effected both better localization of intraperitoneal abscesses and effective percutaneous drainage. Despite these advances, mortality persists, with patients succumbing to the effects of sepsis and eventual multisystem organ failure (MSOF). Clearly, the single, most influential factor in the successful management of intra-abdominal infections is early, accurate diagnosis and treatment. For the abdominal surgeon called upon to manage such infections, a thorough knowledge of the pathophysiology of peritonitis and the diagnostic and therapeutic options available for the treatment of intra-abdominal infections is essential.

■ ANATOMY OF THE PERITONEAL CAVITY

The peritoneal cavity is primarily divided into the greater and lesser sacs, which communicate via the foramen of Winslow. Within the greater sac, a number of areas, due to both anatomic and physiologic factors, are potential sites of fluid accumulation and therefore, abscess formation. These include the right subhepatic space, both right and left subphrenic spaces, the paracolic gutters, and the pelvis (Fig 17–1).

RIGHT SUBHEPATIC SPACE

This space is defined by the inferior surface of the right lobe of the liver, superiorly and the hepatic flexure and transverse mesocolon, inferiorly. It is bound by medially the second portion of the duodenum and the hepatoduodenal ligament, and laterally by the body wall. Posteriorly, this space opens into Morison's pouch, one of the most dependent spaces in the peritoneal cavity during recumbency, marking it a likely site of fluid accumulation and abscess formation.

RIGHT SUBPHRENIC SPACE

This area lies between the right hemidiaphragm and the superior surface of the right lobe of the liver and is bounded medially by the falciform ligament and poste-

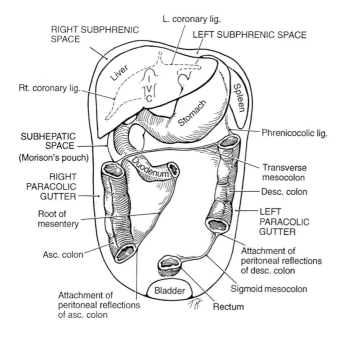

Figure 17–1. Diagram of intraperitoneal spaces.

riorly by the right triangular and coronary ligaments of the liver.

LEFT SUBPHRENIC SPACE

This is an extensive space that extends from above the left lobe of the liver, posterior to the spleen and anteroinferiorly to beneath the left lobe of the liver. The subphrenic component lies between the left hemidiaphragm and left hepatic lobe, and is bounded medially by the falciform ligament. The medial posterior border consists of the left triangular ligament of the liver, while laterally, the space extends between the diaphragm and the spleen. In this lateral aspect, the inferior component also passes between the spleen and kidney. The subhepatic component of the left subphrenic space is defined anteriorly and superiorly by the inferior surface of the left hepatic lobe and posteriorly by the anterior wall of the stomach and gastrohepatic ligament, or lesser omentum. This smaller component freely communicates with the larger subphrenic component around the lateral aspect of the left hepatic lobe.

PARACOLIC GUTTERS

These potential spaces lay between the body wall and on the right, the ascending colon segments and on the left, the descending colon segments. On the left, communication between the gutter and the subphrenic space is limited by the phrenocolic ligament. Inferiorly, communication with the pelvis is prevented by the sigmoid colon. On the right, unhindered communication exists

between the paracolic gutter and the right subphrenic and subhepatic spaces, as well as the pelvis.

LESSER SAC

This space lies posterior to the stomach and gastrohepatic ligament. Superiorly, the space extends behind the caudate lobe of the liver and inferiorly, to the transverse mesocolon. The anterior surface of the pancreas forms much of the posterior border of the lesser sac. Despite the free communication of the lesser and greater sacs through the foramen of Winslow, it is uncommon for infections originating in the greater sac to extend to the lesser space. Instead, infections in this space often originate from the involvement of surrounding organs such as the stomach or pancreas.

PELVIC CAVITY

The pelvic space is the most dependent area of the peritoneal cavity in the upright and semirecumbent positions. Anteriorly, this space is bounded by the urinary bladder and body wall and posteriorly, by the rectum, the bony pelvic wall and the retroperitoneum. In females, the space is subdivided into anterior and posterior compartments by the presence of the uterus. The anterior compartment is the uterovesical pouch, and the posterior compartment, rectouterine pouch. It is this area, immediately anterior to the rectum, that is the most likely location of a pelvic abscess. The proximity of such lesions to both the rectum and vagina readily allows diagnosis by digital palpation, as well as allowing for effective routes for drainage.

■ PHYSIOLOGY OF THE PERITONEAL CAVITY

The peritoneum is a *single* layer of mesothelial cells, with a basement membrane supported by a underlying layer of highly vascularized connective tissue.[1] Though thin, the surface area of the peritoneum is extensive, averaging 1.8 m^2 in the adult male, and is comparable to the surface area of the skin.[2] It has been estimated that a 1 mm increase in the thickness of the peritoneum by fluid accumulation can result in the sequestration of 18 L of fluid, a fact relevant to the massive fluid shifts associated with diffuse peritonitis.[3] The peritoneum covers all of the interior surface of the abdominal wall, diaphragmatic, retroperitoneal and pelvic surfaces which comprise the peritoneal cavity, in addition to the intra-abdominal viscera. In males, the peritoneum forms a closed sac, while in females, it is continuous with the mucous membranes of the fallopian tubes. One-half of the peritoneum, about 1 m^2, functions as a passive, semipermeable membrane to the diffusion of water, electrolytes, and macromolecules. Under normal conditions, <50 mL of sterile fluid is present within the peritoneal cavity. The fluid itself closely resembles lymph fluid and has a low specific gravity, protein content, and <3000 cells per cubic mm. Secreted from the visceral peritoneal surfaces, the fluid is circulated through the peritoneal cavity. The movement of this fluid has been defined by studies such as those conducted by Autio. Contrast material introduced into the peritoneal cavity in the paracecal area primarily transmigrates towards the right subphrenic area and into the pelvis (Fig 17–2).[4] The cephalad movement proceeds along the paracolic gutter and subhepatic spaces. It is thought that the cephalad movement of fluid is produced by the creation of a negative pressure area in the subphrenic space by diaphragmatic motion. Most of the peritoneal fluid is absorbed into the lymphatic circulation via the parietal peritoneal surfaces, with the remainder absorbed through diaphragmatic lymphatics.[5] The clearance of particulate matter, cells and microorganisms contained in peritoneal fluid may be largely dependent upon diaphragmatic lympathics.[6] Localized to the peritoneum overlying the muscular portion of the diaphragmatic surface, intercellular gaps or *stomata* are situated between peritoneal mesothelial cells. The diameter of these stomata can be varied by diaphragmatic stretching and contraction, from 4 to 12 μm.[7,8] In addition, in the presence of inflammation, the patency of the stomata may be increased to augment the clearance function of the diaphragm.[9] Both fluid and substances not amenable to absorption through the peritoneal membrane are channeled via the stomata through fenestrations in the basement membrane, and conveyed

to specialized diaphragmatic lymphatics called *lacunae.* During the respiratory cycle, relaxation of the diaphragm in expiration opens the stomata and promotes rapid filling of the lacunae.[6] At inspiration, contraction of the diaphragm empties the lacunae into efferent lymphatic channels. Negative intrathoracic pressure during inspiration facilitates fluid movement into thoracic lymphatic channels, and the majority of this fluid eventually is delivered to the central circulation via the thoracic duct. Based upon observations in animals, this process of fluid movement and particulate clearance via the diaphragmatic lymphatics is rapid. Following the intraperitoneal injection of bacteria, organisms can be recovered from the right thoracic lymph duct within 6 minutes, and from the blood within 12 minutes.[10]

A number of factors can influence this diaphragmatic clearance mechanism or "pump." In animal models, blockage of the stomata can be effected by the introduction of platelets, or the application of talc to occlude stomata.[11,12] Body positioning also can influence the effectiveness of this effect. Steinberg has noted that placing animals in the head-up position delayed, though did not prevent the appearance of bacteria in the circulation after intraperitoneal injection.[10] Other factors or conditions which affect diaphragmatic motion and function also affect bacterial clearance. Reducing spontaneous respiration using general anesthesia has been observed to decrease particulate clearance from the peritoneal cavity.[13] Similarly, the incidence of bacteremia was observed to be very low in pigs undergoing muscular paralysis and mechanical ventilation.[14] Even the application of positive end-expiratory pressure has been shown to decrease peritoneal bacterial clearance.[15] These effects result from chemical paralysis of the diaphragm and elimination of the "pumping mechanism," as well as the application of positive intrathoracic pressure which impairs thoracic lymphatic flow.

Clearly, this diaphragm mechanism is effective in the clearance of bacteria from the peritoneal cavity, and a primary *local* defense mechanism. However, the benefit of this mechanism, in terms of host survival, is uncertain. It has been observed that both the incidence of bacteremia and mortality have been reduced in a number of animal and human studies, when the diaphragmatic clearance of bacteria was *impaired.*[16] In a rat model, Dumont reported a reduction in both mortality and bacteremia when platelets or scarification were used to block stomata.[12] Skau and associates reported similar results in pigs, by reducing bacteremia after peritoneal contamination using only muscular paralysis and mechanical ventilation.[14] Suggestive clinical observations that the mortality from peritonitis is reduced in patients placed in the semiupright position, an action which probably decreases bacterial absorption via the diaphragm.[17] Maddaus has suggested that the primary

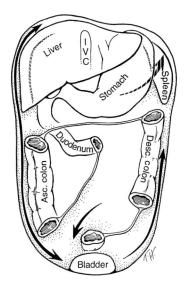

Figure 17–2. Diagram of the flow of fluid within the peritoneal cavity. Note that fluid movement is primarily directed to the subdiaphragmatic spaces and the pelvis.

role of this mechanism is fluid removal from the peritoneal cavity and not the elimination of microorganisms.[16] It is possible that the carriage of bacteria into the systemic circulation may overwhelm systemic defenses, such as the reticuloendothelial system, leading to the high incidence of bacteremia associated with peritonitis.

The second clearance mechanism is by phagocytosis by resident peritoneal macrophages. Dunn and associates have noted that in animals, one-half of the bacteria in an intraperitoneal inoculum are cleared physically via the diaphragmatic lymphatics and another one-third undergo phagocytosis by resident macrophages.[18] These two highly efficient mechanisms probably represent the "first line" of clearance after bacterial contamination.[19] Indeed, it is likely that the sterility of the peritoneal cavity is reestablished and maintained despite many episodes of low inoculum bacterial contamination because of the effectiveness of these local clearance mechanisms. However, if initial clearance is not accomplished, an inflammatory response ensues to facilitate neutrophil recruitment for further bacterial clearance, and localize or contain the infection.

LOCAL RESPONSE TO PERITONEAL INFECTION

The objective of the local response to infection is the removal or containment of microorganisms from the peritoneal cavity. The inflammatory response that occurs within the peritoneal cavity is similar to inflammation that occurs elsewhere in the body. This response is characterized by hyperemia, the influx of fluid, the recruitment of phagocytic cells, and fibrin deposition.

Any noxious stimulus that causes mesothelial or vascular endothelial cell injury is capable of initiating peritonitis. Though endotoxin associated with gram-negative bacteria is considered the classical stimulating agent of peritonitis based upon experimental models of peritonitis, a number of other agents are recognized as capable of inducing similar responses. Wiles has noted that local physiological effects similar to those elicited by endotoxin can be produced by organisms such as gram-positive bacteria, *Bacteroides* species, and yeasts that have no endotoxin, or only biologically inactive forms of endotoxin.[20] This implies that other bacterial products, such as exoenzymes or capsular polysaccharides also act as stimulators of inflammation. In addition, the similarity in systemic response to both anaerobic, gram-negative, and fungal peritonitis, namely fever, hypotension, leukocytosis, platelet aggregation, and shock, suggests that the systemic action of these stimulators is also not direct, but mediated by cytokines such as tumor necrosis factor (TNF) and interleukin-1 (IL-1).[21,22] This would suggest that the overall inflammatory response, both local and systemic is a general one, and not specific for any single infectious agent. Noninfec-

tious irritants such as gastric juice, pancreatic juice, bile salts, urine, and meconium are also well-recognized causes of *sterile* peritonitis and probably initiate the inflammatory process by inciting mesothelial cell damage or direct activation of the complement system. Following activation, the peritoneal inflammatory process is composed of changes in blood flow, the enhancement of bacterial phagocytosis and fibrin deposition to contain or trap bacteria.

ALTERATIONS IN BLOOD FLOW AND VASCULAR PERMEABILITY

An increase in local blood flow and an influx of fluid to the foci of inflammation are the two earliest observed physiological changes. Histamine is the early chemical mediator of these changes, released from tissue mast cells and basophils; bradykinin, a product of the contact activation system, exerts similar effects later in the inflammatory process. The release of histamine is triggered by mesothelial cell injury, though later, antigen-antibody complexes, complement-derived C3a and C5a, and platelet-activating factors also stimulate histamine release. Both histamine and bradykinin cause pain, vasodilatation and increased permeability of the small peritoneal blood vessels.[23] The production of other vasoactive substances such as prostaglandin E2α (PGE2α) and leukotriene C4 (LTC4) are effected by bradykinin and contribute to the observed vascular changes. Normally, the peritoneum allows bidirectional flow of fluid, but with inflammation, there is an unidirectional influx of extracellular fluid into the peritoneal cavity. Depending upon the extent of the peritoneal insult, fluid volumes of 10 L or more may be accumulated in the peritoneal cavity.[24] Following the changes in the microvasculature, the initial fluid that accumulates is a transudate of low protein content. With increasing vascular permeability, the transudation soon is followed by the exudation of copious amounts of fluid rich in immunoglobulins, complement factors, coagulation factors, autocoids, and cytokines.[25] Though this process clearly succeeds in delivering essential humoral mediators of inflammation to the foci of infection, a number of paradoxical effects also occur. Massive third-space fluid shifts and the loss of plasma proteins into the peritoneum can result in hypovolemic shock. In addition, at the local level, the continued accumulation of fluid may eventually impair bacterial phagocytosis by diluting opsonins and impeding neutrophil mobility and migration.[26]

Bacterial Phagocytosis

The central purpose of the local accumulation and interaction of the humoral mediators is the initiation and enhancement of bacterial phagocytosis. Though the membrane attack complex (MAC) produced by the complement system is capable of direct bacterial killing without the involvement of a leukocyte, other humoral mediators are involved in activating both macrophages and neutrophils, modulating leukocyte metabolic activity, chemotaxis, and opsonization of bacteria. The recruitment and accumulation of large numbers of leukocytes to the site of inflammation is accomplished by changes in local blood flow as well as increased margination and adherence of leukocytes to surfaces such as endothelial or mesothelial cells. Bradykinin, anaphylatoxins, platelet-activating factors (PAF), TNF and IL-1 appear to promote these effects.[27] Many of these same substances also promote the migration of neutrophils and macrophages to the sites of microbial invasion. C5a anaphylatoxin possesses the most potent chemoattractant properties, though C3a, C567 complex, kallikrein, IL-1, IL-8 and PAFs also have chemotaxis effects upon neutrophils. By 4 to 6 hours following injury, significant neutrophil influx has occurred and is peaked at about 8 hours.[16] Activated PAF also stimulates platelet aggregation, which may play a role in the platelet sequestration and thrombocytopenia observed in septic shock.

Substances derived from a number of sources influence leukocyte metabolism and the production and release of lysosomal enzymes. Anaphylatoxins increase the oxidative metabolism and stimulate production of lysosomal enzymes in neutrophils and macrophages. Kallikrein induces superoxide anion generation and lysosomal enzyme release in neutrophils. PAFs stimulate similar effects in neutrophils, monomorphonuclear macrophages, as well as platelets, eosinophils and mesangial cells.[28] Large fragments of C3b demonstrate opsonic activity by promoting the recognition and phagocytosis of microorganisms by phagocytic leukocytes.

Fibrin Deposition

Under normal circumstances, intact mesothelial cells maintain fibrinolytic activity within the peritoneal cavity by the secretion of tissue plasminogen activator (t-PA).[29] In the setting of mesothelial cell injury and active inflammation, local fibrinolytic activity is suppressed owing to the loss of plasminogen activator.[30] With high concentrations of fibrinogen present, fibrin deposition readily occurs by activation of the intrinsic pathway.[31,32] Intraperitoneal coagulation is enhanced further by the release of thromboplastin (factor III) from injured mesothelial cells, and surface procoagulant activity from stimulated peritoneal macrophages.[33]

Fibrin deposition appears to play a role in the local inflammatory response. The most credible objective of this process is to isolate or contain contamination and thereby prevent widespread dissemination. At one level, bacteria are entrapped in fibrin matrices.[34] At a larger level, these fibrinous adhesions cause the adherence of loops of intestine and omentum to one another as well as the parietal peritoneal surface, thus creating physical bar-

riers against the spread of bacterial contamination. However, fibrin encasement of bacteria also inhibits phagocytosis by isolating the microbe from the neutrophil.[35]

Abscess Formation

The development of an intraperitoneal abscess is the culmination of the sequestration process described above. The rate of fibrin deposition exceeds the fibrin degradation produced by bacterial enzymes, fibrinolysis and phagocytosis. Within the adhesed mass of viscera, fibrin and bacterial, liquefaction develops from the release of proteolytic enzymes from perishing leukocytes and the action of bacterial exoenzymes. The osmolarity of the developing abscess fluid is high, promoting an influx of water and increasing the internal hydrostatic pressure within the cavity.[3] The abscess capsule, composed of organizing fibrin and adherent adjacent viscera, retards the diffusion of oxygen and nutrients into the abscess and then fosters anaerobic glycolysis. The hypoxic, hypercarbic, and acidic environment that is created significantly impairs both neutrophil and phagocytic function. The high concentration of bacterial products such as cell wall components and enzymes impairs phagocytic function, depletes the local supply of complement, and increases local tissue damage. The presence of necrotic debris also depletes complement and contributes to neutrophil deactivation. Hypoxia and acidosis impair neutrophil migration and killing. Hyperosmolarity inhibits neutrophil release of lysosomal granules and hypercarbia causes leukocyte dysfunction by lowering the cytoplasmic pH.

Peritoneal Healing

The peritoneum appears to heal rapidly after injury. Observations in animal models indicate that the replacement of injured mesothelium occurs over the entire wound simultaneously. Thus, the rate of healing is independent of the size of the peritoneal wound. Within 3 days after injury, the wound is covered by connective tissue cells, and by day 5, these new cells resemble normal mesothelium.[36,37] The source of these new cells is unclear. Possibilities include submesothelial stem cells producing replacement mesothelial cells, differentiation of monocytes and macrophages in the peritoneal fluid into mesothelial cells, and the proliferation of intact mesothelial cells from the peritoneal fluid or wound edges.[3] As noted above, peritoneal injury in the presence of inflammation and infection results in adhesion formation. Following resolution of the inflammation, normal fibrinolytic activity returns as mesothelial cell regeneration nears completion, and fibrinous adhesions are degraded and removed. However, in the setting of severe peritoneal injury or persistent infection, filmy fibrinous adhesions are transformed to fibrous adhesions by the ingrowth of fibroblasts, capillaries, and the deposition of collagen. Resolution of the peritoneal insult allows eventual removal of these fibrous adhesions by phagocytosis and remodeling.

FACTORS INFLUENCING PERITONEAL INFLAMMATION AND INFECTION

Bacterial Virulence

The virulence of contaminating bacteria is influenced by a number of factors. Several organisms are well recognized for their innate ability to produce intra-abdominal infections in humans. As an example, in secondary peritonitis, common fecal pathogens include aerobic coliform bacteria, anaerobic *Bacteroides* species, enterococci, anaerobic and aerobic streptococci, and *Clostridia* species (Table 17–1). In contrast, other organisms such as *Propionibacteria* rarely produce disease. Despite the massive contamination and complexity of the microbial spectrum that occurs with fecal perforation, within 24 to 48 hours, only a few isolates are recovered in peritoneal fluid culture.[38] This indicates that only a few pathogenic bacteria survive to predominate in the infection. In addition, the predominance of a particular microorganism within the local inflammatory process has been shown to vary. In an animal model of a polymicrobial colonic peritonitis, Weinstein demonstrated that *E. coli* and enterococcus were the predominant organisms during the peritonitis phase, while *B. fragilis* predominated during the abscess phase.[39] Another example of unique pathogenicity is the remarkable ability of encapsulated anaerobic bacteria to produce abscess formation, a characteristic attributed to the capsular polysaccharide components. The size of the bacterial inoculum also influences virulence and, as expected, both the ability to produce an infection and the severity of the disease increases with an increasing bacterial dose. The ability to adhere to the mesothelial surface may also enhance the virulence of some organisms such as the *Enterobacteriaceae* and *Bacteroides fragilis*.[40] Experimental models indicate that such organisms are resistant to mechanical removal via peritoneal lavage, which increases the difficulty in clearing these microbes from the peritoneum.

Bacterial *synergism* also potentiates the virulence of a single organism. Polymicrobial infections, specifically combinations of aerobic and anaerobic species, exhibit significantly greater lethality than comparable infections involving a single species of pathogenic bacteria.[41] Aerobic bacteria may benefit anaerobic species by lowering the redox potential of the microenvironment and producing essential nutrients, while anaerobic bacteria may provide the ability to inhibit neutrophil function and to develop antibiotics resistance by inactivation.

Adjuvant Factors

The ability of adjuvant substances to promote infection has been well demonstrated in a number of studies. Adjuvants enhance the virulence of the microorganisms by interference with host defense mechanisms, whether mechanical or cellular. Blood components, hemoglobin, and ferrous iron are the adjuvant factors most studied, to date (Table 17–2). The lethality of *E. coli* is enhanced in vitro by hemoglobin.[42] Whether this effect is the result of the induction of a leukocyte-derived toxin injurious to neutrophils or to the presence of iron which enhances bacterial growth is not clear.[43–46] Fibrin entrapment of bacteria may be both helpful and detrimental to the overall host response. The presence of fibrin may inhibit phagocytic killing of bacteria by activated neutrophils as well as cause premature degranulation of neutrophils as the PMNs attempt to phagocytose fibrin particles.[34,47] The presence of both fibrin and platelets within the peritoneal cavity also may impair physical bacterial clearance by blockage of the diaphragmatic lymphatics.[12] A number of substances originating from the gastrointestinal tract itself have also been shown, in experimental peritonitis, to produce lethal peritonitis. Fecal matter (sterile), bile salts, and gastric mucin have all demonstrated such adjuvant activity.[48,49] Even nonirritant fluid may impair bacterial elimination. Copious amounts of intraperitoneal fluid may diminish phagocytosis by diluting opsonins, or im-

TABLE 17–1. ADJUVANT FACTORS AND POSSIBLE EFFECTS UPON HOST DEFENSES

Adjuvants and Effects on Host Defenses	
Adjuvant Factor	**Effect**
Hemoglobin, ferrous iron	Enhances bacteria-mediated inhibition of neutrophil function, iron source may support bacterial growth
Intraperitoneal fluid	Dilution of opsonins, inhibition of phagocytosis, flooding of diaphragmatic lympatics
Fibrin	Impairment of phagocytosis, premature neutrophil degranulation
Platelets	Occlusion of diaphragmatic lymphatics
Necrotic tissue	Depletion of complement, neutrophil inactivation
Gastric juice, pancreatic juice, urine, meconium	Induces sterile chemical peritonitis
Bile, bile salts	Facilitates bacterial spreading, toxic to neutrophils and peritoneal mesothelial cells
Barium sulfate	Impairs access of phagocytic cells to bacteria
Talc, drains, suture material, cellulose (Gelfoam, Oxycel)	Premature degranulation of neutrophils

Adapted from Wittman DH, Walker AP, Condon RE. Peritonitis and intra-abdominal infection. In: Schwartz S, Shires G, Spencer F (eds), Principles of Surgery, 6th ed. New York, NY: McGraw-Hill; 1991:1449–1483

TABLE 17–2. PERITONEAL ISOLATES AT LAPAROTOMY

Organism	Solomkin et al[a]	Mosdell et al[b]
Gram-negative aerobic and facultative anaerobes		
Escherichia coli	56.8	68.4
Enterobacter species	13.5	6.1
Klebsiella species	15.4	17
Pseudomonas aeruginosa	14.8	19.1
Proteus species	6.2	2.7
Serratia marcescens	1.2	4.1
Morganella morganii	1.2	—
Citrobacter species	3.1	3.4
Others	3.7	7.5
Yeast		
Candida species	18.6	4.1
Gram-positive aerobic and facultative anerobes		
Nonenterococcal steptococci	35.8	25.9
Enterococci	23.5	10.5
Staphylococcus aureus or *S. epidermidis*	10.5	10.5
Anaerobic organisms		
Bacteroides fragilis	22.8	44.5
Other *Bacteroides*	21	—
Clostridium species	17.9	5.8
Peptococci/streptococci	7.4	16
Fusobacterium species	6.2	5.1
Lactobacillus	5.6	—
Eubacterium species	4.3	—
Others	12.4	3.7

[a]Data represent percent of all patients.
[b]Data represent percent of cultures.
Adapted from *Solomkin JS, Dellinger EP, Christou NV, et al. Results of a multicenter trial comparing imipenem/cilastin to tobramycin/clindamycin for intraabdominal infections.* Ann Surg *1990;212:581,* and *Mosdell DM, Morris DM, Voltura A, et al: Antibiotic treatment for surgical peritonitis.* Ann Surg *1991;214:543*

mersing bacteria in solution. This latter event eliminates the surface phagocytic cells required for engulfing and ingesting bacteria.[26] Foreign materials such as barium sulfate, talc, and cellulose or processed collagen probably also impair phagocytosis by causing the premature activation of neutrophils and release of lysosomal enzymes.[50,51] Clearly, a number of substances found in conjunction with peritoneal infection may be detrimental to host defenses and jeopardize the success of eradicating the infection. From a clinical standpoint, a rational approach in the surgical management of peritoneal infection should include attention to meticulous hemostasis, copious lavage to remove adjuvant material, the thorough evacuation of intraperitoneal fluid, and minimizing the use of foreign material such as hemostatic agents and suture material.

SYSTEMIC RESPONSE TO PERITONEAL INJURY OR INFECTION

The systemic response to peritoneal infection emulates the response of the body to other forms of injury, such as trauma or surgery. The development of hypovolemia is a phenomenon central to the systemic response and

probably results from the fluid influx occurring in the peritoneal cavity. The subsequent intravascular volume change leads to a reduction in venous return and cardiac output. Incomplete compensation is obtained with increases in heart rate. Systemic hypotension also may be the result of the secretion of TNF, IL-1, platelet-activating factors, and nitric oxide, which all have vasodilatory effects and may reduce systemic vascular resistance.[21,22] In particular, a significant degree of precapillary shunting may occur in the pulmonary and splanchnic circulation, which leads to a reduction in oxygen delivery and subsequent consumption. Diminished urine flow develops as a result of the effects of increased aldosterone and antidiuretic hormone secretion, the reduced cardiac output, and intrarenal shunting of blood. This is the setting that has been dubbed hyperdynamic or "warm" septic shock, characterized by tachycardia, fever, oliguria, hypotension, and warm extremities. Hemodynamic and oxygen transport measurements would reveal an elevated cardiac output, low peripheral vascular resistance, low arteriovenous O_2 difference, and a high mixed-venous oxygen content. Pulmonary function also is altered in this setting. Abdominal distention secondary to accumulated fluid within the peritoneal cavity and bowel creates mechanical restriction to diaphragmatic mobility and decreases ventilatory volume, creating eventual atelectasis. Ventilation-perfusion mismatching results from both the atelectasis and intrapulmonary shunting due to beta-adrenergic stimulation. Increases in pulmonary vascular permeability also develops as a result of a number of the inflammatory mediators. The accumulation of fluid in the pulmonary interstitium and alveoli decreases pulmonary compliance and increases the work of breathing. Early manifestations of these changes include hyperventilation and the development of a respiratory alkalosis. With the worsening of the pulmonary edema and alveolar collapse, severe hypoxemia will develop, creating the adult respiratory distress syndrome (ARDS).

Tissue metabolism is severely altered during the response to peritonitis. The metabolic rate is increased owing to the increased secretion of catecholamines and cortisol. However, hypovolemia reduces cardiac output. Tissue hypoxia develops as a result of reduced oxygen delivery, owing to both decreased perfusion as well as shunting. Increasing anaerobic glycolysis produces accumulating amounts of lactic acid and acid by-products. Renal and pulmonary clearance of this increased acid load leads to metabolic acidosis, unless perfusion is restored. A significant conversion in substrate metabolism also occurs in peritonitis. Following the early depletion of hepatic glycogen stores, protein catabolism is augmented in the skeletal muscle to release branched-chain amino acids for use by myocytes as an energy source. Other amino acids are released into the circulation to be utilized in hepatic gluconeogenesis as well as the production of acute-phase proteins to support the systemic inflammatory response. Though the body lipolysis rate also is increased, utilization of free fatty acids as an energy source is not efficient in the early septic period. The severe loss in lean body mass that can occur from the net protein catabolism occurs rapidly and is only partially ameliorated by the use of nutritional support.

PERITONITIS

Inflammation of the peritoneum can be caused by a number of etiologic agents including bacteria, fungi, viruses, chemical irritants, and foreign bodies. The sequence of both local and systemic events that occurs following the peritoneal insult represents a relatively constant response to a variety of injurious agents. However, the clinical aspects, specifically, the management of peritonitis, is influenced significantly by the etiology of the infectious process.

Currently, peritonitis is organized into three divisions based upon the source and nature of the microbial contamination. *Primary peritonitis* is defined as an infection, often monomicrobial, of the peritoneal fluid without visceral perforation. Often the source of the bacteria is an *extraperitoneal* source. *Secondary peritonitis*, by far the most common form of peritonitis, refers to peritoneal infection arising from an *intra-abdominal* source, usually a perforation of a hollow viscus. *Tertiary peritonitis* develops following the treatment of secondary peritonitis and represents either a failure of the host inflammatory response, or a superinfection.

CLINICAL PRESENTATION OF PERITONITIS

The respected aphorism that states that the diagnosis of peritonitis is made by clinical evaluation remains true today. Abdominal pain is almost universally the predominant presenting symptom. The historical characteristics of the abdominal pain can vary tremendously depending upon the ultimate cause. For example, the sudden, sharp onset of epigastric pain peculiar to the perforation of an anterior duodenal ulcer can differ markedly from the gradual onset of lower quadrant symptoms characteristic of acute appendicitis. It is beyond the scope of this chapter to describe the variety of presentations of the various causes of peritonitis and the reader is directed to other sections of this book for such information. The pain of fully established peritonitis is constant, burning and aggravated by motion or movement. The extent of the pain may be localized or diffuse, depending upon the area of parietal peritoneum that is inflamed. The abdominal pain typically starts at the site of local peritoneal inflammation and later be-

comes more diffuse as more of the peritoneal surface becomes involved. However, if the site of inflammation is effectively isolated from the parietal peritoneum (eg, covered by loops of intestine or omentum), the initial discomfort may be only minimal in intensity and vague in location. Anorexia is almost always an accompanying symptom. Nausea and possibly vomiting, as well as thirst and oliguria are frequently present.

Typical systemic signs include fever, and diaphoresis. Tachycardia resulting from hypovolemia is frequently present. If septic shock is present, patients may exhibit tachycardia, hypotension, and warm, pink extremities. If severe shock is present, severe hypotension, hypothermia, and cool extremities may be seen. Patients often prefer to remain still and recumbent, a position that yields minimal exacerbation of their pain. The eliciting of tenderness may best be accomplished by percussion followed by direct palpation, a process that yields better localization of the tenderness and less discomfort for the patient. The evoking of rebound tenderness is less helpful. In the setting of generalized peritonitis, abdominal tenderness is diffuse and is often maximal in the region where the peritonitis originated. Bowel sounds are usually markedly diminished or absent and abdominal distention owing to the paralytic ileus is often present. Abdominal wall rigidity due to voluntary guarding and reflex muscle spasm can be extensive. With localized peritonitis, tenderness is focal, and the remainder of the abdomen may be relatively soft and nontender. Ileus may be minimal or even nonexistent.

Physical findings may be concealed or obscured in patients administered analgesics or corticosteroids, or who have altered consciousness from head injury, toxic or metabolic encephalopathy, or spinal injury. In the postoperative patient, the physical examination for suspected peritonitis also is rendered difficult. Incisional tenderness, as well as peritoneal injury secondary to the operation, can muddle the examination of the abdomen. In these situations, the physical evaluation for peritonitis may be rendered unreliable or inconclusive and the diagnosis may depend upon other diagnostic modalities.

In general, routine laboratory and radiographic studies often add little specific information in the evaluation of peritonitis. Leukocytosis, with a predominance of immature neutrophil forms is almost uniformly present. Plain radiographs of the abdomen may reveal obliteration of the peritoneal fat lines and the psoas shadow indicating the presence of peritoneal edema. Air-filled loops of bowel, with thickened, opaque walls may be found when bowel edema and paralytic ileus is present. Free intraperitoneal air, indicative of a perforated viscus, may be found on upright abdominal, lateral decubitus abdominal, or upright chest radiograph.

The role of more elaborate diagnostic studies in peritonitis is limited to those patients presenting with abdominal pain who have *no* immediate, compelling indication for abdominal exploration and (1) may have an extraabdominal or nonsurgical cause for peritonitis such as pyelonephritis or a ruptured ovarian cyst or (2) may have an unreliable physical evaluation such as was noted above. For example, an intravenous pyelogram may be useful in the diagnosis of pyelonephritis, or pelvic ultrasound helpful in evaluating a young female with lower quadrant abdominal pain. Patients with abdominal pain or a question of peritoneal irritation, in whom the abdominal examination may be equivocal or unreliable such as those with head injuries or on corticosteroids, may require computed tomography (CT) to ensure that a significant intra-abdominal process is not overlooked. Though this is a technique the authors have used, we believe it is only useful in very exceptional instances. In general, ultrasonography, CT and especially magnetic resonance imaging (MRI) *should not be routinely used* in patients with acute peritonitis. Exclusive of very exceptional situations, such studies have no role in the evaluation of peritonitis and only contribute unnecessary delay in treatment, and unnecessary increase in cost. In comparison, CT and ultrasonography are both extremely useful in the diagnosis of intraperitoneal abscess, and will be discussed later.

PRIMARY PERITONITIS

Primary peritonitis refers to bacterial infection of the peritoneal cavity originating from an extraperitoneal site, possibly by lymphatic or hematogenous seeding. Representing approximately 1% of all cases of peritonitis, primary peritonitis most commonly occurs in adults with alcoholic cirrhosis and ascites, and in children with nephrotic syndrome or systemic lupus erythematosus.[52,53] Patients with ascites secondary to other causes, such as cardiac failure, malignancy, and autoimmune disorders, are also at high risk for developing this condition.[53–56]

The route by which bacteria are transported to the peritoneal cavity is not known. At present, the most likely explanation appears to be the hematogenous route. This theory is supported by clinical observations in adults of primary peritonitis that occurs simultaneously with urinary tract infections involving the same single organism. In children, primary peritonitis commonly is caused by streptococci, and often is anteceded by an ear or upper respiratory infection. The theory of translocation of enteric bacteria is less favored now, although the predominant pathogens in primary peritonitis in adults today are coliform bacteria. It is possible that bacterial translocation is the route of infection in the minority of patients with primary peritonitis in whom no preceding evidence of bacteremia or concurrent infection can be demonstrated.[57] In females, particularly children, ascending bacterial contamination originating from the genitalia and conducted via the fallopian tubes has been implicated as an alternate route of infection. This may explain the high female:male ratio of primary peritonitis in children with nephrotic syndrome.

While the presence of ascites alone is a risk factor in developing primary peritonitis, the protein content of the ascitic fluid may influence this risk. Runyon has noted that patients with ascites of a low protein concentration (<1 gm/dL) are 10 times more likely to develop primary peritonitis than patients with ascitic fluid with a protein concentration >1 gm/dL.[58] Low-protein ascites is common in patients with cirrhosis and nephrosis, while high protein concentrations can be found in patients with malignant ascites. The incidence of primary peritonitis is lower in the latter group. An explanation of this observation may lie in the concentration of humoral inflammatory factors such as complement and immunoglobulins found in ascitic fluid. Opsonic activity is roughly proportional to the total protein concentration of ascitic fluid.[59] The preserved ability to effectively eliminate bacteria in high-protein ascites may prevent the dissemination of infection following contamination.

The integrity of host immune function also influences the development of primary peritonitis. For example, alcoholic cirrhosis is associated with decreased neutrophil killing and phagocytic activity, and a marked reduction in the hepatic reticuloendothelial clearance of bacteria.[60,61] Further, serum bilirubin concentration has been found to correlate independently with the development of primary peritonitis, which indicates that hepatic insufficiency itself places patients at higher risk for primary peritonitis.[62]

Clinical Presentation

In children, there is a bimodal incidence occurring in neonates and at 4 to 5 years of age. The onset of symptoms is acute and mimics that of secondary bacterial peritonitis, characterized by fever, vomiting, lethargy, and abdominal pain and distention. Abdominal examination yields evidence of peritoneal irritation, although the presence of bowel sounds is variable. In adults, the presentation is more subtle, and up to 30% of patients may be asymptomatic.[12] Presenting symptoms may include low-grade fever, encephalopathy, hepatorenal syndrome, or increasing ascites.

Diagnostic Studies

In children, the diagnosis of primary peritonitis is rarely made prior to operation. The absence of ascites in these children and the clinical presentation suggestive of acute appendicitis often leads to early laparotomy.

In adults, diagnostic paracentesis is the most useful initial study. Fluid should be examined for cell count and differential, pH, and Gram's stain, and aerobic and anaerobic culture. An ascitic fluid neutrophil count of >250 cells/mm³ is strongly indicative of peritonitis.[40] An elevated neutrophil count, in combination with either an elevated arterial-ascitic fluid pH gradient or a low ascitic fluid pH may have a specificity of 97% for peritonitis. Gram's stain of ascitic fluid is quite insensitive in patients with primary peritonitis owing to the low bacterial concentration, although this test is helpful when positive. A stain demonstrating a single type of organism is highly suggestive of primary peritonitis, while a mixed flora of both gram-negative and gram-positive organisms suggests intestinal perforation. Obviously, the presence of gross feces, bile, blood, or vegetable fibers in the aspirated fluid also should promote urgent exploratory laparotomy.

Obtaining positive microbe cultures from ascitic fluid can be difficult owing to the low concentration of bacteria in ascitic fluid. However, because of the 24 to 72 hour delay in obtaining microbiological confirmation of primary peritonitis, a diagnosis of primary peritonitis should be based upon the criteria of *clinical presentation*, the presence of *ascites*, an *elevated ascitic-fluid neutrophil count* and *no indication of visceral perforation*. Plain abdominal radiographs should be obtained in a search for pneumoperitoneum.

Two variants of primary peritonitis have been described. The first is culture-negative neutrocytic ascites (CNNA). It is defined by the presence of an ascitic-fluid neutrophil count of ≥500 cell/mm³, negative ascitic-fluid cultures, absence of an intra-abdominal source of infection, no prior antibiotic treatment within 30 days, and no alternative explanation for the elevated ascitic-fluid polymorphonuclear (PMN) count. The culture negativity seen in these patients may represent a lack of sensitivity of certain culture methods, or reflect the resolution phase of primary peritonitis in which host defenses have eradicated the organism without the help of antibiotics, but with a persistent elevation of the ascitic-fluid neutrophil count. Despite the culture negativity, CNNA patients should be treated aggressively. A second variant is monomicrobial nonneutrocytic bacterascites (MNB). In MNB, the ascitic-fluid culture yields a pure growth of a single organism, but the ascitic-fluid neutrophil count is <250 cell/mm³. Most patients with MNB are asymptomatic, although about one-half of these patients will progress to primary peritonitis.[67] Because of this fact, patients with MNB should be treated only if signs or symptoms of infection occur.

Treatment

Primary peritonitis should be treated aggressively. Adequate drug levels in the ascitic fluid can be achieved by parenteral intravenous administration and intraperitoneal installation of antibiotics is not necessary. Primary peritonitis caused by group A streptococci or *Streptococcus pneumoniae* should be treated with intravenous penicillin G. For other patients, particularly those with cirrhosis or who require empirical therapy, broad-spectrum therapy to cover gram-negative and gram-positive bacteria should be selected. The antibiotics of choice are either a third-generation cephalosporin as a single agent, or a beta-lactamase inhibitor combination. Alternate choices would include a monobactam with an additional agent to cover gram-positive cocci. Because of the demonstrated effectiveness of single-agent therapy, and the 30% incidence of aminoglycoside nephrotoxicity, aminoglycoside antibiotics should be avoided.[68] A recent prospective study indicated that 5 days of antibiotic therapy was equally as effective as a 10 day course.[69] There were no differences between the two treatment regimens, with respect to cure rates or length of hospitalization, although the cost of treatment was reduced by one-half by the abbreviated duration of therapy.

Prognosis

In children with nephrosis, successful treatment results in a survival rate of >90%.[70] Regardless of the antibiotic used, cure rates in excess of 75% can be expected in adults.[69,71] However, the probability of recurrence of primary peritonitis following successful treatment is nearly 50% at 6 months, and 69% at 1 year after treatment.[72] In-hospital mortality is approximately 50%, with deaths primarily the result of liver failure. In addition, the 1 year mortality in these patients, despite successful treatment, approaches 70%. Survival time appears to be shorter in patients with cirrhosis who develop primary peritonitis, when compared to similar patients in whom peritonitis did not develop.[73]

Tuberculous Peritonitis

A chronic form of primary bacterial peritonitis can be caused by *Mycobacterium tuberculosis*. Although this disease is common in undeveloped countries, it is only recently that the incidence of tuberculous peritonitis has increased in the United States and other western countries. This change in the pattern of occurrence may be attributable to a number of causes, including increasing immigration from endemic areas, a resurgence of tuberculosis in urban areas in the United States, and the prevalence of immunocompromised individuals, such as those with acquired immunodeficiency syndrome (AIDS). Although the primary site of infection (lungs, intestine) may no longer be clinically apparent, tuberculous peritonitis, typically, is caused by hematogenous spread. It can even be caused by reactivation of a primary infection that has been dormant for an extended period of time.

Clinical Manifestation. Patients present with complaints of abdominal pain that is often chronic as well as intermittent fever, malaise, anorexia, and weight loss. During the early stages, ascites is a prominent clinical finding. Later, the ascites resolves as dense adhesions form.

Diagnosis. In the early phase, paracentesis yields an ascitic fluid with elevated protein content, lymphocytosis, and a low glucose concentration. Acid-fast bacilli can be cultured from the ascitic fluid.

Diagnostic laparoscopy of laparotomy is recommended if diagnosis cannot be obtained with paracentesis. To minimize exposure, laparoscopy is preferred. Upon visualization, both the visceral and parietal peritoneal surfaces may be completely studded with small white tubercles. In the absence of ascites, characteristic dense fibrinous adhesions extend from the parietal peritoneum. Though these findings are unique, biopsies of the adhesions and collection of peritoneal fluid for acid-fast smear and culture are recommended.

Treatment. Aggressive multidrug chemotherapy against tuberculosis can be instituted immediately while awaiting culture results, and should be continued for a period of 2 years. Surgical management should be reserved for the diagnosis of tuberculous peritonitis or for treatment of complications such as fistula formation or intestinal obstruction.

Peritoneal Dialysis-Associated Peritonitis

With an incidence of approximately one episode per patient-year, peritonitis is the most common and significant complication associated with permanent peritoneal dialysis catheters. Despite aggressive treatment, a mortality rate of up to about 5% is still reported.[74] The incidence of peritoneal dialysis-associated peritonitis (PDAP) is higher in patients receiving chronic ambulatory peritoneal dialysis (CAPD) versus intermittent peritoneal dialysis. Frequent manipulation of the dialysis catheter is the most common underlying cause, although infections also arise from exit-site and tunnel infections. Two-thirds of patients with PDAP are found to have monomicrobial infections from their skin flora, usually *Staphylococcus aureus* or *Staphylococcus epidermidis*. Gram-negative infections are less common, and are associated with recurring episodes of PDAP and previous antibiotic treatment. Virulent organisms such as *Pseudomonas aeruginosa* and fungi are found in a small percentage of cases, but are often difficult to eradicate. The presence of anaerobes or a polymicrobial infection suggests intestinal perforation or intra-abdominal disease, such as acute appendicitis, perforated diverticulitis, or perforated duodenal ulcer.

Clinical Presentation and Diagnosis. Patients often present with low-grade fever, and mild abdominal pain and tenderness. The diagnosis of PDAP typically requires at least *two* of the following features: (1) symptoms of peritonitis,

such as abdominal pain and guarding, (2) cloudy peritoneal dialysate drainage with >100 white cells/mm³ and predominately PMNs, and (3) the presence of microorganisms on Gram's stain or peritoneal fluid culture.[75] Unfortunately, Gram's stain of the dialysate effluent for bacteria have reported positive yields in only 10% to 20% of cases. Cloudy dialysate fluid appears to be the earliest and most reliable sign of PDAP. Additional peritoneal fluid should be obtained for culture and the skin exit site and tunnel examined for signs of infection.

If Gram's stain or culture reveal a polymicrobial gram-negative infection, secondary peritonitis due to appendicitis, perforated duodenal ulcer, or perforated diverticulitis should be suspected. Gastrograffin contrast studies or abdominal CT may aid in confirming the diagnosis.

Management. Early empiric *intraperitoneal* antibiotic therapy should be instituted once the diagnosis is *suspected*. Since the selection of antibiotics should be influenced by the likely organism, a first-generation cephalosporin, such as cephalothin or cefazolin, or vancomycin, may be used as a single agent for gram-positive cocci coverage. Other authors recommend use of dual agents for broad-spectrum therapy combining the cephalosporin with an aminoglycoside such as tobramycin.[76] The antibiotics, as well as heparin, in a dose of 2000 U/L, are added to the dialysate, and the dwell time increased following instillation. The duration of therapy varies with the institution, however a course of 7 days of treatment *after the last positive dialysate culture* is obtained is recommended. Antibiotic selection should be adjusted based upon culture and sensitivity information as it becomes available.

If clinical improvement does not occur, the peritoneal fluid should be cultured again, and the antibiotic therapy altered. Alternatively, consideration can be given to catheter removal at this point. The catheter should also be removed when (1) recurrent episodes of peritonitis involving the same organism occur, (2) fungal or pseudomonal peritonitis is present, (3) persistent skin-site infections occur, and (4) fecal peritonitis has occurred. Catheters removed for fecal or recurrent peritonitis should not be replaced for approximately 3 weeks.[48] On rare occasions when there is no clinical improvement despite catheter removal, exploratory laparotomy may be necessary to drain loculated fluid collections.

SECONDARY PERITONITIS

Secondary peritonitis is the consequence of contamination from an organ within the peritoneal cavity. The majority of these episodes are the result of primary lesions of the stomach, duodenum, small intestine, colon, and appendix.[77] Approximately 10% of cases are caused by complications of abdominal surgery.

Because secondary peritonitis represents such a broad

spectrum of diseases, the mortality ranges from 10% to 40%. Condition-related mortality for limited processes such as perforated duodenal ulcer and perforated appendicitis is usually low, ranging from 0% to 10%. The mortality related to intestinal perforation and diseases of the biliary tract is substantially higher, ranging from 20% to 40%. Postoperative peritonitis resulting from a leaking intestinal anastomosis is associated with a substantial mortality, perhaps approaching 30%.[3]

Clearly, outcome also is influenced by other factors as well. The presence of advanced age, renal, cardiac, hepatic, or pulmonary insufficiency, malignancy and diabetes all increase the mortality associated with bacterial peritonitis, perhaps as much as three-fold.[3] Wittman has noted that even delays of 6 hours prior to obtaining treatment can increase mortality from 10% to 30%.[3]

The clinical presentation of peritonitis has been mentioned earlier. A discussion of the diagnosis and management of individual conditions causing bacterial peritonitis is beyond the scope or intent of this chapter, and the reader is referred to other sections of this work for this information. The following comments regarding the management of secondary peritonitis will focus upon general principles.

Management

Once the clinical diagnosis of secondary peritonitis is made, rapid institution of both physiologic support and aggressive antiinfective therapy are imperative. The primary objectives in the treatment of secondary peritonitis are (1) resuscitation, (2) initiation of antibiotic therapy, (3) elimination of the source of bacterial contamination, (4) reduction of the bacterial inoculum, and (5) continued metabolic support.

Resuscitation. It is an axiom that in all cases of peritonitis, some degree of hypovolemia is present. This is owing to the "third-spacing" of extracellular fluid within the peritoneal cavity, which can sometimes be immense.[24] The rapidity at which resuscitation is accomplished is dependent upon the degree of hypovolemia and the physiologic status of the patient. The acuity of the situation also determines the rate at which fluid resuscitation is conducted. If immediate operation is required, for example, in the setting of intestinal ischemia, preoperative fluid replacement may need to be curtailed in order to avoid potentially fatal delays. In contrast, an elderly patient with perforated sigmoid diverticulitis may better tolerate resuscitation during 2 or 3 hours. The effectiveness of fluid-replacement efforts can be judged by the normalization of pulse rate, blood pressure, and mental status. Placement of a urinary drainage catheter is essential since restoration of urine output is a reliable indicator of adequate fluid resuscitation. Invasive peripheral arterial and central cardiac

pressure-monitoring catheters (ie, Swan-Ganz catheter) should be placed in patients with frank septic shock, advanced age, or cardiac, pulmonary or renal insufficiency to provide more precise determinations of intravascular volume and cardiac output. Supplemental oxygen may be necessary, and in more extreme circumstances, endotracheal intubation and mechanical ventilation may be needed to preserve oxygenation. Nasogastric decompression using a sump tube should be used in the presence of an ileus to prevent pulmonary aspiration, and reduce abdominal distention. Antiacid agents such as H2 blocking agents (eg, ranitidine, or famotidine) or resin binding agents (eg, sucralfate) should be administered to prevent stress gastric ulceration.

Antibiotic Therapy. Antibiotic therapy should be initiated as soon as a clinical diagnosis of peritonitis is obtained, simultaneously with the implementation of resuscitation. The initial selection of antibiotics is empiric. The choice of antibiotics is made with the following considerations: (1) the demonstrated activity of the drug against bacteria that are presumed to be present upon the level of gastrointestinal perforation; and (2) the bactericidal activity of the antibiotic in the infected tissue. The microbial contamination of the peritoneal cavity depends upon which portion of the gastrointestinal tract is involved. Perforations of the esophagus usually involve gram-positive cocci and anaerobes reflective of oral microflora. Under normal circumstances, the stomach and duodenum are colonized by small numbers of lactobacilli and yeast. Perforations of the stomach and duodenum usually result in chemical peritonitis owing to acid injury, rather than from bacterial infection. An exception to this situation is the greater number of gram-negative bacilli found in the upper gastrointestinal tract following the use of antiacid agents such as antacids or H2 blocking agents.[78] Proceeding in an aboral direction, the intestinal flora increases in both species diversity and quantity, as well as the number of anaerobic organisms. The number of bacteria per gram of intraluminal contents in the colon varies from 10^7 in the cecum to 10^{12} in the rectum, with an anaerobe:aerobe ratio of 100:1.[79] Therefore, perforations of the small intestine or colon result in massive polymicrobial contamination. Surprisingly, despite the degree and complexity of bacterial contamination that occurs in fecal perforation, the microbial spectrum recovered at the time of laparotomy is remarkably simple. Though Bennion has demonstrated up to 10 isolates per patient using sophisticated transport and culture techniques, most studies indicate that only 3 to 4 isolates are recovered per patient.[80–83] This reflects the tendency for only a few dominant organisms to survive in bacterial peritonitis. Recently, it was reported that 76% of patients with peritonitis had peritoneal fluid cultures with mixed aerobic and anaerobic bacteria, with *Escherichia coli* and *Bacteroides fragilis* the most common combination.[84]

As noted earlier, this combination of microbes has demonstrated a synergistic effect in animal models, which potentiates the pathogenicity of both bacterial species present. In addition, a number of prospective studies comparing gentamicin and clindamycin versus single-agent therapy with third-generation cephalosporins with poor anaerobic coverage in patients with complicated appendicitis have noted treatment failures associated with *Bacteroides fragilis*.[85–87] Because of these concerns, presumptive therapy should include coverage for *both aerobic gram-negative rods and anaerobic organisms.*

Agents that possess activity directed against aerobic gram-negative bacilli include aminoglycosides, second- and third-generation cephalosporins, monobactams, carbapenems, carboxypenicillins, acylampicillins, and either ampicillin or ticarcillin combined with a β-lactamase inhibitor (ie, sulbactam or clavulanic acid). In vitro studies of anaerobic susceptibility demonstrate no resistance to metronidazole and chloramphenicol, <1% resistance to imipenem-cilastin, ticarcillin-clavulanate, ampicillin-sulbactam, and cefoperazone-sulbactam. In vitro resistance rates to cefoxitin and clindamycin were 8% and 3%, respectively.[88] In terms of achieving adequate minimal inhibitory concentrations (MIC), fortunately, most of the agents listed above achieve high MICs in peritoneal fluid.

Community-Acquired Secondary Peritonitis

For most cases of *community-acquired* bacterial peritonitis (ie, appendicitis, diverticulitis, perforated ulcer disease, perforated ulcers or carcinomas, cholecystitis and cholangitis), a single antibiotic agent with both aerobic and anaerobic activity is a preferred choice. Second- or third-generation cephalosporins or β-lactamase inhibitor combinations would be satisfactory choices, based upon both their efficacy and safety. Clinical cure rates approximating 85% to 95% can be expected using these agents, in combination with definitive surgical intervention. Alternatively, dual-agent therapy, using aztreonam and metronidazole yields clinical cure rates of 80% to 90%.[88] (Table 17–3).

Hospital-Acquired and Severe Secondary Peritonitis

For cases of bacterial peritonitis acquired in a hospital environment, or which occur in patients with advanced age, immunosuppression, malnutrition, or severe debilitation, the risk of more virulent, and potentially resistant, organisms is much greater. In such instances, a potent broad-spectrum agent should be selected. Imipenem-cilastin is an excellent single agent in this setting, unless there is a history of penicillin allergy. Alternatively, multiagent regimens using either metronida-

TABLE 17–3. SUGGESTED ANTIMICROBIAL AGENT THERAPY FOR THE TREATMENT OF ESTABLISHED SECONDARY BACTERIAL PERITONITIS

MILD TO MODERATE INTRA-ABDOMINAL INFECTION
Second- or third-generation cephalosporin
or
β-lactamase inhibitor combination
or
Monobactam + metronidazole

SEVERE INTRA-ABDOMINAL INFECTION WITHOUT RENAL DYSFUNCTION[a]
Carbapenem
or
Fluoroquinolone + metronidazole
or
Aminoglycoside + metronidazole ± ampicillin

SEVERE INTRA-ABDOMINAL INFECTION WITH RENAL DYSFUNCTION[a]
Carbpenem
or
Fluoroquinolone + metronidazole

[a]Includes mild to moderate peritonitis in immunosuppressed patients and hospital-acquired peritonitis in otherwise normal patients.
Adapted from Sawyer MD, Dunn DL: Antimicrobial therapy of intra-abdominal sepsis. Surg Infect *1992;6:545*

zole or clindamycin as the antianaerobe agent may be used. Although a combination using an aminoglycoside as an antiaerobe agent has been a traditional choice in the past, its use is declining. The risk of nephrotoxicity is substantial, particularly in elderly patients and in those with hypotension, or preexisting renal dysfunction. In addition, the attainment of adequate serum levels may require up to 3 to 4 days of administration. For these reasons, a monobactam, aztreonam, or a second- or third-generation cephalosporin are substituted for the aminoglycoside in dual-agent regimens. The selection of an antiaerobe agent definitely should include consideration of institutional antibiotic-resistance patterns when treating complex bacterial peritonitis. Although some experimental data suggests a synergistic effect between enterococcus and gram-negative enteric bacilli, there is no prospective study that has demonstrated a benefit of the addition of an antienterococcal agent to an *empiric* antibiotic regimen for the treatment of bacterial peritonitis. The empiric use of antienterococcal multidrug regimens may be responsible for the alarming emergence of vancomycin-resistant enterococci.

Candida are the most common fungi in intra-abdominal infections and are recovered with especially high frequency in perforations of the upper gastrointestinal system. Although there has been some controversy about the pathogenicity of these infections, it is currently felt that the recovery of fungi in secondary peritonitis as either the only pathogen or a co-pathogen is worthy of treatment, especially in immunocompromised patients. There are primarily two agents currently used in the treatment of significant intra-abdominal fungal therapies, amphotericin B and fluconazole. In nonneutropenic patients, either amphotericin B, 0.5 to 0.6 mg/kg/day or fluconazole 400 mg/day can be used. For severe, life-threatening fungal infections in immunocompromised patients, amphotericin B should be used and doses increased to 0.75 mg/kg/day.

Once antibiotic therapy has begun, changes in individual agents should be based primarily upon clinical progress. Substitutions of antibiotics based solely upon culture and sensitivity data should be discouraged, if the patient is otherwise improving by clinical parameters. Frequent alterations in the antibiotic regimen increases the likelihood of the emergence of resistance organisms.

Duration of Antibiotic Therapy

The duration of antibiotic therapy is determined by the clinical circumstances. Very brief courses of antibiotic therapy may be used when minimal peritoneal soilage and peritoneal inflammation are found at the time of abdominal exploration. Illustrative examples of such instances include acute, nonperforated appendicitis, and traumatic intestinal perforation repaired within 6 hours of injury. In such settings, a regimen approaching that of prophylaxis, using one preoperative dose and two subsequent doses in a period of 24 hours is sufficient.

In the treatment of established bacterial peritonitis, the use of "predetermined" days of treatment should be discouraged. Instead, judgements using the clinical indicators of temperature, white blood count (WBC), and leukocyte differential should be made. In a retrospective review of 2567 patients, Stone reported no recurrent or persistent sepsis occurring in patients with normal temperature, WBC, and differential at the time antibiotic therapy was discontinued.[89] In contrast, if persistent fever or leukocytosis is present at the time therapy is discontinued, the likelihood of recurrent sepsis ranges from 33% to 57%.[90]

Surgical Management

In true secondary peritonitis, surgical control of the infecting organ is the mainstay of treatment. Although the specific operation for each organ that potentially may be involved in secondary peritonitis is beyond the scope of the chapter, essential surgical concepts will be discussed. Operative management primarily should be directed towards the control of the source of contamination. This can be accomplished by closure of the perforation, resection of the perforated viscus, or exclusion of the affected organs from the peritoneal cavity. In most instances, exploration should be carried out through a midline incision, which affords generous exposure and access to the majority of the peritoneal cavity. Limited incisions may be acceptable in cases of localized peritonitis in which the infected organ has been identified prior to operation (ie, appendicitis, acute cholecystitis).

The secondary goal of operative management is to reduce the bacterial inoculum with the intent to prevent recurrent sepsis. Standard intraoperative techniques to accomplish this goal include swabbing and debriding fibrin, blood, and necrotic material, and copious irrigation of the peritoneal cavity are generally accepted and practiced maneuvers. The addition of antibiotics or antiseptic agents to the irrigant solution has not been shown to decrease the mortality of the intraperitoneal infection, although it may decrease the incidence of wound infections.[91,92]

The use of nonstandard surgical techniques to prevent recurrent sepsis remains controversial. *Radical peritoneal debridement* involving the removal of all fibrin and necrotic tissue, including abscess cavity walls was originally proposed by Hudspeth in 1975.[93] Although theoretical justification for this tedious technique exists in the knowledge that fibrin traps bacteria, a randomized prospective trial of this procedure found no difference between the standard operative treatment of local debridement and drainage of abscesses and radical debridement.[94] Radical debridement of fragile serosal surfaces may, itself, cause significant bleeding and fibrin deposition. At present, there is no perceived benefit in the use of this technique.

Continuous postoperative lavage has received renewed interest. Essentially an extension of intraoperative lavage, this technique involves the placement of multiple catheters or closed-suction drains at the time of operation. In the immediate postoperative period, lavage is begun by instilling large volumes of crystalloid solutions (>2L) containing a mixture of antibiotics and heparin. Lavage is conducted on 3 hour cycles for a period of 48 to 72 hours. Studies of this technique conducted to date suggest that the incidence of postoperative abscess formation may be reduced, and in selected patients, mortality can be reduced.[95–97] However, the poor design of the studies conducted to date leaves the question of the efficacy of this technique in preventing recurrent infection unanswered.

Planned repeated laparotomy for generalized peritonitis is a technique developed to prevent recurrent sepsis by repetitive abdominal exploration to deride necrotic material and drain abscesses. This aggressive technique expectantly addresses the limitations in monitoring these severely ill patients for the development of postoperative sepsis and abscess formation. Often, these patients are sedated, on mechanical ventilation, with large wounds and multiple drains, all of which renders clinical examination unreliable. Basic laboratory studies such as WBC and liver-function studies are frequently abnormal, but nonspecific, while CT has diagnostic utility, usually after the first week following surgery. Closure of the abdominal wound using prosthetic mesh, or zipper-type devices prevents intra-abdominal hypertension by avoiding closure of the wound under tension. A European study of this technique noted a significant difference in the mortality rate between patients treated by scheduled, repeat laparotomy (29%) and those undergoing exploration for clinical indications (73%).[98] Wittman has reported on the largest North American experience of this technique with 117 patients. In this group undergoing repeated laparotomy, which they have dubbed "Etappenlovage," actual postoperative mortality was 24%, compared to a predicted rate of 39% based upon Apache II severity scores.[99] Although these results are encouraging, a number of disadvantages have been noted with this technique, including unnecessary reexploration, prolonged periods of mechanical ventilation, longer intensive care–unit stays, and substantial rates of intestinal fistulization.

TERTIARY PERITONITIS

Tertiary peritonitis refers to a persistent diffuse peritonitis usually following the initial treatment of secondary peritonitis. At present, tertiary peritonitis appears to represent both a failure of host responses and superinfection.

The clinical presentation is characterized by low-grade fever, leukocytosis, elevated cardiac output and low systemic vascular resistance. The general metabolism is elevated and these patients are catabolic. Dysfunction of one or more organ systems is a frequent feature of this syndrome. In spite of the indications of occult sepsis, both CT and laparotomy often fail to identify a focal source of infection. Instead, a frequent finding is a diffuse peritoneal infection with a dispersion of fibrinous material over peritoneal surfaces. If superinfection is present, culture data yields two distinct categories of microorganisms: (1) infection with highly virulent gram-negative aerobic bacteria, such as *Pseudomonas* species, and *Serratia* species, with extensive antibiotic resistance characteristics; and (2) infection with low-virulence organisms such as *Staphylococcus epidermidis,* enterococcus, and *Candida* species which are resistant to the initial antibiotic therapy.

Treatment of the highly resistant bacteria is based upon sensitivity information. The use of two agents with different mechanisms of action is advisable. Though enterococci may be sensitive to ampicillin, in this setting, where antibiotic failure may be fatal, treatment with vancomycin is advisable. The presence of *Candida* in peritoneal fluid cultures should be treated with amphotericin B, as discussed previously. In the absence of a focal site of infection such as an intraperitoneal abscess, operative management has a remarkably minor role in the treatment of this entity.

Given the clinical presentation of this disease, the high failure rate of antibiotic therapy, and the failure of peritoneal defense mechanisms to localize infection, it is likely that tertiary peritonitis represents an abnormal host response. Despite evidence of cytokine-mediated systemic symptoms, local defenses are no longer competent. The development of multiorgan failure may be related to a loss of regulation of inflammatory mediators such as TNF and IL-1. At present, investigation into a number of strategies in the treatment of this disease is ongoing.

■ INTRAPERITONEAL ABSCESS

Intraperitoneal abscesses may occur in virtually any location within the peritoneal cavity, even within abdominal viscera. The most common mechanisms by which extravisceral abscesses develop are as residual loculations following diffuse peritonitis, infection of an intraperitoneal fluid collection following laparotomy, and contained leakage from a spontaneous visceral perforation or failed intestinal anastomosis. Visceral abscesses, in contrast, commonly develop from the hematogenous or lymphatic seeding of solid organs, such as the liver, spleen or pancreas.[76] The various sites of extravisceral abscesses essentially reflect the potential spaces within the peritoneal cavity. The most common sites of involvement are the subphrenic spaces, subhepatic spaces, lesser sac, paracolic gutters and pelvis.

The mortality of intraperitoneal abscesses treated without drainage is 100%.[100] Currently, mortality associated with intraperitoneal abscess ranges from approximately 10% to 30%.[101,102]

CLINICAL PRESENTATION

High spiking fevers, mild localized abdominal pain, anorexia, and weight loss compose the classic presentation of an intraperitoneal abscess. However, the clinical findings vary considerably with the site of the abscess, and the presentation is usually only sufficient to prompt suspicion of the presence of an abscess.

Patients with subphrenic abscesses may present with vague, upper quadrant pain, or referred shoulder pain on the involved side. On the left, costal margin tenderness also may be found. Abscesses involving, or extending into, the subhepatic space may cause a more localized pain than is seen in abscesses limited to the subphrenic space. Often, the pain may be exacerbated by coughing or other motion. Localized tenderness is also likely to be a more prominent finding. Interloop abscesses the abscesses occurring in the paracolic gutters are the most likely to present with both an abdominal mass and localized tenderness. This may be due to the proximity of these lesions to the abdominal wall. Pelvic abscesses usually present with vague, lower abdominal pain, but with few abdominal signs. Irritation of the urinary bladder or rectum may produce urgency and frequency, or tenesmus and diarrhea, respectively. Rectal and pelvic examination frequently will identify a tender mass through the anterior rectal wall.

DIAGNOSIS

While the diagnosis of peritonitis is primarily dependent upon clinical findings, the diagnosis of an intraperitoneal abscess may be quite difficult if the evaluation is solely dependent upon the history and physical examination. A number of studies have shown that localized tenderness or a palpable mass can be found by thorough examination in only about one-half of patients with intraperitoneal abscess. In the postoperative patient, physical examination may be of even less diagnostic value. Fry noted that in 143 patients with proven abdominal abscesses, only one-third of patients had localized tenderness sufficient to aid in locating the abscess, and only 10% of patients were found to have a palpable mass.[103]

Plain abdominal radiographs may provide useful information in up to one-half of patients.[104] Findings obtained from these studies that are indicative of intraperitoneal abscesses include (1) an air-fluid level in the upright or decubitus position, (2) the presence of extraluminal gas, and (3) a soft-tissue mass displacing adjacent bowel or other organs. Chest radiographs may demonstrate lower lobe atelectasis or a pleural effusion, if a subphrenic abscess is present.

With the exception of pelvic abscesses, physical examination and plain radiography appear to have limited value in both detecting and locating intraperitoneal abscesses. It is for this reason that both ultrasonography and CT have become mainstays in the diagnosis of intraperitoneal abscesses. Ultrasonography is noninvasive, rapid, inexpensive, and produces no ionizing radiation. In addition, the units are portable, thus allowing studies to be performed at bedside. In experienced hands, ultrasonography has a diagnostic accuracy for intraperitoneal abscess in excess of 90%.[105,106] However, the role for ultrasonography is limited by a number of serious shortcomings. Optimal anatomic resolution is achieved only in the right upper quadrant area and in the pelvis, limiting the sensitivity of this technique. In addition, imaging may be distorted by bowel gas, especially in patients with profound ileus, and by physical impediments to probe movement, such as dressings, open wounds, and stomas. Finally, the quality of the studies that are obtained are extremely dependent upon operator skills and experience.

CT currently is the most accurate modality available for the diagnosis of intraperitoneal abscess. In unselected patients, the diagnostic accuracy rates of up to 95% have been reported.[107,108] CT offers several advantages over ultrasonography, including the ability to image both intraperitoneal and retroperitoneal structures with high anatomic resolution, without interference from bowel gas, dressings, and drains. In addition, CT also offers the opportunity for percutaneous drainage. The major disadvantages of CT is the higher cost, the lack of portability, and the use of ionizing radiation. In addition, the accuracy of the study may be substantially reduced if intraluminal contrast is not used to opacify the bowel. This limits the ability of the radiologist to distinguish between fluid-filled intestine and an intraperitoneal abscess.

Although isotope-imaging techniques using gallium-67 citrate or indium-111, have received much attention in the diagnosis of intraperitoneal abscesses, the application of these techniques in surgical patients is extremely limited.

MANAGEMENT

The management of intraperitoneal abscesses is similar to the management of secondary peritonitis. Immediate attention is given to the resuscitation and general support of the patient. Although the efficacy of antibiotics is severely limited by the conditions created by the abscess, empiric therapy should still be instituted as early as possible. Antibiotic selection also should be directed towards both aerobic and anaerobic pathogens which are likely to be present. The mainstay of treatment is drainage of the abscess, which can be accomplished by either percutaneous or surgical techniques.

PERCUTANEOUS DRAINAGE

The use of percutaneous drainage has become a well accepted, and often, the favored alternative in the treatment of intaperitoneal abscesses. This modality offers several potential advantages, such as fewer complications, reduced hospitalization, avoidance of general anesthesia, and lower costs, when compared to surgical drainage. The anatomic guidance necessary for the placement of closed-system drainage catheters may be provided by CT or, in select situations, ultrasonography. When properly applied, it appears that percutaneous drainage can be performed as safely as surgical drainage, with equal or better success. An early study of the use of percutaneous drainage in draining intraperitoneal abscesses reported a success rate of 86% when the technique was selectively applied.[109] Criteria proposed at that time recommended that only unilocular abscesses with unobstructed access should be treated with these techniques. As experience with this modality has grown, the indications for the use of percutaneous drainage have been considerably broadened. Currently, percutaneous drainage also is considered acceptable in the following situations: (1) multiloculated, or multiple abscesses, (2) abscesses with enteric communication, and (3) the need to traverse normal peritoneum or a solid viscera to reach the abscess. Situations in which percutaneous drainage is unlikely to be successful and therefore, its application contraindicated are ill-defined abscesses, fungal abscesses, infected hematomas, necrotic tumor mass, and interloop abscesses. In these situations, surgical drainage may be the preferred method of management.

Despite a multitude of studies comparing percutaneous with surgical drainage, to date no randomized controlled study of this comparison has been performed. Mortality rates quoted for patients treated with surgical drainage range from 23% to 37%, while those cited for percutaneous drainage range from 11% to 17%. In addition, Deveney noted a significant decrease in mortality from 39% to 21% in the eras before and after the availability of CT and percutaneous drainage.[110] However, the inference that a lower mortality is achieved with percutaneous drainage is inaccurate. Levinson has noted that it is the severity of the illness that determines mortality, not the method of abscess drainage. In 91 patients with postoperative abscesses that underwent drainage, only 1.7% died if the APACHE II score was <15, whereas mortality was 78% if the score was ≥15. The outcome in these patients was independent of the technique of drainage.[111] Further, the lower mortality achieved following the introduction of CT and percutaneous drainage probably reflects the earlier and more specific diagnosis achieved with computed tomography. It may be better to consider the two techniques as complementary. Percutaneous drainage should be used when the likelihood of successful drainage is relatively high, to utilize the potential advantages of this technique. Surgical drainage can be then used for situations in which percutaneous techniques are unlikely to be successful, or previous attempts have failed.

The goal of percutaneous drainage may be either curative or palliative. Complete cures, defined as complete drainage without the need of subsequent surgical drainage, can be expected in 60% to 90% of cases, depending upon the features of the abscess. Palliative drainage, in contrast, provides the control of sepsis and improves both the safety and efficacy of subsequent surgical intervention. For example, Stabile reported upon 19 patients undergoing percutaneous drainage of diverticular abscesses. In this group, sepsis resolved within 72 hours, and 14 patients successfully underwent subsequent single-stage colon resection.[112]

The use of percutaneous drainage in abscesses with suspected or confirmed enteric communication was eschewed owing to concerns of fistula formation and a high failure rate of abscess resolution. However, a number of studies indicate that the percutaneous drainage of these abscesses can be achieved without an undue risk of fistula formation. Jeffrey reported a 90% success rate in appendiceal abscess resolution using percutaneous drainage. Although 40% of patients developed fecal fistulae, these all closed spontaneously within 14 days.[113] In the study cited earlier by Stabile, of 19 patients with diverticular abscesses, only 3 developed fecal fistulae and failed to resolve their sepsis.[112] Even abscesses associated with Crohn's disease have been successfully treated with percutaneous techniques. In this group at high risk for the development of enteric fistulae, many never developed communication with the intestine, and in over one-half of patients who developed fistulae, eventual spontaneous closure occurred.

SURGICAL DRAINAGE

Primary surgical drainage is indicated in any situation in which (1) the abscess is poorly defined or difficult to localize by imaging techniques (eg, interloop abscesses), (2) the abscess material is viscous or extensive necrotic debris is present (eg, pancreatic abscesses), (3) if cancer is present, and (4) the approach for percutaneous drainage requires perforation of a hollow viscus (eg, lesser sac abscesses). Secondary surgical drainage should be performed if either clinical signs of sepsis persist after percutaneous drainage or complete evacuation of the abscess cavity cannot be achieved. Following an initial failure of percutaneous drainage, the decision to proceed with secondary or, in some situations, tertiary attempts to percutaneous drainage should be made jointly by both surgeon and interventional radiologist.

During operation, the abscess wall should be identified, and the cavity aspirated with a needle to confirm the nature of the abscess with the presence of pus. The abscess should then be widely opened and its contents evacuated. Necrotic tissue is debrided and copious irrigation of the cavity is performed. Drains are placed in dependent positions, and externalized via separate incisions, if necessary. If dependent drainage is easily achieved, soft Penrose drains may be used. However, the authors prefer large-bore closed-suction drains which can be affixed to suction if needed. If significant debris is present, large sump-suction drains (eg, Axiom) also should be placed.

MANAGEMENT OF SPECIFIC ABSCESSES

Subphrenic and Subhepatic Abscess

Left-sided abscesses develop following diffuse suppurative peritonitis, perforation of a hollow viscus, acute, severe pancreatitis, and splenectomy. The most common cause of de novo right subphrenic abscesses is spontaneous rupture of a hepatic abscess. Postoperative abscesses may develop following operations of the stomach, or duodenum. Subhepatic collections most commonly occur following gastric or duodenal perforation, and operations involving the stomach. Appendicitis, biliary tract and colon procedures also may be antecedent events. Percutaneous drainage of subphrenic and subhepatic abscesses is successful in up to 80% of cases, although Mueller has noted that the majority of patients require catheter drainage for up to 3 weeks before the abscess is resolved.[114]

If surgical drainage of these abscesses is required, an extraperitoneal approach is preferred. Adherence of the abscess to the peritoneum or diaphragm is a necessary prerequisite for this approach. Subphrenic abscesses of either side and right subhepatic abscesses should be approached via lateral abdominal incisions, dividing the external oblique and transversus abdominus muscles and sparing the rectus sheath. Left subphrenic abscesses may also be approached from a posterior 12th rib incision.

Paracolic Abscess

Abscesses in this area most commonly result from perforations of the colon like those seen in acute appendicitis or sigmoid diverticulitis. On the right, paracolic abscesses may extend inferiorly into the pelvis, and superiorly into both the subphrenic and subhepatic spaces. On the left, superior extension of infection is prevented by the phrenocolic ligament. When clearly visualized by CT, abscesses in this location effectively can be drained using percutaneous techniques. Multiple catheters may be required if synchronous abscesses are also present. Surgical drainage of these lesions should be performed via a midline incision.

Interloop Abscess

These are actually multiple abscesses created by adherent loops of intestine, mesentery, omentum and the abdominal wall. Though superior extension of these abscesses is prevented by the transverse mesocolon, synchronous pelvic abscesses may be found. Because of the ill-defined nature of these abscesses, and the difficulty in locating fluid collections, surgical drainage is the preferred approach. Laparotomy should be performed via a midline incision. During exploration, adherent intestinal loops should be thoroughly mobilized, and the abdomen irrigated with copious volumes of saline.

Pelvic Abscess

Pelvic abscesses may constitute up to 40% of intraperitoneal abscesses and are often the result of perforated sigmoid diverticulitis, perforated appendicitis, pelvic inflammatory disease, or following diffuse peritonitis. Percutaneous drainage of abscesses adjacent to the anterior abdominal wall can be successfully performed using a transabdominal approach. However, abscesses deeper within the pelvis have required translumbar, transciatic and, most recently, transrectal approaches.[115] Some studies have suggested that only 35% to 50% of ab-

scesses can be treated adequately using percutaneous techniques.[116] Surgical drainage can be accomplished easily via a transrectal approach, if the collection is palpable anterior to the rectum. Percutaneous procedures in this setting could be reserved for deep pelvic abscesses that are not palpable.

REFERENCES

1. von Recklinghausen FT. Zur Fettresorption. *Arch Pathol Anat Physiol* 1863;26:172
2. Dixon CT, Rixford EL. Cytologic response to peritoneal irritation in man: a protective mechanism. *Am J Surg* 1934; 25:504
3. Wittman DH, Walker AP, Condon RE. Peritonitis and intraabdominal infection. In: Schwartz S, Shires G, Spencer F (eds), *Principles of Surgery*, 6th ed. New York, NY: McGraw-Hill; 1991:1449–1483
4. Autio V. The spread of intraperitoneal infection. *Acta Chir Scand Suppl* 1981;91:98
5. Flessner MF, Parker RJ, Sieber SM. Peritoneal lymphatic uptake of fibrinogen and erythrocytes in the rat. *Am J Phys* 1983;244:H89
6. Allen L. The peritoneal stomata. *Anat Rec* 1936;67:89
7. Wang NS. The performed stomas connecting the pleural cavity and the lymphatics in the parietal pleura. *Am Rev Respir Dis* 1975;111:12
8. Leak LV, Just EE. Permeability of peritoneal mesothelium: a TEM and SEM study. *J Cell Biol* 1976;70:423a
9. Leak LV. Interaction of mesothelium to intraperitoneal stimulation. *Lab Invest* 1983;48:479
10. Steinberg B. *Infections of the Peritoneum*. New York, NY: Hoeber; 1944
11. Dumont AE, Robbins E, Martelli A, et al. Platelet blockade of particle absorption from the peritoneal surface of the diaphragm. *Proc Soc Exp Biol Med* 1981;167:137
12. Dumont AE, Maas Wk, Iliescu H, et al. Increased survival from peritonitis after blockade of transdiaphragmatic absorption of bacteria. *Surg Gynecol Obstet* 1986;162:248
13. Mengle HA. Effect of anesthetics on lymphatic absorption from the peritoneal cavity in peritonitis: an experimental study. *Arch Surg* 1937;34:389
14. Skau T, Nystrom PO, Ohman L. Bacterial clearance and granulocyte response in experimental peritonitis. *J Surg Res* 1986;40:13
15. Last M, Kurtz L, Stein TA, et al. Effect of PEEP on the rate of thoracic duct lymph flow and clearance of bacteria from the peritoneal cavity. *Am J Surg* 1983;145:126
16. Maddaus MA, Ahrenholz D, Simmons RL. The biology of peritonitis and implications for treatment. *Surg Clin North Am* 1988;68:431
17. Fowler GR. Diffuse septic peritonitis, with special reference to a new method of treatment, namely, the elevated head and trunk posture, to facilitate drainage into the pelvis: with a report of nine consecutive cases of recovery. *Med Rec* 1900;57:617
18. Dunn DL, Borke RA, Knight NB, et al. Role of resident macrophanges, peritoneal neutrophils, and translym-

phatic absorption in bacterial clearance from the peritoneal cavity. *Infect Immun* 1985;49:257

19. Dunn DL, Barke RA, Ewald DC, Simmons RL. Macrophages and translymphatic absorption represents the first line of defense of the peritoneal cavity. *Arch Surg* 1987; 122:105

20. Wiles JB, Cerra FB, Siegel JH, Border JR. The systemic response: does the organism matter? *Crit Care Med* 1980;2:55

21. Tracey KJ, Beutler B, Lowry SF, et al. Shock and tissue injury induced by recombinant human cachetin. *Science* 1986;234:470

22. Dinarello CA. Interleukin-1. *Rev Infect Dis* 1984;6:51

23. Gutman RA, Nixon WP, McRai RL, et al. Effect of intraperitoneal and intravenous vasoactive amines on peritoneal dialysis: study I anephric dogs. *Trans Am Soc Artif Intern Organs* 1976;22:570

24. McLean LD, Mulligan WG, McLean APH, et al. Patterns of septic shock in man: a detailed study of 56 patients. *Ann Surg* 1967;163:866

25. Hau T, Ahrenholz DH, Simmons Rl. Secondary bacterial peritonitis: the biological basis of treatment. *Curr Probl Surg* 1979;16:1

26. Dunn DL, Barke RA, Ahrenholz DH, et al. The adjuvant effect of peritoneal fluid in experimental peritonitis. *Ann Surg* 1984;199:37

27. West NAL. Role of cytokines in leukocyte activation: phagocytic cells. In: Grinstein S, Rotstein OD eds., *Mechanisms of Leukocyte Activation: Current Topics in Membranes and Transport.* New York, NY: Academic Press; 1990:537

28. Corderio RSB, Martins MA, Silva PMR. Proinflammatory activity of platelet-activating factor: pharmacological modulation and cellular involvement. *Prog Biochem Pharmacol* 1988;22:156

29. Hau T, Payne WD, Simmons RL. Fibrinolytic activity of the peritoneum. *Surg Gynecol Obstet* 1979;148:415

30. Raftery AT. Effect of peritoneal trauma on peritoneal fibrinolytic activity and intraperitoneal adhesion formation. *Eur Surg Res* 1981;13:397

31. Thompson JN, Paterson-Brown S, Harbourne T, et al. Reduced human peritoneal plaminogen activating activity: possible mechanism of adhesion formation. *Br J Surg* 1989;76:382

32. Vipond MN, Whawell SA, Thompson JN, Dudley HAF. Peritoneal fibrinolytic activity and intra-abdominal adhesions. *Lancet* 1990;335:1120

33. Sinclair SB, Rotstein OD, Levy GA. Disparate mechanisms of induction of procoagulant activity by live and inactivated bacteria and viruses. *Infect Immun* 1990;58:1821

34. Ahrenholz DH, Simmons RL. Fibrin in peritonitis, I. beneficial and adverse effects of fibrin in experimental *E. coli* peritonitis. *Surgery* 1980;88:41

35. Dunn DL, Simmons RL. Fibrin in peritonitis, III. the mechanisms of bacterial trapping by polymerizing fibrin. *Surgery* 1982;92:513

36. Raftery AT. Regeneration of parietal and visceral peritoneum: a light microscopical study. *Br J Surg* 1973;60:293

37. Raftery AT. Regeneration of parietal and visceral peritoneum: an electron microscopical study. *J Anat* 1973;115:375

38. Sawyer MD, Dunn DL. Antimicrobial therapy of intraabdominal sepsis. *Infect Dis Clin North Am* 1992;6:545

39. Weinstein WM, Onderdonk AB, Bartlett JG, et al. Experimental intra-abdominal abscesses in rats: development of an experimental model. *Infect Immun* 1974;10:1250

40. Zalesnik DF, Kasper DL. The role of anaerobic bacteria in abscess formation. *Ann Rev Med* 1982;33:217

41. Rotstein OD, Pruett TL, Simmons RL. Lethal microbial synergism in intraabdominal infections. *Arch Surg* 1985; 120:146

42. Yull AB, Abrams JS, Davis JH. The peritoneal fluid in strangulation obstruction: the role of the red blood cell and *E. coli* bacteria in producing toxicity. *J Surg Res* 1962; 2:223

43. Hau T, Hoffman R, Simmons RL. Mechanisms of the adjuvant effect of hemoglobin in experimental peritonitis, I. in vivo inhibition of peritoneal leukocytosis. *Surgery* 1978; 83:223

44. Pruett TL, Rotstein OD, Fiegel VD, et al. Mechanism of the adjuvant effect of hemoglobin in experimental peritonitis, VIII. a leukotoxin is produced by Escherichia coli metabolism in hemoglobin. *Surgery* 1984;96:375

45. Ward CG. Influence of iron on infection. *Am J Surg* 1986; 151:291

46. Bullen JJ. The significance of iron in infection. *Rev Infect Dis* 1981;3:1127

47. Rotstein OD, Pruett TL, Simmons RL. Fibrin in peritonitis, V. fibrin inhibits phagocytic killing of *Escherichia coli* by human polymorphonuclear leukocytes. *Ann Surg* 1986; 203:413

48. Rotstein OD. Peritonitis and intra-abdominal abscesses. In: Wilmore DW, Brennan MF, Harken AH, et al. (eds), *Care of the Surgical Patient.* New York, NY: Scientific American; 1992:1–22

49. Cho J, Rotstein OD, Pruett TL, et al. The adjuvant effect of bile salts in experimental peritonitis. *Surg Forum* 1984; 35:231

50. Zimmerli W, Waldvogel FA, Vaudaux P, et al. Pathogenesis of foreign body infection: description and characteristics of an animal model. *J Infect Dis* 1982;146:487

51. Zimmerli W, Lew PD, Waldvogel FA. Pathogenesis of foreign body infection: evidence for a local granulocyte defect. *J Clin Invest* 1984;73:1191

52. Speck WT, Dresdale SS, McMillan RW. Primary peritonitis and the nephrotic syndrome. *Am J Surg* 1974;127:267

53. Hoefs JC, Runyan BA. Spontaneous bacterial peritonitis. *Dis Mon* 1985;31:1

54. Isner J, MacDonald JS, Schein PS. Spontaneous *Streptococcus pneumoniae* peritonitis in a patient with metastatic gastric cancer. *Cancer* 1979;39:2306

55. Runyon BA. Spontaneous bacterial peritonitis with cardiac ascites. *Am J Gastroenterol* 1984;79:796

56. Shesol BF, Rosato EF, Rosato FE. Concommitant acute lupus erythematosus and primary pneumococcal peritonitis. *Am J Gastroenterol* 1975;63:324

57. Bhuva M, Ganger D, Jensen D. Spontaneous bacterial peritonitis: an update on evaluation, management, and prevention. *Am J Med* 1994;97:169

58. Runyon BA. Low-protein-concentration ascitic fluid is predisposed to spontaneous bacterial peritonitis. *Gastroenterology* 1986;91:1343

59. Runyon BA. Patients with deficient ascitic fluid opsonic

activity are pre-disposed to spontaneous bacterial peritonitis. *Hepatology* 1988;8:632

60. Rajkovic IA, Williams R. Abnormalities of neutrophilic phagocytosis, intracellular killing and metabolic activity in alcoholic cirrhosis and hepatitis. *Hepatology* 1986;6:252

61. Rimola A, Soto R, Bory F, et al. Reticuloendothelial system phagocytic activity in cirrhosis and its relation to bacterial infections and prognosis. *Hepatology* 1984;4:53

62. Andreu M, Sola R, Sitges-Serra A, et al. Risk factors for spontaneous bacterial peritonitis in cirrhotic patients with ascites. *Gastroenterology* 1993;104:1133

63. Quenzer RW. Primary peritonitis. In: Fry DE (ed), *Surgical Infections*. Boston, MA: Little, Brown; 1995:309–314

64. Hoefs JC. Diagnostic paracentesis: a potent clinical tool. *Gastroenterology* 1990;98:230

65. Garcia-Tsao G, Conn HO, Lerner E. The diagnosis of bacterial peritonitis: comparison of pH, lactate concentration, and leukocyte count. *Hepatology* 1985;5:85

66. Runyon BA, Canawati HN, Akriviadis EA. Optimization of ascitic fluid culture technique. *Gastroenterology* 1988;95:1351

67. Runyon BA. *Hepatology* 1990;12:710–715

68. Moore RD et al. *Ann Intern Med* 1984;100:352

69. Runyon BA et al. *Gastroenterology* 1991;100:1737–1742

70. Nohr CW, Marshall DG. Primary peritonitis in children. *Can J Surg* 1974;27:179

71. Grange JD, Amiot X, Grange V, et al. Amoxicillin-clavulanic therapy of spontaneous bacterial peritonitis. *Hepatology* 1990;11:360

72. Tito L, Rimola A, Gines P, et al. Recurrence of spontaneous bacterial peritonitis in cirrhosis. *Hepatology* 1988;8:27

73. Tito L, Rimola A, Llach J, et al. Recurrence of spontaneous bacterial peritonitis in cirrhosis; frequency and predictive factors. *Hepatology* 1988;8:27

74. Digenis GE, Abraham G, Savin E, et al. Peritonitis-related deaths in continuous ambulatory peritoneal dialysis (CAPD) patients. *Perit Dial Int* 1990;10:45

75. Vas SI: Peritonitis during CAPD: a mixed bag. *Perit Dial Bull* 1981;1:47

76. Rotstein OD, Meakins JL. Diagnostic and therapeutic challenges of intraabdominal infections. *World J Surg* 1990;14:159

77. Farthman EH, Schoffel U. Principles and limitations of operative management of intraabdominal infections. *World J Surg* 1990;14:210

78. Ruddell WSJ, Axon ATR, Findlay JM, et al. Effect of cimetidine on the gastric bacterial flora. *Lancet* 1980;1:672

79. Stone HH, Kolb LD, Geheber CE. Incidence and significance of intraperitoneal anaerobic bacteria. *Ann Surg* 1975;181:705

80. Bennion RS, Baron EJ, Thompson JE, et al. The bacteriology of gangrenous and perforated appendicitis-revisited. *Ann Surg* 1990;211:165

81. Bennion RS, Thompson JE, Baron EJ, et al. Gangrenous and perforated appendicitis with peritonitis: treatment and bacteriology. *Clin Ther* 1990;12(suppl B):1

82. Gonzenbach HR, Simmen HP, Amgwerd R. Imipenem (N-F-Thienamycin) versus netilmicin plus clindamycin. *Ann Surg* 1987;205:271

83. Hackford AW, Tally FP, Reinhold RB, et al. Prospective study comparing imipenencilastin with clindamycin and gentamicin for the treatment of serious surgical infections. *Arch Surg* 1988;123:322

84. Brook I. A 12 year study of aerobic and anaerobic bacteria in intra-abdominal and postsurgical abdominal wound infections. *Surg Gynecol Obstet* 1989;169:387

85. Baird IM. Multicentered study of cefoperazone for treatment of intra-abdominal infections and comparison of cefoperazone with cefamandole and clindamycin plus gentamicin for treatment of appendicitis and peritonitis. *Rev Infect Disease* 1983;5:S165

86. Berne TV, Yellin AW, Appleman MD, et al. Antibiotic management of surgically treated gangrenous or perforated appendicitis: comparison of gentamicin and clindamycin versus cefamandole versus cefoperazone. *Am J Surg* 1982;144:8

87. Heseltine PNR, Yellin AE, Appleman MD, et al. Perforated and gangrenous appendicitis: an analysis of antibiotic failure. *J Infect Dis* 1983;148:322

88. Sawyer MD, Dunn DL. Antimicrobial therapy of intra-abdominal sepsis. *Surg Infect* 1992;6:545

89. Stone HH, Bourneuf AA, Stinson LD. Reliability of criteria for predicting persistent or recurrent sepsis. *Arch Surg* 1985;120:17

90. Lennard ES, Dellinger EP, Wertz MJ, et al. Implications of leukocytosis and fever at conclusion of antibiotic therapy for intra-abdominal sepsis. *Ann Surg* 1982;195:19

91. Farthman EH, Schoffer U. Principles and limitations of operative management of intra-abdominal infections. *World J Surg* 1990;14:210

92. Noon GP, Beall AC Jr, Jordan GL Jr, et al. Clinical evaluation of peritoneal irrigation with antibiotic solution. *Surgery* 1967;62:73

93. Hudspeth AS. Radical peritoneal debridement for established peritonitis. *Ann Surg* 1975;110:1233

94. Polk HC Jr., Fry, DE. Radical peritoneal debridement for established peritonitis. *Ann Surg* 1980;192:350

95. Hallerback B, Andersson C, Englund N, et al. A prospective randomized study of continuous peritoneal lavage postoperatively in the treatment of purulent peritonitis. *Surg Gynecol Obstet* 1986;163:433

96. Stephen M, Lowenthal J. Continuing peritoneal lavage in high risk peritonitis. *Surgery* 1979;85:603

97. Washington BC, Villalba MR, Lauter CB. Cefamandole-erythromycin-heparin peritoneal irrigation: an adjunct to the surgical treatment of diffuse bacterial peritonitis. *Surgery* 1983;94:576

98. Penninck FM, Kerremans RP, Lauwers PM. Planned relaparotomies in the surgical treatment of severe generalized peritonitis from intestinal origins. *World J Surg* 1983;7:762

99. Wittman DH, Abrahamian C, Bergstein JM. Etappenlavage: advanced diffuse peritonitis managed by planned multiple laparotomies utilizing zippers, slide fastener, and Velcro analogue for temporary abdominal closure. *World J Surg* 1990;14:218

100. Altmeier WA, Culbertson WR, Fullen WD, et al. Intra-abdominal abscesses. *Am J Surg* 1973;125:70

101. Malangoni MA, Shumate CR, Thomas HA, et al. Factors influencing the treatment of intra-abdominal abscess. *Am J Surg* 1983;145:120

102. Hemming A, Davis NL, Robins RE. Surgical versus percutaneous drainage of intraabdominal abscess. *Am J Surg* 1991;161:593

103. Fry DE, Garrison RN, Heitch RC, et al. Determinants of death in patients with intraabominal abscess. *Surgery* 1980;88:517

104. Connell TR, Stephens DH, Carlson HC. Upper abdominal abscess: a continuing and deadly problem. *AJR Am J Roentgenol* 1980;134:759

105. Doust BD, Quiroz F, Stewart JM. Ultrasonic distinction of abscesses from other intraabdominal fluid collections. *Radiology* 1977;125:213

106. Taylor KJW, Wasson JF, De Graff C, et al. Accuracy of grey-scale ultrasound diagnosis of abdominal and pelvic abscesses in 220 patients. *Lancet* 1978;1:83

107. Mueller PR, Simeone JF, et al. Intra-abdominal abscesses: diagnosis by sonography and computed tomography. *Radiol Clin North Am* 1983;21:425

108. Roche J. Effectiveness of computed tomography in the diagnosis of intra-abdominal abscess. *Med J Aust* 1981; 25:85

109. Gerzof SG, Robbins AH, Birkett DA, et al. Percutaneous catheter drainage of abdominal abscesses guided by ultrasound and computed tomography. *AJR Am J Roentgenol* 1979;133:1

110. Deveney CW, Lurie K, Deveney KE. Improved treatment of intra-abdominal abscess: a result of improved localization, drainage and patient care, not technique. *Arch Surg* 1988;123:1126

111. Levinson MA, Zeigler D. Correlation of APACHE II score. drainage technique and outcome in postoperative intra-abdominal abscess. *Surg Gynecol Obstet* 1991;172:89

112. Stabile BE, Puccio E, van Sonnenberg E, et al. Preoperative percutaneous drainage of diverticular abscesses. *Am J Surg* 1990;159:99

113. Jeffrey RB, Tolention CS, Federle MP, et al. Percutaneous drainage of periappendiceal abscesses: review of 20 patients. *AJR Am J Roentgenol* 1987;149:59

114. Mueller PR, Simeone JF, Butch RJ, et al. Percutaneous drainage of subphrenic abscess: a review of 62 patients. *AJR Am J Roentgenol* 1986;147:1237

115. Alexander AA, Eschellman DJ, Nazarian LN, et al. Transrectal sonographically guided drainage of deep pelvic abscesses. *AJR Am J Roentgenol* 1994;162:1227

116. Jaques P, Mauro M, Safrit H, et al. CT features of intra-abdominal abscesses: prediction of successful percutaneous drainage. *AJR Am J Roentgenol* 1986;146:1041

18

Mesenteric Ischemic Disorders

Scott J. Boley ▪ *Ronald N. Kaleya*

Mesenteric ischemic diseases (MID) are the consequence of insufficient blood flow to all or part of the intestines. The causes of ischemic insult vary, but the end result for all ischemic intestinal injuries is similar: a spectrum of bowel injury ranging from completely reversible alterations of intestinal function to transmural hemorrhagic necrosis of the intestinal wall. The clinical syndromes associated with MID depend upon the degree of the ischemic injury and the site and length of intestine affected by the injury. Resulting symptoms and signs vary considerably, making the diagnosis of MID difficult. As awareness of these diseases has heightened, understanding of the pathophysiologic causes and repercussions of intestinal ischemia has increased and diagnostic modalities have improved. A cogent approach to diagnosis and management of these diseases has been formulated.

Mesenteric ischemic disorders can be broadly classified into five types: acute mesenteric ischemia (AMI), chronic mesenteric ischemia (CMI), mesenteric venous thrombosis (MVT), focal segmental ischemia (FSI) of the small intestine, and colonic ischemia (CI). Colonic ischemia is the most common mesenteric vascular disorder, followed by acute mesenteric ischemia. AMI affects all or portions of the small intestine and/or right colon in the distribution of the superior mesenteric artery. CI results from inadequate circulation to part or all of the colon. In chronic mesenteric ischemia, blood flow is unable to meet the increased functional demands of the intestine without loss of tissue viability. On the other hand, FSI affects small segments of the small

intestine and may result in transmural infarction. MUT may be asymptomatic, may cause gastrointestinal hemorrhage or may present with manifestations similar to AMI. These disorders have distinct clinical manifestations and are managed differently.

Ischemic disorders of the intestine can be further divided into those caused by a transient diminution of blood flow, as in most cases of CI, and those resulting from a more permanent interruption of mesenteric blood flow, as in some forms of AMI. Furthermore, mesenteric vascular diseases can be broadly classified into those affecting the superior and/or the inferior mesenteric circulation. In addition, these diseases can be further categorized as acute or chronic, and of arterial or venous origin (Fig 18–1). While the viability of the intestine is not compromised in the chronic forms of MI, blood flow may be insufficient to support the functional demands of the intestine. In contrast, intestinal viability is endangered in the acute forms of mesenteric ischemia. Atherosclerotic narrowing or occlusion of the mesenteric arteries, producing intestinal angina and gradually evolving MVT are the common forms of CI. AMI is much more common than CI, and ischemia of arterial origin is much more frequent than that of venous origin. The arterial forms of AMI include superior mesenteric arterial embolus (SMAE), nonocclusive mesenteric ischemia (NOMI), superior mesenteric artery thrombosis (SMAT), and those cases of FSI resulting from local atherosclerotic emboli or vasculitides. Acute MVT and FSI caused by strangulation obstruction of the small

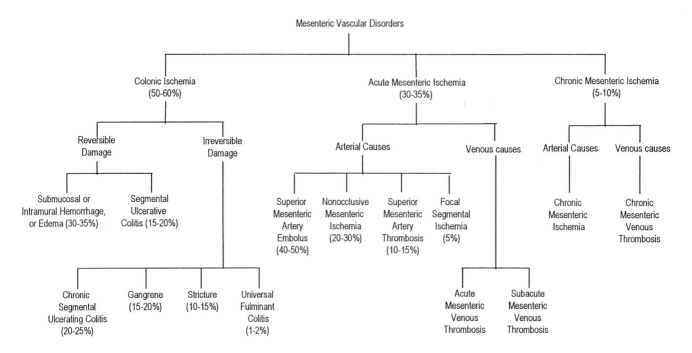

Figure 18–1. Mesenteric ischemic disorders.

intestine or by localized venous thrombosis comprise the venous forms of AMI.

■ MESENTERIC CIRCULATION

The intestines are normally protected from ischemia by an extensive collateral circulation. Communications between the celiac (CA), superior mesenteric (SMA), inferior mesenteric (IMA) and iliac arterial beds are numerous. As a rule, at least two of the major splanchnic vessels must be compromised to produce symptomatic intestinal ischemia. However, occlusion of two of the three vessels occurs frequently without evidence of ischemia, and total occlusion of all three vessels in asymptomatic patients has been observed.

Collateral flow around small arterial branches is made possible by multiple arterial arcades within the colonic mesentery. SMA or IMA occlusions can be bypassed via the arc of Riolan, the central anastomotic artery and/or the marginal artery of Drummond. Additionally, within the bowel wall, a network of communicating submucosal vessels can maintain viability of short segments of the colon where the extramural arterial supply has been compromised. The intestine responds to reduced mesenteric blood flow by redistributing intramural blood flow to the mucosa, especially to the superficial portion.[1,2]

When a major mesenteric artery becomes occluded,

arterial pressure falls distal to the obstruction and collateral pathways open immediately. Initially, acutely decreased perfusion pressure is compensated by local regulatory mechanisms that mitigate the effective flow reduction relative to the perfusion pressure.[3] This physiologic mechanism, termed autoregulation, leads to vasodilation of resistance vessels "downstream" to the occlusion, largely in response to release of local metabolites from the ischemic tissue. Relaxation of vascular smooth muscle in direct response to decreased perfusion pressure causes some of this vasodilation.[4] Experimentally, occlusion of the SMA is followed transiently by increased celiac and inferior mesenteric arterial flow. The increased blood flow through this collateral circulation continues as long as the pressure in the vascular bed distal to the obstruction remains below systemic pressure and is almost always sufficient to maintain intestinal viability. However, autoregulation of flow is maintained only for brief periods of time. With prolonged ischemia, vasoconstriction develops, raising the arterial pressure in the bed distal to the obstruction and thereby reducing collateral flow and potentially compromising bowel viability.

The degree of blood flow reduction tolerable to the bowel without damage is remarkable. No morphologic changes could be identified by light microscopy and there was normal distribution of patent-blue V dye when mesenteric arterial flow was reduced by 75% for 12 hours.[5] These findings may be attributed to the redundancy in the vasculature where only one-fifth of mesenteric capillaries are open at any time and uptake of oxygen occurs only in these open capillaries. When intestinal blood flow is reduced, oxygen extraction is increased, allowing a fairly constant oxygen consumption over a wide range of blood flows. Additionally, the arteriovenous oxygen difference widens as oxygen extraction is enhanced. Therefore, normal oxygen consumption can be maintained with only 20% to 25% of normal blood flow. However, oxygen consumption falls precipitously when increased oxygen extraction can no longer compensate for the diminished blood flow below the critical level.[6]

The colon has an inherently lower blood flow than the small intestine and is, therefore, more sensitive to injury during acute reductions in blood flow. Moreover, experimental studies have shown that motor activity of the colon is accompanied by decreased blood flow. In contrast, blood flow to the small intestine increases markedly during peristalsis and digestion. In addition, the effect of "straining" on systemic arterial and venous pressure in constipated patients provides indirect evidence that constipation may accentuate the adverse circulatory effects of defecation. Geber has postulated that "the combination of normally low blood flow and decreased blood flow during functional activity would seem to make the colon (1) rather unique among all areas of the body where increased motor activity is usually accompanied by an increased blood flow, and (2) more susceptible to pathology."[7] Other factors that decrease colonic blood flow include changes in the environment, digestion, and emotionally stressful situations. Hypothalamic control of gastrointestinal blood flow in the awake cat model suggests that "of the entire gastrointestinal tract, the colon blood flow is most affected by autonomic stimulation."[8]

Ischemic injury occurs when the tissue is deprived of oxygen and other nutrients necessary to maintain cellular metabolism. The severity of this injury is inversely related to blood flow.[9] Several factors contribute to ischemic injury of the bowel, including the state of the general circulation, the extent of collateral blood flow, the response of the mesenteric vasculature to autonomic stimuli, circulating vasoactive substances, local humoral factors, and the normal and abnormal products of cellular metabolism before and after reperfusion of the ischemic segment of intestine. In addition, the functional demands of the bowel as dictated by motor, absorptive, and secretory activities, the intestinal microflora, and the rate of cellular turnover affect the extent and severity of intestinal injury. Because these factors are so diverse and cannot all be controlled simultaneously in the laboratory setting, the contribution of the individual factors does not account for the full and profound pathophysiologic consequences of intestinal ischemia.

■ AMI

Acute mesenteric ischemia has been increasingly diagnosed during the past 30 years, not only because of a heightened awareness of the many clinical syndromes produced by these disorders, but also because the actual incidence has risen. At our large metropolitan medical center, AMI is responsible for approximately 0.1% of all admissions. The rising incidence has been attributed to an aging population in so far as AMI predominantly affects geriatric patients, especially those with serious cardiovascular or other systemic disorders. Similarly, the widespread use of coronary and surgical intensive care units and other extraordinary means of cardiopulmonary support have salvaged patients who previously would have died rapidly of cardiovascular complications. They then develop AMI as a later consequence of primary disease.

TYPES OF AMI

SMAE are responsible for 40% to 50% of episodes of acute mesenteric ischemia. The thrombus embolizes after being dislodged or fragmented from the left atrium or ventricle during a period of dysrhythmia or following cardiac catheterization. Accordingly, many patients with SMAE have had prior peripheral artery emboli, and approximately 20% have other synchronous emboli at the time they are diagnosed as having AMI. Emboli to the superior mesenteric artery (SMA) tend to lodge at points of normal anatomical narrowing that usually occur immediately distal to the origin of a major branch (Fig 18–2). Emboli lodge peripherally in branches of the SMA, or in the SMA itself, distal to the origin of the ileocolic artery in 10% to 15% of patients. These are termed minor emboli. The arterial lumen may be completely occluded by the emboli, but more often the vessel is partially occluded.

Experimental and clinical studies suggest that, at least initially, the collateral circulation can maintain intestinal viability following most acute SMA occlusions. However, arterial vasoconstriction develops both proximal and distal to the embolus even in cases of partial inflow obstruction. This vasoconstriction usually impairs the collateral blood flow sufficiently to cause or exacerbate ischemic injury.

NOMI causes 20% to 30% of episodes of AMI and is thought to result from splanchnic vasoconstriction initiated by vasoactive medications or a period of hypotension. Predisposing factors for NOMI include acute myocardial infarction, congestive heart failure, aortic insufficiency, hepatic diseases, renal diseases, especially in patients requiring hemodialysis,[10,11] and major cardiac or intra-abdominal operations. Frequently, a more immediate precipitating cause such as acute pulmonary

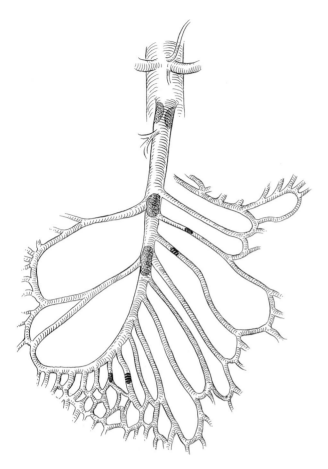

Figure 18–2. Common sites of SMA emboli. Minor emboli distal to the ileocolic branch or in segmental branches are considered minor emboli. All others are major emboli. Thrombosis usually occurs near the origin of the SMA.

edema, cardiac arrhythmia, or shock is present, although the consequent intestinal ischemia may not become manifest until hours or days later.

The incidence of nonocclusive ischemia has declined recently, possibly owing to increased use of systemic vasodilators, such as the calcium channel blocking agents and nitrates. These agents may protect the mesenteric vascular beds from vasospasm and decrease the period of profound hypotension associated with acute myocardial events. In addition, the use of left ventricular assist devices in the treatment of cardiogenic shock, especially following coronary revascularization, has attenuated the profound hypotension associated with left ventricular failure and, presumably, has diminished its effect on the mesenteric circulation.

SMAT occurs at areas of severe atherosclerotic narrowing, most often at the origin of the SMA (Fig 18–2). The acute ischemic episode is commonly superimposed on chronic mesenteric ischemia. Hence, approximately 20% to 50% of these patients have a history of abdominal pain with or without malabsorption and weight loss dur-

ing the weeks to months preceding the acute episode. Additionally, most patients with SMAT have severe and diffuse atherosclerosis with a prior history of coronary, cerebrovascular, or peripheral arterial insufficiency.

PATHOPHYSIOLOGY

A decrease in SMA flow initially produces local mesenteric vascular responses that tend to augment collateral blood flow to the affected intestine. If the lower flow is prolonged, active vasoconstriction develops that may persist even after the primary event causing diminished flow is corrected. Following an acute 50% reduction in SMA blood flow in anesthetized dogs, the mesenteric arterial pressure (MesAP) in the peripheral mesenteric arteries falls to 49% of mean control valves.[12] When the SMA flow is maintained at 50% of normal, the MesAP returns to control values in 1 to 6 hours, while the celiac flow, which initially increases, falls to control levels. The greater fall in mesenteric pressure suggests lowered resistance or vasodilation. However, changes in active resistance cannot be deduced when pressure and flow are changing in the same direction.[13] The increased vascular resistance caused by vasoconstriction ultimately results in decreased collateral perfusion through the celiac system. If the occluder is removed from the SMA as soon as the MesAP rises to control values, the flow through the SMA immediately returns to normal. However, if the SMA occlusion is maintained for 30 to 240 minutes after the MesAP returns to control levels, the flow in the SMA does not return to normal; it remains at 30% to 50% of the control level because arterial vasoconstriction persists despite removal of the inflow obstruction. This decreased flow continues for up to 5 hours of observation. In this manner, mesenteric vasoconstriction plays a significant role in the development of ischemia in both acute occlusive and nonocclusive arterial forms of mesenteric ischemia.

When papaverine is infused directly into the SMA during the 50% flow restriction, the MesAP remains low and increased celiac flow persists throughout 4 hours of observation. The SMA flow returns to normal upon release of the obstruction. Based on these observations, intra-arterial papaverine infusion is recommended in both occlusive and nonocclusive forms of AMI. Intra-arterial papaverine also is recommended for selected patients with acute MVT because venous thrombosis has been shown experimentally to cause arterial spasm.[14]

The onset of abdominal signs and symptoms caused by intestinal ischemia actually may begin after correction of the primary systemic problems in patients with NOMI. The presumption that the bowel injury occurs during the period of diminished cardiac output or hypotension, and that correction of these problems returns the mesenteric blood flow to normal does not adequately explain persistent bowel ischemia when no arterial or venous obstruction is found at laparotomy and cardiac function has been optimized. This paradox can be explained by the experimental observations that an episode of low mesenteric flow, as short as 2 hours in duration, can produce mesenteric ischemia as a result of persistent vasoconstriction that continues after correction of the initial problem. Because vasospasm may persist even after the initial cause of ischemia is corrected, bowel injury continues unless the vasospasm is relieved. An aggressive radiologic and surgical approach to these diseases targets both the cause and the persistent vasospasm.

CELLULAR RESPONSE

Intestinal ischemia induces a spectrum of injury from subtle changes in capillary permeability to transmural necrosis. The final outcome depends on local and systemic factors. There are two related processes responsible for the subsequent intestinal damage: tissue hypoxia and reperfusion injury. Hypoxia occurs during the period of ischemia, whereas reperfusion injury occurs after some flow is reconstituted. As an episode of intestinal ischemia progresses and homeostatic changes occur, one region of bowel may experience hypoxic injury while another undergoes reperfusion-induced damage.

The changes that occur when intestine is deprived of an adequate blood supply are both metabolic and morphologic. Ultrastructural changes occur within 10 minutes, and by 30 minutes extensive changes, including accumulation of fluid between the cells and the basement membranes, are present.[15] The tips of the villi begin to slough and a membrane of necrotic epithelium, fibrin, inflammatory cells, and bacteria accumulates. Later, edema appears, followed by bleeding into the submucosa. Cellular death progresses from the lumen outwards until there is transmural necrosis of bowel wall.[9,16]

A major consequence of bowel ischemia is enhanced transcapillary filtration, interstitial edema, and ultimately, fluid movement into the lumen of the bowel. Comparison of vascular permeability in control intestinal preparations and bowel subjected to 1 hour ischemia with and without subsequent reperfusion indicated that both ischemia and reperfusion increase vascular permeability.[17]

Several endogenous substances, including oxygen free radicals, platelet activating factor, arachidonic acid metabolites, and bacterial endotoxins have been implicated in the pathogenesis of reperfusion injury. These substances are released during small bowel ischemia, and they are felt to be major mediators of intestinal damage. In addition, a rapidly growing body of evidence suggests that oxygen free radicals such as superoxide, hydrogen peroxide, and hydroxyl free radicals, mediate the cellular injury produced by reperfusion of ischemic intestine.

EFFECT ON THE MUCOSAL BARRIER

Although the primary function of the small intestinal mucosa is the absorption of nutrients, it also functions as an important barrier to luminal bacteria and their toxins. The barrier function of the intestinal mucosa is deranged in experimental animals subjected to ischemia. Changes in mucosal permeability induced by ischemia and reperfusion have been studied by measuring the clearance from blood to intestinal lumen of various agents, and by translocation of luminal bacteria to mesenteric lymph nodes. Complete ischemia followed by reperfusion leads to a marked increase in gut mucosal permeability.[18,19] The increment in mucosal permeability is directly related to the extent and duration of the ischemic insult. However, oxygen uptake must be reduced by more than 50% of control values for ischemia reperfusion to increase mucosal permeability.[20]

CLINICAL RESPONSE TO AMI

The response to reduced intestinal blood flow is complicated and the consequences of mesenteric ischemia are only now being fully appreciated. Initially, upon occlusion of the SMA, bowel activity increases markedly. This increased motor function causes rapid bowel evacuation. This activity increases the functional oxygen demands of the affected intestine. Shortly thereafter, bowel motility ceases owing to either the massive sympathetic response to ischemia or as a consequence of local factors associated with the ischemia itself. Within hours, the bowel becomes hemorrhagic and edematous as the capillary integrity is compromised. Intramural hydrostatic pressure rises with increased edema and hemorrhage. In normal bowel, this increased intramural pressure is usually well tolerated, but as perfusion pressure to the edematous bowel decreases, the edema further compromises the marginal blood flow. In addition, lumenal bacteria utilize the limited intestinal oxygen supply and produce toxic metabolites that may exacerbate ischemic injury.

The shift of intravascular volume into the bowel wall causes severe hemoconcentration and hypovolemic shock. Vasoactive mediators and bacterial endotoxins are released from the ischemic bowel into the peritoneal cavity and absorbed into the general circulation, causing a variety of physiologic effects, including cardiac depression, septic shock, and acute renal failure. These effects may contribute to the death of the patient even before there is complete necrosis of the bowel wall.

CLINICAL PRESENTATION

Early identification of AMI requires a high index of suspicion for those patients who have significant risk factors associated with this disease. AMI occurs most frequently in patients >50 years of age who have chronic heart disease and long-standing congestive heart failure, especially those poorly controlled with diuretics or digitalis. Cardiac arrhythmias, especially atrial fibrillation, recent myocardial infarction or hypotension due to burns, pancreatitis, or hemorrhage all predispose the patient to AMI. Previous or synchronous arterial emboli increase the likelihood of an acute SMA embolus. The development of sudden abdominal pain in a patient with any of these risk factors should suggest the diagnosis of AMI.

Acute abdominal pain varying in severity, nature, and location occurs in 75% to 98% of patients with intestinal ischemia. A history of postprandial abdominal pain, in the weeks to months preceding the acute onset of severe abdominal pain occurs in only a small fraction of patients with AMI caused by SMAT and represents an acute thrombosis occurring in patients with CMI. In early AMI, the pain experienced by the patient is markedly out of proportion to the physical findings. Therefore, sudden severe abdominal pain accompanied by rapid and often forceful bowel evacuation, especially with minimal or no abdominal signs, strongly suggests an acute arterial occlusion in the mesenteric circulation.

Unexplained abdominal distention or gastrointestinal bleeding may be the only indications of acute intestinal ischemia, especially in nonocclusive disease, since pain is absent in up to 25% of these patients. Patients surviving cardiopulmonary resuscitation who develop culture-proven bacteremia and diarrhea without abdominal pain should be suspected of having NOMI.[21] Distention, while absent early in the course of mesenteric ischemia, is often the first sign of impending intestinal infarction. The stool contains occult blood in 75% of patients and this bleeding may precede any other symptom of ischemia. Right-sided abdominal pain associated with the passage of maroon or bright-red blood in the stool, although characteristic of CI, also may suggest the diagnosis of AMI.

Although there are no abdominal findings early in the course of intestinal ischemia, as infarction develops, increasing tenderness, rebound tenderness, and muscle guarding reflect the progressive loss of intestinal viability and the presence of transmural gangrene. Significant abdominal findings strongly indicate the presence of infarcted bowel. Nausea, vomiting, hematochezia, hematemesis, massive abdominal distention, back pain, and shock are other late signs that indicate compromise of bowel viability.

DIAGNOSIS

Leukocytosis exceeding 15,000 cell/mm³ occurs in approximately 75% of patients with AMI, whereas about 50% will present with metabolic acidemia. Elevations of serum amylase, phosphate and other serum enzymes, as well as the presence of intestinal alkaline phosphatase and inorganic phosphate in the peritoneal fluid have been described. However, the sensitivity and specificity of these markers of intestinal ischemia have not been established.[22] Leukocytosis, out of proportion to the clinical findings, and an elevated hemoglobin and hematocrit indicating hemoconcentration as a result of fluid loss into the bowel and peritoneal cavity are not specific for AMI, but suggest advanced intestinal necrosis and sepsis.

Before infarction occurs, plain abdominal radiographs are usually normal.[23] As the disease progresses, a pattern of adynamic ileus, a gasless abdomen or small bowel pseudo-obstruction can be noted. Late in the course of the disease, formless loops of small intestine or small intestinal "pinkyprinting" can suggest the diagnosis of AMI. Less commonly, isolated "thumbprinting" of the right colon may be the only indication of AMI. The finding of colonic ischemia confined to the right colon may be the result of disease in the main SMA circulation rather than simply interference with colonic blood flow. Rare findings accompanying all types of bowel infarction include pneumatosis or gas in the portal venous system.

Upper gastrointestinal series can show dilated loops of small intestine with thickened folds, mucosal ulceration, or a scalloped bowel border. These findings are more characteristic of FSI. Duplex scanning has been of some value in identifying portal and superior MVT, and, in a few patients, SMA occlusion. Computed tomography (CT) also has been used to identify arterial and venous thromboses, as well as ischemic bowel, but only in the late stages of the disease. Magnetic resonance imaging (MRI) and positron emission tomography (PET) may, in the future, be helpful in the diagnosis of mesenteric ischemia.

Laparoscopy may be useful for patients whose clinical status precludes angiography.[24] However, laparoscopic examination of the bowel is limited to the serosal surface, making it unreliable for diagnosing early mucosal necrosis at a time when the serosa still appears relatively normal.

Historically, angiography has been limited to identifying arterial occlusions by embolus or thrombosis. Currently, selective angiography is the mainstay of diagnosis and initial treatment of both occlusive and nonocclusive forms of AMI. Four reliable angiographic criteria for the diagnosis of mesenteric vasoconstriction have been identified (Fig 18–3): (1) narrowing of the origins of multiple branches of the SMA; (2) alternate dilatation and narrowing of the intestinal branches (string-of-sausage sign); (3) spasm of the mesenteric arcades; and (4) impaired filling of intramural vessels.[25]

While mesenteric vasoconstriction occurs in hypo-

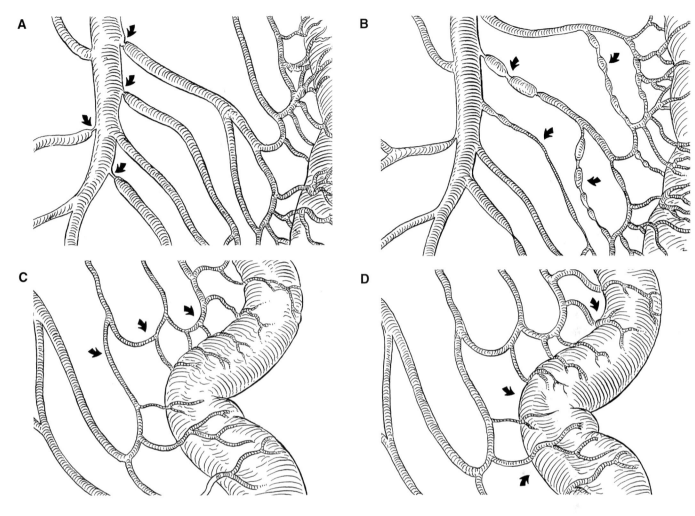

Figure 18–3. Angiographic criterial of AMI. **A.** Narrowing of multiple branches. **B.** Alternate spasm and dilatation of intestinal branches (string-of-sausage sign). **C.** Spasm of arcades; impaired filling of intramural vessels.

tensive patients and in those with pancreatitis, its presence in patients with suspected intestinal ischemia who are not in shock, do not have pancreatitis and are not receiving vasopressors is diagnostic of NOMI. Therefore, if angiography is performed sufficiently early in the disease, patients with occlusive and nonocclusive AMI can be identified before bowel infarction develops, prior to the development of the clinical and radiologic signs that indicate irretrievable bowel infarction.

MANAGEMENT

Patients more than 50 years of age with any of the previously enumerated risk factors for AMI, who develop sudden onset of abdominal pain severe enough to require the attention of a physician, and which lasts for more than 2 hours, should be suspected of having AMI. These patients should be managed according to an ag-

gressive radiologic and surgical algorithm (Fig 18–4). Less absolute indications for inclusion into this protocol include unexplained abdominal distention, colonoscopic evidence of isolated right-sided colonic ischemia, or acidosis with unidentifiable cause. Because the presence of diagnostic clinical or non-angiographic radiologic signs usually indicates irreversible intestinal injury, broad selection criteria are essential if early diagnosis and successful treatment are to be achieved. Some negative studies must be accepted in order to identify and salvage patients who do have AMI.

General Principles of Management

Initial treatment is directed towards correcting the predisposing or precipitating causes of ischemia. Relief of acute congestive heart failure, and correction of hypotension, hypovolemia, and cardiac arrhythmias must precede

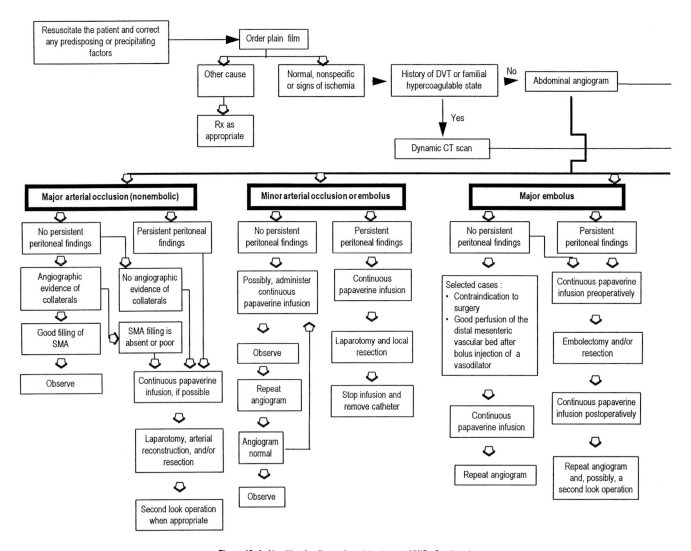

Figure 18–4. Algorithm for diagnosis and treatment of MID. *Continued.*

any diagnostic evaluation. Efforts to improve mesenteric blood flow are futile if low cardiac output, hypovolemia, or hypotension persist. Frequently, patients have septic cardiac parameters, a very low systemic vascular resistance and sequestration of fluid into the "third space." Cardiac performance can best be optimized in these circumstances with the aid of a Swan-Ganz catheter, using serial cardiac profiles to insure maximal systemic perfusion.

After resuscitation is accomplished, plain films of the abdomen should be obtained. These films are not used to establish the diagnosis of AMI, but rather, to exclude other identifiable causes of abdominal pain (eg, a perforated viscus with free intraperitoneal air). A normal plain film does not exclude AMI; indeed, ideally patients will be studied before radiologic signs develop since such findings indicate the presence of infarcted bowel. If no alternative diagnosis is made on the basis of plain abdominal films, selective SMA angiography is

performed. Based on the angiographic findings and the presence or absence of peritoneal signs that persist for more than 20 minutes following a bolus dose of intra-arterial vasodilator, the patient is treated according to the algorithm in Fig 18–4.

Even when the decision to operate has already been made, a preoperative angiogram is necessary for proper management at laparotomy. Relief of mesenteric vasoconstriction is an essential component of the treatment of emboli and thromboses, as well as the nonocclusive "low-flow" states. Intra-arterial infusion of papaverine through the angiography catheter placed percutaneously in the orifice of the SMA is the best method to relieve mesenteric vasoconstriction preoperatively and postoperatively. The drug is infused at a constant rate of 30 to 60 mg/hour in a concentration of 1 mg/mL. The clinical and angiographic response to vasodilator therapy determines the duration of the papaverine infusion.

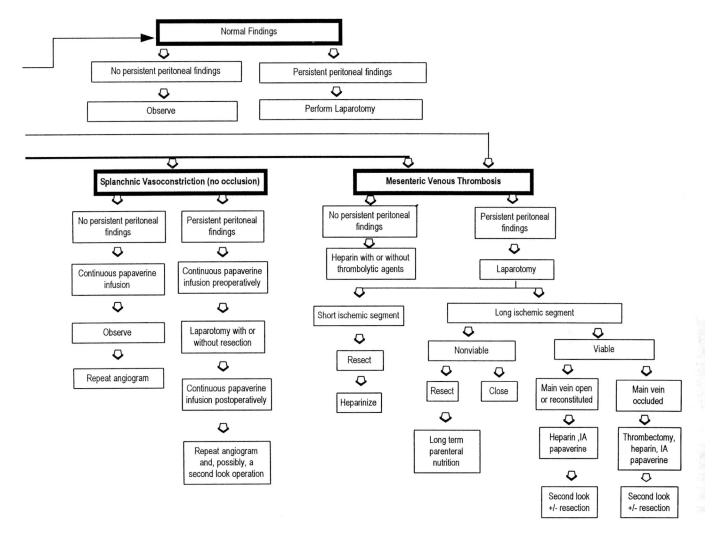

Figure 18–4, cont'd.

Although almost all of the papaverine infused into the mesenteric circulation is cleared during its passage through the liver; under some circumstances, this dose may have adverse systemic effects. Therefore, systemic arterial pressure, heart rate, and cardiac rhythm must be monitored constantly during papaverine infusions. Dislodgement of the catheter from the SMA is the most common cause of hypotension with this level of papaverine infusion. Therefore, hypotension during papaverine infusion should be managed by changing the papaverine infusion to saline followed by a plain abdominal film to confirm the position of the arterial catheter.

Laparotomy is indicated in AMI to restore intestinal arterial flow after an embolus or thrombosis and/or to resect irreparably damaged bowel. Revascularization should precede evaluation of intestinal viability because bowel that initially appears nonviable may show surprising recovery after restoration of adequate blood flow.

After revascularization, intestinal viability can be assessed by several methods. Traditionally, the bowel is placed in warm saline-soaked laparotomy pads and observed during a period of 10 to 20 minutes for return of normal color and peristalsis and the presence or absence of pulsations in the intestinal arteries. The accuracy of this clinical assessment is limited; therefore, more sensitive and specific evaluation requires the use of technological aids. Techniques to assess bowel viability include surface fluorescence,[26] perfusion fluorometry,[27] Doppler measurements of arterial flow,[28] electromyography,[29] surface temperature, serosal pH, surface oxygen consumption and radioisotope uptake determinations. Only Doppler pulse determinations, fluorescence using an ultraviolet light after an intravenous injection of fluorescein, and perfusion fluorometry have gained wide clinical acceptance. Surface fluorescence increases the accuracy of differentiating viable from nonviable bowel; although the equipment is inexpensive and the dye is safe, the technique remains subjective. Perfusion fluorometry is more objective, allows repeated determinations and is more accurate than surface fluorescence. However, the equipment is expensive and only small areas of the bowel can be evaluated at one time. Although Doppler probes are available in most operating rooms, this modality is, again, limited to examining small areas of the intestine. A practical solution is the initial use of surface fluorescence, with either perfusion fluorometry or Doppler examination reserved for evaluation of equivocal areas.

Short segments of bowel that are nonviable or questionably viable after revascularization are resected. If extensive portions of the bowel are involved, only the clearly necrotic bowel is resected and a planned re-exploration (second-look operation) is performed within 12 to 24 hours. The decision to perform a second-look operation is made during the initial celiotomy, if major portions or multiple segments of intestine are of equivocal viability. The purpose of the second-look celiotomy, as proposed by Shaw is "not just to allow a clear definition between dead and live bowel to take place, but also to allow time for the institution of supportive measures which may render more of the bowel viable."[30] Such measures may include optimizing cardiac output, SMA infusion with papaverine, antibiotic therapy, and anticoagulant therapy. Once made, the decision to perform a second-look operation is inviolate and must be done irrespective of the clinical course of the patient. If it is planned, anastomoses need not be made until the time of the re-exploration. Only 18% of second-look procedures have been shown to contribute to patient survival.[31]

If, at the initial laparotomy, there is obvious infarction of all, or most of the small bowel with or without a portion of the right colon, then the surgeon is faced with a philosophical decision. Doing nothing will result in the early death of the patient, whereas resection of all of the involved bowel inevitably will produce short bowel syndrome with its attendant problems and almost certain commitment to life-long parenteral nutrition. Whether these older patients are suitable candidates for such an approach is arguable. A preoperative discussion with the patient and the patient's family concerning this problem is warranted so that an acceptable decision can be reached, if the situation is encountered at surgery.

The use of anticoagulants in the management of AMI remains controversial. Heparin anticoagulation may cause intestinal, submucosal, or intraperitoneal hemorrhage and, except in the case of mesentric venous thrombosis, we have not used it in the immediate postoperative period. However, late thrombosis following embolectomy or arterial reconstruction occurs frequently enough that anticoagulation beginning 48 hours postoperatively seems advisable.

Because of the high incidence of positive blood cultures in patients with AMI, and the clinical and experimental evidence that ischemic bowel permits translocation of intralumenal bacteria,[32] broad-spectrum systemic antibiotics are begun as soon as the diagnosis is entertained and continued throughout the postoperative period. Both systemic and locally administered antibiotics have been shown to improve the survival of ischemic bowel.[33]

Specific Management

SMAE (Fig 18–5). Upon angiographic detection of an SMA embolus, papaverine is infused through the catheter, which is placed selectively in the origin of the SMA,

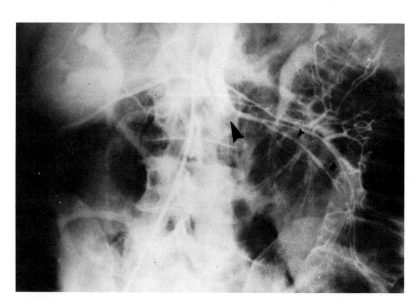

Figure 18–5. Arteriogram showing embolus completely occluding the SMA (*large arrow*) with associated vasoconstriction (*small arrows*) occluding blood flow with distal vasoconstriction.

proximal to the occlusion. The patient then is managed according to the algorithm in Fig 18–4, based on the site of the embolus, the presence or absence of peritoneal signs, the extent of collateral blood flow, and the degree of vasospasm in the vascular beds both proximal and distal to the embolus, as demonstrated by a repeat angiogram following selective intra-arterial injection of 25 mg of tolazoline.

Minor emboli are those in the branches of the SMA or in the SMA distal to the origin of the ileocolic artery. Patients with minor emboli, whose pain is relieved by the vasodilator therapy, can be managed expectantly. Patients with major emboli who are selected for nonoperative therapy must have significant contraindications to surgery, no peritoneal signs, and adequate perfusion of the vascular beds distal to the embolus following initiation of vasodilator therapy. Direct infusion of thrombolytic agents through selectively placed catheters has been used when the SMA was only partially occluded. However, thrombolytic agents may require up to 36 hours to dissolve the embolus,[34] during which time there may be continued ischemia and ultimate necrosis of the bowel. Furthermore, because the extent of injury to the small intestine cannot be monitored during infusion of the thrombolytic agents, we do not recommend their use for AMI.

Embolectomy is always performed before assessing intestinal viability. The embolus is approached directly, or less optimally, through a proximal arteriotomy (Fig 18–6). The proximal SMA is exposed by drawing the transverse colon cephalad and anteriorly, as the small intestine is retracted inferiorly. The inferior leaf of the transverse mesocolon is incised and the proximal SMA is dissected free between the pancreas and the fourth portion of the duodenum. The SMA is exposed for 2 to 3 cm proximal and distal to the origin of the middle colic artery. The SMA is palpated gently to determine the most distal extent of arterial pulsation, or the artery may be examined directly with a Doppler probe to identify the site of the embolus. Once the site of the embo-

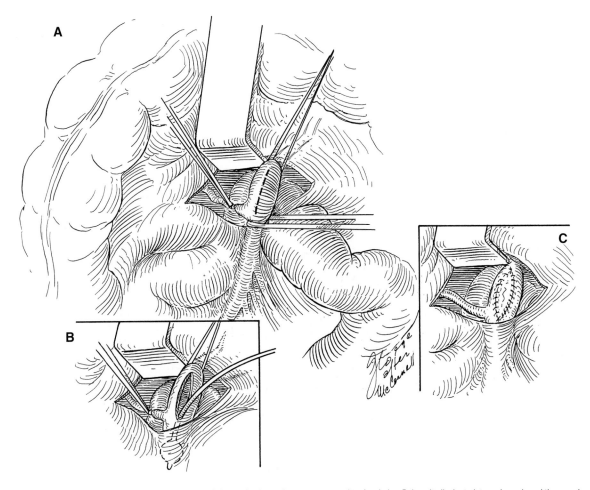

Figure 18–6. Technique of SMA embolectomy. **A.** The artery is isolated at base of mesentery over site of embolus. **B.** Longitudinal arteriotomy is made and the vessel is cleared of debris. **C.** The arteriography is closed primarily or with vein patch (shown). (Redrawn from Boley SJ, et al. In: Nyhus LM (ed), *Surgery Annual.* New York, NY: Appleton-Century-Crofts; 1973.

lus is found, the SMA and its branches are controlled proximally and distally with vessel loops or gentle vascular clamps. These authors use a longitudinal arteriotomy over the embolus or just proximal to it, and the embolus is removed and residual clots are flushed out of the artery by briefly releasing the vessel loops. A balloon embolectomy catheter then is passed proximally and distally to remove all remaining clots. The arteriotomy is closed with or without a vein patch.

Following embolectomy, bowel viability is determined. If no second-look procedure is planned, the papaverine infusion is continued for an additional 12 to 24 hours. An arteriogram then is obtained to exclude persistent vasospasm, prior to removing the arterial catheter. If a second-look procedure is performed, the infusion is continued through this second procedure and until no vasoconstriction is present on a follow-up angiogram.

NOMI. NOMI is diagnosed when the angiographic signs of mesenteric vasoconstriction are seen in a patient who has the clinical picture of mesenteric ischemia and is neither in shock nor receiving vasopressors. The angiographic findings may vary from the previously described local signs to a pruned appearance of the entire mesenteric vasculature (Fig 18–7). A selective SMA infusion of papaverine is begun in all patients with NOMI as soon

as the diagnosis is made. In patients with persistent peritoneal signs, the infusion is continued during and after exploration. At operation, manipulation of the SMA is minimized. Overtly necrotic bowel is resected, and a primary anastomosis is performed only if no second-look procedure is planned. We believe it is better to leave bowel of questionable viability than to perform a massive enterectomy because, frequently, the bowel will improve with supportive measures or demarcate more clearly by the time of the second-look operation.

When papaverine infusion is used as the primary treatment for NOMI, it is continued for approximately 24 hours, after which the infusion is changed to normal saline for 30 minutes prior to a repeat angiogram. Based on the clinical course of the patient and the presence or absence of vasoconstriction on the repeat angiogram, the infusion is either discontinued or maintained for an additional 24 hours. Angiography is repeated daily until there is no radiographic evidence of vasoconstriction (Fig 18–7b) and the clinical symptoms and signs of the patient have resolved. Infusions usually are discontinued after 24 hours, but have been used for as long as 5 days.

When papaverine is used in conjunction with surgery for nonocclusive disease, a second-look operation is frequently necessary. In such cases, the infusion is continued as previously described for second-look operations following embolectomy. The arterial catheter is re-

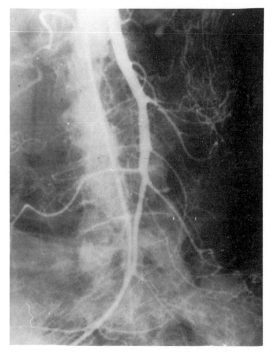
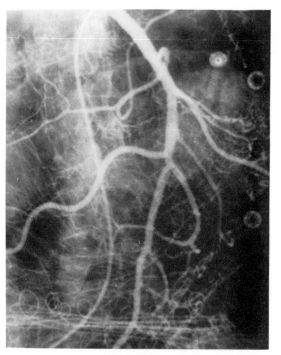

A   **B**

Figure 18–7. Patient with nonocclusive MI managed with papaverine infusion for 3 days. **A.** Initial angiogram showing spasm of main superior mesenteric artery, origins of branches, and intestinal arcades. **B.** Angiogram after 36 hours of papaverine infusion. Study was obtained 30 minutes after papaverine was replaced with saline. At this time the patient's abdominal symptoms and signs were gone. (From Boley SJ, Brandt LJ, Veith FJ: Curr Probl Surg 15:1, 1978)

moved when no angiographic signs of vasoconstriction are seen 30 minutes after cessation of vasodilator therapy.

SMAT. SMAT most often is identified on a flush aortogram showing complete occlusion of the SMA within 1 to 2 cm of its origin. Some filling of the SMA distal to the obstruction via collateral pathways is almost always present. Branches both proximal and distal to the obstruction may show local spasm or diffuse vasoconstriction. Differentiation between thrombosis and an embolus can be difficult and, in such cases, patients are treated initially for SMA embolus. A more difficult problem arises in patients with abdominal pain without abdominal signs and complete occlusion of the SMA on aortogram. In these cases, it is important to differentiate between an acute and a longstanding occlusion, since the latter may be coincidental to an unrelated presenting illness. Prominent collateral vessels between the superior mesenteric and the celiac and/or inferior mesenteric circulations are characteristic of chronic SMA occlusion. If large collaterals are present and there is good filling of the SMA on the late films during the angiogram, the occlusion can be considered to be chronic and the abdominal pain is probably unrelated to mesenteric vascular disease. In the absence of peritoneal signs, such patients are treated expectantly. The absence of collateral vessels, or the presence of collaterals with inadequate filling of the SMA indicates an acute occlusion. In the latter instance, the middle colic artery, which provides collateral flow to the distal SMA from the inferior mesenteric system via the arc of Roilan and central anastomotic artery, is probably occluded, thus interrupting the collateral circulation to an already marginal SMA. Promote intervention is indicated irrespective of the abdominal findings in these cases.

If possible, an angiographic catheter is placed in the proximal SMA and a papaverine infusion is begun. If the origin of the SMA cannot be identified or cannulated at angiography, a small silastic catheter should be advanced proximally into the SMA through a jejunal artery at the time of operative revascularization to treat the associated vasospasm. This catheter is brought out through a separate incision in the abdominal wall and is used for postoperative papaverine infusion.

Revascularization procedures for SMAT are similar to those used for CMI. Reimplantation, thrombectomy and endarterectomy, or some form of bypass graft to the SMA distal to the obstruction, are employed. These are discussed in the section on CMI. Percutaneous balloon and laser angioplasty of the SMA also have been reported.[35] Because there is presently no good method to monitor end organ injury, and because of the danger of re-thrombosis with irreparable bowel loss as was the case

with one of our patients, we do not recommend these techniques for acute SMA occlusions.

COMPLICATIONS

Complications of the angiographic studies and prolonged papaverine infusions have not been excessive. Three of our first 50 patients developed transient acute tubular necrosis following angiography and treatment of mesenteric ischemia. One patient developed arterial occlusions in both lower extremities during a papaverine infusion for an SMA embolus, probably representing synchronous emboli from his primary source of embolization. The SMA catheter, however, could not be excluded as the cause of arterial occlusion. Several patients developed local hematomas at the arterial puncture site, but no major lower extremity vascular occlusions occurred in these cases.

Problems caused by prolonged papaverine infusions have been minimal. Infusions have been used for more than 5 days without significant adverse systemic effects. Fibrin clots on the arterial catheter have been observed commonly, but have not caused any difficulty. Three catheters thrombosed and had to be removed or exchanged. This complication has been avoided subsequently by using continuous infusion pumps to deliver the papaverine solution. Catheter dislodgement requiring repositioning has occurred several times.

Septic complications, including wound infections, pneumonia, intra-abdominal abscesses, and hepatic abscesses are common. Intraoperative and postoperative myocardial infarctions occur frequently in this population with advanced atherosclerotic disease and other predisposing comorbidities. Long intensive care unit stays are the rule, even following early diagnosis of AMI.

Late thrombosis after embolectomy or arterial reconstruction has been minimized by anticoagulating these patients 48 hours after surgery. Earlier anticoagulation is not advised because it may precipitate postoperative bleeding or hemorrhage into the ischemic bowel wall.

RESULTS

Although mortalities of 70% to 90% have been reported through 1980, using traditional methods of diagnosis and therapy, the aggressive approach described above can reduce these catastrophic figures[36–47] (Table 18–1). Of our first 50 patients managed by this approach, 35 (70%) proved to have AMI. Of these, 33 had angiographic signs of ischemia. The remaining two patients had normal angiograms. Of 65 patients from two institutions using this protocol, 36 (55%) survived including 14 of 26 with NOMI, 14 of 23 with SMAE, 4 of 6 with SMAT, and 4 of 6 with superior MUT. Most of the survivors lost no bowel or <3 feet of small intestine.

In a separate review of 47 patients with intestinal is-

TABLE 18–1. MORTALITY RATES FOR ACUTE MESENTERIC ISCHEMIA WITH OR WITHOUT INTRA-ARTERIAL VASODILATOR THERAPY

Ref. No.	Author	No. Patients	Vasodilator Therapy	Survival (%)	Year
41	Levy	62	No	60	1990
42	Battellier	65	No	50	1990
43	Finucane	32	No	34	1989
44	Georgiev	175	No	7	1989
45	Paes	38	No	47	1988
46	Clavien	81	No	29	1986
40	Koveker	39	No	15	1985
37	Clark	27	Yes	48	1984
32	Sachs	49	No	35	1984
47	Rogers	12	No	33	1982
48	Krausz	40	No	22	1978
38	Boley	35	Yes	55	1977

chemia resulting from SMA emboli, a survival rate of 55% was achieved in patients managed according to our aggressive protocol, whereas only 20% of those patients treated by traditional methods survived. Intra-arterial papaverine as the primary treatment was successful in four patients; two of these were not operated upon, and the other two had normal intestine at the time of delayed laparotomy. Of special interest in this study was the observation that two-thirds of patients with SMA emboli placed in the protocol within 12 hours of reporting their pain to their physician, and managed strictly according to this protocol survived.

Using the aggressive approach outlined above, this catastrophic mortality has been reduced substantially. Overall, 50% or more of patients presenting with AMI and treated according to the present algorithm survive, and approximately 70% to 90% lose less than a meter of intestine. Ninety percent of patients with AMI who had angiography but no signs of peritonitis have survived, demonstrating the potential value of early diagnosis. Ideally, all patients with AMI should be studied at a time when the plain films of the abdomen are normal and prior to the development of an acute surgical abdomen. Other published reports of patients in whom vasodilator therapy was not used have had significantly higher mortality rates. Therefore, a wider use of this aggressive protocol for patients at risk for AMI may improve overall results.

■ CMI

CMI results from inadequate perfusion of the midgut during periods of increased oxygen demand. The oxygen requirements of the bowel increase significantly in the postprandial period owing to rises in motility, secretion, and absorption, which are all energy-dependant

functions of the bowel. Although experimental studies have shown increases in mesenteric blood flow following meals, vascular resistance also increases during peristalsis, impairing intramural perfusion. In the normal individual, these changes in blood flow are well tolerated and lead to no untoward effects. However, in patients with impairment of mesenteric circulation resulting from atherosclerotic disease of the vessel supplying the intestines, oxygen requirements often exceed the ability to meet these demands and cause cellular hypoxia. This hypoxic injury is manifested either by ischemic visceral pain and/or abnormalities in gastrointestinal absorption or motility. The pain is similar to that arising in the myocardium, with angina pectoris, or in the calf, with intermittent claudication.

Atherosclerotic involvement of the mesenteric vessels is almost always the cause of this form of intestinal ischemia; however, the various small-vessel diseases such as thromboangiitis obliterans (Buerger's Disease) or polyarteritis nodosa also may produce chronic intestinal ischemia. Although partial or complete occlusion of the celiac artery, the SMA, or the IMA is fairly common, relatively few patients have documented chronic intestinal ischemia. Moreover, there are many patients with occlusion of two or even three of these vessels who remain asymptomatic.

CLINICAL PRESENTATION

The one consistent feature of CMI is abdominal discomfort or pain. Most commonly this occurs 10 to 15 minutes after meals, gradually increasing in severity, finally reaching a plateau and then slowly dissipating during the course of 1 to 3 hours. The pain pattern is so intimately associated with eating that the patients reduce their food intake and typically have weight loss. Bloating, flatulence, and derangements in motility with constipation or diarrhea also occur.

Physical findings are rarely helpful, although the presence of an abdominal bruit has been reported in up to 75% of the patients. Occasionally, the patient will have occult blood in the stool. Weight loss in the setting of occult fecal blood often leads to an evaluation for gastrointestinal malignancy.

DIAGNOSIS

Failure to demonstrate an etiology of postprandial abdominal pain associated with weight loss should strongly suggest CMI. There is no specific or reliable diagnostic test for abdominal angina. The diagnosis must be based on the clinical symptoms, the arteriographic demonstration of occlusion of the splanchnic arteries and, to a great degree, the exclusion of other gastrointestinal diseases.

Angiographic evaluation includes flush aortography

in the frontal and lateral views and selective injections of the SMA, CA, and IMA. The degree of occlusion of the three major arteries can be assessed best on the lateral projections and the collateral circulation. Patterns of flow are best evaluated on the frontal views (Fig 18–8). The presence of prominent collateral vessels not only indicates a significant stenosis of a major vessel but also connotes a chronic process. Stenosis or occlusion of one or more of the major visceral vessels demonstrated on an angiogram does not, by itself, establish the diagnosis of arterial insufficiency.

In the past, a major indication for early surgical intervention was the prevention of acute intestinal infarction. However, more than 75% of the AMI cases are the result of embolus or nonocclusive disease, and in neither condition are prodromal symptoms present, nor has the incidence of intestinal infarction in patients with chronic occlusive disease of the splanchnic vessels been established. Therefore, the fear of impending intestinal infarction is not an indication for operation if there are no other symptoms to warrant it. There is one special case in which reconstruction or bypass of obstructed visceral arteries is recommended in the absence of abdominal pain. This occurs in patients who are undergoing aortic reconstructions for peripheral

vascular disease in whom aortography demonstrates occlusive disease of the SMA or CA and the presence of a large "meandering artery."

MANAGEMENT

The difficulty in establishing an unequivocal diagnosis of CMI, the fragility of elderly patients, and the operative risk for gut revascularization has made the selection of patients for surgery difficult. More recently, balloon angioplasty, which can be performed with much less morbidity, has made it less critical to establish a definitive diagnosis before undertaking treatment.

With no available method for measuring intestinal blood flow accurately, precise criteria to define the need for operative arterial reconstruction are lacking. There is agreement that a patient with the typical pain of abdominal angina and unexplained weight loss, whose diagnostic evaluation has excluded other gastrointestinal diseases, and whose angiogram shows occlusive involvement of at least two of the three major mesenteric arteries, should benefit from revascularization. The issue is less clear if only one major vessel is involved or if the clinical presentation is atypical. Until a quantitative test becomes available, patients with atypi-

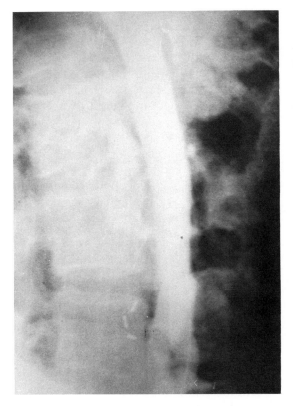 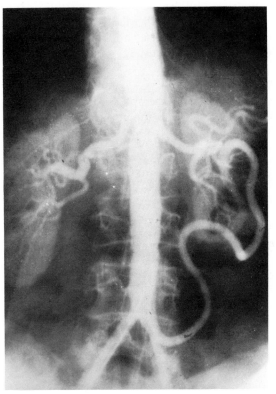

A   **B**

Figure 18–8. Chronic versus acute SMA occlusion. **A.** Lateral projection showing occlusion of major vessels. **B.** Chronic occlusion with large meandering artery.

cal symptoms must continue to be treated expectantly. Revascularization is indicated even if only one vessel is occluded when pain and weight loss does not respond to other treatments and balloon angioplasty is unsuccessful.

Patients suffering from chronic intestinal ischemia are often severely malnourished and may require a period of parenteral alimentation prior to revascularization. Albumin and prothrombin time should be corrected prior to intervention. In addition, vitamin deficiencies may be apparent and supplementation with parenteral folate, vitamin C, vitamin K, thiamine and B12 should be considered if they have lost more than 10% of their lean body weight.

Several procedures have been advocated for the restoration of normal flow and pressure distal to an occlusion of the SMA or CA, including reimplantation, endarterectomy, and bypass. Presently, the preferred procedure is bypass to the SMA distal to the occlusion, although several surgeons believe that both the SMA and CA must be revascularized, if they are both occluded.

Reimplantation

Reimplantation is performed by transecting the artery distal to the occlusion and performing an anastomosis directly to the aorta. This procedure is technically difficult owing to the short length of available vessel and the presence of severe aortic atherosclerotic disease in the region of the take-off of the celiac and SMA trunks. The procedure should be reserved solely for situations in which the aorta is being replaced and the revascularization is being done prophylactically.

Endarterectomy (Fig 18–9)

Endarterectomy has been attempted both through the diseased vessel and through the aorta itself. Both are

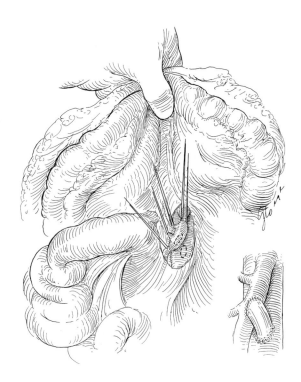

Figure 18–10. Technique of aorta-to-superior mesenteric artery (SMA) bypass. An incision in the retroperitoneum has been made over the aorta and carried superiorly to divide the ligament of Treitz. This provides exposure of the aorta and the SMA in the region of the middle colonic artery. Sites of the anastomoses are shown. Inset left shows fine suture technique of anastomosis. Inset right shows completed bypass. (Redrawn from Boley SJ, Brandt LJ, Veith FJ. *Curr Probl Surg* 1978;15:1)

technically difficult and can result in embolization of atheromatous fragments into the distal visceral and systemic circulation. The transarterial approach is usually unsuccessful because the most proximal extent of the occlusion is difficult to remove safely. The transaortic "trapdoor" endarterectomy requires cross-clamping the aorta in the supraceliac position, which increases the possibility of ischemic injury to the kidneys and distal circulation. Although this approach offers the theoretical advantage of clearing both the visceral and renal vessels and is completely autogenous, the extensive nature of the operation makes it applicable to few patients.

Bypass (Fig 18–10)

Mesenteric bypass from the aorta or the iliac artery to the side of the SMA distal to the occlusion is the procedure of choice. A reversed autologous saphenous vein is the preferred conduit if, after gentle distention, it is at least 5 mm in its smallest diameter. PTFE or knitted dacron are suitable substitutes if the saphenous is unavailable or inadequate.

The ideal site to provide inflow for bypass has been disputed. Because of the mobility of the SMA, grafts originating from the infrarenal aorta may be occluded with the movement of the mesentery of the small intestine. In

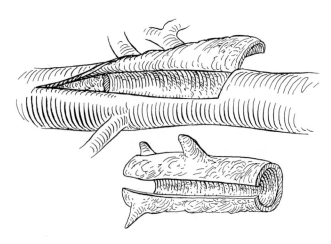

Figure 18–9. Combined visceral and renal endarterectomy with sleeve aortic endarterectomy. (Redrawn from Wylie EJ, et al. *Manual of Vascular Surgery*, vol. 1. New York, NY: Springer-Verlag; 1980:217)

addition, late failure owing to progressive atherosclerotic disease of the infrarenal aorta has led some surgeons to use the supraceliac aorta as the inflow for the graft. Occasionally, it may be necessary to use the iliac artery as the inflow for the graft when dissection of the supraceliac aorta is difficult and the infrarenal aorta is too diseased.

Results

Patency rates with bypass grafts to the SMA and CA have been generally good, and symptomatic relief in properly selected patients has been excellent. Stoney and colleagues have reported poor results with infrarenal bypasses. They attribute this is to an unusual and rapidly progressive form of atherosclerosis that involves the subdiaphragmatic aorta and that occurs more commonly in females and in relatively young subjects. On the basis of their extensive experience, they advocate either an antegrade prosthetic bypass from the supraceliac aorta via a transabdominal approach or a thoracoabdominal retroperitoneal "trapdoor" endarterectomy.[48]

■ FIS

Ischemic insults localized to short segments of the small intestine produce a broad spectrum of clinical features without the life-threatening systemic consequences associated with damage to more extensive portions of the gut. The most frequent causes are atheromatous or small thrombotic emboli, strangulated hernias, blunt abdominal trauma, and segmental venous thrombosis. In the late 1960s, enteric coated thiazide-potassium chloride preparations were shown to cause short ulcerating stenoses secondary to localized venous infarctions. Mesenteric vascular lesions associated with systemic diseases may occur late in the course of the illness or may be the heralding event of the generalized disorder.

CLINICAL FEATURES

FIS usually occurs in the presence of adequate collateral circulation to prevent transmural hemorrhagic infarction. Lesions commonly are infected infarcts, resulting from partial necrosis of the bowel wall with secondary invasion by intestinal bacteria. It tissue necrosis is limited, it may heal completely. Conversely, it may progress as chronic enteritis simulating Crohn's disease or it may cause a stricture resulting in partial or complete intestinal obstruction. Transmural necrosis, complicated by localized peritonitis or perforation, may follow a severe local insult.

CLINICAL PRESENTATION

Preoperative diagnosis of focal segmental ischemia is difficult to make. An antecedent episode of transient pain, trauma, incarcerated hernia, or a known systemic vasculitis can suggest the correct diagnosis. Patients with short segment ischemic bowel injury present differently, depending upon the site and severity of the insult. The acute presentation, seen with transmural necrosis, is marked by sudden onset of abdominal pain that may simulate acute appendicitis. These patients manifest clinical signs of peritonitis and sepsis. Another common presentation is that of chronic enteritis with crampy abdominal pain, diarrhea, occasional fever, and weight loss. This clinical picture is indistinguishable from Crohn's disease of the small intestine. The most common presentation, however, is that of chronic small bowel obstruction, with or without a history of trauma, pain, or hernia incarceration. Intermittent abdominal pain, distention, and vomiting are usually the results of the obstruction. Bacterial overgrowth in the dilated bowel proximal to the obstruction may lead to the metabolic and clinical derangements usually associated with the blind-loop syndrome (ie, anemia, diarrhea, and steatorrhea).

DIAGNOSIS AND MANAGEMENT

The treatment of acute focal segmental ischemia is usually surgical, but some patients without signs of peritonitis can be managed expectantly. In the latter instance, the diagnosis is made by finding small intestinal "pinkyprints" either on plain film or on a small bowel series. Serial studies should demonstrate a changing pattern. Both clinical and roentgenographic findings must resolve or the nonoperative approach is abandoned. Patients who present with chronic enteritis or obstruction should undergo exploration after proper preparation. Limited resection is the procedure of choice for both focal enteritis and obstructing lesions.

■ MVT

MVT is an infrequent, but distinct, form of intestinal ischemia. We now recognize that thrombosis of the superior mesenteric vein can develop slowly with no symptoms, in a more subacute manner with pain, but no intestinal infarction, or acutely with the classic presentation of AMI. Our understanding of the etiology, methods of diagnosis, and management have changed so radically that much of what has been written about MVT is no longer applicable.

In our experience, patients with operative or pathologic confirmation of MVT represented 2 per 100 000 admissions and comprise well under 10% of patients with AMI. Approximately 0.01% of all emergency surgical service admissions to a Dutch hospital were attributable to MVT.[49] While a review of the literature suggests a male predilection of up to 1.5:1,[50,51] our experience has shown no such preference. In a large literature review, the mean age was reported to be 48 years, whereas it was 60 years at our institution.[50] We have attributed these demographic differences to the higher proportion of geriatric patients seen at our medical center as compared to most other institutions.

CLINICAL FEATURES

Although many conditions have been associated with MVT (Table 18–2), previous studies were unable to show an etiological factor in up to 55% of patients. In more recent reports, however, contributing disorders are identified in up to 81% of patients.[51] This discrepancy can be explained by the fact that many of the cases in retrospective reviews occurred before the description of such conditions as antithrombin III, protein S and protein C deficiencies.[52] Therefore, the number of cases of MVT in which no cause can be identified will decrease as thorough hematological investigation is pursued. Hypercoagulable states are especially important and were found in 14 of 16 patients, in one report.[53] In our series, oral contraceptive-related MVT accounted for about 9% of female cases, but only 4% of the total series.[54] This finding is corroborated in a review showing a 5% incidence in the total population, with an 18% incidence in females. The lower incidence of oral con-

traceptive-related episodes in our series possibly reflects the large proportion of geriatric patients seen at our institutions. In addition, a spate of isolated cases relating oral contraceptive use to MVT may skew the composition of cases in the literature.

PATHOPHYSIOLOGY

The location of the initial thrombosis within the mesenteric venous circulation varies with etiology. SMVT secondary to cirrhosis, neoplasm, or operative injury starts at the site of obstruction and extends peripherally, while thromboses caused by hypercoagulable states tend to start in smaller venous branches and propagate towards the major mesenteric veins. Intestinal infarction rarely occurs unless the branches of the peripheral arcades and vasa recta are thrombosed, even when the junction of the portal and superior mesenteric vein is occluded. Inferior mesenteric vein thrombosis leading to infarction has been reported in fewer than 6% of cases of mesenteric venous thrombosis.

When venous drainage from a segment of bowel is compromised, the involved intestine becomes increasingly congested. The bowel becomes edematous, cyanotic, and thickened with intramural hemorrhages. Similar changes subsequently develop in the subjacent mesentery. Arterial pulsations are present up to the bowel wall, but arterial vasoconstriction frequently intervenes, which compromises intramural blood flow in the congested bowel. Later in the disease, transmural infarction occurs and, at this point, it may be impossible to differentiate venous from arterial occlusion. Serosanguineous peritoneal fluid accompanies early hemorrhagic infarction.

CLINICAL MANIFESTATIONS

Presentation

SMVT can present with a sudden acute onset, a subacute onset of weeks to months, or a chronic onset that usually is asymptomatic until late complications occur. As many as 60% of patients have a history of extremity deep-vein thrombosis.[55,56]

Acute Superior MVT

The symptoms and signs of acute SMVT, the classically described form of the disease, are both varied and nonspecific. The disorder has long been known as the "great imitator" of other abdominal disorders. In series that predate angiography and imaging studies, a correct preoperative diagnosis was infrequent. Except for abdominal pain, which was present in more than 90% of patients, no symptoms were pathognomonic of SMVT. Moreover, the duration, nature, severity, and location of the pain varied widely, but typically it was out of proportion to the physical findings. Although in our review

TABLE 18–2. MESENTERIC VENOUS THROMBOSIS: ASSOCIATED CONDITIONS

Hypercoagulable States
  Peripheral deep venous thrombosis
  Neoplasm
  Protein C deficiency
  Protein S deficiency
  Antithrombin III deficiency
  Oral contraceptive use
  Pregnancy
  Polycythema vera
  Thrombocytosis
Inflammation
  Pancreatitis
  Peritonitis (eg, perforated appendicitis or diverticulitis)
  Inflammatory bowel disease
  Pelvic or intra-abdominal abscess
Portal Hypertension
  Cirrhosis
  Congestive splenomegaly
  Following sclerotherapy of varices
Trauma
  Postoperative states
  Following splenectomy
  Blunt abdominal trauma
Other
  Decompression sickness

the mean duration of pain before admission was 5 days, others have reported ranges from 2 weeks to more than 1 month.[57,58] Some of the latter patients would now be reclassified as having the subacute form of SMVT. An initially surprising finding is that survivors had a longer interval, 6 days, before admission than did those patients with fatal outcomes, 4.4 days. We believe that the patients with a more indolent presentation are those who develop less extensive bowel infarction and hence, have a better prognosis.

Other prominent symptoms include nausea and vomiting, which occur in more than 50% of the patients as well as occult fecal blood which also is found in more than 50% of patients. Fifteen percent of patients have lower gastrointestinal bleeding or bloody diarrhea, and an additional 13% have hematemesis. The presence of hematemesis as well as bleeding per rectum should alert the physician to the possibility of a mesenteric ischemic catastrophe, since several cases of MVT presenting as upper gastrointestinal bleeding have been reported.

Initial physical findings in acute SMVT vary greatly, reflecting both different stages and degrees of ischemic injury. Although almost all patients present with abdominal tenderness, and most have decreased bowel sounds and abdominal distention, only 66% manifest overt peritoneal signs. Guarding and rebound tenderness develop later in the course as bowel infarction evolves. The majority of patients with SMVT have temperatures >38°C, but only 25% present with clinical signs of septic shock.

Laboratory studies in all forms of intestinal ischemia have low specificity and/or sensitivity. In our series of 22 patients, only a white blood cell count above 12 000 cu mm, and an increase in the proportion of polymorphonuclear cells were present in more than 66% of patients. Currently, laboratory tests can suggest the diagnosis of intestinal ischemia.

Patients with a personal or family history of deep venous thrombosis or other thrombotic episodes who present with symptoms compatible with MI should undergo evaluation for a hypercoagulable state. The work-up should include antithrombin III, protein S and protein C levels, as well as routine coagulation profiles. Antithrombin III binds to the serine protease portion of thrombin, thereby preventing the conversion of fibrinogen to fibrin. Protein S and C are vitamin K–dependent clotting factors. When activated, protein C, along with its cofactor protein S, inactivate factors V and VIII. In addition, the protein C and S complex may stimulate fibrinolysis, possibly via activation of plasminogen activator. In deficiency states, patients have a tendency to clot. Warfarin therapy is used in these patients because protein C and S are vitamin K–dependent and because antithrombin III deficiency states are heparin resistant.[59]

SUBACUTE SUPERIOR MESENTERIC VENOUS THROMBOSIS

We use the term subacute superior mesenteric vein thrombosis (SMVT) to describe patients who have abdominal pain for several weeks to months without intestinal infarction. Such presentations can be attributed to an extension of the thrombotic process at a rate rapid enough to cause pain, but slow enough to allow the development of venous collaterals before infarction occurs, or they can be attributed to acute thrombosis of only enough venous drainage to produce reversible ischemic injury. The diagnosis usually has been made serendipitously on imaging studies done for other suspected diagnoses, and the pain has subsided spontaneously or after initiation of anticoagulant therapy.

Typically, pain is the only symptom, although some patients have nausea or diarrhea. Physical examination and laboratory tests are usually normal. Pain has been related to meals, in a few patients, but is mostly nonspecific in site and nature. Some patients who start off with this type of presentation do ultimately develop intestinal infarction; hence, the distinction between acute and subacute forms of SMVT may become blurred. Late occurrence of infarction may be the result of recurrent SMVT. Both new and old thromboses have been found at the time of autopsy in nearly 50% of cases with MUT.[60] Moreover, some patients with subacute onset, in which the symptoms subside, may later develop the problems seen with asymptomatic chronic SMVT.

CHRONIC MVT

This term has been applied to patients who have no symptoms at the time of thrombosis. These patients may never develop problems related to SMVT, but those that do have gastrointestinal bleeding from esophageal or intestinal varices.[61] Most have bleeding esophageal varices and all have associated thrombosis of the portal or splenic vein. The physical findings of chronic MVT are those of presinusoidal portal hypertension, if the portal veins are involved. However, when only the superior mesenteric veins are involved there may be no abnormal findings. Laboratory studies with portal or splenic vein involvement also may show hypersplenism with pancytopenia or secondary thrombocytopenia.

DIAGNOSIS

Acute MVT

The absence of any reliable symptoms, signs, or laboratory studies makes a preoperative diagnosis of acute MVT difficult. Moreover, the variability in the course of the disease, with some patients having an indolent course of days to weeks and others having a relatively acute onset and progressive course, further obscures the diagnosis. The continuing difficulty in diagnosing

MVT was graphically described by Anane-Sehaf in his statement, "Perhaps the best overall finding was an uneasy feeling on the part of the examining physician that his patient looks sick but that he could not say why or from what."[62] Hence, in the past, the correct diagnosis has first been made at laparotomy in 90% to 95% of patients. In more recent series, using newer diagnostic modalities, the majority of patients have been diagnosed without or prior to operation.

Roentgenographic and other imaging studies can render a definitive diagnosis of MVT before intestinal infarction occurs. Plain films of the abdomen, if abnormal, almost always indicate bowel infarction. In our series, 75% of patients had abnormal plain films. Of these, 50% showed only a nonspecific ileus pattern, and in only 25% did the study suggest the presence of some form of AMI. Gas in the wall of the bowel or in the portal vein, and free air in the peritoneal cavity are late signs of intestinal infarction.

Barium enemas are of little value since MVT rarely involves the colon. However, when small bowel series have been performed, they have been both specific and sensitive.[63] Characteristic findings include (1) marked thickening of the bowel wall and valvulae conniventes from congestion and edema, (2) separation of loops owing to mesenteric thickening, (3) a long transition zone between involved and uninvolved bowel, with progressive narrowing of the lumen by the thickened wall, and (4) "thumbprints" or pseudotumors.

Selective mesenteric arteriography can establish a definitive diagnosis before bowel infarction and can differentiate venous thrombosis from arterial forms of ischemia. It also can provide access for the administration of intra-arterial vasodilators, if relief of the associated arterial vasoconstriction is deemed important in a specific patient. The angiographic findings of MVT have been determined experimentally and clinically and include (1) demonstration of a thrombus in the superior mesenteric vein (SMV) with partial or complete occlusion, (2) failure to visualize the SMV or portal vein, (3) slow or absent filling of the mesenteric veins, (4) arterial spasm, (5) failure of arterial arcades to empty, and (6) a prolonged blush of the wall of the involved segment. In addition, the angiogram may show reconstitution of venous blood flow proximal to the thrombus. This last finding can be important in therapeutic decisions.

Ultrasonography,[64,65] CT,[66] and MRI[67] have all been used to demonstrate thrombi in the superior mesenteric and portal veins. Ultrasonography is of less value in pure SMVT because overlying gas may prevent good visualization of the vein, but the study can be used as a quick screening test in problem cases. Thickening of the bowel wall and free peritoneal fluid on the sonogram suggest intestinal ischemia.

Gastrointestinal CT scanning can establish the diagnosis in more than 90% of patients with MVT by demonstrating the thrombus, venous collateral circulation, and involved intestine. Specific findings include thickening and persistent enhancement of the bowel wall, enlargement of the SMV, a central lucency in the lumen of the vein caused by the presence of the thrombus, a sharply defined vein wall with a rim of increased density, and dilated collateral vessels in a thickened mesentery (Fig 18–11). These findings are more characteristic of the chronic form of MVT because most of these patients underwent CT for another indication and the mesenteric thrombosis was found serendipitously. Some authors believe that when a diagnosis of MVT is made on CT, little is gained by a subsequent selective mesenteric angiogram. However, the extent of thrombosis is better delineated by angiography, and it provides access for papaverine administration when vasoconstriction is present.

The relative utility of angiography and CT in the patient with acute MVT has not yet been defined. A small number of patients with abdominal findings, diagnosed by imaging techniques, have been treated successfully without angiography or operation. MRI has been used to diagnose MVT in a few patients, although its only apparent advantages are avoidance of ionizing radiation and intravenous contrast.

There have been isolated reports of MVT being diagnosed by various endoscopic methods. Routine gastroduodenoscopy and colonoscopy are rarely valuable since the duodenum and colon are infrequently affected in this disease. However, examination of the proximal jejunum with a long endoscope can suggest the diagnosis, if that portion of the bowel is involved. Laparoscopy may be useful in circumstances where the diagnosis is uncertain. Scintiangiography has been diagnostic of MVT, but it has not been proven clinically reliable.[68]

As previously stated, the correct diagnosis of MVT usually is made at laparotomy. The hallmarks of MVT are serosanguineous peritoneal fluid, dark-red to blue-black edematous bowel, a striking thickening of the mesentery, good arterial pulsations in the involved segment, and thrombi in cut mesenteric veins. At this stage some degree of intestinal infarction has invariably occurred. Thus, as with the other forms of AMI, improved survival will only come from early diagnosis. For this reason, during the past 15 years we have employed the same diagnostic protocol for patients with suspected MVT as for those suspected of having arterial forms of AMI. However, the recent successful nonoperative, pharmacologic treatment of several patients with MVT diagnosed by imaging techniques suggests that, in some patients, this aggressive approach is not necessary.

Today, if patients with suspected AMI have factors suggesting MVT, we first obtain a contrast-enhanced CT. A past history of deep vein thrombosis or a family history of an inherited coagulation defect are examples

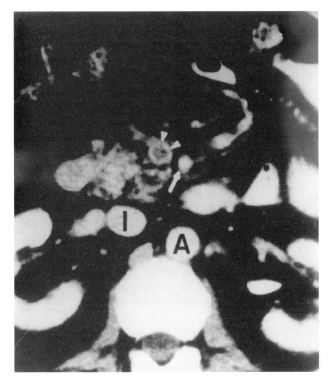

A

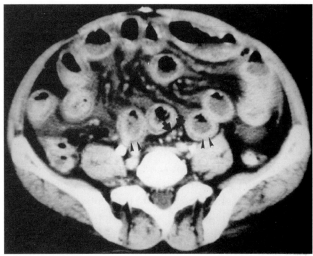

B

Figure 18–11. A. Abdominal computed tomograms with contrast demonstrating enlarged superior mesenteric vein with central luceny in the lumen representing the thrombus. The vein wall is sharply defined with a rim of increased density surrounding the thrombus (*arrows*). **B**. Abdominal contrast CT showing thickening and persistent enhancement of the bowel wall (*small arrows*) and dilated collateral vessels within a thickening mesentery (*large arrows*). (Fig 11b courtesy of Dr. Lawrence Carl.)

of factors that would prompt us to order a CT as the first imaging study. Patients with no predisposition to venous thrombosis are promptly resuscitated and undergo selective mesenteric angiography.

CHRONIC MVT

Since chronic MVT is asymptomatic or presents as gastrointestinal bleeding, the evaluation is directed towards determining the source of hemorrhage. Upper and lower gastrointestinal endoscopy and the same imaging studies used for acute MVT should help establish the diagnosis of chronic MVT, the extent of the thrombosis, and the site of bleeding. Transhepatic splenoportography can be used to better define the extent of the thromboses and varices if necessary, but papaverine enhanced selective SMA angiography is preferable if the portal vein is occluded.

MANAGEMENT

Acute MVT

Until the past few years a diagnosis of MVT mandated prompt laparotomy. However, with the advent of newer methods of diagnosis, MVT is being identified prior to bowel infarction. In addition, nonoperative therapy is proving successful. Therefore, in the small selected group of patients who have no physical findings sug-

gesting intestinal infarction and in whom the diagnosis of MVT has been made by ultrasonography, CT, MRI, or angiography, or a trial of anticoagulent or thrombolytic therapy may prove worthwhile. Heparin and streptokinase have been used successfully in the few case reports of this type of therapy.[69] Immediate operation is indicated should signs of intestinal infarction develop.

All patients, other than the few described above, should have prompt laparotomy. In the past, therapy consisted of resection of infarcted bowel and possibly, the immediate institution of anticoagulant therapy. Although there was previous controversy concerning the value or desirability of anticoagulation, recent studies show a clear benefit to the immediate use of heparin. Of patients who received this therapy, only 13% had recurrence or progression of the disease and only 13% died, compared with a 20% to 25% recurrence rate and a 50% mortality rate for patients who did not receive postoperative anticoagulation. Long-term anticoagulation is accomplished with coumadin.

The extent of bowel resection also has been a subject of disagreement. In past studies, the authors have recommended wide resection beyond the apparently infarcted bowel because the thrombosis often extended beyond the resected mesentery. More recent experience suggests that it is not necessary to sacrifice viable bowel when heparin and second-look operations are used. We believe that only the apparently nonviable bowel should be excised, as determined by clinical evaluation and, if necessary, by administration of fluorescein with examination under ultraviolet light. Although routine second-look operations have been recommended,[70] most surgeons use this procedure selectively.

Therapeutic options are mesenteric venous thrombectomy[71] and intra-arterial papaverine infusion through the SMA angiographic catheter,[72] both of which have been used in only a few patients. The limited experience with these two modalities makes it impossible to define their respective roles in the treatment of MVT. However, their inclusion in our algorithm of management is based upon a rational application of the available information.

If a short ischemic segment of bowel is found, local resection with prompt heparinization should be done. The more difficult problems come when one finds long segments of questionably viable bowel. The angiographic findings then may be essential for making a reasoned decision. If the angiogram demonstrates that the major vein proximal to the thrombus is opened or reconstituted (indicating that blood is flowing through the vein or around the obstruction), then a second-look operation should be performed 12 to 18 hours later. The intervening time is used to improve circulation with papaverine infused into the SMA. In one instance where this situation was noted on opening the abdomen, the surgeon found almost all of the small bowel to be blue. However, at a second look 18 hours later, after infusing papaverine and starting heparin therapy, the entire small bowel was pink and viable. The basis for this therapy is that the MVT has been shown, experimentally, to have an associated arterial spasm, which contributes to the ischemia. Relief of the arterial vasoconstriction may improve the blood supply adequately to preserve viability.

Similarly, if a long segment of questionable bowel is found and the angiogram or operative findings indicate complete thrombosis of the SMV at its junction with the portal vein, with or without extension into the portal vein, then venous thrombectomy is indicated. A second-look operation should be performed after thrombectomy, if the bowel is not clearly viable. Again, heparin therapy is promptly instituted. Intra-arterial papaverine may be beneficial if there appears to be arterial vasoconstriction after thrombectomy. When short segments of bowel are involved, thrombectomy is not indicated, nor is there any evidence that it is advantageous when venous flow is reconstituted around a thrombus. Such an individualized approach to the various possible surgical findings one might encounter is predicated on salvaging the maximum length of bowel.

CHRONIC MVT

Treatment of chronic MVT is directed towards controlling the gastrointestinal bleeding that usually results from esophageal bleeding. Sclerotherapy, various portosystemic shunts, devascularization procedures, and resection of bowel, when bleeding arises from colonic or small intestinal varices all have a place in select patients. No treatment is indicated for patients with asymptomatic chronic MVT in whom the collateral venous drainage is apparently adequate to prevent portal hypertension.

Results

The mortality rate for acute MVT is lower than in other forms of AMI, ranging from 20% to 50%. In our series, it was 32%. The overall recurrence rate has been 20% to 25% but, as discussed previously, falls to 13% to 15% if heparin therapy is instituted promptly when the diagnosis is made.

In the past almost all patients diagnosed with acute MVT had some infarcted bowel. This was true in all patients, in our own series as well. However, the amount of bowel resected was significantly less than in patients with arterial forms of AMI. The mean length of bowel resected in our series was 151 cm., with a range of 43 to 450 cm. There was no correlation between the length of involved bowel and mortality. Ninety-five percent of our patients had segmental involvement of the jejunum and/or ileum, whereas only 5% had involvement of the terminal ileum and right colon.

The natural history of chronic MVT is not known but from postmortem studies, it appears that almost 50% of patients with MVT have no bowel infarction, and most are asymptomatic. The percentage of patients with chronic MVT who develop late gastrointestinal bleeding also has not been determined, but is probably small. As MVT is recognized more frequently on CT scans done for other disorders, our understanding of the end results of this disorder should increase.

■ CI

Before 1950, CI was considered synonymous with colonic infarction or gangrene. Since that time, CI has become recognized as one of the more common disorders of the colon in the elderly and the most common form of ischemic injury of the gastrointestinal tract. Today CI is used to describe a general pathophysiologic process that leads to varied clinical outcomes. The spectrum includes (1) reversible ischemic colopathy (submucosal or intramucosal hemorrhage), (2) reversible or transient ischemic colitis, (3) chronic ischemic ulcerative colitis, (4) ischemic colonic stricture, (5) colonic gangrene, and (6) fulminant universal colitis (Fig 18–1).

PATHOPHYSIOLOGY

What ultimately triggers the episode of CI remains conjectural, in most instances. Whether it is increased demand by colonic tissue, superimposed on an already marginal blood flow, or whether the flow itself is acutely diminished has not been determined. However, because CI is a disease of the elderly, an association with degenerative changes of the mesenteric vasculature has been postulated. Histologically, narrowing of small arteries, arterioles, and veins are evident in colons resected for nonocclusive CI. Autopsy studies also have shown abnormal musculature in the wall of the superior rectal artery in the elderly population, which confirms an age-related alteration in the mesenteric vasculature.[73] In addition, postmortem angiographic studies have revealed an age-related tortuosity of the longer colonic arteries that may cause increased resistance to colonic blood flow, thus predisposing the patient to ischemia.[74]

Despite this suggestive evidence for a vascular or autonomic etiology for CI, most cases have no identifiable etiology. These spontaneous episodes are thought to be the result of local nonocclusive ischemia in association with small vessel disease. Colonic blood flow can be compromised further by alterations in the systemic perfusion. Inadequate systemic perfusion accompanying congestive heart failure, digitalis toxicity, or arrhythmia are rare causes of CI. Many other conditions, spontaneous or iatrogenic, have been associated with CI, although a direct cause-and-effect relationship has not been established (Table 18–3). Two specific and well-recognized exceptions include the development of CI proximal to a potentially obstructing stricture, carcinoma or diverticulitis, and following aortic reconstruction.

CLINICAL FEATURES

The diagnosis of CI usually is made after the period of ischemia has passed and blood flow to the affected segment of colon has returned to normal. Many cases of transient or reversible ischemia are probably missed because the condition resolves before medical attention is sought, or because a barium enema or colonoscopy is not performed early in the course of the disease. Additionally, many cases of CI are misdiagnosed as infectious colitis or inflammatory bowel disease. Thus, no study has yet provided an accurate determination of the incidence of CI.

Several retrospective reviews of older clinical material have revealed many cases of CI that were either undiagnosed or misdiagnosed because the various clinical manifestations of this disorder were not recognized. Us-

TABLE 18–3. CAUSES OF COLONIC ISCHEMIA

Hemodynamic causes
  Cardiogenic shock
  Hemorrhagic shock
  Dysrhythmia
Occlusive causes
  Arterial emboli
  Cholesterol emboli
  Inferior mesenteric artery thrombosis
  Volvulus
  Strangulated hernia
Traumatic causes
  Blunt or penetrating abdominal trauma
  Ruptured ectopic pregnancy
Iatrogenic causes
  Aneurysmectomy
  Aortoiliac reconstruction
  Gynecological operations
  Colonic bypass procedures
  Lumbar aortography
  Coronary angiography or angioplasty
  Colectomy with high ligation of the inferior mesenteric artery
Medications
  Estrogens
  Danazol
  Digitalis
  Vasopressin
  Gold
  Psychotropic drugs
  Cocaine
Vasculitis
  Polyarteritis nodosa
  Systemic lupus erythematosis
  Rheumatoid arthritis and vasculitis
  Takayasu's arteritis
  Thromboangiitis obliterans
Hematological disorders
  Sickle cell anemia
  Protein C and S deficiency
  Antithrombin III deficiency
  Polycythema vera
Other
  Allergy
  Long distance running
  Parasitic infestations

ing the modern clinical, roentgenologic, and pathologic criteria for the diagnosis of colonic ischemia, two retrospective reviews of 154 patients in whom colitis was identified older than 50 years of age revealed that approximately 75% of the patients had probable or definite CI.[75,76] Half of these patients had been erroneously diagnosed as having inflammatory bowel disease.

At Montefiore Medical Center, approximately 50 cases of gastrointestinal ischemia are seen each year and of these cases, 50% to 60% are colonic ischemia. AMI accounts for an additional 30% to 40% of cases, and FSI or chronic MI make up the remainder.[77]

In our experience with more than 300 cases of CI, there is no significant sex predilection. Approximately 90% of patients are above 60 years of age and have other evidence of systemic atherosclerotic disease. This prevalence has been confirmed in other reports.

CI affecting young individuals has been recognized more frequently in case reports or small series. Causes in the younger population include vasculitis (especially systemic lupus erythematosis), medications (estrogens, danazol, vasopression, gold, psychotropic drugs), sickle cell anemia, coagulopathies (thrombotic thrombocytopenic purpura, protein C and protein S deficiency, antithrombin III deficiency, competitive long-distance running and cocaine abuse.[78–90]

CLINICAL PRESENTATION

CI usually presents with the sudden onset of mild, crampy abdominal pain, usually localized to the left lower quadrant. Less commonly, the pain is severe, or conversely, is only elicited retrospectively, if at all. An urgent desire to defecate frequently accompanies the pain and is followed, within 24 hours, by the passage of either bright-red or maroon blood in the stool. The bleeding is not vigorous and blood loss requiring transfusion is so rare that it should suggest an alternative diagnosis. Physical examination may reveal mild to severe abdominal tenderness elicited in the location of the involved segment of bowel.

Any part of the bowel may be affected, but the splenic flexure and descending and sigmoid colon are the most common sites (Fig 18–12). Although specific etiologies, when identified, tend to affect defined areas of the colon, no prognostic implications can be derived from the distribution of the disease. Nonocclusive ischemic injuries usually involve the watershed areas of the colon, the splenic flexure, and the junction of the sigmoid and rectum, whereas ligation of the IMA produces changes in the sigmoid. Similarly, the length of bowel affected varies with the cause. For example, atheromatous emboli result in short segment changes, and nonocclusive injuries usually involve much longer portions of the colon. Depending on the severity and duration of the ischemic insult, the patient may develop fever or leukocytosis. There is usually no acidemia, hypotension, or septic shock. In more severe ischemia, signs of peritonitis may develop.

CLINICAL COURSE

Despite similarities in the initial presentation of most episodes of CI, the outcome cannot be predicted at its onset unless the initial physical findings indicate an unequivocal intra-abdominal catastrophe. The ultimate course of an ischemic insult depends on many factors including (1) the cause (ie, occlusive or nonocclusive), (2) the caliber of an occluded vessel, (3) the duration

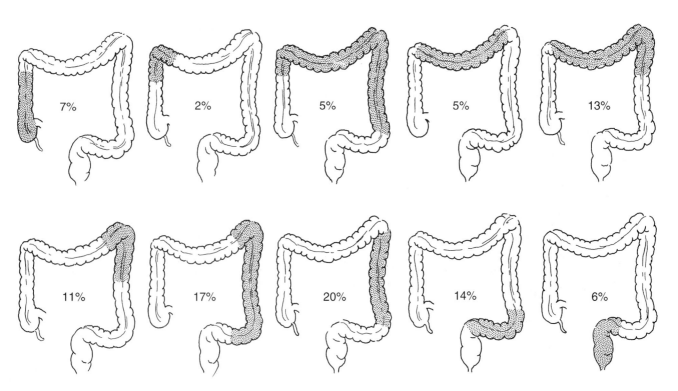

Figure 18–12. Distribution and length of involvement in 300 cases of CI.

and degree of ischemia, (4) the rapidity of onset of ischemia, (5) the condition of the collateral circulation, (6) the metabolic requirements of the affected bowel, (7) the presence and virulence of the bowel flora, and (8) the presence of associated conditions such as colonic distention.

Most commonly, symptoms subside within 24 to 48 hours and clinical, roentgenographic, and endoscopic evidence of healing is seen within two weeks (Fig 18–13). More severe, but still reversible, ischemic damage may take 1 to 6 months to resolve. The majority of patients with reversible disease exhibit only colonic he-

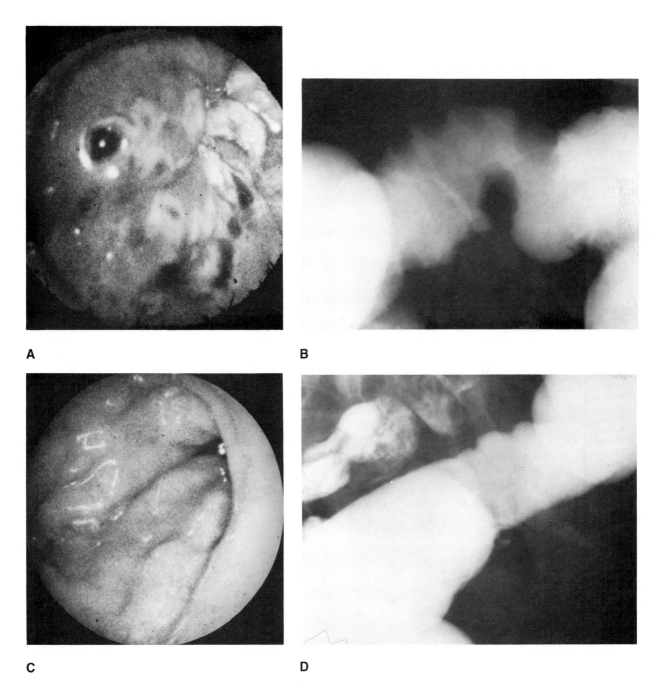

A

B

C

D

Figure 18–13. Ischemic lesion of rectosigmoid. **A**. Sigmoidoscopic appearance of colon at initial examination. Dark nodular mass is a submucosal hemorrhage below which are ulcerations where other areas of hemorrhage have broken down. **B**. Initial barium enema shows typical thumbprints corresponding to submucosal hemorrhages seen at sigmoidoscopy. **C**. Three weeks later, there is complete healing of the rectal mucosa. **D**. Barium enema has returned to normal. (From Littman et al. *Dis Colon Rectum* 1963;6:142)

morrhage or edema, whereas about one-third develop transient colitis. At times, with more severe, yet reversible, ischemia, the entire mucosa may slough as a tube. In half of patients with CI, the ischemic damage is too severe to heal and irreversible disease ultimately develops. In approximately two-thirds of these patients, CI follows a more protracted course, developing into either chronic segmental colitis or ischemic stricture. The remaining one-third develop signs and symptoms of an intra-abdominal catastrophe, such as gangrene with or without perforation, which becomes obvious within hours of the initial presentation.

Patients who develop CI as a complication of shock, congestive heart failure, myocardial infarction, or severe dehydration have a particularly poor prognosis. These patients are typically elderly patients taking digitalis preparations that act as potent splanchnic vasoconstrictors, exacerbating the already compromised colonic perfusion. In one series, these factors were present in 25% of patients with CI. Twelve of 13 patients who presented in shock died.[91]

Because the outcome of an episode of CI usually cannot be predicted, patients must be examined serially for evidence of peritonitis, rising temperature, elevation of white blood cell count or worsening symptoms. Patients with diarrhea or bleeding persisting beyond the first 10 to 14 days usually go on to perforation or, less frequently, a protein-wasting enteropathy. Strictures may develop over weeks to months and may be asymptomatic or produce progressive bowel obstruction. Some of the asymptomatic strictures resolve spontaneously over many months.

DIAGNOSIS

Early and appropriate diagnosis of CI depends upon serial radiographic and/or colonoscopic evaluation of the colon, as well as repeated clinical evaluations of the patient. The more severe cases of CI may be difficult to distinguish from AMI, whereas the less severe cases may present similarly to acute or chronic idiopathic ulcerative colitis, Crohn's colitis, infectious colitis, or diverticulitis. A combination of radiographic, colonoscopic, and clinical findings may be necessary to establish the diagnosis of CI.

In the patient with suspected CI, if abdominal x-rays are nonspecific, sigmoidoscopy is unrevealing and there are no signs of peritonitis, a gentle barium enema or colonoscopy should be performed in the unprepared bowel within 48 hours of the onset of symptoms. The most characteristic finding on barium enema is thumbprinting or pseudotumors (Fig 18–14) and, on colonoscopy, hemorrhagic nodules or bullae during colonoscopy. Hemorrhagic nodules seen at colonoscopy represent bleeding into the submucosa and are equiva-

lent to the thumbprints seen on barium enema. Segmental distribution of these findings, with or without ulceration, is very suggestive of CI. However, the diagnosis of CI cannot be made conclusively on a single study. In fact, persistence of the thumbprints suggests a diagnosis other than CI (eg, lymphoma or amyloidosis).

Repeated radiographic or endoscopic examinations of the colon, together with observation of the clinical course, are necessary to confirm the diagnosis. Segmental colitis associated with a tumor or other potentially or partially obstructing lesion is also characteristic of ischemic disease. The radiographic findings of universal colonic involvement, loss of haustrations, or pseudopolyposis are more typical of chronic idiopathic ulcerative colitis, whereas the presence of skip lesions, linear ulcerations, or fistula suggest Crohn's colitis.

The diagnostic study should be obtained early in the course of the disease because the thumbprinting disappears within days, as the submucosal hemorrhages are either resorbed or evacuated into the colon when the overlying mucosa ulcerates and sloughs. Barium enema or colonoscopy performed 1 week after the initial study should reflect the evolution of the disease, either by a return to normal or by replacement of the thumbprints with a segmental ulcerative colitis pattern.

Caution is warranted if colonoscopy is chosen as the initial study. Distention of the bowel with air to pressures >30 mmHg diminishes colonic blood flow, shunts blood from the mucosa to the serosa, and causes a progressive decrease in the arteriovenous oxygen difference.[92] If intraluminal pressure exceeds 30 mmHg during routine endoscopic examination of the colon,[93] colonoscopy potentially can induce or exacerbate CI. This risk can be minimized by insufflation with carbon dioxide, which increases colonic blood flow at similar pressures. Furthermore, carbon dioxide rapidly is absorbed from the colon, thus decreasing the duration of distention and elevation of the intraluminal pressure.[94]

Biopsies of nodules or bullae identified endoscopically early in the course of CI reveal submucosal hemorrhage, whereas biopsies of the surrounding mucosa usually show nonspecific inflammatory changes.[95] Histologic evidence of mucosal infarction, though rare, is pathognomonic for ischemia. Angiography seldom shows significant occlusions or other abnormalities and is not indicated in patients suspected of having CI. CT may show thickening of the bowel wall, but this finding is not specific for CI.

When the clinical presentation does not allow a clear distinction between CI and AMI, and plain films of the abdomen do not show the characteristic thumbprinting pattern of colonic ischemia, an air enema performed by gently insufflating air into the colon under fluoroscopic

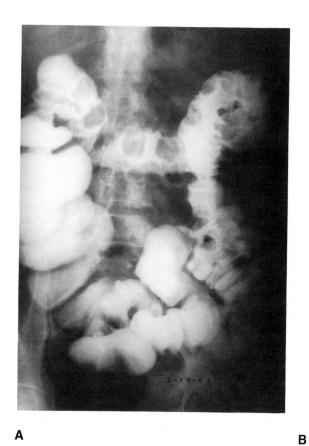

A

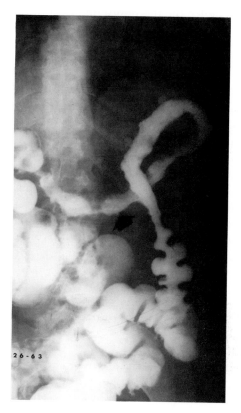

B

C

Figure 18–14. Ischemic changes in transverse colon and splenic flexure. **A**. Initial study shows dramatic "thumbprints" throughout area of involvement. **B**. Eleven days later thumbprints are gone and involved colon has typical appearance of segment colitis including ulcerations (arrow). **C**. Five months after onset there is complete return to normal. Patient was asymptomatic 3 weeks after her illness. (From Boley SJ, et al. Colonic ischemic; reversible ischemic lesion. In: *Vascular Disorders of the Intestine.* New York, NY: Appleton-Century-Crofts; 1971)

observation is obtained. The submucosal edema and hemorrhages that produce the thumbprinting pattern of CI can be accentuated and identified in this manner.

Once the provisional diagnosis of CI is made, a gentle barium enema is performed to determine the site and distribution of the disease, as well as to determine any associated lesion that predisposed to the episode of ischemia (ie, carcinoma, stricture or diverticulitis). If, however, thumbprinting is not observed and the air enema does not suggest the diagnosis of CI, a selective mesenteric angiogram is immediately performed to exclude the diagnosis of AMI. Because AMI progresses rapidly to an irreversible outcome, and optimal diagnosis and treatment of this condition requires angiography, the diagnosis of AMI must be established or excluded prior to a barium study. Residual barium from a contrast study of the colon may obscure the mesenteric vessels and therefore preclude an adequate angiographic examination and intervention.

MANAGEMENT

Acute Management

Once the diagnosis of CI has been established, and the physical examination does not suggest intestinal gangrene or perforation, the patient is treated expectantly. Parenteral fluids are administered and the bowel is placed at rest. Broad-spectrum antibiotics that provide coverage for enterococcus and anaerobic organisms is begun. Antibiotic therapy has been shown to reduce the length of bowel damaged by ischemia, although it will not prevent colonic infarction. Cardiac function is optimized to ensure adequate systemic perfusion. Medications that cause mesenteric vasoconstriction, such as digitalis and vasopressors, should be withdrawn, if possible. Urine output is monitored and maintained with parenteral isotonic fluids. If the colon appears distended, either clinically or radiographically, it can be decompressed with a rectal tube, with or without gentle saline irrigations. Contrary to their efficacy in ulcerative colitis, parenteral corticosteroids are contraindicated because they increase the possibility of perforation and secondary infection. Appropriate management of patients seen during or soon after the ischemic episode requires serial radiographic or endoscopic evaluations of the colon and continued monitoring of the patient.

White blood cell count, hemoglobin and hematocrit measurements should be repeated frequently during the acute episode. Although rarely needed, blood products should be administered according to the requirements of the patient. Serum potassium and magnesium must be monitored, since the levels of these electrolytes may be disturbed by the associated diarrhea and tissue necrosis. Systemic levels of LDH, CPK, SGOT and SGPT may reflect the degree of bowel necrosis, but these serum markers are neither sensitive or specific for CI. Patients having significant diarrhea are begun on parenteral nutrition early. Narcotics should be withheld until it is clear that an intra-abdominal catastrophe is not present and that the patient is clinically improving. Cathartics are contraindicated. No attempt should be made to prepare the bowel for surgery in the acute phase because this may precipitate perforation.

Increasing abdominal tenderness, guarding, rebound tenderness, rising temperature and paralytic ileus during the period of observation suggest colonic infarction. These signs, although not distinct indicators of transmural CI or infarction, dictate the need for expedient laparotomy for resection of the affected segment of colon. At laparotomy, the serosal appearance of infarcted colon ranges from wet tissue paper to mottled, thickened, aperistaltic bowel. The resected specimen should be opened in the operating suite and examined for mucosal injury, and if the margins are involved, additional colon should be removed until the margins appear grossly normal.

Reversible Lesions. In the mildest cases of CI, in which signs and symptoms of illness disappear within 24 to 48 hours, submucosal and intramural hemorrhages are resorbed, and there is complete clinical and radiographic resolution within 1 to 2 weeks (Fig 18–14), no further therapy is indicated. More severe ischemic insults result in necrosis of the overlying mucosa with ulceration and inflammation and the subsequent development of a segmental ulcerative colitis. Varying amounts of mucosa may slough and may ultimately heal during the course of several months. Patients with such protracted healing may be clinically asymptomatic, even in the presence of persistent radiographic or endoscopic evidence of disease. These asymptomatic patients are placed on a high-residue diet and frequent follow-up evaluations are performed to confirm complete healing, the development of a stricture or persistent colitis. Recurrent episodes of sepsis in asymptomatic patients with unhealed areas of segmental colitis usually are caused by the diseased segment of bowel and are an indication for elective resection.

Irreversible Lesions. Patients with persistent diarrhea, rectal bleeding, protein-losing enteropathy or recurrent sepsis for more than 10 to 14 days usually go on to develop perforation. Hence, early resection is indicated to prevent this complication. A polyethylene glycol bowel preparation is administered along with oral and intravenous antibiotics prior to surgery. Again, enemas should not be used to prepare the bowel.

Despite a normal serosal appearance, there may be extensive mucosal injury and the extent of resection should be guided by the distribution of disease as seen on the preoperative studies rather than by the appearance of the serosal surface of the colon at the time of operation. As in all resections for CI, the specimen must be opened at the time of operation to insure normal mucosa at the margins. If, at the time of surgery, the segmental ulcerative colitis involves the rectum, a mucous fistula or Hartmann's procedure with an end colostomy should be performed. The mucous fistula can be fashioned through diseased bowel and, in some cases, this segment will heal sufficiently to allow subsequent restoration of bowel continuity. Local steroid enemas may be helpful in this setting; however, parenteral steroids are, again, contraindicated. A simultaneous proctocolectomy rarely is indicated, except in cases of CI following abdominal aortic replacement.

In those instances in which the patient has had a concurrent or recent myocardial infarction, or if the patient has major medical contraindications to surgery, a trial of prolonged parenteral nutrition with concomitant intravenous antibiotic therapy may be considered as an alternative method of management.

Late Management

Chronic or Persistent Ischemic Colitis.
CI may not manifest clinical symptoms during the acute insult but may still produce chronic segmental colitis. Patients with this form of CI may be misdiagnosed frequently, if not seen during the acute episode. Barium enema studies may show a segmental colitis pattern, a stricture simulating a carcinoma or even an area of pseudopolyposis (Fig 18–15). The clinical course, at this stage of disease, is often indistinguishable from other causes of colitis or stenosis, unless the patient has been followed from the time of the acute episode. Crypt abscesses and pseudopolyposis usually considered histologically diagnostic of chronic idiopathic ulcerative colitis also can be seen in ischemic colitis. Regardless, the de novo occurrence of a segmental area of colitis or stricture in an elderly patient should be considered most likely ischemic and should be treated accordingly.

The natural history of noninfectious segmental colitis in the elderly is that of ischemic colitis; the involvement remains localized, resection is not followed by recurrence, and the response to steroid therapy is usually poor. Patients with chronic segmental ischemic colitis initially are managed symptomatically. Local steroid enemas may be helpful, but parenteral steroids should be avoided. In patients whose symptoms cannot be controlled by medication, segmental resection of the diseased bowel should be performed.

Ischemic Strictures.
Patients with asymptomatic segmental colitis may go on to develop a stenosis or stricture of the colon. Strictures that produce no symptoms should be observed. Some of these will return to normal

in 12 to 24 months with no further therapy. If, however, symptoms of obstruction develop, a segmental resection is required.

Management of Specific Clinical Problems

CI Complicating Abdominal Aortic Surgery.
Mesenteric vascular reconstruction is not indicated in most cases of colonic ischemia, but it may be required to prevent CI during and after aortic reconstruction. Following elective aneurysmectomy, 3% to 7% of patients develop colonoscopic evidence of colonic ischemia.[96,97] The incidence of CI following repair of ruptured aortic aneurysms has been reported to be as high as 60%.[98] Although clinical evidence of this complication occurs in only 1% to 2% of patients, when it does occur it is responsible for approximately 10% of the deaths following aortic replacement.[99] Factors that contribute to the occurrence of postoperative CI include rupture of the aneurysm, hypotension, operative trauma to the colon, hypoxemia, arrhythmias, prolonged cross-clamp time, and improper management of the IMA during aneurysmectomy.

The most important aspect of management of CI following aortic surgery is its prevention. Collateral blood flow to the left colon after occlusion of the IMA comes from the SMA via the arc of Riolan ("the meandering artery") or the marginal artery of Drummond, and from the internal iliac arteries via the middle and inferior hemorrhoidal arteries. If these collateral pathways are intact, postoperative CI can be minimized. Therefore, aortography as well as a full mechanical and antibiotic bowel preparation are essential prior to aortic reconstruction. Aortography is advised to determine the patency of the celiac axis, SMA, IMA, and internal iliac artery is advisable. The presence of a meandering artery does not, in and of itself, allow safe ligation of the IMA, since the blood flow in the meandering artery frequently originates from the IMA and reconstitutes an obstructed SMA. Ligation of the IMA in the latter circumstance can be catastrophic with infarction of the small and large bowel (Fig 18–16a). Ligation of the IMA is safe only when it has been confirmed angiographically that the blood flows in the meandering artery from the SMA to the IMA. Reimplantation of the IMA and revascularization of the SMA is required, therefore, in those instances when the SMA is occluded or tightly stenosed, and the IMA provides inflow to the meandering artery (Fig 18–16b).

Occlusion of both hypogastric arteries on the preoperative arteriogram indicates that the rectal blood flow is dependent upon collateral flow from the IMA or from the SMA via the meandering artery. In this circumstance, reconstitution of flow to one or both hypogastric arteries is desirable at the time of aneurysmectomy (Fig 18–16c).

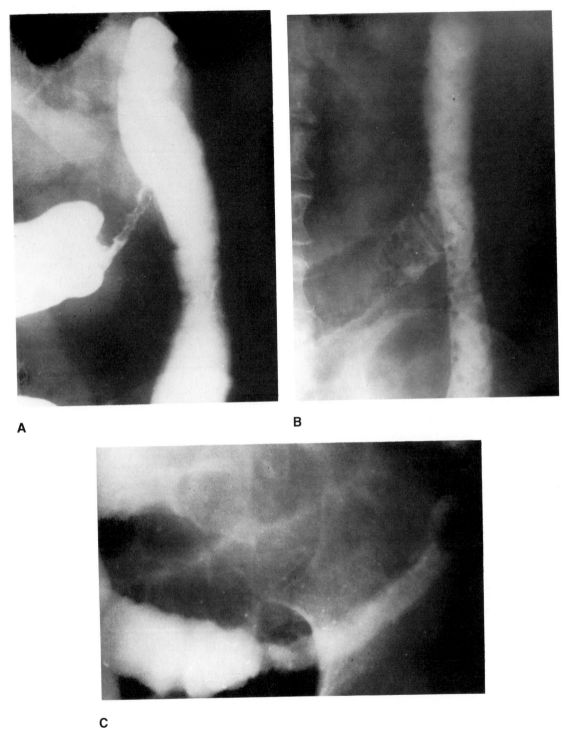

Figure 18–15. Barium enema appearance of irreversible ischemic lesions, of the colon. **A**. Ischemic stricture with characteristics of carcinoma. **B**. Chronic segmental ischemic colitis. **C**. Pseudopolyposis in segment of ischemic colitis. (Courtesy of L Kesner, Buenos Aires, Argentina.)

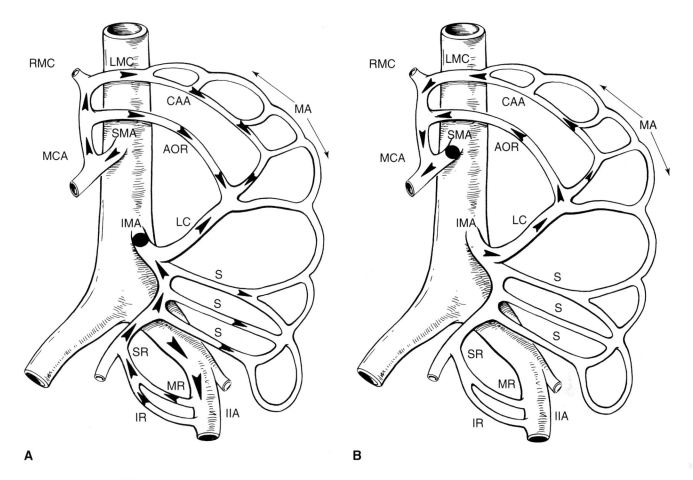

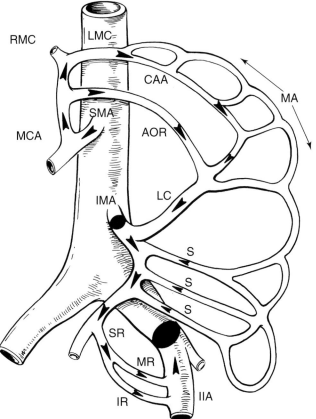

A

B

C

Figure 18–16. Collateral blood flow to the colon. **A.** Collateral blood flow from the marginal artery, arc of Roilan, and internal iliac artery via the inferior and middle rectal arteris to an occluded IMA. **B.** Collateral blood flow from the IMA via the marginal artery and the Arc of Roilan to an occluded SMA. **C.** The entire rectal blood flow dependent on collateral flow due to occlusion of both internal iliac arteris. In this figure, the IMA is also occluded leaving the rectal flow dependent on collateral flow from the SMA via the arc of Roilan and marginal artery and then via the superior rectal vessel to the middle and inferior rectal arteris. (MCA: middle colic artery; RMC: right branch of middle colic artery; LMC: left branch of the middle colic artery; CAA: central anastomotic artery; AOR: arc of Roilan (meandering artery); MA: marginal artery of Drummond; SMA: superior mesenteric artery; IMA: Inferior mesenteric artery; LC: left colic artery; S: sigmoid branches; SR: superior rectal artery; MR: middle rectal artery; IR: inferior rectal artery; IIA: internal iliac artery (hypogastric artery).

At operation, cross-clamp time should be minimized and hypotension must be avoided. If a meandering artery is identified, it should be preserved carefully. Because the serosal appearance of the colon is not a reliable indicator of collateral blood flow, several methods have been suggested to determine the need for IMA reimplantation. Stump pressure in the transected IMA >40 mm Hg or a mean IMA stump pressure to mean systemic blood pressure ratio >0.40 indicates adequate collateral circulation and can be used reliably to avoid IMA reimplantation.[100] Doppler ultrasound flow signals at the base of the mesentery and at the serosal surface of the colon with temporary IMA inflow occlusion also suggest that the IMA can be ligated safely without reimplantation.

Tonometric determination of intramural pH of the sigmoid colon has been used to identify inadequate colonic blood flow during aneurysmectomy.[101,102] A tonometric balloon passed into the sigmoid colon through the anus prior to cross-clamping the aorta enables one to evaluate the effect that occlusion and restoration of aortic flow has on the colonic intramural pH. The intramural pH is a metabolic marker of tissue acidosis, and will reflect any clinically significant ischemia, thus indicating the need for revascularization while the abdomen is open. An abnormal tonometric study of the sigmoid colon, the loss of arterial pulsation, or a decreased transcolonic oxygen saturation following aortic surgery are indications for reimplantation of the IMA. When IMA reimplantation is deemed necessary, the IMA should be excised with a patch of aortic wall (Carrell patch). The patch should be sutured into the side of the aortic prosthesis.

If it is occluded, the SMA can be revascularized by reimplantation into the graft wall, or alternatively, by creating a lateral extension of the prosthesis and performing an end-to-side anastomosis to the SMA. Liberal use of these adjunctive procedures has, in one prospective study, both substantially reduced the incidence of CI and eliminated it as a cause of death following aortic surgery.

The difficulty in accurately assessing CI postoperatively and the significant mortality associated with its occurrence mandates that postoperative colonoscopy be performed in high-risk patients. Patients at high risk for developing postoperative CI following aortic reconstruction are those with ruptured abdominal aortic aneurysms, prolonged cross-clamping time, a patent IMA on preoperative aortography, nonpulsatile flow in the hypogastric arteries at operation, and postoperative diarrhea. In these cases, colonoscopy is performed routinely within 2 to 3 days of the operation, and if CI is identified, therapy is begun before major complications develop. Clinical deterioration indicating progression of the ischemic insult to transmural necrosis necessi-

tates reoperation. These patients should undergo resection and colostomy. Primary anastomosis is contraindicated owing to the potential contamination of the aortic prosthesis in the event of an anastomotic leak. If the rectum is involved, it too must be resected. Every effort should be taken to protect the aortic graft from contamination. As such, the retroperitoneum overlying the graft should be reperitonealized utilizing local tissues or the omentum.

Fulminating Universal Colitis. A rare fulminating form of CI involving all or most of the colon and rectum has been recently identified in a few patients. These patients present with sudden onset of a toxic universal colitis. Bleeding, fever, severe diarrhea, abdominal pain, and tenderness, often with signs of peritonitis, have been present. The clinical course is rapidly progressive. The management of this condition is similar to that of other forms of fulminating colitis. Total abdominal colectomy with an ileostomy is usually required. A second-stage proctectomy has been necessary in some patients within 1 month of the original surgery. The histologic appearance of the resected colon is a combination of ischemic changes, severe ulcerating colitis, and necrosis.

Lesions Mimicking Colon Carcinoma. Ischemic colitis can present with lesions that appear, on barium enema and colonoscopy, as colon carcinoma. Colonoscopy may be able to distinguish the malignant lesions from those resulting from ischemic cicatrization and is advisable when an annular lesion is identified on barium enema. The treatment is local resection with immediate restoration of bowel continuity.

Colitis Associated with Colon Carcinoma. Acute colitis in patients with carcinoma of the colon has been recognized for many years.[103] The colitis is usually, but not always, proximal to the tumor and occurs with and without clinical obstruction. It is of ischemic origin and has the radiologic and endoscopic appearance of ischemic colitis. Clinically, patients may present with symptoms of CI or with symptoms related to the primary cancer, such as crampy pain of a chronic nature, bleeding, or acute colonic obstruction. In most cases, however, the predominant complaints are related to the ischemic episode: sudden onset of mild to moderate abdominal pain, fever, bloody diarrhea, and abdominal tenderness. It is imperative that both the radiologist and surgeon be aware of the frequent association of CI and colon cancer. The radiologist must be careful to exclude cancer in every case of CI, and the surgeon must be careful to examine any colon resected for cancer to exclude the presence of an ischemic process in the area of the anastomosis, since involvement may lead to stricture or a leak.

CI as a Manifestation of AMI. CI localized to the right side of the colon may be a manifestation of AMI. If a thumbprinting pattern or colonoscopy reveals that there is evidence of CI isolated to the right colon, we consider this an indication for selective mesenteric angiography before discharge to evaluate the status of the SMA. Demonstration of a partially or completely obstructed SMA is an indication for revascularization of this artery.

REFERENCES

1. Redfors S, Hallback DA, Haglund U, et al. Blood flow distribution, villous tissue osmolality and fluid and electrolyte transport in the cat intestine during regional hypotension. *Acta Physiol Scand* 1963;57:270–277

2. Lundgren O, Svanik J. Mucosal hemodynamics in the small intestine of the cat during reduced perfusion pressure. *Acta Physiol Scand* 1979;88:551

3. Folkow B. Regional adjustments of intestinal blood flow. *Gastroenterology* 1967;52:423

4. Shephard AP, Granger DN. Metabolic regulation of the intestinal circulation. In: Shepherd AP, Granger DN (eds), Physiology of the Splanchnic Circulation. New York, NY: Raven, 1984:384

5. Boley SJ. Unpublished data

6. Poole JW, Sammartano RJ, Boley SJ. The use of tonometry in the early diagnosis of mesenteric ischemia. *Curr Surg* 1987;44:21–24

7. Geber WF. Quantitative measurements of blood flow in various areas of the small and large bowel. *Am J Physiol* 1960;198:985–989

8. Delaney JP, Leonard AS. Hypothalamic influence on gastrointestinal blood flow in the awake cat. *Fed Proc* 1970;29:260–266

9. Chiu CJ, McArdle AH, Brown R, et al. Intestinal mucosal lesion in low flow states, I: a morphological hemodynamic, and metabolic reappraisal. *Arch Surg* 1970;101:478–483

10. Dahlberg PJ, Kisken WA, Newcomer KL, et al. Mesenteric ischemia in chronic dialysis patients. *Am J Nephrol* 1985;5:327–332

11. Dumazer P, Dueymes JM, Vernier I, et al. Ischemie mesenterique non occlusive chez l'hemodialyse periodique. *Press Med* 1989;18:471–474

12. Boley SJ, Regan JA, Tunick PA, et al. Persistent vasoconstriction: a major factor in nonocclusive mesenteric ischemia. *Curr Topics Surg Res* 1971;3:425–430

13. Selkurt EE, Scibetta MP, Cull TE. Hemodynamics of intestinal circulation. *Circ Res* 1958;6:92–99

14. Laufman H. Significance of vasospasm in vascular occlusion, thesis. Northwestern University Medical School, Chicago, 1948

15. Brown RA, Chiu C, Scott HJ, et al. Ultrastructural changes in the canine ileal mucosal cell after mesenteric artery occlusion. *Arch Surg* 1970;101:290–296

16. Ahren C, Haglund U. Mucosal lesions in the small intestine of the cat during low flow. *Acta Physiol Scand* 1973;88:1–9

17. Granger DN, McCord JM, Parks DA, et al. Xanthine oxidase inhibitors attenuate ischemia induced vascular permeability changes in the cat intestine. *Gastroenterology* 1986;90:80–84

18. Crissinger DK, Granger DN. Mucosal injury induced by ischemia and reperfusion in the piglet intestine: influence of the age and feeding. *Gastroenterology* 1989;97:920–926

19. Parks DA, Grogaard B, Granger DN. Comparison of partial and complete arterial occlusion models for studying intestinal ischemia. *Surgery* 1982;92:896–901

20. Bulkley GB, Kvietys PR, Parks DA, et al. Relationship of blood flow and oxygen consumption to ischemic injury in the canine small intestine. *Gastroenterology* 1985;89:852–857

21. Gaussorgues P, Guerugniand PY, Vedrinne JM, et al. Bacteremia following cardiac arrest and cardiopulmonary resuscitation. *Intensive Care Med* 1988;14:575–580

22. Thompson JS, Bragg LE, West WW. Serum enzyme levels during intestinal ischemia. *Ann Surg* 1990;369–373

23. Smerud MJ, Johnson CD, Stephens DH. Diagnosis of bowel infarction: a comparison of plain films and CT scans in 23 cases. *Am J Roentgenol* 1990;154:99–102

24. Serreyn RF, Schoofs PR, Baetens PR, et al. Laparoscopic diagnosis of mesenteric venous thrombosis. *Endoscopy* 1986;18:249–251

25. Segelman SS, Sprayregen S, Boley SJ. Angiographic diagnosis of mesenteric arterial vasoconstriction. *Radiology* 1974;122:533–540

26. Stolar CJ, Randolph JG. Evaluation of ischemic bowel viability with a fluorescent technique. *J Pediatr Surg* 1978;13:221–225

27. Carter M, Fantini G, Sammartano RJ, et al. Qualitative and quantitative fluorescein fluorescence for determining intestinal viability. *Am J Surg* 1984;147:117–121

28. Shah S, Andersen C. Prediction of small bowel, I viability using Doppler ultrasound. *Ann Surg* 1981;194:97–101

29. Brolin RE, Semmelow JL, Koch RA, et al. Myoelectric assessment of bowel viability. *Surgery* 1987;102:32–38

30. Shaw RS. The "second look" after superior mesenteric arterial embolectomy or reconstruction for mesenteric infarction. In: Ellison EH, Frieser SR, Mulholland JH (eds), *Current Surgical Management*. Philadelphia, PA: WB Saunders; 1965:509

31. Sachs SM, Morton JH, Schwartz SI. Acute mesenteric ischemia. *Surgery* 1982;92:646–653

32. Wells CL. Relationship between intestinal microecology and the translocation of intestinal bacteria. Antonie Van Leeuwenhoek 1990;58:87–93

33. Cohn I, Floyd CE, Dresden CF, et al. Strangulation obstruction in germ-free animals. *Ann Surg* 1962;156:692

34. Vijic I, Stanley J, Gobien RP. Treatment of acute embolus of the superior mesenteric artery by topical infusion of streptokinase. *Cardiovasc Intervent Radiol* 1984;7:94–96

35. Becker GJ, Katzen BT, Dake MD. Noncoronary angioplasty. *Radiology* 1989;170:921–924

36. Clark RA, Gallant TE. Acute mesenteric ischemia: angiographic spectrum. *Am J Roentgenol* 1984;142:555–562

37. Boley SJ, Sprayregan S, Seigelman SS, et al. Initial results

from an aggressive roentgenological and surgical approach to acute mesenteric ischemia. *Surgery* 1977;82: 848–855

38. Hibbard JS, Swenson JC, Levin AG. Roentgenology of mesenteric vascular occlusion. *Arch Surg* 1933;26:20

39. Kovekar G, Reichow W, Becker HD. Ergebnisse der therapie des akuten mesenterialgefassverschlusses. *Langenbecks Arch Chir* 1985;366:536–539

40. Levy PJ, Krausz MM, Manny J. Acute mesenteric ischemia: improved results: a retrospective analysis of 92 patients. *Surgery* 1990;107:373–380

41. Batellier J, Kieny R. Superior mesenteric artery embolism: 82 cases. *Ann Vasc Surg* 1990;4:112–116

42. Finucane PM, Arunachalam T, O'Down J, et al. Acute mesenteric infarction in elderly patients. *J Am Geriatr Soc* 1989;37:355–358

43. Goergiev G. Acute obstruction of the mesenteric vessels: a diagnostic and therapeutic problem. *Khirugiia* 1989;42: 23–29

44. Paes E, Vollmar JF, Hutsehenreiter S, et al. Der Mesenterialinfarkt: Neue Apekte der Diagnosik und therapie. *Chirurgie* 1988;59:828–835

45. Clavien PA, Muller C. Infarctus mesenterique: etude retrospective sur 17 ans. *Schweiz Med Wochenschr* 1986;116: 977–981

46. Rogers DM, Thompson JE, Garrett WV, et al. Mesenteric vascular problems: a 26 year experience. *Ann Surg* 1982; 554–565

47. Krausz MM, Manny J. Acute superior mesenteric arterial occlusion: a plea for early diagnosis. *Surgery* 1978;83: 482–485

48. Cunningham CG, Reilly LM, Stoney R. Chronic visceral ischemia. *Surg Clin North Am* 1992;72:231–244

49. Hansen HJB, Christofferson JK. Occlusive mesenteric infarction: a retrospective study of 83 cases. *Acta Chir Scand* 1976;472(suppl):103–108

50. White R, Boley SJ. Mesenteric venous thrombosis (MVT): an unusual cause of acute mesenteric ischemia. Presented at the 50th Annual Scientific Meeting of the American College of Gastroenterology, Philadelphia, PA; October 9–11, 1985

51. Abdu RA, Zakhour BJ, Dallis DJ. Mesenteric venous thrombosis; 1911–1984. *Surgery* 1987;101:383–388

52. Broekman AW, van Rooyen W, Westerfeld BD, et al. *Gastroenterology* 1988;92:240–242

53. Harward TRS, Green D, Bergen JJ, et al. Mesenteric venous thrombosis. *J Vasc Surg* 1989;9:328–333

54. Kaleya RN, Boley SJ. Mesenteric venous thrombosis. In: Najarian JS, Delaney JP (eds), *Progress in Gastrointestinal Surgery*. Chicago, IL: Year Book Medical; 1989:417–425

55. Clavien PA, Durig M, Harder F. Venous mesenteric thrombosis: a particular entity. *Br J Surg* 1988;75:252–255

56. Clavien PA, Huber O, Mirescu, et al. Contrast enhanced CT scan as a diagnostic procedure in mesenteric ischemia due to mesenteric venous thrombosis. *Br J Surg* 1989; 76:93–94

57. Sack J, Aldrete JS. Primary mesenteric venous thrombosis. *Surg Gynecol Obstet* 1982;154:205–208

58. Matthews J, White RR. Primary mesenteric venous occlusive disease. *Am J Surg* 1971;122:579–583

59. Bertina RM. Hereditary protein S deficiency. *Hemostasis* 1985;15:241–245

60. Johnson CC, Baggenstoss AH. Mesenteric venous occlusion: study of 99 cases of occlusion of veins. *Mayo Clin Proc* 1949;24:628–636

61. Warshaw AL, Gongliang J, Ottinger LW. Recognition and clinical implications of mesenteric and portal vein obstruction in chronic pancreatitis. *Arch Surg* 1987;122: 410–415

62. Anane-Sehaf JC, Blair E. Primary mesenteric venous occlusive disease. *Surg Gynec Obstet* 1975;141:740–742

63. Clemett AR, Chang J. The radiological diagnosis of spontaneous mesenteric venous thrombosis. *Am J Gastroenterol* 1975;63:209–215

64. Kidambi H, Herbert R, Kidami AV. Ultrasonic demonstration of superior mesenteric and splenoportal venous thrombosis. *J Clin Ultrasound* 1986;14:199–201

65. Matos C, Van Gansbeke D, Zalcman M, et al. Mesenteric venous thrombosis: early CT and ultrasound diagnosis and conservative management. *Gastrointest Radiol* 1986; 11:322–325

66. Rosen A, Korobkin M, Silverman PM, et al. Mesenteric vein thrombosis: CT identification. *Am J Roentgenol* 1984; 143:83–86

67. Al Karawi MA, Quaiz M, Clark D, et al. Mesenteric vein thrombosis: noninvasive diagnosis and followup (US + CT) and noninvasive therapy by streptokinase and anticoagulants. *Hepatogastroenterology* 1990;37:507–509

68. Smith RW, Selby JB. Scintiangiographic diagnosis of acute mesenteric ischemia. *Am J Roentgenol* 1979;132:67–69

69. Verbanck JJ, Rutgeerts LJ, Haerens MH, et al. Partial splenoportal and superior mesenteric venous thrombosis: early sonographic diagnosis and successful conservative management. *Gastroenterology* 1984;86:949–952

70. Khodadadi J, Rosencwaig J, Nissim N, et al. Mesenteric venous thrombosis: the importance of a second look. *Arch Surg* 1989;112:315–317

71. Bergentz S, Ericsson B, Hedner U, et al. Thrombosis in the superior mesenteric and portal veins: report of a case treated with thrombectomy. *Surgery* 1974;76:286–290

72. Lanthier P, Lepot M, Mahieu P. Mesenteric venous thrombosis presenting as a neurological problem. *Acta Clin Belg* 1984;29:92–95

73. Quirke P, Campbell I, Talbot IC. Ischaemic proctitis and adventitial fibromuscular dysplasia of the superior rectal artery. *Br J Surg* 1984;71:33–35

74. Binns JC, Issacson P. Age-related changes in the colonic blood supply: their relevance to ischemic colitis. *Gut* 1978;19:384–388

75. Brandt LJ, Boley SJ, Goldberg L, et al. Colitis in the elderly. *Am J Gastroenterol* 1981;76:239–246

76. Wright HG. Ulcerating colitis in the elderly: epidemiological and clinical study of an in-patient hospital population. New Haven, CT: Yale University, 1970. Submitted in thesis for MD degree.

77. Brandt LJ, Boley SJ. Colonic ischemia. *Surg Clin North Am* 1992;72:203–229

78. Ho MS, Teh LB, Goh HS. Ischaemic colitis in systemic lupus erythematosis: report of a case and review of the literature. *Ann Acad Med Singapore* 1987;16:501–505

79. Tedesco FJ, Volpicelli NA, Moore FS. Estrogen and progesterone associated colitis: a disorder with clinical and endoscopic features mimicking Crohn's colitis. *Gastrointest Endosc* 1982;28:247–250

80. Barcewicz PA, Welch JP. Ischemic colitis in young adult patients. *Dis Colon Rectum* 1980;23:109–112

81. Miyata T, Tamechika Y, Torisu M. Ischemic colitis in a 33 year old woman on danazol treatment for endometriosis. *Am J Gastroenterol* 1988;83:1420–1422

82. Schmitt W, Wagner-Thiessen E, Lux G. Ischaemic colitis in a patient treated with glypresin for bleeding oesophageal varices. *Hepatogastroenterology* 1987;34:134–136

83. Wright A, Benfield GF, Felix-Davies D. Ischaemic colitis and immune complexes during gold therapy for rheumatoid arthritis. *Ann Rheum Dis* 1984;43:495–499

84. Gollock JM, Thompson JP. Ischaemic colitis associated with psychotropic drugs. *Postgrad Med J* 1984;26:449–453

85. Gage TP, Gagnier JM. Ischemic colitis complicating sickle cell crisis. *Gastroenterology* 1983;84:171–175

86. Dubois A, Lyonnet P, Cohendy R, et al. Ischemic colitis as a manifestation of Moschkowitz's syndrome. *Ann Gastroenterol Hepatol* 1989;25:19–22

87. Blanc P, Bories P, Donadio D, et al. Colite ischemique et throboses veineuses recidivante par deficit familial en proteine S [Letter]. *Gastroenterol Clin Biol* 1989;13:945

88. Knot E, Tencate J, Bruin T, et al. Antithrombin III metabolism in two colitis patients with acquired antithrombin III deficiency. *Gastroenterology* 1985;89:421–425

89. Heer M, Repond F, Hany A, et al. Acute ischemic colitis in a female long distance runner. *Gut* 1987;28:264–267

90. Fishel R, Hamamoto G, Barbul A, et al. Cocaine colitis: is this a new syndrome? *Dis Colon Rectum* 1985;28:264–267

91. Guttorson NL, Bubrick MP. Mortality from colonic ischemia. *Dis Colon Rectum* 1989;32:469–472

92. Boley SJ, Agrawal GP, Warren AR, et al. Pathophysiological effects of bowel distension on intestinal blood flow. *Am J Surg* 1969;117:226–234

93. Kozarek RA, Ernest DL, Silverman ME. Air pressure induced colon injury during diagnostic colonoscopy. *Gastroenterology* 1980;78:7–11

94. Brandt LJ, Boley SJ, Sammartano RJ. Carbon dioxide and room air insufflation of the colon. *Gastrointest Endosc* 1986;32:324–326

95. Boley SJ, Brandt LJ, Veith FJ. Ischemic disorders of the intestine. *Curr Prob Surg* 1978;15:1–85

96. Ernst CB, Hagihara PF, Daugherty ME, et al. Ischemic colitis incidence following abdominal aortic reconstruction: a prospective study. *Surgery* 1976;80:417–423

97. Zelenock GB, Strodel WE, Knol JA, et al. A prospective study of clinically and endoscopically documented colonic ischemia in 100 patients undergoing aortic reconstructive surgery with aggressive and direct pelvic revascularization comparison with historic controls. *Surgery* 1989;106:771–776

98. Hagihara PF, Ernst CB, Griffen WB. Incidence of ischemic colitis following abdominal aortic reconstruction. *Surg Gynecol Obstet* 1979;149:571–575

99. Kim MW, Hundahl SA, Dang CR, et al. Ischemic colitis following aortic aneurysmectomy. *Am J Surg* 1983;145:392–397

100. Erns CB, Hagihara PF, Daugherty ME, et al. Inferior mesenteric artery stump pressure: a reliable index for safe IMA ligation during abdominal aortic aneurysmectomy. *Ann Surg* 1978;187:641–645

101. Fiddian-Green RG, Amelin PM, Hermann JB. Prediction of the development of sigmoid ischemia on the day of aortic surgery. *Arch Surg* 1986;121:654

102. Poole JW, Sammartano RJ, Boley SJ, et al. The use of tonometry to detect sigmoid ischemia during aneurysmectomy. Presented at the New York Surgical Society; November, 1987

103. Teitjen GW, Markowitz AM. Colitis proximal to obstructing colonic carcinoma. *Arch Surg* 1975;110:1133

19

Abdominal Aneurysms

John J. Ricotta

While abdominal aneurysm remains one of the less common causes of abdominal pain, the dire consequences of delayed diagnosis and management should keep this entity prominent in the differential diagnosis. Aneurysms represent a degeneration of the arterial wall. The multiple potential etiologies of this degeneration include infection, atherosclerosis, increased protease activity within the aneurysm wall,[1,2] and genetically regulated defects in collagen or fibrillin.[3,4] There are three major clinical manifestations of aneurysmal disease: rupture, thrombosis, and embolization. Concern over these complications underlies the rationale for elective treatment of aneurysmal disease.

Clinical options for management of the patient with an abdominal aneurysm include observation, ligation, or resection with bypass. Recently, endoluminal approaches, including the use of stent-anchored grafts, have been applied in selected patients.[5] These new approaches await long-term evaluation, but represent techniques that may significantly change the management of aneurysmal disease in the future.

■ INFRARENAL ABDOMINAL AORTIC ANEURYSM

The infrarenal aorta is the most common site for development of aneurysmal disease. It has been suggested that the hemodynamic forces that result from the lack of major visceral outflow and the configuration of the aortic bifurcation, coupled with a reduced number of elastic lamellae in the vessel wall, explain the increased proclivity of this location to aneurysmal disease.[6] Aortic aneurysms are more common in males (4:1)[7] and often are grouped in kindreds, suggesting a sex-linked inheritance, in some cases.[8,9] The incidence of aortic aneurysms in males >65 years of age is estimated at 2% to 4%,[10,11] an observation that has prompted Scott to suggest a single-screening ultrasound in this age group.[11] Aneurysmal change in the abdominal aorta is often (approximately 10%) accompanied by changes in the iliac vessels, and somewhat less often (5% to 10%), by changes in the popliteal arteries. Conversely, popliteal aneurysms are frequently associated with aortic disease (15% to 20%)[12]; when the former is identified, a search for abdominal aneurysm should be undertaken.

PRESENTATION

The majority of aortic aneurysms are identified as a painless pulsatile mass on physical examination. The threshold size for detection by physical examination is 4 to 6 cm diameter, depending on body habitus. It is important to determine the cephalad extent of the aneurysm whenever possible. In the majority of infrarenal aneurysms, a superior margin can be delineated below the costal margin; if this is not the case, suprarenal extension must be suspected. The lateral margins of the aneurysm are determined by placing the fingers of the examining hands on either side of the mass, and lateral pulsation (in contrast to anterior pulsation) will usually differentiate a true aneurysm from a tortuous aorta. In general, physical examination slightly overestimates aortic diameter.[13]

Symptoms of an expanding or ruptured aortic aneurysm can mimic virtually any abdominal or retroperitoneal process. Most common symptoms are those of back, flank or loin pain from pressure on retroperitoneal structures, nerves, or even spinal cord. This pain may radiate into the thigh or testicle. Abdominal symptoms may mimic peptic disease, pancreatitis, or diverticulitis. As a general rule, the diagnosis of an expanding aneurysm should be considered in any patient who presents with abdominal, back or flank pain, particularly if there is a suggestion of a pulsatile mass. Patients presenting with a history of syncope are particularly worrisome. This often signifies an initial episode of bleeding that temporarily is compensated. These patients usually come to the hospital with stable vital signs and then suddenly deteriorate. If a mass is felt in these cases, urgent surgery is indicated.

Less common presentations of aortic aneurysm include thrombosis or distal embolization, both of which manifest as extremity ischemia. The best known instance of this is the "blue-toe" syndrome. In this situation, small emboli from the aneurysm lodge in the digital vessels producing distal ischemia in the setting of palpable pedal pulses. Less common is profound lower extremity ischemia from thrombosis of the aortic aneurysm itself, or more often, from a larger embolus to one of the major leg vessels. Ischemia also can result from thrombosis of a popliteal aneurysm which may lead indirectly to the discovery of an aortic aneurysm.

DIAGNOSTIC EVALUATION

Imaging studies including plain x-rays, ultrasound, computerized tomography (CT), magnetic resonance imaging (MRI), and angiography all can be used to supplement physical examination. A large number of aneurysms (60% to 70%) contain calcium in their walls that can be seen on abdominal x-rays or lateral spine films (Fig 19–1). However, this is usually not sufficient to accurately measure size. Ultrasound provides the least expensive means to determine aneurysm diameter,[13] the most important determinant of rupture risk, but provides little additional information (Fig 19–2). It usually is used when the initial diagnosis is in doubt, or to follow aneurysm growth when resection is deferred. However, ultrasound alone rarely provides sufficient information to plan operative intervention.

CT scan remains the diagnostic modality of choice in patients who are being considered for aneurysm resection (Fig 19–3).[14] It provides an accurate measure of aneurysm diameter, and wall thickness. In addition, it is useful in evaluating the possibility of retroperitoneal rupture. CT also will demonstrate the proximal and dis-

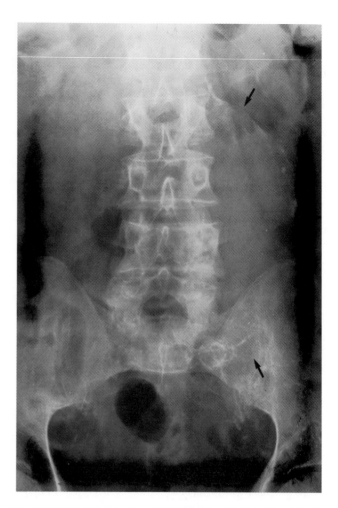

Figure 19–1. Plain abdominal radiograph demonstrating calcification of the aortic wall. Some calcification can be seen in 60% to 70% of aortic aneurysms.

tal extent of aortic disease, the degree of aortic calcification, and the majority of concomitant retroperitoneal (kidney, pancreas) or intra-abdominal processes which may be confused, or coexist, with aneurysmal disease. When contrast is administered, renal size and function can be estimated. Finally, CT provides important information about venous anatomy, particularly anomalies of the vena cava and renal veins (eg, left-sided vena cava, retroaortic left renal vein) which occur in 2% to 5% of patients (Fig 19–3).[15] This study remains the current standard for preoperative evaluation.

MRI shares many of the attributes of CT scanning and also may be used in preoperative evaluation.[16] In general, however, it is less available, more expensive and adds little to CT evaluation. One advantage of MRI is a software adaptation (MR angiography) that allows visualization of flow in the aorta and its branches. At present, however, this remains a potential, rather than real, advantage.

MRI and CT technologies are being developed to

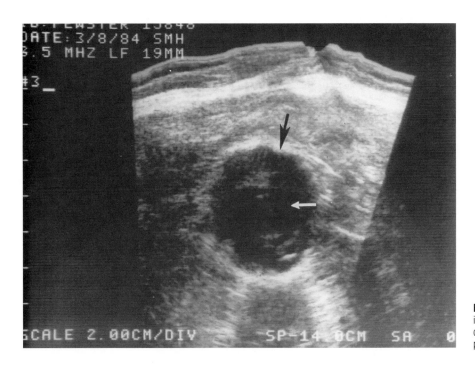

Figure 19–2. Ultrasound demonstrating aortic aneurysm in cross-section. This technique is an inexpensive and accurate method to determine aortic diameter but does not provide the detail available with CT scan.

provide more detailed anatomic information on aortic aneurysm than is currently available.[16,17] These developments are likely to provide new insights into the disease and are proving to be important tools in selecting potential patients for endoluminal intervention. However, these technologies are presently in the developmental stage.

Angiography plays a less important role in the management of patients with aortic aneurysms than it does in other aspects of vascular disease. The major reason for this is that angiography is unable to accurately define arterial diameter (the most important piece of data in management of aneurysmal disease) since it defines only arterial lumen (Fig 19–4A). As a consequence, an-

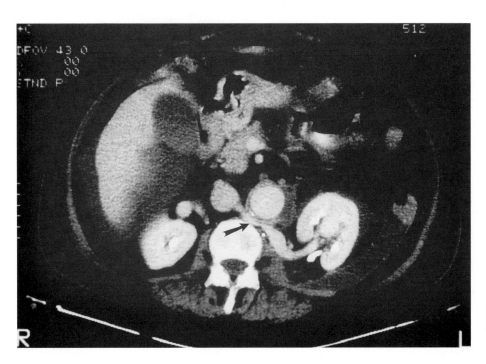

Figure 19–3. CT scan demonstrating a retroaortic left renal vein above an aortic aneurysm. Venous anomalies may occur in 2% to 5% of patients with aortic aneurysms.

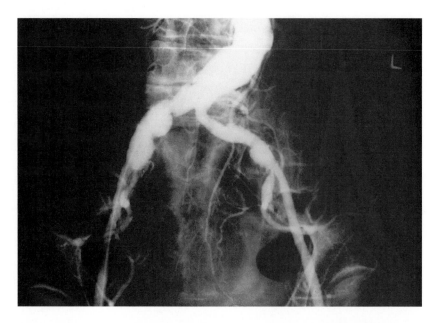

A

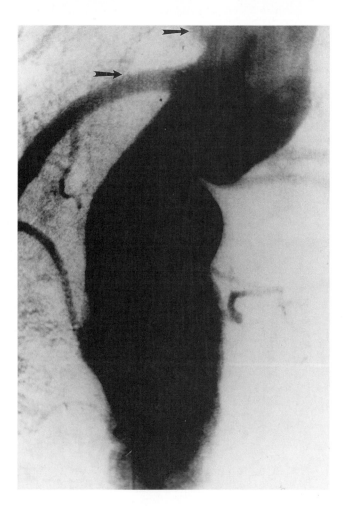

B

Figure 19–4. Angiography of aortic aneurysms. **A**: Anterior view of infrarenal aortic aneurysm extending into the iliac vessels. While luminal diameter is apparent, the true size of the aorta and iliac arteries cannot be determined. **B**: Lateral aortogram of a pararenal aortic aneurysm demonstrating the origins of the celiac and superior mesenteric arteries. In cases of suspected suprarenal extension, lateral aortography is mandatory.

giography is restricted to those cases where the details of arterial lumen are important. These include cases where significant occlusive disease is suspected in the visceral, renal, or distal arterial bed, or where the aneurysm is suspected to extend above the renal vessels (Fig 19–4B). Such patients can be selected on the basis of physical examination, history of hypertension or intestinal angina, or CT findings demonstrating proximal aneurysmal extension or decreased renal size. When angiography is required, it should be detailed enough to provide the appropriate data. Intravenous digital subtraction studies alone are insufficient. Arterial injections are required, including lateral aortography, when the suprarenal aorta and visceral vessels are to be evaluated. When arteriography is performed, attention must be given to the pelvic blood supply (especially the hypogastric vessels) and any abnormal collateral circulation such as the "meandering mesenteric artery" (Fig 19–5).

PREOPERATIVE EVALUATION

The mortality for elective aortic resection remains 2% to 5% in most major series.[18–20] With the exception of technical misadventure, the majority of problems are cardiac, pulmonary, or renal in origin. As a consequence, a thorough evaluation of these three organ systems is required prior to resection. Most pulmonary problems can be identified through a proper history and physical examination. Patients with evidence of significant pulmonary restriction should undergo preoperative pulmonary function tests, with and without bronchodilators. If a productive cough is present, preoperative physiotherapy, with sputum cultures and treatment of any underlying infection, is indicated. Renal evaluation requires baseline electrolytes and creatinine as well as an estimate of renal size and function on CT scan. If abnormalities are suspected, a formal creatinine clearance should be performed. Morbidity and mortality of aneurysm resection rises dramatically with impaired renal function, and routine aortic resection should be considered carefully in patients with moderate to severe renal impairment (creatinine >3.0 mg/dL). In these cases resection may be deferred in aneurysms of modest dimension (eg, <6.5 cm).

The major morbidity and mortality following aneurysm resection is cardiac. The operation itself is associated with significant changes in hemodynamics, with the application and removal of the aortic cross-clamps. Added to this are intraoperative blood loss and postoperative fluid shifts. Accurate assessment of cardiac risk is mandatory. Opinions on the means to achieve this end vary.[21–23] It must be remembered that all patients with aortic aneurysm will have some degree of coronary artery disease and the majority will tolerate aneurysmectomy without adverse events.[24] Routine coronary angiography or stress testing is not likely to be cost effective. The goal of cardiac evaluation is to identify high-risk groups and manage them in one of three ways: (1) defer operation in high-risk patients with smaller aneurysms, (2) increase perioperative monitoring, including preoperative cardiac performance curves, and (3) correct severe coronary ischemia prior to aneurysmectomy by angioplasty or coronary bypass. These goals should be kept in mind when selecting patients for extensive preoperative cardiac evaluation.

Patients with no history of coronary ischemia or congestive heart failure and a normal resting cardiogram have a low incidence of perioperative cardiac events and no further evaluation is needed.[25,26] For the remainder of patients, some assessment of left ventricular function is recommended prior to aneurysmectomy.[27] Coronary reserve is assessed by stress testing or angiography in those patients in whom evidence of ischemia would alter subsequent therapy (vide supra). In some cases, demonstration of coronary disease may have no influence on management and only evaluation of left ventricular (LV) function is required. Such an example would be a patient, 65 years of age, with a history of coronary artery bypass, no current cardiac symptoms,

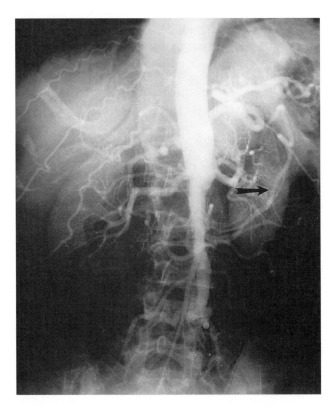

Figure 19–5. Angiogram demonstrating a "meandering mesenteric artery" which is a collateral between the inferior and superior mesenteric circulations. When this is present, occlusive disease at the origin of one of these vessels is present. Lateral angiography to evaluate the superior mesenteric orifice should be performed and reimplantation of a patent inferior mesenteric artery will be required.

and a 7 cm aneurysm. Resection with perioperative monitoring is clearly indicated, a coronary lesion amenable to angioplasty is unlikely to be present, and secondary bypass in such a patient would be inappropriate. In such cases, stress testing or coronary angiography would be superfluous. However, in an older patient with a smaller aneurysm, demonstration of exercise-induced ischemia might result in deferral of operation and, therefore, would be indicated.

Left ventricular function may be assessed by echocardiography or gated blood pool scan. Assessment of coronary reserve involves some application of stress such as treadmill testing, dipyridamole thallium[28] or dobutamine echo.[29] In patients with a history of exercise-induced angina, stress testing is superfluous and one should proceed directly to coronary angiography.[30]

Even with the above guidelines, <10% of patients undergo coronary revascularization prior to aneurysmectomy. The major benefit of screening is to defer surgery in patients without a pressing need for aneurysmectomy or to identify those needing increased intraoperative or preoperative monitoring. Finally, it must be acknowledged that while many centers utilize algorithms based on the assumptions outlined above, there are no prospective randomized studies that unequivocally demonstrate that screening reduces overall morbidity and mortality.

INDICATIONS FOR SURGERY

The mortality of elective aneurysmectomy ranges from 2% to 5%, whereas surgery after rupture continues to result in mortality rates of 50% to 90%.[31–35] This provides the rationale for elective resection. The factor most significantly related to rupture risk is aneurysm size. Risk of rupture begins to rise rapidly as aneurysms exceed 5 cm in diameter. However, even an aneurysm <5 cm in diameter may rupture, with an incidence of approximately 10%. Furthermore, although aneurysm diameter increases at a rate of approximately 0.5 cm/year, changes in diameter may be unpredictable.[36–38] Several authors have attempted to correlate the risk of rupture to relative rather than absolute aneurysm size. The most popular standards against which aneurysm diameter is measured have been the suprarenal aorta and the lumbar vertebral body.[39,40] None of these efforts have proved convincingly superior to absolute diameter. Chronic lung disease and hypertension also have been shown to increase the risk of aneurysm rupture. A computer model, based on the observation of smaller aneurysms, has been developed to predict rupture risk.[41]

As a general rule, aneurysms of >4 cm diameter are considered for resection in patients with low perioperative risk and expectation of 5 year survival. This policy is based on the real (approximately 10%) chance of rup-

ture in this group and the likelihood of significant future growth. In patients at higher operative risk or with diminished life expectancy, the risk of rupture is balanced against these factors. As a guideline, the risk of rupture for aneurysms 6 to 7 cm is 8% to 10% per year. Aneurysms >7 cm are resected, unless operative mortality is judged to exceed 10% or life expectancy is <24 months.

THE OPERATION

Elective Resection

Transabdominal Approach. This is the most common approach for aortic aneurysmectomy. Celiotomy is performed through a midline incision, xiphoid to pubis; although transverse or even paramedian incision have been described by some authors. The abdominal contents are thoroughly evaluated and the retroperitoneum entered by incising the ligament of Treitz and mobilizing the intestine to the right of the patient. It is important to incise the posterior peritoneum close to the bowel wall so that a veil of posterior peritoneum, based on the left of the aorta, is available later for closure (Fig 19–6). Dissection is carried cephalad past the inferior mesenteric vein (running superiorly and medially) until the left renal vein is identified. The retroperitoneal tissue, which is rich in lymphatics, should be clamped and ligated to prevent development of chylous ascites. The inferior mesenteric vein may be ligated without undue concern, although this usually is not required. It is imperative that dissection is carried to the level of the left renal vein so that the aortic clamp may be placed immediately below the renal vessels. If necessary, the left renal vein may be ligated to gain further proximal exposure (Fig 19–7). This should be done as close to the vena cava as possible to allow collateral drainage via the lumbar adrenal and gonadal veins. Alternatively, mobilization of the left renal vein usually suffices. This may require division of the gonadal and adrenal veins. If the left renal vein is not identified, the surgeon must consider the possibility of a retroaortic left renal vein, which occurs in 1% to 3% of cases. If a retroaortic left renal vein is found, posterior mobilization of the aneurysm neck must be done cautiously to avoid venous injury.

Distal control is obtained, prior to circumferential mobilization of the aneurysm neck, to minimize the risk of distal embolization. Control is obtained at the common iliac, external iliac, or femoral levels, depending on the degree of distal aneurysmal involvement. Common iliac control with subsequent tube graft is possible in 40% to 50% of cases, and intra-abdominal placement of the distal anastomosis is possible in >90%. Whenever feasible, the distal anastomosis is performed proximal

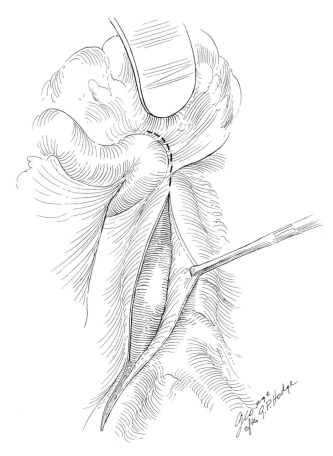

Figure 19–6. Incision of the retroperitoneum with division of the ligament of Treitz and mobilization of the duodenum. The peritoneum should be incised close to the bowel wall, leaving a veil of peritoneum based to the left of the aorta. At the end of the procedure this is closed over the aorta, leaving the mobilized intestine free.

to at least one internal iliac artery to preserve pelvic blood supply. This is usually possible by individually controlling the external and internal iliac vessels separately (Fig 19–8). This is one of the most important points in the operation because of the risk of venous or ureteral injury. Both ureters always should be identified, usually as they cross the iliac bifurcation. The iliac veins and vena cava may be adherent to the aortic bifurcation and iliac vessels. Sharp instruments and blind use of encircling clamps are to be avoided. Most of the posterior mobilization is done with the fingers. Dissection is kept to a minimum, the goal of the surgeon is to isolate the vessel between thumb and index finger so that a clamp can be applied. On occasion this may partially or completely occlude the underlying vein, with no ill effect. At this point, a rapid infusion of 25 gm of mannitol is begun.

Once distal control is achieved, 5000 to 10 000 units of heparin are administered by the anesthetist and the distal vessels are clamped. Only then is proximal dissection begun. The principles of proximal dissection are the same as distal dissection, relying on digital dissection to control the aortic neck. One or two pairs of lum-

bar vessels may be ligated, although this is not always required. When the proximal aorta can be encircled and lifted off the vertebral column between the operator's thumb and index finger (Fig 19–9), the proximal clamp is applied. On occasion, a suitable infrarenal neck cannot be identified, and a suprarenal clamp must be applied. With rare exception, this should be placed at the level of the diaphragm and not between the renal and superior mesenteric vessels. Access to this portion of the aorta is obtained through the gastrohepatic ligament (see section on ruptured aneurysm).

After proximal and distal control is obtained, the aorta is opened anteriorly and to the right of the inferior mesenteric artery (Fig 19–10). Lumbar bleeding is controlled by a gauze pad, and the inferior mesenteric artery orifice examined for evidence of backbleeding; if necessary, this is controlled from within the aneurysm with heavy silk ligatures. Thrombus is serially evacuated and lumbar vessels controlled with mattress sutures of heavy silk (Fig 19–11). The use of mattress sutures obviates problems with calcium around the lumbar orifices. If necessary, the origins of the common iliac vessels are oversewn at this point. A nonporous or preclotted prosthesis is used. The diameter should be equal to that of the aorta at the proximal cuff. The most common error is to select a prosthesis that is too large rather than too small. Therefore the surgeon should resist the temptation to select a large prosthesis and consider "downsizing," particularly if dacron is used.

The proximal anastomosis is now performed using 2-0 or 3-0 monofilament suture. The anastomosis is begun

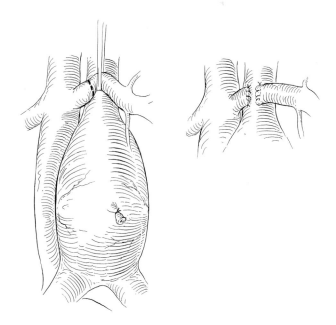

Figure 19–7. Treatment of the left renal vein. If additional proximal exposure is required, the renal vein may be mobilized by dividing the left adrenal or gonadal veins. Alternately, the vein may be ligated (inset) close to the vena cava; in this case, the adrenal and gonadal collaterals must be preserved to allow adequate venous drainage from the kidney.

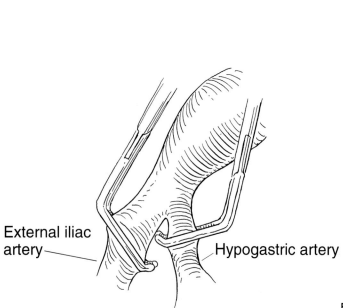

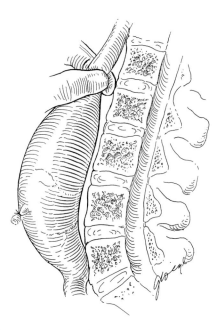

External iliac
artery

Hypogastric artery

Figure 19–8. Distal iliac control: individual clamping of the external and internal iliac vessels facilitates anastomosis to their bifurcation and maintenance of prograde internal iliac perfusion.

Figure 19–9. Proximal aortic control (cross-section). The aortic neck is encircled by the operator's thumb and index finger and lifted off the vertebral column so that a cross-clamp can be applied securely. Usually no lumbar collaterals need be divided to perform this maneuver, although division of a single set of lumbar vessels sometimes is required.

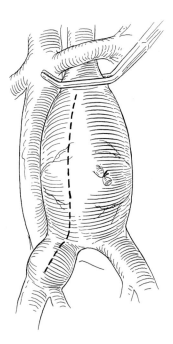

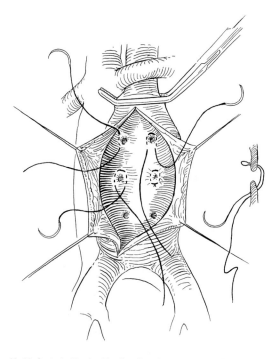

Figure 19–10. Incision of the aortic wall. This is made to the right of the inferior mesenteric artery and continues on the right anterolateral aspect of the vessel. The incision allows reimplantation of the inferior mesenteric artery, if necessary, and avoids the nerve plexus over the aortic bifurcation and the origin of the left common iliac. Disturbances of this plexus increase the incidence of postoperative erectile dysfunction.

Figure 19–11. Control of lumbar bleeding. Use of a mattress technique is preferred to the "figure of eight" (inset). This overcomes problems of calcification at the lumbar orifice by encircling the lumbar vessel itself rather than closing the aorta over it.

posteriorly in the midline and carried up each side with a continuous suture, a parachute technique may be employed (Fig 19–12). Generally, a cuff of aorta suitable for anastomosis is evident. The sides of the aorta may be incised to facilitate exposure, although this is not always necessary. The posterior wall of the aorta is usually left intact, although on occasion complete transection of the aorta facilitates posterior exposure. A relatively normal segment of aorta should be available for proximal anastomosis, even if this requires suprarenal clamping. Often, when the aneurysm neck is pararenal, application of a clamp at the diaphragm allows a tension-free anastomosis immediately below the level of the renal vessels. The needle should proceed from intima to adventitia on the artery and should be drawn cleanly through the vessel without torque or twisting. This may require separate "bites" on the artery and graft. After the proximal anastomosis is completed, it is tested for hemostasis and defects are repaired with felt-buttressed sutures.

The distal anastomoses are completed in a similar manner, beginning posteriorly and proceeding from intima to adventitia on the vessels. The graft is flushed prior to completion of the anastomosis and each limb is re-perfused separately. Hemodynamic effects of declamping are carefully monitored to avoid hypotension. After declamping, hemostasis is secured and the aneurysm wall is closed over the graft by imbrication. Excess wall can be excised, if necessary (Fig 19–13). The retroperitoneum is closed in two layers, if possible. During this closure, the mobilized duodenum is left free and is *not* reattached to its retroperitoneal position (Fig 19–14). The ureters should be visualized during this closure.

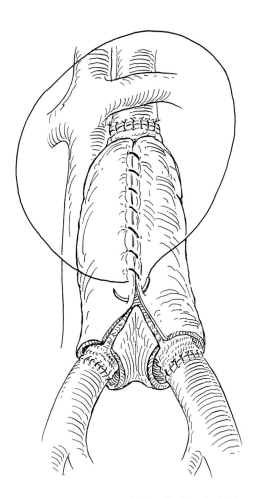

Figure 19–13. Closure of aortic wall over graft. The wall is trimmed or imbricated to produce a tight closure.

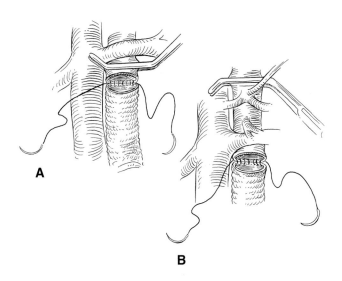

Figure 19–12. A. Proximal aortic suture line that is begun posteriorly. **B.** In this case the aneurysm was close to the renal vessels and a supraceliac clamp was applied while the proximal anastomosis was completed. This usually is not required.

Retroperitoneal Approach. The aorta may be approached through the left retroperitoneum in cases where the patient is obese, has had multiple prior abdominal procedures ("hostile abdomen"), or when visceral aortic control is required.[42–44] Some authors have found that postoperative recovery is more rapid in these cases.[42] The standard retroperitoneal approach is through a flank incision beginning 4 to 5 cm below the umbilicus and extending from the lateral border of the rectus abdominis to the tip of the 12th rib[42] (Fig 19–15). The inferior mesenteric artery must be ligated for exposure, and this approach only provides access to the infrarenal aorta and proximal common iliac arteries; it is not suitable for extensive aneurysms. Exposure of the aorta is anterior to the left kidney, similar to that used with the transabdominal approach.

An extended retroperitoneal approach is taken more proximally through the 10th or 11th interspace and provides access to the supraceliac aorta and visceral vessels without the need for a thoracotomy[45] (Fig 19–15). It is useful in complex aortic reconstruction, suprarenal

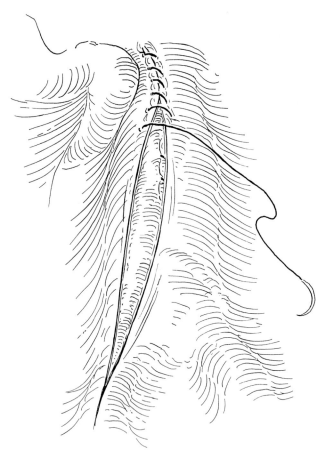

Figure 19–14. Closure of retroperitoneum. This is performed in a single or double layer, taking care to leave the intestine mobile and not to fix it back to the posterior peritoneum.

aneurysm resection, and surgery for recurrent aortic aneurysm.[46] This approach may be associated with significant postoperative intercostal neuralgia and "flank bulge" due to denervation of the lateral abdominal musculature. Generally, it is reserved for more difficult reconstructions. In this approach, dissection proceeds *behind* the left kidney along the posterolateral aspect of the aorta (Fig 19–16). The most important landmark in this approach is the large lumbar vein that drains the left renal vein.[45] This must be divided and ligated early in the procedure.

Reimplanation of the Inferior Mesenteric Artery

On occasion the inferior mesenteric artery is reimplanted into the aortic graft to prevent ischemia to the left colon. A variety of criteria have been applied to determine the need for reimplantation, including size, back pressure, Doppler evaluation of antimesenteric flow, and colonic oxygen tension.[47–49] Practically, this vessel can be safely ligated if there is vigorous back-bleeding from its orifice when the aorta is opened, or if angiography shows an intact collateral circulation from a normal superior mesenteric vessel through the arc of Riolan. Reimplantation is indicated if there is a prior history of colon resection (thus, interrupting collateral circulation), or if angiography indicates that the inferior mesenteric vessel supplies collaterals to a diseased or occluded superior mesenteric system. In addition, large vessels with poor back-bleeding are best reimplanted.

The technique for reimplantation is removal of a "button" of aneurysm wall containing the vessel orifice which is then sewn to the body of the graft using a Carrel patch (Fig 19–17).

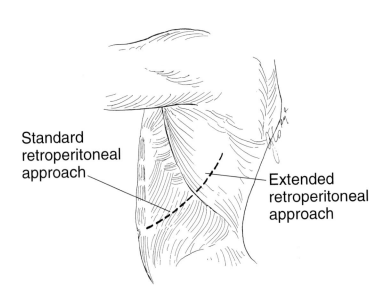

Standard retroperitoneal approach

Extended retroperitoneal approach

Figure 19–15. Contrast between the standard and extended retroperitoneal approach. In the former, the patient's left side is slightly elevated and the incision and dissection is anterolateral to the aorta. In the latter, the patient is rotated with the left flank up; the incision and dissection are directed posterolaterally.

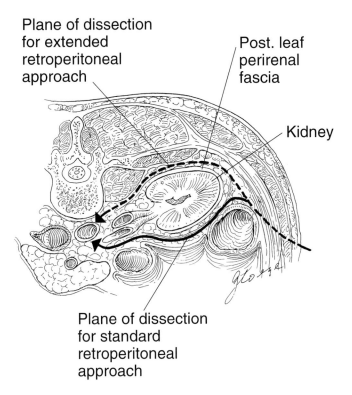

Figure 19–16. Plane of dissection of standard and extended retroperitoneal approach. The standard approach is anterior to the kidney and the aorta is approached anterolaterally. In the extended approach, the left kidney is displaced anteriorly and dissection is along the posterolateral aspect of the aorta. (See text for details).

ILIAC ARTERY ANEURYSM

While aneurysmal disease of the aorta often involves the iliac arteries, isolated iliac artery aneurysms make up only about 1% of all intra-abdominal aneurysms. These aneurysms are often low in the pelvis and are difficult to detect on physical examination. As a consequence, these are usually large at the time of presentation and the incidence of rupture may exceed 50%.[50,51]

Iliac aneurysms present particular challenges because of their proximity to the ureters and iliac veins. These aneurysms are resected using the principles described for aortic aneurysms. Aneurysms >3 cm in size are considered for resection. Whenever possible, prograde flow to the hypogastric artery is maintained.

INFLAMMATORY AORTIC ANEURYSM

This entity often presents with pain that may be confused with an expanding or symptomatic aneurysm. However, the patient is hemodynamically stable and there is no evidence of blood loss. There may be a history of afebrile prodrome, and the erythrocyte sedimentation rate often is elevated. Preoperatively, the diagnosis is suggested by a thickened aortic wall seen on ultrasound or CT scan (Fig 19–18). The thickening is

characteristically anterior and lateral, but does not continue posteriorly. Intraoperatively, there is periaortic inflammation and a "pearl-white" appearance to the aneurysm wall. The duodenum is often densely adherent to the aneurysm neck. The etiology of inflammatory aneurysms is uncertain but histologically, they are characterized by lymphocytic infiltrate in the acute phase, with fibrosis and decreased cellularity in the more chronic condition.[52]

The clinical importance of this process is its involvement of the duodenum, vena cava, and ureters. When the duodenum is involved, aortic control should be gained at the diaphragm, and the aortic wall should be incised without dissection of the duodenum. The process rarely extends above the renal arteries or below the common iliac vessels. Surgical manipulation should be confined to the interior of the aneurysm as much as possible; intraluminal balloon catheters may be preferable to dissection for distal control. Ureteral obstruction may accompany the inflammatory process. While there has been enthusiasm for ureterolysis in these cases,[53] ure-

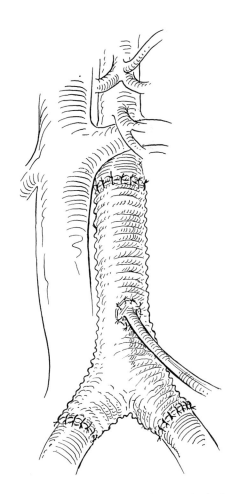

Figure 19–17. Reimplantation of the inferior mesenteric artery using the Carrel technique. (See text for indications for reimplantation).

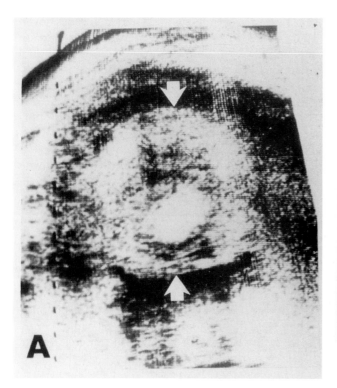

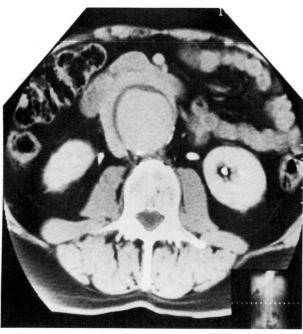

Figure 19–18. Ultrasound (**A**) and CT scan (**B**) showing the thickened wall characteristic of an inflammatory abdominal aneurysm. The inflammation generally is limited to the anterolateral aspects of the aortic wall.

teral stenting and aneurysm resection usually suffice.[54] For unknown reasons, the inflammatory process usually subsides after graft placement, particularly when the aneurysm wall shows a significant lymphocytic infiltrate ("acute" phase).[52]

It has been suggested that the thickened aneurysm wall offers protection against rupture. This has not been proven. There is ample evidence to attest to the danger of aortic rupture in this condition.[53,54] Inflammatory aneurysms should be considered for resection using the same criterion as other aneurysms. Corticosteroids, once suggested for this phenomenon, have no role in management.

AORTIC ANEURYSM WITH HORSESHOE KIDNEY

Horseshoe kidney is found in approximately 1:500 to 1:1000 persons, and its coexistence with aortic aneurysm is even less common. The average vascular surgeon may encounter only a handful of such cases in a career. The diagnosis is suggested by abnormal orientation of renal calyces or pyelography or aortography and by preoperative CT scan. Angiography is indicated prior to aortic resection to identify supernumerary renal arteries which supply the renal isthmus and often arise from the anterior aorta. Aortic resection is best performed us-

ing the retroperitoneal approach, with reimplantation of the renal arteries from within the aorta.[55]

AORTOCAVAL FISTULA

Occasionally an aortic aneurysm may erode into the venous system rather than rupturing into the retroperitoneum or free peritoneal cavity. The resultant arteriovenous fistula can manifest as high-output congestive failure or occasionally, as massive lower extremity edema. More often the only sign of this process is a continuous bruit in the abdomen or back on physical examination. Most aortovenous fistulae are not diagnosed preoperatively.[56,57]

The clinical concerns in the management of aortocaval fistula center around preventing embolization of arterial thrombus to the pulmonary circulation, and control of venous bleeding when the aneurysm is opened. When the diagnosis is made preoperatively, proximal venous control should be obtained before the aortic neck is manipulated and the proximal clamp applied.[58] This is done to prevent venous emboli. Once aortic control is achieved, venous occlusion can be released. Control of venous back-bleeding is achieved by digital pressure, and closure of the fistula proceeds from within the aneurysm wall (Fig 19–19). Even when

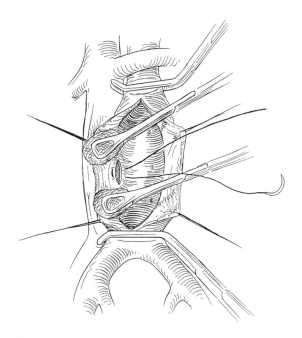

Figure 19–19. Aortocaval fistula. Closure of the fistula is achieved from within the aorta while venous control is obtained by compression of the proximal and distal vein.

this condition is anticipated preoperatively or recognized early on in the operative procedure, mortality rates range from 20% to 50%.

MYCOTIC ANEURYSMS

In the aorta, these aneurysms occur as the result of hematogenous infection, usually of a diseased segment of aorta. The aorta is the second most common site for these aneurysms. While about one-third of clinically bland aneurysms will contain thrombus from which bacteria can be grown, these do not behave clinically in the same way as infected aneurysms.

Patients with a mycotic aneurysm usually demonstrate clinical signs of infection (elevated temperature and leukocyte count) and often complain of back or abdominal pain. The suprarenal and infrarenal aorta may be involved and the aneurysms are often saccular. The most common infective organisms are salmonellae and *Staphylococcus aureus*.[59] These aneurysms require urgent treatment, the goals of which are to prevent hemorrhage, control the infectious process, and maintain arterial perfusion. Broad-spectrum antibiotic coverage is begun preoperatively and later modified, depending on the results of intraoperative cultures. At operation, proximal and distal control is achieved and the periaortic and aortic tissues debrided aggressively to healthy tissue. If the aneurysm is suprarenal, in situ graft replacement is required.[60] If an infrarenal aneurysm is present, and contamination is minimal, in situ replace-

ment is also acceptable. In these circumstances polytetrafluorethylene is used, owing to its increased resistance to infection. If extensive contamination is encountered, and excision with extraanatomic bypass is feasible, this approach is preferred.

Postoperative antibiotics are continued for 2 to 4 weeks or until signs of systemic infection resolve when extraanatomic bypass is performed. For in situ graft placement, 6 to 8 weeks of antibiotics is mandatory, and some authors have suggested lifelong oral antibiotic therapy.

AORTOENTERIC FISTULA

This usually presents as gastrointestinal hemorrhage in a patient with an aortic aneurysm, or more commonly, with an aortic graft.[61] Early diagnosis and a high index of suspicion are the cornerstones of successful management. Diagnosis can be made by endoscopy, CT scan or aortography. The possibility of aortoenteric fistula should be suspected in any patient with an aneurysm or intra-abdominal graft and unexplained gastrointestinal bleeding. Often the initial bleeding episode is relatively minor (''herald bleed'') and results from mucosal erosion rather than frank intraluminal hemorrhage. The most common site of fistula formation is between the proximal aorta and the duodenum or proximal jejunum; however, any level of the gastrointestinal or aortoiliac system can be involved.

Treatment is dependent on the degree of retroperitoneal contamination. When a graft is not in place (primary fistula) and contamination is minimal, resection of the involved intestine and the aneurysm with in situ graft replacement with omental interposition has been successful using criterion similar to those of a mycotic aneurysm; however, such cases are infrequent.[62] More often, there is involvement of the suture line of an aortic graft with false aneurysm formation. In these cases, proximal vascular control, usually at the diaphragm, with graft excision and extraanatomic (axillofemoral) bypass is the appropriate treatment.[63] The intestine is resected and closed primarily. The aortic stump is debrided thoroughly, closed in two layers, and buttressed with omentum. Mortality in these cases remains high.

ANEURYSMS ASSOCIATED WITH INTRA-ABDOMINAL PATHOLOGY

Occasionally aortic aneurysm may coexist with another intra-abdominal condition that requires operation; the most frequent are cholelithiasis and colonic neoplasm. Management of concomitant conditions is controversial and depends on balancing the risk of aneurysm rupture with that of graft infection or complication of the gastrointestinal problem. As a general rule, the symptomatic lesion should be dealt with first and the procedures staged at 6 to 8 week intervals.

When both conditions are asymptomatic and the aneurysm is >5 cm, aneurysmectomy should be performed first. In the case of asymptomatic cholelithiasis, some have advocated cholecystectomy after closure of the retroperitoneum, in order to avoid the occasional problem of postoperative cholecystitis (which may be difficult to identify early after aneurysmectomy).[64] Other authors disagree, however.[65]

When an incidental colonic neoplasm is found at exploration, aneurysmectomy should proceed unless there is a danger of colonic hemorrhage, perforation, or obstruction. This approach obviates the need for resection of unprepared bowel, with possible colonic diversion, and allows appropriate diagnostic evaluation during the recuperative period. Intraoperative clinical staging, including biopsy of suspicious liver nodules, is acceptable; however, the lymphatic drainage of the involved region should be left intact.

RUPTURED AORTIC ANEURYSM

This is a life threatening emergency, with mortality rates in the 50% to 90% range.[32–35] This diagnosis should be considered in any patient with back, flank, or abdominal pain and a pulsatile abdominal mass. Diagnostic work-up is abbreviated and, in most cases, consists of a chest radiograph, electrocardiogram, and blood for cross match. The patient should be taken quickly to the operating room where large-bore intravenous lines are inserted, if this has not been previously done. In hypotensive patients, the abdomen may be draped prior to induction of anesthesia.

Access is gained through a generous midline incision. On occasion, infrarenal control is possible; however, when the hematoma extends to the level of the pancreas or above, control at the diaphragm is in order. If necessary, this is rapidly achieved by manual compression through the gastrohepatic ligament. The left lobe of the liver then is released from its diaphragmatic attachments and retracted to the right (Fig 19–20). Mobilization of the esophagus is unnecessary in most cases. The aorta is identified at its diaphragmatic hiatus and controlled digitally. If possible, the diaphragmatic crural fibers are cut so that the aorta can be isolated. Attempts to place an aortic clamp without clearing the aorta will be fruitless. If proper dissection cannot be accomplished, digital control of the aorta is maintained while the aneurysm is entered.

Anatomy of the retroperitoneum and mesentery often is distorted by hematoma. Every attempt should be made to minimize dissection by approaching the aorta directly anteriorly. With the supraceliac clamp in place

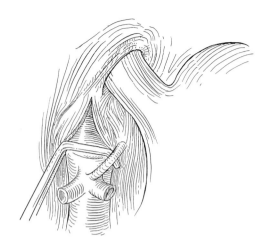

Figure 19–20. Supraceliac control of the aorta is achieved through the gastrohepatic ligament. Initial control is by compression against the vertebral column. Division of the crural fibers allows application of a clamp at this level.

(or digital aortic control by the first assistant), the surgeon enters the aneurysm and digitally identifies the aneurysm neck from within. Using the hand inside the aneurysm for guidance, the aneurysm neck is freed through a combination of sharp and blunt dissection, and an infrarenal clamp is applied. After this, the diaphragmatic clamp is released.

Distal control is obtained in the same fashion, from within the aneurysm. Whenever possible, a tube graft is inserted to minimize dissection and save time. In many cases, distal control is obtained using balloon catheters. If the orifice of the inferior mesenteric artery can be identified, this is preserved for reimplantation unless back-bleeding is profuse. Colonic ischemia is increased in patients with a ruptured aneurysm as the result of perioperative hypotension and disruption of mesenteric collaterals from hematoma. Back-bleeding is often difficult to assess. Consequently, whenever feasible, the inferior mesenteric artery should be reimplanted (vide supra).

Heparin is not used in ruptured aneurysms. To treat distal thrombosis or embolization, balloon embolectomy catheters are passed down both iliofemoral systems prior to unclamping. The remainder of the procedure is identical to the elective operation.

COMPLICATIONS AFTER AORTIC ANEURYSMECTOMY

Major complications particular to aortic aneurysmectomy include hemorrhage, distal ischemia from thrombosis or embolization, renal failure, colonic ischemia, and spinal cord or pelvic ischemia. Hemorrhage is usually related to an intraoperative technical difficulty, either arterial or venous. Venous injuries are particularly difficult to repair and are best avoided, using the principles discussed earlier. When such injuries occur, venous control should be attained by compression (digit or sponge) rather than clamping. The injury then is identified and repaired using vascular suture. Transection of the overlying artery may be required for adequate exposure. Venous ligation may be necessary for hemostasis. Postoperative hemorrhage may be due to dilutional coagulopathy, although technical error always must be excluded. If evidence of hemorrhage persists despite blood-component therapy, or if the patient is unstable, reexploration is performed.

Extremity perfusion should be evaluated prior to leaving the operative suite by palpation and Doppler examination, when necessary. Asymmetric arterial perfusion or absent Doppler pulses are always cause for concern. Transfemoral embolectomy with operative angiography is the procedure of choice when limb ischemia is suspected. Thrombolytic infusions play only a limited role. Prophylactic fasciotomy is performed when ischemia is prolonged (>4 to 6 hrs).

Colonic ischemia is best avoided by reimplantation of the inferior mesenteric artery using the guidelines outlined previously. It usually presents as diarrhea within 12 to 36 hours after aneurysmectomy; stool is hemocult positive and often grossly bloody. Diagnosis is confirmed by flexible sigmoidoscopy. If the ischemia is confined to the mucosa, serial observation is appropriate. If it appears transmural, celiotomy with resection should be performed early to avoid perforation. In these cases, colostomy is required. Mortality rates in these patients are high.

Ischemia of the distal spinal cord and pelvic musculature is a devastating complication with a high mortality.[66,67] It usually results from embolization into the hypogastric circulation or ligation of both hypogastric arteries. Clinical manifestations include motor and sensory loss in the lower extremities, incontinence and gluteal mottling, which may ultimately result in gluteal necrosis. The best treatment is prevention by reimplantation of at least one hypogastric vessel and efforts to avoid embolization of atheromatous debris as described earlier. Renal failure is a serious complication of aortic surgery which may result from intraoperative hypotension, renal artery occlusion or embolization, or inadvertent ureteral ligation. Initial treatment is directed at assuring adequate volume replacement and excluding sources of technical error. Renal artery patency can be evaluated by emergency renal scan and ureteral obstruction can be evaluated by bedside ultrasound examination. Technical problems should be corrected promptly. The mortality rate associated with oliguric or anuric renal failure, particularly after ruptured aneurysm, is prohibitive.[35,68]

■ VISCERAL ANEURYSMS

Aneurysms affecting the visceral arteries are uncommon. They are often seen in a younger population (5th and 6th decade) than abdominal aortic aneurysm. In addition to atherosclerosis, there are a number of etiologies for these aneurysms, including arterial dysplasia, arteritis, infection and periarterial inflammatory processes (eg, pancreatitis). The natural history of most of these lesions is not well documented. Therapeutic decisions are based on minimizing the risk of rupture. This risk is balanced against the consequences of operative intervention.

RENAL ARTERY ANEURYSM

These aneurysms, which are found in >1% of the population,[69–71] have been grouped into four categories by Poutasse: saccular, fusiform, dissecting, and miscellaneous.[70] They are often an incidental finding, an asymptomatic calcification on plain x-ray, or at the time of aortography (Fig 19–21). Saccular aneurysms are usually at a renal artery bifurcation and are often calcified. Fusiform aneurysms may be associated with fibrodysplastic syndromes and with an area of arterial stenosis. Dissecting aneurysms usually present with flank pain from acute thrombosis. Rupture of renal artery aneurysms is rare and probably is related to arterial diameter.

Small (<2 cm) renal artery aneurysms can be observed. Indications for surgery include dissection, renovascular hypertension (documented by lateralizing renal vein renins), and rupture. Prophylactic operation may be indicated in aneurysms >2 cm in diameter which are extrarenal and easily accessible. Ex vivo ("bench surgery") repair has been reported for aneurysms involving the more distal renal branches, but the risks of renal loss associated with complex reconstructions must be balanced against the low rupture rate reported in the literature. Operation includes ligation of the aneurysm with distal renal revascularization, using either saphenous vein or hypogastric artery.

SPLENIC ARTERY ANEURYSMS

These are the most common visceral aneurysms, with an estimated incidence of 0.8%. They are usually saccular and are multiple in 20% of cases. Splenic artery aneurysms are most common in females (4:1) and have been associated with multiparity. Other conditions associated with splenic artery aneurysms include portal hypertension, arterial fibrodysplasia and pancreatitis.[72]

Like aneurysms of the renal artery, most splenic aneurysms are asymptomatic and found as calcifications on plain film or incidentally at angiography. Approximately 20% of these aneurysms present with rupture

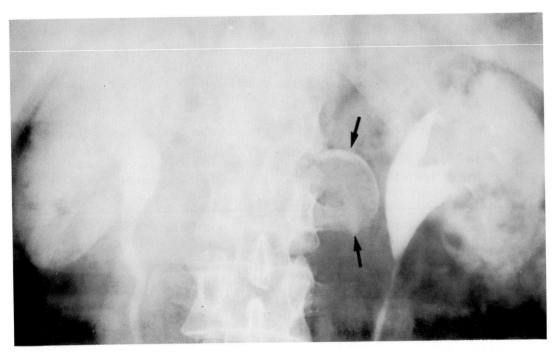

Figure 19–21. Calcified renal artery aneurysm. Asymptomatic visceral aneurysms usually discovered as incidental findings on abdominal radiograph.

which may manifest itself as epigastric or left upper quadrant pain or as abdominal apoplexy. Patients may experience a "double rupture," presenting first with pain and later in shock as the rupture is no longer contained in the lesser sac. The incidence of rupture is markedly increased in gravid females, approaching 90%.

As in renal aneurysmal disease, small (<2 cm) aneurysms may be observed unless they are discovered in a woman of childbearing potential, when resection is warranted. Proximal aneurysms may be ligated and excised. Midsplenic aneurysms are often associated with pancreatitis; the aneurysm is ligated, and the underlying pancreatic process treated appropriately. Aneurysms close to the splenic hilum are treated by splenectomy. In specific cases, catheter embolization or balloon occlusion can be used.[73]

HEPATIC ARTERY ANEURYSMS

These aneurysms are usually solitary and 80% present in the extrahepatic location. Hepatic aneurysms are seen in slightly older patients (6th decade) and the incidence of rupture is 20% to 40%. Rupture may occur into the free peritoneal cavity or into the biliary tree, resulting in hemobilia. Since rupture is associated with a high mortality rate, the primary treatment of these aneurysms is surgical.[74]

Aneurysms of the common hepatic artery can be ligated without reconstruction, but more peripheral aneurysms require concomitant arterial reconstruction. Intrahepatic aneurysm may be treated by catheter thrombosis.

CELIAC ARTERY ANEURYSMS

Aneurysms of the celiac artery are usually due to atherosclerosis or medial degeneration and are associated with aneurysms of the aorta or other splanchnic vessels in 15% to 30% of cases.[73] Most are asymptomatic, although occasionally celiac aneurysms can present as a pulsatile epigastric mass. Aneurysms >2 cm in diameter are usually resected, with reconstruction, particularly of the hepatic artery, whenever possible.

MESENTERIC ANEURYSMS

Aneurysmal disease of the superior and inferior mesenteric vessels, gastric, gastroduodenal and pancreaticoduodenal arteries is rare. They are usually secondary to bacterial endocarditis, arteritides, such as polyarteritis nodosa, or local inflammatory conditions, particularly pancreatitis. The majority of these present with gastrointestinal bleeding or intraperitoneal rupture ("abdominal apoplexy"). Surgery is the treatment of choice. Resection alone is sufficient except in some proximal lesions in which reconstruction with a vein graft is performed. In peripherally located aneurysms, intestinal resection is often required.

REFERENCES

1. Cohen J. Pathogenesis of aortic aneurysms. *Perspec Vasc Surg* 1990;3:101–111

2. Dobrin PB. Pathophysiology and pathogenesis of aortic aneurysms; current concepts. *Surg Clin North Am* 1989; 69:687–703

3. Deak SB, Ricotta JJ, Mariani TJ, et al. Abnormalities in the synthesis of type III procollagen in cultured skin fibroblasts from 2 patients with multiple aneurysms. *Matrix* 1992;12:92–100

4. Tsipouras P, Del Mastro R, Sarfarazi M, et al. Genetic linkage of the Marfan syndrome, ectopia lentis, and congenital contractural arachnodactyly to the fibrillin genes on chromosomes 15 and 5. The International Marfan Syndrome Collaborative Study. *N Engl J Med* 1922;326:905–909

5. Parodi JC, Palmaz JC, Barone HD. Transfemoral intraluminal graft implantation for abdominal aortic aneurysms. *Ann Vasc Surg* 1991;5:491–499

6. Zarins CK, Glagov S. Aneurysms and obstructive plaques: differing local responses to atherosclerosis. In: Bergen JJ, Yao JST (eds), *Aneurysms: Diagnosis and Treatment,* New York, NY: Grune & Stratton; 1982:61–82

7. Taylor LM, Porter JM. Basic data related to clinical decision making in abdominal aortic aneurysms. *Ann Vasc Surg* 1990;1:502–504

8. Tilson MD, Seashore MR. Human genetics of the abdominal aortic aneurysm. *Surg Gynecol Obstet* 1984;158:129–132

9. Adamson J, Powell JT, Greenhalgh RM. Selection for screening for familial aortic aneurysms. *Br J Surg* 1992; 79:897–898

10. Bengtsson H, Bergquist D, Ekberg O, Janzon L. A population based screening of abdominal aortic aneurysms (AAA): *Eur J Vasc Surg* 1991;5:53–57

11. Scott RAP, Ashton HA, Kay DN. Abdominal aortic aneurysms in 4237 screened patients: prevalence, development and management over 6 years. *Br J Surg* 1991; 78:1122–1125

12. Vermillion BD, Kimmins SA, Pace WG, et al. A review of 147 popliteal aneurysms with longterm follow up. *Surgery* 1981;90:1009

13. Quill DS, Colgan MP, Sumner DS. Ultrasonic screening for the detection of abdominal aortic aneurysms. *Surg Clin North Am* 1989;69:713–720

14. Gomes WN, Choyke PL. Preoperative evaluation of abdominal aortic aneurysms: Ultrasound or computed tomography? *J Cardiovasc Surg* 1987;28:159–165

15. Ricotta JJ. Venous anomalies encountered during abdominal aortic reconstruction. In: Ernst CB, Stanley JC (eds.), *Current Therapy in Vascular Surgery II.* Philadelphia, PA: BC Decker; 1991:289–292

16. Tennant WG, Hartnell GG, Baird RN, Horrocks M. Radiologic investigation of abdominal aortic aneurysm disease: comparison of 3 modalities in the staging and detection of inflammatory change. *J Vasc Surg* 1993; 17:703–709

17. Rubin GD, Walker PJ, Dake MD, et al. Three dimensional spiral computed tomographic angiography: an alternative imaging method for the abdominal aorta and its branches. *J Vasc Surg* 1993;18:656–665

18. Hertzer NR, Avellone JC, Farrell CJ, et al. The risk of vascular surgery in a metropolitan community. *J Vasc Surg* 1984;1:13–31

19. Pairolero PC. Repair of abdominal aortic aneurysms in high risk patients. *Surg Clin North Am* 1989;69:755–763

20. Johnston KW. Multicenter prospective study of nonruptured abdominal aortic aneurysm, part II. variable predicting morbidity and mortality. *J Vasc Surg* 1989;9: 437–447

21. Hertzer NR, Beven EG, Young JR, et al. Coronary artery disease in peripheral vascular patients: a classification of 1000 coronary angiograms and results of surgical management. *Ann Surg* 1984;199:223–233

22. Leppo J, Plaja J, Gionet M, et al. Noninvasive evaluation of cardiac risk before elective vascular surgery. *J Am Coll Cardiol* 1987;9:269–276

23. McEnroe CS, O'Donnell TF Jr, Yeager A, et al. Comparison of ejection fraction and Goldman risk factor analysis to dipyridamole-thallium 201 studies in the evaluation of cardiac morbidity after aortic aneurysm surgery. *J Vasc Surg* 1991;11:497–504

24. Roger VL, Ballard DJ, Hallett JW, et al. Influence of coronary artery disease on morbidity and mortality after abdominal aneurysmectomy: a population based study 1971–1987. *J Am Coll Cardiol* 1989;14:1245–1252

25. Hertzer NR. Clinical experience with preoperative coronary angiography. *J Vasc Surg* 1985;2:510–514

26. Golden HA, Whitemore AD, Donaldson MC, Mannick JA. Selective evaluation and management of coronary artery disease in patients undergoing repair of abdominal aortic aneurysms: a 16 year experience. *Ann Surg* 1990;212: 415–423

27. Yeager RA, Moneta GL. Assessing cardiac risk in vascular surgical patients: current status. *Perspect Vasc Surg* 1989; 2:18–39

28. Cutler BS, Leppo JA. Dipyridamole-thallium 201 scintigraphy to detect coronary artery disease before abdominal aortic surgery. *J Vasc Surg* 1987;5:91–100

29. Lalka SG, Sawada SG, Dalsing MC, et al. Dobutamine stress echocardiography as a predictor of cardiac events associated with aortic surgery. *J Vasc Surg* 1992;15:831–842

30. Suggs WD, Smith RB III, Weintraub WS, et al. Selective screening for coronary artery disease in patients undergoing elective repair of abdominal aortic aneurysms. *J Vasc Surg* 1993;18:349–357

31. Hollier LH, Taylor LM, Ochsner JL. Recommended indications for operative treatment of abdominal aortic aneurysms. Report of a subcommittee of the Joint Council of the Society for Vascular Surgery and North American Chapter of the International Society for Cardiovascular Surgery. *J Vasc Surg* 1992;15:1046–1056

32. Bengtsson H, Bergqvist D. Ruptured abdominal aortic aneurysm: a population based study. *J Vasc Surg* 1993;18: 74–80

33. Johansen K, Kohler TR, Nichols SC, et al. Ruptured abdominal aortic aneurysms: the Harborview experience. *J Vasc Surg* 1991;13:240–247

34. Gloviczki P, Pairolero PC, Mucha P, et al. Ruptured abdominal aortic aneurysm: repair should not be denied. *J Vasc Surg* 1992;15:851–859

35. Harris LM, Mangione S, Ricotta JJ. Immunogenicity of the cryopreserved venous allograft in humans: a preliminary report. *Clin Res* 1993;39:660A.

36. Bernstein EF, Chan EL. Abdominal aortic aneurysms in high risk patients: outcome of selective mangement based on size and expansion rate. *Ann Surg* 1984;200:255–263

37. Glimaker H, Holmberg L, Elvin A, et al. Natural history of patients with abdominal aortic aneurysm. *Eur J Vasc Surg* 1991;5:125–130

38. Colin J, Heather B, Walton J. Growth rates of subclinical abdominal aortic aneurysms: implications for review and rescreening programmes. *Eur J Vasc Surg* 1991;5:141–144

39. Louridas G, Reilly K, Perry MD. The role of the aortic aneurysm diameter aortic diameter ratio in predicting the risk of rupture. *S Afr Med J* 1990;78:642–643

40. Ouriel K, Green RM, Donayre C, et al. An evaluation of new methods of expressing aortic aneurysm size: relationship to rupture. *J Vasc Surg* 1992;15:12–20

41. Cronenwett JL, Sargent SK, Wall MH, et al. Variables that affect the expansion rate and outcome of small abdominal aortic aneurysms. *J Vasc Surg* 1990;11:260–269

42. Sicard GA, Allen BJ, Munn JS, Anderson CB. Retroperitoneal vs transperitoneal approach for repair of abdominal aortic aneurysms. *Surg Clin North Am* 1989;69:795–806

43. Cambria RP, Brewster DC, Abbott WM et al. Transperitoneal vs retroperitoneal approach for aortic reconstruction: a randomized prospective study. *J Vasc Surg* 1990;11:314–325

44. Sheppard AD, Tollefson FJ, Reddy DJ, et al. Left flank retroperitoneal exposure: a technical aid to complex aortic reconstruction. *J Vasc Surg* 1991;14:283–291

45. Ricotta JJ, Williams GM. Endarterectomy of the upper abdominal aorta and visceral arteries through an extraperitoneal approach. *Ann Surg* 1980;192:633–638

46. Williams GM, Ricotta JJ, Zinner M, Burdick JF. The extended retroperitoneal approach for the management of extensive atherosclerosis of the aorta and renal vessels. *Surgery* 1980;88:846–855

47. Ernst CB. Prevention of intestinal ischemia following abdominal aortic reconstruction. *Surgery* 1983;93:102

48. Hobson RW II, Wright CB, Rich NM, et al. Assessment of colonic ischemia during aortic surgery by Doppler ultrasound. *J Surg Res* 1976;20:231–235

49. Ouriel KO, Fiore WM, Geary JE. Detection of occult colonic ischemia during aortic procedures. Use of an intraoperative photoplethysmographic technique. *J Vasc Surg* 1988;7:5–9

50. Nachbur BH, Inderbitzi RGC, Bar W. Isolated iliac aneurysms. *Eur J Vasc Surg* 1991;5:375–381

51. Richardson JW, Greenfield LJ. Natural history and management of iliac aneurysms. *J Vasc Surg* 1988;5:165–171

52. Stella A, Gargiulo M, Pasquinelli G, et al. The cellular component in the parietal infiltrate of inflammatory aortic aneurysms. *Eur J Vasc Surg* 1991;5:65–70

53. Boontje AH, van den Dungen JJAM, Blanksma C. Inflammatory abdominal aortic aneurysms. *J Cardiovasc Surg* 1990;31:611–616

54. Lindblad B, Almgreu B, Bergqvist D, et al. Abdominal aortic aneurysm with perianeurysmal fibrosis: experience from 11 Swedish vascular centers. *J Vasc Surg* 1991;13:231–239

55. Crawford ES, Coselli JS, Safi HJ, et al. The impact of renal fusion and ectopia on aortic surgery. *J Vasc Surg* 1988;8:375–383

56. Alexander JJ, Imbembo AL. Aorta-vena cava fistula. *Surgery* 1989;105:1–12

57. Salo JA, Verkkala K, Perhoniemi V, Harjola PT. Diagnosis and treatment of spontaneous aortocaval fistula. *J Cardiovasc Surg* 1987;28:180–183

58. Baker WH, Sharzer LA, Ehrenhaft JL. Aorto caval fistula as a complication of aortic aneurysms. *Surgery* 1972;72:933–938

59. Brown SL, Busuttil RW, Baker JD, et al. Bacteriologic and surgical determinants of survival in patients with mycotic aneurysms. *J Vasc Surg* 1984;1:541–547

60. Reddy DJ, Ernst CB. Infected aneurysms: recognition and management. *Semin Vasc Surg* 1988;1:174–181

61. Sweeney MS, Gadacz TR. Primary aortoduodenal fistula: manifestations, diagnosis and treatment. *Surgery* 1984;91:492–497

62. Daugherty M, Shearer GR, Ernst CB. Primary aortoduodenal fistula: Extra-anatomic vascular reconstruction not required for successful management. *Surgery* 1979;86:399–401

63. Ricotta JJ, Faggioli GL, Stella AM, et al. Total excision and extra-anatomic bypass for aortic graft infection. *Am J Surg* 1991;162:145–149

64. Ouriel K, Ricotta JJ, Adams JT, DeWeese JA. Management of cholelithiasis in patients with abdominal aortic aneurysms. *Ann Surg* 1983;198:717–719

65. Fry RE, Fry WJ, Cholelithiasis and aortic reconstruction: the problem of simultaneous surgical therapy, conclusions from a personal series. *J Vasc Surg* 1986;4:345–350

66. Picone AL, Green RM, Ricotta JJ, et al. Spinal cord ischemia following operations on the abdominal aorta. *J Vasc Surg* 1986;3:94–103

67. Szilagyi DE, Hageman JH, Smith RE, et al. Spinal cord damage in surgery of the abdominal aorta. *Surgery* 1978;83:38

68. Fielding JWL, Black J, Ashton F, Staney G. Ruptured aortic aneurysms: postoperative complications and their aetiology. *Br J Surg* 1984;72:487–491

69. Martin RS III, Meacham PW, Didestreim JA, et al. Renal artery aneurysm: selective treatment for hypertension and prevention of rupture. *J Vasc Surg* 1989;9:26–34

70. Poutasse EF. Renal artery aneurysms. *J Urol* 1974;113:443–449

71. Hupp T, Allenberg JR, Post K, et al. Renal artery aneurysm: surgical indications and results. *Eur J Vasc Surg* 1992;6:477–486

72. Stanley JC, Messina LM, Zelenock GB. Splanchnic and renal artery aneurysms. In: Moore WS (ed), *Vascular Surgery a Comprehensive Review*. Philadelphia, PA: WB Saunders; 1993:435–450

73. Baker KS, Tisnado J, Cho SR, Beachley MC. Splanchnic artery aneurysms and pseudoaneurysms, transcatheter embolization. *Radiology* 1987;163:135–159

74. Miami S, Arpesain A, Giorgelti PL, et al. Splanchnic artery aneurysms. *J Cardiovasc Surg* 1993;34:221–228

20

Lesions of the Mesentery, Omentum, and Retroperitoneum

Oscar J. Hines ▪ *Stanley W. Ashley*

Disorders of the mesentery and omentum rarely are encountered by the clinician. The retroperitoneum is a more common location for disease, but the nature of its anatomy often results in delayed diagnosis. Additionally, many of these disorders present with nonspecific features simulating more common conditions. Since therapeutic trials for these rare diseases are not possible, treatment options are not always clear.

▪ MESENTERY

ANATOMY

Early in fetal development there is a common dorsal mesentery for the entire gastrointestinal tract. Following rotation and return of the intestine to the abdominal cavity, portions of the mesentery retract and fuse with the retroperitoneum, so that the remaining structures include only the small bowel mesentery and transverse and sigmoid mesocolon.

The small intestinal mesentery is a flat, thin, double-layered membrane extending from its posterior attachments at the duodenojejunal flexure to the ileocecal junction. The root of the mesentery is continuous with the peritoneal lining of the posterior abdominal cavity. Its border along the intestine is approximately 40 times longer than its posterior attachment. Between the two layers of the mesentery are the superior mesenteric artery and vein, their tributaries, lymphatic vessels and nodes, and the nerves that supply the jejunum and ileum (Fig 20–1).

The transverse mesocolon extends from the hepatic to the splenic flexures, and, with the greater omentum, serves to restrict the small intestine to the midabdomen. Within this structure are the middle colic artery, vein, and their branches. The sigmoid mesocolon runs along the course of the left iliac artery, and distally toward the rectum. Vessels contained within the sigmoid mesocolon include the inferior mesenteric artery and vein with branches to the inferior mesenteric and superior hemorrhoidal vessels.

MESENTERIC DISEASE

Acute Mesenteric Lymphadenitis

Acute mesenteric lymphadenitis most commonly occurs in children and teenagers, with approximately equal sex distribution. Patients present with complaints of abdominal pain and fever, similar to those of appendicitis. In fact, the diagnosis of mesenteric lymphadenitis is most often made following a laparotomy for appendicitis in which only mesenteric lymphadenopathy is identified.[1]

This disease is associated with acute abdominal pain that localizes to the right lower quadrant. This is likely

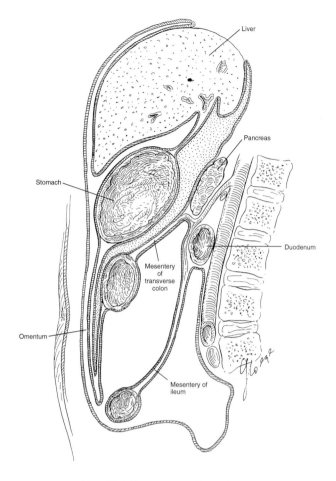

Figure 20–1. The mesentery and its attachments.

because of the greater concentration of lymphatic tissue in the distal small bowel. Peritoneal signs are usually absent, but the patient may manifest slight fever, nausea, vomiting, diarrhea, and elevated white blood cell count. Antecedent or concurrent rhinopharyngitis may be noted.

Although an infectious etiology may never be identified, a variety of agents have been associated with this condition. These include Ebstein-Barr virus, adenovirus, parvovirus, histoplasmosis, giardiasis, tuberculosis, *Salmonella typhus*, and Yersinia. *Yersinia enterocolitica* has been shown to be a cause of combined mesenteric adenitis and intussusception.[2] In areas with a large immigrant or immunosuppressed population, patients with abdominal tuberculosis also may present with acute symptoms.[3]

Since acute mesenteric lymphadenitis may be caused by an infectious agent, nodal histology and cultures are recommended. Additionally, serologic titers may be indicated. In most cases, the disease resolves with hydration and time. However, if an infectious agent is identified, appropriate antimicrobial treatment should be instituted.

Mesenteric Panniculitis

Mesenteric panniculitis, also known as mesenteric lipodystrophy, liposclerotic mesenteritis, mesenteric lipogranuloma, mesenteric variant of Weber-Christian disease, or retroperitoneal xanothgranuloma, is a nonspecific inflammation of the mesenteric adipose tissue. First described in 1955,[4] mesenteric panniculitis is a rare entity occurring in late adulthood, with a median age of 60 years.[5] The disease occurs more commonly in males, with a male-female ratio of 1.8:1. Usually the small intestinal mesentery is involved, but the transverse mesocolon, sigmoid mesentery, omentum or retroperitoneum also may be affected.

The etiology of mesenteric panniculitis has been difficult to determine. Proposed inciting factors include trauma, medications, or immunologic disorders. Although some have suggested that this is a variant of Weber-Christian disease, the evidence for this is negligible. As many as 30% of these patients have had previous abdominal operations.[6] Bacterial infection rarely has been associated with mesenteric panniculitis.

Grossly, mesenteric panniculitis appears as diffuse mesenteric thickening (42%), a solitary mass (32%), or multiple tumors (26%) (Figs 20–2 and 20–3).[5] The mesentery will appear gray to yellow in color, and any discrete masses may appear yellow-orange and have an elastic consistency. The masses may become cystic, filled with oily fluid.[7] On histologic examination, the mesentery is infiltrated with macrophages containing foamy cytoplasm. These cells are distributed in thin, broad, interconnecting bands. Occasionally, calcification or dense fibrosis is apparent in advanced cases.[8]

Patients may be entirely asymptomatic. However, they usually complain of discomfort in the upper abdomen. Other symptoms include anorexia, nausea, vomiting, diarrhea, constipation, and weight loss. Patients rarely will present with signs and symptoms of small bowel obstruction.

Except for an elevated erythrocyte sedimentation rate, laboratory studies are not revealing. Contrast studies may demonstrate a variable number of dilated loops of intestine and a serrated mucosa, suggestive of an inflammatory process. Computed tomographic (CT) scanning has been useful in diagnosing mesenteric panniculitis.[9] Typical findings include an inhomogenous mass in the root of the mesentery which compresses the vascular supply. Magnetic resonance imaging (MRI) demonstrates decreased signal intensity compared to the surrounding tissue in both T1- and T2-weighted images.[9] Although imaging techniques are helpful, biopsy is essential for definitive diagnosis.

The prognosis for patients with mesenteric panniculitis is good. Intervention is necessary only in cases of bowel obstruction. Follow-up of these masses often demonstrates a decrease in size. Patients with persis-

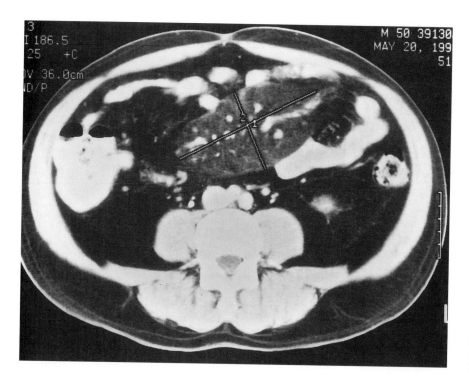

Figure 20–2. A computerized tomography of the abdomen demonstrating the large solitary mass of mesenteric panniculitis.

tent pain may respond to steroids[6] or cyclophosphamide.[10]

Mesenteric Cysts

Mesenteric cysts were first described in 1507.[11] In 1880, Tillaux was the first surgeon to remove a mesenteric cyst successfully.[12] Such cysts are uncommon, accounting for <1 in 100,000 hospital admissions and 1 in 35,000 pediatric admissions.[13] Beahrs has described a variety of mesenteric cyst types including urogenital, enteric, traumatic, gas, mycotic, parasitic, and tuberculous cysts.[14]

Cysts in children usually are congenital, resulting from developmental sequestration of lymphatic vessels.[15] This may be the result of a failure of isolated lymphatics to join the venous system, localized degeneration of lymph nodes, or occult trauma. Since ligation of the thoracic duct does not result in lymphangioma formation, the likelihood that obstruction is an etiology is small.[16] More common in males, these lymphangiomas constitute 29% of mesenteric cysts and are ordinarily (70%) located in the small bowel mesentery. Fifty to sixty percent are found in the ileal mesentery.[17] These lymphangiomas may be unilocular or multilocular. Histologic examination reveals an endothelial lining, foam cells, and a wall containing small lymphatic spaces, lymphoid tissue, and smooth muscle.[18]

Children are more likely to present with acute symptoms, including abdominal pain, anorexia, and vomiting. Additionally, these cysts may be the focus for intestinal obstruction or volvulus with subsequent in-

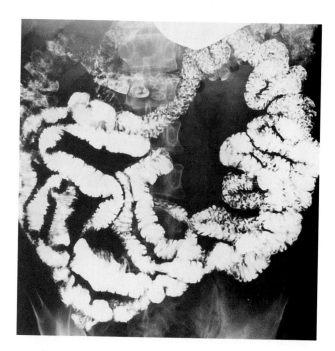

Figure 20–3. A small bowel series demonstrating displacement of the small intestine by the mesenteric panniculitis.

testinal necrosis. Of these patients, 65% have a palpable mass, and evidence of a lymphatic anomaly in other areas should be sought.

Adults more commonly present with vague, poorly localized abdominal pain or nausea. As with children, acute symptoms may occur. Mesenteric cysts are commonly unilocular, and filled with serous fluid. Histologic features include a cuboidal or columnar lining with microvilli, and smooth muscle elements in the wall.[18] The differential diagnosis includes ovarian, pancreatic, renal, or splenic cysts, along with hydronephrosis, hydrops of the gallbladder, intussusception, periappendiceal abscess, and loculated ascites.

The diagnosis of mesenteric cysts is best made by ultrasonography. CT and MRI scanning have been used.[19] Treatment includes surgical excision, preferably by enucleation. Marsupialization, internal drainage, or aspiration are suboptimal and almost always require a second procedure for recurrence. Laparoscopic excision has recently been reported.[20] Mesenteric cysts complicating pregnancy have been successfully removed without fetal demise.[21] Malignant degeneration is rare, with a few cases of sarcoma and adenocarcinoma reported.[22]

Mesenteric Tumors

Primary mesenteric tumors are infrequent.[23] The majority of tumors of the mesentery represent secondary metastases from abdominal organs such as the intestine, or, rarely, from the breast and lung. A large variety of primary tumor types have been found in the mesentery, including neoplasms originating from connective tissue, smooth muscle, adipose, germ cells, epithelium, mesothelium, nerve, and vascular tissue.[23] The two most common types are mesotheliomas and desmoid tumors.

Mesothelioma. Mesotheliomas arise from the lining of the pleura, peritoneum, and pericardium. The three types of peritoneal mesothelial tumors are malignant tubulopapillary mesothelioma, cystic mesothelioma, and benign adenomatoid mesothelioma. Although an association between asbestos exposure and malignant mesothelioma has been established, there is no correlation with benign mesothelioma.[24]

Malignant mesothelioma is an extremely uncommon tumor, with an annual 2.2 cases per million population reported.[25] Peritoneal malignant mesothelioma was first described in 1908[26] and accounts for 20% of all mesotheliomas. Although this tumor has been reported in a child of two years, it usually occurs in males during the fifth and sixth decades.[25] Patients present with symptoms of nonspecific abdominal pain, and may also have signs of bowel obstruction. Ninety percent of patients have ascites; anemia and weight loss also may be apparent.

Cytological examination of peritoneal aspirate has been used for diagnosis and classification with low sensi-

tivity and specificity.[27] An antibody specific for the cytoplasm of mesotheliomas has been generated, and can be used for immunohistochemistry and diagnosis.[28] CT scan and ultrasonography may be employed, but are not able to diagnose mesothelioma definitively. Diagnosis is obtained by biopsy via needle, laparoscopy, or laparotomy.

Grossly, malignant mesothelioma may be mistaken for carcinomatosis. These dense, white nodules eventually coalesce to form plaques extending into surrounding tissues. Metastases can occur in the regional lymph nodes or thoracic cavity. Peritoneal mesotheliomas may be the source of ectopic hormone secretion, including antidiuretic hormone,[29] growth hormone,[30] adrenocorticotropic hormone,[31] or insulin-like hormone.[30] Although histology may reveal epithelial, mesenchymal, or mixed patterns, electron microscopy may be necessary to establish a mesothelial origin. Mesothelial cells will demonstrate microvilli, cytoplasmic tonofilaments, and glycogen-like granules.

Treatment includes a multimodality approach. Surgical intervention has a limited value, but has been used for the purpose of debulking, and for intestinal bypass in the face of obstruction. A multitude of chemotherapeutic regimens have been utilized, with relatively dismal results.[32] Doxorubicin or intracavitary ^{32}P appear to be the most promising.[32,33] Since treatment is not very effective, prognosis for patients with peritoneal malignant mesothelioma is poor, with a median survival rate of 1 year.[34]

In contrast, patients with cystic mesothelioma tend to do quite well. In terms of prognosis, this tumor appears to position between adenomatoid and malignant mesothelioma. Adenomatoid tumors usually are asymptotic and do not recur,[35] whereas malignant mesotheliomas usually are symptomatic and always lethal. Cystic mesothelioma is generally symptomatic and may recur, but is never fatal.

The patient with a cystic neoplasm is usually female, in the fourth or fifth decade, and complains of an abdominal mass and pain. The severity of complaints appears to correlate with the size and location of the cyst. A frequent history of previous abdominal operation, endometriosis, or pelvic inflammatory disease points to a reactive etiology.[36] Definitive diagnosis is made at the time of laparotomy for excision. These lesions are translucent, multicystic masses, lined by flattened, cuboidal, or occasionally, hobnail cells with papillary clusters in the cyst lumina.[37] Again, electron microscopy will demonstrate the microvilli typical of mesothelial cells. Treatment is complete surgical excision. Following excision, 25% of cystic mesotheliomas recur and treatment is reexcision.[37] Adjuvant therapy has little role in the management of these patients.

Desmoid Tumors. The most common primary tumor of the mesentery, desmoid tumors, were first described in

1832.[38] The incidence of desmoid tumors is 2 to 4 per million population and, of these, 8% are mesenteric.[39] There appears to be four peaks of age: 5 years (juvenile), 27 years (fertile), 44 years (middle age), and 68 years (old age). The first two groups predominantly consist of females, while the last two have an equal sex distribution.

These tumors are variable in size, growing as large as 22 kg. The cut surface has a dense consistency, a gray coloring, and may have degenerative cystic changes in the center. Although these tumors have a propensity to invade surrounding tissues, they are not malignant. Histology reveals interwoven bundles of spindle cells with collagen. The central portion of the mass is acellular. Differentiation between desmoid tumors and fibromatose tumors may be difficult. However, desmoid tumors never contain abnormal mitoses or bizarre nuclei. Although not specific to desmoid tumors, sarcolemmal giant cells may be seen. The differential diagnosis includes keloids, neurofibromas, lipomas, dermatofibromas, rhabdomyomas, subacute myositis, and hemangiomas.

Trauma, especially operative trauma, may contribute to the formation of desmoid tumors. A significant number of patients with abdominal desmoid tumors have had previous surgery. Additionally, desmoid tumors have been found in the scars of previous operations. Desmoid tumors with this etiology usually develop within 4 years following the incident.[40]

Estrogen may act as a growth factor. Endogenous estrogen levels have a close correlation with tumor growth rate. Growth of these tumors is slowest in young girls and reaches a maximum at menopause. Estradiol receptors have been documented in desmoid tumor samples, where they appear to be higher than control tissue.[41]

Patients who develop desmoid tumors may have a genetic predisposition. These patients have a disorder similar to Gardner's syndrome, with a variable autosomal dominant inheritance. Forty-eight percent of these patients have concurrent bone malformations, including cortical thickening, exostosis, cystic areas, and compact islands. A significant number of family members also demonstrate bony abnormalities. It has been suggested that independent, but related, genes produce the abnormalities observed in these two syndromes.

Most patients present with complaints of a nontender mass, but, if the tumor is growing into surrounding structures, pain may be evident also. CT and MRI aid in determining the extent of invasion of local structures. Treatment is primarily surgical. Unfortunately, these tumors have a high incidence of recurrence (40%) following operation. Therefore, it is essential that a wide margin be included. Radiotherapy is successful in inducing initial regression; however, excision is often necessary.[42] Of three reported cases of malignant transformation in desmoid tumors, all were associated with local irradiation. Sulindac,[43] indomethacin,[44] and tamoxofen, along with a variety of antineoplastic medications, have been used to treat these patients, with variable results.

■ OMENTUM

ANATOMY

The dorsal mesentery of the stomach expands during the fourth month of gestation to form a large, apron-like fold known as the greater omentum.[45] This structure hangs upon itself, between the greater curvature of the stomach and the transverse colon, and also is referred to as the gastrocolic ligament. It is attached to the duodenum, stomach, spleen, transverse colon, and retroperitoneum. The vascular supply originates from the right and left gastroepiploic arteries. The right side of the omentum may be longer, with a tongue-like extension. The size of the omentum correlates with the size of the patient so that, in obese individuals, the omentum may represent an immense organ. Superiorly, the omentum continues as the gastrosplenic and splenorenal ligaments.

The omentum usually adheres at a site of intra-abdominal inflammation, isolating the focus, and has been termed the "policeman of the abdominal cavity." A rich lymphatic supply probably aids in clearing infection, whereas its vascularity promotes angiogenesis in compromised tissue. Researchers have found that this organ has no inherent properties of movement.[46] It likely functions as a bactericidal structure and aids the containment of the inflammatory process through adhesions.

OMENTAL DISEASE

Omental Torsion and Infarction

First described by Eitel in 1899,[47] torsion of the omentum is a rare entity in which twisting of the omentum results in ischemic necrosis. Torsion can be classified into primary and secondary cases. Primary torsion occurs in males more commonly than in females, with a ratio of 3:2 between 30 and 50 years of age. Because of its greater weight and freedom, the right portion of the omentum is more commonly involved.[48] Secondary torsion usually is the result of an adhesion (bipolar torsion) or hernia.

The involved omentum demonstrates congestion, thrombosis, and hemorrhage. If left untreated, the mass of necrotic tissue may become infected or eventually be the source of adhesions and scarring.

The patient usually presents complaining of the acute onset of moderate to severe pain that localizes to the right lower quadrant. Additionally, the patient may have nausea and vomiting, along with a low-grade fever and mild leukocytosis. Examination will reveal guarding and tenderness. Consequently, the diagnosis of appendicitis may be mistakenly made.

The treatment for omental torsion is complete excision of the involved omentum. In the patient with a preoperative diagnosis of appendicitis and a normal appendix at operation, omental torsion should be considered, especially if free serosanguineous peritoneal fluid is encountered.

Primary infarction of the omentum is rare with no age or sex predilection.[49] The etiology is unknown, but 90% of cases involve the right side of the omentum.[50] Suggested causes include trauma, obesity, cardiac failure, and hypercoagulability. The patients present in much the same manner as those with omental torsion. A midline incision with complete excision of the involved omentum is recommended.

Omental Transposition

The omentum has been employed for reconstruction in virtually every area of the body. Its properties as a vascular and effective immunologic barrier are useful in a variety of situations. The omentum is flexible, allowing it to fill spaces or be spread over large areas. If the omentum is detached from the colon, it will reach the nipple level in 75% of cases, and, when raised on a right gastroepiploic pedicle, it easily will reach the sternal angle and the axilla 70% of the time.[51] The use of the omentum has helped to delineate its vascular anatomy and the techniques for mobilization have been well defined.[52]

In the 19th century, the omentum first was employed to close perforated ulcers.[53] Since then, it has been used to repair vesicovaginal and vesicocolic fistulas,[54] reinforce tracheobronchial anastomoses,[55] treat lymphadema,[56] revascularize the heart[57] and extremities,[58] reconstruct following mastectomy,[59] and repair defects in the bladder and abdominal wall.[60] Since the development of microsurgery, omental free-flaps have been used to repair head and neck defects.[61] Recently, the omentum also has been used to revascularize the brain of stroke patients and patients with cortical blindness from moya-moya disease.[62]

Many have described the use of omental wraps for gastrointestinal anastomoses, particularly for esophageal[63] and rectal anastomoses.[64] The usefulness of the omentum to protect compromised intestinal anastomoses is well established.[65] In one review, a 70% higher survival rate was found using an omental wrap, with compromised anastomoses.[66] Neovascularization by the omentum can be demonstrated by postoperative day 3, and, with severe vascular compromise, the omentum forms a cylinder in areas where ischemic bowel resorbs, maintaining gastrointestinal continuity.

The use of the omentum to protect the bronchial anastomosis in lung transplantation has been instrumental in the success of this procedure.[66a] This practice not only protects the anastomosis, but also helps to reestablish bronchial artery circulation.

The omentum has proven to be an extremely versatile organ. Its attributes have immediate application in a variety of conditions and, when used appropriately, can significantly improve the quality of life of many patients.

Omental Cysts

First described in 1852,[67] omental cysts are rare, accounting for 25% of all abdominal cysts.[68] Sequestration or obstruction of lymphatic vessels likely results in the production of omental cysts, while pseudocysts of the omentum may result from fat necrosis or hematoma. These are found most commonly in children, and usually present as solitary, asymptomatic masses.[69] If the size is large enough, the patient may complain of abdominal pain or symptoms of intestinal obstruction. Rarely, rupture, volvulus, infection, or hemorrhage may result, and the patient will present with an acute abdomen. Diagnosis is usually made at time of operation, but may be aided by abdominal ultrasound. However, even with ultrasound, only 25% of cases are diagnosed preoperatively.[69] Paracentesis may result in the incorrect diagnosis of ascites. Treatment is by surgical excision or marsupialization. Histologic examination should be performed to exclude the extremely rare possibility of malignancy.

Omental Tumors

Primary omental tumors are unusual and carry a poor prognosis. Almost all omental neoplasms represent metastases from tumors, primarily within the abdomen. The first case of an omental tumor was reported in 1942 by Stout and Cassel, and was identified as a hemangiopericytoma.[70] Although the omentum consists primarily of adipose tissue, the majority of these tumors are mesenchymal in nature. The most common benign tumors are leiomyomas, whereas malignant tumors are usually sarcomas, specifically, hemangiopericytomas.[71] In children the most frequent tumor is the cystic lymphangioma.

Patients may present at any age, but most commonly present in the fourth to sixth decade. Omental tumors are slightly more common in males.[71] Although patients may remain symptom free, many present with abdominal pain, distention, nausea, and early satiety. Rarely, the patient may complain of weight loss or diarrhea. Ascites also has been reported. On physical examination, a mobile mass is usually detected; however, in the patient with a malignant lesion, a palpable mass is present in only a third of cases.[71] Leg edema rarely may result from compression of the inferior vena cava.[72]

Although ultrasound may reveal the cystic nature of the lesion, CT scanning is most helpful. CT scan will not only identify the mass, but may also reveal tumor invasion of surrounding structures. Barium enema also may be useful. The finding of a mass that displaces the stomach superiorly and posteriorly, and the transverse colon inferiorly and anteriorly, is pathognomonic of an omental tumor.[73]

Treatment is surgical excision of the mass with adequate margins. Because most of these tumors represent metastases, the surgeon must search for the primary neoplasm. The peritoneum and lung are the most common areas of spread for primary omental tumors. The prognosis for benign disease is excellent; patients who prove to have malignant lesions fare poorly. The median survival is 6 months, and only 10% to 20% are alive at 2 years.[73] Although chemotherapy and radiation treatment have been used, the results are generally poor.

■ RETROPERITONEUM

ANATOMY

The retroperitoneal space is bound by the spine, psoas, and quadratus lumborum muscles posteriorly, the twelfth ribs superiorly, and pelvic brim inferiorly. This region lies between the peritoneum anteriorly and the transversalis fascia posteriorly. Since this space communicates with the mediastinum, perineum, lower extremities and anterior abdominal wall, retroperitoneal disease may extend easily to these structures. Within the retroperitoneum are the adrenals, kidneys, ureters, ovaries, superior vagina, seminal vesicles, vas deferens, bladder, duodenum, ascending and descending colon, upper rectum, pancreas, aorta, inferior vena cava, iliac vessels, and lymphatics.

RETROPERITONEAL DISEASE

Retroperitoneal Hemorrhage

Retroperitoneal hemorrhage and hematoma are largely the result of trauma. Hemorrhage also may be the result of anticoagulant therapy, aortic aneurysm rupture, or translumbar catheterization of the abdominal aorta or inferior vena cava.

Trauma-induced retroperitoneal hematomas usually result from blunt injury. In general, only a third follow penetrating injuries.[74] Approximately 40% of patients with blunt abdominal trauma will develop a retroperitoneal hematoma.[75] Using the Kudsk and Sheldon[76] classification system, 70% are confined to zone III (pelvic), 23% to zone II (lateral), and 7% to zone I (midcentral) (Fig 20–4).[77] The retroperitoneum will accommodate as much as 4000 mL of fluid under a pressure equal to that of the pelvic vessels. Fortunately, as the

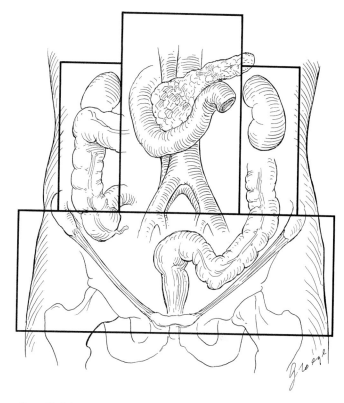

Figure 20–4. Retroperitoneal hematoma classification. Zone 1 = central hematomas; Zone 2 = flank hematomas. Zone 3 = pelvic hematomas.

hematoma expands, the retroperitoneum acts to tamponade hemorrhage. This concept is important when considering management options.

Most patients will complain of pain in the abdomen, flank, or back. If hemorrhage is significant, signs of hypovolemic shock may ensue. If the patient presents 24 hours after injury, a Grey Turner's sign, ecchymosis of the flank, may be present. Laboratory findings may include low hematocrit and hematuria levels. Hyperamylasemia suggests injury to the pancreas or duodenum.

Evaluation of the retroperitoneal hematoma often includes plain films of the abdomen and pelvis. Obliteration of the psoas shadow suggests the presence of a retroperitoneal hematoma. Pelvic films are helpful in evaluating the possibility of bony fracture. In the relatively stable patient, a CT scan, with oral, rectal, and intravenous contrast, is very useful in evaluating the extent of the hematoma, damage to the pancreas, and visceral perforation. If urinalysis reveals more than 30 red cells per high-power field, an intravenous pylography should be performed to evaluate renal injury. Diagnostic peritoneal lavage may be performed in unstable patients, but should be performed through a supraumbilical approach to avoid entering the hematoma.[77]

The management of retroperitoneal hematoma is dependent on the mechanism of injury, the patient's condition, and the anatomy of the hematoma. After proximal and distal control of the aorta and inferior vena cava, hematomas in zone 1 should be opened and explored for vascular injury. Blunt zone 2 injuries may be treated conservatively, if renal evaluation is negative. However, bile staining of the peritoneal fluid or crepitis should alert the surgeon to bile duct or duodenal injury. Penetrating zone 2 hematomas should be explored. As long as groin pulses are present and there is no evidence of bladder injury, zone 3 hematomas should be treated by embolization and pelvic stabilization. Penetrating zone 3 hematomas are best treated operatively.

Retroperitoneal hematoma can be a grave complication of traumatic abdominal injury. The mortality rate ranges from 40% to 70% whereas the morbidity rate is at least 60%.[78,79]

Retroperitoneal Abscess

Retroperitoneal abscesses are the result of infection in neighboring organs or structures. As stated above, with the exception of Gerota's fascia, there are no anatomical barriers limiting the spread of these infections. Consequently, retroperitoneal abscesses are often large, and carry a high mortality. Most commonly, the abscess is the result of diverticulitis, retroperitoneal appendicitis, pancreatitis, pancreatic cancer, biliary tract disease, or perforated ulcer.

The highest incidence of these infections is in patients 30 to 60 years of age.[80] Patients present with complaints of fever, chills, anorexia, and weakness. Pain will be apparent in at least 60% of patients.[81] This may be referred to the lower back, hip, thigh, or knee. Examination often reveals an ill-appearing patient with fever and tachycardia. A psoas sign may be elicited, and a mass may be palpable on abdominal examination.

Laboratory analysis usually reveals a leukocytosis. The urinalysis is frequently normal. Even in patients with perinephric abscess, the urinalysis is normal in a third of cases.[82] Plain x-rays may reveal a pleural effusion, lung atelectasis, an abnormal psoas shadow, or a soft-tissue mass. CT scan is most helpful in diagnosing and evaluating the abscess.

Treatment of a retroperitoneal abscess involves surgical drainage, elimination of the offending source, and antimicrobial therapy. Coliform organisms and *Staphylococcus aureus* are the usual organisms responsible.[83] Rarely, actinomycosis are found.[84] CT-guided drainage may be attempted, but often it is unable to drain these multiloculated collections adequately.

On average, it takes the clinician 12.7 days to diagnose a retroperitoneal abscess.[81] This contributes to the high mortality rate (25% to 50%) associated with this condition.[80]

Retroperitoneal Fibrosis

Retroperitoneal fibrosis is a rare disease involving chronic nonspecific inflammation of the retroperitoneum. In 1905, Albarran first described this process,[85] but it was not accepted as a clinical entity until Ormond's report in 1948.[86] Only 500 cases of this disease have been reported in the literature.[87]

The etiology of retroperitoneal fibrosis is unclear. Only a third of all cases can be linked to an inciting event, while the remainder are of idiopathic origin. It is clear that the diagnosis embodies a variety of conditions with a common pathological presentation.

This disease may be related to an autoimmune phenomena. The syndrome of familial multifocal fibrosclerosis, involving retroperitoneal fibrosis, mediastinal fibrosis, sclerosing cholangitis, Reidel's thyroiditis, and pseudotumor of the orbit, has been described.[88] Additionally, retroperitoneal fibrosis has been linked to scleroderma,[89] Peyronie's disease of the penis, and Dupuytren's contracture of the palmar and plantar fascia.[90]

Recent observations have linked this disorder with atherosclerotic and aneurysmal disease of large vessels.[91] It appears that retroperitoneal fibrosis occurs only in areas of atherosclerotic plaques, and often begins as a mass of fibrotic tissue surrounding the aorta. With time, this mass extends to envelop surrounding tissue and organs. Five to twenty-three percent of abdominal aortic aneurysms are associated with periaortic fibrosis.[92] Ceroid, a by-product of lipoprotein oxidation, leaks through the media, where it acts as an antigen.[93] Patients with clinical and subclinical retroperitoneal fibrosis have been found to have circulating antibody to ceroid, which has been proposed as a marker of disease.

Drug-induced disease is responsible for 12% of cases of retroperitoneal fibrosis.[94] Although a direct causal relationship has been difficult to establish for most medications,[95–103] methysergide, an ergot preparation used for the treatment of migraine headaches, has been clearly implicated.[104] Discontinuation of this drug results in abatement of both subjective symptoms and clinical evidence of the disease.[105]

Finally, a variety of malignant conditions have been associated with retroperitoneal fibrosis, including cancer of the breast, stomach, and prostate, and non-Hodgkin's lymphoma.[94,106] Additionally, trauma, radiation, infection, and previous operation can result in retroperitoneal fibrosis.[107]

Grossly, retroperitoneal fibrosis appears as a solid gray-white dense mass adherent to the retroperitoneum in the midline. It usually encompasses the abdominal aorta and may extend superiorly into the mediastinum. The common iliac arteries may be involved, but the fibrosis rarely continues beyond the pelvic brim.[108] The small intestine and colon are occasionally involved. Histologic examination reveals large collagen bundles accompanied by an inflammatory infiltrate. The tissue is well vascularized with numerous blood vessels.[108]

Most commonly, this process is diagnosed between the ages of 30 and 60 years of age. The incidence is twice as high in men as in women.[94] Patients complain of dull, constant pain localized to the back or flank. Other symptoms include malaise, anorexia, and weight loss. In advanced cases, the patient may present with oliguria and signs of renal failure. A significant number of patients suffer from hypertension: 71% have a diastolic pressure of 90 mm Hg and 53% have a diastolic pressure of 100 mm Hg.[109] Rarely, claudication, secondary to narrowing of the common iliac arteries, may be the presenting complaint.[110] Laboratory evaluation consistently will reveal an elevated erythrocyte sedimentation rate (ESR). Additionally, a normochromic, normocytic anemia and elevated urea nitrogen or creatine often are identified. Six percent of patients will have pyuria or a positive urine culture.[94] If the biliary system is involved, an elevated bilirubin or alkaline phosphatase may be detected.

The diagnosis of retroperitoneal fibrosis is made with IVP (Fig 20–5). The triad of deviation of the middle third of the ureter, hydroureteronephrosis, and extrinsic ureteral compression is pathognomonic for this disease. Ultrasonography and CT scanning (Fig 20–6) may provide useful information, but cannot differentiate between retroperitoneal fibrosis and fibrosis secondary to a malignant condition. Laparotomy with multiple deep biopsies is required to confirm the diagnosis.[94,107]

Traditionally, treatment of retroperitoneal fibrosis has focused on surgical intervention to relieve ureteral obstruction. Any possible inciting agents are discontinued, and some have suggested that, when methysergide is the cause, discontinuation of the drug and monitoring with repeat IVP is adequate. If surgery is chosen, ureterolysis is performed. The ascending and descending colon are reflected medially and, after mobilizing the ureter above and below the mass of fibrosis, it is freed with blunt dissection. The ureter then is placed laterally and held in place by approximating the peritoneum and psoas. Because it is impossible to place the

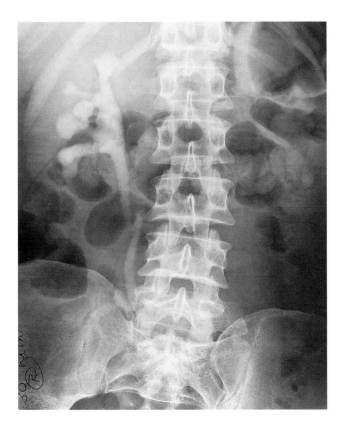

A

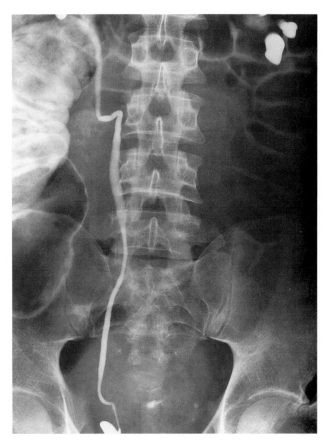

B

Figure 20–5. An IVP **A.** demonstrating hydronephrosis and retrograde pylogram **B.** showing medial displacement of the ureter by retroperitoneal fibrosis. The left ureter is severely obstructed by the fibrosis resulting in delayed filling.

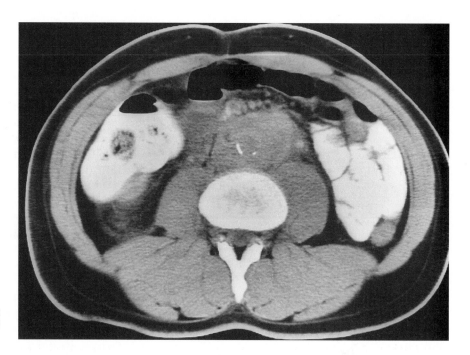

Figure 20–6. A computerized tomograph demonstrating a central mass of retroperitoneal fibrosis encasing the aorta.

entire length of the ureter inside the peritoneum, wrapping the ureter in omentum has been advocated.[111] A 15% to 20% recurrence of ureteral obstruction has been described with surgical intervention. If the ureter is torn, a double J stent is placed and the area is drained.

Because of the high recurrence rate after operation, a nonoperative approach, based on steroid treatment, has been advocated.[112] After initial steroid bolus, long-term prednisolone therapy has been very effective in reducing ureteral obstruction, in mild cases. Steroids also have been recommended in patients who represent poor surgical candidates. Finally, azathioprine may have some role in the treatment of retroperitoneal fibrosis.

The prognosis is good for most patients. Five year survival rates of 86% to 100% have been reported, except in cases where fibrosis is extensive. However, those presenting with disease related to malignancy may succumb within a matter of months.

Retroperitoneal Tumors

Primary neoplasms of the retroperitoneum may arise from the mesoderm, neuroectoderm, or embryonic remnants.[113] These origins account for 75%, 24%, and 1% of primary retroperitoneal tumors, respectively. Lymphomas constitute 30% of all primary retroperitoneal tumors and usually are treated by chemotherapy. The remainder of neoplasms in this location arise from major retroperitoneal organs.

Retroperitoneal Sarcomas. Constituting only 0.7% of adult cancers, soft-tissue sarcomas are rare.[113] Of these, only

15% to 20% are retroperitoneal.[114] These tumors arise from tissues of the epithelium and extraskeleton. Fibrosarcoma and liposarcoma are by far the most common retroperitoneal sarcomas.[115] Others include the leiomyosarcoma, hemangiopericytoma, and rhabdomyosarcoma.

Retroperitoneal sarcomas can occur at any age, but most commonly develop between 40 and 60 years of age. Incidence is equal between the sexes.[115] Although these tumors originate from a variety of tissues, they usually behave in a similar pattern. The retroperitoneal space is deep and can accommodate large masses before detection. As a result, tumors are often large at the time of diagnosis.

Retroperitoneal tumors are often locally aggressive, invading along multiple tissue planes, blood vessels, and nerves. Metastases are hematogenous, and are found, in decreasing incidence, in the lung, liver, bladder, and bone.[116] Lymphatic spread is unusual. Histologic grade and DNA ploidy are major prognostic factors.[117,118] Low-grade sarcomas demonstrate 2 to 10 mitoses/10 high-power fields, while high-grade sarcomas show more than 10 mitoses/10 high-power fields. The TNMG system is used for staging, indicating the size of the primary tumor (T), the involvement of lymph nodes (N), the presence of metastasis (M), and the type and grade of the tumor (G) (Table 20–1).

Three-fourths of patients complain of pain and 60% will have constitutional complaints of anorexia and weight loss.[115] Additionally, a third will have fever, suggesting tumor necrosis. Genitourinary symptoms, ve-

TABLE 20–1. SCHEMATIC OF THE STAGING OF SOFT TISSUE SARCOMAS BY TNMG

T	Primary tumor	
	T1 Tumor <5 cm	
	T2 Tumor ≥5 cm	
	T3 Tumor that grossly invades bone, major vessel, of major nerve	
N	Regional lymph nodes	
	N0 No histologically verified metastases to regional lymph nodes	
	N1 Histologically verified regional lymph node metastasis	
M	Distant metastasis	
	M0 No distant metastasis	
	M1 Distant metastasis	
G	Histologic grade of malignancy	
	G1 Low	
	G2 Moderate	
	G3 High	
Stage I		
Stage Ia		
G1T1N0M0	Grade 1 tumor <5 cm in diameter with no regional lymph nodes or distant metastases	
Stage Ib		
G1T2N0M0	Grade 1 tumor ≥ 5 cm in diameter with no regional lymph nodes or distant metastasis	
Stage II		
Stage IIa		
G2T1N0M0	Grade 2 tumor <5 cm in diameter with no regional lymph nodes or distant metastases	
Stage IIb		
G2T2N0M0	Grade 2 tumor ≥5 cm in diameter with no regional lymph nodes or distant metastases	
Stage III		
Stage IIIa		
G3T1N0M0	Grade 3 tumor <5 cm in diameter with no regional lymph nodes or distant metastases	
Stage IIIb		
G3T2N0M0	Grade 3 tumor ≥5 cm in diameter with no regional lymph nodes or distant metastases	
Stage IIIc		
Any GT1GT2N1M0	Tumor of any grade or size (no invasion) with regional lymph nodes but no distant metastases	
Stage IV		
Stage IVa		
Any GT3N0N1M0	Tumor of any grade that grossly invades bone, major vessel, or major nerve with or without regional lymph node metastases but without distant metastases	
Stage IVb		
Anny GTNM	Tumor with distant metastases	

(From Russell WO, et al. Cancer 40:1562–1570, 1977.)

nous thrombosis, lower-extremity edema, pleural effusion, peripheral nerve disorders, and intra-abdominal bleeding may complicate the presentation. Large vascular tumors may sequester platelets and produce bleeding disorders.

Since these tumors grow to considerable size before presentation, the clinician will find a palpable mass in most patients. Laboratory studies are not usually very helpful, but imaging techniques are valuable preoperatively.[119] Plain x-rays are relatively nonspecific. An IVP can be helpful if it demonstrates displacement and rotation of the kidney and ureter found in 85% to 93% of cases. Angiography and venography rarely are employed, but may be useful in cases of suspected intravascular invasion. Ultrasonography can be revealing, but is inadequate in 30% of cases because of signal interference from intraluminal gas. CT is by far the most useful tool. It is reliable and usually can characterize the extent of the tumor and surrounding organ involvement. Contrast CT studies may obviate the need for IVP. Additionally, CT-guided needle biopsy is particularly useful in obtaining a preoperative tissue diagnosis.[120] The major limitation of the CT scan is the inability of this test to assess local infiltration. Consequently, CT evaluation is not able to predict tumor resectability.[121]

The treatment for these tumors is surgical.[122] To date, there is no evidence that adjuvant therapy improves survival. Radiotherapy, chemotherapy, or phototherapy have not been shown to effect outcome.[116] Intraoperative radiotherapy may prove useful.[123] A transperitoneal approach is used for greatest exposure and en bloc resection is essential. Frozen sections are used to guide the surgeon in establishing tumor-free margins. To perform complete resection, excision of surrounding organs en bloc with the tumor may be necessary.

When complete resection is accomplished, 5 year survival rates vary between 32% and 100%.[115] Overall survival, including partial resection, is 11% to 50% at 5 years and 10% to 20% at 10 years. Follow-up to evaluate recurrent disease should be performed on a regular basis. At least 50% of patients will demonstrate local recurrence and one-third will have distant metastases. Overall, reexploration for recurrence is not very effective. Patients usually succumb to the local invasive effects of the tumor, including renal and intestinal obstruction, perforation, and fistula formation.

■ SUMMARY

When considering lesions of the mesentery, omentum, and retroperitoneum, the clinician must have a high index of suspicion. The rarity, anatomy, and nonspecificity of these disorders often leads to incorrect and untimely diagnosis. The expertise of the surgeon is often required, but, as described, the treatment is sometimes controversial and unproven. When confronting these conditions, an unrestricted differential diagnosis will best serve the patient and clinician.

REFERENCES

1. Gilmore OJA, Browett JP, Griffin PH, et al. Appendicitis and mimicking conditions: a prospective study. *Lancet* 1975;2:421

2. Hervás JA, Alberti P, Bregante JI, et al. Chronic intussusception associated with Yersenia enterocolitica mesenteric adenitis. *J Ped Surg* 1992;27:1591

3. Lambrianides AL, Ackroyd N, Shorey BA. Abdominal tuberculosis. *Br J Surg* 1980;67:887

4. Crane JT, Aguilare MJ, Grimes OF. Isolated lipodystrophy. a form of mesenteric tumour. *Am J Surg* 1955;900:169

5. Kipfer RE, Moertal CG, Dahlim D. Mesenteric lipodystrophy. *Ann Intern Med* 1974;80:582

6. Durst AL, Freund H, Rosenmann E, Birnbaum D. Mesenteric panniculitis: review of the literature and presentation of cases. *Surgery* 1977;81:203

7. Bashir MS, Abbott CR. Mesenteric lipodystrophy. *J Clin Pathol* 1993;46:872

8. Monohan DW, Poston WK, Brown GJ. Mesenteric panniculitis. *South Med J* 1989;82:782

9. Kawashima A, Fishman EK, Hruban RH, et al. Mesenteric panniculitis presenting as a multilocular cystic mesenteric mass: CT and MR evaluation. *Clin Imaging* 1993;17:112

10. Bush RW, Hammar SP, Rudolph RH. Sclerosing mesenteritis: response to cyclophosphamide. *Arch Intern Med* 1986;146:503

11. Braquehage J. Des kystes du mesentery. *Arch Gen* 1892;170:291

12. Tillauz PJ. Cyste duu mesentere un homme: Ablation par la gastromie: quersion. *Revue de Therapeutiques Medico-Chirurgicale Paris* 1880;47:479

13. Kurtz RJ, Heiman TM, Beck AR, Holt J. Mesenteric and retroperitoneal cysts. *Ann Surg* 1986;203:109

14. Beahrs OH, Judd ES, Dockerty MB. Chylous cysts of the abdomen. *Surg Clin North Am* 1950;30:1081

15. Kosir MA, Sonnino RE, Gauderer MWL. Pediatric abdominal lymphangiomas: a plea for early recognition. *J Ped Surg* 1991;26:1309

16. Caropreso PR. Mesenteric cysts: a review. *Arch Surg* 1974;108:242

17. Chung MA, Brandt ML, St-Vil D, Yazbech S. Mesenteric cysts in children. *J Ped Surg* 1991;26:1306

18. Takiff H, Calabria R, Yin L, Stabile BE. Mesenteric cysts and intra-abdominal cystic lymphangiomas. *Arch Surg* 1985;120:1266

19. Tos PR, Olmsted WW, Moser RP Jr., et al. Mesenteric and omental cysts: histologic classification with imaging correlation. *Radiology* 1987;164:327

20. Mackenzie DJ, Shapiro SJ, Gordon LA, Ress R. Laparoscopic excision of a mesenteric cyst. *J Laparoendo Surg* 1993;3:295

21. Gast MJ, Jacobs AJ, Goforth G, Martin CM. Mesenteric cysts in pregnancy: a case report. *J Repro Med* 1989;34:179

22. Tykka H, Koivuniemi A. Carcinoma arising in a mesenteric cyst. *Am J Surg* 1975;129:709

23. Ganzaaleez-Crussi F, Soteloo-Avila C, deMello DE. Primary peritoneal, omental, and mesenteric tumors in childhood. *Sem Diag Pathol* 1986;3:122

24. Kannerstein M, Churg J. Peritoneal mesothelioma. *Hum Pathol* 1977;8:833

25. Asensio JA, Goldblatt P, Thomford NR. Primary malignant peritoneal mesothelioma. *Arch Surg* 1990;125:1477

26. Miller J, Wynn H. A malignant tumor arising from the endothelium of the peritoneum and producing mucoid ascitic fluid. *J Pathol Bacteriol* 1908;12:267

27. Behbehani AM, Hunter WJ, Chapman AL, Lin F. Studies of a human mesothelioma. *Hum Pathol* 1982;13:862

28. Donna A, Betta PG, Bellingeri D, Marchesi A. New marker for mesothelioma: an immunoperoxidase study. *J Clin Pathol* 1986;33:961

29. Perks WH, Stanhope R, Green M. Hyponatremia and mesothelioma. *Br J Dis Chest* 1979;73:89

30. Anderson N, Lokich JJ. Mesenchymal tumors associated with hypoglycemia: a case report and review of the literature. *Cancer* 1979;44:785

31. Knight RA, Ratcliffe JG, Besser GM. Tumor ACTH concentrations in ectopic ACTH syndrome and in control tissues. *Proc R Soc Med* 1971;64:1266

32. Karakousis CP, Seddiq M, Moore R. Malignant mesotheliomas and chemotherapy. *J Surg Oncol* 1980;15:181

33. Rogoff EE, Hilaris BS, Huvos AG. Long term survival in patients with malignant peritoneal mesothelioma treated with irradiation. *Cancer* 1973;32:656

34. Plaus WJ. Peritoneal mesothelioma. *Arch Surg* 1988;123:763

35. Hanrahan JB. A combined papillary mesothelioma and adenomatoid tumor of the omentum: report of a case. *Cancer* 1963;16:1497

36. Ross MJ, Welch WR, Scully RE. Multilocular peritoneal inclusion cysts (so called cystic mesothelioma). *Cancer* 1989;64:1336

37. Katsube Y, Mukai K, Silverberg SG. Cystic mesothelioma of the peritoneum: a report of five cases and review of the literature. *Cancer* 1982;50:1615

38. Macfarlane J. Clinical reports on the surgical practice of the Glasgow Royal Infirmary. Glasgow, Scotland: D Robertson, 1832:63–6

39. Reitamo JJ, Scheinin TM, Häyry P. The desmoid syndrome: new aspects in the cause, pathogenesis, and treatment of the desmoid tumor. *Am J Surg* 1986;151:230

40. Reitamo JJ. *The Desmoid Tumour.* [Academic dissertation] Helsinki, Finland: *University of Helsinki;* 1980

41. Häyry P, Reitamo JJ, Vihko R, et al. The desmoid tumor, III. a biochemical and genetic analysis. *Am J Clin Pathol* 1982;77:681

42. Miralbell R, Suit HD, Phil D, et al. Fibromatoses: from postsurgical surveillance to combined surgery and radiation therapy. *Int J Radiat Oncol Biol Phys* 1990;18:535

43. Belliveau P, Graham AM. Mesenteric desmoid tumor in Gardner's syndrome treated by sulindac. *Dis Colon Rectum* 1984;27:53

44. Waddell WR, Gerner RE. Indomethacin and ascorbate inhibit desmoid tumors. *J Surg Oncol* 1980;15:85

45. Lockwood CB: The development of the great omentum and transverse mesocolon. *J Anat Physiol* 1984;18:257

46. Walker FC. The protective function of the greater omentum. *Ann R Coll Surg Engl* 1963;33:282

47. Eitel GG. Rare omental torsion. *NY Med Rec* 1899;55:715

48. Brady SC, Kliman MR. Torsion of the greater omentum or appendices epiploicae. *Can J Surg* 1979;22:79

49. Croffot DD. Spontaneous segmental infarction of the greater omentum. *Am J Surg* 1980;139:262

50. Epstein LI, Lempke RE. Primary idiopathic segmental infarction of the greater omentum. *Ann Surg* 1968;167:437

51. Das SK. The size of the human omentum and methods of lengthening it for transplantation. *Br J Plast Surg* 1976; 29:170

52. Alday ES, Goldsmith HS. Surgical technique for omental lengthening. *Surg Gynecol Obstet* 1972;135:103

53. Bennett WH. A case of perforating gastric ulcer in which the opening, being otherwise intractable, was closed by means of an omental plug: recovery. *Lancet* 1896;2:310

54. Walters W. An omental flap in transperitoneal repair of recurring vesicovaginal fistulas. *Surg Gynecol Obstet* 1937;64:74

55. Dubois P, Choiniere L, Cooper JD. Bronchial omentoplasty in canine lung allotransplantation. *Ann Thorac Surg* 1984;38:211

56. Goldsmith HS, deSantos R. Omental transposition in primary lymphedema. *Surg Gynecol Obstet* 1967;125:607

57. Carter MJ. The use of the right gastroepiploic artery in coronary artery bypass grafting. *Aust NZ J Surg* 1987;57:317

58. Casten DF, Alday ES. Omental transfer for revascularization of the extremities. *Surg Gynecol Obstet* 1971;132:301

59. Fix RJ, Vasconez LO. Use of the omentum in chest-wall reconstruction. *Surg Clin North Am* 1989;69:1029

60. Samson R, Pasternak BM. Current status of surgery of the omentum. *Surg Gynecol Obstet* 1979;143:437

61. Jurkiewicz MJ, Nahai F. The omentum: its use as a free vascularized graft for reconstruction of the head and neck. *Ann Surg* 1982;195:756

62. Miyamoto S, Kikuchi H, Karasawa J, et al. Study of the posterior circulation in moya moya disease 2: visual disturbances and surgical treatment. *J Neurosurg* 1986;65:454

63. Goldsmith HS, Kiely AA, Randall HT. Protection of intrathoracic oesophageal anastomoses by omentum. *Surgery* 1968;63:464

64. Lanter B, Mason R. Use omental pedicle graft to protect low anterior colonic anastomosis. *Dis Colon Rectum* 1979;22:448

65. Dockendorf BL, Frazee RC, Matheny RO. Omental pedicle graft to improve ischemic anastomoses. *Southern Med J* 1993;86:628

66. Adams W, Ctercteko G, Bilouus M. Effect of an omental wrap on the healing and vascularity of compromised intestinal anastomoses. *Dis Colon Rectum* 1992;35:731

66a. Cooper JD, Pearson FG, Patterson GA, et al. Technique of successful lung transplantation in humans. *J Thor Card Surg* 1987;93:173

67. Gaidner WT. A remarkable cyst in the omentum. *Trans Path Soc Lond* 1852;3:1851

68. Walker AR, Putman TC. Omental mesenteric, and retroperitoneal cysts: a clinical study of 33 new cases. *Ann Surg* 1973;178:13

69. Hebra A, Brown MF, McGeehin KM, Ross AJ. Mesenteric, omental and retroperitoneal cysts in children: a clinical study of 22 cases. *South Med J* 1993;86:173

70. Stout AP, Cassel C. Hemangiopericytoma of the omentum. *Surgery* 1942;11:578

71. Schwartz RW, Reames M, McGrath PC, et al. Primary solid neoplasms of the greater omentum. *Surgery* 1991; 109:543

72. Okajima Y, Nishikawa M, Ohi M, et al. Primary liposarcoma of the omentum. *Postgrad Med J* 1993;69:157

73. Mahon DE, Carp NZ, Goldhahn RT, Schmutzler RC. Primary leiomyosarcoma of the greater omentum: case report and review of the literature. *Am Surg* 1993;53:160

74. Feliciano DV. Management of traumatic retroperitoneal hematoma. *Ann Surg* 1990;211:109

75. Allen RE, Eastman BA, Halter BL, Conolly WB. Retroperitoneal hemorrhage secondary to blunt trauma. *Am J Surg* 1969;118:558

76. Selivanov V, Chi HS, Alverdy JC, et al. Mortality in retroperitoneal hematoma. *J Trauma* 1984;24:1022

77. Hubbard SG, Bivins BA, Sachatello CR, Griffen WO. Diagnostic errors with peritoneal lavage in patients with pelvic fractures. *Arch Surg* 1979;114:844

78. Goins WA, Lewis J, Brathwaite CEM, James E. Retroperitoneal hematoma after blunt trauma. *Surg Gynecol Obstet* 1992;174:281–290

79. Hölting T, Buhr HJ, Richter GM, et al. Diagnosis and treatment of retroperitoneal hematoma in multiple trauma patients. *Arch Ortho Trauma Surg* 1992;111:323

80. Harris LF, Sparks E. Retroperitoneal abscess: case report and review of the literature. *Dig Dis Sci* 1980;25:392

81. Crepps JT, Welch JP, Orlando R. Management and outcome of retroperitoneal abscesses. *Ann Surg* 1987;205:276

82. Altemeier WA, Alexander JW. Retroperitoneal abscess. *Arch Surg* 1961;83:512

83. Stevenson EOS, Ozeran RS. Retroperitoneal space abscesses. *Surg Gynecol Obstet* 1969;128:1202

84. Daniglus GF, Rush BF. Retroperitoneal abscesses. a clinical study. *Arch Surg* 1961;83:322

85. Albarran J. Rétention rénale par périuretèrite; libération externe de l'uretère. *Assoc FrUrol* 1905;9:511

86. Ormond JK. Bilateral ureteral obstruction due to envelopment and compression by inflammatory retroperitoneal process. *J Urol* 1948;59:1072

87. Gilkeson GS, Rice JR. Retroperitoneal fibrosis. the forgotten connective tissue disease. *NC Med J* 1989;50:192–194

88. Comings DE, Skubi KB, Van Eyes J, Motulsky AG. Familial multifocal fibrosclerosis. Findings suggesting that retroperitoneal fibrosis, mediastinal fibrosis, sclerosing cholangitis, Reidel's thyroiditis, and pseudotumor of the orbit may be different manifestations of a single disease. *Ann Intern Med* 1967;66:884

89. Mansell MA, Watts RWE. Retroperitoneal fibrosis and scleroderma. *Postgrad Med J* 1980;56:730

90. Pang J, Vicary FR, Beck ER. Primary retroperitoneal and mediastinal fibrosis. *Postgrad Med J* 1983;59:450

91. Mitchinson MJ. Chronic periaortitis and periarteritis. *Histopathology* 1984;8:589

92. Sethia B, Darke SG. Abdominal aortic aneurysm with retroperitoneal fibrosis and ureteric entrapment. *Br J Surg* 1983;70:434

93. Parmus DV, Mitchinson MJ. Serum antibodies to oxidized

LDL and ceroid in chronic periaortitis. *J Pathol* 1987; 151:57A

94. Koep L, Zuidema GD. The clinical significance of retroperitoneal fibrosis. *Surgery* 1977;81:250

95. Bowler JV, Ormerod IE, Legg NJ. Retroperitoneal fibrosis and bromocriptine [letter]. *Lancet* 1986;2:466

96. Pierce JR Jr., Trostle DC, Warner JJ. Propranolol and retroperitoneal fibrosis [letter]. *Ann Intern Med* 1981; 95:244

97. Johnson JN, McFarland J. Retroperitoneal fibrosis associated with stenolol [letter]. *Br Med J* 1980;280:864

98. Lewis CT, Molland EA, Marshall VR, et al. Analgesic abuse, ureteric obstruction, and retroperitoneal fibrosis. *Br Med J* 1975;2:76–78

99. Kinder CH. Retroperitoneal fibrosis. *J R Soc Med* 1979; 72:485

100. Jeffries JJ, Lyall WA, Bezchlibnyk K, et al. Retroperitoneal fibrosis and haloperidol [letter]. *Am J Psychiatry* 1982;139:1524

101. Ahmad S. Methyldopa and retroperitoneal fibrosis. *Am Heart J* 1983;105:1037

102. Critchley JA, Smith MF, Prescott LF. Distalgesic abuse and retroperitoneal fibrosis. *Br J Urology* 1985;57:486

103. Laakso M, Arvala I, Tervonen S, Sotarauta M. Retroperitoneal fibrosis associated with sotalol. *Br Med J* 1982; 285:1085

104. Graham JR, Suby HI, Le Compte PR, Sadowsky NL. Fibrotic disorders associated with methysarside therapy for headache. *N Engl J Med* 1966;270:359

105. Elkind AH, Friedman AP, Bachman A, et al. Silent retroperitoneal fibrosis associated with methysergide therapy. *JAMA* 1968;206:1041

106. Dlabal PW, Mullins JD, Coltman CA Jr. An unusual manifestation of non-Hodgkin's lymphoma: fibrosis masquerading as Ormond's disease. *JAMA* 1980;243:1161

107. Webb AJ, Dawson-Edwares P. Malignant retroperitoneal fibrosis. *Br J Surg* 1967;54:505

108. Mitchenson MJ. The pathology of idiopathic retroperitoneal fibrosis. *J Clin Pathol* 1970;23:681

109. Pryor JP, Castle WM, Dukes DC, et al. Do beta adreno-ceptor blocking drugs cause retroperitoneal fibrosis? *Br Med J* 1983;287:639

110. Shortland GJ, Archer TJ, Webster JHH. Intermittent claudication caused by retroperitoneal fibrosis. *Br J Surg* 1986;73:156

111. Carini M, Selli C, Rizzi M, et al. Surgical treatment of retroperitoneal fibrosis with omentoplasty. *Surgery* 1982; 91:137

112. Higgins PM, Bennet-Jones DN, Naich PF, Aber GM. Non-operative management of retroperitoneal fibrosis. *Br J Surg* 1988;75:573

113. Bek V. Primary retroperitoneal tumors. *Neoplasma* 1970; 17:253

114. Parkinson MC, Chabrel CM. Clinicopathological features of retroperitoneal tumours. *Br J Urol* 1984;56:17

115. Stower MJ, Hardcastle JD. Malignant retroperitoneal sarcoma: a review of 32 cases. *Clin Oncol* 1982;8:257

116. Van Dam PA, Lowe DG, McKenzie-Gray B, Shepherd JH. Retroperitoneal soft tissue sarcomas: a review of the literature. *Obstet Gyn Survey* 1990;45:670

117. Felix EL, Wood DK, Das-Gupta TK. Tumors of the retroperitoneum. *Curr Probl Cancer* 1982;6:1

118. Kreicbergs A, Tribukait B, Willems J, Bauer HC. DNA-flow analysis of soft tissue tumors. *Cancer* 1987;59:128

119. Davidson AJ, Hartman DS. Imaging strategies for tumors of the kidney, adrenal gland, and retroperitoneum. *CA* 1987;37:151

120. Balfe DM, McClennan BL. CT of the retroperitoneum in urosurgical disorders. *Surg Clin North Am* 1982; 62:919

121. Pistolesi GF, Procacci C, Caudana R, Bergamo et al. CT criteria of the differential diagnosis in primary retroperitoneal masses. *Eur J Radiol* 1984;4:127

122. McGrath PC, Neifeild JP, Lawrence WJR, et al. Improved survival following complete excision of retroperitoneal sarcomas. *Ann Surg* 1984;200:200

123. Sindelar WF, Hoekstra HJ, Kinsella TJ. Surgical approaches and techniques in intraoperative radiotherapy for intraabdominal, retroperitoneal, and pelvic neoplasm. *Surgery* 1988;103:247

21

The Adrenal Glands

Gary R. Peplinski ▪ *Jeffrey A. Norton*

Adrenal surgery requires a knowledge of adrenal anatomy, development, and hormonal physiology. The diagnosis of many adrenal disorders mandates a high index of clinical suspicion. Diagnostic testing does not always indicate a definitive cause, and radiologic localization may be unrevealing. Consequently, the management of adrenal disorders may not be straightforward. Surgery plays a prominent role in treating most adrenal abnormalities and perioperative considerations can greatly influence operative success and outcome.

Eustachius first described the adrenal glands in 1563. Clinical syndromes of inadequate and excessive production of adrenal hormones subsequently were recognized by several prominent investigators, including adrenal insufficiency, by Thomas Addison in 1855, hypercortisolism by Harvey Cushing in 1932, and hyperaldosteronism by Jerome Conn in 1952. Charles Brown-Sequard first performed adrenalectomies in animals and demonstrated that the adrenal glands are necessary for life.

This chapter introduces adrenal endocrinology from a surgical perspective.

▪ ANATOMY AND EMBRYOLOGY

The adrenal glands are situated in the retroperitoneum and cap the superomedial aspect of each kidney anteriorly (Fig 21–1). The normal gland is 3 to 5 cm long, 2 to 3 cm wide, 0.5 cm thick, and weighs 3 to 6 gm.[1] The adrenal glands are firm in consistency and can be distinguished from the surrounding structures by palpation. Each gland is circumscribed by a fibrous connective tissue capsule and enveloped in areolar perirenal fat. Grossly, the normal adrenal cortex appears bright yellow, and the normal adrenal medulla appears red-brown in color. The right adrenal gland is pyramidal in shape, abutting the posterolateral perimeter of the inferior vena cava, the posterior right lobe of the liver, and the undersurface of the right diaphragmatic crus. The left adrenal gland is crescenteric in shape, bordering the posterior aspect of the gastric cardia, pancreas, splenic vessels, and left renal vein on its anterior surface, and resting upon the left diaphragmatic crus posteriorly. It is close to the aorta medially.[2] The dissection of large or invasive tumors is complicated by the proximity of important structures, such as the aorta and inferior vena cava. Several different surgical approaches to exposure of the adrenal glands have been devised to permit safe resection.

The adrenal glands are highly vascular and derive their arterial supply from several different sources. Numerous small arteries enter each gland along the perimeter, arising from the inferior phrenic arteries superiorly, directly from the aorta medially, and from the renal arteries inferiorly (Fig 21–1).[2] The arteries form a vascular plexus within the capsule and give rise to medullary arterioles, which bridge the cortex to supply the medulla directly, and cortical arterioles, which perfuse the cortex and empty into the medullary venous si-

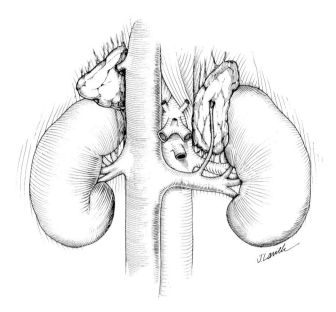

Figure 21–1. Adrenal anatomy. The adrenal glands lie in a central location deep within the retroperitoneum, capping the superior aspect of each kidney. The arterial blood supply is derived from the inferior phrenic arteries superiorly, directly from the aorta medially, and from the renal arteries inferiorly. Venous blood of the right gland drains directly into the vena cava via a wide short vein. The left adrenal vein courses medially to drain into the left renal vein, although rarely, it may drain to the vena cava or the inferior phrenic vein.

nusoids.[1] The direct flow of venous blood from the cortex to the medulla results in high cortisol concentrations bathing the medullary cells. Cortisol activates phenylethanolamine-N-methyltransferase (PNMT), a medullary enzyme that methylates norepinephrine to form epinephrine.[3] As a consequence, the adrenal glands produce high levels of epinephrine as compared to extraadrenal chromaffin tissues, which predominantly secrete norepinephrine.

Venous drainage of the glands is more constant. A wide, short (5 mm) central vein drains venous blood from the medial right adrenal gland directly into the vena cava at its posterolateral perimeter.[2] When the gland is enlarged, the right adrenal vein is difficult to access. Meticulous dissection is warranted around this vein, which is a potentially life-threatening source of hemorrhage. The left adrenal vein exits anteriorly from the left adrenal gland and courses medially to drain into the left renal vein. Rarely, it may drain into the vena cava or the inferior phrenic vein.

Lymphatic vessels are present in the capsule and connective tissue around the larger blood vessels. No lymphatic vessels are identified within the gland parenchyma.[1] In humans, the adrenal cortex has no known innervation. The parenchymal cells of the adrenal medulla are innervated directly by splanchnic nerves containing preganglionic sympathetic neurons that arise from the celiac and renal plexuses. These nerve fibers

stimulate the cells to secrete epinephrine and norepinephrine.[3] Thus, the adrenal medulla is a site of integration between the neurologic and endocrine systems.

Microscopically, three concentric zones are defined in the adrenal cortex: the zona glomerulosa, a thin layer adjacent to the capsule; the zona fasciculata, a thick middle layer; and the zona reticularis, a thin inner layer bordering the medulla.[1] The cells of the cortex are arranged in cords which are separated by capillaries and sinuses. Stimulation by adrenocorticotropin hormone (ACTH) causes hyperplasia of the adrenal cortex, a reversible compensatory increase in the number of cortical cells, and production of greater amounts of cortisol. Conversely, lack of ACTH stimulation results in atrophy of the cortex, a decrease in the number and size of cortical cells, and a reduction in cortisol production.

The medulla represents 10% of the total weight of the gland. It is composed of two cell types, each of which can produce either epinephrine or norepinephrine.[1] These catecholamines are present in numerous granules within each cell and react with chromium salts; thus, the name *chromaffin* cells. Cells are arranged in short, interconnected cords surrounded by blood vessels.

The embryological derivation of adrenal tissue is of importance to the surgeon since tumors may occur in ectopic locations. Cells of the adrenal cortex and medullary have different embryologic origins. The cortex develops from coelomic mesoderm near the urogenital ridge in the fourth to sixth week of life and differentiates into an outer definitive cortex and an inner fetal zone by the eighth week.[4] During gestation, the fetal zone produces steroids that are metabolized by the placenta into estrogens, and it gradually involutes after birth. Differentiation of the three cortical zones is not complete until age 3. Accessory adrenocortical tissue may be found surrounding the adrenal gland, in the kidney, ovary, broad ligament, or testis (Fig 21–2).[5] The medulla originates from ectodermal neural crest cells in the thoracic region that migrate ventrolateral to the aorta to form the primitive sympathetic ganglia.[4] These cells give rise to the celiac, mesenteric, and renal sympathetic ganglia. Medullary cells migrate along the adrenal vein until contact is made with the primitive adrenal cortical cells that surround the medullary cells. Pheochromocytomas may develop anywhere along this path of migration, particularly in the periaortic paraganglia at the level of the kidney, in the organ of Zuckerkandl located to the left of the aortic bifurcation near the origin of the inferior mesenteric artery, in the bladder, mediastinum, neck, and anal or vaginal areas (Fig 21–2).[5] Complete abdominal exploration of these areas is necessary during resection of pheochromocytomas since there is a high incidence of bilaterality and extraadrenal tumors. The incidence of functioning extraadrenal cortical tissue is much lower.

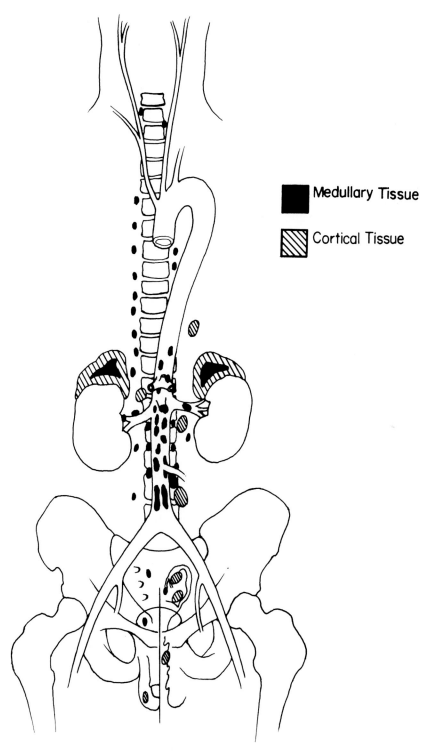

Figure 21–2. Sites of extraadrenal cortical and medullary tissues. Adrenal tumors may arise at any site along the route of developmental migration of adrenal cells. The incidence of functioning extraadrenal pheochromocytomas is very high as compared to functioning extraadrenal cortical tissue. Complete abdominal exploration for ectopic pheochromocytomas is mandatory.

ADRENAL CORTEX

PHYSIOLOGY

The adrenal cortex manufactures several different steroids which are essential for life. Although numerous steroids have been extracted from the adrenal gland, only a few are normally secreted.[3] Steroid hormones are synthesized from cholesterol, which is derived from the circulating blood or produced within the cortical cells from acetate. It is stored in the esterified form. The rate-limiting reaction in steroid synthesis is the conversion of cholesterol to pregnenolone, which requires nicotinamide ademine dinucleotide phosphate (NADPH) and oxygen.[3] It occurs within mitochondria. A number of reactions then can occur in both the mitochondria and the smooth endoplasmic reticulum that commits pregnenolone to one of three pathways leading to the formation of glucocorticoids, mineralocorticoids, or sex steroids (Fig 21–3).

Cortisol

The cells of the zona fasciculata primarily produce glucocorticoids. Cortisol accounts for most of the glucocorticoid activity. Hydroxylation of pregnenolone or progesterone by the enzymes 17α-hydroxylase and then 21-hydroxylase, produces 11-deoxycortisol which, in turn, is hydroxylated at the C-11 position to generate cortisol (Fig 21–3). Approximately 10 to 30 mg of cortisol is produced each day by normal adult adrenal glands; with maximal stimulation, the glands can produce approximately 200 mg of cortisol per day.[3,6]

Cortisol circulates in the plasma, bound primarily to cortisol-binding globulin (CBG), also known as transcortin, an α-globulin produced by the liver. Unbound cortisol represents the physiologically active steroid. During states of increased cortisol production, CBG-binding capacity is exceeded, excessive cortisol binds weakly to albumin, and the level of unbound, unmetabolized (free) cortisol in the urine increases sharply.[3] CBG is increased in patients receiving estrogen therapy or oral contraceptives and during pregnancy and hyperthyroidism. Therefore, the measured total plasma cortisol level is increased in these conditions, but the free cortisol level is maintained at normal levels. The plasma half-life of cortisol is about 90 minutes. The liver metabolizes cortisol to inactive compounds that are conjugated to glucuronide and excreted in the urine.[3] The levels of free (unmetabolized) cortisol and 17-hydroxysteroids in a 24 hour urine sample may be measured to diagnose hypercortisolism.

Cortisol has a diverse repertoire of effects, including metabolic, immunosuppressive, connective tissue, renal, gastric, vascular, and psychoneural actions.[3] The effects of active vitamin metabolites are antagonized, and calcium absorption from the gut is decreased. Chronic, high-dose steroid therapy may lead to euphoria initially, then paranoia and depression. The carbohydrate-sparing and antiinsulin effects of cortisol are well known. Glucocorticoids promote the conversion of amino acids to carbohydrates and increase glycogen storage in the liver. Peripheral protein catabolism, which provides amino acids for gluconeogenesis in the liver, results in muscle wasting and weakness. The glucocorticoid-induced inhibition of glucose transport into muscle and adipose tissues results in a state of glucose intolerance. This antiinsulin effect also contributes to hyperglycemia, with a compensatory hyperinsulinemia. Cortisol also induces lipolysis and the redistribution of fat to truncal areas, with an increase in total body fat.

Glucocorticoids have profound immunosuppressive and antiinflammatory effects. Hematopoiesis is stimulated, but the numbers of circulating lymphocytes, monocytes, eosinophils, and basophils are reduced as these cells are redistributed from the vascular compartment into the lymphoid tissues. Glucocorticoids interfere with the margination, adherence, and diapedesis of neutrophils by antagonizing migration inhibitory factor.[3] Cortisol stabilizes lysosomal membranes, thereby inhibiting the release of enzymes. As a result of these immunosuppressive effects, infections and abscesses do not produce classical clinical signs; a high index of suspicion must be maintained and diagnosed infections must be treated aggressively.

Collagen formation and fibroblast activity is hindered, resulting in impaired wound healing.[3] Connective tissue is reduced in quantity and strength. These are important factors that alter postoperative wound management in the patient on steroids. Nonabsorbable sutures or clips in the skin usually are left in place postoperatively for longer periods of time.

Stimulation by cholinergic neurons or serotonin causes the paraventricular peptidergic neurons of the hypothalamus to release corticotropin-releasing hormone (CRH), which reaches the anterior pituitary via the hypophysial portal system and stimulates the secretion of ACTH into the systemic circulation. ACTH binds to high-affinity receptors on adrenocortical cells, increases intracellular cyclic-AMP concentrations, and induces the synthesis and secretion of cortisol. Peak plasma cortisol concentrations occur between 4 and 8 AM and levels nadir at 8 PM to midnight. Of the endogenous corticosteroids, only free cortisol suppresses the transcription of the ACTH gene in the pituitary and the production of CRH in the hypothalamus (Fig 21–4).[3] Thus, measurement of plasma ACTH levels provides a clue as to the etiology of hypercortisolism. Exogenously administered dexamethasone is also a potent inhibitor of ACTH secretion. With chronic supraphysiologic concentrations of cortisol, the adrenal cortex undergoes disuse atrophy, and conversely, the gland hy-

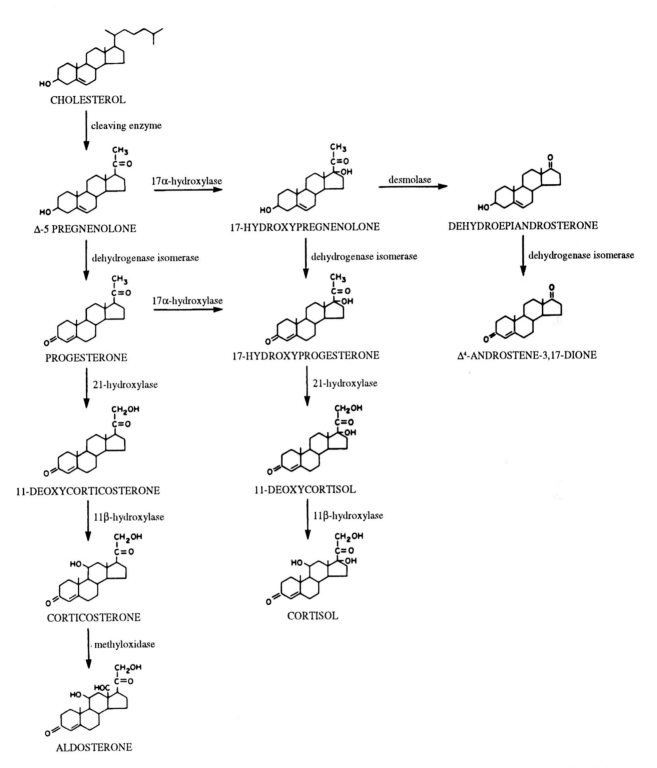

Figure 21–3. Adrenocortical steroid biosynthesis. Adrenal cortical steroid hormones are synthesized from cholesterol, which is derived from the circulating blood or produced within the cortical cells. The rate-limiting reaction in steroid biosynthesis is the conversion of cholesterol to pregnenolone. The zona glomerulosa lacks the enzyme 17α-hydroxylase and therefore, produces aldosterone exclusively.

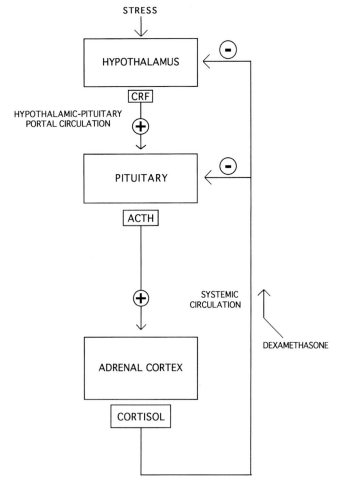

Figure 21–4. The hypothalamic-pituitary-adrenal biofeedback system. The hypothalamus releases CRH into the hypophysial portal system which stimulates the secretion of ACTH from the anterior pituitary. ACTH induces the synthesis and diurnal secretion of cortisol with peak plasma cortisol concentrations occurring between 4 AM and 8 AM. Cortisol and exogenously administered glucocorticoids are potent inhibitors of ACTH secretion. ACTH secretion may be enhanced despite supraphysiologic cortisol levels under conditions of stress.

pertrophies as ACTH secretion rises. Conditions of stress, including surgery, trauma, hemorrhage, pain, pyrogens, exercise, and acute anxiety all enhance ACTH secretion despite supraphysiologic glucocorticoid levels.[3] If atrophy of the adrenal glands exists, endogenous cortisol will not be generated in sufficient amounts acutely in response to ACTH under these circumstances. Adrenal crisis ensues if glucocorticoids are not administered, which may result in death of the patient.

Aldosterone

Unlike the other two cortical zones, the zona glomerulosa lacks the enzyme 17α-hydroxylase. In these adrenocortical cells, pregnenolone therefore is converted to progesterone, which is hydroxylated and methyloxi-

dated to form aldosterone, the major mineralocorticoid hormone (Fig 21–3). The normal adult adrenal glands produce 0.05 to 0.15 mg of aldosterone each day.[3]

Aldosterone circulates weakly bound to plasma proteins, and >90% of aldosterone is inactivated during a single pass through the liver. Metabolites are conjugated to glucuronide and excreted in the urine. Its half-life is about 15 minutes.[3] Measurement of urinary aldosterone metabolites is not routinely performed clinically. An elevated plasma aldosterone level is one criteria for the diagnosis of aldosteronism.

The major stimulus for aldosterone secretion is activation of the renin-angiotensin system. A decreased renal tubular sodium or chloride load in the region of the macula densa, decreased renal artery perfusion pressure, or increased sympathetic stimulation causes the juxtaglomerular (JG) cells of the kidney to release renin. Renin converts angiotensinogen, an α-globulin synthesized in the liver, to angiotensin I. This, in turn, is converted to the very potent angiotensin II by angiotensin-converting enzyme, primarily in the pulmonary vascular endothelium. Angiotensin II is an extremely potent arteriolar vasoconstrictor. It binds to receptors in the adrenal cortex and stimulates the synthesis and secretion of aldosterone, causes secretion of antidiuretic hormone and ACTH, and stimulates thirst. Angiotensin II has a half-life of 1 to 3 minutes and is inactivated by angiotensinases.[3] In primary aldosteronism, the plasma renin activity is low, whereas, in secondary aldosteronism, the plasma renin activity is high. In addition to the renin-angiotensin system, ACTH enhances aldosterone secretion by stimulating the conversion of cholesterol to pregnenolone and thereby driving the cortical biosynthetic pathways. Small changes in the serum potassium concentration also greatly influence aldosterone synthesis and secretion; increases in the serum potassium concentration augment aldosterone production and the converse is also true.

Aldosterone is an important regulator of electrolyte balance and intravascular volume.[3] Aldosterone increases the exchange of intratubular potassium and hydrogen ions for sodium in the distal tubules of the kidney. Sodium reabsorption is increased, which expands the extracellular volume compartment, in part accounting for the hypertension that is observed clinically. Continued potassium excretion leads to progressive depletion of body potassium stores and hypokalemia, a situation that is worsened by concomitant diuretic administration to treat the hypertension. Loss of hydrogen ions by urinary excretion and migration into potassium-depleted cells results in a metabolic alkalosis. The urine is dilute, and urine pH is neutral to alkaline as the result of excessive ammonium and bicarbonate ion excretion, in compensation for the metabolic alkalosis. Sodium reabsorption, and potassium and hydrogen ion excretion also are stimulated in the epithelial cells of sweat glands, salivary glands, and gastrointestinal tract.[3]

Sex Steroids

Cells of the zona reticularis convert pregnenolone to hydroxypregnenolone and then to dehydroepiandrosterone (DHEA) (Fig 21–3). A sulfated derivative of DHEA and androstenedione are the major sex steroids produced by the adrenal cortex. Adrenal androgen production rises during puberty and contributes to adrenarche. However, DHEA and androstenedione are biologically weak androgens, with little intrinsic biological activity, until converted to the potent sex steroids, testosterone and estrogen, in extraadrenal tissues.[3] The primary site of sex steroid production is in the gonad. Signs of excessive androgen production include hirsutism, virilization, acne, and menstrual irregularity. ACTH stimulates the synthesis of adrenal androgens.

■ DISORDERS

HYPERCORTISOLISM

Excessive production of each of the adrenal hormones produces a distinct clinical syndrome. In 1932, Harvey Cushing described eight patients with truncal obesity, hypertension, fatigability, weakness, amenorrhea, hirsutism, purple-colored abdominal striae, edema, glucosuria, osteoporosis, and basophilic tumors of the pituitary gland.[7] This constellation of signs and symptoms is now known as Cushing's syndrome and, when the etiology is a pituitary adenoma, it is called Cushing's disease. Cushing's syndrome is rare, with an estimated annual incidence of 10 per million population.[8] The most common cause of Cushing's syndrome today is the iatrogenic administration of steroids for unrelated disorders. Endogenous hypercortisolism is caused by excessive cortisol production by the adrenal glands, and it is either pituitary-dependent or pituitary-independent.

Approximately 70% of cases of Cushing's syndrome associated with endogenous hypercortisolism can be attributed to the overproduction of ACTH by the pituitary, which results in bilateral adrenal hyperplasia (Cushing's disease). Adrenal hyperplasia is a reversible, compensatory increase in the number of cells in the gland in order to increase cortisol production.[9] The adrenal gland enlarges to approximately twice its normal size, weighing 6 to 8 gm. Increased production of ACTH usually results in macronodular (3 cm nodules) adrenal hyperplasia.[10] The cause is a pituitary adenoma that produces excessive ACTH relative to the level of circulating cortisol, independent of the cortisol biofeedback system (Fig 21–4). Pituitary-dependent adrenal hyperplasia (Cushing's disease) affects women three times more frequently than men, with the onset of symptoms in the third or fourth decade.

In 10% to 15% of patients with Cushing's syndrome associated with endogenous hypercortisolism, "ectopic" sources of ACTH overproduction may arise from extrapituitary tumors. Oat cell bronchogenic carcinoma is the most common tumor, but bronchial carcinoid tumors, epithelial carcinoma of the thymus, thymic carcinoids, pancreatic endocrine tumors, medullary carcinoma of the thyroid, pheochromocytomas, carcinoids of the alimentary tract, adenocarcinomas of the ovary, and pancreatic cystadenomas producing ACTH have all been reported.[11-15] Finding the source of the ACTH production is difficult in some cases, and the underlying neoplasms may be very aggressive cancers that are difficult to treat. Most occult, clinically inapparent ectopic ACTH-secreting tumors are in the chest and are usually bronchial or thymic carcinoids.[14,16] The onset of hypercortisolism is usually rapid, and patients may not exhibit many of the classical Cushingoid symptoms and signs. A hypokalemic metabolic alkalosis is frequently present. Grossly, the adrenal glands enlarge from 2 to 10 times their normal size with weights of 12 to 30 gm.[10] Microscopically, bilateral hyperplasia of the adrenocortical tissue is noted.

In approximately 10% to 20% of cases of endogenous hypercortisolism, cortisol overproduction is a result of a primary adrenal abnormality. Adrenal adenoma, carcinoma, or autonomously functioning hyperplastic nodules, either in pigmented micronodular adrenal hyperplasia or macronodular adrenocortical hyperplasia, may be the cause of Cushing's syndrome.[10] Pigmented micronodular (1 to 5 mm nodules) adrenal hyperplasia usually occurs in glands of normal weight and the nodules tend to function autonomously.[17,18] This entity is observed most frequently in infants and children.[19] Massive macronodular adrenocortical hyperplasia is a newly described, pituitary-independent form of hypercortisolism in which patients have markedly enlarged, autonomously functioning adrenal glands.[18,20]

The most common primary adrenal cause of endogenous hypercortisolism is a solitary adrenal adenoma that secretes cortisol independent of ACTH control. Adenomas are benign neoplasms; microscopic examination reveals adrenal cells that appear normal.[9] The tumors are unilateral in about 80% of cases, and are associated with atrophy of the surrounding and contralateral adrenocortical tissues. Ectopic functional adrenocortical tissue is rare, although cases have been reported, including adenomas arising in the spinal intradural space.[21,22] Syndromes of hypercortisolism and primary aldosteronism may be produced by adrenocortical adenomas, but adrenogenital syndromes are rare and, in many cases, are actually misdiagnosed carcinomas.[23] An adenoma is usually <5 cm in diameter and weighs <100 gm. Larger tumors have a greater chance of being carcinomas, as do tumors which produce androgens and exhibit increased mitoses, pleomorphism, and necrosis.[23] The most common presentation of an adrenocortical neoplasm in adults is Cushing's syndrome. The prognosis is much worse with adrenal carcinomas, and more aggressive treatment and follow-up is warranted.

Clinical Manifestations

Abnormalities of menstruation, obesity, hypertension, osteoporosis, and diabetes are the most common symptoms and signs in patients with hypercortisolism. These are also very nonspecific, and a high index of clinical suspicion is necessary for diagnosis. Progressive weight gain is seen in almost all patients, and redistribution of fat occurs, producing the classic "moon" facies, "buffalo" hump, and truncal obesity. Mild hypertension is usually caused by excessive mineralocorticoid production.[10] Osteoporosis may be severe enough to precipitate pathologic fractures and vertebral body collapse resulting in kyphosis. Weakening and rupture of collagen fibers in the dermis promotes easy bruisability and cutaneous striae, which are more suggestive of Cushing's syndrome. Wound healing is prolonged. Muscle weakness is common, the result of muscle wasting and hypokalemia, and extremities appear thin due to muscle wasting.[10] Prominent weakness and hypokalemia suggests ectopic ACTH production or an adrenocortical carcinoma. Emotional lability is common, varying from irritability to depression and even frank psychosis. Signs of increased androgen production, including acne, hirsutism, and oligomenorrhea, are evident if ACTH levels are increased. Signs of virilization, including a deep voice, alopecia, and clitoromegaly, are more consistent with an adrenocortical carcinoma. Impaired immunity in patients with Cushing's syndrome results in more frequently life-threatening common infections, such as diverticulitis and cholecystitis, and also in opportunistic infections which may be fatal.[10] In children, obesity or growth arrest along with short stature are common presenting signs of Cushing's syndrome.[24] Without treatment, these features will worsen until a major sequela brings the individual to medical attention.

Diagnosis

The diagnosis of Cushing's syndrome depends on the demonstration of increased plasma cortisol levels and the inability to suppress endogenous cortisol production with dexamethasone (Table 21–1). The diagnosis is easier to exclude than to confirm. Although the diurnal cortisol rhythm is abnormal in Cushing's syndrome, a single random cortisol level determination is not very

TABLE 21–1. DIAGNOSIS OF HYPERCORTISOLISM

TEST	EXCLUDES	SUPPORTS
Midnight plasma cortisol level	<2 μg/dL	>2 μg/dL
24 hour urinary free cortisol level	<100 μg	>100 μg
Plasma cortisol level after overnight dexamethasone test	<5 μg/dL	>5 μg/dL*
Low-dose dexamethasone test		
Plasma cortisol level	<5 μg/dL	>5 μg/dL
24 hour urinary free cortisol level	<30 μg	>30 μg
24 hour urinary 17-hydroxysteroids	<3 mg	>3 mg

*The false-positive rate is approximately 30%, and patients who suffer from obesity, alcoholism, or an acute illness or who are taking estrogens or phenytoin have an increased risk of a false-positive result.[8,26–29]

useful.[25] However, a midnight plasma cortisol level of <2 μg/dL is inconsistent with the diagnosis of Cushing's syndrome. Urinary free (unmetabolized) cortisol levels correlate directly with plasma-free cortisol levels and a 24 hour urinary value >100 μg is diagnostic of Cushing's syndrome.[10] False positive and false negative results occur in <5%.

The overnight dexamethasone suppression test usually is employed initially in order to test the suppressability of the cortisol biofeedback mechanism (Fig 21–4).[26] Dexamethasone is a synthetic glucocorticoid that is more potent than cortisol in ACTH suppression. An oral dexamethasone dose of 1 mg is given at 11 PM, and at 8 AM the following morning the plasma is collected and the cortisol level is measured. It is normally <5 μg/dL (Table 21–1). Increased levels are observed in patients with endogenous hypercortisolism. There is a 3% false-negative rate. However, the false-positive rate is approximately 30%, and patients who suffer from obesity, alcoholism, or an acute illness, or who are taking estrogens or phenytoin have an increased incidence of false-positive results.[27–29] The diagnosis of hypercortisolism is essentially excluded by a normal 24 hour urinary free cortisol test and a normal overnight dexamethasone suppression test.[8] The definitive test of adrenal suppressability is the low-dose dexamethasone test, wherein 0.5 mg of dexamethasone is given orally every 6 hours for two consecutive days. Elevated plasma cortisol levels and/or 24 hour urinary levels of 17-hydroxysteroids or free cortisol indicate an abnormality (Table 21–1).

Localization

Once Cushing's syndrome has been established, the etiology of the hypercortisolism and the location of the pathology must be determined (Table 21–2). The first objective is to distinguish pituitary-dependent from pituitary-independent conditions. This may be accomplished with biochemical tests and radiologic imaging

TABLE 21–2. LOCALIZATION OF THE ETIOLOGY OF HYPERCORTISOLISM[17,30,32,33]

TEST	PITUITARY	ECTOPIC TUMOR	ADRENAL TUMOR	MICRONODULAR HYPERPLASIA
Adrenal CT or MR	Normal or bilateral hyperplasia	Normal or bilateral hyperplasia	Unilateral mass	Normal
Plasma ACTH level	Normal or mildly increased	Normal to greatly increased	Low or undetectable	Low or undetectable
High-dose dexamethasone test	Suppression	No suppression	No suppression	No suppression
Petrosal sinus sampling petrosal:peripheral ACTH ratio	>3.0	<3.0	<3.0	<3.0
CRH test plasma ACTH:cortisol ratio	Increased	No increase	No increase	No increase

studies. Occasionally, interventional radiologic procedures are required to clarify unrevealing or equivocal results.

The response of cortisol production to the high-dose dexamethasone suppression test (2 mg given orally every 6 hours for 2 days) is the classic biochemical test used to distinguish pituitary-dependent from pituitary-independent forms of Cushing's syndrome. In patients with pituitary adenomas, the 24 hour urine free cortisol and/or 17-hydroxysteroid levels are suppressed to <50% of basal levels. Failure to suppress cortisol production supports the diagnoses of an ectopic ACTH-producing tumor, an adrenal neoplasm, or primary adrenal bilateral nodular hyperplasia (Table 21–2).[10] The test has an overall accuracy of 95%.[30] Continuous dexamethasone infusion intravenously for 7 hours had a diagnostic accuracy of 98% in one study, and may be a more convenient test.[31]

Alternatively, the metyrapone stimulation test can be used to localize the abnormality.[5] Metyrapone is an inhibitor of the enzyme 11β-hydroxylase. Cortisol precursors accumulate with the compensatory increase in ACTH secretion after metyrapone is administered; 750 mg is given orally every 4 hours for 6 doses. Most patients with a pituitary adenoma demonstrate an increase in ACTH secretion and therefore, an increase in measured urinary 17-hydroxysteroid levels in response to metyrapone. Patients with an ectopic ACTH-producing tumor or a primary adrenal abnormality causing hypercortisolism will not exhibit an increase in urinary 17-hydroxysteroids following metyrapone since the pituitary is suppressed. The metyrapone test will also identify forms of nodular adrenal hyperplasia which may be pituitary-dependent, since in these cases there will be increased urinary 17-hydroxysteroid levels.

The CRH test can differentiate pituitary Cushing's disease from ectopic ACTH production and has more recently replaced the metyrapone test.[32] A dose of 1 μg/kg of CRH given intravenously results in increased plasma levels of ACTH and cortisol in >90% of patients with Cushing's disease (Table 21–2). No ACTH or cortisol increase is observed in over 95% of cases of ectopic ACTH production.[33] The CRH test is as accurate as the high-dose dexamethasone suppression test and the use of both tests together improves diagnostic accuracy even more.[33,34]

Other laboratory tests may provide supportive evidence for the localization of the abnormality responsible for the hypercortisolism. An adrenal adenoma suppresses ACTH production, and its diagnosis is suggested by only modest rises, or even a decrease in baseline urinary 17-ketosteroids (<10 mg/day), or plasma DHEA sulfate levels along with disproportionately increased baseline 17-hydroxysteroid or free cortisol levels in the urine. The plasma ACTH level is usually high-normal (100 pg/mL) or elevated (up to 500 pg/mL) in patients with ACTH producing tumors, but is low or undetectable in patients with adrenal tumors (Table 21–2).[5] Ectopic ACTH-producing tumors may produce extremely high plasma levels (>1000 pg/mL).[10] In patients with autonomous bilateral nodular adrenal hyperplasia, the plasma ACTH level is normal or suppressed. Notably, hypokalemia occurs in only 10% of patients with Cushing's disease, while nearly all patients with ectopic ACTH-producing tumors exhibit hypokalemia. Some have severe hypokalemia with muscle weakness.[35]

High resolution computed tomography (CT) scanning of the adrenals will detect adrenal abnormalities, with a sensitivity of >95%. If both adrenal glands appear enlarged, adrenal hyperplasia is likely, whereas a unilateral mass implies an adrenal tumor (Table 21–2).[20,36–39] Thus, CT can be used to identify primary adrenal causes of hypercortisolism. The detection of a unilateral adrenal mass with a suppressed contralateral gland suggests a unilateral adrenal tumor as the cause of the hypercortisolism, and greatly simplifies the evaluation.[10]

All patients with a presumed diagnosis of Cushing's

disease should have a sellar CT or magnetic resonance imaging (MRI) scan. Pituitary tumors with diameters of 5 to 10 mm may be recognized, but the more common pituitary microadenoma cannot be detected reliably. MRI with gadolinium is slightly better than CT in detecting adenomas, but it still misses microadenomas.[40]

In some cases, the cause of Cushing's syndrome is not clear from the biochemical studies discussed above. Additionally, abdominal CT may reveal only bilateral adrenal enlargement and sellar CT or MRI may not detect an abnormality in the pituitary. In these patients, further studies are needed to localize the abnormality causing the hypercortisolism.

Petrosal sinus sampling is the single best test to distinguish pituitary from ectopic Cushing's syndrome and to localize the half of the pituitary gland with the adenoma.[40] Simultaneous bilateral inferior petrosal sinus samples for ACTH levels and peripheral venous specimens for plasma ACTH levels are collected prior to and following CRH administration. A ratio of peak inferior petrosal sinus to peripheral plasma ACTH levels >3.0 after CRH administration has a sensitivity and specificity of 100% in discerning pituitary adenomas (Table 21–2). Furthermore, the pituitary microadenoma will be localized correctly to one-half of the gland in a majority of patients.[40] This method of distinguishing pituitary-dependent from pituitary independent forms of Cushing's syndrome may not be the primary study of choice, since it is invasive, more costly than the biochemical tests, and not widely available. However, petrosal sinus sampling is indispensable in definitely localizing or excluding a pituitary cause of hypercortisolism in patients with borderline or equivocal biochemical and radiologic results.

If the evaluation suggests a primary adrenal cause of Cushing's syndrome, then surgical therapy is planned based on the adrenal pathology. As discussed above, high-resolution CT is very sensitive for detecting adrenal abnormalities. Since the most common primary adrenal cause of hypercortisolism is a unilateral adrenal adenoma, a CT demonstrating a small unilateral adrenal mass with a suppressed contralateral gland may be enough evidence for adrenalectomy, if this finding is consistent with biochemical testing. However, CT scanning lacks specificity. Adrenocortical carcinoma and pheochromocytoma also may present as a unilateral adrenal mass on CT. Furthermore, patients with primary micronodular hyperplasia have normal appearing adrenal glands on abdominal CT scan. MRI enhances specificity by examining the signal intensity of the adrenal abnormality on the T2-weighted image.[37,41] Adenomas appear darker than the liver on the T2-weighted MRI. Carcinomas, both primary adrenocortical and metastatic, appear as bright as, or slightly brighter than, the liver, while pheochromocytomas appear three times brighter than the liver on the T2-weighted MRI.[41]

[^{131}I]iodomethylnorcholesterol (NP-59) scintigraphy may further distinguish adrenal adenoma, carcinoma, and hyperplasia.[42] Labeled-iodomethylnorcholesterol successfully localizes functional adrenocortical adenomas even when they are not identified by CT or MRI, since adenomas take up the tracer and produce an image.[43] Carcinomas do not take up tracer.[44] An adenoma, which results in an intense unilateral image, may be distinguished from bilateral hyperplasia, in which both glands are imaged.[45] In addition, uptake in both adrenal glands supports the diagnosis of bilateral disease, as in patients with primary micronodular hyperplasia.[46,47] This test also may be useful in identifying ectopic rests of cortical tissue in the rare event that hypercortisolism recurs after bilateral adrenalectomy. However, several days are needed for enough radioisotope to accumulate to produce an image, and the study is not widely available.

Tests to localize ectopic ACTH-producing tumors are dictated by clinical suspicion. Small-cell carcinoma of the lung, bronchial carcinoid tumors, and thymic carcinoid tumors are the three most common sources of ectopic ACTH production.[10] Chest CT scanning, chest MRI, and bronchoscopy may be required.[14,15] Additional tests to exclude other neoplasms include abdominal CT and MRI scanning to detect pancreatic, ovarian, and adrenal neoplasms, measurement of urinary catecholamines to screen for pheochromocytoma, and measurement of plasma calcitonin levels to exclude medullary carcinoma of the thyroid.[48–50] Suspicious lesions should undergo fine-needle aspiration with radioimmunoassay for ACTH in the aspirate.[51]

Table 21–2 summarizes the radiologic studies used to localize the abnormality in patients with hypercortisolism. Once the diagnosis of hypercortisolism is confirmed (see Table 21–1), then a CT scan of the adrenals may reveal a unilateral adrenal mass with a suppressed contralateral gland. This finding greatly simplifies the evaluation and suggests a unilateral adrenal tumor as the cause of the hypercortisolism. If no adrenal mass is observed on CT, the plasma level of ACTH is low, and urinary cortisol levels do not suppress with the high-dose dexamethasone test, primary pigmented micronodular adrenal hyperplasia must be excluded by either petrosal sinus sampling or iodomethylnorcholesterol scanning.[10] An abdominal CT, revealing a large unilateral adrenal mass along with a hypertrophied contralateral adrenal cortex and increased plasma ACTH levels, suggests a pheochromocytoma that is secreting ACTH; 24 hour urinary catecholamines, vanylmadelic acid (VMA), and metanephrine levels should be measured.[10] If the high-dose dexamethasone test produces equivocal results, then petrosal sinus sampling will distinguish between pituitary and ectopic sources of ACTH production in nearly every case.[40] The CRH test and metyrapone test can be used in conjunction with the high-dose dexamethasone test, especially if petrosal sinus sampling is not available.[33,34]

Management

The goal of therapy is to eliminate cortisol hypersecretion. The treatment for patients with hypercortisolism resulting from a unilateral adrenal adenoma is total surgical excision of the involved gland to eliminate the source of the autonomous cortisol production. The prognosis is excellent. A successful operation is curative and no other therapy is necessary.[52] The operation usually is accomplished using a posterior or laparoscopic approach for tumors that are <4 cm in diameter. Larger tumors and those that appear malignant on the T2-weighted MRI require an anterior approach.[41] Details regarding the surgical procedure are presented later in this chapter. It is important that all patients undergoing such a procedure for an adrenal adenoma are treated perioperatively with stress steroid doses, since any remaining adrenal tissue usually is atrophied. Mineralocorticoid replacement is not necessary. Steroids are tapered postoperatively over 6 months to 2 years.[52] Benign tumors >50 to 100 gm may require careful follow-up with clinical evaluation for hormone abnormalities, CT scanning, and/or MRI. Adrenalectomy for Cushing's syndrome secondary to an adrenal adenoma during pregnancy is safe and significantly may reduce fetal loss, premature labor, and maternal morbidity.[53,54]

Patients with the radiographic appearance of bilateral adrenal hyperplasia have ACTH- or CRH-producing tumors in the pituitary or in an "ectopic" location or, rarely, they may have a primary adrenal cause of hypercortisolism. In the former cases, surgical removal of the tumor is the ideal treatment. With pituitary lesions, transsphenoidal resection of tumors <1 cm in diameter is the primary therapy. This results in cure in 50% to 90% of cases.[55]

Ectopic tumors producing ACTH may occur in a variety of locations and usually are treated surgically after localization, with the exception of most small cell carcinomas of the bronchus.[14] The appropriate operation depends upon the specific tumor and the extent of disease. Oat cell carcinoma of the lung causes over 60% of all cases of ectopic ACTH production and often only palliative chemotherapy or radiation therapy can be offered. Bilateral adrenalectomy to control the symptoms of hypercortisolism is suitable for patients with tumors that cannot be localized despite exhaustive efforts and for patients with unresectable but stable metastatic disease with a prognosis for relatively long survival.[16,50]

Rarely, biochemical testing and/or petrosal sinus sampling will unequivocally suggest a primary adrenal cause for hypercortisolism, and abdominal CT, MRI,

and [131I]iodomethylnorcholesterol scintigraphy will reveal no focal adrenal neoplasm. These patients have primary micronodular adrenal hyperplasia or massive macronodular adrenal hyperplasia.[17,18] Bilateral adrenalectomy is curative.[18]

Adrenocortical carcinoma as a cause of Cushing's syndrome is suggested by biochemical testing, which unequivocally suggests a primary adrenal cause for the hypercortisolism, a unilateral adrenal lesion >6 cm on CT scan, a T2-weighted MRI intensity that appears as bright as or slightly brighter than the liver, and no uptake of trace with [131I]iodomethylnorcholesterol scintigraphy.[10] These lesions require aggressive surgical resection and careful follow-up. Complete management is discussed in detail later in this chapter. Despite the laboratory and radiologic tests available, in some patients, the source of ACTH overproduction may remain occult. If the hypercortisolism is severe and medical management is ineffective, then bilateral adrenalectomy may be indicated in order to ameliorate the signs and symptoms of hypercortisolism.[16]

ALDOSTERONISM

In 1956, Conn first described the signs and symptoms of excessive and inappropriate aldosterone secretion, most notably hypokalemia in association with hypertension.[56] In *primary* aldosteronism, the adrenal gland autonomously produces excessive aldosterone. The most common cause is an aldosterone-producing adrenocortical adenoma (Conn's syndrome), followed by idiopathic adrenocortical hyperplasia (IAH).[56–58] Adrenocortical carcinoma only rarely presents solely with primary aldosteronism.[59,60] Hypokalemia and weakness are more severe in these patients.[61] Rarely, hyperaldosteronism is the result of an enzymatic defect of cortisol biosynthesis, with a resultant increase in the mineralocorticoid 11-deoxycorticosterone (Fig 21–3).[5] Licorice contains a sodium-retaining agent called glycyrrhizinic acid which produces a syndrome that mimics primary aldosteronism, but with normal aldosterone levels.[5] Primary aldosteronism is observed in women twice as often as men, usually between the ages of 30 and 50. Approximately 1% of unselected hypertensive patients have primary aldosteronism.[62] *Secondary* aldosteronism implies that the adrenal gland is appropriately producing excessive aldosterone as a result of activation of the renin angiotensin system by an extraadrenal-initiating stimulus. Overproduction of renin may be owing to renal artery stenosis from atherosclerosis or fibromuscular hyperplasia, severe arteriolar nephrosclerosis, or the rare renin-producing juxtaglomerular cell tumor.[5] Intravascular hypovolemia in edematous states, such as cirrhosis, congestive heart failure, or nephrotic syndrome, also will cause increased renin production with consequent aldosteronism. Aldosteronism is a normal physiologic response during pregnancy.[3]

Clinical Manifestations

Patients complain of muscle weakness, muscle cramps, fatigue, headaches, and polyuria.[62] Hypokalemia accounts for the neuromuscular symptoms. Headaches are attributed to hypertension, which is usually not severe and is caused by elevated levels of mineralocorticoid metabolites and by extracellular volume expansion.[63–65] Secondary cardiac effects, such as left ventricular enlargement and cardiac arrhythmias, are not uncommon. In cases of long duration, nephropathy, azotemia, congestive heart failure, and edema may become evident.

Diagnosis

The diagnosis of aldosteronism is suspected in a non-edematous, hypertensive patient with persistent hypokalemia who has not been receiving potassium-wasting diuretics (furosemide, ethracrynic acid, or thiazides).[62] The degree of hypokalemia is related to the duration and severity of excess aldosterone secretion, and the potassium level is usually <3.9 mEq/L.[66] Laboratory studies also may reveal hypernatremia, metabolic alkalosis, and hypomagnesemia. Urine specific gravity is decreased and an impaired ability to concentrate the urine is apparent after an overnight concentration test. The 24 hour urinary excretion of potassium is >30 mEq in most patients.[10] Tests of glucocorticoid and androgen secretion are normal. Plasma renin activity distinguishes primary from secondary aldosteronism, since it is suppressed in the former and elevated in the latter.

Specific criteria for the diagnosis of aldosteronism are (1) diastolic hypertension without edema, (2) a low plasma renin activity level that fails to increase appropriately during volume depletion, and (3) an elevated plasma aldosterone level that does not suppress appropriately during volume expansion (Table 21–3).[62] Volume depletion is brought about by a low-sodium diet or an upright posture, which produces a relative hypovolemia, since the kidneys are most dependent in a supine position. Because suppressed renin activity occurs in approximately 25% of patients with essential hypertension, lack of suppression of aldosterone secretion also must be demonstrated during volume expansion, which is brought about with a high-salt diet. The plasma aldosterone to renin ratio is usually >30.[10] A very high aldosterone level is consistent with adrenocortical carcinoma, as is a greatly elevated deoxycorticosterone level.[61]

A suppression test using captopril is also helpful in diagnosing primary aldosteronism.[67] Patients are administered a morning dose of 25 mg of captopril orally and, 2 hours later, blood is collected and plasma aldosterone and cortisol levels are measured. With essential hyper-

TABLE 21–3. DIAGNOSIS AND EVALUATION OF PRIMARY ALDOSTERONISM[61,66–70]

ESTABLISHMENT OF DIAGNOSIS

Nonedematous diastolic hypertension (>90 mm Hg)
Hypokalemia without diuretics
    Serum potassium level <3.9 mEq/L
    24 hour urine potassium >30 mEq
Plasma aldosterone level:renin activity ratio >30
Captopril Test
    Plasma aldosterone level >15 ng/dL
    Plasma aldosterone level:renin activity ratio >50

EVALUATION OF ETIOLOGY

	IAH	ALDOSTERONOMA
Serum 18-hydroxy-corticosterone	<90 ng/dL	>100 ng/dL
Adrenal CT	Normal	Mass (>7–10 mm)
Iodocholesterol scan	Bilateral, symmetric uptake	Focal uptake
Adrenal vein sampling for aldosterone	Elevated aldosterone levels in both adrenal veins; Adrenal vein aldosterone levels are each greater than a simultaneous peripheral sample	Elevated aldosterone level in ipsilateral adrenal vein; Contralateral adrenal vein aldosterone level is equivalent to a simultaneous peripheral sample

tension and in normal patients, aldosterone levels will be low and renin activity will be increased. No change in aldosterone levels or renin activity is observed in patients with primary aldosteronism; the postcaptopril aldosterone level is usually >15 ng/dL and the aldosterone to renin ratio is more than 50 (Table 21–3).[67]

Localization

Once primary aldosteronism is diagnosed, the etiology must be determined. The main differentiation is between a functional adrenocortical adenoma and IAH (Table 21–3). The treatment of each condition differs significantly and differentiation between adenoma and IAH is not possible solely by clinical history or laboratory findings. Adrenocortical neoplasms usually produce serum levels of 18-hydroxycorticosterone >100 ng/dL, whereas in IAH, levels are <90 ng/dL. However, these values are not absolute and do not always discriminate between the two conditions.

Localization of an aldosterone-producing tumor by abdominal CT scanning is successful in most patients with primary aldosteronism. Difficulty arises in approximately 10% to 25% of cases because tumors smaller than 7 to 10 mm may not be imaged,[68–72] and CT cannot determine whether an adenoma or IAH is the cause of hyperaldosteronism in patients with multiple bilateral adrenal nodules.[73] Furthermore, 42% of patients with IAH have adrenal glands that appear normal rather than diffusely enlarged, on CT scan.[71] CT findings must be correlated with endocrinologic studies for proper interpretation.[74] Evaluation of the adrenal glands in patients with primary aldosteronism by MRI appears to be less effective than CT, at the present time.[72] In addition, radiologic evidence of a tumor does not indicate whether it produces aldosterone in quantities significant enough to account for the clinical syndrome. Further studies are needed in these patients to discriminate between the two conditions.

[131I]iodomethylnorcholesterol (NP-59) scintigraphy discriminates between aldosteronomas and IAH and indicates functional tumors. NP-59 localizes functionally active adenomas, which take up tracer 64% of the time. The sensitivity may be increased to 88% by suppression with dexamethasone prior to the scan.[68] In IAH, both glands show symmetrical uptake of tracer. Additionally, adrenal carcinomas usually show no uptake of tracer. However, NP-59 uptake is related to the adenoma volume, and there is a poor correlation between NP-59 uptake and the ability of an adenoma to secrete aldosterone.[75]

In order to definitively determine whether primary hyperaldosteronism is caused by an adenoma or by IAH, adrenal vein sampling for aldosterone and cortisol is employed.[70] Adrenal vein sampling by the percutaneous transfemoral route with simultaneous bilateral adrenal vein catheterization may demonstrate a two- to three-fold increase in plasma aldosterone concentration or an increase in the ratio of aldosterone to cortisol on the side with the adenoma. Bilateral samples must be obtained simultaneously. Administration of ACTH during the vein catheterization will further increase aldosterone levels in the adrenal veins of patients with aldosteronomas. Cortisol levels should be measured at the same time to eliminate the possible increase in aldosterone concentration from stress or ACTH stimulation. If the aldosterone levels are similar in each adrenal vein and greater than peripheral venous aldosterone levels, IAH is suggested. Although this is an invasive procedure, the sensitivity is 96%, which is better than CT scanning and adrenal scintigraphy.[57,70,73]

Management

An aldosterone-secreting adenoma is managed surgically by resecting the involved adrenal gland. Electrolyte correction is important preoperatively. This is greatly facilitated by the use of spironolactone, an aldosterone antagonist. Clinical assessment for evidence of cardiac failure and renal insufficiency is necessary in long-standing cases. A posterior or the newly described laparoscopic approach almost always is indicated, since tumors are usually small in size. Successful surgical resection results in resolution of hypertension and elec-

trolyte disturbances in patients with a correct preoperative diagnosis of aldosteronoma. However, up to 30% of patients will develop recurrent hypertension within 2 to 3 years after resection.[65,76] A good preoperative clinical response to spironolactone predicts a better cure rate.[77] Age >50 years, male sex, and associated macronodules in the adrenals predict an increased risk of persistent postoperative hypertension.[78] Nonoperative candidates can be treated medically with dietary sodium restriction, calcium channel blockers, and spironolactone. Chronic therapy in men may result in gynecomastia, decreased libido, and impotence.

IAH is usually treated medically with spironolactone, triamterene, amiloride, or nifedipine.[64,76] Patients who are misdiagnosed as having solitary aldosteronomas and who undergo unilateral adrenalectomy experience no improvement in symptoms. This underscores the importance of distinguishing between aldosteronism caused by an aldosteronoma versus IAH preoperatively.

VIRILIZATION AND FEMINIZATION

Excessive production of dehydroepiandrosterone (DHEA) and androstenedione by the adrenal gland produces symptoms and signs of hirsutism, oligomenorrhea, acne, and virilization. Hirsutism is defined as the excessive development of fine hair on the face, back, and arms. Virilization consists of clitoromegaly, a deepened voice, and balding. DHEA and androstenedione are converted to testosterone in the peripheral tissues, and elevated testosterone levels account for the androgenic effects.[3] Hypersecretion of adrenal androgens may be "pure" or "mixed," and is associated with overproduction of other adrenocortical hormones, including cortisol and aldosterone. Feminization, caused by increased estrogen levels, results in gynecomastia, decreased libido, and impotence in males, and irregular menses or dysfunctional uterine bleeding in females.[5,8] Increased estrogen levels may be associated with hypercortisolism.

In infants, excessive adrenal androgen production may result from a deficiency of an enzyme in cortisol biosynthesis. Low cortisol levels result in high ACTH levels and adrenal hyperplasia, with shunting of intermediates into the androgen biosynthetic pathway. C-21 hydroxylase deficiency is most common, with or without an associated salt-losing condition owing to aldosterone deficiency.[5] The condition is treated by the daily administration of glucocorticoids and mineralocorticoids.

In children and adults, virilization associated with Cushing's syndrome increases the likelihood of adrenocortical carcinoma. Pure adrenal virilization may be caused by an adrenocortical adenoma or carcinoma.[79,80] Adrenal adenomas that secrete excessive androgens are rare, and only occasionally will adrenal hyperplasia cause virilization. Hyperestrogenism also may be caused by an adrenal adenoma or carcinoma. Several other disorders may cause virilization and feminization and, in all cases, radiologic evaluation of both adrenal glands is indicated in order to exclude an adrenal tumor.

The diagnosis of virilization or feminization of adrenal origin is confirmed by elevated plasma DHEA, testosterone, or estrogen levels and increased 24 hour urinary excretion of 17-ketosteroids and 17-hydroxysteroids. Failure of dexamethasone administration to suppress elevated urinary 17-ketosteroid levels supports the diagnosis of an adrenal tumor causing the syndrome, and excludes congenital adrenal hyperplasia or ovarian tumors as etiologic possibilities.[5] Abdominal CT scanning localizes the lesion. Neoplasms are resected surgically via a transperitoneal approach because these tumors may be malignant.

ADRENOCORTICAL CARCINOMA

Cancer of the adrenal cortex is a rare but aggressive malignancy, accounting for 0.05% to 0.2% of all cancers.[81] The neoplasm arises in women twice as often as men, usually in the third to fifth decades of life. However, children also may develop adrenal cancer. Another peak in the incidence of adrenocortical carcinoma is observed in children <6 years of age, and girls are affected twice as often as boys.[10] Adrenocortical carcinoma is more common than adenoma in children. The right adrenal gland is affected with the same frequency as the left adrenal gland, and tumor weights between 100 and 5000 gm are common. Pathogenesis may be related to loss of heterozygosity at loci on the short arm of chromosome 11.[82,83]

Determining the malignant potential of adrenocortical carcinomas may be perplexing, especially in neoplasms weighing between 50 and 100 gm. Necrosis, hemorrhage, cells with large nuclei, hyperchromatism, and enlarged nucleoli are all consistent with malignancy.[9] Venous invasion, more than 20 mitoses per 50 high-powered fields, aneuploidy, abnormal production of androgens, and 11-deoxysteroids predict a poorer outcome.[9,84–87] The only absolute indication of malignancy is nodal or distant metastases. Immunostaining may distinguish adrenal neoplasms from other cancers, especially renal cell carcinoma, which does not stain positive with vimentin, but adrenocortical carcinoma and adrenal adenomas stain similarly.[88]

Adrenocortical carcinoma is staged surgically as follows[89–91]:

Stage I: T1, N0, M0-Tumor ≤5 cm without evidence of local invasion or metastases

Stage II: T2, N0, M0-Tumor >5 cm without evidence of local invasion or metastases

Stage III: T3, N0, M0-Any size tumor invading locally into periadrenal fat, or T1 or T2, N1, M0 any size tumor without local invasion with nodal metastases only

Stage IV: T3 or T4, N1, M0-Any size tumor with invasion into periadrenal fat or adjacent organs and lymph node metastases, or Any T, Any N, M1-any tumor with distant metastases.

Clinical Manifestations

About 70% of patients have advanced disease at the time of presentation, usually stage III or IV.[60,90] Patients present in a majority of cases with signs and symptoms of Cushing's syndrome, primary hyperaldosteronism, or a combination of syndromes, depending on the biologically active hormones secreted by the tumor.[60] Virilization is observed in only 10% of adrenocortical carcinomas, and feminization in only 12%.[30] High estrogen levels may be produced and may cause vaginal bleeding even in postmenopausal women.[92] Functional adrenocortical carcinomas occur more frequently in women. In approximately 30% of cases, adrenocortical carcinomas produce no hormones. Patients then present with the nonspecific signs of abdominal pain, increased abdominal girth, weight loss, weakness, and anorexia. Children with adrenocortical carcinoma present with virilization, precocious puberty, or Cushing's syndrome.[93–97] In children, the most common cause of hypercortisolism is an adrenocortical carcinoma.

Diagnosis

An adrenocortical carcinoma should be suspected in patients with Cushing's syndrome and concomitant evidence of virilization or elevated urinary levels of 17-ketosteroids or DHEA sulfate.[98] Any adrenal mass >6 cm in diameter on abdominal CT scan also must be regarded as suspicious. [^{131}I]iodomethylnorcholesterol scintigraphy usually reveals no uptake of tracer; however, unilateral tracer uptake cannot be interpreted to represent a definite benign lesion since a well differentiated cortisol-secreting adrenocortical carcinoma also may display intense uptake of tracer.[99] Adrenal cancers appear as bright as, or slightly brighter than, the liver on the T2-weighted MRI.[41] CT and MRI of the abdomen, as well as the chest, is required to adequately define the extent of the mass and to exclude metastatic pulmonary lesions.[41,100,101] Bony metastases are ruled out by a preoperative bone scan.

Management

Complete resection of all gross tumor at the initial surgery is the best opportunity for cure. Tumor that is not removed at the initial surgery is unlikely to be eradicated. Resection of locally invasive stage III neoplasms decreases functional tumor burden and possible complications from mass effect.[10] Either an anterior approach or a thoracoabdominal incision is required in order to gain adequate exposure for the extent of resection. Invasion of adjacent organs, including the kidney, liver, pancreas, bowel, or diaphragm, necessitates resection of part or all of the involved tissues en bloc. The function of the contralateral kidney must be confirmed by CT with intravenous contrast or by an intravenous pyelogram prior to nephrectomy. A complete preoperative bowel preparation is indicated for lesions that might involve the bowel. Right adrenal neoplasms also may involve the inferior vena cava, sometimes extending to the right atrium. Cardiopulmonary bypass may be necessary to resect such tumors.[102,103] Study of the inferior vena cava with intravenous contrast or ultrasonography in order to assess blood flow may be valuable, if the cava seems involved by, or compressed by, a right adrenal mass. Intraoperative ultrasound to evaluate tumor involvement of the inferior vena cava is helpful and may even change operative management in situations where preoperative studies are inconclusive or unexpected intraoperative findings arise.[104]

Although patients with stage I and stage II disease can be cured by complete surgical resection of the tumor,[105] many patients are unable to undergo curative surgery.[60,89,90,106] Debulking as much of the primary tumor as possible, to minimize the amount of residual functional tissue and to reduce complications from mass effect, may be beneficial, if the primary tumor cannot be completely excised. The overall 5 year survival is approximately 10% to 20%.[106]

Patients need close follow-up after definitive resection. Hormones that are elevated preoperatively should be measured periodically, including plasma 11-deoxycortisol, DHEA, and deoxycorticosterone, urinary levels of free cortisol, and 17-ketosteroids.[8] CT and MRI are used to detect local recurrences and metastases.[101] Adrenocortical carcinoma most often metastasizes to lymph nodes, lung, liver, bone, and brain.[107] Resection of lesions metastatic to the liver, lungs, and brain has produced prolonged remissions.[108–113] Some patients with slow-growing adrenocortical metastases that produce hormones may benefit from a near total resection, if complete resection of the metastases cannot be achieved.[112,114] However, no cures have been reported in patients with recurrent adrenocortical cancer who have undergone aggressive surgery.[112] Radiation therapy is appropriate for patients with painful bony metastases and possibly local abdominal recurrences, although length of survival is not changed.[60,111,115] The only partially effective chemotherapeutic agent is mitotane.[116] A partial response is observed in <33% of patients and few complete responses have been reported.[106,112,117–121] Measuring blood levels of the drug to maintain an appropriate concentration may improve the response and survival rates.[122] However, the therapeutic window is narrow, and moderate to severe toxic effects are common.[121] Adverse reactions include anorexia, nausea, vomiting, and diarrhea in 79% of cases; depression, dizziness, tremors,

headache, confusion, and weakness in 50%; and skin rash in 15%.[116] Hypercortisolism is well treated by mitotane, but its antitumor effects are disappointing. Earlier diagnosis and improved adjuvants may lead to better results with adrenocortical carcinoma.[123]

ACUTE ADRENOCORTICAL INSUFFICIENCY

The surgeon most commonly encounters situations of perioperative steroid insufficiency when operating on patients with medical conditions requiring steroid therapy, in transplant recipients, and in endocrine surgery. Perioperative management must be modified in these patients. Rarely, unsuspected adrenal insufficiency may be observed in traumatized, severely burned, and critically ill patients.[6,124–127] Acute adrenal insufficiency in the postoperative or traumatized patient is a rare event that can be life-threatening if unsuspected, but easily treated, once diagnosed. Signs and symptoms of acute adrenal insufficiency often are obscured by normal postoperative processes. Furthermore, unnecessary exogenous steroid administration poses special problems with regards to immunity and wound healing, especially in the critically ill patient.

The most frequent cause of acute adrenal insufficiency is the rapid withdrawal of steroids from patients on chronic steroid administration.[5] However, acute adrenal insufficiency in the postoperative or traumatized patient may result from bilateral adrenal hemorrhage.[125] Bilateral adrenal hemorrhage may occur in association with overwhelming sepsis (Waterhouse-Friderichsen syndrome). Adrenal hemorrhage also has been reported during pregnancy, following idiopathic adrenal vein thrombosis, as a complication of venography, in the coagulopathic critically ill patient and rarely, from a benign adrenocortical adenoma.[6,128] Anticoagulant administration is the most frequent cause of postoperative adrenal insufficiency.[125–127] There is no indication for operative intervention in these circumstances, unless exsanguinating hemorrhage is imminent. Mitotane, which inhibits steroid biosynthesis, also can induce adrenal insufficiency during severe stress.

The major signs and symptoms of adrenal insufficiency are weakness, fever, hypotension, nausea, vomiting, and abdominal pain.[124] In the intensive care–unit setting, high cardiac output with low systemic vascular resistance and hypotension are observed. This clinical picture is similar to that of a septic patient and may be obscured by volume replacement and the use of pressors.[6] Hemorrhage from the adrenal causes distention of the fibrous adrenal capsule and symptoms of flank pain, nausea, and vomiting. These symptoms appear most frequently between days 7 and 10 after initiating anticoagulant therapy and may precede signs and symptoms of adrenal insufficiency by 3 to 5 days.[6,125] All these signs and symptoms are very nonspecific, and the condition is difficult to discriminate from other processes in the postoperative patient; therefore, a high index of clinical suspicion must be maintained.[125] Early recognition and treatment are important, since lethargy eventually deepens into somnolence and hypovolemic shock ensues. Intensive hemodynamic support may keep a patient alive for weeks. However, if adrenal insufficiency is not recognized and treated appropriately, the unavoidable outcome is death.[6,125]

Plasma levels of cortisol are usually at least twice the normal value in the immediate postoperative or posttraumatic period, with a return to normal levels in 4 to 5 days, if no complications arise. A plasma-free cortisol level <15 μg/dL in the immediate postoperative or posttraumatic period should raise the suspicion of adrenal insufficiency.[6,124] Other laboratory tests are usually not useful in establishing a diagnosis.[125,127] The cosyntropin stimulation test is very helpful in diagnosing acute adrenal insufficiency in postoperative, traumatized, or critically ill patients.[124,129] A dose of 250 μg of cosyntropin, a synthetic ACTH analogue, is administered intravenously. Plasma levels of cortisol are collected at 30 and 60 minutes and are compared to pretest baseline plasma cortisol levels. The cortisol level should increase by at least 7 μg/dL after cosyntropin administration, with peak cortisol levels greater than 18 μg/dL.[6,124] Failure of the plasma level of cortisol to increase appropriately implies adrenal insufficiency. Glucocorticoid coverage may be provided during the test by using dexamethasone (2 to 4 mg every 8 to 12 hours), since it will not interfere with evaluation of adrenal function by cosyntropin. Abdominal CT or ultrasonography may detect adrenal hemorrhage and confirm an equivocal diagnosis.[125,126]

Once recognized, treatment is to immediately restore adequate glucocorticoid levels and to continue correcting electrolyte and fluid deficits. An intravenous infusion of 5% glucose in normal saline should be initiated, and an intravenous bolus of 100 mg of hydrocortisone is administered. Dexamethasone is discontinued and a continuous cortisol infusion is started at a rate of 10 mg/hr. A dose of 50 mg of cortisone acetate is given intramuscularly as a precaution against the accidental termination or infiltration of the cortisol drip. At these doses, a maximal glucocorticoid effect is observed and additional mineralocorticoid administration is unnecessary. Aggressive volume resuscitation of hypovolemic shock is essential. With prompt treatment, the symptoms and hemodynamic status of the patient usually improve dramatically.[6,124,125] Stress steroid doses are tapered as the clinical condition of the patient improves.

Prevention of adrenal crisis is critical in certain patients. Patients on steroid therapy with chronic suppression of the hypothalamic-pituitary-adrenal axis can-

not acutely produce the endogenous steroids necessary during stress, infection, shock, injury, severe burns, or routine surgery.[6,124,125] The steroid dose, as well as the duration of therapy, are the prime determinants of the functional integrity of the adrenal gland. Stress doses of steroids must be given perioperatively to avoid an adrenal crisis in anyone who has been receiving supraphysiologic doses of steroids for a prolonged period, and in patients who have had complete withdrawal of long-term, high-dose steroid therapy within the preceding year. The usual regimen is 100 mg of hydrocortisone, or the equivalent, before surgery, during the operation, and postoperatively. Larger doses of glucocorticoids provide no increased benefit physiologically, and mineralocorticoid administration is unnecessary. Postoperatively, in most patients, the steroid dose may be tapered quickly to the preoperative regimen.[5]

In patients with an adrenal tumor causing Cushing's syndrome, the contralateral adrenal gland undergoes disuse atrophy from lack of stimulation by ACTH, and these patients also may require perioperative stress doses of steroids. Steroids are continued postoperatively on a tapered regimen, until the adrenal gland fully recovers, which may take up to 2 years.[52] Transplant recipients typically receive large doses of steroids at the initial transplant procedure and often are maintained on some dose of steroids indefinitely. They require additional steroid administration for subsequent surgical procedures.

■ ADRENAL MEDULLA

PHYSIOLOGY

The naturally occurring catecholamines (epinephrine, norepinephrine, and dopamine) are synthesized from the amino acid tyrosine, which is sequentially hydroxylated to form dihydroxyphenylalanine (dopa), decarboxylated to form dopamine, and hydroxylated to form norepinephrine.[5] Only cells of the adrenal medulla and specific neurons of the central nervous system synthesize epinephrine through the N-methylation of norepinephrine by PNMT. Glucocorticoids produced in the adrenal cortex induce PNMT activity.[5] The rate-limiting step in catecholamine biosynthesis is the initial hydroxylation of tyrosine by the tyrosine hydroxylase enzyme. Catecholamines are stored within chromaffin granules in the cytoplasm of adrenomedullary cells. The majority of this is epinephrine.[3] This represents an important physiologic reserve of catecholamines that is instantaneously released by exocytosis during intense stimulation.

The adrenal medulla represents an interface between the autonomic nervous system and the endocrine system. Release of acetylcholine from preganglionic sympathetic neurons that synapse directly on the adrenal medullary cell causes fusion of the chromaffin granules and cell membrane. This releases catecholamines into the blood.[5] ACTH does not regulate catecholamine production.

The half-life of epinephrine is 2 minutes. Circulating catecholamines are metabolized in the liver and kidney by O-methylation. This is catalyzed by the enzyme catechol-O-methyltransferase (COMT). Metabolism of epinephrine and norepinephrine results in the metanephrines and 4-hydroxy-3methoxymandelic or vanylmadelic acid (VMA). Homovanillic acid (HVA) is the end product of dopamine metabolism.[5] Measurement of these metabolites in the urine is useful in diagnosing pheochromocytomas.

The effects of catecholamines are observed seconds after release, as compared to the more prolonged effects, during the course of hours and days, that characterize most other endocrine processes. Furthermore, mental anticipation of physiologic stress results in increased sympathoadrenal activity. Cathecholamines increase metabolic rate by stimulating the breakdown and mobilization of stored fuels to make substrates available for cellular consumption.[130] Catecholamines, acting at alpha receptors, stimulate vasoconstriction in the subcutaneous, mucosal, splanchnic, and renal vascular beds. Mobilization of substrates and circulatory support by the sympathoadrenal system is especially important during traumatic injury and shock. Cardiac effects, through β_1 receptors, include increased heart rate and enhanced contractility.[5] Bronchodilation is induced by catecholamine interaction with β_2 receptors. The urinary bladder is relaxed, while its sphincter tone is increased. Furthermore, catecholamines influence the secretion of several other hormones, including insulin, glucagon, renin, calcitonin, parathormone, thyroxine, gastrin, erythropoietin, and progesterone.[130] Hypoglycemia, in particular, results in a marked increase in adrenal medullary epinephrine secretion, accounting for many of the associated clinical manifestations.

PHEOCHROMOCYTOMA

Tumors which arise from chromaffin cells located within the adrenal medulla or sympathetic ganglia are called pheochromocytomas.[131] These tumors synthesize, store, and release catecholamines. Most pheochromocytomas secrete both epinephrine and norepinephrine, and secretion is not associated with neural stimulation. Pheochromocytomas also may produce other hormones, including ACTH, somatostatin, calcitonin, oxytocin, and vasopressin. ACTH secretion may cause concomitant Cushing's syndrome, but production of other hormones is usually not clinically significant.[132–136] Chemodectomas which arise from the

carotid body, ganglioneuromas derived from postganglionic sympathetic neurons, neuroblastomas, and ganglioneuroblastomas also secrete catecholamines and may produce similar clinical syndromes.[5]

Approximately 80% of pheochromocytomas occur as a unilateral, solitary lesion within the adrenal medulla, 10% are bilateral within the adrenal medullae, and 10% are extraadrenal.[137] In children, 25% are bilateral and 25% are extraadrenal.[131] The right adrenal gland is more often involved than the left.[138,139] The tumors are highly vascular, deriving their blood supply from any regional artery.

Ten % of pheochromocytomas occur in extraadrenal sites and may develop anywhere along the path of migration of the ectodermal neural crest cells.[140] Tumors are usually located within the abdomen at the celiac, superior mesenteric, or inferior mesenteric ganglia (Fig 21–2). The most common extraadrenal site is the organ of Zuckerkandl, located to the left of the aortic bifurcation, near the origin of the inferior mesenteric artery. One percent of extraadrenal tumors are found within the thorax, in association with the paravertebral sympathetic ganglia; <1% are found within the neck; and 1% are located within the urinary bladder.[141,142] Ectopic pheochromocytomas arising within the heart also have been reported.[143] Extraadrenal tumors are more likely to be malignant.[144] They secrete norepinephrine exclusively.

Pheochromocytomas are inherited as an autosomal dominant trait in 5% of cases. The neoplasm also occurs in multiple endocrine neoplasia (MEN) type IIa and type IIb, von Recklinghausen's neurofibromatosis, and von Hippel-Lindau disease. Loss of heterozygosity of chromosomes 1p, 3p, 17p, and 22q may be involved in the evolution of pheochromocytomas.[149] Bilateral tumors are common in these disorders.[150] Members of MEN type IIa and IIb kindreds should be screened periodically by measuring 24 hour urinary catecholamine levels.[151] In these individuals, pheochromocytoma should always be excluded or resected prior to thyroid or parathyroid surgery.

Pheochromocytomas most commonly weigh approximately 100 gm and are 3 to 5 cm in diameter.[152] Grossly, the tumors have a tan or gray appearance and a soft consistency. The incidence of malignancy, as determined by local invasion of surrounding tissues or metastatic disease, ranges from 5% to 46%.[131,139,151,153–155] Histologically, the distinction between benign and malignant lesions is unreliable. Extension of tumor cells into the cortex, capsular invasion, vascular invasion, and obvious nuclear pleomorphism may be observed in benign neoplasms.[9] Secondary tumors at sites where chromaffin cells are not normally present and visceral metastases are the only known true indicators of malignancy.[156] Larger tumor size, greater weight, increased necrosis, increased nuclear DNA ploidy, increased number of mitoses, and decreased neuropeptide Y expression in tumors also may indicate malignancy.[9,157-162]

Clinical Manifestations

The majority of cases of pheochromocytoma are sporadic and occur most commonly in young and middle-aged adults[5]; there may be a slight female preponderance. The most common clinical manifestation is hypertension, the pattern and severity of which may be related to the amount and specific type of catecholamine secreted.[163] However, the predominant catecholamine cannot be predicted from the clinical syndrome observed. In approximately 60% of cases, elevated blood pressure is sustained and responds poorly to conventional medical therapy; in addition, half of these patients will have hypertensive crises. The other 40% experience only episodic hypertensive paroxysms. In children, 90% have sustained hypertension.[164] For a given patient, symptoms are usually similar with each attack, often including the sudden onset of headache, diaphoresis, palpitations, and apprehension.[130] It may last from a few minutes to several hours. The attacks are sporadic and, with time, increase in frequency, duration, and severity. Sudden death from hypertensive crises, myocardial infarctions, and cerebrovascular accidents have been reported in patients with pheochromocytomas. Occasionally, activity that displaces the abdominal contents may provoke an attack.[5] Changes in blood flow and tumor necrosis with the sudden release of catecholamines may partially explain these occurrences. Urination may also initiate a paroxysm if the pheochromocytoma is located within the bladder wall. Urinary catecholamine levels usually are not dramatically elevated, since most tumors present early and are small. Hematuria is common and the tumor often can be visualized with cystoscopy.[142] While only 0.1% of the hypertensive population harbors a pheochromocytoma, it is a correctable cause of hypertension and may be fatal if not diagnosed or treated appropriately.[131,138]

Other symptoms and signs also are observed. Evidence of increased metabolic rate, such as sweating and weight loss, are common. Diminished intravascular volume and blunted sympathetic responses produce orthostatic hypotension.[130] These factors are also important contributors to the hypotension that develops during surgery or traumatic injury. Sinus tachycardia, cardiac arrhythmias, angina, and even acute myocardial infarction may occur.[130] Carbohydrate intolerance is present in >50% of patients.

Certain medications induce the release of catecholamines directly from the tumor. Severe and occasionally fatal paroxysms have been precipitated by opiates, histamine, ACTH, saralasin, and glucagon. Methyldopa, tricyclic antidepressants, and guanethidine augment the effects of catecholamines and should be avoided.[5]

Diagnosis

Suspicion of a pheochromocytoma is confirmed by measuring the free catecholamine, metanephrine, and VMA levels in a 24 hour urine sample obtained with the patient at rest.[165,166] The yield is increased if urine collection is initiated during a crisis. Urinary excretion of >100 ng of total free catecholamines, 25 ng of epinephrine, 75 ng of norepinephrine, 1.3 mg of total metanephrines, or 7.0 mg of VMA over 24 hours is diagnostic of a pheochromocytoma.[5] Urinary levels usually are elevated several times above the normal values. The test has a sensitivity of approximately 97% and a specificity of about 91%. False-positive results may be obtained during periods of hypoglycemia, stress, or exertion, or from the ingestion of exogenous catecholamines (methyldopa, levodopa, sympathomimetic amines), monoamine oxidase inhibitors, or propranolol. Measurement of plasma catecholamine levels are unreliable and useful only in the occasional patient with a very suggestive history and borderline urinary assay results.[167] A plasma norepinephrine level >2000 pg/mL may be diagnostic for a pheochromocytoma in nonstressed patients.[168] Measurement of a random urine sample for metanephrines has a false negative rate of 5%.

Given the reliable urinary assays, provocative tests rarely are used today to diagnose pheochromocytomas. In patients with borderline urinary catecholamine levels, the clonidine suppression test is very useful.[137,168-173] In a quiet environment, while the patient is lying supine, blood samples are collected for plasma epinephrine, norepinephrine, and total catecholamine levels for 30 minutes. An oral dose of 300 µg of clonidine is given and another blood sample is obtained 3 hours later. Clonidine markedly reduces plasma catecholamine levels into the normal range in normal patients and those with essential hypertension, but has little effect on levels in patients with pheochromocytomas. There is an approximate 1% false-positive rate and a 1% false-negative rate.[174] An overnight variant of the clonidine test, in which urinary catecholamine levels are measured, is an alternative diagnostic study.[173] The clonidine test essentially has replaced the glucagon test. Glucagon given intravenously will substantially increase blood pressure and the plasma catecholamine level only in patients with pheochromocytomas.[5] However, the test is potentially life-threatening and only should be used cautiously in a closely monitored setting. A patient in a hypertensive crisis will respond to phentolamine (5-mg bolus intravenously after a 0.5-mg test dose) with a reduction of blood pressure of at least 35/25 mm Hg within 10 minutes, which also may support the diagnosis of a pheochromocytoma.[130] Finally, plasma levels of chromogranin A are increased in any condition in which excessive catecholamines are produced, and measurement of plasma chromogranin A levels may be useful as a confirmatory, but not diagnostic, test for pheochromocytoma.[175]

Localization

Localization of a pheochromocytoma is usually very successful with CT scanning and/or MRI.[176–180] Tumors as small as 1 cm in diameter can be detected, and the sensitivities of the two tests are equivalent.[181] On the MR T2-weighted image, pheochromocytomas appear three times as bright as the liver (Fig 21–5).[182] Adrenal arteriography and venography are not indicated. If an abdominal CT or MRI scan does not reveal the tumor, chest CT and MRI scans should be obtained, since tumors may occur in the thorax.

Extraadrenal pheochromocytomas also may be localized by a radionuclide scintiscan utilizing ^{131}I-metaiodobenzylguanine (MIBG), an agent that resembles norepinephrine and is concentrated in adrenergic tissues by amine uptake.[183] Thus, the scan relies upon functioning tissues.[184] The overall sensitivity is 87%, with a specificity of virtually 100%.[183–186] False-positive results are rare. False-negative results occur approximately 15% to 20% of the time and seem to be more common in patients with multiple tumors and metastatic disease.[165,181,187–189] Intraoperative radionuclear scanning may detect pheochromocytomas and metastases in patients treated preoperatively with ^{131}I-MIBG.[190] Positron emission tomography (PET), after the administration of 2-[fluorine-18]-fluoro-2-deoxy-D-glucose (FDG), may be helpful in localizing pheochromocytomas that fail to image with MIBG.[191]

Management

Successful treatment of a pheochromocytoma requires complete surgical excision of the tumor in order to eliminate the life-threatening clinical symptoms and to eradicate any possibility of malignant degeneration.[10] Successful surgical treatment is reliant upon meticulous perioperative care.

The goal of preoperative management is to establish stable α-adrenergic blockade.[130] This usually is accomplished with phenoxybenzamine, an α receptor blocker, at a starting dose of 10 mg every 12 hours. The dose is increased and the interval of administration is reduced every few days until blood pressure is controlled and paroxysms do not occur. Almost all patients experience orthostatic hypotension when a therapeutic dose is reached. The intravascular volume in these patients tends to be reduced markedly as the body attempts to compensate for the hypertension produced by the vasoconstrictive α-adrenergic activity of the catecholamines secreted by the tumor. Additionally, sympathetic responses are blunted. Patients must be advised to drink fluids liberally and to use caution when sitting up or

standing. Symptomatic patients may require hospitalization preoperatively. The intravascular volume returns to normal levels after approximately 14 days of therapy with α-adrenergic blockade[192]; however, we generally find that approximately 7 days are adequate. This simple therapy has resulted in a dramatic improvement in the intraoperative management of patients.[165,166,193] In children undergoing resection of a pheochromocytoma, preoperative normalization of blood pressure and symptoms is associated with fewer intraoperative and postoperative complications.[194]

Other preoperative medications to induce α-adrenergic blockade have also been used with stress. Prazosin, a selective α1 antagonist, controls blood pressure and paroxysms at a dose of 1 to 5 mg every 6 hours.[130] Tyrosine hydroxylase, the rate-limiting step in catecholamine biosynthesis, can be inhibited competitively by the drug metyrosine, at a dose of 250 mg four times each day. Catecholamine production is reduced by metyrosine and this drug may be used to treat hypertensive crises.[195,196] Nifedipine with phenoxybenzamine, or nicardipine alone, are agents useful to control blood pressure lability.[197,198]

Once α-adrenergic blockade has been achieved, β blockade may be initiated 1 week prior to surgery to control tachycardia and catecholamine-induced arrhythmias.[10] A reasonable starting dosage schedule using propranolol is 10 mg three to four times each day. Administration of β-adrenergic receptor blockers without alpha blockade may cause a paradoxical increase in blood pressure by antagonizing β receptor-mediated vasodilatation in skeletal muscle.

Lactic acidosis can often be demonstrated in patients with pheochromocytoma.[130] This is caused by the metabolic effects of catecholamines, as well as the decreased perfusion from vasoconstriction.[199] Arterial blood pH should be measured and corrected in all patients before the induction of anesthesia. During the operative procedure, continuous monitoring of the electrocardiogram, the blood pressure via an arterial line, and the central venous pressure is paramount. A Swan-Ganz catheter may be required to follow pulmonary capillary wedge pressures, in the setting of cardiac disease, to optimize performance. Adequate fluid replacement is crucial. Intraoperative hypotension is managed with volume resuscitation rather than intravenous pressors. Acute episodes of hypertension and arrhythmias are most likely to occur during the induction of anesthesia, intubation, or during manipulation of the tumor. Intravenous phentolamine or nitroprusside are administered to control elevated blood pressure. Propranolol may be given for tachycardia or ventricular ectopy. These measures have substantially reduced the mortality and morbidity for surgical resection of pheochromocytoma.

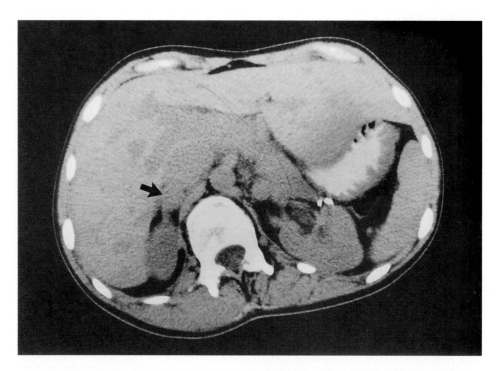

A

Figure 21–5. CT and MRI of a pheochromo-cytoma. **A**. This CT scan demonstrates a solid 1.5 cm right adrenal mass (*arrow*). Note the close proximity of the inferior vena cava that is abutting the anterior aspect of the mass. The differential diagnosis includes adrenal adenoma, adrenocortical carcinoma, and pheochromocytoma. **B**. T2-weighted MRI im-age of the same patient, at approximately the same level as the CT scan, confirms a 1.5 cm mass arising in the right adrenal area (*arrow*). The mass has the high signal intensity typical of a pheochromocytoma. The right adrenal gland was surgically resected and pathologic analysis revealed a 1.5 × 1.2 × 1.1 cm pheochromocytoma in the adrenal medulla.

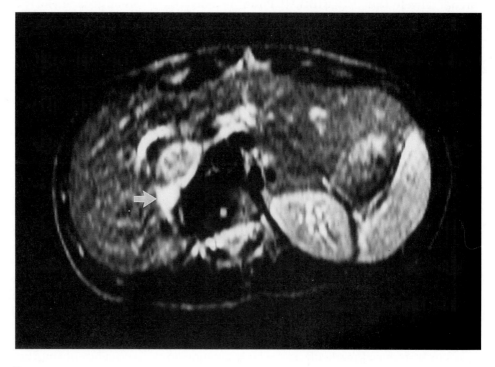

B

Resection of a pheochromocytoma is accomplished from the anterior, transperitoneal approach through a midline incision (discussed in detail later in this chapter). The incidence of bilateral, extraadrenal, and metastatic disease mandates thorough visualization and palpation of the entire abdomen, with special attention given to both adrenals, the renal hila, and periaortic ganglia. A Kocher maneuver is performed to explore the lesser sac. Gaining control of the venous drainage from the tumor is important. Minimal handling of the tumor directly until this is accomplished will decrease the chance of catecholamine release and resultant paroxysmal blood pressure swings and arrhythmias.

Debate has arisen about whether patients with MEN type IIa or IIb should undergo bilateral adrenalectomy.[200–202] Some believe that almost all patients with these syndromes either have, or will develop, bilateral adrenomedullary pheochromocytomas, if followed long enough.[150,200] Others maintain that the incidence of bilateral disease is significantly less, 52% in one study, and the risk of acute adrenal insufficiency after bilateral adrenalectomy is unacceptably high at approximately 23%.[201,202] Recurrence of tumor in the contralateral gland may not occur for 12 years.[202] Therefore, unilateral adrenalectomy may be indicated in select patients with MEN syndromes, if the contralateral adrenal gland appears normal by preoperative studies and by intraoperative examination. Indefinite follow-up of these patients with repeated urinary screening tests is essential.[151] Pheochromocytomas are usually benign and do not recur in patients with MEN syndromes after complete surgical resection.[153,154]

After a successful operation, urinary catecholamine excretion returns to normal in about 1 week. Measurement of 24 hour urinary catecholamine levels after that time may indicate whether residual or metastatic disease is present. Complete excision of a pheochromocytoma results in >95% 5 year survival and cure of the hypertension in 75% of patients. Hypertension that recurs in the remaining 25% of patients is usually well controlled by standard therapy for essential hypertension.[10]

Recurrence of tumor was generally believed to be less than 10%. However, recent studies indicate that there may be an increased potential for malignancy, as defined by recurrent or metastatic disease, which in some series approaches 50%.[153,154] Pathologic analysis of the tumor is unreliable in predicting malignancy.[153] Metastases may develop from 0.2 to 28.7 years after surgery, and 5% of recurrent disease is detected each year in the first 9 years after resection. Males are more likely to develop recurrent tumors. These results emphasize the need for close, long-term follow-up after surgery for pheochromocytoma.[154,155] Measurement of urinary catecholamines, the clonidine suppression test, CT, MRI, and MIBG scans may be required on a yearly basis.[153,154] MIBG imaging usually is able to detect recurrent disease. Bone scintigraphy may be more sensitive than MIBG scans for imaging bony metastases.[203,204] Surgical resection of localized or solitary recurrences or metastases should be attempted, if possible, including metastatic liver and lung lesions.[205,206] A patient with a malignant pheochromocytoma has an overall 5 year survival rate of between 36% and 60%, and patients usually expire within 3 years after the discovery of metastatic disease.[205,207–209]

In cases of unresectable locally invasive tumor, widespread metastatic disease, or poor medical condition rendering the patient inoperable, long-term medical management is the only option. Hypertension may be controlled by the chronic administration of adrenergic antagonists.[207] Metyrosine also can be added. Painful bone metastases may have a good response to radiation therapy.[210] Soft tissue masses respond well to >4000 cGy of radiation.[159] Standard chemotherapy regimens include doxorubicin and streptozocin or BCNU and doxorubicin. They have not been effective in treating malignant pheochromocytomas.[206,209,211–213] Attempts to utilize ^{131}I-MIBG to treat malignant tumors have not been successful.[214–217] Treatment with chemotherapeutic agents responsive against neuroblastomas may be more efficacious in treating pheochromocytomas.[218–222]

■ INCIDENTAL ADRENAL MASS

The management of a patient with an asymptomatic adrenal mass is a new problem that has arisen with the more widespread availability of high-resolution CT scanners.[223] Unexpected adrenal masses are detected on 0.6% of abdominal CT scans.[224,225] The goal of evaluation is to determine if the tumor is malignant or functionally active.[226] Benign, nonfunctional adrenal adenomas do not require surgical resection.

Evaluation of the patient begins with a careful history and physical examination to determine whether signs or symptoms of excessive adrenal function are present.[10] Evidence of Cushing's syndrome, hypertension, hypokalemia, virilization, feminization, or weight change must be sought. Additionally, indications of an occult malignancy must be pursued. Multiple blood pressure measurements are recorded and the serum potassium level is measured in order to exclude an aldosterone-producing tumor.[10] Laboratory studies are obtained based upon the clinical suspicion of hypercortisolism, aldosteronism, virilization, pheochromocytoma, adrenocortical carcinoma, or disease metastatic to the adrenal.[98] Pheochromocytomas may demonstrate only episodic hypertension and a few patients with Cushing's syndrome may not have clinically apparent signs or symptoms.[227] Therefore, 24 hour urine levels of catecholamines, VMA, metanephrines, and free cortisol must be measured in every pa-

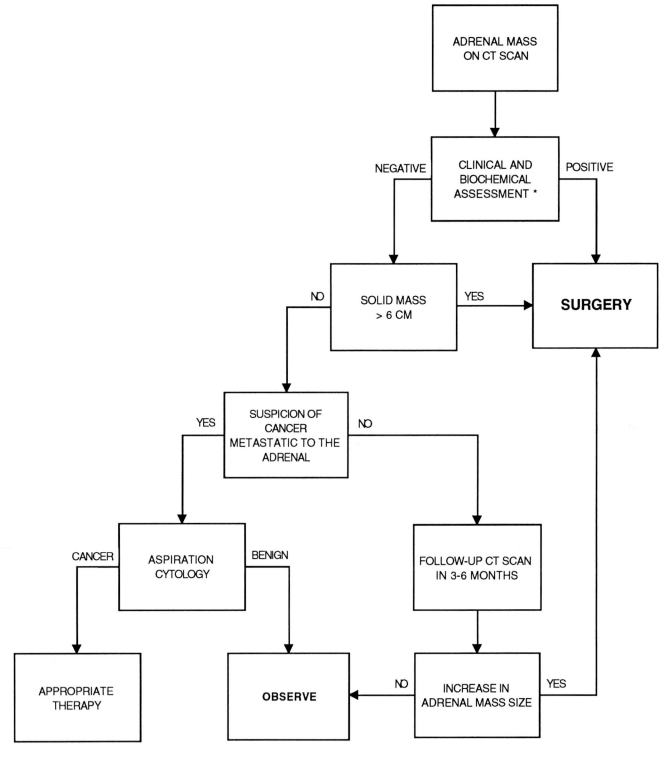

Figure 21–6. Evaluation of an incidentally discovered adrenal mass. Surgical resection of an incidentally discovered adrenal mass is indicated when the mass is >6 cm in diameter on CT scan, displays increased signal intensity on T2-weighted MRI images consistent with adrenocortical carcinoma or pheochromocytoma, indicates functional capacity based on clinical history and biochemical assessment, or enlarges on serial CT scans.
*Clinical assessment includes a history and physical examination to exclude symptoms and signs of hypercortisolism, hypertension, virilization, feminization, or weight change; biochemical assessment includes measurement of 24 hour urinary catecholamines, VMA, metanephrine, and free cortisol levels, and the measurement of the serum potassium level.

tient with an adrenal mass. One must keep in mind that a great majority of incidentally discovered tumors are nonfunctioning benign adenomas. Although 20% of adrenocortical carcinomas are nonfunctioning, they represent <1% of cases.[107,114] Therefore, additional tests should be obtained only if there is clinical evidence of excessive adrenal hormone secretion.

The size of the lesion on CT scan is the best basis for discrimination between nonfunctioning benign and malignant tumors.[226] The incidence of cancer in solid adrenal lesions >6 cm is 35% to 98%.[98] Most adrenocortical adenomas are <4 cm in diameter.[176,223,228] However, a small lesion cannot be ignored, since small adrenocortical carcinomas are possible and are more curable than larger tumors.[89,229,230] Repeat abdominal CT scanning is required within 3 to 6 months for all unresected masses, in order to assess the growth of the lesion.[228] All CT scans also should be analyzed for evidence of metastatic lesions, although CT cannot determine whether a solitary adrenal lesion is benign or malignant.[231] MRI may provide additional information with T2-weighted images. On the T2-weighted MRI image, both primary adrenocortical and metastatic carcinomas appear as bright as, or slightly brighter than, the liver and pheochromocytomas appear three times brighter than the liver. Adenomas appear darker than the liver.[41,176,182,232,233] Adrenal cysts have low signal intensity on both T1- and T2-weighted images, much like an adenoma.[234] [131I]iodomethylnorcholesterol scintigraphy may identify the functional activity of an adrenocortical lesion.

Fine-needle aspiration of the lesion in question can result in life-threatening sequelae, if the lesion is an unsuspected pheochromocytoma.[235] Furthermore, aspiration cytology cannot distinguish between benign and malignant adrenal neoplasms and should not be used to evaluate nonfunctioning adrenal masses. Needle biopsy may be helpful in confirming suspected metastatic adrenal lesions.[236–239] MRI or measurement of urinary catecholamines is necessary before fine-needle aspiration is attempted.

Surgical resection of an incidentally discovered adrenal mass is indicated when the mass is >6 cm in diameter on CT, displays increased signal intensity on T2-weighted MRI images consistent with adrenocortical carcinoma or pheochromocytoma, or indicates functional capacity based on clinical history and/or biochemical assessment (Fig 21–6).[41,232] Lesions that are large or suspected to be malignant should be approached through a standard midline laparotomy incision or a thoracoabdominal incision. Small, apparently benign lesions that are functionally active may be resected using a posterior or laparoscopic approach. Approximately 5% of patients with incidentally discovered adrenocortical masses may actually have subclinical Cushing's syndrome that is recognized only by laboratory test results.[227] All patients should

undergo preoperative biochemical assessment as discussed above. Patients with evidence of hypercortisolism must receive perioperative stress doses of steroids or acute adrenal insufficiency may result.[240] A pheochromocytoma must be ruled out or diagnosed prior to surgery, since preoperative preparation is critical (Fig 21–6).

In one prospective study of 10 patients with operable, early-stage nonsmall-cell lung cancer and a unilateral adrenal lesion, adrenalectomy confirmed benign adrenal lesions after nondiagnostic fine-needle aspirations in 6 patients, who then underwent curative resection of the lung cancer. Survival in these patients was significantly greater than in the patients with metastatic adrenal lesions who were treated with chemotherapy.[238] Therefore, adrenalectomy may play a role in excluding malignant adrenal lesions and thus, in indicating appropriate therapy in some select patients with early-stage lung cancers and unilateral adrenal lesions.

Every patient with an adrenal mass that is not removed surgically should be reexamined clinically for new signs or symptoms and reevaluated by CT scan within 3 to 6 months to assess growth of the mass. The development of new clinical symptoms or signs requires laboratory investigation as discussed above. Increase in the size of the mass on CT scan mandates surgical resection.[98]

■ ADRENALECTOMY

Anatomically, the adrenal glands are located centrally within the body, deep in the retroperitoneum near the junction of the thorax and abdomen. Consequently, the surgical approach and exposure for adrenalectomy or resection of an adrenal mass may pose difficulties. Surrounding structures including the aorta, inferior vena cava, kidneys, pancreas, splenic vessels, and liver, intimately appose the adrenal glands. Adrenal tumors may extend into these surrounding structures, including the inferior vena cava. Therefore, several approaches have been devised to gain adequate exposure for dissection of the gland and associated masses, as well as to gain control of the vasculature. The greatest potential for intraoperative mortality during adrenalectomy is uncontrollable, exsanguinating hemorrhage arising from the venous outflow, when exposure is inadequate.

INDICATIONS

Surgical resection is the primary treatment for adrenal tumors that are functionally active or suspected to be malignant. Adrenal masses may be resected by using an anterior approach through a standard midline laparotomy incision, through a thoracoabdominal incision, by using a posterior approach, or laparoscopically. One or both adrenals may be removed using any of these approaches. The approach that is chosen depends on the suspected pathology and size of the adrenal lesion. Small lesions that are thought to be benign may be resected using a posterior approach or the newly described laparoscopic technique.[241,242] Larger masses and those that may be malignant generally should be resected using an anterior approach in order to gain sufficient exposure and to explore adequately the entire abdomen. A very large lesion often requires a thoracoabdominal incision, especially if adrenocortical carcinoma, which may invade surrounding structures that need to be resected, is suspected.

Table 21–4 summarizes the specific indications for adrenalectomy.

Anterior Approach

The anterior approach for adrenalectomy is mandatory whenever optimum exposure is required or when exploration of the entire abdomen is necessary. Therefore, this approach is used in patients with adrenal tumors >4 cm in diameter, or in patients with possibly malignant tumors of any size, such as pheochromocytoma or adrenocortical carcinoma.

A midline incision is commonly used, with the patient in the supine position with a transverse roll beneath the thoracic spine (Fig 21–7). For very large adrenal masses, a thoracoabdominal incision may provide better exposure (Fig 21–8). In this instance, the patient is placed in the lateral decubitus position with the involved side superiorly.

Once the peritoneum is entered, abdomen is explored for evidence of metastatic disease. Suspicious le-

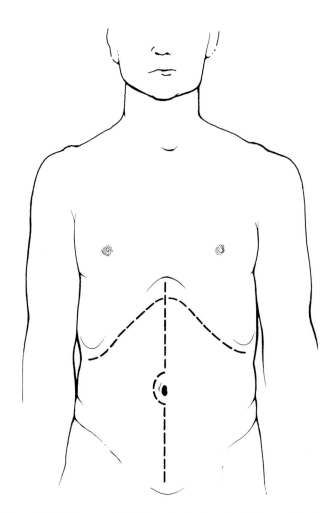

Figure 21–7. Anterior approach. Midline exploratory laparotomy incision or bilateral subcostal incision. Most commonly, the adrenals are approached anteriorly by using either one of these incisions. This approach allows thorough exploration of the entire abdomen, as well as good exposure of both adrenals.

TABLE 21–4. INDICATIONS FOR ADRENALECTOMY

UNILATERAL ADRENALECTOMY	APPROACH
Cortical adenoma causing Cushing's syndrome	Posterior or laparoscopic
Aldosteronoma	Posterior or laparoscopic
Pheochromocytoma, sporadic	Anterior
Pheochromocytoma, MEN IIa or MEN IIb*	Anterior or laparoscopic
Adrenocortical carcinoma	Anterior or thoracoabdominal
Virilizing or feminizing tumor	Anterior
Incidental solid mass >6 cm	Anterior or thoracoabdominal

BILATERAL ADRENALECTOMY	APPROACH
Pheochromocytoma involving both adrenals	Anterior
Primary pigmented micronodular adrenal hyperplasia	Posterior or laparoscopic
Massive macronodular adrenal hyperplasia	Posterior or laparoscopic
Severe Cushing's syndrome caused by an occult ACTH producing tumor which is unresponsive to medical management	Posterior or laparoscopic

*Bilateral adrenalectomy is required if tumors are identified in both adrenals.

sions should be biopsied or excised. To proceed with resection of the right adrenal gland, the retroperitoneal space is entered behind the liver. The entire right lobe of the liver is mobilized by dividing the coronary and triangular hepatic ligaments with cautery or scissors. The right lobe of the liver then is retracted anteriorly and medially. The right adrenal gland can be identified by its position of resting upon the kidney and being posterolateral to the inferior vena cava (Fig 21–9). To identify the inferior vena cava caudal to the tumor, the hepatic flexure of the colon is reflected inferiorly and medially, after dividing its peritoneal attachments, uncovering the duodenum. A Kocher maneuver is performed so that the second portion of the duodenum, which rests upon the superior kidney, can be reflected medially. It is important to ligate the adrenal vein early during an operation for a pheochromocytoma so that further handling of the neoplasm will not result in cat-

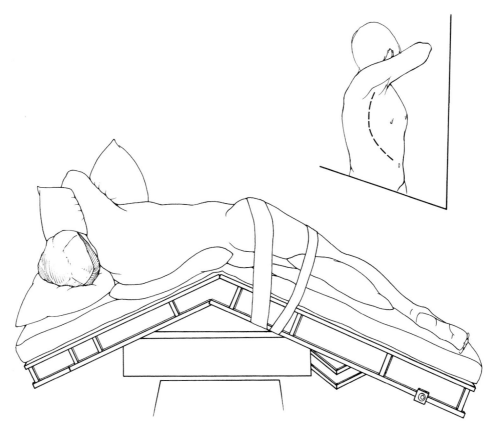

Figure 21–8. Thoracoabdominal incision. Complete resection of adrenal masses that may invade local structures requires adequate exposure. While the standard midline laparotomy may be adequate in most cases, very large adrenal neoplasms are resected more easily in entirety via a thoracoabdominal incision, with the patient in the lateral decubitus position.

echolamine surges and blood pressure fluctuations. Additionally, with large tumors, early ligation of the right adrenal vein eliminates the risk of life-threatening hemorrhage from tearing the vein as the tumor is dissected free. The vena cava is identified easily and careful dissection along its posterolateral border will allow identification of the right adrenal vein, which is usually near the superior margin of the right adrenal. The vein is ligated with 2-O silk suture and divided (Fig 21–9).

Once the adrenal vein is ligated, a plane can be developed on the avascular lateral aspect of the tumor to allow a hand beneath it for handling and palpation of the adrenal gland. The arterial vessels are clipped and divided sequentially, beginning at the superolateral aspect of the gland and continuing medially. The medial vessels arise directly from the aorta and care must be taken to securely clip these arteries.

Alternatively, the right adrenal gland may be approached inferior to the liver by retracting the liver superiorly and mobilizing the hepatic flexure of the colon, as described above. However, with this approach, exposure of the adrenal gland is more limited and control of the venous outflow is more difficult to

achieve. Therefore, we do not recommend this subhepatic approach.

Resection of the left adrenal gland requires mobilization of the spleen and left colon. The lateral peritoneal attachments of the left colon are freed, initially. Then the spleen is scooped out from the left upper quadrant medially and the avascular attachments between the spleen and diaphragm are divided (Fig 21–10). The spleen, stomach, pancreatic tail, and left colon are retracted medially en bloc to the superior mesenteric vessels. The left adrenal gland is exposed splendidly in this manner. Similar to a right adrenalectomy, the left adrenal vein is ligated and divided first, and then the arterial vessels are clipped and divided sequentially, beginning at the superolateral aspect of the gland and continuing medially (Fig 21–10). Again, an avascular plane can be developed from the lateral aspect of the gland.

An alternative approach to the left adrenal gland involves entering the lesser omental space, retracting the stomach superiorly, entering the retroperitoneum along the inferior border of the pancreas, mobilizing the distal pancreas from its posterior attachments, and

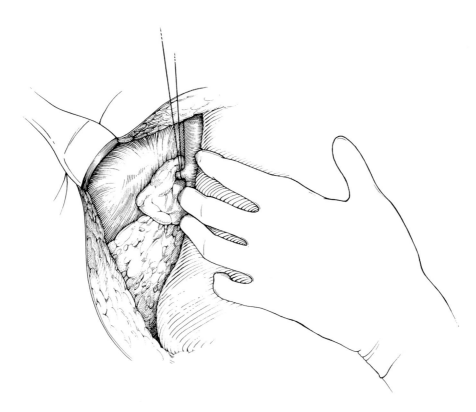

Figure 21–9. Anterior approach: right adrenalectomy. The right adrenal gland is clearly exposed by dividing the attachments of the right hepatic lobe and retracting the liver anteriorly and medially. Mobilizing the hepatic flexure of the colon and Kocherizing the duodenum provides additional exposure of the inferior vena cava caudal to the adrenal. The inferior vena cava is identified easily, and careful dissection along its posterolateral border will reveal the right adrenal vein.

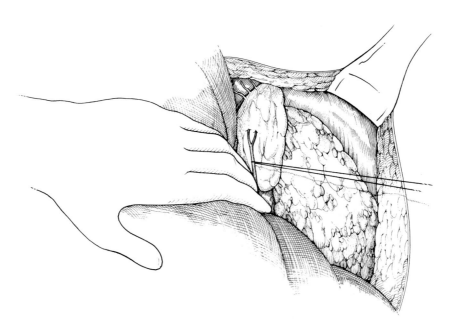

Figure 21–10. Anterior approach: left adrenalectomy. The left adrenal gland is exposed optimally by taking down the splenic flexure of the colon, mobilizing the spleen from the left upper quadrant, and reflecting the spleen, tail of the pancreas, stomach, and colon medially. The left adrenal vein is identified exiting the anterior aspect of the gland and coursing medially.

retracting the pancreas superiorly to expose the left adrenal gland. This approach provides less exposure and is not recommended.

Very large adrenal masses pose difficult problems as a result of their size and vascularity, with the inherent potential for hemorrhage. With very large adrenal masses, the adrenal vein is not easily identified for early ligation and division. Under this circumstance, the tumor must be dissected away from intimate structures in order to gain adequate exposure of the vein. If the vein is involved with tumor, the vena cava may need to be partially resected. Control of the venous effluent as early as possible remains of prime importance.

Postoperatively, parenteral narcotics are required, initially, for pain control. A nasogastric tube or gastric tube usually is placed during surgery; this is removed and the diet is advanced as bowel function returns. If a thoracoabdominal incision is used, a chest tube also is indicated.

Posterior Approach

A posterior approach for excision of either adrenal gland is advantageous because there is less postoperative pain and a faster recovery, when compared with the anterior approach. The peritoneal space is not violated and bowel function is preserved postoperatively. A preoperative bowel preparation is not required. This strategy is most suitable for adrenal tumors measuring <4 cm in diameter. Control of either adrenal vein from the posterior aspect of the gland becomes increasingly more difficult as tumor size increases. A posterior approach is not appropriate for excision of pheochromocytomas, adrenal tumors >4 cm in diameter, adrenal carcinoma, or if concomitant intra-abdominal pathology is present.

The patient is situated in a prone, jack-knifed position upon two vertically placed soft rolls after induction of general anesthesia (Fig 21–11). This positioning allows ample space in order to carry out the procedure on either side. In addition, the abdominal contents fall away from the retroperitoneum. A curvilinear skin incision is made that begins three fingerbreadths from the midline at the tenth rib and is extended inferiorly and increasingly more lateral to a maximum of four fingerbreadths from the midline at its most inferior extent, the superior border of the posterior iliac crest (Fig 21–11). The incision is deepened through the subcutaneous fat and latissimus dorsi muscle until the posterior lamella of the lumbodorsal fascia is exposed. This fascial layer is incised longitudinally to uncover the underlying sacrospinalis muscle. Multiple lumbar vessels and cutaneous nerves are ligated and divided. The sacrospinalis muscle is retracted medially and its attachments to the eleventh and twelfth ribs are divided. Both ribs are dissected subperiosteally with ligation of the intercostal

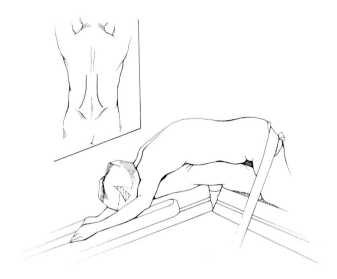

Figure 21–11. Posterior approach: patient positioning and skin incisions. After general anesthesia is induced, the patient is placed in the prone position on two vertically placed rolls, and the table is hyperextended at the waist. A curvilinear skin incision is made that begins three fingerbreadths from the midline at the tenth rib and is extended inferiorly and increasingly more lateral to a maximum of four fingerbreadths from the midline at its most inferior extent, the superior border of the posterior iliac crest.

arteries and veins. Each rib is cut as far medially as possible. The intercostal nerve is carefully retracted superiorly. The middle and anterior lamellae of lumbodorsal fascia are incised in order to enter the retroperitoneum; retroperitoneal fat and Gerotas fascia are identified. For increased exposure, the pleura is pushed bluntly up the diaphragm superiorly. The diaphragm is divided to the level of the tenth rib between clips or by using cautery. If the pleural cavity is inadvertently entered, this is remedied at the time of wound closure by placing a #16 red rubber catheter into the pleural space, running a size O silk suture on each side of the catheter to close the pleural defect, and quickly withdrawing the catheter during maximal hand ventilation while pulling up on the silk sutures.

Once the retroperitoneal space is entered, the kidney is retracted inferiorly to optimally expose the suprarenal area (Fig 21–12). For both the right and left adrenals, the arterial supply is first controlled by clipping and ligating the numerous arterial vessels that course posteriorly (superficially from the posterior viewpoint) and enter the gland along its superior and medial margins. The adrenal vein, which lies more deeply with respect to the arteries, is ligated as it is encountered. For the right adrenal gland, careful identification of the right adrenal vein coursing from its medial surface to the inferior vena cava is mandatory. The short, fat, right adrenal vein must be securely, but gently, ligated with 2-O silk suture and divided. When the gland is enlarged, the right adrenal vein may be more difficult

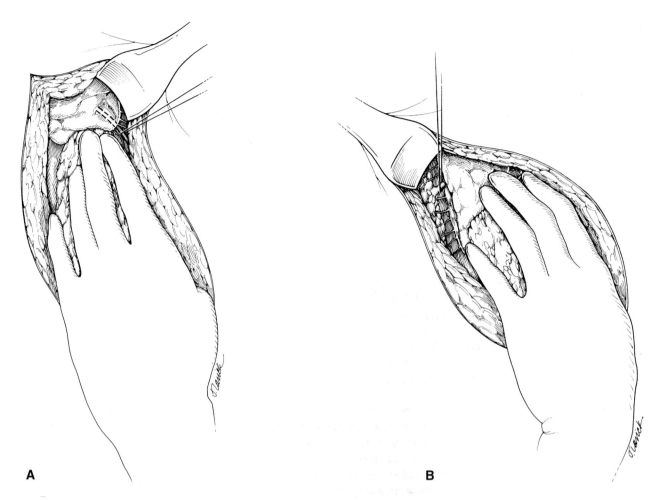

A   **B**

Figure 21–12. Posterior approach: left (**A**) and right (**B**) adrenalectomy. Retroperitoneal fat and Gerotas fascia is immediately obvious upon entrance into the retroperitoneal cavity. The kidney is identified easily. Gentle retraction of the kidney inferiorly provides exposure of the suprarenal area and the adrenal gland. The adrenal arteries appear more superficial from the posterior viewpoint, and these are ligated in a circumferential manner initially. The adrenal vein lies deep with respect to the arteries, when viewed posteriorly. Dissection proceeds until the vein is encountered, at which time it is promptly ligated and divided.

to access. Meticulous dissection with minimal retraction is warranted around this vein, which is a potentially life threatening source of hemorrhage. The gland is freed circumferentially from its lateral to medial aspect. The inferior border of the gland is dissected last to maintain attachment to the kidney and inferior retraction of the gland (Fig 21–12). The left adrenal gland has a longer, deeper vein that courses anteromedially to enter the renal vein. The left adrenal vein is more difficult to access from the posterior approach than the right, since the left lies deep, obscured by the left adrenal gland when viewed from the back. The entire left adrenal gland initially is mobilized circumferentially, and its vein is ligated and divided last (Fig 21–12).

Wound closure consists of reapproximation of the diaphragm, repair of any pleural defects, reapproximation of the anterior and then middle lamellae of the lumbodorsal fascia, and reapproximation of the skin edges.

Postoperatively, patients require parenteral pain medication until pain is controlled by oral analgesics. A clear liquid diet may be started as soon as the patient is fully awake from anesthesia and, if tolerated, advanced to a normal diet by the following morning.

Laparoscopic Adrenalectomy

The recent widespread development of laparoscopic techniques has invoked great enthusiasm for minimally invasive, less morbid surgical procedures. Adrenalectomy has been no exception, and modern surgeons must be familiar with the laparoscopic approach for excision of the adrenal glands.[241,242] Advantages appear to include decreased postoperative pain, a shorter postoperative rehabilitation period, and more cosmetically acceptable incisions. Because laparoscopic adrenalectomy avoids an open anterior transperitoneal approach, it may result in a faster return of bowel function and possibly shorter postoperative hospitalization. However, certain circumstances still may mandate traditional open approaches. Adrenalectomy for a nonfamilial pheochromocytoma requires exploration of the entire abdomen, which may be executed best by intraoperative palpation and visualization. Excision of large malignant tumors, especially those that invade adjacent tissues, appear to pose too great a risk for a laparoscopic approach. Patients who have undergone previous abdominal surgery may have extensive intraperitoneal adhesions that could prevent safe entrance into the peritoneum and the maneuvering of laparoscopic instruments. Morbid obesity, as seen in patients with Cushing's syndrome, also may be a relative contraindication for laparoscopic surgery, since maneuvering instruments through a thick abdominal wall may be more challenging. Finally, expertise in open adrenalectomy is necessary for the laparoscopic surgeon, since encountering unexpectedly difficult dissections with laparoscopy will require conversion to an open procedure to complete the resection appropriately, and to promptly rectify any intraoperative laparoscopic complications.

Laparoscopic adrenalectomy is most ideal for small adrenal masses thought not to be pheochromocytomas, in an otherwise normal gland. It may be the procedure of choice for patients with aldosteronomas. General anesthesia is induced, a urinary catheter and nasogastric tube are placed for decompression of the bladder and bowel, and the patient is placed in the lateral decubitus position, with the affected side superiorly (Fig 21–13). The decubitus positioning allows intraperitoneal contents to fall away from the entry sites of the laparoscopic instruments. The surgeon stands at the back of the patient with the first assistant at the opposite side of the table. Two monitors are placed at the head of the table, one on each side. The camera apparatus and video cassette recorder are placed under one monitor while the insufflation equipment is placed under the other.

The first goal is to gain access to the peritoneal cavity in order to insufflate with carbon dioxide gas. Four ports eventually will be placed equidistantly in a transverse line from the posterior axillary line to the lateral edge of the rectus sheath between the costal margin and iliac crest (Fig 21–13). An insufflator initially is introduced into the peritoneum at the lateral edge of the rectus sheath (at approximately the midclavicular line), two fingerbreadths below the costal margin. This may be accomplished using three different techniques: (1) blind insertion of an insufflator needle percutaneously through a transverse 1 cm incision while retracting anteriorly on the abdominal wall, (2) a semi-open approach, in which a transverse incision is made in the skin and carried down through the subcutaneous tissue to the peritoneum; a needle insufflator then is placed blindly through the peritoneum, or (3) an open approach, in which the peritoneum is in-

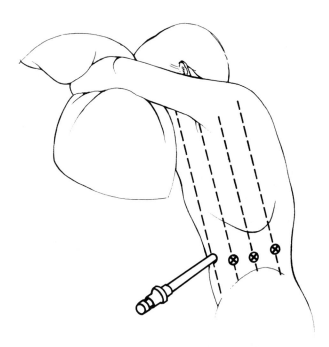

Figure 21–13. Laparoscopic adrenalectomy: patient positioning and port insertion. After general anesthesia is induced, a nasogastric tube and a urinary catheter are placed. The patient is placed in the lateral decubitus position with the affected side superiorly. The abdomen is insufflated and four laparoscopic ports are inserted approximately two fingerbreadths below the costal margin at the midclavicular, anterior axillary, midaxillary, and posterior axillary lines. The table then is hyperextended at the waist.

cised, and a port is placed under direct vision into the peritoneal cavity; purse-string sutures are fastened around the port. The open approach for insufflation is most advantageous in that definitive intraperitoneal entry is confirmed, blind perforation of viscera is nearly eliminated, carbon dioxide gas flows more quickly through the larger port than the smaller-caliber insufflation needle, and closure of the fascia is more definite. Carbon dioxide gas then is insufflated, beginning at a low rate of 2 L/min and then increasing to 9 L/min. Intraperitoneal insufflation is confirmed by low insufflation pressures, lack of subcutaneous air, distension of the abdomen, and tympany over the abdominal cavity. When a pressure of 15 mm Hg is reached and the abdomen is sufficiently distended, trocars and ports then may be placed. If the percutaneous or semi-open insufflation approach is used, the insufflation needle is withdrawn and a trocar with a safety shield is inserted through the same wound into the peritoneum, while retracting the abdominal wall superiorly; this is not necessary if an open approach is used initially. The trocar is withdrawn with the port in place, the insufflator tubing is connected to the port, and carbon dioxide insufflation continues. The videoscope is inserted through the port. The entry site into the peritoneum and surrounding visceral are visualized to assess hemorrhage or injury.

The anterolateral abdominal wall is viewed next to continuously watch placement of the next two ports. The position for the next most lateral port is identified at the anterior axillary line (Fig 21–13), a 1 cm transverse incision is made, and a trocar with a safety shield is advanced slowly through the tissues with a twisting motion. Care is taken not to plunge the trocar through the abdominal wall. The entire procedure is viewed continuously, using the videoscope, to ensure that the trocar enters at the appropriate place and does not damage viscera upon piercing the peritoneum. The trocar is removed and the port is left in place. A one-way valve in the port prevents any leak of carbon dioxide. The third port is placed in the same manner at the next lateral position, near the midaxillary line (Fig 21–13).

Exploration of the peritoneal cavity is performed by visualizing all four quadrants of the abdomen and the pelvis with the videoscope. The videoscope then is placed through the middleport. A fan retractor is placed through the most medial port for retraction of viscera medially, anteriorly, and superiorly. The operating instruments, which consist of grasping forceps, dissecting forceps, and an irrigation/suction apparatus enter the abdomen through the lateral ports. The operating table then is hyperextended at the waist so that abdominal viscera are displaced away from the area of dissection.

The principles of laparoscopic adrenalectomy are very similar to those of the open anterior approach. For a right adrenalectomy, entrance to the retroperitoneum is gained behind to the liver. The triangular liga-

ment and hepatocolic ligament are dissected using cautery and scissors, and the fan retractor is used to retract the right lobe of the liver anteriorly and medially. The hepatic flexure of the large bowel is mobilized using blunt and sharp dissection, which results in the colon falling, medially and anteriorly, away from the retroperitoneum. The adrenal gland then is identified posterolateral to the inferior vena cava and superior to the kidney (Fig 21–14). Once the retroperitoneum is entered, a fourth and final port is placed at the posterior axillary line under direct vision, as described above (Fig 21–13). The right adrenal gland is freed from its attachments using blunt dissection through both lateral ports, and the arteries are clipped and ligated. The right adrenal vein is carefully doubly clipped and ligated (Fig 21–14). The videoscope follows the adrenal gland as it is carried out the lateral port with grasping forceps. A bag can be utilized to prevent spillage of the glandular tissue. The adrenal bed is checked carefully for hemostasis and irrigated. Finally, the retractor and videoscope are withdrawn.

The left adrenal gland is resected in a similar manner. The patient is placed in the right lateral decubitus position. Ports are placed, as described above, in mirror image on the left side. The spleen initially is mobilized by dividing its lateral attachments using cautery and scissors in order to reflect it medially. Once sufficiently mobilized, the spleen, tail of the pancreas, and stomach fall anteriorly and superiorly, owing to the positioning. The fan retractor is placed through the most medial port to assist in providing greater exposure (Fig 21–15). The

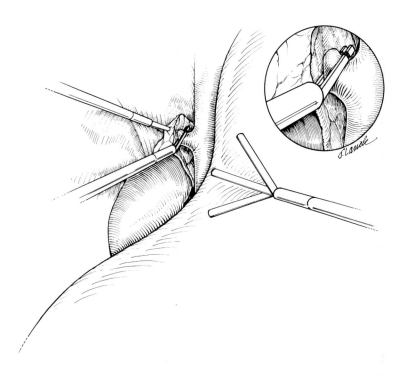

Figure 21–14. Right laparoscopic adrenalectomy. The right lobe of the liver is freed by incising ligamentous attachments, using cautery or blunt dissection. The fan retractor, placed through the medial port, retracts the liver anteriorly and medially. Mobilization of the hepatic flexure of the colon provides better exposure of the adrenal gland. A grasping forceps holds the adrenal gland, while a dissecting forceps is used to free the gland from the surrounding tissues. Arteries are clipped as they are encountered. The adrenal vein is gently doubly clipped and divided last.

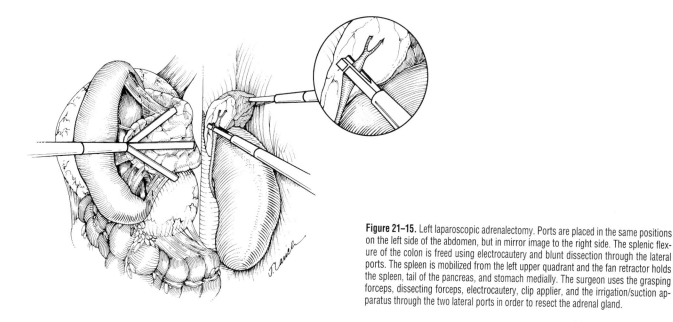

Figure 21–15. Left laparoscopic adrenalectomy. Ports are placed in the same positions on the left side of the abdomen, but in mirror image to the right side. The splenic flexure of the colon is freed using electrocautery and blunt dissection through the lateral ports. The spleen is mobilized from the left upper quadrant and the fan retractor holds the spleen, tail of the pancreas, and stomach medially. The surgeon uses the grasping forceps, dissecting forceps, electrocautery, clip applier, and the irrigation/suction apparatus through the two lateral ports in order to resect the adrenal gland.

splenic flexure of the colon is mobilized using the same techniques as above, allowing the colon to fall inferiorly and anteriorly, away from the retroperitoneum. The remainder of the procedure is identical to a laparoscopic right adrenalectomy in that the gland is mobilized from surrounding tissues, arteries are clipped and divided as they are encountered, and the left adrenal vein is clipped and divided last (Fig 21–15).

At the conclusion of the procedure, the abdomen is desufflated and the ports are withdrawn. Closure consists of placing one or two simple interrupted sutures through the fascial defects. A long-acting local anesthetic, such as bupivacaine, may be injected subcutaneously at the port sites to aid in controlling immediate postoperative pain. The skin edges are then reapproximated. The urinary catheter and nasogastric tube may be removed in the operating room after closure.

Postoperatively, patients usually require only oral pain medications. A clear liquid diet may be started as soon as the patient is fully awake from anesthesia and, if tolerated, advanced to a normal diet by the following morning.

Postoperative Hormone Replacement

For certain conditions, replacement of glucocorticoids and/or mineralocorticoids is necessary after adrenalectomy. Patients with an adrenal tumor causing Cushing's syndrome must receive glucocorticoids postoperatively. Hydrocortisone may be administered at a maintenance dose of 12–15 mg/m^2 each day. A normal response to the ACTH stimulation test suggests that glucocorticoid therapy may be withheld, but this may not occur for approximately 2 years postoperatively.[52] Mineralocorticoid replacement is not necessary in these patients. Patients who undergo bilateral adrenalectomy require both glucocorticoid therapy as well as mineralocorticoid replacement (fludrocortisone 100 micrograms/d). No postoperative hormonal therapy is necessary in a patient undergoing resection of an aldosteronoma, unilateral pheochromocytoma, a nonfunctional adrenal cancer, or a virilizing tumor.

Complications

Surgical resection of the adrenal glands is subject to potential complications that may arise as a consequence of any surgical procedure, including bleeding, infection, and incisional hernias. Hemorrhage as a result of tearing the adrenal vein may be significant if not controlled promptly and is potentially life threatening. Adrenal insufficiency is a sequela that may occur more commonly after adrenalectomy than after other surgical procedures. A high clinical index of suspicion must be maintained for diagnosis in the postoperative patient, as discussed previously, and treatment must be instituted promptly. Adrenal insufficiency is prevented by administering stress doses of steroids perioperatively, in select patients. The pleural space may be entered inadvertently when using a posterior approach or thoracoabdominal incision. If recognized intraoperatively, this is easily resolved as described above. A significant pneumothorax postoperatively, which increases in size or causes respiratory symptoms, is treated with tube thoracostomy. Mortality for adrenalectomy is minimal when performed by an experienced surgeon.

REFERENCES

1. Ross MH, Reith EJ. Histology: a text and atlas. New York, NY: Harper & Row, JB Lippincott; 1985:581–589

2. Clemente CD. Anatomy: a regional atlas of the human body, 3rd ed. Baltimore, MD: Urban & Schwarzenberg; 1987

3. Gill GN. The adrenal gland. In: West JB (ed), *Physiologic Basis of Medical Practice.* Baltimore, MD: Williams & Wilkins; 1991:820–832

4. Moore KL. *Before We are Born: Basic Embryology and Birth Defects.* Philadelphia, PA: WB Saunders; 1983:176–178

5. Loriaux DL. The adrenal glands. In: Becker KL (ed), *Principles and Practice of Endocrinology and Metabolism.* Philadelphia, PA: JB Lippincott, 1990:571–708

6. Sheridan RL, Ryan CM, Tompkins RG. Acute adrenal insufficiency in the burn intensive care unit. *Burns* 1993; 19:63–66

7. Cushing H. The basophil adenomas of the pituitary body and their clinical manifestations (pituitary basophilism). *Bulls Johns Hopkins Hosp* 1932;50:137

8. Loriaux DL, Cutler GB. Diseases of the adrenal glands. In: Kohler PO (ed), *Clinical Endocrinology.* New York, NY: John Wiley and Sons; 1986:167–238

9. Page DL, DeLellis RA, Hough AJ. Tumors of the adrenal.(monograph) In: *Atlas of Tumor Pathology,* Washington, D.C.: AFIP; 1986

10. Norton JA, Levin B, Jensen RT. Cancer of the endocrine system: the adrenal gland. In: DeVita VT Jr., Hellman S, Rosenberg SA (eds), *Cancer: Principles and Practice of Oncology.* Philadelphia, PA: JB Lippincott; 1993:1352–1371

11. Brown WH. A case of pluriglandular syndrome. *Lancet* 1928;2:1022

12. Christy NP. Adrenocorticotrophic activity in plasma of patients with Cushing's syndrome associated with pulmonary neoplasms. *Lancet* 1961;1:85

13. Liddle GW, Island D, Meador CK. Normal and abnormal regulation of corticotropin secretion in man. *Recent Prog Horm Res* 1962;18:125

14. Vincent JM, Trainer PJ, Reznek RH, et al. The radiologic investigation of occult ectopic ACTH-dependent Cushing's syndrome. *Clin Radiol* 1993;48:11–17

15. Pass HI, Doppman JL, Nieman L, et al. Management of the ectopic ACTH syndrome due to thoracic carcinoids. *Ann Thorac Surg* 1990;50:52–57

16. Zeiger MA, Pass HI, Doppman JD, et al. Surgical strategy in the management of nonsmall cell ectopic adrenocorticotropic hormone syndrome. *Surgery* 1992;112:994–1001

17. Grant CS, Carney JA, Carpenter PC, van Heerden JA. Primary pigmented nodular adrenocortical disease: diagnosis and management. *Surgery* 1986;100:1178–1184

18. Zeiger MA, Nieman LK, Cutler GB, et al. Primary bilateral adrenocortical causes of Cushing's syndrome. *Surgery* 1991;110:1106–1115

19. Travis WD, Tsokos M, Doppman JL, et al. Primary pigmented nodular adrenocortical disease. *Am J Surg Pathol* 1989;13:921–930

20. Doppman JL, Nieman LK, Travis WD, et al. CT or MR imaging of massive macronodular adrenocortical disease: a rare cause of autonomous primary adrenal hypercortisolism. *J Comput Assist Tomogr* 1991;15:773–779

21. Kepes JJ, O'Boynick P, Jones S, et al. Adrenal cortical adenoma in the spinal canal of an 8-year old girl. *Am J Surg Pathol* 1990;14:481–484

22. Mitchell A, Scheithauer BW, Sasano H, et al. Symptomatic intradural adrenal adenoma of the spinal nerve root: report of two cases. *Neurosurgery* 1993;32:658–662

23. Hough AJ, Hollifield JW, Page DL, Hartmann WH. Diagnostic factors in adrenal cortical tumors. *Am J Clin Pathol* 1979;72:390

24. Thomas CG Jr, Smith AT, Griffith JM. Hyperadrenalism in childhood and adolescence. *Ann Surg* 1984;199:538

25. Tourniaire J, Chalendar D, Rebattu B, et al. The 24-h cortisol secretory pattern in Cushing's syndrome. *Acta Endocrinol* 1986;112:230–237

26. Pavlatos FC, Smilo RP, Forsham PH. A rapid screening test for Cushing's syndrome. *JAMA* 1965;193:720

27. Willenbring ML, Morley JE, Niewoeher CB, et al. Adrenocortical hyperactivity in newly admitted alcoholics: prevalence, course and associated variables. *Psychoneuroendocrinology* 1984;9:415

28. Chrousos GP, Vingerhoeds A, Brandon D, et al. Primary cortisol resistance in man: a glucocorticoid receptor-mediated disease. *J Clin Invest* 1982;69:1261

29. Chrousos GP, Schuermeyer TH, Doppman J, et al. Primary cortisol resistance: a family study. *J Clin Endocrinol Metab* 1983;56:1243

30. Weiss ER, Rayjis SS, Nelson DH, Bethune JE. Evaluation of stimulation and suppression tests in the etiological diagnosis of Cushing's syndrome. *Ann Intern Med* 1969; 71:941

31. Biemond P, de Jong FH, Lamberts SWJ. Continuous dexamethasone infusion for seven hours in patients with Cushing's syndrome: a superior differential diagnostic test. *Ann Intern Med* 1990;112:738–742

32. Chrousos GP, Schuermeyer TH, Doppman J, et al. Clinical applications of corticotropin-releasing factor. *Ann Intern Med* 1985;102:344

33. Nieman LK, Chrousos GP, Oldfield EH, et al. The ovine corticotropin-releasing hormone stimulation test and the dexamethasone suppression test in the differential diagnosis of Cushing's syndrome. *Ann Intern Med* 1986; 105:862–867

34. Grossman AB, Howlett TA, Perry L, et al. CRF in the differential diagnosis of Cushing's syndrome: a comparison with the dexamethasone suppression test. *Clin Endocrinol* 1988;29:167–178

35. Howlett TA, Drury PL, Perry L, et al. Diagnosis and management of ACTH-dependent Cushing's syndrome: comparison of the features in ectopic and pituitary ACTH production. *Clin Endocrinol* 1986;24:699

36. Epstein AJ, Patel SK, Petasnick JP. Computerized tomography of the adrenal gland. *JAMA* 1979;242:2791

37. Roubidoux M, Dunnick NR. Adrenal cortical tumors. *Bull NY Acad Med* 1991;67:119–130

38. Remer EM, Weinfeld RM, Glazer GM, et al. Hyperfunctioning and nonhyperfunctioning benign adrenal cortical lesions: characterization and comparison with MR imaging. *Radiology* 1989;171:681–685

39. Doppman JL, Travis WD, Nieman L, et al. Cushing's syndrome due to primary pigmented nodular adrenocortical

disease: findings at CR and MR imaging. *Radiology* 1989; 172:415–420

40. Oldfield EH, Doppman JL, Nieman LK, et al. Petrosal sinus sampling with and without corticotropin-releasing hormone for the differential diagnosis of Cushing's syndrome. *N Engl J Med* 1991;325:897–905

41. Doppman JL, Reining JW, Dwyer AJ, et al. Differentiation of adrenal masses by magnetic resonance imaging. *Surgery* 1987;102:1018–1026

42. Fig LM, Gross MD, Shapiro B, et al. Adrenal localization in the adrenocorticotropic hormone-independent Cushing's syndrome. *Ann Intern Med* 1988;109:547–553

43. Geatti O, Fig L, Shapiro B. Adrenal cortical adenoma causing Cushing's syndrome: correct localization by functional scintigraphy despite nonlocalizing morphological imaging studies. *Clin Nucl Med* 1990;15:168–171

44. Schteingart DE, Seabold JE, Gross MD, Swanson DP. Iodocholesterol adrenal tissue uptake and imaging in adrenal neoplasms. *J Clin Endocrinol Metab* 1981;52:1156

45. Bierwaltes WH, Sisson JC, Shapiro JC, Shapiro B. Diagnosis of adrenal tumors with radionucleide imaging. *Spec Topics Endocrinol Metab* 1984;6:1

46. McArthur RB, Bahn RC, Hayles AB. Primary adrenocortical nodular dysplasia as a cause of Cushing's syndrome in infants and children. *Mayo Clin Proc* 1982;57:58

47. Donaldson MDC, Grant DB, O'Hare MJ, Shackleton CH. Familial congenital Cushing's syndrome due to bilateral nodular adrenal hyperplasia. *Clin Endocrinol* 1981;14:519

48. Imura H. Ectopic hormone syndrome. *Clin Endocrinol Metab* 1980;9:235

49. Davis CJ, Hoplin GF, Welbourn RB. Surgical management of the ectopic ACTH syndrome. *Ann Surg* 1982;246:1966

50. Jex RK, van Heerden JA, Carpenter PC, Grant CS. Ectopic ACTH syndrome. *Am J Surg* 1985;149:276

51. Doppman JL, Loughlin T, Miller DL, et al. Identification of ACTH-producing intrathoracic tumors by measuring ACTH levels in aspirated specimens. *Radiology* 1987;163:501

52. Doherty GM, Nieman LK, Cutler GB Jr, et al. Time to recovery of the hypothalamic-pituitary-adrenal axis after curative resection of adrenal tumors in patients with Cushing's syndrome. *Surgery* 1990;108:1085–1090

53. Bevan JS, Gough MH, Gillmer MDG, Burke CW. Cushing's syndrome in pregnancy: the timing of definitive treatment. *Clin Endocrinol* 1987;27:225–233

54. Pricolo VE, Monchik JM, Prinz RA, et al. Management of Cushing's syndrome secondary to adrenal adenoma during pregnancy. *Surgery* 1990;108:1072–1078

55. Nakane T, Kuwayama A, Watanabe M, et al. Long-term results of transsphenoidal adenomectomy in patients with Cushing's disease. *Neurosurgery* 1987;21:218–222

56. Conn JW. Presidential Address, part I. painting background, II. primary aldosteronism, a new clinical syndrome. *J Lab Clin Med* 1972;9:264

57. McLeod MK, Thompson NW, Gross MD, Grekin RJ. Idiopathic aldosteronism masquerading as discrete aldosterone-secreting adrenal cortical neoplasms among patients with primary aldosteronism. *Surgery* 1989;106:1161–1168

58. Carey RM, Sen S, Dolan LM, et al. Idiopathic hyperaldosteronism: a possible role for aldosterone-stimulating factor. *N Engl J Med* 1984;311:94

59. Tenschert W, Maurer R, Vetter H, Vetter W. Primary aldosteronism by carcinoma of the adrenal cortex. *Klin Wochenschr* 1987;65:428

60. Cohn K, Gottesman L, Brennan M. Adrenocortical carcinoma. *Surgery* 1986;100:1170–1177

61. Arteaga E, Biglieri EG, Kater C, et al. Aldosterone-producing adrenocortical carcinoma: preoperative recognition and course in three cases. *Ann Intern Med* 1984; 101:316

62. Melby JC. Diagnosis of hyperaldosteronism. *Endocrinol Metabol Clin North Am* 1991;20:247–255

63. Gomez-Sanchez CE, Montgomery M, Ganguly A, et al. Elevated urinary excretion of 18-oxocortisol in glucocorticoid-suppressible aldosteronism. *J Clin Endocrinol Metab* 1984;59:1022

64. Brown RD, Hollifield JW. Endocrine hypertension. In: Kohler PO (ed), *Clinical Endocrinology*. New York, NY: John Wiley and Sons; 1986:239–262

65. Favia G, Lumachi F, Scarpa V, D'Amico DF. Adrenalectomy in primary aldosteronism: a long-term follow-up study in 52 patients. *World J Surg* 1992;16:680–684

66. Weinberger MH, Grim CE, Hollifield JW, et al. Primary aldosteronism: diagnosis, localization and treatment. *Ann Intern Med* 1979;90:386

67. Lyons DG, Kern DC, Brown RD, et al. Single dose captopril as a diagnostic test for primary aldosteronism. *J Clin Endocrinol Metab* 1983;57:892

68. Guerin CK, Wahner HW, Gorman CA, et al. Computed tomographic scanning versus radioisotope imaging in adrenocortical diagnosis. *Am J Med* 1983;75:653

69. Falke THM, Strake L, Shaff MI, et al. MR imaging of the adrenals: correlation with computed tomography. *J Comp Assit Tomogr* 1986;10:242–253

70. Geisinger MA, Zelch M, Bravo E, et al. Primary hyperaldosteronism: comparison of CT, adrenal venography, and venous sampling. *Am J Roentgenol* 1983;141:299

71. Dunnick NR, Leight GS Jr, Roubidoux MA, et al. CT in the diagnosis of primary aldosteronism: sensitivity in 29 patients. *Am J Roentgenol* 1993;160:321–324

72. Ikeda DM, Francis IR, Glazer GM, et al. The detection of adrenal tumors and hyperplasia in patients with primary aldosteronism: Comparison of scintigraphy, CT, and MR imaging. *Am J Roentgenol* 1989;153:301–306

73. Doppman JL, Gill JR Jr, et al. Distinction between hyperaldosteronism due to bilateral hyperplasia and unilateral aldosteronoma: reliability of CT. *Radiology* 1992;184:677–682

74. Radin DR, Manoogian C, Nadler JL. Diagnosis of primary hyperaldosteronism: Importance of correlating CT findings with endocrinologic studies. *Am J Roentgenol* 1992;158:553–557

75. Nomura K, Kusakabe K, Maki M, et al. Iodomethylnorcholesterol uptake in an aldosteronoma shown by dexamethasone-suppression scintigraphy: relationship to adenoma size and functional activity. *J Clin Endocrinol Metab* 1990;71:825–830

76. Alder GK, Williams GH. Primary aldosteronism. In: Krieger DT, Bardin CW (eds), *Current therapy in endocrinology and metabolism*. Toronto, Canada: BC Decker; 1985:116–121

77. Auda SP, Brennan MF, Gill JR. Evolution of the surgical management of primary aldosteronism. *Ann Surg* 1980; 191:1

78. Obara T, Ito Y, Okamoto T, et al. Risk factors associated with postoperative persistent hypertension in patients with primary aldosteronism. *Surgery* 1992;112:987–993

79. Gabrilove JL, Seman AT, Sabet R, et al. Virilizing adrenal adenoma with studies on the steroid content of the adrenal venous effluent and a review of the literature. *Endocr Rev* 1981;2:462

80. Gabrilove JL, Frieberg EK, Nicolis GL. Peripheral blood steroid levels in Cushing's syndrome due to adrenocortical carcinoma or adenoma. *Urology* 1983;22:576

81. Hutter AM, Jr., Kayhoe DE. Adrenal cortical carcinoma. *Am J Med* 1966;41:572

82. Yano T, Linehan M, Anglard P, et al. Genetic changes in human adrenocortical carcinomas. *J Natl Cancer Inst* 1989; 81:518–523

83. Henry I, Grandjovans S, Couillin P, et al. Tumor-specific loss of 11p15.5 alleles in del 11p13 Wilms tumor and in familial adrenocortical carcinoma. *Proc Natl Acad Sci USA* 1989;86:3247–3251

84. Weiss LM. Comparative histologic study of 43 metastasizing and nonmetastasizing adrenocortical tumors. *Am J Surg Pathol* 1984;8:163

85. Weiss LM, Medeiros LJ, Vickery AL. Pathologic features of prognostic significance in adrenocortical carcinoma. *Am J Surg Pathol* 1989;13:202–206

86. Hosaka Y, Rainwater LM, Grant CS, et al. Adrenocortical carcinoma: nuclear deoxyribonucleic acid ploidy studied by flow cytometry. *Surgery* 1987;102:1027–1034

87. O'Hare MJ, Monaghan P, Neville AM. The pathology of adrenocortical neoplasia: a correlated structural and functional approach to the diagnosis of malignant disease. *Human Pathol* 1979;10:137

88. Wick MR, Cherwitz DL, McGlennen RC, Dehner LP. Adrenocortical carcinoma, an immunohistochemical comparison with renal cell carcinoma. *Am J Pathol* 1986;122:343

89. Sullivan M, Boileau M, Hodges CV. Adrenal cortical carcinoma. *J Urol* 1978;120:660–665

90. Henley DJ, van Heerden JA, Grant CS, et al. Adrenal cortical carcinoma—a continuing challenge. *Surgery* 1983;94: 226–231

91. Macfarlane DA. Cancer of the adrenal cortex. *Ann R Coll Surg* 1958;23:155–186

92. Singer F. Adrenal carcinoma presenting with postmenopausal vaginal bleeding. *Obstet Gynecol* 1991;78: 569–570

93. Jones GS, Shah KJ, Mann JR. Adreno-cortical carcinoma in infancy and childhood: a radiological report of ten cases. *Clin Radiol* 1985;36:257

94. Daneman A, Chan HSL, Martin J. Adrenal carcinoma and adenoma in children: a review of 17 patients. *Pediatr Radiol* 1983;13:11

95. Neblett W, Frexes-Steed M, Scott HW. Experience with adrenocortical neoplasia in childhood. *Am J Surg* 1987; 53:117

96. Ribeiro RC, Sandrini Neto R, Schell MJ, et al. Adrenocortical carcinoma in children: a study of 40 cases. *J Clin Oncol* 1990;8:67–74

97. Chudler RM, Kay R. Adrenocortical carcinoma in children. *Urol Clin North Am* 1989;16:469–479

98. Ross NS, Aron DC. Hormonal evaluation of the patient with an incidentally discovered adrenal mass. *N Engl J Med* 1990;323:1401–1405

99. Pasieka JL, McLeod MK, Thompson NW, et al. Adrenal scintigraphy of well-differentiated (functioning) adrenocortical carcinomas: potential surgical pitfalls. *Surgery* 1992;112:884–890

100. Baker ME, Spritzer C, Blinder R, et al. Benign adrenal lesions mimicking malignancy on MR imaging: report of two cases. *Radiology* 1987;163:669

101. McClennan BL. Oncologic imaging: staging and follow-up of renal and adrenal carcinoma. *Cancer* 1991;67: 1199–1208

102. Cheung PSY, Thompson NW. Right atrial extension of adrenocortical carcinoma: surgical management using hypothermia and cardiopulmonary bypass. *Cancer* 1989;64:812–815

103. Moul JW, Hardy MR, McLeod DG. Adrenal cortical carcinoma with vena cava tumor thrombus requiring cardiopulmonary bypass for resection. *Urology* 1991;38: 179–183

104. Long JP, Choyke PL, Shawker TA, et al. Intraoperative ultrasound in the evaluation of tumor involvement of the inferior vena cava. *J Urol* 1993;150:13–17

105. Richie JP, Gittes RF. Carcinoma of the adrenal cortex. *Cancer* 1980;45:1957–1964

106. Luton JP, Cerdas S, Billaud L, et al. Clinical features of adrenocortical carcinoma, prognostic factors and the effect of mitotane therapy. *N Engl J Med* 1990;322: 1195–1201

107. Didolkar MS, Bescher RA, Elias EG, Moore RH. Natural history of adrenal cortical carcinoma: a clinicopathologic study of 42 patients. *Cancer* 1981;47:2153–2161

108. Hajjar RA, Hickey RC, Samaan NA. Adrenal cortical carcinoma: a study of 32 patients. *Cancer* 1975;35:549

109. Appelqvist P, Kostiainen S. Multiple thoracotomy combined with chemotherapy in metastatic adrenal cortical carcinoma: a case report and review of the literature. *J Surg Oncol* 1983;24:1–4

110. Potter DA, Strott CA, Javadpour N, Roth JA. Prolonged survival following six pulmonary resections for metastatic adrenal cortical carcinoma: a case report. *J Surg Oncol* 1984;25:273–277

111. Percarpio B, Knowlton AH. Radiation therapy of adrenal cortical carcinoma. *Acta Radiol Ther Physiol Biol* 1976; 15:288

112. Jensen JC, Pass HI, Sindelar WF, Norton JA. Recurrent or metastatic disease in select patients with adrenocortical carcinoma. *Arch Surg* 1991;126:457–461

113. Kwauk S, Burt M. Pulmonary metastases from adrenal cortical carcinoma: results of resection. *J Surg Oncol* 1993;53:243–246

114. Hogan TF, Gilchrist KW, Westring DW, Citrin DL. A clinical and pathological study of adrenocortical carcinoma. *Cancer* 1980;45:2880

115. Markoe AM, Serber W, Micaily B, Brady LW. Radiation therapy for adjunctive treatment of adrenal cortical carcinoma. *Am J Clin Oncol* 1991;14:170–174

116. Gutierrez ML, Crooke ST. Mitotane (o, p-DDD). *Cancer Treat Rev* 1980;7:49

117. Bodie B, Novick AC, Pontes JE, Straffon RA, et al. The Cleveland Clinic experience with adrenal cortical carcinoma. *J Urol* 1989;141:257–260

118. Venkatesh S, Hickey RC, Sellin RV, et al. Adrenal cortical carcinoma. *Cancer* 1989;64:765–769

119. Decker RA, Elson P, Hogan TF, et al. Eastern Cooperative Oncology Group study 1989: mitotane and adriamycin in patients with advanced adrenocortical carcinoma. *Surgery* 1991;110:1006–1013

120. Haak HR, Van Seters AP, Moolenaar AJ. Mitotane therapy of adrenocortical carcinoma. *N Engl J Med* 1990; 322:758

121. Bukowski RM, Wolfe M, Levine HS, et al. Phase II trial of mitotane and cisplatinum in patients with adrenal carcinoma: a Southwest Oncology Group study. *J Clin Oncol* 1993;11:161–165

122. Van Slooten H, Moolenaar AJ, Van Seters SP, Smeek D. Treatment of adrenocortical carcinoma with o, p-DDD: prognostic implications of serum levels monitoring. *Eur J Clin Oncol* 1984;20:47

123. Bates SE, Shieh CY, Mickley La, et al. Mitotane enhances cytotoxicity of chemotherapy in cell lines expressing a multidrug resistance gene (mdr-1/P-glycoprotein) which is also expressed adrenocortical carcinomas. *J Clin Endocrinol Metab* 1991;73:18–29

124. Claussen MS, Landercasper J, Cogbill TH. Acute adrenal insufficiency presenting as shock after trauma and surgery: three cases and review of the literature. *J Trauma* 1992;32:94–100

125. Jacobson SA, Blute RD Jr, Green DF, et al. Acute adrenal insufficiency as a complication of urological surgery. *J Urol* 1986;135:337–340

126. Ting W, Nosher JL, Scholz PM, Spotnitz AJ. Bilateral adrenal hemorrhage after an open heart operation. *Ann Thorac Surg* 1992;54:357–358

127. Hardwicke MB, Kisly A. Prophylactic subcutaneous heparin therapy as a cause of bilateral adrenal hemorrhage. *Arch Int Med* 1992;152:845–847

128. Anderson WM, Timberlake GA. Massive retroperitoneal hemorrhage from an asymptomatic adrenal cortical adenoma. *Am Surg* 1989;55:299–302

129. Mohler JL, Michael KA, Freedman AM, et al. The evaluation of postoperative function of the adrenal gland. *Surg Gynecol Obstet* 1985;161:551–556

130. Bravo EL, Gifford RW Jr. Pheochromocytoma. *Endocrinol Metab Clin North Am* 1993;22:329–341

131. Cryer PE. Phaeochromocytoma. *Clin Endocrinol Metab* 1985;14:203

132. Perry RR, Nieman LK, Cutler GB, et al. Primary adrenal causes of Cushing's syndrome: diagnosis and surgical management. *Ann Surg* 1989;210:59–68

133. Spark RF, Connolly PB, Gluckin DS, White R, et al. ACTH secretion from a functioning pheochromocytoma. *N Engl J Med* 1979;301:416

134. Berelowitz M, Szabo M, Barowsky HW, et al. Somatostatin-like immunoactivity and biological activity is present in human pheochromocytoma. *J Clin Endocrinol Metab* 1983;56:134

135. Weinstein RS, Ide LF. Immunoreactive calcitonin in pheochromocytomas. *Proc Soc Exp Biol Med* 1980;165:215

136. Ang VTY, Jenkins JS. Neurohypophysical hormones in the adrenal medulla. *J Clin Endocrinol Metab* 1984;58:688

137. Gifford RW, Bravo EL, Manger WM. Diagnosis and management of pheochromocytoma. *Cardiology* 1985;72:186

138. Beard CM, Sheps SG, Kurland LT, et al. Occurrence of pheochromocytoma in Rochester, Minnesota, 1950 through 1979. *Mayo Clin Proc* 1983;58:802

139. Remine WH, Chong GC, van Heerden JA, et al. Current management of pheochromocytoma. *Ann Surg* 1974; 179:740

140. Cooper MJ, Helman LJ, Israel MA. Molecular biology and the pathogenesis of neuroblastoma and pheochromocytoma. *Cancer Cells* 1989;7:95–99

141. Zimmerman ID, Biron RE, MacMahon HE. Pheochromocytoma of the urinary bladder. *N Engl J Med* 1953;249:25

142. Thrasher JB, Rajan RR, Perez LM, et al. Pheochromocytoma of urinary bladder: contemporary methods of diagnosis and treatment options. *Urology* 1993;41:435–439

143. Orringer MB, Sisson JC, Glazer G, et al. Surgical treatment of cardiac pheochromocytomas. *J Thorac Cardiovasc Surg* 1985;89:753

144. Melicow MM. One hundred cases of pheochromocytoma (107 tumors) at the Columbia Presbyterian Medical Center, 1926–1976. *Cancer* 1977;40:1987

145. Irvin GL, Fishman LM, Sher JA. Familial pheochromocytoma. *Surgery* 1983;94:938–940

146. Glowniak JV, Shapiro B, Sisson JC, et al. Familial extra-adrenal pheochromocytoma. *Arch Intern Med* 1985;145: 257–261

147. Loughlin KR, Gittes RF. Urological management of patients with von Hippel-Lindau's disease. *J Urol* 1986;136: 789

148. Nakagawara A. Malignant pheochromocytoma with ganglioneuroblastomatous elements in a patient with von Recklinghausen's disease. *Cancer* 1985;55:2794

149. Khosia S, Patel VM, Hay ID, et al. Loss of heterozygosity suggests multiple genetic alterations in pheochromocytomas and medullary thyroid carcinomas. *J Clin Invest* 1991;87:1691–1699

150. Lips KJM, Van der Sluys Veer J, Struyvenberg A, et al. Bilateral occurrence of pheochromocytoma in patients with multiple endocrine neoplasia syndrome type 2a (Sipple's syndrome). *Am J Med* 1981;70:1051

151. Casanova S, Rosenberg-Bourgin M, Farkas D, et al. Phaeochromocytoma in multiple endocrine neoplasia type 2a: survey of 100 cases. *Clin Endocrinol* 1993;38:531–537

152. Sutton MGS, Sheps SG, Lie JT. Prevalence of clinically unsuspected pheochromocytoma: review of a 50 year autopsy series. *Mayo Clin Proc* 1981;56:354

153. Beierwaltes WH, Sisson JC, Shapiro B, et al. Malignant potential of pheochromocytoma. *Proc of American Association of Cancer Research (Proc Amer Assoc Cancer Res)* 1986; 27:617

154. Scott HW, Halter SA. Oncologic aspects of pheochromocytoma: the importance of follow-up. *Surgery* 1984; 96:1061

155. Proye C, Vix M, Goropoulos A, et al. High incidence of malignant pheochromocytoma in a surgical unit: 26

cases out of 100 patients operated from 1971 to 1991. *J Endocrinol Invest* 1992;15:651–663

156. Sherwin RP. Present status of the pathology of the adrenal gland in hypertension. *Am J Surg* 1964;107:136

157. Lewis PD. A cytophotometric study of benign and malignant pheochromocytomas. *Virchows Arch* 1971;9:371

158. Hosaka Y, Rainwater LM, Grant CS, et al. Pheochromocytoma: nuclear deoxyribonucleic acid patterns studied by flow cytometry. *Surgery* 1986;100:1003

159. Sheps SG, Jiang NS, Klec GG, van Heerden JA. Recent developments in the diagnosis and management of pheochromocytoma. *Mayo Clin Proc* 1990;65:88–95

160. Helman LJ, Cohen PS, Ayerbuch SD, et al. Neuropeptide Y expression distinguishes malignant from benign pheochromocytoma. *J Clin Oncol* 1989;7:1720

161. Grouzmann E, Gicquel C, Pluin PF, et al. Neuropeptide Y and neuron specific enolase levels in benign and malignant pheochromocytomas. *Cancer* 1990;66:1833–1835

162. Medeiros LJ, Wolf BC, Balogh K, Federman M. Adrenal pheochromocytoma. A clinicopathologic review of 60 cases. *Hum Pathol* 1985;16:k580

163. Ito Y, Fujimoto Y, Obara T. The role of epinephrine, norepinephrine, and dopamine in blood pressure disturbances in patients with pheochromocytoma. *World J Surg* 1992;16:759–764

164. Manger WM, Gifford RW. Pheochromocytoma. New York, NY: Springer-Verlag; 1977

165. Hanson MW, Feldman JM, Beam CA, et al. Iodine [131]-labelled metaiodobenzylguanidine scintigraphy and biochemical analyses in suspected pheochromocytoma. *Arch Intern Med* 1991;151:1397–1402

166. Samaan NA, Hickey RC, Shutts PE. Diagnosis, localization and management of pheochromocytoma. *Cancer* 1988;62:2451–2460

167. Duncan MW, Compton P, Lazarus L, Smythe GA. Measurement of norepinephrine and 3,4-dihydroxyphenylglycol in urine and plasma for the diagnosis of pheochromocytoma. *N Engl J Med* 1988;319:136–142

168. Sjoberg RJ, Simcic KJ, Kidd GS. The clonidine suppression test for pheochromocytoma: a review of its utility and pitfalls. *Arch Int Med* 1992;152:1193–1197

169. Karlberg BE, Hedman L. Value of the clonidine suppression test in the diagnosis of pheochromocytoma. *Acta Med Scan* 1986;714:15

170. Brandstetter K, Krause U, Beyer W. Preliminary results with the clonidine suppression test in the diagnosis of pheochromocytoma. *Cardiology* 1985;72:157

171. Karlberg BE, Hedman L, Lennquist S, Pollace T. The value of the clonidine-suppression test in the diagnosis of pheochromocytoma. *World J Surg* 1986;10:753

172. Bravo EL, Tarazi RC, Fouad FM, et al. Clonidine suppression test: a useful aid in the diagnosis of pheochromocytoma. *N Engl J Med* 1981;305:623

173. MacDougall IC, Isles CG, Stewart H, et al. Overnight clonidine suppression test in the diagnosis and exclusion of pheochromocytoma. *Am J Med* 1988;84:993–1000

174. Taylor HC, Mayes D, Anton AH. Clonidine suppression test for pheochromocytoma: examples of misleading results. *J Clin Endocrinol Metab* 1986;63:238

175. Cryer PE, Wortsman J, Shah SD, et al. Plasma chromogranin A as a marker of sympathochromaffin activity in humans. *Am J Physiol* 1991;260:E243–E246

176. Reinig JW, Doppman JL. Magnetic resonance imaging of the adrenal. *Radiologe* 1986;26:186–190

177. Dunnick NR, Doppman JL, Gill JR Jr, Strott CA, Keiser HR, Brennan MF. Localization of functional adrenal tumors by computed tomography and venous sampling. *Radiology* 1982;142:429

178. Welch TJ, Sheedy PF, van Heerden JA, et al. Pheochromocytoma: value of computed tomography. *Radiology* 1983;148:501

179. Radin DR, Ralls PW, Boswell WD Jr, et al. Pheochromocytoma: detection by unenhanced CT. *Am J Roentgenol* 1986;146:741

180. Greenberg M, Moawad AH, Wieties BM, et al. Extraadrenal pheochromocytoma: Detection during pregnancy using MR imaging. *Radiology* 1986;161:475

181. Velchik MG, Alavi A, Kressel HY, Engelman K. Localization of pheochromocytoma: MIBG, CT and MRI correlation. *J Nucl Med* 1989;30:328–336

182. Fink IJ, Reinig JW, Dwyer AJ, et al. MR imaging of pheochromocytomas. *J Comput Assist Tomogr* 1985;9:454

183. Shapiro B, Copp JE, Sisson JC, et al. Iodine-131 metaiodobenzylguanidine for the locating of suspected pheochromocytoma: experience in 400 cases. *J Nucl Med* 1985;26:576

184. Fischer M, Galanski M, Winterberg B, Vetter H. Localization procedures in pheochromocytoma and neuroblastoma. *Cardiology* 1985;72:143

185. Swenson SJ, Brown MJ, Sheps SG, et al. Use of ^{131}I-MIBG scintigraphy in the evaluation of suspected pheochromocytoma. *Mayo Clin Proc* 1985;60:299

186. Koizumi M, Endo K, Sakahara H, et al. Computed tomography and ^{131}I-MIBG scintigraphy in the diagnosis of pheochromocytoma. *Acta Radiologica Diag* 1986;27:305

187. Lynn MD, Shapiro B, Sisson JC, et al. Pheochromocytoma and the normal adrenal medulla: improved visualization with I-123 MIBG scintigraphy. *Radiology* 1985;156:851

188. Cheung PSY, Thompson NW, Dmuchowski CF, Sisson JC. Spectrum of pheochromocytoma in the ^{131}I-MIBG era. *World J Surg* 1988;12:546–551

189. Gouch IR, Thompson NW, Shapiro B, Sisson JC. Limitations of ^{131}I-MIBG scintigraphy in locating pheochromocytomas. *Surgery* 1985;98:115

190. Proye CAG, Carnaille BM, Flament JBE, et al. Intraoperative radionuclear ^{125}I-labeled metaiodobenzylguanidine scanning of pheochromocytomas and metastases. *Surgery* 1992;111:634–639

191. Shulkin BL, Loeppe RA, Francis IR, et al. Pheochromocytomas that do not accumulate metaiodobenzylguanidine: localization with PET and administration of FDG. *Radiology* 1993;186:711–715

192. Stenstrom G, Kutti J. The blood volume in pheochromocytoma patients before and during treatment with phenoxybenzamine. *Acta Med Scand* 1985;218:381

193. Stenstrom G, Haljamae H, Tisell LE. Influence of preoperative treatment with phenoxybenzamine on the incidence of adverse cardiovascular reactions during

anaesthesia and surgery for phechromocytoma. *Acta Anaesthesiol Scand* 1985;29:797

194. Turner MC, Lieberman E, DeQuattro V. The perioperative management of pheochromocytoma in children. *Clin Pediatr* 1992;31:583–589

195. Perry RR, Keiser HR, Norton JA, et al. Surgical management of pheochromocytoma with the use of metyrosine. *Ann Surg* 1990;212:621–628

196. Imperato-McGinley J, Gautier T, Ehlers K. Reversibility of catecholamine-induced dilated cardiomyopathy in a child with a pheochromocytoma. *N Engl J Med* 1987; 316:793

197. Chimori K, Miyazaki S, Nakajima T, Muira D. Preoperative management of pheochromocytoma with the calcium-antagonist nifedipine. *Clin Ther* 1985;7:372

198. Proye C, Thevenin D, Cecat P, et al. Exclusive use of calcium channel blockers in preoperative and intraoperative control of pheochromocytomas: hemodynamics and free catecholamine assays in ten consecutive patients. *Surgery* 1989;106:1149–1154

199. Bornemann M, Hill SC, Kidd GS. Lactic acidosis in pheochromocytoma. *Ann Intern Med* 1986;105:880

200. Carney JA, Sizemore GW, Sheps SG. Adrenal medullary disease in multiple endocrine neoplasia, type 2. *Am J Clin Path* 1976;66:279–290

201. Cance WG, Wells SA Jr. Multiple endocrine neoplasia type IIa. *Curr Probl Surg* 1985;22:1

202. Lairmore TC, Ball DW, Baylin SB, Wells SA Jr. Management of pheochromocytomas in patients with multiple endocrine neoplasia type 2 syndromes. *Ann Surg* 1993; 217:595–603

203. Shulkin BL, Shen SW, Sisson JC, Shapiro B. Iodine 131 MIBG scintigraphy of the extremities in metastatci pheochromocytoma and neuroblastoma. *J Nucl Med* 1987;28:315

204. Lynn MD, Braunstein EM, Wahl RL, et al. Bone metastases in pheochromocytoma: comparative studies of efficacy of imaging. *Radiology* 1986;160:701

205. Lewi HJE, Reid R, Mucci B, et al. Malignant phaeochromocytoma. *Br J Urol* 1985;57:394

206. Brennan MF, Keiser HR. Persistant and recurrent pheochromocytoma: the role of surgery. *World J Surg* 1982;6:397

207. van Heerden JA, Sheps SG, Hamberger B, et al. Pheochromocytoma: current status and changing trends. *Surgery* 1982;91:367

208. Guo JZ, Gong LS, Chen SX, et al. Malignant pheochromocytoma: diagnosis and treatment in fifteen cases. *J Hypertens* 1989;7:261–266

209. Scott WH, Reynolds V, Green N, et al. Clinical experience with malignant pheochromocytoma. *Surg Gynecol Obstet* 1982;154:801

210. James RE, Baker HL, Scanlon PW. The roentgenological aspects of metastatic pheochromocytoma. *Amer J Roentgenology* 1972;115:783

211. Feldman JM. Treatment of metastatic pheochromocytoma with streptozotocin. *Arch Intern Med* 1983;143:1799

212. Gross DJ, Schlank E, Ipp E. Streptozotocin therapy for malignant pheochromocytoma. [Letter to the editor] *Arch Intern Med* 1985;145:368

213. Feldman JM. In reply to a letter to the Editor by Gross DJ, Schlank E, Ipp E. *Arch Intern Med* 1985;145:368

214. McEwan A, Shapiro B, Sisson JC, et al. Radioiodobenzylguanidine for the scintigraphic location and therapy of adrenergic tumors. *Semin Nucl Med* 1985;15:132

215. Krempf M, Lumbroso J, Mornex R, et al. Use of [131]In-iodobenzylguanidine in the treatment of malignant pheochromocytoma. *J Clin Endocrinol Metab* 1991;72: 455–461

216. Feldman JM, Frankel N, Coleman RE. Platelet uptake of the pheochromocytoma-scanning agent ^{131}I-metaiodobenzylguanidine. *Metabolism* 1984;33:397

217. Vetter H, Fischer M, Muller-Rensing R, et al. [^{131}I]-metaiodobenzylguanidine in treatment of malignant pheochromocytomas. *Lancet* 1983;2(8341):107

218. Goldstein DS, Stull R, Eisenhofer G, et al. Plasma 3,4-dihydroxyphenylalanine (Dopa) and catecholamines in neuroblastoma or pheochromocytoma. *Ann Intern Med* 1986;105:887

219. Keiser HR, Goldsteins DS, Wade JL, et al. Treatment of malignant pheochromocytoma with combination chemotherapy. *Hypertension* 1985;7:1:18

220. Auerbuch S, Steakley C, Gelmann E, et al. Malignant pheochromocytoma: Treatment with a combination of cyclophosphamide, vincristine and darcarbazine. *Proceedings of the American Society of Clinical Oncology* 1987;6:241

221. Auerbach SD, Steakley CS, Young RC. Malignant pheochromocytoma: effective treatment with a combination of cyclophosphamide, vincristine and dacarbazine. *Arch Intern Med* 1988;109:267–273

222. Finklestein JZ, Klemperer MR, Evans A, et al. Multiagent chemotherapy for children with metastatic neuroblastoma: a report from children's cancer study group. *Med Pediatr Oncol* 1979;6:179

223. Aso Y, Homma Y. A survey on incidental adrenal tumors in Japan. *J Urol* 1992;147:1478–1481

224. Glazer HS, Weyman PJ, Sagel SS, et al. Nonfunctioning adrenal masses: Incidental discovery on computed tomography. *Am J Roentgenol* 1982;139:81

225. Prinz RA, Brooks MH, Chuchill R, et al. Incidental asymptomatic adrenal masses detected by computed tomographic scanning: is operation required? *JAMA* 1982; 248:701

226. Copeland PM. The incidentally discovered adrenal mass: diagnosis and treatment. *Ann Intern Med* 1983;98: 940

227. McLeod MK, Thompson NW, Gross MD, et al. Sub-clinical Cushing's syndrome in patients with adrenal gland indidentalomas: pitfalls in diagnosis and management. *Am Surg* 1990;56:398–403

228. Belldegrun A, Hussain S, Seltzer SE, Loughlin KR, Gittes RF, Richie JP. Incidentally discovered mass of the adrenal gland. *Surg Gynecol Obstet* 1986;163:203

229. Tang CK, Gray GF. Adrenocortical neoplasms: prognosis and morphology. *Urology* 1975;5:691–695

230. Bradley EL. Primary and adjunctive therapy in carcinoma of the adrenal cortex. *Surg Gynecol Obstet* 1975; 141:507–511

231. Hussain S, Belldegrun A, Seltzer SE, Richie JP, Gittes RF, Abrams HL. Differentiation of malignant from benign

adrenal masses: predictive indices on computed tomography. *Am J Roentgenol* 1985;144:61

232. Reinig JW, Doppman JL, Dwyer AJ, et al. Distinction between adrenal adenomas and metastases using MR imaging. *J Comput Assist Tomogr* 1985;9:898

233. Reinig JW, Doppman JL, Dwyer AJ, Frank J. MRI of indeterminate adrenal masses. *Am J Roentgenol* 1986;147: 493

234. Aisen AM, Ohl DA, Chenevert TL, et al. MR of an adrenal pseudocyst: magnetic resonance imaging 1992; 10:997–1000

235. McCorkell SJ, Miles NL. Fine-needle aspiration of catecholamine-producing adrenal masses: a possibly fatal mistake. *Am J Roentgenol* 1985;145:113

236. Katz RL, Shirkhoda A. Diagnostic approach to incidental adrenal nodules in the cancer patient. *Cancer* 1985;55:1995

237. Gaboardi F, Carbone M, Bozzola A, Galli L. Adrenal incidentalomas: what is the role of fine needle biopsy? *Int J Urol Nephrol* 1991;23:197–207

238. Ettinghausen SE, Burt ME. Prospective evaluation of unilateral adrenal masses in patients with operable non-small-cell lung cancer. *J Clin Oncol* 1991;9:1462–1466

239. Reyes L, Parvez Z, Nemoto T, Regal AM, Takita H. Adrenalectomy for metastasis from lung carcinoma. *J Surg Oncol* 1990;44:32–34

240. Huiras CM, Pehling GB, Caplan RH. Adrenal insufficiency after operative removal of apparently nonfunctioning adrenal adenomas. *JAMA* 1989;261:894–898

241. Gagner M, LaCroix A, Bolte E. Laparoscopic adrenalectomy in Cushing's syndrome and pheochromocytoma [letter]. *N Engl J Med* 1992;327:1033

242. Gagner M, LaCroix A, Prinz RA, Bolte E, Albala D, et al. Early experience with laparoscopic approach for adrenalectomy. *Surgery* 1993;114:1120–1125

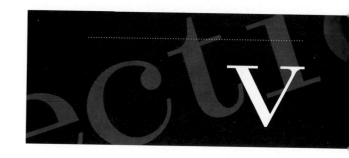

V

ABDOMINAL TRAUMA

22

Blunt and Penetrating Abdominal Trauma

Robert A. Read ▪ *Ernest E. Moore* ▪ *Frederick A. Moore* ▪ *Jon Burch*

Civilian trauma remains the fourth leading cause of death in the United States and the most frequent cause of mortality in persons under 45 years of age. More than half of these trauma-related deaths are the result of motor vehicle accidents. Other common causes include falls, gunshot or stab wounds, poisonings, burns, and drownings. In 1985, nonfatal injuries accounted for nearly 25 million hospitalizations and an estimated 75 to 150 billion dollars of direct and indirect costs to our society. Abdominopelvic trauma accounts for a large fraction of this tragic loss of life and continues to be a distressingly frequent cause of preventable death. Peritoneal signs in these patients can be subtle and frequently unreliable, secondary to distracting pain from associated injuries or decreased sensorium owing to intoxicants or head injury. Although 75% to 90% of patients with abdominal gunshot wounds require emergency laparotomy, only 25% to 35% of patients with stab wounds and 15% to 20% of patients following blunt trauma require operative intervention. Additionally, as many as one-third of these patients who require urgent abdominal exploration have an initial benign physical examination.

Favorable outcome of these critically injured patients demands an integrated multidisciplinary team effort beginning at the injury scene and continuing through rehabilitation. The team is comprised of emergency medical technicians (EMT), emergency department personnel, trauma surgeons, and a myriad of ancillary support and consulting services. Initial management is dictated by the patient's immediate physiologic requirements for survival (ie, the ABCs: airway, breathing, and circulation), and is often initiated before the establishment of specific diagnosis. Multiple life-threatening injuries often coexist, requiring rapid triage with simultaneous diagnostic and therapeutic interventions. The trauma surgeon must assume ultimate responsibility for the injured patient, assimilating key diagnostic results and orchestrating specific management, implemented by trauma team members. The purpose of this chapter is to discuss the management of abdominal injuries within this framework, provide rationale for a current management plan, and anticipate evolving policy changes. However, while this chapter is primarily concerned with abdominal trauma, it is not possible to separate out a single system in the injured patient. A general approach, as well as specific organ approaches, are provided.

▪ INJURY PATTERNS

Various traumatic insults will produce similar patterns of organ-specific injury. A working knowledge of these patterns and factors that influence their presentation is helpful in the evaluation and treatment of multisystem-injured patients. Further, a general understanding of the potential spectrum of response to specific patterns of injury and host characteristics that influence this response is helpful in predicting patient outcome.

INJURY MECHANISM

The biomechanics of blunt and penetrating injuries have been studied extensively in recent years. Blunt injuries are thought to result from a combination of crushing, deforming, stretching, and shearing forces. The magnitude of these forces is directly related to the mass of the objects involved, the rate of their acceleration or deceleration, and their relative direction on impact. Injury results when the sum of these forces exceeds the cohesive strength of the tissues and organs involved. The injuries produced are a constellation of contusions, abrasions, fractures, and tissue and organ ruptures.

Penetrating injuries from firearms are related to the ballistics of the weapon, the trajectory of the missile, and the tissues or organs involved. The wounding potential of a projectile is determined largely by its kinetic energy on impact and its efficiency of energy dissipation in tissue. The kinetic energy of a missile is proportional to its mass and velocity ($KE = 1/2$ mass $\times$ velocity^2). An increase in the mass of a given missile by a factor of 2 results in doubling its kinetic energy, whereas the same increment in its velocity results in four times the kinetic energy. This observation has led to the oversimplified classification of low-, medium-, and high-velocity weapons, defined as those with velocities <1000 ft/sec, 1000 to 2000 ft/sec, and >2000 ft/sec, respectively. The efficiency of energy dissipation in tissue of a given projectile is determined both by its physical characteristics and its pattern of flight. For a given missile velocity, a soft lead or hollow-tip projectile, prone to mushrooming, fragmentation, and tumbling, is considerably more destructive than a fully jacketed spiraling projectile. The tissue damage produced is related to the interaction of the dissipated energy and physical properties of the involved tissue and organs. A shotgun fires a group of pellets that disperse as a function of distance, or range and length, or taper of the gun barrel. Shotguns vary in the number and size of pellets per load, but at close range the aggregate kinetic energy represents the wounding potential. Low-velocity weapons are thought to produce injury predominately by direct crush and tearing mechanisms, whereas high-velocity missiles also induce tissue cavitation. The extent of the cavitation effect is related to the rate of energy dissipation, organ density, and elasticity. Solid, inelastic organs such as liver, spleen, and brain are considerably more susceptible to these effects than relatively pliant lung and skeletal muscle.

HOST CHARACTERISTICS

The musculoskeletal system provides considerable protection from most traumatic insults. Abdominal injuries associated with rapid deceleration at points of maximum fixation include tears of the jejunum at the ligament of Treitz, the terminal ileum, and other points of adhesion. Other host-related factors thought to influence the response to trauma include age and preexisting disease. For a given injury, it has been observed that patients more than 70 years of age experience a mortality rate approximately five times that of younger adults. This difference in mortality has been attributed to diminished physiologic reserve, as well as to more fragile tissue with aging. Additional comorbid factors include acute ethanol intoxication, which reduces the physiologic response to stress and may alter the injury pattern.

SPECIFIC INJURY PATTERNS

Patterns of injury can be generally divided into those resulting from blunt trauma versus penetrating wounds. Serious blunt injuries most commonly represent energy transfer to underlying visceral and vascular structures in the anatomic region sustaining direct impact. Specific examples of these patterns are listed in Table 22–1. Penetrating injuries, on the other hand, typically follow the tract or trajectory of the inflicting instrument and thus, involve contiguous structures. Examples of penetrating injury patterns are listed in Table 22–2.

INITIAL EVALUATION AND RESUSCITATION

Triage at the emergency department entrance is an important component of early trauma management requiring the sound judgement of an experienced individual, often the emergency department charge nurse or emergency physician. Initial management of the critically injured patient demands simultaneous evaluation and treatment. Rapid assessment of vital functions is done while an empiric sequence of life-saving therapeutic and diagnostic procedures is initiated, as dictated by the physiologic status of the patient (Fig 22–1).

TABLE 22–1. BLUNT ABDOMINAL AND PELVIC INJURY PATTERNS

Direct Impact Injuries	Associated Regional Injuries
Lower right rib fractures	Liver disruption
Lower left rib fractures	Splenic disruption
Midepigastric contusion	Duodenal perforation
	Pancreatic fracture
Lumbar transverse process fracture	Renal injury
Pelvic fracture	Bladder rupture
	Urethral injury

TABLE 22–2. PENETRATING ABDOMINAL AND PELVIC INJURY PATTERNS

Most Conspicuous Wound	Associated Injuries
Liver	Diaphragm
Portal vein	Common bile duct
	Hepatic artery
SMA	Pancreas
	Left renal artery
	Abdominal aorta
Spleen	Diaphragm
	Stomach
Stomach	Pancreas
	Spleen
Duodenum	Pancreas
	Vena cava
	Common bile duct
Rectum	Bladder

PRIMARY SURVEY (LIFE-SUSTAINING PRIORITIES)

The physiologic requirements of the patient govern initial resuscitation. The fundamental goal is to reestablish adequate oxygen supply to vital organs. Tissue oxygen delivery is largely determined by blood oxygen content, circulating blood volume, and cardiac output. The first priorities are to secure a patent airway and optimize ventilation. Following blunt trauma, cervical spine immobilization is imperative while establishing a patent airway. The pleural space may need to be evacuated of blood and air to facilitate ventilation. For patients in persistent shock, tube thoracostomies are inserted before a chest radiograph is obtained. Blood from the thorax should be collected in sterile containers with isotonic saline for later autotransfusion.[1]

Once a secure airway has been established, the next priority is to enhance cardiovascular performance. Initially, hypotension is assumed to be the result of acute blood loss and is treated with rapid volume infusion.

Intravascular volume restitution is initiated with crystalloid administration via large-bone peripheral intravenous catheters. Refractory hypotension despite rapid crystalloid infusion suggests active bleeding or myocardial dysfunction. Cardiogenic shock is further characterized by distended neck veins or a persistently elevated central venous pressure (CVP)>15 cm H_2O. However, in patients with mixed pathology, cardiac dysfunction may be masked until hypovolemia is corrected. Tension pneumothorax is the most frequently source of postinjury cardiogenic shock. The next most common cause is myocardial contusion following blunt trauma, and pericardial tamponade following penetrating thoracic wounds.

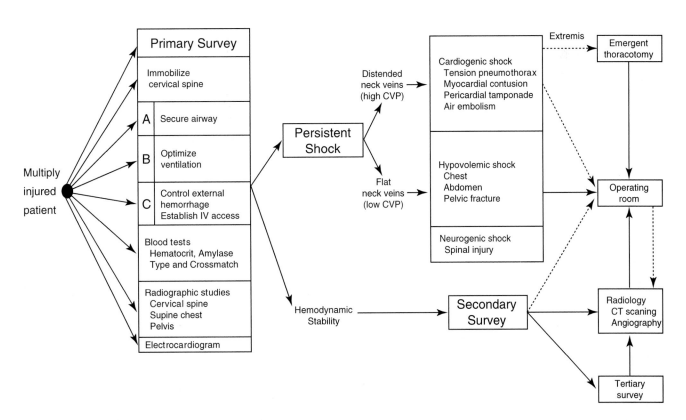

Figure 22–1. The initial emergency department trauma evaluation and resuscitation is a coordinated sequence of simultaneous diagnostic and therapeutic maneuvers undertaken in response to the injuries and physiologic status of the patient.

SECONDARY SURVEY (TRIAGE DECISION-MAKING)

The second echelon of emergency department management encompasses a detailed assessment of the overall condition of the patient and identification of potential life-threatening injuries (Fig 22–1). Emergency medical technicians, ambulance personnel, and flight nurses often provide important clues that suggest occult injury, and they should be queried before leaving the emergency department. In blunt trauma, the type of impact, vehicular damage, use of restraining devices, and condition of the other victims are helpful observations. For penetrating wounds, a description of the weapon and the amount of blood lost at the scene may be useful.

A rapid but systemic physical examination is essential to perform, and to document in the medical record. Patients are completely disrobed, examined for spinal injuries, and then rolled for inspection of their flanks and back. Important, but frequently neglected, aspects of the physical examination include detailed neurologic function, peripheral pulses, rectal examination for blood and sphincter tone, and inspection of the perineum, back and axillae. A lateral cervical spine radiograph is obtained following major blunt trauma to the upper torso, neck or head. The cervical spine is assumed to be unstable until all seven cervical and first thoracic vertebral bodies are visualized and a reliable, nontender physical examination is obtained. Splinting long-bone fractures decreases pain and minimizes additional soft-tissue damage and blood loss. Prompt insertion of a nasogastric tube decompresses the stomach. The tube should be placed orally when midfacial fractures exist, in order to minimize the risk of passage into the cranial vault.[2] Blood in the gastric aspirate may be the only sign of an otherwise occult injury of the stomach or duodenum. A Foley catheter empties the bladder, may demonstrate hematuria, and permits monitoring of urinary output.

Occult regions of major hemorrhage include the pleural spaces, the abdomen, the retroperitoneum, and skeletal fractures. A chest radiograph is the most reliable screen for thoracic fractures, and mediastinal and intrathoracic bleeding. The chest film also helps confirm the position of the central venous catheter and the endotracheal, nasogastric, and thoracostomy tubes. Initial abdominal examination of the multisystem injured patient is notoriously unreliable in detecting acute intraperitoneal hemorrhage or visceral perforation. Intoxication, head injury, or pain from associated fractures often mask peritoneal irritation resulting in a false-negative examination in 20% to 50% of acutely injured patients.[3] Similarly, contusion of the abdominal wall musculature, acute gastric dilation, and referred pain from spinal process fractures, lower rib fractures, and pelvic fractures often result in false-positive physical examination.[4] Diagnostic peritoneal lavage (DPL) remains the most expedient and reliable method of identifying significant intraperitoneal hemorrhage.[5,6] The sensitivity of DPL for significant intraperitoneal blood exceeds 98%.[7] However, the specificity is only 86%. Plain abdominal radiographs are primarily helpful in mapping bullet trajectory or characterizing pelvic fractures following blunt trauma. Patients who are hemodynamically stable may be evaluated by computed tomography (CT) of the abdomen for the presence of free fluid or air in the peritoneal cavity. CT scans also can identify solid organ injury.

TERTIARY SURVEY (RE-EVALUATION AND DISPOSITION)

The third echelon in the management of trauma patients consists of a compulsive and systematic re-evaluation after all life- and limb-threatening injuries have been cared for and toxic or metabolic derangements have been corrected. This process frequently occurs 12 to 24 hours after admission. Patients are systematically re-examined for occult injuries not evident on presentation owing to the urgency of other life-threatening priorities or alterations in consciousness from pain, injury, and intoxicants. Increasing abdominal pain and tenderness suggest an occult bowel perforation or pancreatic injury. The signs and symptoms of significant occult injuries are, at times, difficult to discern from the distracting pain of strains, contusions, and abrasions. Following a detailed re-examination and survey of pertinent diagnostic studies (ie, repeat hematocrit, serum amylase, chest radiograph), plans are made for appropriate disposition and follow-up. These may include physical therapy and rehabilitation, further diagnostic studies, alcohol detoxification facilities, or simply a return visit to the primary physician's office.

■ DIAGNOSTIC ADJUNCTS

DIAGNOSTIC PERITONEAL LAVAGE

Initial physical examination of the abdomen often fails to detect significant intra-abdominal injury in the context of multisystem trauma. Delay in diagnosis results in increased morbidity and mortality, prolonged hospitalization, and ultimately, in greater healthcare costs. The introduction of diagnostic peritoneal lavage (DPL)[6] in 1965 provided a safe and inexpensive method to rapidly identify life-threatening intraperitoneal injuries. Despite the widespread popularity of CT scanning in the United States and ultrasonography in Europe and Japan, we believe DPL remains an integral part of the evaluation of the critically injured patient.

There are three fundamental methods of introducing the DPL catheter into the peritoneal cavity. The closed approach consists of inserting the catheter in a blind percutaneous fashion. The major problem with this approach is uncontrolled depth of penetration, which renders the underlying intraperitoneal or retroperitoneal structures at risk for perforation. Unfortunately, the currently available Seldinger wire techniques in adults have been suboptimal because of inadequate lavage return. The open procedure, traversing the abdominal wall under direct visualization, is safer, but more time consuming, and introduces air into the peritoneal cavity. We prefer the semiopen technique performed at the infraumbilical ring as a compromise; this approach is quick, easy, and extremely reliable. The same procedure can be used in the patient with a major pelvic fracture because the enlarging anterior hematoma is limited by the infraumbilical ring. Before introducing the DPL catheter, the stomach and bladder are decompressed with a nasogastric tube and a Foley catheter, respectively. The periumbilical area is shaved, prepped with povidone-iodide solution, and draped sterilely. The area is infiltrated generously with local anesthesia (1% xylocaine without epinephrine). A gently curved incision is made to one side of the umbilicus, at the level of the infraumbilical ring (Fig 22–2). The advantages of making the incision at this site include relative avascularity, paucity of preperitoneal fat, and greater adherence of the peritoneum, resulting from obliteration of the umbilical arteries and urachus. The incision is carried down to the linea alba, ensuring meticulous hemostasis. A 5-mm incision is made in the linea alba, and the free edges are grasped with towel clips. While elevating the abdominal wall by traction on the towel clips, a standard dialysis catheter with its trocar is inserted into the peritoneal cavity toward the pelvis. Once the peritoneum is entered, the trocar is withdrawn and the catheter directed towards the pelvic floor. The tap is considered positive if >10 mL of gross blood is aspirated. Otherwise, 1 L (15 mL/kg in children) of warmed 0.9% sodium chloride is infused. If the clinical condition permits, the patient is rolled from side to side to enhance intraperitoneal sampling. The saline bag then is lowered to the floor for the return of lavage fluid by siphonage. A minimum 75% recovery of lavage effluent is required for the test to be considered valid. The fluid is sent for laboratory analysis of red blood cell (RBC) and white blood cell (WBC) counts, lavage amylase (LAM) and lavage alkaline phosphatase (LAP) levels, and examination for the presence of bile.

The criteria for positive DPL are outlined in Table 22–3. In the context of blunt abdominal trauma, significant visceral damage is encountered in >90% of patients in whom the RBC count exceeds 100,000/mm^3, but in <2% of those in whom the count is under 20,000/mm^3. RBC counts between 20 and 100,000/mm^3, however, may reflect serious injury in 15% to 35% of cases and merit further diagnostic evaluation; our current preference is abdominal CT scanning or intraoperative laparoscopy. Occasionally, an elevated WBC count (>500/mm^3), LAM, or LAP will signal an

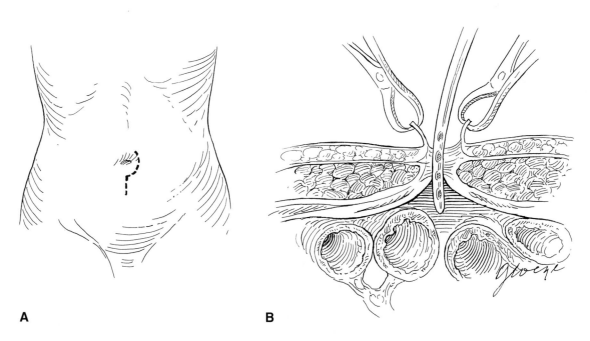

A   **B**

Figure 22–2. Diagnostic peritoneal lavage. **A**. The semiopen diagnostic peritoneal lavage is performed through a gently curved periumbilical incision, allowing access to the inferior portion of the umbilical ring. **B**. The free edges of the incised midline fascia are elevated with towel clips to minimize injury to the underlying viscera during introduction of the lavage catheter.

TABLE 22–3. CRITERIA FOR POSITIVE DPL FOLLOWING BLUNT ABDOMINAL TRAUMA

Index	Positive	Equivocal
Aspirate		
Blood	>10 mL	—
Fluid	Enteric Contents	—
Lavage		
Red Blood Cells	>1 000 000/mm^3	>20 000/mm^3
White Blood Cells	>1 000 000/mm^3	>500/mm^3
Enzyme	Amylase >20 IU/L and Alkaline Phosphatase >3 IU/L	Amylase >20 IU/L or Alkaline Phosphatase >3 IU/L
Bile	Confirmed biochemically	—

otherwise occult intestinal injury. The contents of perforated viscus evoke a migration of leukocytes into the peritoneal cavity, but this response may be delayed for at least 3 hours postinjury. Conversely, an isolated WBC count exceeding 500/mm^3, in a DPL done promptly after injury, is often nonspecific. We repeat the DPL in 4 hours if the initial WBC count is elevated, and perform a laparotomy if the count remains elevated. A LAP >3 IU/L is more accurate than lavage WBC count in the detection of small bowel injury. From a series of nearly 2 000 DPLs performed over a 4 year period, we found that, in an otherwise negative DPL, a LAM >20 IU/L combined with a LAP >3 IU/L was 97% specific for small bowel perforation. Serial or repeat DPLs are also valuable in multisystem injured patients who develop signs of hypovolemia or unexplained blood loss during extensive diagnostic or therapeutic interventions such as head CT, aortography, or pelvic angiography.

DPL does have inherent limitations and a morbidity rate of about 1%. The serious complications occur most frequently using the closed technique and include perforations of the small bowel, mesentery, bladder, and retroperitoneal vascular structures. Previous abdominal surgery, a gravid uterus, and massive obesity are relative contraindications for DPL. However, the only absolute contraindication is an existing indication for laparotomy. In patients with previous midline abdominal incisions, DPL can be performed through a left lower quadrant transverse incision, although this is technically more challenging. Moreover, intra-abdominal adhesions can loculate both the lavage fluid and free blood, increasing the risk of a false-negative study. Thus, the DPL is only useful if positive in the patient with previous extensive abdominal surgery. Finally, DPL does not sample the intact retroperitoneum and may not adequately reflect isolated hollow visceral or diaphragmatic perforations.

CT

CT plays an important role as a diagnostic adjunct in the early evaluation of abdominal and pelvic injuries. The limitations of this diagnostic modality center on its timely completion, availability of experienced radiologists, equipment variability, patient cooperation, the necessity for oral and intravenous contrast–enhancement agents, and costs. Early studies comparing CT with DPL demonstrated that while CT scan is more specific than DPL, several injuries to the gastrointestinal tract were missed by CT and detected by DPL.[8] More recent experience with modern scanners has demonstrated an overall CT accuracy of 92% to 98%.[9–11] In addition, CT has the unquestionable virtue of injury specificity. Clearly, select patients with isolated and self-limiting injury to the liver or spleen can be managed expectantly, based primarily on CT scanning.[8]

We believe CT should complement DPL in the evaluation of blunt abdominal trauma. Four groups of patients are particularly suitable for CT scanning: (1) patients with delayed (>12 hours) presentation who are hemodynamically stable and do not have overt signs of peritonitis; (2) patients in whom DPL results are equivocal and repeated physical examination is unreliable or untenable (eg, those who required prolonged anesthesia for neurosurgical or orthopedic procedures; patients with an altered mental status from head injury, drugs, or alcohol; or patients with spinal cord injury); (3) patients in whom DPL is difficult to perform (eg, patients with morbid obesity, portal hypertension, or previous laparotomies); and (4) patients at high risk for retroperitoneal injuries in whom DPL is unremarkable (eg, the unrestrained, intoxicated driver who strikes the steering column or a patient with postinjury hypermylasemia). Additionally, CT is valuable for defining the extent and configuration of complex pelvic fractures. However, it must be emphasized that CT scanning may not demonstrate blunt pancreatic fractures in the first 6 hours postinjury and cannot be relied on for the early detection of hollow visceral perforation.

DIAGNOSTIC ULTRASOUND

Quality ultrasound machines have become portable, and their role in the initial evaluation of blunt abdominal trauma is expanding. Diagnostic ultrasound is currently used routinely in emergency departments in Japan and Germany.[12] Ultrasonography can demonstrate the presence of free intraperitoneal fluid as well as locate solid organ hematomas. The procedure is particularly appealing for the injured pregnant patient, owing to its relatively limited hazard from radiation or contrast media. Ultrasonography, however, is limited in the assessment of solid organ fractures and is relatively poor for acute hollow visceral perforation. Moreover, the accuracy of ultrasonography is operator dependent and can be compromised by the presence of lower rib fractures, extensive soft-tissue injuries, or dressings. In one comparative study, Gruessner and associates found DPL superior to ultrasonography and concluded that the studies should be viewed as complementary rather than competitive.[13] However, with more sophisticated equipment (and resolution of territorial dispute with radiology), ultrasonography could largely supplant the role of DPL in the emergent evaluation of the critically injured. For example, work is in progress to generate three-dimensional computer reconstructions of ultrasound images.

LAPAROSCOPY

With the advent and development of new technology, diagnostic laparoscopy will no doubt have a role in the evaluation as well as definitive treatment of the acutely injured. In the past, laparoscopy was limited by the time required to perform the examination, the need for specialized equipment, and the necessity for general anesthesia. At this moment, there are several studies confirming the utility of laparoscopy done under local anesthesia in the emergency department to identify diaphragmatic injuries and quantitate the amount of intraperitoneal blood.[14-16] Presently, however, the major limitation is performing a comprehensive examination of the entire abdomen and pelvis, particularly the posterior recesses and retroperitoneum. However, enthusiasm for laparoscopy will continue with the advent of more sophisticated equipment and the potential for therapeutic intervention.

■ BLUNT ABDOMINAL TRAUMA

Our management plan for patients with significant abdominal trauma is outlined in Fig 22–3. Patients who present with overt peritonitis or massive hemoperitoneum are intubated, volume loaded, and transferred emergently to the operating room for abdominal exploration. Those patients who present following a high-energy transfer injury, particularly when intoxicated or with a concurrent head injury, undergo prompt DPL during their initial evaluation. A positive DPL in these high-risk patients mandates emergent abdominal exploration. Hemodynamically stable patients who have equivocal DPL results (20 000 to 100 000 RBC/mm^3) undergo abdominal CT scan to rule out major solid organ injury. Major spleen and liver injuries in adult patients are explored and lesser injuries are observed. Patients who are hemodynamically stable following low-energy transfer injury are evaluated by abdominal CT scanning and observed if grade <III solid visceral in-

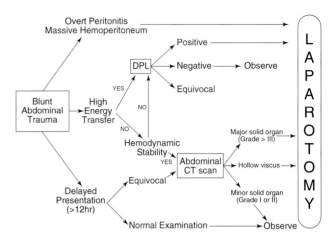

Figure 22–3. Decision algorithm for the initial evaluation of blunt abdominal trauma in the adult. Diagnostic peritoneal lavage plays a central role in the evaluation of these severely injured patients. CT is a valuable adjunctive examination for the relatively low-risk patient.

juries are confirmed. Alternatively, if the CT scan is not available, or there are multiple patients, DPL is used as the initial screening test with positive results further characterized by CT scanning. Those who present >12 hours following trauma are either observed or evaluated with an abdominal CT, depending on their initial physical examination and associated injuries. This diagnostic algorithm provides a general guideline for initial evaluation; as more information becomes available, this algorithm is modified as needed to include additional diagnostic studies or therapeutic interventions. These interventions might include (1) x-ray studies of the spine, chest and pelvis, (2) head CT scan, (3) intravenous pyelography, (4) retrograde cystourethrography, (5) contrast duodenography, or (6) diagnostic or therapeutic angiography.

The decision algorithm also is modified for pregnant or pediatric patients. Pregnancy alters both the susceptibility to blunt injury and the physiologic response to injury. The gravid uterus occupies the pelvis and lower abdomen and, hence, is vulnerable to a variety of insults from direct blows or seat belt injuries. These insults result in a spectrum of injuries from minor soft-tissue contusions to uterine wall disruption or placental abruption and potential exsanguination, as well as fetal loss. Thus, the significance of relatively minor injuries mandates an aggressive posture in the early evaluation of such women. We routinely use DPL (open technique) in pregnant patients while simultaneously evaluating the gravid uterus with ultrasound, noninvasive fetal monitoring, or amniocentesis.[17,18]

Hemodynamic instability, uterine rupture, placental abruption, fetal distress, and a bloody amniocentesis are indications for emergent abdominal exploration and uterine evacuation, with the rare possibility of hysterectomy.

The evaluation of pediatric trauma affords special challenges to the clinician owing to the size and unique physiology of these children. The elasticity of the lower rib cage and the relative large size of the abdominal cavity increase the susceptibility to intra-abdominal injury. On the other hand, the injury pattern encountered in the pediatric population and the greater potential for spontaneous hemostasis warrants a more selective approach. Liver and spleen injuries are common and frequently amenable to nonoperative management, whereas significant pancreatic fractures and intestinal perforations are infrequent.[19] Despite these facts, we maintain an aggressive attitude toward abdominal evaluation because of the limited physiologic reserve of children. Grossly positive DPLs in hemodynamically stable children are evaluated further by CT scan to verify solid organ injury that may be managed expectantly. However, early abdominal exploration is done for hemodynamic instability, need for ongoing blood transfusions, and a positive peritoneal lavage by enzymes.

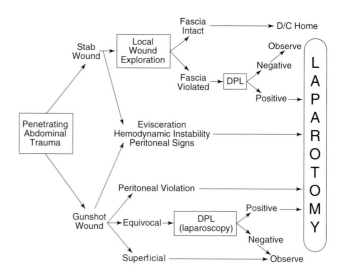

Figure 22–4. Decision algorithm for the evaluation of penetrating abdominal trauma in the adult.

■ PENETRATING ABDOMINAL TRAUMA

The initial management of patients with penetrating abdominal trauma can be simplified to (1) aggressive resuscitation, (2) directed physical examination, and (3) related diagnostic studies and therapeutic interventions (Fig 22–4). Hemodynamic stability, the nature of the penetrating object, and location of wounds are key factors in the decision algorithm. Patients presenting with massive hemoperitoneum or persistent hemodynamic instability are promptly intubated, volume loaded, and transported emergently to the operating room for abdominal exploration. Hemodynamically stable patients, on the other hand, are managed according to injury mechanism.

Civilian (low-energy) gunshot wounds to the anterior abdomen enter the peritoneal cavity in 80% of patients and result in significant visceral injury in 95% of patients. Thus, laparotomy is performed for gunshot wounds violating the peritoneum, as determined by physical examination and corroborated with biplanar abdominal roentgenograms that demonstrate missile trajectory. Bullets entering the upper abdomen may penetrate the chest, resulting in concomitant intrathoracic injuries. Similarly, bullets may traverse the abdomen and enter the retroperitoneal space, thereby endangering major abdominal vessels, bowel, and kidneys. When no exit site appears on the patient and the bullet cannot be seen on torso roentgenograms, transvascular embolization should be considered. If the bullet tract is tangential and appears superficial in the abdominal wall, pa-

tients can be managed individually, based on diagnostic peritoneal lavage or laparoscopy.

Stab wounds to the anterior abdomen are managed selectively. Patients who present with significant hemodynamic instability or obvious life-threatening wounds are promptly transported to the operating room for abdominal exploration. The remaining patients who present with hemodynamic stability are evaluated initially in the emergency department. Although two-thirds of these patients present with wounds that enter the peritoneum, less than half result in visceral injury that necessitate operative repair. Unless evisceration exists, violation of the peritoneum cannot be ascertained by gross appearance of the wound site, and blind probing may be misleading. Formal wound exploration with local anesthesia, in the emergency department, is the most reliable means for establishing the depth of penetration and hence, the need for further evaluation. DPL is performed in all patients with suspected or proven penetration of the peritoneal cavity.[20] While there is some controversy, most authorities agree that 100 000 RBC/mm^3 is an indication for laparotomy. Because of the proportionally higher number of isolated gastrointestinal perforations following a stab wound; however, peritoneal lavage has a 5% false-negative rate. Thus, all patients with a negative lavage are admitted for at least 24 hours of observation and undergo prompt exploration if signs of peritoneal irritation ensue. Fortunately, most injuries missed by initial DPL involve the stomach or small bowel. These usually are recognized within 6 to 12 hours and are associated with little excess morbidity.

Penetrating flank wounds pose unique diagnostic problems. These wounds are associated with retroperitoneal injury to the colon, duodenum, kidney, and major vascular structures. Accordingly, life-threatening injuries may exist in the face of hemodynamic stability and a negative DPL. The triple contrast (oral/intravenous/rectal) CT scan has been useful in this situation and most surgeons maintain a low threshold for early abdominal exploration if, by the scan, the wound tract appears to be in proximity to a significant retroperitoneal structure.

Preoperative broad-spectrum antibiotics are indicated for penetrating abdominal wounds because of the relatively high incidence of distal ileal or colonic perforations. The optimal antimicrobial agent has not been established, but a number of single agents provide effective activity against anaerobic as well as aerobic bacteria. Tetanus prophylaxis should be administered according to standard guidelines established for contaminated wounds.

■ OPERATIVE MANAGEMENT

The resolve to perform urgent surgery is a pivotal emergency room triage decision made by the trauma surgeon. The operating room in many hospitals is not immediately adjacent to the emergency department and may be removed further if the patient must undergo evaluation in the radiology department. Thus, the timing of patient transport to the operating room is crucial and depends on the injury mechanism, the physiologic status of the patient and response to resuscitation, the results of critical diagnostic studies and appropriate consultation, and the availability of an operating room. The emergency department stay for a patient in refractory shock following an abdominal gunshot wound should be brief (eg, 10 to 15 minutes) whereas a stable patient sustaining multisystem blunt trauma may remain in the emergency department or radiology department for some time. Premature triage to the OR may lead to an unnecessary laparotomy and delayed evaluation of life or limb-threatening extra-abdominal injuries. However, an undue delay in the emergency department may result in physiologic deterioration leading to irreversible shock and coagulopathy. Transfer to the operating room should be done by experienced personnel prepared to manage acute emergencies en route. Common errors include inadequate airway management, insecure lines and tubes, and insufficient patient monitoring. Each hospital should establish protocols to ensure timely, efficient, and safe patient transport from the emergency department resuscitation suite to an operating suite.

ORGANIZATION OF THE TRAUMA OPERATING ROOM

Although organization of the operating room is generally the prerogative of anesthesiologists, the trauma surgeon is ultimately responsible for the patient and should assist in providing an optimal environment for ongoing resuscitation and definitive surgical treatment. A specific operating room suite should be designated for trauma. Unique features of this room should include ample space to accommodate special equipment and additional personnel, supplementary cabinet space for trauma instruments, auxiliary lighting for multiteam operations, a large writing board to record key laboratory data, and speaker telephones to facilitate communication with the laboratory, blood bank, and consultants.

Adequate monitoring is critical for the patient with persistent shock undergoing urgent surgery. A CVP catheter should be placed for serial readings and a Swan-Ganz catheter inserted as soon as feasible in patients with extensive injuries. An arterial cannula provides constant blood pressure readings as well as access for blood gas determinations to ascertain acid-base, ventilatory, and oxygen transport status. Core temperatures should be monitored continuously and hypothermia minimized by infusing all fluids via warmers and heating gases from the ventilator. The ECG should be displayed and the pulse rate made audible. Urinary output and thoracostomy drainage should be channeled into receptacles that indicate the volume accumulated. All these indices are important in the ongoing assessment of the patient. The more visible and accessible they are to the surgeon and anesthesiologist, the better the team effort.

■ SPECIFIC INJURIES

DIAPHRAGMATIC INJURY

The diaphragm can be injured as the result of either blunt or penetrating trauma. Penetrating injuries below the nipples have an approximate 30% incidence of diaphragmatic injury. Blunt injuries occur from massive increases in intra-abdominal pressure resulting in lacerations that radiate laterally from the central tendon. Physical findings vary from asymptomatic to life-threatening cardiac and pulmonary instability owing to herniation of visceral contents into the chest. If a ruptured spleen herniates into the chest, it can masquerade as a pulmonary laceration with hemorrhage from a chest tube thoracostomy and a normal diagnostic peritoneal lavage. At the other extreme, a totally asymptomatic patient may harbor a diaphragmatic injury that goes unnoticed until years later when gradual herniation of abdominal viscera into the chest leads to pulmonary compromise, symptoms of visceral herniation, or strangulation of the stomach or intestines.

Direct operative repair of penetrating injuries to the diaphragm is important to prevent late sequelae of chronic herniation. A two-layer closure with interrupted mattress sutures, using nonabsorbable material, usually is accomplished easily.

Blunt injuries are often more challenging because they can extend to include the entire diaphragm. If the disruption occurs near the lateral attachment to the rib cage, direct suturing to the ribs may be necessary. Since the heart and lung are immediately behind the laceration, care must be taken to avoid injury to these organs during suture placement. One useful technique is to place one layer of tagged, interrupted horizontal mattress sutures well back from the edges of the laceration. These tagged sutures then are used to lift the repair away from the heart and lung and a second layer of running suture is used to close the laceration. The tagged sutures then are tied, providing a two-layer closure with nonabsorbable suture. Occasionally, when the defect is very large, synthetic mesh is required to buttress the repair or to patch the defect. If diaphragmatic injuries are detected more than four weeks after injury, they should be approached through a thoracotomy so that adhesions to the lung and pleura can be lysed. Diaphragmatic dysfunction is common after repair of large blunt injuries and may require prolonged ventilatory support.

HEPATIC INJURIES

The liver is the most frequently injured intra-abdominal organ, and more than 85% of hepatic wounds can be managed by simple hemostatic techniques. Gauze packing will terminate active hemorrhage from most superficial hepatic wounds. For continued surface bleeding, electrocautery argon beam coagulation and topical hemostatic agents are generally effective. Prophylactic perihepatic drainage is not necessary for these minor parenchymal lacerations.[21]

The first priority with severe hepatic bleeding is to resuscitate the patient. Pringle's maneuver (temporary occlusion of the porta hepatis, ie, portal vein, hepatic artery, and common bile duct) and tight liver packing are critical maneuvers to attenuate blood loss. Although human liver tolerance to warm ischemia was traditionally considered to be minutes, the safe period is now considered to be in excess of an hour. Failure of Pringle's maneuver to slow bleeding is the result of a hepatic vein–retrohepatic vena caval tear or an aberrant derivation of the lobar hepatic artery. In Michel's anatomic study, a left hepatic artery arose from the left gastric artery in 25% of patients and was the primary artery for the left lobe in 12%. Similarly, a right hepatic artery originated from the superior mesenteric artery in 17% of patients and was the principle lobar artery in 12%. Such accessory hepatic arteries do not lie within the porta hepatis, and, therefore, must be occluded separately. If hepatic vascular inflow occlusion is successful,

the liver should then be mobilized to allow adequate inspection of the extent of injury.

Adequate liver mobilization is imperative for surgical repair of complex liver injuries. The liver is mobilized by dividing the falciform ligament to the diaphragm, incising the peritoneal attachments between the left and right lobe of the liver and the diaphragm, and incising the right and left triangular ligaments to expose the hepatic veins and inferior vena cava. Mobilization is completed by incising the gastrohepatic ligament and the retroperitoneum along the caudate lobe, which exposes the retrohepatic vena cava on the left. These maneuvers allow the liver to be pulled up into the midline wound for surgical repair of parenchymal and vascular injuries. The fracture sites then are explored systematically by tractotomy, with individual ligation of the divided intrahepatic blood vessels and bile ducts.

If individual vessel ligation and packing do not achieve adequate hemostasis after release of inflow occlusion, selective hepatic artery ligation (SHAL) should be considered. This procedure is usually safe because the lobar portal vein provides sufficient oxygen to the dearterialized hepatic tissue until collaterals are functional. Failure to control hemorrhage after an effective Pringle's maneuver implies hepatic vein injury. If bleeding persists, the choice is whether to proceed with hepatic resection or use abdominal packing. Packing is clearly preferred if there is refractory coagulopathy, hypothermia, extensive bilobar injuries, other life-threatening injuries, or lack of blood bank support.[22] Reoperation is planned within 24 hours for removal of the packs and additional hepatic debridement. Packs should be removed early because they increase intra-abdominal pressure, which may compromise splanchnic and renal perfusion, and because the collected blood serves as a good medium for bacterial proliferation.

Hepatic lobectomy following trauma is formidable, with a mortality that exceeds 50%. Liver anatomy is variable, and the surgeon must be familiar with the prevalent anomalies of the hepatic arteries, hepatic veins, and biliary duct system (Fig 22–5). Common bile duct drainage via a T tube is not beneficial following major hepatic resection, but drainage of the perihepatic area is important because of the high incidence of postoperative bile leaks.

Retrohepatic vena cava injury is rare and constitutes the only immediate indication for hepatic lobectomy in the adult. Vena cava injury usually occurs at its junction with a major hepatic vein following blunt trauma. The typical clue to such an injury is failure of Pringle's maneuver, corroborated by the outpouring of desaturated blood with mobilization of the liver. Most authorities recommend hepatic vascular exclusion by placement of retrohepatic vena cava shunt. We prefer a balloon shunt introduced via the saphenofemoral junction for this

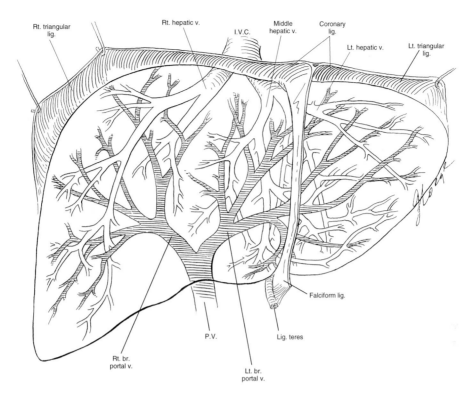

Figure 22–5. Surgical anatomy of the liver: (1) inferior vena cava; (2) right hepatic vein; (3) middle hepatic vein; (4) left hepatic vein; (5) portal vein; (6) right branch of portal vein; (7) left branch of portal vein; (8) right triangular ligament; (9) coronary ligament; (10) left triangular ligament; (11) falciform ligament; (12) ligamentum teres.

purpose (Fig 22–6).[23] However, despite these adjuncts, the mortality continues to exceed 80% in adults. In the child, neither a shunt nor hepatic lobectomy is necessary because the confluence of the major hepatic veins and vena cava is more extrahepatic; consequently, repair can be done by direct exposure and patient salvage is greater.

SPLENIC INJURIES

Operative management of the injured spleen has changed radically over the past decade. Once regarded as "mysterii pleni organon," the spleen now is considered an important immunologic factory as well as reticuloendothelial filter. Although the risk of postsplenectomy sepsis is greatest in the child under 2 years of age, the asplenic adult is clearly vulnerable. This danger of overwhelming sepsis has prompted the current enthusiasm for splenic salvage procedures. The risk of complications of splenorrhaphy, however, must not exceed the risk of total splenectomy. Spleen repair is attempted only if (1) the patient is hemodynamically stable and has no other immediate life-threatening injuries; (2) the spleen is amenable to repair; and (3) the surgeon is familiar with salvage techniques.[24]

The most important feature of splenorrhaphy is mobilization. The spleen must be freed by incision of its superior (phrenicolienal) and lateral (lienorenal) peritoneal attachments. These ligaments are essentially avascular and can be divided without direct visualization. The inferior (lienocolic) ligament may contain sizable blood vessels and therefore, should be divided and ligated prior to the other ligaments to facilitate splenic mobility. A plane then is developed posterior to the pancreas with blunt finger dissection. Once mobile, the spleen is rotated medially into the abdominal wound for complete inspection.

Small capsular avulsions are controlled with electrocautery or Argon beam coagulation, and topical hemostatic agents are applied to the denuded parenchyma. Deep parenchymal lacerations require individual vessel ligation; if bleeding persists, interlocking mattress sutures are placed. The thickened capsule in the child permits direct suturing; however, bolsters usually are needed in the adult (Fig 22–7). Major splenic fractures should be managed by anatomic resection. The spleen is composed of autonomous vascular compartments based on secondary diversions of the splenic artery. In 85% of patients, the splenic artery bifurcates into two primary branches, supplying the superior and inferior lobes. The lobar arteries further divide into cephalic and caudal segments. Segmental arterial ligation produces demarcation at the avascular intersegmental

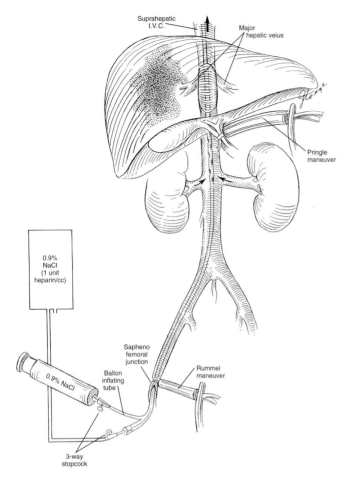

Figure 22–6. Retrohepatic vena caval or hepatic venous injuries are isolated with balloon-tipped Moore-Pilcher shunt introduced via the sapheno-femoral junction. Hepatic arterial and portal venous inflow are controlled with a Pringle's maneuver. The balloon is inflated with saline in the retrohepatic cava at the level of the hepatic veins.

ESOPHAGUS, STOMACH AND SMALL BOWEL WOUNDS

Stomach and small bowel perforations are second in frequency only to liver following penetrating abdominal wounds. Although blunt gastric rupture is rare, proximal jejunal and distal ileal disruptions occur after abrupt deceleration, particularly against lap-belt restraints. The most important feature of operative management is complete inspection of the gastrointestinal tract and adjacent mesentery. Failure to visualize the posterior aspect of the stomach or duodenum with an anterior gastric wound is a common oversight and may lead to serious complications from a missed perforation. In general, the number of perforations following a gunshot wound is even. An odd number suggests a missed exit wound, although occasionally the bullet comes to rest within the gut lumen or makes a tangential wound. The mesenteric border of the bowel must be exposed to exclude perforation when a hematoma is present.

Primary repair of the stomach and small bowel usually is safe because of the rich blood supply and relatively modest bacterial content. All defects in the gut should be identified before embarking on repair of an apparently isolated injury. Intestinal wounds should be temporarily sealed with noncrushing clamps while

plane, permitting amputation of the ischemic portion (Fig 22–8). Hemostasis of the cut end of viable spleen then is controlled with sutures and topical agents. Occasionally, splenic artery ligation is necessary to control bleeding, but there is an immunologic penalty from this maneuver.

Splenectomy remains the optimal management when the spleen is pulverized or the patient has other life-threatening injuries. The splenic artery and vein should be ligated individually. Reimplantation of the splenic tissue restores some of the immune function lost with splenectomy. We section the removed spleen into five fragments (40×40×3 mm) and enclose them in greater omental pouches. The left upper quadrant is not drained following splenorraphy or splenectomy, unless for a concurrent pancreatic injury. Because of the risk of overwhelming pneumococcal sepsis, all patients undergoing loss of >50% of their spleen should be given polypneumococcal vaccine postoperatively.

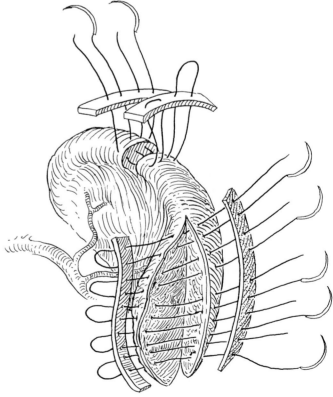

Figure 22–7. Repair of a damaged spleen can be accomplished using mattress sutures over Teflon pledgets.

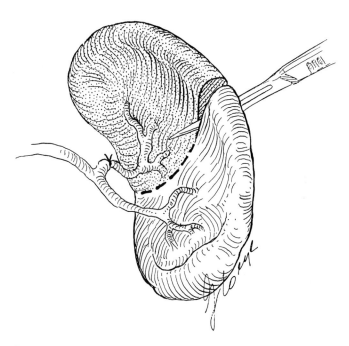

Figure 22–8. Following ligation of the superior pole splenic vessels, there is clear demarcation of ischemic tissue, allowing anatomic resection.

awaiting formal closure to avoid additional peritoneal contamination. Simple perforations of the stomach and the small bowel should be closed with standard techniques in either one or two layers. Two adjacent holes usually are connected, and the bowel closed transversely to avoid narrowing the lumen. Minimal debridement is required after stab injuries and low-energy gunshot wounds, but devitalized tissue from high-energy insults must be removed. Mesenteric bleeding should be controlled by individual vessel ligation, as close to the bowel as possible. If questionable areas of viability or multiple perforations are found in a short segment of small bowel, the segment should be resected and the ends anastomosed. In rare cases of extensive ischemic gut caused by proximal superior mesenteric artery injury, the remaining viable bowel ends can be brought out as temporary enterostomies.

Injuries to the intra-abdominal esophagus should be adequately debrided and repaired in two layers over a nasogastric tube or dilator. In addition, the repair should be buttressed with a full thickness diaphragmatic pedicle flap, a Thal fundal patch, or a Nissen fundoplication. If significant narrowing will result from a primary repair of the intra-abdominal esophagus, a Thal fundal patch coupled with a Nissen fundoplication is performed over a number 50 to 60 French esophageal dilator. A nasogastric tube should always be left in place until a barium esophagram is performed 10 to 14 days after operation to verify healing without leak. If a small

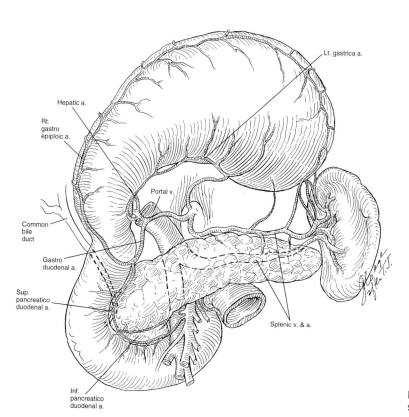

Lt. gastrica a.

Hepatic a.

Rt. gastro epiploic a.

Portal v.

Common bile duct

Gastro duodenal a.

Sup. pancreatico duodenal a.

Splenic v. & a.

Inf. pancreatico duodenal a.

Figure 22–9. Anatomic relations of the pancreas and duodenum demonstrating adjacent organs and important nearby vascular structures.

leak is present, serial esophagrams should be performed until it has resolved.[25]

DUODENUM AND PANCREAS TRAUMA

Anatomic and physiologic complexities of the duodenum and pancreas (Figure 22–9) have prompted a variety of operative techniques for their treatments. Overlooked or underestimated injuries may lead to disastrous complications; whereas, inappropriately aggressive management can result in permanent morbidity or death at surgery. Blunt duodenal injury usually is caused by abrupt deceleration, crushing the retroperitoneal duodenum against the spine or causing a blowout of the air-filled, closed duodenal loop. The most common site for nonpenetrating pancreatic disruption is the area overlying the vertebral column. Prompt recognition is essential for successful treatment of pancreaticoduodenal injuries. Complete examination of these structures in imperative during celiotomy if there is (1) history of rapid deceleration, (2) blood in the nasogastric aspirate, (3) blood or bile staining of the midline retroperitoneum, or (4) wounds penetrating the upper midabdomen. A generous Kocher maneuver is performed to expose the pancreatic head and first two portions of the duodenum, and the lesser sac is opened widely through the gastrocolic omentum to examine the body and tail of the pancreas and third portion of the duodenum. Visualization of the fourth portion of the duodenum is facilitated by division of the ligament of Treitz.

Limited duodenal contusions are best left alone when discovered at laparotomy. Most hematomas will reabsorb within 1 to 2 weeks. Placement of a gastrostomy and feeding jejunostomy tube should be considered for extensive contusions where delayed resolution of the hematoma is anticipated. Limited perforations and simple lacerations of the duodenum are closed primarily using standard suture techniques. Presumptive drainage is not used for these minor defects.

Extensive duodenal injuries may require one of a variety of patch and bypass procedures for safe closure. These procedures vary from a side-to-side patch duodenojejunostomy to gastrojejunostomy with duodenal exclusion and attempted closure of duodenum, to Roux-en-Y duodenojejunostomy with duodenal resection or division (Fig 22–10). Care must be taken to identify the duodenal ampulla. Extension resectional procedures (ie, pancreaticoduodenectomy) are performed only for massive combined pancreaticoduodenal injuries. Management of complex duodenal injuries, or those associated with pancreatic injuries, particularly when recognized late, is controversial. Some authorities believe suction decompression of the duodenum is important, either via transpyloric nasogastric tube, tube duodenostomy, or retrograde tube jejunostomy. We favor exclusion for precarious duodenal injuries.[26] A gastrotomy is made on the greater curvature of the antrum through which the pylorus is closed with a 2-0 polypropylene purse-string suture. A side-to-side gastrojejunostomy then is completed using the gastrotomy (Fig 22–11). Specific indications for these protective measures include (1) free perforation with delay in surgery of >24 hours, (2) injury involving >75% of the wall in the first or second portion of the duodenum, and (3) associated injuries of the pancreatic head or distal common bile duct. A feeding jejunostomy should be placed for early postoperative enteral feeding in patients with high-risk duodenal wounds.[27]

Operative decisions for pancreatic trauma are based on injury site and status of the ductal system. Most injuries are superficial contusions and lacerations, and main duct integrity is not in question. Peripancreatic drainage is routine for such minor lesions because disrupted parenchyma and peripheral ducts may result in a fistula. Closed suction catheters are effective for removing pancreatic juice, and fistulas usually resolve with adequate drainage. Location dictates the management of deep fractures or penetrating wounds with suspected ductal violation. Major injuries in the body and tail of the pancreas warrant distal resection.[28] Removal of this portion of the gland is not associated with endocrine deficiency, and the spleen can be preserved with little additional effort. Roux-en-Y internal drainage of the distal pancreas is not recommended since it is frequently complicated by fistula and secondary infection. Surgical treatment of injuries to the right side of the superior mesenteric vein is generally

A

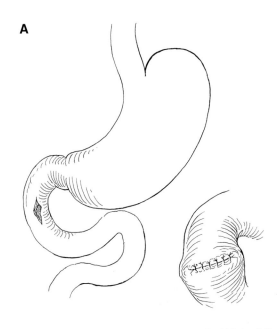

Figure 22–10. Procedures used in the management of duodenal injuries. **A.** The majority of duodenal injuries can be managed by simple primary repair using a one- or two-layer suture techniques. *Continued*

B

C

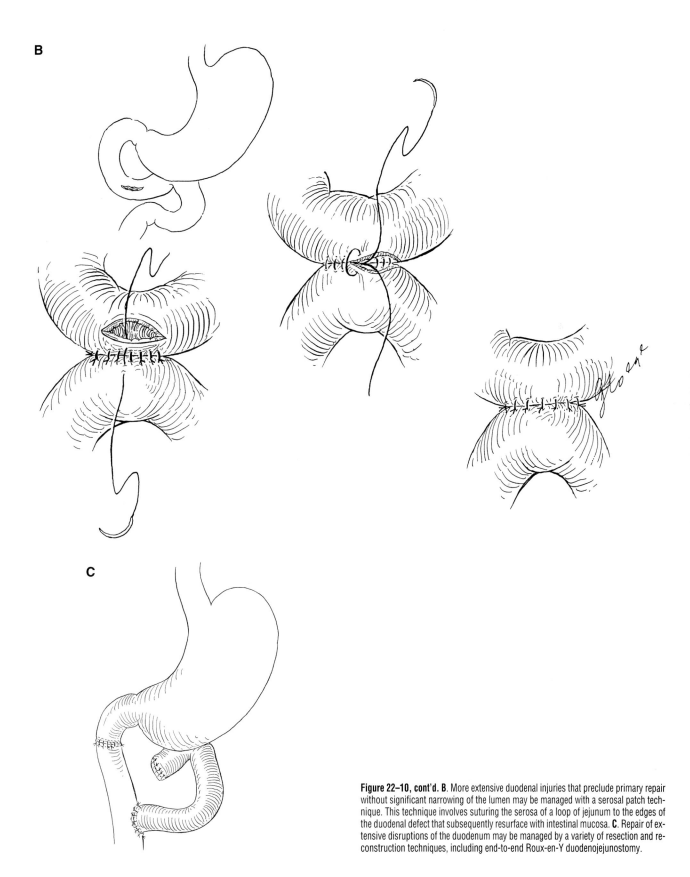

Figure 22–10, cont'd. B. More extensive duodenal injuries that preclude primary repair without significant narrowing of the lumen may be managed with a serosal patch technique. This technique involves suturing the serosa of a loop of jejunum to the edges of the duodenal defect that subsequently resurface with intestinal mucosa. **C**. Repair of extensive disruptions of the duodenum may be managed by a variety of resection and reconstruction techniques, including end-to-end Roux-en-Y duodenojejunostomy.

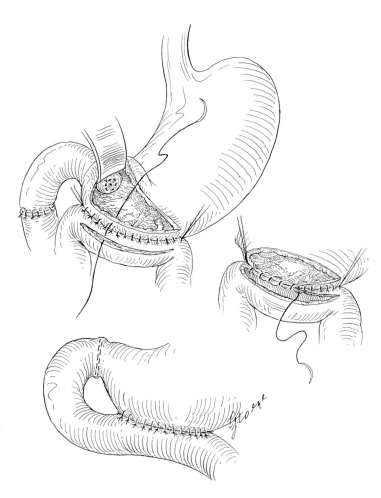

Figure 22–11. A. Pyloric exclusion and gastrojejunostomy for protection of severe duodenal injuries that have been closed primarily. The pylorus is sutured closed through a dependent distal gastrotomy. A gastrojejunostomy then is fashioned to a proximal loop of jejunum. **B.** An alternative method of pyloric exclusion using an intestinal stapling device to occlude the proximal duodenum. A gastrojejunostomy then is performed between the dependent stomach and the proximal jejunum.

conservative. Because ductal integrity is the critical factor, intraoperative pancreatography may be used to define the status of the duct. Options for pancreatic head trauma with ductal involvement include anterior Roux-en-Y pancreaticojejunostomy, pancreatic division with Roux-en-Y drainage of both segments, pancreaticoduodenectomy, or external drainage. The latter, simpler approach is preferred for most injuries, accepting the risk of a controlled pancreatic fistula. The others involve greater operative risk and potential complications. Early postoperative nutrition via jejunostomy is an important adjunct; jejunal administration of a defined elemental diet with low fat content and neutral pH has minimal stimulatory effects on the pancreas.

COLONIC WOUNDS

The most frequent cause of colon injuries are penetrating wounds. However, blunt disruptions and hemorrhagic contusions can result from high-energy transfer. Operative management of colon perforation has changed dramatically during the last 25 years. The practice of mandatory colostomy, adopted from military experience, has given way to a selective policy of primary colon repair. Pri-

mary closure of the intraperitoneal colon can be achieved safely in at least 70% of patients in the civilian setting.[29] Criteria for primary repair are (1) <6 hour interval from injury, (2) less than two associated intraperitoneal injuries, (3) absence of hemorrhagic shock, and (4) an otherwise stable patient. Although some suggest that right-sided colon injuries can be treated more aggressively then left-sided ones, this theory has not been substantiated. Exteriorization of the sutured colon is a viable alternative to colostomy when the factors listed above preclude safe intraperitoneal repair. The exteriorized segment will heal in 75% of patients, sparing the added morbidity of colostomy closure. Attention to technical details enhances the success of exteriorization. These details include (1) adequate debridement and meticulous suturing, using resection when injury is extensive, (2) wide mobilization of the involved colon segment to prevent obstruction and tension on the suture line, (3) maintaining the exteriorized repair in a moist, clean environment, and (4) delaying intraperitoneal return of the colon until at least postoperative day 7.

If the surgeon believes primary repair or exteriorization is ill-advised because of clinical or technical reasons, colostomy is clearly appropriate.[30] The colostomy and nonfunctional mucous fistula should exit close to each other on the abdominal wall to facilitate subsequent takedown and closure. When the colonic wound permits, a loop colostomy is considered adequate. If the colon must be divided for technical reasons, the distal colon can be simply stapled rather than fashioning a mucous fistula, especially if the distal colon is too short to bring out. The skin and subcutaneous tissue should be left open after fascia closure to reduce the risk of wound infection.

RECTAL INJURIES

Rectal injury is usually a result of gunshot wounds or bone fragmentation from major pelvic fractures. These injuries are at high risk for septic complications owing to the heavy bacterial load contaminating a hematoma in the poorly vascularized soft tissue of the pelvis. Fecal diversion with a proximal colostomy is mandatory for all full-thickness rectal defects.

The patient should be placed in the lithotomy position on the operating table to provide adequate exposure of the perineum and the abdomen. The abdomen is explored through a midline laparotomy and associated intraperitoneal injuries are managed as indicated. Proximal vascular isolation of the distal aortal or common iliac vessels is obtained before entering any significant pelvic hematoma. The retrorectal space is opened to the level of the coccyx, and devitalized tissue is debrided. Ideally, the rectal wound is closed, although most unrepaired rectal injuries deep in the pelvis heal adequately. Retrograde methylene blue injection or intraoperative rectosigmoidoscopy may help identify lesions difficult to visualize directly. Adequate drainage of these wounds is critical, using sump or penrose drains placed in the presacral space and brought out through the perineum anterior to the tip of the coccyx. Total fecal diversion is established with a proximal colostomy. When possible, a loop sigmoid colostomy is constructed with the distal limb stapled (Fig 22–12). A large Foley catheter is then placed through a small temporary colostomy in the distal limb to facilitate evacuation of colonic and rectal contents by copious irrigation with saline and antibiotic solution.

MAJOR ABDOMINAL VASCULAR INJURIES

Vascular trauma is responsible for most deaths following penetrating abdominal wounds. The most lethal injuries are those in the retrohepatic vena cava,[31,32] visceral aorta,[33] and main portal vein.[32,34] Blunt trauma usually involves the venous system; the abdominal aorta rarely is disrupted, and injury here may dissect later.[35] Although the diagnosis of major abdominal vascular injury is occasionally subtle because of retroperitoneal tamponade,

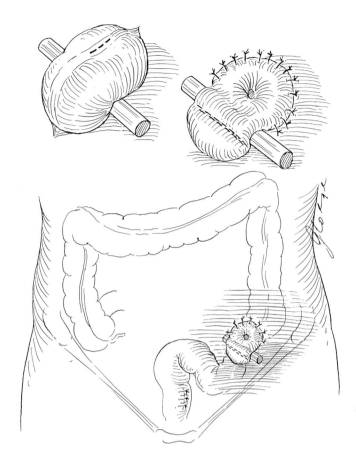

Figure 22–12. Sigmoid loop colostomy for rectal injury. Staple closure of the distal limb assures complete fecal diversion.

these patients typically arrive at the hospital in shock. Successful treatment demands quick recognition and prompt resuscitation with adequate volume replacement, including blood, followed by ample vascular exposure to allow rapid control of the hemorrhage.

Operative preparation of the patient includes the chest and upper legs to facilitate access for proximal and distal vascular control. Sterile equipment should include a variety of vascular clamps, tourniquets, and shunts that allow temporary nontraumatic vessel occlusion. Visceral rotation is valuable for operative exposure of major intra-abdominal vascular wounds.[36] Left peritoneal reflection is carried out for midline and left-sided supramesocolic hematomas. With mobilization of the left aspect of the colon, spleen, stomach, and distal pancreas in a plane deep to the pancreas, optimal exposure of the suprarenal aorta, celiac axis, proximal superior mesenteric artery, and left renal vessels is obtained (Fig 22–13). For right-sided supramesocolic hematomas, reflection of the ascending colon, duodenum, and pancreatic head provides a wide view of the infrahepatic vena cava, portal venous system, and right renal vessels (Fig 22–14). Proximal vascular control for inframesocolic or pelvic bleed-

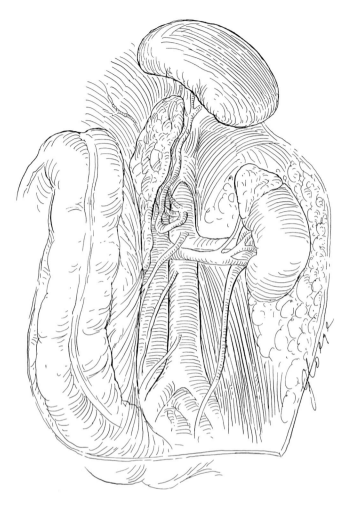

Figure 22–13. Left medial visceral rotation for exposure of left-sided retroperitoneal structures, including the left kidney, aorta, and major visceral vessels.

ing is better obtained via right visceral rotation because of the position of the vena cava and iliac veins. Anterior penetrating vascular wounds usually have a posterior component, which may be tamponaded temporarily by adjacent soft tissue so that both sides must be inspected for entrance and exit sites.

Abdominal Aortic Injuries

Abdominal aortic injuries should be closed by lateral arteriorrhaphy when feasible. For large-caliber gunshot wounds, autogenous vein patching may be appropriate, but for complete transection, synthetic graft interposition is used, even in the face of contamination. Extra-anatomic bypass is not warranted for intestinal contamination because of the critical status of most patients with this injury. Extension damage of the celiac trunk can usually be treated by ligation because of the rich collateral circulation. However, occlusion of the superior mesenteric artery (SMA) proximal to the middle colic branch requires reconstruction. Autogenous saphe-

nous vein grafting may be necessary either as an interposition or in the form of a bypass from the aorta to the SMA; a second-look procedure is recommended for most cases.

Inferior Vena Cava Wounds

Vena cava injuries should be repaired primarily, even if luminal diameter is compromised, although a vein patch may be necessary for extensive injuries.[37] The fear of pulmonary emboli following repair has not been confirmed.[38] For massive tissue loss, infrarenal cava ligation can be done with little hemodynamic change; careful postoperative treatment minimizes long-term sequelae. Abrupt occlusion of the suprarenal cava, however, may have serious consequences, including renal impairment from venous hypertension. Reconstruction can be accomplished by panel saphenous vein interposition or synthetic grafting.[39]

Portal Vein Injuries

Portal vein bleeding can be controlled temporarily by digital pressure, but definitive repair at the confluence of the superior mesenteric and splenic veins may necessitate division of the pancreas. With severe injuries, portal vein ligation is a reasonable alternative that is

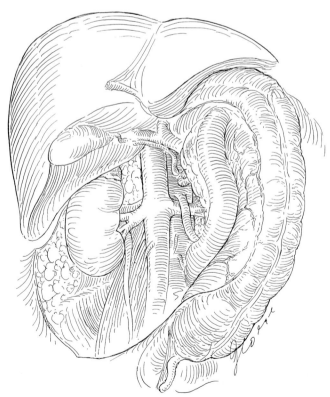

Figure 22–14. Right medial visceral rotation for exposure of right kidney, intrahepatic vena cava, and distal aorta.

tolerated by >80% of patients.[32,34] A second-look procedure should be done 24 hours later, and portosystemic shunting should be performed, if bowel viability is jeopardized

Iliac Arterial and Venous Injury

Iliac arterial and venous injury caused by penetrating wounds of blunt injury, including pelvic fractures, is serious because of the lack of tamponade in the pelvis and extensive interconnecting collaterals.[40] The common and external iliac arteries should be repaired and the proximal hypogastric artery may be transposed to the external iliac for reconstruction. Although venorrhaphy is preferred, iliac veins are generally ligated if major injury has caused a loss of substance. Temporary packing may be required for presacral and deep pelvic venous bleeding. Occasionally, bilateral internal iliac arteriography may be used to localize a major bleeding point, which then can be controlled by surgical ligation or embolization through the catheter.

UROLOGIC TRAUMA

Renal Trauma

Operative management of renal parenchymal trauma is generally limited. Minor injuries (contusions and shallow parenchymal fractures without contrast extravasation) represent 70% of blunt renal injuries and require no surgical intervention. Intermediate injuries (parenchymal laceration through corticomedullary junction with contrast extravasation) account for 20% of blunt trauma. Although somewhat controversial, kidney salvage appears greatest with initial nonsurgical care of these lesions.[6,41] Major injuries (shattered kidneys, renal artery occlusion) clearly mandate prompt exploration. Similar classification and management decisions pertain to penetrating wounds. Although penetrating renal injuries are usually more severe than those following blunt trauma, nearly 60% can be treated nonsurgically.[42] Contrast extravasation, if confined within Gerota's (renal) fascia, does not warrant immediate surgery.

Renovascular Trauma

Renovascular trauma is infrequent, and kidney salvage following complete renal artery occlusion is poor.[43,44] On the other hand, revascularization has been successful 12 to 19 hours after injury, supporting an aggressive attempt despite late recognition.[44] Renal artery thrombectomy alone frequently results in early thrombosis. The damaged vessel should be resected and a reanastomosis performed or an aorta-renal bypass graft inserted. The right renal vein should be reconstructed, whereas the left vein usually can be ligated, if done medial to the entrance of a patent gonadol vein.[34]

Ureteral Disruption

Ureteral disruption usually occurs with penetrating wounds but occasionally may result from blunt avulsion.[45,46] Suspected ureteral injury may be evaluated intraoperatively with a 5-mL intravenous injection of indigo-carmine or methylene-blue, with the physician observing the area for leak of bluish urine. Ureteral contusion also may occur from gunshot wounds. Despite an innocuous appearance, contusions have a small risk of subsequent necrosis with urinary fistula formation.[47] Ureteral repair is accomplished by various techniques, depending on the level of injury, upper, middle, or lower third.[46]

In most cases, injuries to the upper two thirds of the ureter can be repaired by uretero-ureterostomy after debridement of the injured area. Uretero-ureterostomy is performed by spatulating the ureter ends, and anastomosing them over a J stent with interrupted full-thickness sutures of 5.0 chromic. Ureteropelvic injuries should be treated by nephrostomy and stenting of the repair. Major disruption of the vesicoureteral junction of the lower one-third of the ureter requires submucosal replantation of the ureter into the bladder using 4.0 chromic interrupted sutures. If long segments of ureter are damaged, a transureterostomy may be required. The proximal end of the transected ureter is passed through a retroperitoneal tunnel and anastomosed to the side of the opposite ureter. With all ureteric surgery, dissection must be kept to a minimum to insure an adequate blood supply. Drainage is mandatory in such cases.

Bladder Perforations

Bladder perforations may be either intraperitoneal or extraperitoneal.[48] The less common intraperitoneal rupture is usually at the dome, where the bladder is weakest. These injuries usually are explored transperitoneally, repaired in two layers, and drained by a suprapubic cystostomy. Most extraperitoneal bladder injuries are the result of pelvic fracture,[49] with the smaller lesions managed by urethral drainage alone.[48] Larger injuries are exposed from the inside after cystostomy and repaired with 2/0 chromic sutures. If the injury is near the trigone, indigo-carmine is used to ensure patency of the ureters, and stents are placed. The cystostomy is done in two layers and a suprapubic cystostomy tube is placed, followed by drainage of the extravessicle space.

Although definitive management is a low priority, these injuries are frequently debilitating owing to secondary impotence, incontinence, and stricture formation.[50] Posterior urethral injury usually is associated with pelvic fracture, whereas anterior tears most often are caused by straddle injury falls. Suprapubic cystostomy is performed initially for all major urethral injuries. Primary reconstruction is advocated for anterior tears, but delayed repair generally is preferred for posterior lesions.[51] The secondary urethroplasty, is needed, is done after 3 to 6 months.

GYNECOLOGIC TRAUMA

Injury to the normal female reproductive organs is rare and usually results from penetrating wounds. Most injuries to the uterus and adnexa can be treated with simple suture repair. Hysterectomy is occasionally necessary for lower segment injuries complicated by major hemorrhage.

Unfortunately, trauma during pregnancy is not rare.[17,18] The mother must take priority over the fetus in operative decision-making, and the best assurance for saving the fetus is maternal survival. If the mother is hemodynamically stable, preoperative real-time sonography is valuable in identifying placental separation, as well as to ascertain the physiologic status of the fetus. Hysterectomy is usually unnecessary but is justified for uncontrolled uterine hemorrhage or if the gravid uterus interferes with surgical treatment of associated injuries.

REFERENCES

1. Jurkovich GJ, Moore EE, Medina G. Autotransfusion in trauma—a pragmatic analysis. *Am J Surg* 1984;148:782
2. Frenstad JD, Martin SH. Lethal complication from insertion of nasogastric tube after severe baseline skull fracture. *J Trauma* 1982;22:190
3. Marx JA, Moore EE, Jorden RC, et al. Limitations of CT scanning in the evaluation of acute abdominal trauma—a prospective comparison with peritoneal lavage. *J Trauma* 1985;25:933
4. Miller RD, Robbins TO, Tong MJ, et al. Coagulation defects associated with massive blood transfusions. *Ann Surg* 1971;174:794
5. Moore JB, Moore EE, Markovchick VC, et al. Diagnostic peritoneal lavage for abdominal trauma: superiority of the open technique at the infraumbilical ring. *J Trauma* 1981;21:570
6. Root HD, Hauser CW, McKinley CR, et al. Diagnostic peritoneal lavage. *Surgery* 1965;57:633
7. Fisher RP, Berverlin BC, Engrav LH, et al. Diagnostic peritoneal lavage: fourteen years and 2,586 patients later. *Am J Surg* 1978;136:701
8. Fabian TC, Mangiante EC, White TJ, et al. A prospective study of 91 patients undergoing both computed tomography and peritoneal lavage following blunt abdominal trauma. *J Trauma* 1986;26:602–608
9. Meyer DM, Thal ER, Weigelt JA, et al. Evaluation of computed tomography and diagnostic peritoneal lavage in blunt abdominal trauma. *J Trauma* 1986;29:1168
10. Kearney PA Jr, Vahey T, Burney RE, et al. Computed tomography and diagnostic peritoneal lavage in blunt abdominal trauma: their combined role. *Arch Surg* 1989;124:344
11. Peitzman AB, Makaroun MS, Slasky BS, et al. Prospective study of computed tomography in initial management of blunt abdominal trauma. *J Trauma* 1986;26:585
12. Furtschegger A, Egender G, Jaske G. The value of sonography in the diagnosis and follow-up of patients with blunt abdominal trauma. *Br J Urol* 1988;62:110
13. Gruessner R, Mentges B, Duber C, et al. Sonography vs. peritoneal lavage in blunt abdominal trauma. *J Trauma* 1989;29:242–245
14. Ivatury RR, Simon RJ, Weksler B, et al. Laparoscopy in the evaluation of the intrathoracic abdomen after penetrating injury. *J Trauma* 1992;33:101–108
15. Livingston DH, Tortella BJ, Machiedo GW, et al. The role of laparoscopy in abdominal trauma. *J Trauma* 1992;33:471–475
16. Zantut LF, Rodrigues AJ, Birolini D. Laparoscopy as a diagnostic tool in the evaluation of trauma. *Panam J Trauma* 1990;2:6–11
17. Esposito TJ, Gens DR, Smith LG, et al. Trauma during pregnancy: a review of 79 cases. *Arch Surg* 1991;126:1073–1078
18. Neufield JDG, Moore EE, Marx JA, et al. Trauma in pregnancy. *Emerg Med Clin North Am* 1987;5:623–632
19. Oldham KT, Guice KS, Ryckman F, et al. Blunt liver injury in childhood: evolution of therapy and current perspective. *Surgery* 1986;100:542
20. Feliciano DV, Bitondo CG, Steed G, et al. 500 open taps on lavages in patients with abdominal stab wounds. *Am J Surg* 1985;148:772
21. Moore EE. Critical decision-making in management of acute hepatic injury. *Am J Surg* 1984;148:712
22. Feliciano DV, Mattox KL, and Jordan GL. Intra-abdominal packing for control of hemorrhage: a reappraisal. *J Trauma* 1981;21:285
23. Pilcher DB, Harman PK, Moore EE. Retrohepatic vena cava balloon injuries—a continuing challenge. *J Trauma* 1977;17:837
24. Pickhardt B, Moore EE, Moore FA, et al. Operative splenic salvage in the adult—a decade perspective. *J Trauma* 1989;29:1386
25. Popovosky J. Perforations of the esophagus from gunshot wounds. *J Trauma* 1984;24:337
26. Vaughan GD, Frazier OH, Graham DY, et al. The use of pyloric exclusion in the management of severe duodenal injuries. *Am J Surg* 1977;134:785
27. Moore EE, and Moore FA. Immediate enteral nutrition following multisystem trauma—a decade experience. *Am Coll Nutr* 1991;10:633
28. Cogbill TH, Moore EE, Morris JA Jr, et al. Distal pancreatectomy for trauma: a multicenter experience. *J Trauma* 1991;31:1600
29. Shannon FL, Moore EE. Primary colon repair—a safe alternative. *Surgery* 1985;95:851
30. Burch JM, Feliciano DV, Mattox KL. Colostomy and drainage for civilian rectal injuries: is that all? *Ann Surg* 1988;209:600
31. Kashuk JL, Moore EE, Millikan JS, et al. Major abdominal vascular trauma: a unified approach. *J Trauma* 1982;22:672
32. Peterson SR, Sheldon GF, Lim RC. Management of portal vein injuries. *J Trauma* 1979;19:616

33. Millikan JS, Moore EE. Abdominal aortic trauma—critical factors in determining mortality. *Surg Gynecol Obstet* 1985; 160:313

34. Pachter HL, Spencer FC, Jofstetter SR, et al. Experience with the finger fracture technique to achieve intrahepatic hemostasis in 75 patients with severe injuries of the liver. *Ann Surg* 1983;197:771

35. Lassonde J, Laurendeau F. Blunt injury of the abdominal aorta. *Ann Surg* 1981;194:745

36. Bascaglia LC, Blaisdell WF, Lim RC. Penetrating abdominal vascular injuries. *Arch Surg* 1969;99:764

37. Millikan JS, Moore EE, Steiner E, et al. Complications of tube thoracostomy for acute trauma. *Am J Surg* 1980;9:591

38. Rich NM, Hughes CW, Baugh JH. Management of venous injuries. *Ann Surg* 1970;171:724

39. Rosaria MD, Rumsey EW, Arakalki G, et al. Blood microaggregation and ultrafilters. *J Trauma* 1978;18:498

40. Millikan JS, Moore EE, Van Way CW, et al. Vascular trauma in the groin: contrast between iliac and femoral injuries. *Am J Surg* 1981;142:695

41. Peterson NE. Intermediate-degree blunt renal trauma. *J Trauma* 1977;17:425

42. Whitney RF, Peterson NE. Penetrating renal injuries. *Urology* 1976;7:7

43. Barlow B, Gandhi R. Renal artery thrombosis following blunt trauma. *J Trauma* 1980;20:614

44. Turner WW, Snyder WH, Fry WJ. Mortality and renal salvage after renovascular trauma—a review of 94 patients treated in a 20 year period. *Am J Surg* 1983;146:848

45. Carlton CE, Scott RJ, Guthrie AG. The initial management of ureteral injuries. *J Urol* 1971;105:335

46. Pitts JC, Peterson NE. Penetrating injuries of the ureter. *J Trauma* 1981;21:978

47. Cass AS, Ureteral contusion with gunshot wounds. *J Trauma* 1984;24:59

48. Richardson JR, Leadbetter GW. Nonoperative treatment of the ruptured bladder. *J Urol* 1975;114:213

49. Weems WL. Management of genitourinary injuries in patients with pelvic fractures. *Ann Surg* 1979;189:717

50. Morehouse DD, MacKinnon KJ. Management of prostato-membranous urethral disruption: thirteen years' experience. *J Urol* 1980;123:173

51. McAninch JW. Traumatic injuries to the urethra. *J Trauma* 1981;21:291–296

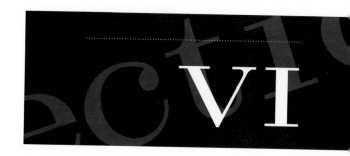

ESOPHAGUS

23

Gastroesophageal Reflux and Hiatal Hernia

Jeffrey H. Peters ■ *Tom R. DeMeester*

■ THE EVOLUTION OF SURGICAL THERAPY FOR GASTROESOPHAGEAL REFLUX DISEASE

From a historical perspective gastroesophageal reflux disease (GERD) was not recognized as a significant clinical problem until the mid 1930s, and was not identified as a precipitating cause for esophagitis until after World War II.[1] Initially, the symptoms of gastroesophageal reflux were associated with a hiatal hernia. This led to the conclusion that the hernia itself was the cause of the symptoms. It seemed reasonable to attempt to correct these symptoms by surgically reducing the hernia with simple closure of the crura. The result of this first surgical effort was uniform failure. The reasons for failure were elusive because of ignorance regarding the pathophysiology of gastroesophageal reflux disease and its relationship to a hiatal hernia. This ignorance was the result of the lack of esophageal function studies and the difficulty of performing rigid endoscopy. Consequently, the anatomical abnormality of a hiatal hernia became the indication for operation and, as our current day knowledge would predict, the results were dissatisfying.

Phillip Allison was the first to link the symptomatology of hiatus hernia to the occurrence of gastroesophageal reflux. This contribution encouraged surgeons to improve the function of the cardia rather than simply reducing the hernia. The Allison repair, introduced in 1951, represented the first effort in this direction.[2] Allison emphasized the need to place the gastroesophageal junction in its normal intra-abdominal position in order to improve its function. Although the repair was associated with a high incidence of recurrence, Allison justly received credit for initiating the modern era of antireflux surgery.[3]

The experience with the Allison repair demonstrated that relief from the symptoms of reflux occurred in those patients whose gastroesophageal junction remained in the intra-abdominal position. The problem was that in 50% of patients, the hernia recurred. Consequently, surgeons were stimulated to develop procedures designed to place and anchor the lower esophagus more effectively in the intra-abdominal position. Initially, these operations consisted of various forms of gastropexy in which an intra-abdominal esophagus was achieved by pulling the stomach down in the abdomen, whether it was herniated or not, and attaching it to the anterior abdominal wall or to any posterior peritoneal structure that seemed strong enough to maintain it there. The design of the gastropexy operation placed the stomach and esophagus on a great deal of continual tension which was further stressed by the normal respiratory and swallowing movements. Consequently, dislodgement of the gastropexies occurred with the return of reflux symptoms.[4,5] The most popular of these operations was the Hill procedure, which anchors the gastroesophageal junction posteriorly to the median arcuate ligament.[6]

787

With the exception of the Hill procedure, these operations did not stand the test of time and were gradually abandoned as more durable methods were sought to achieve an intra-abdominal esophagus. One of these was the Belsey Mark IV repair[7] and the other the Nissen fundoplication.[8,9] Both procedures incorporate a portion of the distal esophagus into the stomach to assure that it will be affected by changes in intra-abdominal pressure transmitted by the gastric conduit. The Belsey Mark IV procedure is, in essence, a partial fundoplication, or an enveloping of the distal esophagus with the gastric fundus over 280°, while the Nissen is a complete fundoplication, or a 360° enveloping of the distal esophagus by the gastric fundus.

With wider application of the Nissen procedure, it became evident that a successful Nissen fundoplication is not simply a matter of wrapping the stomach around the lower esophagus and sewing it in place. Rather, a good deal of judgment and experience is required to determine how tight and how long to make the fundoplication, what portion of the stomach should be used and what conditions preclude the use of the operation. Consequently, Nissen fundoplications have contributed to a number of severe postoperative complications.[10] Most can be attributed to surgical technique and inaccurate selection of patients for operation. If the fundoplication is constructed too long or performed as a wrap rather than an enveloping of the esophagus by the fundus, permanent dysphagia, or odynophagia, may result. Such a fundoplication precludes physiologic belching and vomiting. Instead of performing the operation properly, surgeons began to introduce a variety of partial fundoplications to avoid these problems. They are usually constructed by covering either the anterior or the posterior wall of the distal esophagus with the stomach. This necessitates suturing the fundus of the stomach to the esophagus as the primary and most important portion of the procedure. This suture line is subject to a great deal of stress, and as a consequence, has a limited durability. Although the partial fundoplication operations are successful in preventing reflux and permitting physiologic belching when they remain intact, they disrupt with a distressing frequency.

The most durable of the partial fundoplication procedures is the Belsey Mark IV operation. In this procedure, the attachment of the esophagus to the stomach is more extensive than that advocated for the other partial fundoplications, and the procedure is performed transthoracically, so that the esophagus can be adequately mobilized to construct the repair without undue tension. In situations where the esophagus has shortened, aggressive mobilization does not give a tension-free repair, and disruption or withdrawal of the repair into the chest is the rule, giving rise to the symptoms of recurrent heartburn or dysphagia. Recognition of this problem stimulated the development of an esophageal lengthening technique, by making a tube about the diameter of the esophagus and 5 cm in length along the lesser curvature of the stomach, and constructing a Belsey type partial fundoplication over the tube. This procedure is called a Collis Belsey repair in honor of Dr. J. Leigh Collis who designed the gastroplasty and Dr. Ronald Belsey who designed the antireflux repair.[11]

The main drawback of the Belsey Mark IV procedure is that, when universally applied by surgeons with varied skills, the antireflux protection achieved is not as predictable as with a complete Nissen fundoplication. This situation occurs because the Belsey procedure is difficult to teach and communicate and has less margin for error. In experienced hands, the success of the Belsey operation appears similar to that of the Nissen procedure.

These historical lessons have allowed improvements in antireflux surgery to the point that excellent results can be achieved in the majority of patients given proper patient selection and the meticulous performance of the appropriate procedure. It is hoped that in this era of minimally invasive surgery, mistakes of the past will not be repeated by those who are unfamiliar with the pathophysiology of the disease and history of antireflux surgery.

■ PATHOPHYSIOLOGY

ETIOLOGY OF INCREASED ESOPHAGEAL EXPOSURE TO GASTRIC JUICE

There are three known causes of increased esophageal exposure to gastric juice in patients with gastroesophageal reflux disease. The first is a mechanically incompetent lower esophageal sphincter. This cause accounts for about 60% to 70% of gastroesophageal reflux disease.[12] The identification of this cause is important, since it is the one etiology that antireflux surgery is designed to correct. The other two causes are inefficient esophageal clearance of refluxed gastric juice and abnormalities of the gastric reservoir that augment physiologic reflux. Conceptually, the antireflux mechanism in man can be thought of as a pump, the esophagus; a valve, the lower esophageal sphincter (LES); and a reservoir, the stomach. Because antireflux surgery is directed principally at restoring the function of a defective valve, the status of the other two components should be assessed prior to undertaking surgical therapy.

The Lower Esophageal Sphincter

The lower esophageal sphincter can fail if it has inadequate pressure, a short overall length, or an abnormal abdominal length, that is, the portion of the sphincter exposed to the positive pressure environment of the abdomen as measured by manometry.[13] Clinically, mechanical failure of the lower esophageal sphincter is identified by esophageal manometry if the pressure is <6 mm Hg, the overall length <2 cm, or the abdominal length <1 cm. The probability of increased exposure to gastric juice is 69% to 76% if one component of the sphincter is abnormal, 65% to 88% if two components are abnormal, and 92% if all three are abnormal.[12] This indicates that failure of one or two of the components of the sphincter may be compensated for by the clearance function of the esophageal body. Failure of all three sphincter components inevitably leads to increased esophageal exposure to gastric juice.

The most common reason for a mechanically defective lower esophageal sphincter is inadequate sphincter pressure.[12] The explanation for the reduced pressure is most likely the result of an abnormality of myogenic function. This is supported by two observations. First, the location of the lower esophageal sphincter, in the positive pressure environment of the abdomen, is not a major factor in the genesis of the sphincter pressure, since a positive pressure can still be measured when the abdomen is opened surgically and the distal esophagus is held freely in the surgeon's hand and exposed to atmospheric pressure.[14] Second, Biancini and his associates have shown that the distal esophageal sphincter's muscle response to stretch is reduced in patients with an incompetent cardia.[15] This suggests that sphincter pressure depends on the length-tension characteristics of its smooth muscle. Surgical fundoplication has been shown to restore the mechanical efficiency of the sphincter to normal by correcting the abnormal length-tension characteristics.

Although an inadequate pressure is the most common cause of a mechanically defective sphincter, the efficiency of a sphincter with normal pressure can be nullified by an inadequate abdominal length or an abnormally short overall resting length (Fig 23–1).[16] An adequate abdominal length is important is preventing reflux caused by increases in intra-abdominal pressure that exceed our sphincter pressure. An adequate overall length is important in providing the resistance to reflux caused by increases in intragastric pressure over sphincter pressure that occurs independent of increases in intra-abdominal pressure. Therefore, patients with a low sphincter pressure, or those with a normal pressure but a short abdominal length, are unable to protect against reflux caused by fluctuations of intra-abdominal pressure that occur with daily activities or changes in body position. Patients with a low sphincter pressure or those with a normal pressure but short overall length are unable to protect against reflux related to independent increases in gastric pressure caused by outlet obstruction, aerophagia, gluttony or altered pressure volume relationship of the stomach as occurs in various gastropathies. In this situation, reflux can occur whenever an increase in gastric pressure exceeds the sphincter pressure that is necessary to provide competency for the overall length of sphincter present. Persons who have a short overall length on a resting motility study are at a disadvantage in protecting against normal fluctuations is gastric pressure secondary to eating, and suffer postprandial reflux. This situation occurs because with normal dilation of the stomach sphincter, length becomes shorter and, if short in the resting state, there is very little tolerance for further shortening before incompetency occurs.

Resistance to the reflux of gastric juice into the esophagus is brought about by the combined effects of pressure, and the overall length of the sphincter can be determined by summing the effects of the radial pressures extended over the entire length of the sphincter. This measurement, called the sphincter pressure vector volume (SPVV) can be quantitated by three-dimensional computerized imaging of four or more vector pressures, measured at all points along the sphincter length, and calculating the volume of this image (Fig 23–2).[17,18] Vector volume measurements are, at present, the most accurate measure of sphincter competence, and are markedly abnormal with severe disease. It must be remembered that even if the SPVV is normal, the sphincter can still be defective if its abdominal length is inadequate.

Esophageal Clearance

The second component of the antireflux mechanism in man is effective esophageal pump.[19] Ineffective esophageal pumps can result in an abnormal esophageal exposure to gastric juice in individuals who have a mechanically effective lower esophageal sphincter and normal gastric function but are unable to clear physiologic reflux episodes. This situation is relatively rare, and ineffectual clearance is more apt to be seen in association with a mechanically defective sphincter, where esophageal body function deteriorates from repetitive inflammation and augments the esophageal exposure to gastric juice by prolonging the duration of each reflux episode.

Four factors important in esophageal clearance are gravity, esophageal motor activity, salivation, and anchoring of the distal esophagus in the abdomen.[20,21] The loss of any one of these factors can augment esophageal exposure to gastric juice by contributing to ineffective clearance. The loss of gravity accounts for one reason why reflux episodes are more prolonged in the supine position. In this position, esophageal clearance depends almost completely on the peristalsis of the esophageal body. The bulk of refluxed gastric juice is cleared from the esophagus by a primary peristaltic

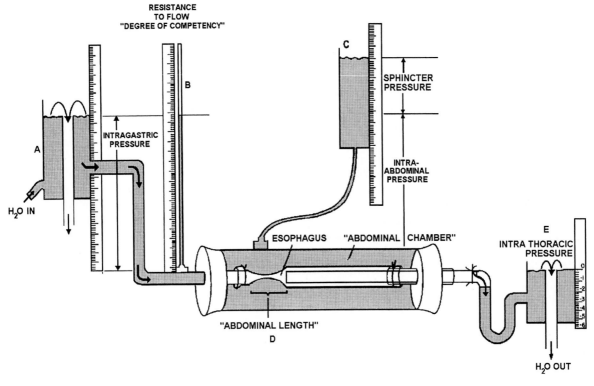

A

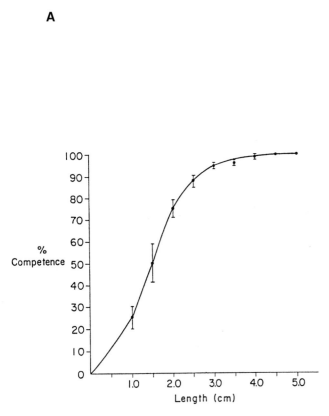

B

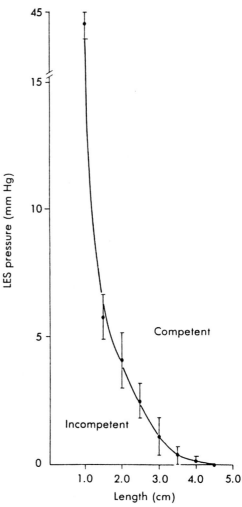

C

Figure 23–1. A. Schematic drawing of the in vitro model used to study the mechanics of the intra-abdominal esophagus. **B.** Effect of length on the competency of the intra-abdominal esophagus. **C.** Interrelationship between intrinsic tone and length to the competency of the intra-abdominal esophagus.

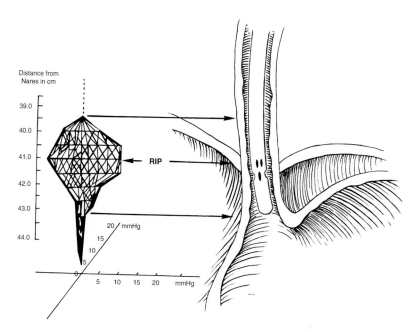

Figure 23–2. Computerized three-dimensional imaging of lower esophageal sphincter. A catheter with four to eight radial side holes is withdrawn through the gastroesophageal junction. For each level of the pullback, the radially measured pressures are plotted around an axis representing gastric baseline pressure. When a stepwise pullback technique is used, the respiratory inversion point (RIP) can be identified.

wave initiated by a pharyngeal swallow. Secondary peristaltic waves, although able to be initiated by either distention of the esophagus or a drop in the intraesophageal pH, have been shown, on ambulatory motility studies, to be uncommon and have a more minimal role in clearance than previously thought (Fig 23–3).[22] The esophageal contractions initiated by a drop in esophageal pH rarely have a normal peristaltic pattern and usually have a broad-based, powerful, and synchronous pattern. They reduce the efficiency of esophageal clearance by encouraging the regurgitation of refluxed material into the pharynx, predisposing the patient to aspiration. They also may cause chest pain that is commonly confused with angina pectoris.

Manometry of the esophageal body can detect failure of esophageal clearance by analyzing the contraction amplitude and speed of wave progression through the esophagus. The work of Kahrilas and Dodds has shown that the amplitude of an esophageal contraction required to clear the esophagus of barium varies according to the level.[23] Lower segments require a greater amplitude than upper segments, and inadequate amplitude results in ineffective clearance.

Salivation contributes to esophageal clearance by neutralizing the minute amount of acid that is left following a peristaltic wave.[24] Return of esophageal pH to normal is significantly longer if salivary flow is reduced, such as after radiotherapy, and shorter if saliva is stimulated by sucking lozenges. Saliva production also may be increased by the presence of acid in the lower esophagus. When this occurs, the patient experiences excessive mucous in the throat. Clinically, this is referred to as

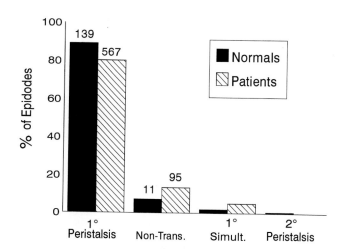

Figure 23–3. Peristaltic sequence analysis of 24 hour ambulatory motility studies in normal volunteers and patients with gastroesophageal reflux.

"water brash."[25] The reduction in saliva flow during the night also contributes to the prolongation of reflux episodes while asleep in the supine position.

The presence of a hiatal hernia also can contribute to an esophageal propulsion defect owing to loss of anchorage of the esophagus in the abdomen, resulting in a reduced efficiency of acid clearance (Fig 23–4).[20,26] Sloan and Kahrilas have shown that complete esophageal emptying without retrograde flow as achieved in 86% of test swallows in control subjects without a hiatal hernia, 66% in patients with a reducing hiatal hernia, and only 32% in patients with a nonreducing hiatal hernia.[27] Impaired clearance in patients with nonreducing hiatal hernias is one of the ways a hiatal hernia contributes to the pathogenesis of gastroesophageal reflux disease.

The Gastric Reservoir

The third component of the antireflux mechanism in man is a properly functioning reservoir, or stomach. Abnormalities of the gastric reservoir that increase esophageal exposure to gastric juice include gastric dilation, increased intragastric pressure, a persistent gastric reservoir, and increased gastric acid secretion. The effect of gastric dilation is to shorten the overall length of the lower esophageal sphincter, resulting in a decrease in the sphincter resistance to reflux.[13] This is analogous to the shortening of a balloon neck on inflation. Excessive gastric dilation in patients with gastroesophageal reflux disease commonly results from aerophagia owing to an unconscious increase in pharyngeal swallowing in an

effort to improve esophageal clearance. Such dilation accounts for the symptom of bloating often seen in these patients. Each pharyngeal swallow results in the propulsion of 1 to 2 cc of air into the stomach. This occurs in chronic gum chewers, patients with decreased saliva secondary to Sjorgen's syndrome or previous head and neck radiation, and patients who have altered esophageal motor function and require multiple pharyngeal swallows to propel food into the stomach.

Increased intragastric pressure occurs from the outlet obstruction or deinervation of the gastric fundus and body from a vagotomy or neuropathy secondary to diabetes or systemic sclerosis. The latter condition interferes with the normal active relaxation of the stomach.[28] In these abnormalities, the increase in intragastric pressure, owing to alteration in the pressure volume relationship, occurs independently from increases in intraabdominal pressure and can overcome the sphincter resistance, resulting in reflux.

Delayed gastric emptying increases the exposure of the esophagus to gastric juice by accentuating physiologic reflux by the presence of a persistent gastric reservoir. It is most commonly caused by gastric atony secondary to myogenic abnormalities from diffuse neuromuscular disorders, such as diabetes, anticholinergic medications, and postviral infections.[29] Nonmyogenic causes are vagotomy, antropyloric dysfunction, and duodenal dismotility. Delayed gastric emptying also can result in increased exposure of the gastric mucosa to bile and pancreatic juice refluxed from the duodenum into the stomach, with the development of gastritis.[30]

Gastric hypersecretion can increase esophageal exposure to gastric acid juice by the physiologic reflux of increased volumes of concentrated gastric acid. Barlow has shown that 28% of patients with increased esophageal exposure to gastric juice, measured by 24 hour pH monitoring, have gastric hypersecretion.[31] He showed, however, that a mechanically defective sphincter was more important than gastric hypersection in the development of complications of the disease. This indicates that, from a therapeutic perspective, treatment of a patient with severe complications should be directed at correction of the mechanically defective sphincter rather than the suppression of acid. In this respect, GERD differs from duodenal ulcer disease, since the latter is specifically related to gastric hypersection.

THE CONCEPT OF TRANSIENT RELAXATION OF THE LOWER ESOPHAGEAL SPHINCTER

Transient relaxations of the LES (TRLESs) can be detected in both normal subjects and patients with gastroesophageal reflux disease, and have been proposed as a mechanism underlying increased esophageal acid exposure.[32] These transient relaxations can be corre-

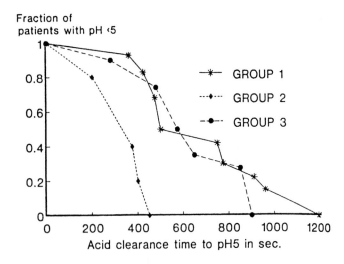

Figure 23–4. Acid clearance in subjects with hiatal hernia and symptoms of GERD (group 1), subjects with no hiatal hernia but symptoms of GERD (group 2), and subjects with hiatal hernia but no symptoms of GERD (group 3). The y-axis shows the number of patients who persist with esophageal pH <5. The acid clearance time to ≥pH 5 is significantly faster in group 2 (symptomatic, no hiatal hernia) compared with group 1 (symptomatic, hiatal hernia) and group 3 (asymptomatic, hiatal hernia). Groups 1 and 3 have similar acid clearance times. (From Mittal RK, Lange RC, McCallum RW. Identification and mechanism of delayed esophageal acid clearance in subjects with hiatus hernia. *Gastroenterology* 1987;92:130–135)

lated to esophageal acid exposure and have been detected by short-term simultaneous monitoring of esophageal pH, pharyngeal and esophageal body motor activity, and the pressure within the LES. Fundamental to this concept is that reflux occurs only when the LES relaxes inappropriately to zero (Fig 23–5). Transient relaxation of the LES is a normal physiologic event that occurs with pharyngeal swallowing and probably accounts for a physiological reflux event, if no peristaltic wave of the esophageal body follows. The cause of inappropriate TRLESs is poorly understood, although gastric distention has been proposed as the major stimulus.

Several features of TRLESs raise doubt as to their importance as the major mechanism underlying GERD.

First, relaxations are suppressed in the supine period and during sleep. This makes it difficult to explain why supine reflux episodes are commonly seen in patients with GERD.[32] Second, correlation of the frequency of TRLESs occurring in association with reflux episodes is greatest in patients with a mechanically normal LES, such as normal subjects, and in patients with uncomplicated GERD. As the severity of GERD progresses, particularly in association with a mechanically deficient LES, the association of TRLESs with esophageal acid exposure becomes uncommon. Finally, recent data in which LES was monitored via a gastrostomy, rather than the usual transpharyngeal catheter, showed that more than half of the observed TRLESs may result as artifact from pharyngeal stimulation by the measuring catheters.[33] Taken together, these data indicate that while TRLESs may account for the majority of physiologic reflux episodes, they are unlikely to be responsible for severe pathologic reflux seen in patients with complicated GERD.

THE NATURAL HISTORY OF GASTROESOPHAGEAL REFLUX DISEASE

Studies on the natural history of GERD are difficult to perform because of the mobility of modern society. Those studies that have been done indicate that most patients have limited disease responsive to simple lifestyle, dietary habits, and medical therapy and do not go on to develop complications. Investigations of the natural history of GERD in the absence of esophagitis have demonstrated return of symptoms in the majority of patients following cessation of medical therapy.[34] Furthermore, progression to a more severe form of the disease occurs in 10% to 20% of patients.[35] Increasingly, GERD is recognized as a chronic disease requiring lifelong medical treatment to prevent symptomatic recurrence, with the potential for progressive esophageal injury and end organ dysfunction. Surgery provides the only known means of altering the natural history of the disease.

The Swiss population tends to be less mobile and their lifestyle is highly organized. Thus, physicians at the University of Laussanne, Switzerland have been able to longitudinally follow a large number of patients with reflux esophagitis. In the Laussanne region, the prevalence of esophagitis at endoscopy rose from 190 per 100 000 population, in 1970, to 1058 per 100 000 in 1980. While the major reason for this increase is likely the wider availability and use of upper endoscopy, the increased consumption of alcohol, tobacco, large fatty meals, and perhaps, even antisecretory agents may have played a role. Savary and colleagues have investigated the natural history of grades 1 to 3 esophagitis in 701 patients receiving medical therapy, including omeprazole (Fig 23–6). Forty-six percent of patients had an isolated episode of esophagitis, 31% had recurrent episodes of

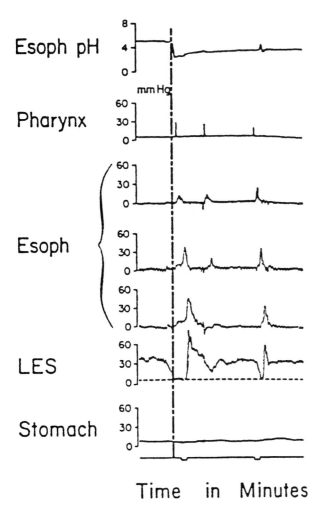

Figure 23–5. Gastroesophageal reflux associated with a transient LES relaxation in a patient with reflux esophagitis. Before acid reflux, resting LES pressure was stable at about 30 mm Hg above intragastric pressure (*broken line*). Reflux of acid into the esophagus occurred during a transient LES relaxation that was not related to swallowing. Reflux occurred only when the LES relaxed completely so that its pressure equaled intragastric pressure. After acid reflux, three swallow-induced peristaltic sequences were recorded in the body of the esophagus. (From Dodds WJ, Dent J, Hogan WJ, et al. Mechanisms of gastroesophageal reflux in patients with reflux esophagitis *N Engl J Med* 1982;307:1547–1552)

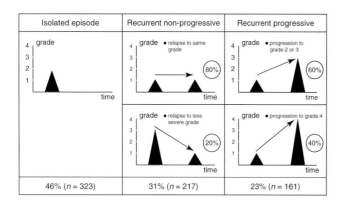

Figure 23–6. The natural history of erosive esophagitis in patients with GERD. This study was carried out in Lausanne, Switzerland, with a relatively fixed population of patients who underwent serial endoscopy over the course of several years. (From Ollyo JB, Monnier P, Fontolliet C, et al, *Gullett* 1993;3(suppl):3–10)

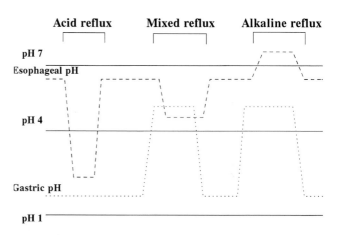

Figure 23–7. Diagrammatic representation of the criteria used for the simultaneous analysis of gastric (*broken line*) and esophageal (*dotted line*) pH. Esophageal reflux is a decrease in the esophagus pH to <4 associated with an acid gastric pH. Mixed refluxes are characterized by a decrease in esophageal pH from the baseline to a value >4 associated with increases in the gastric pH to >4. Alkaline refluxes are those with increases of esophageal pH to >7 associated with an increase in the gastric pH to >4. (From Fiorucci S, Santucci L, Chiucchiu S, Morelli A. Gastric Acidity and Gastroesophageal Reflux Patterns in Patients with Esophagitis. *Gastroenterology* 1992;103:855–861)

esophagitis but no increase in their severity, and 23% developed recurrent and progressive mucosal damage.

At present, there is no reliable method to identify which patients will develop progressive disease. Although the concept of endoscopic surveillance has largely centered upon those patients with Barrett's esophagus, it seems prudent to suggest intermittent upper endoscopy as a means to detect patients with progressive or recurrent disease. Patients who fall into these categories should be offered early antireflux surgery as a means to prevent the development of the irreversible complication of Barrett's esophagus or the progressive deterioration of esophageal function.

DEVELOPMENT OF COMPLICATIONS OF INCREASED ESOPHAGEAL EXPOSURE TO GASTRIC JUICE— THE IMPORTANCE OF ALKALINE REFLUX

Reflux of alkaline duodenal contents into the stomach and esophagus is increasingly recognized as an important pathophysiologic factor in GERD. Pure alkaline reflux, that is, increased esophageal exposure to gastric juice with a pH >7, is an uncommon although well-documented event, occurring almost exclusively after cholecystectomy or surgical disruption of the antral pyloric mechanism. The vast majority of patients reflux either pure acid gastric juice or a mixture of gastric and duodenal juice. Pellegrini and his associates investigated reflux patterns by simultaneously monitoring antral, fundic, and esophageal pH in 67 patients with symptoms suggestive of GERD and no previous history of gastric surgery.[36] Patients were classified as acid,

acid/alkaline, or alkaline refluxers based upon the characterization of their reflux episodes (Fig 23–7).[37] Forty-two percent of the patients were found to have acid reflux, 40% had acid/alkaline reflux, and 18% had alkaline reflux. Fiorucci performed a similar study using just a fundic and esophageal probe and related the type of reflux episode to the severity of esophagitis.[37] He found that severe esophagitis was related to a high prevalence of acid, alkaline, or mixed reflux episodes (Fig 23–8).[37] He further showed that patients who had mixed reflux episodes had a higher average gastric pH, suggesting that the mixed reflux episodes were the result of duodenogastric regurgitation (Fig 23–9).[37]

Recognition of Alkaline Gastroesophageal Reflux

The term alkaline gastroesophageal reflux is somewhat of a misnomer since the pH in the lower esophagus rarely exceeds 8. By convention, alkaline reflux is said to be present when there is excessive esophageal exposure to a pH >7, owing to repetitive rises in esophageal pH to >7 during a time when the gastric pH is >4. The quantification of this exposure is based on six measurements: the percentage of total, upright, and supine time the esophagus has a pH >7; number of episodes that pH of the esophagus exceeds 7; number of episodes lasting longer than 5 minutes; and longest episode the pH remained above 7.[38] Normal values for these six components have been derived from 50 asymptomatic control subjects. The upper limits of normal were established at the 95th percentile. If a patient's values are above this level, he or she is considered abnormal for the component measured. The six components are combined into

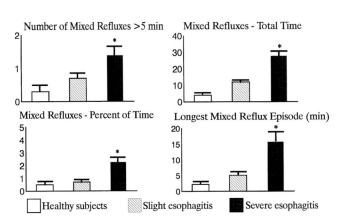

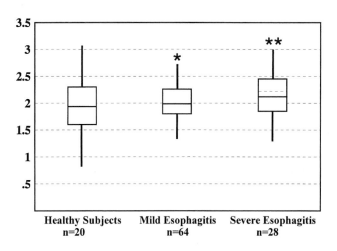

Figure 23–8. Pattern of mixed reflux in healthy subjects, patients with mild esophagitis, and patients with severe-complicated esophagitis. *P<.01 vs both healthy subjects and patients with mild esophagitis. (From Fiorucci S, Santucci L, Chiucchiu S, Morelli A. Gastric Acidity and Gastroesophageal Reflux Patterns in Patients with Esophagitis. *Gastroenterology* 1992;103:855–861)

Figure 23–9. Box - Whisker plots of gastric pH and gastric acidity in healthy subjects and patients with mild esophagitis or severe-complicated esophagitis. Gastric pH was determined from 540 individual pH values obtained by determining the mean of 2-minute intervals. Postprandial pH values (2 hours) were not considered. Mean 18 hour gastric pH was significantly higher in patients with severe esophagitis than in healthy subjects (P<.001) or patients with mild esophagitis (P<.01). *P<.01 vs severe esophagitis; **P<.001 vs healthy subjects. (From Fiorucci S, Santucci L, Chiucchiu S, Morelli A. Gastric Acidity and Gastroesophageal Reflux Patterns in Patients with Esophagitis. *Gastroenterology* 1992;103:855–861).

one expression of the overall esophageal alkaline exposure, by calculating a composite alkaline pH score.[39]

The presence of increased esophageal exposure to pH >7 must be interpreted carefully. Increased exposure in this pH range can be caused by abnormal calibration of the pH recorder, the presence of dental infection which increases salivary pH,[40] the presence of esophageal obstruction resulting in static pools of saliva with an increase in pH secondary to bacterial overgrowth,[41] or the regurgitation of a mixture of gastric and duodenal juice that results in the pH of the esophagus to rise above 7. When using a properly calibrated probe, in the absence of dental infections or esophageal obstruction, the percent time the pH is measured above 7 has been shown to correlate with the concentration of bile acids continuously aspirated from the esophagus during a 24 hour period.[42]

Recently, it has been shown that gastric juice with a pH of 1.5 must contain at least 70% of duodenal juice in order to raise the pH >7 (unpublished data) and less if some saliva is present. However, it appears difficult to measure an abnormal esophageal exposure to pH >7 in the absence of excessive amounts of duodenogastric reflux. It is important to understand that increased esophageal exposure to pH >7 only infers increased esophageal exposure to duodenal juice (bile and/or pancreatic juice). When present, it represents only the tip of the iceberg of the total time the esophagus actually is exposed to duodenal contents.

Newer tests that can directly measure the compo-

nents of duodenal juice in the esophagus have shown that reflux episodes containing components of duodenal juice can occur when the esophageal pH remains in its normal range of 4 to 7, or even when the esophageal pH drops below 4 as in acid reflux episodes. Data from 24 hour esophageal aspiration studies indicate that, compared to normal subjects, abnormal amounts of bile are detected in patients with proven acid reflux during the postprandial and supine periods (Fig 23–10).[43] Studies using a fiberoptic probe, which recognizes intraluminal bilirubin as a marker of duodenal juice, have shown that bile, and hence, duodenal juice, is commonly present in the refluxate independent of its pH. Thus, the measurement of increased esophageal acid exposure does not exclude the reflux of components of duodenal juice. In general, there appears to be a direct relationship between the degree of duodenal juice present in the refluxate and the severity of mucosal injury (ie, refluxing a mixture of duodenal and gastric juice is worse than gastric juice alone). Patients with Barrett's esophagus, for example, had a significantly higher amount of bilirubin in their refluxate than patients with uncomplicated reflux disease. The latter group showed higher amounts of bilirubin than normal subjects, but the increase is not statistically significant (Fig 23–11). The refluxing of a high percentage of duodenal juice with gastric juice in Barrett's esophagus is presumably owing to excessive duodenogastric reflux present in these patients. When the mixed gastric and duodenal juice is refluxed into the esophagus, there is little

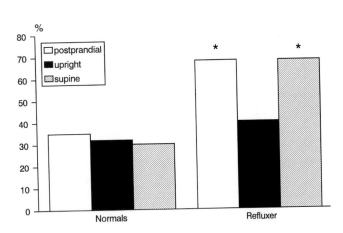

Figure 23–10. Percentage of subjects with bile on esophageal aspiration during postprandial, upright and supine period in normals and patients with reflux disease (*P<.01 vs normals).

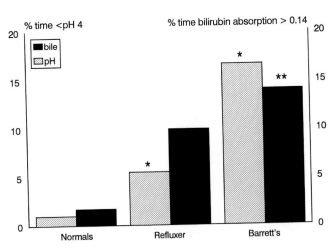

Figure 23–11. Esophageal acid and duodenal juice exposure expressed as percentage total time pH <4 and percentage total time bilirubin absorption >0.14 in normals, patients with reflux disease and patients with Barrett's esophagus. *P<.03 and **P<.01 vs. normals.

change in the esophageal pH and, consequently, minimal heartburn. Despite the lack of symptoms, mucosal damage still appears, probably from activated pancreatic enzymes.

Duodenogastric Reflux as the Cause of Increased Esophageal Alkaline Exposure

Several authors have demonstrated concomitant increases in duodenogastric reflux in patients with symptomatic gastroesophageal reflux disease.[44–46] Combined esophageal and gastric pH monitoring has shown that the alkaline component is probably the result of excessive reflux of duodenal contents through the stomach and into the distal esophagus. In normal subjects, 24 hour gastric pH monitoring with multiple gastric probes has shown that elevations in antral pH typically occur in the early hours of the morning and progress from the pylorus into the proximal stomach.[47] Aspiration has confirmed the presence of bile during the same time periods when elevation in gastric pH was noted.[48,49] Consequently, the reflux of a limited amount of duodenal content into the stomach, particularly in the early morning hours, is a normal physiological event.[50,51]

Excessive reflux of duodenal contents into the stomach occurs after cholecystectomy, pyloromyotomy, pylorectomy, antrectomy, or gastroenterostomy. The typical symptom complex includes epigastric pain, nausea, and bilious vomiting. Peristomal gastritis often is seen and may progress to intestinalization of the gastric mucosa and possibly even malignant change.[52,53] Abnormal duodenogastric reflux also is known to occur as a primary disease process, owing to disordered motility of the antropyloro-duodenal complex. When excessive duodenogastric reflux occurs in a patient with a mechan-

ically defective lower esophageal sphincter, increased esophageal exposure to components of duodenal juice can be expected to occur. Further, this exposure may occur at the normal pH interval of the esophagus, resulting in very few symptoms (Fig 23–12).

Consequences of Increased Esophageal Alkaline Exposure

The complications of gastroesophageal reflux result from the damage inflicted by gastric juice on the esophageal mucosa or respiratory epithelium and changes caused by their subsequent repair and fibrosis. Complications of reflux are esophagitis, stricture, and Barrett's esophagus and the complication from repetitive aspiration is progressive pulmonary fibrosis. The observation that complications of gastroesophageal reflux can occur in patients with a mechanically normal sphincter and that some patients who have a mechanically defective sphincter can be free of complications indicates that factors other than a mechanically defective sphincter, such as the composition of the refluxed gastric juice, are important in the development of the complications.

The prevalence of reflux complications (ie, esophagitis, stricture, and Barrett's esophagus) are related to the presence of a mechanically defective sphincter and an increased esophageal exposure to both acid and alkalinity (Fig 23–13).[54] Further, the severity of the complications are significantly higher in patients with acid/alkaline reflux, as compared with those patients with only acid reflux (Fig 23–14). These estimations come from measuring an increase in esophageal exposure to pH >7 and pH <4 and represent the most severe forms of mixed reflux. In other patients, the esophagus is exposed to mixed reflux, but the degree of the duo-

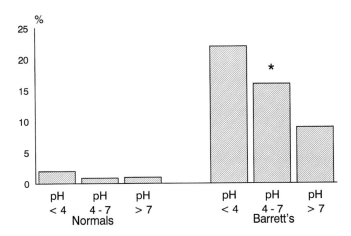

Figure 23–12. Median percentage time of pH <4, pH 4 to 7, and pH <7 spent at bilirubin absorbance >0.14 in normals and patients with Barrett's esophagus. * P <.01 vs normals.

denal component is not sufficient to push the esophageal exposure of pH >7 to abnormal levels.

Differences of opinion exist as to what ingredient in the refluxed gastric or duodenal juice produces the mucosal injury. Components from both have been implicated. Our current knowledge regarding the noxious component in the refluxed juice is based on the elegant studies of Johnson and Harmon.[55] Hydrogen ion injury to the esophageal squamous mucosa occurs mainly at a pH below 2. It results in injury to the mucosal barrier, but rarely produces mucosal lesions or inflammatory changes. In an acid refluxate, the enzyme pepsin appears to be the major injurious agent. Reflux of bile and pancreatic enzymes into the stomach can either protect or augment esophageal mucosal injury. For instance, in a patient whose gastric acid secretion maintained an acid environment, the presence of bile salts would attenuate the injurious effect of pepsin, and the acid gastric environment would inactivate the trypsin. Such a patient would have bile-containing acid gastric juice that, when refluxed into the esophagus, would injure the mucosal barrier and the epithelial cells, but would be less caustic than the reflux of acid gastric juice containing pepsin. In contrast, a patient with significant duodenogastric reflux may create an alkaline intragastric environment that supports optimal trypsin activity and encourages the dissolution of bile salts with a high pk_a that potentiate the enzyme's effect. Reflux of this juice into the esophagus causes severe esophagitis. Hence, duodenogastric reflux and the acid secretory capacity of the stomach interrelate by altering the pH and enzymatic activity of the refluxed juice to modulate the injurious effects of the enzymes on the esophageal mucosa.[56]

Similarly, the disparity in injury, or mucosal barrier abnormalities, caused by acid and bile alone, as op-

posed to esophagitis caused by pepsin and trypsin, explains the poor correlation between severity of heartburn and mucosal pathology. The reflux of acid gastric juice contaminated with duodenal juice can readily break the esophageal mucosal barrier, irritate nerve endings in the papillae close to the luminal surface, and cause severe heartburn. The bile salts in the duodenal juice inhibit pepsin, the acid pH environment of the stomach inactivate trypsin, and thus the patient has severe heartburn with little or no gross evidence of esophagitis. In contrast, the patient who refluxed alkaline gastric juice may have minimal heartburn because of the reduction of hydrogen ions in the refluxed juice, but has endoscopic esophagitis owing to bile salt potentiation of trypsin activity on the esophageal mucosa. This suggests that the combination of duodenogastric reflux and gastroesophageal reflux may be more detrimental than gastroesophageal reflux alone.

The Sequelae of Mucosal Injury

When the composition of the refluxed gastric juice is such that sustained or repetitive esophageal injury occurs, two sequelae can result. First, a luminal stricture can develop from submucosal and eventually, intramural fibrosis. Second, a Barrett's esophagus can develop when replacement of destroyed squamous mucosa by a peculiar form of healing with columnar epithelium occurs.[57] The columnar epithelium is resistant to acid and is associated with the alleviation of the complaint of heartburn. Endoscopically, the Barrett's

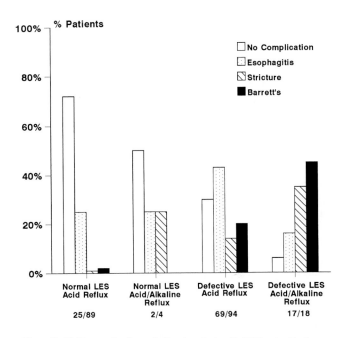

Figure 23–13. The severity of complications in patients with GERD and acid reflux or acid/alkaline reflux with and without a mechanically defective LES.

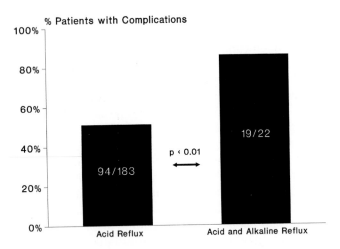

Figure 23-14. Prevalence and severity of esophageal mucosal injury in patients with only acid reflux and acid/alkaline reflux.

changes can be quiescent or associated with complications of esophagitis, stricture, Barrett's ulceration, and dysplasia. Clinical evidence suggests that the complication associated with Barrett's may be the result of the continuous injury and repair from refluxed alkalinized duodenogastric juice.[46] The most important complication is the development of dysplastic changes in the Barrett's epithelium that initiates the progression to adenocarcinoma. The incidence of this occurring in patients with Barrett's esophagus is yet to be determined, but is predicted to be between 0.5% and 10%.[58]

It appears that the healing of the mucosal lesions by Barrett's metaplasia can occur at any time during the course of the disease and is not an event that occurs only in patients with severe longstanding disease. As columnar epithelial healing occurs, it gives the impression that the metaplasia is advancing into the area of inflammation, as a slow progressive process. This may not be so; rather, the whole process may occur suddenly. An esophageal stricture can be associated with severe esophagitis or Barrett's esophagus.[59] In the latter situation, it occurs at the site of maximal inflammatory injury (ie, the columnar-squamous epithelial interface). Patients who have a stricture in the absence of Barrett's esophagus should have the presence of gastroesophageal reflux documented before the etiology of the stricture is ascribed to reflux esophagitis. In patients with normal acid exposure, the stricture may be owing to a drug-induced chemical injury resulting in the lodgment of a capsule or tablet in the distal esophagus.[60] In such patients, dilation usually corrects the problem of dysphagia. Heartburn, which may have occurred only because of the chemical injury, need not be treated. It is also possible for drug-induced injuries to occur in patients who have underlying esophagitis and

a distal esophageal stricture secondary to gastroesophageal reflux. In this situation, a long string-like stricture progressively develops as a result of repetitive caustic injury from capsule or tablet lodgment on top of an initial reflux stricture. These strictures are often resistant to dilation.

When the refluxed gastric juice is of sufficient quantity, it can reach the pharynx with the potential for pharyngeal tracheal aspiration, causing symptoms of repetitive cough, choking, hoarseness, and recurrent pneumonia.[61] This is often an unrecognized complication of gastroesophageal reflux disease, since either the pulmonary or the gastrointestinal symptoms may predominate in the clinical situation and focus the physician's attention on one to the exclusion of the other. Studies have identified three factors that are important in the pulmonary complication of reflux. First, the loss of respiratory epithelium secondary to the aspiration of gastric contents can take up to seven days to heal and may give rise to a chronic cough between episodes of aspiration. When studied during this time the cough may not be related to a reflux episode. Second, the presence of an esophageal motility disorder is observed in 75% of patients with reflux-induced aspiration and is believed to promote the aboral movement of the refluxate toward the pharynx. Finally, if the pH in the cervical esophagus is below 4 for 3% of the time, the respiratory symptoms have a high probability of being caused by aspiration.[62] Caution must be exerted in treating the patient with an abnormal motility disorder by surgery, since a component of their aspiration may be retained esophageal secretions and their cough will persist.

■ DIAGNOSIS

DEFINITION AND SYMPTOMS OF THE DISEASE

Gastroesophageal reflux is a common disease that accounts for approximately 75% of esophageal pathology. It is now recognized as a chronic disease requiring life-long medical therapy. Antireflux surgery is the only effective and long-term therapy and is the only treatment that is able to modify the natural history of recurrent progressive reflux esophagitis. Despite the common prevalence of gastroesophageal reflux disease, it can be one of the most challenging diagnostic and therapeutic problems in benign esophageal disease. A contributing factor to this is the lack of a universally accepted definition of the disease.[63]

The most simplistic approach is to define the disease by its symptoms. However, symptoms thought to be indicative of gastroesophageal reflux disease, such as heartburn or acid regurgitation, are very common in the general population and many individuals consider them to be normal and do not seek medical attention. Even when excessive, these symptoms are not specific for gastroesophageal reflux. They can be caused by other diseases such as achalasia, diffuse spasm, esophageal carcinoma, pyloric stenosis, cholelithiasis, gastritis, gastric or duodenal ulcer, and coronary artery disease. We recently assessed the reliability of the symptoms of heartburn and regurgitation in the diagnosis of gastroesophageal reflux disease in 161 patients referred for surgical therapy with these complaints. Only 65% of these patients had objective evidence of reflux on 24 hour pH monitoring, 7% had normal esophageal exposure to gastric juice, although manometry demonstrated an esophageal motor disorder. The remaining 28% had no detectable esophageal pathology. The overall sensitivity and specificity of the typical symptoms of heartburn and regurgitation to diagnose GERD were 64% and 58%, respectively. Thus, symptoms alone are not a reliable means of detecting this disease. Further, atypical symptoms of gastroesophageal reflux such as nausea, vomiting, postprandial fullness, chest pain, choking, chronic cough, wheezing, asthma and hoarseness are common, if not more common than typical symptoms. Failure to recognize such symptoms can result in pulmonary complications, such as bronchiolitis, recurrent pneumonia, and idiopathic pulmonary fibrosis. Extensive cardiac evaluation is commonplace in the presence of chest pain, although a normal coronary angiogram rarely results in the recognition of GERD as a possible explanation for the patient's symptoms. The issue is further confused by the fact that gastroesophageal reflux disease can coexist with cardiac and pulmonary disease.

An alternative definition for GERD is the presence of endoscopic esophagitis. Using this criteria for diagnosis assumes that all patients who have esophagitis have excessive regurgitation of gastric juice into their esophagus. This is true in 90% of patients, but in 10%, the esophagitis is caused by other etiologies, the most common being unrecognized chemical injury from drug ingestion.[60] In addition, the definition leaves undiagnosed those patients who have symptoms of gastroesophageal reflux, but do not have endoscopic esophagitis.

A third approach to define gastroesophageal reflux disease is to measure the basic pathophysiologic abnormality of the disease, that is, increased exposure of the esophagus to gastric juice. In the past, this was inferred by the presence of a hiatal hernia, later by endoscopic esophagitis, and more recently, by a hypotensive lower esophageal sphincter pressure. The development of a miniaturized pH electrode and data recorder allowed measurement of esophageal exposure to gastric juice by calculating the percent time the pH was <4 during a 24

hour period. This provided an opportunity to objectively identify the presence of the disease and stimulated a rational step-by-step approach to determining the cause for the abnormal esophageal exposure to gastric juice. We have recently come to realize that some patients with excessive duodenogastric reflux can regurgitate gastric juice with a pH of 5 or more into the esophagus. Most patients in whom this occurs also will have abnormal esophageal exposure to gastric juice with a pH <4, and are mixed acid and alkaline refluxers. A few will reflux only alkalized gastric juice and will require an esophageal probe sensitive to bile in order to detect duodenal juices.

PREOPERATIVE ASSESSMENT OF PATIENTS WITH GASTROESOPHAGEAL REFLUX DISEASE

24 Hour Ambulatory pH Monitoring

The most direct method of measuring increased esophageal exposure to gastric juice is by an indwelling pH electrode.[38,64] Prolonged monitoring of esophageal pH is performed by placing a pH probe 5 cm above the manometrically measured upper border of the distal sphincter for 24 hours. Such measurement quantitates the actual time the esophageal mucosa is exposed to gastric juice, measures the ability of the esophagus to clear refluxed acid, and correlates esophageal acid exposure to the symptoms of the patient. A 24 hour period is necessary so that measurements are made during one complete circadian cycle. This timeframe allows for measuring the effect of a physiologic activity, such as working, eating, or sleeping, on the reflux of gastric juice into the esophagus (Fig 23–15).

It is important to emphasize that 24 hour esophageal pH monitoring should *not* be considered a test for reflux, but rather, a measurement of the esophageal exposure to gastric juice. The measurement is expressed by the time the esophageal pH was below a given threshold during the 24 hour period. This single assessment, although concise, does not reflect how the exposure has occurred; that is, did it occur in a few long episodes or several short episodes? Consequently, two other assessments are necessary: the frequency of the reflux episodes and their duration.

The units used to express esophageal exposure to gastric juice are: (1) cumulative time the esophageal pH is below a chosen threshold, expressed as the percent of the total, upright, and supine monitored time; (2) frequency of reflux episodes below a chosen threshold, expressed as number of episodes per 24 hours; and (3) duration of the episodes expressed as the number of episodes >5 minutes per 24 hours and the time in minutes of the longest episode recorded.[65] Normal values for these six components of the 24 hour record at each whole number pH threshold were derived from 50

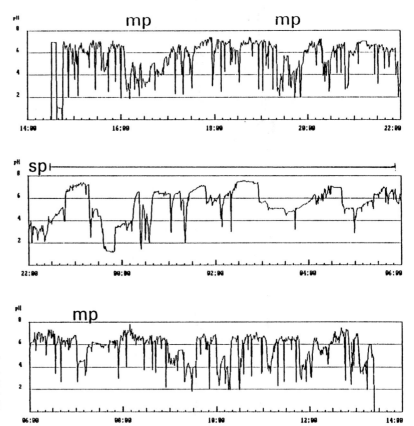

Figure 23–15. Strip chart display of a 24 hour esophageal pH monitoring study in a patient with increased esophageal acid exposure. MP=meal period; SP = supine period. (From DeMeester TR, Stein HJ, Fuchs KH. Physiologic diagnostic studies. In: Zuidema GD, Orringer MB (eds). *Shackelford's Surgery of the Alimentary Tract.* 3rd ed. vol I. Philadelphia, PA: WB Saunders; 1991:119)

asymptomatic control subjects. The upper limits of normal were established at the 95th percentile. Fig 23–16 shows the median and the 95th percentile of the normal values for each component. Patient values are shown in black. If the values are outside the 95th percentile of normal subjects, the patient is considered abnormal for the component measured. Most centers use pH 4 as the threshold. Using this threshold, there was a uniformity of normal values for the six components from centers throughout the world, when compared at a Zurich conference.[66] The normal values for the six components are shown in Table 23–1. This comparison indicated that esophageal acid exposure can be quantitated, and that normal individuals have similar values despite nationality or dietary habits.

To combine the results of the six components into one expression of the overall esophageal acid exposure below a pH threshold, a pH score was calculated by using the standard deviation of the mean of each of the six components, measured in the 50 normal subjects, as a weighing factor.[67] By accepting an abstract zero level two standard deviations below the mean, the data measured in normal subjects could be treated as though it had a normal distribution (Fig 23–17). Thus, any measured patient value could be referenced to this zero point and in turn be awarded points based on whether

it was below or above the normal mean value for that component. The formula used for performing the calculation illustrated in Fig 23–14 was:

$$\text{Component score} = \frac{\text{Pt Value} - \text{Mean}}{\text{SD}} + 1$$

This formula was used to score each of the six components of the 24 hour pH record obtained from the 50 normal subjects. The score for each component was added to obtain a composite score for each of the 50 normal subjects and the upper level of a normal score was established at the 95th percentile. The upper limits of normal for the composite score for each whole number pH threshold is shown in Table 23–2. The median and 95th percentile for the composite score for each whole number pH threshold also can be expressed graphically (Fig 23–18). An IBM compatible program to perform this function is available (Gastrosoft, Inc, 1350 Walnut Hill Lane, Suite 145, Irving, Texas 75038).

When evaluated in a test population with an equal distribution of normal healthy subjects and patients with the classical reflux symptoms and a defective sphincter, 24 hour esophageal pH monitoring had a sensitivity and specificity of 96%. This gave a predictive value of a positive and a negative test of 96% and an overall accuracy of 96%. Based on these studies and extensive clinical experience, 24 hour esophageal pH monitoring has emerged as a gold standard for the diagnosis of gastroesophageal reflux disease.[68]

Stationary Manometry

Esophageal manometry is a widely used technique to examine the motor function of the esophagus and its sphincters.[69] At present, it is the most accurate method for assessing the function of the lower sphincter and body of the esophagus.[70] In patients with symptomatic gastroesophageal reflux disease, manometry of the esophageal body can identify a mechanically defective lower esophageal sphincter and failure of esophageal clearance.

Esophageal manometry is performed using electronic pressure-sensitive transducers or water-perfused catheters with lateral side holes attached to transducers outside the body.[71] A train of five pressure-sensitive transducers or water-perfused catheters are bound together with the transducers or lateral openings placed at 5 cm intervals from the tip and oriented radially at 72° from each other around the circumference of the catheter. A special catheter assembly consisting of four pressure-sensitive transducers at the same level, oriented at 90° to each other, is of special use in assessing three-dimensional vector volume of the lower esophageal sphincter. Occasionally, other specially designed catheters may be used to assess the upper sphincter.

As the pressure-sensitive station is brought across the gastroesophageal junction, a rise in pressure on the gastric baseline identifies the beginning of the lower esophageal sphincter. The respiratory inversion point is identified when the positive excursions that occur with breathing in the abdominal cavity change to negative deflections in the thorax. The respiratory inversion point serves as a reference point at which the amplitude of lower esophageal sphincter pressure and the length of the sphincter exposed to abdominal pressure are measured. As the pressure-sensitive station is withdrawn into the body of the esophagus, the upper border of the lower esophageal sphincter is identified by the drop in pressure to the esophageal baseline. The pressure, abdominal length, and overall length of the sphincter are determined from these measurements (Fig 23–19). To account for the asymmetry of the sphincter (Fig 23–20), the measurement is repeated with each of the five transducers and the average values for sphincter pressure above gastric baseline, overall sphincter length, and abdominal length of the sphincter are calculated.

Table 23–3 shows the values for these parameters in 50 normal volunteers, without subjective or objective evidence of a foregut disorder. The level at which incompetence of the lower esophageal sphincter occurs was defined by comparing the frequency distribution of these values in the 50 healthy volunteers to a population of similarly studied patients with symptoms of gastroesophageal reflux disease.[12] The presence of increased esophageal exposure to gastric juice was assessed by 24 hour esophageal pH monitoring in each patient. Based on these studies, a mechanically defective sphincter is identified by having one or more of the following characteristics: an average lower esophageal sphincter pressure of <6 mm Hg, an average length exposed to the positive pressure environment in the abdomen of ≤1 cm, and an average overall sphincter length of ≤2 cm. Compared to the normal volunteers, these values are below the 2.5 percentile for sphincter pressure and overall length, and abdominal length.

More recently, it has been shown that the resistance of the sphincter to reflux of gastric juice is determined by the integrated effects of radial pressures extended over the entire length, resulting in a three-dimensional computerized imaging of sphincter pressures.[18] The volume circumscribed by this three-dimensional figure integrates sphincter pressure and length into one number (the sphincter pressure vector volume, SPVV) which is a quantitative measure of sphincter resistance to gastric contents. A calculated SPVV less than the 5th percentile, or <1212 is an indication of a mechanically defective sphincter.

In a study of 50 normal volunteers and 150 patients with increased esophageal exposure to gastric juice and various degrees of esophageal mucosal injury, the calculation of the sphincter pressure vector volume increased the ability of manometry to identify a mechanically defective sphincter compared with standard techniques.[18] This was particularly so in patients without mucosal injury and borderline sphincter abnormalities (Fig 23–21). Three-dimensional lower esophageal sphincter manometry and calculation of the vector volume should, therefore, become the standard technique to assess the barrier function of the lower esophageal sphincter in patients with GERD. Patients with GERD and an SPVV below the 5th percentile of normal or a deficiency of one, two, or all three mechanical components of a lower esophageal sphincter on standard manometry have a pathophysiologic defect of their antireflux barrier that a surgical antireflux procedure is designed to correct.

To assess the relaxation and postrelaxation contraction of the lower esophageal sphincter, a pressure transducer is repositioned within the high pressure zone, with a distal transducer located in the stomach and the proximal transducer within the esophageal body. Ten wet swallows (5 cc water) are performed. The normal pressure of the lower esophageal sphincter should drop to the level of gastric pressure during each wet swallow.

The function of the esophageal body is assessed with

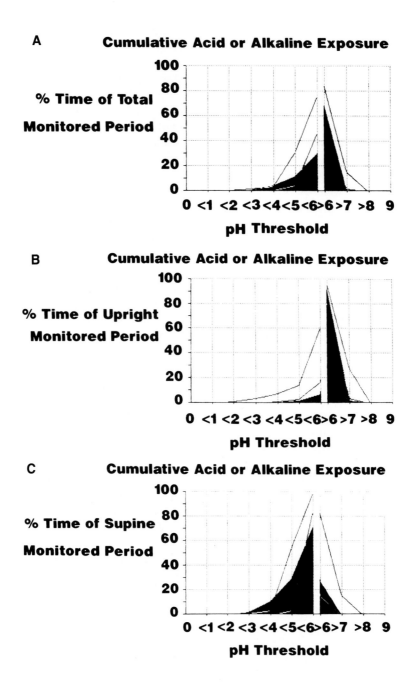

Figure 23–16. Gastric display of esophogram showing the median and 95th percentile levels in 50 normal individuals, using whole pH values above, and below 6 as thresholds. The black area represents measurements made in the patient. The lower line shows the median, and the upper line shows the 95th percentile value for the 50 normal subjects. When the black area exceeds the 95th percentile line for a given pH threshold, the patient has an abnormal value for the component measured. **A.** Percent cumulative exposure for total time. **B.** Percent cumulative exposure for upright time. **C.** Percent cumulative exposure for supine time. *Continued*

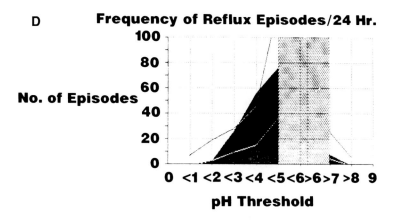

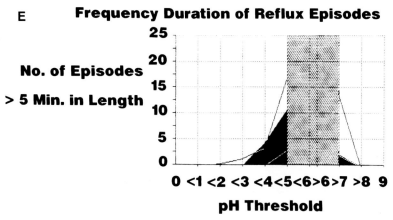

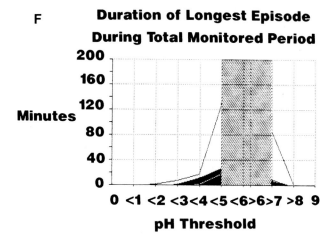

Figure 23–16, cont'd. D. Number of episodes. **E**. Number of episodes >5 minutes in length. **F**. Length of longest episode.

TABLE 23–1. NORMAL VALUES FOR ESOPHAGEAL EXPOSURE TO PH <4 (n=50)

Component	Mean ± SD	95%
Total time	1.51 ± 1.36	4.45
Upright time	2.34 ± 2.34	8.42
Supine time	0.63 ± 1.0	3.45
Number of episodes	19.00 ± 12.76	46.90
Number >5 minutes	0.84 ± 1.18	3.45
Longest episode	6.74 ± 7.85	19.80

(From DeMeester TR, Stein HJ. Gastroesophageal reflux disease. In: Moody FG, Carey LC, Jones RS, et al (eds), Surgical Treatment of Digestive Disease. 2nd ed. Chicago, IL: Year Book Medical; 1989:65–108

TABLE 23–2. NORMAL COMPOSITE SCORE FOR VARIOUS pH THRESHOLDS

pH Threshold	Upper Level of Normal Value (95th Percentile)
<1	14.2
<2	17.37
<3	14.10
<4	14.72
<5	15.76
<6	12.76
>7	14.90
>8	8.50

(From DeMeester TR, Stein HJ. Gastroesophageal reflux disease. In: Moody FG, Carey LC, Jones RS, et al (eds), Surgical Treatment of Digestive Disease, 2nd ed. Chicago, IL: Year Book Medical; 1989:65–108)

the 5 pressure transducers located in the esophagus. To standardize the procedure, the most proximal pressure transducer is located 1 cm below the well-defined cricopharyngeal sphincter. By this method, a pressure response throughout the whole esophagus can be obtained on one swallow. The study consists of recording ten wet swallows. Amplitude, duration, and morphology of contractions following each swallow are calculated at all recorded levels of the esophageal body. The delay between the onset or peak of esophageal contractions at the various levels of the esophagus is used to calculate the speed of wave propagation. The relationship of the esophageal contractions following a swallow are classified as peristaltic or simultaneous.

24 Hour Ambulatory Manometry

The development of miniaturized electronic pressure transducers and portable digital data recorders with large storage capacities has made ambulatory monitoring of esophageal motor function during an entire circadian cycle possible.[72] The broad clinical application of this new technology in a large number of asymptomatic normal volunteers and patients with primary esophageal motor disorders or GERD provides new insights into esophageal motor function in health and disease under a variety of physiologic conditions.[73] In both normal volunteers and symptomatic patients, esophageal motor activity increases with the state of consciousness and focus on eating activity, that is from the supine, to the upright, to meal periods. In the normal situation, there is a higher prevalence of nonperistaltic contractions than appreciated on stationary manometry.

Compared to standard manometry, ambulatory esophageal manometry provides a more than 100-fold larger database for the classification and quantitation of abnormal esophageal motor function and leads to a change in the diagnosis in a substantial portion of patients with symptoms suggestive of a primary esophageal

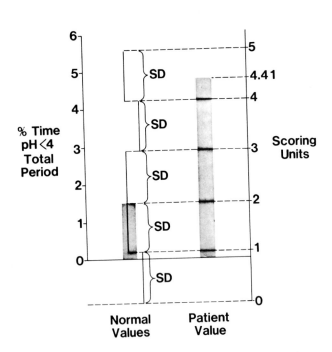

Figure 23–17. Concept of using the standard deviation as the scoring unit to score the component percent time pH <4 for the total period. Note the establishment of an abstract zero point 2 SD below the mean value for total-period acid exposure measured in normals (see Table 23–1). Theoretically, this allows scoring the measurement in patients as though the normal values were parametric. By this method, a patient who had a total acid exposure below pH 4 of 4.8 percent would have a score for this component of 4.41.

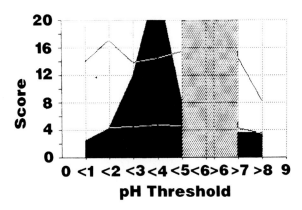

Figure 23–18. The composite score used to express the overall acid exposure at various pH thresholds. The lower line represents the median score, and the upper line the 95th percentile of 50 normal subjects. The black area represents the composite score for various pH thresholds derived from the six components used to measure esophageal acid exposure in the patient in Fig 23–2. The score is abnormal (above the 95th percentile line) for the pH threshold of 3 and 4.

motor disorder (Fig 23–22). In patients with nonobstructive dysphagia the circadian esophageal motor patterns are characterized by an inability to organize the motor activity into peristaltic contractions during a meal period (Fig 23–23).[74] This finding can be used to provide a new classification of motility disorders in regards to when they may give rise to dysphagia (Fig 23–24). In patients with noncardiac chest pain, ambulatory motility monitoring can document a direct correlation of abnormal esophageal motor activity with the symptom and shows that the abnormal motor activity immediately preceding the pain episodes is characterized by an increased frequency of simultaneous double- and triple-peaked high-amplitude and long contractions. In patients with GERD ambulatory motility monitoring shows that the contractility of the esophageal body deteriorates with increasing severity of esophageal mucosal injury, compromising the clearance function of the esophageal body (Fig 23–25). Ambulatory esoph-

ageal manometry will replace standard manometry in the assessment of esophageal body function and has the potential to improve the diagnosis and management of patients with esophageal motor abnormalities.

Video Roentgenography and Endoscopy

Endoscopy and biopsy are necessary to assess for the presence of complications of GERD (ie, esophagitis, stricture, and Barrett's esophagus).[75] Esophagitis is graded from 1 to 4; reddening of the mucosa without ulceration is scored as grade 1. The sensitivity of detecting grade 1 esophagitis endoscopically varies depending on the observer. Its presence may be confirmed by biopsy that shows mucosal infiltration with polymorphs, lymphocytes, eosinophils, and the recently described balloon cells.[76] The extension of the relative height of the mucosal papillae and hyperplasia of the basal zone are further evidence of mucosal injury.[77] These microscopic signs, while providing cor-

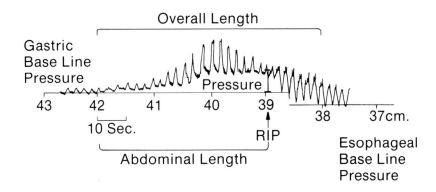

RIP = Respiratory Inversion Point

Figure 23–19. Sample manometric measurement of the lower esophageal sphincter. The distances are measured from the nares. (From Zaninotto G, DeMeester TR, et al, *Am J Surg* 1988, 155:105, with permission).

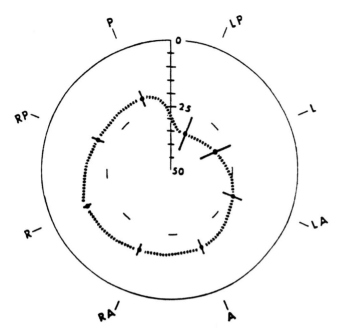

Figure 23–20. Radial configuration of the lower esophageal sphincter. A = anterior; L = left; LA = left anterior; LP = left posterior; P = posterior; R = right; RA = right anterior; RP = right posterior. (From Winans CS. Manometric asymmetry of the lower esophageal high pressure zone. *Dig Dis Sci* 1977;22:348–354)

roborative evidence, do not prove the presence of increased exposure to gastric juice because they also can occur from other forms of injury.[78,79] Grade 2 esophagitis is identified by the presence of linear ulcerations lined with granulation tissue that bleeds easily when touched. Grade 3 esophagitis represents a more advanced stage, when the ulcerations coalesce leaving islands of epithelium, which, on endoscopy, appear as a "cobblestone" esophagus. Grade 4 esophagitis is the presence of a stricture. Its severity can be assessed by the ease of passing a 36-French (Fr) endoscope. When a stricture is observed, the severity of the esophagitis above it should be recorded. The absence of esophagitis above a stricture suggests a drug-induced injury or a neoplasm as a cause for the stricture. The latter always should be considered and is ruled out only by tissue biopsies.

Barrett's esophagus is suspected at endoscopy when there is difficulty in visualizing the squamocolumnar junction at its normal location and by the appearance of a redder, more luxuriant mucosa than is normally seen in the lower esophagus. Its presence is confirmed by the finding of columnar epithelium with intestinalization on microscopic inspection of the biopsy. The roentgenographic definition of gastroesophageal reflux varies, depending on whether the reflux of barium is spontaneous or induced by various maneuvers. In only about 40% of patients with classic symptoms of GERD is spontaneous reflux of barium observed by the radiologist (ie, reflux of barium from the stomach into

the esophagus with a patient in the upright position).[70] In most patients who show spontaneous reflux of barium on roentgenography, the diagnosis of increased esophageal acid exposure is confirmed by 24 hour esophageal pH monitoring. Therefore, the roentgenographic demonstration of spontaneous regurgitation of barium into the esophagus in the upright position is a reliable indicator that reflux is present. Failure to see this does not, however, indicate the absence of disease.

TESTS OF DUODENOGASTRIC FUNCTION

Esophageal disorders are frequently associated with abnormalities of the stomach and duodenum. Abnormalities of the gastric reservoir or increased gastric acid secretion can be responsible for increased esophageal exposure to gastric juice. Reflux of alkaline duodenal juice, including bile salts, pancreatic enzymes, and bicarbonate, is thought to have a role in the pathogenesis of esophagitis and complicated Barrett's esophagus. Furthermore, functional disorders of the esophagus often are not confined to the esophagus alone, but are associated with functional disorders of the rest of the foregut (ie, stomach and duodenum). Tests of duodenogastric function that are helpful to investigate esophageal symptoms include gastric-emptying studies, gastric acid analysis, and the use of cholescintigraphy for the diagnosis of pathologic duodenogastric reflux. The single test of 24 hour gastric pH monitoring can be used to identify gastric hypersecretion and imply the presence of duodenogastric reflux and delayed gastric emptying.

Gastric Emptying

Gastric emptying studies are performed with radionuclide labeled meals. Emptying of solids and liquids can be assessed simultaneously when both phases are marked with different tracers. After ingestion of a labeled standard meal, gamma camera images of the stomach are ob-

TABLE 23–3. NORMAL MANOMETRIC VALUES OF THE DISTAL ESOPHAGEAL SPHINCTER (n=50)

Parameter	Mean	Mean −2 SD	Mean +2 SD	Median	2.5%[a]	97.5%[a]
Pressure (mm Hg)	13.8 ± 4.6	4.6	23.0	13.0	5.8	27.7
Overall length (cm)	3.7 ± 0.8	2.1	5.3	3.6	2.1	5.6
Abdominal length (cm)	2.2 ± 0.8	0.6	3.8	2.0	0.9	4.7

[a] % denotes percentile.
(From DeMeester TR, Stein HJ. Surgical treatment of gastroesophageal reflux disease. In: Castell DO (ed), The Esophagus. Boston: Little, Brown; 1992:579–625)

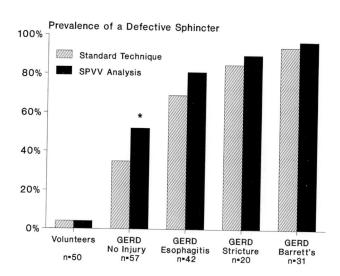

Figure 23–21. Comparison of standard manometric techniques and SPVV analysis in the identification of a mechanically defective lower esophageal sphincter. *P <.05 vs. standard manometry. (From Stein HJ, DeMeester TR, et al., *Ann Surg* 1991;214:380)

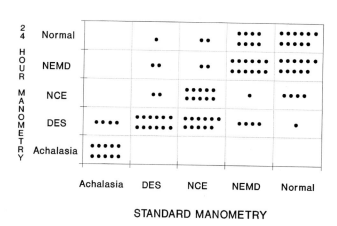

STANDARD MANOMETRY

Figure 23–22. Classification of esophageal motility disorders on standard and ambulatory 24 hour manometry in 78 patients. NEMD: nonspecific esophageal motility disorders; NCE: nutcracker esophagus; DES: diffuse esophageal spasm. (From DeMeester TR, Stein HJ. Surgery for esophageal motor disorders. In: Castell DO (ed), *The Esophagus*. Boston: Little, Brown; 1992:412)

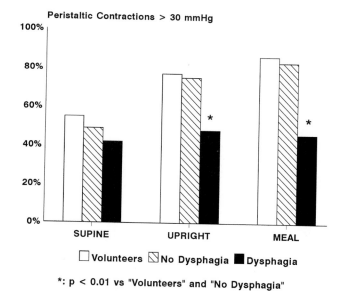

*: p < 0.01 vs "Volunteers" and "No Dysphagia"

Figure 23–23. Frequency of peristaltic contractions with an amplitude >30 mm Hg during supine, upright, and meal periods, showing that patients with nonobstructive dysphagia are unable to organize their esophageal contractions with increasing states of awareness from sleep (supine) to alertness (upright) to focus on eating (meals). (From Stein HJ, DeMeester TR. Indications, technique, and clinical use of ambulatory 24 hour esophageal motility monitoring in a surgical practice. *Ann Surg* 1993;217(2):128–137)

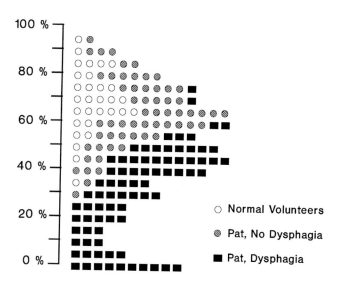

Figure 23–24. Prevalence of "effective contractions" (ie, peristaltic contractions) with an amplitude >30 mm Hg, during meal periods in individual normal volunteers, patients without dysphagia and patients with nonobstructive dysphagia.

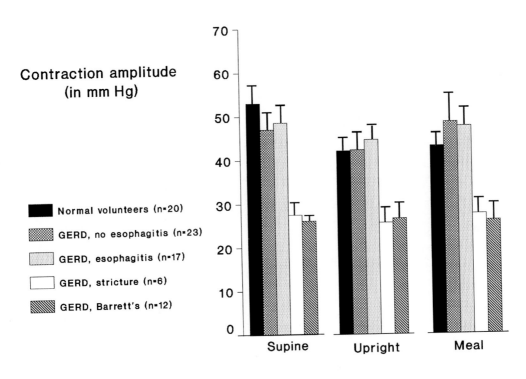

A

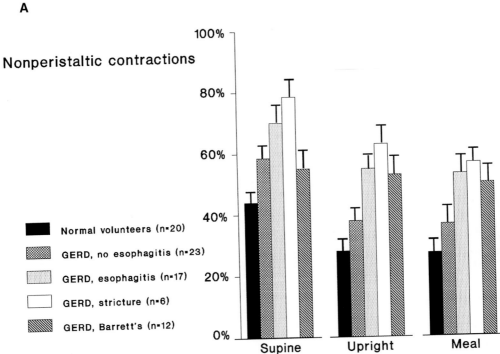

B

Figure 23–25. A. Median contraction amplitude and **B**. frequency of nonperistaltic contractions on 24 hour ambulatory esophageal motility monitoring in patients with gastroesophageal reflux disease (GERD) and various degrees of mucosal injury. Normal volunteers (n = 20); GERD, no esophagitis (n = 23); GERD, esophagitis (n = 17); GERD, stricture (n = 6); GERD, Barrett's esophagus (n = 12). (From Stein HJ, Eypasch EP, DeMeester TR, et al. Circadian esophageal motor function in patients with gastroesophageal reflux disease. *Surgery* 1990;108:769–778)

tained in 5 to 15 minute intervals for 1.5 to 2 hours. After correction for decay, the counts in the gastric area are plotted as percentage of total counts at the start of the imaging. The resulting emptying curve can be compared with data obtained in normal volunteers. Normal subjects will empty 59% of a meal within 90 minutes.

Gastric Acid Analysis

The gastric secretory state usually is evaluated by determination of the titrable gastric acid in aspirated gastric juice. Interdigestive or basal gastric acid secretion (BAO) is measured in the fasting state and varies between 0 to 5 mMol/hr in normal volunteers. The maximal secretory capacity (MAO) of the stomach, which reflects the available parietal cell mass, is calculated following stimulation of gastric acid secretion with pentagastrin or histamine. Acid hypersecretors have a BAO >5 mMol/hr and an MAO >30 mMol/hr.

Cholescintigraphy

Scintigraphic hepatobiliary imaging is performed after intravenous injection of 5 uCi of technetium 99m (^{99m}Tc) imminodiacetic acid derivates such as disofenin (DISIDA). Gamma camera images of the upper abdomen, including the gallbladder and stomach, are obtained at 5 minute intervals for 60 minutes. Imaging is continued for an additional 30 minutes after stimulation of gallbladder contraction with 20 mg/kg of synthetic C-terminal octapeptide of cholecystokin (CCK).

Duodenogastric reflux is demonstrated as an increase of radioactivity in the stomach in the sequential images. The clinical value of this test is limited owing to its short duration and a relatively high false-positive rate in normal volunteers.[50]

24 Hour Gastric pH Monitoring

Monitoring is performed during a complete circadian cycle with a pH electrode placed 5 cm below the manometrically located lower esophageal sphincter.[51] The patient is fully ambulatory during the test and is encouraged to perform normal daily activity. The gastric pH profile is assessed separately for the meal, postprandial period, and fasting period. The latter is divided into the time spent upright and supine.

The interpretation of continuous gastric pH recordings is more difficult than that of esophageal pH recordings. This situation arises because the gastric pH environment is determined by a complex interplay of acid and mucous secretion; ingested food; swallowed saliva; regurgitated duodenal, pancreatic, and biliary secretions; and the effectiveness of the mixing and evacuation of the chyme. Using 24 hour gastric pH monitoring to evaluate the gastric secretory state is based on studies showing that a good correlation exists between increased basal acid output on standard gastric acid analysis and a left shift on the frequency distribution graph of gastric pH recordings during the supine fasting period (Fig 23–26). The evaluation of gastric emptying by

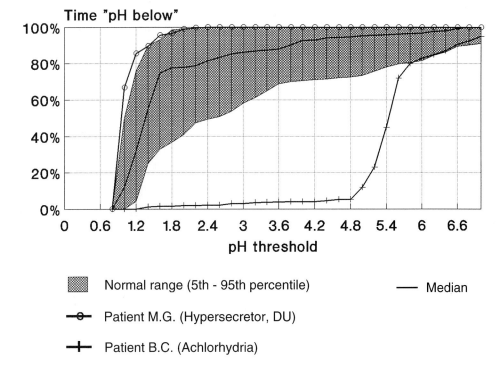

Figure 23–26. Cumulative frequency distribution of recorded gastric pH values during the supine period. The *shaded area* represents the 5th and 95th percentiles of 50 healthy volunteers; the *solid line* shows the median. Patient MG has a markedly left shift in pH profile out of the normal range, suggesting gastric acid hypersecretion. Patient BC has a right shift in pH profile, indicating hypochlorhydria. DU = duodenal ulcer. (From Stein HJ, De-Meester TR. Integrated ambulatory foregut monitoring in patients with functional foregut disorders. In: Nyhus LM (ed), *1992 Surgery Annual*, part 1, volume 24. Stamford, CT: Appleton & Lange; 1992:168)

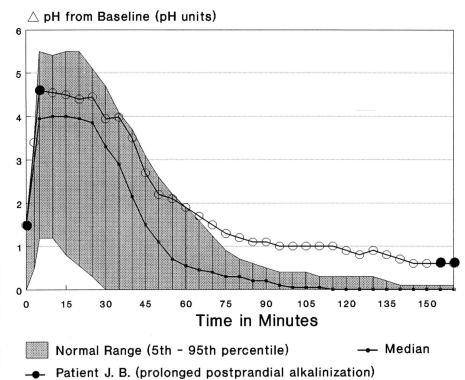

△ pH from Baseline (pH units)

Figure 23–27. Postprandial alkalinization measured by gastric pH monitoring. The *shaded area* represents the 5th and 95th percentile of 50 healthy volunteers; the *solid line* shows the median. Patient JB showed a markedly prolonged postprandial alkalinization, suggesting delayed gastric emptying. (From Stein HJ, De-Meester TR. Integrated ambulatory foregut monitoring in patients with functional foregut disorders. In: Nyhus LM (ed), *1992 Surgery Annual*, part 1, volume 24, Stamford, CT: Appleton & Lange; 1992:170)

24 hour gastric pH monitoring is based on studies demonstrating a good correlation between the emptying of a solid meal and the duration of the postprandial plateau and decline phase of the gastric pH record (Fig 23–27). Using 24 hour gastric pH monitoring to evaluate duodenogastric reflux is based on the observation that reflux of alkaline duodenal juice into the stomach can alkalinize the gastric pH environment. The measurement is not straightforward because the effect of meals and reduction in acid secretion can result in changes in gastric pH that mimic alkaline reflux episodes. To overcome this problem, computerized measurements of the number and height of alkalinizing peaks, baseline pH, postprandial pH plateau, and pattern of pH decline from the plateau can be used to identify the probability of duodenogastric reflux. The results are presented as an overall score that indicates the likelihood of pathologic duodenogastric reflux. Initial data indicate that this approach has a higher sensitivity and specificity for the diagnosis of pathologic duodenogastric reflux than scintigraphic methods.

Combined 24 hour esophageal and gastric pH monitoring recently has been introduced. Using this technique, excessive alkaline duodenogastric and alkaline gastroesophageal reflux can be identified in symptomatic patients. The combined tracings often can identify simultaneous gastric and esophageal alkalinization,

suggesting a duodenal origin for the esophageal alkaline exposure.

Integrated Ambulatory Foregut Monitoring

Recently, integrated ambulatory foregut monitoring consisting of 24 hour esophageal and gastric pH monitoring, and ambulatory motility has been introduced.[80] This monitoring allows an evaluation of the foregut function during one 24 hour period in a physiologic outpatient environment, with only minor discomfort to the patient. This technology may replace the series of laboratory tests currently required to thoroughly evaluate foregut function and give surgeons the ability to evaluate complex foregut problems in their own offices. Integrated monitoring of foregut function therefore has the potential of giving surgical therapy for functional abnormalities of the foregut a more scientific basis than was previously possible.

■ SURGICAL TREATMENT

INDICATIONS FOR ANTIREFLUX SURGERY

Before proceeding with an antireflux procedure in a patient suspected of having GERD, it is necessary to confirm that the patient's symptoms are caused by esopha-

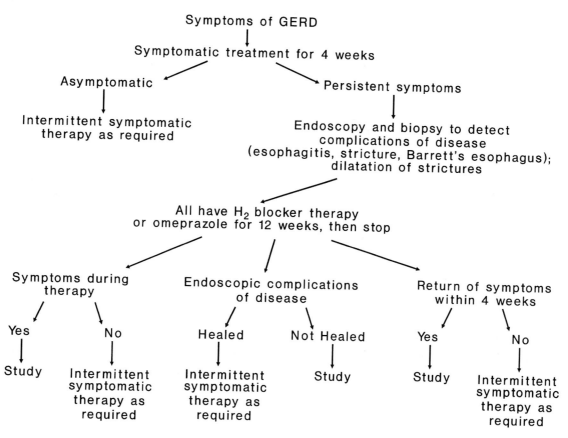

Figure 23–28. Algorithm showing medical management and indications for functional studies (ie, 24 hour pH monitoring and manometry) in patients with symptoms of GERD.

geal exposure to gastric juice secondary to a mechanically defective lower esophageal sphincter. Esophageal function studies (ie, 24 hour esophageal pH monitoring and esophageal manometry) are required for such confirmation. As outlined in the algorithm in Fig 23–28, esophageal function studies should be done if the patient has persistent symptoms or unimproved esophageal mucosal injury after 8 to 12 weeks of acid suppression therapy. Patients who respond to a course of medical therapy but have recurrence of symptoms within 4 weeks after cessation of therapy also should be studied since they are prone to drug dependency.

The requirements to proceed with an antireflux procedure in such patients are:

1. Persistent or recurrent symptoms and/or complications after 8 to 12 weeks of intensive acid suppression therapy
2. Increased esophageal exposure to gastric juice documented by 24 hour esophageal pH monitoring
3. Presence of a mechanically defective lower esophageal sphincter on manometric studies
4. Adequate esophageal body motor function

If 24 hour esophageal pH monitoring is normal in a patient with unequivocal endoscopic esophagitis, the possibilities of alkaline, drug-induced, or retention esophagitis should be considered. Patients with increased esophageal exposure juice in whom the sphincter is manometrically normal should be evaluated for a gastric or esophageal cause of reflux. Approximately 40% of these patients will have gastric acid hypersecretion and respond to more aggressive antisecretory therapy. Patients with increased esophageal acid exposure, a mechanically defective sphincter, and no complications of the disease should be given the option of surgery as a cost effective alternative.[81]

The presence of endoscopic esophagitis in a symptomatic patient with a mechanically defective LES should raise the question of surgical therapy, because these patients are prone to a relapse of their symptoms while receiving medical therapy.[82,83] If the patient responds symptomatically to medical therapy but endoscopic esophagitis persists, surgery should be performed. Without surgery, these patients can progress to develop a stricture or Barrett's esophagus while on therapy and will lose esophageal body function while on therapy because reflux of alkalized gastric contents continues through the mechanically defective sphincter.[84] In this situation, an antireflux procedure corrects the mechanically defective sphincter, heals the esophagitis, and prevents the formation of a stricture or Barrett's esophagus.

FACTORS TO CONSIDER BEFORE ANTIREFLUX SURGERY

Before proceeding with an antireflux operation, several factors should be evaluated. First, the propulsive force of the body of the esophagus should be evaluated by esophageal manometry to determine if it has sufficient power to propel a bolus of food through a newly reconstructed valve.[23] Patients with normal peristaltic contractions do well with a 360° Nissen fundoplication. When peristalsis is absent, severely disordered, or the amplitude of the contraction is below 20 mm Hg, the Belsey two-thirds partial fundoplication is the procedure of choice.

Second, anatomic shortening of the esophagus can comprise the ability to do an adequate repair without tension and leads to an increased incidence of breakdown or thoracic displacement of the repair (Fig 23–29). Esophageal shortening is identified radiographically by a sliding hiatal hernia that will not reduce in the upright position or that measures >5 cm between the diaphragmatic crura and gastroesophageal junction on endoscopy. When present, the motility of the esophageal body must be evaluated carefully and, if adequate, a gas-

troplasty should be performed. In patients who have a motility study that shows the absence of contractility or more than 50% interrupted or dropped contractions or a history of several failed previous antireflux procedures, esophageal resection should be considered as an alternative.

Third, the surgeon should specifically query the patient for complaints of epigastric pain, nausea, vomiting, and loss of appetite. In the past, these symptoms were accepted as part of the reflux syndrome, but we now realize that they can be the result of excessive duodenogastric reflux which occurs in about one-third of patients with gastroesophageal reflux disease.[54] This problem is most pronounced in patients who have had previous upper gastrointestinal surgery, particularly cholecystectomy, although this is not always the case.[85] In such patients, the correction of only the incompetent cardia may result in a disgruntled individual who continues to complain of nausea and epigastric pain on eating. In these patients, 24 hour pH monitoring of the stomach may help to detect and quantitate duodenogastric reflux.[51] The abnormality can also be documented with a ^{99m}Tc-HIDA scan if excessive reflux of radionucleotide from the duodenum into the stomach can be demonstrated.[50] Antireflux surgery may reduce duodenogastric reflux by improving the efficiency of gastric emptying. If the symptoms of duodenogastric reflux persist after antireflux surgery, the administration of sucralfate may relieve the persistent complaint of nausea and epigastric pain. In a few patients, this may give inadequate relief and eventually, a bile diversion procedure may be necessary.

Fourth, approximately 30% of patients with proven gastroesophageal reflux on 24 hour pH monitoring will have hypersecretion on gastric analysis[31]; 2% to 3% of patients who have an antireflux operation will develop a gastric or duodenal ulcer. These factors may modify the proposed antireflux procedure in patients with active ulcer disease or documentation of previous ulceration by the addition of a highly selective vagotomy.

Fifth, delayed gastric emptying is found in approximately 40% of patients with GERD and can contribute to symptoms after an antireflux repair.[86] Usually, however, mild degrees of delayed gastric emptying are corrected by the antireflux procedure and only in patients with severe emptying disorders is there a need for an additional gastric procedure.

PRINCIPLES OF SURGICAL THERAPY

The primary goal of antireflux surgery is to safely reestablish the competency of the cardia by mechanically improving its function while preserving the ability of the patient to swallow normally, to belch to relieve gaseous distention, and to vomit when necessary. Regardless of

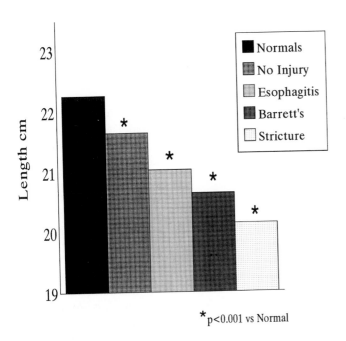

*p<0.001 vs Normal

Figure 23–29. Length of esophagus in patients with GERD compared with normal subjects. Esophageal length progressively shortens as complications of the disease become more severe.

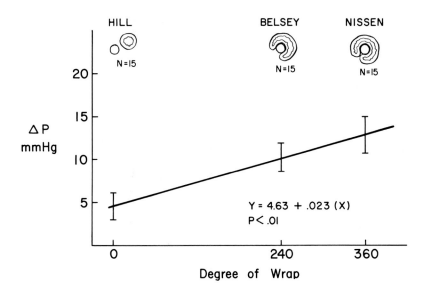

Figure 23–30. Relationship between the augmentation of sphincter pressure above preoperative pressure (ΔP) and the degree of gastric fundic wrap. (From DeMeeser TR. Transthoracic antireflux procedure. In: Nyhus LM, Baker FJ (eds), *Mastery of Surgery.* Boston: Little, Brown; 1984:384)

the choice of procedure, this goal can be achieved if attention is paid to five principles in reconstructing the cardia.

First, the operation should restore the pressure of the distal esophageal sphincter to a level twice the resting gastric pressure (ie, 12 mm Hg for a gastric pressure of 6 mm Hg, and its length to at least 3 cm). This restoration can be achieved by buttressing the distal esophagus with the fundus of the stomach. Preoperative and postoperative esophageal manometry measurements have shown that the resting sphincter pressure and the overall sphincter length can be surgically augmented over preoperative values, and that the change in the former is a function of the degree of gastric wrap around the esophagus (Fig 23–30).

Second, the operation should place an adequate length of the distal esophageal sphincter in the positive pressure environment of the abdomen by a method that ensures its response to changes in intra-abdominal pressure. The permanent restoration of 1.5 to 2 cm of abdominal esophagus in a patient whose sphincter pressure has been augmented to twice resting gastric pressure will maintain the competency of the cardia over various challenges of intra-abdominal pressure. Fig 23–31 shows that all three of the popular antireflux procedures increase on average the length of the sphincter exposed to abdominal pressure by an average of 1 cm. However, when poorly performed an operation can result in a reduction of the length of abdominal sphincter. Increasing the length of sphincter exposed to ab-

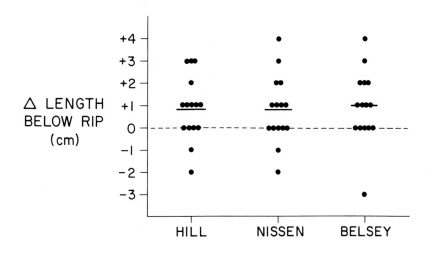

Figure 23–31. Increase in abdominal sphincter length expected after the three major antireflux procedures. On the average, all the procedures increase the length by 1 cm. However, it is possible for the procedure actually to decrease the length. (From DeMeester TR. Gastroesophageal reflux disease. In: Moody FG, Carey LC, et al (eds), *Surgical Treatment of Digestive Disease.* Chicago, IL: Year Book Medical; 1985:147)

dominal pressure will improve competency only if it is acted on by challenges of intra-abdominal pressure. Thus, the creation of a conduit that will ensure the transmission of intra-abdominal pressure changes around the abdominal portion of the sphincter is a necessary aspect of surgical repair. The fundoplication in the Nissen and Belsey repairs serves this purpose.

Third, the operation should allow the reconstructed cardia to relax on deglutition. In normal swallowing a vagally mediated relaxation of the distal esophageal sphincter and the gastric fundus occurs. The relaxation lasts for approximately ten seconds and is followed by a rapid recovery to its former tonicity. To ensure relaxation of the sphincter, three factors are important: (1) only the fundus of the stomach should be used to buttress the sphincter since it is known to relax in concert with the sphincter, (2) the fundoplication should be properly placed around the sphincter and not incorporate a portion of the stomach or be placed around the stomach itself, since the body of the stomach does not relax with swallowing, and (3) damage to the vagal nerves during dissection of the thoracic esophagus should be avoided because it may result in failure of the sphincter to relax.

Fourth, the fundoplication should not increase the resistance of the relaxed sphincter to a level that exceeds the peristaltic power of the body of the esophagus. The resistance of the relaxed sphincter depends on the degree, length, and diameter of the fundoplication and on the variation in intra-abdominal pressure. A 360° fundoplication should be no longer than 2 cm and constructed over a 60-Fr bougie. This will ensure that the relaxed sphincter will have an adequate diameter with minimal resistance that easily can be overcome by esophageal body contractions of normal amplitude. This is not necessary when constructing a partial fundoplication.

Fifth, the operation should ensure that the fundoplication can be placed in the abdomen without undue tension and maintained there by approximating the crura of the diaphragm above the repair. Leaving the fundoplication in the thorax converts a sliding hernia into a paraesophageal hernia with all the complications associated with that condition.[88] Maintaining the repair in the abdomen under tension predisposes to an increased incidence of recurrence. This occurs in patients who have a stricture or Barrett's esophagus and is probably owing to shortening of the esophagus from the inflammatory process. This problem can be resolved by using a gastroplasty to lengthen the esophagus and constructing a partial fundoplication.

PRIMARY ANTIREFLUX REPAIRS

The Nissen Fundoplication

The most common antireflux procedure is the Nissen Fundoplication. The procedure can be performed through the abdomen or the chest and more recently, either open or through a laparoscope. Rudolph Nissen described the procedure as a 360° fundoplication around the lower esophagus for a distance of 4 to 5 cm. Although this provided good control of reflux, it was associated with a number of side effects that have encouraged modifications of the procedure, as originally described. These include taking care to use only the gastric fundus to envelope the esophagus in performing the fundoplication, sizing the fundoplication with a 60-Fr bougie, and limiting the length of the fundoplication to 1 to 2 centimeters.[89] The essential elements necessary for the performance of a transabdominal fundoplication are common to both the laparoscopic and open procedures and include the following:

1. Crural dissection, identification and preservation of both vagi, and the anterior hepatic branch
2. Circumferential dissection of the esophagus
3. Crural closure
4. Fundic mobilization by division of short gastric vessels
5. Creation of a short, loose fundoplication by enveloping the anterior and posterior walls of the fundus around the lower esophagus

The Laparoscopic Approach. Laparoscopic fundoplication has become commonplace and may soon replace traditional open Nissen fundoplication as the procedure of choice.[90,91] The patient should be placed supine, in a modified lithotomy position, with the table elevated 30° to 45°. The knees should be only slightly flexed. If the legs are sharply flexed at the knees, they will interfere with the mobility of the instruments during the course of the procedure. The surgeon, working with both hands, is best placed between the patient's legs, allowing the right- and left-handed instruments to approach the hiatus from the respective upper abdominal quadrants. A semi-Fowler's or head-up position is used to displace the transverse colon and small bowel inferiorly, keeping them from obstructing the view of the video camera. Five 10-mm ports are used (Fig 23–32). The camera is placed above the umbilicus, one-third of the distance to the xiphoid process. In most patients, placement of the camera in the umbilicus will not allow adequate visualization of the hiatal strictures, once dissected. Two lateral retracting ports are placed in the right and left anterior axillary lines, respectively. The right-sided liver retractor is best placed immediately subcostal in the right anterior axillary line. This allows an acute angle toward the left lateral segment of the liver and thus, the ability to push the instrument toward the operating table, lifting the liver. A second retraction port is placed at the level of the umbilicus, in the left anterior axillary line. The right-

structures. Laparoscopic fundoplication begins with exposure of the esophageal hiatus. A fan retractor is placed into the right anterior axillary port, and positioned to hold the left lateral segment of the liver towards the anterior abdominal wall. These authors prefer to use a table retractor to hold this instrument, once properly positioned. Trauma to the liver should be meticulously avoided, because subsequent bleeding will obscure the field. Mobilization of the left lateral segment by division of the triangular ligament is not necessary.

A Babcock clamp is placed into the left anterior axillary port and the stomach is retracted toward the patient's feet. This maneuver exposes the esophageal hiatus (Fig 23–33). Commonly, a hiatal hernia will need to be reduced. An atraumatic clamp should be used, and care taken not to grasp the stomach to vigorously, as gastric perforations can occur.

The key to the hiatal dissection is identification of the right crus (Fig 23–34). Metzenbaum-type scissors and

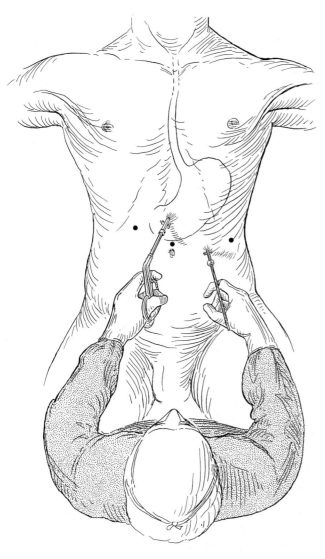

Figure 23–32. Patient positioning and trocar placement for laparoscopic antireflux surgery. The patient is placed with the head elevated 45° in the modified lithotomy position. The surgeon stands between the patient's legs.

and left-handed trocars are placed in the right and left midclavicular lines, 2 to 3 inches below the costal margin. Placing the operating trocars on either side of the midline allows triangulation between the camera and the two instruments, avoiding the difficulty associated with the instruments being in direct line with the camera. The falciform ligament hangs low in many patients and provides a barrier around which the left-handed instrument must be manipulated. Most recently, we have placed a 12-mm trocar in the left midclavicular position to allow the use of a large clip applier to divide the short gastric vessels. One of the most important and occasionally, the most difficult elements of laparoscopic surgery is adequate retraction and safe exposure of the necessary

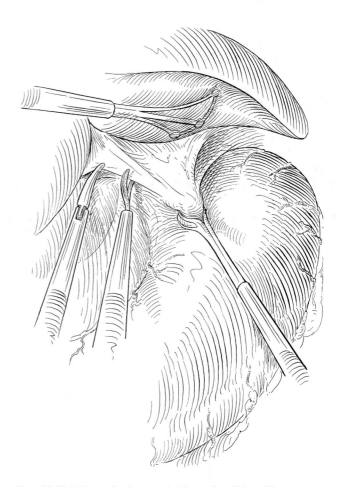

Figure 23–33. Initial retraction for exposure of the esophageal hiatus. A fan retractor is placed below the left lateral segment of the liver to retract it anteriorly. A Babcock clamp is placed on the esophageal fat pad and retracted toward the patient's feet to expose the phrenoesophageal membrane.

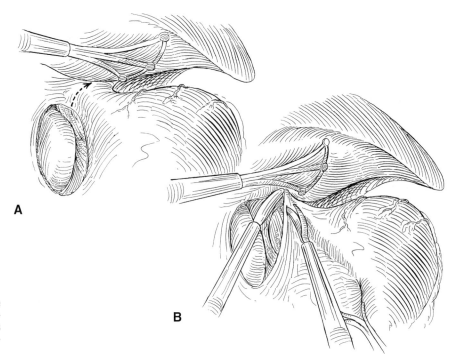

Figure 23–34. Dissection of the diaphragmatic crura is the key to safe exposure of the esophagus. **A**. The gastrohepatic omentum is incised above the hepatic vagal branches and the right crus exposed. **B**. The dissection is carried anteriorly toward the superior portion of the left crus.

fine grasping forceps are preferred for dissection. In all except the most obese patients, there is a very thin portion of the gastrohepatic omentum overlying the caudate lobe of the liver. Dissection is begun by incision of this portion of the gastrohepatic omentum above the hepatic branch of the anterior vagal nerve. A large, left hepatic artery arising from the left gastric artery will be present in ≤25% of patients. It should be identified and avoided. Once opened, the outside of the right crus will become evident. The peritoneum overlying the anterior aspect of the right crus is incised with scissors and electrocautery. The medial portion of the right crus leads into the mediastinum, and is entered by blunt dissection with both instruments. At this juncture, the esophagus usually becomes evident. The right crus is retracted laterally and the posterior or right vagus is identified and dissected away from the esophagus for a distance of 3 to 4 cm. The anterior or left vagus is left undisturbed.

Meticulous hemostasis is critical. Blood and fluid tends to pool in the hiatus and is difficult to remove. Irrigation should be kept to a minimum. Care must be taken not to injure the phrenic artery and vein as they course above the hiatus. Lifting the esophagus with a blunt-tipped grasper placed within the esophageal hiatus underneath the organ, the dissection is carried inferiorly and laterally, exposing the medial and lateral aspects of the right crus. A large hiatal hernia often makes this portion of the procedure easier as it accentuates the diaphragmatic crura. On the other hand, dissection of a large mediastinal hernia sac can be difficult.

Following dissection of the right crus, attention is turned toward the angle of His and a complete dissection of the lateral and inferior aspect of the left crus and the fundus of the stomach. This dissection is the key maneuver allowing circumferential mobilization of the esophagus. Failure to do so will result in difficulty encircling the esophagus, particularly if approached from the right. Division of the attachments of the fundus to the diaphragm and crura is a crucial part of the dissection. Repositioning of the Babcock retractor toward the fundic side of the stomach facilitates retraction for this portion of the procedure.

The esophagus is mobilized by careful dissection of the anterior and posterior soft tissues within the hiatus. This can be the most difficult aspect of laparoscopic antireflux surgery, largely because the instruments are angled cephalad into the mediastinum and not toward the right or left. Circumferential dissection of the esophagus is further hampered by the limited exposure of the laparoscopic procedure. Gentle blunt dissection, from both right and left is necessary. From the patient's right side, the esophagus should be retracted anteriorly with the surgeon's left-hand instrument allowing posterior dissection with the right hand, and vice versa for the left-sided dissection. In the presence of severe esophagitis

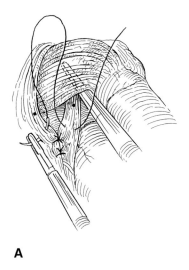

A

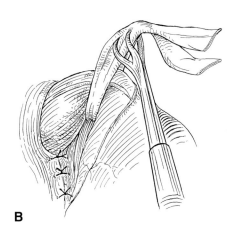

B

Figure 23–35. A. A Penrose drain is placed around the esophagus to facilitate exposure. **B.** Closure of the diaphragmatic crura. The esophagus is displaced anteriorly and to the left and three to four sutures of 2-0 silk are placed to approximate the crura.

and transmural inflammation with or without esophageal shortening, esophageal dissection may be particularly difficult. Following this dissection, a grasper is passed via the surgeon's left-handed port behind the esophagus and over the left crus. A Penrose drain is placed around the esophagus to facilitate crural closure (Fig 23–35A).

The crura are dissected inferiorly for a distance of 2 to 3 centimeters. The esophagus is held anterior and to the left and the crura approximated with 3 to 4 interrupted 0 silk sutures, starting just above the aortic decussation and working anterior (Fig 23–35B). Because space is limited, it is necessary to use the surgeon's left-handed (nondominant) instrument as a retractor, facilitating placement of single bites through each crus with the surgeon's right hand. We prefer extracorporeal knot tying using a standard knot pusher, although tying within the abdomen is perfectly appropriate.

Complete fundic mobilization allows construction of

a tension-free fundoplication. Removal of the liver retractor and placement of a second Babcock forceps through the right anterior axillary port facilitates retraction during division of the short gastric vessels. The gastrosplenic omentum is suspended anteroposteriorly, in a clothesline fashion via both Babcock forceps and the lesser sac entered approximately one-third the distance down the greater curvature of the stomach. Short gastric vessels are dissected sequentially, double clipped and divided. An anterior-posterior rather than medial to lateral orientation of the vessels is preferred, with the exception of those close to the spleen. With caution and meticulous dissection the fundus can be completely mobilized, in most patients.

Following complete mobilization of the fundus, a Babcock clamp is placed through the left-handed operating port and passed behind the esophagus to grasp the posterior wall of the fundus (Fig 23–36). It is

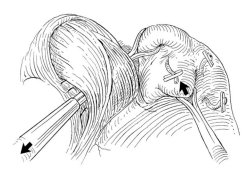

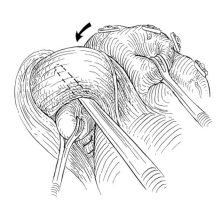

Figure 23–36. Creation of the fundoplication. A Babcock clamp is placed behind the esophagus and the posterior fundus of the stomach is grasped and brought to the right. Careful attention must be paid to grasping the posterior portion of the stomach and not the anterior wall to avoid twisting of the stomach.

brought gently behind the esophagus to the right side. The anterior wall of the fundus is brought anterior to the esophagus above the supporting Penrose drain. Both posterior and anterior fundic lips are manipulated to allow the fundus to envelope the esophagus without twisting. The laparoscopic visualization has a tendency to exaggerate the size of the posterior opening that has been dissected. Consequently, the space for the passage of the fundus behind the esophagus may be tighter than thought and the fundus relatively ischemic when brought around. If the right lip of the fundoplication has a bluish discoloration, the stomach should be returned to its original position and the posterior dissection enlarged. Once adequately placed, both lips of the fundoplication are held in place with an instrument through the left-sided retracting port that then frees the surgeon's left-hand trocar. A 60-Fr bougie is passed to properly size the fundoplication, and it is sutured using a single U stitch of 2-0 Prolene buttressed with felt pledgets (Fig 23–37). The most common error is an attempt

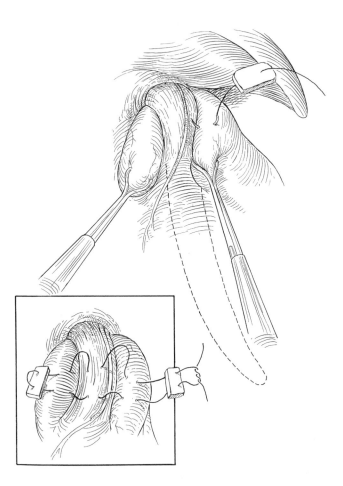

Figure 23–37. Fixation of the fundoplication. The fundoplication is sutured in place with a single U stitch of 2-0 Prolene pledgeted on the outside. A 60-Fr mercury-weighted bougie is passed through the gastroesophageal junction prior to fixation of the wrap to assure a floppy fundoplication.

to grasp the anterior portion of the stomach to construct the fundoplication rather than the posterior fundus. The esophagus should lie comfortably in the untwisted fundus prior to suturing. Two anchoring sutures of 3-0 silk are placed above and below the U stitch to complete the fundoplication. When finished, the suture line of the fundoplication should be facing in a right anterior direction. The abdomen is irrigated, hemostasis assured, and the bougie replaced with a nasogastric tube. Failure of the nasogastric tube to pass easily into the stomach indicates a potential obstruction at the cardia and should be investigated.

Transabdominal Open Nissen Fundoplication. Excellent exposure of the esophageal hiatus is paramount in performing an open procedure (Fig 23–38). This can be achieved by utilizing a specialized retractor constructed by welding a Weinberg retractor to a Balfour handle. This retractor is placed under the liver down to the esophageal hiatus. The operating table is placed in a reverse Trendelenburg position and the retractor is lifted cephalad in a 45° angle and secured to an overhead bar attached to the table. This elevates the anterior chest wall and lifts the liver out of the way. The wound is retracted laterally with a Balfour retractor. Without this exposure, careful dissection of the hiatus is difficult, time consuming, and dangerous.

The esophageal hiatus is approached by dividing the gastrohepatic ligament in the area where it is thin and usually transparent. The cephalad portion of the gastrohepatic ligament is divided and the incision carried superiorly over the anterior surface of the esophagus and down the left crus of the esophageal hiatus.

The esophagus is dissected circumferentially within the posterior mediastinum by blunt finger dissection. A soft rubber drain is passed around the esophagus, excluding the posterior or right vagal trunk. While retracting on the rubber drain, the loose fibroareolar tissue within the hiatus is divided to clearly identify the medial surface of the right and left crus.

The procedure continues with mobilization of the gastric fundus by dividing the short gastric vessels. The proximal third of the greater curvature is freed. One can appreciate how these vessels, if not divided, force the surgeon to construct the fundoplication with a portion of the body of the stomach rather than the fundus. The esophageal hiatus is closed by retracting the esophagus to the left, and approximating the right and left crura with interrupted 0 silk sutures. Care is taken not to place the uppermost sutures on the right side in the fascia of the diaphragm, since this will result in a constriction of the hiatus and dysphagia. When complete, the hiatus should freely admit a fingertip adjacent to the esophagus.

Construction of the fundic wrap completes the pro-

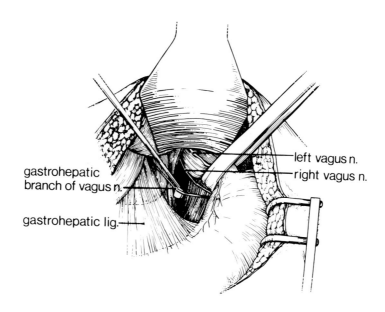

gastrohepatic
branch of vagus n.

gastrohepatic lig.

left vagus n.
right vagus n.

A

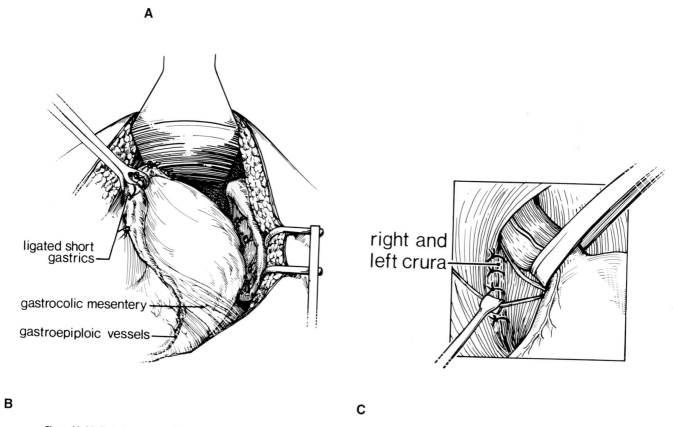

ligated short
gastrics

gastrocolic mesentery

gastroepiploic vessels

right and
left crura

B

C

Figure 23–38. Technique of transabdominal Nissen fundoplication. **A.** Completed hiatal dissection done through the transabdominal approach showing the vagal nerves, position of the rubber drain around the esophagus, and the right and left crus. **B.** The mobilized gastric fundus after division of the short gastric vessels. Some of these vessels can take a retroperitoneal course, tethering the fundus of the stomach posteriorly. **C.** The closed esophageal hiatus. Notice that the esophageal body has been displaced anteriorly by the approximation of the right and left crura. *Continued*

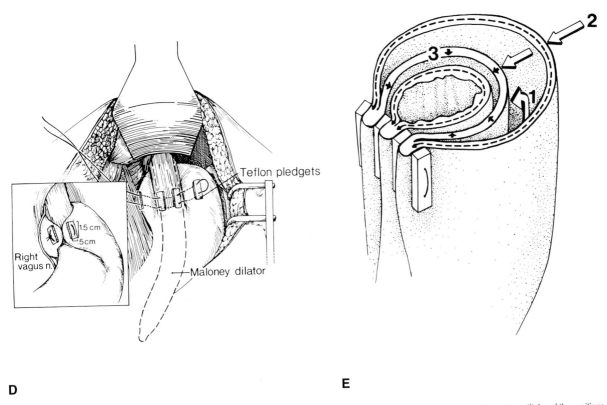

D

E

Figure 23–38, cont'd. D. Construction of the fundoplication by the transabdominal approach illustrating the placement of the horizontal mattress stitch and the positions of the pledgets. The wrap is formed over a 60-Fr bougie with enough space left over to allow the passage of an index finger through the wrap adjacent to the bougie. Inset: the completed fundoplication. **E.** Schematic cross-section of a Nissen fundoplication done with 1.5 × 0.5 cm pledgets illustrating how the pledgets compress the stomach and esophagus together and how intragastric (1), intra-abdominal pressure (2), and gastric fundic muscle tone (3) are transmitted to the sphincter.

cedure. The pad of areolar tissue that lies on the anterior surface of the gastroesophageal junction is removed to allow proper identification of the junction and encourage the fusion of the fundic wrap to the esophagus. The freed posterior wall of the fundus is pulled between the right vagal trunk and the posterior wall of the esophagus. A 60-Fr bougie is passed by the anesthesiologist into the stomach, and the anterior wall of the fundus is pulled across the anterior wall of the esophagus. This results in enveloping the distal esophagus between the anterior and posterior fundic wall. We prefer a short wrap secured with Teflon pledgets and permanent monofilament sutures. The suture is tied with a single throw to approximate the two lips of the fundic wrap around the esophagus containing the 60-Fr bougie. When drawn together, the fundic wrap should be large enough to accept the insertion of the surgeon's index finger alongside the esophagus containing the 60-Fr bougie. If the surgeon is unable to insert his finger or feels tight bands over his finger, the wrap is too tight, and the left end of the horizontal U stitch must be replaced more laterally and inferiorly on the anterior wall of the fundus. This enlarges the internal diameter of the wrap. If there is excessive space, the

wrap is too floppy, and the left or anterior end of the U stitch must be replaced more medially and superiorly on the anterior wall of the fundus. This reduces the internal diameter of the wrap. When the wrap is of proper size, and the limbs of the U stitch are tied securely, the bougie is removed.

Transthoracic Nissen Fundoplication. The indications for performing an antireflux procedure by a transthoracic approach are as follows:

1. A patient who has had a previous hiatal hernia repair. In this situation, a peripheal circumferential incision in the diaphragm is made to provide simultaneous exposure of the upper abdomen. This allows safe dissection of the previous repair from both the abdominal and thoracic sides of the diaphragm.
2. A patient who requires a concomitant esophageal myotomy for achalasia or diffuse spasm.
3. A patient who has a short esophagus, which is usually associated with a stricture or Barrett's esophagus. In this situation, the thoracic approach is preferred in order to obtain maxi-

mum mobilization of the esophagus in order to place the repair without tension below the diaphragm.

4. A patient with a sliding hiatal hernia that does not reduce below the diaphragm during a roentgenographic barium study in the upright position. This can indicate esophageal shortening and, again, a thoracic approach is preferred for maximum mobilization of the esophagus.

5. A patient who has associated pulmonary pathology. In these patients, the nature of the pulmonary pathology can be evaluated and the proper pulmonary surgery, in addition to the antireflux repair, can be performed.

6. An obese patient. In these patients, the abdominal repair is difficult because of poor exposure, whereas the thoracic approach gives better exposure and allows a more precise repair.

The hiatus is approached transthoracically through a left posterior lateral thoracotomy incision in the sixth intercostal space (ie, over the upper border of the seventh rib). For patients who have a failed antireflux repair and are undergoing a second procedure, the seventh intercostal space is preferred (ie, above the superior border of the eighth rib). This approach allows better exposure of the abdomen through the diaphragm incision. When necessary, the diaphragm is incised circumferentially 2 to 3 cm from the chest wall for a distance of approximately 10 to 15 cm. An adequate fringe of diaphragm must be preserved along the chest wall of reapproximation of the muscle. The operation is made easier if the anesthetic is delivered through a double-lumen endotracheal tube and the left lung is selectively deflated.

The first step in the operation is to mobilize the esophagus from the level of the diaphragm underneath the aortic arch. Care is taken not to injure the vagal nerves. There are usually two arteries that arise from the proximal descending thoracic aorta and pass over the left lateral surface of the esophagus to the left main stem bronchus. They are the left superior and inferior bronchial arteries. These are ligated individually and represent the cephalad extension of the esophageal mobilization. In addition to these arteries, there are two or three esophageal arteries coming directly from the distal descending thoracic aorta to the lower third of the esophagus. They also are ligated and divided. One need not worry about ischemic necrosis of the esophagus with this degree of dissection. There is sufficient blood supply through the intrinsic arterial plexus of the esophagus, fed by the inferior thyroid artery in the neck and branches of the right bronchial artery in the thorax, to maintain the integrity and prevent ischemic necrosis of the muscle. Mobilization up to the aortic arch is usually

necessary to place the reconstructed cardia of a shortened esophagus into the abdomen without undue tension. Failure to do this is one of the major causes for subsequent breakdown of a transthoracic repair and return of symptoms. The second step of the operation is to free the cardia from the diaphragm. It is the most difficult portion of the transthoracic approach. To accomplish this, it is *not* necessary to make an incision through the central tendon of the diaphragm or to enlarge the hiatus by dividing the crura. With experience, this portion of the operation can be completed through the hiatus. The dissection is started by gaining access into the abdominal cavity through the phrenoesophageal membrane along the anterior border of the left crus, close to the wall of the stomach, away from the gastric vessels. It can be difficult to find the right tissue plane, since the properitoneal fat tends to protrude through the incision once the superior leaf of the membrane has been divided. Persistence and dissection above the protruding properitoneal fat will eventually be rewarded with entry into the free peritoneal space. Entry into the abdominal cavity is easier when a hiatal hernia is present.

The proper stance of the surgeon at the operating table will aid him in the dissection of the hiatus. He should stand adjacent to the patient, facing the head of the table. The left index and middle fingers are placed through the diaphragmatic hiatus into the abdominal cavity, with the palm of the hand facing the patient's feet. The surgeon's line of vision is down and backward under his left axilla. With judicial use of the left thumb, index, and middle fingers, the surgeon is able to spread the hiatal tissues and guide the dissection, done with the scissors in his right hand. In this position, the left hand also is used to retract the esophagus and protect the vagal trunks. Although the description of this stance sounds somewhat awkward, its use greatly facilitates the most difficult part of the operation. In fact, the stance is quite natural and would be assumed eventually by any surgeon who, on numerous occasions, has experienced the struggle of freeing the cardia from the hiatus through a transthoracic approach.

When all the attachments between the cardia and diaphragmatic hiatus are divided, the fundus and part of the body of the stomach are drawn up through the hiatus into the chest. This requires dividing 4 to 6 short gastric arteries supplying the proximal stomach. When the stomach is brought up into the chest, the vascular fat pad that lies on the anterior lateral surface of the cardia is excised in a manner similar to that described for the abdominal approach (Fig 23–39). The third step of the procedure is the placement of the crural sutures used to close the hiatus. To do so the stomach is placed back into the abdomen and the mobilized esophagus is retracted anteriorly to expose the posterior limbs of the right and left crus. Usually there is a decussation of mus-

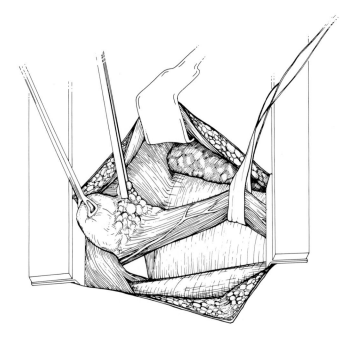

Figure 23–39. Transthoracic antireflux procedure through a left posterolateral thoracotomy, showing mobilization of the esophagus and freeing of the cardia from the diaphragmatic hiatus. The fundus of the stomach is drawn through the hiatus into the chest with a Babcock clamp. The forceps is on the vascular fat pad at the cardioesophageal junction. (From DeMeester TR. Transthoracic antireflux procedures. In: Nyhus LM, Baker RJ (eds), *Mastery of Surgery*. Boston: Little, Brown; 1984:385)

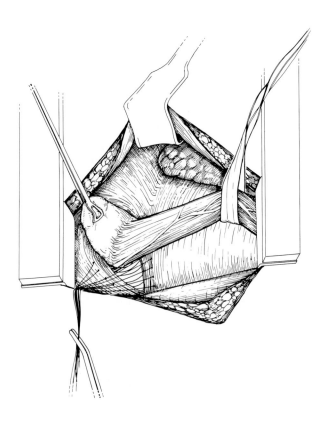

Figure 23–40. Transthoracic antireflux procedure, showing the vascular fat pad removed and anterior retraction of the esophagus, with placement of the crural sutures for closure of this hiatus posteriorly. (From DeMeester TR. Transthoracic antireflux procedures. In: Nyhus LM, Baker RJ (eds), *Master of Surgery*. Boston: Little, Brown; 1984:386)

cle fibers from the right crus around the aorta, but occasionally, the aorta lies free within the enlarged hiatus. In either situation, the first crural stitch is placed close to the aorta, taking a generous bite of crural muscle. Traction on this first suture elevates the crura toward the surgeon and facilitates the placement of subsequent crural stitches. Each stitch should incorporate the fascia from the periphery of the central tendon that blends with the muscle fibers of the right crus. Approximately six sutures, placed 1 cm apart, are necessary to approximate the crura adequately and reduce the size of the hiatus. To insert the most anterior crural stitch, it is often necessary to push the esophagus posteriorly against the previously placed sutures and pass a stitch through the right crus, anterior to the esophagus, then bring it posterior to the esophagus and through the left crus. The crural sutures are not tied until the reconstruction of the cardia is complete (Fig 23–40).

The fourth step of the operation is to construct the fundoplication. The fundus of the stomach is withdrawn through the hiatus into the chest. The wrapping of the fundus around the distal esophagus is performed in a manner similar to that described for the abdominal approach. As in the abdominal approach, the distal esophagus is invaginated into the stomach by placing the fundus lip between the posterior or right vagal nerve and the esophageal body (Fig 23–41). A 60-Fr. bougie is passed by the anesthesiologist into the stomach to size the wrap (Figure 23–42). The technique used to secure the wrap is similar to that described in the transabdominal approach (Figure 23–43).

When complete, the fundoplication is placed into the abdomen by compressing the fundic ball with the hand and manually maneuvering it through the hiatus. Resistance to placing the repair into the abdomen can result from the shoelace obstruction of the previously placed crural sutures. Opening the crural sutures, like loosening the laces of a shoe, relieves the obstruction and aids in placing the reconstructed cardia into the abdomen. Once in the abdomen, the fundoplication should remain there, and a gentle up-and-down motion on the diaphragm should not encourage it to emerge

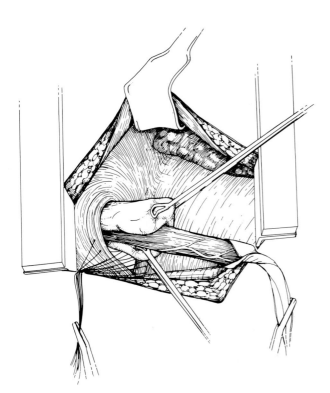

Figure 23–41. Construction of a Nissen 360° gastric fundic wrap, showing the fundus of the stomach brought up through the hiatus anterior to the esophagus. (From DeMeester TR. Transthoracic antireflux procedures. In: Nyhus LM, Baker RJ (eds), *Mastery of Surgery*. Boston: Little, Brown; 1984:388)

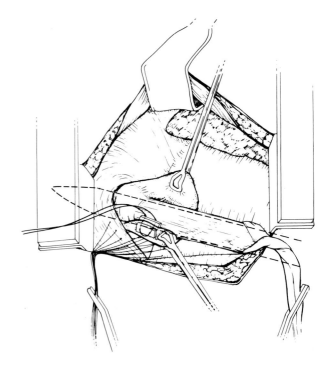

Figure 23–42. Continued construction of a Nissen 360° gastric wrap, showing placement of the U stitch with the Teflon pledgets in the right lateral lip of the fundic wrap. The esophagus and stomach have been rotated to the right for easier placement of this suture. When the suture has been placed, a 60-Fr bougie is passed into the stomach to allow accurate sizing of the wrap and to allow identification of the posterior border of the gastroesophageal junction. (From DeMeester TR. Transthoracic antireflux procedures. In: Nyhus LM, Baker RJ (eds), *Mastery of Surgery*. Boston: Little, Brown; 1984:389)

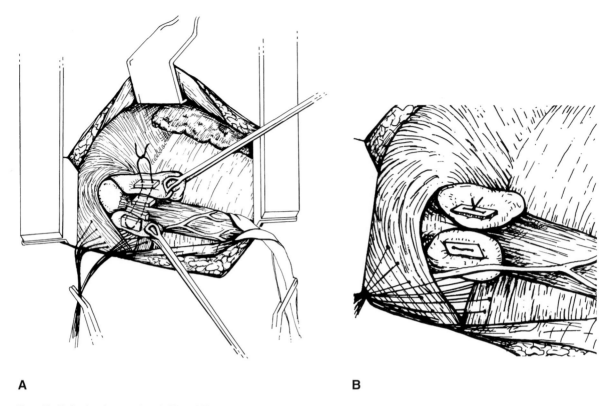

A

B

Figure 23–43. Continued construction of a Nissen 360° gastric fundic wrap, showing the position of the U stitch and the four Teflon pledgets. The stomach and esophagus have been rotated to the right for easier placement of the U stitch, which is tied over 1.5 to 0.5-cm Teflon pledgets. The stomach and esophagus have been rotated to the right to demonstrate the U stitch. The inferior or right lip of the wrap should lie between the right vagus nerve and the esophageal wall. (Redrawn from De-Meester TR. Transthoracic antireflux procedures. In: Nyhus LM, Baker RJ (eds), *Mastery of Surgery.* Boston: Little, Brown; 1984:390)

back through the esophageal hiatus into the chest. If the repair remains in the abdomen unaided, the previously placed crural sutures are tied.

If the fundoplication tends to ride up through the hiatus, tension on the repair is too great, usually owing to inadequate mobilization of the esophagus. If there has been complete mobilization and the fundoplication still tends to ride up through the hiatus, the branches of the left vagus nerve to the left pulmonary plexus can be divided in an effort to reduce the tension. If, after this maneuver, the tendency to ride up through the hiatus persists, a Collis gastroplasty is done. If a short wrap of 1 to 2 cm is used and the esophagus has been adequately mobilized, the need for a Collis gastroplasty becomes a serious consideration in only about 10% of the repairs. This, however, will vary depending on how long the referring gastroenterologist persists in treating these patients.

At the completion of the procedure, a nasogastric tube should be able to be passed, without guidance from the surgeon, directly into the stomach to ensure that there has been no angulation of the distal esophagus. A chest tube for drainage of the pleural cavity is properly placed and the chest incision closed.

Belsey Mark IV Partial Fundoplication

In the presence of altered esophageal motility, where the propulsive force of the esophagus is not sufficient to overcome the outflow obstruction of a complete fundoplication, a partial fundoplication may be indicated. The Belsey Mark IV repair is the prototype of such a partial fundoplication and consists of a 270° gastric fundoplication performed through the chest. The dissection of the Belsey Mark IV and the transthoracic Nissen operations are the same, differing only in the technique of constructing the gastric fundoplication (Fig 23–44).

To perform the Belsey Mark IV reconstruction antireflux procedure, the esophagus is mobilized up to the aortic arch, the cardia is dissected free of the hiatus and the fundus of the stomach is brought up through the hiatus, as described for the transthoracic Nissen procedure. The partial fundoplication is held in place by two rows of three horizontal mattress sutures placed equidistantly between the seromuscular layers of the stomach and the muscular layers of the esophagus. Each suture should obtain a firm grip of the esophageal muscle fibers by passing down to, but not through, the muscularis mucosa. The first row of sutures is placed 1.5 cm

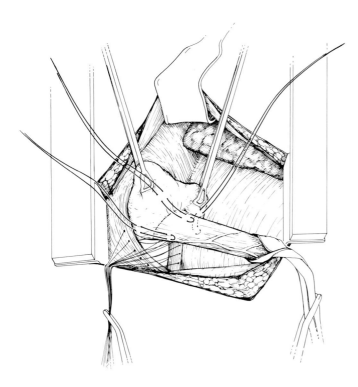

A

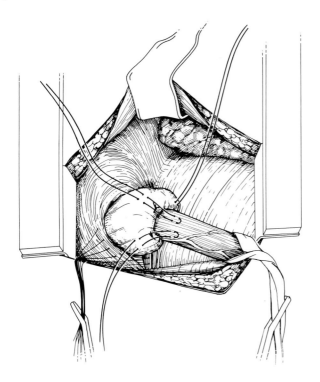

Figure 23–44. A. Construction of a Belsey 240° gastric fundic wrap showing placement of the first row of sutures 1.5 cm above the gastroesophageal junction. Particular attention must be given to placement of the right lateral suture. **B**. Continued construction of the Belsey 240° gastric fundic wrap showing placement of the second row of sutures 1.5 to 2.0 cm above the previously tied sutures of the first row. *Continued*

B

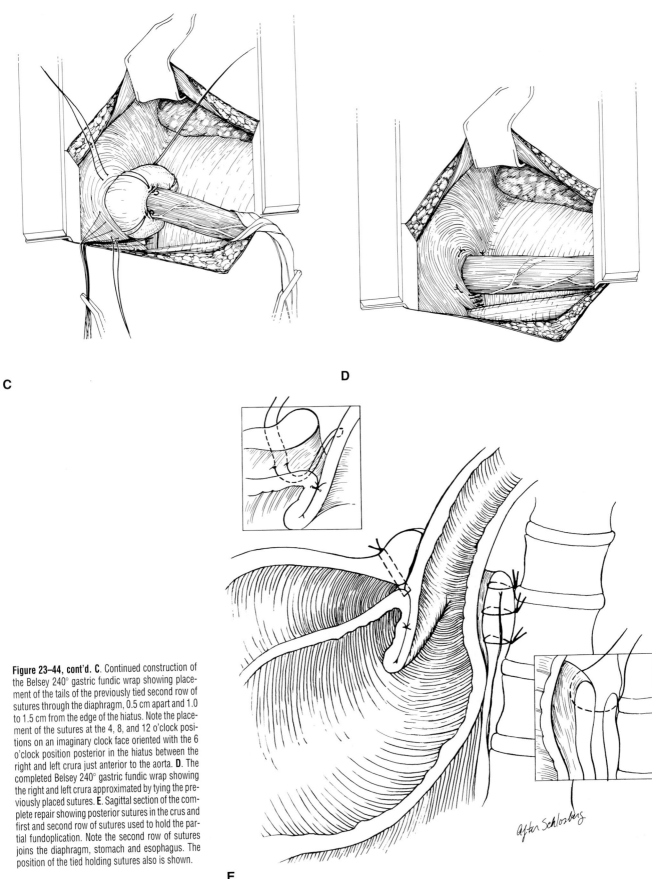

C

D

Figure 23–44, cont'd. C. Continued construction of the Belsey 240° gastric fundic wrap showing placement of the tails of the previously tied second row of sutures through the diaphragm, 0.5 cm apart and 1.0 to 1.5 cm from the edge of the hiatus. Note the placement of the sutures at the 4, 8, and 12 o'clock positions on an imaginary clock face oriented with the 6 o'clock position posterior in the hiatus between the right and left crura just anterior to the aorta. **D**. The completed Belsey 240° gastric fundic wrap showing the right and left crura approximated by tying the previously placed sutures. **E**. Sagittal section of the complete repair showing posterior sutures in the crus and first and second row of sutures used to hold the partial fundoplication. Note the second row of sutures joins the diaphragm, stomach and esophagus. The position of the tied holding sutures also is shown.

after Schlosberg

E

above the external gastroesophageal junction and is tied only tightly enough to obtain tissue apposition without disrupting the muscle fibers of the esophagus. It is important to remember that the hiatus is approached surgically from the left lateral position. To construct the fundoplication over the anterolateral two-thirds of the esophagus, it is necessary that the far right suture be placed in the right lateral wall of the esophagus. This is out of the surgeon's view and requires rotating the esophagus before placement of the suture. A common mistake is placing this suture too far anteriorly, resulting in an anterolateral fundoplication displaced to the left. This is a less effective gastric wrap and can result in an incompetent cardia.

A second row of sutures is placed 1.5 to 2.0 cm above the first row, using the position of the previously placed sutures in the first row as a guide. Once again the sutures in the second row are tied carefully to achieve tissue apposition without strangulation. The tails of these sutures are not cut, but are separately rethreaded on a large thin Ferguson needle and passed 0.5 cm apart from each other through the diaphragm from the abdominal to the thoracic surface, 1.0 cm from the edge of the hiatus. The diaphragmatic sutures are placed at the 4, 8, and 12 o'clock positions, oriented with the 6 o'clock position placed posteriorly between the right and left crus just anterior to the aorta. It is important to place the right lateral, or 4 o'clock suture, correctly to avoid the common error of putting this stitch too far anteriorly, in the 1 or

2 o'clock position, and ending with an anterolateral fundoplication displaced to the left. These sutures must be carefully placed to avoid injury to the abdominal structures. Belsey has popularized the spoon retractor to aid in their placement. The needle is guided along the inner surface of the spoon prior to passing it through the diaphragm. This avoids the possibility of snagging loose omental tissue.

The reconstructed cardia is pushed gently through the hiatus and placed in the abdomen. It is not dragged down into the abdomen by pulling on the diaphragmatic sutures, but rather placed into the abdomen by compressing the fundic ball with the hand and manually maneuvering it through the hiatus as described for the transthoracic Nissen procedure. Once in the abdomen, the cardia should remain there without tension on the holding sutures. As with the transthoracic Nissen repair, a gentle up-and-down motion of the diaphragm should not allow the repair to emerge back through the esophageal hiatus. If it does, the tension on the repair is too great, and the problem is managed as described previously for the transthoracic Nissen procedure. If the repair remains in the abdomen unaided, the previously placed crural sutures are tied. The holding sutures then are tied, approximating the knot against the previously tied knot now located under the diaphragm, so as to avoid any redundancy in the suture between the repair and the diaphragm. An additional safety factor of the double-knot technique is that if one of the tails of the holding sutures breaks while it is being tied, it is not nec-

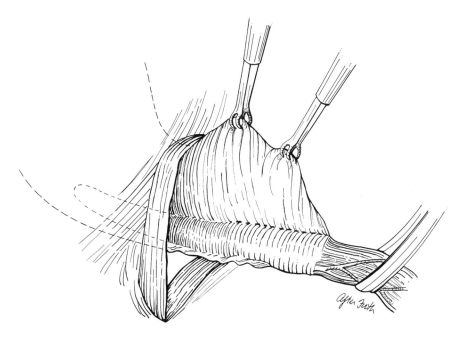

Figure 23–45. A. Construction of a Collis gastroplasty. A 48-Fr bougie is passed into the stomach. The *dotted line* indicates the site of division of the gastric wall for construction of the gastric tube in continuity with the esophagus. *Continued*

A

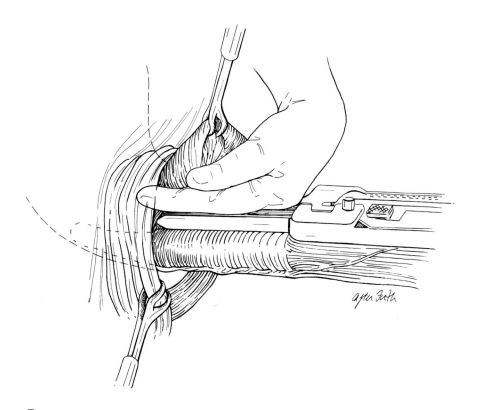

B

Figure 23–45, cont'd. **B**. Continued construction of the Collis gastroplasty. The stomach is divided with a GIA stapler. Traction is exerted on the greater curvature side of the fundus before closing the jaws of the stapler. This ensures that the gastric tube closely approximates the diameter of the indwelling 48-Fr bougie throughout its length. **C**. After stapling and division of the stomach, a 5-cm gastric tube is formed along the proximal portion of the lesser curvature. This effectively lengthens the esophagus and allows the construction of a Belsey partial fundoplication that can be placed below the diaphragm without tension.

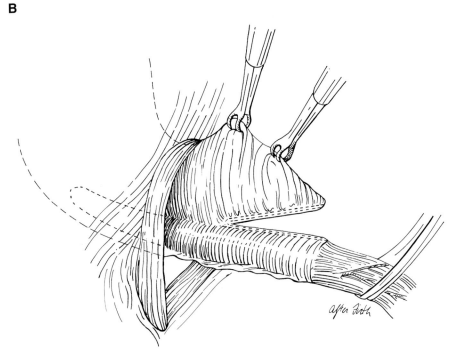

C

TABLE 23–4. IMPROVEMENT OF THE PRIMARY SYMPTOM RESPONSIBLE FOR SURGERY AFTER THE VARIOUS TAILORED ANTIREFLUX PROCEDURES

	No. of Patients Cured	No. of Procedures Failed	% Cured
TAN/LN (n=49)	44	5	90
TTN (n=20)	19	1	95
Belsey (n=7)	4	3	57
Collis-Belsey (n=9)	8	1	88
Total (n=85)	75	10	89

(From Kauer WKH, Peters JH, Ireland AP, et al. A tailored approach to antireflux surgery. J Thorac Cardiovasc Surg 1995;110:141–147)
TAN = Transabdominal Nissen
TTN = Transthoracic Nissen
LN = Lap Nissen

essary to take the repair down, pull the stomach back up into the chest, and insert a new suture. Simple anchoring of the single remaining tail to the diaphragm is sufficient to hold the cardia in position. This technique also prevents tying the sutures too tight and causing necrosis of the incorporated esophageal tissue.

In patients with a short esophagus secondary to a stricture, Barrett's esophagus or a large hiatal hernia, the esophagus is lengthened with a Collis gastroplasty (Fig 23–45). The gastroplasty lengthens the esophagus by constructing a gastric tube along the lesser curvature. This allows a tension-free construction of a Belsey Mark IV or Nissen fundoplication around the newly formed gastric tube, with placement of the repair in the abdomen. Because of the absence of peristalsis in the gastric tube, most surgeons prefer to combine the gastroplasty with a 280° Belsey Mark IV fundoplication rather than a 360° Nissen fundoplication.

Results of Primary Antireflux Surgery

Antireflux surgery is different from the surgery to extirpate a diseased organ whose function is of no concern, since it will be destroyed with its removal. Rather, antireflux surgery is designed to improve the function of an organ that will remain in the patient (ie, to provide complete and permanent relief of all symptoms and complications of gastroesophageal reflux secondary to an incompetent cardia). Successful surgery for antireflux disease requires tailoring of the surgical approach to the patient's underlying physiology. Poor results are frequently based on an inappropriate procedure performed without consideration of underlying physiologic and anatomic abnormalities. Options include open and laparoscopic Nissen fundoplication, transthoracic approaches, partial fundoplications such as the Belsey Mark IV and esophageal lengthening procedures. There authors recently reviewed the results of 136 patients undergoing antireflux surgery in which such a tai-

lored approach was used (Table 23–4). Tailoring of the surgical approach in patients with advanced disease resulted in an outcome similar to that of patients with normal esophageal length and contractility. We believe patients considered for antireflux surgery should undergo physiologic testing and the choice of surgical procedure tailored to the findings.

In the majority of patients who have good esophageal contractility and normal esophageal length, the Nissen fundoplication is the procedure of choice for a primary antireflux repair. Experience and randomized studies have shown that the Nissen fundoplication is an effective and durable antireflux repair with minimal side effects, while providing relief of reflux symptoms in 91% of patients over 10 years (Fig 23–46).[89] This is accomplished by restoring normal mechanical characteristics to a defective lower esophageal sphincter (Fig 23–47). Comparison of Nissen fundoplication to both symptomatic and continuous medical therapy in a recent Veterans Administration cooperative trial resulted in the conclusion that surgery was superior to medical therapy in every outcome measure used (Fig 23–48).[92] Furthermore, these results were consistent across the spectrum of institutions and surgical expertise encountered in this multi-institutional study, refuting arguments suggesting antireflux surgery is only appropriate in the hands of esophageal specialists.[93] Although this study has been criticized as not including modern medical therapy, such as proton pump inhibitors, it is unlikely that improvements in medical therapy will result in different conclusions, particularly in the era of laparo-

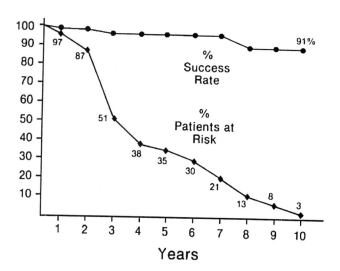

Figure 23–46. Actuarial success rate of the Nissen fundoplication in the control of reflux symptoms. The numbers on the lower curve represent the patients at risk for each subsequent yearly interval from which the actuarial curve was calculated. (From DeMeester TR, Bonavina L, Albertucci M. Nissen fundoplication for gastroesophageal reflux disease—evaluation of primary repair in 100 consecutive patients. *Ann Surg* 1986; 204:15)

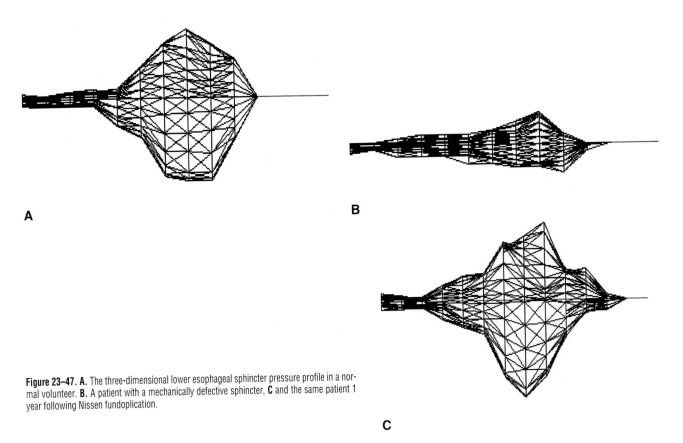

A

B

Figure 23–47. A. The three-dimensional lower esophageal sphincter pressure profile in a normal volunteer. **B.** A patient with a mechanically defective sphincter, **C** and the same patient 1 year following Nissen fundoplication.

C

scopic fundoplication.[94] In addition, when data from this study were subjected to sophisticated analysis of the costs associated with therapy, antireflux surgery proved more cost effective than long term medical therapy in patients under 59 years of age.[95]

SURGICAL THERAPY OF COMPLICATED REFLUX DISEASE

The Problem of Barrett's Esophagus

The condition whereby the tubular esophagus is lined with columnar epithelium rather than squamous epithelium was first described by Norman Barrett in 1950. He incorrectly believed it to be congenital in origin. It is now realized that it is an acquired abnormality, occurs in 7% to 20% of patients with GERD, and represents a peculiar form of healing of the mucosal ulceration produced in this disease. It also is understood to be distinctly different from the congenital condition in which islands of mature gastric columnar epithelium are found in the upper half of the esophagus. In the spectrum of GERD, Barrett's esophagus stands out as being associated with profound mechanical deficiency of the lower esophageal sphincter, severe impairment of esophageal body function, and the market esophageal acid exposure. Gastric hypersecretion occurs in 44% of patients.

The typical complications of Barrett's esophagus include ulceration in the columnar lined segment, stric-

ture formation, and a dysplasia cancer sequence. Ulceration is unlike the erosive ulceration of reflux esophagitis, in that it more closely resembles peptic ulceration in the stomach or duodenum and has the same propensity to bleed, penetrate, or perforate. The strictures found in Barrett's esophagus occur at the squamocolumnar junction, and are typically higher than peptic strictures in the absence of Barrett's. The risk of adenocarcinoma developing in Barrett's mucosa is variously estimated at 1 in 50 to 1 in 400 patient years of follow-up. By conservative estimates, this represents a risk 40 times that of the general population. Most adenocarcinomas of the esophagus arise in Barrett's esophagus. Conversely, about one-third of all patients with Barrett's esophagus present with malignancy.

The development of complications is believed to be related to the reflux of gastric juice, mixed with duodenal juice secondary to the concomitant excessive duodenogastric reflux. Nearly 60% of patients with complications of Barrett's esophagus had abnormal esophageal alkaline exposure compared with 6% of patients without complications. The columnar mucosal insensitivity and the higher pH of the mixed reflux may be the reason why tissue damage may continue without worsening of the patient's symptoms.

The approach to the patient with suspected Barrett's

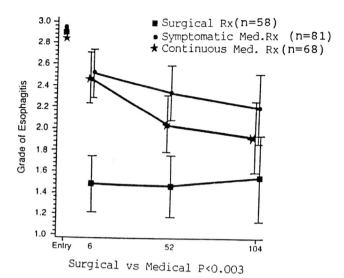

Figure 23–48. Grade of esophagitis in patients with gastroesophageal reflux during a 2-year study. Values are mean ± 2 SE. Three groups are represented: (1) continuous medical therapy (*stars*), (2) intermittent medical therapy for symptoms only (*circles*), and (3) surgical treatment (*squares*). Mean scores were significantly lower in the surgical therapy group when compared with either medical therapy group, P <.003. (From Spechler SJ. Department of Veterans Affairs Gastroesophageal Reflux Study Group. Comparison of medical and surgical therapy for complicated gastroesophageal reflux disease in veterans. *N Engl J Med* 1992;326:789)

esophagus begins with an upper gastrointestinal barium contrast roentgenogram and endoscopy. The esophagogram may show a hiatus hernia that, if it fails to reduce in the upright posture, may indicate a shortened esophagus. It also may show a high esophageal stricture or a penetrating ulcer. Endoscopically, Barrett's esophagus is recognized by the appearance of gastric-type mucosa extending 2 cm or more into the tubular esophagus. Shorter segments of Barrett's mucosa have been discovered by biopsy and are prone to the same risks of cancer. The columnar mucosa may be in the form of a tongue, and need not be circumferential. The endoscopic diagnosis must be confirmed histologically. To avoid sampling errors, we recommend performing at least two biopsies for every 1 cm interval along the length of the Barrett's segment. The most important feature is to identify the presence of intestinalization of the mucosa and whether dysplasia has occurred, and if so, whether of high or low grade.

Patients with a low risk of developing complications and whose symptoms are readily controlled by medication are suitable for medical therapy. H2 blockers and omeprazole often bring symptomatic improvement, especially if hypersecretion of acid is an etiologic factor. Objective healing of ulcers and stabilization of strictures is not as reliably achieved. The value of prokinetic agents, such as bethanechol or cisapride, is usually minimal because of the loss of esophageal body function. The chief problem with medical treatment is that acid

reduction therapy does nothing to correct the underlying mechanically defective sphincter and, therefore, does nothing to reduce the reflux of neutralized gastric juice or the prevention of aspiration. The symptomatic relief may allow tissue damage to progress unnoticed, so that advancement of the disease continues to occur. For this reason, surgery is appropriate earlier in the course of the disease, when it is first evident that the esophagitis is resistant to healing by usual measures.

In uncomplicated Barrett's esophagus, the loss of esophageal body function still can occur, but the patients are less often referred for surgery. More often, patients with complicated Barrett's esophagus are referred for surgery and the status of esophageal function renders it necessary to modify the operative strategy. These include esophageal body shortening, loss of peristaltic propulsive force, stricture formation, and a large penetrating ulcer.

In these circumstances, it is wiser to use a transthoracic approach, since it allows thorough mobilization of the infra-aortic esophagus and provides the option for performing a Collis gastroplasty, if shortening of the esophagus persists despite full mobilization. It also puts the surgeon in the best position to deal with mediastinal inflammation secondary to a penetrating ulcer, where there is a risk of creating a full-thickness defect in the esophageal wall after mobilization. If this occurs, esophageal replacement is usually necessary.

Since Barrett's esophagus is a premalignant condition, there are strong theoretic grounds for stopping the progress towards malignancy by performing antireflux surgery. Regression of Barrett's epithelium after surgery has not often been reported, and when reported, the cause may have been an artefact related to surgical relocation of the esophagogastric junction. Despite the lack of regression, there is a growing body of evidence to attest to the ability of fundoplication to protect against dysplasia and invasive malignancy. Although some cancers have developed after antireflux surgery, the absence of preexistent dysplasia or the efficacy of the operative procedure in reducing 24 hour esophageal acid exposure to normal has not been documented. A long-term registry maintained on patients with Barrett's esophagus, free of dysplasia on entry, recently reported that the development of dysplasia and cancer in patients healed medically was 19.7% and 1.3%, respectively, whereas in those treated by fundoplication, dysplasia emerged in only 3.4%, and no cancers developed. This information has been used to recommend surgery as a prophylactic measure in patients with a segment of Barrett's mucosa free of dysplasia. It is unknown what effect antireflux surgery has when dysplasia is already present. The situation is more clear when high-grade dysplasia is discovered at biopsy. If this is confirmed by two knowledgeable pathologists, an

esophagectomy is recommended, since 50% of the operative specimen from these patients will show early invasive carcinoma.

Stricture

The development of a stricture while on acid suppression therapy, in a patient with a mechanically defective
sphincter, represents a failure of medical therapy, and
is an indication for a surgical antireflux procedure.
Prior to surgery, a malignant etiology of the stricture
should be excluded and the stricture progressively dilated up to a 60-Fr bougie. Three factors become important in the management of these patients: (1) their
response to dilation, (2) an assessment of esophageal
length by endoscopy or barium swallow, and (3) adequacy of esophageal contractility on motility studies. If
dysphagia is relieved and the amplitude of esophageal
contractions and the length of the esophagus is adequate, a total fundoplication can be performed. In a
patient with adequate esophageal length in whom dysphagia persists or esophageal contractility is compromised, a partial fundoplication should be done. If, in either of these situations, the esophagus is shortened by
the disease process, a gastroplasty and partial fundoplication should be performed (Fig 23–35). When
esophageal acid exposure is normal in a patient with a
stricture, the etiology is most likely owing to a drug-induced injury, and dilation is commonly all that is necessary.

Atypical Reflux Symptoms

Chronic respiratory symptoms such as chronic cough,
recurrent pneumonias, episodes of nocturnal choking,
waking up with gastric contents in the mouth, or soilage
of the bed pillow also may indicate the need for surgical
therapy. The chest roentgenogram in patients suffering
from repetitive pulmonary aspiration secondary to gastroesophageal reflux often shows signs of pleural thickening, bronchiectasis, and chronic interstitial pulmonary fibrosis. If 24 hour pH monitoring confirms the
presence of increased esophageal acid exposure and
manometry shows a mechanical defect of the lower esophageal sphincter and normal esophageal body motility, an antireflux procedure can be done with an expected good result. However, these patients usually
have a nonspecific motor abnormality of the esophageal
body that tends to propel the refluxed material towards
the pharynx. In some of these patients, the motor abnormality will disappear following a surgical antireflux
procedure. In others, the motor disorder will persist
and contribute to postoperative aspiration of swallowed
saliva and food. Consequently, the results of an antireflux procedure in patients with a motor disorder of the
esophageal body are variable.

Chest pain may be an atypical symptom of gastro-

esophageal reflux and is often confused with coronary
artery disease. Fifty percent of patients in whom a cardiac etiology of the chest pain has been excluded will
have increased esophageal acid exposure as a cause of
the episode of pain. An antireflux procedure provides
relief of the chest pain with greater constancy than will
occur with medical therapy.

Dysphagia, regurgitation and/or chest pain on eating,
in a patient with normal endoscopy and esophageal function, can be an indication for an antireflux procedure.
These symptoms usually are related to the presence of a
large paraesophageal hernia, intrathoracic stomach, or a
small hiatal hernia with a narrow diaphragmatic hiatus. A
Schatzki ring may be present with the latter. All these conditions are identified easily with an upper gastrointestinal
roentgenographic barium examination done by a knowledgeable radiologist. These patients may have no heartburn, since the lower esophageal sphincter is usually normal and reflux of gastric acid into the esophagus does not
occur. The surgical repair of the hernia usually includes
an antireflux procedure because the competency of the
cardia has a high probability of being destroyed by the
surgical dissection. If a Schatzki ring is identified in a patient with dysphagia, a hiatus hernia, a normal size of hiatus, and normal esophageal acid exposure, then dilation
with a 60-Fr dilator is usually effective therapy and surgery
is not required.

Scleroderma

Gastroesophageal reflux in association with sclerader-
ma is a particularly difficult situation owing to the complete absence of the lower esophageal sphincter and
contractility in the distal esophagus. Intensive medical
therapy should be used initially, until symptoms or severe esophagitis can no longer be controlled. When this
occurs, a Belsey Mark IV partial fundoplication in association with a gastroplasty can be done with the expectation that this will reduce esophageal acid exposure
but not return it to normal. The gastroplasty is added
because of the shortening of the esophagus that occurs
as a consequence of the disease. About 50% of the patients receive excellent to good results with this approach. If the esophagitis is severe or there has been a
previous failed antireflux procedure and the disease
is associated with delayed gastric emptying, a gastric
resection with Roux-en-Y esophagojejunostomy and a
Hunt-Lawrence pouch provides the best option.

Previous Gastric Surgery

The presence of a mechanically defective sphincter after vagotomy and gastric resection or pyloroplasty can
allow reflux of gastric and pancreaticobiliary secretions
into the esophagus. This problem usually is manifested
by symptoms of regurgitation and pulmonary aspiration. Heartburn may be present. Endoscopic esophagi-

tis can occur and is usually mild. Medical therapy designed to control both acid and alkaline reflux usually fails, and a bile-diverting procedure, without reconstruction of the cardia, is of little benefit in preventing the symptoms of aspiration and may contribute to delayed gastric emptying. A simple antireflux procedure may be difficult when a gastric resection has been done. In this situation, the proper surgical therapy usually requires a gastric resection with a Roux-en-Y esophagojejunostomy and a Hunt-Lawrence pouch.

Reflux in Association with Esophageal Motor Disorders

The presence of reflux esophagitis after balloon dilation for achalasia that persists despite medical therapy is an indication for early surgical intervention, since esophagitis in the presence of a severe motility disorder progresses rapidly to stricture formation. A Belsey Mark IV partial fundoplication should be done in this situation because its low outflow resistance makes it particularly suitable to an esophageal body that has no propulsive activity. Once a stricture has developed under these conditions, esophageal resection and a colon interposition are usually necessary to reestablish alimentation. In this situation, a vagal sparing esophagectomy should be done since postoperative function of the reconstructed foregut is much improved if the vagal function is preserved.

REMEDIAL SURGERY FOR FAILED ANTIREFLUX REPAIRS

Failure of an antireflux procedure occurs when the patient, after the repair, is unable to swallow normally, experiences upper abdominal discomfort during and after meals, and has recurrence or persistence of reflux symptoms. The assessment of these symptoms and the selection of patients who need further surgery is a challenging problem.[96–98] Functional assessment of patients who have recurrent, persistent, or emergent new symptoms following a primary antireflux repair is critical to identify the cause of failure. A retrospective analysis of patients requiring reoperation after a previous antireflux procedure showed that misplacement of the fundoplication around the stomach is the most frequent cause for failure.[99] This situation is followed by partial or complete breakdown of the fundoplication, herniation of the repair into the chest, and construction of a too tight or too long fundoplication (Table 23–5). Attention to the technical details during construction of the primary procedure will avoid these failures, in most instances. The critical role of preoperative esophageal function tests, before the initial procedure, is emphasized by the fact that 10% of these patients had antireflux procedure for a misdiagnosed underlying esophageal motor disorder.

The preferred surgical approach to a patient who has had a previously failed antireflux procedure is through

TABLE 23–5. REASONS FOR FAILURE OF PRIMARY ANTIREFLUX PROCEDURES

Finding	Number
Wrap around stomach	19
Delayed breakdown	13
Repair in chest	11
Too long or too tight Nissen	4
Operative damage to lower esophagus	4
Unsuspected primary motor disorder	5
Ineffective but intact repair	5

a left thoracotomy with a peripheral circumferential incision in the diaphragm, to provide for simultaneous exposure of the upper abdomen and safe dissection of the previous repair from both abdominal and thoracic sides of the diaphragm. Patients who have recurrence of heartburn and regurgitation without dysphagia and good esophageal motility are most amenable to reoperation and can be expected to have an excellent outcome. When dysphagia is the cause of failure, the situation is more difficult to manage. If the dysphagia occurred immediately following the repair, it is usually the result of a technical failure, most commonly owing to a misplaced fundoplication around the upper stomach. Re-repair is usually satisfactory. When dysphagia is associated with poor motility and multiple previous repairs, serious consideration should be given to esophageal resection and replacement. It should be kept in mind that with each redo surgery the esophagus is damaged further and the chances of preserving function becomes less. Also, blood supply is reduced and ischemic necrosis of the esophagus can occur after several previous mobilizations.

■ HIATAL HERNIAS

With the advent of clinical roentgenology, it became evident that a hiatal hernia was a relatively common abnormality and was not always accompanied by symptoms. Three types of esophageal hiatal hernias were identified: (1) the sliding hernia (type I), characterized by an upward dislocation of the cardia in the posterior mediastinum (Fig 23–49); (2) the rolling of paraesophageal hernia (type II), characterized by an upward dislocation of the gastric fundus alongside a normally positioned cardia (Fig 23–50); and (3) the combined sliding-rolling or mixed hernia (type III), characterized by an upward dislocation of both the cardia and the gastric fundus (Fig 23–51). The end stage of a type I or II hernia occurs when the whole stomach migrates up into the chest by rotating 180° around its longitudinal axis

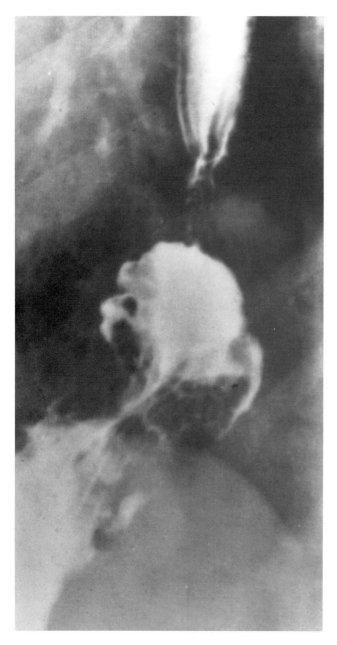

Figure 23–49. Roentgenogram of a type I sliding hiatal hernia. (From DeMeester TR, Bonavina L. Paraesophageal hiatal hernia. In: Nyhus LM, Condon RE (eds), *Hernia*, 3rd ed. Philadelphia, PA: JB Lippincott; 1989:684)

with the cardia and pylorus as fixed points. In this situation, the abnormality usually is referred to as an intrathoracic stomach (Fig 23–52).

INCIDENCE AND ETIOLOGY

The true incidence of a hiatal hernia in the overall population is difficult to determine because of the absence of symptoms in a large number of patients. When roentgenographic examinations were done in response to gastrointestinal symptoms, the incidence of a sliding hiatal hernia was seven times more frequent than a paraesophageal hernia. The age distribution of patients with paraesophageal hernias is significantly different from that observed in sliding hiatal hernias. The former patient has a median age of 61, whereas the latter is 48 years of age. Paraesophageal hernias are more likely to occur in women by a ratio of four to one.

Structural deterioration of the phrenicoesophageal membrane, in the course of time, may explain the higher incidence of hiatal hernias in the older age group (Fig 23–53).[100] These changes involve thinning of the upper fascial layer of the membrane (supradiaphragmatic continuation of the endothoracic fascia) and loss of elasticity in the lower fascial layer (infradiaphragmatic continuation of the transversalis fascia). Consequently, the membrane yields to stretching in the cranial direction owing to persistent intra-abdominal pressure. The upper fascial layer is formed only by loose connective tissue and is of little importance. The lower fascial layer is thick,

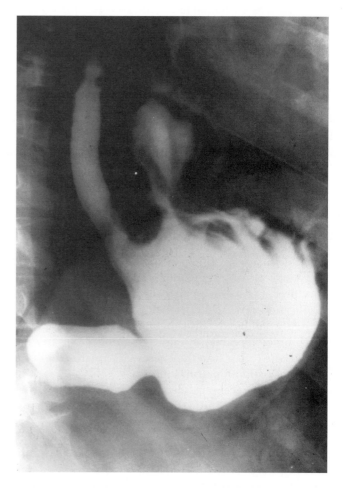

Figure 23–50. Roentgenogram of a type II rolling or paraesophageal hernia. (From DeMeester TR, Bonavina L. Paraesophageal hiatal hernia. In: Nyhus LM, Condon RE (eds), *Hernia*, 3rd ed. Philadelphia, PA: JB Lippincott; 1989:685)

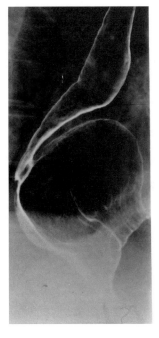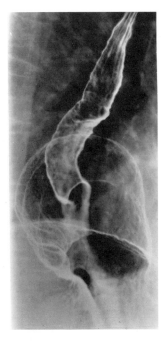

Figure 23–51. Roentgenogram of a type III combined sliding-rolling or mixed hernia. (From DeMeester TR, Bonavina L: Paraesophageal hiatal hernia. In: Nyhus LM, Condon RE (eds), *Hernia,* 3rd ed. Philadelphia, PA: JB Lippincott; 1989:685)

tion present in sliding hiatal hernias also can be present. Both are caused by gastroesophageal reflux secondary to an underlying mechanical deficiency of the cardia. The symptoms of dysphagia and postprandial fullness, in patients with a paraesophageal hernia, are explained by the compression of the adjacent esophagus by a distended cardia, or twisting of the gastroesophageal junction by the torsion of the stomach that occurs as it becomes progressively displaced in the chest.[103]

About one-third of patients with a paraesophageal hernia complain of hematemesis owing to recurrent bleeding from ulceration of the gastric mucosa.[102] Respiratory complications frequently are associated with a paraesophageal hernia and consist of dyspnea from mechanical compression and recurrent pneumonia from aspiration.[102] Intermittent esophageal obstruction can develop in patients with an intrathoracic stomach owing to the rotation that has occurred as the organ migrates into the chest. Conversely, many patients with paraesophageal hiatal hernia are asymptomatic or complain of very minor symptoms.

The condition is life-threatening in one-fifth of patients in that the hernia can lead to sudden cata-

stronger, and of more importance. It divides into an upper and lower leaf, approximately 1 cm, before attaching intimately with the esophageal adventitia.[100] Owing to stretching in the cranial direction from intra-abdominal pressure, the attachment of the lower leaf protrudes upward and can frequently be identified in the thoracic cavity. These observations suggest that the development of a hiatal hernia appears to be a phenomenon related to age and is secondary to repetitive upward stretching of the phrenicoesophageal membrane, owing to up and down movements of the esophagus during swallowing and the upward pushing of the membrane by intra-abdominal pressure. A paraesophageal hernia, rather than a sliding hernia, develops when there is a defect, perhaps congenital, in the esophageal hiatus anterior to the esophagus.[101] The persistent posterior fixation of the cardia to the preaortic fascia and the median arcuate ligament is the only essential difference between a sliding and a paraesophageal hernia. When an anterior defect in the hiatus occurs, in association with a loss of fixation of the cardia, a mixed or type III hernia develops.

SYMPTOMS

The clinical presentation of a paraesophageal hiatal hernia differs from that of a sliding hernia.[102] There is usually a higher prevalence of symptoms of dysphagia and postprandial fullness with paraesophageal hernias, but the typical symptoms of heartburn and regurgita-

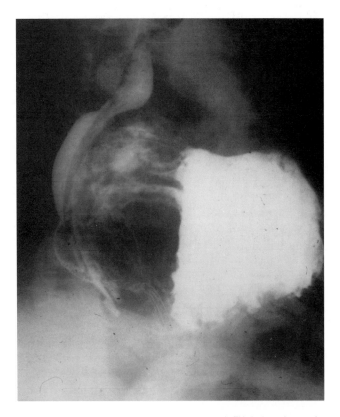

Figure 23–52. Roentgenogram of an intrathoracic stomach. This is the end stage of a large hiatal hernia regardless of its initial classification. Note that the stomach has rotated 180° around its longitudinal axis with the cardia and pylorus as fixed points. (From DeMeester TR, Bonavina L. Paraesophageal hiatal hernia. In: Nyhus LM, Condon RE (eds), *Hernia,* 3rd ed. Philadelphia, PA: JB Lippincott; 1989:686)

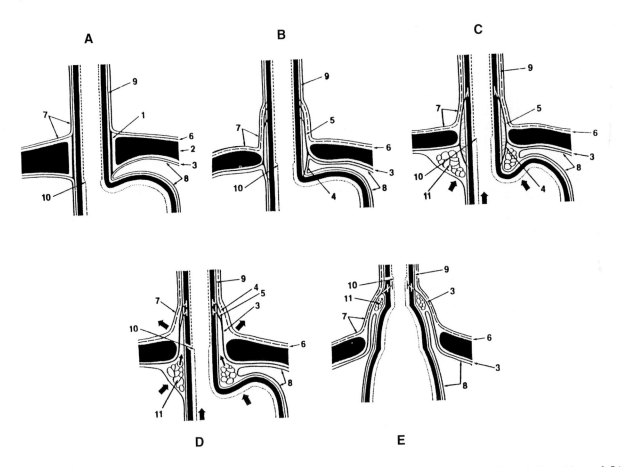

Figure 23–53. Changes in the anatomy of the phrenoesophageal membrane over time based on the dissection of 163 human cadavers from the fetal period to age 75 years. **A.** Fetus; **B.** Newborn and small infants and young adults 20 to 30 years of age; **C.** Old adults 55 to 70 years of age; **D.** Old adults in transition to a hiatal hernia; **E.** Old adults with hiatal hernia. In the fetus, the membrane is closely attached to the adventitia of the esophagus. In neonates, children and young adults, the membrane is slightly stretched. In old adults, loose connective tissue develops in the lower fascial layer. In old adults in transition to hiatal hernia, the lower fascial tissue is pushed cranially to form the developed hernia shown in (E). *Broad arrows* indicate direction of stretch owing to intra-abdominal pressure and movement of the esophagus during swallowing. 1. phrenoesophageal membrane; 2. diaphragmatic crus; 3. lower fascial tissue; 4. lower leaf of lower fascial layer; 5. upper leaf of lower fascial layer; 6. upper fascial layer; 7. pleura; 8. peritoneum; 9. esophageal adventitia; 10. gastroesophageal epithelial junction; 11. subperitoneal fat. (From DeMeester TR, Bonavina L. Paraesophageal hiatal hernia. In: Nyhus LM, Condon RE (eds), *Hernia,* 3rd ed. Philadelphia, PA: JB Lippincott; 1989:687)

strophic events, such as excessive bleeding or volvulus with acute gastric obstruction or infarction.[102] With mild dilation of the stomach, the gastric blood supply can be markedly reduced, causing gastric ischemia, ulceration, perforation, and sepsis.

The symptoms of sliding hiatal hernias are usually the result of functional abnormalities associated with gastroesophageal reflux and include heartburn, regurgitation, and dysphagia. These patients have a mechanically defective lower esophageal sphincter, giving rise to reflux of gastric juice and to the symptoms of heartburn and regurgitation. The symptom of dysphagia occurs from the presence of mucosal edema, Schatzki's ring, stricture, or the inability to organize peristaltic activity in the body of the esophagus as a consequence of the disease. There are a group of patients with hiatal hernias unassociated with the reflux disease who have dysphagia without any obvious endoscopic or manometric explanation. Video barium roentgenograms have shown the cause of dysphagia in these patients to be an obstruction to the passage of the swallowed bolus by diaphragmatic impingement on the herniated stomach. Manometrically, this is reflected by a double-humped high-pressure zone at the gastroesophageal junction caused by diaphragmatic impingement of the herniated stomach and the true distal esophageal sphincter. These patients usually have a mechanically competent sphincter, but the impingement of the diaphragm on the stomach can result in propelling the contents of the supradiaphragmatic portion of the stomach up the esophagus and into the pharynx, resulting in patient complaints of regurgitation and aspiration, often confused with typical GERD. Surgical reduction of the hernia results in relief of the dysphagia in 91% of patients.

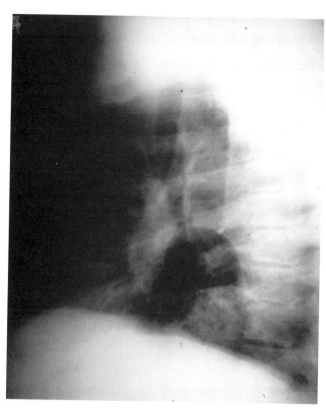

Figure 23–54. Lateral chest roentgenogram showing a posterior mediastinal air-fluid level in a gas bubble, indicating the presence of a paraesophageal hernia. (From De-Meester TR, Bonavina L. Paraesophageal hiatal hernia. In: Nyhus LM, Condon RE (eds), *Hernia*, 3rd ed. Philadelphia, PA: JB Lippincott; 1989:688)

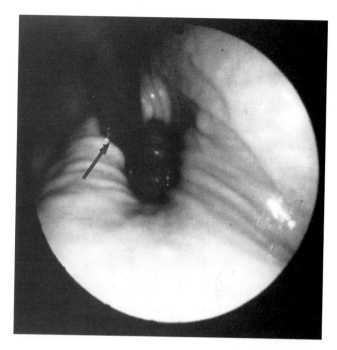

Figure 23–55. Endoscopic view through a retroflexed fiberoptic gastroscope showing the shaft of the scope (*arrow*) coming down through a sliding hernia. Note the gastric rugal folds extending above the impression caused by the crura of the diaphragm. (From DeMeester TR, Bonavina L. Paraesophageal hiatal hernia. In: Nyhus LM, Condon RE (eds), *Hernia*, 3rd ed. Philadelphia, PA: JB Lippincott; 1989:689)

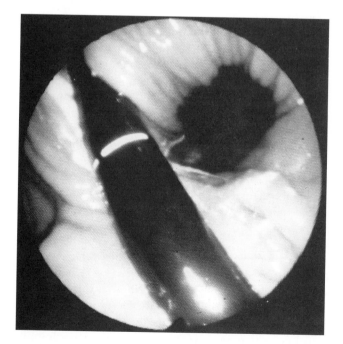

Figure 23–56. Endoscopic view through a retroflexed fiberoptic gastroscope showing the shaft of the scope coming down through the gastroesophageal junction adjacent to a separate orifice of the paraesophageal hernia into which the gastric rugal folds ascend. (From DeMeester TR, Bonavina L. Paraesophageal hiatal hernia. In: Nyhus LM, Condon RE (eds), *Hernia*, 3rd ed. Philadelphia, PA: JB Lippincott; 1989:689)

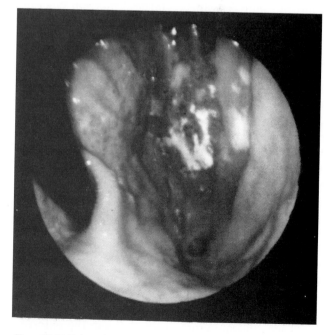

Figure 23–57. Endoscopic view through a retroflexed fiberoptic gastroscope showing the shaft of the scope entering a hernia about midway up the side of a mixed hiatal hernial pouch that extends high into the thorax. (From DeMeester TR, Bonavina L. Paraesophageal hiatal hernia. In: Nyhus LM, Condon RE (eds), *Hernia*, 3rd ed. Philadelphia, PA: JB Lippincott; 1989:689)

DIAGNOSIS

A roentgenogram of the chest with the patient in the upright position can diagnose a hiatal hernia, if it shows an air-fluid level behind the cardiac shadow (Fig 23–54). This presentation usually is caused by a paraesophageal hernia or an intrathoracic stomach. The accuracy of the upper gastrointestinal barium study in detecting a paraesophageal hiatal hernia is greater than for a sliding hernia, since the latter often can reduce spontaneously. The paraesophageal hiatal hernia is a permanent herniation of the stomach into the thoracic cavity, so that a barium swallow provides the diagnosis in virtually every case. When seen, attention should be focused on the position of the gastroesophageal junction to differentiate it from a type II hernia.

Fiberoptic esophagoscopy is very useful in the diagnosis and classification of a hiatal hernia because of the ability to retroflex the scope. In this position, a sliding hiatal hernia can be identified by noting a gastric pouch lined with rugal folds extending above the impression caused by the crura of the diaphragm (Fig 23–55), or measuring at least 2 cm between the crura, identified by having the patient sniff, and the squamous columnar junction on withdrawal of the scope.[20] A paraesophageal hernia is identified on retroversion of the scope by noting a separate orifice adjacent to the gastroesophageal junction into which gastric rugal folds ascend (Fig 23–56). A sliding-rolling or mixed hernia can be identified by noting a gastric pouch lined with rugal folds above the diaphragm, with the gastroesophageal junction entering about midway up the side of the pouch (Fig 23–57).

PATHOPHYSIOLOGY

It has been assumed for a long time that a sliding hiatal hernia is associated with an incompetent distal esophageal sphincter, whereas a paraesophageal hiatal hernia constitutes a pure anatomical entity and is not associated with an incompetent cardia. Accordingly, surgical therapy has been directed toward restoration of the physiology of the cardia in patients with a sliding hernia, and simply reducing the stomach into the abdominal cavity and closing the crura for a paraesophageal hernia.

In the past three decades, there has been an increased interest in the physiology of the gastroesophageal junction and its relationship to the various types of hiatal hernias. Physiologic testing with 24 hour esophageal pH monitoring has shown increased esophageal exposure to acid gastric juice in 60% of the patients with a paraesophageal hiatal hernia, compared with the observed 71% incidence in patients with a sliding hiatal hernia. No relation was found between the symptoms experienced by the patient with a paraesophageal hernia and the competency of the cardia (Table 23–6). Thus, it now

TABLE 23–6. SYMPTOMS IN 15 PATIENTS WITH A PARAESOPHAGEAL HERNIA COMPARED WITH RESULTS OF 24 HOUR ESOPHAGEAL pH MONITORING

Status	Positive	Negative
Heartburn	6 of 9	4 of 6
Regurgitation	6 of 9	3 of 6
Dysphagia	6 of 9	4 of 6
Postprandial fullness	8 of 9	3 of 6
Bleeding	4 of 9	1 of 6

(From DeMeester TR, Bonavina L. Paraesophageal hiatal hernia. In: Nyhus LM, Condon RE (eds), Hernia. 3rd ed. Philadelphia, PA: JB Lippincott; 1989:684–693)

is recognized that paraesophageal hiatal hernia can be associated with pathologic gastroesophageal reflux.[102]

Physiological studies have shown that the competency of the cardia depends on an interrelationship of distal esophageal sphincter pressure, its length exposed to the positive-pressure environment of the abdomen, and its overall length. A deficiency in any one of these manometric characteristics of the sphincter is associated with incompetency of the cardia, regardless of whether a hernia is present.[20,102,104] Patients with a paraesophageal hernia who have incompetent cardias have been shown to have a distal esophageal sphincter with normal pressure, but a shortened overall sphincter length and its displacement outside the positive pressure environment of the abdomen (Fig 23–58).[102] In a sliding hernia, even though the sphincter appears to be within the chest on a roentgenographic barium study, it still can be exposed to abdominal pressure because of the surrounding hernia sac that functions as an extension of the abdominal cavity (Fig 23–59).[20] A high insertion of the phrenoesophageal membrane into the esophagus gives adequate length of the distal esophageal sphincter exposed to abdominal pressure. A low insertion gives inadequate length. The importance of the anatomic length of esophagus within the hernia sac has been emphasized by Bombeck, Dillard, and Nyhus[104] in their careful dissections of the hiatus. They showed that, in 55 patients who underwent postmortem dissection, there were 8 who had a hiatal hernia, 5 of whom had no evidence of esophagitis and, therefore, a competent cardia. In these five patients, the phrenoesophageal membrane inserted 2 to 5 cm with a mean of 3.6 cm above the gastroesophageal junction. The other three patients had evidence of esophagitis and, therefore, an incompetent cardia. In these patients, the membrane inserted 0 to 1 cm with a mean of 0.5 cm above the gastroesophageal junction. This difference was significant and emphasized the importance of an adequate length of intra-abdominal esophagus in maintaining competency of the cardia, even in the presence of a hiatal hernia.

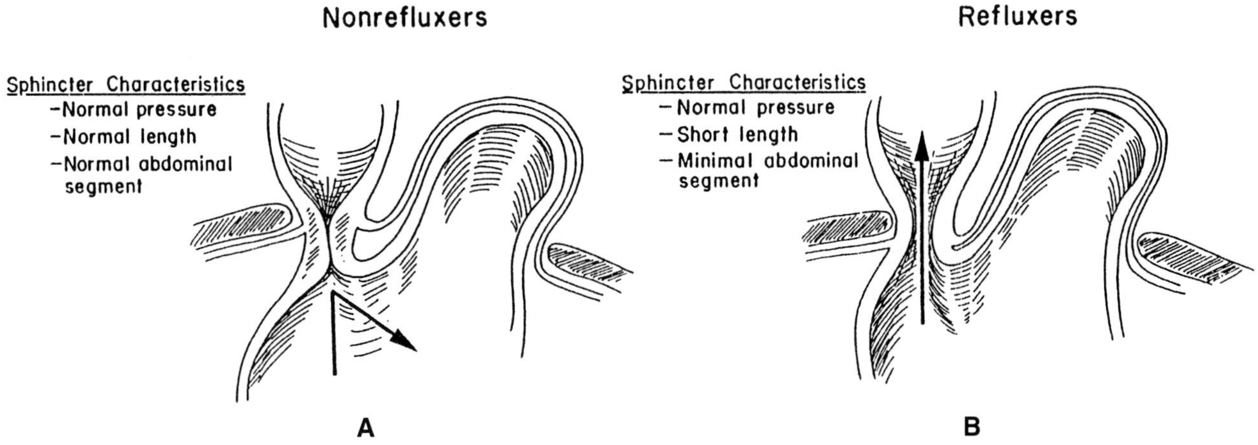

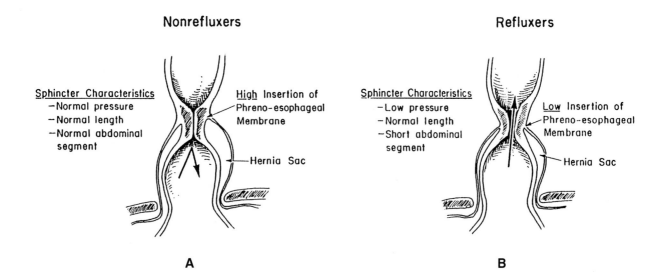

Figure 23–58. Schematic diagram of the anatomic and manometric difference between patients with a paraesophageal hiatal hernia with reflux and those without it, based on a 24 hour esophageal pH monitoring. (From DeMeester TR, Bonavina L. Paraesophageal hiatal hernia. In: Nyhus LM, Condon RE (eds). *Hernia*, 3rd ed. Philadelphia, PA: JB Lippincott; 1989:690)

In contrast to a paraesophageal hernia where the sphincter remains fixed in the abdomen, in a mix type III hernia, the sphincter moves extraperitoneally into the thorax through the widened hiatus along with a portion of the lesser curvature of the stomach and cardia and forms part of the wall of the hernia sac. Consequently, the lower esophageal sphincter lies outside the abdominal cavity and is unaffected by its environmental pressures. The loss of normal esophageal fixation that occurs in a type I sliding hernia or a type III mixed hernia results in the body of the esophagus being less able to carry out its propulsive function. This situation contributes to a greater exposure of the distal esophagus to refluxed gastric juice when components of an incompetent cardia are present.

The cause for a mechanical incompetency of the cardia is similar, regardless of the type of hernia, and is identical in patients who have an incompetent cardia and no hiatal hernia.

THERAPY

The presence of a paraesophageal hiatus hernia is an indication for surgical repair. The catastrophic life-threatening complications of bleeding, infarction, and perforation that are part of the natural history of the hernia in about 25% of patients drive its surgical correction, even in the elderly who have a shorter life expectancy.

In the classic report of Skinner and Belsey, 6 of 21

Figure 23–59. Schematic diagram of the anatomic and manometric difference between patients with a sliding hiatal hernia with reflux and those without it, based on 24 hour esophageal pH monitoring. (From DeMeester TR, Bonavina L. Paraesophageal hiatal hernia. In: Nyhus LM, Condon RE (eds). *Hernia*, 3rd ed. Philadelphia, PA: JB Lippincott; 1989:691)

patients with a paraesophageal hernia, treated medically because of minimal symptoms, died from the complications of strangulation, perforation, exsanguinating hemorrhage, or acute dilation of the herniated intrathoracic stomach. These catastrophes occurred without warning. With this in mind, patients with a paraesophageal hernia are counseled to have electric repair of their hernia, regardless of the severity of their symptoms or the size of the hernia. If surgery is delayed and repair is done on an emergency basis, there is a 19% operative mortality,[105] compared with <1% for an elective repair.[106]

Based on pathophysiologic studies on patients with a paraesophageal hiatal hernia, the repair of paraesophageal hernia should include an antireflux procedure to correct the sphincter characteristics associated with a mechanically incompetent cardia. This procedure is particularly necessary when the operation is performed on an urgent basis without preoperative studies. If time permits, preoperative evaluation with 24 hour esophageal pH monitoring and esophageal manometry allows the identification of patients with competent cardia. Such patients are candidates for a simple anatomic repair, provided it can be done without surgical dissection of the cardia. If dissection of the cardia is necessary, an antireflux procedure should be added to the repair. Operative repair of sliding hiatal hernias are driven by symptoms of, or complications of, GERD, unless the patient is determined to have impingement of the stomach by the diaphragm as a cause of symptoms, as discussed above.

REFERENCES

1. Allison PR. Peptic ulcer of the esophagus. *J Thorac Surg* 1946;15:308
2. Allison PR. Reflux esophagitis, sliding hiatus hernia and the anatomy of repair. *Surg Gynecol Obstet* 1951;92:419
3. Allison PR. Hiatus hernia: a 20 year retrospective survey. *Ann Surg* 1973;178:273
4. Boerema I. Gastropexia anterior geniculata for sliding hiatus hernia and cardiospasm. *J Int Coll Surg* 1958;29:533
5. Nissen R. Gastropexy as the lone procedure in the surgical repair of hiatus hernia. *Am J Surg* 1956;92:389
6. Hill LD, Tobias JA. An effective operation for hiatal hernia: an eight year appraisal. *Ann Surg* 1967;166:681
7. Baue AE, Belsey RHR. The treatment of sliding hiatus hernia and reflux esophagitis by the Mark IV technique. *Surgery* 1967;62:396
8. Nissen R. Eine einfache Operation zur Beeinflussung der Refluxoesophagitis. *Schweiz Med Wochenschr* 1956;86:590
9. Nissen R. Gastropexy and 'fundoplication' in surgical treatment of hiatus hernia. *Am J Dig Dis* 1961;6:954
10. Negre JB. Hiatus hernia: Post-fundoplication symptoms: do they restrict the success of Nissen fundoplication? *Ann Surg* 1983;198:698
11. Pearson FG, Cooper JD, Patterson GA, et al. Gastroplasty and fundoplication for complex reflux problems. *Ann Surg* 1987;206:473–480
12. Zaninotto G, DeMeester TR, Schwizer W, et al. The lower esophageal sphincter in health and disease. *Am J Surg* 1988;155:104–111
13. Bonavina L, Evander A, DeMeester TR, et al. Length of the distal esophageal sphincter and competency of the cardia. *Am J Surg* 1986;151:25–34
14. DeMeester TR. What is the role of the intraoperative manometry? *Ann Thorac Surg* 1980;30:1–4
15. Biancani P, Zabinsky MP, Behar J. Pressure, tension, and force of closure of the human lower esophageal sphincter and esophagus. *J Clin Invest* 1975;56:476–483
16. DeMeester TR, Wernly JA, Bryant GH, et al. Clinical and in vitro analysis of gastroesophageal competence: a study of the principles of antireflux surgery. *Am J Surg* 1979; 137:39–46
17. Bombeck CT, Vaz O, DeSalvao J, et al. Computerized axial manometry of the esophagus. *Ann Surg* 1987;206:465
18. Stein HJ, DeMeester TR, Naspetti R, et al. Three-dimensional imaging of the lower esophageal sphincter in gastroesophageal reflux disease. *Ann Surg* 1991;214:374–384
19. Joelsson BE, DeMeester TR, Skinner DB, et al. The role of the esophageal body in the antireflux mechanism. *Surgery* 1982;92:417–424
20. DeMeester TR, Lafontaine E, Joelsson BE, et al. The relationship of a hiatal hernia to the function of the body of the esophagus and the gastroesophageal junction. *J Thorac Cardiovasc Surg* 1981;82:547–558
21. Helm JF, Riedel DR, Dodds WJ, et al. Determinants of esophageal acid clearance in normal subjects. *Gastroenterology* 1983;85:607–612
22. Bremner RM, Hoeft SD, Constatini M, et al. Pharyngeal swallowing: the major factor in clearance of esophageal reflux episodes. *Ann Surg* 1993;218:364–370
23. Kahrilas PJ, Dodds WJ, Hogan WJ. Effect of peristaltic dysfunction on esophageal volume clearance. *Gastroenterology* 1988;94:73–80
24. Helm JF, Dodds WJ, Pelc LR, et al. Effect of esophageal emptying and saliva on clearance of acid from the esophagus. *N Engl J Med* 1984;310:284–288
25. Helm JF, Dodds WJ, Hogan WJ. Salivary responses to esophageal acid in normal subjects and patients with reflux esophagitis. *Gastroenterology* 1982;93:1393–1397
26. Mittal RK, Lange RC, McCallum RW. Identification and mechanism of delayed esophageal acid clearance in subjects with hiatus hernia. *Gastroenterology* 1987;92:132
27. Sloan S, Kahrilas PJ. Impairment of esophageal emptying with hiatal hernia. *Gastroenterology* 1991;100:596–605
28. Davenport HW. *Physiology of the Digestive Tract*, 5th ed. Chicago, IL: Year Book Medical; 1982:52–69
29. McCallum RW, Berkowitz DM, Lerner E. Gastric emptying in patients with gastroesophageal reflux. *Gastroenterology* 1981;80:285–291
30. Kaye MD, Showalter JP. Pyloric incompetence in patients with symptomatic gastroesophageal reflux. *J Lab Clin Med* 1974;83:198–206
31. Barlow AP, DeMeester TR, Ball CS, et al. The significance of the gastric secretory state in gastroesophageal reflux disease. *Arch Surg* 1989;124:937–940

32. Mittal RK, McCallum RW. Characteristics of transient lower esophageal sphincter relaxation in humans. *Am J Physiol* 1987;252:636

33. Mittal RK, Stewart WR, Shirmer BD. Effect of a catheter in the pharynx on the frequency of transient lower esophageal relaxations. *Gastroenterology* 1992;103:1236–1240

34. Pace F, Santalucia F, Porro GB. Natural history of gastro-oesophageal reflux disease without esophagitis. *Gut* 1991; 32:845–848

35. Ollyo JB, Monnier P, Fontolliet C, et al. The natural history, prevalence and incidence of reflux esophagitis. *Gullet* 1993;3(suppl):3–10

36. Pellegrini CA, DeMeester TR, Wernly JA, et al. Alkaline gastroesophageal reflux. *Am J Surg* 1978;135:177–184

37. Fiorucci S, Santucci L, Chiucchiu S, et al. Gastric acidity and gastroesophageal reflux patterns in patients with esophagitis. *Gastroenterology* 1992;103:855–861

38. DeMeester TR, Wang CI, Wernly JA, et al. Technique, indications, and clinical use of 24 hour esophageal pH monitoring. *J Thor Cardiovasc Surg* 1980;79(5):656–667

39. Jamieson JR, Stein HJ, DeMeester TR, et al. Ambulatory 24-hour esophageal pH monitoring: normal values, optimal thresholds, specificity, sensitivity, and reproducibility. *Am J Gastroenterol* 1992;87(9):1102–1111

40. Jaervinen V, Meurman JH, Hyvaerinen H, et al. Dental erosion and upper gastrointestinal disorders. *Oral Surg Med Pathol* 1988;65(3):298–303

41. DeVault KR, Georgeson S, Castell DO. Salivary stimulation mimics esophageal exposure to refluxed duodenal contents. *Am J Gastroenterol* 1993;88(7):1040–1043

42. Stein HJ, Feussner H, Kauer W, et al. 'Alkaline' gastroesophageal reflux assessment by ambulatory esophageal aspiration and pH monitoring. *Am J Surg* 1994. (In press).

43. Kauer WKH. Langzeitrefluxaspirationstest - eine neue Methode zur qualitativen und quantitativen Refluatanalyse bei "nicht saurem" Reflux. Munich, Germany: Technical University of Munich: 1994. Thesis. (Submitted).

44. Singh S, Bradley LA, Richter JE. Determinants of esophageal 'alkaline' pH environment in controls and patients with gastro-oesophageal reflux disease. *Gut* 1993;34(3): 309–316

45. Stein HJ, Hoeft S, DeMeester TR. Functional foregut abnormalities in Barrett's esophagus. *J Thorac Cardiovasc Surg* 1993;105(1):107–111

46. Attwood SE, DeMeester TR, Bremner CG, et al. Alkaline gastroesophageal reflux: implications in the development of complications in Barrett's columnar-lined lower esophagus. *Surgery* 1989;106(4):764–770

47. Fuchs KH, DeMeester TR. Intragastric pH pattern analysis in patients with duodenogastric reflux. *Dig Dis Sci* 1990;8:(suppl 1)54–59

48. Gotley DC, Ball DE, Ownen RW, et al. Evaluation and surgical correction of esophagitis after partial gastrectomy. *Surgery* 1992;111:29–36

49. Gotley DC, Morgan AP, Ball D, et al. Composition of gastro-oesophageal refluxate. *Gut* 1991;32:1093–1099

50. Stein HJ, Hinder RA, DeMeester TR. Clinical use of 24-hour gastric pH monitoring vs. o-diisopropyl iminodiacetic acid (DISIDA) scanning in the diagnosis of pathologic duodenogastric reflux. *Arch Surg* 1990;125(8):966–970

51. Fuchs KH, DeMeester TR, Hinder RA, et al. Computerized identification of pathologic duodenogastric reflux using 24-hour gastric pH monitoring. *Ann Surg* 1991; 213(1):13–20

52. Ritchie WP. Alkaline reflux gastritis: an objective assessment of its diagnosis and treatment. Ann Surg 1980;92: 288–298

53. Offerhaus GJ, Tersmette AC, Tersmette KW, et al. Gastric, pancreatic and colorectal carcinogenesis following remote peptic ulcer surgery. *Mod Pathol* 1989;1:352–356

54. Stein HJ, Barlow AP, DeMeester TR. Complications of gastroesophageal reflux disease: role of the lower esophageal sphincter, esophageal acid and acid/alkaline exposure, and duodenogastric reflux. *Ann Surg* 1992;216: 35–43

55. Harmon JW, Johnson LF, Maydonovitch CL. Effect of acid and bile salts in the rabbit esophageal mucosa. *Dig Dis Sci* 1981;26(2):65–72

56. Harmon JW, Doang T, Gadacz TR. Bile acids are not equally damaging in the gastric mucosa. *Surgery* 1978; 84(1):79–86

57. DeMeester TR. Barrett's esophagus. *Surgery* 1993;113: 239–240

58. Sarr MG, Hamilton SR, Marone GC, et al. Barrett's esophagus: its prevalence and association with adenocarcinoma in patients with symptoms of gastroesophageal reflux. *Am J Surg* 1985;149:187–193

59. Zaninotto G, DeMeester TR, Bremner CG, et al. Esophageal function in patients with reflux induced strictures and its relevance to surgical treatment. *Ann Thorac Surg* 1989;47:362–370

60. Bonavina L, DeMeester TR, McChesney L, et al. Drug-induced esophageal strictures. *Ann Surg* 1987;206: 173–183

61. Pellegrini CA, DeMeester TR, Johnson LF, et al. Gastroesophageal reflux and pulmonary aspiration: incidence, functional abnormality, and results of surgical therapy. *Surgery* 1979;86:110–119

62. Patti MG, Debas HT, Pellegrini CA. Clinical and functional characterization of high gastroesophageal reflux. *Am J Surg* 1993;165:163–168

63. DeMeester TR, Stein JH. Gastroesophageal reflux disease. In: FG Moody, LC Carey, RC Jones, et al. (eds), *Surgical Treatment of Digestive Disease*, 2nd ed. Chicago, IL: Year Book Medical; 1989

64. DeMeester TR, Johnson LF, Joseph GJ, et al. Patterns of gastroesophageal reflux in health and disease. *Ann Surg* 1976;184:459–470

65. Johnson LF, DeMeester TR. Twenty-four hour pH monitoring of the distal esophagus: a quantitative measure of gastroesophageal reflux. *Am J Gastroenterol* 1974;62:325–332

66. Emde C, Garner A, Blum A. Technical aspects of intraluminal pH-metry in man: current status and recommendations. *Gut* 1987;23:1177–1188

67. Johnson LF, DeMeester TR. Development of 24-hour intraesophageal pH monitoring composite scoring. *J Clin Gastroenterol* 1986;8:52–58

68. Fuchs KH, DeMeester TR, Albertucci M. Specificity and sensitivity of objective diagnosis of gastroesophageal reflux disease. *Surgery* 1987;102:575–580

69. Castell DO, Richter JE, Dalton CB (eds). *Esophageal Motility Testing.* New York, NY: Elsevier; 1987

70. Battle WS, Nyhus LM, Bombeck CT. Gastroesophageal reflux: diagnosis and treatment. *Ann Surg* 1973;177: 560–565

71. Winans CS. Manometric asymmetry of the lower esophageal high pressure zone. *Dig Dis Sci* 1977;22:348–354

72. Eypasch EP, DeMeester TR, Stein JH, et al. A new technique to define and clarify esophageal motor disorders. *Am J Surg* 1990;159:144–152

73. Stein HJ, Eypasch EP, DeMeester TR. Circadian esophageal motor function in patients with gastroesophageal reflux disease. *Surgery* 1990;108:769–778

74. Stein HJ, DeMeester TR, Singh S, et al. Assessment of primary esophageal motor disorders with ambulatory 24-hour monometry. Presentation 1994 Western Surgical Association Annual meeting. Seattle, WA

75. Johnson LF, DeMeester TR, Haggitt RC. Endoscopic signs for gastroesophageal reflux objectively evaluated. *Gastrointest Endosc* 1976;22:151–155

76. Jessurun J, Yardley JH, Giardiello FM, et al. Intracytoplasmic plasma proteins and distended esophageal squamous cells (balloon cells). *Mod Patho* 1988;1(3):175–181

77. Ismail-Beigi F, Pope CE. Distribution of histological changes of gastroesophageal reflux in the distal esophagus in man. *Gastroenterology* 1975;66:1109–1113

78. Johnson LF, DeMeester TR, Haggitt RC. Esophageal epithelial response to gastroesophageal reflux: a quantitative study. *Am J Dig Dis* 1978;23:498–509

79. Attwood SEA, Smyrk TC, Barlow AP, et al. The sensitivity and specificity of histologic parameters in the diagnosis of gastroesophageal reflux disease. In: Little AG, Ferguson MK, Skinner DB (eds), *Diseases of the Esophagus, vol II, Benign Diseases.* Mount Kisco, NY: Futura; 1990:73–83

80. Stein HJ, DeMeester TR. Integrated ambulatory foregut monitoring in patients with functional foregut disorders. In: Nyhus LM (ed). *1992 Surgery Annual, part 1, vol 24.* Stamford, CT: Appleton & Lange; 1992:161–180

81. Fuchs KH, DeMeester TR. Cost benefit aspects in the management of gastroesophageal reflux disease. In: Siewert JR, Hölscher AH (eds), *Diseases of the Esophagus.* New York, NY: Springer Verlag; 1988:857–861

82. Hetzel DJ, Dent J, Reed WD, et al. Healing and relapse of severe peptic esophagitis after treatment with omeprazole. *Gastroenterology* 1988;95:903

83. Lieberman DA. Medical therapy for chronic reflux esophagitis: long-term follow-up. *Arch Intern Med* 1987;147: 1717–1720

84. Salzman M, Barwick K, McCallum RW. Progression of cimetidine-treated reflux esophagitis to a Barrett's stricture. *Dig Dis Sci* 1982;27(2):181

85. Tolin RD, Malmud LS, Stelzer F, et al. Enterogastric reflux in normal subjects and patients with Billroth II gastroenterostomy: measurement of enterogastric reflux. *Gastroenterology* 1979;77:1027

86. Schwizer W, Hinder RA, DeMeester TR. Does delayed gastric emptying contribute to gastroesophageal reflux disease? *Am J Surg* 1989;157:74

87. Lind JF, Duthie HL, Schlegal JR, et al. Motility of the gastric fundus. *Am J Physiol* 1961;201:197

88. Richardson JD, Larson GM, Polk HC. Intrathoracic fundoplication for shortened esophagus: treacherous solution to a challenging problem. *Am J Surg* 1982;143:29

89. DeMeester TR, Bonavina L, Albertucci M. Nissen fundoplication for gastroesophageal reflux disease—evaluation of primary repair in 100 consecutive patients. *Ann Surg* 1986;204:9

90. Weerts JM, Dallemagne B, Hamoir E, et al. Laparoscopic Nissen fundoplication; detailed analysis of 132 patients. *Surg Laparosc Endosc* 1993;3:359–364

91. Hinder RA, Fillipi CJ. The technique of laparoscopic Nissen fundoplication. *Surg Laparosc Endosc* 1993;3:265–272

92. Spechler SJ. Department of Veterans Affairs Gastroesophageal Reflux Study Group: Comparison of medical and surgical therapy for complicated gastroesophageal reflux disease in veterans. *N Engl J Med* 1992;326(12): 786–792

93. Richter JE. Surgery for reflux disease: reflections of a gastroenterologist. *N Engl J Med* 1992;326(12):825–827 (Editorial).

94. Dunnington GL, DeMeester TR. Department of Veterans Affairs Gastroesophageal Reflux Study Group: outcome effect of adherence to operative principles of Nissen fundoplication by multiple surgeons. *Am J Surg* 1993;166:654–659

95. Coley CM, Barry MJ, Spechler SJ, et al. Initial medical vs. surgical therapy for complicated or chronic gastroesophageal reflux disease (GERD): a cost effective analysis. *Gastroenterology* 1993;104(4, part 2):A138

96. Little AG, Ferguson MK, Skinner DB. Reoperation for failed antireflux operations. *J Thorac Cardiovasc Surg* 1986;91:511

97. Siewert JR, Isolauri J, Feussuer M. Reoperation following failed fundoplication. *World J Surg* 1989;13:791

98. Stirling MC, Orringer MB. Surgical treatment after the failed antireflux operation. *J Thorac Cardiovasc Surg* 1986; 92:667

99. Peters JH, DeMeester TR. Lessons of failed antireflux repairs. In: Peters JH, DeMeester TR (eds), *Minimally Invasive Surgery of the Foregut.* Quality Med Publishing; 1994:188–196

100. Eliska O. Phreno-oesophageal membrane and its role in the development of hiatal hernia. *Acta Anat* 1973;86:137

101. Kleitsch WP. Embryology of congenital diaphragmatic hernia, I. esophageal hiatus hernia. *Arch Surg* 1958;76: 868–873

102. Walther B, DeMeester TR, Lafontaine E, et al. Effect of paraesophageal hernia on sphincter function and its implication on surgical therapy. *Am J Surg* 1984;147: 111–116

103. Dalgaard JB. Volvulus of the stomach. *Acta Chir Scand* 1952;103:131–153

104. Bombeck TC, Dillard DH, Nyhus LM. Muscular anatomy of the gastroesophageal junction and role of the phrenoesophageal ligament. *Ann Surg* 1966;164:643

105. Postlethwait RW. *Surgery of the Esophagus.* New York, NY: Appleton-Century-Crofts; 1979:195–255

106. Skinner DB, Belsey RHR. Surgical management of esophageal reflux and hiatus hernia: long-term results with 1030 patients. *J Thorac Cardiovasc Surg* 1967;53:33–54

24

Benign Disorders of the Esophagus

David W. McFadden ▪ *Michael J. Zinner*

The principal function of the esophagus is to move food from the mouth while avoiding retrograde passage of esophageal or gastric contents. Prograde transport is an active process; retrograde flow is passive. Disturbances of these basic functions can arise from either benign or malignant causes; in either case, the net effects often are distressing and debilitating for the sufferer.

Disorders of the esophagus are associated with a variety of signs and symptoms, including dysphagia, odynophagia, heartburn, regurgitation, vomiting, chest pain, aspiration pneumonitis, hoarseness, or bleeding. A thorough history and physical examination can identify the cause of esophageal symptoms in nearly 90% of patients. Disorders of the esophagus are common; more than one-third of the United States population reports at least occasional heartburn.[1] A rational approach to esophageal symptoms and the management of benign esophageal diseases are the goals of this chapter.

▪ ANATOMY AND PHYSIOLOGY

Anatomically, the esophagus is a muscular, tubular structure, 25 cm in length, that is secured by an upper esophageal sphincter (UES) at the level of C5-C6 in the neck and, in the abdomen, by the lower esophageal sphincter (LES) around the esophageal hiatus of the diaphragm. Its lumen is lined with squamous epithelium, and it possesses no serosal layer. The proximal 5% of the esophagus is composed of striated muscle. The middle 35% to 40% is mixed striated and smooth muscle, and the distal 50% to 60% of the esophagus is entirely smooth muscle. The inner esophageal muscle layer is circular, continuous, and of uniform thickness throughout. The outer longitudinal muscle begins below the cricopharygeus muscle, resulting in a posterior triangular region called Laimer's triangle. Distal to this area, the outer muscular coat is continuous and of uniform thickness.

Innervation of the esophagus is both sympathetic, with branches from multiple sympathetic ganglia, and parasympathetic, with branches from the vagus nerves. The vagus nerves diverge to form plexuses that encompass the thoracic esophagus and then coalesce into right and left vagal trunks that lie anterior and posterior to the esophagus at the diaphragmatic hiatus. Submucosal, or Meissner's, neural plexuses are sparse in the esophagus, whereas a rich supply myenteric, or Auberach's, plexuses provide the remainder of intrinsic esophageal innervation.

The arterial supply of the esophagus is segmental with little overlap, making devascularization and ischemia serious concerns of the esophageal surgeon. The cervical esophagus is supplied by branches of the inferior thyroid artery, as well as variable branches from the common carotid, subclavian, and ascending pharyngeal arteries. In the chest, branches from the aorta, intercostal arteries and bronchial arteries supply the esophagus. The short, intra-abdominal segment is supplied by branches of the left gastric, short gastric, and left inferior phrenic arteries.

Esophageal venous drainage is composed of the fine intraepithelial channels that drain into subepithelial superficial venous plexus. These, in turn, drain into deep submucosal veins. The superficial and deep systems anastomose with the gastric system at the gastroesophageal junction. These connections allow porta-systemic venous shunting in the case of portal hypertension with resultant esophageal varices. Adventitial veins communicate with the deep intrinsic veins via venous perforators, and drain into the inferior thyroidal, deep cervical, vertebral, and peritracheal veins in the neck; the azygous, hemizygous, and intercostal veins in the chest; and the gastric venous systems in the abdomen.

The lymphatic drainage of the esophagus comprises two networks, a mucosal and a muscular system. The drainage of the proximal two-thirds of the esophagus is primarily proximal, with the distal third draining distally. The rich lymphatic channels may drain directly into adjacent lymph nodes or may travel longitudinally for some distance prior to penetrating to the local lymph nodes.

The basic function of the esophagus is food transport. The food must first be prepared into a bolus by the mouth and transferred to the esophageal inlet. Swallowing initiates the transport function of the esophagus. The act of swallowing is complex, involving extremely fine motor control, as evidenced by the nerve fiber to muscle fiber ratio of approximately 1. This ratio is comparable to that seen in the extraocular muscles. The cell bodies of the responsible nerve fibers lie in the cranial nerves (trigeminal, facial, hypoglossal), the nucleus ambiguous, and spinal segments. The response requires afferent sensory input and cannot be implemented in an anesthetized oropharynx or without a sufficient food bolus.

The UES is anatomically both pharynx and esophagus. A zone of maximal pressure exists that is approximately 1 cm in length corresponds to the location of the cricopharyngeal muscle. The IES lies in the state of tonic contraction, with a resting pressure that is difficult to determine. This difficulty exists because UES pressure is altered by most testing methods. UES pressures are augmented by inspiration (presumably to prevent air swallowing), phonation, panting, recumbence, intraluminal stimulation or distention, and stress. Its nadirs are during sleep and anesthesia, at approximately 10 mm Hg.

The involuntary swallow response is initiated by the voluntary act of moving the food bolus to the back of the tongue. The UES relaxes and a peristaltic contraction passes down the esophagus at 2 to 4 cm/sec, delivering the food bolus to the stomach in 4 to 8 seconds. This is primary peristalsis, initiated by a swallow and effectively stripping the esophagus from proximal to distal. The longitudinal muscle of the esophagus also contracts at the onset of peristalsis, effectively shortening the esophagus by 2 to 2.5 cm. The organization of peristalsis in the striated portion of the esophagus is controlled by the medullary swallowing center via the vagus nerves. The smooth muscle portion of the esophagus is partially controlled in a similar fashion, but the vagal role is more complex. The vagus nerves appear to facilitate peristalsis in this area, since the intramural neurons are capable of organizing peristalsis. Vagal stimulation or cooling also affects smooth muscle activity.

Secondary peristalsis is like primary peristalsis in so far as it is orderly and sequential, but it is initiated by luminal distention, continues until the esophagus is cleared, and can occur without extrinsic innervation. Secondary peristalsis is coordinated by myenteric plexuses. The vagal nerves appear to modulate the excitatory cholinergic neurons with these plexuses, but not the inhibitory nonadrenergic, noncholinergic neurons.

The LES has an average maximal axial length of 31 mm. Two components exist, including short semicircular transverse muscle clasps that terminate on the anterior and posterior gastric walls, and long oblique loops to the stomach. Biochemical evidence exists that this circular muscle is different from other circular muscle of the gastrointestinal tract. It has a lower resting potential, increased passive diffusion of potassium, and higher intracystolic concentrations of calcium and inositol phosphates. The diaphragmatic crura probably play an augmentary role in LES tone, especially during inspiration.

Resting LES pressure range between 10 to 30 mm of Hg and are influenced by many extrinsic factors. Relaxation of the LES is mediated by vagal preganglionic and postganglionic nonadrenergic, noncholinergic nerves. LES relaxations occur as the neural inhibitory front passes along the esophagus, leading to esophageal peristalsis and LES relaxation. The LES also intermittently relaxes unassociated with swallows. These brief relaxations may represent a physiologic response to gastric distention and allow gas venting.

■ DIAGNOSTIC TECHNIQUES

RADIOLOGY

Many tests have been developed to improve the visualization of the esophagus, including computed tomographic (CT) scans, magnetic resonance imaging (MRI), nuclear medicine studies, and endoscopic ultrasound. Despite these advances, the barium swallow remains the standard radiographic evaluation. The barium swallow is composed of four parts. The first is the double-contrast study used for visualization of the distended esophagus and its mucosal surfaces. This allows identification of small neoplasms as well as different forms of esophagitis. The disadvantages include poor visualization of the gastroesophageal junction, which may allow small hiatal hernias, mucosal rings, and peptic strictures to be underdiagnosed. This disadvantage is compensated by the full-column technique that clearly defines these three pathologic conditions as well as more severe forms of esophagitis, circumferential lesions, and contour deformities. However, milder forms of esophagitis, esophageal varices, and small neoplasms still may be missed. Mucosal and relief films may reveal these otherwise occult lesions. Finally, fluoroscopic observation of the quality and rate of radiograph changes in essential for adequate functional assessment of the esophagus. Normally, several longitudinal folds travel the length of the collapsed esophagus and extrinsic compressions are visible from the aortic arch, left main stem bronchus, and the heart. The tubular esophagus terminates in the vestibule, which is the junction between the esophagus and stomach. This is a bell-shaped area that is partially intra-abdominal, and it is where the squamocolumnar junction lies.

CT scanning is useful in the evaluation of intramural lesions, extrinsic abnormalities, wall thickness, adenopathy, and neoplastic spread. MRI may play a similar role in staging of esophageal malignancies, but its exact role remains undetermined. Nuclear medicine studies assist in defining transit dysfunction and emptying and reflux disorders.

Endoscopic ultrasonography has been recently introduced and may prove valuable in evaluating mucosal, intramural, and extramural disease. The esophagus has five echogenically distinct layers corresponding to the specific histologic layers. The location of a lesion within these layers can be identified endoscopically, allowing accurate preoperative staging. Nodal involvement can also be assessed.

ENDOSCOPY

Flexible fiberoptic endoscopy has developed into one of the mainstays of esophageal diagnosis and therapy. It allows for direct visualization of the esophageal mucosa and submucosal vascular pattern. Biopsies of suspicious lesions and intervention for certain disease states are also possible. Endoscopically, the esophagus begins as a slit-like orifice approximately 15 to 20 cm from the incisors. As the endoscope is passed distally, the esophagus will distend easily with insufflation. It is lined with a pale pink-white squamous epithelium that is translucent, allowing observation of the submucosal vascular pattern. The squamocolumnar junction is the junction of the pale lining of the esophagus and the reddish-pink columnar lining of the stomach. This is seen as a wavy line called the Z line or ora serrata. Extrinsic compression usually is recognized at the level of the aortic arch and left mainstream bronchus.

MANOMETRY

Esophageal manometric evaluation has become essential in the diagnosis of dysphagia, odynophagia, noncardiac chest pain, gastroesophageal reflux, and diffuse gastrointestinal diseases. Recent technologic advances have led to the development of solid-state transducers that can simultaneously sense 360° circumferentially. These advances, coupled with new computer software, allow for (1) studying patients over longer periods of time; (2) studying patients in the more physiologic upright position; and (3) integration of multiple simultaneous transducer readings into one three-dimensional representation of the esophagus and its sphincters. Current catheters are <5 mm in diameter, and are inserted transnasally and advanced approximately 60 cm. This maneuver assures that the entire pressure-sensing complex is in the stomach. The station pull-through technique is used to assess the lower esophageal pressure. This involves a slow stepwise withdrawal of the catheter in 0.5 cm increments, with resting at each station for 3 to 5 respirations, to allow for adequate time for equilibration and pressure measurement. Once the tracing is noted to arise above baseline, the LES has been entered. The response of the LES to a swallow then is evaluated by a dry swallow, followed by a sip of 5 cc of water. Normally, LES pressure should relax to within 2 mm Hg of the resting gastric pressure.

As the catheter advances into the thoracic esophagus and exits the LES, the pressure tracing drops and flattens out to a point of no further change. Importantly, low LES may be associated with gastroesophageal reflux and high pressures associated with dysphagia, but absolute diagnostic numbers do not exist.

Esophageal body manometry allows assessment of the strength and duration of the peristaltic activity. Complete studies include evaluation of the smooth muscle in the distal esophagus as well as the proximal striated musculature. Body positioning, age, bolus size, transducer location, and catheter size all affect the reproducibility and comparability of the study. Abnormal findings include simultaneous, nontransmitted, triple-peaked, and retrograde contractions. Very weak (<30 mm Hg) and very strong (>180 mm Hg) are also abnormal. The latter are found in only 2.5% of normal patients, but are seen in 48% of patients with noncardiac chest pain.

Manometric evaluation, formerly the sole domain of the barium swallow, has recently become possible for the UES. The UES is asymmetric with the highest pressures noted anteriorly and posteriorly complicating evaluation in one position. The muscle is striated and responds rapidly, often in less than one second. It is also stimulated by movement of the catheter; therefore the station pull-through technique is used, pausing for 15 to 30 seconds at each station to allow for equilibration. Accurate evaluation requires computer analysis of pharyngeal peristalsis and UES-pharyngeal coordination.

pH MONITORING, AMBULATORY PRESSURE MONITORING AND PROVOCATIVE TESTING

A variety of electrodes are available for clinical usage in ambulatory monitoring of esophageal function. Newer models are capable of sampling up to eight times per minute with a resolution of 01. pH units. The electrode should be positioned 5 cm above the upper border of the LES. The most reproducible results are obtained when patients are studied for 24 hours and the total time below a pH of 4.0 is determined. The time below a pH of 4.0 is called the reflux time or acid exposure time, and <3% is considered normal. The pH of 4.0 is somewhat arbitrary, but has some clinical grounds in that proteolytic enzymes are inactive at a pH >4.0 and patients begin to report symptoms at a pH of <4.0. Symptoms such as heartburn and regurgitation are not very reliable since patients with profound endoscopic findings of reflux may be asymptomatic, whereas others with severe heartburn and regurgitation may have cholelithiasis, dyspepsia, or peptic ulcer disease. Atypical symptoms such as angina-like chest pain or pulmonary symptoms are often the presenting symptoms of reflux disease. Monitoring pH can be useful in correlating reflux and symptoms. Gastroesophageal reflux is discussed in Chapter 23. Nonsurgical medical management is listed in Table 24–1.

Attempts to increase the changes of capturing esophageal dysmotility during episodes of chest pain have included ambulatory esophageal monitoring. Although initiated with a great hope for success, the results over-all have been disappointing, with only a small percentage of patients reporting pain in association with esophageal contractile abnormalities. Provocative tests also have been used. Acid perfusion (Bernstein test), edrophonium chloride, bethanecol, ergonavine maleate, treadmill testing, food ingestion, and psychologic stressors have all been used. Currently, acid infusion, edrophonium, and balloon distention are safe and reproducible tests for evolving esophageal pain in patients with noncardiac chest pain. A summary of esophageal motility disorders is seen in Table 24–2.

■ ACHALASIA

Willis first described and treated achalasia over three centuries ago, using a whalebone and sponge dilator to overcome "cardiospasm" in a patient. In 1929, Hurst coined the term achalasia, meaning a failure to relax. The major points of controversy in this disorder to be discussed are (1) whether forceful dilation or surgery should be the preferred methods of treatment, and (2) whether an antireflux procedure is required with operation.[26]

Achalasia has a poorly understood neurogenic basis. Myenteric ganglion cell degeneration and associated chronic inflammation of the esophageal smooth muscle are usually seen. Neurotropic infectious disorders, possibly viral, are considered likely etiologic agents, but a cause and effect relationship is unproven. The similarity to the esophageal disorder seen in Chagas' disease, caused by the *Trypanosoma cruzi* organism, is remarkable.[27]

Both sexes are equally affected in the age range of 25 to 60 years, and the disease most commonly affects Caucasians. Clinically, patients present with dysphagia, regurgitation, and weight loss. All patients have solid food dysphagia, and most have dysphagia for liquids as well. Patients often complain about fullness or gurgling in the chest. Emotional stress and rapid eating worsen the dysphagia. Postural maneuvers, such as walking while eating, chin thrusting with neck extension, and posterior extension of the shoulders may be used to alleviate the symptoms. Regurgitation of food is described by 60% to 90% of patients. Nocturnal choking or regurgitation with food or saliva found on the pillows are commonly described; aspiration pneumonia is seen in up to 10% of patients. Chest pain and heartburn, unresponsive to either nitrates or antacids, is described in nearly one-half of patients. Achalasia is also a premalignant disease. Approximately 7% of patients develop squamous cell carcinoma of the esophagus after 15 to 25 years.[27]

Plain radiologic investigations may reveal a widened mediastinum, an air-fluid level in the chest, absence of the gastric air bubble, and evidence of previous pulmonary aspiration. Barium swallows reveal failure or delayed esophageal clearance. The barium may "wash"

TABLE 24–1. MEDICAL MANAGEMENT OF GASTROESOPHAGEAL REFLUX DISEASE

1. Elevate head of bed, on blocks, by 6–12 inches
2. If overweight, lose weight
3. Stop smoking
4. Avoid heavy ethanol ingestion
5. Reduce meal size
6. Do not eat or drink less than two hours before bedtime
7. Eat less fat
8. Avoid tight clothing
9. Avoid certain foods, including chocolate, coffee, tea, cola beverages, citrus drinks, tomato juice, and peppermint or spearmint candy
10. Certain drugs may aggravate GERD and are to be avoided if possible, including: theophylline, diazepam, narcotics, anticholinergics, calcium channel blockers, progesterone (certain oral contraceptives)
11. Avoid lifting or heavy exercise for two hours after eating

TABLE 24–2 ESOPHAGEAL MOTILITY DISORDERS[28,29]

DISORDER	SYMPTOMS	MANOMETRY	THERAPY
Achalasia	Dysphagia, chest pain, regurgitation	Aperistalsis, incomplete LES contraction, simultaneous contractions	Esophagomyotomy +/− Belsey procedure; pneumatic dilation
DES	Chest pain, often substernal dysphagia	Normal peristalsis, simultaneous contractions in >10% wet swallows	Smooth muscle relaxants (nitrates, calcium channel blockers); long myotomy if dysphagia main symptom
Nutcracker esophagus, or high amplitude peristaltic contraction	Chest pain, asymptomatic, dysphagia; major cause of noncardiac chest pain	High amplitude (>180 mm Hg) peristaltic contractions	Smooth muscle relaxants; *rarely* long myotomy
Nonspecific esophageal motility disorder	Chest pain, asymptomatic, dysphagia	Variable; rarely high amplitude spontaneous, repetitive or simultaneous contractions	Address GERD if present

back and forth with repetitive nonperistaltic contractions. The LES opens partially, intermittently, and is not synchronized with swallowing.[28] Once filled, the esophageal body is dilated with maximal dilation found distally. The barium column tapers to a point, or "bird's-beak" where the tapered end point represents the nonrelaxing LES (Fig 24–1). Early in the disease, dilation may be absent rendering fluoroscopy essential for diagnosis. Late in the disease the esophagus assumes a sigmoid appearance (Fig 24–2).

Endoscopy is necessary to rule out malignancy with "pseudoachalasia," as well as to survey for malignant change in longstanding cases of the achalasia. The LES does not open normally with insufflation but the endoscope usually passes through easily. If there is difficulty in traversing the LES, benign or malignant stricture should be considered.[29] Once the endoscope has traversed the LES, a search for the rare association of hiatal hernia (4%) and achalasia is performed, because of the increased incidence of esophageal perforation in these patients upon pneumatic dilation.

Manometric evaluation is mandatory in suspected achalasia patients. Findings include (1) absence of peristalsis, (2) incomplete or abnormal LES relaxation, (3) elevated LES pressures, and (4) elevated intraesophageal pressure relative to gastric pressures. An absence of distal esophageal peristalsis is an absolute requirement for diagnosis. Elevated LES resting pressures are found in 60% of patients.[28–30]

TREATMENT OF ACHALASIA

Recently, pharmacologic depressions of LES pressure have been reported with the use of oral nitrates and calcium channel blockers. If tolerated, these agents should be given a therapeutic trial, but in general, the results have been poor. Intrasphincteric injections of botulinum toxin is also gaining success as a temporary treatment modal-

ity.[16] Presently there are two methods used for treatment of achalasia: pneumatic dilation and esophageal myotomy with or without antireflux procedure. The indications for, and effectiveness of, the two techniques remain controversial. Only one randomized prospective trial comparing these two treatments have been published.[28,29]

The aim of esophageal dilation is to weaken or rupture the circular muscle fibers of the LES by forceful stretch. The minimal effective pressures that are required are 250 to 300 mm Hg. Other than pain, perforation is the most common complication, occurring in 2% to 5% of patients. Success rates depend on the type of dilation (pneumatic 46% to 90%, mean 80%, hydrostatic 65% to 76%, mean 67%), length of follow-up, and number of dilations required.[28]

Surgery for achalasia has been performed since 1903, and is associated with success rates of 65% to 99%, with a mean of 87%.[29] The only published prospective comparison of surgery to dilatation was reported by Csendes and associates.[31] With a mean follow-up of 62 months, surgical relief was seen in 95% of patients versus 65% after dilatation. The relief of dysphagia was greater and more rapidly achieved in surgical patients, but was not severe. Statistically, it appears that myotomy is the superior treatment for achalasia.[31–33] Nevertheless, the need for a general anesthetic and the pain and disability of a thoracotomy have placed this more effective option into the background.

The second controversy is the need for an antireflux procedure at the time of myotomy. A review of over 5000 surgical patients found that the addition of an antireflux procedure did not lower the postoperative incidence of gastroesophageal reflux disease (GERD) if the myotomy was performed through the chest (7.7% without antireflux procedure, 7.3% with antireflux procedure). If the myotomy is performed via laparotomy, the addition of an antireflux operation halved the risk of postoperative GERD (7.4% with versus 13.2% without).[27] Several au-

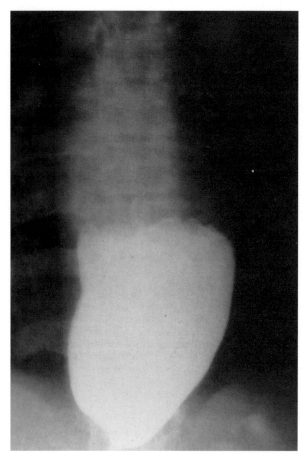

Figure 24–1. Barium column ending in a "bird's-beak." A classic picture of achalasia.

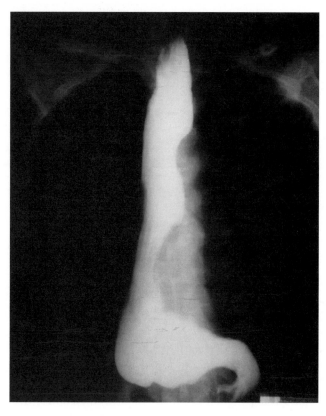

Figure 24–2. Late achalasia. Sigmoid shape to esophagus.

thors recommend a simultaneous Belsey procedure because it does not represent a full wrap, and may not elevate LES pressure to the range where dysphagia or obstruction occurs.[32]

We prefer to perform the esophageal myotomy through a left posterolateral thoracotomy, using the 7th interspace or the bed of the resected 8th rib. The esophagus is mobilized, the vagus nerves protected, and the esophagogastric junction is gently lifted into the chest without dividing its hiatal attachments. A longitudinal myotomy is performed on the left anterolateral surface (Fig 24–3A), with the incision deepened through the encircling muscles down to, but not into, the mucosa. The incision extends inferiorly across the GE junction, with the gastric extension being <1 cm (Fig 24–3B). Proximally, it extends past the areas of thickened esophagus, guided also by preoperative manometry. Usually a myotomy of 5 to 10 cm is required. After myotomy, the muscular wall is dissected laterally for 180°, allowing the mucosa to protrude freely (Fig 24–3C). A Belsey procedure, performed over a 42-French (Fr) dilator, with indwelling

nasogastric tube, then is performed. Hemostasis, closed chest drainage with a 30- to 36-Fr chest tube, and standard chest closure completes the operation. If mucosal perforation occurs during myotomy, suture repair with placement of the Belsey wrap over the injury usually will suffice. With these techniques, good to excellent results should be expected in 85% to 95% of patients, and reoperation required in <3%.

Transabdominal esophageal myotomies rarely are performed, primarily because of the limited surgical exposure and the increased risk of GERD postoperatively. A distal 5 to 7 cm length of esophagus usually can be visualized, via caudad retraction of the gastroesophageal junction, with a posteriorly placed penrose drain. The addition of a loose or "floppy" Nissen fundoplication is recommended, given the reported higher risks of postoperative gastroesophageal reflux.[27]

Minimally invasive techniques still are being developed, but preliminary data are encouraging.[34] The lack of a thoracotomy or laparotomy may facilitate surgical referrals for these patients.

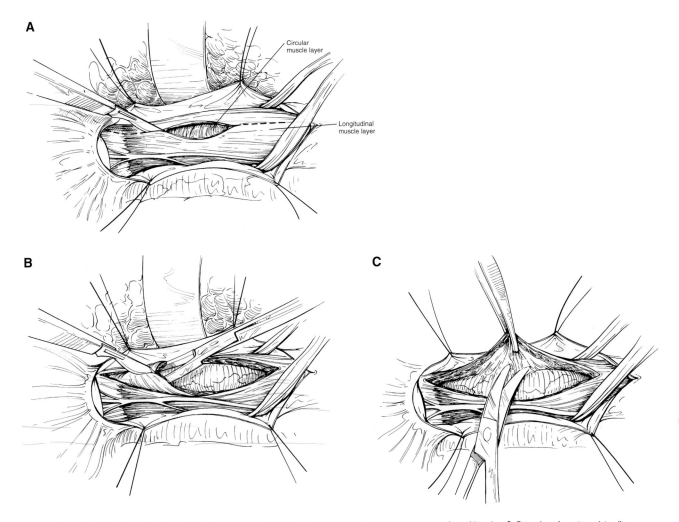

Figure 24–3. Esophageal myotomy. **A.** Incision along longitudinal muscles. **B.** Incision just across gastroesophageal junction. **C.** Extension of myotomy laterally.

■ DIFFUSE ESOPHAGEAL SPASM

Diffuse esophageal spasm (DES) is the most commonly named diagnosis in a group of ill-defined esophageal disorders that are characterized by episodic chest pain and dysphagia.[28,29] Manometrically, high-amplitude or tertiary spastic esophageal muscle contractions are seen frequently. Other diagnoses in this group include segmental esophageal spasm, presbyesophagus, hypertensive distal esophageal "nutcracker" esophagus. Many questions exist concerning the diagnosis, significance, and treatment for these conditions and some consider them the esophageal equivalent of irritable bowel syndrome. Surgery infrequently is indicated or successful unless the overwhelming complaint is dysphagia.[28]

Diffuse esophageal spasm was first described over a century ago, and its cause remains unknown. The esophageal muscle is hypertrophied, but histologically normal. Symptoms are precipitated by stress and ingestion of cold liquids. Chest pain correlates poorly with the abnormal esophageal contractions, leaving the physiological basis of the pain obscure. Manometry is needed to confirm the diagnosis.[29] A number of manometric abnormalities are described; the most consistent and ratified finding is simultaneous esophageal contractions in the distal two-thirds of the esophagus occurring after more than 10% of wet swallows.[30] Barium esophagography may show irregular areas of narrowing and dilatation, colorfully alluded to as multiple pseudodiverticulosis, "shish kebab," "corkscrew," and "rosary bead" esophagus.[29]

Treatment is usually pharmacologic, using calcium channel antagonists. Nitrates can be used if GERD is not present; LES pressure, which is frequently normal in DES, is lowered by these medications, but symptomatic improvement is usually no better than placebo. At best, severity, but not frequency, of chest pain may be relieved.

Endoscopic esophageal dilatation is of unproven value. Surgically, long esophageal myotomies, performed to the level of the aortic arch (Fig 24–3), result in excellent symptomatic improvement in 49% to 86% (mean 67%) of patients whose prominent symptoms are dysphagia.[35] If the predominant symptom is chest pain, surgical results are poor. Few studies exist, however, with more than 15 patient and long-term (>5 year) follow-ups. Surgical controversy exists as to the need for simultaneous antireflux procedures. If the myotomy extends onto the gastric wall, or if preoperative symptoms or manometry suggested low LES pressure, than the addition of a Belsey procedure should be strongly considered.[28,29]

Nutcracker esophagus, or symptomatic esophageal peristalsis, may be the most common esophageal motility disorder. Approximately 28% to 45% of patients with noncardiac chest pain will be found to have this diagnosis. Often exertionally related, and less associated with dysphagia (50% to 70% of patients), the central chest pain of nutcracker esophagus is associated with high amplitude peristalsis. Mean amplitudes of >150 mm Hg are seen in affected patients, versus 80 to 100 mm Hg in the general population.[29] Striking physiologic and psychologic similarities also exist between nutcracker esophagus and irritable bowel syndrome.[29] Pain response to treatment is usually no different than seen with placebo, and one large series of more than 100 patients found no need for surgical referral of any patients.[28]

Cricopharyngeal hypertension or spasm is associated with GERD in 3% of patients, and also is seen with pharyngeal inflammatory processes or cancer. Cricopharyngeal discoordination can be caused by incomplete relaxation (cricopharyngeal achalasia), delayed relaxation, or premature contraction.[28] Associated symptoms are dysphagia, regurgitation, pulmonary aspiration, and cricopharyngeal diverticulum formation. Although dilatation may be helpful, cricopharyngeal myotomy usually is required.

■ DIVERTICULA OF THE ESOPHAGUS

Although uncommon, the practicing surgeon should expect to see several esophageal diverticula during his or her career. A useful classification is based upon location (cricopharyngeal, midesophageal, epiphrenic), recognizing that most upper and lower diverticula are pulsion pseudodiverticula (not containing all layers of the esophageal wall), whereas the midesophageal variety are usually traction and true. In the former, increased intraluminal pressures secondary to abnormal esophageal motility push the mucosa and submucosa through a muscular defect in the wall of the esophagus creating pulsion diverticula. Traction diverticula are created by extraluminal forces that pull the full thickness of the esophagus out, creating a true diverticulum.

PHARYNGOESOPHAGEAL (ZENKER'S) DIVERTICULUM

Recognized since 1764 but still poorly understood, Zenker's diverticula are mucosal outpouchings occurring through the triangular bare area (Killian's triangle) between the cricopharygeus muscle and the inferior pharyngeal constrictor muscle. Most Zenker's diverticula occur on the left side and project caudally. Only 50% of patients demonstrate improper coordination between UES relaxation and the cricopharyngeus muscle.[36] Three basic hypotheses for the origin of this diverticulum exist: (1) tonic UES contraction; (2) failure of the UES to relax and (3) lack of coordination of UES and pharyngeal contractions. The difficulty in identifying the cause lies in the asymmetric nature of the pharyngoesophageal junction, the rapidity of swallowing in this area, and the inherent difficulty in obtaining accurate manometric and cineradiographic studies.

Clinically, the diverticula rarely are seen before 30 years of age, and most commonly after 50 years of age. Many are merely incidental findings on barium esophagram. Dysphagia is the dominant symptom. Pathological gastroesophageal reflux is seen in 40% of patients. Aspiration is described in 40% of patients, and other symptoms include a "lump" in the throat, gurgling sounds during swallowing, coughing, choking, bad breath, and weight loss. Squamous cell cancer is found in 0.4% of diverticula, with a mean duration of symptoms of 17 years prior to diagnosis. Cervical webs occur in 50% of the patients and can be a cause of dysphagia postoperatively if not dealt with intraoperatively. Barium swallows are diagnostic. Rigid esophagoscopy, once considered forbidden, has been replaced by the safer fiberoptic techniques.[28]

Treatment is surgical and is indicated in most symptomatic patients. It should almost always consist of cricopharyngeal myotomy. The operation should be performed through an incision placed anterior and parallel to the left sternocleidomastoid muscle, although some authors use a lower transverse incision (Fig 24–4A). Local anesthesia can be used in the unfit patient. The myotomy should extend about 1 cm proximal to the pouch and 3 to 5 centimeters distal to the pouch (Figs 24–4B and 24–4C). A myotomy will suffice for small diverticula. In the case of large diverticula (>4 cm), the surgeon should either suspend the diverticulum superiorly from the prevertebral fascia, using 2-0 permanent sutures, to facilitate its prograde drainage (diverticulopexy) or resect it using a line stapling device placed perpendicular to the axis of the esophagus (Fig 24–5).[36] If resection is performed, we use a 50-Fr esophageal dilator to prevent esophageal narrowing. In all cases, the neck is drained with closed-suction catheters. Success is seen in over 90% of patients, most

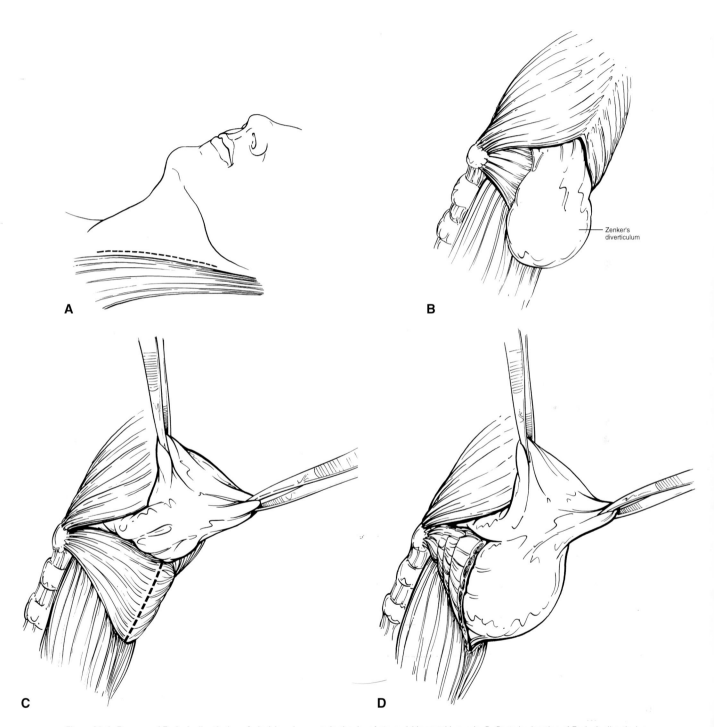

Figure 24–4. Exposure of Zanker's diverticulum. **A.** Incision along anterior border of sternocleidomastoid muscle. **B.** Posterior location of Zanker's diverticulum. **C.** Cricopharangeal myotomy. **D.** Suspension of diverticulum.

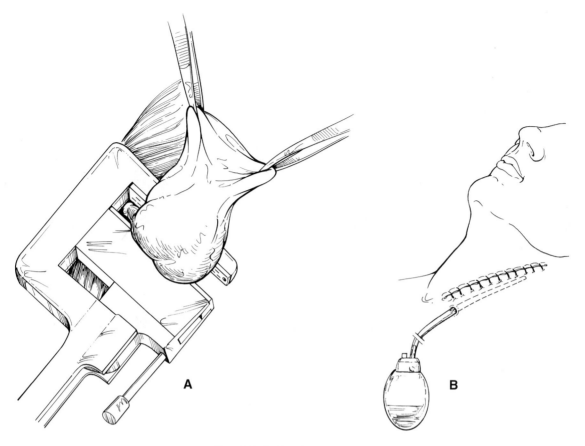

Figure 24–5. Excision of Zanker's diverticulum.

of whom can be discharged within 48 hours of surgery. Success rates fall to 70% if a myotomy is not performed.[28]

MIDESOPHAGEAL DIVERTICULUM

First described by Mondiere in 1833, midesophageal diverticula are usually traction and true, with diverticular secondary to an inflammatory process of the mediastinum. Historically, the cause was achalasia or DES, which may also have associate mideosphageal false diverticula.[37] Midesophageal diverticula are acquired and rarely seen in childhood, with a reported range of 38 to 74 years of age. They are frequently incidental findings on barium esophagram, and are most commonly found at the level of the carina. Symptoms include dysphagia, regurgitation, aspiration, and chest pain. Rarely is surgery indicated specifically for traction diverticular unless treatment of the underlying disorder is unsuccessful or symptoms (bleeding, bronchoesophageal fistula, abscess) are refractory. In these rare cases, esophageal manometry should be performed to rule out occult motility disorders. Thoracotomy is performed with excision of the diverticulum

and any associated inflammatory mass. A pedicle of pleura or muscle is interposed between the esophagus and tracheobronchial tree.[36] Rarely is coincident pulmonary resection required. In the presence of motility disorders and small midesophageal diverticula, myotomy should suffice.

EPIPHRENIC DIVERTICULUM

Epiphrenic diverticula are invariable of the pulsion type. They appear in the elderly, are within 10 cm of the GE junction, usually lie on the right side (Figs 24–6, 24–7, and 24–8), and are multiple in 19% of cases. Men are affected twice as often as women. Epiphrenic diverticula are one-fifth as common as Zenker's diverticula. Symptoms are dysphagia, regurgitation, or the underlying esophageal disease. Aspiration and pneumonia are well described in these patients.[37]

An underlying functional or mechanical obstruction usually is discovered and usually is achalasia, hypercontracting LES, or diffuse spasm. Hiatal hernia requires diverticulectomy with esophageal myotomy; repair is indicated if present.[36,37]

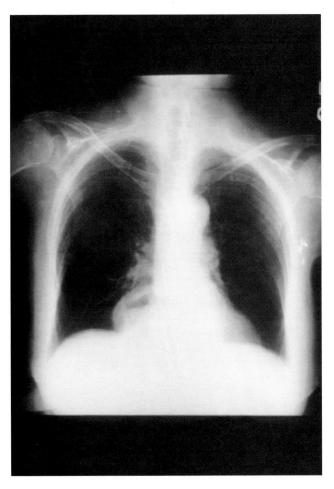

Figure 24–6. PA chest x-ray of epiphrenic diverticulum.

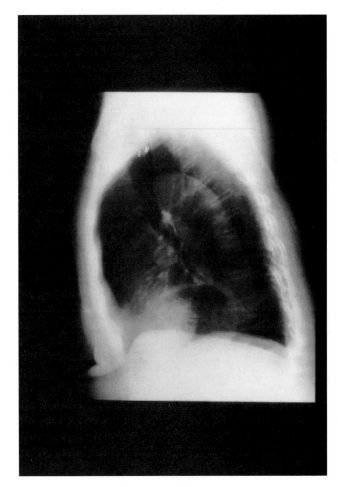

Figure 24–7. Lateral chest x-ray of epiphrenic diverticulum.

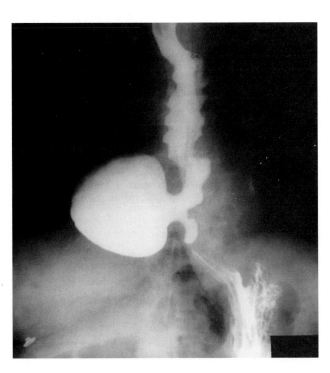

Figure 24–8. Barium swallow of epiphrenic diverticulum.

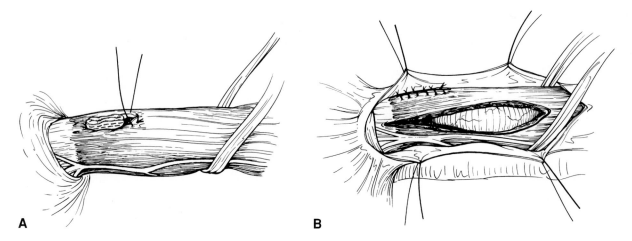

Figure 24–9. Exposure and excision of epiphrenic diverticulum.

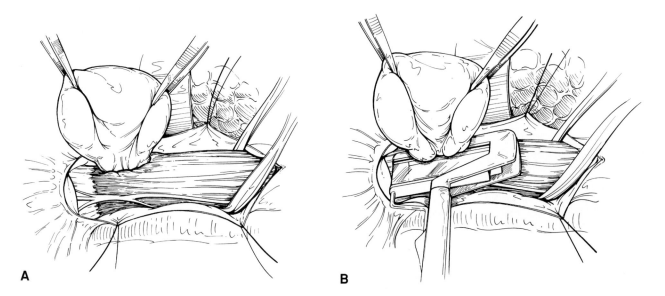

Figure 24–10. A. Closure of muscle over neck of diverticulum. **B.** Lateral longitudinal myotomy across gastroesophageal junction following excision of diverticulum. An antireflux procedure often follows this step.

The surgical approach is through a long 7-8th interspace left posterolateral thoracotomy. The left lower lobe is mobilized by dividing the inferior pulmonary ligament. The use of a double lumen endotracheal tube is helpful. The diverticular sac is dissected careful to avoid rupture and spillage (Fig 24–9A), then excised in the presence of a 50-60 French esophageal dilator (Fig 24–9B). The muscle is then closed over the excised neck of the sac (Fig 24–10A). Diverticulopexy also has been recommended by some authors for large-mouthed diverticular whose excision would narrow the esophageal lumen. Standard procedures then are performed for associated achalasia (Fig 24–10B), hiatal hernia, or DES. These usually include a myotomy and/or a Belsey antireflux procedure. Drainage and closure are as previously described.

SCLERODERMA

Scleroderma is a collagen-vascular disease that affects smooth muscle and has a penchant to cause dysfunction of the distal third of the esophagus and LES. Between 75% to 85% of affected patients will have clinical or manometric evidence of esophageal involvement. Patients are typically white, female, and 30 to 50 years of age.[38]

Clinical manifestations include dysphagia and heartburn. Symptoms may be less impressive than manometric or endoscopic findings, suggesting some degree of sensory impairment. GERD may be severe, and both Barrett's esophagus and esophageal cancer have been described in these patients.

Radiographic studies reveal a dilated esophagus that may have intraluminal air. Although emptying is normal in the standing position, barium will remain in the esophagus for hours in the supine posture. Almost one-third of patients have peptic stricture, and hiatal hernia may be seen. Manometry reveals low to absent LES pressure, weak distal esophageal peristalsis, and normal upper esophageal pressures and motility.[38]

No effective treatment exists. Medical therapy for symptoms of GERD is recommended (Table 24–1). Strictures are more refractory in scheroderma patients and frequent dilatation often is required. Because of the loss of esophageal peristalsis, the Belsey procedure appears to have better results than the Nissen fundoplication because of its lesser augmentation of LES pressure. The esophagus frequently is shortened, and a Collis gastroplasty is required to permit the gastric wrap.[9,11] Surgical results are good if the disease is approached prior to the development of nondilatable strictures.

TABLE 24–3 ESOPHAGEAL PERFORATIONS

	CERVICAL	THORACIC	ABDOMINAL
Frequency	25%	60%	15%
Pain	70%	90%	60%
Fever	30%	80%	50%
Crepitus	55%	14%	0%
Dysphagia	35%	6%	0%
Common causes	Penetrating trauma, endoscopy, foreign body	Endoscopy dilatation, trauma, spontaneous	Periesophageal surgery, spontaneous
Treatment	Primary repair with drainage	Repair with drainage; resection or diversion in complicated cases	Repair at time of injury; resection or diversion in complicated cases
Onset	Subacute	Rapid	Subacute

ESOPHAGEAL PERFORATIONS

Esophageal perforation remains one of the most devastating perforations of the gastrointestinal tract. Success is inversely proportional to delay in recognition and onset of treatment. Boerhaave's recognition of spontaneous rupture of the esophagus in 1724 was followed by more than two centuries of inability to treat properly. It was not until the mid 1940s that drainage and repair were performed successfully. Common etiologies and locations of perforation are summarized in Table 24–3. Most series reveal that 60% of patients have iatrogenic perforations, 25% have traumatic perforations, and 15% have spontaneous perforations.[39] The location of perforations reveals that 25% are in the cervical esophagus, 60% in the thoracic esophagus, and 15% in the abdominal esophagus.

CERVICAL PERFORATIONS

Cervical perforations usually occur posteriorly where the esophageal wall is thinnest.[39] Eventual dissection of contaminants may lead to mediastinitis, but early symptoms are neck stiffness and ache, bloody regurgitation, and subcutaneous emphysema. Diagnosis is confirmed by gastrograffin swallow, or direct operative inspection.

Exploration is performed through an anterior oblique neck incision. The perforation is identified, conservatively debrided, and closed with a single layer of 3-0 monofilament nonabsorbable suture. Drainage of the neck and superior mediastinum is performed with a closed-suction catheter. Antibiotics against oral flora are used perioperatively for 5 days, at which time a water soluble contrast radiographic examination should reveal healing. Oral liquids are begun and the patient discharged if the drain reveals no leakage of ingested material.[40]

Occasionally the perforation cannot be located at the time of the operation. We then use wide drainage of the neck and superior mediastinum, intravenous antibiotics, and keep the patient fasted for 7 days, at which time a contrast esophagogram is performed.

■ THORACIC PERFORATION

Perforations of the thoracic esophagus result in direct, immediate contamination of the mediastinum. The thin mediastinal pleura is ruptured easily by the inflammatory process, leading to contamination of the pleural pace and a pleural effusion, usually on the left side. Gastric contents are drawn up into the cavity by negative intrathoracic pressure, exacerbating the contamination. The clinical presentation is insolvent and catastrophic, with pain, sepsis, and dyspnea predominating.

Water-contrast agent esophagography is recommended unless a major risk of aspiration, concurrent respiratory injury, or fistula is present, at which time thin barium should be used (Fig 24–11). In suspected perforations where the plain radiographic contrast studies are negative, CT scanning may demonstrate periesophageal or mediastinal air, abscess cavity or a direct communication.[39]

The surgical treatment of thoracic esophageal perforations consists of closure of the esophageal rent, and wide mediastinal and pleural debridement and drainage. For lesions in the upper two-thirds of the esophagus, a right posterolateral 5th or 6th space thoracotomy can be used. For lower lesions, we prefer a left 6th or 7th interspace posterolateral thoracotomy. If treated early, suture of the esophagus with two layers, an inner absorbable and an outer nonabsorbable, will suffice.[40] Most authors routinely add a buttress or flap of mediastinal pleura, muscle, or pericardial fat pad to secure the closure. At least two large (36 Fr) chest tubes are placed in the mediastinum and pleural spaces. The perforation is unlikely to heal primarily if it is old (>24 to 48 hours). A variety of ingenious methods of handling the esophagus have been described (Table 24–4). A simple approach is to insert a large T tube into the esophagus with suturing of the esophagus around it. This creates a controlled esophageal-cutaneous fistula. Wide drainage is performed as described above, and the tube usually can be removed in 4 to 6 weeks. Nutrition is maintained by intravenous methods or preferably, by enteral tubes placed via laparotomy or laparoscopy. As with all thoracic perforations, broad intravenous antibi-

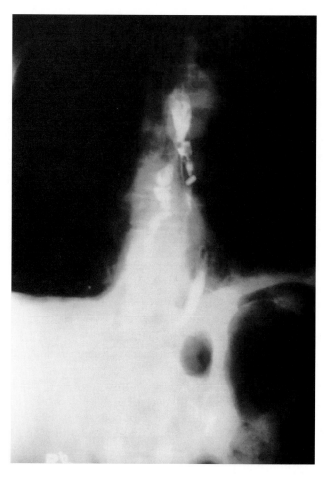

Figure 24–11. Esophageal perforation in the mediastinum following attempted dilatation of esophageal stricture. Note that there are two channels of barium.

otic coverage is recommended, as are intravenous hyperalimentation and the use of oral antifungal agents. Mediastinal irrigation with antibiotic-containing saline solution is recommended by some authors.[40]

A clinical dilemma exists when the perforation is proximal to a diseased esophagus. Repairs will not heal in the presence of distal mechanical or functional obstruction. In these tragic circumstances, we proceed with esophagectomy, cervical esophagostomy, and placement of a decompressive gastronomy and a feeding jejunostomy. Preoperative recognition of this combination of problems is selected stabile patients with minimum contamination has led some authors to recommend transhiatal esophagectomy. In the others, preservation of the entire stomach will facilitate subsequent reconstruction, usually performed 3 to 6 months later.

Cameron has applied several criteria for nonoperative management of thoracic esophageal perforations with selected success.[41] The criteria include a contained mediastinal leak with free drainage back into the eso-

TABLE 24–4. ESOPHAGEAL PERFORATION: SURGICAL MANAGEMENT OF OPTIONS

1. Primary closure with or without autologous tissue reinforcement (pleura, muscle, pericardial fat pad, omentum, gastric wall [Thal patch]). Thoracostomy tube drainage is required.
2. Drainage alone: works best in neck; also an option in old thoracic perforations with widespread contamination.
3. T tube drainage: creates controlled fistula; useful when primary repair is doubtful. Use at least a 20-Fr tube.
4. Resection: necessary in malignancy, distal stricture patients. Transhiatal resection with cervical anastomosis recommended if minimal contamination. If unstable or widely soiled, use cervical esophagostomy and gastrostomy tube-reconstruct later.
5. Exclusion and diversion: usually consists of cervical esophagostomy, ligation of GE junction, and gastrostomy tube. Mandates second major operation, many patients never swallow normally after esophagostomy.
6. Intraluminal stents: consider in advanced malignancies, tracheoesophageal fistulas.

phagus, minimal symptoms, and little or no signs of systemic sepsis. Important associated criteria to be considered include no food intake between injury and diagnosis, recent perforation, and lack of tumor or distal obstruction. Nonoperative therapy is applied best for instrumental cervical perforations, small perforations after dilatation of peptic strictures, achalasia, or variceal sclerosis (in whom periesophageal fibrosis may limit spread of contamination), and late-diagnosed perforations in patients with minimal symptoms.[39] Treatment is hyperalimentation, broad-spectrum antibiotics, and careful serial patient evaluation.[41]

In the patient with malignant perforation and/or a limited life span, consideration of an expansile metal stent should be made. Recent data supports their use in malignant esophageal fistulas and contained perforations.[42]

■ ABDOMINAL PERFORATIONS

Abdominal perforations usually are associated with periesophageal surgical procedures, such as vagotomy or splenectomy.[39] Usually these injuries are recognized, and direct suture closure is generally possible and safe. Occasionally, instrumental or spontaneous perforations occur in the abdominal esophagus. If spontaneous, and a normal distal esophagus and GE function are identified, then suture repair with either a Thal fundic patch or omental buttress will suffice. Placement of periesophageal drainage, gastrostomy and jejunostomy tubes, and copious peritoneal irrigation is performed along with the use of broad-spectrum antibiotics.

If the abdominal perforation is proximal to a tumor or fixed stricture, we proceed with transhiatal esophagectomy, cervical esophagectomy, and enteral tubes, as

described above in the section on thoracic perforations. Reconstruction is usually deferred for 3 to 6 months to allow resolution of sepsis and inflammation.

REFERENCES

1. Sontag SJ. The medical management of reflux esophagitis. *Gastroenterol Clin North Am* 1990;19:683
2. Dehn TCB. Surgery for uncomplicated gastroesophageal reflux. *Br J Surg* 1992;33:293
3. Ott DJ, Gelfand DW, Wu WC, et al. Radiologic evaluation of dysphagia. *JAMA* 1986;256:2718
4. Hill LD, Aye RW, Ramel S. Antireflux surgery. *Gastroenterol Clin North Am* 1990;19:745
5. Stein HJ, DeMeester TA. Indications, technique, and clinical use of ambulatory 24-hour esophageal motility monitoring in a surgical practice. *Ann Surg* 1993;217:128
6. Mercer CD, Hill LD. Surgical management of peptic esophageal stricture. *J Thorac Cardiovasc Surg* 1986;91:371
7. Zaninotto G, DeMeester TR, Bremner CG, et al. Esophageal function in patients with reflux-induced strictures and its relevance to surgical treatment. *Ann Thorac Surg* 1989;47:362
8. Henderson RD, Henderson RF, Marryat GV. Surgical management of 100 consecutive esophageal strictures. *J Thorac Cardiovasc Surg* 1990;99:1
9. Pearson FG, Cooper JD, Patteson GA, et al. Gastroplasty and fundoplication for complex reflux problems. *Ann Surg* 1987;206:473
10. Eastridge CE, Pate JW, Mann JA. Lower esophageal ring: experiences in treatment of 88 patients. *Ann Thorac Surg* 1984;37:103
11. Ellis FH, Gibb SP. Esophageal reconstruction for complex benign esophageal disease. *J Thorac Cardiovasc Surg* 1990;99:192
12. DeMeester TR, Johansson KE, Franze I, et al. Indications, surgical technique, and long-term functional results of colon interposition or bypass. *Ann Surg* 1988;208:460
13. Wright C, Cuschiere A. Jejunal interposition for benign esophageal disease. *Ann Surg* 1987;205:54
14. DeMeester TR. Barrett's esophagus. *Surgery* 1993;113:239
15. DeMeester TR, Attwood SEA, Smyrk TC, et al. Surgical therapy in Barrett's esophagus. *Ann Surg* 1990;212:528
16. Streitz JM, Ellis JH, Gibb SP, et al. Adenocarcinoma in Barrett's esophagus. *Ann Surg* 1991;213:122
17. Williamson WA, Ellis FH, Gibb SP, et al. Effect of antireflux operation on Barrett's mucosa. *Ann Thorac Surg* 1990;49:537
18. Menguy R. Surgical management of large periesophageal hernia with complete intrathoracic stomach. *World J Surg* 1988;12:415
19. Ferguson MK. Periesophageal hernia. In: Cameron JL (ed), *Current Surgical Therapy*. 4th ed. St Louis, MO: Mosby Year Book; 34:1992
20. Baue AE, Belsey RHR. The treatment of sliding hiatus hernia and reflux esophagitis by the Mark IV technique. *Surgery* 1967;62:396
21. DeMeester TR, Bonavina L, Albertucci M. Nissen fundo-

plication for gastroesophageal disease. *Ann Surg* 1986; 204:9

22. Stirling MC, Orringer MB. Continued assessment of the combined Collis-Nissen operation. *Ann Thorac Surg* 1989; 47:224

23. Vander Salm TJ. Gastroesophageal reflux. In: Cutler BS, Dodson TF, Silva WE, Ander Salm TJ, eds. Manual of clinical problems in surgery. Boston, MA: Little Brown; 91:1984

24. DeMeester TR, Stein HJ. Gastroesophageal reflux disease. In: Moody FG, Carey LC, Jones RS, et al. (eds), *Surgical Treatment of Digestive Disease*, 2nd ed. Chicago, IL: Year Book Medical; 63:1990

25. Stuart RC, Dawson K, Keeling P, et al. A prospective randomized trial of Angelchik prosthesis versus Nissen fundoplication. *Br J Surg* 1989;76:86

26. Ferguson MK. Achalasia: Current evaluation and therapy. *Ann Thorac Surg* 1991;52:336

27. Andreollo NA, Earlam RJ. Heller's myotomy for achalasia: is an added antireflux procedure necessary? *Br J Surg* 1987;74:765

28. Chakkaphak S, Chakkaphak K, Ferguson MK, et al. Disorders of esophageal motility. *Surg Gynecol Obstet* 1991; 273:325

29. Stuart RC, Hennessy TPJ. Primary motility disorders of the esophagus. *Br J Surg* 1989;76:111

30. Little AG, Skinner DB, Chen WH, et al. Physiologic evaluation of esophageal function in patients with achalasia and diffuse esophageal spasm. *Ann Surg* 1986;203:500

31. Spencer J. Achalasia cardia: dilation or operation? *Gut* 1993;34:148

32. Little AG, Soriano A, Ferguson MK, et al. Surgical treatment of achalasia: results with esophagomyotomy and Belsey repair. *Ann Thorac Surg* 1988;45:489

33. Bonavina L, Nosadina A, Bardini R, et al. Primary treatment of esophageal achalasia. *Arch Surg* 1992;127:222

34. Pellegrini C, Wetter LA, Palti M, et al. Thorascopic esophagomyotomy. *Ann Surg* 1992;216:29

35. Henderson RD, Ryder D, Marryat G. Extended esophageal myotomy and short total fundoplication hernia repair in diffuse esophageal spasm: five-year review in 34 patients. *Ann Thorac Surg* 1987;43:25

36. Peters JH. Diverticula of the esophagus. In: Cameron JL (ed), *Current Surgical Therapy*, 4th ed. St Louis, MO: Mosby Year Book Medical; 20:1992

37. Streitz JM, Glick ME, Ellis FH. Selective use of myotomy for treatment of epiphrenic diverticula. *Arch Surg* 1992; 127:585

38. Richter JE. Motility disorders of the esophagus. In: Yamada T, Alpers DH, Owyang C, et al. (eds), *Textbook of Gastroenterology*. Philadelphia, PA: JB Lippincott; 1992: 1113

39. Pate JW, Walker WA, Cole FH, et al. Spontaneous rupture of the esophagus: a 30-year experience. *Ann Thorac Surg* 1989;47:689

40. Jones WG, Ginsberg RJ. Esophageal perforation: a continuing challenge. *Ann Thorac Surg* 1992;53:534

41. Cameron JL, Kieffer RF, Hendrix TR, et al. Selective nonoperative management of contained intrathoracic esophageal perforations. *Ann Thorac Surg* 1979;27:404

42. Knyrim K, Wagner HH, Bethge N, Keymling M, Vakil N. A controlled trial of an expansile metal stent for palliation of esophageal obstruction due to inoperable cancer. *N Engl J Med* 1993;329:1302

43. Csendes A, Braghetto I, Korn O, Cortes C. Late subjective and objective evaluations of antireflux surgery in patients with reflux esophagitis: analysis of 215 patients. *Surgery* 1989;105:374

25

Cancer of the Esophagus

Manson Fok ▪ *John Wong*

Carcinoma of the esophagus generally is considered an extremely aggressive tumor with poor prognosis. In recent years, with an improved standard of surgical technique and perioperative care, substantial reduction of operative morbidity and mortality has been achieved in experienced centers. The chance of cure has improved, and when cure is not possible, good-quality palliation is obtained. Recent proliferation of nonoperative treatments for palliation also has altered the once pessimistic prospect for patients afflicted by this dreaded disease.

■ HISTORICAL BACKGROUND

An esophageal growth causing swallowing disability and death was first described in western literature by Galen in the 2nd century, and was again documented as a cause for dysphagia by Avicenna in the 10th century. In early Chinese literature, a patient who had esophageal cancer was described as "one suffers in autumn, and does not live to see the coming summer." This depiction of the disease is still reasonably true in modern time.

Surgery for esophageal cancer began in 1877, when Czerny carried out the first successful resection of a cervical esophageal cancer and the patient lived for over a year. However, not until 1913 was the first successful resection of a thoracic esophageal cancer performed.[1] This was only possible because of the development in the field of anesthesia of differential positive pressure chambers for ventilation.[2] During the early part of this century,

reestablishment of feeding with or without esophageal resection was by gastrostomy, interposition of a plastic tube, skin tube, or a presternal conduit using the greater curvature of the stomach. The first successful one-stage resection of a thoracic esophageal cancer and reconstruction, using the whole stomach, was described by Ohsawa in 1933. Since then, surgery for the esophagus has entered into the modern era, and it is now possible to carry out a primary resection and anastomosis with acceptable operative morbidity and mortality risks.

■ EPIDEMIOLOGY

The incidence of esophageal cancer in western countries is low. In the United States, the yearly incidence is 6.0 per 100 000 population for males, and 1.6 per 100 000 in females.[3] For squamous cell carcinoma, the incidence is higher among blacks than whites. In low-incidence areas, a close relationship has been demonstrated between esophageal cancer, smoking, and alcohol consumption. For example, relatively higher incidences of esophageal cancers are found in sporadic areas in Scotland among the main whisky distilling areas.[4] The combined attributable risk of alcohol and tobacco consumption for esophageal cancer is more than 80% in northern France and northern Italy.[5]

In Asia and Africa, esophageal carcinoma is much more prevalent and is the sixth most common cause of cancer deaths in adult males (Fig 25–1). In Africa, a

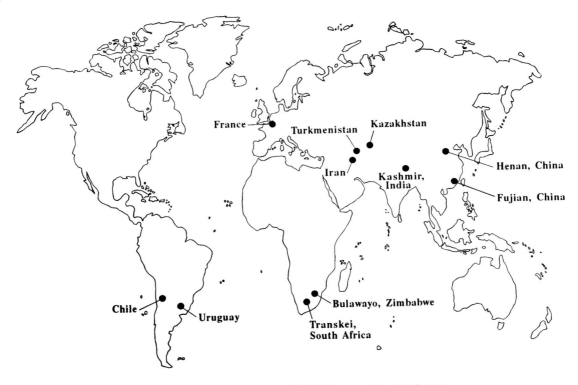

Figure 25–1. Map of the world showing high-incidence areas of esophageal cancer

high incidence of esophageal cancer is reported in Zimbabwe, Kenya, and in the homeland state of Transkei, South Africa.[6] The highest incidence of esophageal cancer is found in the southern shore of the Caspian Sea in Iran, through Central Asia of the Commonwealth of Independent States and Mongolia, across to northern China. In the Henan and Shanxi provinces of northern China, the age-adjusted mortality rate from esophageal cancer is 161/100 000 in men and 103/100 000 in women. It is the second most common cause of cancer death in adult males following lung cancer.[7] The death rate from esophageal cancer is 100 times higher than in the lowest risk area of China.[8] Within this "Asian esophageal cancer belt" there are common epidemiological factors peculiar to these regions. Mass population screening in countries like Iran and China using balloon exfoliative cytology have identified chronic esophagitis and severe dysplasia of the middle-third of the esophagus, in the absence of reflux disease, as predisposing conditions for the development of squamous cell carcinomas.[9] The occurrence of chronic esophagitis among the general population is high. In Kashmir, India, which also falls within this cancer belt and has an esophageal cancer incidence of 43.6/100 000 population, chronic esophagitis was found in 75% and dysplasia in 7.5% of otherwise apparently healthy individuals.[10]

Food habits and lifestyle are identified cultural factors related to the high incidence of chronic esophagi-

TABLE 25–1. RISK FACTORS IN THE DEVELOPMENT OF ESOPHAGEAL CARCINOMA

DIETARY
  Pickled vegetables, preserved meat and salted dry fish high in nitrosamine and other N-nitroso compounds
  Food contaminated by fungus (*geotrium candidum,* Fusarium species)
  Food and beverage consumed at high temperature
  Micronutrient deficiency (vitamin A, B12, C, E, beta-carotene)
  Trace element deficiency (cobalt, copper, molybdenum, zinc)

ACQUIRED
  Tobacco smoking
  Tobacco chewing
  Alcohol
  Chronic esophagitis
  Chronic dysplasia
  Barrett's esophagus
  Achalasia
  Lye corrosive stricture
  Other aerodigestive malignancy

HEREDITARY
  Tylosis

tis and esophageal cancers (Table 25–1). This includes the habit of drinking beverages at high temperature, which causes thermal injury to the esophageal mucosa,[11] and the regular consumption of dietary items containing substantial amounts of N-nitroso compounds, such as preserved fish and vegetables.[12] Dietary deficiencies in vitamin A, zinc, and molybdenum also have been implicated as likely dietary factors.[13] Beta-carotene has a protective role in cancer development, and low levels of beta-carotene have been found in patients with esophageal cancers, as well as among their relatives.[14]

Patients with other aerodigestive malignancies have an increased risk of developing squamous cell carcinoma of the esophagus, presumably because both malignancies involve exposure to similar environmental carcinogens. The overall incidence of synchronous or metachronous esophageal cancer in patients with primary head and neck cancer is 3% to 7%.[15] Patients with lye corrosive stricture of the esophagus and long-standing achalasia also have increased risks for esophageal cancer.

A genetic role in the development of esophageal cancer is unlikely, except in association with certain rare genetic disorders. Tylosis is an uncommon disease that has an autosomal dominant transmission with a high degree of penetrance. It is characterized by hyperkeratosis of the palms and soles. First described by Howel-Evans et al. in 1958,[16] the disease has a strong association with the development of squamous esophageal carcinoma. One possible link is a common mitogen for epithelial cells, such as elevated levels of epidermoid growth factor receptor, which was isolated in various genetic disorders affecting the epidermis, and in many malignant tumors, including esophageal cancer.[17]

■ PATHOPHYSIOLOGY

ANATOMY OF THE ESOPHAGUS

The esophagus is a tubular organ that begins at the level of the cricopharyngeus and descends through the thorax slightly to the left of the midline, curving forward in its lower part, away from the vertebral column, and piercing the diaphragm at the level of the 10th thoracic vertebra. A short transabdominal course ends at the gastric cardia. A functional high-pressure zone at the esophagogastric junction constitutes the lower esophageal sphincter, which prevents reflux of gastric acid into the lower esophagus.

In its mediastinal course, lying anterior to the esophagus are the trachea, bronchi, pulmonary veins, pericardium, and left atrium, with the pleura and the lungs laterally, and the vertebral column and the thoracic aorta posteriorly. Separating the esophagus from the

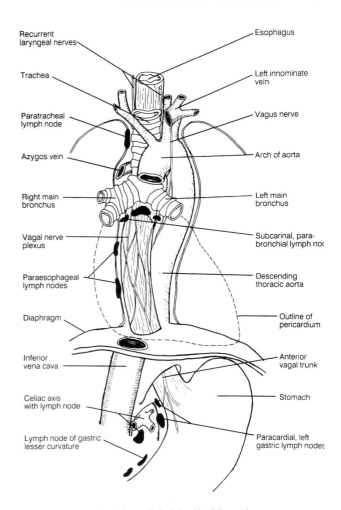

Figure 25–2. Anatomical relationship of the esophagus

vertebral column are the thoracic duct, azygos and hemiazygos veins, and the posterior intercostal arteries (Fig 25–2). Tumor spread within the esophagus is primarily subepithelial, and may appear as a submucosal plaque, satellite nodule, or as an extension from the main tumor. Further spread is by direct infiltration of adjacent organs, via the lymphatic channels to the regional lymph nodes, and via the blood-borne route to distant locations such as the lung, liver, kidney and brain.

PATHOLOGY

Among the high incidence areas of Asia and Africa, up to 80% of esophageal carcinomas are of squamous cell type; the majority of these tumors are located in the middle or lower portion of the thoracic esophagus. About 15% of carcinomas are located at the cardia, of which adenocarcinomas predominate. There is evidence of a rising incidence of cancer of the cardia and adenocarcinoma of the esophagus, especially among white males over 50 years of age. The increase is presumed to be associated with the rising incidence of Barrett's esophagus in western communities. In the 1970s, adenocarcinoma of the esophagus constituted 7% of all esophageal cancers, including the cardia. Recent surveys have shown a dramatic increase, with adenocarcinoma now constituting more than 40% of esophageal cancers.[18] In some western centers, the prevalence of adenocarcinoma of the esophagus may equal or even outnumber the prevalence of patients with squamous cell carcinoma.[19]

Barrett's Esophagus

Described first by Norman Barrett more than 40 years ago,[20] the disease is characterized by the presence of columnar epithelium metaplasia, which extends >3 cm into the distal tubular esophagus. Commonly, the Barrett's mucosa extends upward and interdigitates with the stratified squamous esophageal mucosa, which may extend to involve the entire length of the esophagus (Fig 25–3).

Three types of columnar epithelium are described. The most common is the intestinal type; the junctional type has mucosa similar to the gastric cardia, and the fundic type resembles the mucosa of the gastric body and fundus. Barrett's esophagus is diagnosed in 8% to 20% of patients examined endoscopically for symptoms of gastroesophageal reflux, and in 44% of patients with peptic stricture of the esophagus.[21] Prevalence rate of Barrett's esophagus in 14 898 patients undergoing endoscopy was 7.4/1000.[22]

Barrett's esophagus is considered a premalignant condition and patients should be followed up systemat-

ically. A progression from low-grade through high-grade dysplasia to adenocarcinoma is common. Prospective studies show a variable prevalence of adenocarcinoma in patients with Barrett's esophagus, from 5% to 46%, with an average of 13%.[23,24] Its incidence ranged between 1/52 and 1/441 patient years, or equivalent to a 30- to 125-fold increased risk of esophageal cancer compared with the general population. This risk of adenocarcinoma in Barrett's esophagus increases in relation to the length of columnar-lined epithelium. Smoking and male gender are additional risk factors.[25] The disease is uncommon in Asians and blacks.

Barrett's carcinoma accounts for 24% of the surgically treated adenocarcinomas of the esophagus and cardia in western countries, and may occur in patients after previous antireflux operation.[26] Regular follow-up of patients with Barrett's esophagus by endoscopic and histologic surveillance is recommended generally, although the benefits of an intensive surveillance program remain unproven and its cost-effectiveness is questionable. However, endoscopic surveillance permits detection of carcinoma at an early stage, with improved long-term survival after resection.[27]

Adenocarcinoma in Barrett's esophagus develops within an area of specialized columnar epithelium at the squamocolumnar junction in 85% of patients, and within 2 cm of the squamous epithelium in the remainder[28] (Fig 25–3). Hence, particular attention should be paid to this narrow squamocolumnar epithelial border during endoscopic surveillance. In the absence of dysplasia, the risk of cancer development is low, and endoscopic surveillance can be carried out biannually. In the presence of low-grade dysplasia, continue medical treat-

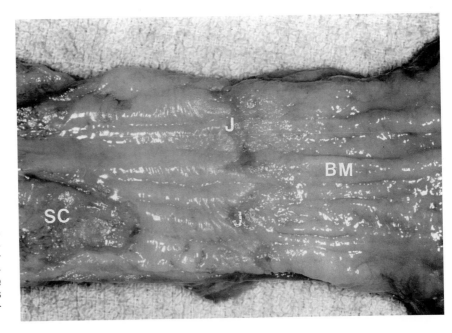

Figure 25–3. Barrett's mucosa (BM) extending into the distal esophagus. Adenocarcinoma is most likely to develop in the squamocolumnar junction (J) between the normal stratified squamous epithelium and the columnar metaplasia. A careful inspection of this junctional zone during endoscopic surveillance is important, especially if there is known dysplasia. In this specimen, there is a squamous cancer (SC) of the middle esophagus, which is by comparison more common in Asian patients.

ment and endoscopy should be carried out at 12 month intervals. High-grade dysplasia has substantial risk of malignancy, and is considered a carcinoma in-situ. These patients should be treated as if they have cancer, and resection is recommended. Multifocal carcinomas also are found in resected specimens of patients with severe dysplastic changes. If these patients are to be followed up with endoscopic examination, the intervals should be from 3 to 6 months. For resection, a subtotal esophagectomy should be performed with the removal of all the columnar-lined mucosa, since recurrent adenocarcinoma from the residual, abnormal mucosa is possible.

Additional parameters to identify patients at risk for malignant degeneration may include the use of flow cytometry to identify multiple aneuploid population,[29] and the assessment of tumor suppressor gene p53.[30] Their presence in dysplastic patients are indications for closer surveillance.

Tumor Biology and Markers

Cancer develops from genetic alterations that disrupt the control of cell growth and differentiation. On the molecular level, the loss of heterozygosity on chromosome 17P has been identified to occur at high frequency in esophageal cancer, and this loss may inactivate a tumor-suppressor gene causing cancer development.[31] Point mutation in the p53 gene, which is one of the tumor-suppressor genes, also has been found to occur frequently in squamous esophageal cancers.[32]

The presence of aneuploidy indicates genomic instability within the tissue that is related to tumorigenesis. The DNA distribution pattern measured by flow cytometry is shown to be a significant and independent prognostic factor in esophageal cancer. The presence of an aneuploid tumor cell population is associated with an aggressive clinical course, with higher rate of lymph node metastasis and higher frequency of recurrence than those with diploid tumors.[33] The 5 year survival of patients with diploid tumors is 20% to 30%, while there are no 5 year survivors reported for aneuploid tumors.[34] This finding is independent of lymph node metastases. The evaluation of the DNA content can be a valuable guide in selecting patients for adjuvant therapy.

Among the immunomarkers, squamous cell carcinoma-related antigen (SCC-RA) is probably the most sensitive for esophageal cancer. Positive sera has been isolated in 50% of patients, and its positivity increases with tumor growth, invasion, and metastases.[35] Epidermal growth factor receptor (EGF-R) is another immunomarker commonly studied, and its expression is related directly to tumor aggressivity. Cancers that strongly express EGF-R metastasize to lymph nodes more frequently than those which faintly express EGF-R.[36]

Histological indicators of favorable prognosis include the presence of abundant lymphocytes and polymor-

phonuclear leukocyte reactions within the tumor, and the presence of a fibrotic stroma[37], and poor prognosis is associated with lymph node metastases, venous invasion, tumor necrosis and the lack of peritumor fibrosis.[38]

■ DIAGNOSIS AND EVALUATION

SYMPTOMS, SIGNS AND DIFFERENTIAL DIAGNOSIS

In over 85% of patients with esophageal carcinoma, the presenting symptom is dysphagia, which initially is for solids and later progresses to liquids as the obstruction becomes complete. However, dysphagia may not be apparent until half of the esophageal lumen has become obliterated. Other common symptoms include regurgitation, cough, and weight loss. Moderate to severe weight loss occurs in as many as 40% of patients on presentation. Pain is a less frequent complaint and may indicate tumor infiltration to the mediastinum. Hoarseness is the result of recurrent laryngeal nerve palsy and usually affects the left side. General examination may reveal evidence of weight loss, muscle wasting, and dehydration. Examination of the chest may show the presence of pneumonia from aspiration, or the development of a tracheoesophageal fistula. Metastatic cervical lymphadenopathy occurs in 14% of patients on presentation, while 10% of patients will have metastases to solid organs (Table 25–2).

In Asia, where esophageal cancer is prevalent, over 90% of adult male patients over 55 years of age presenting with progressive onset of dysphagia will have esophageal carcinoma. Therefore, it is imperative to exclude the presence of a neoplasm when there is complaint of swallowing difficulty. In western countries, benign causes of dysphagia are also common. This includes dysphagia from reflux esophagitis which often is associated with a sliding-type hiatal hernia, and Barrett's esophagus. Neuromuscular causes of dysphagia include achalasia, diffuse esophageal spasm, and "nutcracker" esophagus. Benign neoplasms, such as an adenomatous polyp or a leiomyoma of the esophagus, are rare causes. Occasion-

TABLE 25–2. COMMON SYMPTOMATOLOGY OF ESOPHAGEAL CARCINOMA[a]

Dysphagia	Cough on swallowing
Regurgitation	Dyspnea
Weight loss	Neck mass
Cough	Hemoptysis
Pain	Hematemesis
Hoarseness	Tarry stool
Anorexia	

[a]in descending order of frequency

TABLE 25–3. DIFFERENTIAL DIAGNOSIS OF DYSPHAGIA

LOCAL CAUSES
  Intraluminal
    Foreign body
  Intramural
    Achalasia
    Diffuse esophageal spasm
    Reflux esophagitis
    Barrett's esophagus
    Esophageal (peptic) stricture
    Lye corrosive stricture
    Plummer-Vinson syndrome
    Pharyngeal pouch
    Diverticulum
    Benign neoplasm
    Malignant neoplasm
    Instrumental perforation
    Boerhaave's syndrome
  Extraluminal
    Retrosternal goiter
    Mediastinal tumor
    Mediastinal lymphadenopathy
    Thoracic aortic aneurysm
    Hiatus hernia
GENERAL CAUSES
  Myasthenia gravis
  Muscular dystrophy
  Bulbar palsy
  Poliomyelitis
  Scleroderma, SLE, rheumatoid arthritis
  Hysteria

noma is between 74% and 97%.[39] Reports indicate that barium swallow is less efficient in screening for adenocarcinoma in patients with Barrett's esophagus, with as much as 60% of the carcinoma remaining undetected by radiography,[40] however, this could be related to relative size and stage.

Fluoroscopically guided films taken at different angles are required in order to detect early lesions. Usually, anteroposterior, lateral, left and right anterior oblique projections are necessary. The barium-swallow study can determine the location and length of tumor, and may reveal the presence of submucosal secondaries. The relationship of the tumor to the whole thoracic cavity and the tracheal bifurcation is useful in deciding the operative approach (Fig 25–4). Deformity of the esophageal axis, such as tortuosity, angulation, and deviation are signs indicating an advanced tumor with fixation and retraction from infiltration of the adjacent organs (Fig 25–5).

Fiberoptic endoscopy allows direct visualization of the tumor and biopsy for histologic confirmation and typing. The yield of fine-needle aspiration cytology and multiple endoscopic biopsies is 90% to 100% (Fig 25–6). However, early mucosal or submucosal lesions can be missed on endoscopy because they may appear as small inconspicuous erosions, nodules, or plaques that may be flat, slightly raised, or depressed. To facilitate the detection of early esophageal cancer, vital staining

ally, dysphagia is the result of extrinsic compression of the esophagus by a mediastinal neoplasm or structures such as a retrosternal goiter, aortic arch aneurysm, mediastinal lymph nodes of neoplastic or tuberculosis origin, or from a rolling-type hiatal hernia (Table 25–3).

INVESTIGATION

The biologic behavior of esophageal carcinoma is characterized by submucosal spread, rapid transmural invasion of the esophageal wall, early spread to the regional lymph nodes, and distant dissemination. Usually, the clinical assessment significantly underestimates the extent of disease. A general physical examination may reveal evidence of nutritional depletion resulting from the dysphagia, and the presence of metastasis to lymph nodes or solid organs. For accuracy, examination of the cervical lymph nodes should not be confined to physical examination, but should include an ultrasound examination as well.

Barium Swallow and Endoscopy

A double-contrast, full-column barium swallow is very useful; the sensitivity in detecting an esophageal carci-

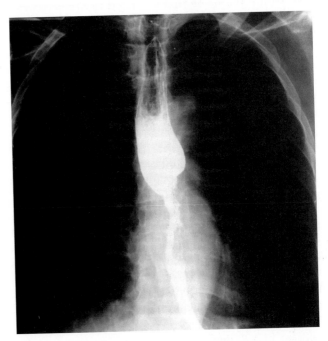

Figure 25–4. Barium swallow showing a middle third esophageal cancer in relationship to the trachea, vertebra, and diaphragm. Tumor is evidenced by an irregular, narrowed esophageal lumen, with a "shoulder" or "apple-core" appearance, and with dilatation of the partially obstructed proximal esophagus.

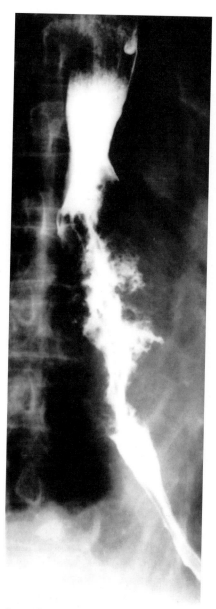

Figure 25–5. A barium swallow showing an advanced esophageal cancer with angulation and sinus formation into the mediastinum.

of the esophagus can be performed via the endoscope. Commonly, a solution of 1% to 2% Lugol's iodine or 1% toluidine-blue is used. Lugol's iodine will stain the glycogen content of the normal nonkeratinizing squamous epithelium, while the dysplastic mucosa remains unstained and can be biopsied selectively. Toluidine-blue has a strong affiliation for nuclear DNA and will stain neoplastic or dysplastic epithelium blue while leaving the squamous epithelium unstained.

For advanced tumor, the macroscopic appearance can be exophytic-polypoidal, ulcerative, diffusely infiltrating, or in combinations. It is important to examine carefully

the esophagus proximal to the tumor, since upward submucosal spread is common and satellite lesions may arise at some distance from the primary lesion. At times, a diffuse dysplastic area is seen around the tumor; the changes represent a form of "field cancerization" and is an ominous sign of an aggressive tumor (Fig 25–7).[41]

Flexible bronchoscopy is useful in detecting vocal cord paralysis, which occurs when a tumor invades into the left recurrent laryngeal nerve at its transmediastinal path between the esophagus and trachea. Advanced unresectable disease is evident by tumor compression, deviation of the tracheobronchial tree, or actual visible tumor infiltration on bronchoscopy.[42]

Computed Tomography and Endoscopic Ultrasound

Prognosis in esophageal cancer depends on the depth of tumor infiltration (T), presence of regional lymph node metastases (N), and distant metastases (M). Tumor staging is based on the 1987 TNM classification of the Union Internationale Contre le Cancer (Table 25–4).[43] In the present TNM classification, the primary tumor is staged as T1 to T4. T1 is when the tumor has invaded into the lamina propria or submucosa; T2 is when the muscularis propria is invaded. When the tumor has invaded the adventitia and adjacent structures, it is classified as T3 and T4, respectively. N0 and N1 lymph node staging depends on the absence or presence of regional lymph node metastasis. Similarly, M0 and M1 staging depends on the absence or presence of distant metastasis. Preoperative determination of wall penetration and lymph node status to determine resectability has been limited in the past because of the inaccuracy of standard radiography, endoscopy, computed tomography (CT) and magnetic resonance imaging (MRI) studies.

Barium study and upper endoscopy provide information of the luminal involvement by the tumor, but provide little information of its radial extension, which is important to know when considering resectability. Therefore, for the staging of tumors, CT scan and endoscopic ultrasonography (EUS) are used. Both CT and EUS are useful for the staging of the locoregional disease, while CT can, in addition, stage distant metastasis.

EUS is highly effective in determining the depth of primary cancer invasion; the accuracy of detecting intramural and transmural invasion in T staging is over 85% (Fig 25–8).[44–46] CT on the other hand, has difficulty in assessing T1 tumors and a tendency to overstage T3 and wrongly stage T4 tumors. The reliability of CT in staging infiltration is subject to controversy. Infiltration of adjacent organs is based on the degree of contact between the tumor and organs such as the aorta, presence of displacement or indentation of the tracheobronchial tree, and the absence of fat planes between the tumor

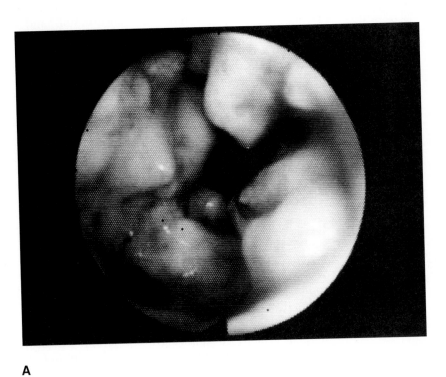

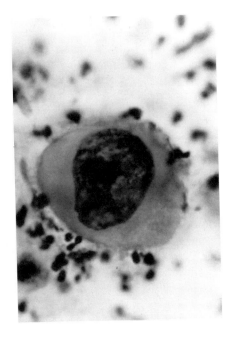

B

A

Figure 25–6. A. An endoscopic view of an advanced cancer of the middle third esophagus. **B**. Cytological examination of the esophageal cancer confirming malignancy. The accuracy of this examination is about 90%.

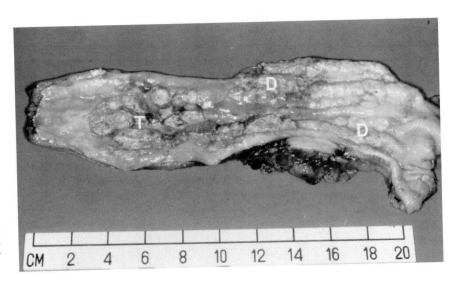

Figure 25–7. Specimen of an esophageal cancer showing diffuse dysplasia (D) around the tumor (T), and extending well beyond the margin of the primary cancer. This "field-cancerization" is a sign of aggressive tumor with poor prognosis.

TABLE 25–4. STAGING FOR ESOPHAGEAL CARCINOMA[a]

Stage 0	Tis	N0	M0
Stage I	T1	N0	M0
Stage IIA	T2	N0	M0
	T3	N0	M0
Stage IIB	T1	N1	M0
	T2	N1	M0
Stage III	T3	N1	M0
	T4	any N M0	
Stage IV	any T any N	M1	

T: Depth of primary tumor involvement. Tis: *carcinoma in situ*, T1: *invading lamina propria or the submucosa*, T2: *invading the muscularis propria*, T3: *invading the adventitia*, T4: *Invading adjacent structures*. N: Regional lymph nodes involvement. N0: *none*, N1: *regional nodes involved*. M: Distant metastasis. M0: *none*, M1: *distant metastasis present*.
[a]According to the classification of the Union Internationale Contre le Cancer (UICC: TNM Classification of malignant tumors. 4th edition. Hermanek P, Sobin LH (eds). Springer-Verlag, Berlin. 1987).

and the pericardium, the latter being unreliable in patients who are emaciated[39,47] (Fig 25–9). Interpretation of infiltration by CT is often subjective, and the comparative accuracy of CT staging of T3 and T4 tumors is inferior to that of EUS.[48,49]

Another limitation of CT is its inability to detect involvement of periesophageal lymph nodes. The size of the lymph node does not accurately reflect tumor involvement. Small lymph nodes may harbor tumor cells, whereas enlarged nodes may be chronic inflammatory. Often, enlarged nodes adjacent to the esophageal cancer are indistinguishable from contiguous tumor spread. The overall accuracy of CT in the detection of regional lymph node involvement averages around 50%.[39,40,47] For EUS, the overall accuracy of N staging is between 73% and 93%.[44,50] Although lymph nodes as small as 3 mm are detected by EUS, the differentiation of benign from malignant nodes remains problematic. On ultrasound, malignant nodes tend to be more spherical in shape, are sharply defined, and hypoechoic.[51] However, determination of malignancy based on these criteria remains rather subjective.

EUS is not appropriate for staging distant metastases or intra-abdominal lymph node metastases, since its focus is restricted to a 5-cm tissue penetration. The accu-

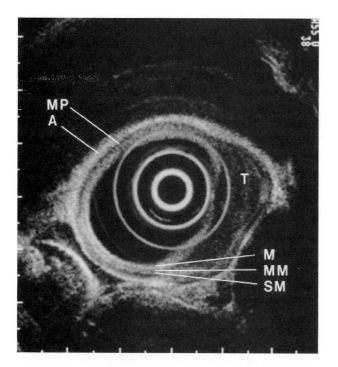

Figure 25–8. Endoscopic ultrasound (EUS) of an esophageal tumor (T) showing its penetration into the depth of the esophageal wall. Five layers of the normal esophageal wall is seen on EUS. The first, third and fifth layers are echogenic and these are respectively, the mucosa (M), submucosa (SM) and the adventitia (A). While the interweaning muscularis mucosa (MM) (second layer) and the muscularis propria (MP) (fourth layer) are hypoechoic. *Courtesy of Dr. Yoko Murata, Institute of Gastroenterology, Tokyo Women's Medical College.*

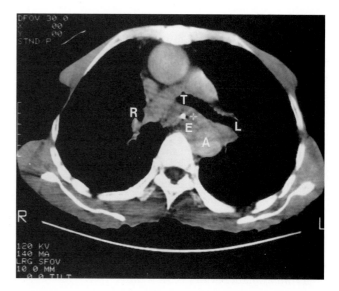

Figure 25–9. A computer axial tomography showing a T4 esophageal tumor in the mediastinum. There is displacement of the tracheobronchial tree, and loss of the fat plane between the tumor and the descending thoracic aorta (A) suggestive of infiltration to these organs. (T: trachea, L: left main bronchus, R: right main bronchus, E: esophagus)

racy of EUS in staging celiac lymph nodes involvement is 68%, compared with 82% for staging by CT scan.[46,48] CT scan is also more appropriate than EUS for M staging of solid organ, such as in metastases to the liver and the lung. The reported accuracy of CT is between 87% and 100%.[39]

An additional limitation of EUS is its inability to pass the endoscope through a stenotic tumor, which is reported in 37% to 65% of cases examined.[46,51,52] Unfortunately, most stenotic tumors are advanced stage III or IV lesions, where the need for accurate tumor staging is more important in determining its resectability. The recent development of finer-caliber probes, such as the 8-mm diameter E-probe (Olympus Tokyo, Japan), or the 3.4-mm diameter catheter probe (UM-1W, Olympus), may overcome the difficulties described.

With the advent of minimally invasive surgery, the use of laparoscopy and thoracoscopy may be valuable in staging tumor spread and thus, would obviate the need of performing a laparotomy or thoracotomy for unresectable lesions, although a general anesthesia still would be required.[53]

■ TREATMENT

OVERVIEW

Esophageal cancer remains a lethal disease, with a 5 year survival rate of 20% in unselected patients after resection.[54] The management of esophageal cancer largely depends on the stage of disease at presentation. Although subtle symptoms may develop in early stage tumor, presentation is usually delayed until the onset of dysphagia, by which time the patients will have either advanced local disease or distant metastases that preclude, for the majority, a cure at initial diagnosis, and where palliation becomes the only appropriate aim of treatment. Therefore, management has been focused on providing expedient palliation of the dysphagia, with low risk.

The optimal treatment of patients with esophageal cancer is still a subject of debate. For many decades, the lack of comparable alternative treatment for esophageal cancer has made resection an unrivaled treatment form, despite the high risk and poor survival associated with it. In recent years, reports of success with radiotherapy and chemotherapy as alternative primary treatments or as adjuvant therapy to surgery have had an increasing influence on nonoperative therapies in the overall treatment strategy for patients with esophageal cancers.

From available evidence, it is unlikely that any single treatment protocol is applicable to all patients. Treatment should be multidisciplinary, with contributions and support from the oncologists, radiotherapists, surgeons and other health workers. The choice of therapy is dependent on its morbidity and mortality risk, the quality of palliation, the risk of recurrence, and the availability and experience of the particular discipline at the institution where treatment is offered.

OPERATIVE TREATMENT

Surgical therapy remains the mainstay therapy for patients with resectable esophageal carcinoma who are fit for major operation. For favorable lesions, both squamous and adenocarcinoma can be cured by surgical resection. The 5 year survival rate after resection for cancers limited to the mucosa was over 80% and was 55% for tumors extending to the submucosa.[55] The frequency of lymph node metastases increases significantly once the tumor has bridged into the submucosa, thereby reducing the favorable outcome. Recently, successful endoscopic mucosal resection as alternative treatment for lesions confined to the mucosa, with good long-term survival and the avoidance of an open operation, has been reported.[56]

Whether radical en bloc resection that includes systematic mediastinectomy and extensive lymph node dissection can prolong survival in a more advanced stage tumor that has penetrated the esophageal wall or has metastasized to regional lymph nodes, is still controversial.[57] However, in the presence of incurable disease, resection can offer superior palliation compared to other nonoperative treatment modalities, with restoration of normal swallowing in over 90% of patients.[58] In prospective randomized analysis of the quality of palliation, significant difference was found in favor of surgery, both in the lower incidence of stricture formation and the improved efficacy of swallowing when compared with radiotherapy. The incidence of esophageal stricture, both benign and malignant, was 16% after surgery and was 50% after radical radiotherapy.[59]

In experienced centers, the 30 day mortality of esophageal cancer operation is less than 5%. The 5 year survival after curative resection is between 20% and 35%,[60,61] and is 5% after palliative resection.[62,63] For patients free of lymph node metastasis, 5 year survival may be as high as 60%, whereas it was 10% to 20% for patients with positive metastatic lymph nodes[37,62] (Fig 25–10).

Choice of Operation

The type of operation depends mainly upon the location and extent of the primary tumor, and whether a transthoracic resection, if required, is possible in view of the cardiopulmonary proficiency of the patient (Table 25–5). The objectives of resection are to extirpate the primary tumor and its involved lymphatic drainage, to obtain adequate proximal and distal resection margins, and to remove any adjacent expendable soft tissue that has been infiltrated.[64] Resection is followed by recon-

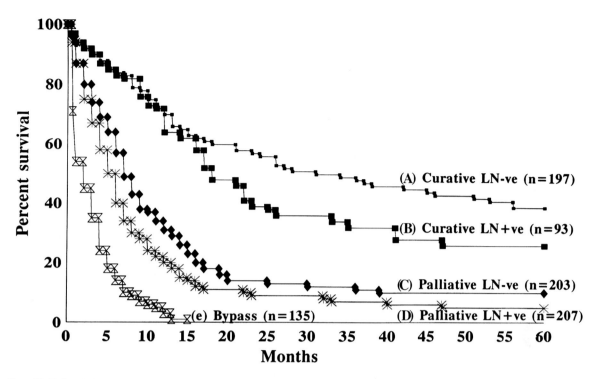

Figure 25–10. Cumulative survival curves of 700 patients operated on for esophageal carcinoma at the Department of Surgery, The University of Hong Kong. Survival was significantly better for patients who underwent curative resection (**A,B**) as compared with patients who underwent palliative resection (**C,D**). Survival was also longer in patients without lymph node metastasis (LN-ve) as compared with patients with metastatic lymph nodes (LN+ve) (a versus b, c versus d = significant).

TABLE 25–5. CHOICE OF OPERATION

RESECTION
  Cervical esophagus
    Pharyngolaryngoesophagectomy
    Free jejunal transfer
  Superior mediastinal
    Split sternum esophagectomy
    Three-phase esophagectomy
  Middle and lower third
    Lewis-Tanner operation
    Transhiatal esophagectomy
    Three-phase esophagectomy
    Esophagectomy (left thoracotomy approach)
  Cardia
    Transhiatal esophagectomy
    Esophagogastrectomy (left thoracoabdominal approach)
    Esophagogastrectomy (abdominal right-chest approach)
    Abdominal gastrectomy

BYPASS
  Kirschner gastric bypass
  Colon bypass
  Jejunum bypass

struction with the use of a suitable esophageal substitute organ, such as the stomach, colon, or jejunum, to reconstitute the food passage.

For cancers located at the cervical esophagus, resection will involve a laryngectomy, partial pharyngectomy, total esophagectomy with a blunt dissection of the thoracic esophagus, and the establishment of a terminal tracheostomy (Fig 25–11).[65] Alternately, radiotherapy may be preferred because of the 10% mortality associated with an operation of such magnitude, and the possible preservation of voice, if not already impaired by tumor involvement of the recurrent laryngeal nerve. For cancers localized to the cricopharyngeus, free intestinal transplant is increasingly used to replace the resected portion of the upper esophagus. Although it is time consuming and necessitates microvascular anastomosis, the free jejunal loop can provide good functional results while avoiding the risks of a mediastinal dissection.[66] However, late complications, such as stricture formation, were higher for free jejunal graft compared with the traditional gastric pull-up.[67] Another alternative to reconstruct the pharynx and upper esophagus is to use the pectoralis major myocutaneous flap after its tuberization.[68]

For carcinoma of the thoracic inlet, resection can be carried out by a combined cervical and thoracic approach, as advocated by McKeown,[69] or with a median

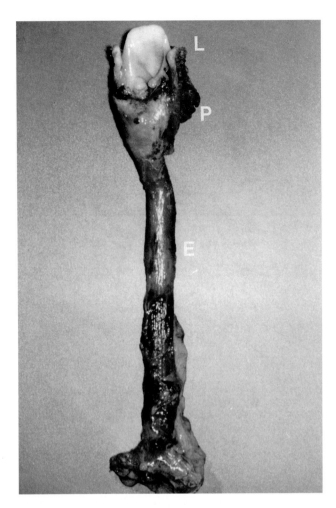

Figure 25–11. Specimen of a pharyngolaryngoesophagectomy operation for a post-cricoid carcinoma of the esophagus. The larynx (L), pharynx (P), and the whole esophagus (E) are included. Resection is followed by reconstruction with a pharyngogastric anastomosis made in the neck, using a gastric substitute that has been brought up via the orthotopic or retrosternal route.

sternotomy together with a blunt dissection of the thoracic esophagus as advocated by Ong.[70] The latter procedure allows adequate exposure and preservation of the great vessels in the superior mediastinum to prevent their inadvertent injury, while tumor dissection can be done under vision.[71] The avoidance of a thoracotomy may reduce cardiopulmonary disturbance.

The majority of squamous cell carcinomas are located in the middle portion of the thoracic esophagus. For its extirpation, both the thoracic and abdominal part of the esophagus are removed. The most common approach is the Lewis-Tanner operation, described independently by Ivor Lewis, in 1946, and Norman Tanner, in 1947.[72,73] The operation begins with an abdominal phase where the substitute organ, such as the stomach, is prepared. This is followed by a

right posterolateral thoracotomy that permits access to all parts of the thoracic esophagus and allows for a systematic dissection and resection of the tumor, together with the mediastinal lymph nodes and thoracic duct. The stomach then is advanced cephalad for reconstruction with the proximal esophagus at the apex of the pleural cavity. A sufficient proximal resection margin is obtained without the need of an additional neck incision (Fig 25–12). Alternately, a resection via the left thoracic approach also can be carried out[74]; however, the exposure of the upper thoracic esophagus may be compromised by the overlying arch of the aorta.

Transhiatal Versus Transthoracic Resection

Most surgeons experienced in both thoracotomy and nonthoracotomy technique do not see a clear superiority of one method over the other, and no advantage has been demonstrated by a controlled trial.

While traditionalists have long held that the best treatment for esophageal cancer is an efficient esophagectomy with wide tissue clearance in potentially curable patients as a means of improving survival,[75] an increasing number of surgeons favor a transhiatal resection of the esophagus, which involves a posterior mediastinal blunt (blind) dissection without the need for a thoracotomy. The theoretical advantage of the transhiatal resection is a lower operative risk. A low hospital mortality rate of 2.4% was reported for patients with adenocarcinoma of the esophagus who underwent transhiatal resection,[76] although the incidence of respiratory complications was not less compared with transthoracic resection. A low hospital mortality rate of 1.3% also is possible with resection via the transthoracic approach.[77] Proponents of the transhiatal resection adhere to the concept that the biologic behavior of the tumor, rather than the magnitude of the resection, principally determines the survival.[78] This was justified by demonstrating comparable survival for patients with transhiatal and transthoracic resections.

Transhiatal resection is preferred in patients with impaired respiratory function and strong contraindication for a thoracotomy. However, the approach does not appear to be associated with significant decrease in postoperative complications. But there is an increased risk of injury to the azygos vein and the esophageal branches of the thoracic aorta, which may cause major hemorrhage. Additionally, tearing of the membranous trachea or injury to the left recurrent laryngeal nerve, which may cause hoarseness, can occur. The latter occurs in about 12% of patients.[79] Thus, the transhiatal approach is contraindicated in midthoracic tumor, unless it is shown to be at an early stage, especially when the tumor is located above the trachea bifurcation. An esophageal tumor of the upper or lower esophagus, however, can be dis-

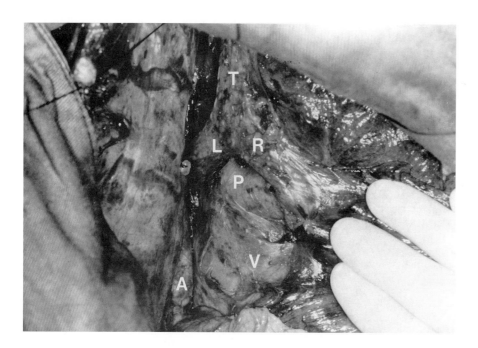

A

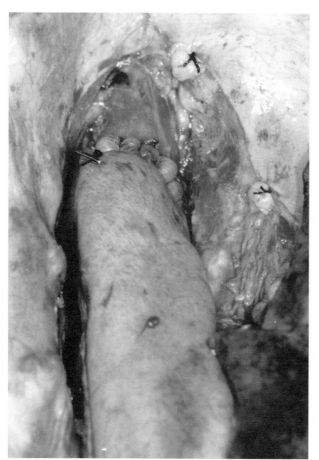

B

Figure 25–12. A. A posterolateral view of the mediastinal dissection in a Lewis-Tanner operation for carcinoma of the middle and lower third esophagus. The tumor and the esophagus have been removed together with the paratracheal, carinal, parabronchial lymph nodes, the connective tissues in the mediastinum and the thoracic duct. (T: trachea, L: left main bronchus, R: right main bronchus, P: pericardium, V: right pulmonary vein, A: descending thoracic aorta). **B**. View of the completed operation with the hand-sewn anastomosis made between the stomach and the divided proximal esophagus at the apex of the right pleural cavity.

sected mostly under vision with adequate exposure, via the enlarged diaphragm hiatus, where mobilization by blunt dissection involves only the removal of the remaining normal esophagus.

Minimally Invasive Surgery

Minimal invasive surgery (MIS) using thoracoscopy or mediastinoscopy is a new development of surgery for the esophagus. Videoscopic-directed thoracoscopy has been used extensively for lung biopsy, pleurodesis and pleurectomy, excision of peripheral lung tumors, sympathectomy and vagotomy, resection of esophageal leiomyoma, and esophageal myotomy for achalasia.[80,81] For patients with esophageal carcinoma who are at high risk for thoracotomy because of poor lung function, videoscopic surgery is a possible alternative. Using thoracoscopy, a subtotal endoscopic esophagectomy can be performed safely under visual guidance. The avoidance of a thoracotomy should improve postoperative respiratory function and expedite recovery.[82]

Operative mediastinoscopy also can substitute for the traditional blunt mediastinal dissection, so that the esophagus is dissected under endoscopic control. However, owing to its limited view to the periesophageal organs, only small tumors above the bifurcation can be resected safely by this technique.[83]

Notwithstanding its appeal, it remains to be proven whether a smaller incision can offset the inherent disadvantages of the procedure. These include an increased morbidity and mortality risk, especially at the learning phase, a long anesthesia with single-lung ventilation, and inadequate radical lymph node dissection of the mediastinum, which can possibly decrease the chances of cure. It is likely that MIS eventually will be applicable only to a few, select early-staged patients.

Ultraradical Lymphadenectomy

A standard lymph node dissection would include the removal of the paratracheal, parabronchial, carinal, paraesophageal, and posterior mediastinal lymph nodes in the mediastinum, and the paracardial, left gastric, and lymph nodes along the gastric lesser curvature in the abdomen (Fig 25–2).

An ultraradical lymphadenectomy (synonymous with extended-lymphadenectomy or three-field lymphadenectomy) incorporates the standard mediastinal and abdominal lymph node dissection with extension to include a bilateral cervical lymphadenectomy, the dissection of the upper mediastinal lymph nodes, and the celiac, retropancreatic and subhepatic lymph nodes in the abdomen. The neck dissection includes the removal of the supraclavicular, internal jugular, and paraesophageal nodes.[60] In Japanese patients with squamous cancer of the thoracic esophagus, the reported incidence of lymph node metastasis in the thoracocervical transitional region is 26%.

Prospective uncontrolled studies comparing the ultraradical lymphadenectomy with conventional two-field lymphadenectomy showed significantly improved 5 year survival rates when neck dissection was performed (49% versus 34%, respectively).[84] Recurrence rate was 64% for patients who underwent limited lymphadenectomy, 37% for patients with block dissection of mediastinal lymph nodes, and 22% for patients with ultraradical lymphadenectomy of pericardiac, mediastinal, and bilateral neck.[84,85] However, many of these studies are flawed by non-comparable patient groups. The efficacy of ultraradical lymphadenectomy can only be determined by future randomized trials.

Extensive node dissection is time consuming and increases postoperative mortality. The incidence of recurrent laryngeal nerve injury for patients with and without extended lymphadenectomy was 40% and 12%, respectively,[86] whereas the incidence of postoperative pulmonary complications was 35% and 18%, respectively.[87]

Arguments against the ultraradical lymphadenectomy procedure, again, are that it is the biology and staging of the tumor rather than the nature or radicality of the operation that chiefly influences the survival rate in esophageal cancer.

Esophageal Substitute

The stomach is the most widely used and preferred organ for esophageal replacement after esophagectomy for cancer. The gastric substitute can be expeditiously prepared, and is mobilized based on the right gastric and right gastroepiploic arcades. Depending on the type of operation, the stomach is divided from the esophagus near the angle of His on the lesser curvature (Fig 25–13A). Thus, the gastric substitute made is brought up to the apex of the right pleural cavity in the Lewis-Tanner operation or alternately, to the neck, either orthotopically, retrosternally, or subcutaneously, to be anastomosed to the proximal divided esophagus in the three-phase esophagectomy, or by the transhiatal approach. Only a single anastomosis is required to reconstruct the food passage. However, up to 50% of patients may complain of postprandial fullness, with acid or bile regurgitation especially on supine position.[88] We have found that it is essential to drain the vagotomized stomach with a pyloroplasty to prevent gastric outlet obstruction, which occurs in approximately 13% of undrained stomachs (Fig 25–13B). Delayed gastric drainage contributes to postoperative morbidity from aspiration pneumonia and significantly prolongs the patient's recovery.[89]

The alternate use of the colon as an esophageal substitute may offer a better quality of palliation with less postprandial symptoms. Either the left or right side of the colon can be used. Compared with the stomach, preparation of the colon is more tedious and reconstruction necessitates three anastomoses. An isoperi-

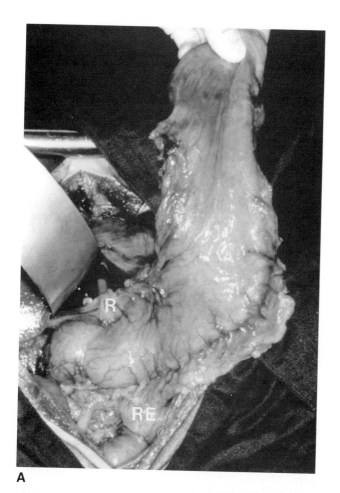

A

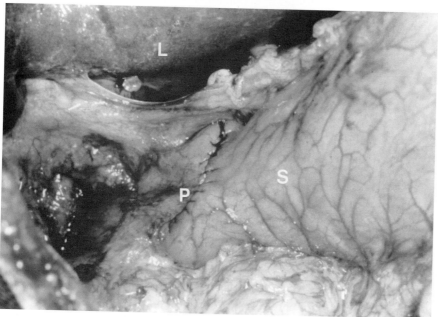

B

Figure 25–13. A. The prepared stomach tube that is based on the right gastric (R) and right gastroepiploic (RE) arcades for its blood supply. The stomach is ready to be brought up to the chest or to the neck for anastomosis with the proximal divided esophagus. **B**. A close-up view of the pylorus showing the pyloroplasty which was done to facilitate gastric drainage for the vagotomized stomach. (S = stomach, P = pyloroplasty, L = liver).

staltic colonic loop is prepared by using the right colon based on the middle colic vessels, and for the left colon, based on the ascending branch of the left colic vessels. Care is taken to preserve the marginal arcades and the communicating arch between the main branches (Fig 25–14). Anastomoses then are made between the interposed colon and the cervical esophagus proximally, the stomach or small bowel distally, with a third anastomosis to reestablish colon continuity. Although technically more demanding and time consuming, some surgeons prefer using the colon because of its durability and functional advantages over the stomach.[90] Controlled trials are not available to establish these claims.

Anastomotic Leakage

An overall fall in operative mortality in recent years can be attributed to a significant reduction in preventable technical complications, such as anastomotic leakage,

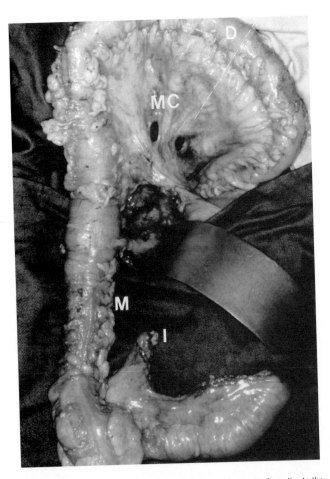

Figure 25–14. Preparation of the right colon for interposition as an alternative to the stomach. The terminal ileum is used for anastomosis with the esophagus, both of which have similar luminal size. The blood supply to the right colonic loop is by the middle-colic arcade (MC). Careful preservation of the marginal arcade (M) and flush-ligation of the right colic and ileo-colic (I) vessels are necessary to ensure good vascular supply to the loop. The divided distal end of the colonic loop (D) is anastomosed to the stomach or to the small bowel.

which should occur in less than 5% of anastomoses.[91] However, a leakage rate of 20% still is regarded as the acceptable average, and high leakage rates are still not infrequently reported.[92]

Since approximately half of these anastomotic leakages have fatal outcome, a significant reduction in the incidence of this preventable complication can decrease postoperative mortality significantly. The location of the anastomosis (chest or neck) and the methods employed (hand-sewn or stapled) are probably less important than their accurate application (Fig 25–15).

From a review of the experience of 59 surgical centers, the leakage rate of intrathoracic esophageal anastomoses was 11%, and was consistently less than the 19% incidence of cervical esophageal anastomotic leaks.[93] However, there are many reports of a much higher mortality rate for a thoracic anastomotic leak as compared with a cervical leak. The claimed advantage of a cervical anastomosis is irrelevant if the anastomotic leakage rate is low.[94]

The hand-sewn anastomosis, using a single-layer continuous technique, has been shown consistently to have better results compared with double-layer anastomosis or stapled anastomosis, because of the lower incidence of fibrotic stricture formation (Fig 25–16).[95,96] Although the leakage rate for hand-sewn anastomosis varies, a low incidence rate similar to that for the stapled anastomosis can be achieved.[97] Histologic evaluation in bowel anastomosis has shown more complete epithelialization and less inflammation in hand-sewn anastomosis, whereas a higher level of collagen formation was found in stapled anastomoses.[98] The apparent ease of the stapled anastomosis is offset by the higher tendency to stricture formation and less complete healing as compared with the hand-sewn anastomosis.

Surgical Bypass

The main aim of a bypass operation is to obtain effective palliation similar to that obtained with resection. However, the problems of performing major surgery on patients with advanced malignancy are reflected in high operative mortality rates of close to 40%.[99] With the availability of accurate imaging for preoperative tumor staging, more of these patients diagnosed with advanced disease and expected short survival are being treated by nonoperative means (Fig 25–10).

The most common procedure for bypass operation is the Kirschner operation. Repopularized by Ong in 1973,[100] the stomach is used as the substitute organ, and is brought to the neck via a retrosternal or subcutaneous tunnel to be anastomosed to the divided cervical esophagus. The abdominal esophagus is anastomosed to a loop of small bowel. An intrathoracic gastric bypass also is described for patients who initially undergo exploratory thoracotomy with intention to re-

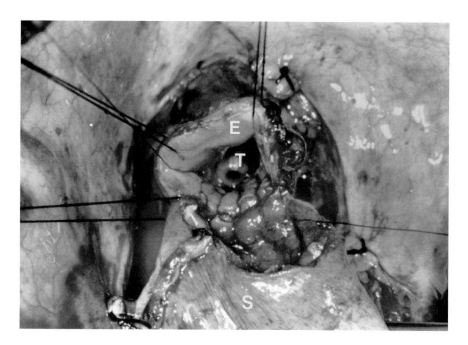

A

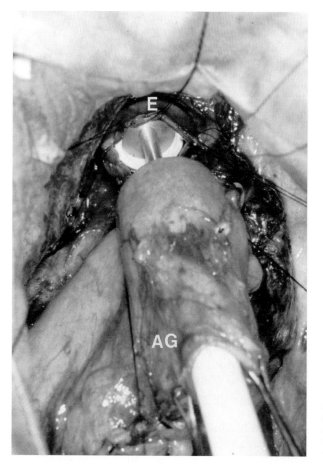

Figure 25–15. A. The construction of an esophagogastric anastomosis in the right chest using a single layer continuous hand-sewn technique with an absorbable 4-0 Maxon suture (polyglyconate, Davis and Geck, Cyanamid, Gosport, UK). The posterior wall is near completion. (E: esophagus, S: stomach, T: gastric suction tube). **B**. The construction of an esophagogastric anastomosis in the right chest using a circular stapler. The device is passed through an anterior gastrotomy (AG), through the apex of the gastric tube, into the esophagus (E).

B

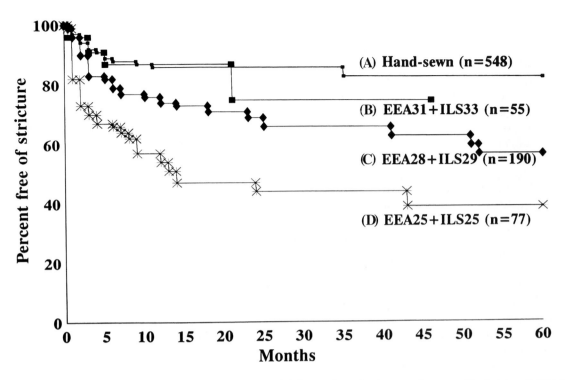

Figure 25–16. The comparative incidence of stricture formation between the single layer continuous hand-sewn anastomoses and the stapled anastomoses according to stapler sizes. Significantly less stricture is seen with hand-sewn anastomoses (**A**) compared with anastomoses made by circular staplers (**B,C,D**). Also, significantly more strictures occurred when the smaller size staplers are used (**D** versus **B,C**). EEA (Autosuture, U.S. Surgical Corporation), ILS (Ethicon Ltd., Edinburgh, UK).

sect, but are found to have disease that is extensive and therefore, unsuitable for resection. Under this circumstance, a bypass procedure should not add significantly to the morbidity and mortality risks of the operation.[99] If the stomach is not available for use because of disease, previous surgery or insufficient length, the colon or the jejunum also can offer good symptomatic relief of dysphagia.

NONOPERATIVE TREATMENT

Radiotherapy

The role of radiotherapy as the definitive treatment for esophageal cancer always has been unclear. Even with a radical dose of radiotherapy (50 to 65 Gy), treatment failure from locoregional recurrence may occur in up to 80% of patients.[101] The 5 year survival rate after radiotherapy for operable cancers is 14% and 4% for inoperable lesions.[102,103] Efforts to improve survival by varying the dosage of radiotherapy or changing the techniques have not had a significant impact. Proponents of radiotherapy argue that despite these dismal results, patients treated by radiotherapy have similar survival rates to surgically treated patients with similar disease stage, but avoid the associated operative mortality.

Initial improvement of dysphagia with radiotherapy can be expected in more than three-quarters of patients. However, the median duration of relief is only 3 to 6 months,[104,105] with up to 75% of patients requiring subsequent dilatation or other treatment such as laser or intubation, to maintain adequate swallowing.[103] The relief of dysphagia until death is expected in less than 40% of patients.[104] The combined use of external-beam irradiation with intracavitary irradiation may have better control of locoregional recurrence, but it also has increased risk of stricture and fistulation.[106]

In an attempt to improve the poor results of radiotherapy, chemotherapeutic agents, such as Cisplatin, 5-fluorouracil, and mitomycin-C, have been added as radiation sensitizers to enhance the therapeutic results of radiotherapy. Improved results have been reported from nonrandomized studies showing improved survivals from combined chemoradiotherapy compared with historical controls treated by radiotherapy alone,[107] or with radiotherapy and surgery.[108]

However, preliminary results from randomized trials comparing radiotherapy alone with chemoradiotherapy did not show significant differences in survival, while substantially more toxicities were noted from the combined treatment.[109]

Adjuvant Radiotherapy

After resection of esophageal carcinoma, complete eradication of the cancer is achieved in less than half of treated patients, with locoregional recurrence as a common cause of failure. Recognizing the limitations of surgery, there has been much interest in combining radiotherapy with surgery to accomplish a more effective locoregional control of the cancer.

Although complete resolution of tumors with preoperative radiotherapy has been reported in a small proportion of patients, 15% to 50% of patients have unresectable lesions after radiotherapy.[110,111] Prospective, randomized controlled trials on preoperative radiotherapy, using a total dose of 35 to 45 Gy radiation, revealed no differences in tumor resectability, curability, tumor penetration, lymph node metastasis, and operative mortality rates compared with control patients.[112–114] Furthermore, preoperative radiotherapy has not been shown to prolong survival.[62] Preoperative radiotherapy also can add to the risk of surgery because of radiation injury to the heart and lungs. In addition, with preoperative radiotherapy, there is an increased risk of tumor metastases to the lymph nodes outside of the irradiated field, and a possible role of radiation-induced immunodeficiency is suggested.[115]

Radiotherapy given after resection has been shown to enhance local control of the residual disease, but has not demonstrated any improvement of survival in nonrandomized studies.[116,117] Prospective studies of patients given radiotherapy after curative resection of squamous esophageal carcinoma did not demonstrate any survival benefits compared with the control group.[118] Our prospective randomized controlled study showed that postoperative radiotherapy was associated with increased morbidity and death caused by radiation injury to the esophageal substitute, early appearance of metastatic disease, and reduced overall survival compared with the surgery-alone group. The sole benefit from radiotherapy was in the prevention of tracheobronchial recurrence in patients with known residual mediastinal disease after palliative resection, and in whom the risk of symptomatic recurrence is high.[119]

Adjuvant Chemotherapy and Chemoradiotherapy

Efforts to improve the survival of patients with esophageal carcinoma have combined both local and systemic therapy in the treatment protocol. Currently, three modes of combined local-systemic therapies are under study: preoperative chemotherapy, preoperative chemoradiotherapy, and chemoradiotherapy without surgery. Phase II studies on preoperative chemotherapy or chemoradiotherapy have shown a tumor response rate of 40% to 60%,[120–122] with a complete pathologic response rate of 0% to 40%.[123,124] Response is highest with combined preoperative chemotherapy and radiotherapy.

However, not all patients submitted to combined therapy have their treatment completed, and as much as 73% of patients never reach the resection stage after chemoradiotherapy.[110] In a prospective study, minimal response to preoperative chemotherapy was reported in 38% of patients, while disease progression was observed in another 19% of patients.[125] The delay of definitive surgery in this large percentage of patients, as a result of ineffectual treatment, is a major concern.

The commonly used chemotherapeutic agents are Cisplatin, 5-fluorouracil, mitomycin, bleomycin, vinblastine and vincristine, in various combinations, with or without concurrent 30 to 55 Gy radiation therapy.[122,123] Preoperative adjuvant chemotherapy is usually given as a single or double treatment cycle over a period of 6 to 8 weeks. Hence, a longer duration of treatment and hospitalization compared with surgery-alone patients often is needed.

The incidence of toxicity from preoperative adjuvant therapy can be substantial and death from the toxicity has been reported to be around 2% to 7%.[123,125,126] Most reports did not show any significant increase of operative morbidity and mortality for patients who subsequently underwent resection after preoperative adjuvant therapy,[123] although increased postoperative respiratory complication was associated with the use of bleomycin.[109,126]

While many phase II studies on preoperative chemotherapy or chemoradiotherapy have reported improved survival compared with historic controls, some large series showed no improvement of survival compared with the surgery-alone groups.[110,127] Prospective studies on multimodality therapy showed a nonoperative rate after neoadjuvant therapy of 24% for patients who were initially assessed to have resectable lesions, compared with 7% in the surgery-alone group.[126] Schlag reported a significantly greater perioperative morbidity and mortality risk with preoperative chemotherapy.[125] Overall, there was no survival benefit demonstrated in patients with adjuvant chemotherapy using Cisplatin, bleomycin or 5-fluorouracil, compared with surgery-alone patients.[125,126] Our preliminary results of a prospective randomized controlled trial of preoperative chemotherapy using Cisplatin and 5-fluorouracil showed an overall response rate of about 50% (Fig 25–17), without overall improved survival. Survival benefits only occurred to patients with early-stage cancers.[128]

More results from prospective randomized studies are needed to determine whether there are any overall benefits with preoperative adjuvant therapy. It is also imperative to identify the subset of patients who are likely to respond to treatment rather than apply it to all patients, many of whom will not benefit from the added therapy and are open to the many side effects.

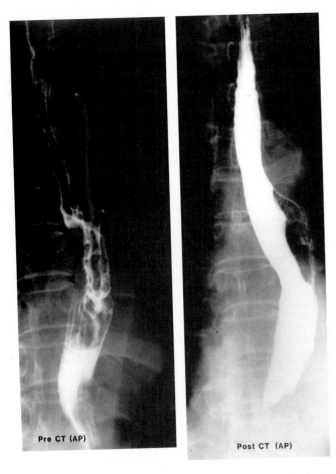

Figure 25–17. Barium swallow showing good tumor response to preoperative adjuvant chemotherapy. Two cycles of Cisplatin and 5-fluorouracil infusion at three weekly intervals were given. (Pre-CT: pre-chemotherapy, Post-CT: post chemotherapy).

Other Nonoperative Therapy for Palliation

At least a quarter of patients with esophageal carcinoma are not suitable for surgery because of advanced disease or because of age, infirmity, or concurrent medical illnesses. Alternative, efficient, cost-effective, rapid and safe methods of restoring and maintaining swallowing ability are needed. The aim of these palliative therapies is to reestablish swallowing and to stabilize the body weight, since dysphagia and loss of weight are the leading symptoms that reduce the quality of life of the patient.

These options for palliation include dilatation, external radiotherapy, brachytherapy, prosthetic intubation, and laser photoablation. In selected patients, possible additional procedures include thermal destruction by electrocautery, chemical destruction by injection of alcohol or other sclerosants, hyperthermia, and photodynamic therapy. Choosing one technique over the other is based on consideration of availability, expertise, efficacy, complication, the acceptance of the patient, and cost.

Brachytherapy, Laser Therapy and Intubation With brachytherapy, a close cooperation between the endoscopist and radiotherapist is essential. The esophageal tumor first is dilated under fluoroscopic guidance. An 8-mm diameter afterloading catheter then is accurately placed at the tumor under fluoroscopy. The selection unit is connected to the catheter, and iridium-192 wires are afterloaded into the catheter. A dose of 10 to 15 Gy is delivered with a circumferential distance of approximately 1 cm. The technique can be coupled with external-beam irradiation. Relief of dysphagia is achieved in 70% of patients.[129]

For laser therapy, a neodymium yttrium-aluminum-garnet (Nd:YAG) laser system is used. Laser energy is delivered via quartz fiber through fiberoptic endoscopy to the tumor in a retrograde manner; 50 to 100 watt power for 0.7 to 1.0 second pulse duration is normally used. A free laser beam tip is preferred over the contact laser tip. Vaporization and cavitation of the tumor is carried out under direct vision, and any bleeding points can be easily controlled because of the excellent coagulation property of the YAG laser. Treatment is limited to the exophytic area of the tumor to avoid perforation of the esophageal wall, since penetration of the laser energy continues for a few mm beyond the visual zone of photoablation. Although laser therapy offers good palliation, repeated sessions are needed every 3 to 6 weeks in order to maintain luminal patency. With progression of the tumor, further treatment often becomes increasingly time consuming and uncomfortable to the patient.

Both brachytherapy and laser therapy are more likely to allow for an early return to normal swallowing as compared with other methods of treatment. Prospective randomized comparison of brachytherapy and laser have shown similar degrees of palliation with relief of dysphagia in 75% to 81% of patients at 2 months.[130] A prospective study comparing laser and intubation also demonstrated superior quality of palliation with laser in terms of improved swallowing ability.[131] Only 11% of patients undergoing intubation could manage a normal diet, as opposed to 33% in the laser treated group,[132] with the majority of remaining patients limited to taking soft or semisolid diets. The risk of perforation was greater with intubation, 13% compared with laser therapy, 2%.

Intubation with a prosthetic stent is an attractive alternative to laser therapy because it can provide a more lasting palliation after a single procedure. This feature is important in patients with expected short survival and in patients who live a long distance from the hospital. Intubation also is indicated for infiltrative stenotic type of tumors, long tumors or when the obstruction is mainly extrinsic compressive. Stenting is especially useful in sealing off a fistula into the tracheobronchial tree. A variety of commercially available stents and custom-made stents from polyvinyl tubing are used. Commercially available tubes are made of biocompatible material such as silicon rubber that will remain inert for years. Certain tubes are reinforced with a spiral metal wire in their walls to prevent extrinsic tumor compression, while tubes with a self-expanding balloon in its shaft are used to obliterate a tracheo-esophageal fistula (Fig 25–18). These tubes usually have an inner diameter of 10 mm to 15 mm, with the size and length of the tube having a direct bearing on its patency rate.

The technique of insertion involves the dilatation of the tumor with Savary-Gilliard dilators, followed by the insertion of the tube using the pulsion method, either endoscopically or under fluoroscopic guidance. The widened funnel at the top of the tube prevents its distal migration, while the flanges distally prevent proximal displacement. Perforation is related to the need for rapid dilation of the tumor for stent insertion. Other complications include reflux esophagitis, which occurs when the tube is placed across the cardia. Airway obstruction is evident in 30% of patients when the tube is placed at the level of the trachea. For this reason, and because of complaints of a foreign-body sensation, tumors at the cervical esophagus cannot be stented.

The use of self-expanding metal stents offers a new option in palliation. Compressed into a small-delivery catheter, the stent is placed into the tumor under fluoroscopic guidance, and once released, the stent opens to its maximal diameter during a 24 hour period. The avoidance of dilation of the tumor substantially decreases the risk of perforation. Two types of stents are currently used, one is a coated or uncoated wallstent and the other is a Z stent with a silicon membrane. Unlike a conventional esophageal tube, the metal stent does not have a widened funnel and hence, should cause less compression on the airway. Thus, it is also applicable for cervical tumors. Unfortunately, initial experiences with metal stents have reported significant complications.[133,134] These include incomplete expansion, stent migration, and tumor ingrowth into the metal mesh, which causes luminal obstruction (Fig 25–19). Expansion of the stent can be facilitated by balloon dilators. Migration of the stent is a potential hazard because, unlike a plastic stent, metal stents once placed, cannot be removed. With better stent design and materials, many of the current problems with metal stents should be solved. However, a great deal of development and assessment of the metal stent is needed before it can be incorporated as part of the standard treatment for esophageal cancers.

Electrocautery, Ethanol Injection and Photodynamic Therapy

A bipolar electrocoagulation probe (BICAP, ACMI-Circon) can be used to debulk tumors from the esophageal wall by electrocoagulation. Positioned under fluoroscopic control, the tumor is coagulated using 50 watt power at 10 to 20 seconds duration. Since contact with the tumor is less precise, the treatment is associated with high failure rates and serious complications. Perforation of the esophageal wall may occur especially for noncircumferential tumors. However, with experience, the BICAP probe can be relatively safe to use, and can give a similar palliative effect as laser therapy. The comparative cost of equipment is much less.[135] The BICAP probe also may be applicable for very high esophageal lesions.

Local injection of sclerosant offers an easy and inexpensive alternative method of palliation. Using absolute alcohol, tumor necrosis after local injection was found to be as effective as when using laser therapy, at a much reduced cost.[136]

In photodynamic therapy, a hematoporphyrin derivative such as Photofrin II (dihematoporphyrin ether) is used. The photosensitizer is selectively retained by neoplastic and reticuloendothelial tissues which, when exposed to the argon-pump dye laser, catalyzes a photochemical reaction to release free oxygen radicals responsible for cell death and tumor necrosis. In multicenter studies, up to an 80% response rate has been reported, especially when the lesion is small.[137] However, effective cell lysis occurs only for cancer cells excited by the laser light delivered via quartz fibers through a gastroscope. Hence, tumors in the outer esophageal wall and in the regional lymph nodes are not treated. Furthermore, side effect of treatment can be substantial.

■ CONCLUSION

The results of resection in the treatment of esophageal cancer have improved in recent years. Even without ad-

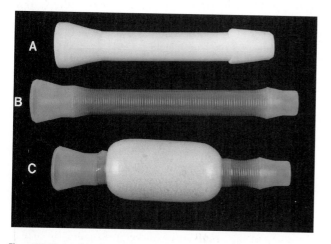

Figure 25–18. A variety of prosthetic esophageal tubes is available for intubation. The Atkinson tube (Key Med, Southend, UK) is made of silicon rubber and has a wide proximal funnel and distal flanges to prevent tube migration. (**A**). The tube made by Wilson Cook (Wilson Cook Medical Inc., Bloomington, IN, USA) has a spiral metal wire in its wall to prevent tumor compression and narrowing of its lumen (**B**). A low-pressure sponge balloon in the shaft can obliterate a tracheo-esophageal fistula. (**C**).

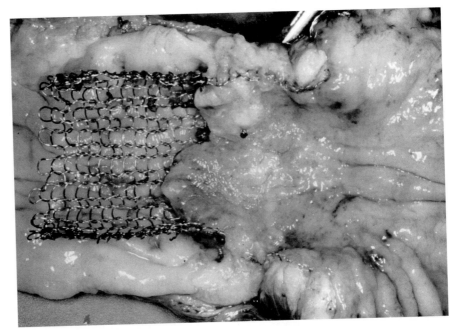

Figure 25–19. Tumor ingrowth into the meshwork of a metal stent causing obliteration of its lumen.

ditional treatment, mortality rates have dropped significantly and survival rates have increased because of avoidance of surgical complications. Further improvements can be expected with the careful identification and exclusion of the very high-risk patient, the elimination of technique-related complications, and improved perioperative care through results gained from prospective controlled studies. Extended survival also is possible with the proper selection and application of adjuvant therapy to patients who are most likely to benefit from these treatments, without adding unnecessary discomfort and toxicity to nonresponders. For patients with unresectable tumors, effective nonoperative therapy can provide meaningful quality of palliation for the remaining short period of survival.

REFERENCES

1. Hurt R. Surgical treatment of carcinoma of the oesophagus. *Thorax* 1991;46:528–535
2. Sauerbruch F. Ueber die Ausschaltung der schadlichen Wirkung des Pneumothorax bei intrathorakalen Operationen. *Zentralbl Chir* 1904;31:146–149
3. Waterhouse J, Shanmugaratnam K, Muir C, et al. *Cancer Incidence in Five Continents*, vol 4. JARC scientific publication no. 42. Lyon, France: IARC; 1982;390–397
4. Kemp IW, Clarke K, Kinlen LJ. Oesophageal cancer and distilleries in Scotland. *Br Med J* 1992;304:1543–1544
5. Negri E, La Vecchia C, Franceschi S, et al. Attributable risks for oesophageal cancer in northern Italy. *Eur J Cancer* 1992;28:1167–1171
6. Burrell RJ. Oesophageal cancer among Bantu in the Transkei. *J Natl Cancer Inst* 1962;28:495–514
7. Huang GJ. Epidemiology of esophageal cancer in China. In: Siewert JR, Holscher AH (eds), *Diseases of the Esophagus*. Berlin, Germany: Springer-Verlag; 1988:3–5
8. Yang CS. Research on esophageal cancer in China: a review. *Cancer Res* 1980;40:2633–2644
9. Wahrendorf J, Chang-Claude J, Liang QS, et al. Precursor lesions of oesophageal cancer in young people in a high-risk population in China. *Lancet* 1989;2:1239–1241
10. Khuroo MS, Zargar SA, Mahajan R, et al. High incidence of oesophageal and gastric cancer in Kashmir in a population with special personal and dietary habits. *Gut* 1992;33:11–15
11. De Stefani E, Munoz N, Esteve J, et al. Mate drinking, alcohol, tobacco, diet, and esophageal cancer in Uruguay. *Cancer Res* 1990;50:426–431
12. Cheng KK, Day NE, Duffy SW, et al. Pickled vegetables in the aetiology of oesophageal cancer in Hong Kong Chinese. *Lancet* 1992;339:1314–1318
13. Munoz N, Wahrendorf J, Bang LJ, et al. The effect of riboflavine, retinol, and zinc on prevalence of precancerous lesions of esophageal cancer in Henan province. *Lancet* 1985;2:11–14
14. Smith AH, Waller KD. Serum beta-carotene in persons with cancer and their immediate families. *Am J Epidemiol* 1991;133:661–671
15. Atabek U, Mohit-Tabatabai MA, Rush BF, et al. Impact of esophageal screening in patients with head and neck cancer. *Am Surg* 1990;56:289–292
16. Howel-Evans W, McConnell RB, Clarke CA, et al. Carcinoma of the esophagus with keratosis palmaris et plantaris (tylosis). *Q J Med* 1958;27:413–429
17. Marger RS, Marger D. Carcinoma of the esophagus and tylosis. A lethal genetic combination. *Cancer* 1993;72:17–19
18. Alpern HD, Buell C, Olson J. Increasing percentage of

adenocarcinoma in primary carcinoma of the esophagus. *Am J Gastroenterol* 1989;84:574

19. DeMeester TR, Attwood SEA, Smyrk TC, et al. Surgical therapy in Barrett's esophagus. *Ann Surg* 1990;212:528–542

20. Barrett NR. Chronic peptic ulcer of the oesophagus and "oesophagitis". *Br J Surg* 1950;38:175–182

21. Kruse P, Boesby S, Bernstein IT, et al. Barrett's esophagus and esophageal adenocarcinoma: endoscopic and histologic surveillance. *Scand J Gastroenterol* 1993;28:193–196

22. Barrett's esophagus: epidemiological and clinical results of a multicentric survey. (GOSPE) *Int J Cancer* 1991;48: 364–368

23. Stein HJ, Siewert JR. Barrett's esophagus: pathogenesis, epidemiology, functional abnormalities, malignant degeneration, and surgical management. *Dysphagia* 1993;8: 276–288

24. Skinner DB, Walther BC, Riddell RH, et al. Barrett's esophagus: comparison of benign and malignant cases. *Ann Surg* 1983;198:554–565

25. Menke-Pluymers MB, Hop WCJ, Dees J, et al. The Rotterdam esophageal Tumor Study Group. Risk factors for the development of an adenocarcinoma in columnar-lined (Barrett) esophagus. *Cancer* 1993;72:1155–1158

26. Li H, Walsh TN, Hennessy TP. Carcinoma arising in Barrett's esophagus. *Surg Gynecol Obstet* 1992;175:167–172

27. Streitz JM Jr., Andrews CW Jr., Ellis FH Jr.. Endoscopic surveillance of Barrett's esophagus. Does it help? *J Thorac Cardiovasc Surg* 1993;105:383–387

28. Nishimaki T, Holscher AH, Schuler M, et al. Histopathologic characteristics of early adenocarcinoma in Barrett's esophagus. *Cancer* 1991;68:1731–1736

29. Reid BJ, Blount PL, Rubin CE, et al. Flow-cytometric and histological progression to malignancy in Barrett's esophagus: prospective endoscopic surveillance of a cohort. *Gastroenterology* 1992;102:1212–1219

30. Ramel S, Reid BJ, Sanchez CA, et al. Evaluation of p53 protein expression in Barrett's esophagus by two-parameter flow cytometry. *Gastroenterology* 1992;102:1220–1228

31. Wagata T, Ishizaki K, Imamura M, et al. Deletion of 17p and amplification of the int-2 gene in esophageal carcinomas. *Cancer Res* 1991;51:2113–2117

32. Hollstein MC, Peri L, Mandard AM, et al. Genetic analysis of human esophageal tumors from two high incidence geographic areas: frequent p53 base substitutions and absence of ras mutations. *Cancer Res* 1991;51:4102–4106

33. Tsutsui S, Kuwano H, Mori M, et al. A flow cytometric analysis of DNA content in primary and metastatic lesions of esophageal squamous cell carcinoma. *Cancer* 1992;70: 2586–2591

34. Bottger T, Storkel S, Stockle M, et al. DNA image cytometry: a prognostic tool in squamous cell carcinoma of the esophagus? *Cancer* 1991;67:2290–2294

35. Ikeda K. Clinical and fundamental study of a squamous cell carcinoma related antigen (SCC-RA) for esophageal squamous cell carcinoma. *Nippon Geka Gakkai Zasshi* 1991; 92:387–396

36. Yano H, Shiozaki H, Kobayashi K, et al. Immunohistologic detection of the epidermal growth factor receptor in human esophageal squamous cell carcinoma. *Cancer* 1991; 67:91–98

37. Panis Y, Gayet B, Flejou JF, et al. Five-year survivors after radical operation for oesophageal carcinoma: influence of pathological findings. *Br J Surg* 1992;79(suppl):S93–S94

38. Theunissen PHMH, Borchard F, Poortvliet DCJ. Histopathological evaluation of oesophageal carcinoma: the significance of venous invasion. *Br J Surg* 1991;78: 930–932

39. Reeders JWAJ, Bartelsman JFWM. Radiological diagnosis and preoperative staging of oesophageal malignancies. *Endoscopy* 1993;25:10–27

40. Chernin MM, Amberg JR, Kogan FJ, et al. Efficacy of radiologic studies in the detection of Barrett's esophagus. *AJR Am J Roentgenol* 1986;147:257–260

41. Caletti GC, Ferrari A, Fiorino S, et al. Staging of esophageal carcinoma by endoscopy. *Endoscopy* 1993;25:2–9

42. Cheung HC, Siu KF, Wong J. A comparison of flexible and rigid endoscopy in evaluating esophageal cancer patients for surgery. *World J Surg* 1988;12:117–122

43. Hermanek P, Scheibe O, Spiessl B, Wagner G (eds). *UICC: TNM-Classification of Malignant Tumor.* 4th ed. New York, NY: Springer-Verlag; 1987

44. Dittler HJ, Siewert JR. Role of endoscopic ultrasonography in esophageal carcinoma. *Endoscopy* 1993;25:156–161

45. Dittler HJ, Bollschweiler E, Siewert JR. What is the value of endosonography in the preoperative staging of esophageal carcinoma? *Dtsch med Wschr* 1991;116:561–566

46. Fok M, Cheng SW, Wong J. Endosonography in patient selection for surgical treatment of esophageal carcinoma. *World J Surg* 1992;16:1098–1103

47. Picus D, Balfe DM, Koehler RE, et al. Computed tomography in the staging of esophageal carcinoma. *Radiology* 1983;146:433–438

48. Tio TL, Cohen P, Coene PP, et al. Endosonography and computed tomography of esophageal carcinoma. *Gastroenterology* 1989;96:1478–1486

49. Ziegler K, Sanft C, Zeitz M, et al. Evaluation of endosonography in TN staging of oesophageal cancer. *Gut* 1991;32:16–20

50. Grimm H, Hamper K, Binmoeller KF, et al. Enlarged lymph nodes: malignant or not? *Endoscopy* 1992;24:320–323

51. Murata Y, Muroi M, Yoshida M, et al. Endoscopic ultrasonography in the diagnosis of esophageal carcinoma. *Surg Endosc* 1987;1:11–16

52. Hordijk ML, Zander H, van Blankenstein M, et al. Influence of tumor stenosis on the accuracy of endosonography in preoperative T staging of esophageal cancer. *Endoscopy* 1993;25:171–175

53. Watt I, Stewart I, Anderson D, et al. Laparoscopy, ultrasound and computed tomography in cancer of the oesophagus and gastric cardia: a prospective comparison for detecting intra-abdominal metastases. *Br J Surg* 1989;76: 1036–1039

54. Ellis FH Jr. Carcinoma of the esophagus. *CA Cancer J Clin* 1983;33:264–281

55. Kato H, Tachimori Y, Watanabe H, et al. Superficial esophageal carcinoma: surgical treatment and the results. *Cancer* 1990;66:2319–2323

56. Inoue H, Endo M, Takeshita K, et al. Endoscopic resection of early-stage esophageal cancer. *Surg Endosc* 1991; 5:59–62

57. DeMeester TR, Stein HJ. Surgical therapy for cancer of the esophagus and cardia. In: Castell DO (ed.), *The Esophagus*. Boston, MA: Little, Brown; 1992;299–342

58. Watson A. A study of the quality and duration of survival following resection, endoscopic intubation and surgical intubation in oesophageal carcinoma. *Br J Surg* 1982;69:585–588

59. O'Rourke IC, McNeil RJ, Walker PJ, et al. Objective evaluation of the quality of palliation in patients with oesophageal cancer comparing surgery, radiotherapy and intubation. *Aust N Z J Surg* 1992;62:922–930

60. Ellis FH Jr. Treatment of carcinoma of the esophagus or cardia. *Mayo Clin Proc* 1989;64:945–955

61. Akiyama H, Tsurumaru M, Kawamura T, et al. Principles of surgical treatment for carcinoma of the esophagus. *Ann Surg* 1981;194:438–446

62. Collard JM, Otte JB, Fiasse R, et al. Five-year survival after resection of the oesophagus for cancer. *Br J Surg* 1992;79(suppl):S94–95

63. Wong J. Esophageal resection for cancer: the rationale of current practice. *Am J Surg* 1987;153:18–24

64. Wong J. Management of carcinoma of oesophagus: art or science? *J R Coll Surg Edinb* 1981;26:138–149

65. Ong GB, Lee TC. Pharyngogastric anastomosis after oesophago-pharyngectomy for carcinoma of the hypopharynx and cervical oesophagus. *Br J Surg* 1960;48:193–200

66. Peracchia A, Bardini R, Ruol A, et al. Cancer of the hypopharynx and cervical esophagus. *Ann Chir* 1991;45:313–318

67. Schusterman MA, Shestak K, de Vries EJ, et al. Reconstruction of the cervical esophagus: free jejunal transfer versus gastric pull-up. *Plast Reconstr Surg* 1990;85:16–21

68. Lam KH, Wei WI, Lau WF. Avoiding stenosis in the tubed greater pectoral flap in pharyngeal repair. *Arch Otolaryngol* 1987;113:428–431

69. McKeown KC. The surgical treatment of carcinoma of the oesophagus. A review of the result in 478 cases. *J R Coll Surg Edinb* 1985;30:1–14

70. Ong GB, Lam KH, Lam PHM, et al. Resection for carcinoma of the superior mediastinal segment of the esophagus. *World J Surg* 1978;2:497–504

71. Orringer MB. Partial median sternotomy: anterior approach to the upper thoracic esophagus. *J Thorac Cardiovasc Surg* 1984;87:124–129

72. Lewis I. The surgical treatment of carcinoma of the oesophagus with special reference to a new operation for growths of the middle third. *Br J Surg* 1946;34:18–31

73. Tanner NC. The present position of carcinoma of the oesophagus. *Postgrad Med J* 1947;23:109–139

74. Huang GJ, Wang LJ, Liu JS, et al. Surgery of esophageal carcinoma. *Semin Surg Oncol* 1985;1:74–83

75. Skinner DB. En bloc resection for neoplasms of the esophagus and cardia. *J Thorac Cardiovasc Surg* 1983;85:59–71

76. Finley RJ, Inculet RI. The results of esophagogastrectomy without thoracotomy for adenocarcinoma of the esophagogastric junction. *Ann Surg* 1989;210:535–543

77. Ellis FH Jr, Gibb SP, Watkins E Jr. Esophagogastrectomy. A safe, widely applicable, and expeditious form of palliation for patients with carcinoma of the esophagus and cardia. *Ann Surg* 1983;198:531–540

78. Orringer MB. Transhiatal esophagectomy without thoracotomy for carcinoma of the thoracic esophagus. *Ann Surg* 1984;200:282–288

79. Fok M, Law SYK, Stipa F, et al. A comparison of transhiatal and transthoracic resection for oesophageal carcinoma. *Endoscopy* 1993;25:660–663.

80. Donnelly RJ, Page RD, Cowen ME. Endoscopy assisted microthoracotomy: initial experience. *Thorax* 1992;47:490–493

81. Pellegrini C, Wetter LA, Patti M, et al. Thoracoscopic esophagomyotomy. *Ann Surg* 1992;216:291–299

82. Cuschieri A, Shimi S, Banting S. Endoscopic oesophagectomy through a right thoracoscopic approach. *J R Coll Surg Edinb* 1992;37:7–11

83. Buess G. Thoracoscopic dissection of the esophagus. *Surg Endosc* 1992;6:150–151

84. Kato H, Watanabe H, Tachimori Y, et al. Evaluation of neck lymph node dissection for thoracic esophageal carcinoma. *Ann Thorac Surg* 1991;51:931–935

85. Sasaki K, Tanaka Y, Ueki H, et al. The significance of the extensive systematic lymphadenectomy for thoracic esophageal carcinoma. *Nippon Geka Gakkai Zasshi*. 1989;90(9):1605–1608

86. Kuwano H, Tsutsui S, Nagamatsu M, et al. Clinical evaluation of systematic lymph node dissection for the intrathoracic esophageal carcinoma. *Nippon Geka Gakkai Zasshi* 1989;90:1609–1611

87. Tsurumaru M, Akiyama H, Udagawa H, et al. Evaluation of the collo-thoraco-abdominal dissection for the intrathoracic esophageal carcinoma. *Nippon Geka Gakkai Zasshi* 1989;90:1612–1615

88. Wang LS, Huang MH, Huang BS, et al. Gastric substitution for resectable carcinoma of the esophagus: an analysis of 368 cases. *Ann Thorac Surg* 1992;53:289–294

89. Fok M, Cheng SWK, Wong J. Pyloroplasty versus no drainage in gastric replacement of the esophagus. *Am J Surg* 1991;162:447–452

90. DeMeester TR, Johansson KE, Franze I, et al. Indications, surgical technique, and long-term functional results of colon interposition or bypass. *Ann Surg* 1988;208:460–474

91. Watson A. Oesophageal neoplasms. *Curr Opin Gastroenterol* 1990;6:590–596

92. Dewar L, Gelfand G, Finley R, et al. Factors affecting cervical anastomotic leak and stricture formation following esophagogastrectomy and gastric tube interposition. *Am J Surg* 1992;163:484–489

93. Muller JM, Erasmi H, Stelzner M, et al. Surgical therapy of oesophageal carcinoma. *Br J Surg* 1990;77:845–857

94. Lam TCF, Fok M, Cheng SWK, et al. Anastomotic complications after esophagectomy for cancer: a comparison of neck and chest anastomoses. *J Thorac Cardiovasc Surg* 1992;104:395–400

95. Zieren HU, Muller JM, Pichlmaier H. Prospective randomized study of one- or two-layer anastomosis following oesophageal resection and cervical oesophagogastrostomy. *Br J Surg* 1993;80:608–611

96. Wong J, Cheung HC, Lui R, et al. Esophagogastric anastomosis performed with a stapler: the occurrence of leakage and stricture. *Surgery* 1987;101:408–415

97. Fok M, Ah-Chong AK, Cheng SW, et al. Comparison of a single layer continuous hand-sewn method and circular stapling in 580 oesophageal anastomoses. *Br J Surg* 1991; 78:342–345

98. Dziki AJ, Duncan MD, Harmon JW, et al. Advantages of handsewn over stapled bowel anastomosis. *Dis Colon Rectum* 1991;34:442–448

99. Lam KH, Wong J, Lim STK, et al. Intrathoracic gastric bypass for carcinoma of oesophagus found unresectable at exploration. *Br J Surg* 1982;69:71–73

100. Ong GB. The Kirschner operation—a forgotten procedure. *Br J Surg* 1973;60:221–227

101. Beatty JD, DeBoer G, Rider WD. Carcinoma of the esophagus: pretreatment assessment, correlation of radiation treatment parameters with survival, and identification and management of radiation treatment failure. *Cancer* 1979;43:2254–2267

102. Earlam RJ, Cunha-Melo JR. Oesophageal squamous cell carcinoma: II. A critical review of radiotherapy. *Br J Surg* 1980;67:457–461

103. Earlam RJ, Johnson L. 101 oesophageal cancers: a surgeon uses radiotherapy. *Ann R Coll Surg Engl* 1990;72:32–40

104. Leslie MD, Dische S, Saunders MI, et al. The role of radiotherapy in carcinoma of the thoracic oesophagus: an audit of the Mount Vernon experience 1980–1989. *Clin Oncol* 1992;4:114–118

105. Wara WM, Mauch PM, Thomas AN, et al. Palliation for carcinoma of the esophagus. *Radiology* 1976;121:717–720

106. Agrawal RK, Dawes PJ, Clague MB. Combined external beam and intracavitary radiotherapy in oesophageal carcinoma. *Clin Oncol* 1992;4:222–227

107. Coia LR, Engstrom PF, Paul A. Nonsurgical management of esohageal cancer: report of a study of combined radiotherapy and chemotherapy. *J Clin Oncol* 1987;5:1783–1790

108. Leichman L, Herskovic A, Leichman CG, et al. Nonoperative therapy for squamous cell cancer of the esophagus. *J Clin Oncol* 1987;5:365–370

109. Araujo CMM, Souhami L, Gil RA, et al. A randomized trial comparing radiation therapy versus concomitant radiation therapy and chemotherapy in carcinoma of the thoracic esophagus. *Cancer* 1991;67:2258–2261

110. Parker EF, Reed CE, Marks RD, et al. Chemotherapy, radiation therapy, and resection for carcinoma of the esophagus. Long-term results. *J Thorac Cardiovasc Surg* 1989;98:1037–1044

111. Popp MB, Hawley D, Reising J, et al. Improved survival in squamous esophageal cancer. *Arch Surg* 1986;121:1330–1335

112. Gignoux M, Roussel A, Paillot B, et al. The value of preoperative radiotherapy in esophageal cancer: results of a study of the EORTC. *World J Surg* 1987;11:426–432

113. Launois B, Delarue D, Campion JP, et al. Preoperative radiotherapy for carcinoma of the esophagus. *Surg Gynecol Obstet* 1981;153:690–692

114. Huang GJ, Gu XZ, Wang LJ, et al. Experience with combined preoperative irradiation and surgery for carcinoma of esophagus. *Jpn J Cancer Res* 1986;31:159

115. Maeta M, Koga S, Andachi H, et al. Preoperative radiotherapy and intra-abdominal metastasis of the lymph node in the surgical treatment of carcinoma of the thoracic esophagus. *Surg Gynecol Obstet* 1987;165:235–238

116. Sunagawa M, Endo M. Clinical evaluation of adjuvant radiotherapy and chemotherapy for esophageal carcinoma. *Gan To Kagaku Ryoho* 1988;15:1634–1639

117. Nishiyama K, Kagami Y, Ikeda H, et al. Radiation therapy of esophageal cancer: radical radiotherapy and radiotherapy in combination with surgery. *Gan To Kagaku Ryoho* 1982;9:2077–2083

118. Teniere P, Hay JM, Fingerhut A, et al. Postoperative radiation therapy does not increase survival after curative resection for squamous cell carcinoma of the middle and lower esophagus as shown by a multicenter controlled trial. *Surg Gynecol Obstet* 1991;173:123–130

119. Fok M, Sham JST, Choy D, et al. Postoperative radiotherapy for carcinoma of the esophagus: a prospective, randomized controlled study. *Surgery* 1993;113:138–147

120. Forastiere AA. Treatment of locoregional esophageal cancer. *Semin Oncol* 1992;19:57–63

121. Katlic MR, Wilkins EW Jr, Grillo HC. Three decades of treatment of esophageal squamous carcinoma at the Massachusetts General Hospital. *J Thorac Cardiovasc Surg* 1990;99:929–938

122. Kelsen D. Neoadjuvant therapy of esophageal cancer. *Can J Surg* 1989;32:410–414

123. Orringer MB, Forastiere AA, Perez-Tamayo C, et al. Chemotherapy and radiation therapy before transhiatal esophagectomy for esophageal carcinoma. *Ann Thorac Surg* 1990;49:348–355

124. Wolfe WG, Vaughn AL, Seigler HF, et al. Survival of patients with carcinoma of the esophagus treated with combined-modality therapy. *J Thorac Cardiovasc Surg* 1993; 105:749–756

125. Schlag PM. Randomized trial of preoperative chemotherapy for squamous cell cancer of the esophagus. *Arch Surg* 1992;127:1446–1450

126. Nygaard K, Hagen S, Hansen HS, et al. Pre-operative radiotherapy prolongs survival in operable esophageal carcinoma: a randomized, multicenter study of pre-operative radiotherapy and chemotherapy. The second Scandinavian trial in esophageal cancer. *World J Surg* 1992;16:1104–1110

127. Poplin E, Fleming T, Leichman L, et al. Combined therapies for squamous-cell carcinoma of the esophagus: a Southwest Oncology Group study (SWOG-8037). *J Clin Oncol* 1987;5:622–628

128. Fok M, Wong J. Adjuvant chemotherapy and radiotherapy: the Hong Kong experiences. Presented at the panel symposium on *Multimodal Treatment of Advanced Esophageal Cancer*. 33rd World Congress of Surgery of the International Society of Surgery; August 1993.

129. Bader M, Dittler HJ, Ultsch B, et al. Palliative treatment of malignant stenoses of the upper gastrointestinal tract using a combination of laser and afterloading therapy. *Endoscopy* 1986;18:27–31

130. Low DE, Pagliero KM. Prospective randomized clinical trial comparing brachytherapy and laser photoablation for palliation of esophageal cancer. *J Thorac Cardiovasc Surg* 1992;104:173–179

131. Carter R, Smith JS, Anderson JR. Laser recanalization

versus endoscopic intubation in the palliation of malignant dysphagia: a randomized prospective study. *Br J Surg* 1992;79:1167–1170

132. Loizou LA, Grigg D, Atkinson M, et al. A prospective comparison of laser therapy and intubation in endoscopic palliation for malignant dysphagia. *Gastroenterology* 1991;100:1303–1310

133. Schaer J, Katon RM, Ivancev K, et al. Treatment of malignant esophageal obstruction with silicone-coated metallic self-expanding stents. *Gastrointest Endosc* 1992;38:7–11

134. Bethge N, Knyrim K, Wagner HJ, et al. Self-expanding metal stents for palliation of malignant esophageal obstruction—a pilot study of eight patients. *Endoscopy* 1992;24:411–415

135. McIntyre AS, Morris DL, Sloan RL, et al. Palliative therapy of malignant esophageal stricture with the bipolar tumor probe and prosthetic tube. *Gastrointest Endosc* 1989;35:531–535

136. Angelini G, Pasini AF, Ederle A, et al. Nd:YAG laser versus polidocanol injection for palliation of esophageal malignancy: a prospective, randomized study. *Gastrointest Endosc* 1991;37:607–610

137. Kato H, Kito T, Furuse K, et al. Photodynamic therapy in the early treatment of cancer. *Gan To Kagaku Ryoho* 1990;17:1833–1838

26

Surgical Procedures to Resect and Replace the Esophagus

David J. Sugarbaker ▪ *Malcolm M. DeCamp* ▪ *Michael J. Liptay*

▪ HISTORICAL PERSPECTIVES

ESOPHAGECTOMY

The history of surgical resection of the esophagus for malignancy parallels advances made in the performance of safe intrathoracic operations. Resection of the cervical esophagus was first described by Billroth in 1871.[1] Torek performed the first resection of a thoracic esophageal cancer in 1915.[2] A left thoracotomy approach was performed with the use of an external rubber tube to connect a proximal esophagostomy to a gastrostomy (Fig 26–1). The patient lived for 17 years following surgery. Unfortunately, the next 23 patients did not survive, and it was not until 1933, when Ohsawa reported the first thoracic resection and primary esophagogastric anastomosis, that esophagectomy became accepted therapy.[3] In 1938, Adams and Phemister reported the first transthoracic esophageal resection and reconstruction in the United States (Fig 26–2).[4]

Since that time, several prominent practitioners of 20th century surgery have refined these pioneering techniques to produce an array of surgical approaches, degrees of resection, and choices of conduits used for reconstruction. This chapter outlines the available surgical therapies for esophageal resec-

tion and reconstruction for both malignant (the most common scenario) and benign disease. A rationale for the selection of the various approaches and a description of the perioperative management of specific issues is provided.

ESOPHAGEAL CANCER: CHANGING EPIDEMIOLOGY

Esophageal cancer typically affects patients in late middle age (50 to 70 years). Until recently squamous cell carcinoma has dominated clinical series, accounting for 80% to 90% of all esophageal cancers.[5] It is more common in blacks than Caucasians and males more than females. Alcohol and tobacco abuse are independent risk factors associated with the majority of cases presenting in North America and Western Europe.[5]

Over the past decade there has been a recognized increase in the incidence of adenocarcinoma of the esophagus. Recent series show the prevalence of adenocarcinoma to be over 50% in some areas of the United States.[6–8] This changing etiology appears to be related, in part, to the increase in lower esophageal and gastroesophageal (GE) junction tumors associated with Barrett's esophagus.[9] With the increased prevalence of adenocarcinoma of the esophagus, a recognized increased incidence of esophageal cancer in Caucasian males has been noted.[10]

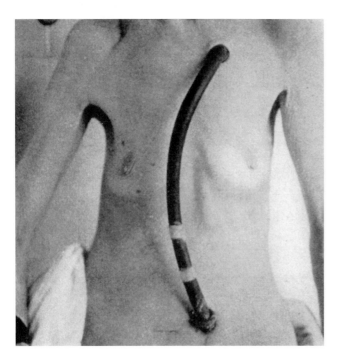

A

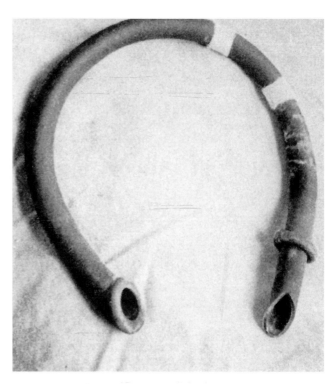

B

Figure 26–1. A. Depiction of Torek's first patient after esophageal resection. The rubber tube connected the lower end of the esophagus with a gastrostomy. The patient lived 17 years after the surgery and died at age 80. **B**. Removable rubber tube conduit with beveled ends. (From Torek F. The operative treatment of carcinoma of the esophagus. *Ann Surg* 1915;61:385)

Esophageal cancer remains an aggressive malignancy for which single-modality therapy has had limited success. Accounting for 1% of all cancers diagnosed in the United States, approximately 12 000 to 13 000 patients will be diagnosed with esophageal cancer in 1996.[11] Despite the efforts of surgeons, medical oncologists, and radiotherapists, <10% of diagnosed patients will live 5 years.[11]

Historical results of surgical resection alone have provided 5-year survival rates of 15% to 35%.[12] Reported series have demonstrated the feasibility of preoperative induction therapy using chemotherapy and radiation therapy. Acceptable toxicity with no significant increase in operative mortality and a 20% to 30% complete response rate have yielded superior survival in selected patients.[13–16]

The debate on the precise roles of surgery, radiotherapy, and chemotherapy in the treatment of esophageal carcinoma continues. The argument for

inclusion of surgical treatment in all patients with resectable disease is based on the superior palliation attained, acceptable morbidity and mortality, and the opportunity for *in vivo* assessment of tumor response to induction therapy by pathologic staging at resection.

The role of surgery in the treatment of esophageal cancer as single-modality therapy is limited to those patients who present with early stage disease, or those felt to have resectable lesions but who are not acceptable candidates for chemotherapy. The most important prognostic factors identified relating to survival in patients with localized disease are depth of tumor invasion (T stage) and nodal status (N stage).[17,18] Advances in multimodality treatment of the disease highlight the need for accurate pretreatment staging to stratify homogenous cohorts to treatment protocols appropriate for their specific stage of disease.

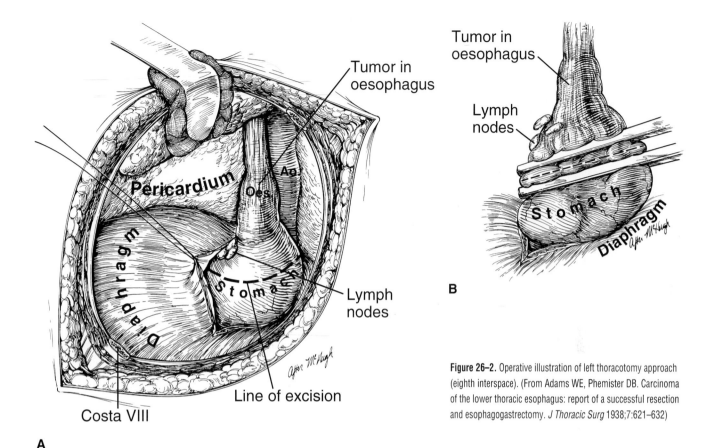

A

Figure 26–2. Operative illustration of left thoracotomy approach (eighth interspace). (From Adams WE, Phemister DB. Carcinoma of the lower thoracic esophagus: report of a successful resection and esophagogastrectomy. *J Thoracic Surg* 1938;7:621–632)

■ SELECTION OF OPERATIVE APPROACH FOR CANCER

When contemplating surgical resection for esophageal carcinoma the choice of operative approach should be based on four factors: (1) surgical intent (curative or palliative), (2) anatomic location of the tumor (cervical or upper, middle and lower thoracic), (3) the preferred method of esophageal replacement and reconstruction (gastric pull-up, colonic or jejunal interposition), and (4) whether surgery alone will be offered or a combination including chemotherapy and/or radiation will be used.[19]

The first consideration involved in determining the operative approach is whether a curative or a palliative procedure will be performed. If distant metastases are excluded, the most critical information remains the accurate staging of locoregional disease.

NONINVASIVE STAGING TECHNIQUES

Several noninvasive means have been used to aid in clinical staging. These include computed tomography (CT),

magnetic resonance imaging (MRI) and, most recently, endoesophageal ultrasound (EUS). Each technique has its limitations and none provide pathologic information on tumor extent, fixation, or nodal status.

CT scanning is excellent in assessing the presence of distant metastatic spread of tumor in the chest (lungs) or abdomen (liver, adrenals, nonperigastric lymph nodes).[20] Overall accuracy of CT in predicting T stage and extension to mediastinal structures is in the range of 80% to 85% when correlated with resected specimens.[21] Nodal predictive accuracy falls to less than 69%,[21] and one report found the sensitivity of predicting celiac nodal involvement to be only 48%.[22] MRI scanning adds little to the information gained with CT scans and has a virtually identical accuracy rate when compared to pathologic staging of the resected specimen.[23]

The recently adopted use of preresectional EUS has improved the accuracy of tumor staging in nonobstructing cases to 80% to 90% (Fig 26–3).[24] The sensitivity for nodal involvement is reported as between 85% to 95%. The accuracy of predicting nodal status by this method is adversely affected by a 21% to 44% inability

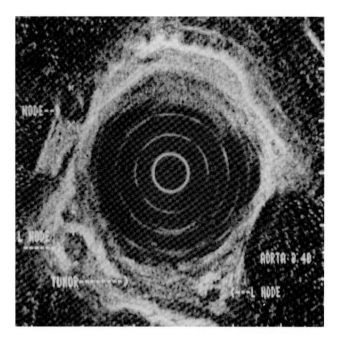

Figure 26–3. Endoesophageal ultrasound image of an adenocarcinoma of the esophagus (T3) and multiple lymph nodes suspicious for metastatic disease (N1). (From Van Dam J. Endosonographic evaluation of the patient with esophageal carcinoma. *Chest Surg Clin North Am* 1994;4:269–284)

to pass the EUS probe owing to high-grade malignant obstruction. In evaluable cases, accuracy reaches 70% to 86%.[24] Combinations of EUS and cross-sectional imaging can improve accuracy in assessment of esophageal wall penetration by tumor and nodal status, with an 86% accuracy in the prediction of stage of disease.[25]

Over two-thirds of patients with esophageal malignancy present with nodal involvement (Fig 26–4).[26] With the growing interest in multimodality studies utilizing induction chemotherapy and/or radiotherapy in the treatment of esophageal carcinoma, accurate disease staging at protocol enrollment is of paramount importance.

With advances in video-assisted thoracoscopic surgery, as well as video-laparoscopy, it is now possible to evaluate for nodal involvement histologically, using a minimally invasive surgical technique. Pretreatment pathologic staging creates more homogenous cohorts of patients and enhances comparative trials. In addition, high-risk patients can be definitively identified, thus justifying more intensive therapy.[27]

THORACOSCOPIC AND LAPAROSCOPIC (MINIMALLY INVASIVE) STAGING OF ESOPHAGEAL CARCINOMA

Thoracoscopic staging of esophageal cancer can provide accurate information on depth of tumor invasion and adherence to other mediastinal structures. In addition, a systematic pathologic staging of paraesophageal

lymph node stations is feasible. Laparoscopy allows for evaluation of the stomach, liver, and celiac and portal regions for nodal disease. This evaluation is critical because up to 35% of patients with upper thoracic lesions will have associated subdiaphragmatic nodal disease (Fig 26–4).[26,28]

Our preference is to perform minimally invasive surgical staging, prior to selection of a treatment strategy, on all patients with newly diagnosed esophageal cancer. In addition to thoracoscopy and laparoscopy, the surgeon also should perform his own endoscopy to inspect the lesion. A bronchoscopy also is indicated in the presence of all upper and middle lesions, or in any case of suspected subcarinal adenopathy. Those patients found to have resectable disease without lymph node involvement may proceed with immediate definitive resection.

Thoracoscopic Staging Procedure

A nasogastric tube is inserted in all patients at the time of induction of general anesthesia to evacuate built-up secretions in the often obstructed proximal esophagus. Double-lumen endotracheal intubation is used to allow for a right-sided approach, with single left-lung ventilation. The patient is positioned in the full left lateral decubitus position and a 12-mm port is introduced in the seventh interspace, in the midaxillary line. Two or three other trocars are inserted under direct camera vision (Fig 26–5),[20] one in the third posterior intercostal space medial to the scapula and another in the fourth interspace along the anterior axillary line, forming a baseball diamond around the camera port.[20]

With the lung deflated and retracted superomedially, the right hemithorax is inspected and the mediastinal pleura is opened along the length of the esophagus with electrocautery; this allows for inspection of the esophageal adventitia for evidence of transmural invasion by the primary tumor. If necessary, the azygous vein can be divided using an endoscopic stapler, allowing for ease of dissection of the esophagus and surrounding nodes. The subcarinal nodes, as well as intrathoracic periesophageal nodes, are biopsied and histologically examined (Fig 26–6).[20] The nodes are sampled at multiple levels, even if they appear grossly normal. Hemostasis is confirmed, and the ports are removed and skin closed, leaving one chest tube in place through the camera port hole. If the tumor is well below the aortic arch or at the GE junction, a left thoracoscopic approach may be indicated, with attention paid to the nodal stations evaluable on the left side, including the aortopulmonary window, subcarinal space, inferior pulmonary ligament, and associated periesophageal nodes. A similar three-port approach is used, although less of the esophagus is evaluable. A left-sided thoracoscopy is valuable when CT or EUS suggest sus-

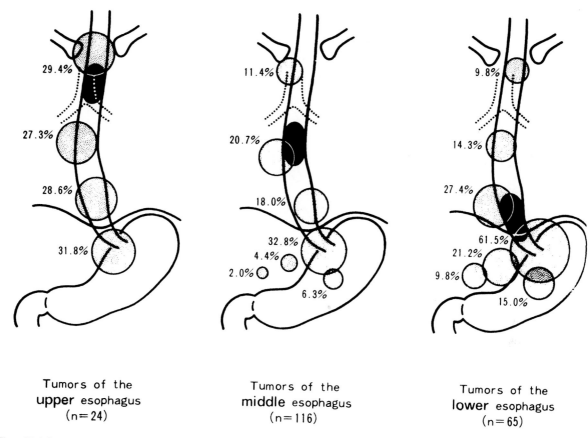

Tumors of the
upper esophagus
(n=24)

Tumors of the
middle esophagus
(n=116)

Tumors of the
lower esophagus
(n=65)

Figure 26–4. Percentages of lymph node involvement by station grouped by location of esophageal tumor. (From Akiyama H, Tsurumaru M, Kawamura T, Ono Y. Principles of surgical treatment for carcinoma of the esophagus: analysis of lymph node involvement. *Ann Surg* 1981;194:438–446)

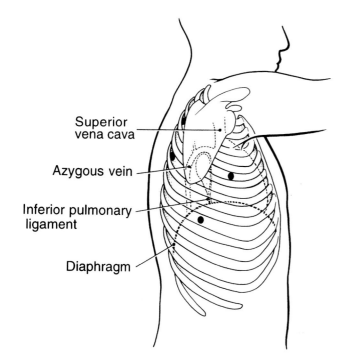

Superior
vena cava

Azygous vein

Inferior pulmonary
ligament

Diaphragm

Figure 26–5. Surface landmarks for port placements have been chosen by their spatial relationships to internal landmarks. The camera port is generally in the seventh intercostal space, midaxilllary line. Instrument ports are in the third, fourth, and fifth interspaces. This provides excellent access to the azygous vein, inferior pulmonary ligament, and mediastinal bed of the esophagus. (From Jaklitsch MT, Harpole DH, Healey EA, Sugarbaker DJ. Current issues in the staging of esophageal cancer. *Semin Radiol Oncol* 1994;4(3):135–145).

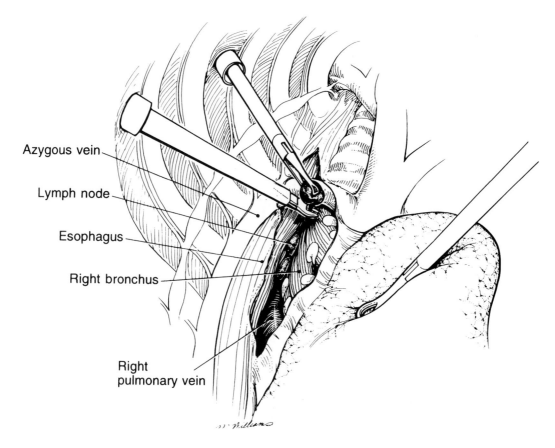

Azygous vein

Lymph node

Esophagus

Right bronchus

Right
pulmonary vein

Figure 26–6. View through the camera of the sampling of an azygous node. The mediastinal pleura overlying the esophagus has been opened, and the deflated lung retracted anteriorly. The entire node is removed by gentle traction with an endoscopic forceps while a hemostatic clip is placed at the pedicle. (From Jaklitsch MT, Harpole DH, Healey EA, Surgarbaker DJ. Current issues in the staging of esophageal cancer. *Semin Radiol Oncol* 1994;4(3):135–145)

picious lesions restricted to the left chest or involving the left lung.

Laparoscopic or Minilaparotomy Staging Procedure

Following the thoracoscopic evaluation, the patient is placed supine, and a staging laparoscopy or minilaparotomy is performed under the same anesthetic. A 12-mm telescope port is placed in the superior umbilical area under direct vision, followed by the insertion of two dissecting ports in each upper quadrant. The upper abdomen is examined systematically for the presence of liver metastases or evidence of cirrhosis, any evidence of peritoneal gastrohepatic ligament, or subdiaphragmatic direct extension of disease, as well as direct extension onto the wall of the stomach. Retractors aid in the examination of the undersurface of the liver, caudate lobe, and pouch of Douglas. The gastrohepatic ligament is divided, and biopsies are taken of the perigastric and celiac nodes, regardless of their gross appearance. Portal nodes may be sampled, if they appear grossly abnormal.

After histologic assessment of their biopsied tho-racic and upper abdominal lymph nodes, patients found to have resectable disease without evidence for nodal involvement proceed directly to esophagectomy. In those patients with positive nodal disease or advanced primary tumors (T3, T4), a feeding jejunostomy and central venous infusion port are inserted for enteral feeding and preoperative chemotherapy. The importance of the early institution of supplemental nutrition in these often nutritionally depleted patients cannot be overemphasized.

CURATIVE VERSUS PALLIATIVE STRATEGIES

There is considerable debate over whether an extended or en bloc resection of the esophagus with all mediastinal and upper abdominal nodal stations removed adds any benefit to overall survival compared to simply removing the esophagus without a systematic nodal dissection or wide margins.[17,29] With a growing interest in the use of neoadjuvant therapy, a complete resection is necessary to assess the efficacy of the induction therapy in attacking cancer cells in the primary tumor as well as in involved nodes.

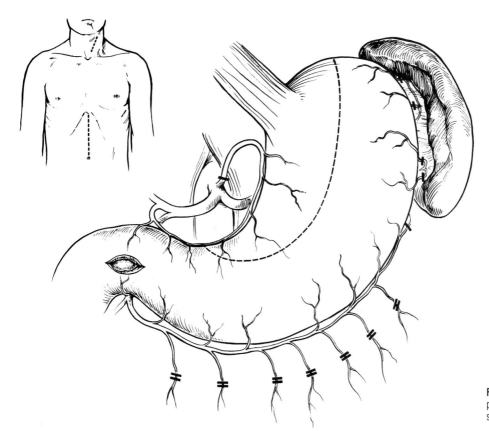

Figure 26–7. The stomach is mobilized as a pedicle based on the right gastroepiploic vessels. *Inset:* Incisions illustrated.

Palliative Therapy

Transhiatal esophagectomy (THE) accomplishes removal of the entire thoracic esophagus in a safe manner, without the morbidity of a thoracotomy. No attempt is made to resect the mediastinal nodes or other potentially contiguous structures involved with tumor, although they may be sampled. For this reason, we do not use the THE for patients in whom complete resection would be potentially curative. We do favor this technique for esophagectomy in cases of benign disease, carcinoma in situ or in patients for whom induction therapy is contraindicated.

Transhiatal esophagectomy was first described by Denk in 1913,[30] and first used to resect an esophageal carcinoma by Gray Turner in 1933, using a two-stage procedure and a skin tube as an esophagogastric conduit.[31] With the advent of endotracheal anesthesia and one-lung ventilation, this approach gave way, in most instances, to the transthoracic routes of esophageal resection and reconstruction. Orringer and Sloan reintroduced the technique in 1978, citing a potential decrease in perioperative morbidity and mortality by avoiding a thoracotomy.[32] A review of Orringer's 16-year experience with THE in 583 cases demonstrated a 5% in-hospital mortality for the procedure.[33]

Transhiatal Esophagectomy Technique. The operative technique of THE begins with placing the patient in a supine position with the neck extended to the right side, exposing the left sternocleidomastoid muscle. The procedure is performed through left cervical and upper abdominal incisions (see Fig 26–7). The resection and reconstruction proceed in three phases beginning with the intra-abdominal component, followed by the mediastinal esophageal dissection and the cervical dissection and gastroesophageal anastomosis.

Abdominal Dissection. An upper midline incision is made from xiphoid to umbilicus. Upon entering the peritoneal cavity a general exploration is performed. If occult liver or peritoneal metastases are encountered, the procedure is terminated with the insertion of a jejunostomy tube for feeding, because the mean survival for stage IV esophageal cancer patients is <6 months. If nodal enlargement is confined to the celiac and perigastric region, most surgeons would include these regions in their dissection and proceed with the planned procedure. The mobilization and preparation of the gastric conduit is described in detail below in the three-hole technique.

After mobilization of the stomach, based on the right gastroepiploic and right gastric arteries, the esophageal

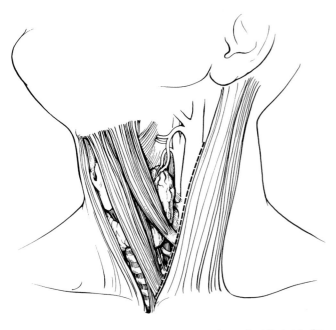

Figure 26–8. Anatomic structures of the left neck below platysma level. The incision line along the medial border of the sternocleidomastoid muscle is shown. Division of the omohyoid muscle along with ligation of the middle thyroid vein allows for exposure of the underlying esophagus.

hiatus is enlarged and the back end of a Deever retractor is inserted and lifted upwards. Care should be taken to position the stationary "upper hand" retractors at each costal margin to provide exposure. The left lobe of the liver is mobilized from the diaphragm and gently retracted rightward. A Penrose rubber drain is placed around the lower esophagus and used for traction purposes. With the Penrose drain providing downward traction, the distal esophagus is mobilized cephalad under direct vision. Palpation through the enlarged hiatus should allow for evaluation of the middle mediastinal esophagus and for confirmation of its resectability.

The most difficult area of dissection, as with all approaches for esophageal malignancy, will be the area surrounding the tumor. Local extension to involve the pleura, inferior pulmonary ligament, or posterior pericardium can be readily handled via the transhiatal approach. Many surgeons would discourage the transhiatal approach to any tumor in the upper third region because the close proximity of the membranous trachea and mainstem bronchi make blunt or blind dissection hazardous. After evaluation from the abdominal approach suggests tumor resectability, attention is now paid to the cervical dissection.

Cervical Dissection. The left cervical incision is made along the anteromedial border of the sternocleidomastoid muscle and dissection carried through the platysma, and the omohyoid muscle is divided. The middle thy-

roid vein is ligated to allow for medial rotation of the thyroid and trachea to expose the underlying esophagus (Fig 26–8). The sternocleidomastoid and carotid sheath are reflected laterally and the trachea is reflected gently, medially. The use of self-retaining metal retractors should be avoided during this dissection in an attempt to prevent injury to the recurrent laryngeal nerve. Using mostly blunt finger dissection, the posterior cervical esophagus is dissected free of the prevertibral fascia and the anterior cervical esophagus is freed from the trachea in the tracheoesophageal groove. A Penrose drain again is used to encircle the esophagus and provide countertraction. By keeping the fingers against the esophagus, the superior portion usually can be mobilized to the level of the carina.

Transhiatal Dissection. The transhiatal dissection is performed initially from the abdominal incision. The cardia and lower third of the esophagus can usually be dissected under direct vision. Care is taken to identify and control feeding arteries to the esophagus from the aorta with clips or ligation because these may result in significant bleeding if torn.

An attempt is made now to create a dissection plane posterior to the esophagus, with the finger tips against the posterior esophagus approaching from the abdominal incision and the cervical incision (Fig 26–9). This works best with a two-team approach. Blunt mobilization of the circumference of the thoracic esophagus then is accomplished. Care is taken not to compress the posterior heart excessively with the dissection because profound hypotension may result. The cervical esophagus is then elevated with the Penrose drain to allow for division with a GIA stapler. A long Penrose drain is sutured to the distal transected esophagus and both are pulled down through the esophageal hiatus. The Penrose drain is detached from the distal esophagus and sutured to the gastric fundus to aid in transhiatal passage to the neck. The gastroesophageal area then is divided along the lesser curvature with multiple firings of the GIA stapler, and the specimen is removed from the field. The stomach then is passed through the esophageal bed and an esophagogastric anastomosis performed as outlined in the techniques below.

Prior to wound closure, the mediastinum is evaluated for hemostasis and the pleurae are evaluated for violation and the need for chest tube placement. A feeding jejunostomy tube is routinely inserted using a small red Robnell catheter secured 10 cm from the ligament of Treitz via a Witzell technique.

Bypass Procedures. Various surgical attempts have been described to restore swallowing in those patients with severe dysphagia and advanced or unresectable esophageal carcinomas. The retrosternal stomach has been

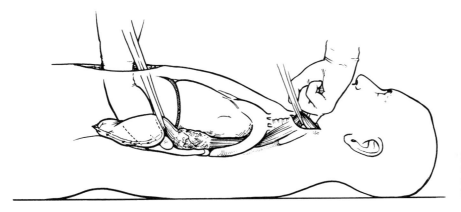

Figure 26–9. The blunt dissection progresses from above and below keeping fingers close to the esophageal wall posteriorly. Note the Penrose drains providing countertraction.

the most commonly described bypass conduit in recent series. Perioperative mortality and morbidity with this procedure, in these patients, is excessive. Reported series cite operative mortality rates exceeding 20%, with major morbidity in >50% of the patients. Median survival for patients bypassed was between 5 and 6 months.[34,35] For these reasons, many surgeons have abandoned this approach to those patients felt to have unresectable esophageal carcinomas in favor of palliative radiation, stent placement, dilatation or supportive care only.

Curative Intent

Curative surgery requires mediastinal dissection under direct vision with inclusion of regional nodal stations. The specific transthoracic approaches are based on tumor location. When possible, surgical therapy is standardized to include dissection of all lymph node stations in the mediastinum, periesophageal, and celiac stations.

SELECTION OF APPROACH BASED ON TUMOR LOCATION

Once the patient has been selected for a curative surgical approach, the next consideration is the anatomic location of the tumor. The esophagus may be divided into four segments for this purpose. The *cervical esophagus* extends from the cricopharyngeus muscle to the thoracic inlet. The *thoracic esophagus* is considered in three portions. The *upper third* extends from the thoracic inlet to the aortic arch. The *middle third* extends from the arch to the inferior pulmonary vein. Lastly the *lower-third* lesions are located between the inferior pulmonary vein and the cardia. The operative approach selected is that which will provide the best exposure to the tumor location.

Surgical Approach to Cervical Lesions

Czerny reported the first successful resection of the cervical esophagus in 1877.[36] The surgical treatment of cervical esophageal tumors can be a challenging endeavor

and a combined-discipline approach most often is required, involving thoracic surgery, otolaryngology, and occasionally, plastic surgery. Many head and neck oncologists advocate primary radiotherapy for these lesions, reserving resection for treatment failures. In resecting lesions grossly involving only the cervical esophagus superior to the thoracic inlet, a combined-team approach with otolaryngology, omitting the thoracotomy, is utilized. The cervical incision is performed along the medial border of the sternocleidomastoid muscle, and the lesion is evaluated for resectability. If nodal metastases or tumor are found to be fixed to the spine or neck vessels, the operation is aborted and palliative radiotherapy should be considered. If the lesion is found to be resectable, a two-team approach may aid in decreasing operative time by simultaneous dissection of the cervical esophagus and gastric conduit mobilization (as described below). The neck excision may be extended across the midline for greater exposure. The larynx often is involved and is removed en bloc with the cervical esophagus, along with the paraesophageal lymph nodes bilaterally. Bilateral radical neck dissection is morbid and is not performed routinely. A functional neck dissection, sparing the sternocleidomastoid muscle, jugular vein, and spinal accessory nerve is preferred. After tumor mobilization laterally and from the prevertebral fascia, the trachea is transected at a point in the lower neck leaving enough length to permit construction of a permanent tracheostomy. At this point, the ventilation tubing is switched to the tracheal opening and the hypopharynx is divided. Traction on the specimen upwards is used to aid in encircling the lower cervical esophagus with a Penrose drain, and blunt dissection of the upper thoracic esophagus is performed along with transhiatal mobilization from the abdominal end. The gastric neoesophagus is elevated to the neck, and the GE junction transected to deliver the specimen off the field. The pharyngogastrostomy is constructed using a single-layer, interrupted, hand-sewn technique with nonabsorbable suture. The cervical tracheostomy is constructed above the sternal notch, if possible. On occasion, the amount resected precludes this, and a mediastinal tracheostomy then should be considered.

Alternative conduits for restoration of gastrointestinal continuity include the colon interposition (described below). Jejunal free grafts and the construction of various myocutaneous flaps for complicated laryngopharyngoesophageal malignancies based on microvascular and plastic surgical techniques will not be addressed here, but should be considered in complicated settings.

Surgical Approach to Lesions Below the Thoracic Inlet

Three-hole Esophagectomy. McKeown introduced a three-incision esophagectomy in the 1960s.[37] His approach utilized an abdominal incision to mobilize the stomach followed by a right thoracotomy and right cervical incision to remove the esophagus and perform an esophagogastric reconstruction in the neck.

In the setting of a multimodality protocol approach to esophageal cancer, accurate pathologic information on nodal involvement, and a complete resection of all tumor is critical. Maximal local control and pathologic evaluation of tumor response to induction therapies are obtained with the technique described.

For tumors of the middle esophagus and all esophageal cancers below the thoracic inlet treated with induction chemoradiation, we prefer to use a right thoracotomy approach first, to allow for mobilization of the tumor and the intrathoracic esophagus along with a complete mediastinal and periesophageal nodal dissection. This is followed by a repositioning of the patient and an upper midline abdominal incision to mobilize the stomach for an eventual left cervical esophagogastrostomy.

Brigham Three-Hole Esophagectomy Technique

Right Posterolateral Thoracotomy. The right posterolateral thoracotomy incision provides excellent exposure to the entire intrathoracic esophagus, as well as the subcarinal space aorta, trachea, and both mainstem bronchi.

The procedure begins with a preanesthetic passage of a nasogastric tube to allow for decompression of the proximal esophagus, followed by insertion of a left double-lumen tube to allow for deflation of the right lung during esophageal dissection. The patient then is placed in the left lateral decubitus position and a fifth interspace posterolateral thoracotomy incision is made dividing the latissimus muscle as caudally as possible. The serratus anterior is preserved (Fig 26–10). The pleural cavity is entered, and the inferior pulmonary ligament is divided while the right lung is allowed to deflate. The deflated lung is retracted superomedially to allow for exposure of the posterior mediastinal pleura overlying the esophagus. T4 tumors adherent to unresectable mediastinal structures may be discovered at this stage of the operation and a palliative procedure, such as bypass or stenting, should be considered in these cases.

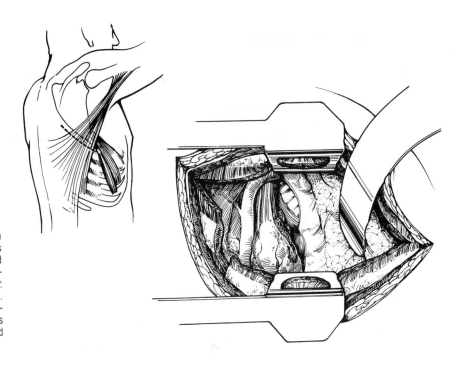

Figure 26–10. The right chest has been entered through the fifth interspace. A piece of the posterior sixth rib has been "shingled" to aid in exposure. The lung is retracted anteromedially and the mediastinal pleura has been incised posteriorly to expose the esophageal tumor. *Inset.* The patient is placed in the left lateral decubitus position. The *dotted line* marks the skin incision for a right posterolateral thoracotomy. The latissimus muscle is divided as caudally as possible and the serratus muscle is spared and reflected medially.

After assessment of the tumor reveals it to be resectable, an en bloc esophagectomy is begun. The mediastinal pleura is incised along the upper border of the vertebral bodies, extending from the upper border of the thoracic inlet down to the esophageal hiatus, using sharp dissection. The esophagus is mobilized along with its surrounding tissues at a point superiorly away from the tumor to allow for passage of a Penrose rubber drain around the esophagus to provide countertraction during the dissection. The azygous vein is divided at a point near its caval confluence and is reflected anteriorly (Fig 26–11). Superiorly, the tracheoesophageal plane is developed with finger dissection to a level above the thoracic inlet. Traction is applied to the Penrose drain and the superior thoracic esophagus is freed up into the neck (Fig 26–12). Any remaining nodal tissue is included with the specimen. Care is taken to avoid injury to the left recurrent laryngeal nerve unless it is involved with tumor, in which case it is sacrificed as part of the en bloc resection. After the esophagus is dissected free superior to the tumor, the Penrose drain is loosely knotted and pushed superiorly to the left side of the thoracic inlet to aid in the cervical dissection (Fig 26–13). The

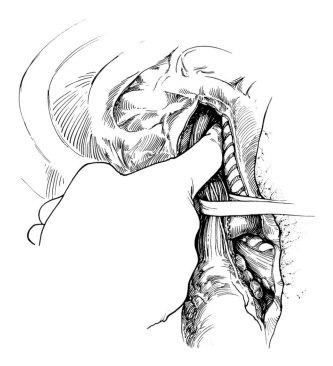

Figure 26–12. With countertraction applied to the Penrose drain encircling the esophagus above the tumor, blunt finger dissection is used to develop the tracheoesophageal plane to and above the thoracic inlet.

dissection proceeds between the aorta and esophagus, and esophageal arterial branches are divided. A Penrose drain encircling the esophagus distal to the tumor is placed, providing countertraction for the lower dissection. The thoracic duct is identified near the esophageal hiatus and ligated. Pericardium intimately associated with the tumor is removed, as well as any adherent pleura along both sides of the mediastinum. A 2-cm rim of the diaphragm is incised circumferentially around the esophageal hiatus. The lower Penrose drain is loosely tied and pushed down onto the GE junction, below the diaphragm, to facilitate the abdominal dissection (Fig 26–14). The completely mobilized intrathoracic esophagus is left in place while a thoracostomy tube is placed through a site inferior to the incision along the anterior and midaxillary line. The chest is closed, and the patient is repositioned supine for the upper abdominal and left neck explorations.

Upper Abdominal Dissection. Our preferred method for esophageal replacement and reconstruction is mobilization of the stomach based on the right gastroepiploic and distal right gastric arterial supply. All patients should have a full colonic bowel prep preoperatively, in case the need arises for a colonic interposition graft for esophageal reconstruction.

The patient is repositioned supine with arms tucked in at the sides. The head is turned to the right for ex-

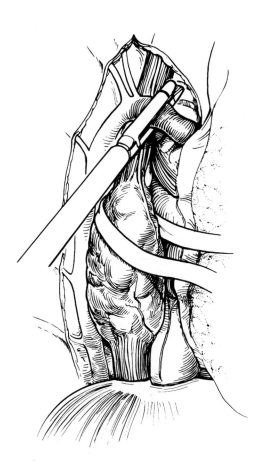

Figure 26–11. The esophagus has been isolated circumferentially at a point superior to the tumor and encircled with a Penrose drain. An endostapling device is used to divide the azygous vein near its caval connection.

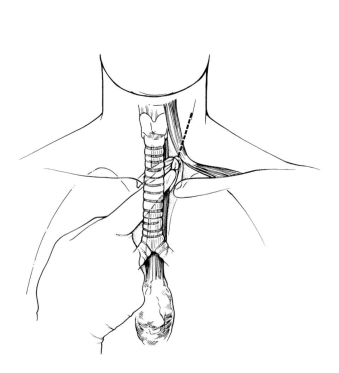

Figure 26–13. The knotted Penrose drain is pushed up through the thoracic inlet and left to lie beneath the omohyoid muscle on the left side of the neck.

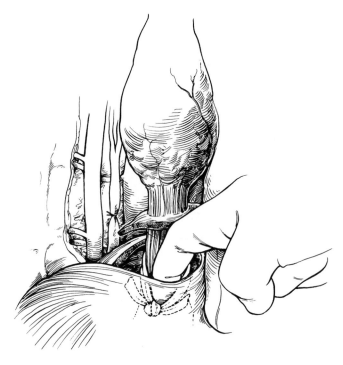

Figure 26–14. The lower Penrose drain is pushed down onto the GE junction below the diaphragm. The thoracic duct is shown ligated and a rim of the diaphragmatic hiatus encircles the lower esophagus.

posure of the left neck. The field is prepped and draped from chin to pubis.

The abdomen is entered through an upper midline incision, the xiphoid process may be resected to provide maximal exposure to the esophageal hiatus. A general exploration of the abdomen is conducted paying particular attention to the liver and upper abdomen for signs of metastases. The suitability of the stomach for a conduit is assessed. Exposure is attained with the aid of a large Balfour self-retaining retractor in the midline, as well as an "upper-hand" type self-retaining retractor for elevation of the rib cages. The triangular ligament of the left lobe of the liver is divided with electrocautery to allow for the left lobe of the liver to be reflected laterally, exposing the hiatus (Fig 26–15).

The stomach now is mobilized, beginning at the greater curvature near the hiatus. We do not routinely perform a splenectomy. The first of approximately four short gastric vessels between the spleen and stomach are carefully identified and sequentially dissected with a right-angle clamp and doubly ligated with sutures or clips and divided (Fig 26–16). The "transition zone" area along the greater curvature, where the left and right gastroepiploic arterial branches terminate, is identified, and great care is taken to continue this dissection at a distance of at least 2 cm away from the right gastroepiploic artery descending along the greater curva-

ture towards the pylorus through the lesser omentum and gastrocolic ligament. Division of the omentum is carried out between clamps, with extreme care to preserve the right gastroepiploic arcade because this will provide the main blood supply to the gastric conduit. The pyloroduodenal area is approached cautiously, avoiding excessive traction which may result in injury to the gastroepiploic vein as it inserts into the middle colic vein. Hemorrhage can be annoying and control of it may ultimately compromise the venous drainage of the repositioned stomach. The right gastroepiploic arcade is freed to its origin from the gastroduodenal artery.

After complete mobilization of the greater curvature, the stomach may be elevated superiorly and to the right. After sharp dissection of any gastropancreatic fibrous attachments, the fold containing the left gastric artery and coronary vein is exposed and ligated with an endostapler near its take off from the celiac axis (Fig 26–17). The gastrohepatic ligament then is divided and a Kocher maneuver is performed. The peritoneal attachments of the posterior duodenum are freed from the second portion to the superior mesenteric vessels. This usually provides enough mobility to allow the pylorus to reach the level of the esophageal hiatus.

We routinely perform a pyloromyotomy to avoid the uncommon but frustrating complication of delayed gastric emptying in the neoconduit (Fig 26–18). A pyloro-

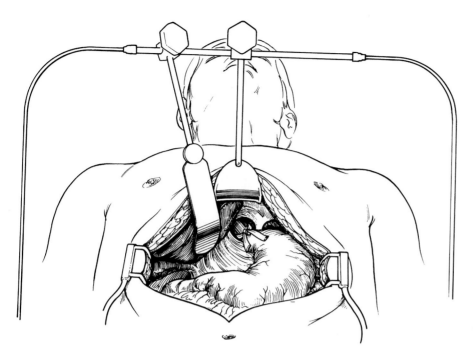

Figure 26–15. Exposure achieved by upper midline laparotomy. The large Balfour retractor is on the lateral abdominal walls and the upper hand retractor reflects the liver to the right exposing the hiatus and lower Penrose drain around the GE junction.

plasty also is acceptable, but has the disadvantages of shortening the gastric length and of an additional suture line.

An endostapling device divides the right gastric artery and lesser omental fatty tissue just above the incisura. The stomach is now ready for conduit creation by the use of a GIA stapler. Beginning at the lateral GE junction on the greater curvature side, the stapler is fired three to four times along the lesser curvature to create the gastric tube to be brought to the neck (Fig 26–19). Perigastric lymph nodes along the lesser curvature with, and celiac lymph nodes proximal to, the divided left gastric artery remain as part of the specimen. The staple line along the lesser curvature may be oversewn with a continuous layer of absorbable suture.

Occasionally the esophageal hiatus requires enlargement with two opposite radial incisions of 1 to 2 cm in length to allow for passage of the stomach through the mediastinum, as well as to avoid venous congestion of the vascular pedicle at the hiatus. At this point, attention is directed at mobilization of the cervical esophagus through a left neck incision.

Left Cervical Approach. An oblique incision along the medial border of the left sternocleidomastoid muscle is used with division of the platysma and deep cervical fascia by electrocautery. The sternocleidomastoid muscle is reflected laterally along with the carotid sheath. The left middle thyroid vein and, on occasion, the inferior thyroid vessels are divided to improve exposure (Fig 26–20). No effort is made to dissect out

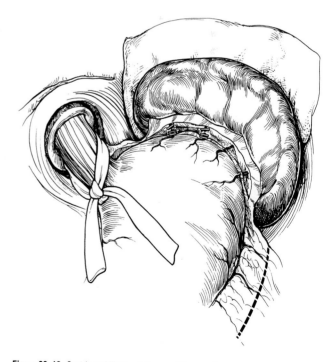

Figure 26–16. Gastric mobilization is begun at the superior greater curvature near the hiatus. A rolled Miculitz pad is placed behind the spleen to aid in exposure. The short gastric vessels between the spleen and the stomach are divided and the transition zone between the left and right gastroepiploic arteries is identified. Mobilization proceeds at least 2 cm away from the right gastroepiploic arcade (*dotted line*).

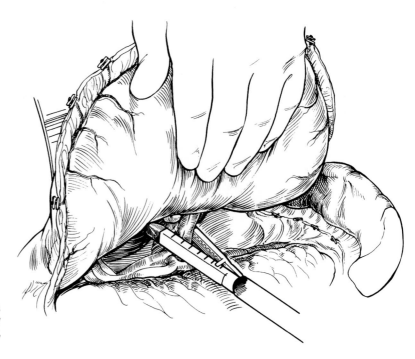

Figure 26–17. After the greater curvature is mobilized the stomach is reflected superiorly and to the right, exposing the left gastric artery and coronary vein. These are ligated and divided with an endostapler, near their origin, from the celiac axis.

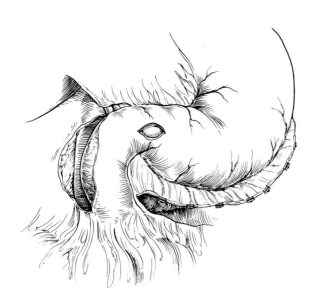

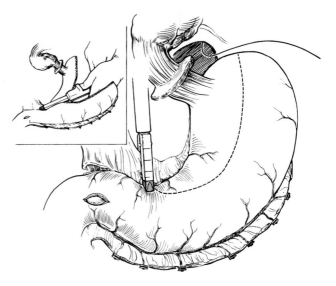

Figure 26–18. A Kocher maneuver to mobilize the duodenum and a pyloromyotomy are performed.

Figure 26–19. The right gastric artery and lesser omentum are divided with an endostapling device. *Inset:* A GIA stapler divides the stomach along the lesser curvature creating the gastric conduit.

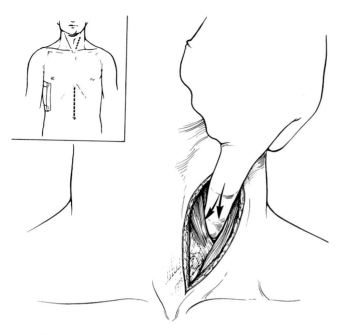

Figure 26–20. Left cervical incision with sternocleidomastoid muscle reflected laterally. Finger dissection beneath omohyoid muscle develops plane to the knotted Penrose drain. *Inset:* The patient is placed supine for the neck and abdominal incisions (*outlined*).

the left recurrent laryngeal nerve because this does not aid the mobilization. Traction or placement of self-retaining retractors below the sternocleidomastoid muscle is avoided. The prevertebral fascia and tracheoesophageal groove are dissected bluntly, and gentle finger dissection is used to identify the knotted Penrose drain to allow countertraction for further dissection. After sufficient mobilization, the cervical esophagus is divided with a stapling device (Fig 26–21). The specimen is delivered next through the abdominal wound. A long silk suture is tied to the cervical end of the specimen and the esophagus is pulled down through the hiatus (Fig 26–22). The silk is attached to the tip of a Foley catheter with a 30-cc balloon, and the catheter is delivered down through the hiatus (Fig 26–23). The end of the Foley catheter is inserted into the camera tip of an arthroscopy drape. The balloon is inflated with 30 cc of saline and tied into the drape. The stomach now is placed into the folded-up arthroscopy drape near the Foley tip, insuring the proper axial orientation of the stomach (Fig 26–24). The drainage end of the Foley catheter is pulled up to the cervical wound and connected to wall suction (Fig 26–25). With this maneuver, the bag collapses around the neoesophagus and the suction of the bag drags the stomach atraumatically into the neck. When the proximal end has reached a suitable position in the neck, the plastic bag is removed through the cervical incision and discarded. Intraven-

ous glucagon (1 mg) may relax the stomach and facilitate its comfortable passage into the neck.

Anastomosis Construction. Our preferred anastomotic technique utilizes a hand-sewn interrupted, full-thickness single layer of nonabsorbable suture. The anastomosis is an end-to-side esophagogastrostomy performed on the anterior surface of the stomach. The gastrotomy is made 4 to 6 cm distal to the fundus and away from the lesser curvature staple line. The posterior row is placed before the knots are tied inside the lumen. A silastic sump tube is inserted in the superior fundus and left to exit the neck through the wound. The avoidance of the nasogastric tube in this setting leads to improved comfort and pulmonary toilet postoperatively. A Jackson-Pratt drain is placed in the lower cervical area through a separate incision to lie near the thoracic inlet (Fig 26–26). Alternatively, a stapled anastomosis may be used as described below.

After completion of the esophagogastric anastomosis, the cervical and abdominal wounds are closed. If a feeding jejunostomy tube was not inserted previously for nutrition during induction therapy, a red Robnell catheter is inserted in the jejunum 10 cm distal to the ligament of Treitz and secured with a Witzell suture technique prior to closure of the abdominal incision.

Stapled Cervical Gastroesophagostomy. After insuring an adequate length of gastric conduit is present to create a tension-free anastomosis, the stapled esophagogastric anastomosis is a quick and safe technique when properly performed. Our preferred stapled technique constructs a functional end-to-end esophagogastric anastomosis approximating the distal side of the esophagus with the anterior wall of the stomach (Fig 26–27). After a stab wound is made on the anterior stomach wall, staying well away from the lesser curvature staple line, the limbs of a GIA stapling device each are inserted into the stomach opening and esophageal end, respectively. The stapler is fired and Allis clamps are used to approximate the free stomach wall end with the free superior esophageal wall. A TA linear stapler is used to reapproximate these tissues beneath the clamps. After trimming the excess tissue from the stapler, suture reinforcement is usually unnecessary.

In our experience an EEA stapled anastomosis should be avoided because these are associated with a high occurrence of nondilatable strictures.

Alternative Anastomotic Techniques (Hand-Sewn). The choice of anastomotic technique between stapled or hand-sewn (number of layers and suture material used) is one of personal preference and experience. In a review of the world esophageal surgical literature, similar overall leak rates in the range of 12% were reported for single-

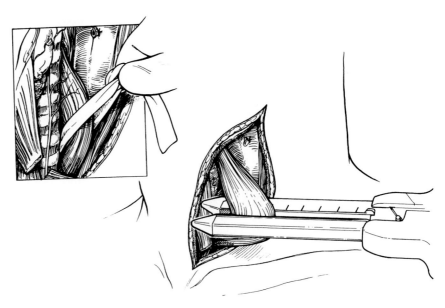

Figure 26–21. A GIA stapler is used to divide the cervical esophagus. Note the ligated middle thyroid vein and divided omohyoid muscle. *Inset:* Traction is placed on the Penrose drain around the cervical esophagus.

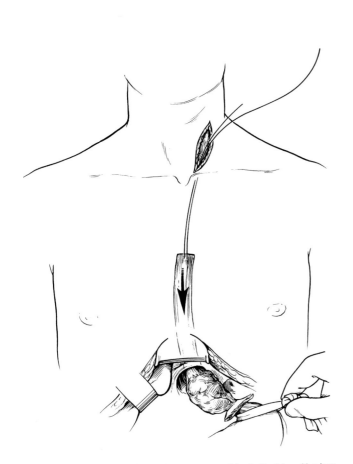

Figure 26–22. The specimen is removed through the abdominal incision with a long heavy silk suture attached to the end of the esophagus.

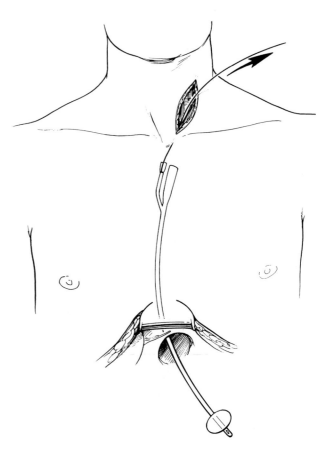

Figure 26–23. The heavy silk is tied to the port of a 30-cc balloon Foley catheter and is pulled up partially through the neck incision.

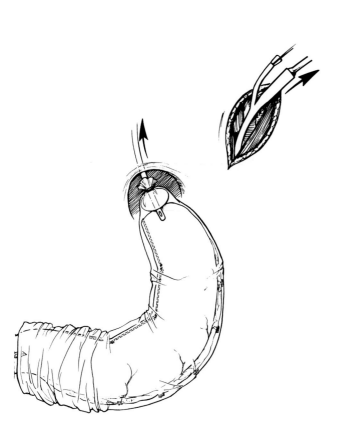

Figure 26–24. An arthroscopy camera bag is tied around the Foley catheter balloon and the gastric conduit is placed in the folded up arthroscopy bag insuring the proper axial orientation. *Inset*: A Yankauer suction is attached to the Foley catheter to collapse the bag around the neoesophagus.

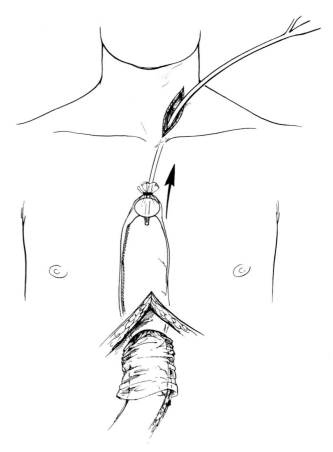

Figure 26–25. The gastric conduit is atraumatically pulled through the posterior mediastinum into the cervical wound.

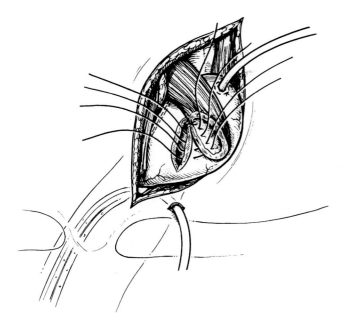

Figure 26–26. The esophagogastric anastomosis is performed with a single layer of full-thickness interrupted, nonabsorbable sutures. The silastic sump drain is shown emanating from the fundus of the gastric conduit. A Jackson-Pratt drain is shown positioned alongside the gastric conduit inferiorly and exiting from a separate stab wound above the clavicle.

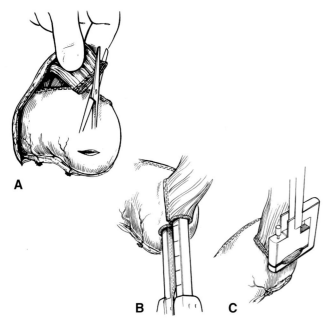

Figure 26–27. A and **B**. The stapled functional end-to-end anastomosis is performed using the GIA stapler to approximate the side of the esophagus to the anterior wall of the stomach. **C**. The TA linear stapler then is used to close the defect between the two free walls.

layer, hand-sewn anastomoses (3648 cases) as well as for the two-layer technique (5078 cases).[38]

Excellent results have been reported for various techniques of hand-sewn anastomoses. Rather than adherence to specific suture material or number of layers, results appear to be related more to careful handling of tissue and precise placement of sutures to appose the mucosal layers without tension. A single layer of running 5 to 0 steel wire,[39,40] interrupted two-layer technique using inverted silk sutures,[41] and a two-layer anastomosis of a running, absorbable inner layer and interrupted silk outer layer[42] have all yielded excellent functional results with minimal complications.

Although conflicting reports exist on the decreased morbidity and mortality associated with a cervical anastomotic leak compared to one in the thorax, most surgeons in the United States would agree that the cervical anastomotic leak is a less devastating problem.

Alternative Surgical Approaches

Ivor Lewis Approach. In 1946, Ivor Lewis described a new approach for lesions of the middle third of the esophagus.[43] It was originally presented as a two-stage procedure in which an abdominal exploration with gastric mobilization and placement of a feeding jejunostomy tube was followed a few weeks later by a right thoracotomy and thoracic esophageal resection with esophagogastric anastomosis in the apex of the right chest.

This procedure has become accepted by many surgeons as one of the standard approaches today for lesions of the mid and lower esophagus. The only major modification is a one-stage approach. Lewis favored a single-layer, end-to-side interrupted silk suture technique for construction of the esophagogastric anastomosis, and he tacked the stomach to the posterior mediastinum to prevent torsion (Fig 26–28). Although this approach remains a safe and effective technique for lesions of the mid and lower esophagus, our preference is for the three-hole approach for these lesions based upon the decreased morbidity associated with anastomotic leaks in the neck compared to the chest, as well as the ability to obtain a wider proximal esophageal margin.

Left Thoracotomy Approach (Lower-Third Lesions). For tumors of the lower 10 cm of esophagus and those involving the GE junction, a left thoracotomy or thoracoabdominal approach provide excellent exposure. If there is any consideration of submucosal tumor extension or proximal Barrett's changes, a three-hole approach should be considered.

The preoperative preparation is similar to that of the other approaches to esophagectomy, with a nasogastric tube inserted before induction of anesthesia and a double-lumen endotracheal tube placed to allow for collapse of the left lung during the esophageal dissection. The patient is positioned with the left arm suspended forward and at a 60° angle with the left side elevated.

The incision is begun posterolaterally below the tip of the scapula over the seventh rib to allow for entrance to the chest in the sixth intercostal space. It is then carried down across the costal margin medially. The degree of extension in the upper midline abdomen varies, but it is rarely necessary to use more than a few centimeters length inferiorly.

The latissimus muscle is divided with electrocautery and similarly the serratus muscle is divided medially. The ribs are counted from beneath the raised scapula and the intercostal muscles are divided just superior to the seventh rib. The pleura is entered and the costal margin is divided medially with a rib cutter. The internal mammary artery and vein are ligated deep and slightly lateral to the costal margin. The left lung is deflated and reflected superomedially.

The diaphragm is incised next in a circumferential manner 2 cm from its insertion into the rib cage. A peripheral circumferential incision is used for ease of closure, as well as to avoid phrenic nerve injury and to preserve diaphragmatic muscle function (Fig 26–29). The phrenic nerve innervates the middle of the diaphragm and sends radiating branches to the periphery of the muscle. Radial incisions in the diaphragm are associated with a high rate of postoperative paralysis and dysfunction.

The exposure of the thoracic esophagus is obtained by

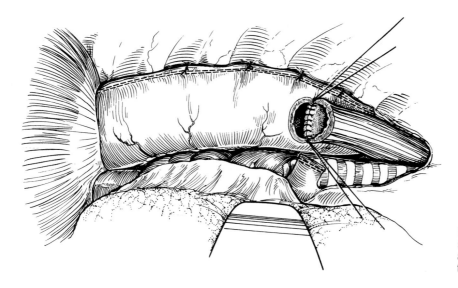

Figure 26–28. View through a right thoracotomy incision showing an esophagogastric end-to-side anastomosis in the apical right chest. Note the tacking sutures from stomach to the posterior chest wall to avoid torsion.

incising the inferior pulmonary ligament to the inferior pulmonary vein, using sharp dissection. The area of the tumor is evaluated to assess resectability and nodal involvement. The esophagus is liberated by incising the mediastinal pleura from just below the aortic arch to the hiatus. The vagus nerves are divided as they appear below the hilum of the lung along the body of the esophagus.

Using blunt finger dissection, the esophagus is encircled first with the surgeon's finger then followed by a Penrose drain to allow for countertraction. As the esophagus and tumor are mobilized, two to three arterial branches from the aorta are ligated with hemoclips. The aortopulmonary, subcarinal, inferior pulmonary ligament, and periesophageal lymph nodes routinely are dissected with the specimen.

A 2- to 3-cm cuff of diaphragm may be resected around the esophageal hiatus to insure adequate margins. This also aids in the eventual gastric mobilization into the chest. The thoracic duct is identified and doubly ligated at this level.

The abdomen is explored for evidence of metastatic disease. The mobilization of the stomach is performed in a similar manner to that described in the three-hole technique. Careful attention to the right gastroepiploic arcade along the greater curvature of the stomach is imperative to the viability of the gastric neoconduit.

A splenectomy is not performed routinely for cancers of the lower esophagus and GE junction. However, if a portion of the gastric cardia appears involved, or there is direct extension of tumor into the spleen, then a splenectomy easily can be added to the en bloc resection. If this is desirable, then prior to mobilization of the short gastric vessels, the spleen is retracted medially and the lienophrenic ligament divided. The lienocolic ligament then is divided, and the splenic artery and vein are

identified near the tail of the pancreas. The vessels are ligated individually with silk ties. The spleen now is attached only by the short gastric vessels. By carefully elevating the spleen into the field, division of these vessels between the spleen and fundic greater curvature is made easier.

The celiac nodes are involved in >60% of patients with lower esophageal tumors.[26] This may lead to left gastric artery encasement by tumor, and great care should be exercised during that part of the dissection because hemorrhage can be difficult to control safely. After the gastric mobilization is completed, plans for the definitive resection are made, emphasizing an at least 10-cm proximal margin of esophagus to palpable tumor. A 6-cm margin along the stomach is the goal distally.

The gastric tube is constructed with several firings of a GIA stapling device across the superior fundus to include the lesser curvature down to the incisura in the specimen, along with the celiac nodes. If the GE junction or a portion of the cardia is involved with tumor, the length of available stomach conduit may prohibit a cervical anastomosis, unless a segment of colon or jejunum is used as an interposition (see below). The proximal esophagus is divided with a GIA stapler as well and the specimen is removed from the field. The staple line along the fundus of the stomach tube is oversewn with a running layer of 3 silk. After a Kocher maneuver and pyloromyotomy or pyloroplasty are performed as described above, the stomach tube then is passed through the enlarged esophageal hiatus. An esophagogastric reconstruction is the preferred method, with an anastomosis performed under the aortic arch. A cervical level reconstruction is possible, although difficult, if enough length is available. If this is the case, the

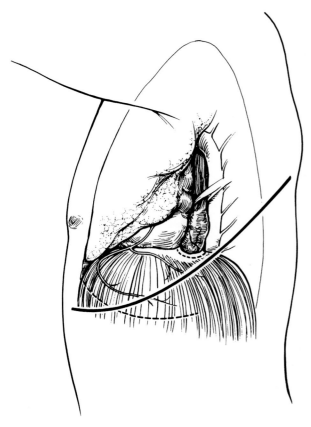

Figure 26–29. Left thoracoabdominal approach; *dotted lines* delineate the circumferential diaphragmatic incision as well as the hiatal margin incision. A Penrose drain encircles the esophagus above the tumor.

residual esophagus is dissected bluntly beneath the aorta, with the balance of the dissection performed via the left neck. A left cervical incision along the medial edge of the sternocleidomastoid muscle is used to expose the cervical esophagus, as described above. A stapled or hand-sewn end-to-side esophagogastrostomy is performed at either level, depending on the surgeon's preference.

On rare occasions, an intrathoracic supraaortic anastomosis is necessary. Poor exposure makes this a technically challenging anastomosis. In most cases the stomach will reach the neck for a safer and easier anastomosis.

A major source of postoperative morbidity with the left thoracic approach is the divided costochondral junction. Great care must be taken to reapproximate these firmly because patients often complain bitterly of pain from the rubbing together of the two costochondral edges if approximated too loosely. The union can be secured with permanent suture, wire, or a miniplate with bone screws. An alternative strategy is to resect 1 to 2 cm of each costochondral edge to prevent any contact of the two edges after wound closure.

ALTERNATE METHODS OF RECONSTRUCTION

Colonic Interposition

The stomach is the preferred organ of use for the restoration of gastrointestinal continuity. However, previous gastric surgery, scarring from severe ulcer disease, or extensive involvement with tumor may preclude its use and require the use of the colon as an alternative conduit. Several reasons account for the colon being a less desirable primary choice. The vascular supply of the colon is more tenuous with fewer collaterals than the stomach. In addition, the procedure requires the construction of three anastomoses in an often already nutritionally depleted host.

In situations where the stomach is not a suitable conduit, the colon can be used to restore gastrointestinal continuity. To decrease operative time, a two-team approach may be utilized. The isoperistaltic left colon is preferred by many experienced thoracic surgeons.[40,44,45] Colonic interposition bypass grafts of the unresected esophagus are not recommended, owing to the previously cited high mortality and morbidity[45] in malignant disease and the late complications from a retained, excluded esophagus in benign situations. The approach most often used in cases of attempted curative resection would be the three-hole technique in all but the most distal lesions, where a left thoracotomy approach may provide better exposure.

The preoperative preparation should include a complete bowel prep with adequate hydration. A preoperative arteriogram is obtained in all cases to define anomalous anatomy and plan the colon procurement. The right colon has been noted to have a higher incidence of anomalous arterial supply and venous drainage.[46] Because of the reliable supply based on the left colic artery, the left colon is the conduit of choice in most cases.

The standard sequence follows as described above for the three-hole technique. A fifth interspace right thoracotomy is performed and the esophagus and tumor are mobilized fully. The chest then is closed after the insertion of two chest tubes and the patient returned to the supine position. An upper midline abdominal incision, usually to below the xyphoid, is performed and a careful search for metastatic disease is undertaken. If none is found, the colon is mobilized at both hepatic and splenic flexures. The lateral peritoneal attachment of the left colon is divided along the white line of Toldt, and a careful inspection of the arterial supply to the left colon follows. Particular attention is paid to the integrity of the marginal artery of Drummond at the splenic flexure. A palpable pulse should be present in the left colic artery as well as the marginal artery and middle colic artery branches (Fig 26–30). The vessels are isolated with the aid of transillumination of the mesentery, avoiding the marginal artery. A vascu-

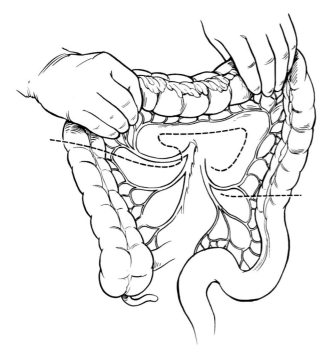

Figure 26–30. The mobilized colon is elevated and the arterial supply and venous drainage are examined. The arterial and venous ligation sites and the mesenteric incision lines are illustrated for an isoperistaltic conduit based on a left colic arterial supply.

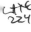

lar clamp may be placed on the branch of the middle colic artery supplying the left colon to aid in evaluation of the marginal artery. In most cases of malignancy, a long conduit is harvested to provide for a cervical esophagocolic anastomosis.

Prior to division of the colon and conduit isolation, the GE junction is approached and the cardia and lesser curvature dissected free with division of the fibers of the phrenoesophageal ligament and gastrohepatic ligament. The stomach is divided using the 4.8-mm GIA stapling device, using the method described above to include the lesser curvature nodes in the specimen. A pyloromyotomy also is performed. At this point, the colon is isolated for transfer into the bed of the resected esophagus.

After the surgeon is convinced there is satisfactory blood supply to the eventual colonic conduit, the marginal artery is ligated distal to both branches of the left colic artery. The middle colic artery is divided well proximal to its branch point into left and right segments. An adequate length for a tension free interposition is critical. The colon is divided with a GIA stapler, and the conduit is placed in the left upper quadrant wrapped in warm moist gauze, taking care not to twist or kink the left colonic artery pedicle.

The colocolonic anastomosis to restore continuity of the large bowel is performed in the standard fashion. We prefer the stapled side-to-side technique (functional end-to-end). The mesenteric defect between the right colon and sigmoid should be closed to avoid internal hernias; however, caution should be taken to avoid too tight a closure thus compromising pedicle flow. During this time, the second team can ready the cervical esophagus. A left neck incision is made along the medial border of the sternocleidomastoid as described above, and the cervical esophagus is encircled with a Penrose drain.

The esophagectomy is completed as described, and the conduit is positioned to restore intestinal continuity (Fig 26–31). The colon can be placed in either an orthotopic, transhiatal position (lying in the esophageal bed) or it may be brought retrosternally. Our preference is the orthotopic, posterior mediastinal interposition. This provides the most direct route to the cervical esophagus and avoids the acute angulation of the retrosternally placed graft at the diaphragm and thoracic inlet. The cologastric anastomosis is constructed on the posterior surface of the stomach, one-third of the distance down from the fundus (8 to 12 cm below the diaphragm). The stomach is reflected to the right, and a posterior gastrotomy incision is made. Using this method, the colon is placed in an isoperistaltic interposition; thus, the distal end of the left colon conduit is opened and the anastomosis is performed. Hand-sewn or stapled anastomotic techniques are equally acceptable. Care is taken not to torque the vascular pedicle during the process. The specimen may be removed from either the abdominal or cervical incision. The proximal esophagocolic anastomosis is performed using different colored sutures on each side to prevent colonic torsion. We prefer a single-layer technique using interrupted nonabsorbable suture, although stapled anastomoses using the EEA or functional end-to-end techniques are acceptable.

Prior to the completion of the cervical anastomosis, the colonic mesentery and mucosa are examined and blood supply is assessed carefully. If there is any evidence of venous engorgement or vascular insufficiency, the graft should be examined in the neck and abdomen at the pedicle's origin and diaphragmatic hiatus for compression or kinking. If blood flow remains a concern and no obvious source of mechanical problem can be found, the thoracotomy incision may need to be re-explored to rule out torsion of the interposition graft.

After vascular integrity is confirmed, the colonic conduit is gently straightened in the posterior mediastinum by mild traction at the diaphragmatic hiatus to avoid the complication of late intrathoracic redundancy. Redundant colon graft below the diaphragm is well tolerated.[40] The graft is sutured to the left crus of the diaphragm at the hiatus using absorbable, seromuscular, interrupted sutures in a two-thirds circumferential fashion. This prevents herniation of other intraperitoneal structures around the conduit (para "neoesophageal"

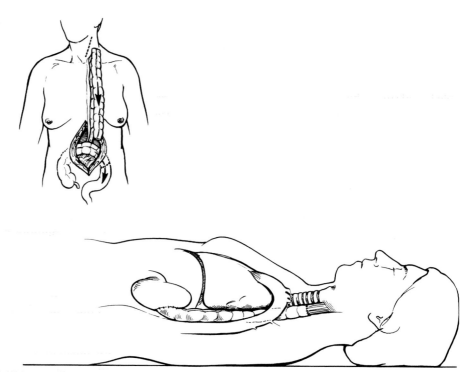

Figure 26–31. Lateral view of colonic conduit in posterior mediastinal esophageal bed. Cervical esophagocolonic and posterior cologastric anastomoses are shown. *Inset.* Neck incision marked and left colon conduit mobilized on anterior chest wall, based on marginal artery pedicle of left colonic artery and placed in isoperistaltic position.

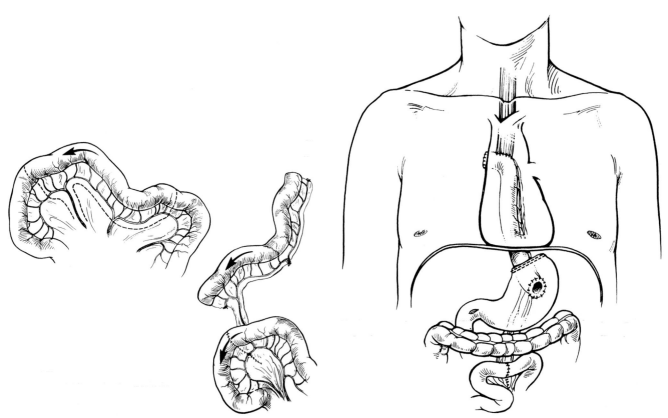

Figure 26–32. A. The jejunum is prepared in an isoperistaltic fashion (*arrows*) based on a distal mesenteric branch and proximal marginal arcade. The *dotted line* illustrates the line of resection of mesentery and the division of vessels. **B**. After dividing the mesentery and preserving the pedicle, jejunal continuity is restored and the mesenteric defect closed.

Figure 26–33. Jejunal interposition graft to reconstruct the lower esophagus. An end-to-side esophagojejunostomy is performed to avoid tension on the vascular pedicle. A posterior jejunogastric anastomosis avoids tortuosity of the conduit while an 8- to 12-cm segment of the jejunal graft situated below the hiatus aids in the control of reflux.

hernia). Care must be taken to avoid injury or compromise of the left colic vascular pedicle.

Alternatively, the right colon may be used for an isoperistaltic conduit as well. The disadvantages include the increased caliber size of the cecum and more variable blood supply based on the right colic artery or right branch of the middle colic artery, depending on the vascular anatomy. Some surgeons have recommended inclusion of the ileocecal valve in the conduit, since it enables a better size match between the ileum and esophagus at the proximal anastomosis.[47]

Jejunal Interposition

Replacement of the esophagus with a jejunal interposition for malignancy is reserved as a last resort, in most cases. Difficulty in fashioning a conduit of sufficient length to provide for adequate margins is the most significant obstacle. The pedicled jejunal graft rarely can reach above the aortic arch without the use of a free graft relying on a microvascular anastomosis, making the procedure more complex and prone to complication.

The usual approach for the jejunal interposition is through a left thoracoabdominal incision which affords the best exposure to the distal esophagus.[48] After dissecting the esophageal segment and assessing the length needed for interposition, an isoperistaltic graft is prepared on its vascular pedicle (Fig 26–32), and the jejunum is divided with GIA staplers. The jejunum may be

reconstituted via a stapled or hand-sewn technique. The graft is brought retrocolic and posterior to the stomach to lie in the esophageal bed (Fig 26–33). An end-to-side esophagojejunal anastomosis is constructed. The jejunogastric anastomosis is performed on the posterior stomach away from the gastric staple line. The hiatus is tacked to the jejunum to avoid torsion and herniation of peritoneal contents.

■ RECONSTRUCTION FOR BENIGN DISEASE

TRANSHIATAL ESOPHAGECTOMY

Several methods have been described in the treatment of benign esophageal disorders that require total or partial esophagectomy. In most settings, we prefer the transhiatal approach with cervical esophagogastrostomy. The excellent functional results and low perioperative mortality and morbidity achievable with this approach make it our approach of choice for achalasia with megaesophagus or severe neuromotor dysfunction, benign strictures from reflux or caustic ingestions, and occasionally for severe, recurrent GE reflux. There is considerable debate about whether one should remove the entire esophagus for a short segment stricture that may easily be handled by a partial esophagectomy with either a thoracic esophagogas-

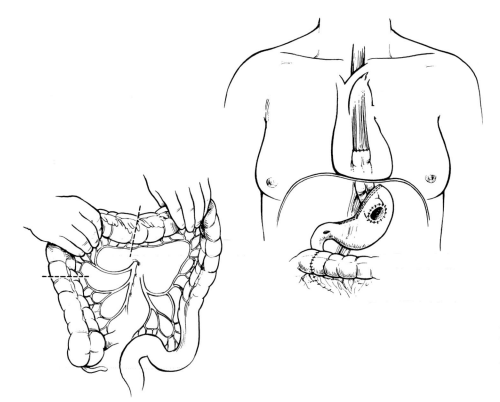

Figure 26–34. The conduit is passed behind the stomach through the hiatus and an end-to-end intrathoracic esophagocolic anastomosis constructed. The cologastric anastomosis is performed on the posterior gastric wall away from the gastric staple line and with 8 to 10 cm of intra-abdominal colon situated below the hiatus to aid in reflux prevention. *Inset:* Preparation of a short segment transverse colon conduit based on the middle colic vessels.

trostomy or short segment colon or jejunal interposition. Our results have been similar to those reported in the literature regarding the occurrence of regurgitation, dysphagia from anastomotic stricture, and postprandial diarrhea.[33] Most often these problems are managed easily with head-of-the-bed elevation at night, outpatient dilatation, and opiates, respectively. The occurrence of reflux with symptoms after an intrathoracic anastomosis is generally believed to be more frequent and may result in more severe complications than with the cervical technique. For these reasons, the cervical anastomosis is the procedure of choice when possible.

SHORT SEGMENT COLON INTERPOSITION

The stomach may be unsuitable for esophageal reconstruction in the setting of a benign distal esophageal disease not amenable to conservative therapy. In these instances, a left thoracoabdominal approach with the use of a short segment colon interposition has been used with success. The most common colonic conduit is the transverse colon based on the middle colic artery. Using a similar preparation technique to that of the long colon, the short segment is mobilized in an isoperistaltic position based on the middle colic artery and vein (Fig 26–34). The conduit segment is brought posterior to the stomach through the hiatus and an end-to-end esophagocolic anastomosis performed through the left chest. The cologastric anastomosis is performed as described previously, end-to-side on the posterior gastric surface. A short or long segment colon interposition has been described for benign lesions either based on the left, right, or middle colic artery.[40] The jejunum is a suitable option for replacement of the distal esophagus with the most common indication being complications associated with GE reflux, either in the form of an nondilatable stricture or esophagitis refractory to medical and antireflux interventions.

■ COMPLICATIONS OF ESOPHAGEAL SURGERY

Esophageal surgery involving resection and reconstruction can be a very morbid procedure with a significant operative mortality, especially in the case of malignancy. Advances in perioperative care including anesthetic techniques and nutrition have enabled mortality rates for resection of esophageal cancer to fall to between 5% to 10% in experienced hands.[33,49]

Vigilant postoperative care is critical to achieve an uneventful recovery. However, when complications do arise, prompt recognition may have a significant effect on outcome. The following is a brief list of common complications associated with esophageal resection and their recognition and treatment.

PULMONARY COMPLICATIONS

Pulmonary complications are the most common problems encountered in esophagectomy patients. Pneumonia resulting from aspiration or retained secretions can be life threatening. Smoking cessation preoperatively, adequate pain control with aggressive pulmonary toilet (including the liberal use of bedside flexible bronchoscopy) and early ambulation are the cornerstones of preventive therapy. Long-term management postoperatively includes aspiration precautions consisting of head-of-bed elevation, frequent small meals, and allowing time for the conduit to empty prior to retiring.

ANASTOMOTIC LEAK

Anastomotic leak rates have been quoted in several large collective series to be near 12%, regardless of the method of suturing or the use of mechanical staplers.[50] Leaks in the neck from a cervical anastomosis can be treated usually with either observation or opening of the cervical wound and packing with gauze dressings. Most cervical anastomoses will seal in 1 to 2 weeks with this conservative approach. Thoracic anastomoses pose a more difficult problem because a significant leak can lead to mediastinitis and sepsis. Small contained leaks noted on follow-up barium swallow can be observed initially, especially if well drained by the chest tubes. An uncontrolled thoracic leak or one associated with signs of sepsis requires emergent reexploration of the thoracotomy for wide pleural and mediastinal drainage and possible revision of the anastomosis and flap coverage with either a pericardial fat pad, intercostal muscle, or omentum. In the case that reanastomosis is not possible owing to tension or uncontrolled infection, the esophagus is exteriorized through the neck and the stomach is closed, returned to the abdomen and drained with a gastrostomy.

CONDUIT NECROSIS

Infrequently, the gastric conduit or colonic graft become ischemic and necrose. The treatment is emergent excision of the graft or conduit with esophageal diversion via a cervical esophagostomy and a feeding jejunostomy, if not already in place. No attempt at reconstruction is made until recovery from the ischemic/septic insult is complete.

ANASTOMOTIC STRICTURE

Stricture of the cervical esophagogastrostomy requiring dilatation occurs in up to 40% of the patients at some point postoperatively. Patients with previous anastomotic leaks are likely to require dilatation. These strictures most commonly respond to one or two outpatient dilatations. A careful upper endoscopy is mandatory to rule out recurrent tumor as the cause in late strictures.

GASTROESOPHAGEAL REFLUX

Reflux or postprandial regurgitation to a mild degree are common complaints in postesophagectomy patients. The importance of upright posture after eating has been demonstrated. With gastric conduits the routine use of pyloroplasty with resection can aid in emptying of the vagotomized stomach. Reflux is less of a reported problem in colonic anastomoses.[40,51]

COLONIC DYSMOTILITY—REDUNDANCY PARTIAL OBSTRUCTION

In long colon grafts, the colon tends to become redundant eventually, leading to intermittent obstruction of food boluses as the result of kinking. This can be minimized by assuring that the intrathoracic portion of the colon graft is straight and any redundant colon noted at the time of surgery is placed below the diaphragm, before anchorage of the conduit to the hiatus.

■ CONCLUSIONS

As evident by the many approaches for esophageal resection and replacement presented in this text, no single technique is suitable for all patients. The only requirements for safe esophageal surgery are careful patient selection, meticulous dissection and hemostasis, precision in constructing anastomoses and diligent perioperative care.

The advantages of the three-hole technique described include the ease and safety of a cervical neo-esophageal anastomosis, initial intrathoracic dissection via the right chest to assess resectability and gross response to induction therapies. The use of the Penrose drains at the thoracic inlet and the esophageal hiatus facilitate ease of dissection in the subsequent cervical and abdominal phases. The gastric conduit utilizes only one anastomosis, and the functional results are excellent in most cases.

With the increasing role of induction therapy, "complete resection" to include all nodal stations for postresectional pathologic evaluation of disease stage and the response to preoperative chemoradiation in protocol settings is crucial to increasing our understanding of the biologic behavior of esophageal cancer and improving survival in patients afflicted with this deadly malignancy.

REFERENCES

1. Bilroth T. Notes concerning the resection of the esophagus. *Arch Clin Chir* 1871;13:65
2. Torek F. The operative treatment of carcinoma of the esophagus. *Ann Surg* 1915;61:385
3. Ohsawa T. The surgery of the esophagus. *Arch Jpn Chir* 1933;10:605
4. Adams WE, Phemister DB. Carcinoma of the lower thoracic esophagus: report of a successful resection and esophagogastrectomy. *J Thorac Surg* 1938;7:621–632
5. Schottenfeld D. Epidemiology of cancer of the esophagus. *Semin Oncol* 1984;11:92–100
6. DeMeester TR, Attwood SE, Smyrk TC, et al. Surgical therapy in Barrett's esophagus. *Ann Surg* 1990;212: 528–542
7. Alpern HD, Buell C, Olson J. Increasing percentage of adenocarcinoma in primary carcinoma of the esophagus. *Am J Gastroenterol* 1989;84:574
8. Kirby TJ, Rice TW. The epidemiology of esophageal carcinoma: the changing face of a disease. *Chest Surg Clin North Am* 1994;4(2):217–225
9. Kruse P, Boesby S, Bernstein IT, Andersen IB. Barrett's esophagus and esophageal adenocarcinoma: endoscopic and histologic surveillance. *Scand J Gastroenterol* 1993;28: 193–196
10. Rusch VW, Levine DS, Haggitt R, Reid BJ. The management of high grade dysplasia and early cancer in Barrett's esophagus. *Cancer* 1994;74:1225–1229
11. Parker SL, Tong T, Bolden S, Wingo PA. Cancer Statistics. 1996. CA 1996;46:5–27
12. Nishihira T, Nakano T, Mori S. Adjuvant therapies for cancer of the thoracic esophagus. *World J Surg* 1994;18: 388–398
13. Forastiere AA, Orringer MB, Perez-Tamayo C, et al. Preoperative chemoradiation followed by transhiatal esophagectomy for carcinoma of the esophagus: final report. *J Clin Oncol* 1993;11:1118–1123
14. Naunheim KS, Petruska P, Roy TS, et al. Preoperative chemotherapy and radiotherapy for esophageal carcinoma (discussion). *J Thorac Cardiovasc Surg* 1992;103: 887–893
15. Gill PG, Denham JW, Jamieson GG, et al. Patterns of treatment failure and prognostic factors associated with the treatment of esophageal carcinoma with chemotherapy and radiotherapy either as sole treatment or followed by surgery. *J Clin Oncol* 1992;10:1037–1043
16. Popp MB, Hawley D, Reising J, et al. Improved survival in squamous esophageal cancer: preoperative chemotherapy and irradiation. *Arch Surg* 1986;121:1330–1335
17. Skinner DB. En bloc resection for neoplasms of the esophagus and cardia. *J Thorac Cardiovasc Surg* 1983;85: 59–71
18. Abe S, Tachibana M, Shiraishi M, Nakamura T. Lymph node metastasis in resectable esophageal cancer. *J Thorac Cardiovasc Surg* 1990;100:287–291
19. Sugarbaker DJ, DeCamp MM. Selecting the surgical approach to cancer of the esophagus. *Chest* 1993;103 (suppl):410S–414S
20. Jaklitsch MT, Harpole DH, Healey EA, Sugarbaker DJ.

Current issues in the staging of esophageal cancer. *Semin Radiat Oncol* 1994;4(3):135–145

21. Inculet RI, Keller SM, Dwyer A, Roth JA. Evaluation of noninvasive tests for the preoperative staging of carcinoma of the esophagus. *Ann Thorac Surg* 1985;40:561–565

22. Van Overhagen H, Lameris JS, Berger MY, et al. Improved assessment of supraclavicular and abdominal metastases in oesophageal and gastro-esophageal junction carcinoma with the combination of ultrasound and computed tomography. *Br J Radiol* 1993;66:203–208

23. Siewart JR, Holscher AH, Dittler HJ. Preoperative staging and risk analysis in esophageal carcinoma. *Hepatogastroenterology* 1990;37:382–387

24. Van Dam J. Endosonographic evaluation of the patient with esophageal carcinoma. *Chest Surg Clin North Am* 1994; 4(2):269–284

25. Botet JF, Lightdale CJ, Zauber AG, et al. Preoperative staging of esophageal cancer: comparison of endoscopic US and dynamic CT. *Radiology* 1991;181:419–425

26. Akiyama H, Tsurumaru M, Kawamura T, Ono Y. Principles of surgical treatment for carcinoma of the esophagus: analysis of lymph node involvement. *Ann Surg* 1981;194:438–446

27. Krasna MJ, McLaughlin JS. Thoracoscopic lymph node staging for esophageal cancer. *Ann Thorac Surg* 1993;56:671–674

28. Ellis FH Jr, Watkins E Jr, Krasna MJ, et al. Staging of carcinoma of the esophagus and cardia: a comparison of different staging criteria. *J Surg Oncol* 1993;52:231–235

29. Orringer MB. Transhiatal esophagectomy without thoracotomy for carcinoma of the thoracic esophagus. *Ann Surg* 1984;200:282–288

30. Denk W. Zur Radikaloperation des Oesophaguskarfzentralbl. *Chirugie* 1913;4:1065

31. Turner GG. Excision of the thoracic esophagus for carcinoma with construction of an extrathoracic gullet. *Lancet* 1933;2:315

32. Orringer MB, Sloan H. Esophagectomy without thoracotomy. *J Thorac Cardiovasc Surg* 1978;76:643–654

33. Orringer MB, Marshall B, Stirling MC. Transhiatal esophagectomy for benign and malignant disease. *J Thorac Cardiovasc Surg* 1993;105:265–276

34. Orringer MB. Substernal gastric bypass of the excluded esophagus: results of an ill-advised operation. *Surgery* 1984;96:467–470

35. Conlan AA, Nicolaou N, Hammond CA, et al. Retrosternal gastric bypass for inoperable esophageal cancer: a report of 71 patients. *Ann Thorac Surg* 1983;36:396–401

36. Czerny J. Neue Operationen Vorlaufige Mitteilung. *Zentralbl Chir* 1877;4:433

37. McKeown KC. Total three-stage esophagectomy for cancer of the esophagus. *Br J Surg* 1976;63:259–262

38. Muller JM, Erasmi H, Stelzner M, et al. Surgical therapy of esophageal carcinoma. *Br J Surg* 1990;77:815

39. Skinner DB. Esophageal reconstruction. *Am J Surg* 1980; 139:810–814

40. Belsey RB. Reconstruction of the esophagus with left colon. *J Thorac Cardiovasc Surg* 1965;49:33–55

41. Mathisen DJ, Grillo HC, Wilkins EW Jr., et al. Transthoracic esophagectomy: a safe approach to carcinoma of the esophagus. *Ann Thorac Surg* 1988;45:137–43

42. Akiyama H. Surgery for carcinoma of the esophagus. *Curr Probl Surg* 1980;17:101

43. Lewis I. The surgical treatment of carcinoma of the esophagus: with special reference to a new operation for growths of the middle third. *Br J Surg* 1946;34:18–31

44. Wilkins EW, Burke JF. Colon esophageal bypass. *Am J Surg* 1975;129:394–400

45. DeMeester TR, Johansson KE, Franze I, et al. Indications, surgical technique, and long term functional results of colon interposition or bypass. *Ann Surg* 1988;208(4):460–474

46. Ventemiglia R, Khalil KG, Frazier OH, Mountain CF. The role of preoperative mesenteric arteriography in colon interposition. *J Thorac Cardiovasc Surg* 1977;74:98–104

47. Wain JC. Long segment colon interposition. *Semin Thorac Cardiovasc Surg* 1992;4:336–341

48. Wright C, Cuschieri A. Jejunal interposition for benign esophageal disease. Technical considerations and long-term results. *Ann Surg* 1987;205:54–60

49. Huang GJ, Wang LJ, Liu JS, et al. Surgery of esophageal carcinoma. *Semin Surg Oncol* 1985;1:74–83

50. Bardini R, Asolati M, Ruol A, et al. Anastomosis. *World J Surg* 1994;18:373–378

51. DeMeester TR, Barlow AP. Surgery and current management for cancer of the esophagus and cardia: part II. *Curr Probl Surg* 1988;25:535–605

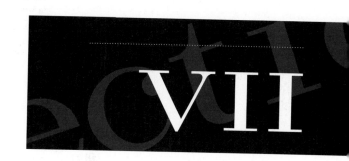

STOMACH AND DUODENUM

27

Diverticula, Volvulus, Superior Mesenteric Artery Syndrome, and Foreign Bodies

N.J. Cheshire ▪ *G. Glazer*

▪ DIVERTICULA OF THE STOMACH AND DUODENUM

The increasingly frequent use of contrast radiology, fiber optic endoscopy and computed tomography (CT) to screen for and investigate upper gastrointestinal pathology has resulted in a sharp increase in the detection of upper gastrointestinal diverticula. Previous studies, based on clinical and operative findings, suggested that diverticula of the stomach and duodenum were extremely rare. This discrepancy illustrates one of the most important features of upper gastrointestinal diverticula—they are almost invariably asymptomatic and rarely require surgical intervention.

GASTRIC DIVERTICULA

Diverticula of the stomach can be classified as true and false. Differentiation between the two types is usually obvious to the surgeon at operation, but radiological appearances may cause diagnostic difficulty.

False diverticula are usually a result of benign ulceration causing deep penetration (Fig 27–1) or a localized perforation (Fig 27–2). For example, other causes include necrotic neoplasms and external traction from adhesions. When explored at operation, it is important

to understand that these diverticula may not consist of any identifiable gastric wall.

True, or primary, gastric diverticula are rarer than their false counterparts. They may be multiple and are usually composed of all layers of the gastric wall. Etiology is uncertain, but they are probably congenital. True gastric diverticula account for about 3% of all gastrointestinal diverticula.

Incidence

In a review of 412 true gastric diverticula in the literature, 165 were diagnosed during approximately 380 000 routine barium meal examinations, an incidence of 0.04%.[1] However, in a personal series by Meerhoff and associates 30 diverticula were detected in 7500 radiological examinations, an incidence of 0.4%.[2] Although these figures vary by a factor of 10, it is unlikely that they represent real differences in the incidence of gastric diverticulosis, since small lesions are missed easily and reports from radiological series are very dependent on the operator.

Presentation

Diverticula may present at any age, but most occur in adults between 20 and 60 years of age (80% of Palmer's

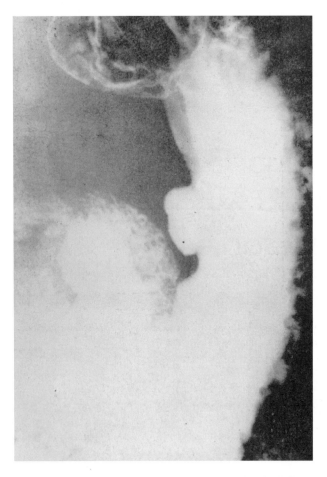

Figure 27–1. Deep lesser curve gastric ulcer, may be confused with a diverticulum on upper gastrointestinal studies.

shape. The size of the aperture between the gastric lumen and the diverticulum is also variable: large defects may be sufficient to admit one or two fingers at operation, while the smallest may be barely visible and allow only the introduction of a fine probe. In most cases, the ostium is between 2 to 4 cm in diameter. The size of the opening is associated with the development of complications; large-necked, open diverticula allow gastric contents to pass in and out of the sac without stagnation, and in these cases, the risk of complications is low. When the lumen is small, however, food residues may be retained and bacterial overgrowth may precipitate inflammatory changes. In addition, diverticula with small apertures easily may be missed on x-ray screening because of the inability of contrast medium to enter the sac.

Complications

Complications of gastric diverticula are rare. Stasis with bacterial overgrowth can cause acute diverticulitis, and perforation may occur in severe cases. Alternatively, erosion of local blood vessels by the inflammatory process may cause hemorrhage and hematemesis. Bleeding associated with perforation, causing hemoperitoneum also have been described.[5] Large juxtacardiac lesions have long been recognized as causes of dysphagia, but recently a rare case of adult pyloric outflow obstruction secondary to a gastric diverticulum was published.[6] Less commonly, malignant neoplasms and the presence of

series).[1] In children lesions are most often primary diverticula and are prone to develop complications; for example, a 4 month old child was successfully operated for a diverticulum of the stomach, that had strangulated through the mesocolon.[3] More recently, a bleeding fundal diverticulum causing hematemesis in a child was reported.[4]

Pathology

Gastric diverticula occur most commonly around the posterior aspect of the cardia, (Fig 27–3) on the right side. In Meeroff's study, 80% of patients had juxtacardiac diverticula while the remainder were mostly juxtapyloric (Fig 27–4). Palmer reported his collected series of 342 gastric diverticula: 259 were in the posterior proximal part of the stomach (73%), 31 in the antrum (Fig 27–5), 29 in the body, 15 in the pylorus, and 8 in the fundus.

Gastric diverticula vary greatly in size but most measure between 1 to 6 cm in diameter and are saccular in

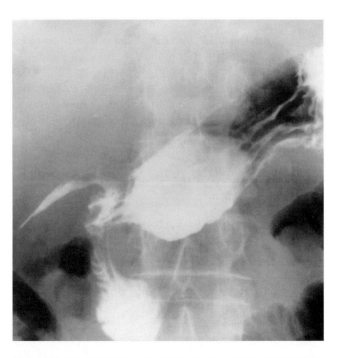

Figure 27–2. Localized perforation of a pyloric ulcer. The contained contrast may appear to be in a diverticulum.

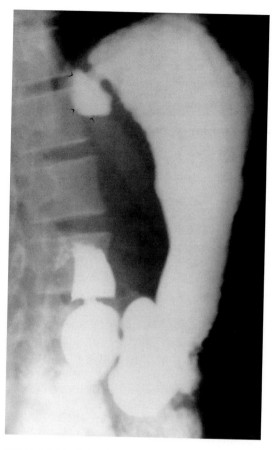

Figure 27–3. Lateral view of a gastric diverticulum (*arrow*) during upper gastrointestinal contrast study; the lesions occur most commonly around the cardia, on its posterior surface.

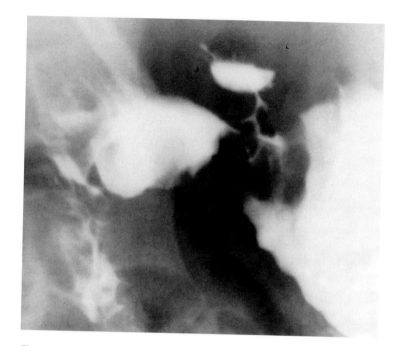

Figure 27–4. Diverticulum in the pyloric channel (*arrow*).

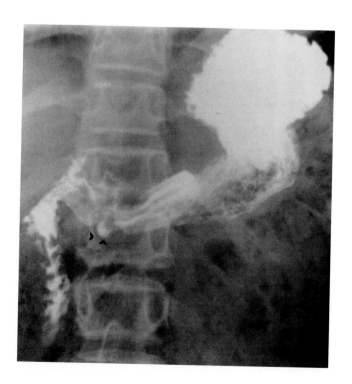

Figure 27–5. Antral diverticulum (*arrow*).

foreign bodies and enteroliths within diverticula have been recorded.

Diagnosis

The vast majority of gastric diverticula produce no symptoms unless one of the aforementioned complications supervene. Therefore, most are incidental findings during investigations for upper gastrointestinal disease. Discovery of a diverticulum, in the absence of other pathology, can present difficulty; it is possible that, in some patients, a large gastric diverticulum distended with food debris may cause epigastric fullness and discomfort, but in the absence of specific complications, surgical excision of diverticula rarely provides symptomatic relief.

Diverticula most often are discovered on upper gastrointestinal contrast studies and appear as well-circumscribed, smooth, evenly rounded projections from the gastric lumen. Contrast may pool at the bottom of the sac, with an air bubble above it when the patient is in the erect position (Fig 27–4 and Fig 27–5).

Diverticula arising from the anterior or posterior wall may easily be missed unless a double-contrast technique is used and the patient is examined in all positions between the extreme Trendelenburg and the erect position. Small diverticula may be mistaken for a large penetrating gastric ulcer, or vice versa. Differentiation often depends on the site of the lesion, since juxtacardiac ulcers are rare. Other differential diagnoses on barium meal include carcinoma of the cardia, hiatus hernia, diverticulum of the terminal portion of the esophagus, and cascade stomach.

On CT scanning, gastric diverticula usually are demonstrable if the patient is given oral contrast. If contrast is not given, or if the diverticulum does not fill, CT appearances may mimic an adrenal tumor.[7]

Artefacts may be seen that mimic the appearance of an intraluminal gastric diverticulum on barium-meal examination.[8] These artefacts appear to have occurred in relatively unprepared patients, suggesting that they are related to an interaction between the barium and retained gastric fluid. In fact, unlike the duodenum, there have been no examples of pathologically verified gastric intramural diverticulum.

Endoscopy is most valuable in making a differential diagnosis among abnormalities seen on barium-meal examination.

Treatment

Most diverticula of the stomach are asymptomatic. When found during the course of investigations of dyspeptic symptoms, in the absence of other pathology, it may be tempting to undertake surgical treatment. If complications of the diverticulum are not present, such surgery is unlikely to relieve the symptoms of the patient. Surgical management is indicated only when complications such as those described above have developed, when there is an associated lesion present that requires surgical treatment, or when the diagnosis is uncertain and laparotomy is deemed advisable as a last resort.

A case can be made for elective excision of an asymptomatic large diverticulum with a narrow ostium (in circumstances analogous to the treatment of narrow-necked hernias), since such a lesion has a high probability of developing diverticulitis in the future.

Operative Technique

Surgical treatment of gastric diverticula depends on the position of the lesion in the stomach and presence or absence of associated pathology.

If the diverticulum is near the cardia, it is displayed by mobilizing the upper half of the greater curvature of the stomach and reflecting the body and cardia to bring the posterior gastric wall into view (Fig 27–6). A careful dissection in this rather inaccessible area, including division of any adhesions that tether the sac to the pancreas or to the stomach wall itself, and a certain amount of traction on the diverticulum will be necessary before the neck of the pouch is identified clearly. The diverticulum then is amputated and the stump closed in two layers of catgut. Alternatively, a linear stapling device can be employed to close the base.

If there is difficulty in finding the diverticulum at laparotomy, Heijboer and Nieuwenhuizen advise cross-clamping the antrum and filling the stomach with saline solution via a nasogastric tube.[9]

Diverticula of the lesser and greater curvatures of the stomach can be excised simply and the gap repaired. Excision is preferable to inversion of the sac, followed by closure of the defect in the gastric wall, since the risk of recurrence or intraluminal complications is reduced. Inversion and closure might be carried out in poor-risk patients or when technical difficulty prevents excision and suture. Complete relief of symptoms following this simple inversion procedure has been reported in two patients.[10]

Diverticula of the pyloric region may well be treated best by performing a partial gastrectomy, which may be necessary if there is an associated gastric lesion.

Laparoscopic approaches to the treatment of gastric diverticula have not been reported at the time of writing, but no doubt this approach, perhaps using an endoscopically introduced stapler, may be feasible in some cases.

DUODENAL DIVERTICULA

Like their gastric counterparts, diverticula of the duodenum are classified as primary or secondary. The ma-

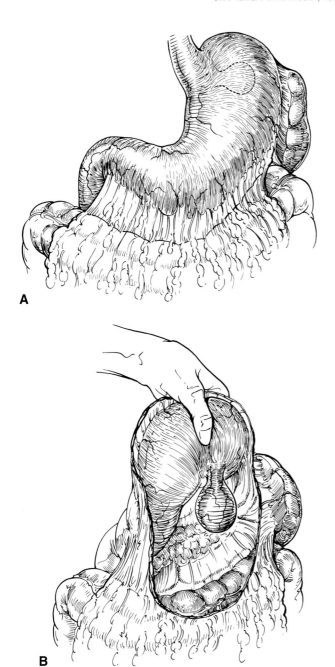

A

B

Figure 27–6. Gastric diverticulum at the cardia. **A**. With the stomach in situ. **B**. Mobilization of the upper greater curvature by division of the short gastric vessels to allow rotation of the stomach.

Incidence

In one series, between 1914 and 1960, at the Henry Ford Hospital, in Detroit, MI, an incidence of just over 1% in more than 1 million consecutive barium-meal examinations was found.[11] However, postmortem examinations suggest that the condition occurs much more frequently. Ackerman (1943), by making plaster of Paris casts of the duodenum in 50 cadavers selected at random, found 11 specimens with diverticula, an incidence of 22 percent.

In a review of the literature on duodenal diverticula, of nine published studies reporting over 2900 postmortem examinations, the reported incidence ranged from 2.2% to 22% with an average of 8.6%.[13] Of 11 radiological studies, of a total of approximately 90 000 examinations, the incidence varied from 0.016% to 5%, with an average of 1.7%. A more modern study of 451 barium meals, in patients more than 65 years of age, many in a geriatric unit, demonstrated 39 duodenal diverticula, an incidence of 8.5 percent.[14]

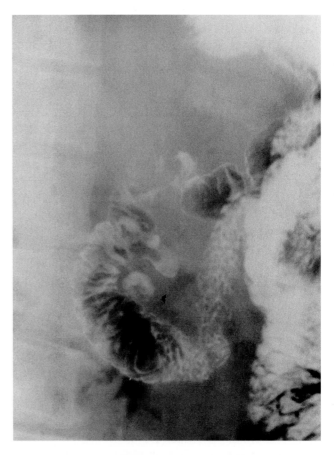

Figure 27–7. Duodenal diverticulum in the most common position, in the second part of the duodenum arising from the concave border of the bowel (*arrow*).

jority of the secondary or false diverticula are the result of chronic duodenal ulceration, the so-called prestenotic diverticulum. Therefore, discussion will be concerned solely with the primary type.

By far the majority of primary duodenal diverticula are solitary (about 90%), and most occur in the second part of the duodenum (about 80%), commonly on its concavity in the region of the ampulla of Vater (Fig 27–7).

Presentation

Duodenal diverticula are rare before 30 years of age and most cases are diagnosed in patients between 50 and 65 years of age. The frequency in the two sexes is equal.

Pathology

Primary duodenal diverticula are essentially mucosal outpouchings and therefore, are devoid of muscle. The neck of most duodenal diverticula arise from the second part of the duodenum (Fig 27–7), although they may be found in the third or fourth portion (Fig 27–8). The position of the fundus and the body of the diverticulum is variable and depends on the size of the lesion. Most lie in the retroperitoneum, with a large proportion situated on the concave medial surface of the gut, close to the common bile and pancreatic ducts. In these cases, the neck of the diverticulum often opens into the duodenum close to the papilla. The sac may lie alongside, extend behind, or even penetrate into the pancreas and occasionally, the common bile duct and the duct of Wirsung may open into the diverticulum itself.

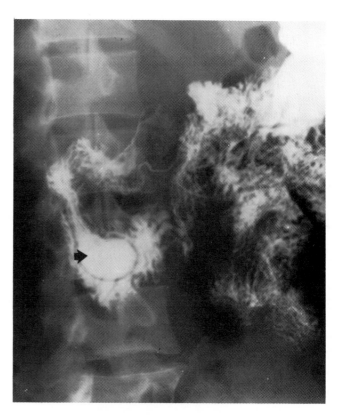

Figure 27–9. Unusual diverticulum arising from the lateral side of the duodenum.

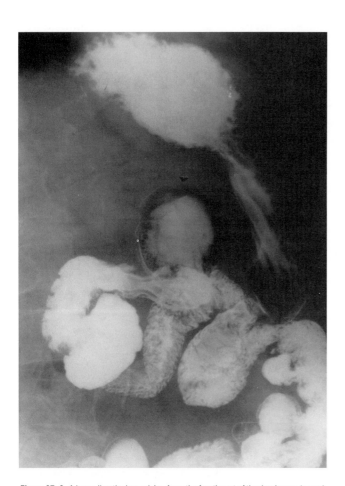

Figure 27–8. A large diverticulum arising from the fourth part of the duodenum (*arrow*) in a patient who also has jejunal diverticulosis.

A more unusual case, where the neck of the diverticulum arises from the convex side of the duodenum, is shown in Fig 27–9. In some cases, these appearances are suggested on barium study when the fundus of a diverticulum originating on the medial border of the bowel projects over the lateral border of the duodenum, giving a false impression of a laterally arising neck.

Although unusual, duodenal diverticula may be "inverted," with the sac visible in the lumen of the duodenum (Fig 27–10). In 1964[15] six cases of intraluminal duodenal diverticula were collected and reported, bringing the total of reported cases at that time to fourteen. A recent review of this subject was given by Abdel-Hafiz and his colleagues.[16]

Clinical Manifestations

The great majority of duodenal diverticula are asymptomatic. In one series of 1064 patients with this condition, only one had a serious complication (diverticulitis and common duct obstruction) that necessitated operation.[11] Five others resulted in diverticulectomy (0.5%), but all had additional upper gastrointestinal abnormalities. When symptoms do occur, they are usually the result of the complications of this condition, although in some instances, distention of the pouch may produce symptoms that are indistinguishable from those caused

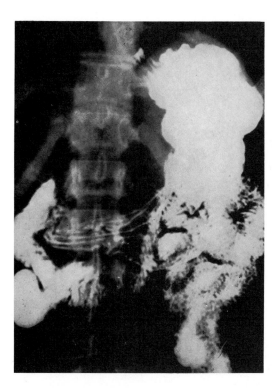

Figure 27–10. Intraluminal duodenal diverticulum.

by peptic ulcer, cholecystitis, or pancreatitis. This diagnosis may be implied by the retention of barium in the sac for 6 or more hours during radiological investigation.

The most common complications of duodenal diverticula have been well reviewed.[17–19] These complications can be conveniently divided into those related to pressure on adjacent structures, and those caused by inflammation. Jaundice, cholangitis, acute and chronic pancreatitis, and duodenal obstruction can result from mechanical compression by a duodenal diverticulum, whereas diverticulitis, ulceration with hemorrhage, perforation, abscess, and internal fistula occur as inflammatory sequelae. Endoscopic biliary manometry has been used to demonstrate abnormalities in the function of the sphincter of Oddi in association with periampullary duodenal diverticula and suggested that these abnormalities, rather than simple pressure effects, may account for some of the biliary and pancreatic disease seen in patients with these lesions.[20] Despite this, however, a case has been described of acute pancreatitis secondary to papillary obstruction by an intraluminal duodenal diverticulum.[21]

An interesting cause of perforation of duodenal diverticula is stercoral ulceration caused by the presence of a stone in the diverticulum. Such a stone also may pass down the lumen of the gut before impacting and producing enterolith ileus. Less spectacularly, but more commonly, duodenal diverticula may impair the investigation of upper gastrointestinal disease by preventing endoscopic retrograde cholangiopancreatography (ERCP) examination.

Preoperative diagnosis invariably is based on an upper gastrointestinal barium-meal series and fibre optic duodenoscopy. A careful search must always be made for other pathologic conditions that possibly may be responsible for the signs and symptoms.

Treatment

Surgery for diverticula of the duodenum is indicated only when there are complications producing symptoms. Such complications are so rare that in spite of a professional lifetime of interest in gastrointestinal diverticula, Professor Harold Ellis, writing in the previous edition of this book, claims never to have operated on a diverticulum in this situation. This is a common experience that we share.

The removal of a diverticulum adjacent to the ampulla of Vater may be difficult. Injury to the ampulla and subsequent interference with the drainage of bile or pancreatic secretion may lead to jaundice, pancreatitis, or even the development of a duodenal fistula. Consequently, diverticula found on routine examination of the upper gastrointestinal tract should be left alone. Those that are associated with vague upper abdominal symptoms demand a thorough investigation to eliminate other causes. Even if these are negative, and the diverticulum is the only abnormality found in a patient with persistent symptoms, surgical excision must be approached with caution and some skepticism; in one report >50% of patients treated by operation were entirely relieved of their symptoms.[19]

When surgery is undertaken for a diverticulum of the second part of the duodenum, the operation involves mobilization of the bowel by Kocher's maneuver (incising the peritoneum along the convex aspect of the duodenum) and reflection of the gut medially and to the left, thus exposing the thin-walled sac and the yellow lobulated head of the mobilized pancreas (Fig 27–11). The diverticulum is dissected out from the retroperitoneal tissues surrounding it, taking care to avoid damage to the terminal portions of the nearby common bile and pancreatic ducts. The fundus is grasped with tissue forceps to provide traction and the dissection proceeds to isolate the pedicle. Once sufficiently freed up, the sac is opened to expose the papilla of Vater and thus, avoid damage to it. The diverticulum then is excised flush with the duodenal wall. The resulting enterotomy is sutured transversely in two layers.

In some cases, where closure of the bowel wall may impinge on the lower end of the bile duct, it is a sensible precaution to open the supraduodenal portion of the common bile duct and insert a long T tube down the

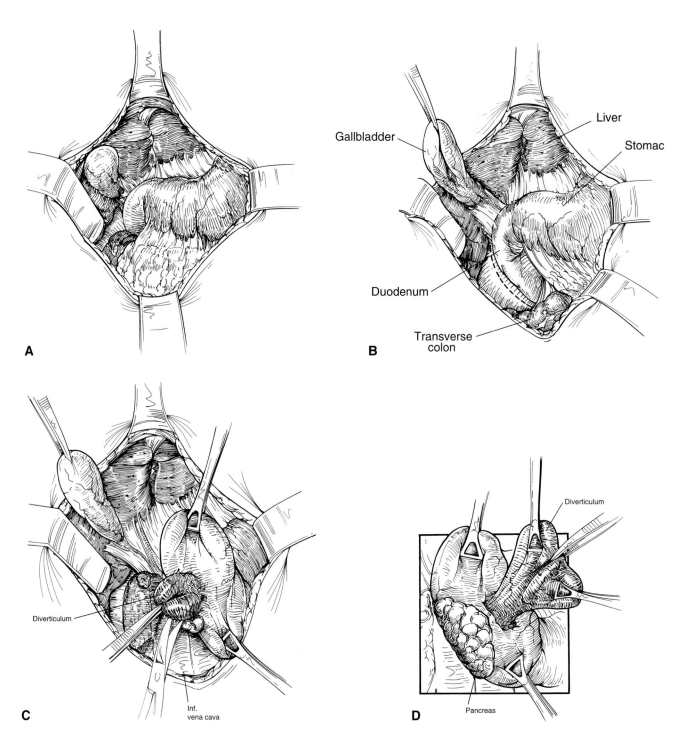

A

B

Gallbladder

Liver

Stomac

Duodenum

Transverse
colon

C

Diverticulum

Inf.
vena cava

D

Diverticulum

Pancreas

Figure 27–11. A and **B**. Exposure of the duodenum and incision (*dotted line*) for Kocher's maneuver. **C** and **D**, Operation to expose a diverticulum of the second part of the duodenum. (Adapted from Madden JL. Excision of duodenal diverticulum. In: *Atlas of Technics in Surgery,* 2nd ed. New York, NY: Appleton-Century-Crofts; 1964:320

duct into the duodenum before attempting closure of the defect. The tube serves as a useful guide during the dissection, especially when the common duct opens into the sac. The T tube is left in situ for 10 days postoperatively.

Diverticula arising from the third or fourth part of the duodenum may be approached through the transverse mesocolon, taking care to avoid the right colic artery or injury to the pancreatic substance (Fig 27–12). The sacs of diverticula of the third and fourth parts of the duodenum may lie deep to the pancreas or actually be incorporated into pancreatic tissue. Although simple excision and closure usually are feasible (and constitute the treatment of choice), alternative procedures may be used. Simple inversion of the diverticulum and closure of the muscle defect obviate danger of leakage, but partial duodenal obstruction or bleeding may occur. If dissection of the sac is difficult and there is possibility of injury to the common bile duct, pancreatic duct, or duodenal blood supply, a Roux-en-Y diverticulojejunostomy may be necessary. In difficult cases of peri-Vaterian or intrapancreatic diverticula, duodenotomy and inversion of the sac from the luminal aspect of the bowel have been advised.

A novel method was reported in a patient with a 6-cm diameter diverticulum extending upwards behind the pancreas, making dissection from the outside difficult and hazardous.[22] After opening the anterior wall of the duodenum, the sac was packed with ribbon gauze through its luminal orifice, and a circular mucosal incision was made around the mouth of the diverticulum, developed between the mucosal and serosal layers of the duodenum and extended into the retropancreatic tissues. This allowed the diverticulum to be excised intact. The diathermy incision in the duodenal wall was closed in two layers and the anterior duodenotomy closed transversely.

Despite ingenious approaches such as this, resection can still be difficult, especially when the biliary anatomy is disturbed. It has been suggested that common bile duct obstruction in cases where the ampulla enters a duodenal diverticulum was managed best by choledochoduodenostomy as opposed to any direct surgical assault on the diverticulum.[23]

■ GASTRIC VOLVULUS

Gastric volvulus was first described by Berti in 1866 at autopsy on a 60 year old woman who had died of high, closed-loop bowel obstruction.[24] Berg carried out the first recorded successful operation on a patient with this condition in 1896,[25] and Rosselet demonstrated radiological diagnosis of the condition in 1920.[26] Buchanan published a collective review of 33 cases in 1930,[27] and, by 1952, Dalgaard had analyzed the results of 150 patients collected from previously published papers.[28] In 1971, Wastell and Ellis reported eight examples and reviewed the literature of over 200 cases.[29] In recent years the condition, although still uncommon, has been reported more and more frequently, probably as a consequence of the increased frequency of upper gastrointestinal investigations. In particular, it has become recognized (through radiology) that chronic volvulus may occur without symptoms.

PATHOLOGY

The stomach is normally secured at the esophageal hiatus proximally and by the peritoneal attachments of the second part of the duodenum distally. The lesser curvature is anchored by the left gastric vessels and the gastrohepatic ligament, whereas the greater curvature is held less firmly by the short gastric vessels and the peritoneal attachments of the spleen and transverse colon, the gastrosplenic and gastrocolic ligaments. In autopsy studies, it was shown that the normal stomach cannot be rotated through 180° unless one or both of the latter two attachments are divided; the pylorus becomes approximated to the cardia when the stomach is full, thus making rotation easier.[28] It is a common observation that symptoms of volvulus appear after eating a large meal.

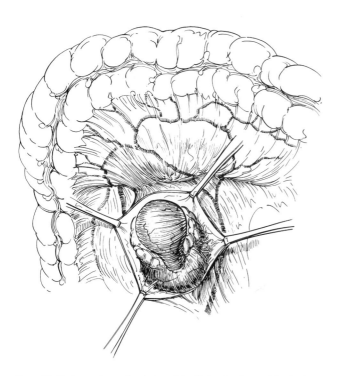

Figure 27–12. Approach to a diverticulum of the third or fourth part of the duodenum through the transverse mesocolon. Care must be taken to avoid injury to the right and middle colic vessels. (after Kidd)

When gastric volvulus occurs in the absence of associated abnormality or disease within the abdominal cavity, it is termed "idiopathic." This usually occurs only when there is considerable lengthening of the attachments of the stomach to the parietes.

In approximately 75% of cases, gastric volvulus is associated with, or secondary to, some other pathological factor. The following conditions often are found:

1. Hiatus hernia: congenital or acquired
2. Other diaphragmatic hernias resulting from trauma or congenital defects
3. Eventration of the left diaphragm, either idiopathic or after phrenic nerve injury
4. Pyloric obstruction that produces chronic dilatation of the stomach
5. Adhesions

In one series, one patient underwent surgery for radiologically diagnosed gastric volvulus almost 50 years after open cholecystectomy.[29] At operation, the omentum had gathered into a ball adherent to the laparotomy scar and was acting as the apex of an easily reduced volvulus of the stomach. Gastropexy was performed with complete recovery.

An example of organoaxial volvulus after highly selected vagotomy for pyloric stenosis has been reported.[30] At operation, the greater curvature of a grossly dilated stomach was adherent to the anterior edge of the liver, with the combination of gastric dilatation and adhesions sufficient to produce the gastric torsion.

In a classification of volvulus of the stomach, several factors must be taken into consideration, and the classification is therefore a mixed one of type, extent, direction, severity, and etiology.

Type

An organoaxial volvulus (Figs 27–13, 27–14, and 27–15) is one that occurs around a line from the pylorus to the esophagogastric junction.

A mesenterioaxial volvulus (Figs 27–16 and 27–17) occurs around the axis that runs from the center of the greater curvature of the stomach to the porta hepatis. This line is approximately at right angles to that for an organoaxial volvulus.

Organoaxial volvulus occurs more commonly than mesenterioaxial volvulus. In a review of over 200 cases, 59% were organoaxial, 29% were mesenterioaxial, 2% were combined, and the remaining 10% were not classified.[29]

Extent

The whole stomach may be implicated (total), or only part of the stomach involved (partial). Most cases of total gastric volvulus are organoaxial, as are the majority of acute cases. This type usually is associated with di-

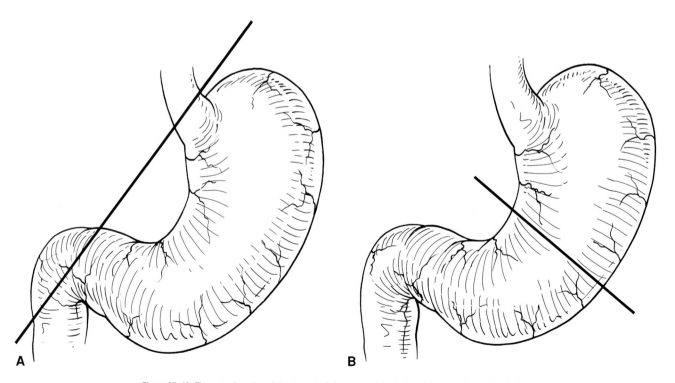

Figure 27–13. The axes of rotation of the stomach. **A.** In organoaxial volvulus. **B.** In mesenterioaxial volvulus.

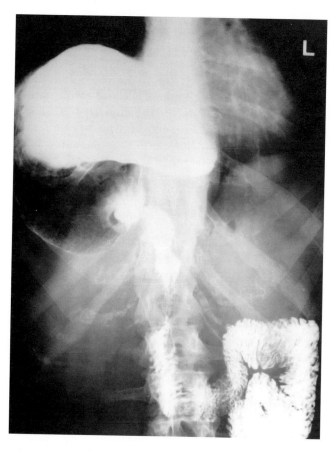

Figure 27–14. Contrast study showing organoaxial volvulus of the whole stomach.

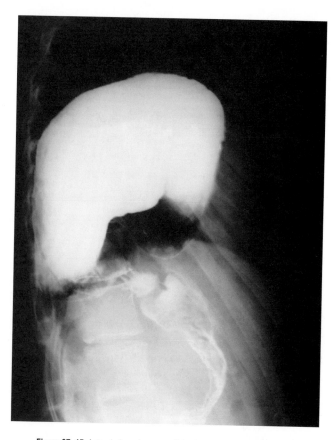

Figure 27–15. Lateral view of organoaxial volvulus seen in Figure 27–14.

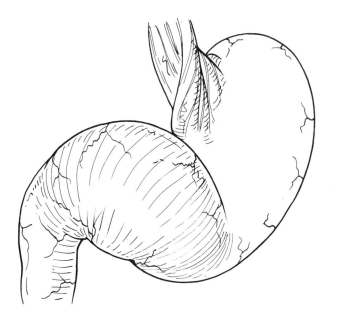

Figure 27–16. Approximation of the cardia and pylorus in the full stomach facilitates rotation. The drawing shows conditions predisposing to mesenterioaxial volvulus.

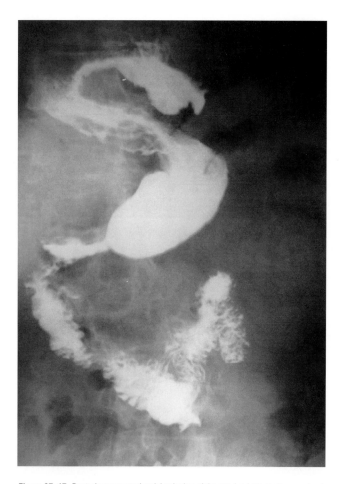

Figure 27–17. Posterior mesenterioaxial volvulus of the proximal stomach on contrast study (see text for definition of direction).

aphragmatic hernia or eventration. The mesenterioaxial volvulus, in contrast, is more often idiopathic and partial in extent, often being limited to the mobile distal portion of the stomach. Fig 27–17 shows a partial volvulus of the proximal part of the stomach.

Direction

By convention, an organoaxial volvulus, in which the transverse colon comes to lie in front of the stomach, and a mesenterioaxial volvulus, in which the pylorus passes in front of the stomach, are both termed "anterior." This type is much more common than the posterior type. This is as expected on anatomic grounds because, for posterior rotation to occur in the organoaxial type, the transverse colon must pass behind the stomach, elongating or tearing the mesocolon as it does so. It is not surprising, therefore, that a posterior type of volvulus was present in only 8 of the 93 organoaxial cases reviewed.[29] However, in 10 to 47 mesenterioaxial cases, rotation commencing with the forward displace-

ment of the splenic region of the fundus had occurred (Fig 27–17). Such cases are classified as posterior.

Severity

The volvulus may be acute when it occurs as an abdominal emergency, and either obstruction or actual strangulation of the stomach (or both) can occur. Gangrenous change is uncommon because of the widely anastomosing blood supply to the stomach and is more prone to occur in the organoaxial type; in one series, gangrene occurred in 7 of the 25 cases of acute gastric volvulus.[31]

More commonly, in clinical practice, the volvulus is chronic or recurrent. In Wastell and Ellis' review, 60% of the mesenterioaxial and 64% of the organoaxial cases from previous publications were recorded as acute.[29] This obvious discrepancy between cases reported and clinical experience is probably the result of a bias in reporting of acute volvulus, with its often dire consequences, and considered more worthy of publication than asymptomatic chronic volvulus.

Etiology

The classification of these cases as idiopathic or secondary has already been described.

CLINICAL MANIFESTATIONS

Gastric volvulus may occur at any age. In both men and women, the peak incidence occurs in the fifth decade, and the distribution is relatively normal. Two examples have been reported of intrathoracic organoaxial volvulus occurring in the first week of life; both neonates had a large lax esophageal hiatus and absence of the gastrocolic ligament.[32] Forty-nine previous case reports in children under 12 have been reported, of which 26 occurred in the first 12 months of life and 11 in the first month. Another series reported 10 cases in children, four of whom were under 1 year of age, and one was premature.[33] The incidence is approximately the same in both sexes.

Chronic volvulus may be symptomless and an incidental finding on a barium-meal examination, chest x-ray, CT, or magnetic resonance imaging (MRI). If symptoms occur, they usually consist of mild, upper abdominal discomfort with features that are impossible to differentiate from peptic ulcer or calculus disease of the gallbladder. Pain or bloating during meals or shortly thereafter may occur, and can be followed by retching and vomiting. However, if the stomach becomes very distended, it may obstruct the esophagogastric junction and thus prevent belching or vomiting. This may be relieved when the patient lies down, since the swallowed gas can then leave the pylorus. Symptoms resulting from an associated pathology, such as hiatus hernia, may be present, or the patient may complain of breathlessness if there is a marked degree of eventration of the diaphragm or a large paraesophageal hernia.

Acute volvulus presents a striking clinical picture, first described in 1904 by Borchardt, who emphasizes three main features: (1) severe epigastric pain and distention, (2) vomiting followed by violent retching with an inability to vomit, (3) difficulty or inability to pass a nasogastric tube.[34] In classical cases, the sequence of pathological events that produce this picture is believed to begin with pyloric occlusion (causing the incessant vomiting characteristic of high obstruction), followed by obstruction of the cardia (producing inability to vomit or to pass a stomach tube). In the more severe cases, this is followed by distention of the stomach with gas and fluids in a closed-loop type of obstruction.

In a study of 25 cases of acute gastric volvulus, it was suggested that three additional findings are of prime importance:

1. Minimal abdominal signs when the stomach is in the thorax
2. A gas-filled viscus in the lower part of the chest or the upper abdomen shown by chest radiography, especially when associated with a paraesophageal hiatus hernia
3. Obstruction at the site of the volvulus as demonstrated by emergency upper gastrointestinal barium studies[31]

Gangrene occurred in 7 of the 25 cases (28%) in this series, and the distinctive features of gastric volvulus with strangulation included gastrointestinal bleeding, acute cardiorespiratory distress, and shock.[31] Most cases of acute gastric volvulus are organoaxial, and associated with eventration of the diaphragm, paraesophageal hiatus hernia, or traumatic diaphragmatic hernia.

TREATMENT

Chronic Volvulus

When symptoms of chronic recurrent volvulus are disabling, operative measure may be undertaken to correct the underlying abnormality. Careful investigation of the patient to identify an associated lesion that may also need treatment, particularly hiatus hernia, or accompanying conditions, such as peptic ulcer or biliary disease, must be undertaken.

At operation, a careful search is made for adhesive bands, abnormal ligamentous laxity, associated peptic ulcer or tumor, diaphragmatic hernia, or the presence of eventration of the diaphragm. The stomach may well be in a normal position at the time of operation, but the volvulus can be reproduced by twisting the stomach in the appropriate direction.

Treatment must be directed towards the type of volvulus found.

Primary Volvulus. In primary volvulus with no obvious cause, some form of gastropexy must be considered by tacking the anterior wall of the stomach to the parietal peritoneum of the abdominal wall.

Volvulus Resulting From Other Conditions. If the volvulus is a result of some other condition, correction of the primary defect may be adequate, such as repair of a diaphragmatic hernia or of a traumatic defect in the diaphragm, or division of bands that obstruct or sling up the stomach.

Volvulus Resulting From Non-Operable Conditions. In this third situation, volvulus results from some other condition that does not lead itself readily to surgical correction. Examples are eventration of the diaphragm or abnormal ligamentous laxity. Under these circumstances, a partial gastrectomy will be curative, but this is a radical operation for such a condition. A simpler procedure is the colonic displacement operation.[35] An account of the operation is as follows (Fig 27–18):

"Carefully separate the stomach from the transverse colon by dividing the gastrocolic omentum from duodenum to the gastric fundus. Any adhesions of the ascending colon or the hepatic and splenic flexures of the colon are divided. When this is completed, and provided there is an average length of mesocolon, the whole mobilized transverse colon and greater omentum can now be made to rise and fill the left subphrenic area without tension. A simple gastropexy will not give a far greater chance of success . . . As the subphrenic space is now filled with colon, the upward pulling force and the direct drag on the greater curve of the stomach is eliminated and so there is a greatly reduced chance of recurrent volvulus."[35]

Gastrojejunostomy is advocated as a simple method of preventing recurrence of gastric volvulus, because anastomosis to the fixed point of the gastrojejunal junction tethers the untwisted stomach.[36]

In patients unfit for laparotomy, insertion of a percutaneous endoscopic gastrostomy (PEG) tube, using upper gastrointestinal endoscopy to locate the site of the stomach on the anterior abdominal wall, has been described by some authors. However, two cases of gastric volvulus in handicapped patients being fed through gastrostomy tubes have been described, and it has been suggested that the additional anchor site provided by the tube may, in some circumstances, predispose to twisting of the stomach.[37] This may be prevented by using two percutaneously inserted gastrostomy tubes to prevent recurrent volvulus in an unfit patient.[38] Gastrostomy tubes may be safely removed after sufficient

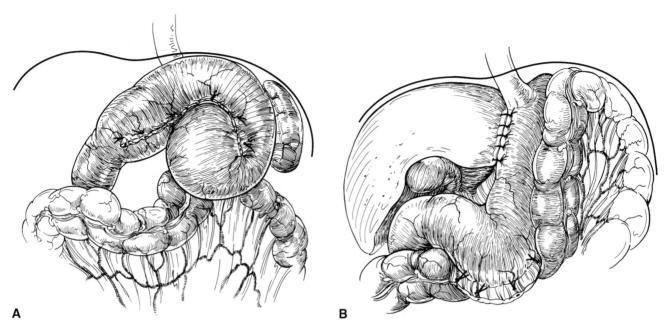

A

B

Figure 27–18. Principles of the colonic displacement operation described by Tanner. (From Tanner NC. Chronic and recurrent volvulus of the stomach with late results of colonic displacement. *Am J Surg* 1968;115:505)

time has passed to allow the stomach to adhere to the anterior abdominal wall.

Laparoscopy has been used to reduce and fix an organoaxial volvulus associated with hiatus hernia.[39] Techniques such as this may become important in the treatment of gastric volvulus in patients unfit for more major surgery, but at the time of writing, experience is limited.

Acute Volvulus

Acute volvulus can sometimes be reduced by the passage of a nasogastric tube, but more frequently, a tube cannot be passed and immediate operation is mandatory. The volvulus is reduced surgically. If gastric necrosis has taken place, local excision, subtotal gastrectomy, or total resection will be required, depending on the extent of the ischemic injury. If the stomach is viable, attention is directed to the correction of any underlying condition that may have been a precipitating factor. However, in a patient at extremely high risk, a temporary gastrostomy may be the safest and quickest procedure at this stage.

■ SUPERIOR MESENTERIC ARTERY SYNDROME

Rokitansky in 1842 was the first to postulate that the third part of the duodenum might be compressed and obstructed by the superior mesenteric artery. Sixty-five years later, Bloodgood went on to suggest that this con-

dition could be treated surgically by duodenojejunostomy.[40] However, the first successful operation was not recorded for another three years.[41] In 1921, Wilkie published a classic article on this subject, giving a detailed account of the pathologic features of the condition and advocated duodenojejunostomy as the most certain method of treatment. It is of interest that he found evidence of chronic peptic ulceration in 35 of the 135 patients upon whom he operated. It was Wilkie who coined the term "chronic duodenal ileus," a misnomer, since this is a mechanical obstruction rather than a paralytic condition, as implied by the term ileus.

In succeeding decades, the condition was blamed for a large number of vague upper gastrointestinal symptoms, and the syndrome fell into some disrepute. However, a masterly review of the subject presented 281 examples collected from previous publications of both acute and chronic obstruction of the duodenum by the superior mesenteric artery and suggested the term "vascular compression of the duodenum."[42] The condition also has been called duodenal ileus, gastromesenteric ileus, arteriomesenteric duodenal compression syndrome, and Wilkie's disease. At the time of writing, there is still no consensus on terminology. However, Harold Ellis has suggested that the most appropriate term is the superior mesenteric artery (SMA) syndrome. This term will be used in the ensuing description.

Acute onset of the SMA syndrome was described by a number of authors when plaster body casts and hip spicas were in common use in orthopedic practice. The first example of this was described by Willett in 1878—a fatal case that followed application of a plaster of Paris jacket in a case of spinal scoliosis.[43] This association has unfortunately added to the confusion of terminology; in 1950 Dorph called the condition the "cast syndrome,"[44] while Hall, in 1974, pointed out that acute obstruction could occur in patients after trauma, requiring bedrest in the supine position, without plaster, particularly if there had been rapid loss of weight after trauma.[45] He termed this "the cast syndrome incognito"!

Recent reviews of the subject include a report of 10 examples and a review of 125 cases,[46] and a study from Westminster Hospital, London.[47]

ANATOMY

One of the consequences of man's erect posture is that the superior mesenteric artery comes off the aorta at a more acute angle than it does in four-legged animals. The third part of the duodenum passes through this angle, hitched up at its junction with the fourth part by the suspensory ligament of Treitz (Fig 27–19). The posterior limb of this angle is formed by the lumbar vertebrae, the paravertebral muscles, and the aorta; the anterior limb is formed by the superior mesenteric vessels and sometimes, by one of their first two branches in the transverse mesocolon. The narrowest part of the angle, above the duodenum, contains the uncinate process of the pancreas and the left renal vein. In normal individuals, the superior mesenteric artery frequently grooves the anterior surface of the duodenum, and occasionally, compression is produced by the middle colic artery.

In a normal person, the mass of fat and lymphatic tissue around the origin of the superior mesenteric artery is believed to protect the duodenum from compression. The syndrome occurs almost invariably in thin patients. Factors that may precipitate obstruction are sudden weight loss (consider in anorexia nervosa), rapid growth in height, an increased lordosis, a short mesentery, or a high attachment of the ligament of Treitz. Recent reports have highlighted the frequency of the condition in traumatic quadriplegic patients, many of whom lose weight rapidly and may be positioned supine for prolonged periods; two reviews describe eight young patients (10 to 20 years) who developed SMA syndrome after traumatic brain injury.[48,49] As described above, immobilization of an orthopedic patient in the hyperextended position, and application of a plaster cast in the treatment of scoliosis or vertebral injury are other precipitating factors. Less commonly, a variation of the

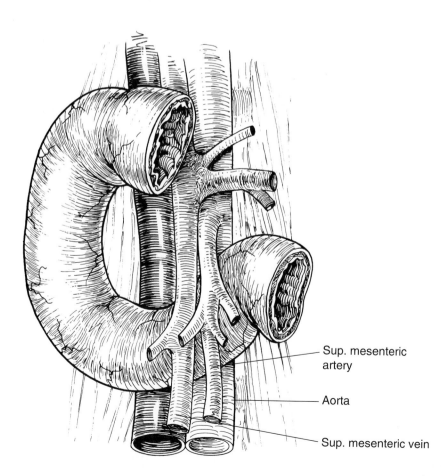

Figure 27–19. Important anatomy in the SMA syndrome. The third part of the duodenum can be seen lying in the angle between the superior mesenteric artery and the aorta.

Sup. mesenteric artery

Aorta

Sup. mesenteric vein

SMA syndrome has been described in association with an abdominal aortic aneurysm,[50] while the syndrome was found in a patient with a traumatic pseudoaneurysm of the superior mesenteric artery.[51]

Measurement of the aortomesenteric angle at abdominal angiography has demonstrated that this angle is more acute in patients with the SMA syndrome than in control subjects, because the distance is reduced between the aorta and the superior mesenteric artery.[52] This angle also may now be measured by using color duplex doppler techniques.

CLINICAL MANIFESTATIONS

The SMA syndrome tends to affect young adults most commonly. Approximately three-quarters of patients are between 10 and 39 years of age, and 60% are female.

The clinical picture may have either a chronic or an acute presentation.

Chronic Vascular Compression

Chronic vascular compression usually presents with epigastric pain with fullness and bloating after meals. Vomiting commonly may occur and provides relief from pain and bloating. Characteristically, the vomit contains the remains of the previous meal. Oddly, these symptoms are often intermittent, with periods of weeks, or even months, between attacks. Symptoms may be relieved by posture; patients may lie on the left side or assume the knee-chest position. A history of this is of value in the diagnosis.

Clinical examination most often reveals a thin patient of asthenic build. On occasion, epigastric tenderness and visible gastric peristalsis may be detected.

Acute Superior Mesenteric Artery Syndrome

Acute SMA syndrome is less common but may present as a surgical emergency. There may be a precipitating factor, such as those described above, or the condition may occur postoperatively; development has been described following a number of procedures, including ligation of a patent ductus arteriosus, total colectomy, abdominal aortic aneurysm repair, and nephrectomy.

Other cases have no obvious precipitating factor and may occur merely as an acute upper gastrointestinal obstruction.[53] Of the 281 collected cases reviewed, 32 patients had symptoms for less for 1 month.[42] The symptoms are similar to those already described for the chronic syndrome, with the exceptions that the vomiting is invariably present and symptoms are persistent and severe. Physical examination often reveals the presence of gastric dilatation with an audible splash, and the presence of visible persitalsis. The severity of this condition is demonstrated by the fact that the patient may have severe alkalosis, hy-

pokalaemia, and uremia, and even gangrene and perforation of the distended stomach.[54,55]

INVESTIGATIONS

A positive diagnosis is often made during barium-meal screening because of the presence of constant dilatation of the proximal duodenum with marked "to and fro" peristalsis, delay in the passage of contrast material, and evidence of a characteristic vertical linear extrinsic pressure defect in the third portion of the duodenum (Fig 27–20). If the patient is placed in the prone position, the duodenal retention often disappears almost completely. In the chronic case, the condition is often intermittent in nature, and for this reason, the absence of typical x-ray signs in one examination does not exclude the existence of the syndrome. Radiological evidence of occlusion will be most manifest during an attack, and therefore, in clinically suspected cases, repeated examinations are essential, if possible during an attack. Hy-

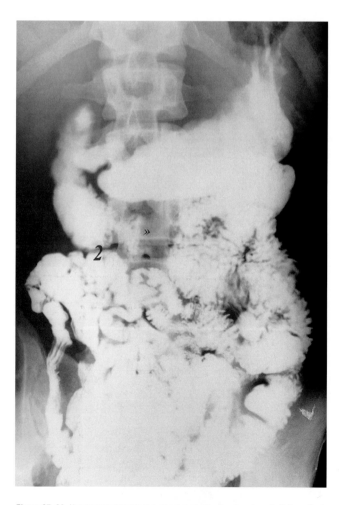

Figure 27–20. Upper gastrointestinal contrast study showing the characteristic vertical, linear, extrinsic pressure defect (*arrow*) in the third part of the duodenum.

potonic duodenography has been advocated as being superior to conventional barium-meal studies; three patients were reported with negative barium meal–study results in whom the diagnosis of duodenal ileus (confirmed at operation) was made at duodenography.[52] In recent years, CT scanning has proved to be of some value of the diagnosis of this condition.[56] We have experience with one patient in whom the condition was clinically apparent but barium-meal findings were equivocal. CT scanning, after ingestion of oral contrast, demonstrated the compressed duodenum between the aorta and SMA (Fig 27–21). The patient was successfully treated operatively.

During radiological examination of suspected cases, there may be coexisting abnormalities, and indeed, a high incidence of duodenal ulcer.[42,57]

DIFFERENTIAL DIAGNOSIS

The symptom complex may suggest a peptic ulcer, biliary disease, or chronic pancreatitis, and these may need to be excluded by specific investigations. Demonstration of obstruction in the third part of the duodenum strongly suggests the diagnosis since causes of obstruction in this region are uncommon, although they include cysts and tumors of the pancreas or duodenum, enlarged lymph nodes at the base of the mesentery, retroperitoneal neoplasms, adhesions, and Crohn's disease affecting the duodenojejunal region.

TREATMENT

Conservative treatment is successful in most cases associated with orthopedic conditions. Treatment usually involves little more than removal of the plaster cast and mobilization of the patient. Modern orthopedic surgery can treat most conditions by open reduction and fixation to allow this mobilization or to prevent the complication in the first place. In severe cases, where options are limited, nasogastric tube decompression of the stomach with intravenous feeding may be required.

In cases of chronic SMA syndrome, a trial of conservative treatment can be used in the first instance. Initial nasogastric tube decompression of the stomach may be required, after which the patient should be advised to turn into the prone or knee-elbow position after meals to facilitate gastric emptying. Prokinetic agents also may be employed to assist in gastric emptying.

It was previously believed that weight gain, with increase in the size of the fat pad lying between the aorta and duodenum, would then increase the aortomesenteric angle and improve gastric emptying. While such resolution of the obstruction undoubtedly can occur, a CT and anthropometric study suggests that this is not a consequence of fat deposition in the aortomesenteric angle.[56]

If the patient fails to respond to these simple measures, the operation of choice is duodenojejunostomy, a relatively simple procedure with good late results. At laparotomy, dilatation of the duodenum up to the level of the superior mesenteric pedicle can be verified. If this is not obvious, about 200 mL of saline solution can be instilled through a nasogastric tube to confirm dilatation of the duodenum and retention of fluid above the vascular pedicle.

The transverse colon is drawn through the wound and elevated, thus exposing the prominent, bulging second and third parts of the duodenum (Fig 27–22). The peritoneum over this area is incised and the third part of the duodenum freely mobilized. The first loop of the jejunum, approximately 7.5 to 10 cm from the ligament

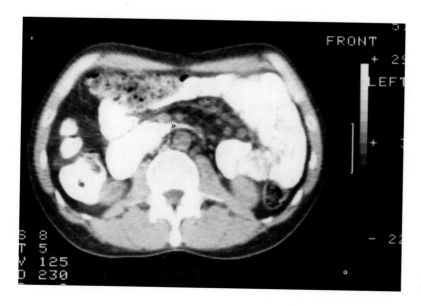

Figure 27–21. CT scan through the upper abdomen after ingestion of oral contrast in a patient with equivocal findings on barium meal. The compressed duodenum can be seen between the SMA anteriorly and the aorta posteriorly (*arrow*).

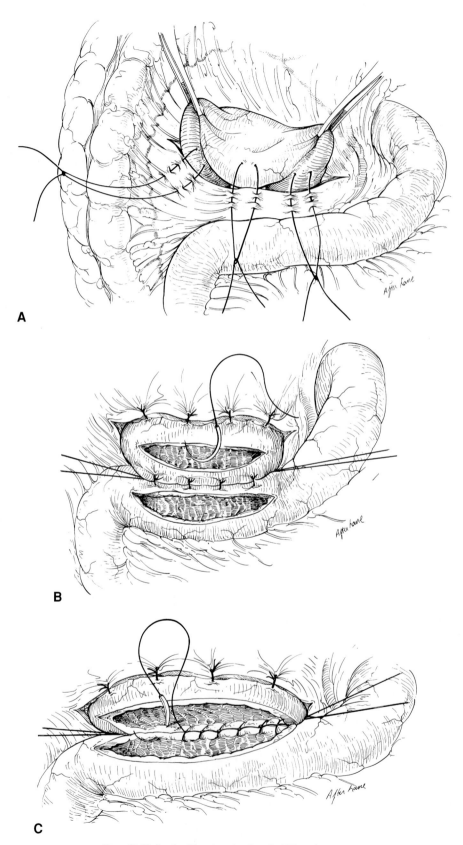

Figure 27–22. Duodenojejunostomy to relieve the SMA syndrome.

of Trietz, then is brought over to the right and anastomosed to the mobilized duodenum, very much as in the performance of a gastrojejunostomy. At the completion of the operation, the anterior and posterior margins of the mesocolon are stitched to the duodenum to obliterate any dangerous gaps in the mesentery. The stoma should be at least 5 cm wide and the anastomosis performed with 2/0 chromic catgut.

Gastrojejunostomy plays no part in the treatment of chronic SMA syndrome; the results of this operation in the past were disappointing. In contrast, in a collected review of 50 duodenojejunostomies for this condition only four failures were found.[58]

■ FOREIGN BODIES OF THE ESOPHAGUS, STOMACH, AND DUODENUM

A variety of foreign bodies in the upper part of the alimentary tract may come to the attention of the general surgeon. Most objects can be left to pass spontaneously through the rectum, but occasionally, perforation, ulceration, or obstruction may occur.

Foreign bodies can be classified as (1) swallowed (accidental or deliberate) foreign bodies and food, (2) bezoars: trichobezoars, phytobezoars, and other concretions, and (3) transmurally introduced foreign bodies.

SWALLOWED FOREIGN BODIES

Swallowing, either accidentally or deliberately, is by far the most common way in which foreign materials enter the gastrointestinal tract. Children, especially toddlers, are the worst offenders, although other special categories include mentally retarded persons, psychiatric patients, and prisoners (Fig 27–23, Fig 27–24, and 27–25).

The swallowed objects include almost every known object, such as bones, pins, coins, thermometers, toys, knives, forks, spoons, screws, and nails. Dentures may be swallowed and, indeed, patients who have complete dentures are themselves more likely to swallow foreign material because of the diminished tactile sensation within the mouth. Mentally ill patients may repeatedly ingest large numbers of foreign bodies; the world record still seems to be held by a manic-depressive patient who had 2533 foreign bodies removed in laparotomy.[59]

A relatively new hazard is the ingestion of balloons or condoms containing smuggled drugs. The balloon may produce intestinal obstruction, and rupture of the balloon followed by absorption of the contained drugs has led to death in some patients. The plain x-ray films of the abdomen in such cases may show the typical appearance of a uniformly oblong balloon, usually with a

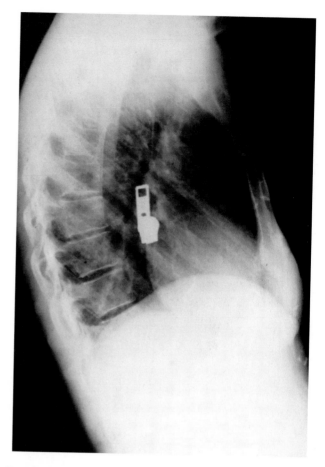

Figure 27–23. A large zipper ingested accidentally. This will probably pass through the gastrointestinal tract.

cresenteric air cap at one end, where air is trapped within the balloon.

A number of factors influence outcome after ingestion of foreign bodies. It is important to appreciate that any object that can be swallowed can traverse the normal gastrointestinal tract. As may be expected, spontaneous passage is especially likely to occur when the object is small, smooth, and round. Impaction is more likely to occur when the foreign material is long, large, and sharp. Open safety pins are particularly dangerous.

The normal points of relative constriction along the gastrointestinal tract represents the sites of possible obstruction of a foreign body. After an object passes the cricopharyngeus muscle, there are two sites of narrowing in the esophagus. One is at the bifurcation of the trachea and the area of compression by the aorta, and the second is at the esophagogastric junction. In about 10% of patients who present with impacted foreign bodies in the esophagus, a preexisting stricture will cause the obstruction.

Ordinarily, if a foreign body will pass through the cardiac end the esophagus, it may be expected to pass read-

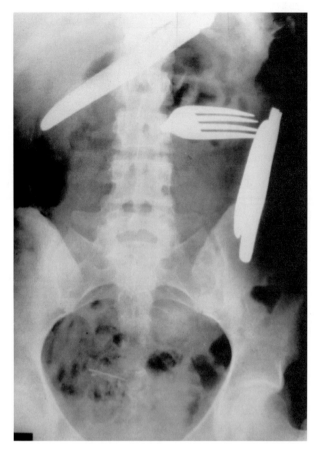

Figure 27–24. Items of cutlery and a cut-throat razor swallowed by a psychotic patient. Items of this size require operative removal.

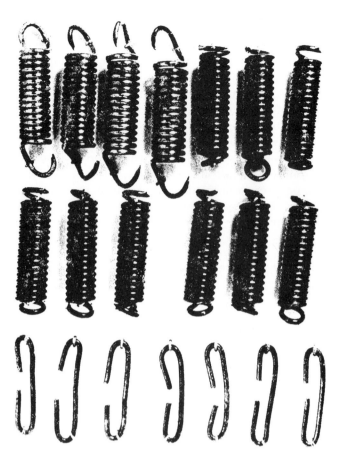

Figure 27–25. Bedsprings removed from the stomach of a 28 year old prisoner. (Presented to the Museum of the Westminster Medical School, London by Mr. IR Rosin, OBE, of Salisbury, Zimbabwe).

ily through the entire gastrointestinal tract. The pylorus, however, may impede passage, and the presence of a duodenal ulcer may compound this problem.

Beyond the pylorus, the next most common point of obstruction is the second or proximal part of the third portion of the duodenum, where relatively long objects, such as a hairgrip (hairpin) or a long needle, may be unable to negotiate the curve.

The ileocaecal region is the next point of possible impaction. The area of the peritoneal reflection in the pelvis impedes passage, as does the anal sphincter.

It may take many days before the foreign body passes spontaneously. In one series, of 69 foreign bodies that were voided, the average time of passage from mouth to anus was 5 days, with a range of 1 to 37 days.[60] In a study of 660 examples of ingested foreign bodies in children, 205 objects had to be removed endoscopically from the esophagus. Of the remainder, operation was needed in only 6% of the cases. The transit time averaged 4.8 days for blunt objects, 5.8 days if one end of an object was pointed, and 7 days if both ends were sharp.

ESOPHAGEAL FOREIGN BODIES

Clinical Manifestations

The symptoms caused by impaction of a foreign body in the esophagus are variable. Smooth objects, even if large, may occasionally cause no symptoms. Usually, however, the patient complains of choking, dysphagia, and retrosternal or cervical discomfort or pain. Obstruction and overflow of ingested liquids or foodstuffs may produce cough, dyspnea, and expectoration of frothy sputum. Foreign bodies retained for long periods commonly cause pressure necrosis with perforation of the esophagus or hemorrhage. If not removed early, sharp objects may puncture the esophagus and cause mediastinitis. Perforation into surrounding structures may take place, and the object may actually migrate completely through the esopahgus. Disastrous perforation into the trachea, pleura, lung, and even heart has been reported. The most common manifestation, that of mediastinitis, is accompanied by fever and often by surgical emphysema in the neck as air dissects superiorly.

Treatment

Although removal of an occasional small, smooth object in the distal portion of the esophagus may be delayed for a few hours to allow for possible spontaneous passage into the stomach, most objects, especially those which are large or sharp, should be removed endoscopically as soon after diagnosis as possible. Use of the flexible esophagogastroscope has certainly made the procedure easier and safer, although the rigid instrument is preferred if the object is large or difficult to grasp. A general anesthetic usually will be required for rigid esophagoscopy and in all young children. The foreign body is grasped with a forceps or a snare and brought up against the end of the esophagoscope, with the instrument, forceps, and foreign body removed simultaneously.

FOREIGN BODIES IN THE STOMACH AND DUODENUM

Clinical Manifestations

Swallowed foreign bodies that reach the stomach or duodenum are usually asymptomatic and progress down the alimentary tract until passed spontaneously without discomfort, unless pyloric obstruction is present. Some patients, however, complain of vague abdominal discomfort, and those with multiple, long-standing foreign bodies (Figs 27–24 and 27–25) may have a sense of heaviness and discomfort in the epigastrium, as well as anorexia. If the object becomes impacted, high obstructive symptoms may occur. Perforation is fortunately rare. Hematemesis or melena may accompany impaction of a foreign body and, occasionally, the object may migrate through the wall of the stomach or duodenum and perforate another structure. Additionally, it actually may fistulate through the abdominal wall.

Diagnosis

Diagnosis can usually be made from the history and plain x-ray films of the abdomen, and can be confirmed by endoscopy.

Treatment

If the swallowed object can traverse the esophagogastric junction, then, in the great majority of cases, it is likely to pass through the alimentary canal without causing further harm. The spontaneous passage of 827 foreign bodies in a series of 834 patients has been observed.[62]

If a conservative management policy is to be undertaken, daily examination of the abdomen, together with a plain abdominal x-ray film, is indicated to detect untoward manifestations and to watch the progress of the foreign body through the gastrointestinal tract. It is a wise policy to admit to the hospital, for closer observation, patients who have swallowed open safety pins or irregular, jagged objects.

The availability of the flexible gastroscope means that many objects now can be removed by gastroscopy. If an object is pointed or jagged, extraction through the esophagus may be dangerous and a sheath may be needed to protect the esophagus during removal. Snares and a number of ingenious devices have been used successfully to close safety pins within the stomach for safe withdrawal through the esophagus.

Indications for active treatment may be listed as follows: (1) failure of the object to progress through the gastrointestinal tract, or evidence of impaction on serial x-ray films, (2) signs of penetration or actual perforation, (3) long, large, pointed or jagged objects are most unlikely to move on (Fig 27–24), (4) the accumulation of large numbers of foreign bodies (Fig 27–25), (5) evidence of gastrointestinal tract hemorrhage.

If surgical removal of a foreign body is undertaken, an x-ray film of the abdomen should be obtained immediately before laparotomy to verify that the position of the foreign body has not changed. If the foreign body is in the stomach, it may readily be found by palpating the stomach between the fingers and may be extracted through a small gastric incision. If the object is in the duodenum, it is preferable to manipulate it back into the stomach before removal.

Slender, pointed objects, such as pins and needles, are best removed by pushing the sharp end through the wall of the stomach or duodenum after a purse-string suture has been placed around this point. The protruding end of the object is then grasped with forceps, and as the object is withdrawn, the suture is tightened and tied (Fig 27–26).

A large gastric incision must be used for multiple foreign bodies, and care should be taken to ensure that all the objects are removed. If necessary, an additional x-ray film is obtained before closure of the abdomen.

BEZOARS

Bezoars are concretions of foreign material found in the stomach and intestines. They occur infrequently in man, but are more common in other animals, particularly goats and sheep. For centuries, bezoars were considered to be potent antidotes against snake venom and other poisons, and were also supposed to prevent depression. The clinical application of bezoars in modern surgical practice is, however, severely limited!

Bezoars may be classified as trichobezoars (hair balls), phytobezoars (made up of vegetable material), and other concretions (made up of various ingested chemical substances).

Trichobezoars

Trichobezoars consist of a matted mass of ingested hair that may form a perfect cast of the stomach (Fig 27–27).

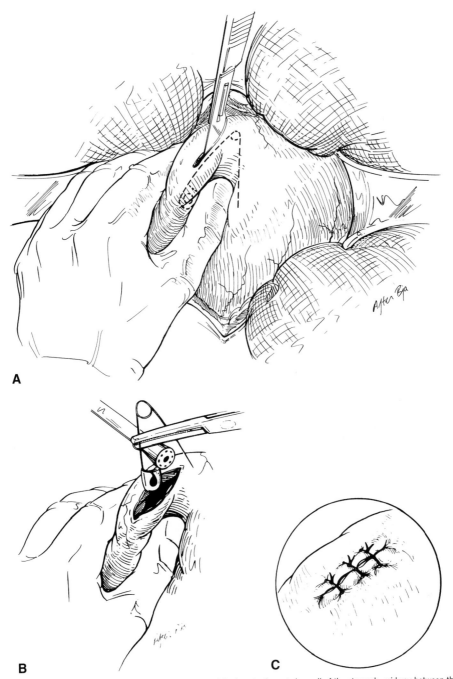

Figure 27–26. Gastrotomy for removal of a foreign body. **A.** Lesion is gripped firmly onto the anterior wall of the stomach, midway between the greater and lesser curves, and a small incision is made at one end. **B.** The pin is grasped through the opening with forceps and drawn out. Contamination is minimized by the hand of the surgeon holding the gastrotomy and the assistant using the sucker. **C.** The gastrotomy is closed in layers *Continued*

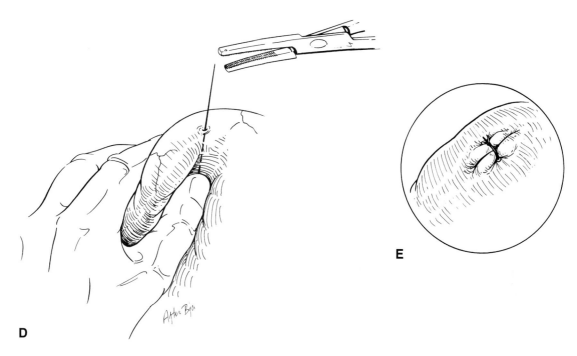

D

E

Figure 27–26, cont'd. D. Pins and needles may be removed by transgastric manipulation and pushed through the stomach wall without incision. **E**. A single suture has been used to close the pin hole.

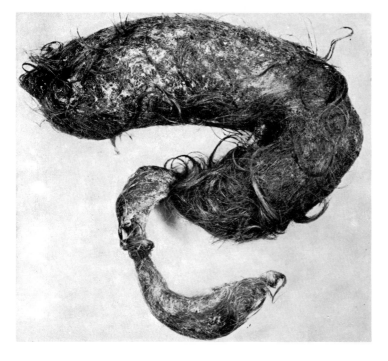

Figure 27–27. Trichobezoar forming a cast of the stomach.

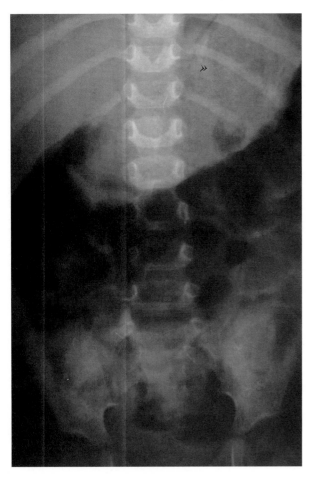

Figure 27–28. Whorled appearance of a trichobezoar in the stomach (*arrow*).

On occasion, the mass may project into the duodenum and rarely, it may extend throughout the bowel (the "Rapunzel Syndrome"). Usually, the mass is dark greenish-brown or black and has a slimy surface and an offensive odor. They are usually encountered in young girls. In a review of bezoars, more then 80% occurred in patients under 30 years of age and more than 90% were in women.[63,64] The etiology is trichopagy (hair swallowing) and seems to be less common in societies where very long hair in young women is no longer fashionable. About 10% of patients show some degree of mental disturbance.

Phytobezoars

A phytobezoar consists of a compact concretion of vegetable material. About three-quarters of reported cases are the result of ingestion of the persimmon, but other fruits and vegetables with high fiber and cellulose content may be responsible. Phytobezoars of other material (eg, orange pith) may be found in patients who have undergone gastric surgery, particularly partial gastrec-

tomy; presumably, the decreased motility and digestive capability of the stomach allows formation of these accumulations of vegetable material.

Other Concretions

Other concretions are relatively unusual and account for <5% of reported cases. Magnesium and sodium carbonate concretions were reported when these substances were widely used to treat peptic ulcer diseases, as were concretions of bismuth carbonate, when bismuth was used as contrast for radiological investigations. Modern, orally ingested drug delivery systems also may be associated with such pharmacobezoar formation: one bezoar was described that was of sustained release theophylline in a patient who had taken an overdose of her medication.[65] The presence of this mass resulted in delayed absorption of the toxin and the death of the patient. In another case report, a bezoar consisting of the slow-release nifedipine delivery system was described.[66]

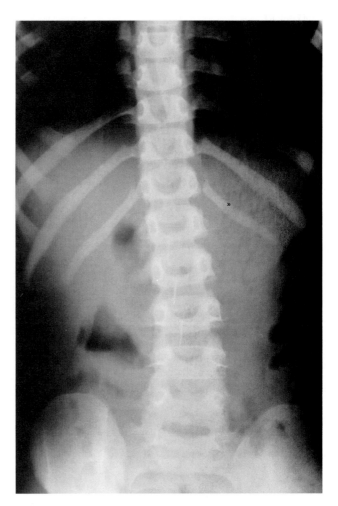

Figure 27–29. Stippled appearance of a trichobezoar in the stomach.

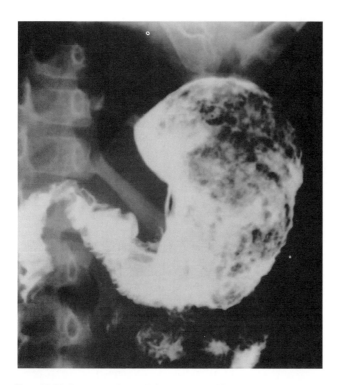

Figure 27–30. Appearance of the trichobezoar in Fig 27–29 after ingestion of oral contrast.

Clinical Features

The majority of bezoars cause upper abdominal pain, loss of weight, and anorexia. The characteristic finding is a mobile epigastric mass that has a whorled or stippled appearance on plain abdominal x-ray (Figs 27–28 and 27–29). A barium-meal examination outlines the foreign body (Fig 27–30), which also may be visualized at gastroscopy.

Complications

As well as causing epigastric discomfort and pain, bezoars may produce ulceration (resulting in gastrointestinal hemorrhage), perforation, and intestinal obstruction. Intestinal obstruction is the most common complication. The frequency of complications appears to vary with the type of bezoar; trichobezoars have been associated with gastrointestinal tract hemorrhage in 6% of cases, but were complicated by obstruction in 10%, while phytobezoars have been associated with a 15% incidence of hemorrhage and a 25% incidence of obstruction.[63] In the former, the obstruction is usually consequent upon detachment of a portion of a hair ball that has extended into the duodenum, broken off, and traveled downward until it becomes impacted in the terminal ileum. In contrast, phytobezoars, which are often multiple, probably pass intact through the pylorus to become impacted in the small bowel.

Management

Because of the high incidence of complications, bezoars should always be removed from the stomach. In some cases, small bezoars, composed mainly of food substances, can be fragmented through the fiber optic endoscope; the fragments then will pass spontaneously through the bowel. Recently, a laser-based endoscopic lithotripsy device has been used to break up gastric bezoars, with excellent early results.[67] The dissolution of five phytobezoars by the enzyme cellulase, all dissolved within three days, has also been reported.[68] A combination of endoscopic fragmentation and enzymatic dissolution has been used to successfully treat five cases.[69] The latter study also demonstrated that all five patients treated had normal gastric motility and acid production, factors that it has previously been suggested may be abnormal in patients who develop gastric bezoars.

Large bezoars, particularly hair balls, may not be amenable to any treatment other than open surgical removal by means of a gastrotomy. However, the successful use of extracorporeal shock-wave lithotripsy to treat a large, hard gastric bezoar that could not be removed endoscopically, in an 8 year old child, has recently been described.[70]

In the operative treatment of phytobezoars, it is important to remember that because these concretions are often multiple, both the stomach and the remainder of the intestine must be searched carefully to ensure complete removal of all foreign bodies. Trichobezoars often extend through the pylorus into the duodenum, and special care should therefore be taken to ensure extraction of the entire mass.

TRANSMURAL MIGRATION

Occasionally, foreign bodies enter the stomach or duodenum by migration as a result of trauma or ulceration. Such incidents have been reported in gunshot wounds or other penetrating injuries in which the missile had not been removed from the peritoneal cavity at the time of the initial incident and subsequently ulcerated into the gut lumen. Laparotomy packs, swabs, and surgical instruments, inadvertently left within the abdominal cavity, may also behave in such a manner, but, not unnaturally, such accidents are not commonly reported. The most common type of foreign body that reaches the bowel by transmural migration is a gallstone.

REFERENCES

1. Palmer ED. Gastric diverticula (collective review). *Surg Gynecol Obstet* 1951;92:417
2. Meeroff M, Gollan JRM, et al. Gastric diverticulum. *Am J Gastroenterol* 1967;47:189

3. Sinclair N. Congenital diverticulum of the stomach in an infant. *Br J Surg* 1929;17:182

4. Benhamou PH, Lenaerts C, Canareli JP, et al. Diverticulum of the stomach in children. Apropos of a case of congenital diverticulum. *Ann Paediatr Paris* 1989;36(7): 476–478

5. Ward WW, Oca CF, et al. Massive hemoperitoneum due to gastric diverticulum. *JAMA* 1966;196:798

6. Hale PC, O'Flynn WR. Late presentation of a congenital gastric diverticulum causing pyloric obstruction. *Postgrad Med J* 1992;68(798):296–298

7. Chaulin B, Damoo B, Verdeil C, et al. Gastric diverticulum mimicking adrenal mass: x-ray computed tomographic findings. *J Radiol* 1992;73(6–7):389–393

8. Shackelford GD. Barium collections in the stomach mimicking intraluminal diverticula. *AJR Am J Roentgenol* 1982; 139:805

9. Heijboer MP, Nieuwenhuizen LN. Gastric diverticula. *Neth J Surg* 1980;32:16

10. Young HB. Juxta-oesophageal diverticula of the stomach. *Br J Surg* 1962;50:150

11. Whitcomb JG. Duodenal diverticulum: a clinical evaluation. *Arch Surg* 1964;88:275

12. Ackerman W. Diverticula and variations of the duodenum. *Ann Surg* 1943;117:403

13. Jones RW, Merendino KA. The perplexing duodenal diverticulum. *Surgery* 1960;48:1068

14. Pearce VR. The importance of duodenal diverticula in the elderly. *Postgrad Med J* 1980;56:777

15. Heilbrum N, Boyden EA. Intraluminal duodenal diverticula. *Radiology* 1964;82:887

16. Abdel-Hafiz A, Birkett DH, et al. Congenital duodenal diverticula: a report of three cases and a review of the literature. *Surgery* 1988;104:74

17. Eggert A, Teichmann W, et al. The pathologic implication of duodenal diverticula. *Surg Gynecol Obstet* 1982; 154:62

18. Manny J, Muga M, et al. The continuing clinical enigma of duodenal diverticulum. *Am J Surg* 1981;142:596

19. Neill SA, Thompson NW. The complications of duodenal diverticula and their management. *Surg Gynecol Obstet* 1965;120:1251

20. Takaaki J, Kodama T, Akaki H, et al. Relationship between juxtapapillary duodenal diverticula and biliopancreatic disease—evaluation by endoscopic biliary manometry. *Nippon Shokakibyo Gakkai Zasshi* 1992;89(5):1270–1278

21. Hartley RH, Barlow AP, Kilby JO. Intraluminal duodenal diverticulum: an unusual of acute pancreatitis. *Br J Surg* 1993;80(4):488

22. Slater RB. Duodenal diverticulum treated by excision of mucosal pouch only. *Br J Surg* 1971;58:198

23. Scudamore CH, Harrison RC, et al. Management of duodenal diverticula. *Can J Surg* 1982;25:311

24. Berti A. Singolare attotigliamento dell'esofago col duodeno seguita da rapida morte. *Gaz Med Ital* 1866;9:139

25. Berg J. Zwei falle von Axendrehung des Magens; Operation; Heilung. *Nord Med Ark* 1897;30:1

26. Rosselet DJ. Contribution a l'etude du volvulus de l'estomac. *J Radiol Electrol* 1920;4:341

27. Buchanan J. Volvulus of the stomach. *Br J Surg* 1930;18:99

28. Dalgaard JB. Volvulus of the stomach: case report and survey. *Acta Chir Scand* 1952;103:131

29. Wastell C, Ellis H. Volvulus of the stomach: a review with a report of 8 cases. *Br J Surg* 1971;58:557

30. Kaushik SP. Gastric volvulus following highly selective vagotomy: a case report. *Br J Surg* 1979;66:574

31. Carter R, Brewer LA, et al. Acute gastric volvulus. *Am J Surg* 1980;140:99

32. Idowu J, Aitken DR, et al. Gastric volvulus in the newborn. *Arch Surg* 1980;115:1046

33. Youssef SA, Lorenzo DI, et al. Volvulus gastrique chez l'enfant. *Chir Pediatr* 1987;28:32

34. Borchardt M. Zur pathologie und therapie des magenvolvulus. *Arch FJ Chir* 1904;74:243

35. Tanner NC. Chronic and recurrent volvulus of the stomach with late results of colonic displacement. *Am J Surg* 1968;115:505

36. Farkas AG, Celestin LR. Gastrojejunostomy: a simple method of treatment of gastric volvulus. *Ann R Coll Surg Engl* 1986;68:107

37. Alawadi A, Chou S, Soucy P. Gastric volvulus—a late complication of gastrostomy. *Can J Surg* 1991;34(5):485–486

38. Ghosh S, Palmer KR. Double percutaneous endoscopic gastrostomy fixation: an effective treatment for recurrent gastric volvulus. *Am J Gastroenterol* 1993;88(8):1271–1272

39. Koger KE, Stone JM. Laparoscopic reduction of acute gastric volvulus. *Am Surg* 1993;59(5):325–328

40. Bloodgood JC. Acute dilation of the stomach: gastromesenteric ileus. *Ann Surg* 1907;46:736

41. Stavely AL. Chronic gastromesenteric ileus. *Surg Gynecol Obstet* 1910;11:288

42. Barner HB, Sherman CD. Vascular compression of the duodenum. *Surg Gynecol Obstet* 1963;117:103

43. Willett A. Fatal vomiting following application of plaster-of-Paris bandage in case of spinal curvature. *St. Bart's Hosp Rep* 1878;14:333

44. Dorph MA. The cast syndrome. *N Engl J Med* 1950;243:440

45. Hall LW. The cast syndrome incognito. *Am J Surg* 1974; 127:371

46. Akin JT, Gray SW, et al. Vascular compression of the duodenum: presention of 10 cases and review of the literature. *Surgery* 1976;79:515

47. Jones PA, Wastell C. Superior mesenteric artery syndrome. *Postgrad Med J* 1983;59:376

48. Roth EJ, Fenton LL, Gaebler-Spira DJ, et al. Superior mesenteric artery syndrome in acute traumatic quadriplegia: case reports and literature review. *Arch Phys Med Rehabil* 1991;72(6):417–420

49. Philip PA. Superior mesenteric artery syndrome: an unusual cause of intestinal obstruction in brain injured children. *Brain Inj* 1992;6(4):351–358

50. Sostek M, Fine SM, Harris TL. Duodenal obstruction by abdominal aortic aneurysm. *Am J Med* 1993;94(2): 220–221

51. Rappaport WD, Hunter GC, McIntyre KE, et al. Gastric outlet obstruction caused by traumatic pseudoaneurysm of superior mesenteric artery. *Surgery* 1990;108(5):930–932

52. Lukes PJ, Rolny P, et al. Diagnostic value of hypotonic duodenography in superior mesenteric artery syndrome. *Acta Chir Scand* 1978;144:39

53. Vohra R, Saini L, et al. "Duodenal ileus" presenting as acute upper gastrointestinal obstruction. *Aust NZ J Surg* 1982;52:512

54. Kennedy RH, Cooper MJ. An unusually severe case of the cast syndrome. *Postgrad Med J* 1983;59:539

55. Lundell L, Thulin A. Wilkie's syndrome—a rarity? *Br J Surg* 1980;67:604

56. Santer R, Young C, Rossi T, et al. Computed tomography in superior mesenteric artery syndrome. *Pediatr Radiol* 1991;21(2):154–155

57. Wilkie DPD. Chronic duodenal ileus. *Br J Surg* 1921;9:204

58. Lee CS, Mangla JC. Superior mesenteric artery compression syndrome. *Am J Gastroenterol* 1978;70:141

59. Chalk SG, Foucar HO. Foreign bodies in the stomach. *Arch Surg* 1928;16:494

60. Henderson FF, Gaston EA. Ingested foreign body in the gastrointestinal tract. *Arch Surg* 1938;36:66

61. Spitz L. Management of ingested foreign bodies in childhood. *Br Med J* 1971;4:469

62. Clerf LH. Foreign bodies in the gastrointestinal tract. *Surg Clin North Am* 1934;14:77

63. DeBakey ME, Ochsner A. Bezoars and concretions. A comprehensive review of the literature with an analysis of 303 collected cases and a presentation of 8 additional cases. *Surgery* 1939;5:132

64. DeBakey ME, Ochsner A. Bezoars and concretions: a comprehensive review of the literature with an analysis of 303 collected cases and a presentation of 8 additional cases. *Surgery* 1938;4:934

65. Bernstein G, Jehle D, Bernaski E, et al. Failure of gastric emptying and charcoal administration in fatal sustained release theophylline overdose: pharmacobezoar formation. *Ann Emerg Med* 1992;21(11):1388–1390

66. Prisant LM, Carr AA, Bottini PB, et al. Nifedipine GITS (gastrointestinal therapeutic system) bezoar. *Arch Int Med* 1991;151(9):1868–1869

67. Huang YC, Guo ZH, Gu Y, et al. Endoscopic lithotripsy of gastric bezoars using a laser ignited mini-explosive device. *Chin Med J Engl* 1990;103(2):152–155

68. Lee SP, Holloway WD. The medical dissolution of phytobezoars using cellulase. *Br J Surg* 1977;64:403

69. Tohdo H, Haruma K, Kitadai Y, et al. Gastric emptying and bezoars in Japanese. Report of five cases. *Dig Dis Sci* 1993;38(8):1422–1425

70. Benes J, Chmel J, Jodl J, et al. Treatment of gastric bezoars by extracorporeal shock wave lithotripsy. *Endoscopy* 1991;23(6):346–348

28

Duodenal Ulcer and Peptic Ulceration

David Johnston ▪ *Iain Martin*

The past twenty years have seen a revolution in the treatment of peptic ulcers of the stomach and duodenum. There are now a large number of very potent acid-suppressing drugs such as the H2 receptor antagonists and the proton pump inhibitors that can control, but not cure, the ulcer diathesis in the vast majority of patients. More recently, the realization that *Helicobacter pylori* may have a fundamental role in the pathogenesis of peptic ulceration has led to therapeutic strategies aimed at eradicating this bacterium and curing the disease. As a result of these advances and the fact that, in the Western world at least, peptic ulceration is becoming less common, elective surgery for uncomplicated duodenal and gastric ulcer has virtually disappeared. Added to this are recent surgical advances in the field of minimally invasive therapy; laparoscopic vagotomy and suture of perforated duodenal ulcer are now viable practical procedures.

As a result of all these changes and developments, discussing surgery for duodenal and gastric ulcer is now more difficult than it was 20 years ago when open surgery was the only long-term effective therapy.

In Europe and North America, surgery for peptic ulceration has largely become the surgery of complicated ulceration: hemorrhage, perforation, and gastric outlet obstruction, and even in this area, interventional endoscopy and minimally invasive therapy have an increasing role. One of the major problems confronting the practicing surgeon is the rapidity of development of these new therapeutic strategies. In the past, long-term results were available for all forms of treatment; these

data are not available for the 1990s and consequently the best we can do is to interpret the data from the 1970s and 1980s in the light of what we think ought to happen. Consequently, for instance, the belief that whenever possible, treatment of emergency cases with bleeding or perforated ulcer should be accompanied by definitive ulcer curing surgery may no longer be appropriate. As a result of this and other clinical problems, there is perhaps more, not less, need for further well conducted clinical trials.

Although the incidence of peptic ulceration has decreased dramatically, paradoxically the number of deaths from complicated ulceration has not decreased yet. It will be interesting to see whether the death rate from complicated ulcers in an increasingly elderly population can be reduced in the 1990s.

▪ DUODENAL ULCER

DIAGNOSIS

History

The patient usually complains of epigastric pain, the features of which are known to every medical student: characteristically episodic, the pain is felt in the center of the epigastrium and slightly to the right, may radiate through to the back, is relieved by food and antacids, and comes on when the patient is hungry. The pain will often wake the patient at 2 o'clock in the morning and is seldom very severe unless some major complication

941

has occurred. The patient is more likely to be male than female and often there is a strong family history of duodenal ulceration.

Unfortunately patients do not read medical textbooks! Hence the history may differ greatly from the description given above. For example, the site of the pain may be as low as the umbilicus or in the lower chest. Its nature or severity may lead one to suspect biliary tract pathology. In consequence, it is seldom possible to be certain of the diagnosis of duodenal ulceration on the basis of history alone; patients whom we are clinically certain have duodenal ulceration frequently turn out to have a gastric ulcer or even gastric cancer. In surgical out-patient clinics in Britain, the most common organic causes of upper abdominal pain are gallstones, peptic ulceration, and reflux esophagitis, but carcinoma of the stomach and pancreas and functional dyspepsia are also common.

Physical Signs

Physical examination of the abdomen is usually normal, but valuable signs may be present and, in addition, signs of concomitant illness also may be detected. There may be tenderness in the epigastrium. The painful area in the abdomen is usually constant and does not move with respiration.

On rare occasions, a duodenal ulcer may form a palpable tumor. However, it is difficult to feel such a tumor unless the patient is very thin. It cannot be distinguished from a neoplastic mass.

When obstruction of the stomach presents, as a result of a stenosing ulcer near the pylorus, the dilated hypertrophied stomach may be visible and palpable through a thin abdominal wall. Peristalsis may be visible as the powerful musculature of the antrum attempts to overcome the obstruction. If the patient is shaken bodily, a succussion splash may be audible. This is, in the words of Sir James Walton, "the stomach you can hear, the stomach you can see and the stomach you can feel."

In the general examination of the patient, one should look for carious teeth, gingivitis, tattooing and signs of excessive use of tobacco or alcohol. Pallor and anemia may be present as a result of hemorrhage, acute or chronic. A rectal examination should never be omitted.

Assessment of the Patient

The diagnosis of duodenal ulceration should be confirmed by fibre optic endoscopy. Barium examination can no longer be recommended as the first line of investigation. It is vital that every patient with new dyspeptic symptoms, who is more than 40 years of age, be investigated prior to initiating treatment, if early stage gastric neoplasms are not to be missed. If duodenal ulceration is found, antral biopsies should be taken to ascertain the presence or absence of H pylori infection.

If the presence of duodenal ulceration is confirmed, the first line treatment is medical. Most (>97%) ulcers are associated with H pylori infection, and the treatment of choice for these ulcers is a regimen designed to both heal the ulcer and eradicate H pylori. The exact nature of such a regimen varies considerably and, to date, the most effective combination of drugs has yet to be determined; it is beyond the remit of this chapter to discuss the many regimes available. H pylori–negative ulcers should provoke a little more diagnostic thought, particularly if there is no history of nonsteroidal anti-inflammatory drug (NSAID) ingestion; rarer causes of duodenal ulceration such as Crohn's disease, lymphoma, carcinoma of the pancreas, the Zollinger-Ellison syndrome, or hypercalcemia should be considered, particularly if the ulcer does not respond rapidly to medical therapy.

ELECTIVE SURGERY

Indications

The indications for surgical therapy remain the same as they always were, namely failure of medical treatment or the occurrence of the complications of hemorrhage, perforation, or pyloric stenosis. What has changed is that medical treatment is nearly always successful in healing the ulcer. The H2 receptor antagonists such as cimetidine and ranitidine can heal 90% of ulcers in routine clinical practice. The proton pump inhibitors, such as omeprazole, will heal almost 100% of duodenal ulcers; intragastric pH is increased to more than three for the majority of the day. Omeprazole is expensive and, in many parts of the world, is not licensed for long-term use. The major defect with both proton pump inhibitors and H2 receptor antagonists is that when treatment stops, within 1 year 70% to 90% of patients will suffer a relapse of their ulcer. Until recently, the only medical alternative was long-term therapy with H2 receptor antagonists at a maintenance dose, which is inconvenient for the patient and expensive for the health care institutions.

The 1990s have seen the advent of combined anti-acid/antibiotic regimens increasingly based on the use of a proton pump inhibitor, designed to eliminate H pylori. These regimens can heal almost all duodenal ulcers and if the bacterium is eliminated from the stomach, long-term cure may be the result. It seems that, maybe, the medical "Holy Grail" is within our grasp, but it is not yet completely achieved: long-term results (5 to 10 years) are eagerly awaited.

Despite these advances, there are still a few patients who should be considered for surgical therapy. Unfortunately, these patients are often young men who both smoke and drink too heavily for the health of their duodenal mucosa. These patients are far from ideal candidates for surgery and, if the surgeon is less rigorous than he should be in selecting patients for surgical intervention, he will unfortunately end up with a group of patients who complain as bitterly about the surgery and its aftermath as they did preoperatively about the symptoms of their duodenal ulcer!

Choice of Operation for Duodenal Ulcer

Having thus selected the minority of patients with duodenal ulcer who need surgical treatment and seem likely to benefit from it, the next question is, which operative procedure should be used?

The answer to that question is not simple. It depends on a consideration of the physiology of the stomach, of current published clinical results of various operative procedures—bearing in mind that results from surgeons with a specialist interest and expertise bear little resemblance to average results across the country, the patient on whom we are considering operating and very importantly the skill and type of practice of the surgeon. With that last point in mind, it should be said that with the vastly reduced numbers of patients undergoing elective peptic ulcer surgery, there is no longer a place for the nonspecialist surgeon in this field.

In this era of modern effective medical therapy, the dictum *primum non nocere* is more important than ever. Since medical therapy can heal most ulcers, recurrent ulceration should no longer be regarded as the one criterion by which operations for duodenal ulcer should be compared. Rather, each patient should be offered an "ideal" operation based on the criteria outlined in Table 28–1. This "ideal" operation should be measured against a set of well-defined and weighted criteria (Table 28–2). In the 1990s, with modern pylorus-preserving surgery, the objectives are zero mortality, no side effects and a relatively low incidence of recurrent ulceration (10% to 15%, 10 years after operation), rather than an aggressive approach designed to cure all ulcers at considerable cost in terms of operative risk and side effects, by methods such as vagotomy with antrectomy.

The 1990s have seen an explosion of interest in minimally invasive therapy and unsurprisingly, many surgeons are applying these technical advances to the treatment of duodenal ulceration. Unfortunately, the philosophy that should underlie successful laparoscopic surgery, that the technique and technology should be developed to suit a particular operation rather than the operation being chosen to suit the techniques available, has not always been applied. Lessons learned during the past 50 years, from Dragstedt's first vagotomies onwards, have been ignored, in the stampede by some surgeons to apply minimally invasive techniques. We believe that the factors that influenced the choice of operation before the explosion of interest in laparoscopic surgery should still govern the choice of a laparoscopic operation for duodenal ulcer today.

TABLE 28–1. THE MAIN FACTORS TO BE CONSIDERED WHEN CHOOSING AN ELECTIVE OPERATION FOR DUODENAL ULCER

1. Operative mortality (and postoperative morbidity)
2. Incidence of recurrent ulceration after 5 to 10 years
3. Side effects of operation (dumping, diarrhea, etc.)
4. Long-term metabolic consequences after 5 to 30 years
   Loss of weight
   Anemia, iron deficiency/megaloblastic
   Tuberculosis
   Bone disease, osteomalacia, osteoporosis
5. Incidence of gastric carcinoma after 15 to 30 years
6. Relative ease or difficulty of second-salvage operation if the first operation should fail
7. Who will perform the operation?

Vagotomy or Gastrectomy?

Partial Gastrectomy. Resection of two-thirds of the stomach is obsolete in the treatment of duodenal ulcer. Somewhat paradoxically, in controlled trials, no other procedure has been shown to yield significantly better results than partial gastrectomy[1,2] and, after 5 to 8 years of follow-up, the patient's Visick grades were as good as after vagotomy with antrectomy or a drainage procedure. Nevertheless, partial gastrectomy should no longer be used in the elective surgical treatment of duodenal ulcer, because, even in expert hands, the patient is three to six times more likely to die of the operation than if treated by highly selective vagotomy (HSV). The postoperative morbidity is significantly greater than after HSV, there is appreciable weight loss (mean 5kg) and metabolic sequelae are not infrequent. Dumping is significantly more common with partial gastrectomy than after HSV. More than 20 years after operation the risk of gastric carcinoma is three to six times greater than expected,[3,4] probably because of the chronic gastric mucosal reaction[5–7] elicited by the excessive enterogastric reflux.

Even in cases of bleeding, perforated or stenosing duodenal ulcer, partial gastrectomy should now hardly ever be used. It still occasionally has a place as a salvage operation for recurrent ulceration after vagotomy.

Selective Vagotomy with a Drainage Procedure

Selective vagotomy with a drainage procedure (SV and D) is now seldom, if ever, used in the surgical treatment of duodenal ulcer. It has an honorable place in the history of surgery for duodenal ulcer because its proponents, such as Griffith in the United States and Burge, Kennedy, Hedenstedt, Grassi and de Miguel in Europe, showed that SV and D was followed by a lower incidence of diarrhea than was truncal vagotomy with a drainage procedure (TV and D) and that the technique of selective vagotomy permitted complete vagal denervation of

TABLE 28–2. EVALUATION OF AN OPERATION FOR PEPTIC ULCER: ENDPOINTS AND THEIR TIMING; THE SCORING SYSTEM OR THERAPEUTIC INDEX

Endpoint	Definition	Timing[a]	Weight or Score[b]
Operative Death	The patient dies as a result of the operation	0 to 3 months	50
Recurrent ulcer	Ulcer seen endoscopically or at reoperation	5 to 10 years	5
Side effects			
Severe	Side effects are so bad that both patient and doctor regard the operation as a failure	2 to 5 years	6
Moderate	Side effects mar the outcome and cannot be avoided	2 to 5 years	2
Mild	Symptoms can be controlled to a large extent by care with diet or way of life	2 to 5 years	0.5
None	Perfect result	2 to 5 years	0
Long term effects			
Very severe	Carcinoma of the stomach, pulmonary tuberculosis, osteomalacia or osteoporosis or patient becomes a postgastric surgery cripple with massive weight loss, anemia and malnutrition	5 to 30 years	10
Moderate	Moderate weight loss, marked anemia	5 to 30 years	5
Mild	Mild weight loss, mild anemia	5 to 30 years	1
None	Perfect result	5 to 30 years	0

[a]Time that must elapse before an endpoint can be said to be absent
[b]This is a numerical expression of the relative importance of the endpoint compared to recurrent ulceration which is arbitrarily given a weight of 5.

the parietal cell mass in almost all patients, in contrast to truncal vagotomy. Subsequent prospective randomized controlled trials confirmed these findings.[8–10] However, selective vagotomy is a complete gastric vagotomy which, like truncal vagotomy, denervates the antral mill and makes the use of a drainage procedure necessary. Thus, it still involves damage to the gastric reservoir function and has been superseded by highly selective vagotomy (HSV), which possesses all of its advantages and few of its disadvantages. Selective vagotomy and drainage has been compared with HSV in several prospective controlled trials.[11–14] Neither procedure emerged as a clear-cut winner of the contest. Although the incidence of recurrent ulceration after HSV was higher, overall, a greater proportion of patients enjoyed good results after HSV than after SV and D.

Though obsolete in the treatment of duodenal ulcer, SV and D may still have a place in the surgical treatment of prepyloric gastric ulcer because, when used for this condition, the incidence of recurrent ulceration after HSV is >20% at 5 years, and the use of either SV and D pyloroplasty or antrectomy seems preferable.

Thus, the choice of elective operation for duodenal ulcer is from three operative procedures: vagotomy with a drainage procedure, vagotomy combined with antrectomy, and highly selective vagotomy.

Vagotomy Combined with Antrectomy

This operation is highly effective in curing duodenal ulcers, with a recurrent ulceration rate of 1%, 5 to 10 years after operation.[15–17] This is because the operation removes the two principal drives to gastric acid secretion:

the vagal-cholinergic pathway and gastrin release from the antrum. The vagotomy itself may be selective or truncal in type. Although there is no reason to divide the hepatic and celiac fibers of the vagus, in practice, truncal vagotomy usually is employed. Similarly the antrectomy often amounts to a 50% gastrectomy. Finally, the reconstruction can take the form of the Billroth I or Billroth II variety; the former is more popular although there is little hard evidence that it confers any advantage over the Billroth II linkup.

Vagotomy combined with antrectomy has been in widespread clinical use for 35 to 40 years, particularly in North America,[18] so that its clinical results are well documented.[15,16,19] As stated in the preceding paragraph, its great advantage is the low incidence of recurrent ulceration, 1%, 5 to 10 years after operation. However, even in the hands of expert surgeons, the operative mortality is 1% and may approach 2% in some series. Postoperative morbidity is considerable, principally owing to gastric stasis or anastomotic leakage. On followup, side effects such as early dumping, diarrhea and bilious vomiting are relatively common[1] and metabolic sequelae are not rare. For these reasons, the patient may have to pay a heavy price for the 99% certainty of not having a recurrent ulcer. Prospective comparisons of vagotomy and antrectomy with HSV are dealt with later in this chapter.

Truncal vagotomy with a drainage procedure

Truncal vagotomy and pyloroplasty (TV and P) is still the most commonly used operation for duodenal ulceration in Britain. Yet, in many ways, it is the worst opera-

TABLE 28–3. PERCENTAGE INCIDENCE OF SIDE EFFECTS AFTER DIFFERENT ELECTIVE OPERATIONS FOR DUODENAL ULCER

Symptom	Polya partial gastrectomy (n=107)	Truncal vagotomy with antrectomy (n=116)	Truncal vagotomy with gastrojejunostomy (n=119)	Truncal vagotomy with pyloroplasty (n=161)	Selective vagotomy with drainage (n=85)	Highly Selective Vagotomy (n=212)
Early Dumping	22	9	18	12	20	2
Diarrhea	7	23	26	22	16	5
Bile vomiting	13	14	15	10	7	3
Epigastric fullness	37	36	40	37	38	23
Nausea	23	17	13	18	26	9
Food Vomiting	6	10	4	4	—	2
Late Dumping	1	4	6	2	—	2
Flatulence	20	23	18	20	—	9
Heartburn	8	16	20	13	14	18
Dysphagia	0	0	1	1	2	2

(Data from the Leeds and York gastric follow up clinics)

tive procedure that has been used in the treatment of duodenal ulceration since World War II. This unselective type of vagotomy is needlessly aggressive and damaging, and destruction of the pyloric sphincter is simply unnecessary. It is not surprising, therefore, that in the Leeds-York study,[20] V and P yielded Visick grade I + II results in just 64% of male patients 2 years after operation; results in women were even worse. This prompted Goligher to write that V and P had not fulfilled its promise and was not the obvious first choice in the surgical treatment of duodenal ulcer. Similar trials in the United States also showed that TV and D yielded inferior results to partial gastrectomy or vagotomy and antrectomy.[2,19,21]

The results of TV and D may be summarized as follows: operative mortality, 0.7%; incidence of recurrent ulceration, 10% (3% to 30%); with dumping, diarrhea and bile vomiting occurring frequently (Table 28–3). Slight weight loss and anemia also are seen.[22] According to Stalsberg and Taksdal, carcinoma of the stomach becomes a significant risk to any patient who has undergone gastrojejunostomy for benign peptic ulceration more than 20 years previously.[3] It has been suggested that truncal vagotomy with gastrojejunostomy (TV and GJ) leads to an increased risk of gastric carcinoma; this is an important consideration for any center where TV and D has been widely used in the treatment of duodenal ulceration.[7]

The question of which drainage procedure to use with truncal vagotomy has been answered by two trials, both of which showed very similar results.[8,23] Both centers found virtually identical results after the two drainage procedures: bile vomiting was a little more common after GJ than P and recurrence was slightly more common after TV and P than after TV and GJ. Hence, the choice of drainage procedure should be dic-

tated by the condition of the duodenum; when the ulcer is large and the duodenum friable, GJ should be preferred to P. There is also a slight, theoretical advantage in favor of GJ, in that it can be dismantled if side effects attributable to it become troublesome, whereas pyloric reconstruction is not so straightforward. Although that may be so, TV permanently weakens the motility of the antrum, so that closure of a GJ stoma frequently leads to severe gastric stasis.[24] It also must be remembered that bile reflux into the stomach is much more copious after TV and GJ than after TV and P, so that the risk of chronic gastritis, intestinal metaplasia and even gastric carcinoma may be greater, in the long term, after TV and GJ than after TV and P.

Highly Selective Vagotomy

Although either partial gastrectomy or vagotomy combined with a drainage procedure could cure the majority of duodenal ulcers, it was apparent from the mid 1960s that the results of the established operations were far from ideal because of the large proportion of patients suffering from sequelae of the operation, notably dumping and diarrhea. At this time, vagotomy combined with a pyloroplasty was the most popular surgical option for the treatment of duodenal ulcer; selective vagotomy, despite its initial promise, never became widely accepted. There was no doubt that truncal vagotomy was an effective treatment for duodenal ulcer, but the necessity of vagally denervating the other abdominal viscera, together with the drainage procedure, caused much of the associated morbidity. Therefore, to improve the results of peptic ulcer surgery, an operation was needed that not only had a low incidence of recurrent ulceration but, and probably more importantly, also fewer sequelae, particularly dumping, diarrhea, bile vomiting, and epigastric fullness.

With respect to the vagal denervation of the rest of the abdominal viscera, it has been shown that by preserving the celiac branches of the vagus, the incidence of the explosive postvagotomy diarrhea that so crippled many patients after vagotomy could be reduced. However, it was also recognized that many of the postgastric surgery sequelae were a consequence of the destruction of an intact pyloric sphincter mechanism, be it by gastric resection or drainage procedure. Several authors demonstrated that after vagotomy and drainage the drainage procedure was a major cause of these side effects,[24] the mechanism for this being either the permissive effect upon duodenogastric reflux or the fact that the stomach is rendered totally and permanently incontinent, allowing rapid and uncontrolled gastric emptying. The importance of an integrated and intact antral, pyloric, and proximal duodenal function in reducing the side effects of gastric surgery was appreciated by several authors early in the 1960s.[25,26] In an elegant study Carlsson and his associates demonstrated, in dogs, using cineradiography, the importance of an intact antrum in gastric function and the controlled propulsion of chyme into the duodenum.[27]

The permissive effect of a drainage procedure, particularly gastroenterostomy, upon duodenogastric reflux has long been recognized. The "malevolent gall" of Silen[6] is known to have toxic short-term and long-term sequelae. In the short term, it causes a chronic gastritis with recognized specific histological features thought to be responsible for some of the symptoms after gastric surgery (epigastric pain, bile vomiting, heartburn, etc.[28]). The long-term sequelae are more controversial, but it is likely that long-term exposure of the gastric mucosa to excessive duodenogastric reflux increases the risk of gastric cancer. Certainly, after long-term follow-up (>20 years) there is an increased incidence of gastric cancer in patients who have previously undergone gastric surgery for benign disease.[29] Patients who have undergone a Billroth I–type resection would appear to have a lower incidence of gastric cancer than those patients who have undergone a Billroth II–type resection, perhaps because the latter operation more frequently is associated with excessive duodenogastric reflux than the former. Several studies in animals, including recent work from this Department, have shown an association between duodenogastric reflux and subsequent gastric cancer.[30,31] Thus, although not proven beyond doubt, it is likely that decreasing the quantity of duodenogastric reflux will decrease the incidence of gastric cancer following surgery for peptic ulcer. Decreasing duodenogastric reflux certainly will reduce the incidence of its associated side effects.

Thus, to improve the results of surgery for peptic ulceration, two things needed to be avoided. First, the vagal denervation of any viscera other than the parietal cell mass and second, the destruction, either functionally by denervation or mechanically by pyloroplasty or resection, of the antropyloric segment of the stomach.

Ferguson treated a series of patients in whom he combined a vagotomy preserving the nerve supply to the antrum and pylorus with a segmental gastric resection, with apparently good short-term results.[32] Others, in an attempt to preserve an intact pylorus, developed a pylorus-preserving gastrectomy in dogs[26,33]; although the pyloric ring of muscle was preserved, the vagal innervation was not. There followed much debate as to whether the concept of a pylorus-preserving gastrectomy was possible and, if possible, how much of the antrum should be left in situ. Maki described good results with the pylorus-preserving gastrectomy with denervated pylorus in patients with gastric ulceration.[34] However, others have not been able to duplicate these results and it seems likely that stasis would remain a major problem if an intact, but denervated, pylorus and prepyloric stomach were left in situ.

The First Clinical Studies. In 1969, almost simultaneously, Amdrup working in Copenhagen and Johnston in Leeds introduced to clinical practice a vagotomy confined to the parietal cell mass without a concomitant drainage procedure.[35,36] The name given by Johnston to the operation was *highly selective vagotomy*, whereas Amdrup who mapped out the distal border of the parietal cell mass termed the procedure *parietal cell vagotomy.*

Although these two papers described the first use of vagotomy confined to the parietal cell mass without a drainage procedure, Holle in Munich[37] had been treating patients using a very similar operative technique with the notable difference that he routinely added a pyloroplasty or segmental gastric resection. Holle termed the operation *selective proximal vagotomy* and continued to use this operation with good clinical results.[38]

Both Johnston and Amdrup believed that a drainage procedure would not be required because retained antral and pyloric vagal innervation would ensure adequate and controlled gastric emptying. The procedure itself was not new, having been described in dogs by Griffith and Harkins in Seattle 12 years previously.[39]

The operation was received with a good deal of controversy, for several reasons, but most notably because it disregarded the principles that Nyhus had layed down for dealing with the antrum in the course of surgery for peptic ulceration.[40] Many surgeons still had memory of the revenge reaped by the antrum after the ill conceived antral exclusion operations for peptic ulceration. Because of this, Nyhus proposed that if the antrum be retained in the course of gastric surgery it

should be well drained
should remain in the acid stream
should be vagally denervated.

There is no doubt that the antrum remains in the acid stream after highly selective vagotomy and, if the hypothesis of Amdrup and Johnston is correct, it should be well drained. The main controversy regarded the necessity of antral denervation.

The principles of Nyhus were based upon work carried out in prepared canine gastric pouches. In such pouches, the demonstration of vagally mediated gastrin secretion is straightforward,[40] but, when the antrum remains within the acid stream, the vagal release of gastrin is extremely difficult to demonstrate.[41] As was mentioned above, the disastrous results of the antral exclusion operation lay behind much of the fear that surgeons had of leaving innervated antrum in situ. The evidence that, in man, a well-drained antrum that remained within the acid stream would release an excessive quantity of gastrin was very limited.

At the time, Johnston first introduced highly selective vagotomy, he postulated that, far from the excessive incidence of recurrent ulceration that Nyhus might have predicted, the incidence of recurrent ulceration may well be extremely low for the following reasons.

■ There is evidence that celiac and hepatic fibers of the vagi may actually inhibit gastric secretion
■ Acid within the duodenum inhibits gastric secretion partly by means of a vagal mechanism.[42]
■ Truncal vagotomy destroys the inhibition of gastric secretion brought about by the instillation of fat into the duodenum.[43]

Thus, highly selective vagotomy would preserve these inhibitory mechanisms and hence, would better serve to protect the duodenum from exposure to excessive levels of acidity.

The Results of HSV. The following paragraphs detail the results of highly selective vagotomy reported during the early 1970s onwards.

Mortality. By the mid 1970s highly selective vagotomy had proved itself to be a very safe operation. In 1975 Johnston reported the results of a postal questionnaire sent to all surgeons known to be using highly selective vagotomy at that time.[44] Data was received on 5539 patients treated electively for duodenal ulceration by highly selective vagotomy. Overall, there were 17 operative deaths, giving an operative mortality of 0.31%. The causes of the reported deaths were as follows:

Cardiorespiratory   8
Pulmonary embolism   2

Hemorrhage   2
Lesser-curve necrosis 5

Thus, the operative mortality of highly selective vagotomy was significantly lower than that of any other of the commonly used operations for the surgical treatment of duodenal ulceration and, although the control data is not matched, it is likely, given the large numbers that this reflects, a real difference. Lesser-curve necrosis would appear to be a specific complication of highly selective vagotomy occurring in approximately 1 in 500 cases, causing death in approximately 1 in 1000 patients.

Morbidity (Postoperative). Aside from the common and non-operation-specific morbidity, such as respiratory infection, the complication that initially caused most concern was the incidence of gastric stasis. In Johnston's survey, it was found that 0.7% of patients developed evidence of early gastric stasis but that only 1 in 7 of these patients required reoperation because of this.[44] Late gastric stasis requiring the addition of a drainage procedure occurred in a further 0.5% of patients. Thus, a total of 0.6% of patients (1 in every 167) will require reoperation because of gastric stasis; this is certainly no higher than the incidence of troublesome gastric stasis after other operations for peptic ulceration.

Diarrhea. One of the original hopes that was entertained when highly selective vagotomy was introduced was that the incidence of troublesome postvagotomy diarrhea would be greatly reduced, if not abolished altogether. Has this hope been fulfilled? The simple answer is a resounding yes. Almost without fail every reported series detailing the clinical course of patients after highly selective vagotomy has shown a very low incidence of diarrhea and the virtual absence of severe diarrhea (Table 28–4). There is no doubt that these figures are in sharp contrast with those seen after either truncal or selective vagotomy.

Dumping. Highly selective vagotomy, because it preserves the intact and innervated antropyloric region, maintains gastric continence and, hence, is associated with a very low incidence of dumping. Again, the hopes have been fulfilled. In marked contrast to either vagotomy and drainage or partial gastrectomy, the incidence of dumping after operation consistently has been found to be very low (Table 28–4). These figures should be compared to those reported in the Leeds/York trial of elective surgery for duodenal ulcer (Table 28–3), the results of which are typical of those seen after operations other than highly selective vagotomy.

Other Symptoms. The incidences of other symptoms after highly selective vagotomy are also very low. This has led

TABLE 28–4. THE INCIDENCE OF DIARRHEA AND DUMPING AFTER HIGHLY SELECTIVE VAGOTOMY: THE WORLD WIDE EXPERIENCE.

Year	First Author	Number of HSV	Number with dumping	Severe dumping	Number with diarrhea	Severe diarrhea
1982	Busman	229	3	0	4	0
1988	Byrne	244	2	0	2	0
1982	De Miguel	158	9	0	13	0
1984	Donahue	40	2	0	0	0
1986	Enskog	306	7	0	33	0
1984	Garey	509	0	0	0	0
1987	Hoffman	135	18	3	12	0
1986	Jordan	100	17	0	0	0
1983	Knight	258	23	0	17	0
1975	Kronborg	50	3	0	4	1
1986	Herrington	131	2	0	3	0
1983	Gonzalez	829	14	0	37	0
1979	Nilsell	52	2	0	2	0
1986	Rossi	51	0	0	0	0
1987	Von Holstein	100	0	0	6	0
1984	Stoddard	59	1	1	3	0
TOTAL		3251	103	4	136	1
TOTAL (%)		100%	3.2%	0.12%	4.2%	0.03%

several to question the incidence of symptoms other than diarrhea and dumping after highly selective vagotomy and ask how many of these symptoms are specific to highly selective vagotomy and not found in a control group of patients who have not undergone gastric surgery.[11,12] Two studies have clearly addressed this question and the results of both agree closely. The first was the work of Salaman and associates.[45] Salaman studied the gastrointestinal symptoms of patients undergoing herniorraphy and found that their spectrum of Visick grades was identical to that in a matched group of patients after highly selective vagotomy.

Muller, in a much larger and more detailed series, compared the symptoms experienced by 415 patients 5 years after highly selective vagotomy with those symptoms found in 561 age- and sex-matched control subjects (blood donors).[46] The first finding of Muller was that the Visick grade pattern of patients after highly selective vagotomy was almost identical to that seen in the normal controls, the only significant difference being in the percentage of patients graded Visick IV. However this difference was entirely owing to patients with recurrent ulceration after highly selective vagotomy. The symptoms most frequently encountered in the control patients were those of dyspepsia (pain and epigastric fullness) and gastroesophageal reflux. Two percent of the control group experienced dumping-like symptoms and 4% complained of diarrhea. Muller concluded: (1) the Visick grade pattern 5 years after highly selective vagotomy is almost identical with that of healthy controls, (2)

dull pain, epigastric fullness, and reflux symptoms are not specific symptoms after highly selective vagotomy, (3) the separation between Visick grades I and II should be abandoned since it is of no clinical importance and (4) highly selective vagotomy has virtually no specific long-term sequelae except recurrent ulceration.

Long-Term Nutritional Consequences of Highly Selective Vagotomy. If highly selective vagotomy has no specific symptomatic sequelae, other than recurrent ulceration, what then of its longer term nutritional consequences?

Weight Loss. There is no evidence of any long-term weight loss after highly selective vagotomy. Indeed, in almost all reported series there is a general increase in the body weight of patients after highly selective vagotomy.[17,47–50] This experience is mirrored in this Department, Blackett reporting a mean weight gain of 2.5 kg after an average of 9 years following selective vagotomy.[51] Other operations for peptic ulceration are associated with a significant decrease in fat absorption; this does not appear to be the case after highly selective vagotomy. In a study from this Department, Edwards reported that after highly selective vagotomy there was no significant increase in fecal fat excretion compared to levels measured before operation, but there were significant increases both after truncal and selective vagotomy and drainage, compared to both unoperated controls and patients after highly selective vagotomy.[52] Thus, there is no evidence that highly selective vagotomy causes any long-term weight loss, although in itself this is very crude index of overall nutritional status.

Anemia. There has been no series in which the mean hemoglobin has fallen after highly selective vagotomy. Our experience in the Department of Surgery at Leeds General Infirmary found the mean hemoglobin to be static, with a mean of 6% of patients with subnormal hemoglobin levels.[51] Despite this normal hemoglobin, there was a tendency for the mean serum iron to fall after highly selective vagotomy; however the proportion of patients with low serum iron did not increase with time. The situation with regard to serum vitamin B_{12} is more complex. Meikle reported a decreased level of intrinsic factor within the gastric juice after highly selective vagotomy.[53] This decrease in intrinsic factor is reflected in lower mean serum vitamin B_{12} levels compared to values measured before operation,[48,51] but there is no evidence of subsequent pernicious anemia, indeed it is likely that the levels of serum B_{12} never fall to subnormal levels.

Although there are few really long-term follow-up studies of patients after highly selective vagotomy, there is no evidence of any longer term nutritional sequelae, such as osteoporosis, being a clinical problem. It is extremely unlikely, given the combined facts that these patients are nutritionally replete and that there are no more patients with a poor functional outcome than would be seen in an unoperated control of patients, that these problems will become apparent.

Other Long-Term Sequelae of Highly Selective Vagotomy. What of the other sequelae traditionally associated with partial gastrectomy or vagotomy and drainage? For example, both tuberculosis and gastric cancer have been reported as being more common after partial gastrectomy and perhaps, also after vagotomy and drainage. As to tuberculosis, there is no evidence of highly selective vagotomy and predisposing to tuberculosis; indeed, given that, for the great majority of the day after the highly selective vagotomy, the luminal contents of the stomach have a pH level <3 units,[54] it is very unlikely that tuberculosis will pose a problem.

The problem of an increased risk of gastric cancer after previous gastric surgery for benign disease is more thorny. There is now little doubt that there is an increased risk of gastric cancer in the gastric remnant following partial gastrectomy, with the risk being greater after a Polya-type of operation as opposed to the Billroth I procedure.[29] However, the problem is that this increased risk only becomes apparent after many years (>20 yrs) of follow up, and it is likely that the differences from previous reports that suggest a decreased or similar incidence as compared to control subjects are the results of discrepancies in the length of follow-up. The picture regarding vagotomy and drainage is much less clear, owing to few suitably large long-term follow-up studies. As would be expected, an association between vagotomy and pyloroplasty or gastroenterostomy and gastric carcinoma has been reported,[3,7] but the exact magnitude of the increased risk, if any, is unclear. There is no evidence of any increase in risk of gastric cancer after highly selective vagotomy; the few reported cases are no more than case reports. One can, however, postulate as to whether it is likely that after long-term follow-up there will be an increased risk. First, it is probable that excessive duodenogastric reflux plays a role in the pathogenesis of stump cancer, this observation based on both epidemiological and experimental evidence.[55] We know that after highly selective vagotomy duodenogastric reflux is not increased and hence it is unlikely that this factor will increase the risk of gastric cancer after highly selective vagotomy.[56] Second, in the presence of a high intragastric pH, there may be bacterial overgrowth leading to increased levels of nitrosamines, which are powerful carcinogens, within the gastric lumen: however, after highly selective vagotomy the intragastric pH is not particularly low.[54,57]

Finally, highly selective vagotomy preserves normal gastric emptying and, hence, the gastric stasis often seen after vagotomy and drainage is not a feature. For these reasons we do not believe that there will be an increased incidence of gastric carcinoma after highly selective vagotomy. While realizing that, at present, this is pure speculation and will have to await long-term follow-up studies for verification, in an elegant study, albeit in a rat model, Diament, working in this department, failed to show an increased incidence of gastric cancer after highly selective vagotomy.

Summary. The evidence available to date suggests strongly that the only significant long-term sequelae of highly selective vagotomy is recurrent ulceration; hence the long-term evaluation of highly selective vagotomy in the treatment of duodenal ulceration will largely and almost exclusively be determined by the long-term evaluation of the incidence, mortality, complication, and response to treatment of recurrent ulceration after highly selective vagotomy. Therefore, recurrent ulceration is discussed in depth in the following paragraphs.

Recurrent Ulceration after HSV for Duodenal Ulceration. There is no doubt that the Achilles heel of HSV is recurrent ulceration; there is considerable variation in the reported incidences of recurrent ulceration after HSV, with an average of 10% to 12% 5 to 10 years after operation (Table 28–5). The important finding is that recurrent ulceration after HSV is not inevitable and is not related to any identifiable factor such as high acid output.[58,59] The majority of recurrent ulcers after HSV for duodenal ulceration occur as a result of incomplete vagal denervation of the parietal cell mass. The majority of recurrences can be avoided by the surgeon; this is reflected in the experience of our own department where the incidence of recurrent ulceration varies from 5% to >30% depending upon the surgeon who performed the operation. In Adami's study,[60] after 10 years of follow-up, the mean incidence of recurrent ulceration was 17%, but one surgeon had an incidence of recurrent ulceration of 6% compared to 46% for one other surgeon. The incidence of recurrent ulceration is directly related to measures of the completeness of vagotomy, such as peak acid output to insulin 1 to 2 weeks after operation; Kronborg and Madsen reported an incidence of recurrent ulceration of 22% 1 to 4 years after HSV, but 58% of the vagotomies were incomplete on insulin testing.

Operative Technique. When carrying out HSV a number of pointers should be remembered in order to reduce the frequency of incomplete denervation of the parietal cell mass. First, access must be good and the use of a mechanical substernal retractor to improve access to the

TABLE 28–5. RECURRENT ULCERATION AFTER HSV FOR DUODENAL ULCERATION

Year	First Author	Number of HSV	Number of RU	RU-Perf	RU-Haem
1979	Nilsell	118	17	0	0
1981	Poppen	170	35	0	2
1982	Hollinshead	70	4	0	0
1982	Busman	229	22	0	1
1983	Lunde	605	59	1	2
1983	Knight	285	20	0	0
1984	Stoddard	59	5	0	0
1985	Graffner	405	57	0	2
1986	Rossi	25	2	0	0
1986	Herrington	131	10	0	0
1986	Enskog	326	42	0	0
1987	Hoffman	135	32	0	1
1987	Stael von Holstrein	100	18	0	0
1987	Jordan	100	9	0	0
1988	Byrne	244	25	0	0
1990	Macintyre	283	49	1	3
1990	Koruth	57	3	0	0
TOTAL		3342	409	2	11
TOTAL (%)			12%	0.5%	2.5%

esophagus is essential. Another important retractor is the stomach itself, whose greater curvature should be mobilized by division of the gastrocolic omentum, but with careful preservation of the gastroepiploic arterial arcade. The esophagus should be cleared of all fibers for 5 to 6 cm above the cardia[61]; thus, when Hallenbeck cleared just 1 to 2 cm of esophagus, the incidence of recurrent ulceration was 28% compared to <10% when 6 cm of esophagus was cleared of all vagal fibers. Likewise, Kronborg and Madsen cleared only 1 to 2 cm of esophagus and reported an incidence of recurrent ulceration of 22% to 28%.[13] Much time and care must be devoted to this portion of the operation. The borderline between the acid-secreting parietal cell mass and the antrum is, on average, 6 to 9 cm from the pylorus; therefore, to be sure of vagally denervating the distal parietal cells, the vagotomy should be extended to 5 to 6 cm from the pylorus but, at the same time, 1 or 2 major branches of the nerves of Latarjet are preserved. If the vagotomy is extended to within 6 cm of the pylorus, 98% of vagotomies will be complete.[62] Some surgeons strongly advocate the division of either the right gastroepiploic artery or clearance of the distal greater curve. This is done on the basis of the work of Rosati,[63] who demonstrated that some vagal fibers may enter the parietal cell mass via the gastroepiploic arcade. Despite this, we have never used this technique and have a low frequency of incomplete vagotomies and a low incidence of recurrent ulceration (DJ, 6% at 10 years). Likewise, Matheson has not employed the Rosati vari-

ant of HSV, and yet has reported a very low incidence of recurrent ulceration after HSV (5% at 12 years).[64]

Intraoperative Tests for Completeness of Vagotomy. The use of intraoperative tests for completeness of vagotomy is fully discussed in *Vagotomy in Modern Surgical Practice*.[65–68] They may be of use in the training of surgeons and also may produce a psychological benefit in inducing the surgeon to try harder to spend more time to secure a complete vagotomy. They are, however, tedious, not always technically satisfactory and, if the Grassi test is used, may involve opening the stomach. Some of the surgeons who have produced the best results with HSV have not used intraoperative testing. However, it seems logical to use some form of quality control when using a new technique (vide infra, laparoscopic vagotomy), either in the form of intraoperative testing or a postoperative test such as the insulin test or modified sham feeding.

Natural History and Treatment. As recurrent ulceration after HSV is virtually its only specific long-term complication,[60] both the incidence and behavior of these recurrent ulcers will greatly influence the overall evaluation of HSV in the long term.

Standard surgical teaching states that recurrent ulceration following surgery for peptic ulceration is associated with a high morbidity and is an indication for reoperation in the majority of cases: is this still for recurrent ulceration after HSV for duodenal ulceration? On the basis of both data from our department and that from the literature, both described below, we should suggest that the majority of recurrent ulcers presenting after HSV for duodenal ulcer behave in a benign fashion, are treated easily without reoperation, and should not, in most cases, be regarded as absolute failures of treatment.

In our department, since 1969, 990 patients have undergone HSV for duodenal ulceration, either elective or emergency. Of these 990 patients, 100 developed endoscopically proven recurrent ulceration. Of these 100 patients, 1 presented with perforation and 10 with hemorrhage. There was no ulcer-related mortality. Of the 100 patients, only 9 had an eventual poor outcome (Visick grade IV). The vast majority could be successfully treated medically, even in patients whose ulcers were relatively resistant to medical therapy preoperatively.

This relatively benign course of recurrent ulceration is reflected in the literature (Table 28–5). Of more than 3300 patients treated by HSV, operative mortality was 0.12% with just one death from recurrent ulceration. Although in these series, 42% of patients underwent reoperation for recurrent ulceration, later figures suggest that most, if not all, recurrent ulcers after HSV now can be treated medically and few, if any, now need a further operation. Thus, although in the past recurrent ulceration has been regarded as an absolute failure of treatment, this is no longer the case.

Highly Selective Vagotomy Compared in Prospective Trials to Other Ulcer Operations

HSV versus SV and D. HSV has been compared with SV and D in several prospective trials.[11–14] The results have tended to favor HSV, mainly because early dumping was significantly more common after SV and D than HSV. In Kronborg & Madsen's trial, no fewer than 22% of patients developed recurrent ulceration after HSV, and yet the remainder (78%) were either in Visick grade I or II, whereas after SV and D, only 68% of patients were graded Visick I or II, despite a lower incidence of recurrent ulceration. In the other two trials, there was no difference in the incidence of recurrent ulceration between HSV and SV and D.

HSV versus TV and D. Stoddard conducted one of the earliest trials of this kind. Side effects were significantly more common after TV and D than after HSV.[70] He concluded that the results of HSV were superior. After 4 to 8 years of follow-up, the results continued to favor HSV because the side effects were fewer and the incidence of recurrent ulceration was about 10% in both groups.[71]

A large multicenter trial of HSV compared to TV and D was carried out in Manchester.[72] The results of this trial were much less favorable towards HSV, mainly because of recurrent ulceration; the incidence in the HSV group was 21% compared to 8% after TV and D. The trial, however, involved a large number of surgeons and no form of vagotomy quality control was used.

An elegant prospective trial of TV and P versus HSV was carried out by Matheson and colleagues in Aberdeen.[73,74] All 140 patients were operated upon by one experienced surgeon and subsequently reviewed by two independent physicians who were unaware of the surgery performed. With almost 100% follow-up at 5 years, there was no mortality, but side effects were more common after TV and D than after HSV. Four of 70 patients (5.7%) developed recurrent ulceration after TV and D compared with just one recurrent ulcer after 69 HSV procedures (1.4%). Matheson and colleagues concluded that although technically more demanding than TV and D, HSV yielded superior clinical results; this was the same conclusion drawn from the Sheffield study.[71]

Although two further patients in the Aberdeen study developed later recurrent ulceration giving an incidence of recurrent ulceration 12 years after HSV of 5.3%, no fewer than 12 of the patients in the TV and P group had required reoperation for side effects.[74]

Some important lessons can be learned from the results of this excellent trial. The first is that when HSV is performed well, by a skilled and motivated surgeon, the incidence of recurrent ulceration at 12 years can be as low as 5%. A similar conclusion can be drawn from the results of Jordan's trial (vide infra). The second conclusion is that, when performed well, the incidence of recurrent ulceration after HSV is the same as that seen after TV and P. The final lesson is that, when performed correctly, the results of HSV are better than TV and D in the elective surgical treatment of duodenal ulceration.

HSV Versus Vagotomy with Antrectomy. Such trials are of great interest because they compare the most aggressive with the most physiological surgical approach to the elective surgical treatment of duodenal ulceration. Vagotomy with antrectomy (V and A) could confidently be predicted to emerge the victor with regard to recurrent ulceration because surgical ablation of both the vagal and gastrin drives to acid secretion results in an incidence of recurrent ulceration of 1%. By contrast, when antrectomy is omitted the incidence of recurrent ulceration after any form of vagotomy is between 5% and 15%. The question, therefore, is whether the predictably low incidence of recurrent ulceration after V and A is outweighed by the advantages of HSV in terms of operative risk, side effects, and metabolic consequences.

Six prospective trials of HSV versus V and A have been conducted,[15,17,75–80] and we have previously reviewed the results of these trials.[81] The results of these trials are in fairly good agreement: postoperative morbidity was significantly greater and gastric retention and weight loss significantly more common after V and A than after HSV. Recurrent ulceration was more common after HSV than after V and A (10% vs 1.5%), but the number of reoperations was similar in both groups. Patients were significantly more likely to have a perfect result after HSV than after V and A.

Which Operation for Duodenal Ulcer? From the data presented above we think that in the 1990s the operation of choice for duodenal ulceration is HSV. Although the incidence of recurrent ulceration is higher than the "belt and braces" approach of V and A, the price paid in increased side-effects is greater than the cost of the extra recurrent ulcers. There is no evidence that the incidence of recurrent ulceration after a *properly* performed HSV is any higher than after TV and D or SV and D. The caveat to this statement is that the surgeon must be well trained and meticulous in his technique; unfortunately, with decreasing numbers of patients, meeting these training requirements outside specialized centers is becoming increasingly difficult.

Laparoscopic Surgery for Duodenal Ulceration

> What experience, and history teach is this—that people and governments never have learned anything from history, or acted on principles deduced from it. Philosophy of History, GWF Hegel, 1770–1831.

The laparoscope was ignored by most gastroenterological surgeons until the development of laparoscopic cholecystectomy in 1987. When the first reports started to appear in major journals,[82] surgeons rapidly appreciated that minimally invasive surgery may have a role in the management of elective and emergency peptic ulcer disease. The following paragraphs review the status of the world literature with regards to laparoscopic surgery for peptic ulcer disease. Because we are at such an early stage with regards to laparoscopic general surgery the following reports are rather brief. What is apparent is that several exciting approaches may offer the patient long-term ulcer cure without the need for an open operation. As with the open operation, large long-term studies are needed before any accurate conclusions can be drawn, but even at this stage it is apparent that laparoscopic surgery for peptic ulcer is more than just a passing gimmick.

Elective Laparoscopic Surgery for Duodenal Ulcer. Already a multitude of techniques have been described and, unfortunately, as Hegel pointed out 150 years ago (vide supra) the tendency for man to ignore the lessons of the past persists amongst surgeons eager to apply their newfound dexterity with the laparoscope.

Bilateral Truncal Vagotomy Without a Drainage Procedure. Despite the realization by Dragstedt early in his experience of the untoward consequences of bilateral truncal vagotomy without a drainage procedure, the operation has appealed to laparoscopic surgeons because of its simplicity. Murphy and colleagues described its use in 4 patients without clinical gastric stasis.[83] However, there is no reason to suppose that the long-term results of this procedure will be any more satisfactory than those reported historically after open operation. Balloon dilatation of the pylorus has been suggested as an alternative to a drainage procedure, but clinical results are awaited. Laser energy was used to produce a pyloromyotomy in dogs to provide a drainage route for Pietrafitta,[84] but again no clinical results are available.

Laparoscopic Anterior HSV with Posterior Truncal Vagotomy Without a Drainage Procedure. The operation of anterior HSV was first described by Hill and Barker in 1978 as an attempt to simplify the operation of HSV.[85] There have, however, been no long-term clinical studies of patients after this operation. Kum and colleagues have described one patient who had this procedure performed laparoscopically.[86]

Laparoscopic Anterior Seromyotomy with Posterior Truncal Vagotomy. Anterior seromyotomy with posterior truncal vagotomy was first used by Taylor with apparently good clinical results.[87] Therefore, it was natural that laparoscopic surgeons would employ this technique since it lends itself well to laparoscopic surgery. Voeller used pigs to demonstrate the feasibility of this approach and, at the same time, Katkhouda was using this technique in human subjects, without complication.[88,89] The results in the first ten patients were described as good with no recurrent ulceration 1 year after the paper was published (comment at the IIIrd World Congress of Endoscopic Surgery, Bordeaux, June 1992). Katkhouda must be congratulated for measuring gastric secretion and the response to insulin hypoglycemia both before and after operation, although the decreases in insulin-stimulated acid secretion were small. If we use our previous experience with insulin-stimulated acid secretion after operation and the incidence of subsequent recurrent ulceration we have seen after HSV, the incidence of recurrent ulceration with this group of patients may well be more than 30% at 5 to 10 years. Again, larger numbers of patients with longer follow-up is required before the value of this approach can be assessed.

Linear Gastrectomy with Posterior Truncal Vagotomy. This operation utilizes a linear stapler to remove a strip of stomach from the anterior gastric wall to achieve a vagotomy, akin to that achieved by anterior seromyotomy.[90] The operation is unattractive; it opens the stomach with a very long resulting suture line, and is costly. It has little to commend it.

Laparoscopic HSV. This operation is technically one of the most complex and time-consuming laparoscopic procedures contemplated but it has been performed in a few patients with apparently good results (IIIrd World Congress of Endoscopic Surgery, Bordeaux, June, 1992). There is, to date, no publication describing its results in humans, but Josephs has shown that it can be performed in pigs with good results in terms of the apparent completeness of the vagotomy (Congo-red test).[91] Further evaluation is eagerly awaited, but already two leading surgical groups have abandoned this operation as too time consuming.[92] This having been said, others are now realizing that HSV has proved itself as the correct operation for elective duodenal ulcer at open operation and is the correct laparoscopic operation. Groups from Belgium and, in particular, Katkhouda

(France and California) have recently presented encouraging results at surgical meetings during 1994.

In summary, the choice of operation for duodenal ulceration should not be determined by the technical approach but by the same considerations that have been applied over the past 30 years, namely safety and long-term results. By these criteria, no operation has yet surpassed HSV.

■ GASTRIC ULCER

It was fashionable until recently to stress the differences between gastric (GU) and duodenal (DU) ulcers. Today, one is more inclined to emphasize their similarities: both are peptic ulcers, both respond well to histamine H2 receptor antagonists and to vagotomy.

CLASSIFICATION

Gastric ulcers are often divided into three categories according to Daintree Johnson's classification[93]:

- Type I: Gastric ulcer on the lesser curvature
- Type II: Combined gastric and duodenal ulceration
- Type III: Prepyloric ulcer

This system is both difficult to remember and quite arbitrary, in the sense that there is no proof that the three "types" of ulcer have different etiologies or that they require specific and different methods of treatment. For example, according to this system, prepyloric ulcers are distinguished sharply from "ordinary" lesser curve gastric ulcers, on the grounds that they are associated with higher levels of acid secretion, are more akin to duodenal ulcers, and are treatable surgically like duodenal ulcers (by vagotomy), whereas type I ulcers are held to be associated with "hypoacidity" and are to be treated by partial gastrectomy. This is obfuscating nonsense, or, more diplomatically, not in accordance with the facts.

The fact is that we do not fully understand the pathogenesis of gastric ulceration, and until we do, such rigid systems of classification are inappropriate, serving only to cloak our ignorance. The possibility that *a gastric ulcer may be malignant* must never be forgotten. Thus, a prepyloric ulcer may not behave like a duodenal ulcer, for the simple reason that it is not benign. It may not behave like a duodenal ulcer in any case: for example, in several series, the incidence of recurrent ulceration has been found to be significantly higher (20%) after TV or HSV for prepyloric ulcer than after TV or HSF for duodenal ulcer (5% to 10%).[94,95] Even an ulcer that heals with medical treatment with cimetidine or ranitidine may be malignant,

and for that reason *all* patients who are treated medically for benign gastric ulceration *must* be followed up and re-endoscopy done after 6 to 8 weeks, when accurate biopsy of the ulcer or the scar (if the ulcer has healed) should be done. Thus, although most gastric ulcers—even large ones—are benign, they should be assumed to be malignant until they have been proved to be benign, and such proof must rest not merely on the evidence of a few initial biopsies, which may be unrepresentative (ie, false-negative), but on the evidence obtained by means of repeated endoscopy and the taking of multiple biopsy specimens. This point is stressed because the patient's prognosis is relatively good if gastric carcinoma is diagnosed promptly at the stage of ulcer-cancer, the 5 year survival rate after radical partial or total gastrectomy being in the range of 40% to 70%, whereas the prognosis of the common, more advanced type of gastric carcinoma remains dismal.

Let us assume now that the gastric ulcer is indeed benign and chronic, not acute. The definition of an acute ulcer (gastric erosion) is that it is confined to the mucosa and submucosa, whereas a chronic gastric ulcer has, by definition, penetrated the muscle coat of the stomach. What do we know about such a chronic gastric ulcer?

PATHOGENESIS

Gastric ulceration is more common in the elderly than in the young, amongst unskilled or manual workers, than amongst professionals and in cigarette smokers than in nonsmokers. Most drugs that are taken for arthritis, such as aspirin, cortisone, and indomethacin, render the gastric mucosa more vulnerable to autodigestion by acid and pepsin.

It is part of the mythology of gastric ulceration that the patients with such ulcers have hypoacidity or hyposecretion of acid. Therefore, it is said that the use of vagotomy in the surgical treatment of such patients is illogical. The facts are different. Patients with gastric ulcer do not have hypoacidity because acid concentrations in their stomachs are normal. Nor are they, as a group, hyposecretors of acid.[96,97] It should be borne in mind that such patients are often 50 to 80 years of age and that acid output declines with age. Moreover, they tend to be thin; thus, whereas the "average" DU patient is a male of 44 years, weighing about 70 kg, the average GU patient is almost as likely to be female as male, is 56 years of age, and weighs 57 kg. Since acid output is directly proportional to body weight and to lean body mass, patients with GU would be expected to secrete less acid than the heavier, younger DU patients.[97] Adequate control data on the acid outputs of normal people, matched for age, sex, weight, and social class with patients with GU, are lacking, but extrapolation from what information we do possess about normal people suggests that acid outputs in patients with gastric ulcer are, in most cases, well within the normal range.[96–99] Only a few patients, with ulcers high on the lesser curve, may have low acid outputs. In patients with GU, in Leeds, mean peak acid output (PAO) to pentagastrin is about 22 mmol/hr, which is normal. This figure, however, is an underestimate of the patients' true acid output, because some acid is inevitably lost via the pylorus, some is neutralized by alkaline juice refluxing from the duodenum (such reflux is greater than normal in patients with gastric ulcer[100]), and some disappears from the lumen of the stomach into the gastric wall, by the process of "backdiffusion" of hydrogen ions.[101,102] In summary, acid output is not low in most patients with gastric ulcer, rather, it is normal.

Once it is accepted that acid output is not low, but normal, in most patients with gastric ulcer, it becomes easy to understand why cimetidine, ranitidine and omeprazole are so successful in healing benign gastric ulcers (at least temporarily), and vagotomy is seen to be a logical method of surgical treatment for gastric ulcer. Vagotomy, after all, is almost universally used in the surgical treatment of patients with duodenal ulcer, the majority of whom also secrete normal, not high, levels of hydrochloric acid.[99]

The classical Dragstedt theory of the etiology of gastric ulceration incriminated antral stasis, excessive release of gastrin, and hypersecretion of acid, but his theory is no longer tenable in its entirety.[103,104] Gastrin levels are indeed high, but acid output is normal, and few patients with gastric ulcer can be shown to have gastric stasis.[105] The contending theory, which is associated with the names of Du Plessis and Capper, that bile refluxing from the duodenum breaks the gastric mucosal barrier and facilitates autodigestion by acid and pepsin, seems more convincing but cannot be the full explanation either, because gastric ulcers are rare in the vicinity of a gastroenterostomy stoma, where there is no lack of bile, and gastritis is common.[106,107] Most patients with a gastroenterostomy, however, have also undergone vagotomy or partial gastrectomy; consequently outputs of acid and pepsin are low, and thus any attack on the vulnerable mucosa near the stoma is likely to be feeble.

It is probably futile to search for a single cause of gastric ulceration. In any individual patient, it is more likely that various combinations and permutations are factors. There is certainly something abnormal about the pyloric antireflux mechanism in many patients with gastric ulcer: pressure within the pylorus has been found to be abnormally low,[108] and reflux of duodenal content into the stomach is significantly greater than in normal people.[56,100,106,107] Such reflux of bile salts and lysolecithin is thought to break the gastric mucosal barrier, produce gastritis, release gastrin, and render the gastric mucosa more vulnerable to the action both of irritant drugs and of the patient's own acid and pepsin.[109] Gastric ulcers tend to form where the concentration of acid and pepsin is highest, at the junction of the parietal cell mass and the alkaline mucosa of the pyloric gland area or antrum.[110] The crucial role of hydrochloric acid in the pathogenesis of gastric ulcer was a recurrent theme in Dragstedt's writings.[103,104,111] The importance of acid and pepsin is shown also by the fact that where there is no acid, there is no (benign) ulcer,[112] and that acid has been shown to potentiate the harmful effects of alcohol, aspirin, and bile on the gastric mucosa.[102]

Penetration of the gastric mucosal defenses by acid-peptic attack thus seems to be the final common pathway. Hence, as a working hypothesis, it follows that a surgical operation that is designed to cure gastric ulceration should ideally (1) reduce the output of acid and pepsin, (2) prevent or reduce reflux of bile into the stomach, (3) ensure that gastric stasis does not occur, and (4) preserve the gastric reservoir in its entirety.

CHOICE OF TREATMENT

It used to be taught that whereas duodenal ulceration was primarily a medical condition, gastric ulceration was primarily surgical. This was because the *cumulative* mortality and morbidity of prolonged medical treatment for gastric ulcer were higher than the cumulative mortality and morbidity of surgical treatment.[123,124] Medical treatment often failed to secure healing of the ulcer permanently, the pathologic process continued, and the ulcer extended, leading to hemorrhage or perforation in patients who were older and less fit generally than patients with duodenal ulcer, and in whom the mortality of such complications was about 20%. Another cause for mortality among patients treated medically, the presence of an ulcer-cancer, was sometimes missed.

Currently, a greater proportion of patients with gastric ulcer can be treated medically than was formerly the case. Indeed, Morgan and associates reported that all benign gastric ulcers healed in response to 3 months' treatment with cimetidine.[125] The presence of carcinoma must first be excluded, as described previously. The patient then can be treated with cimetidine, ranitidine, omeprazole, De-Nol, or other cytoprotective agents such as sucralfate or misoprostol, and a further endoscopy with biopsies is carried out 6 to 8 weeks later. If the ulcer heals, medical treatment with maintenance doses of these drugs is continued. The patient may require additional antacids and should be advised to obtain adequate rest and regular meals, to give up cigarettes and alcohol, and, if possible, to avoid drugs such as aspirin and indomethacin, which might damage the gastric mucosa.

The *cumulative* menace that the presence of chronic benign gastric ulcer represents to a life and health of a patient over many years must still be appreciated, however. The patient should therefore be followed up regularly, and if the ulcer recurs on more than one occasion, surgical treatment usually should be advised.

CHOICE OF ELECTIVE OPERATION FOR GASTRIC ULCER

Billroth I Partial Gastrectomy (BIPG)

This operative procedure has been widely used in the treatment of gastric ulceration for more than a century, and it is still considered by most surgeons to be the operation of choice.[115,126] However, the results of the largest controlled trial suggest that HSV combined with excision of the ulcer yields better functional results than does Billroth I gastrectomy.[116]

There is no doubt that in the elective surgical treatment of gastric ulcer, BIPG provides superior results to those of vagotomy with a drainage procedure (V and D). The evidence for and against the use of V and D for gastric ulcer was comprehensively reviewed by Forrest and Duthie.[117,118] These authors found that the mean operative mortality of V and D (1.5%) was little less than the mean mortality of partial gastrectomy (PG) (2%). PG was more effective than V and D in curing the ulcer, with a mean incidence of recurrent ulceration after PG of approximately 4%, compared with 10% (range, 2% to 20%) after V and D. De Miguel, for example, followed up 67 patients for 5 to 10 years after selective V and P for GU and found that no fewer than 19% of them had developed recurrent ulceration.[119] In contrast, Cade and Allan followed up 58 patients for a mean period of 7.5 years after truncal V and P with excision of the ulcer and found that 96% of them achieved very good results, while only two developed recurrent ulceration.[120] Perhaps, therefore, excision of the ulcer helps to prevent recurrence. In Copenhagen, Madsen and Schousen[95] reviewed 215 patients 9 to 15 years after TV and P for gastric ulcer; operative mortality was 2%, and the incidence of recurrent ulceration was 8% for GU alone, 0% for GU and DU, and 13% for prepyloric ulcer. After TV and D and excision of the ulcer for GU, mainly at the incisura or on the lesser curve (type 1), Johnson and Giercksky reported a mortality of 1.3% in elective cases and an incidence of recurrence of 13%; they noted that patients with negative insulin tests tended to do well.[121] Kronborg also showed that the risk of recurrent ulceration after TV and P for GU was related significantly to incompleteness of the vagotomy, as judged by the acid response to insulin in the early postoperative period; when PAO (to insulin) minus BAO was greater than 1 mmol/hr, the incidence of recurrence was 30%, whereas when PAO1−BAO was nil, the incidence of recurrence was only 5.5%.[122]

Review of the literature thus shows that although the mean incidence of recurrent ulceration after V and D for GU is about 10% (which is similar to the incidence of recurrence after V and D for DU) the risk of recurrence is considerably less than 10% if the vagotomies are complete, and perhaps, if the ulcer is excised in addition to vagotomy.

Two prospective, controlled trials of TV and D versus BIPG in the treatment of gastric ulceration showed that BIPG yielded better results than TV and D, although the difference between the two procedures was not statistically significant in either trial.[113,114] In Duthie's trial, 78% of patients achieved good-to-excellent results 5 years after BIPG, whereas only 68% of patients achieved such results after TV and P. In Madsen's trial, 95% of patients achieved good results after BIPG and 78% had good results after TV and P.

Although the results of BIPG are good, as a report from Bristol has confirmed they are probably not as good as is widely believed.[115] The operative mortality of 2%, half of which is specific to the gastric resection, owing to hemorrhage, sepsis, or anastomotic leakage with peritonitis, is, for the 1990s, unacceptably high. When BIPG was subjected to blind assessment in the course of a controlled trial in Sheffield, no fewer than 5 of the 29 patients (18%) developed recurrent ulceration during 5 to 12 years of follow-up, 1 patient died of hemorrhage owing to recurrent ulceration, and of the 21 patients who did *not* develop recurrent ulceration and who were assessed a mean of 8 years after operation, only 13 (62%) were found to be enjoying a really good quality of life (Visick grades I and II).[116] The remaining patients were in suboptimal health owing to a wide variety of symptoms, such as dumping, vomiting, and abdominal discomfort (Tables 28–2 and 28–4). Thus, although generally fairly good, the results of BIPG for gastric ulcer provide no grounds for complacency; there is certainly room for improvement.

Determined attempts have been made in the past 20 years to find alternatives to BIPG for the treatment of gastric ulcer. TV and D, as we have seen, offers no real advantage, although it may still be a better choice than BIPG in unfit, elderly patients or in the treatment of massive hemorrhage from gastric ulcer. A Billroth II resection, likewise, yields results that are no better than those of Billroth I. Three other operative procedures, however, are worthy of consideration: the very conservative distal gastrectomy described by de Miguel, the Maki pylorus-preserving gastrectomy, and HSV with excision of the ulcer.

de Miguel's Distal Antrectomy

As mentioned previously, de Miguel found a 19% incidence of recurrent ulceration in the long term after selective vagotomy and pyloroplasty for gastric ulcer, and therefore, sought other methods that might yield better results.[119] Reasoning that many of the indifferent clinical results after BIPG might be owing to loss of gastric reservoir capacity, and also that the antropyloric region might, in some way, be involved in the pathogenesis of gastric ulcer (as Burge had suggested previously), de Miguel has advocated the use of a very conservative variant of the Billroth I procedure, which consists of distal antrectomy, pylorectomy, and excision of the ulcer, followed by a gastroduodenal (BI) anastomosis.[127] Only about a quarter of the stomach is removed. He has reported the results of 46 of these procedures, performed for gastric ulcer alone with a follow-up of 5 to 10 years. There was no operative mortality, not a single case of recurrent ulceration, and 90% of patients achieved good (Visick grades I and II) clinical results. These are impressive figures, from an author who has always analyzed his data rigorously. They lend further support to the idea that a Billroth I resection should be very conservative in its extent—removing at most 30% to 50% of the stomach—rather than the 60% to 70% gastric resection that was formerly performed in the treatment of duodenal ulcer. De Miguel's challenging ideas should be tested by prospective trials.

Maki's Pylorus-Preserving Gastrectomy

This is a variant of BIPG, a hemigastrectomy with excision of the ulcer, in which the pylorus and 1 to 2 cm of prepyloric stomach are preserved.[34,128] Although good clinical results have been obtained by its originators in Japan, Liavag and colleagues in Oslo have reported a 17% incidence of failure owing either to recurrent ulceration (11%) or to gastric retention (6%), after a 5 to 7 year follow-up of 47 patients; the remaining patients enjoyed excellent results. Dumping and diarrhea, in particular, were completely eliminated.[129]

It is interesting that all five recurrent ulcers in Liavag's series were situated in the short prepyloric segment of stomach: perhaps an anastomosis so close to the pylorus predisposed to gastric stasis and so to recurrence in these patients. If the Maki procedure is to be used at all, the preoperative endoscopic assessment must be of the highest quality because the procedure must be confined to patients with type I lesser curve gastric ulcers, and patients with prepyloric or pyloroduodenal ulceration excluded. The anastomosis must be performed impeccably, with minimal inversion of tissue. Great care must be taken not to leave too long a segment of stomach proximal to the pylorus because this segment is vagally denervated and, if more than 2 cm long, leads to gastric stasis. Nevertheless, further trial of the Maki operation seems justifiable, under controlled conditions, provided that these preconditions are met.

Highly Selective Vagotomy with Excision of the Ulcer

Use of HSV in the treatment of GU is based on the hypothesis that a GU, like a DU, is a peptic ulcer. It is produced by *normal*, not low, amounts of pepsin breaching a gastric mucosal barrier that has been weakened by various factors. Our hypothesis was that if acid-peptic attack could be blunted by the use of HSV, the ulcer would heal, and the patient would reap the benefit of having a complete stomach, with an intact antropyloroduodenal segment, rather than having just half a stomach and no pylorus, as is the case after Billroth I partial gastrectomy.[130] A further advantage of HSV compared with BIPG or V and D is that it actually reduces the concentration of bile acids in the stomach,[56] perhaps because it increases intragastric pressure and speeds gastric emptying of liquids.[131,132] Thus, the ulcer-healing effect of HSV may be the result of a strengthened gastric mucosal defense, as well as to a weakened acid-peptic attack.

Our own policy, since 1969, has thus been to treat all patients coming to elective operation for gastric ulcer by HSV and excision (HSV-E) (or occasionally merely biopsy) of the ulcer.[130] The series is not quite consecutive, however, because a few patients had to be excluded owing to technical difficulties or suspicion that the ulcer was malignant. An up-to-date account of the operative technique has been published.[133] HSV for GU is certainly more difficult to perform than HSV for DU because edema and fibrosis in the base of the ulcer may obliterate the plane of dissection along the lesser curvature. Since the parietal cell mass is proximal to the ulcer, however,[110] it may not be necessary to clear the lesser curvature as far distally as the incisura: it may be sufficient to perform the usual dissection on the esophagus and to clear the lesser curvature as far as the upper margin of the ulcer. Certainly, to date, this proximal variant of HSV has yielded percentage reductions in acid output as great as those found after standard HSV, while the clinical results also have been as good as after standard HSV.

Results of HSV and Ulcer Excision for Gastric Ulcer Alone. One hundred and sixteen patients with type I gastric ulcer were treated by HSV-E between 1969 and 1990, with one operative death (1%).

Acid Secretion. The insulin test was positive in only 7% of patients; peak response to pentagastrin (PAOPg) was reduced by 67% at 1 week, and by 80% at 1 to 5 years after HSV, reductions that are greater than we reported after HSV for DU (approximately 50%).

Fecal Fat Excretion. This was measured on a metabolic ward and was found to be normal after HSV but significantly elevated after BIPG.

Bodyweight. Before operation, patients with GU lost an average of 5 kg in weight. After HSV, significant weight gain of about 4 kg occurred, whereas after BIPG body weight did not increase; in fact, a further small decrease in weight was found.

Recurrent Ulceration. The incidence of recurrent ulceration was 13% by life table analysis after a 10 year follow-up. Most of the recurrences were diagnosed in the first year after operation. Four of ten patients with recurrence underwent reoperation in the form of partial gastrectomy, with good results in each, whereas six responded to the medical treatment.

Overall Results (Visick). About 80% of patients have achieved very good clinical results after HSV for gastric ulcer, which is superior to the results recorded after BIPG in this department. Results after 18 emergency procedures were similar to the results of elective surgery, and patients with high lesser curve ulcer fared as well as others.

The Visick grades after HSV seem unimpressive but represent high marks for the Leeds Gastric Follow-Up Clinic. Likewise, in Cardiff, Salaman and colleagues noted that Visick grades were as good after HSV (for DU) as after herniorrhaphy, but that only about 85% to 90% of patients from either group achieved Visick grade I or II results.[45] There is a lot of dyspepsia in the apparently normal population, and the achievement of good (ie, I and II) Visick grades in all patients with peptic ulcer is thus an unattainable ideal, at least according to the stringent criteria used in York and Leeds.

To sum up, this 20 year experience of HSV for gastric ulcer at the Leeds General Infirmary has shown that the operative mortality is about the same as that of BIPG, but the patients suffer from fewer side effects of operation, eat better, and gain more weight than patients who have undergone BIPG. The 13% incidence of recurrent ulceration is probably higher than after BIPG, but most patients with recurrence achieved good results after receiving further treatment. HSV should not be used in the treatment of prepyloric or pyloric ulcers, but it is suitable for all gastric ulcers situated on the lesser curvature from 3 cm proximal to the pylorus right up to near the cardia. The importance of doing multiple, accurate preoperative biopsies and of excising the ulcer by a transgastric approach via a gastrotomy on the greater curvature is emphasized. Even healed ulcers should be excised because malignant ulcers may heal temporarily with medical treatment, and we have had several examples of exactly that occurrence in our own practice.

Similar results to ours were reported by Jorde and associates, who treated 72 patients with gastric ulcer by HSV-E with no operative mortality and 10% recurrent ulceration after a 5 year follow-up.[135] They made the interesting observation that, compared with SV and P-E, which they had previously used to treat 137 patients with GU, HSV-E led to less gastric stasis, less gastritis, less dysplasia, and *presumably*, less risk of carcinoma. Among 71 patients with type I GU who had been treated with HSV-E, Heberer and Teichmann reported that the incidence of *symptomatic* recurrent ulceration was 8% after a 5 year follow-up, but that the total incidence of recurrence (ie, symptomatic and silent) by endoscopic surveillance was 17.5%; most of the recurrences responded well to further medical treatment.[136] Heberer and Teichmann believed that HSV with excision or biopsy of the ulcer provided acceptable treatment both for type I GU and for combined GU and DU, but that it should not be used for pyloric or prepyloric ulcer because of a recurrence rate that ranged from 16 to 44 percent; we would agree with their conclusions.

Highly Selective Vagotomy (Selective Proximal Vagotomy) with Pyloroplasty

It was Professor Holle of Munich who first introduced vagotomy of the proximal stomach (SPV) into clinical practice in the mid 1960s, but he insisted that SV had to be accompanied by a pyloroplasty or an antrectomy, which, in our opinion, negates many of its advantages.[37] Holle and Bauer reported 124 patients with gastric ulcer who were treated by SPV during a 10 year period, with an operative mortality, in elective cases, of 0.8% and an incidence of recurrent ulceration of 2.4%.[137] The long-term functional results were good in 80% of patients, fair in 12%, and poor in 8%. These results were not as good as the results of SPV for duodenal ulcer in Holle's practice (90%, good; 6%, fair; and 4%, poor). Holle and Bauer remarked, "The reduction of clinical symptoms in duodenal ulcer is impressive, but the effect on gastric ulcer is less remarkable. We attribute this, in particular, to the high average age and the number of concomitant diseases in the gastric group."[137] Nevertheless, Holle's results in patients with gastric ulcer are quite impressive, and no doubt a good deal is owed to his meticulous operative technique, which results in very little response to insulin stimulation after operation. In his series, BAO was reduced from a mean of 1.4 mmol/hr before operation to 0.1 mmol HCl per hour, MAO from 12 to 1 mmol/hr, and the peak response to insulin from 11.3 to 0.8 mmol/hr. The lesson seems clear: if Holle's excellent clinical results are to be emulated, his efficient vagal denervation of the parietal cells must first be reproduced. Holle also stressed the need for efficient gastric emptying (which is why he adds a pyloroplasty) and in our opinion the addition of pyloroplasty to HSV also might have advantages in the minority of patients with gastric ulcer who have demonstrable gastric stasis before operation. In the majority of patients, however, no such stasis is evident, and since HSV speeds gastric emptying of liquids, there seems little logic in adding a drainage procedure that leads to greater abnormalities in the pattern of gastric emptying and produces symptoms of dumping.

Prospective Controlled Trials of HSV and BIPG for Gastric Ulcer

In a scientific sense, an acknowledged weakness of our own work has been that we have treated an almost consecutive series of patients by means of HSV, without prospective comparison with gastric resection. Such a comparison has been made, however, by other surgeons.

A multicenter study in North Germany found an incidence of recurrent ulceration of 20% after HSV, compared with 5% after BIPG. In that trial, a relatively small number of HSV procedures were performed by quite a large number of surgeons, many of whom had not previously had much experience with HSV for gastric ulcer. Hence, the poor results after HSV are perhaps not surprising, and the trial was by no means unbiased, because the surgeons, an uncontrolled variable, were presumably more experienced in the performance of gastric resection than in the performance of HSV for gastric ulcer.

A larger trial, carried out in one center, was reported by Duthie and colleagues from Sheffield.[117] Fifty-six patients with gastric ulcer alone (type I) were allotted in a random manner either to HSV-E (HSV with excision) or to BIPG. There was no operative mortality. Fifty-four patients (96%) were followed up for a mean period of 8 years (5 to 12 years). Four deaths occurred during follow-up in each group. There was no ulcer-related deaths during follow-up in the HSV group but, in the BIPG group, one patient died of hematemesis owing to recurrent ulceration, and another patient died 1 month after suffering a severe melena, the cause of which was not defined. In the HSV group, six patients developed recurrent ulceration, of whom three did well on medical treatment with cimetidine and three underwent gastric resection, with good results. In the BIPG group, five patients developed recurrent ulceration, of whom only two eventually achieved good results, one died, and two had poor long-term results. In the HSV group, all patients who did not develop recurrent ulceration achieved good (Visick grades I and II) clinical results, whereas only 62% of patients without recurrence in the BI group achieved such good clinical results. The side effects of operation were much more frequent after BIPG than after HSV. The final clinical status of all the patients from either group was that 95% of patients eventually achieved good results after HSV, whereas only 60% of patients achieved good results after BIPG.

This paper by Duthie and colleagues is historic because it is the first controlled trial to show that BIPG can no longer be regarded as the automatic treatment of choice for benign lesser curve gastric ulcer.[116] The numbers of patients, although fairly small, were relatively large for a trial of surgery for gastric ulcer, and follow-up was commendably complete and prolonged. A disturbing feature was the high incidence of recurrent ulceration in both groups of patients, which is difficult to explain. Perhaps patients who require elective operation for gastric ulcer in these days of potent medical agents form a relatively resistant group, who may fare less well after operation than patients who formerly underwent BIPG. Many of them, for example, are receiving medication on a long-term basis for rheumatic conditions. Another possible explanation for the high incidence of recurrence after HSV is that the operations were carried out by all grades of surgical staff, and although many patients did not undergo postoperative insulin tests, the incidence of incomplete vagotomy in those who did have insulin tests was about 30 percent.

If HSV is to be used more widely in the treatment of gastric ulcer, it seems important that the surgeon who operates should have performed many HSVs for duodenal ulcer. Ulcer excision should be carried out by a transgastric approach from a gastrotomy sited parallel to the greater curvature (a proximal to the antrum), because attempts to excise the ulcer by a wedge excision from the lesser curvature aspect inevitably endanger the nerves of Latarjet and are likely to lead to antral stasis and thus to recurrent ulceration. As stated previously, patients with pyloric or prepyloric ulcer should not be treated by HSV but by vagotomy and antrectomy.

■ HEMORRHAGE FROM PEPTIC ULCER

GENERAL CONSIDERATIONS

The following remarks are confined to the subject of bleeding from chronic gastric or duodenal ulcer. About 30 000 patients per year are admitted to hospital in Britain with severe upper gastrointestinal hemorrhage, and the mortality remains high, with about 3500 deaths each year.[138–140] Chronic peptic ulceration accounts for about 50% of such cases. There seems to have been no significant improvement since the introduction of the H2 receptor antagonists, perhaps because of the widespread use of cigarettes and of nonsteroidal anti-inflammatory agents (NSAIDs) in an aging population.[141]

Until the late 1980s there was one major difference between the operative treatment of hemorrhage from peptic ulcer and the operative treatment of hemorrhage from peptic ulcer and the operative treatment of perforation: the use of a definitive ulcer-curing operation was regarded as mandatory in patients with hemorrhage, whereas in patients with perforation it is optional. This concept has recently been challenged by the widespread availability of potent antisecretory drugs such as ranitidine and omeprazole, and the combination of nondefinitive surgery and drug therapy has been advocated. However, the data from the literature do not support the widespread use of this approach without further careful evaluation, preferably within the context of controlled trials. A study coordinated from Birmingham, England compared definitive surgery with simple underrunning and ranitidine therapy.[142] The mortality in both groups was high, 26% after conservative surgery and 19% after definitive surgery. However, the main difference between the two groups was in the incidence of fatal rebleeds, with no fewer than 6 (10%) in the conservative group and none after conventional surgery. However, this study cannot be regarded as definitive. In Leeds, we are selectively using more conservative therapy; the important point to make is that the bleeding point must be well underrun with a strong nonabsorbable suture and, if possible, the bleeding point excluded from the lumen of stomach or duodenum. Following simple underrunning the patient must be placed on the most potent anti-acid therapy available, currently a proton pump inhibitor, such as omeprazole. This having been said, the surgical treatment of bleeding peptic ulcer is still one of definitive therapy in the majority of cases; the surgeon should weigh up the risks and benefits of each approach for every individual case and not adopt a blanket approach.

Clearly, in the surgical treatment of these shocked, high-risk patients the presence of an expert surgeon may mean the difference between life and death. Thus, although it is customary for registrars or senior registrars to deal with many of these emergency cases in the middle of the night, the chances of the patient are likely to be significantly improved if a consultant surgeon takes a close personal interest in the case and performs the operation personally.

These comments apply to patients who require emergency surgery. However, in the 1990s, a higher proportion of patients will be treated without operation, by means of injection, laser, or coagulation applied to the ulcer via the endoscope. At the same time, potent antisecretory agents such as ranitidine or omeprazole will be administered, in the hope that recurrent bleeding will thereby be diminished.

After admission to the hospital, the patient should be transfused with blood until, ideally, the skin becomes warm and pink, the blood pressure stable, the central venous pressure positive, and the urinary output good. Naturally, this ideal state cannot always be achieved if the bleeding continues. If the bleeding stops, at least four units of blood should be kept in the blood bank, in case of recurrence of bleeding. The patient should be watched very carefully at this stage, both by physician and surgeon, who should visit several times a day.

It is now more than 30 years since Sir Francis Avery Jones showed the advantages of care in a combined medical and surgical unit, where the mortality was only 6.3%.[143] The advantages of a team approach and of a special unit devoted to the care of patients with gastrointestinal hemorrhage were again highlighted by Hunt, Hansky and Korman from Melbourne, who adopted an aggressive policy of endoscopy within 12 hours of admission, early surgery in most patients with gastric ulcer, and in patients ≥60 years of age with duodenal ulcer, and intensive care for all poor-risk and postoperative patients.[144] This policy led to a significant decrease in mortality from bleeding peptic ulcer, from 8% to 4%, while in the high-risk group of patients >60 years of age, mortality decreased from 13% to 8%.

The source of bleeding should be pinpointed within a few hours of the admission of the patient to hospital by means of esophagogastroduodenoscopy (OGD), supplemented, if necessary, by emergency angiography or double contrast barium meal examination. However, in the case of hemorrhage from chronic peptic ulcer, an expert endoscopist should be able to see the lesion in at least 95% of cases. The history alone may be misleading because cirrhotic patients may bleed not from varices but from acute or chronic peptic ulceration, and patients with a history of peptic ulcer may be bleeding from Mallory-Weiss tears at the cardia or from other lesions. It is disappointing that the more accurate diagnosis of these patients by means of OGD in recent years so far has not been followed by any convincing evidence of clinical benefit,[145,146] however there is good evidence that interventional endoscopy is now decreasing the need for emergency operation[147] and it is likely that during the next few years this may be reflected in lower overall mortality. Surgical mortality from severe hemorrhage has not diminished significantly, remaining obstinately at between 10% and 14%. In the few cases in whom angiography proves necessary, it may be possible to secure cessation of the hemorrhage by the local infusion of vasopressin or by embolizing the bleeding vessel with Gelfoam.[148] It should be emphasized that such measures are seldom used and their effectiveness is, at best, variable.

MANAGEMENT

Once the patient is resuscitated and the source of hemorrhage identified, the surgeon is left with two crucial decisions: first, whether and when to operate, and second, which operation to perform.

To Operate or Not to Operate?

The aim is to avoid operating on all patients who would recover with medical treatment, but to operate on all patients who, if treated medically, would bleed again to a dangerous extent. Furthermore, if surgical treatment is undertaken, it should be performed at the optimal time, and the safest operative procedure should be used, by a highly skilled surgeon. Obviously, such a degree of perfection is clinically unattainable, but a clear appreciation of the principles of management, based on an understanding of risk factors, will at least prevent many deaths.

The most important risk factor is the emergency operation itself, which has a mortality of about 10%, 10 to 20 times the mortality of elective operation for peptic ulcer. The factor of emergency operation is, in reality, a cluster of adverse factors, which includes advanced age, concomitant disease, continued bleeding, and shock on the part of the patient, and at times inexperience on the part of the surgeon, anesthetist, and nurses. Hence, if an emergency case can be converted into an elective or semielective one, the operative mortality is reduced from 10% to 1% or 2%. Thus, the timing of surgical intervention is vital.

The age and general condition of the patient are important factors to consider. Rebleeding in patients >60 years of age is very dangerous, increasing mortality sixfold,[149] and so, if any elderly patient is admitted to hospital with severe bleeding and then stops bleeding and is resuscitated, there is much to be said for operating in a semiemergency fashion before he or she bleeds again. In the face of severe comorbidity, such as cardiac failure or chronic obstructive airways disease, mortality can be as high as 50%.[149] Under 50 years of age, patients' cardiovascular systems are more resilient and rebleeding is much less likely to be fatal.[150]

The amount and rate of hemorrhage are of prognostic significance,[151] so if patients are admitted in shock after a recent hematemesis, they are obviously at high risk and require intensive care and very often operative intervention when they are fit enough to withstand the operation. Transfusion of more than 10 units of "old" bank blood within 24 hours is associated with a high mortality. Thus, if bleeding does not stop, an operation should be performed long before 10 units of blood have been transfused.

Patients in whom endoscopy shows the presence of a chronic gastric ulcer, particularly a large ulcer, are at high risk and the threshold for operative intervention should be low.[152]

An elegant study from Birmingham has taken and applied these clinical factors and combined them to derive a policy for the management of bleeding peptic ulcers, and whether early or delayed operative intervention is most appropriate.[150] Patients <60 years of age can be managed for longer in a conservative manner; two rather than one rebleeds are an indication for surgery or a maximum blood replacement of 6 rather than 4 units of blood in 24 hours. This policy is safe, there were no deaths in the Birmingham series, but it should not be used as an absolute and rigid guide, particularly in

patients with gastric ulceration. However, patients > 60 years of age, who, in fact, constitute the main problem, should be offered surgery early. The mortality was 2% in the early arm of the Birmingham trial compared to 13% in the delayed arm; the criteria for early intervention were one rebleed, more than 4 units of blood required in 24 hours, and endoscopic stigmata. Early intervention is particularly appropriate for elderly patients with large gastric ulcers and endoscopic stigmata. Indeed, there is much to be said in that group for not waiting for even one rebleed.

Endoscopic Stigmata Indicating Risk of Further Hemorrhage
In most patients, gastrointestinal bleeding does not recur and mortality is low, but in 20% to 30% of patients, hemorrhage will either continue or will recur, with a subsequent mortality of 10% to 30%. Hence, it is important to try to predict which patients will rebleed. In 1978 Foster and his colleagues at St. James's Hospital in Leeds pointed out the importance of "visible-vessel" active hemorrhage at the time of endoscopy and other endoscopic stigmata of recent bleeding as predictors of recurrent bleeding.[153] Depending on the exact criteria used, between 50% and 100% of ulcers with visible vessels will rebleed.[153–156] Hence, early endoscopy, within 24 hours of admission, is of value in pinpointing the source of hemorrhage and in separating patients into high-risk and low-risk groups. It is easy to miss small, high gastric ulcers at operation or to miss a gastric lesion coexisting with an obvious duodenal ulcer. Because their treatment is different, endoscopy is also necessary when it is suspected that esophageal varices may be the course of the hemorrhage. Likewise, surgeons want to know whether they are dealing with acute hemorrhagic gastritis, rather than varices or chronic peptic ulcer. For these reasons the use of early endoscopy is desirable, despite the lack of supporting evidence from controlled trials.

Drug Therapy
Bed rest and careful monitoring are necessary, at first. If urgent surgery is not planned and vomiting has stopped, free intake of oral fluids and a light diet should be encouraged.[157]

Cimetidine, Ranitidine, and Omeprazole. Most controlled trials have yielded little evidence that the use of H2 receptor antagonists prevents rebleeding or saves lives.[158–160] However, in a study of 100 patients with moderate or severe hemorrhage, Hoare and associates found that in patients with gastric ulcer only 2 or 14 who received cimetidine experienced rebleeding, whereas 10 of the 19 who received placebo experienced rebleeding ($p < 0.05$), and only 1 patient on cimetidine required emergency surgery, whereas 8 receiving placebo required emergency surgery—again, a significant difference.[161] This little-quoted paper is important because it is just those patients who were studied—those in the older age group, with more severe hemorrhage, and with gastric rather than duodenal ulceration—who are at particular high risk of rebleeding and who are likely to die if they should require emergency surgery. Regarding the mechanism whereby H2 blockers prevent rebleeding in gastric ulcer, Hoare suggested that, since acid output is lower in GU than in DU patients, the rise in intragastric pH may be greater after treatment with cimetidine, and this, in turn, may help blood to clot in the stomach and prevent lysis of clot. In patients with duodenal ulcer, the rise in pH may not be sufficient. Support for the belief that the use of H2 receptor antagonists can reduce the incidence of rebleeding comes from two meta-analyses.[162,163] The data regarding the use of proton pump inhibitors such as omeprazole is not as mature as that for the H2 receptor antagonists, but some interesting trends are developing. Although, when compared to placebo, the use of omeprazole has not been shown to reduce short-term rebleeding in the largest study to day.[164] There was a significant reduction in the endoscopic stigmata of recent bleeding, suggesting that omeprazole may be having some effect. Indeed, one smaller study did demonstrate a significant reduction in rebleeding in the omeprazole-treated patients.[165] Almost as important, several authors have now demonstrated that for patients with *H pylori*–positive bleeding duodenal ulcers, early therapy to eradicate the *H pylori* using a combination of omeprazole and antibiotics is more effective than only omeprazole in preventing rebleeding in the medium term.[166,167] Therefore, where available, patients with bleeding peptic ulcers should be treated with omeprazole and where indicated *H pylori* eradicated as soon as possible.

Tranexamic Acid. Excessive fibrinolytic activity occurs in patients with bleeding peptic ulcer. Tranexamic acid has antifibrinolytic activity and has been shown to reduce both requirements for blood transfusion and the need for emergency surgery.[168–171] The drug should be given orally and does not seem to affect fibronolysis in the peripheral blood. Despite its possible therapeutic benefit, tranexamic acid is not widely used.

Somatostatin. Somatostatin raises intragastric pH to about 7, reduces splanchnic blood flow, and may be superior to cimetidine in preventing rebleeding.[172]

Nonsurgical Methods for Arresting Hemorrhage and Preventing Rebleeding

The cause of death in most of these patients is recurrent bleeding. This comes not from the entire ulcer but from an eroded artery, the endoscopist's "visible vessel," in the base of an ulcer. If this artery could be sealed, by endoscopic means, the need for emergency surgery might be reduced, and this would certainly result in a reduction in overall mortality.

Ever since the pioneering work of Fruhmorgen and associates[173] and Kiefhaber and associates[175] with laser photocoagulation of the bleeding point, there has been an explosion of interest in endoscopic methods of arresting hemorrhage, whether by means of laser,[156,175–178] diathermy,[179–181] or injection of adrenaline (epinephrine)[182] or alcohol.[183] The results are conflicting, as might be expected. Thus, MacLeod and associates found that relatively few patients (45 out of 640) were suitable for treatment with the laser.[156] Some trials have suggested that use of lasers reduced the incidence of rebleeding, but Krejs and associates alloted 174 patients with active bleeding to treatment with, or without, the neodymium-yttrium aluminum garnet (Nd:YAG) laser and found more rebleeding in the laser-treated patients and just as great a need for urgent surgery.[178] They concluded that the use of Nd:YAG laser did not benefit the patients. Rutgeers and associates reported that use of multipolar electrocoagulation yielded similar results to the Nd:YAG laser, namely, an 86% to 88% success rate in stopping bleeding and 14% mortality with either method.[184] Johnston and associates, however, found that the heater probe yielded superior results to those of the YAG laser.[179,180]

Thus, at present, it is by no means clear what endoscopic method is best. Johnston suggests that the hemorrhage should be stopped initially by injections or the heater probe, or both, while simultaneous use of potent antacid-pepsin agents and antifibrinolytic agents may diminish rebleeding.[180] There is now sufficient evidence that definitive endoscopic therapy can reduce the incidence of rebleeding; it is the method that remains controversial.[164,185–187] It is our belief that all patients with peptic ulcers with stigmata of recent hemorrhage should be offered endoscopic therapy. It seems important that the understandable enthusiasm for such methods should not lead to undue procrastination and avoidance of operative intervention in patients who need it urgently.

Selection Of Operative Procedure

Bleeding Duodenal Ulcer. In a review of the world literature on bleeding peptic ulcer between 1957 and 1967, Alexander-Williams found a mean operative mortality of 15% after 1088 partial gastrectomies, and a mean operative mortality of 8% after 513 truncal vagotomies combined with pyloroplasty and underrunning of the bleeding point.[188] Somewhat surprisingly, the incidence of rebleeding was no greater after TV and P than after PG (14%). Lyndon, in this department, reviewed the literature for the ensuing decade and found a mortality of 16% after 1197 partial gastrectomies and a mortality of 9% after 1260 TV and Ps [Lyndon, unpublished]. For these reasons, although such data no doubt contain some bias, most surgeons now favor the use of under-running of the bleeding point, followed by truncal vagotomy with a drainage procedure. The main criticism of such a policy is the incidence of rebleeding, but it should be remembered that any mortality from re-bleeding is included in the overall mortality, which is nearly twice as high after partial gastrectomy as it is after V and P.

Preoperative Preparation. In practice, then, what we do is make the diagnosis, get the patient into as good condition as possible, and, once operative treatment has been decided upon, assemble the strongest team of surgeons, anesthetist, and theater sister that can be mustered. If the patient is in the high-risk category, the intensive care unit is warned that it may have to look after this patient after operation. The patient's stomach is emptied by means of a wide-bore tube. Induction of anesthesia can be as hazardous in these patients as in patients with ruptured aortic aneurysm because the onset of muscular relaxation may be associated with profound hypotension, which may quickly progress to cardiac arrest or dangerous arrhythmia; hence, the need both for an experienced anesthetist and for bringing the patient to the theater adequately transfused, as shown by the central venous pressure. It is the elderly patients, particularly those with hypertension or ischemic heart disease, who are most at risk for periods of transient hypotension and anoxia. In all shocked patients, it is vital to have at least one and preferably two wide-bore intravenous cannulae securely in place before operation and to have plenty of blood available. The fresher the blood the better, and it should be warmed. A single intramuscular injection of cephalosporin or ampicillin is given with the premedication to guard against sepsis because the alimentary tract is sure to be opened and contamination of the peritoneal cavity and of the wound is inevitable. The incidence of wound infection is over 30%, if such antibiotic cover is omitted.[189]

Operative Technique: Truncal or Highly Selective Vagotomy? The abdomen is opened quickly through a midline incision. The diagnosis of duodenal ulceration is confirmed and the stomach palpated carefully for the presence of a gastric ulcer that might have been missed at endoscopy (this easily happens when the stomach is full of blood clot). Assuming that the diagnosis is one of duodenal ulceration alone, the next step is to perform a duodenotomy and underrun the bleeding point. The bleeding point must be underrun by a number of strong nonabsorbable sutures, taking deep bites to encircle the vessel well.

There is no evidence from the literature to suggest that, even with modern antisecretory medication, a definitive acid-reducing operation should not be performed at the time of operation for bleeding duodenal ulcers and, by this stage, we usually will have decided whether to perform a truncal V and P or an HSV. Truncal V and P should be the standard method of surgical treatment in these emergency conditions and, certainly if the patient is shocked, elderly, or still actively bleeding, there is no doubt that the vagotomy should be truncal in type. However, quite often at operation the bleeding is either found to have stopped or is quickly brought under control. If, in addition, the patient is relatively young (<60), not obese, and generally fit, the operative risk should not be much greater than that of an elective procedure, we therefore prefer to perform an HSV, which takes about 30 minutes longer than a truncal vagotomy. These considerations determine the extent of the duodenotomy incision because, if TV and P is planned, a wide gastroduodenotomy incision can be made across the pylorus, whereas, if the intention is to perform an HSV, the incision in the duodenum should stop at the pylorus. The ulcer is exposed, the bleeding point identified and underrun with several X stitches of 0 Mersilene or other nonabsorbable material, mounted on a strong atraumatic needle that is capable of penetrating the thick fibrous base of the ulcer without breaking. The stomach, now emptied of blood clots, is examined again for any sign of gastric ulceration. The gastroduodenotomy incision then is sutured transversely as a Heinecke-Mikulicz pyloroplasty and a rapid truncal vagotomy is performed.

We excise 3 to 5 cm from each vagal trunk and clear the lower 5 cm of esophagus of all vagal fibers, but in view of the emergency circumstances spend only about 5 minutes or so on the vagotomy, whereas we would normally take two or three times as long. In contrast, when HSV is to be used, we suture the duodenotomy incision as it was made, longitudinally, apposing the cut surfaces edge-to-edge without inversion.[190] In 5 patients out of a personal series of 25, the duodenotomy was found to give inadequate access to a deeply penetrating duodenal ulcer and so the incision had to be extended across the pylorus. In each patient, the incision then was sutured longitudinally, so that the distal antrum and pyloric sphincter were reconstituted.[190] None of these patients developed gastric retention. We use HSV in about 30 percent of patients with massive hemorrhage and TV and P in 70 percent. This proportion obviously reflects my special interest and is not advocated for general adoption. There was no operative mortality on our unit after HSV in 90 patients with bleeding peptic ulcer, and although 3 patients experienced rebleeding, none required reoperation. After TV and P in 50 patients, the operative mortality was

12%, which doubtless reflects the selection of higher risk patients for truncal vagotomy.

Bleeding Gastric Ulcer

Partial gastrectomy, often of the Billroth I variety, is still the most commonly used procedure, but the operative mortality is high, ranging from 5% to 50%, with a mean of approximately 20%.[151,188,191] McArdle and Tilney, for example, reviewed the results of surgery for peptic ulcer in the Western Infirmary, Glasgow, between 1970 and 1972. While the mortality of elective surgery was low, the mortality of emergency partial gastrectomy was appalling, since no fewer than 18 of the 39 patients died after that procedure, a 46% mortality. The operative mortality of emergency partial gastrectomy for bleeding *gastric* ulcer was 54%. Rogers, Murray and associates have reported that the mortality of emergency PG for GU at the same hospital fell to 26% in the period 1977 to 1985.[54] Even though one would like to think that it might be that these figures, which are from a teaching center, must be completely atypical of Britain as a whole, sadly it is not so. Thus, in a survey of all hospital admissions for bleeding gastric and duodenal ulcer of two teaching hospitals in Nottingham in 1976 and 1977, Dronfield and associates reported that the operative mortality after emergency partial gastrectomy for duodenal ulcer was 44%, and for gastric ulcer, 21%.[139] Hence, if we accept that the main objective, or endpoint, of this type of surgery is that the patient should survive and walk out of the hospital (in this context, recurrent ulceration hardly matters, as it can be dealt with on its merits), the continued use of emergency partial gastrectomy must be called into question.

Several reports suggest that it is much safer to underrun the bleeding point, biopsy or excise the ulcer, and then perform a vagotomy, which of course is usually truncal in type, but this procedure may occasionally be highly selective.[130,151,192–194] Certainly, in an elderly, unfit patient with an ulcer high on the lesser curve, such a policy has much to commend it. Where possible, we excise the gastric ulcer in toto, but if it is large we often leave the base of the ulcer adhering to the pancreas or other viscera and merely take several biopsy specimens.[130] If the ulcer seems likely to be malignant, a partial gastrectomy should obviously be performed, but it is somewhat unusual for a malignant ulcer to precipitate emergency surgery of this nature.

REFERENCES

1. Goligher FE, Pulvertaft CN, et al. Five to eight year results of Leeds/York controlled trial of elective surgery for duodenal ulcer. *Br Med J* 1968;2:781–786
2. Postlethwait RW. Five year follow up results of operations for duodenal ulcer. *Surg Gynecol Obstet* 1973;137:387
3. Stalsberg H, Taksdal S. Stomach cancer following gastric surgery for benign conditions. *Cancer* 1971;ii:1175
4. Schrumpf E, Stadaas J, et al. Mucosal changes in the gastric stump 20–25 years after partial gastrectomy. *Cancer* 1977;ii:467
5. Lawson HH. Effect of duodenal contents on the gastric mucosa under experimental conditions. *Cancer* 1964;1:469
6. Silen W. Malevolent gall. *Surgery* 1972;71:311–312
7. Watt PC, Patterson C, Kennedy TL. Late morality after vagotomy and drainage for duodenal ulcer. *BMJ* 1984;288:1335
8. Kennedy T, Connell AM, et al. Selective or truncal vagotomy? Five year results of a double blind prospective randomised controlled trial. *Br J Surg* 1973;60:944
9. Kennedy T, Johnston GW, et al. Pyloroplasty versus gastrojejunostomy. Results of a double blind, randomized controlled trial. *Br J Surg* 1973;60:949
10. Kronborg O, Malmstrom I, et al. A comparison between the results of truncal and selective vagotomy in patients with duodenal ulcer. *Scand J Gastroenterol* 1970;5:519
11. Kennedy T, Johnston GW et al. Proximal gastric vagotomy. Interim results of a randomized controlled trial. *BMJ* 1975;2:301
13. Kronborg O, Madsen P. A controlled randomized trial of highly selective vagotomy versus selective vagotomy and pyloroplasty in the treatment of duodenal ulcer. *Gut* 1975;16:268
14. Amdrup BM, Andersen D, et al. The Aarhus County vagotomy trial. I, an interim report on primary results and incidence of sequelae following parietal cell vagotomy and selective gastric vagotomy in 748 patients. *World J Surg* 1978;2:85
15. Sawyers JL, Herrington JL, et al. Proximal gastric vagotomy compared with vagotomy and antrectomy and selective gastric vagotomy and pyloroplasty. *Am Surg* 1977;186:510
16. Sawyers JL, Herrington JL. Vagotomy and antrectomy, In: Nyhus LM, Wastell C (eds), *Surgery of the Stomach and Duodenum.* Boston, MA: Little Brown; 1977:343–369
17. Jordan PH, Thornby J. Should it be parietal cell vagotomy or selective vagotomy antrectomy for the treatment of duodenal ulcer? *Ann Surg* 1987;205:572
18. Farmer DA, Smithwick RH. Hemigastrectomy combined with section of the vagus nerves. *N Engl J Med* 1952;247:1097
19. Jordan PH, Condon RE. A prospective evaluation of vagotomy-pyloroplasty and vagotomy-antrectomy for treatment of duodenal ulcer. *Ann Surg* 1970;172:547
20. Goligher JC, Pulvertaft CN, et al. Five to eight year results of truncal vagotomy and pyloroplasty for duodenal ulcer. *BMJ* 1972;1:7
21. Jordan PH. A follow up report of a prospective evaluation of vagotomy-pyloroplasty and vagotomy-antrectomy for treatment of duodenal ulcer. *Ann Surg* 1974;180:259
22. Wheldon EJ, Venables CW, et al. Late metabolic sequelae of vagotomy and gastroenterostomy. *Cancer* 1970;i:437
23. Kennedy F, Mackay C, et al. Truncal vagotomy and

drainage for chronic duodenal ulcer disease, a controlled trial. *BMJ* 1973;2:71

24. McKelvey STD. Gastric incontinence and postvagotomy diarrhea. *Br J Surg* 1970;57:741

24. Stoddard CI, Smallwood R, et al. The immediate and delayed effects of different types of vagotomy on human gastric myoelectrical activity. *Gut* 1975;16:165

25. Friesen SR, Rieger E. A study of the role of the pylorus in the prevention of the dumping syndrome. *Ann Surg* 1960; 151:517

26. Killen DA, Symbas PN. Effect of preservation of the pyloric sphincter during antrectomy and postoperative gastric emptying. *Am J Surg* 1962;104:836

27. Carlson HC, Code CF, Nelson RA. Motor action of canine gastroduodenal ulceration: a cineradiographic, pressure and electrical study. *Am J Dig Dis* 1966;11:155

28. Keighley MRB, Asquith P, et al. The importance of an innervated and inhet antrum and pylorus in preventing postoperative duodenogastric reflux and gastritis. *Br J Surg* 1975;62:845

29. Levin B. Gastric cancer. *Curr Opin Gastroenterol* 1989;5: 859–864

30. Diament R. Unpublished data. 1989

31. Taylor PR, Hanley DC, Filipe MI, Mason RC. What factor is responsible for malignant change in the rat stomach following truncal vagotomy and gastroenterostomy. In: Reed PI, Hill MJ (eds), *Gastric Carcinogenesis*. Amsterdam, Netherlands: Elsevier; 1988.

32. Ferguson DJ, Billings H, Swensen D, et al. Segmental gastrectomy with innervated antrum for duodenal ulcer. *Surgery* 1960;47:548–556

33. Flynn PJ, Longmire WP. Subtotal gastrectomy with pyloric sphincter preservation. *Surg Forum* 1960;10:185

34. Maki T, Shiratori T, et al. Pylorus-preserving gastrectomy as an improved operation for gastric ulcer. *Surgery* 1967; 61:838

35. Amdrup E, Jensen HE. Selective vagotomy of the varietal cell mass preserving innervation of the undrained antrum. *Gastroenterology* 1970;59:522

36. Johnston D, Wilkinson AR. Highly selective vagotomy without a drainage procedure in the treatment of duodenal ulcer. *Br J Surg* 1970;57:289

37. Holle F, Hart W: Neue Wege tee chirurgie des gastroduodenalulkus. *Met Klin* 1967;62:441

38. Holle F. Adequate selective proximal vagotomy with pyloroplasty as nonresective surgery for peptic ulcer disease: a 20 year review. *Int Surg* 1983;68:295–298

39. Griffith CA, Harkins HN. Partial gastric vagotomy: an experimental study. *Gastroenterology* 1957;32:96

40. Nyhus LM, Chapman ND, Devito RW, Harkins HN. The control of gastrin release: an experimental study illustrating a new concept. *Gastroenterol* 1960;39:582–589

41. Janowitz HD, Hollander F. The exocrine-endocrine partition of enzymes in the digestive tract. *Gastroenterology* 1951;17:591–592

42. Code CF, Watkinson G. The importance of vagal innervation in the regulatory effect of acid in the duodenum on gastric secretion of acid. *J Physiol London* 1955;130: 233–236

43. Johnston D, Duthie HL. Effect of fat in the duodenum on gastric acid secretion before and after vagotomy in man. *Scand J Gastroenterol* 1969;4:561–567

44. Johnston D. Operative morality and postoperative morbidity of highly selective vagotomy. *BMJ* 1975;4:545

45. Salaman JR, Harvey J, et al. Importance of symptoms after highly selective vagotomy. *BMJ* 1981;283:1438

46. Muller C, Engelke MD, Fiedler L, et al. How do clinical results after proximal gastric vagotomy compare with the Visick grade pattern of healthy controls. *World J Surg* 1983;7:610–615

47. Amdrup E, Jensen HE, Johnston D, Walker BE, Goligher JC. Clinical results of parietal cell vagotomy (highly selective two to four years after operation. *Ann Surg* 1974; 180:279–284

48. Busman DC, Munting JDK. Results of highly selective vagotomy in a nonuniversity teaching hospital. *Br J Surg* 1982;69:620–624

49. Enskog L, Rydberg B, Adami HO, et al. Clinical results 1–10 years after highly selective vagotomy in 306 patients with prepyloric and duodenal ulcer disease. *Br J Surg* 1986;73:357–360

50. Stael von Holstein C, Graffner H, Oscarson J. One hundred patients ten years after parietal cell vagotomy. *Br J Surg* 1987;74:101–103

51. Blackett RL, Johnston D. Recurrent ulceration after highly selective vagotomy for duodenal ulcer. *Br J Surg* 1981;68:705

52. Edwards UP, Lyndon PJ, et al. Fatal fat excretion after truncal, selective and highly selective vagotomy for duodenal ulcer. *Gut* 1974;15:521

53. Meikle DD, Bull J, Callender ST, Truelove SC. Intrinsic factor secretion after vagotomy. *Br J Surg* 1977;64:795–797

54. Rogers MJ, Holmfield JHM, Primrose JN, et al. A prospective comparison of the effects of placebo, ranitidine and highly selective vagotomy on 24 hr ambulatory intragastric pH in patients with duodenal ulcer. *Br J Surg* 1988; 75:961–965

55. Reed PI, Hill MJ (eds). *Gastric Carcinogenesis*. Amsterdam, Netherlands: Elsevier; 1988

56. Dewar EP, King RFG, et al. Bile acid and lysolecithin concentrations in the stomach of patients with gastric ulcer before operation and after treatment by highly selective vagotomy, Billroth I partial gastrectomy and truncal vagotomy and pyloroplasty. *Br J Surg* 1983;70:401

57. Johnston D, Wilkinson AR, et al. Serial studies of gastric secretion in patients after highly selective (parietal cell) vagotomy without a drainage procedure for duodenal ulcer. II, the insulin test after highly selective vagotomy. *Gastroenterology* 1973;64:12

58. Madsen P, Kronborg O. Recurrent ulcer 5–15 years after highly selective vagotomy without drainage and selective vagotomy with pyloroplasty. *Scand J Gastroenterol* 1980; 15:193

59. Johnston D, Blackett RL. Recurrent peptic ulcers. *World J Surg* 1987;11:274

60. Adami HO, Enander L-K, et al: Recurrence 1 to 10 years after highly selective vagotomy in prepyloric and duodenal ulcer disease. *Ann Surg* 1984;199:393

61. Hallenbeck GA, Gleysteen IJ, et al. Proximal gastric vagotomy: effects of two operative techniques on clinical and gastric secretory results. *Ann Surg* 1976;184:435

62. Johnson AG, Baxter HK. Where is your vagotomy incomplete? Observations on operative technique 1977;64: 583–586

63. Rosati I, Serantoni C, et al. Extended proximal vagotomy: observations on a variant in technique. *Chir Gastroenterol* 1976;10:33

64. Koruth NM, Dua KS, Brunt PW, Matheson NA. Comparison of highly selective vagotomy with truncal vagotomy and pyloroplasty: results at 8–15 years. *Br J Surg* 1990;77:70–72

65. Muhe E, Muller C, et al. Five year results of a prospective multicentre trial of proximal gastric vagotomy. In: Baron JH, et al (eds), *Vagotomy in Modern Surgical Practice*. London, England: Butterworth, 1982:176–186

66. Grassi G. A new test for complete nerve section during vagotomy. *Br J Surg* 1971;58:187–189

67. Burge H, Vane JR. Method for testing for complete nerve section during vagotomy. *BMJ* 1958;1:615–618

68. Baron JH, Alexander-Williams J, et al (eds), *Vagotomy in Modern Surgical Practice*. London, England: Butterworths; 1982

69. Muller C, Lieberman-Meffert D, Allgower M. The different outcome of duodenal and pyloric channel ulcers after proximal gastric vagotomy. *Scand J Gastroenterol* 1984; 19(suppl 92):210–214

70. Stoddard CI, Vassilakis JS, et al. Highly selective vagotomy or truncal vagotomy and pyloroplasty for chronic duodenal ulceration: a randomized prospective clinical study. *Br J Surg* 1978;65:793

71. Stoddard CI, Johnson AG, Duthie HL. The four to eight year results of the Sheffield Trial of elective duodenal ulcer surgery—highly selective or truncal vagotomy? *Br J Surg* 1984;71:779

72. Koffman CG, Hay DO, et al. A prospective randomized trial of vagotomy in chronic duodenal ulceration: 4-year follow up. *Br J Surg* 1983;70:342

73. Fraser AG, Brunt PW, et al. A comparison of highly selective vagotomy with truncal vagotomy and pyloroplasty, one surgeon's results after 5 years. *Br J Surg* 1983;70:485

74. Dua K, Koruth NM, et al. Is highly selective vagotomy a good operation for duodenal ulcer? A longer look at the operation. *Gut* 1987;28:1374

75. Jordan PH. An interim report on parietal cell vagotomy versus selective vagotomy and antrectomy for treatment of duodenal ulcer. *Am Surg* 1979;189:643

76. Dorricott NO, McNeish AR, et al. Prospective randomized multicenter trial of proximal gastric vagotomy or truncal vagotomy and antrectomy for chronic duodenal ulcer: interim results. *Br J Surg* 1978;65:152

77. DeVries BC, Eeftinck M, et al. Prospective randomized multicenter trial of proximal gastric vagotomy or truncal vagotomy and antrectomy for chronic duodenal ulcer: results after 5–7 years. *Br J Surg* 1983;70:701

78. Koo I, Lam SK, et al. Proximal gastric vagotomy, truncal vagotomy with drainage and truncal vagotomy with antrectomy for chronic duodenal ulcer. *Ann Surg* 1983; 197:265

79. Gleysteen IJ, Condon RE, et al. Prospective trial of proximal gastric vagotomy. *Surgery* 1983;94:15

80. Donahue PE, Nyhus LM, et al. Proximal gastric vagotomy versus selective vagotomy with antrectomy: results of a prospective randomized clinical trial after four to twelve years. *Surgery* 1984;96:585

81. Johnston D. Surgery for duodenal ulcer in 1984: Highly selective vagotomy with intact pylorus or vagotomy with antrectomy? *Int Med Spec* 1984;5:55

82. Dubois F, Icard P, Berthelot G, Levard H. Coelioscopic cholecystectomy. *Ann Surg* 1990;211:60–63

83. Murphy JJ, McDermott EW. Laparoscopic truncal vagotomy without drainage for the treatment of chronic duodenal ulcer. *Ir Med J* 1991;1:25–26

84. Pietrafitta JJ, Schultz LS, Graber JN, Hickok DF. Laser laparoscopic vagotomy and pyloromyotomy. *Gastrointest Endosc* 1991;3:38–43

85. Hill GL, Barker MCJ. Anterior highly selective vagotomy with posterior truncal vagotomy: a simple technique for denervating the parietal cell mass. *Br J Surg* 1978;65:702–705

86. Kum CK, Goh P. Laparoscopic posterior truncal vagotomy and anterior highly selective vagotomy—a case report. *Singapore Med J* 1992;33:302–3

87. Taylor TV, Gunn AA, MacLeod DAD, MacLennan I. Anterior lesser curve seromyotomy with posterior truncal vagotomy in the treatment of chronic duodenal ulcer. *Lancet* 1982;2:160–163

88. Voeller GR, Pridgen WL, Mangiante EC. Laparoscopic posterior truncal vagotomy and anterior seromyotomy: a porcine model. *J Laparoendosc Surg* 1991;1:375–378

89. Katkhouda N, Mouiel J. A new technique of surgical treatment of chronic duodenal ulcer without laparotomy by videocoelioscopy. *Am J Surg* 1991;161:361–364

90. Hannon JK, Snow LL, Weinstein LS. Linear gastrectomy: an endoscopic staple-assisted anterior highly selective vagotomy combined with posterior truncal vagotomy for treatment of peptic ulcer disease. *J Laparoscendosc Surg* 1992;2:254–257

91. Josephs LG, Arnold JH, Sawyers JL. Laparoscopic highly selective vagotomy. *J Laparoendosc Surg* 1992;2:151–153

92. Cuschieri A. Laparoscopic vagotomy: gimmick or reality? *Surg Clin North Am* 1992;72:357–367

93. Johnson HD. Etiology and classification of gastric ulcers. *Gastroenterology* 1957;33:121

94. Andersen S, Hostrup H, et al. The Aarhus County Vagotomy Trial. II, an interim report on reduction of acid secretion and ulcer recurrence rate following varietal cell vagotomy and selective gastric vagotomy. *World J Surg* 1978;2:91

95. Madsen P, Schousen P. Long term results of truncal vagotomy and pyloroplasty for gastric ulcer. *Br J Surg* 1982; 69:651

96. Baron JH. Studies of basal and peak acid output with an augmented histamine test. *Gut* 1963;4:136

97. Baron JH. Lean body mass, gastric acid and peptic ulcer. *Gut* 1969;10:637

98. Baxter JN, Grime IS, et al. Effect of truncal vagotomy and pyloroplasty and of highly selective vagotomy alone on gallbladder emptying dynamics: a prospective study. *Gut* 1984;27:A578

99. Wormsley KG, Grossman MK. Maximal histalog test in control subjects and patients with peptic ulcer. *Gut* 1965;6:427

100. Rhodes J, Barnardo SE, et al. Increased reflex of bile into the stomach in patients with gastric ulcer. *Gastroenterology* 1969;57:241

101. Davenport HW. Is the apparent hyposecretion of acid by patients with gastric ulcer a consequence of a broken barrier to the diffusion of hydrogen ions into the gastric mucosa? *Gut* 1965;6:513

102. Davenport HW. Destruction of the gastric mucosal barrier by detergents and urea. *Gastroenterology* 1968;54:175

103. Dragstedt LR. A concept of the etiology of gastric and duodenal ulcers. *Gastroenterology* 1956;30:208

104. Dragstedt LR. On the cause of gastric and duodenal ulcers. *J R Coll Surg Edinb* 1971;16:251

105. Griffith GH, Coven GM, et al. Gastric emptying in health and in gastroduodenal disease. *Gastroenterology* 1968;54:1

106. Du Plessis DJ. Pathogenesis of gastric ulceration. *Cancer* 1965;1:974

107. Capper WM. Factors in the pathogenesis of gastric ulcer. *Ann R Coll Surg Engl* 1967;40:21

108. Fisher RS, Cohen S. Pyloric sphincter dysfunction in patients with gastric ulcer. *N Engl J Med* 1973;288:273

109. Lawson HH. The effect of the duodenal contents on the gastric mucosa. *S Afr J Surg* 1965;3:79

110. Oi M, Oshida K, et al. The location of gastric ulcer. *Gastroenterology* 1959;36:45

111. Dragstedt LR, Owens FM. Supradiaphragmatic section of the vagus nerves in the treatment of duodenal ulcer. *Proc Soc Exp Biol Med* 1943;53:152

112. Schwartz K. Ueber penetrierende Magen-und jejunalgeschwur. *Beitr Klin Chir* 1910;67:96

113. Duthie HL, Kwong NK. Vagotomy of gastrectomy for gastric ulcer. *BMJ* 1973;4:79

114. Madsen P, Kronborg O, et al. Billroth I gastric resection versus truncal vagotomy and pyloroplasty in the treatment of gastric ulcer. *Acta Chir Scand* 1976;142:151

115. Thomas WEG, Thompson MH, et al. The long-term outcome of Billroth I partial gastrectomy for benign gastric ulcer. *Am Surg* 1982;195:189

116. Reid DA, Duthie HL, et al. Late follow-up of highly selective vagotomy with excision of ulcer compared with Billroth I gastrectomy for treatment of benign gastric ulcer. *Br J Surg* 1982;69:605

117. Forrest APM. Gastric ulcer. In: Alexander-Williams J, Cox AG (eds), *After Vagotomy*. London, England: Butterworths; 1969

118. Duthie HL. Vagotomy for gastric ulcer. *Gut* 1970;11:540

119. de Miguel J. Recurrence of gastric ulcer after selective vagotomy and pyloroplasty for chronic uncomplicated gastric ulcer: a 5–10 year follow-up. *Br J Surg* 1975;62:875

120. Cade D, Allan D. Longterm follow-up of patients with gastric ulcer treated by vagotomy, pyloroplasty and ulcerectomy. *Br J Surg* 1979;66:46

121. Johnson JA, Giercksky KE. Gastric ulcer treated with ulcerectomy, vagotomy, and drainage. *World J Surg* 1980;4:463–470

122. Kronborg O. Truncal vagotomy and drainage for gastric ulcer. In: Baron JH, et al (eds), *Vagotomy in Modern Surgical Practice*. London, England: Butterworths; 1982

123. Littman A (ed), The Veterans Administration Cooperative Study on Gastric Ulcer. *Gastroenterology* 1971;61:565

124. Nielson I, Amdrup E, et al. Gastric ulcer. II, surgical treatment. *Acta Chir Scand* 1973;139:460

125. Morgan AG, McAdam WAF, et al. Cimetidine: an advanced in gastric ulcer treatment. *BMJ* 1978;2:1323

126. Greenall M, Lehnert T. Vagotomy or gastrectomy for elective treatment of benign gastric ulceration. *Dig Dis Sci* 1985;30:353

127. de Miguel J. Pylorectomy and prepyloric antrectomy for gastric ulcer. *Br J Surg* 1979;66:48

128. Sekine T, Sato T, et al. Pylorus preserving gastrectomy for gastric ulcer one to nine year follow-up study. *Surgery* 1977;55:92

129. Teigan T, Liavag I, et al: Pylorus-preserving gastric resection for gastric ulcer. A 5–7 year follow-up. *Acta Chir Scand* 1978;144:249

130. Johnston D, Humphrey CS, et al. Treatment of gastric ulcer by highly selective vagotomy without a drainage procedure: an interim report. *Br J Surg* 1972;59:787

131. Stadaas J, Aune S. Intragastric pressure/volume relationship before and after vagotomy. *Acta Chir Scand* 1970;136:611

132. Wilbur BG, Kelly KA, Effect of proximal gastric, complete gastric and truncal vagotomy on canine gastric electrical activity, motility and emptying. *Ann Surg* 1973;178:295

133. Johnston D. Highly selective vagotomy with excision of the ulcer for gastric ulceration. In: Dudley HAF (ed), *Rob and Smith's Operative Surgery*. 4th ed. London, England: Butterworths; 1973:349–352

135. Jorde R, Johnson IA, et al. An endoscopic study of ulcer recurrence and mucosal changes following vagotomy and excision of gastric ulcer. *Acta Chir Scand* 1987;153:297

136. Heberer G, Teichmann RK. Recurrence after proximal gastric vagotomy for gastric, pyloric and prepyloric ulcers. *World J Surg* 1987;11:283

137. Holle F, Bauer H. SPV and pyloroplasty in ulcer disease. In: Holle F, Andersson S (eds): *Vagotomy-Latest Advances*. Berlin, Germany: Springer-Verlag; 1974:198

138. Forrest IAN, Finlayson NDL. The investigation of acute upper gastrointestinal hemorrhage. *Br J Hosp Med* 1974;12:160

139. Dronfield MW, Atkinson M, et al. Effect of different operation policies on mortality from bleeding peptic ulcer. *Cancer* 1979;1:1126

140. Editorial: Bleeding ulcer: scope for improvement? *Cancer* 1984;1:715

141. Christensen A, Bonsfield R, et al. Incidence of perforated and bleeding peptic ulcers before and after the introduction of H2 receptor antagonists. *Ann Surg* 1988;207:4

142. Poxon VA, Keighley MR, Dykes PW, et al. Comparison of minimal and conventional surgery in patients with bleeding peptic ulcer: a multicentre trial. *Br J Surg* 1991;78:1344–1345

143. Jones FA. Haematemesis and melena with special reference to causation and to the factors influencing the mortality from bleeding peptic ulcers. *Gastroenterology* 1956;30:166

144. Hunt PS, Hansky J, et al. Mortality in patients with hematemesis and melena: a prospective study. *BMJ* 1979; 1:1238

145. Dronfield MW, McMurray MB, et al. A prospective randomized study of endoscopy and radiology in acute upper-gastrointestinal tract bleeding. *Cancer* 1977;1:1167

146. Conn HO. To scope or not to scope. *N Engl J Med* 1981; 304:967

147. Williams RA, Varhny A, Davis IP, Wilson SE. Impact of endoscopic therapy on outcome of operation for bleeding peptic ulcers. *Am J Surg* 1993;166:714–715

148. Ring EJ, Oleagan IA, et al. Interventional radiology in gastrointestinal hemorrhage. In: Berk JE (ed): *Developments in Digestive Disease*. Philadelphia, PA: Lea & Febiger; 1977:59–72

149. Branicki FJ, Coleman SY, Pritchett CI, et al. Emergency surgical treatment for non-variceal bleeding of the upper part of the gastrointestinal tract. *Surg Gynecol Obstet* 1991;172:113–120

150. Morris DL, Hawker PC, Brearley S, et al. Optimal timing of operation for bleeding peptic ulcer: a prospective randomized trial. *BMJ* 1984;288(1):277–280

151. Schiller KFR, Truelove SG, et al. Haematemesis and melaena, with special reference to factors influencing the outcome. *BMJ* 1970;2:7

152. Chua CL, Feyara PR, Low CH. Relative risks of complications in giant and non-giant gastric ulcers. *Am J Surg* 1992;164:94–97

153. Foster DN, Miloszewski KJA, et al. Stigmata of recent hemorrhage in diagnosis and prognosis of upper gastrointestinal bleeding. *BMJ* 1978;2:1173

154. Griffith WI, Neumann DA, et al. The visible vessel as an indicator of uncontrolled or recurrent gastrointestinal hemorrhage. *N Engl J Med* 1979;300:1411

155. Storey DW, Boulos PB, et al. Proximal gastric vagotomy after five years. *Gut* 1981;22:702

156. MacLeod IA, Mills PR, et al. Neodymium yttrium aluminum garnet laser photo coagulation for major hemorrhage for peptic ulcers and single vessels. *BMJ* 1983;286:345

157. Meulengracht E. Fifteen years experience with free fading of patients with bleeding peptic ulcer. *Arch Int Med* 1947,80:697

158. Pickard RG, et al. Controlled trial of cimetidine in acute upper gastrointestinal bleeding. *BMJ* 1979;1:661–662

159. La Brooy SJ, Misiewicz II, et al. Controlled trial of clinetidine in upper gastrointestinal hemorrhage. *Gut* 1979; 20:892

160. Carstensen HE, Bulow S, et al. Cimetidine in severe gastroductal hemorrhage: a randomized controlled trial. *Scand J Gastroenterol* 1980;15:103

161. Hoare AM, Jones EL, Hawkins CF. Cimetidine for ulcers recurring after gastric surgery. *BMJ* 1978;i:1325–1326

162. Collins R, Langman M. Treatment with histamine H2 antagonists in acute upper gastrointestinal hemorrhage.

Implications of randomized trials. *N Engl J Med* 1985; 313:660–666

163. Jones SC, Axon AT. Bleeding peptic ulcer—endoscopic and pharmacological management. *Postgrad Med J* 1991; 67:606–612

164. Daneshmend TK, Hawkey CJ, Langman MJ, et al. Omeprazole versus placebo for acute upper gastrointestinal bleeding: randomized double blind controlled trial. *BMJ* 1992;304:143–147

165. Brunner G, Chang I. Intravenous therapy with high doses of ranitidine and omeprazole in critically ill patients with bleeding peptic ulcerations of the upper intestinal tract and open randomized controlled trial. *Digestion* 1990;45:217–225

166. Labenz I, Borsch G. Role of *helicobacter pylori* eradication in the prevention of peptic ulcer bleeding relapse. *Digestion* 1994;55:19–23

167. Jaspersen D, Koerner T, Schorr W, et al. *Helicobacter pylori* eradication reduces the rate of rebleeding in ulcer hemorrhage. *Gastrointest Endosc* 1995;41:5–7

168. Cormack F, Chakrabarti RR, et al. Tranexamic acid in upper gastrointestinal hemorrhage. *Lancet* 1973;1: 1207

169. Biggs JC, Hugh TB, et al. Tranexamic acid and upper gastrointestinal haemorrhage—a double-blind trial. *Gut* 1976;17:729

170. Engqvist A, Brostrom O, et al. Tranexamic acid in massive hemorrhage from the upper gastrointestinal tract: a double-blind study. *Scand J Gastroenterol* 1979;14:839

171. Barer D. Ogilvie A, et al. Cimetidine and tranexamic acid in the treatment of acute upper-gastrointestinal-tract bleeding. *N Engl J Med* 1983;308:1571

172. Kayasseh L, Keller U, et al. Somatostatin and cimetidine in peptic ulcer haemorrhage—a randomized controlled trial. *Cancer* 1980;1:844

173. Fruhmorgen P, Bodem F, et al. Endoscopic laser coagulation of bleeding gastrointestinal lesions. *Gastrointest Endosc* 1976;23:73

174. Kiefhaber P, Nath G, et al. Endoscopic control of massive gastrointestinal hemorrhage by irradiation with a high-power neodymium YAG laser. *Prog Surg* 1977;15:140

175. Vallon AG, Cotton PB, et al. Randomized trial of endoscopic argon laser photo coagulation in bleeding peptic ulcers. *Gut* 1981;22:228

176. Rutgeers P, Vantrappen G, et al. Controlled trial of YAG laser treatment of upper digestive hemorrhage. *Gastroenterology* 1982;83:410

177. Swain CP, Bown SG, et al. Controlled trial of neodymium YAG laser photo coagulation in bleeding peptic ulcer. *Laser Surg Med* 1983;3:111

178. Krejs GF, Little KH, et al. Laser photo coagulation for the treatment of acute peptic ulcer bleeding: a randomized controlled clinical trial. *N Engl J Med* 1987;316: 1618

179. Johnston JH, Sones JQ, et al. Heater probe is superior to YAG laser in clinical endoscopic treatment of major bleeding from peptic ulcer. *Gastrointest Endosc* 1985; 31:175

180. Johnston JH. Endoscopic haemoshsis for bleeding peptic ulcer. *Gastrointest Endosc* 1987;33:260

181. Brearley S, et al. Pre-endoscopic bipolar diathermy coagulation of visible vessels using a 3.2 mm probe-a randomized clinical trial. *Endoscopy* 1987;19:160

182. Leung OW, et al. Endoscopic injection of adrenaline in bleeding peptic ulcer. *Gastrointest Endosc* 1987;33:73

183. Asaki S, Nishimura T, et al. Endoscopic haemostasis of gastrointestinal hemorrhage by local application of absolute alcohol: a clinical study. *Tohoku J Exp Med* 1983; 141:373

184. Rutgeers P, Vantrappen G, et al. Neodymium YAG laser photocoagulation versus multi polar elKtrocoagulation for the treatment of severely bleeding ulcers: a randomized comparison. *Gastrointest Endosc* 1987;33:199

185. Sacks HS, Chalmers TC, Blum AL, et al. Endoscopic hemostasis-an effective therapy for bleeding peptic ulcers. *JAMA* 1990;264:494–499

186. Henry D, Cook D. Meta-analysis workshop in upper gastrointestinal hemorrhage. *Gastroenterology* 1991;100: 1481–1482

187. Koelz HR. Die Kurativetherapie des Ulcus ventriculi and des Ulcus duodeni. In: Blum AL, Bauerfield P (eds), *Ulkusalmanch 2.* Heidelberg: Springer Verlag; 1990

188. Alexander-Williams J. In: Alexander-Williams J, Cox AG (eds), *After Vagotomy,* London, England: Butterworth; 1969:325

189. Keighley MRB, Burdon DW. *Antimicrobial Prophylaxis in Surgery.* London, England: Pitman; 1979:59–61

190. Johnston D: Division and repair of the sphincteric mechanism at the gastric outlet in emergency operations for bleeding peptic ulcer. *Ann Surg* 1977;186:723

191. McArdle CS, Tilney NL. Surgery for peptic ulcer disease. Operative complications and immediate morality. *J R Coll Surg Edinb* 1976;21:285

192. Foster RA, Hicock DF, et al. Changing concepts in the surgical treatment of massive gastroduodenal hemorrhage. *Ann Surg* 1965;161:968

193. Dorton HE: Vagotomy, pyloroplasty, and suture for bleeding gastric ulcer. *Surg Gynecol Obstet* 1966;122:1015

194. Hegarty MM, Grime RT, et al. The management of upper gastrointestinal tract hemorrhage. *Br J Surg* 1973; 60:275

SELECTED READING

Aadland E, Berstad A, et al. Effect of cimetidine on pentagastrin stimulated gastric secretion before and after proximal gastric vagotomy for duodenal ulcer. *Scand J Gastroenterol* 1979;13:679

Amdrup BM, Griffth CA. Selective vagotomy of the varietal cell mass: part 1; with preservation of the innervated antrum and pvlorus. *Ann Surg* 1969;170:207

Buckler KG. Effects of gastric surgery upon gastric empting in cases of peptic ulceration. *Gut* 1967;8:137

Bushkin FL, Wickborn G, et al. Postoperative alkaline reflux gastritis. *Surg Gynecol Obstet* 1974;138:933

Christiansen J, Jensen H-E, et al. Prospective controlled vagotomy trial for duodenal ulcer: primary results, sequelae, acid secretion and recurrence rates. *Ann Surg* 1981;193:49

Clark CG, Fresini A, et al. Proximal gastric vagotomy or truncal vagotomy and drainage for chronic duodenal ulcer? *Br J Surg* 1986;73:298

Clark CG, Karamanolis D, et al. Preference for proximal gastric vagotomy combined with cholecystectomy. *Br J Surg* 1984;71:185

Clave RA, Gaspar MR. Incidence of gall bladder disease after vagotomy. *Am J Surg* 1969;118:169

Colmer MR, Owen GM, et al. Pattern of gastric emptying after vagotomy and pyloroplasty. *BMJ* 1973;2:448

Cowie AG, Clark CG. The lithogenic effect of vagotomy. *Br J Surg* 1972;59:363

Cox AG, Bond MR, et al. Aspects of nutrition after vagotomy and gastrojejunostomy. *BMJ* 1964;1:465

de Miguel J: Late results of proximal gastric vagotomy without drainage for duodenal ulcer: 5–9 year follow-up. *Br J Surg* 1982;69:7

Debas HT, Konturek SJ, et al. Proof of a pyloro-oxyntic reflex for stimulation of acid secretion. *Gastroenterology* 1974; 66:526

Debas HT, Yamagishi T. Evidence for a pyloro-cholKystic reflex for gallbladder contraction. *Ann Surg* 1979;190:170

Debas HT, Yarnagishi T. Evidence for a pyloro-pancreatic reflex for pancreatic exocrine secretion. *Am J Physiol* 1978; 234:E468

Dewar EP, King RFG, et al. Bile acid and lysolecithin concentrations in the stomach in patients with duodenal ulcer before operation and after treatment by highly selective vagotomy, partial gastrectomy or truncal vagotomy and drainage. *Gut* 1982;23:569

Fletcher DM, Clark CG. Changes in canine bile-flow and composition after vagotomy. *Br J Surg* 1969;56:103

Fletcher DM, Clark CG. Gall-stones and gastric surgery. A review. *Br J Surg* 1968;55:895

Fritz ME, Brooks FP. Control of bile flow in the cholecystectomized dog. *Am J Physiol* 1963;204:825

Gear MWL. Proximal gastric vagotomy versus long-term maintenance treatment with cimetidine for chronic duodenal ulcer. *BMJ* 1983;1:98

Gledhill T, Buck M, et al. Cimetidine or vagotomy? Comparison of the effects of proximal gastric vagotomy, cimetidine and placebo on nocturnal intragastric acidity and acid secretion in patients with cimetidine-resistant duodenal ulcer. *Br J Surg* 1983;70:704

Goodman AJ, Johnson AG, et al. Effect of preoperative response to H2 receptor antagonists on the outcome of highly selective vagotomy for duodenal ulcer. *Br J Surg* 1987;74:897

Gorey TF, Lennon F, et al. Highly selective vagotomy in duodenal ulceration and its complications: a 12-year review. *Ann Surg* 1984;200:181

Grassi G. The results of highly selective vagotomy in our experience (787 cases). *Chir Gastroenterol* 1977;11:51

Hansen JH, Knigge V. Failure of proximal gastric vagotomy for duodenal ulcer resistant to cimetidine. *Lancet* 1984;2:84

Hoffman I, Jensen H-E, et al. Retrospective 14–18 year follow-up after varietal cell vagotomy. *Br J Surg* 1987;74:1056

Humphrey CS, Johnston D et al. Incidence of dumpting after truncal and selective vagotomy with pyloroplasty and highly selective vagotomy without drainage procedure. *BMJ* 1972; 3:785

Itoh T, Idezuki Y, et al. Incidence of gallstone formation following gastrectomy for gastric carcinoma. Abstract II, 10th World Congress CICD, 1988

Jensen H-E, Amdrup E. Follow-up of 100 patients five to eight years after varietal cell vagotomy. *World J Surg* 1978;2:525

Johnson FE, Boyden EA. The effect of double vagotomy on the motor activity of the human gallbladder. *Surgery* 1952; 32:591

Johnston D, Humphrey CS, et al. Vagotomy without diarrhea, *BMJ* 1972;3:788

Johnston D, Lyndon PI, et al. Highly selective vagotomy without a drainage procedure in the treatment of hemorrhage, perforation and pyloric stenosis due to peptic ulcer. *Br J Surg* 1973;60:790

Johnston D: A therapeutic index (scoring system) for the evaluation of operations for peptic ulcer. *Gastroenterology* 1976; 70:433

Jones FA. Haematemesis and melaena with special reference to bleeding peptic ulcers. *BMJ* 1943;1:689

Jordan PH. A prospective study of parietal cell vagotomy and selective vagotomy-antrectomy for treatment of duodenal ulcer. *Ann Surg* 1976;183:619

Knight CD, van Harden IA, et al. Proximal gastric vagotomy: update. *Ann Surg* 1983;197:22

Liavag I, Roland M. A seven-year follow-up of proximal gastric vagotomy: clinical results. *Scand J Gastroenterol* 1979;14:49

Lyndon PI, Greenall MJ, et al. Serial insulin tests over a five-year period after highly selective vagotomy. *Gastroenterology* 1975;69:1188

MacGregor IL, Parent J et al. Gastric emptying of liquid meals and pancreatic and biliary secretion after subtotal gastrectomy of truncal vagotomy and pyloroplasty in man. *Gastroenterology* 1977;72:195

Makey DA, Tovey FL, et al. Results of proximal gastric vagotomy over 1–5 years in a district general hospital. *Br J Surg* 1979;66:39

Malagelada OR, Go VLW, et al. Altered pancreatic and biliary function after vagotomy and pyloroplasty. *Gastroenterology* 1974;66:22

Narbona Arnau B, Charlo T, et al. Proximal gatric vagotomy. A prospective study of 829 patients with 4-year follow up. *Acta Chir Scand* 1983;149:69

Nyhus LM, Wastell C (eds): Surgery of the Stomach and Duodenum, 4th ed Boston, MA: Little, Brown; 1984

Parkin GJS, Smith RB, et al. Gall bladder volume and contractility after truncal, selKtive and highly selective (parietal cell) vagotomy in man. *Ann Surg* 1973;178:581

Pickard WR, Mackay C. Early results of surgery in patients considered cimetidine failures. *Br J Surg* 1984;71;67

Pickford I, Craven JL, Hall R, et al. Endoscopic examination of the gastric remnant 31–39 years after subtotal gastrectomy for peptic ulcer. *Gut* 1984;25:393

Primrose IN, Axon A I R, et al. Highly selective vagotomy and duodenal ulcers that fail to respond to H2 receptor antagonists. *BMJ* 1988;296:1031

Protell RL, Rubin CE, et al. The heater probe-a new endoscopic method for stopping massive gastrointestinal bleeding. *Gastroenterology* 1978;74:257

Rudick I, Hutchinson ISF. Effects of vagal nerve section on the biliary system. *Cancer* 1964;1:579

Sapala MA, Sapala IA, et al. Cholelithiasis following subtotal gastrectomy with truncal vagotomy. *Surg Gynecol Obstet* 1979; 148:36

Shaffer EA. The effect of vagotomy on gall bladder action and bile composition in man. *Ann Surg* 1982;195:413

Shunt PS, Francis JK, et al. Reduction in mortality from upper gastrointestinal hemorrhage. *Med J Aust* 1983;2:552

Shunt RH, Vincent D, et al. Comparison of medical and surgical reduction in intragastric acidity in duodenal ulcer. *Gut* 1980;21:A455

Smith RB, Edwards UP, et al. Effect of vagotomy on exocrine pancreatic and biliary secretion in man. *Am J Surg* 1981; 141:40

Stoddard CI, Brown BH, et al. Effects of varying the extent of vagotomy on the myoelectrical and motor activity of the stomach in man. *Br J Surg* 1973;60:307

Taylor TV. Postvagotomy and cholecystectomy syndrome. *Ann Surg* 1981;194:625

Tompkins RE, Kraft AR, et al. Clinical and biochemical evidence of increased gallstone formation after complete vagotomy. *Surgery* 1972;71:196

Uvnas B: The part played by the pyloric region in the cephalic phase of gastric secretion. *Ach Physiol Scand* 1942; 4(suppl):13

Wastell C, Colin I, et al. Prospectively randomized trial of proximal gastric vagotomy either with or without pyloroplasty in treatment of uncomplicated duodenal ulcer. *BMJ* 1977;2:851

Wastell C, Ellis H: Fatal fat excretion and stool color after vagotomy and pyloroplasty. *BMJ* 1966;1:1194

29

Gastric Ulcers

Edward Passaro, Jr. ■ *Bruce E. Stabile*

At the turn of the century gastric ulcer was a disease seen primarily in young women. Now, nearly a century later, the disease is found almost exclusively in the elderly, in both men and women. Furthermore, whereas a hundred years ago, gastric ulcers came to the attention of clinicians because of perforation, now this complication is much less common. These and other features point out the vagaries of a disease about which we know very little.

While the incidence of duodenal ulcer disease has decreased in the last three decades, the incidence of gastric ulcer has remained unchanged or has increased slightly. The estimated incidence is approximately 0.3 per thousand per year, with a peak occurring between the fifth and seventh decades of life. Distribution between the sexes is equal. Mortality and hospitalization rates for gastric ulcer have not decreased as it has for duodenal ulcer disease. The reasons for this are not entirely known; however, in part, they may be related to an aging population and, at least in the United States, to the widespread use of nonsteroidal anti-inflammatory agents (NSAIDs), which cause injury to the gastric mucosa.

■ PATHOGENESIS

As yet, there is no understanding of the mechanisms of gastric ulcer formation. It is probably a heterogeneous disorder, and some patients may be genetically suscep-

tible to ulcer formation. For example, gastric ulcers have been associated with blood group A.

Gastric ulcers are almost always associated with gastritis. Gastritis is thought to precede the ulcer because it does not improve or heal following ulcer healing. A gastric ulcer can be thought of as a point in the progression of a gastric mucosal disorder ranging from chronic gastritis to overt malignancy. However, while chronic gastritis is common, only a small percentage of patients with gastritis go on to develop a gastric ulcer. In select patients, the ulcer may appear as a discreet lesion in one area of the gastritis.

An alternative theory of gastric ulcer formation stresses abnormal gastric motility with resultant reflux of duodenal contents into the stomach. Powerful cytotoxic agents such as bile acids, and lysolecithin from the duodenum, are thought to injure the gastric mucosa and disrupt the barrier mechanism. Reflex of duodenal contents into the stomach is a common finding, particularly in the elderly. However, few of these patients develop a gastric ulcer. Reflux of duodenal contents persists in such patients despite subsequent healing of a gastric ulcer.

Acid secretion in patients with gastric ulcer is thought to be low. However, clinical studies indicate that patients with gastric ulcer secrete near normal levels of gastric acid for their age group. The associated gastritis is believed to be responsible for allowing secreted hydrogen ion to back diffuse into the tissue. Whether such ions engage in gastric ulcer formation is still unknown.

Epidemiological studies have identified a number of agents as contributors to gastric ulcer formation. These include tobacco use, alcohol abuse, dietary factors, aspirin, and other NSAIDs.

Cigarette smoking is a potent factor in gastric ulcer formation; tobacco products, when present both in the blood and in the saliva of smokers, cause ulcers to develop more frequently than in nonsmokers. These products prevent ulcers from healing, thereby causing frequent recurrence.

NSAIDs appear to be the most common cause of gastric ulcer formation because of their widespread use, which often is unaccompanied by appropriate antacid prophylaxis.

Among 500 consecutive patients referred for endoscopic examination, gastric ulcers were more common in women taking NSAIDs (25%) than in those who did not (7%).[1] In addition to gastric ulcers, gastric erosions were three times as common in patients taking NSAIDs. Bleeding was twice as common among those taking NSAIDs (40%) compared to those who did not (20%). NSAIDs allow hydrogen ions to enter the mucosa and inhibit its normal healing and cytoprotective mechanisms. Their widespread use in a progressively aging population is considered a major reason why the incidence of gastric ulcer formation has not decreased. Active gastric ulcers are estimated to occur in approximately 10% of patients taking NSAIDs.

NSAIDs-related ulcers are peculiar in other ways. Currently, attention has focused on the presence of the organism *Heliobacter pylori* and its role in gastric ulcer formation (vide infra). However, patients with NSAIDs-related gastric ulcers are found to have less histological evidence of gastritis and a lower prevalence of *H pylori* (53% vs 83%).[2] This suggests that in gastric ulcer formation, NSAID acts directly on the mucosa, and not through associated mechanisms. NSAID-related gastric ulcers respond better to prostaglandin replacement therapy (misoprostol) than to treatment with conventional therapy.[3]

It is difficult to interpret the role of *H pylori* in gastric ulcer disease because many individuals may harbor the organism, yet only a few ever develop gastric ulcer disease. *H pylori* is present in about 10% of healthy individuals under the age of 30, in 50% of individuals between 50 to 65 years of age, and in 75% of those more than 65 years of age. The reason for this distribution is unknown.

It is clear, however, that almost all gastric ulcers are associated with some form of chronic active gastritis. In turn, *H pylori* is the major determinant in the development and propagation of the gastritis. Thus, when *H pylori* is eradicated, the gastritis resolves.

Quantitative studies of *H pylori* infection show that gastric ulcers, particularly those located in the upper half of the stomach, are associated with a very heavy infestation of *H pylori*.[5] The high colonization level is associated with recalcitrant active gastric ulcers. More than half of gastric ulcer patients with a persistent ulcer 7 years later had heavy colonization of *H pylori*, while those who had healed ulcers during this time period had none present.

Some strains of *H pylori* are known to secret toxins capable of causing changes in both mucin and cell growth.[4] The role of this and other *H pylori* virulence factors in gastric ulcer formation is unknown. Whether *H pylori* is the cause or the effect of gastric mucosal disease remains controversial. However, preliminary studies do seem to relegate it to a causative and precipitating event in the development of gastric disease.

Current medical therapy directed at eradicating *H pylori* consists of bismuth subsalicate liquid or tablets four times a day for a month, tetracycline or amoxicillin four times a day, and metronidazole three times a day. However, such therapy is both cumbersome and expensive. Since the relapse rate is high (80%), treatment is reserved for those ulcers that are chronic or recurrent.

■ SYMPTOMS

The principal symptom is deep-seated epigastric pain. Unlike duodenal ulcer pain, which occurs two hours after a meal and is relieved by eating, gastric ulcer pain is exacerbated by eating and occurs a half-hour or so after meals. These episodes are longer in duration and more severe in nature than those associated with duodenal ulcer pain. Consequently, patients tend to eat less or avoid meals entirely. As such, an appreciable weight loss is associated with gastric ulcer attacks. Anorexia and vomiting are also commonly associated with gastric ulcers. Patients with duodenal ulcers are anxious to eat because food relieves their symptoms, whereas patients with gastric ulcers tend to do the opposite. Additionally, gastric ulcers impair the gastric antral mechanism, thereby causing gastric stasis and vomiting.

In many patients with both duodenal ulcer and gastric ulcer, the characteristic symptoms are less defined. Since the diseases tend to overlap, it is often difficult, if not impossible, to distinguish the type of ulcer based on the described symptoms of the patient.

■ PHYSICAL EXAM

On physical examination, diffuse epigastric tenderness to palpation is present. Gastric ulcer pain to palpation is in the epigastrium, or slightly to the left of the midline.

■ TEST

Patients considered to have a gastric ulcer are best evaluated by early upper gastrointestinal endoscopy. A barium upper gastrointestinal series offers no advantages and is much more hazardous in elderly patients because of possible gastric retention, vomiting, and aspiration. Endoscopy can be done safely and expeditiously, decompresses the stomach of any secretions, accurately assesses the extent and degree of any associated gastritis, and allows for excellent characterization of the ulcer and its location. Additionally, endoscopy facilitates biopsy of the ulcer and, therefore, defines the diagnosis early in clinical course of a patient.

The only pertinent laboratory tests are those related to bleeding, a common and feared complication of gastric ulcers. These tests include hemoglobin, hematocrit, reticulocyte counts, bleeding and clotting times, and a Schilling test for vitamin B-12 stores in patients having an extensive atrophic gastritis. Several stool samples should be examined for the presence of blood.

■ MEDICAL THERAPY

The primary form of treatment for gastric ulcer disease is H2 receptor antagonist therapy because of its safety, convenience, and efficacy. There is very little difference in healing rates between any of the H2 receptor antagonists. In patients not taking NSAIDs, approximately 60% healed by 4 weeks and 80% to 90% by 8 weeks. Large ulcers, >3 cm in diameter, heal more slowly and may require 12 or more weeks.

Increased acid suppression is not associated with increased healing rates. Gastric ulcer healing rates depend more on the duration of therapy than on the degree of acid inhibition. In practice, a benign gastric ulcer that does not heal in 4 to 6 weeks is treated by extending the treatment for another 4 weeks, rather than increasing the dose of the H2 receptor antagonist. Ulcers that do not heal with H2 receptor antagonist therapy can be healed by using the proton pump blocker, omeprazole.

A big limitation of current medical therapy is the re-currence rate. A third of patients will have had a recurrence within 6 months, regardless of the agent used. In a series of 16 studies with different treatment modalities, the recurrence rate was 50% (238/475) after approximately 1 year of follow-up.[6] These results are similar to the 42% recurrence rate after 2 years observed in a large Veterans Administration cooperative trial conducted before the advent of H2 receptor antagonist therapy.[7] The addition of omeprazole to the clinician's armamentarium has not significantly changed the ulcer recurrence rate.[8]

Giant gastric ulcers (3 cm) have been regarded as a particularly virulent form of the disease, since they are intractable to conventional medical therapy and are complicated by increased tendencies to bleed and perforate. In these cases, early surgical treatment is recommended.[9]

Favorable results in treating gastric ulcers with H2 receptors blockers prompted use of this therapy for treatment of giant ulcers. However, the number of patients studied thus far has been small, with those chosen for study having uncomplicated giant ulcers.

In the largest and best documented study to date, giant gastric ulcers were defined as a particular subset of ulcers more virulent and more likely to require operation than their smaller counterparts.[10] Sixty-two patients with giant ulcers were compared to 476 patients with benign, smaller gastric ulcers studied in the same time period. Most giant ulcers were to the left of the incisura (75%), and only 13% were prepyloric, as compared to the 34% of smaller ulcers. More importantly, as shown in Tables 29–1, 29–2, and 29–3, in patients with giant ulcers, severe hemorrhage was greater ($p < .009$), penetration into the pancreas, liver, and mesocolon was more frequent ($p < .0001$), and the proportion of patients with microscopic evidence of malignancy was greater ($p = .013$). While some would suggest that the data, derived from an Asian population in Singapore, is not comparable to that among Caucasians in the Occident, there is no data available that there are demonstrable and significant differences between these populations.

Certain reports suggest a more benign course for giant gastric ulcers; however, we believe that the available data favors a more virulent course.

TABLE 29–1. ULCER PATIENTS WITH SEVERE HEMORRHAGE

Ulcer Type	Total No. of Patients	No. Patients with Severe Hemorrhage (BP<100 mm Hg Systolic)
Nongiant ulcers	476	127
Giant ulcers	62	27

BP = blood pressure
From Chua CL, Jeyaraj PR, Low CH. Relative risks of complications in giant and nongiant gastric ulcers. Am J Surg 1992;164:94–98

TABLE 29–2. ULCER PENETRATION OF CONTIGUOUS STRUCTURES

	Pancreas	Liver/Mesocolon/Colon
Giant ulcer	19	3[a]
Operated on	42	
Nongiant ulcer	9	3[b]

[a]These patients also had penetration into pancreas.
[b]These patients had no pancreatic involvement.
From Chua CL, Jeyaraj PR, Low CH. Relative risks of complications in giant and nongiant gastric ulcers. Am J Surg 1992;164:94–98

TABLE 29–3. PROPORTION OF BENIGN AND MALIGNANT ULCERS

Ulcer Type	Histologically Benign	Microscopic Evidence of Malignancy	Prevalence (%)
Giant ulcers	62	9	13
Nongiant ulcers	476	15	3

From Chua CL, Jeyaraj PR, Low CH. Relative risks of complications in giant and non-giant gastric ulcers. Am J Surg 1992;164:94–98

■ SURGICAL TREATMENT

INDICATIONS

Fewer patients are referred for elective operation of gastric ulcer disease. As a result, patients are seen on an emergency basis, and probably under dire circumstances. Thus, now more than ever, the surgeon should have a clear idea of the situations he is most likely to encounter, and what constitutes an appropriate course of action. While this section attempts to provide some of this information, the increasing use of both endoscopic and laparoscopic techniques may profoundly change future surgical treatment plans.

The great variation in size, characteristic (shallow with irregular edges, or sharply "punched out" with a circular rim), and location of gastric ulcers has not yet been appreciated. In dealing with peptic ulcer disease, gastric ulcers are thought to have the same uniformity of size and location as duodenal ulcers. This is not the case at all, because the stomach obviously presents a greater area in which ulcers can develop and because the mechanism of gastric ulcer formation in the various parts of the stomach are different. Thus, treatment of ulcers in various parts of the stomach is different, for practical anatomic reasons as well as therapeutic ones.

LOCATION AND CHARACTERISTICS

Lesser Curvature Ulcers

The most common ulcer found is located at or near the incisura, at the boundary between healthy parietal cell mucosa and/or gastritis or antral mucosa. These ulcers have sharp, well-defined edges (punched out), and the crater is deep. Because of the proximity of the left gastric artery and its branches, bleeding from ulcers in this location can be serious.

Endoscopic control of bleeding ulcers by heater probes, or by injection therapy is effective in stopping the bleeding and converting an emergency into a deliberately urgent or elective operation. Endoscopic control should be attempted in all patients since the risk/benefit ratio is exceedingly favorable. When these efforts fail and an urgent operation is required, the usual approach is to palpate the ulcer through the ventral wall and to make an incision using electrocautery parallel and approximately 2 cm away from the lesser curvature. After evacuation of blood from the stomach, a finger is inserted into the ulcer crater to stop the bleeding. Most bleeding will stop when pressure is applied in this manner. The vessel then can be suture-ligated for hemostasis.

If, on the other hand, a larger deeper ulcer is palpated in this region, and the preoperative bleeding is brisk, then it is unwise to perform a gastrotomy to evacuate the stomach. Such an ulcer is likely to have eroded into a major branch of the left gastric artery. Dislodging a clot in or about the ulcer may provoke bleeding, which may not be controllable from the luminal aspect. Rather, we divide the stomach quickly at the pylorus and raise it cephalad and to the left (Fig 29–1). This procedure permits rapid and easy access to the left gastric artery shortly after it branches off from the aorta. A vascular clamp is placed across the vascular pedicle and the stomach is returned to its usual position and evacuated. By releasing the clamp at the pylorus, we ensure that all bleeding has stopped. With the stomach clear and decompressed, we proceed from the pylorus along the lesser curvature, dividing the branches of the left gastric artery as we encounter them distal to the vascular clamp, and individually suture-ligate them until the lesser curvature is free of all vascular attachments. The vascular clamp then can be slowly released to check for hemostasis.

Under these circumstances, we advise that a distal hemigastrectomy incorporating the ulcer be done. The most efficient method is to mark the proximal point of resection on the lesser curvature with a suture (Fig 29–2). The distal point on the greater curvature is marked with two parallel noncrushing (Glassman) clamps inserted to the length of the diameter of the duodenum. The stomach, contained between the non-crushing clamps, is divided, and a GIA Stapler is applied (Fig 29–3), in the line A–B.

Two cartridges are generally required. We then over-sew the staple line with a running absorbable suture to secure hemostasis (Fig 29–4) and imbricate it with a running non-absorbable suture which approximates serosa to serosa. After aligning the distal end of the stomach to the duodenum with temporary stay sutures, we carry out a one-layer running suture with a large (0) absorbable material, first closing the posterior wall, then positioning a nasogastric tube over the suture line into the duodenum and closing the anterior layer over it. The anastomosis then can be done rapidly and is attended by fewer complications. This technique results in earlier gastric emptying than the more traditional two-layer closure. A truncal vagotomy is indicated if there is coexistent or past duodenal ulcer disease.

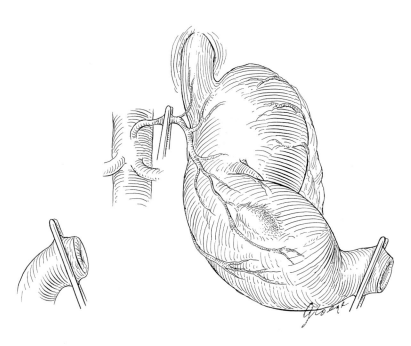

Figure 29–1. Stomach is divided at pylorus, raised and displaced to left.

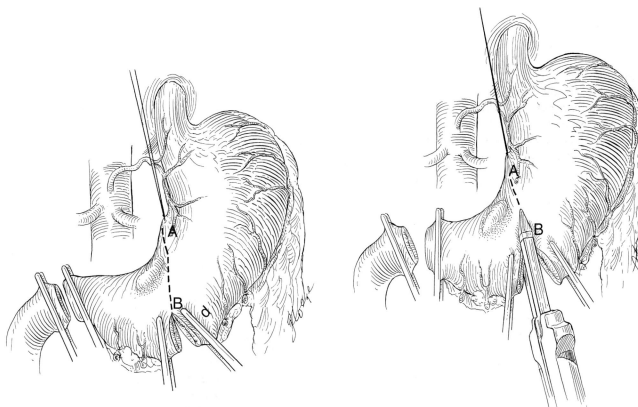

Figure 29–2. A silk suture on the lesser curvature marks the proximal point of resection. Noncrushing clamps are inserted into the stomach from the greater curvature to the distance (d), the approximate diameter of the duodenum.

Figure 29–3. A GIA stapler is applied along the line from A to B.

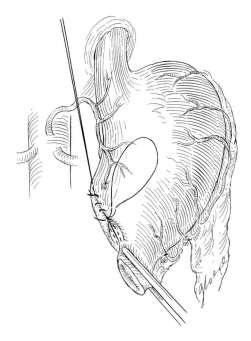

Figure 29–4. The staple line is oversewn with a running absorbable suture to secure hemostasis.

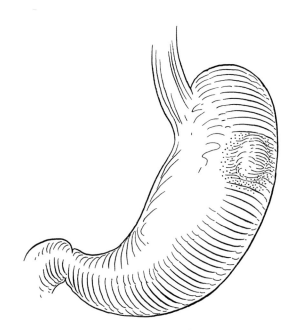

Figure 29–5. High greater curvature.

Greater Curvature Ulcers

These ulcers have a greater area of surrounding gastritis and one should always be concerned with malignant changes, even if the preoperative biopsies do not show it. When the ulcer is high in the greater curvature, a distal resection incorporating the ulcer may not be feasible (Fig 29–5). A wide wedge resection of the ulcer and frozen section histologic determination is advisable. More distal greater curvature ulcers will often incorporate the transverse colon in the inflammatory process. In more advanced cases, a gastrocolic fistula develops. Gastric cancers ensuing in such ulcers will present in this fashion. The colon should be well prepared when operation is necessary in this location. The best approach is to enter the lesser sac to either side and some distance from the area of inflammation until the ulcer and surrounding area of inflammation and/or fistula are located. The stomach then can be bluntly dissected from the colon, and any defect in the colon can be repaired primarily. The gastric ulcer can be removed in the distal gastrectomy.

Posterior Wall Ulcers

These ulcers tend to be large fundic ulcers which, despite their size, produce few symptoms (Fig 29–6). They are discovered late, generally when there are signs of acute and chronic blood loss. In our experience, patients tend to be elderly and may have been taking large quantities of aspirin and/or NSAIDs. Erosion or dense attachment to the pancreas is common. After opening the lesser sac widely, the stomach is lifted to disclose the portion of the posterior wall adherent to the pancreas. The perimeter of the ulcer should be palpated and if possible, packed away from the surrounding tissues. To free the stomach from the ulcer, a finger is insinuated between the stomach and the pancreas in an accessible site and the gastric wall is bluntly dissected from the ulcer base along the perimeter. This is possible since the ulcer rim is fibrotic and relatively avascular. The defect in the back wall of the stomach is closed with a running suture to prevent spillage into the field.

Because of inflammation, the ulcer bed is sealed from the pancreas and need not be drained. However, we have encountered deeper ulcers penetrating into branches as well as the main pancreatic duct itself. These are treated by bringing a Roux-en-Y jejunal limb up to the ulcer rim and sewing it with running sutures along the perimeter.

Because of the size and location of these ulcers, it is not possible to perform a distal resection that incorporates the ulcer. We have excised the gastric edges of the ulcer back to healthy tissue and then primarily repaired the gastrostomy.

Paraesophageal Ulcers

Patients with ulcers in this location experience dysphagia and reflux esophagitis early. The ulcers are small and sharply circumscribed and most often are located on the lesser curvature at, or immediately distal to, the cardioesophageal junction (Fig 29–7). The ulcers re-

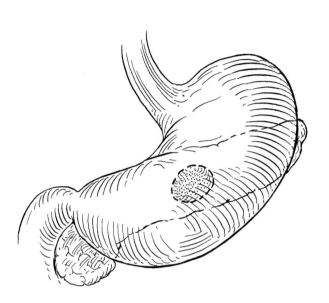

Figure 29–6. Posterior wall ulcer.

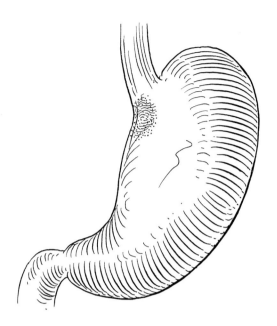

Figure 29–7. Peroesophageal ulcer.

spond poorly to medical therapy and careful biopsies are needed to exclude malignancy. Attempts to excise the ulcer in this region are attended by a high rate of leakage and subsequent sepsis or esopheageal obstruction. If adequate biopsies have been obtained from these relatively small ulcers, the best approach is to leave the ulcer in place and do an antrectomy (Kelling-Madelener procedure). The ulcer heals within 3 weeks. While antrectomy is particulary effective (98%) cure for this and other forms of gastric ulcer, we have yet to understand the mechanism.

Ulcers in Hiatal Hernia

These ulcers can be found in the herniated portion of the stomach or at the margin of the hernia where it drapes over the crus of the diaphgram (Fig 29–8). The latter is thought to occur because of the ischemic changes produced by the displaced stomach. In either case, the hernias are difficult to visualize at endoscopy, which is usually done for chronic gastrointestinal bleeding. Ulcers in the sac can erode into contiguous structures and have even been reported to erode into the heart.

The surgical approach to these ulcers is difficult. The stomach should be lavaged carefully preoperatively to eliminate both secretions and air. At operation, great difficulty is encountered in trying to reduce the hernia because of adhesions and inflammation. The short gastric arteries leading up to the herniated stomach should be divided, and the herniated stomach gradually pulled and replaced into the abdomen as far as possible. Enlarging the hiatal orifice will allow for better visualiza-

tion of the ulcer in the hernia. If it cannot be seen, a finger is inserted into the hernia and the stomach wall is followed until the ulcer is identified. If possible, the ulcer is bluntly dissected from its attachment to the sac and the stomach is completely reduced. The gastric defect is closed, the ulcer base excised or cauterized, and a repair of the hernia is done. In these instances, we have used vagotomy and pyloroplasty as treatment.

When the ulcer is found at the edge of the crus, the inflammatory response is greater than when the ulcer penetrates into the pancreas or liver; thus, it is not amenable to blunt dissection. For this reason, after defining the extent of the attachment, we have cut the stomach along the perimeter of the ulcer to free the stomach from the crus of the diaphragm. The tissue on the crus can be more carefully excised under direct vision.

These ulcers are large and relatively shallow and in keeping with ischemic changes in that part of the stomach. We have treated them by excision of the involved area and repair of the hiatal defect.

Prepyloric Ulcers

These ulcers are the subject of much debate. Although clinically they simulate duodenal ulcer disease, operations that are effective for duodenal ulcers, such as highly selective vagotomy, are ineffective for prepyloric ulcers. These ulcers are difficult to manage medically and tend to be small and sharply punched out, producing severe inflammation in the area (Fig 29–9). In women taking NSAIDs, they are particulary prone to perforate, whereas in others they generally cause bleed-

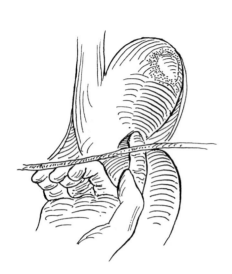

Figure 29–8. Hiatal henia ulcer.

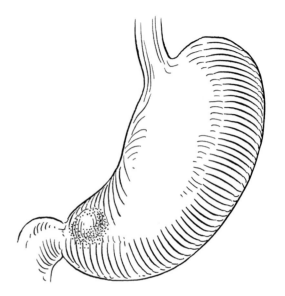

Figure 29–9. Prepyloric ulcer.

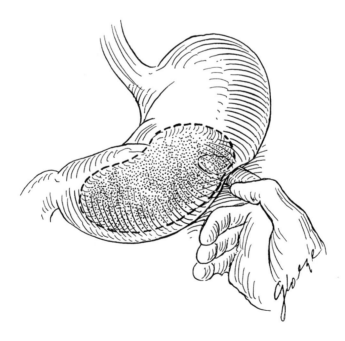

Figure 29–10. Giant ulcer.

ing. The inflammation of the distal antrum produces functional, if not mechanical, obstruction in about a third of the patients.

Vagotomy and distal gastrectomy is the treatment of choice for these ulcers, since vagotomy and pyloroplasty is either not possible or hazardous because of the inflammation in the area. The usual landmarks identifying the pylorus may be distorted or obliterated. Before attempting to dissect the stomach down to the duodenum, it is advisable to make a distal gastrostomy and identify the level of the duodenal mucosa and to palpate and note the distance of the papilla from the pylorus. The dissection should not proceed exclusively extraluminal, since injury to the common bile duct, hepatic artery, and ampulla of Vater has occurred because of grossly distorted anatomy caused by the inflammatory process. Injuries to these important structures result in very high morbidity and mortality.

Once the antrum has been cleared down to the duodenum and resected, we favor a gastroduodenostomy reconstruction as described above.

Giant Ulcers (3 cm)

Controversy continues as to whether these ulcers are more virulent than other gastric ulcers. We believe that they are. Most occur in elderly patients who present with little or no history of peptic ulcer disease. As noted previously, three-fourths of these ulcers are found to the left of the incisura, and commonly erode into the pancreas and liver (Fig 29–10). Penetration into these organs cannot be readily discerned at endoscopy since the ulcer base appears "dirty" and ill-defined. Occasionally, the biopsy report will disclose hepatocytes or pancreatic acinar tissue. Since the ulcers are broad and flat rather than deep, reaching adjacent tissues with the biopsy forceps is relatively easy. Bleeding is common because of the penetration. Treatment is similar to that for posterior wall ulcers noted above.

Despite the advent of new and powerful antacid drugs, gastric ulcer recurrence remains common after any form of medical therapy. The widespread use of NSAIDs has resulted in more complicated forms of this disease. Additionally, the experience of individual surgeons with this disease has decreased, and gastric ulcer surgery now poses a greater challenge than ever. The operation is dictated by both the size and location of the ulcer. When possible, a definitive procedure, such as removal of the ulcer and gastric antrum, is preferred because it will prevent recurrence.

REFERENCES

1. Bellary SV, Issacs PET, Lee FI. Upper gastrointestinal lesions in elderly patients presenting for endoscopy: relevance of NSAID usage. *Am J Gastroenterol* 1991; 86:961–964

2. Lane L, Marin-Sorensen M, Weinstein WM. Nonsteroidal anti-inflammatory drug associated gastric ulcers do not require helicobacter pylori for their development. *Am J Gastroenterol* 1992;87:1398–1402

3. Agarwal NM, Roth S, Graham DY, et al. Misoprostol compared with sucralfate in the prevention of nonsteroidal anti-inflammatory drug induced gastric ulcer. *Ann Int Med* 1991;115:195–200

4. Figura N, Guglielmetti P, Rossolini A, et al. Cytotoxin production by campylobacter pylori strains isolated from patients with peptic ulcers and from patients with chronic gastritis only. *J Clin Microbiol* 1989;27:225

5. Maaroos HI, Kekki M, Sipponen P, et al. Grade of helicobacter pylori colonization chronic gastritis and relative risks of contracting high gastric ulcers: a seven year follow-up. *Scand J Gastroenterol* 1991;26(suppl 186): 65–72

6. Wolosin JD, Gertler SL, Peterson WL, et al. Gastric ulcer recurrence: follow-up of a double-blind placebo-controlled trial. *J Clin Gastroenterol* 1989;11(1):12–16

7. Sun DC, Stempien SJ. The Veterans Administration Cooperative Study on gastric ulcer: site and size are determinants of outcome. *Gastroenterology* 1971;61(suppl 2): 576–584

8. Lauritsen K. Relapse of gastric ulcer after healing with omeprazole and cimetidine. *Scand J Gastroenterol* 1989;24: 557–560

9. Herrington JL, Sawyer JL. Gastric ulcer. *Curr Probl Surg* 1987;24:759–865

10. Chua CL, Jeyaraj PR, Low CH. Relative risks of complications in giant and nongiant gastric ulcers. *Am J Surg* 1992;164:94–98

30

Complications of Peptic Ulcer

Haile T. Debas ▪ *Sean J. Mulvihill*

The incidence of peptic ulcer disease has declined during the past 30 years, both in Europe and the United States. The reasons for this decline are not completely understood. Fig 30–1 shows hospitalization rates for duodenal and gastric ulcer in 5928 Federal acute-care hospitals in the United States from 1970 through 1978.[1] A marked fall in hospital admissions for peptic ulcer occurred during this time period. An even more striking fall has taken place in elective operations for peptic ulcer. A major reason for the decline in elective ulcer surgery was the introduction of powerful and effective anti-ulcer drugs, in particular the histamine H2-receptor antagonists and the hydrogen-potassium ATPase (proton-pump) blockers. Despite this change in the rate of elective surgery, neither the incidence nor the need for surgery for the emergent complications of ulcer (perforation, bleeding, and obstruction) have changed significantly during the past 15 to 20 years. This is illustrated in Fig 30–2, which shows the rates of elective and emergent operations for peptic ulcer in a Veteran's Administration Medical Center.[2] Similar trends have been observed in tertiary referral medical centers and national registries in the United States and Scandinavia.[3–6]

The introduction of effective drug therapy for peptic ulcer coincided with the introduction of highly selective vagotomy (HSV), an effective and physiologically-based operation. This operation also is known as proximal gastric vagotomy or parietal cell vagotomy. One of the great advantages of HSV over other ulcer operations is the relative absence of long-term side effects.[7,8] HSV can now be performed laparoscopically without a large abdominal incision, with little postoperative pain, and a short period of hospitalization and recovery.[9] It is possible that the availability of this new, minimally invasive approach will revive interest in elective surgical treatment of patients with peptic ulcers refractory to medical treatment.

The complications of peptic ulcer include perforation, penetration into adjacent organs with or without fistula formation, bleeding, and obstruction. These complications can occur in the setting of either duodenal or gastric ulceration. Gastric outlet obstruction is a complication that occurs much more frequently in duodenal than gastric ulcer. Conversely, the potential for malignancy, either because of misdiagnosis or malignant degeneration of an ulcer, exists almost exclusively in gastric, and not duodenal, ulcer. Malignant degeneration of a benign gastric ulcer is rare and the rate of misdiagnosis of an ulcerated cancer as a benign ulcer has decreased since the advent of flexible endoscopy and biopsy. However, the problem has not been eliminated and, in the United States, carcinoma has been found in about 3% of resected gastric ulcers.[10–12]

The most important advance in our understanding of the pathophysiology of peptic ulcer disease in recent years has been the recognition of the role of the bacterium, *Helicobacter pylori* (*HP*).[13,14] This small spiral organism is uniquely suited to survive in the hostile environment of the stomach. One of its most important adaptive features is the expression of urease, which, through the breakdown of urea, creates a locally buffered environment.[15] This feature may protect *HP* from gastric acid. Microscopically, *HP* resides in the mucous-gel layer

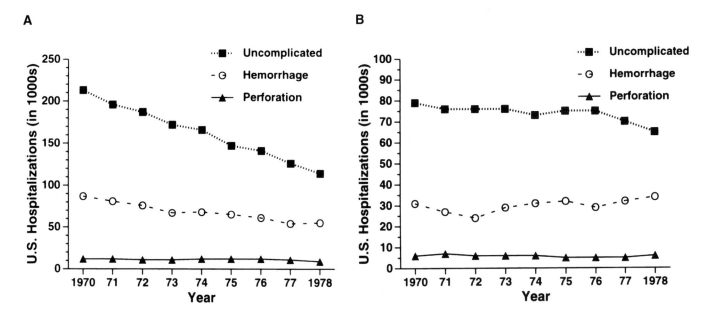

A

B

Figure 30–1. Trends in hospitalization for peptic ulcer disease and its complications over time. A dramatic decline in admissions for uncomplicated duodenal ulcer (**A**) has occurred. This is also true, to a lesser extent, for gastric ulcer (**B**). In contrast, the rates of hospitalization for emergent complications of duodenal and gastric ulcer, including bleeding and perforation, have remained stable. (Data derived from Elashoff and Grossman[1])

Figure 30–2. Trends in operation rates for peptic ulcer disease in a veterans' hospital. A marked decline in the rate of elective surgery has occurred, but the rates of operations for complications of ulcer have remained relatively stable. (From McConnell DB, Baba GC, Deveney CW. Changes in surgical treatment of peptic ulcer disease within a veterans' hospital in the 1970s and the 1980s. *Arch Surg* 1989;124:1164–1167)

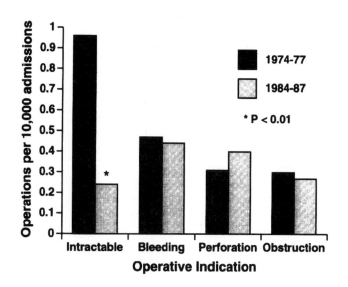

of the surface epithelium and in the crypts of gastric glands. *HP* is nearly universally present in patients with a duodenal ulcer and in the majority of patients with gastric ulcer.[14] The observation that eradication of *HP* reduces the incidence of long-term ulcer recurrence by 80% to 90% is strong evidence of its crucial role in the pathogenesis of peptic ulcer.[16–18] The mechanism of this effect is not fully understood, but may include stimulation of gastrin release, inhibition of somatostatin release, interruption of inhibitory vagal reflexes, and inhibition of gastroduodenal bicarbonate secretion.[14] The significance of this new knowledge to the surgeon is that all patients requiring operative treatment of ulcer disease should first undergo *HP* eradication. The eradication of *HP* may result in a future decline in the incidence of the emergent complications of peptic ulcer. At present, however, there are no data to support this prediction.

A second recent advance in understanding of the pathophysiology of peptic ulcer is recognition of the role of defects in angiogenesis. Angiogenesis is under the regulatory control of peptides growth factors and plays a crucial role in the development of solid tumors.[19,20] In peptic ulcer, basic fibroblast growth factor has recently been shown to stimulate angiogenesis and promote ulcer healing.[21,22] This process may be exploited therapeutically in the future as a means for improving mucosal defense.

■ PERFORATION

INCIDENCE

The incidence of perforated peptic ulcer is approximately 7 to 10 cases per 100 000 population per year.[23] Perforation is present in about 7% of patients hospitalized for peptic ulcer disease, and is the first manifestation of the disease in about 2% of patients with duodenal ulcer. It is estimated that, after the diagnosis of duodenal ulcer, 0.3% of patients perforate annually in the first 10 years. Whether eradication of *HP* will reduce this incidence is as yet unknown. In the duodenum, the ulcers that perforate are located anteriorly, and the aphorism that "anterior ulcers perforate, posterior ones bleed" is as relevant today as ever. In contrast, gastric ulcers may perforate freely through either the anterior or posterior wall. In 5% to 10% of cases, a "kissing ulcer" may be present on the posterior wall of the duodenum opposite the one that perforates anteriorly.[24] In a patient presenting with a perforated duodenal ulcer, the presence of significant concomitant hemorrhage should suggest the presence of a "kissing ulcer."

RISK FACTORS FOR PERFORATION

A strong association has been observed between the use of nonsteroidal anti-inflammatory agents (NSAIAs) and perforation of gastric and duodenal ulcers. The use of these drugs appears to be the major precipitating factor in currently treated patients.[25] A second risk factor for perforation is immunosuppression, particularly among transplant patients treated with steroids.[26–28] Other factors include increasing patient age, chronic obstructive lung disease, major burns, and multiple organ system failure.

CLINICAL PRESENTATION

The patient with a perforated duodenal ulcer classically presents with abrupt onset of epigastric pain, with or without radiation to the shoulders. Generalized peritonitis supervenes within hours, and the patient lies motionless to minimize abdominal pain. On examination, the patient appears critically ill, anxious, and diaphoretic. Respirations are shallow. Tachycardia is nearly universal. The abdomen is flat or scaphoid, with board-like rigidity. Clear signs of diffuse peritoneal irritation are usually present, and bowel sounds are diminished or absent. Liver dullness to percussion may be replaced by tympany.[29] Fever is usually present.

These classic features may be absent in several circumstances. In the very young or aged, the immunosuppressed, the quadriplegic, and the comatose patient, perforation may present in a much more subtle manner. The clinical diagnosis of perforation is also difficult in early postoperative period, especially after an unrelated abdominal procedure. The classic presentation can be modified when gastric juice flows down the paracolic gutters, simulating acute appendicitis on the right side and acute sigmoid diverticulitis on the left. At other times, a perforated duodenal ulcer simulates a perforated gallbladder in acute cholecystitis, with the accumulation of bilious fluid near the gallbladder and duodenum. Acute pancreatitis may closely mimic the presentation of perforated ulcer, but is usually distinguished by the absence of board-like rigidity and pneumoperitoneum, and the presence of marked hyperamylasemia. Elevated serum amylase levels, however, do not exclude the diagnosis of perforated ulcer, as peritoneal absorption of amylase can occur.[30] Perforated ulcer rarely is associated with acute hypotension. If present, this sign should suggest other diagnoses, such as ruptured abdominal aortic aneurysm, myocardial infarction, or mesenteric ischemia.

CLINICAL ASSESSMENT AND RESUSCITATION

Appropriate laboratory evaluation of patients with suspected perforation includes a complete blood count, serum electrolytes, and amylase. Patients presenting late following perforation may require assessment of renal function with a serum creatinine and pulmonary function and acid-base balance with an arterial blood gas. Leukocytosis with a left shift is usually present, but may be absent in the immunosuppressed or elderly patient. Serum amylase is most commonly normal, but elevated levels less than three times normal are occasionally encountered. Liver function tests are usually normal. Unless the presentation is delayed, serum electrolytes and renal function are normal.

A chest radiograph and supine and left decubitus abdominal films should be obtained.[31] Free air in the peritoneal cavity is seen in 70% of patients (Fig 30–3). The absence of free air, therefore, does not exclude the diagnosis. When perforation is suspected, but pneumoperitoneum is absent, an upper gastrointestinal study with water soluble contrast may establish the diagnosis (Fig 30–4). With clear-cut signs of peritonitis, however, such contrast studies are unnecessary.

Initial management includes the insertion of a nasogastric tube, intravenous hydration, and monitoring of urine output via a bladder catheter. Intravenous antibiotics, usually a broad-spectrum cephalosporin or, for more seriously ill patients, combination therapy with ampicillin, gentamicin, and metronidazole are instituted. Central hemodynamic monitoring is indicated in unstable patients or those with significant cardiopulmonary disease. Prolonged efforts to establish a diagnosis and resuscitate these patients are counterproductive, as early operation is warranted. The main goal of initial management should be to promptly reestablish intravascular fluid volume in order to decrease the risk of anesthesia induction.

SURGICAL TREATMENT

Ideally, the patient with a perforated ulcer should be operated on within the hour of presentation. Delay in treatment, especially >24 hours, increases mortality and morbidity rates, and length of hospitalization.[32] The usual approach is to explore the abdomen via a supraumbilical midline incision. Ordinarily, the perforation is immediately apparent in the anterior duodenal bulb. If not, the presence of fibrinous exudate and bile-stained fluid suggest the diagnosis. If an anterior duodenal perforation is not found, a thorough search should be undertaken to identify the source of the leak. Specific sites to be examined include both the anterior and posterior walls of the stomach from the gastroesophageal junction to the pylorus, the remainder of the duodenum, and the proximal jejunum. The lesser sac must be entered, either through the gastrohepatic or gastrocolic ligaments, to adequately exclude an occult perforation in the posterior gastric wall.

Perforated Duodenal Ulcer

If a duodenal perforation is found, it should be closed with full-thickness interrupted silk sutures and reinforced with an omental onlay. If the ulcer edges are edematous, the perforation is closed with a Graham patch. Following ulcer closure, a decision must be made whether to add a definitive acid-reductive procedure. In the past, definitive procedures were reserved for patients with chronic ulcer disease, as determined either by history or by operative findings. Recent experience

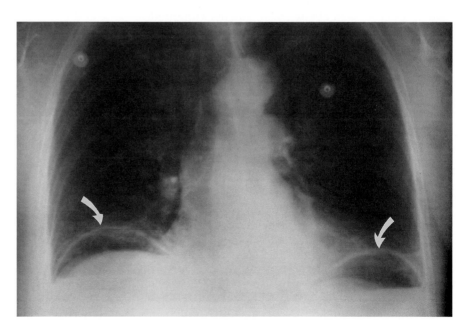

Figure 30–3. A chest radiograph showing pneumoperitoneum in a patient with perforated duodenal ulcer. The *arrows* point to free intra-abdominal air beneath the right and left hemidiaphragms.

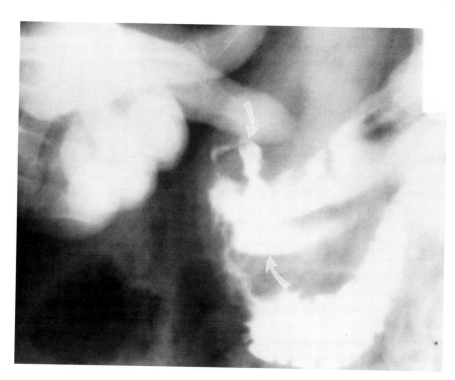

Figure 30–4. Upper gastrointestinal contrast study with water soluble material in a patient with perforated duodenal ulcer. The *arrows* delineate extravasation of contrast material.

from three continents, however, suggest that proximal gastric vagotomy should be routinely applied whether or not the ulcer is chronic.[33–39] These studies show that neither morbidity nor mortality is increased with the addition of proximal gastric vagotomy, but the ulcer recurrence rate and the need for subsequent operation is reduced substantially (Table 30–1). A definitive ulcer procedure should not be performed if the patient is unstable, if the perforation is more than 24 hours duration, or gross abdominal contamination with food or purulent material is present.

Perforated Gastric Ulcer

In perforated gastric ulcer, the main options include simple closure after four-quadrant biopsy, excision and primary closure, or gastric resection. Factors influencing operative choice include patient age and general condition, the location of the ulcer, the degree of peritoneal contamination, and the presence of malignancy on frozen section biopsy. For ulcers located in the distal stomach, antrectomy both removes the ulcer and provides definitive therapy. Benign ulcers in unstable or elderly patients may be treated with excision and closure or closure with omental patch. Ulcers high on the lesser curvature should be excised and closed. If excision is not possible, the ulcer margins should be biopsied before closure with omental patch.

The Case of the "Kissing Ulcer"

When perforation of a duodenal ulcer is accompanied by overt gastrointestinal bleeding, a concomitant posterior ulcer should be suspected.[24] In these patients, the duodenum is opened through the anterior perforation for suture control of the posterior bleeding ulcer. An acid-reductive procedure is mandatory. The two alternatives are truncal vagotomy or proximal gastric vagotomy. Even with the latter procedure, pyloroplasty may be necessary to prevent duodenal narrowing. Failure to recognize and treat a concomitant posterior ulcer may lead to severe hemorrhage requiring reoperation in the early postoperative period. The mortality of this complication is as high as 50%.[24]

Management of Delayed Presentation

Occasionally patients present late (>24 hours after perforation). In this group of patients, nonoperative management may be considered if (1) the patient is hemodynamically stable, (2) generalized peritonitis is absent, and (3) water soluble contrast examination shows no free leak into the peritoneal cavity. Management of these patients includes nasogastric suction, intravenous histamine H2-receptor antagonists, broad-spectrum intravenous antibiotics, and close clinical observation. Operation should be immediately considered if clinical deterioration occurs. These patients are susceptible to the development of subphrenic or subhepatic abscess.

TABLE 30–1. DEFINITIVE SURGERY FOR PERFORATED DUODENAL ULCER: RESULTS OF PROSPECTIVE TRIALS COMPARING PROXIMAL GASTRIC VAGOTOMY (PGV) TO ULCER CLOSURE ALONE

Trial	Operative Mortality (%)	Ulcer Recurrence (%)
Boey, et al[34]		
Closure alone (n=39)	0	36.6
PGV + closure (n=39)	0	10.8[a]
Christiansen, et al[35]		
Closure alone (n=25)	4	52
PGV + closure (n=25)	4	16[a]
Wara, et al[39]		
Closure alone (n=56)	5.3	29[a]
PGV + closure (n=67)	4.5	20.7

[a]Statistically significant compared with closure alone.

This complication usually can be managed with percutaneous catheter drainage. Previous retrospective studies have suggested a more liberal use of nonoperative management, even in early perforation, as long as no free leak is identified and diffuse peritonitis is absent.[40,41] A recent randomized, prospective trial from Hong Kong confirms that nonoperative management is safe in selected patients.[42] Caution should be exercised in application of this approach to the elderly, frail patient. Only one-third of patients more than 70 years of age were successfully managed nonoperatively in the Hong Kong series, compared with nearly 80% of those 40 to 70 years of age, and 100% of those younger than 40 years of age. Elderly patients are less able to tolerate complications related to failure of the nonoperative approach, and early operation may be preferable.

Laparoscopic Approaches to Perforated Ulcers

Recent developments in minimally invasive surgery now allow a laparoscopic approach to the patient with perforated duodenal ulcer.[43–45] With proper trocar placement and exposure, the perforation can be identified readily, in most cases. The perforation is closed with intracorporeal suturing in a manner identical to open surgery. The closure is reinforced with an omental patch, which is secured with additional sutures. The optimal patient position to perform this procedure is low lithotomy, with the surgeon standing between the legs of the patient. In addition to the camera port, three additional ports usually are required for retraction of the liver and suturing. Following closure of the perforation, the abdomen is irrigated and aspirated to evaluate contaminated peritoneal fluid. Special attention is paid to the pelvis and subphrenic spaces. Depending on the experience of the surgeon, a proximal gastric vagotomy or Taylor procedure (anterior seromyotomy and posterior truncal vagotomy) may be performed. The early enthu-

siasm for the Taylor procedure has lessened as technical skills have improved, and today, proximal gastric vagotomy is preferred in the United States.

Techniques of Proximal Gastric Vagotomy

Whether performed open or laparoscopically, the principal steps in proximal gastric vagotomy are the same. The operation is begun by identifying the distal extent of the vagotomy, about 6 cm proximal to the pylorus. The terminal vagal branches in the "crow's foot" innervating the pylorus and antrum are spared. The vagal branches from the anterior nerve of Latarjet to the fundus and body of the stomach in the anterior leaflet of the gastrohepatic ligament are divided, along with small vessels from the left gastric arcade. This dissection is continued proximally to include the distal 5 cm of esophagus, with reflection of the anterior vagal trunk to the right. A similar dissection is performed in the posterior leaflet of the gastrohepatic ligament, with preservation of the posterior nerve of Latarjet and posterior vagal trunk. With complete dissection of the distal esophagus, small branches to the cardia of the stomach are divided. The final step is closure of the de-serosalized lesser curvature with interrupted seromuscular sutures. The completed procedure is shown in Fig 30–5. Technical factors in this operation, such as the extent of esophageal denervation, have direct impact on its success. Denervation of only the distal 1 to 2 cm of esophagus, for example, results in an ulcer recurrence rate of 15% to 25%, whereas denervation of 5 to 7.5 cm of esophagus reduces this rate to 7%.[46]

■ PENETRATION AND FISTULA FORMULATION

INCIDENCE

The true incidence of penetration is unknown, but about 15% to 20% of intractable ulcers will be found at operation to have penetrated beyond the wall of the duodenum.[47] The posterior wall may be the pancreas, the gastrohepatic ligament, the prevertebral fascia, the gallbladder, or the common bile duct. In rare circumstances, penetration may terminate in the formation of a fistula either into the gallbladder or common bile duct, in the case of a duodenal ulcer, or into the transverse colon, in the case of a gastric ulcer. In extremely rare circumstances, following a previous Billroth II gastrectomy, a recurrent ulcer may cause a gastrojejunocolic fistula.[48,49]

CLINICAL PRESENTATION

The single most important symptom that suggests that an ulcer has penetrated through the wall of the duodenum is middle back pain, usually in the region of the

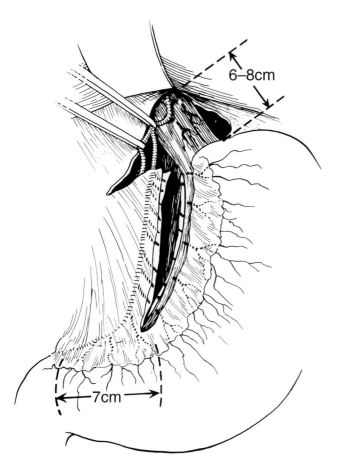

Figure 30–5. Technique of proximal gastric vagotomy. Important technical features include preservation of innervation to the pylorus and distal 6 cm of antrum, complete division of the gastrohepatic ligament in the fundus and body of the stomach, and denervation of at least the distal 5 cm of esophagus.

first lumbar vertebra. In addition, patients begin to obtain progressively less relief of symptoms with antacids or H2-receptor antagonists. This presentation is typical in penetration from both duodenal and gastric ulcers.

Fistula Formation

No characteristic symptoms can be ascribed to gastroduodenobiliary fistulas. When a gastrocolic or gastrojejunocolic fistula develops, however, diarrhea and halitosis become prominent symptoms. The cause of diarrhea in gastrocolic fistula differs from that in gastrojejunocolic fistula. Gastrocolic fistulas, which are rare complications of benign gastric ulcer, tend to be large in size, and food, fluids, as well as gastric acid secretion is dumped into the transverse colon, causing diarrhea. In a gastrojejunocolic fistula, however, the fistula into the colon is small, often no larger than a pinhole. This can make the fistula difficult to demonstrate on upper gastrointestinal barium contrast radiographs. The cause of diarrhea in a gastrojejunocolic fistula is jejunitis owing to bacterial reflux from the colon into the jejunum. Broad-

spectrum antibiotics are effective in controlling the diarrhea, at least temporarily.

CLINICAL ASSESSMENT

Endoscopy may suggest penetration when the ulcer crater is deep. Giant gastric ulcers with uneven base are likely to be benign ulcers that have penetrated into the pancreas. These giant ulcers often present emergently with frank perforation or bleeding, and usually require surgical management.[50] Barium studies of the upper gastrointestinal tract, particularly with lateral views, will often show the penetration. A very rare radiological sign of penetration is the finding of a "double pylorus." This occurs when a duodenal or gastric ulcer forms a contained perforation that subsequently drains into the antrum or the duodenum, respectively.[51] Penetration of an ulcer into the pancreas is suggested by the presence of hyperamylasemia.

The tell-tale sign of the presence of a fistula into the gallbladder or common bile duct is the presence of air in the biliary tree. Both endoscopy and upper gastrointestinal series are effective means of documenting the presence of a fistula either into the biliary tree or into the transverse colon.

MANAGEMENT

Penetration indicates intractability and is an indication for elective operation if the ulcer cannot be healed with the use of proton pump blockers and eradication of *HP*. The surgical options are vagotomy (truncal or proximal gastric) or vagotomy and antrectomy. Many surgeons, believing that penetration represents unusually severe virulence of ulcer disease, prefer vagotomy and antrectomy to proximal gastric vagotomy. However, conclusive data to support this preference does not exist.

If vagotomy and antrectomy is to be performed for a penetrating duodenal ulcer, the surgeon must carefully assess the duodenum for two structural complications of chronic ulcer before embarking on resection. The first is to examine how severely the first portion of the duodenum has become scarred or is involved in an inflammatory mass. Transection of this type of duodenum is likely to result in a difficult duodenal stump to close or to anastomose. Foregoing the option of resection at this stage is the best prevention of a blown duodenal stump or a leaking gastroduodenal anastomosis. The second structural change that must be assessed is the severity of the foreshortening of the first portion of the duodenum. In severe ulcer disease, the shortening can be so marked that the ampulla of Vater is close to the pylorus. In this setting, it is possible to damage the common bile duct or the ampulla during duodenal transection. The experienced surgeon will avoid antrectomy when either of these unfavorable anatomic circumstances are encountered. Our choice in this setting is to perform PGV. Truncal vagotomy and gastrojejunostomy (avoiding pyloroplasty) is another option, but this procedure may result in the undesirable sequelae of dumping and diarrhea.

Penetrating Gastric Ulcer

The treatment of choice of a penetrating benign gastric ulcer is antrectomy with gastroduodenal anastomosis. The base of such an ulcer, which is usually large, is the pancreas. In performing antrectomy, the base of the ulcer is left undisturbed and the stomach is separated by sharp dissection circumferentially around the edges of the perforation. In type I gastric ulcer, prospective trials suggest that the long-term ulcer recurrence rate is not improved by the addition of vagotomy to distal gastrectomy.[52] It is not necessary to add truncal vagotomy to the antrectomy unless the ulcer is prepyloric. Patients with prepyloric ulcers, however, often have an acid secretory profile that resembles those with duodenal ulcer, and the addition of vagotomy is thought to provide additional protection.

Penetration and Biliary Fistula

When a fistula has formed between a duodenal ulcer and the gallbladder or the common bile duct, vagotomy and antrectomy with gastrojejunal anastomosis excludes the fistula and effectively treats the ulcer disease. This procedure, however, is only possible if the proximal duodenum can be transected and the duodenal stump closed safely. If this is not possible, a direct attack on the fistula with cholecystectomy and T tube drainage of the common bile duct, closure of the duodenal fistula with omental patch re-enforcement, and either PGV or truncal vagotomy with gastrojejunostomy is indicated.

Gastrocolic Fistula

A gastrocolic fistula owing to benign gastric ulcer is best treated by a one-stage resection of the antrum and involved transverse colon with gastroduodenal anastomosis and colocolostomy. Preoperative mechanical and antibacterial bowel preparation is necessary. Colostomy is not warranted except in the unusual case with an associated abscess.

Gastrojejunocolic Fistula

The patient with gastrojejunocolic fistula is often nutritionally depleted. Preoperative preparation requires total parenteral nutrition, broad-spectrum antibiotics to control diarrhea, and therapy with an H2-receptor antagonist or a proton pump blocker. Following an adequate bowel preparation, a one-stage resection of the gastrojejunocolic fistula is performed with gastrojejunal or gastroduodenal anastomosis, jejunojejunostomy, and colocolostomy. In the past, the operative treatment of a gastrojejunocolic fistula was staged, with a divided colostomy in the proximal transverse colon as the initial procedure to control diarrhea and a subsequent resection of the fistula. This approach is no longer necessary, as improvements in preoperative correction of fluid, electrolyte, and nutritional deficits have made a one-stage procedure safe for most patients.

■ BLEEDING

INCIDENCE

In the United States, bleeding is four times more common than perforation as a complication of duodenal ulcer. It is estimated that about 150 000 patients per year in the United States are hospitalized for bleeding ulcers.[3,5] This rate has been relatively constant over the last 20 to 30 years. About 20% of patients with duodenal ulcer bleed during the course of their disease.[53] Bleeding appears to be more common in patients with duodenal ulcer than gastric ulcer. Bleeding is apt to be more serious when it occurs in the elderly and when it is from gastric ulcer. Patients with peptic ulcer disease account for approximately one-half of all patients hospitalized for upper gastrointestinal tract hemorrhage.[54] Unfortunately, although drug therapy with H2-antagonists and omeprazole has decreased the number of patients presenting for elective surgery with intractable ulcers, no decline has been observed in patients presenting with complications such as bleeding.[3,5,6]

RISK FACTORS

Nonsteroidal Antiinflammatory Agents

As with perforation, the use of NSAIAs is a major factor associated with ulcer hemorrhage, and the proportion of patients with this risk factor appears to be increasing.[55,56] More than 50% of patients with upper gastrointestinal tract bleeding have a history of current use of NSAIAs, most of which are over-the-counter medications.[56] The risk of this complication is higher in the elderly population, in those with prior gastrointestinal symptoms, and in those treated for short periods with NSAIAs.[57] In patients prophylactically treated with 300 mg/day of aspirin to prevent transient ischemic attacks, the relative risk of upper gastrointestinal tract bleeding is 7.7-fold higher than in those receiving placebo treatment.[58] This risk is increased an additional 2-fold with higher doses of aspirin.

Other NSAIAs are also associated with increased risks of upper gastrointestinal tract bleeding due to ulcer.[59] In a recent study of 1144 elderly patients, the use of nonaspirin NSAIAs was strongly associated with peptic ulcer bleeding. The relative risk of bleeding, compared to age- and sex-matched controls, was 4.5 (95% confidence interval 3.6 to 5.6). The risk was greater with some agents, such as indomethacin (relative risk 11.3) and naproxen (relative risk 9.1), than others such as ibuprofen (relative risk 2.0).[59]

Corticosteroids

The role of corticosteroids in the development of peptic ulcer, with or without hemorrhage, has been controversial. Recent reviews suggest that an independent causal association does not exist, and that the concomitant use of NSAIAs is a more important risk factor.[60] The combined use of corticosteroids and NSAIAs raises the risk of upper gastrointestinal tract hemorrhage 10-fold.[61] Population studies using the Medicaid Prescribing and Clinical Database suggest that the risk of upper gastrointestinal tract hemorrhage associated with corticosteroids alone is low, approximately 2.8 events per 10 000 patient-months of exposure.[62]

The Critically Ill

Another patient group at major risk for peptic ulcer hemorrhage are the critically ill patients, especially those requiring intensive care unit treatment. After cardiac surgery, for example, the incidence of this complication is approximately 0.4%.[63] Most of these patients prove to have duodenal ulcer. These ulcers are often large or multiple. A large, Canadian multihospital cohort study found an incidence of clinically important gastrointestinal bleeding among patients in intensive care units of 1.5%, with a mortality rate of 48%.[64] The main risk factors identified in this group of critically ill patients were pulmonary failure and coagulopathy. This is a group in whom ulcer prophylaxis is warranted.

Helicobacter Pylori

Curiously, the prevalence of *HP* in patients with bleeding ulcers appears to be 15% to 20% lower than in those with nonbleeding ulcers. Nonetheless, eradication of *HP* is important in reducing the long-term risk of ulcer recurrence and rebleeding.[65,66]

...TION

...tic ulceration is most common in pa... ...ecade of life. The clinical manifesta- ...g on the amount of hemorrhage. ...atures are hematemesis, melena, ...xperimentally with as little as 50 ...ed into the upper gastroin- ...erally indicates blood ...ents bleed

amination, but certain features are helpful. About 75% of patients with a prior history of peptic ulcer disease prove to have ulcer as the etiology of their bleeding.[68] Sudden onset of bleeding following an episode of retching or vomiting suggests a Mallory-Weiss tear. Evidence of cirrhosis from the history or physical examination suggests the possibility of variceal hemorrhage, but a significant fraction of these patients prove to have ulcers as the etiology. For an accurate diagnosis of the bleeding source, upper gastrointestinal endoscopy must be performed.

INITIAL RESUSCITATION

The patient with massive bleeding should be immediately resuscitated with intravenous fluid and blood replacement via large-bore intravenous catheters. A careful assessment of estimated blood loss should be made based on intravascular volume deficit. Hypotension in the absence of preexisting cardiac disease indicates significant blood loss, often in the range of 25% of blood volume. More subtle evidence of blood loss can be detected by the presence of tachycardia of postural changes. Blood transfusion sufficient to maintain a hemoglobin concentration near 10 gm/dL should be given. A bladder catheter is placed to monitor urine output. A central venous catheter is useful for hemodynamic monitoring in patients presenting with shock. In the most seriously ill, continuous monitoring of arterial blood pressure is indicated via a radial arterial catheter. Inadequate volume resuscitation is a common error made by those inexperienced with management of patients with upper gastrointestinal hemorrhage. Vasoactive pressor agents such as dopamine and norepinephrine have little role in this situation, except in the elderly, in whom hypovolemic shock may be compounded by cardiac failure. In the younger patient, however, persistent hemodynamic instability usually is associated with inadequate volume resuscitation.

A nasogastric catheter should be placed to determine the presence of blood in the stomach. Absence of blood, but the presence of bile, in the stomach suggests that the bleeding site is not the stomach or duodenum. In this situation, colonoscopy is preferable to upper endoscopy as the initial diagnostic test. Monitoring of nasogastric tube output with intermittent lavage may help in the assessment of the character of the bleeding and whether recurrent bleeding occurs. Continuous gastric aspiration also may lessen the risk of aspiration in the confused or comatose patient.

The role of acid suppression with histamine H2 restrate important clinical benefit in reducing blood loss or mortality. Similarly, use of the inhibitory peptide, somatostatin, or its analog, octreotide, have failed to benefit patients with bleeding peptic ulcer in controlled trials[71] although benefit has been observed in uncontrolled reports.[72]

PATIENT ASSESSMENT

Certain clinical characteristics are useful in predicting the risk of death and rebleeding, allowing selection of high-risk patients for intensive care unit monitoring. Table 30–2 delineates factors shown to be predictive of high rates of ulcer rebleeding and patient mortality. Previously healthy patients with only "coffee ground" emesis, absence of melena or hematochaezia, absence of hemodynamic instability, and hemoglobin concentration >12 gm/dL are unlikely to have major blood loss or rebleed and may be managed with short-stay observation or even outpatient follow-up alone.[73,74]

ROLE OF ENDOSCOPY

Endoscopy has several useful roles in the patient with upper gastrointestinal hemorrhage, and it should be employed in most patients. First, endoscopy generally differentiates the source of bleeding accurately as owing to diffuse gastritis, variceal, Mallory-Weiss tear, or peptic ulcer. This information has benefit in treatment planning, especially regarding surgery. Second, the endoscopic appearance of the peptic ulcer has significant prognostic implications. In the patient with minor hemorrhage, the finding of a clean-based ulcer or a flat, pigmented spot predicts a low rate of recurrent hemorrhage, in the range of 2%. These patients are candidates for early oral feeding and discharge.[75] Conversely, the finding of a visible vessel or fresh clot in the ulcer base predicts a high rate of rebleeding.[76,77] Similarly, large ulcers (>1 cm diameter) have high rates of recurrent bleeding.[78,79] Finally, although studies published in the early 1980s suggested that early endoscopy did not impact subsequent patient outcome,[80,81] this view has changed with the advent of therapeutic endoscopy. It is now clear that endoscopic control of peptic ulcer hemorrhage reduces the need for surgery and mortality.[82,83]

INDICATIONS FOR SURGERY

Surgery is indicated in patients with persistent or recurrent hemorrhage (Table 30–3). Some evidence suggests that early surgery is preferable, especially in the elderly population.[84,85] In most hospitals with therapeutic endoscopists, however, surgery is reserved for patients in whom endoscopic control is either not initially possible or for those who rebleed. The number of patients requiring surgery appears to be decreasing as increasingly effective endoscopic therapy has become available.[86] It is estimated that, today, about 10% of patients with bleeding ulcers require urgent surgery because of failure of endoscopic control.[54] Prolonged efforts at endoscopic control, however, are inappropriate, especially in high-risk patients. It remains unclear how to best treat the patient with successful initial endoscopic control of a lesion with a high predicted rebleeding rate. Although some of these patients will not rebleed, semi-elective surgical treatment in a stable patient is clearly safer than emergency surgery in an unstable patient with a major rebleed. Decision-making in this situation must be individualized and collaborative.

SURGICAL TREATMENT

Gastric Ulcer

For bleeding gastric ulcer, resection of the ulcer via distal gastrectomy is the preferred approach (Table 30–4). Reconstruction may be via either a Billroth I gastroduodenostomy or Billroth II gastrojejunostomy, depending on the extent of the resection and the duodenal anatomy. Vagotomy is unnecessary, as randomized trials have shown no benefit in reducing long-term recurrence rates in patients with typical type I gastric ulcers.[52] The pathophysiology of ulcers in these patients is believed to be related more to diminished mucosal resistance than to increased acid secretion. Patients with prepyloric ulcers, however, more closely mimic the pathophysiology of patients with duodenal ulcer, and

TABLE 30–2. FACTORS PREDICTIVE OF RECURRENT HEMORRHAGE OR DEATH IN PEPTIC ULCER DISEASE

Patient age >60 years
Comorbid cardiac, pulmonary, hepatic, or neoplastic disease
Presence of shock at presentation
Presence of visible vessel or fresh clot in the ulcer at endoscopy
Gastric ulcer
Persistent hematemesis
Significant hematochaezia

TABLE 30–3. INDICATIONS FOR SURGERY IN BLEEDING PEPTIC ULCER

Hemodynamic instability owing to hemorrhage
>4 units transfusion in first 24 hours
Failure of endoscopic control of bleeding site
Persistent hemorrhage beyond 48 hours
Recurrent hemorrhage during the same hospitalization

TABLE 30–4. PREFERRED SURGICAL APPROACHES TO BLEEDING PEPTIC ULCER

Ulcer Type	Preferred Approach	Alternate Approach
Duodenal ulcer	Vagotomy, pyloroplasty, suture ligation	PGV + duodenotomy and suture ligation Vagotomy and antrectomy
Type I gastric ulcer	Distal gastrectomy	Ulcer excision, vagotomy, pyloroplasty
Prepyloric ulcers Type IV gastric ulcer	Vagotomy, antrectomy Distal gastrectomy with esophagogastro-jejunostomy	

vagotomy is an important maneuver to decrease ulcer recurrence rates.

Gastrectomy for bleeding gastric ulcer is accomplished through an upper midline laparotomy. A self-retaining retractor aids in exposure. The gastrocolic ligament is divided, and the stomach is bimanually palpated to aid in identification of the ulcer and exclude the presence of a mass suggestive of carcinoma. A longitudinal gastrotomy is made overlying the suspected site of the ulcer and gross blood and clots are evacuated. The mucosa is carefully inspected and all ulcers are identified. At this point, the extent of resection required to incorporate all of the ulcers is determined.

An alternative, acceptable strategy to gastric resection is ulcer excision and closure followed by vagotomy and pyloroplasty. This ensures that rebleeding from the ulcer will not occur and, like gastrectomy, provides a specimen for histologic evaluation to exclude the presence of malignancy. In the unstable patient, four-quadrant biopsy and suture ligation of the bleeding gastric ulcer may be considered.

A special problem is the high-lying gastric ulcer, near the gastroesophageal junction. These type IV ulcers are uncommon in the United States, but are prevalent in South America.[87] Preferred management of these patients includes resection of the distal stomach and a tongue of lesser curvature that incorporates the ulcer. If the resection is near the gastroesophageal junction, reconstruction should be undertaken via a Roux-Y esophagogastrojejunostomy to avoid narrowing the gastric inlet (Csendes procedure).[88,89]

Duodenal Ulcer

The preferred approach to the patient with a bleeding duodenal ulcer is longitudinal pyloroduodenotomy through an upper midline incision (Table 30–4). Immediate control of hemorrhage is achieved by digital pressure on the ulcer base through the pyloroduo-

denotomy. Figure-of-eight sutures are applied at the cephalad and caudad aspect of the ulcer, to incorporate the underlying gastroduodenal artery. A U stitch is placed in the ulcer base to occlude potential transverse pancreatic branches from the gastroduodenal artery (Fig 30–6). After ensuring that hemostasis is complete, a search is made in the bulb and prepyloric stomach for additional ulcers. If present, these are oversewn. The pyloroduodenotomy is closed as a Heineke-Mikulicz pyloroplasty in one layer.[90] A bilateral truncal vagotomy completes the procedure. Identification of vagal trunks is simplified with the use of caudad traction on the sling made by the hepatic vagal branches and the left gastric artery at its celiac origin, after division of the phrenoesophageal membrane.[91] The anterior trunk, which may have multiple branches below the diaphragm, is readily apparent as a taut "bowstring" on the anterior surface of the esophagus. The posterior trunk is found in the plane between the esophagus and the right crus of the diaphragm. As with the anterior trunk, the posterior trunk is made much more readily apparent with caudad

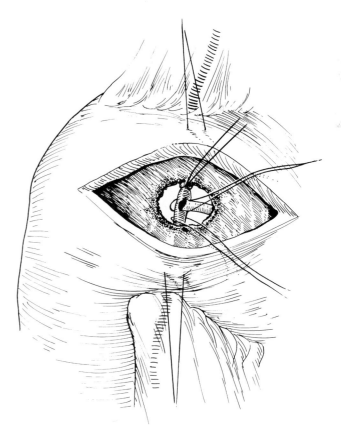

Figure 30–6. Technique of suture control of bleeding duodenal ulcer. Through a longitudinal pyloric incision, figure-of-eight sutures are placed at the cephalad and caudad aspect of the ulcer deep enough to occlude the gastroduodenal artery. An additional U stitch is placed to control small transverse pancreatic branches from the gastroduodenal artery.

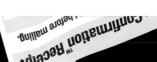

traction on the celiac branches of the vagus and the origin of the left gastric artery.

Occasionally, the bleeding site is found distal to the duodenal bulb. In these cases, the pyloroduodenotomy is extended to expose the bleeding site. After suture ligation of the bleeding ulcer, the pyloroduodenotomy is closed as a Finney pyloroplasty (Fig 30–7). Truncal vagotomy is performed.

A recent randomized trial comparing minimal surgery (suture control of the bleeding site alone) plus antisecretory agents versus conventional surgery (vagotomy and pyloroplasty or gastrectomy) was terminated early because of the high rebleeding and mortality rates observed in the minimal surgery group.[92] Definitive operative inhibition of acid and pepsin secretion is a crucial aspect of treatment of these high-risk patients. Truncal vagotomy is the simplest and most effective technique in the emergency setting. Recent reports of proximal gastric

vagotomy in the setting of upper gastrointestinal bleeding appear promising; however this operation is more technically demanding and time consuming.[93,94]

Vagotomy and antrectomy have been proposed as an alternative to vagotomy and pyloroplasty in the management of patients with bleeding duodenal ulcer. This alternative has the advantage of lower rebleeding rates and lower long-term ulcer recurrence rates. Prior studies have documented higher operative morbidity and mortality with this approach, thus it has not been employed routinely. However, a recent multicenter prospective randomized trial from France suggests that the addition of resection does not increase morbidity in currently treated patients and provides additional protection against ulcer recurrence.[95] In this trial, 59 patients requiring emergency surgery for massive, persistent, or recurrent bleeding were randomized to oversew of the ulcer, truncal vagotomy, and drainage and 61 were randomized to distal gastric resection with or without vagotomy. Recurrent bleeding occurred in 17% of those treated with vagotomy and drainage, but only 3% of those treated with resection. Operative mortality rates were 22% and 23%, respectively. Further examination of this issue is required, but it is possible that general advances in patient care may now make resection as safe as vagotomy and pyloroplasty, even in the emergency setting.

PROGNOSIS

Although bleeding from ulcers ceases spontaneously in about 80% of patients, it remains a serious problem, with an overall mortality rate of 6% to 7%.[70,85,86] This rate has remained relatively constant during the past 30 years. The mortality rate in patients treated for bleeding gastric ulcer is twice that of patients with bleeding duodenal ulcer. This is likely related to the higher incidence of gastric ulcer in the elderly, who often have significant comorbid illness. Patients more than 60 years of age have a 20-fold greater risk of death from bleeding peptic ulcer than younger patients.[79,97] Few patients today die of exsanguination. Instead, the majority of deaths are due to organ system failure caused by the bleeding episode. Operative mortality, in most series, averages 5% to 10% for duodenal ulcer and 15% for gastric ulcer.

Risk of Rebleeding

Patients who have bled from peptic ulcers have a significant risk for rebleeding, both in the short-term and in long-term follow-up. In 10 to 15 year follow-up, about half of medically treated patients with bleeding peptic ulcer suffer recurrent hemorrhage.[98] In the short term, if rebleeding is to occur, it usually will do so within 3 days.[99] Table 30–5 summarizes the endoscopic findings predictive of ulcer rebleeding.

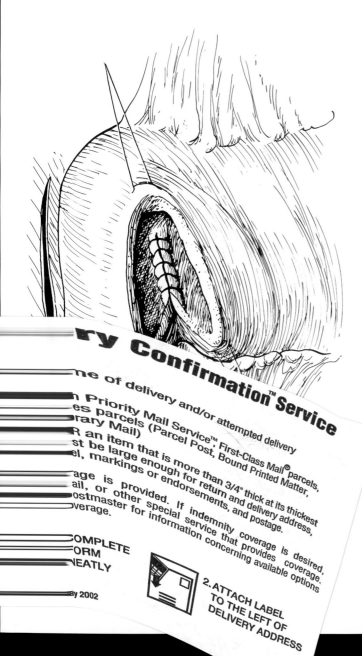

TABLE 30–5. ENDOSCOPIC PROGNOSTIC FACTORS IN BLEEDING PEPTIC ULCER

Endoscopic Finding	Rebleeding Rate (%)	Mortality Rate (%)
Clean base, flat spot	5–10	0–3
Adherent clot	20–25	7
Visible vessel	40–50	11
Active bleeding	50–60	11

(From Laine L, Peterson WL. Bleeding peptic ulcer. N Eng J Med 1994;331(1):717–727

Following surgery, rebleeding is uncommon, but this risk is dependent on the operation performed. Suture control of the bleeding site alone has a high rate of rebleeding. The addition of definitive ulcer procedures, such as vagotomy, reduces this rate. Overall, rebleeding occurs in about 10% of surgically treated patients. Rebleeding is an important cause of postoperative morbidity and mortality.

■ OBSTRUCTION

INCIDENCE

Chronic duodenal or channel ulcers are responsible for 80% of cases of gastric outlet obstruction. This complication is less frequent than either bleeding or perforation. Most of these patients have a history of chronic peptic ulcer symptoms. Pyloric obstruction occurs in 2% to 4% of patients with chronic duodenal ulcer, particularly in those in whom a "clover deformity" has occurred. Gastric outlet obstruction may sometimes be caused by edema surrounding an ulcer. Such obstruction will often respond to 7 to 10 days of conservative management. However, even in the responders, the long-term prospects are not good, and 75% of these patients end up requiring surgical treatment in the subsequent 1 to 2 years.

CLINICAL PRESENTATION

The usual presentation of gastric outlet obstruction is with symptoms of progressively worsening early satiety. Most patients have a several-year history of peptic ulcer disease. Vomiting then develops, usually following several months of symptoms of early satiety. Vomiting typically occurs after dinner and is nonbilious, consisting of semidigested food eaten that day or the previous day. As the obstruction worsens, vomiting may occur at any time. With time, the patient loses weight and may even become cachectic. Some patients present with weight loss without significant history of vomiting. This suggests the presence of malignancy.

Severe protracted vomiting, if it occurs, causes severe dehydration and a typical pattern of electrolyte and acid-base disturbance characterized by hypochloremic, hypokalemic metabolic alkalosis. When such a disturbance becomes established, the patient paradoxically excretes acidic urine as the kidney exchanges H^+ for Na^+ in an attempt to conserve extracellular fluid volume.

Physical examination typically shows a patient with variable degrees of weight loss and dehydration. The characteristic sign on physical examination is the presence of a "succussion splash," elicited by gently shaking the patient from side to side while auscultating over the stomach.

CLINICAL ASSESSMENT

A nasogastric tube should be inserted early to prevent aspiration. A large volume of foul-smelling, nonbilious fluid may be aspirated from the stomach. The hematocrit is usually elevated, indicating dehydration. Electrolyte determination may show severe hypokalemia, hypochloremia, and elevated bicarbonate, suggesting metabolic alkalosis. The urine is concentrated with a high specific gravity and an acid pH. Upper gastrointestinal endoscopy should be performed to rule out malignancy. At endoscopy, the stomach is dilated and contains a large volume of fluid. The pylorus is narrowed and irregular, and the endoscope cannot be passed into the duodenum. The gastric rugae may be hypertrophied. Multiple biopsies and brushings are obtained from the pylorus and the pyloric channel to exclude underlying pyloric malignancy. Barium examination of the upper gastrointestinal tract usually shows a large and atonic stomach, the fluid within which may cause flocculation of the barium. A small amount of barium normally enters the duodenum, demonstrating a severely scarred and distorted duodenal bulb. The barium is retained in the stomach for several hours.

PREOPERATIVE MANAGEMENT

The initial goals of management are to institute nasogastric suction, correct the blood volume and the electrolyte and metabolic disturbances, reduce acid secretion with intravenous H2-receptor antagonists, and initiate nutritional support. A Foley catheter may be required to monitor urine output. The hypokalemic, hypochloremic metabolic alkalosis is best corrected by administering intravenous normal saline solution containing potassium chloride (KCl). When the hypokalemia is severe and more than 20 mEq of KCl per hour needs to be infused, cardiac rhythm should be monitored continuously. Rarely will central venous monitoring be necessary, but if it is, the administration of large quantities of KCl centrally must be avoided. The administration of sodium chloride solution usually will reverse the metabolic alkalosis. In rare cases with severe alkalosis, intravenous infusion of isotonic solution of dilute hydrochloric acid may be required. Nutritional support may be provided by a central venous line or enterally via a laparoscopically placed jejunostomy feeding tube.

The optimum timing for surgical intervention is when the fluid deficit and electrolyte and metabolic disturbances are corrected, and when nutritional repletion is evident by positive nitrogen balance. Many surgeons believe that nasogastric suction of 7 to 10 days is useful to restore tone of the gastric musculature. The obstructed stomach is nearly always colonized by bacteria. Hence, it is useful to obtain culture of the nasogastric aspirate, and to perform gastric lavage with saline the night before surgery and to instill into the stomach nonabsorbable broad-spectrum antibiotics (neomycin and erythromycin-base) several hours before operation. Broad-spectrum antibiotics also should be given intravenously in the perioperative period.

OPERATIVE MANAGEMENT

The abdomen is entered through an upper midline incision. The first portion of the duodenum should be assessed carefully for severity of the ulcer disease, particularly for the presence of an inflammatory mass. Only then can the surgeon choose the safest procedure to perform. The choice of operation is between vagotomy and antrectomy and vagotomy and drainage. If the duodenum appears unsafe for transaction, vagotomy and gastroenterostomy should be performed. Although truncal vagotomy usually is done in this setting, the authors prefer HSV with gastrojejunostomy. If the disease in the duodenal bulb is not severe, many surgeons prefer to perform vagotomy and antrectomy, believing that this operation is not only more effective in preventing recurrence, but may reduce the incidence of prolonged postoperative gastric atony that is often seen after truncal vagotomy and drainage. After antrectomy, whenever possible, intestinal continuity should be established by gastroduodenal, rather than by gastrojejunal, anastomosis. Whatever procedure the surgeon chooses to perform, it is wise to establish a tube-feeding jejunostomy. When the stomach is markedly atonic and dilated, a tube gastrostomy should be placed to prevent the need for prolonged postoperative nasogastric suction.

The Difficult Duodenal Stump

A devastating postoperative complication of Billroth-II gastrectomy is a blown duodenal stump. The best policy is to prevent the complication by avoiding gastrectomy when the duodenal bulb is severely diseased. However, on occasion the surgeon may not discover the severity of the duodenal inflammation before the transection. Faced with this dilemma, one needs to decide whether a safe closure can be achieved using special surgical techniques or whether a controlled duodenal fistula should be accepted. When in doubt, it is prudent to construct a controlled duodenal fistula.

One technique for closure of a difficult duodenal stump is the Nissen technique. This method is suitable when the problem is caused by a posterior penetrating ulcer. The duodenal stump is closed with a continuous absorbable suture. The anterior wall of the duodenum then is sutured with interrupted 3-0 silk sutures to the pancreatic capsule at the inferior edge of the ulcer penetration. The closure then is reinforced by covering it with omentum.

When a decision is made to create a controlled duodenal fistula, a 20-Fr or 24-Fr Foley catheter is inserted into the duodenal stump and the duodenum closed around it with a 2-0 silk purse string. This is reinforced with omentum. Additionally, drains are placed in the subhepatic space. It must be stressed again that it is best to prevent having to do this by judiciously avoiding operation on the duodenal bulb that is severely scarred or involved in an inflammatory mass.

POSTOPERATIVE MANAGEMENT

The major postoperative problem following uncomplicated surgery for obstruction is delayed gastric emptying. Adequate gastric emptying will be restored in most patients within 5 to 10 days. However, in a few patients, particularly in those with long-standing pyloric obstruction, delayed gastric emptying could last for weeks and rarely for months, hence, the advisability of placing a gastrostomy and feeding jejunostomy. If gastric emptying persists beyond 10 to 14 days, a gastrograffin swallow is obtained to rule out a mechanical obstruction. After 3 weeks, flexible gastroscopy may be performed safely to examine the anastamosis. In most instances, the problem is gastric atony and not mechanical anastomotic obstruction. The cause of the prolonged gastric ileus is uncertain, but may be related to intramural edema from the prolonged obstruction. Prokinetic agents are notoriously unsuccessful in improving emptying, and a tincture of time may be the only solution. During the entire time of poor gastric emptying, adequate nutrition is maintained via jejunostomy. The use of omeprazole per jejunostomy significantly reduces gastric secretion and gastrostomy tube losses. If gastric secretion is excessive, the gastrostomy fluid can be returned into the intestine via jejunostomy.

REFERENCES

1. Elashoff JD, Grossman MI. Trends in hospital admissions and death rates for peptic ulcer in the United States from 1970 to 1978. *Gastroenterology* 1980;78:280–285

2. McConnell DB, Baba GC, Deveney CW. Changes in surgical treatment of peptic ulcer disease within a veterans hospital in the 1970s and the 1980s. *Arch Surg* 1989;124:1164–1167

3. Gustavsson S, Kelly KA, Melton L, Zinsmeister AR. Trends in peptic ulcer surgery: a population-based study in Rochester, Minnesota, 1956–1985. *Gastroenterology* 1988;94(3):688–694

4. Gustavsson S, Nyren O. Time trends in peptic ulcer surgery, 1956 to 1986. A nation-wide survery in Sweden. *Ann Surg* 1989;210(6):704–709

5. Kurata JH, Corboy ED. Current peptic ulcer time trends: an epidemiological profile. *J Clin Gastroenterol* 1988;10(3):259–268

6. Makela J, Laitinen S, Kairaluoma, MI. Complications of peptic ulcer disease before and after the introduction of H2-receptor antagonists. *Hepatogastroenterology* 1992;39(2):144–8

7. Soper NJ, Kelly KA, van Heerden JA, Ilstrup DM. Long term clinical results after proximal gastric vagotomy. *Surg Gynec Obstet* 1989;169(6):488–94

8. Jordan PH Jr., Thornby J. Twenty years after parietal cell vagotomy or selective vagotomy antrectomy for treatment of duodenal ulcer: final report. *Ann Surg* 1994;220(3):283–93

9. Zucker KA, Bailey RW. Laparoscopic truncal and selective vagotomy for intractable ulcer disease. *Semin Gastrointest Dis* 1994;5(3):128–139

10. Theenold S, Wetteland P. Ulcer-carcinoma of the stomach in a 10-year biopsy series: a follow-up study of 19 patients. *Arch Pathol Microbiol Scand* 1962;56:155

11. Smith FH, Jordan SM, Gastric ulcer: a study of 600 cases. *Gastroenterology* 1948;11:575

12. Farinati F, Cardin F, Di Mario F, et al. Early and advanced gastric cancer during follow-up of apparently benign gastric ulcer: significance of the presence of epithelial dysplasia. *J Surg Oncol* 1987;36(4):263–7

13. NIH Consensus Development Panel. *Helicobacter pylori* in peptic ulcer disease. *JAMA* 1994;272:65–69

14. Graham DY, Go MF. *Helicobacter pylori*: current status. *Gastroenterology* 1993;105(1):279–82

15. Marshall BJ, Barrett LJ, Prakash C, et al. Urea protects *Helicobacter (Campylobacter) pylori* from the bactericidal effect of acid. *Gastroenterology* 1990;99(3):697–702

16. Graham DY, Lew GM, Klein PD, et al. Effect of treatment of *Helicobacter pylori* infection on the long-term recurrence of gastric or duodenal ulcer. A randomized, controlled study. *Ann Int Med* 1992;116(9):705–8

17. Hentschel E, Brandstatter G, Dragosics B, et al. Effect of ranitidine and amoxicillin plus metronidazole on the eradication of *Helicobactor pylori* and the recurrence of duodenal ulcer. *N Eng J Med* 1993;328(5):308–12

18. Forbes GM, Glaser ME, Cullen DJ, et al. Duodenal ulcer treated with *Helicobacter pylori* eradication: seven-year follow-up. *Lancet* 1994;343(8892):258–60

19. Folkman J. The role of angiogenesis in tumor growth. *Semin Cancer Biol* 1992;3(2):65–71

20. Folkman J, Shing Y. Angiogenesis. *J Biol Chem* 1992;267(16):10931–4

21. Szabo S, Folkman J, Vattay P, et al. Accelerated healing of duodenal ulcers by oral administration of a mutein of basic fibroblast growth factor in rats. *Gastroenterology* 1994;106(4):1106–11

22. Folkman J, Szabo S, Stovroff M, et al. Duodenal ulcer: discovery of a new mechanism and development of angiogenic therapy that accelerates healing. *Ann Surg* 1991;214(4):414–25

23. Watkins RM, Dennison AR, Collin J. What has happened to perforated peptic ulcer? *Br J Surg* 1984;71(10):774–6

24. Stabile BE, Hardy HJ, Passaro E Jr. "Kissing" duodenal ulcers. *Arch Surg* 1979;114(10):1153–6

25. Gunshefski L, Flancbaum L, Brolin RE, Frankel A. Changing patterns in perforated peptic ulcer disease. *Am Surg* 1990;56(4):270–4

26. Spanos PK, Simmons RL, Rattazzi LC, et al. Peptic ulcer disease in the transplant recipient. *Arch Surg* 1974;109(2):193–7

27. Cates J, Chavez M, Laks H, et al. Gastrointestinal complications after cardiac transplantation: a spectrum of diseases. *Am J Gastroenterol* 1991;86(4):412–6

28. Feduska NJ, Amend WJ, Vincenti F, et al. Peptic ulcer disease in kidney transplant recipients. *Am J Surg* 1984;148(1):51–7

29. Felix W Jr., Stahlgren LH. Death by undiagnosed perforated peptic ulcer: analysis of 31 cases. *Ann Surg* 1973;177(3):344–51

30. Rogers FA. Elevated serum amylase: a review and an analysis of findings in 1000 cases of perforated peptic ulcer. *Ann Surg* 1961;153:228–233

31. Paster SB, Brogdon BG. Roentgenographic diagnosis of pneumoperitoneum. *JAMA* 1976;235(12):1264–7

32. Svanes C, Lie RT, Svanes K, et al. Adverse effects of delayed treatment for perforated peptic ulcer. *Ann Surg* 1994;220(2):168–75

33. Boey J, Lee NW, Koo J, et al. Immediate definitive surgery for perforated duodenal ulcers: a prospective controlled trial. *Ann Surg* 1982;196(3):338–44

34. Boey J, Branicki FJ, Alagaratnam TT, et al. Proximal gastric vagotomy: the preferred operation for perforations in acute duodenal ulcer. *Ann Surg* 1988;208(2):169–74

35. Christiansen J, Andersen OB, Bonnesen T, Baekgaard N. Perforated duodenal ulcer managed by simple closure versus closure and proximal gastric vagotomy. *Br J Surg* 1987;74(4):286–7

36. Jordan PH Jr. Proximal gastric vagotomy without drainage for treatment of perforated duodenal ulcer. *Gastroenterology* 1982;83(1, pt 2):179–83

37. Hay JM, Lacaine F, Kohlmann G, Fingerhut A. Immediate definitive surgery for perforated duodenal ulcer does not increase operative mortality: a prospective controlled trial. *World J Surg* 1988;12(5):705–9

38. Sawyers JL, Herrington J Jr. Perforated duodenal ulcer managed by proximal gastric vagotomy and suture plication. *Ann Surg* 1977;185(6):656–60

39. Wara P, Kristensen ES, Sorensen FH, et al. The value of parietal cell vagotomy compared to simple closure in a selective approach to perforated duodenal ulcer: operative morbidity and recurrence rate. *Acta Chirurg Scand* 1983;149(6):585–9

40. Berne TV, Donovan AJ. Nonoperative treatment of perforated duodenal ulcer. *Arch Surg* 1989;124(7):830–2

41. Keane TE, Dillon B, Afdhal NH, McCormack CJ. Conservative management of perforated duodenal ulcer. *Br J Surg* 1988;75(6):583–4

42. Crofts TJ, Park KG, Steele RJ, et al. A randomized trial of nonoperative treatment for perforated peptic ulcer. *N Eng J Med* 1989;320(15):970–3

43. Champault GG. Laparoscopic treatment of perforated peptic ulcer. *Endosc Surg Allied Technol* 1994;2(2):117–8

44. Darzi A, Carey PD, Menzies-Gow N, Monson JR. Preliminary results of laparoscopic repair of perforated duodenal ulcers. *Surg Laparosc Endosc* 1993;3(3):161–3

45. Mouret P, Francois Y, Vignal J, et al. Laparoscopic treatment of perforated peptic ulcer. *Br J Surg* 1990;77(9).

46. Hallenbeck GA, Gleysteen JJ, Aldrete JS, Slaughter RL. Proximal gastric vagotomy: effects of two operative techniques on clinical and gastric secretory results. *Ann Surg* 1976;184(4):435–42

47. Norris JR, Haubrich WS. The incidence and clinical features of penetration in peptic ulceration. *JAMA* 1961; 178:386

48. Blumen LJ, Weber JM. Gastrojejunocolic fistula secondary to benign ulcer. *JAMA* 1970;214(13):2335–6

49. Hodgson J, Medina OF, Teodorescu M, Messe AA. Modern concepts in the management of gastrojejunocolic fistula. *Mt Sinai J Med* 1975;42(3):239–44

50. Morrow CE, Mulholland MW, Dunn DH, et al. Giant duodenal ulcer. *Am J Surg* 1982;330–331

51. Polloni A, Marchi S, Bellini M, et al. Double pylorus: report of two cases and review of the literature. *Ital J Gastroenterol* 1991;23(6):360–3

52. Rehnberg O. Antrectomy and gastroduodenostomy with or without vagotomy in peptic ulcer disease: a prospective study with a 5-year follow-up. *Acta Chirurg Scand* 1983; 515(suppl):1–63

53. Fry J. Peptic ulcer: a profile. *BMJ* 1964;2:809

54. Laine L, Peterson WL. Bleeding peptic ulcer. *N Engl J Med* 1994;331(11):717–27

55. Griffin MR, Piper JM, Daugherty JR, et al. Nonsteroidal anti-inflammatory drug use and increased risk of peptic ulcer disease in elderly persons. *Ann Int Med* 1991; 114(4):257–63

56. Wilcox CM, Shalek KA, Cotsonis G. Striking prevalence of over-the-counter nonsteroidal anti-inflammatory drug use in patients with upper gastrointestinal hemorrhage. *Arch Int Med* 1994;154(1):42–6

57. Gabriel SE, Jaakkimainen L, Bombardier C. Risk for serious gastrointestinal complications related to use of nonsteroidal anti-inflammatory drugs: a meta-analysis. *Ann Int Med* 1991;115(10):787–96

58. Shorrock CJ, Langman MJS, Warlow C. Risks of upper GI bleeding during TIA prophylaxis with aspirin. *Gastroenterology* 1992;102(4):A165

59. Langman MJ, Weil J, Wainwright P, et al. Risks of bleeding peptic ulcer associated with individual non-steroidal anti-inflammatory drugs. *Lancet* 1994;343(8905):1075–8

60. Guslandi M, Tittobello A. Steroid ulcers: a myth revisited. *BMJ* 1992;304(6828):655–6

61. Piper JM, Ray WA, Daugherty JR, Griffin MR. Corticosteroid use and peptic ulcer disease: role of nonsteroidal anti-inflammatory drugs. *Ann Int Med* 1991;114(9):735–40

62. Carson JL, Strom BL, Schinnar R, et al. The low risk of upper gastrointestinal bleeding in patients dispensed corticosteroids. *Am J Med* 1991;91(3):223–8

63. Lebovics E, Lee SS, Dworkin BM, et al. Upper gastrointestinal bleeding following open heart surgery: predominant finding of aggressive duodenal ulcer disease. *Dig Dis Sci* 1991;36(6):757–60

64. Cook DJ, Fuller HD, Guyatt GH, et al. Risk factors for gastrointestinal bleeding in critically ill patients. Canadian Critical Care Trials Group. *N Eng J Med* 1994;330(6): 377–81

65. Laine L. Eradication of *Helicobacter pylori* reduces gastric and duodenal ulcer recurrence. *Gastroenterology* 1992; 103(5):1695–6

66. Graham DY, Hepps KS, Ramirez FC, et al. Treatment of *Helicobacter pylori* reduces the rate of rebleeding in peptic ulcer disease. *Scand J Gastroenterol* 1993;28(11):939–42

67. Daniel WA Jr., Egan S. The quantity of blood required to produce a tarry stool. *JAMA* 1939;113:2232

68. Cotton PB, Rosenberg MT, Waldram RP, Axon AT. Early endoscopy of oesophagus, stomach, and duodenal bulb in patients with haematemesis and melaena. *Br Med J* 1973;2 (865):505–9

69. Collins R, Langman M. Treatment with histamine H2 antagonists in acute upper gastrointestinal hemorrhage. Implications of randomized trials. *N Eng J Med* 1985;313(11): 660–6

70. Daneshmend TK, Hawkey CJ, Langman MJ, et al. Omeprazole versus placebo for acute upper gastrointestinal bleeding: randomised double blind controlled trial. *BMJ* 1992;304(6820):143–7

71. Christiansen J, Ottenjann R, Von AF. Placebo-controlled trial with the somatostatin analogue SMS 201-995 in peptic ulcer bleeding. *Gastroenterology* 1989;97(3):568–74

72. Jenkins SA, Taylor BA, Nott DM, et al. Management of massive upper gastrointestinal haemorrhage from multiple sites of peptic ulceration with somatostatin and octreotide—a report of five cases. *Gut* 1992;33(3):404–7

73. Bordley DR, Mushlin AL, Dolan JG, et al. Early clinical signs identify low-risk patients with acute upper gastrointestinal hemorrhage. *JAMA* 1985;253(22):3282–5

74. Harland R, Neilson D. Criteria for selective admission of patients with haematemesis. *J R Soc Med* 1992;85(1):26–8

75. Laine L, Cohen H, Brodhead J, et al. Prospective evaluation of immediate versus delayed refeeding and prognostic value of endoscopy in patients with upper gastrointestinal hemorrhage. *Gastroenterology* 1992;102(1):314–6

76. Griffiths WJ, Neumann DA, Welsh JD. The visible vessel as an indicator of uncontrolled or recurrent gastrointestinal hemorrhage. *N Eng J Med* 1979;300(25):1411–3

77. Wara P. Endoscopic prediction of major rebleeding—a prospective study of stigmata of hemorrhage in bleeding ulcer. *Gastroenterology* 1985;88(5, pt 1):1209–14

78. Waring JP, Sanowski RA, Sawyer RL, et al. A randomized comparison of multipolar electrocoagulation and injection sclerosis for the treatment of bleeding peptic ulcer. *Gastrointest Endosc* 1991;37(3):295–8

79. Branicki FJ, Coleman SY, Fok PJ, et al. Bleeding peptic ulcer: a prospective evaluation of risk factors for rebleeding and mortality. *World J Surg* 1990;14(2):262–9

80. Conn HO. To scope or not to scope. *N Eng J Med* 1981; 304(16):967–9

81. Peterson WL, Barnett CC, Smith HJ, et al. Routine early endoscopy in upper-gastrointestinal-tract bleeding: a randomized, controlled trial. *N Eng J Med* 1981;304(16): 925–9

82. Sacks HS, Chalmers TC, Blum AL, et al. Endoscopic hemostasis: an effective therapy for bleeding peptic ulcers. *JAMA* 1990;264(4):494–9

83. Cook DJ, Guyatt GH, Salena BJ, Laine LA. Endoscopic therapy for acute nonvariceal upper gastrointestinal hemorrhage: a meta-analysis. *Gastroenterology* 1992;102(1): 139–48

84. Cochran TA. Bleeding peptic ulcer: surgical therapy. *Gastroenterol Clin North Am* 1993;22(4):751–78

85. Morris DL, Hawker PC, Brearley S, et al. Optimal timing of operation for bleeding peptic ulcer: prospective randomised trial. *BMJ* 1984;288(6426):1277–80

86. Bown S. Bleeding peptic ulcers. *BMJ* 1991;302(6790): 1417–8

87. Csendes A, Braghetto I, Smok G. Type IV gastric ulcer: a new hypothesis. *Surgery* 1987;101(3):361–6

88. Csendes A, Lazo M, Braghetto I. A surgical technic for high (cardial or juxtacardial) benign chronic gastric ulcer. *Am J Surg* 1978;135(6):857–8

89. Csendes A, Braghetto I, Calvo F, et al. Surgical treatment of high gastric ulcer. *Am J Surg* 1985;149(6):765–70

90. Weinberg JA. Treatment of the massively bleeding duodenal ulcer by ligation, pyloroplasty and vagotomy. *Am J Surg* 1961;102:158–167

91. Roberts JP, Debas HT. A simplified technique for rapid truncal vagotomy. *Surg Gynecol Obstet* 1989;168(6): 539–41

92. Poxon VA, Keighley MR, Dykes PW, et al. Comparison of minimal and conventional surgery in patients with bleeding peptic ulcer: a multicentre trial. *Br J Surg* 1991;78(11): 1344–5

93. Falk GL, Hollinshead JW, Gillett DJ. Highly selective vagotomy in the treatment of complicated duodenal ulcer. *Med J Aus* 1990;152(11):574–6

94. Miedema BW, Torres PR, Farnell MB, et al. Proximal gastric vagotomy in the emergency treatment of bleeding duodenal ulcer. *Am J Surg* 1991;161(1):64–6

95. Millat B, Hay JM, Valleur P, et al. Emergency surgical treatment for bleeding duodenal ulcer: oversewing plus vagotomy versus gastric resection, a controlled randomized trial. French Associations for Surgical Research. *World J Surg* 1993;17(5):568–73

96. Walt RP, Cottrell J, Mann SG, et al. Continuous intravenous famotidine for haemorrhage from peptic ulcer. *Lancet* 1992;340(8827):1058–62

97. Branicki FJ, Boey J, Fok PJ, et al. Bleeding duodenal ulcer: a prospective evaluation of risk factors for rebleeding and death. *Ann Surg* 1990;211(4):411–8

98. MacLeod IA, Mills PR. Factors identifying the probability of further haemorrhage after acute upper gastrointestinal haemorrhage. *Br J Surg* 1982;69(5):256–8

99. Northfield TC. Factors predisposing to recurrent haemorrhage after acute gastrointestinal bleeding. *Br Med J* 1971;1(739):26–8

31

Tumors of the Stomach

Richard D. Rosin

Benign tumors of the stomach are rare and are found at routine endoscopy and occasionally, during postmortem examinations. They make up <2% of all gastric neoplasms. Occasionally, they may present by their complications, such as pain, bleeding, and gastric outlet obstruction. The only cause for concern is that some of them have potential for malignant transformation. There are three major types of benign tumors found in the stomach (Table 31–1). Epithelial tumors account for 75%, with mesenchymal and miscellaneous tumors each making up about half of the other 25%.

▪ EPITHELIAL POLYPS

Two distinct types of epithelial polyps are recognized: hyperplastic (regenerative) and adenomatous. The latter have the potential to undergo malignant change.

Hyperplastic polyps are distributed throughout the entire stomach, are usually multiple, and <2 cm in diameter. They are five times as common as adenomatous polyps. Endoscopically, they are small smooth protuberances, usually found on the gastric folds. They may well undergo spontaneous regression. Microscopically, the cells in the dilated cystic glands are identical to those of the surrounding stomach epithelium (Fig 31–1).

Adenomatous polyps are usually single, most commonly situated in the antrum, and are usually >2 cm in diameter. They may be sessile, pedunculated, or villous. When larger than 2 cm, between one-third and one-half of these tumors will become malignant. Histologically, the cells are hyperchromatic, with elongated nuclei of uniform architecture (Fig 31–2).

MANAGEMENT OF GASTRIC POLYPS

The management of gastric polyps depends greatly on (1) the histologic appearance of the polyps at biopsy, and (2) whether they are symptomatic. If possible, a single polyp should be removed endoscopically in preference to biopsy, since this will assist the pathologist in his diagnosis.

If a polyp is symptomatic, it should be removed. Removal is performed best by endoscopy, using either a snare or a laser. If neither method is possible, the polyp or polyps can be removed at gastrectomy. Diffuse polyposis can mask a frank carcinoma, and frozen section examination is necessary. If polyps show histologic evidence of carcinoma in situ, wedge excision will suffice. However, in the case of invasive carcinoma, a formal gastric resection is necessary.

If asymptomatic polyps are found by chance at endoscopic examination, biopsy should be done to exclude in situ or invasive carcinoma. If the polyps are >2 cm in diameter, they should be removed with the use of a snare or a laser because of their propensity for malignant change. Once proven to be benign, annual endoscopic examination is sufficient. If multiple polyps are present, examination at 6 month intervals is needed. Factors influencing the outcome of epithelial polyps are listed in Table 31–2.

TABLE 31–1. CLASSIFICATION OF BENIGN TUMORS

EPITHELIAL POLYPS
    Hyperplastic
    Adenomatous

MESENCHYMAL TUMORS
    Leiomyoma
    Fibroma
    Neurogenic
    Lipoma
    Vascular
    Osteoma and osteochondroma

MISCELLANEOUS TUMORS
    Heterotopic pancreas
    Inflammatory pseudotumors
    Hamartomatous in Peutz-Jeghers polyp
    Cyst

TABLE 31–2. FACTORS INFLUENCING OUTCOME OF EPITHELIAL POLYPS

Appearance	Management
SIZE	
<2 cm	Observe
>2 cm	Remove
NUMBER	
Single more likely to be malignant	Remove
Multiple usually hyperplastic	Observe
SHAPE	
Pedunculated	Observe
Sessile/villous	Remove
LOCATION	
Adenomatous found in antrum	Remove
Hyperplastic randomly distributed	Observe

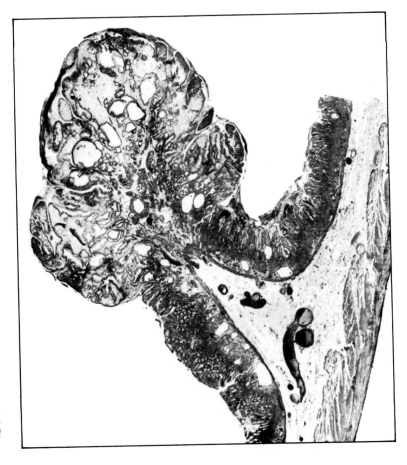

Figure 31–1. Topography of a hyperplastic polyp. Note the cystic glands. (x7) (From Tomasulo J. Gastric polyps: histologic types and their relationship to gastric carcinoma. *Cancer* 1971;27:1346, with permission of the American Cancer Society)

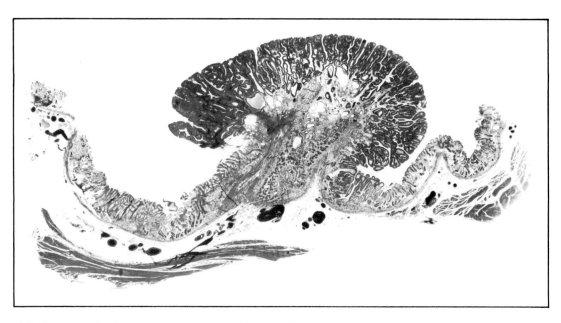

Figure 31–2. Adenomatous polyp. (Low power topography, *x7*) (From Tomasulo J. Gastric polyps: histologic types and their relationship to gastric carcinoma. *Cancer* 1971;27:1346, with permission of the American Cancer Society)

All symptomatic gastric polyps should be removed endoscopically, if possible. Surgical excision, if necessary, should be carried out by the least radical operation that will permit complete removal. Excisional biopsy is necessary for asymptomatic polyps >2 cm, but polyps smaller than this, if shown to be benign by biopsy, may be kept under regular endoscopic observation. It is our practice to remove benign polyps that cannot be removed endoscopically by laparoscopic excision.

■ MESENCHYMAL TUMORS

Leiomyomas are the most common of the benign mesenchymal tumors, and they are followed next in frequency by the fibroma group. Since these tumors are remarkably similar in their macroscopic appearance and clinical behavior, they can be described together. According to Palmer, mesenchymal tumors constitute one-eighth of all benign gastric neoplasms.[1] Palmer's list of the different types of mesenchymal tumors and their relative frequency are given in Table 31–3.

HISTOPATHOLOGY

Mesenchymal tumors, usually single, well-circumscribed, and roughly spheroidal, are located in the submucosa. The overlying mucosa can be ulcerated, and frank bleeding is a common presentation, particularly so with schwannomas, in which the ulcer typically extends deep into the tumor (Fig 31–3). Their size can range from a few millimeters to many centimeters. Usually, the subserosal types assume the large size. They are usually found in the antrum, although leiomyomas and fibromas also are often found near the gastroesophageal junction.

Degeneration in the form of cystic change, myxoid degeneration, calcification, and even ossification can occur. Malignant transformation is a complication, but the evidence for this change is largely anecdotal. If a benign mesenchymal tumor recurs, or if metastases develop after the tumor has been excised, it is probable that the tumor was malignant from the outset, and the histology should be carefully reviewed. Malignant transformation may occur especially in vascular tumors, if they are left untreated.

It is often difficult to distinguish between benign mesenchymal neoplasms and low-grade sarcomas, particularly with certain types of vascular tumors. Usually these tumors present in adults, and their incidence in men and women appears to be equal, although schwannomas are found more often in women.

The most common symptoms are those caused by bleeding: melena, or anemia due to occult gastrointestinal blood loss. Dyspepsia may occur, although the reason is obscure, unless there is ulceration of the neoplasm. Occasionally, a pedunculated tumor may prolapse through the pylorus and cause outlet obstruc-

TABLE 31–3. INCIDENCE OF MESENCHYMAL TUMORS

Tumor	Autopsy Series		Gastric Tumors of All Types		Benign Nonepithelial Gastric Tumors	
	No. of Tumors/ No. of Autopsies	(%)	No.	(%)	No.	(%)
Leiomyoma	70/38,222	0.18	82/5194	1.58	158/273	57.90
	23/50[a]	46.00[a]				
Fibroma	24/32,268	0.07	13/4445	0.29	59/269	21.90
Neurogenic:						
Schwannoma	3/18,276	0.02	5/4806	0.10	10/200	5.00
	106/1500[a]	7.10[a]				
Neurofibroma	0/32,268	0	1/4445	0.02	4/269	1.49
Vascular	—	—	9/10,079	0.09	9/123	7.30
Lipoma	14/47,780	0.03	—	—	20/317	6.30

[a]Data derived from detailed autopsy studies.
From Palmer ED. Benign intramural tumors of the stomach: A review with special reference to gross pathology. Medicine (Baltimore) 1951;30:81, with permission.

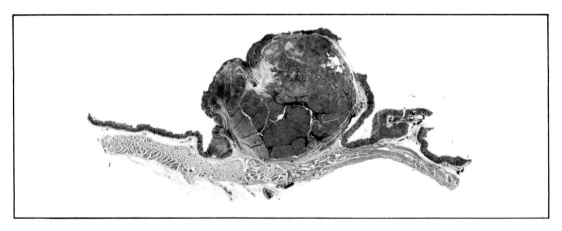

Figure 31–3. Cross-section typical ulcerated submucosal leioyoma.

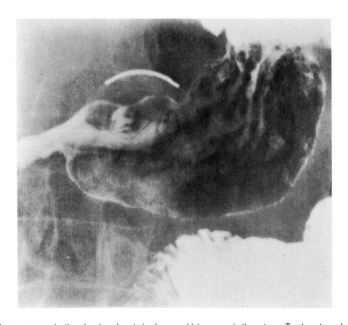

Figure 31–4. Barium x-ray examination showing ulcerated submucosal leiomyoma in the antrum. Treatment was by partial gastrectomy.

tion. In the older age group, the very large tumors may appear first as a palpable abdominal mass. However, the most common method of presentation is incidental discovery at laparotomy, endoscopy, or radiological examination.

DIAGNOSIS

The majority of mesenchymal tumors can be demonstrated with a double-contrast barium-meal examination, and they will be seen as rounded sessile or pedunculated masses (Fig 31–4). Ulceration of the overlying mucosa may appear as an irregular surface or possibly, as a grossly visible crater in the contour of the tumor. A submucosal lipoma has a smooth and well-circumscribed contour that typically changes shape during peristalsis.

Upper gastrointestinal endoscopy is a more sensitive investigation and also permits biopsy. Each tumor has a different appearance. Leiomyomas tend to be firm, and the overlying mucosa frequently is ulcerated. Many of the neurogenic tumors and fibromas, however, also have this appearance. Lipomas and the submucous angiomas are softer and more compressible and will bleed more profusely when biopsy is performed. Endoscopy also helps differentiate these tumors from other conditions such as epithelial polyps, trichobezoars, varices, hematomas, chronic peptic ulceration, heterotopic pancreatic rests. Menetrier's disease, postoperative inflammatory granulomas, inflammatory pseudotumors, and carcinomas.

Differentiation of one type of mesenchymal neoplasm from another can be difficult, not only because they may appear similar, but also because biopsy may not provide a specific diagnosis, especially if only superficial tissue has been taken. The use of the spiked biopsy forceps and careful application of these to the side of the tumor enhance the taking of a deeper biopsy specimen.

MANAGEMENT

Since it is usually difficult to differentiate between benign and malignant mesenchymal tumors, both should be excised, if the patient is well enough to undergo surgery. A possible exception might be made for the asymptomatic patient with submucosal lipoma, which should be followed up by regular endoscopy and biopsy.

For benign mesenchymal tumors, radical resection is unnecessary and either segmental resection or enucleation via a gastrostomy should suffice. For lesions in the body of the stomach, antral gastrostomy and excision of this tumor from within the stomach, followed by oversewing of the mucosa, is preferred. If the tumor is situated at the cardia where segmental resection may be difficult, this method also may be used. Histologic examination using frozen section is mandatory in every case.

MISCELLANEOUS TUMORS

The differential diagnosis of benign gastric tumors includes aberrant rests of pancreatic tissue located in the wall of the stomach. As with mesenchymal tumors of the stomach, these tumors are usually asymptomatic, although occasionally, patients present with symptoms such as epigastric pain, outlet obstruction, and frequently, hemorrhage. The exact incidence is unknown, although it has been stated that they are as frequent as benign mesenchymal tumors.[2]

These pancreatic rests usually are found in the antrum or in the prepyloric region of the stomach. They are typically rubbery, discrete submucosal lesions up to 3 cm in diameter. The tumor may have an umbilicated appearance, which is, in fact, a central ductal orifice that communicates with a filiform ductal system to the pancreatic acini that form the tumor. The processes that affect the pancreas, for example, pancreatitis and the formation of cysts, can also affect these rests. Rarely, ulceration and frank bleeding are an indication of malignant change.[3] Once the diagnosis has been made, usually by endoscopy, surgical excision is the accepted form of treatment.

■ INFLAMMATORY PSEUDOTUMORS

Inflammatory pseudotumors are also described as inflammatory fibroid polyps, eosinophilic granuloma, eosinophilic gastritis, and gastric submucosal granuloma with eosinophilic infiltration. Macroscopically, they can appear as either polypoid or infiltrative lesions and usually are located in the antrum. The polypoid type can be soft or rubbery to palpation and may be several centimeters in size. In both types, the overlying mucosa is commonly ulcerated. These tumors can be mistaken easily for carcinomas. Histologically, there is inflammation with connective tissue and vascular proliferation as well as a predominantly eosinophilic cell infiltrate (Figs 31–5, and 31–6).

The patient may complain initially of abdominal pain, melena, anemia, or vomiting owing to pyloric obstruction, but usually there are no specific symptoms. Recognition of these tumors is important because they mimic malignancy. After they have been recognized and their benign nature has been confirmed, they should be treated conservatively, if possible by endoscopic excision.

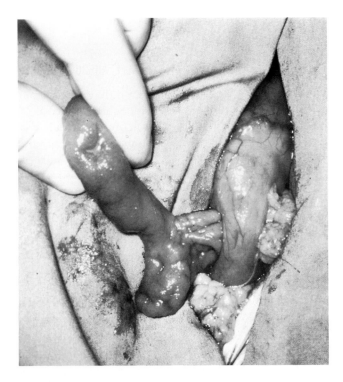

Figure 31–5. Inflammatory pseudotumor of the stomach, polypoid form. Lesion has been removed through a gastrostomy incision. Treatment was by simple polypectomy.

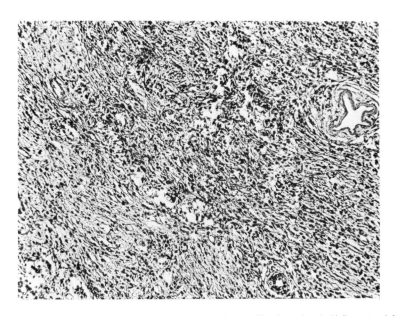

Figure 31–6. Microscopic appearance of inflammatory pseudotumor showing connective tissue proliferation and marked inflammatory infiltrate. (x 125)

■ PEUTZ-JEGHER'S POLYPS

Peutz-Jegher's polyps are nonmalignant malformations or hematomas representing focal overgrowth, and they may occur occasionally in the stomach. Malignancy may occur as a rare event in this syndrome, either in degenerating polyps or de novo in the nonpolypoid mucosa. It is unknown whether Peutz-Jegher's syndrome predisposes patients to the development of gastrointestinal carcinoma. Peutz-Jegher's polyps should be removed only if they are symptomatic. Symptoms are the same as those of other benign gastric polyps and they can usually be removed at endoscopy.

■ CYSTIC TUMORS

Cystic tumors in the stomach are rare,[1] and they comprise a heterogeneous group of developmental anomalies and infective, posttraumatic, or neoplastic lesions.

■ CARCINOMA OF THE STOMACH

Outside of Japan, carcinoma of the stomach is usually at an advanced stage by the time of diagnosis, with infiltration beyond the submucosa, into or through the gastric wall. To a patient, diagnosis of cancer of the stomach often signifies impending death. In fact, even among the medical profession, there is widespread belief that this diagnosis implies hopelessness. This attitude is a great deterrent to progress and is a sad one— cancer of the stomach can be a curable disease. Fortunately, there have been recent rapid advances in the science and earlier diagnosis of this disease, which is encouraging for the future.

HISTORICAL BACKGROUND

Avicenna (980–1037) gave the first account of cancer of the stomach. The first detailed paper on malignant lesions of the stomach, however, was written by Morgagni in 1761. Pean (1879) performed the first gastric resection for cancer. Two years later Billroth carried out the first successful pyloric resection, and 16 years later, in 1897, Schlatter carried out the first successful total gastrectomy. The first detailed description of the lymphatic drainage of the stomach, which influenced the extent of gastric resection, was given by Cuneo in 1906. Five years later, in 1911, Polya described his partial gastrectomy, which he admitted was based on von Hacker's description of an end-to-end gastrojejunostomy.

The recommendation for more radical operations was given by McNeer and associates in 1951 after they had reviewed 92 postmortem specimens following partial gas-

trectomy for carcinoma.[4] In half of the cases, they found recurrence in the gastric remnant, and therefore advised radical total gastrectomy with partial pancreatectomy and splenectomy. However, a study at the Mayo Clinic of the late results following total gastrectomy in 170 cases in which 78% had involved nodes showed a 5 year survival of 18%.[5] Only 10% of patients with a malignant lesion in the distal part of the stomach lived for 5 years. These researchers concluded that total gastrectomy was not the operation of choice for all gastric carcinomas.

Recently, there has been renewed interest in the etiology of cancer of the stomach, its early diagnosis, results of medical and surgical treatment in various subgroups, the geography of stomach cancer, gastric ulcer and cancer risk, the importance of resection margins and lymph node involvement, and the possible use of oncogenes in future studies. The concept of early gastric cancer and screening for it has been widely published by the Japanese. One of the most remarkable facts in the whole field of cancer treatment is the difference in the results of treatment of stomach cancer reported by the Japanese and those reports emanating from Europe, North America and Australia. The Japanese reports are optimistic, revealing significant improvements in the resectability rate, in resections for cure, and in both 5 and 10 year survival rates. Reports from the rest of the world remain pessimistic.

INCIDENCE AND PATHOLOGY

Despite the decline in the incidence of gastric carcinoma in recent years,[6] it remains the most common cause of death from malignant disease worldwide. There is a great variation in the incidence, both internationally and nationally. In the United Kingdom, in 1980, there were 10 900 deaths from gastric carcinoma with an annual mortality of 22.1 per 100 000.[7] This compares with a world standardized rate of 100.2 for males from Nagasaki City, Japan, and 11.1 for males from Connecticut, in the United States, during the period 1973 to 1977. These figures reflect large regional variations. Coggan and Acheson, using age-standardized incidence rates per 100 000 per year, analyzed data from twenty countries for males and females.[8] They emphasized differences of more than twenty-fold between the highest rates in the world in Japan and the lowest recorded rates from Dakar, Senegal. In most countries, gastric cancer incidence has been steadily declining during the past 40 years. It is said to be the sixth most common cause of cancer death in the United States, with 24 000 new cases occurring in 1980. Although it still remains a problem in that country, the death rate has decreased from 30 per 100 000 in 1930 to 8 per 100 000 in 1980. This decline is steepest in older persons and in Caucasians. This unexplained decrease of highly lethal malignancy is particularly striking when considered in such countries as Japan (78 per 100 000) and Chile (70 per 100 000).

The fact that migrant populations from high-to-low incidence countries show a significant decrease in the occurrence of gastric cancer clearly suggests that its cause must be environmental. The first generation of migrants have higher risks of stomach cancer than do natives of the host countries. It might well be that the migrant population diet disappears as the groups are assimilated into their new culture.

One study in Norway suggested that gastric cancer was not declining in Norwegians over a 25 year period.[9] These authors, however, failed to take account of the 20% overall increase in population and the greater proportion of elderly people. This oversight illustrates how important it is when performing epidemiologic studies to standardize for age.

Despite very large international differences in the incidence of gastric cancer, the male to female ratio shows little geographic variation. Such a remarkably constant pattern, irrespective of absolute level of incidence, suggests that whatever the many factors responsible for the international variation may be, they affect men and women in a similar manner throughout the world. The sex ratio given for the Western world indicates the incidence of gastric cancer to be twice as high in men as in women.

The disease is seen most frequently between the ages of 50 and 70, with a peak age of about 60 for both sexes. Gastric cancer is rare under 30 years of age. Most observers suggest age-related differences in tumor behavior. In a study of 1778 gastric carcinomas, the percentage of diffuse carcinomas decreased with increasing age, while incidence of the intestinal type increased markedly up to 50 years (29.6%).[10] In those patients older than 70 years, the proportion was 61.5%. Since intestinal-type cancers occur more commonly in the antrum, gastric carcinoma limited to the antrum was seen much more frequently in those more than 70 years of age than in younger patients. However, the age-corrected 5 year survival rates did not differ between any of the four age groups studied. In a study of gastric cancer in the elderly (69 to 90 years), elderly patients had the same morbidity and mortality from surgery for gastric cancers as patients under 65 years of age.[11] The authors concluded that if aggressive preoperative and postoperative care can be given, gastric resection should not be withheld in the elderly purely on the grounds of age. Seven of eighteen patients were alive after 2 years, and 6 survived longer than 3 years (33%).

In studies in a small group of young patients (17 patients aged 40 years or less), the patients were divided into two groups according to the presence or absence of endocrine immunohistochemical markers for serotonin, gastrin, somatostatin, carcinoembryonic antigen (CEA), beta-hyman chorionic gonadotropin (β-HCG), and alphafetoprotein.[12] Those patients testing positive for endocrine markers survived longer (four of eight were alive at 25 to 56 months after diagnosis) than those in the nonendocrine group. However, the authors warned that their results must be interpreted with caution since the groups were small and the majority of the patients were Hispanic.

Two studies reinforced the clinical impression that tumors of the cardia are becoming more common. Patterson and colleagues studied all pathology reports of adenocarcinoma of the stomach or lower esophagus during the periods 1951 to 1955 and 1981 to 1985.[13] Analysis revealed that during the latter period there was an increase in carcinomas of the upper portion of the stomach to 39% in all cases, compared with 18% seen earlier. The main reduction was seen in carcinomas of the middle third or body of the stomach. Similarly, Meyers and associates studied 255 consecutive patients between 1953 and 1983 with 100% follow-up.[14] They found that carcinomas of the proximal esophagogastric junction and fundic areas have increased significantly over the last four decades from 21% to 44% and that this increase was accompanied by a significant decrease in antral carcinomas, from 60% to 30%. Interestingly, patients with antral carcinoma were significantly more likely to be black (64% vs 36%). These authors also noted that the overall survival rate did not change during the 30 years studied.

PREDISPOSING FACTORS

Certain conditions have been shown to be associated with an increased risk of malignancy. With the development of effective treatment and consequent increase in survival, the increased incidence of carcinoma in patients with pernicious anemia was noted in the 1950s.

The risk has now been quantified at being four to six times that of the general population.[15,16] Screening of patients with pernicious anemia has been undertaken and results of one study of 80 patients showed 33 cases of dysplasia, three of which were severe. The same study identified one early gastric carcinoma.[17]

The long-term effects of gastric surgery also have shown an increased risk of carcinoma in the remnant 15 or more years after gastrectomy for benign disease.[18] There is also evidence that gastric carcinoma increases after vagotomy and pyloroplasty.[19]

In the United States and Western Europe, stomach cancer is twice as frequent in the lower as in the higher socioeconomic groups. Increased stomach cancer rates have been associated with a number of occupational groups, including coal miners, farmers, pottery workers, rubber workers, and workers who process timber. Whether these occupations truly are associated with increased gastric cancer risk or whether they merely reflect the socioeconomic characteristics of these employees is not clear.[20] Familial occurrence of gastric cancer is rare, and the association between gastric cancer and blood group A is probably just a tenuous relationship.[21] The risk ratio for gastric cancer in persons with blood group A compared with blood group O, however, is only a modest 2:1. Also, in several large studies from the Scandinavian countries, it was found that there is no correlation between gastric cancer and blood group A.

The relationship between atrophic gastritis and gastric cancer has been postulated for many years.[22] It appears that atrophic gastritis is commonly associated with gastric malignancy. It does not follow, however, that atrophic gastritis is a precursor lesion to gastric carcinoma. In the older age group, in which gastric cancer occurs, approximately 80% to 95% of individuals exhibit some degree of atrophic gastritis. Thus, a larger percentage of older patients without stomach cancer have atrophic gastritis, making untenable the hypothesis that atrophic gastritis is a precursor of gastric cancer. Correa and his associates have studied subjects in the high-incidence region of Columbia for almost 20 years and report that the high incidence of precursor lesions, chronic atrophic gastritis, intestinal metaplasia, and dysplasia that are seen as sequential stages in the precancerous process, are strongly related to changes in gastric chemistry and rise linearly with pH, nitrate and nitrite values in the gastric juice.[23]

Many researchers have postulated that diet generally is deemed the main factor in gastric cancer etiology. A high-risk diet is one low in animal fat and animal proteins, high in complex carbohydrates, high in grains and tubers, low in salads and fresh green leafy vegetables, low in fresh fruits, especially citrus types, and, finally, high in salt.[24] There is certainly a high incidence in patients who smoke and drink alcohol. Forman and associates made the surprising discovery that there is no correlation between salivary nitrate and nitrite concentrations and the incidence of gastric cancer.[25] This study pointed out, however, that this relationship could be the result of an association between consumption of vitamin C, which is a nitrite scavenger of other protective factors in vegetables, and the consumption of nitrate. Also published were results showing that in Britain the risk of gastric cancer cannot be correlated with the nitrate content of the water supply in over 200 urban areas.[26] In an unpublished study on men producing nitrate fertilizers, and who thus were exposed to unusually large amounts of nitrates, their mortality from gastric cancer was almost identical to that of other men in the same part of Britain not exposed to similar high levels of nitrate. A case cohort from Hawaii of diet and stomach cancer confirmed the significantly protective value of fruits and vegetables.[27]

Infection with *Helicobacter pylori* has been linked with chronic atrophic gastritis, an inflammatory precursor of gastric adenocarcinoma.[28] A nested case-control study was used to study whether *H pylori* infection increases the risk of gastric carcinoma. From a cohort of 128 992 persons followed since the mid 1960s at a health maintenance organization, 186 patients with gastric carcinoma were selected as case patients and were matched according to age, sex and race with 186 control subjects without gastric carcinoma. Stored serum samples collected during the 1960s were tested for IgG antibodies to *H pylori* by enzyme-linked immunosorbent assay. Data on cigarette use, blood group, ulcer disease, and gastric surgery were obtained from questionnaires administered at enrollment. Tissue sections and pathology reports were reviewed to confirm the histologic results. The mean time between serum collection and the diagnosis of gastric carcinoma was 14.2 years. Of the 109 patients with confirmed gastric adenocarcinoma (excluding tumors of the gastroesophageal junction), 84% had been infected previously with *H pylori*, as compared with 61% of the matched control subjects (odds ratio, 3.6; confidence interval, 1.8 to 7.3). Tumors of the gastroesophageal junction were not linked to *H pylori* infection, nor were tumors in the gastric cardia. *H pylori* was a particularly strong risk factor for stomach cancer in women (odds ratio, 18) and blacks (odds ratio, 9). A history of gastric surgery was independently associated with the development of cancer (odds ratio, 17; $P=.03$), but a history of peptic ulcer disease was negatively associated with subsequent gastric carcinoma (odds ratio, 0.2; $P=.02$). Neither blood group nor smoking history affected risk. In conclusion, it was stated that infection with *H pylori* is associated with an increased risk of gastric adenocarcinoma and may be a co-factor in the pathogenesis of this malignant condition.

PREMALIGNANT CONDITIONS

A premalignant condition is a histologic change in healthy mucosa that places the mucosa at risk of malignancy. The changes within the stomach that are associated with malignancy are atrophic gastritis, intestinal metaplasia, dysplasia, and gastric polyps.

Gastritis has been classified as types A and B.[29] Type A, which is associated with pernicious anemia, involves the body and fundus and leaves the antral mucosa intact. It appears to be autoimmune in origin. Type B involves principally the antrum and appears to be environmental in origin. Both types are implicated in the development of gastric carcinoma of the intestinal type, but the much higher incidence of type B makes it numerically more important. The presence of intestinal metaplasia around or adjacent to gastric carcinomas has been recognized since the initial work by Morson.[30]

This has been shown to be true in both early and advanced lesions. Hypermetaplasia has been classified by the complement of small intestinal enzymes that can be demonstrated on the cells and by the type of mucin secreted.[31] The sulphomucin-secreting incomplete metaplasia is seen in association with gastric carcinoma and is regarded as the probable premalignant form. Dysplasia appears to be the common precursor of malignant change and is common to normal foveolar epithelium and intestinal metaplasia.

Gastric polyps already have been described and classified. Although the risk of malignant transformation is highest in adenomatous polyps (38%), hyperplastic polyps do carry a small risk.

Controversy exists concerning the association between gastric ulcer and malignancy.[32,33] Data from the United States support the hypothesis that gastric cancer commonly ulcerates but that benign gastric ulcers rarely, if ever, become cancers. The usual incidence given for gastric ulcers that become malignant is 3%, but in Japan it has been suggested that there is a much higher correlation between chronic gastric ulcer and cancer.[34] In general it appears that now, even in Japan, the risk of gastric cancers occurring in conjunction with gastric ulcer disease is small. Data was analyzed on 121 gastric ulcers diagnosed as benign on gastroscopic biopsy and cytologic evidence at the initial examination, and six years later, 78 patients were reexamined clinically and with multiple endoscopic biopsies. Gastric cancer had developed in only one, and this was not at the site of the previous gastric ulcer.

PROGNOSTIC FACTORS

Growth factors continue to be investigated. A tissue culture study showed expression of epidermal growth factor (EGF) and insulin-like growth factor-1 in gastric cancer cell lines, and both promoted cell growth in the cell-line cultures.[36] Gastrin further enhanced the stimulated growth produced by EGF and insulin-like growth factor-1. Overexpression and co-expression of EGF and EGF receptor identified a gastric cancer subgroup that was more deeply invasive; such expression may be used as a prognostic marker.[37]

The importance of the histopathological type of the tumor as a parameter for recurrence and for prognosis of gastric cancers has been pointed out in a study of 4 419 patients who underwent surgery in Aichi Cancer Center during 23 years, from 1965 to 1987.[38] Correlation of initial recurrence site and the histology of the tumor was examined by the categorical discriminate analysis in 617 patients. Among these patients, 62% of liver metastasis was caused by well-differentiated type of cancers (71% of peritoneal recurrence was poorly differentiated type of cancers). Cox's regression tree

type analysis was performed for 2 893 cases with curative gastrectomy, and the maximum difference in risk ratio was observed where the tumor microscopically penetrated the serosal layer of the stomach. Difference of the prognosis owing to histopathological type of the tumor appeared after correction of the S and N factors and, in the early stages, poorly differentiated type had better prognosis than well-differentiated type of cancers. In more advanced cases, well-differentiated type of tumors had a much better prognosis than poorly differentiated type of cancers. With these results, this study suggested that the consideration of histopathological type of the tumor should be implemented as an important parameter for the evaluation of prognosis of gastric cancers.

PATHOLOGY

When the term gastric cancer is used, it refers to adenocarcinomas of the stomach, which comprise 95% of the malignant tumor of this organ (Fig 31–7). Several factors have important clinical significance in the evaluation of the pathology of gastric cancers. The gross appearance, site, and degree of local invasion of the tumor all bear on prognosis, as do the histologic features. Fifty years ago, the German pathologist Bormann classified the macroscopic appearance into five types (Table 31–4).[39] The classic description of Bormann has been adapted by others.[40] Most authors have taken into account the shape of the tumor, extent of invasiveness, and degree of ulceration. The value of detailed descriptive macroscopic classifications, however, is limited to the small proportion (>8%[41]) of circumscribed polypoid tumor with a good prognosis. Size appears to be important when considering the prognosis; tumors <4 cm in maximum dimension are associated with a distinctly better prognosis.[42] One study showed that 80% of patients with carcinomas <2 cm in diameter survived for 5 years.[43] The macroscopic classification adopted by the Japanese Research Society for Gastric Cancer avoids needless descriptive verbosity.[44]

HISTOLOGICAL CLASSIFICATION

Attempts to categorize gastric carcinomas precisely on purely morphologic features are difficult because of their heterogeneous morphology. This difficulty no doubt results from their multifocal and polyclonal origin. Both Lauren and Mulligan proposed histogenetic systems of classification, with Lauren's system becoming the most widely accepted in the West.[45,46] A more detailed classification has been proposed by Jaas.[47] However, adenocarcinoma may be classified according to the degree of histologic differentiation. Although not an independent prognostic variable, this fact is important since the prognosis is worse in the

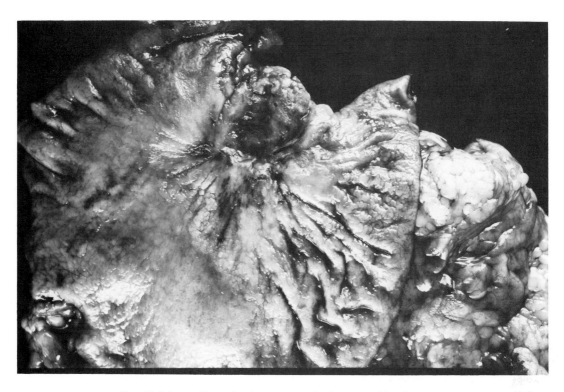

Figure 31–7. Large malignant ulcerating tumor occupying the antrum and the pylorus.

poorly differentiated lesions. Border's classification grades cells from grade I (well differentiated) to grade IV (anaplastic).

In Lauren's system, two categories are described: intestinal and diffuse. These correspond to the differentiated and undifferentiated categories used by other histopathologists. In high-incidence areas such as Finland, 50% to 60% of gastric carcinomas are of intestinal type, whereas in low-incidence areas, their proportion falls to <40%. Lauren regarded 14% of gastric carcinomas as unclassifiable into either category. There is no doubt that many tumors show both intestinal and diffuse features. Ming has described a functional classification, dividing gastric carcinomas into those with an expanding and those with an infiltrative growth pattern.[41] These also correspond closely with the intestinal and diffuse types, respectively. Lymphocytic infiltration of the stoma in and around the periphery of the tumor often is found in the intestinal type but not in diffuse adenocarcinoma. Intestinal metaplasia also is found in the adjacent mucosa in the majority of cases of the intestinal type of carcinoma.

There is some epidemiologic evidence suggesting that intestinal type of cancer of the stomach is related to environmental influences, while diffuse carcinoma occurs in a younger age group and is determined more by genetic predisposition.[48]

There is considerable disparity between the survival of patients with stomach cancer in Japanese and Western series. Although early diagnosis, a higher incidence of intestinal type of tumors, and the use of radical surgery in Japan may explain some of the difference, a major contributing factor may be the extensive and meticulous surgical and pathological staging of gastric cancer in Japan. Several reports from the United States, Japan and Europe have demonstrated the significant prognostic impact of advancing T stage (Fig 31–8). Table 31–5 sets out the AJCC staging of gastric cancer described in 1988. The Japanese Research Society for Gastric Cancer defines the primary tumor stage based on the depth of invasion and the presence and extent of serosal (S) invasion. The SO classification is further divided into M (mucosa), SM (submucosa) and PM (muscularis propria) components. The SS (subserosa) and S1 tumors were reclassified to further stratify the degree and type of serosal invasion. SS alpha is a subserosal tumor with expansive growth, SS beta is a subserosal tumor with intermediate growth and SS gamma is a subserosal tumor with infiltrating growth. S2 and S3 are now defined as se (cancer cells exposed to the peritoneal cavity), si (cancer cells infiltrating neighboring tissue), or sei (coexistence of se and si).

The Japanese staging system extensively classifies 18 lymph node regions into four N categories depending

TABLE 31–5. PHNS STAGING SYSTEM

P FACTOR
- P0   No evidence of peritoneal spread
- P1   Peritoneal spread limited to supracolic area; includes greater omentum, not diaphragm
- P2   Small numbers of nodules below mesocolon or diaphragm
- P3   Numerous nodules below mesocolon or on diaphragm

H FACTOR
- H0   No metastases to liver
- H1   Metastases limited to one lobe
- H2   Small number of metastases to both lobes
- H3   Many metastases to both lobes

N FACTOR
- N0   No lymph node involvement
- N1   Group 1 involvement
- N2   Group 2 involvement
- N3   Group 3 involvement
- N4   Extending beyond group 3

S FACTOR
- S0   No penetration to serosa
- S1   Minimal involvement of serosa
- S2   Obvious involvement of serosa
- S3   Obvious involvement of serosa and neighboring organs

TABLE 31–4. GROSS MORPHOLOGY OF GASTRIC CARCINOMAS

Type	Bormann, 1926	Morson and Dawson, 1979	Kajitani, 1971
I	Polypoid or fungating	Nodular	Localized
II	Ulcerated with elevated borders	Ulcerating	Intermediate
III	Ulcerated and infiltrating gastric wall	Fungating	
IV	Diffusely infiltrating	Linitis plastica Superficial	Infiltrative
V	Unclassifiable		

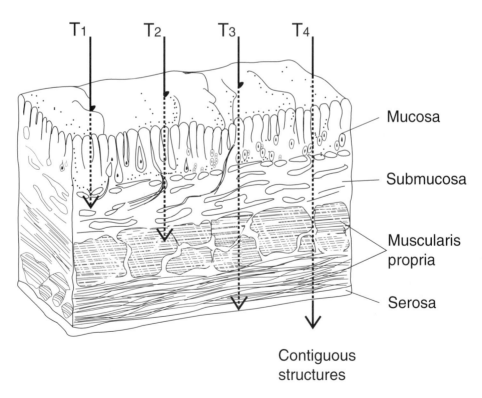

Figure 31–8. Definition of T stage based on depth of penetration of the gastric wall.

on their relation to the primary tumor and anatomic location. The careful and complete resection of the operative specimen often may be performed by the attending surgeon. Involvement with N1 and N2 lymph node groups represents regional disease, which is encompassed by en bloc resection of second echelon lymph nodes. N3 and N4 lymph nodes are considered distant metastases.

Descriptive Pathological Classification

This author favors the macroscopic classification adopted by the Japanese Research Society for Gastric Cancer as already described. Cancer of the stomach, however, still is classified as carcinoma in a polyp, proliferative type, sessile or ulcerating type, atrophic or leather-bottle type, and mucous carcinoma.

Squamous carcinoma of the stomach is rare. Callery and associates reported a study of four patients with a detailed analysis of histogenesis.[49] While some criticized classification of squamous lesions of the stomach as being mere extensions of carcinomas of the esophagus, there is little doubt that, in at least two of their cases, the tumor originated within the stomach from squamous metaplasia in damaged gastric epithelium. Mori and associates described three primary squamous tumors of the stomach with a detailed review of the histological features.[50]

Carcinoid of the stomach is more common, but only 2% of all carcinoid tumors arise in the stomach, compared with 70% in the appendix and 20% in the ileum and cecum.

It must be remembered that carcinoma of the stomach is not always a primary lesion. Walker and associates reported three patients in whom primary gastric carcinoma of the linitis plastica type was initially confidently diagnosed.[51] All three patients, however, had been treated for breast carcinoma and, in two of the patients, the disease was bilateral. A review of the original histopathology showed infiltrating nodular breast carcinoma of a similar type to that seen in the stomach. In one case the response to Tamoxifen was encouraging.

PATTERN OF SPREAD AND PROGNOSIS

The routes of spread for gastric carcinoma are similar to those for other gastrointestinal lesions. They include spread in the submucosa to adjacent organs via lymphatic channels, and transperitoneal and hematogenous spread.

The extension of an advanced tumor in a lateral direction is clearly not confined to early gastric cancers. Diffuse cancers may be expected to extend widely in the submucosa and individual cancer cells may be found several centimeters from the main tumor in an apparently healthy stomach. Cancers of the intestinal type appear to extend only a few millimeters from the main tu-

mor. Margins of a minimal clearance of 4 cm measured in situ are required for intestinal type of cancers and a minimum of 8 cm for diffuse cancers. It was suggested by Gall and Hermanek that improvements in prognosis of patients are partly owing to this approach.[52] Penetration of the cancer through the submucosa into deeper aspects of the stomach wall has long been known to be associated with altered prognosis. In most studies performed outside Japan, <5% of gastric cancers are limited to the mucosa and submucosa. The 5 year prognosis for early gastric cancer is in excess of 90% in Japanese reports but as low as 60% in some European reports.[53]

Regional lymph node invasion appears to be present in at least 60% of patients. The overall 5 year survival rate of approximately 50%, if local tumor infiltration is ignored, falls to approximately 20% if lymph nodes are involved. The prognosis is proportional to the number of nodes involved. Lymph node invasion is not, however, a totally independent variable. The incidence of lymph node invasion increases as the depth of the tumor penetration occurs. Furthermore, lymph node invasion is more prevalent in carcinomas that arise from the proximal third of the stomach compared with those arising from the distal third.

As might be expected, patients with hepatic metastases have a short survival rate. The Japanese Research Society for Gastric Cancer has related the degree of hepatic involvement as follows: H1, metastases confined to one lobe; H2, two or three metastases in right and left lobes; H3, many metastases in both lobes. Okuyama and associates reported that 95% of patients with hepatic metastases will die within 12 months if the primary tumor remains unresected.[54] In this study, no further improvement in survival was seen in patients in whom gastrectomy alone was performed, although an improved prognosis was found in those patients with resection of the primary tumor and resection of liver metastases or hepatic arterial chemotherapy or both.

When cancer has reached the peritoneal surface of the stomach, malignant cells may be freely released into the general peritoneal cavity and give rise both to peritoneal deposits and to tumors in the pelvis. The pelvic peritoneum may become studded with growth or large masses may form there because of cells gravitating downward. Ovarian Krukenberg tumors may be mistaken for primary growths of the ovaries. In every case of malignant disease or cysts of the ovaries, the stomach should be examined carefully at exploratory operation for any evidence of primary growth.

DNA PLOIDY PATTERNS OF GASTRIC CARCINOMA

Gastric mucosa is normally composed of predominantly diploid cells. In cancer, four patterns are recognized: (1) diploid mode, 68%; (2) heteroploid mode, 15%;

(3) diploid and heteroploid modes, 13%; and (4) mosaic of several heteroploid modes, 4%. Both early and advanced cancers can be shown to contain polyploid cells, particularly as the cancer reaches an advanced state. Diffuse cancers and well-differentiated intestinal type carcinomas are mainly unimodal, either diploid or heteroploid.[55] However, poorly differentiated cancers can be mosaic types. The polyploid nature of these tumors reflects their inability to form a normal structural pattern.

In 125 gastric carcinomas, the nuclear DNA content was determined by flow cytology from Formalin-fixed and paraffin-inverted tissues of surgical specimens.[56] The carcinomas were of intestinal mixed type (n=85) and diffuse type (n=40). DNA-aneuploidy was found in 46% of the intestinal type and in 42% of the mixed type, but only in 15% of the diffuse type carcinomas (P<.01). The total rate of DNA-aneuploidy was 34%. Carcinomas localized in the cardia were more frequently DNA-aneuploid than tumors in other locations (P<.01). DNA-aneuploid carcinomas had metastasized more frequently to regional lymph nodes (P<.05), whereas no correlations with tumor stage and cytological/histological grade were detected. In 94 patients, follow-up data were available. DNA-aneuploidy was associated with a statistically significant poorer prognosis when compared with DNA-diploid tumors only in advanced gastric carcinomas with lymph node metastases (P=.0488), and in the subgroup of advanced intestinal and mixed-type tumors (P=.0289).

STAGING

As more sophisticated combined-modality approaches have been utilized in the treatment of gastric cancer, staging has become more important. Staging ideally should involve all independent prognostic variables. To date, most of the proposed staging schemes have dealt only with pathologic features of the resected specimen and the spread of the tumor found at surgery. The host response, as yet, has not been fully taken into account.

Two basic staging schemes have been developed. American and European studies have extended the TNM Scheme outlined initially by Kennedy in 1970.[57] Four grades of tumor penetration were identified, T1 through T4. Perigastric lymph node invasion in the immediate vicinity of the primary tumor was graded as N1. N2 describes those tumors in which perigastric nodes were involved at a distance from the primary tumor. Metastatic disease was defined as absent M0 or absent M1. A revision of the TNM System was promulgated by the American Joint Committee for Cancer Staging in 1977.[58] T1 classification was confined to mucosal and submucosal lesions, T2 involved muscle coats as far as the subserosa, T3 the serosa, and T4 spread to involve contiguous structures. Nodal involvement was classified

more precisely in terms of distance from the primary tumor and introduced the N3 grade to take account of groups of nodes involved around the aorta, retropancreatic, hepatoduodenal, and mesenteric regions. Account also was taken of residual tumor (R classification), in which R0 indicated no residual tumor after surgical excision, R1 microscopic evidence of residual tumor after surgery, and R2 macroscopic evidence of residual tumor.

The Japanese Research Society for Gastric Cancer has approached cancer staging in an alternative way.[44] Four factors are used, namely, the grade of peritoneal dissemination (P factor), the presence of hepatic metastases (H factor), lymph node involvement (N factor), and serosal invasion (S factor). These grades are similar in structure to the TNM grades of severity. Under the PHNS Staging System, parametric analysis has shown that the most important factor in determining the prognosis is the S factor, which is clearly related to the depth of cancer penetration into the stomach wall (Table 31–5).

At a meeting of the World Health Organization on Gastric Cancer held in Munich in September, 1993, a classification revolving around R for residual tumors was suggested by Maruyama.[59] He suggested that the lymph node status be designated D. Thus, there would be R0, R1 and R2 ± D0, D1, and D2.

CLINICAL MANIFESTATIONS

The clinical features depend on the length of history, age of the patient, and situation, extent, and type of growth. In its earliest stage, cancer of the stomach gives rise to few constitutional disturbances. Those tumors situated at the inlet or outlet of the stomach are associated with mild dyspeptic symptoms before producing symptoms of obstruction. Growths occurring in the body of the stomach may be clinically silent until the end, or may produce vague symptoms such as anorexia or epigastric discomfort.

The most common symptoms in patients with cancer of the stomach are epigastric pain and indigestion, anorexia, weigh less, vomiting or hematemesis, melena, dysphagia, abdominal mass, diarrhea, and steatorrhea. There are no pathognomonic symptoms of early cancer of the stomach, and the so-called classic clinical manifestations are usually those of an advanced tumor. The vagueness of the early symptoms is one of the reasons for late diagnosis. Three common clinical types, however, are recognized: insidious, obstructive, and gastric ulcer.

Insidious Type

This tumor is the most difficult type to diagnose because of the vagueness of the initial symptoms. This vagueness is chiefly a result of the position of the growth in the body of the stomach and because there is little or no interference with gastric function in the early stages. However, hematemesis or melena, which can be quite dramatic, and acute perforation can occur. The early symptoms in these insidious types include epigastric pain or discomfort, anorexia, nausea, weight loss, and anemia.

Obstructive Type

Symptoms in this type vary according to whether the growth is situated at the cardia or at the pylorus. Features common to both types are associated with obstruction. If the growth occurs at or near the esophagogastric junction, the patient usually complains of increasing dysphagia, first with solid foods and later with fluids. Weight loss is excessively rapid once growth encroaches on the narrow inlet of the stomach. When the pyloric region is the seat of cancer, the late symptoms are those of pyloric stenosis. It is often impossible to determine by the symptoms alone whether obstruction is owing to growth or to ulcer. The early symptoms of this type often mimic those of peptic ulceration.

Peptic Ulcer Type

Approximately one-third of patients with cancer of the stomach present with a history of peptic ulcer that has existed for some years before the discovery of the malignant tumor. Some of these patients are treated primarily by medical measures for chronic gastric ulcers.

None of the symptoms discussed unequivocally indicate gastric cancer. Unless the clinician is aware of the possibility, it is possible that the patient will be treated empirically for ulcer disease or not treated at all. In advanced tumors, the major presenting finding can be a palpable mass, ascites, metastases to superficial nodes, or jaundice. By the time physical signs of gastric cancer are present, patients are incurable.

INVESTIGATION

The importance of early recognition of cancer to the stomach cannot be overemphasized. Early detection is dependent on a high index of suspicion on the part of the general population as well as the doctor. Simple routine blood tests are likely to give normal results in patients with early cancer of the stomach. The erythrocyte sedimentation rate (ESR) is nonspecific and, even if elevated, is only a vague clue suggesting need for further investigation.

The accepted sequence of diagnostic procedures in suspected gastric cancer is as follows:

1. Careful physical examination for pathologic findings amenable to biopsy, such as palpable lymph nodes or liver
2. Upper gastrointestinal tract radiologic studies with double contrast to establish the site of abnormality within the stomach (Fig 31–9)
3. Endoscopy with biopsy and cytology
4. Diagnostic laparoscopy
5. Diagnostic and/or therapeutic laparotomy

Other procedures that may be of ancillary use include computed tomography (CT) scanning, ultrasonography, tumor markers, endoscopic ultrasonography (EUS), and magnetic resonance imaging (MRI).

There has been great debate as to which of the two main diagnostic tools, that is, barium-meal examination and gastroscopy, is superior. The two methods of examination are, in fact, complementary. In Western countries, panendoscopy has been considered to give far better diagnostic yields. Some Western endoscopists have presented extreme arguments that radiology is unnecessary, but such arguments have not been substantiated by a strict comparison of x-ray examination and endoscopy.[60] The advantage of endoscopy is the obtaining of tissue biopsy or exfoliative cytology. If the tumor mass is exophytic, endoscopy is usually successful in establishing a tissue diagnosis. In 24 of 26 such patients (92%), Winawer and associates obtained positive biopsy or cytologic brush pathology.[61] In 24 patients with infiltrative gastric cancer, however, the diagnosis was made in only 50%. Other factors mitigating against the success of endoscopic biopsy include tumors <3 cm in diameter, location at the cardia or on the lesser curve,

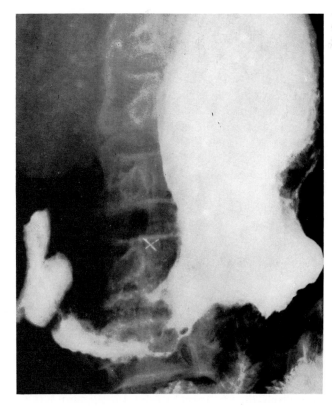

Figure 31–9. Carcinoma of the antrum of the stomach.

and recurrent tumors. In such unfavorable situations, lavage cytology may increase the accuracy of brush cytology or biopsy.

The predictability of whether a gastric cancer is resectable before laparotomy is still a difficult task. Tiller and associates evaluated CT scanning in 40 patients with fairly advanced gastric carcinoma and found 72.5% accuracy in correct staging and 80% accuracy in correct estimation of resectability.[62] Despite these results, exploratory laparotomy wisely was considered essential for evaluation of the operability of the gastric carcinoma. Laparotomy could have been avoided in patients with proximal gastric cancer only with clear CT demonstration of organ infiltration, locally, or large lymph node metastases. Cook and colleagues studied 37 patients who underwent preoperative CT scanning, as well as operative evaluation of their tumors.[63] Nineteen patients (51%) were found to have more extensive disease than predicted, and of six patients predicted to have widespread disease by CT scanning, three were found at operation to have the disease confined to the stomach or regional lymph nodes. Therefore, a significant percentage of patients whose disease was thought to be unresectable on scanning, in fact had potentially resectable lesions.

Hopes of better methods for predicting surgical outcome come from EUS. Heyder and Lux claim accurate assessment of the depth of penetration of the tumor i00n the esophagus and stomach,[64] and Yasuda and associates reported that submucosal tumors are easily detected even if the deposit is <5 mm.[65] Aibe and his associates have used enhancement of the ultrasonic image by a 10% oil-in-water type emulsion and have warned that although enlargement of lymph nodes can be detected, histological examination of the removed enlarged lymph nodes does not always confirm that the enlargement is the result of To cancer.

MRI of a diffusely infiltrating gastric carcinoma has been reported by Winkler and colleagues,[67] but lack of widespread availability of such machines may limit its usefulness, initially. Furthermore, no clear-cut results are available to suggest whether this technique will provide accurate prediction of resectability.

TUMOR MARKERS AND ONCOGENES

Heptner and associates emphasized the importance of monoclonal antibodies to the neoantigens CA 19-9, CA 50, CA 12-5, as well as the existing spectrum of oncofetal antigens.[68] Although monoclonal antibodies are useful research tools, most of them are not sensitive enough to be used in vivo for the detection of gastric carcinoma. Janssen and associates recommended measuring preoperatively the ESR, serum IgG, complement 4 (C4) fraction, C1 inhibitor (C1 INH), and CEA.[69] Discriminant analysis predicted presence or absence of metastases in 75% of cases, and preoperative prediction of nonsurvival reached 94% during follow-up.[38] The expression of blood group-related antigens A, B, H type 2, Lewis type 1 (Lewis(a) [Le(a)] and Lewis(b) [Le(b)], Lewis type 2 (Lewis(x) [Le(x)] and Lewis(y) [Le(y)]), syalyated Le(a) (CA 19-9), and sialyated Le(x) (CSLEX1), was analyzed sequentially, with immunohistochemical methods, in early gastric cancer, intestinal metaplasia, and uninvolved gastric mucosa obtained from 35 surgical specimens of patients who underwent gastrectomy. The high incidence of the inappropriate expression of Lewis type 1 antigens and the deletion of H and Lewis type 2 antigens was observed similarly in patients with cancer and intestinal metaplasia. The acquisition of CA 19-9 and CSLEX1 and the deletion of B antigen frequently were found in intestinal type of cancer and in all types of intestinal metaplasia. The simultaneous deletion of A antigen was detected only in the combination of intestinal type of cancer and incomplete-type intestinal metaplasia. Thus, this study showed that similar changes of tissue antigenicities exist in early gastric cancer and intestinal metaplasia.

One study compared CEA with CA 19-9 for the detection of local recurrences and distal metastases after complete resection of gastric carcinoma.[70] The aim of this study was to compare carcinoembryonic antigen (CEA) with CA 19-9 for the detection of local recurrences and distant metastases after complete resection of gastric carcinoma. At least one postoperative measurement of CEA and CA 19-9 was performed in 54 patients. Among these, 32 had recurrence (59%) with median follow up of 618 days.

Significantly higher sensitivity was observed for CA 19-9 in comparison with CEA (68.8% vs 38.2%, respectively). Increased CEA plasma level never preceded the diagnosis of recurrence, while increasing CA 19-9 preceded diagnosis in 13 patients (40.6%) from 1 to 22 months (median=4.5 months). Increasing the normal range of CA 19-9 to 80 UI/mL ($2.5 \times N$) raises the specificity to 100% compared with acceptable sensitivity (53.1%). This study shows that CA 19-9, compared with CEA, allows diagnosis of recurrence more often and earlier in the follow up of resected gastric cancer.

Intracellular estradiol (E_2) has been found in 44% of 52 male patients and in 20% of 34 female patients with gastric carcinoma.[71] These findings suggest that hormonal factors may be involved. Hormonal therapy with tamoxifen has been tried with conflicting results. Wu and associates showed that estrogen receptors (ER) were present in 50% of cases of Chinese patients with gastric cancers. More recently, they found the amplification of c-erbB-2 oncogene. Its over-expression correlated with the advancement of lung, ovarian, breast, and gastric cancers. In addition, estrogen has been found to inhibit the expression of c-erbB-2 through ER in breast cancer cell lines. A hypothesis is that the same event may occur in ER-positive gastric cancer cell. Thus, patients with gastric cancers whose tumors are positive for both ER and c-erbB-2 gene expression may benefit from estrogen therapy rather than tamoxifen therapy. Oncogene expression is increasingly recognized in human cancer. This work is at a very early stage and is not of use in the clinical situation at the present time.

Lemoine and associates demonstrated the abnormal expression of c-erbB-2 proto-oncogene and EGF receptor in a significant number of retrospectively studied, formalin-fixed, paraffin-embedded specimens of gastric cancer.[73] They suggested that their technique could be used to analyze archive material for which survival data were available, and that it may prove to be a more accurate determinant to prognosis than conventional tissue typing. Some proof of their hypothesis was provided when Yonemura and his associates examined tissue obtained from 260 cancers.[74] Expression of erbB-2 protein correlated with serosal invasion, lymphatic, and lymph node invasion with a significantly worse prognosis. They claimed to show that erbB-2 protein expression is an important independent prognostic indicator. A smaller study by revealed expression of erbB-2 in none of twenty early cancers, 5.8% of advanced cancers, and 25% of metastatic gastric cancers, thereby suggesting that oncogene alterations occur late, during the stage of tumor progression metastases.[75] Ranzini and associates came to the same conclusions in their report from Italy of a study of gene expression in 50 gastric cancer patients.[76] Protooncogene expression was absent from precursor lesions such as chronic active gastritis and from all early gastric cancers. It was present only in advanced or metastatic tumors.

Twenty-four Japanese patients with alpha-feta protein-screening gastric cancer were followed for 10 to 14 years.[77] These patients had a dismal prognosis, which was significantly worse then expected from the state of the disease. Most patients died from the early development of liver metastases. The recurrence of this type of gastric cancer is high in the United States (15%) but lower in Japan (5%), which may contribute, in part, to the worse results obtained by surgical resection in the United States.

SCREENING

Because of the extent of the gastric cancer problem in some countries, there has been interest in developing techniques of screening for detection of early lesions. This approach has been the most highly developed in Japan. The Japanese have demonstrated the value of mass surveys for gastric carcinoma in their particular population. The use of mass upper gastrointestinal sur-

veys and the gastrocamera has made possible earlier detection of lesions than is possible with the usual methods in the rest of the world. The aim of screening programs is to decrease mortality, and the Japanese have succeeded in doing this. Screening procedures in Japan have increased the yield of lesions confined to the mucosa or submucosa from 3.8% in 1955 to 34.5% in 1966, with a corresponding survival rate of 90.9%.[78] The Japanese mass screening program has shown that early diagnosis is possible. However, mass screening would not be cost-effective in areas with a lower incidence of gastric cancer. Therefore, the identification and screening of high-risk groups must be developed.

SURGICAL MANAGEMENT

Since the stomach is not vital to a relatively normal life span, the surgical procedure can involve anything up to and including a total gastrectomy, removal of the omentum, removal of the spleen, removal of the distal portion of the esophagus, removal of the proximal portion of the duodenum, and even simultaneous removal of a portion of the transverse colon. Lesser resections of the stomach are anatomically, surgically, and oncologically possible, and the extent of resection can be determined partly by the extent of the lesion and partly by knowledge of its usual pathways of extension.

Surgery provides the only possibility of a cure. Preoperative proof of diagnosis and staging should be carried out, but laparotomy should be seen as the essential prerequisite to rational decisions regarding resectability. Before resection, operative staging should be undertaken. This staging demands an assessment of the extent of tumor, depth of invasion, extent of lymph node involvement, presence and extent of peritoneal deposits, and presence of hepatic metastases. Curative resection should be attempted only on tumors limited to the stomach and neighboring lymph nodes, although the presence of fixity to surrounding structures does not preclude a resection, if these structures can be removed en bloc with the primary tumor. A lesion in the distal two-thirds of the stomach requires a subtotal gastrectomy with en bloc removal of the spleen and omentum. The pancreatic tail should not be resected unless it or the retropancreatic nodes are involved. A 5cm clearance of the tumor is required in all resections, and frozen-section histology should be used.

Many experts have now agreed that radical surgery can be performed with preservation of the pancreas and spleen. This approach reduces the morbidity while still removing as many lymph nodes as when en bloc resection is performed.

Pathologic staging is an essential part of the operative strategy. This approach demands that a histologic definition of the state of the resection lines, the depth of invasion, and the extent of lymphatic involvement is available for all resected cases. The Japanese experience would suggest that an R1 resection with removal of the N1 and N2 nodes is a desirable approach, but it may be that the more radical R2/R3 procedures would improve prognosis.

Keighley and associates have related patient survival to preaortic or hepatic hilar node involvement.[79] Median survival when these nodes were involved and apparently resected was 4.5 months, which is only marginally longer than that of patients having a palliative resection without extensive lymphadenectomy. They also address the question of how often N4 nodes (preaortic nodes) are involved. They have suggested that aggressive surgery is not worthwhile in patients with positive N4 nodes. However, Scott and associates stated that radical surgery with lymphatic node dissection of the hepatoceliac glands can be a worthwhile endeavor in gastric carcinoma.[80] They have an operative mortality rate of 9.6%, with an average survival rate of 2.87 years and a 5 year survival rate of 16%.

The importance of the resection-line clearance in stomach cancer has been emphasized in a prospective multicenter study from the British Stomach Cancer Group.[81] Of 390 patients with resected gastric cancers, 85 (22%) had disease at the resection margin, 32 at the esophagus, 20 at the gastric margin, and 17 at the duodenum. Six patients had microscopic disease at both incision margins. When resection margin clearance was achieved, a significantly increased overall survival was found. Their study emphasized that microscopic disease of the resection line influenced long-term survival and that surgeons must ensure that resection lines are clear.

Surgical results for early gastric cancer from a general hospital in Japan have been reported by Abe and associates.[82] The surgeons involved in this study were nonspecialists, and the aim of their paper was to examine whether the 5 year survival of 90% attainable in specialist centers in Japan was actually being attained in district general hospitals. This survival rate, in fact, proved possible. Only seven total gastrectomies were performed in 140 patients.

Palliative procedures should not be overlooked. Gastric lavage is indicated in cases of pyloric obstruction, not only to decompress the stomach but also to relieve pain and colicky spasms and to improve the general condition of the patient. If the tumor is nonresectable at laparotomy, it may be possible to perform a gastrojejunostomy or exclusion gastrectomy. Occasionally, in the elderly, a jejunostomy would be the only procedure possible. Newer palliative procedures, such as laser resection of inoperable gastric lesions at the esophagogastric junction or pylorus, may be beneficial in alleviating obstruction. Intubation of the gastric carcinoma is very rarely indicated and gives poor palliation.

The aim of curative surgery in gastric cancer is the complete removal of all tumor bulk, both macroscopically and microscopically (RO resection).[83] The operative strategy should consider the location of the tumor, its histological character (Lauren classification), and the stage of disease according to the TNM classification. Lymphadenectomy of compartments I and II does not increase operative morbidity and mortality if performed routinely, but seems to increase long-term survival in patients with stages II and IIIa disease. Routine removal of the spleen does not lead to better results. Gastrectomy in locally advanced gastric cancer with combined resection of adjacent organs can prolong survival in the absence of peritoneal disseminating or distant metastases if RO resection is achieved. The indication for gastrectomy of patients with an incurable stage of disease (peritoneal dissemination, distant metastases) should be determined after considering the individual status of the patient and the surgical risk involved. In such cases, gastrectomy can be performed as a so-called ultima ratio resection with the aim of palliation.

Laparoscopic assessment may be the best way forward for determining operability and staging. Ultrasonography of the liver can be performed laparoscopically at this staging procedure.

RADIATION THERAPY

Radiation alone has been shown to have curative potential in a very small percentage of patients with resected but residual or unresectable localized disease. Its greatest benefit is achieved when used in combination with chemotherapy.[84] In some centers, intraoperative radiotherapy for gastric cancer has been used.

CHEMOTHERAPY

Although surgery is the only documented curative treatment for gastric cancer, chemotherapy in this disease may be of great benefit, with response rates of between 40% and 50% being recorded with combination chemotherapy. Schein has analyzed this difficult field, which included studies with 5-fluorouracil, Adriamycin (doxorubicin), and mitomycin C (FAM) used as outpatient treatment.[85] Twenty-six of 62 patients (42%) with advanced and accessible gastric cancer had a partial remission. The overall median duration of response was 9.5 months, but the median survival of patients who responded was 14 months, with 6 of 26 alive for >2 years. Median survival of patients who failed to respond was 3.5 months from the start of treatment. Trials were carried out using FAM with cisplatin at the Mayo Clinic.[5] In this trial, 17 patients with advanced disease were treated and a response rate of 53% was obtained. This response rate included 18% in which a complete response was described. Randall and associates pointed out the dangers of gastrointestinal hemorrhage and perforations during chemotherapy.[86] They emphasized that early operative intervention is essential for reduction of morbidity and mortality, and reported four cases in which delay in diagnosis and surgery resulted in three deaths.

Prediction of sensitivity to chemotherapy is an attractive aim, and Maehara and associates reported on the succinate dehydrogenase inhibition test in vitro using six different antitumor drugs against gastric carcinoma tissues obtained at the time of surgery.[87] A decrease in enzyme activity <50% of control cells in tissue culture, and an exposure of 3 days, was taken as a partial response. They found that 63% of poorly differentiated gastric adenocarcinomas were sensitive to >3 antitumor drugs but that the sensitivity was only 19% in well-differentiated tissues.

At the present time, there is no evidence that adjuvant cytotoxic chemotherapy improves survival for patients with carcinoma of the stomach. There may be a place for combination radiotherapy and chemotherapy following surgical resection. Most gastric carcinomas that recur after surgery do so within an area that may be encompassed by radiation fields of the gastric bed; thus, locoregional failures might be reduced by this approach. Preliminary studies indicate that radiotherapy and cytotoxic chemotherapy may be combined in this situation without undue toxicity. Use of intraperitoneal chemotherapy in the adjuvant setting may well have a place for those patients whose tumor has penetrated the serosa. It also would seem to be effective in patients with small peritoneal deposits.

A randomized trial of adjuvant chemotherapy versus placebo in operable stomach cancer recruited 249 patients from the West Midlands region of Great Britain between 1976 and 1980.[88] A cancer registry survey identified a further 1261 suitable concurrent cases. Trial patients were compared with the 960 nontrial cases from participating districts. Only 493 (51%) nontrial cases passed all of the prospective trial selection criteria for entry. Stage and fitness caused the majority of exclusions and were also highly prognostic. A univariate analysis comparing eligible patients within the trial showed the two groups to be balanced for the significant independent prognostic factors of the trial. However, differences in patient age and the surgery performed indicate that recruitment may have been influenced by unknown selection factors. This survey highlights the difficulty of retrospective selection and confirms the need for randomized controls. Data available from specialist registries may be used to help develop new protocols and to verify and extend trial results.

In our own unit and at the Royal Marsden hospital, pilot studies on chemotherapy using epirubicin, cis-platin and 5-fluorouracil, the latter given by continuous intravenous infusion daily, showed definite response with some complete responders.[89] Epirubicin 50 mg/m^2 is given three times weekly by bolus intravenous injection. Cisplatin 16 mg/m^2 intravenously in 1L of normal saline with 20 mmol KCL and 10 mmol of magnesium sulphate is infused over four hours together with Manitol 20% 100 mL. 5-fluorouracil 20 mg/m^2 over 24 hours by continuous intravenous infusion daily by Hickman line is commenced four hours before the first course of cisplatin.

■ SARCOMA OF THE STOMACH

Malignant mesenchymal tumors comprise 1% to 3% of all malignant lesions of the stomach. The extranodal variety of gastric lymphoma is probably the most common, followed by the benign and malignant smooth muscle cell tumors. Other types of sarcomatous lesions of the stomach seldom are seen and tend to be clinical curiosities. These include fibrosarcoma, angiosarcoma, and hemangiopericytoma. Neurofibrosarcomas are not mesenchymal tumors, since they arise from neuroectoderm. However, they also occur in the stomach.

An association has been shown between colonization of gastric mucosa by *H pylori*, acquisition of mucosa-associated lymphoid tissue (MALT) and an occurrence of primary B-cell gastric MALT lymphoma. Hussell and associates investigated the immunological response of cells from three low-grade primary B-cell multiple lymphomas to *H pylori*-type NCTC 11637 and 12 isolates of *H pylori* from patients without lymphomas.[90] After co-culture of tumor cells with bacteria, cells were examined for phenotypic evidence of activation and proliferation, and were supernatantly assayed to detect tumor-derived immunoglobulin and interleukin-2 (IL-2). Neoplastic B cells and nonneoplastic T cells proliferated, and IL-2 receptor expression by most cells in the cultures was increased with stimulating strains of *H pylori*. There were also increases in tumor immunoglobulin and IL-2 release when activation and proliferation were seen in response to stimulating bacteria. Removal of T cells from the tumor-cell suspension reduced proliferation and IL-2 receptor expression. In comparison, no responses were seen in cells from high-grade gastric MALT lymphomas or low-grade B-cell gastric MALT lymphomas of other sites. The response of low-grade B-cell MALT lymphomas to stimulating strains of *H pylori* is dependent on *H pylori*-specific T cells and their products, rather than on the bacteria themselves.

Certain features of primary low-grade B-cell gastric lymphoma of MALT suggest that the tumor is antigen responsive. Given the close association between gastric MALT lymphoma and *H pylori*, these organisms might be evoking the immunological response, and eradication of *H pylori* might inhibit the tumor. In six patients in whom biopsies showed histologic and molecular genetic evidence of low-grade gastric B-cell MALT lymphoma with *H pylori*, it was eradicated in five, with repeated biopsies showing no evidence of lymphoma. These results suggest that eradication of *H pylori* causes regression of low-grade B-cell gastric MALT lymphoma, and that anti-*H pylori* treatment should be given for this lymphoma.[91]

LYMPHOID TUMORS OF THE STOMACH

Lymphomatous tumors of the stomach are most commonly found in association with systemic malignant lymphoma. In 1961, Dawson and associates laid down the minimum criteria for acceptance of a gastric lymphoma as a primary neoplasm.[20] These criteria are as follows:

1. There is no palpable superficial lymphadenopathy at presentation.
2. No enlargement of mediastinal nodes is disclosed on chest x-ray examination.
3. The white cell count is normal.
4. At laparotomy, the bowel lesion predominates, the only obviously affected lymph nodes are those immediately related.
5. The liver and spleen appear free of tumor.

Since then, a stricter definition of a primary gastric lymphoma should include a normal mediastinal CT scan and normal bone marrow examination.

In systemic lymphoma, it is difficult to compare accurately the incidence of primary gastric lymphoma with that of secondary involvement of the stomach, since different series use different criteria for the diagnosis. Gastrointestinal lymphomatous involvement in systemic lymphoma may be as high as 32% of cases and even up to 43% at postmortem examination.[92] In comparison, the same authors found that primary gastrointestinal lymphoma accounted for only 9% of all cases of lymphoma.

In view of the difficulty in distinguishing primary from secondary gastric lymphoma, as well as terminologic differences and diagnostic difficulties, it is impossible to determine the true incidence of gastric lymphoma in the world. Everyone agrees that it is much less common than gastric carcinoma. The incidence of primary gastric lymphoma, when compared with that of primary gut lymphomas in general, reveals that the stomach is the most favored site. With regard to the distribution of lymphoma within the stomach, most authors agree that the pyloric antrum is the most common site, followed by the body, and then the cardia.[93] Some authors, however, have found a higher incidence in the body than in the antrum.[94]

Differential Diagnosis

Two conditions can be mistaken for lymphoma of the stomach. They are lymphoid hyperplasia and systemic lymphoma.

Characteristics

Rosenberg and associates found a male-to-female ratio of 1.7:1. When lymphomas of all portions of the gastrointestinal tract are considered, there is no sex predominance.[95] They also reported that of 1269 patients with primary lymphoma of all sites, only 21 were black. Lymphomas of the stomach are found in all age groups.

Pathology

Macroscopically, by the time the lesions are discovered, most are ≥10 cm, in 50% of patients (Fig 31–10). They tend to spread within the submucosal planes, sparing the muscular coat until late in the course. About 25% of patients have more than one focus of lymphoma in the stomach. Between one-third and one-half of patients have been reported to have mucosal ulceration, and the mucosal rugae may be hypertrophic, with deep ulceration. None of the gross characteristics of lymphoma are pathognomonic of this particular lesion, and it may be confused with carcinoma of the stomach.

Histopathologic Classification

The Kiel classification is probably based on a more accurate understanding of normal lymphocytic maturation than any of the other classifications currently in use (Table 31–6). One criticism of this classification is that it does not readily accommodate some of the more recently recognized variants of T-cell lymphomas, but neither does any other classification.

The whole field of non-Hodgkin's lymphoma is in a rapid state of flux as new immunologic markers become available for T and B cells and their precursors, for histocytes, and for other lymphoid-related cells such as dendritic and interdigitating reticulum cells. Most authorities believe that the majority of non-Hodgkin's lymphomas are of B-cell origin. This fact is well established for nodal lymphomas, but accurate immunohistochemical labeling and gene rearrangement studies still require fresh unfixed tissue. There have been few such studies on gastric and other gut lymphomas for a categorical statement on the proportion of T- and B-cell tumors originating there.[96]

Immunoblastic Lymphoma

This high-grade lymphoma is typically found in adults. A characteristic feature is its diffuse patterns of infiltration, with extensive surface ulceration and destructive invasion of the muscularis propria, often over a broad front with a relatively well-defined advancing margin. This destructive invasion of muscularis propria leads to

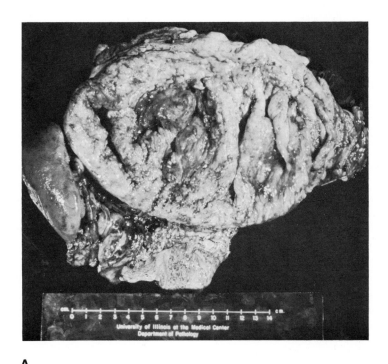

A

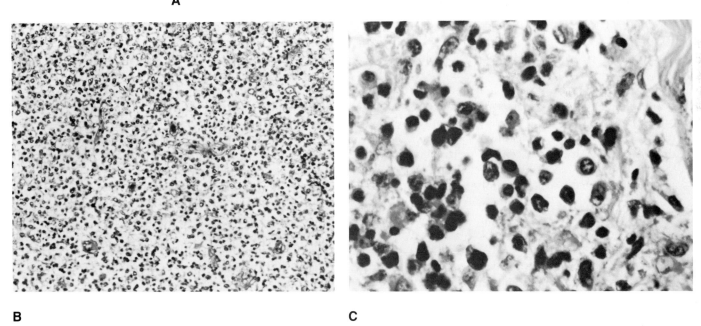

B   **C**

Figure 31–10. A. Gross specimen of lymphoma of stomach with submucosal infiltration and a nodular-appearing area of mucosa. Uninvolved spleen seen in the right upper corner of the picture. Low-power (**B**) and high-power (**C**) magnification. **C**. Atypical lymphoid cells with hyperchromatism, disorderly arrangement, and occasional notching; some muscle fibers can be seen in the right upper corner.

TABLE 31–6. SIMPLIFIED KIEL CLASSIFICATION OF NON-HODGKIN'S LYMPHOMAS

Low-grade	High-grade
Lymphocytic	Centroblastic
Lymphoplasmacytoid	Immunoblastic (including plasmacytoid differentiation)
Plasmacytoma (extra-medullary)	Lymphoblastic: B type (Burkitt) T type (convoluted)
Centrocytic	Other
Centroblastic/centrocytic (follicular and/or diffuse)	Tumors of uncertain histogenesis

fissuring ulceration, which almost certainly accounts for the high incidence of perforation. The tumor masses may be multiple but are always sharply circumscribed. Lymph node metastases are common in this form of lymphoma and produce discrete foci of tumor in the nodes in a similar manner to carcinomatous deposits. The depth of invasion into the stomach wall and the presence of lymph node metastases are prognostic factors.

Centrocytic Lymphoma

This type of lymphoma was described by Lennert in 1981[97] and accounted for approximately 20% of the total number of gastric lymphomas.[98] As with most of the subtypes of lymphomas, it is a tumor of adults. It may be a local disease or part of multiple lymphomatous polyposis. In the latter case, it is likely that large parts of the bowel, including the small and large intestines, will be involved.[99] The lymph nodes show a characteristically diffuse infiltrate. It is in the centrocytic lymphomas and the lymphomas of centroblastic or centrocytic morphology that the so-called lymphoepithelial lesions, which are said to be diagnostic of gastrointestinal lymphomas, are seen.

Lymphoplasmacytoid Lymphoma

This is a low-grade lymphoma accounting for 12% of the total primary gastric lymphomas in Levison and Shepherd's series.[96] It is also a tumor of adults and exists as a histologic and behavioral spectrum, rather than as a sharply defined entity. Lymphoplasmacytoid lymphomas are relatively slow-growing tumors, tend to be superficial, and have a low incidence of lymph node involvement. At the malignant end of the spectrum, a larger proportion of cells are immunoblastic in appearance, with relatively fewer lymphoplasmacytoid cells, which are, however, still the predominant cell type. The tumors at this end of the spectrum may show extensive infiltration and a higher incidence of lymph node involvement.

Lymphoblastic Lymphoma

Lymphoblastic lymphoma is classically seen in the ileocecal region in children; however, it has been reported to occur in the stomach. The tumor is usually very advanced at presentation, with extensive infiltration through all layers of the stomach wall. Unlike immunoblastic lymphoma, however, it is remarkably nondestructive. Although deeply invading and widely permeating, there is little destruction of the muscularis propria. Another peculiarity is that it seldom invades mesenteric lymph nodes, which may be uninvolved, although surrounded by infiltrating tumor cells. Even after radical surgery, recurrence is common, and early widespread dissemination, especially within the peritoneal cavity, is problematic.

Malignant Lymphoma with Eosinophilia

This tumor is easily misdiagnosed as a reactive lesion, especially eosinophilic gastroenteritis or Hodgkin's disease, since the blast type of lymphoma cells are commonly binucleate. When it spreads to involve nodes, there are fewer and thus, much more obvious eosinophils associated with the tumor cells.

Staging

Patients with a lymphoma of the stomach have a more favorable prognosis than those with carcinoma. Staging should be based on the TNM classification, although the Ann Arbor Staging System of extranodal lymphoma also can be applied.

Clinical Manifestations

Epigastric pain is the most common symptom and is present in approximately 80% of patients. This pain can be relieved by H2 antagonists. In approximately 50% of patients, the presenting symptom is an epigastric mass. Although weight loss occurs, patients do not appear to be as cachectic as those with carcinoma of the stomach. Gastrointestinal hemorrhage is an uncommon symptom; however, occult blood loss occurs in >50% of patients. Because of the gross nature of lymphoma of the stomach, obstruction is uncommon, but perforation, as mentioned, is higher in carcinoma of the stomach.

Investigations

Only biopsy and histologic examinations will confirm the diagnosis of lymphoma. A barium-meal examination may show an irregular filling defect of diffuse infiltrating irregularities in the wall of the stomach that resembles linitis plastica. Multiple superficial ulcerations and a giant hypertrophic mucosal fold can sometimes be seen. If giant hypertrophic rugae are present, they will be indistinguishable from benign hypertrophic gastritis. Since lymphomas are usually submucosal, cytologic examination is not useful unless there is ulceration of the mucosa. A definitive diagnosis is made at endoscopy, at which time multiple deep biopsy specimens should be taken. CT scanning and endoscopic ultrasonography may be helpful.

Treatment

All patients with a presumptive preoperative diagnosis of lymphoma of the stomach should undergo exploratory laparotomy, unless there is evidence of diffuse systemic involvement or strong medical contraindications. An abnormal liver ultrasound or epigastric mass should not exclude an exploratory laparotomy. As usual, routine preoperative tests, as well as bone marrow aspiration and biopsy, should be performed. Aortic lymphangiography may be of help for anatomic location, but is probably unnecessary.

At laparotomy all intra-abdominal viscera are thoroughly examined for the presence of metastases. If the lesion is situated in the antrum or the body of the stomach, distal subtotal radical gastrectomy is performed. When the lesion is situated proximally near the cardiac end of the stomach, total gastrectomy is probably the operation of choice. The spleen is removed at all operations, and needle biopsy specimens are taken from the liver. Nodes from the paraaortic areas should be examined histologically. If the stomach is diffusely involved, frozen section examination of the resection margins is mandatory.

Radiation therapy has been used as the main method of treatment in some centers following histologic proof of the disease. Resection of the stomach, however, is probably preferable for removal of bulk disease. The use of postoperative irradiation after resection is debatable. If recurrence occurs, irradiation probably should be used, and if there is invasion of the line of resection (which should not happen if frozen section examinations are performed), irradiation is indicated. Lymphocytic lymphomas are highly radiosensitive, but the reticulum cell type of lymphosarcoma is relatively radioresistant.

Chemotherapy

If the lymph nodes are positive, or if there is evidence of systemic disease, chemotherapy should be used. Complete response rates for the numerous treatment programs in the literature vary from 13% to 69%. The four best programs for treating these lymphomas are mechlorethamine, Oncovin (vincristine), procarbazine, prednisone (MOPP), cyclophosphamide (Cytoxan), Oncovin methotrexate, leucovarin, ara-C (cytarabine) (COMLA), cyclophosphamide, hydroxydounomycin/doxorubicin (Adriamycin), Oncovin, prednisone and bleomycin, Adriamycin (doxorubicin), cyclophosphamide, Oncovin, prednisone (BACOP). These regimens should be used for non-Hodgkin's lymphoma.

Prognosis

Stobbe and associates observed that 40% to 50% of their patients survived 5 years despite positive nodes when the lesions were otherwise amenable to resection.[100] Another review of 153 cases gave a 5 year survival rate for curative resection at 34% and curative resection plus radiotherapy at 43.5%, rising to 73.4% for node-negative cases.[101] In this series, patients who did not undergo extensive gastric resection survived <5 years. There have been sporadic reports of improvement in survival with the use of adjuvant chemotherapy following gastric resection, but no series is large enough to show statistical significance.

PRIMARY PLASMACYTOMA OF THE STOMACH

Primary gastric plasmacytoma arising from lymphoid tissue is rare. In most cases reported, patients have been >40 years of age, with a long history of symptoms similar to those of peptic ulcer disease. Tumors have usually been situated in the antrum and distal part of the body of the stomach.

Macroscopically, tumors resembled lymphoma, with diffuse involvement in the wall that resembles carcinoma, with regional lymph nodes involvement possible.

If there is diffuse bony involvement, the diagnosis of plasmacytoma of the stomach must be entertained. Histologically, the appearance is of mature and immature plasmacytes in dense conglomerations.

Treatment is by total gastrectomy, but even following surgery, prognosis is poor. Since the tumor is radiosensitive, postoperative adjuvent radiotherapy is advised.

Lymphoma of the stomach may present as a primary lesion, or it may be part of the involvement of the systemic lymphoma. There is no definite etiologic agent for tumors of the lymphoreticular system in the stomach. Resection is the treatment of choice in primary lymphoma of the stomach. If the nodes are positive, either radiotherapy or chemotherapy should be used postoperatively.

MALIGNANT SMOOTH MUSCLE TUMORS OF THE STOMACH

The incidence of smooth muscle sarcoma is lower than that of lymphoma, and malignant smooth muscle tumors make up approximately 1% to 3% of all malignant lesions of the stomach. The most common malignant smooth muscle tumor is the leiomyosarcoma. Leiomyoblastoma, which is another variant of smooth muscle tumor of the stomach, is also recognized.[102]

Leiomyoblastoma

This tumor is a myogenic tumor that most commonly arises in the stomach. It either can be benign or malignant. There is considerable disagreement among pathologists as to its origin and the criteria for differentiating a malignant from a benign lesion. One study found

7 of 22 leiomyoblastomas to be malignant.[103] Metastases from leiomyoblastoma do occur, but the incidence is relatively low. Collective cases indicate the incidence of metastases to be approximately 16%. Any tumor >10 cm is considered malignant. Although the majority are benign, they should be considered as potentially malignant and treated accordingly.

Pathology. Ninety percent of leiomyoblastomas are situated in the body or antrum of the stomach (Fig 31–11), in sharp contrast in leiomyosarcoma, which usually occurs in the body and fundus of the stomach. The growth of the tumor may be intragastric or outside the stomach. At times, both these growth patterns can be present without much involvement of the intramural portion of the stomach, resulting in its hourglass appearance. The mucosa overlying the tumor may be ulcerated. Necrosis and hemorrhage within the tumor do not necessarily signify a malignant lesion. The tumor is usually soft and rubbery, and well circumscribed but without any definite capsule. The surface may be lobulated and there may be gross infiltration of the surrounding tissues. Histologically, the predominant features are large round or polygonal pleomorphic cells. The nucleus usually is situated at the center of the cell, with a clear zone of cytoplasm surrounding it. A reticuloid pattern surrounding the individual cells or groups of cells may be found. Mitoses are rare, but the number of mitotic figures have a high correlation with the malignant character of this tumor. In frozen sections, it may well be confused with adenocarcinoma.

Clinical Manifestations. Leiomyoblastomas are more common in men than in women, and the mean age for occurrence is 57 years, which is a decade older than that for leiomyosarcomas. The duration of symptoms varies from a few days to several years. The most common clinical presentation, occurring in about 50% of patients, is of gastrointestinal hemorrhage. This can be manifested by hematemesis, melena, or chronic blood loss resulting in anemia. If pain is present, it is similar to that of peptic ulcer disease and can be associated with vomiting. Approximately 25% of patients have an abdominal mass and weight loss. Tumors near the pylorus of the stomach may first be seen as gastric outlet obstruction.

Investigation. Double-contrast barium-meal examination will demonstrate mucosal ulceration in 10% of patients. The majority of lesions appear as filling defects

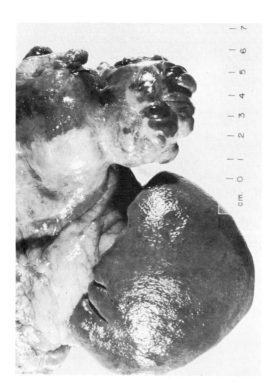

A

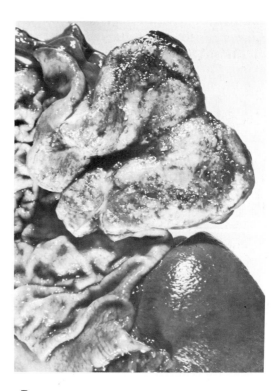

B

Figure 31–11. A. Gross specimen of leiomyoblastoma of stomach with lobular appearance. **B**. Cut surface of tumor with small areas of hemorrhage and necrosis. *Continued*

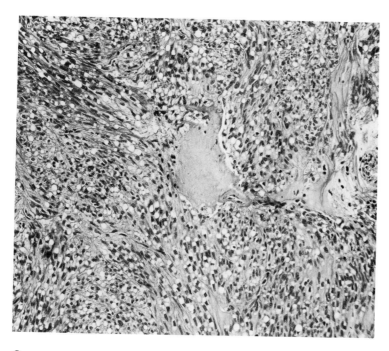

C

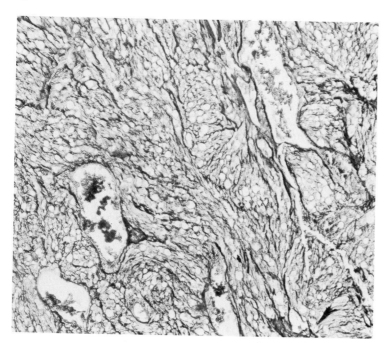

D

Figure 31–11, cont'd. C. Microscopic picture of leiomyoblastoma. Cells have centrally placed nuclei with paranuclear clear zone of cytoplasm. Myofibrils in tumor cells are usually absent. **D**. Reticulum stain with reticular fibers surrounding individual cells or small groups of cells.

in the wall of the stomach without any mucosal abnormality. Definitive diagnosis is made by endoscopy and biopsy.

Treatment. Treatment is surgical, and a distal subtotal gastrectomy is the operation of choice. If the lesion is in the fundus or cardiac end of the stomach, proximal gastroesophagectomy is performed. Combination chemotherapy is given to those patients in whom metastases is found at operation. The usual regimen includes cyclophosphamide, docarbazine, dimethyltriazenoimidazole, carboxaminde (DTIC), vincristine, and doxorubicin. Cisplatin has been used in isolated cases. Research protocols using chemotherapy intraperitoneally are also underway.

Prognosis. Since <15% of these tumors are malignant, the prognosis is excellent, although late metastases can occur. In view of this prolonged follow-up, regular endoscopy is indicated.

Leiomyosarcoma
Leiomyosarcomas account for approximately 1% of all malignant tumors of the stomach but about 30% to 40% of malignant mesodermal tumors.

Pathology. Macroscopically, leiomyosarcoma resembles leiomyoma and leiomyoblastoma of the stomach. Tumor size varies from 1 to 20 cm in diameter. The tumor is often necrotic, giving a soft, cystic appearance. Areas of focal hemorrhage are common. In one-half of cases, the mucosa covering the tumor is ulcerated. As stated previously, in 75% of cases the tumor is situated in the upper part of the body or in the fundus of the stomach. Involvement of the posterior wall of the stomach is much more common, and the tumor may spread into the gastrohepatic ligament or into the omentum. It is devoid of any capsule, although it has a smooth surface. Like leiomyoblastoma, the tumor may be either intragastric or exogastric, with considerable extension into the muscular wall of the stomach. Perforation of these tumors into the lesser sac is well documented.

Histology. Most leiomyosarcomas are composed of spindle-shaped cells with varying amounts of cytoplasm. Myofibrils are easily identifiable, in contrast to leiomyoblastomas. Half of the tumor cells may be polygonal or plump in configuration. Reticular fibers are found around individual cells or groups of cells. Anaplastic spindle cells, resembling cells of muscular origin, and fatty changes like those seen in liposarcoma are common features.

Clinical Manifestation. Patients with these tumors are usually younger than patients with malignant epithelial tumors of the stomach. Most are in their fifth or sixth decade. The main clinical presentation, like leiomyoblastoma, is gastrointestinal bleeding. The reported incidence of bleeding ranges from 50% to 75%, with chronic anemia observed in about 55% of patients. Less than half of patients have epigastric pain at initial presentation, and about one-third have epigastric masses. Weight loss is noted in only 10% of patients, in contrast to patients with adenocarcinoma. The tumor initially may present as acute peritonitis secondary to perforation.

Diagnosis. As for leiomyoblastoma of the stomach, a double-contrast barium-meal examination will probably show a filling defect with either smooth or ulcerative mucosa. Extrinsic pressure on the stomach also may be evident. The situation of the tumor is helpful in distinguishing its nature. Endoscopy will show a submucosal mass with possible ulceration. Multiple biopsies are required to establish the diagnosis of leiomyosarcoma, and these should be as deep as possible.

Treatment. Subtotal radical gastrectomy is used for distal lesions and proximal gastroesophagectomy for lesions situated in the fundus or near the esophagogastric junction. Whole lymph node clearance is performed as for adenocarcinoma of the stomach. Adjuvant chemotherapy has been advised using the same drugs as for leiomyoblastomas.

Prognosis. Approximately 20% of patients will be found to have metastases at operation. A further 20% will develop metastases within 18 months. Close follow-up is indicated since metastases can occur even after a long interval. McNeer and Berg reported a 53.8% crude 5 year survival rate,[104] and Burgess and associates gave a 5 year survival rate of 50% and a 10 year survival rate of 35%.[105] Patients who underwent resection for cure had survival rates of 62% and 45% at 5 and 10 years, respectively. The prognosis, therefore, seems better than that for patients with lymphoma of the stomach.

The Department of Surgery, Cancer Institute Hospital, Tokyo, Japan reported 76 patients with smooth muscle tumors of the stomach (18 leiomyomas, 58 leiomyosarcomas).[106] They stated that advanced age, short duration of illness, region of the middle portion of the stomach, large tumor size and ulcerative tumor were suggestive of pathological malignancy. They found that male sex, symptomatic patients, and larger tumor size were suggestive of poor prognosis. The rate of curative surgery was 94.8% for 58 patients with leiomyosarcoma. The cumulative 5 year survival rate after curative operation was 74.9% for all patients with leiomyosarcoma. Regardless of resecting method, all patients with a tumor <5 cm in diameter lived without any indication of recurrence. Four of the 58 patients with leiomyosarcoma had regional lymph node metastases and died <5 years after operation.

MISCELLANEOUS MALIGNANT MESENCHYMAL TUMORS OF THE STOMACH

Fibrosarcoma, hemangiopericytoma, rhabdomyosarcoma, liposarcoma, neurofibrosarcoma, and angiosarcoma are all described, although their occurrence is rare. Neurofibrosarcoma (schwannoma) is also found in the stomach, but since it arises from the Schwann cells of the nerve sheath, it is not a sarcomatous lesion.

Fibrosarcoma

Most fibrous tissue tumors of the stomach are benign. They are usually situated in the antrum and can involve the mucosa, with subsequent mucosal ulceration. They are thought to be variants of leiomyosarcoma.

Hemangiopericytoma

These tumors are as rare in the stomach as in other parts of the body. Only 10% of all tumors reported have been malignant. They arise from blood vessels of the stomach and may be solitary or multiple. Metastases to lymph nodes may occur. They may arise in the retroperitoneum and involve the stomach, or alternatively, they may arise in the stomach and involve the surrounding structures. Commonly they metastasize to the regional lymph nodes and have great propensity for local recurrence following resection. Treatment is surgical, implying radical resection and lymph node clearance.

Rhabdomyosarcoma

Rhabdomyosarcoma is a malignant tumor arising from the skeletal muscle. It has a tendency to metastasize to regional lymph nodes, as well as to the lung and liver. It is extremely rare and should be treated by radical gastrectomy with adjuvant chemotherapy.

Liposarcoma

Only four cases of liposarcoma of the stomach have been reported since 1887.[107]

Kaposi's Sarcoma

A 10% incidence of visceral involvement in Kaposi's sarcoma has been reported. Most of the lesions have been in the gastrointestinal tract. Gastric lesions usually resemble dermal lesions and are hemorrhagic and small. The tumors may be multiple and are usually situated in the submucosa, but mucosal ulceration is a possibility. Typically, these tumors are composed of elongated

cells with numerous capillaries; foci of recent hemorrhage and deposition of hemosiderin pigment are seen around the tumor. Wide resection in the form of either distal subtotal gastrectomy or proximal gastroesophagectomy should be performed.

With the increase in acquired immune deficiency syndrome (AIDS) and its relationship to an increased incidence of cutaneous Kaposi's sarcoma, there may well be a rise in incidence of gastrointestinal Kaposi's sarcoma in the future. A patient with human T cell leukaemia/lymphoma virus type I (HTLV-1) who subsequently developed gastric lymphoma was described by Kubonishi and associates.[108]

Neurofibrosarcoma

At initial presentation, the patient with neurofibrosarcoma has a mass in the wall of the stomach. Invasion of the mucosa, the outer structure, and the retroperitoneum also is found. Pain usually is present in the epigastric region. The diagnosis is made either at endoscopic examination or laparotomy. Radical resection should be performed unless there is evidence of other visceral metastases. Organs involved by direct extension of the tumor should be resected en bloc.

REFERENCES

1. Palmer ED. Benign intramural tumors of the stomach: a review with special reference to gross pathology. *Medicine*, 1951;30:81
2. Eklof O. Benign tumors of the stomach and duodenum. *Acta Chir Scand* 1962;291(suppl):1
3. Rosai J. *Ackerman's Surgical Pathology*, 7th ed. St. Louis, MO: CV Mosby; 1988
4. McNeer G, Berg JW. The clinical behavior and management of primary malignant lymphoma of the stomach. *Surgery* 1951;46:829
5. Scott HW, Adkins RB, Sawyer JL. Results of an aggressive surgical approach to gastric carcinoma during a 23 year period. Surgery 1985;97:57
6. McCreadie M, Coates M, Ford JM. Epidemiology of alimentary cancers in New South Wales 1973–1982. *Aust NZ J Surg* 1990;60:93–98
7. OPCS, 1980
8. Coggan D, Acheson E. Cancer of the stomach. *Br Med Bull* 1984;40:335
9. Maartmann-Mol H, Hartweit F. On the reputed decline in gastric carcinoma: study from Western Norway. *Br Med J* 1985;290:103
10. Hermanek P. Gastrointestinal carcinoma—are there age-related differences in tumor behaviour? *Hepatogastroenterology* 1986;81:747
11. Edelman DS, Russin DJ, Wallack MK. Gastric cancer in the elderly. *Am Surg* 1987;53:170
12. Radi MJ, Fenoglio-Preiser CM, et al. Gastric carcinoma in the young: a clinicopathological and immunohistochemical study. *Am J Gastroenterol* 1986;81:747

13. Patterson IM, Easton DF, et al. Changing distribution of adenocarcinoma of the stomach. *Br J Surg* 1987;74:481

14. Meyers WC, Damicono RJ, Jr, et al. Adenocarcinoma of the stomach: changing patterns over the last four decades. *Am Surg* 1987;205:1

15. Zanchek W, Grable E, et al. Occurrence of gastric cancer among patients with pernicious anemia at the Boston City Hospital. *N Engl J Med* 1955;252:1103

16. Hitchcock C. The value of achlorhydria as a screening test for gastric cancer: a ten year report. *Gastroenterology* 1955; 29:621

17. Stockbrugger RW, Menon GG, et al. Endoscopic screening in patients with pernicious anemia, in Cotton P (ed), *Early Gastric Cancer*. Welwyn Garden City, UK: Smith, Kline & French Laboratories; 1982:59–63

18. Farrands PA, Blake JRS, et al. Endoscopic review of patients who have had gastric surgery. *Br Med J* 1983;286:755

19. Ellis DJ, Kingston RD, et al. Gastric ulceration and previous peptic ulceration. *Br J Surg* 1979;66:117

20. Dawson IMP, Cornes JS, Morson BC. Primary malignant lymphoid tumors of the gastrointestinal tract. *Br J Surg* 1961;49:80

21. Aird I, Benthall HH, Roberts JAF. A relationship between cancer of the stomach and the ABO blood groups. *Br Med J* 1953;1:799

22. Editorial. Gastric ulcer or cancer? *Lancet* 1985;i:202

23. Correa P, Haenszel W, Cuello C, et al. Gastric precancerous process in a high risk population: cross-sectional studies. *Cancer Res* 1990;50:4731–4736

24. Correa P. Carcinoma of the stomach. *Proc Nutr Soc* 1985;46:111

25. Forman D, Al-Dabbagh S, Doll R. Nitrates, nitrites and gastric cancer in Great Britain. *Nature* 1985;313:620

26. Beresford J. Risk of gastric cancer is negatively correlated with nitrate content of water supply. *Int J Epidemiol* 1985;14:57

27. Chang YC, Nagasue N, et al. Clinicopathologic features and long-term results of alpha-fetoprotein-producing gastric cancer. *Am J Gastroenterol* 1990;85:1480–1485

28. Parsonnet J, Friedman GD, et al. *Helicobacter pylori* infection and the risk of gastric carcinoma. *N Engl J Med* 1991;16:325(16):1127–1131

29. Strickland RG. A reappraisal of the nature of significance of chronic atrophic gastritis. *Am J Digest Dis* 1973;18:426

30. Morson BC. Intestinal metaplasia of the gastric mucosa. *Br J Cancer* 1955;9:356

31. Jass JR, Filipe MI. A variant of intestinal metaplasia associated with gastric carcinoma: a histochemical study. *Histopathology* 1979;3:191

32. Moertel CG. The stomach. In: Holland JH, Frei E, III (eds), *Cancer Medicine*. Philadelphia, PA; Lea & Febiger; 1973:1527–1541

33. Oota K. On the nature of the ulcerative changes in early carcinoma of the stomach. *Geneva Monogr* 1986;3:141

34. Piper DW (ed): *Stomach Cancer*. Geneva, Switzerland: UICC Technical Report Series; 1978:31

35. Polleg A, Jacobsen CD. Gastric ulcer and risk of cancer—a five year follow-up study. *Acta Med Scand* 1986;216:105

36. Durrant LG, Watson SA, Hall A, et al. Co-stimulation of gastrointestinal tumor cell growth by gastrin, transforming growth factor-alpha and insulin-like growth factor-1. *Br J Cancer* 1991;1:67–70

37. Lee EY, Wang TC, Clouse RE, et al. Gastric carcinoma, epidermal growth factor, and epidermal growth factor receptor [letter]. *Gastroenterology* 1991;100:289

38. Sakamoto J, Kito T, Yamamura Y, et al. Importance of the histopathological type of the tumor as a parameter for recurrence and for prognosis of gastric cancers. *Nippon Geka Gakki Zasshi* 92(a);1082–1085

39. Bormann R. Hambuch der Spezielin. In: Henke F, Lubarsch O (eds), *Pathologische Anatomie und Histologie*. Berlin, Germany: Springer; 1926

40. Morson and Dawson, 1979.

41. Ming SC. Gastric carcinoma. A pathological classification. *Cancer* 1979;39:2475

42. Comfort MW, Grey HK, et al. Small gastric cancer. *Arch Intern Med* 1954;94:513

43. Monafo WW, Krause GL, Medina JG. Carcinoma of the stomach: morphological characteristics affecting survival. *Arch Surg* 1962;85:754

44. Kajitani T. Gastric Cancer. In: *Modern Surgery*. Tokyo, Japan: Nakayana Shoten; 1971: 20–26

45. Lauren P. The two histological main types of gastric carcinoma: diffuse and so-called intestinal type carcinoma. *Acta Pathol Microbiol Scand* 1965;64:31

46. Mulligan RM. Histogenesis and biological behavior of gastric carcinoma. In: Sommers S (ed), *Path Annal*, vol 7. New York, NY: Appleton-Century-Crofts; 1972:349–415

47. Jass JR. Role of intestinal metaplasia in the histogenesis of gastric carcinoma. *J Clin Pathol* 1980;33:801

48. Grabiec J, Owen DA. Carcinoma of the stomach in young persons. *Cancer* 1985;56:388

49. Callery CD, Sanders MM, et al. Squamous cell carcinoma of the stomach: a study of four patients with comments on histogenesis. *J Surg Oncol* 1985;29:166

50. Mori M, Iwashita A, Enjoji M. Squamous cell carcinoma of the stomach—report of three cases. *Am J Gastroenterol* 1986;81:339

51. Walker Q, Bilous M, et al. Breast cancer metastases masquerading as primary gastric carcinoma. *Aust NZ J Surg* 1986;56:395

52. Gall FP, Hermanek P. New aspects in the surgical treatment of gastric carcinoma—a comparative study of 1636 patients operated on between 1969 and 1982. *Eur J Surg Oncol* 1985;3:219

53. Fielding JWL, Ellis DJ, et al. Natural history of early gastric cancer: results of a 10 year regional survey. *Br Med J* 1980;281:965

54. Okuyama K, Isono K, et al. Evaluations of treatment for gastric cancer with liver metastasis. *Cancer* 1985;55:2498

55. Hattori T, Hosokawa Y, et al. Analysis of DNA ploidy patterns of gastric carcinomas of Japanese. *Cancer* 1986;54:1591

56. Baretton G, Carstensen O, Schardey M, et al. DNA-ploidy and survival in gastric carcinomas: a flow-cytometric study. *Virchows Arch A* 1991;418:301–309

57. Kennedy BJ. TNM classification for stomach cancer. *Cancer* 1970;26:971

58. American Joint Committee for Cancer Staging and End

Results Reporting: *Manual for Staging of Cancer.* Chicago, IL: The Committee; 1972

59. Maruyama M, Sasaki T, et al. Studies on computer processing of information concerning the endoscopic diagnosis of the gastrointestinal tracts, I. Modification of IRD and practical coding. *Gastrointest Endosc* 1983;25:17

60. Maruyama M, Sasaki T, et al. Studies on computer processing of information concerning the endoscopic diagnosis of the gastrointestinal tracts, I. modification of IRD and practical coding. *Gastrointest Endosc* 1983;25:17

61. Winawer SJ, Melamed M, Sherlock P. Potential of endoscopy, biopsy, and cytology in the diagnosis, and management of patients with cancer. *Clin Gastroenterol* 1976; 5:575

62. Tiller J, Roder R, et al. CT in advanced gastric carcinoma—is exploratory laparotomy avoidable? *Eur J Radiol* 1986;6:181

63. Cook AO, Levine BA, et al. Evaluation of gastric adenocarcinoma: abdominal computed tomography does not replace coelotomy. *Arch Surg* 1986;121:603

64. Heyder N, Lux G. Malignant lesions of the upper gastrointestinal tract. *Scand J Gastroenterol* 1986;21(suppl 123):47

65. Yasuda K, Nakajima M, Kawai K. Endoscopic ultrasonography in the diagnosis of submucosal tumor of the upper digestive tract. *Scand J Gastroenterol* 1986;21(suppl 123):59

66. Aibe T, Ho Y, et al. Endoscopic ultrasonography of lymph nodes surrounding the upper gastrointestinal tract. *Scand J Gastroenterol* 1986;21(suppl 123):166

67. Winkler ML, Hricak H, Higgins CB. MR imaging of diffusely infiltrating gastric carcinoma. *J Comput Assist Tomogr* 1987;11:337

68. Heptner G, Domschke W. The role of tumor markers in the diagnosis and management of gastrointestinal cancer. *Hepatogastroenterology* 1986;33:140

69. Janssen CW, Maartmann-Moe H, Terje R. Concentrations of proteins and ESR in patients with different histologic types of gastric carcinomas. *Eur J Surg Oncol* 1987;13:207

70. Ychou M, Tuszinski T, Pignon JP, et al. Stomach adenocarcinomas: comparison between CA 19-9 and carcinoembryonic antigen for the diagnosis of recurrences after surgical treatment. *Gastroenterol Clin Biol* 1992;16(11): 848–852

71. Nishi K, Tokunega KNA, et al. Immunohistochemical study of intracellular oestradiol in human gastric cancer. *Cancer* 1987;59:1328

72. Wu CW, Lui Wy, P'eng FK, et al. Hormonal therapy for stomach cancer. *Med Hypotheses* 1992;39(2):137–139

73. Lemoine NR, Jain S, et al. Amplification and over-expression of the EGF receptor and c-erb B-2 protooncogenes in human stomach cancer. *Br J Cancer* 1991;63:601–608

74. Yonemura Y, Ninomiya I, et al. Evaluation of immunoreactivity for erb B-2 protein as a marker of poor short term prognosis in gastric cancer. *Cancer Res* 1991;3:1034–1038

75. Tsujino T. Alterations of oncogenes in metastatic tumors of human gastric carcinomas. *Br J Cancer* 1990;62:226–230

76. Ranzani GN, Pellegata NS, et al. Heterogeneous protooncogene amplification correlates with tumor progression and presence of metastases in gastric cancer patients. *Cancer Res* 1990;50:7811–7814

77. Charing, et al.

78. Prola JC, Kobayashi S, Kirsner JB. Gastric Cancer: some recent improvements in diagnosis based upon the Japanese experience. *Arch Intern Med* 1969;124:238

79. Keighley MRB, Moore J, et al. Incidence and prognosis of N4 mode involvement in gastric cancer. *Br J Surg* 1984; 71:863

80. Scott HW, Adkins RB, Sawyers JL. Results of an aggressive surgical approach to gastric carcinoma during a 23 year period. *Surgery* 1985;97:57

81. British Stomach Cancer Group. Resection line disease in stomach cancer. *Br Med J* 1984;289:601

82. Abe S, Ogawa Y, et al. Early gastric cancer—results in a general hospital in Japan. *World J Surg* 1984;8:308

83. Haring R, Germer CT, Diermann J. Multivisceral and extended resection in tumor surgery: stomach cancer. *Langenbecks Arch Chir Suppl Kongressbd* 1992;55–60

84. Nordmann E, Kanppinen C. The value of megavolt therapy in carcinoma of the stomach. *Strahlentherapie* 1972; 144:635

85. Schein PS. Chemotherapy of gastric carcinoma. *Eur J Surg Oncol* 1987;13:3

86. Randall J, Oberd MC, Blackledge GRP. Hemorrhage and perforation of gastric neoplasms during chemotherapy. *Ann R Coll Surg Engl* 1986;68:286

87. Maehara Y, Anai H, et al. Poorly differentiated human gastric carcinoma is more sensitive to antitumor drugs than is well differentiated carcinoma. *Eur J Surg Oncol* 1987; 13:203

88. Ward LC, Fielding JW, Dunn JA, et al. The selection of cases of randomised trials: a registry survey of concurrent trial and non-trial patients. The British Stomach Cancer Group. *Br J Cancer* 1992;66(5):943–950

89. Findlay M, Cunningham D. Chemotherapy of carcinoma of the stomach. *Cancer Treatment Rev* 1993;18:29–44

90. Hussell T, Isaacson P, Crabtree J, et al. The response of cells from low-grade B-cell gastric lymphomas of mucosa-associated lymphoid tissue to *Helicobacter pylori. Lancet* 1993;342:571

91. Wotherspoon A, Doglioni C, Diss T, et al. Regression of primary low-grade B-cell gastric lymphoma of mucosa-associated lymphoid tissue type after eradication of *Helicobacter pylori. Lancet* 1993;342:575

92. Hermann R, Panahon AM, et al. Gastrointestinal involvement in non-Hodgkin's lymphoma. *Cancer* 1980;46:215

93. Lim FE, Hartman AS, et al. Factors in the prognosis of gastric lymphoma. *Cancer* 1977;39:1715

94. Salmela H. Lymphosarcoma of the stomach. A clinical study of 39 cases. *Acta Chir Scand* 1968;134:567

95. Rosenberg SA, Diamond HD, et al. Lymphosarcoma: a review of 1269 cases. *Medicine* 1961;40:31

96. Levison DA, Shepherd NA. Pathology of gastric lymphomas and smooth muscle tumors. In: Preece P, Cuschieri A, Wellwood J (eds), *Cancer of the Stomach.* Orlando, FL: Grune & Stratton; 1985

97. Lennert K. Histopathology of non-Hodgkin's lymphomas (based on the Kiel classification). Berlin, Germany: Springer; 1981

98. Moore I, Wright DH. Primary gastric lymphoma—a tumor of mucosa-associated lymphoid tissue: a histological and

immunohistochemical study of 36 patients. *Histopathology* 1984;8:1025

99. Blackshaw AJ. Non-Hodgkin's lymphomas of the gut. In: Wright R (ed), *Recent Advances in Gastrointestin Pathology.* Philadelphia, PA: WB Saunders; 1980:213–240

100. Stobbe JA, Dockerty MB, et al. Primary gastric lymphoma and its grades of malignancy. *Am J Surg* 1966;122:10

101. Hockey MS, Powell J, et al. Primary gastric lymphoma. *Br J Surg* 1987;74:483

102. Stout AP. Tumors of the stomach. In: *Atlas of Tumor Pathology,* Fascicle 21. Washington, DC: Armed Forces Institute of Pathology; 1953.

103. Smithwick W III, Blescekler JL, et al. Leiomyoblastoma: behaviour and prognosis. *Cancer* 1969;24:996

104. McNeer G, Berg JW. The clinical behavior and management of primary malignant lymphoma of the stomach. *Surgery* 1959;46:829

105. Burgess JN, Dockerty MB, et al. Sarcomatous lesions of the stomach. *Am Surg* 1971;173:758

106. Yuasa N, Takagi K, Ota H, et al. Clinical study of 76 cases of smooth muscle tumor of the stomach. *Nippon Geka Gakki Zasshi* 1992;93(3):248–256

107. Shokouh-Amiri MH, Hansen CP, Muesgaard F. Liposarcoma of the stomach. *Acta Chir Scand* 1986;152:389

108. Kubonishi J, Kaibata M, et al. Gastric lymphoma associated with human T-cell leukaemia virus type 1. *Arch Intern Med* 1987;147:603

SELECTED READINGS

Abe M, Yabumoto E, et al. Intraoperative radiotherapy of gastric cancer. *Cancer* 1980;45:40

Bancheck W, Grable E, et al. Occurrence of gastric cancer among patients with pernicious anemia at the Boston City Hospital. *N Engl J Med* 1955;252:1103

Broders AC. Carcinoma: grading and practical application. *Arch Pathol* 1926;2:376

Chyou PH, Nomura AMY, Hankin JH, et al. A case-cohort study of diet and stomach cancer. *Cancer Res* 1990;50: 7501–7504

Gunderson LL, Sosin H. Adenocarcinoma of the stomach—areas of failure in a preoperation series. *Int J Radiat Oncol Biol Phys* 1982;8:1

Haas JF, Schottenfield D. Epidemiology of gastric cancer. In: Lopkin M, Good RA (eds), *Gastrointestinal Tract Cancer.* Sloan-Kettering Cancer Series. New York, NY: Plenum Medical; 1978

Lofeld RJLF, Willems I, Flendrig JA, et al. *Helicobacter pylori* and gastric carcinoma. *Histopathology* 1990;17:537–541

Schildberg FW, Stangl MJ. Surgical treatment of early stomach cancer. *Langenbecks Arch Chir Suppl Kogressbd* 1992; 118–122

Schlag PM. Stomach cancer: multimodality therapy—reliable and new developments. *Langenbecks Arch Chir Suppl Kongressbd* 1992;147–151

Selikoff IJ. Cancer risk of asbestos exposure. In: Hiatt HH, Watson JD, Winsten JA (eds), *Origins of Human Cancer*, Book C. Cold Spring Harbour, NY: Cold Spring Harbour Laboratory; 1977:1765–1784

Tomasulo J. Gastric polyps: Histologic types and their relationship to gastric carcinoma. *Cancer* 1971;27:1346

Winawer SJ, Sherlock P, Hajdu SI. The role of upper gastrointestinal endoscopy in patients with cancer. *Cancer* 1976;37:440

32

Complications Following
Gastric Operations

David I. Soybel ■ *Michael J. Zinner*

The purpose of this chapter is to provide an overview of the recognition, evaluation, and management of acute and late complications that follow operations on the stomach and duodenum. Since vagotomy is an important component of many of these operations, the early and late complications of vagal denervation also are presented. The incidence of operations on the stomach and duodenum has been decreasing, largely owing to the declining need for surgical intervention in patients with acid-peptic disease. Experience with complications of these operations also has declined. Of the intraoperative and early complications that follow vagotomy and gastric procedures, it may be said that the best way to minimize complications is to anticipate them. However, the late complications of these procedures often result from disturbances in gastrointestinal motility and mucosal function that are direct consequences of the operation that was planned. Such functional disturbances will occur, to a greater or lesser degree, in every patient. It remains difficult to predict which of these patients will develop incapacitating symptoms. Thus, late complications cannot necessarily be anticipated or avoided in any given patient. The surgeon should explain the incidence and natural history of such complications to the patient before the initial operation is performed. Attention to this detail is not only part of the obligation to obtain informed consent, but increases the likelihood that such patients

will return to the surgeons who know them best for evaluation and management of their postoperative complications.

■ VAGOTOMY COMPLICATIONS

As discussed in the previous chapter, denervation of the acid-secreting mucosa of the stomach can be accomplished by means of three types of vagotomy. *Truncal vagotomy* (TV) denervates the entire stomach, biliary tract, pancreas, small intestine, and proximal colon. *Selective gastric vagotomy* (SV) preserves hepatobiliary and celiac branches, but denervates the motor and acid secretory apparatus of the entire stomach. *Highly selective (proximal gastric or parietal cell) vagotomy* (HSV) denervates the acid secretory apparatus and motor fibers to the corpus and fundus, but preserves all other branches, including those to the gastric antrum. Truncal and selective forms of vagotomy require that some form of drainage procedure be performed in order to avoid gastric stasis. Highly selective vagotomy need not be accompanied by a drainage procedure, since coordinated antral and pyloric motor functions are preserved. The complications associated with these different forms of vagotomy may be divided into those occurring at the time of operation, those occurring shortly after operation, and those occurring in time.

OPERATIVE COMPLICATIONS OF VAGOTOMY

Complications that occur during the operation are usually the result of errors in technique. These are listed in Table 32–1. These complications usually are recognized at the time of operation and recommended approaches to their management are outlined in Table 32–1. Splenic injury has been reported in up to 4% of patients, but is not nearly so common, at present. Often, it occurs owing to injudicious placement of retractors in the left upper quadrant by inexperienced assistants. Use of the mechanical retracting devices (Bookwalter, "upperhand") seems to minimize it. Splenic injury also can occur from undue traction on the greater curvature of the stomach or when the spleen is large and the vagotomy is being attempted for a second time. Local measures for hemostasis and splenorrhaphy usually are adequate for management. Splenectomy is rarely required, unless the procedure is being performed emergently and time under anesthesia must be minimized.

Laceration of the distal esophagus or disruption of the esophagogastric junction are rare and almost always preventable complications. They can be lethal unless recognized immediately. Laceration of the esophagus may occur when the surgeon is attempting to dissect out the posterior vagal trunk. The safest way to identify this trunk is to approach it after the anterior vagus has been cut. This permits the posterior vagal trunk to become taut, like a bow string. The surgeon, standing on the patient's right, places his right index finger to the left and posterior to the esophageal wall, with the finger directly in contact with the anterior surface of the aorta. As the finger curls around the esophagus, it penetrates the pancreaticogastric fold of peritoneum, and the taut posterior vagal trunk becomes palpable. However, if the surgeon's finger penetrates the fold too anteriorly, the posterior esophageal wall, which has no serosa, may be injured and even entered. The tear is thus located on the right posterolateral wall of the esophagus. The tear is visualized by placing two 1 inch Penrose drains around the esophagus and rotating it anteriorly. The tear is repaired in two layers, with interrupted fine 4-0 silk sutures. The mucosal layer is repaired first, followed by reapproximation of the muscle layer. A Nissen fundoplication, serving as a patch, can be added if there are concerns about the repair or its blood supply. Drainage of the left upper quadrant is not recommended. An entire disruption of the esophagogastric junction is very rare, but must be managed aggressively, usually with resection of the injured tissues and reanastomosis of the distal esophagus and gastric fundus. Left thoracotomy may be required for optimal exposure of the esophagus. Since such injuries are more likely to occur when revagotomy is being attempted, approaches to the vagi at the previously undissected level at the diaphragm may be useful.

In the event that the complication is not recognized at the time of surgery but is delayed, the patient will complain of severe upper abdominal and chest pain and may have evidence of mediastinal air or left-sided atalectasis and pleural effusion.[1] Esophagram, using water soluble contrast material, is performed to verify the diagnosis. Immediate exploration, closure, and drainage is required under these circumstances. Antibiotic therapy is begun as soon as the diagnosis is suspected and maintained postoperatively until signs of sepsis are gone.

EARLY POSTOPERATIVE COMPLICATIONS OF VAGOTOMY

The recognized early complications include (1) gastric atony and delayed emptying despite an adequate drainage procedure (TV or SV), (2) dysphagia or even achalasia, (3) functional gastric outlet obstruction owing to excessive denervation of the antral-pyloric region by HSV, and (4) necrosis of the lesser curvature of the stomach, owing to devascularization during HSV.

Gastric Atony With Delayed Gastric Emptying

This complication, not uncommon after truncal, selective, or highly selective vagotomy, occurring in about 10% of patients.[2] It is less frequent in patients undergoing HSV, but still can occur in up to 3%.[2, 3] Normally, the pace-setting potentials that regulate peristalsis in the distal stomach and pylorus are located in the gastric

TABLE 32–1. INTRAOPERATIVE COMPLICATIONS OF VAGOTOMY

Complication	Management
Injury to the spleen	Avitene/gelfoam, splenorrhaphy, splenectomy (rarely needed)
Laceration of distal esophagus	Repair, fundoplication (Nissen) patch
Esophagogastric disconnection	Resection of fragmented tissues, possibly esophagogastrectomy
Disruption of crural sling	Repair
Pneumothorax	Observation and repeat CXR if asymptomatic and <15%; otherwise tube thoracostomy.
Liver Trauma	
Hematoma	Observation
Tear	Pressure, omental tongue for deep lacerations or parenchymal avulsions
Pancreas trauma	Drainage (somatostatin)
Colon injury (Splenic flexure)	Repair if spillage minimal and injury <50% of circumference; resection and reanastomosis if injury extensive but spillage minimal; diverting colostomy otherwise
Vascular Injuries	
Phrenic vein	Suture ligation
Left hepatic vein	Repair if possible, suture ligation if not possible
Thoracic duct	Suture ligation and drainage
Left gastric artery	Suture ligation

corpus, on the greater curvature. The absence of coordinated peristalsis appears to be attributable to the loss of this single dominant pacemaker, which leads to appearance of several ectopic pacemakers in the myenteric plexus.[4] The result is gastric dilatation and ineffective gastric propulsion of solids. The dominant symptoms are nausea and bloating, occasionally abdominal distention. When gastric atony is severe, as it is in a little less than 1% of patients, the patient may describe vomiting of partially digested food that was eaten hours or even days previously. Nevertheless, basic nutritional needs frequently can be met through ingestion of liquids. In such cases, plain films and barium studies will reveal a large stomach that is retaining air and fluid. Endoscopically, the gastric outlet or stoma is patent. A solid-phase radionuclide gastric emptying study will be highly abnormal. Bezoars also may contribute to this clinical picture, occurring in as many as 12% of patients with gastric atony.[5]

In most cases, nasogastric decompression and time will resolve gastric atony and delayed gastric emptying. Prokinetic medications have been used in this setting, including metaclopramide, cisapride, and erythromycin. In general, the experience with these drugs has been disappointing.[6,7] Of these medications, the authors' experience has been that cisapride is of some use in hastening return of gastric emptying. It should be prescribed before recommending surgical therapy. Since vagal innervation cannot be restored, the principal goal of surgery is to reduce the reservoir capacity of the gastric remnant and avoid bile reflux. In a series of 40 patients treated at the Mayo clinic,[8] extensive distal gastric resection or near subtotal resection of the stomach and Roux-en-Y reconstruction led to excellent/good results in 23 patients, and some improvement in 4 patients. Of note, 13 patients did not improve. Eckhauser and associates reported similar results, in a series of 15 patients.[6]

Dysphagia

Dysphagia is uncommon, but may occur in 2% or more of patients following vagotomy.[9,10] Rarely, the dysphagia is nearly complete and imitates achalasia.[9] This symptom does not always follow the surgical procedure immediately. Often, the patient has no trouble while in the hospital. The dysphagia may appear up to 4 weeks after discharge. Occasionally, esophageal dilatation is required.[10] The complication remains difficult to explain. It is the impression of some surgeons that this complication is more common after HSV, an operation that requires more extensive dissection in the area of the gastroesophageal junction. Trauma to the distal esophagus and is attachments at the level of the diaphragm may be involved. Studies in humans undergoing any of the three types of vagotomy have not demonstrated consis-

tent changes in the mechanism of the lower esophageal sphincter, either in its competence or ability to relax with primary peristalsis.[11,12]

Evaluation of this condition, if it persists, must be complete. Included in the diagnostic studies are barium swallow under fluoroscopy, upper endoscopy, and esophageal manometry studies. Mechanical and malignant causes must be excluded. The differential diagnosis of post-vagotomy dysphagia is outlined in Table 32–2. If other causes are excluded, and the possibility of postvagotomy dysphagia seems likeliest, the natural course of the condition is to resolve in time. Patients with severe symptoms may require bougienage. However, dilatations should not be performed until the diagnostic evaluation has been completed. A number of medications, especially nitrites and calcium channel blockers such as nifedipine, are currently under investigation for medical management of achalasia.[13,14] Their usefulness in this setting of postvagotomy dysphagia is not known.

Antral-Pyloric Stasis after Extensive HSV

As discussed in an earlier chapter, a key part of the HSV operation is the selection of the distal extent of denervation. In some cases, the denervation may be so extensive as to interrupt motor fibers of the antrum, leading to stasis and ineffective emptying of chyme through the pylorus. The major symptoms are bloating, nausea, and vomiting. The likelihood that such symptoms will resolve nonoperatively may depend on the extent of scarring in the pyloric region. If scarring is significant, with deformity of the duodenal bulb and pylorus, symptoms of stasis will probably persist. Prokinetic agents may be tried in this setting. Severe and persistent stasis may be amenable to endoscopic dilatation.[15] If there is marked deformity of the pyloroduodenal region, or if endoscopic approaches have failed, a drainage procedure should be performed. A Finney-type pyloroplasty often works well in the setting of marked scarring. If there is any question about the safety of dissecting the pyloric region, a gastrojejunostomy may be performed.

TABLE 32–2. CAUSES OF DYSPHAGIA IN POSTGASTRIC SURGERY PATIENTS

Carcinoma—primary or recurrent
Sutures at esophageal hiatus
Hematoma
Gastric bezoar
Paraesophageal hernia
Late stricture owing to reflux acid or alkaline gastritis
Extrinsic mass lesions—mediastinal cysts, retroperitoneal cyst or mass
Esophageal diverticulum
Motility disorders
Unexplained (idiopathic)

Necrosis of the Lesser Curvature of the Stomach after HSV

This complication usually is recognized between 24 and 72 hours postoperatively. The chief complaints are sudden, severe upper abdominal pain, with tenderness, rigidity, and shock. The complication of lesser-curve necrosis is extremely rare after HSV, less than 30 cases having been reported. Although the devascularization that accompanies HSV may be involved, other factors such as gastric distention, underlying atherosclerosis, and inadvertent injury by operating instruments may play more important roles. The complication may be more common when HSV is combined with Nissen fundoplication.[16] The management of this devastating complication is resection of the necrotic area, if it is localized, with closure and reinforcement with an omental patch. Extensive necrosis may require a near total or total gastrectomy.

LATE COMPLICATIONS OF VAGOTOMY

The recognized late complications include (1) diarrhea, (2) reflux esophagitis, with or without stricture, and (3) cholelithiasis.

Postvagotomy Diarrhea

Although changes in bowel habits are common after any abdominal operation, persistent diarrhea is a well-established consequence of vagotomy. In the Vanderbilt experience, persistent diarrhea has been observed in about 25% of patients undergoing TV, in 3% undergoing SV, and <1% undergoing HSV.[17] The etiology of this complication remains unclear. Factors that have been implicated include (1) gastric alkalinization, which leads to colonization of the upper GI tract with coliforms and other intestinal bacteria, (2) alterations in receptive relaxation and gastric emptying through the pylorus, resulting in disturbances in the timing of emptying of gas, liquid, and chyme into the intestine, and (3) alterations in emptying of bile into the duodenum. The latter set of disturbances is particularly intriguing. Studies performed by Allen and associates have indicated that patients with postvagotomy diarrhea have higher levels of fecal bile acids than do control patients.[18,19] Furthermore, oral cholestyramine, an agent that binds bile acids intraluminally, significantly reduces stool volumes in patients with postvagotomy diarrhea.[19]

In most patients, symptoms improve over the course of 6 months to 1 year. In perhaps 1% to 2% of patients, the diarrhea is disabling.[17] The diarrhea is characterized by frequent watery stools, often explosive and nocturnal. Meals are not necessarily provocative of such episodes. The medical management of this symptom would include simple dietary changes, including an increase in dietary fiber and decreasing dietary lactose intake. Opiates and, in difficult cases,

cholestyramine are useful in reducing frequency and severity of episodes. Octreotide, the long-acting somatostatin analogue, has not been consistently beneficial.[20] In some cases, it may be detrimental, owing to inhibition of pancreatic exocrine function with resulting malabsorption.

In cases refractory to medical management, the goal of surgical therapy is to reduce intestinal transit times. The recommended procedure (Fig 32–1) is construction of a 10 to 15 cm antiperistaltic jejunal loop, interposed 100 cm to the ligament of Treitz (or gastrojejunostomy, if the prior procedure involved a Bill-

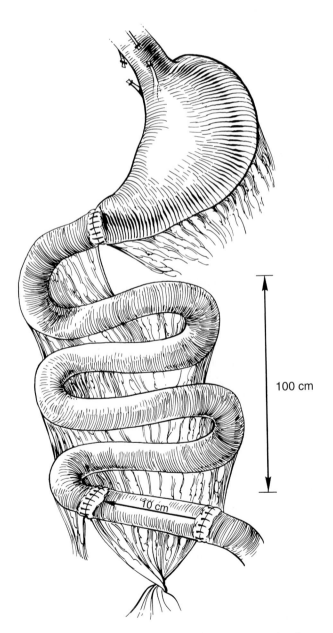

100 cm

10 cm

Figure 32–1. Remedial operation for postvagotomy diarrhea. (Redrawn from Sawyers JL. Management of postgastrectomy syndromes. *Am J Surg* 1990;159:8)

roth II reconstruction). In one recent series of 19 patients with severe symptoms refractory to medical management, 14 of these procedures achieved good or excellent results. The overall experience, however, has not been as encouraging. Cuschieri[21] recently described good results with an operation devised originally by Sadowski in experimental studies in dogs. The procedure involves extraction of a 10 cm segment of the terminal ileum, located 20 to 30 cm from the ileocecal valve. Ileal continuity is restored by end-to-end anastomosis. The ileal segment is opened along its antimesenteric border, rotated to an antiperistaltic position, and sutured as an onlay just proximal to the anastomosis. This operation appears to have promise for patients in whom the reversed jejunal segment would not be feasible.

Postvagotomy Reflux Esophagitis

This complication should be extremely rare. It has been described as occurring when an inexperienced surgeon, in mobilizing the vagi, causes injury to the right crura and attachments of the gastroesophageal junction. The duodenogastric reflux, caused by the drainage procedure accompanying the vagotomy, and the loss of lower esophageal sphincter function act in concert to promote reflux and stricturing at the gastroesophageal junction.

Postvagotomy cholelithiasis

While some controversy remains, it is generally accepted that vagotomy predisposes to the development of gallstones. The effects of vagotomy on biliary tract motility and bile composition are under active investigation. However, there is clinical evidence to suggest that the hepatic branches of the anterior vagal trunk play a role in regulating gallbladder motility and preventing stone formation. Ihasz and Griffith studied 53 patients who had undergone **selective** vagotomy and pyloroplasty.[22] As assessed by preoperative and postoperative oral cholecystography, there were no alterations in gallbladder size or emptying function, and gallstones were found in 2 patients. In a comparison group of 91 patients who had undergone **truncal** vagotomy, the gallbladder was distended in 46; of these 46, the gallbladder emptied poorly in 30, and 9 patients had gallstones. In the remaining 45 patients, gallbladder size and emptying were normal and gallstones were found in 1 patient. Some, but not all, clinical studies of patients who have undergone TV have demonstrated increases in gallbladder size under resting conditions and documented close to two-fold increases in the expected incidence of gallstones.[22,23] The indications for surgery are symptoms of biliary colic or complications such as cholecystitis, choledocholithiasis, cholangitis, or pancreatitis.

■ POSTGASTRECTOMY COMPLICATIONS

As discussed by Drs. Herrington and Sawyers in previous editions of this chapter, complications after operations on the stomach and duodenum may be divided into two categories: (1) those occurring in the early postoperative period and related to pathologic anatomy and to operative misadventures (Table 32–3), and (2) long-term sequelae arising from physiological alterations caused by the operation (Table 32–4). Also included in this latter category are chronic obstructive problems in different regions of the upper gastrointestinal tract that are involved in the reconstruction when the stomach is removed.

EARLY POSTGASTRECTOMY COMPLICATIONS

Bleeding

Intragastric Bleeding. Intraluminal blood loss is observed frequently following gastric resection. Bloody aspirates in the nasogastric tube usually resolve within 24 to 48 hours and are rarely a cause for significant decreases in circulating blood volume. Gross and continuous bleeding can occur, however, and arises from blood vessels in the anastomosis. When gastric resection has been performed for a bleeding duodenal ulcer, the ulcer bed itself may be responsible for such postoperative bleeding. Reoperation for persistent bleeding should be considered in such cases of persistent bleeding, especially

TABLE 32–3. COMPLICATIONS OF GASTRECTOMY IN THE PERIOPERATIVE PERIOD

Bleeding
    Intragastric
    Intraperitoneal
Gastrointestinal leaks
    Duodenal stump
    Gastroduodenostomy
    Gastroenterostomy
    Pyloroplasty
Obstruction
    Gastroduodenostomy
    Gastroenterostomy
    Afferent jejunal loop
    Efferent jejunal loop
Hepatobiliary pancreatic
    Jaundice
    Pancreatitis
    Common Bile Duct Injury
Miscellaneous
    Intraperitoneal Abscess
    Omental Infarction
    Gastrostomy complications
    Necrosis of gastric remnant
    Inadvertent gastroileostomy

TABLE 32–4. LATE POSTGASTRECTOMY DISTURBANCES

Syndromes of Ulcer Recurrence
    Recurrent ulcer
    Gastrojejunocolic fistula
Mechanical Disorders
    Chronic afferent loop obstruction
    Chronic efferent loop obstruction
    Internal hernia
    Jejunogastric intussusception
    Late gastroduodenal obstruction
Pathophysiologic Disorders
    Blind loop syndrome
    Postvagotomy diarrhea
    Alkaline reflux gastritis
    Early dumping syndrome
    Late dumping syndrome
    Gastric atony
    Roux stasis
Malabsorption and Nutritional Disturbances
Miscellaneous Complications
    Bezoar formation
    Small gastric remnant
    Carcinoma of the gastric remnant

has been used, it is not unreasonable to consider conversion to a Billroth II gastrojejunostomy. Theoretically, taking the ulcer out of the stream of chyme should reduce risk of bleeding and may promote healing. The timing of such a reoperation is a matter of judgement. Consideration to reoperation should be given, if the quantity of bleeding exceeds three units.

Intraperitoneal Bleeding. Postoperative intraperitoneal bleeding following gastrectomy may be the result of operative injury to different organs. Bleeding most commonly is observed from omental vessels that may have been controlled inadequately or from injuries to the spleen caused by instruments or traction. Traction on the liver can also be a source of bleeding complications. Infrequent sources of bleeding are inadequately ligated gastric or gastroepiploic vessels. Occasionally, vessels located just below the diaphragm have been injured during the vagotomy and will be a source of bleeding. As above, the decision to reoperate should be made expeditiously, based on clinical signs such as increased pulse,

when the initial surgery has been performed only within the last 2 or 3 days. If the bleeding occurs more than 5 or 6 days following the initial operation, endoscopy and endoscopically applied coagulation or injection of epinephrine may be effective. However, an endoscopic approach should be undertaken only by the most experienced endoscopists, with special attention to avoiding overinsufflation of a fresh anastomosis. In most cases, an operative approach will be safer.

If surgery is required to stop persistent bleeding, the gastric remnant is entered through a transverse incision, several centimeters above the anastomosis (gastroduodenostomy or gastrojejunostomy). Clots are evacuated and the gastric pouch irrigated with saline solution. The bleeding site usually is visualized as a pumping arteriole on the gastric side of the anastomosis, often located on the side of the lesser curvature. A figure-of-eight suture (2-0) will provide control of the bleeding.

If the source of the bleeding is a postbulbar duodenal ulcer that was actively bleeding before the surgery, access can be gained to the site by use of an anterior duodenotomy placed beyond the Billroth I anastomosis. The ulcer crater is obliterated using 2-0 silk figure-of-eight sutures. If the ulcer is located adjacent to a Billroth I anastomosis, it is usually necessary to take down the anastomosis and securely transfix the ulcer bed with figure-of-eight sutures. If, despite these maneuvers, bleeding cannot be controlled, the gastroduodenal ulcer should be isolated and ligated, above and below the duodenum (Fig 32–2). When a Billroth I reconstruction

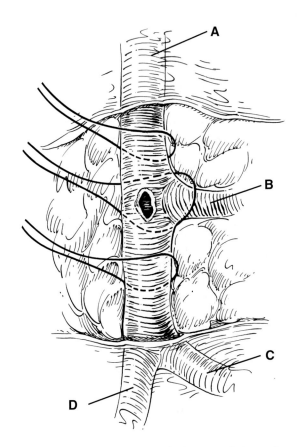

Figure 32–2. Proper suture ligation of gastroduodenal artery complex in posterior penetrating duodenal ulcer. Branches of the complex are A: gastroduodenal; B: transverse pancreatic; C: right gastroepiploic; D: superior pancreaticoduodenal. (Redrawn from Berne CJ, Rosoff L. Peptic ulcer perforation of the gastroduodenal artery complex. *Ann Surg* 1969;169:143)

lowered blood pressure, and abdominal distention. Hypotension and evidence of shock mandate early exploration. The exploration of the operated area should be systematic, including spleen, short gastric vessels, liver, diaphragm, lesser sac, omentum, gastric and gastroepiploic vessels. Splenic salvage may be considered in selected cases in which small lacerations of fractures are responsible for bleeding. If deep or multiple areas of injury are present or if the patient is in shock, total splenectomy is safest.

Suture Line Leaks

Duodenal Stump. Leakage of a duodenal stump following gastrectomy and Billroth II reconstruction is serious. If not recognized and managed expeditiously, it can be life threatening. This complication occurs in 1% to 4% of patients undergoing Billroth II anastomosis.[24] The mortality rate associated with this complication has decreased markedly, from >50% in the 1950s, to about 10% in the 1960s and 1970s, to <5% currently.[24] Although the complication is not always avoidable, certain patients may be at higher risk for it than others. Such patients would include those with extensive inflammation surrounding the pylorus and duodenal bulb. However, in some patients, the extent of inflammation and scarring may not be appreciated until the patient has been committed to gastrectomy by division of the stomach or even until the duodenum has been transected. The difficult duodenum has been discussed in the previous chapter. When the duodenum cannot be closed without significant tension, the closure may be performed around a soft red rubber catheter (Fig 32–3a) as recommended by Welch and Rodkey.[25,26] When the closure comes together without too much tension, but seems insecure due to surrounding inflammation or to incapability of the tissues to hold sutures or staples, the closure can be reinforced by bringing up a tongue of omentum. In this setting, one approach for decompression of the duodenal stump and afferent limb is the placement of a lateral duodenostomy (Fig 32–3b). In this case, our preference is to use a 16 Fr T tube. It should be emphasized that the indications for "end" duodenostomy are not strictly comparable to those for lateral duodenostomy: the former is used when the stump cannot be closed and the latter is used when the stump can be closed but, for other reasons, the closure seems insecure. Alternatives for management of the difficult duodenum are discussed in the previous chapter. In many cases, the duodenum made "difficult" by scarring owing to acid-peptic disease can be recognized before a commitment has been made a gastrectomy. In these cases, vagotomy and gastroenterostomy may be the safest alternative.

A duodenal stump leak often occurs when a large

(2.5 cm) ulcer has deeply penetrated the posterior wall of the duodenum. Typically, the relationships of the duodenum, pancreas, and bile duct have been distorted by inflammation and scarring. Other factors implicated in the occurrence of such leaks are (1) excessive use of suture, leading to devascularization of the stump, (2) localized infection due to accumulation of hematoma or fluid, (3) post-operative pancreatitis, and (5) obstruction of the afferent loop (Fig 32–4). Breakdown usually occurs between postoperative days 2 and 5. The dominant symptom is pain, associated with high fever and shock. In some cases, a subtler clinical picture develops over several days. Pain, fever, and leukocytosis are mild; jaundice may develop. A duodenal leak can be demonstrated by aspiration of biliary content in a right upper quadrant fluid collection, which is visualized by computerized tomography (CT) or ultrasound. A dynamic mode for imaging such leaks is the technetium 99m (^{99m}TC)-labeled HIDA scan.

Treatment consists of prompt and adequate closed-suction drainage of the right upper quadrant. Small and localized fluid collections presenting with mild symptoms may be managed successfully by percutaneous, radiologist-guided approaches for drainage. In cases where the fluid collection is large or poorly contained, operative drainage is safest. It is uncommon to be able to close such leaks primarily. In addition to closed-suction drains, effective decompression of the stomach is required and placement of a feeding jejunostomy in the efferent limb is recommended. The goal is to create a controlled fistula to the skin and prevent stimulation of biliary and pancreatic secretions by food/chyme passing through the stomach. Broad-spectrum antibiotics usually are required until the fluid collection is fully drained and fever and signs of sepsis have abated. Follow-up CT scans are helpful in assessing the effectiveness of drainage.

Use of somatostatin and its long-acting analogue, octreotide, deserves special mention in this setting. A number of anecdotal reports and prospective studies, some randomized, have demonstrated that octreotide can significantly reduce output from enterocutaneous fistulas.[27–30] These reports have rarely included patients with duodenal stump leak, but have included those with fistulas arising from upper GI tract sources (gastric, pancreatic, biliary). The overall improvements in care have been related to decreases in fistula output and, possibly, earlier closure of fistulas. The actual rate of spontaneous closure does not seem to be influenced by administration of the drug. Higher output fistulas (>500cc/day) are not necessarily less responsive to octreotide.[31] Failure of fistulas to close is more often associated with infection in the tract, inadequate drainage, presence of foreign bodies, or distal obstruction. Thus, although not uniformly endorsed, the use of octreotide

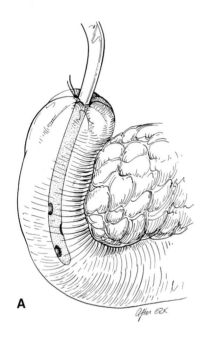

A

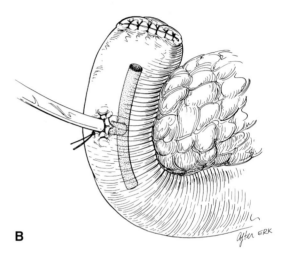

B

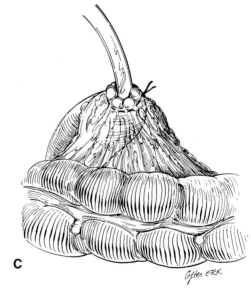

C

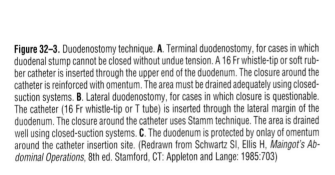

Figure 32–3. Duodenostomy technique. **A**. Terminal duodenostomy, for cases in which duodenal stump cannot be closed without undue tension. A 16 Fr whistle-tip or soft rubber catheter is inserted through the upper end of the duodenum. The closure around the catheter is reinforced with omentum. The area must be drained adequately using closed-suction systems. **B**. Lateral duodenostomy, for cases in which closure is questionable. The catheter (16 Fr whistle-tip or T tube) is inserted through the lateral margin of the duodenum. The closure around the catheter uses Stamm technique. The area is drained well using closed-suction systems. **C**. The duodenum is protected by onlay of omentum around the catheter insertion site. (Redrawn from Schwartz SI, Ellis H, *Maingot's Abdominal Operations*, 8th ed. Stamford, CT: Appleton and Lange: 1985:703)

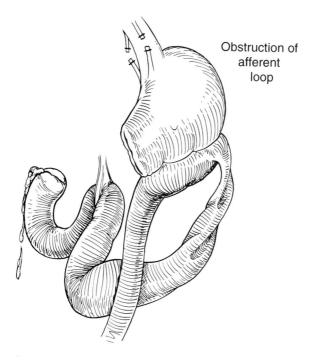

Obstruction of afferent loop

Other Causes of Stump Leakage

1. Severe disease of duodenal bulb
2. Excessive suture closure of stump
3. Bleeding about pancreatic bed
4. Post operative pancreatitis
5. Localized infection and sepsis

Figure 32–4. Causes of leakage from the duodenal stump after Billroth II reconstruction.

has been associated with more rapid resolution of upper gastrointestinal (GI) tract fistulas. Starting with 50 mcg given subcutaneously every 8 hours, dose can be increased to 200 mcg, if necessary. Immediate responses in the first 48 hours after starting the drug have been associated with high rates (>70%) of spontaneous resolution. Anecdotal reports, and our own experience, have suggested that the drug is useful in reducing fistula output following duodenal stump blow-out as well.

Billroth I Gastroduodenostomy. Such leaks are more likely to occur when the anastomosis is performed in the presence of severe scarring and inflammation of the duodenum. In patients properly selected for a Billroth I reconstruction, the complication should be rare. When they occur, such leaks present with moderate or mild symptoms, fever, and leukocytosis. In some cases, the first manifestation is leakage of bile-stained fluid through the upper portion of the incision. The fistula often is localized in the upper abdomen and does not always require reoperation. Expectant management includes (1) search for and control of exacerbating fac-

tors such as distal obstruction, (2) serial evaluation of the fluid cavity by CT scan, (3) antibiotics until drainage is well established and signs of sepsis are resolved, (4) intravenous hyperalimentation, initially, with subsequent enteral alimentation provided by feeding catheters placed well beyond the anastomosis, and (5) use of octreotide.

The main indications for surgery are peritonitis, sepsis, or inability to control accumulation of fluid intraperitoneally. If reoperation becomes necessary, the anastomosis should be carefully inspected. A small rent may be reinforced with omental patch and wide drainage. A large disruption should be managed by conversion to a Billroth II or Roux-en-Y reconstruction. In these cases, closure of the duodenal stump can be reinforced with omentum. Placement of a lateral duodenostomy would not be unreasonable.

Billroth II Gastrojejunostomy. This complication is highly unusual. As above, small leaks may sometimes be managed expectantly. Uncontrolled leaks are managed operatively. If the anastomotic rent is small, it may be reinforced with omentum. If the leak is large, the anastomosis should be taken down and the gastric margin excised back to healthy tissue. A new gastrojejunostomy or Roux-en-Y reconstruction then is performed.

Obstruction Syndromes

Stomal Obstruction (Billroth I or Billroth II). Stomal obstruction in the early postoperative period is not uncommon following Billroth I, Billroth II, or Roux-en-Y reconstructions. The cause is usually edema of the anastomosis, although loss of vagal innervation may play a role. Such blockages can result in distention of the gastric remnant with food and fluid. In most cases, nasogastric suction and hydration through intravenous fluids will lead to resolution of the obstruction after several days.

Prolonged obstruction, as evidenced by failure of an endoscope or swallowed barium to pass through the stoma, most commonly reflects improper surgical technique. In some cases, the obstruction may result from extensive scarring of the duodenum and reflect poor judgement in having chosen a Billroth I reconstruction. When prolonged obstruction follows a Billroth II reconstruction, the cause may be inflammatory adhesions causing the efferent loop to kink just below the anastomosis. Very rarely, both the afferent and efferent loops, or the stoma itself, can be distorted by such adhesions. Extensive fat necrosis, inflamed omentum, pancreatitis, postoperative bleeding, or anastomotic leak also may contribute to prolonged obstruction of the stoma.

In general, the patient can begin to tolerate oral feedings between postoperative days 3 and 6. If the initial attempts to eat result in nausea, bloating and vomiting, the nasogastric tube is reinserted and decompression is carried out for several days. A barium study can be performed as early as postoperative day 7, unless there are concerns of anastomotic leak. Poor emptying of the contrast material will mandate continued nasogastric suction and intravenous fluids. Sometimes, a small-bore feeding tube can be passed under fluoroscopy in order to initiate enteral feeding. If not, parenteral nutrition is indicated.

Patients with prolonged obstruction symptoms may require reoperation. It is uncommon for such anastomoses to be amenable to endoscopic or operative dilatation. If a Billroth I reconstruction is involved, the anastomosis should not simply be revised. However, attempts to take the anastomosis down and simply oversew the duodenal stump carries an appreciable risk for devascularization and stump leak. Perhaps the safest alternative is to leave the anastomosis intact and to perform an antecolic side-to-side gastrojejunostomy along the distal greater curvature of the gastric remnant.

If a Billroth II reconstruction is involved, the operative findings will dictate the solution to the problem of obstruction. If the stoma or efferent limb are kinked by adhesions, it may suffice to lyse the adhesions. Under these circumstances, a feeding jejunostomy is recommended. If either the afferent or efferent limbs are found to be herniating into the lesser sac (Fig 32–5), they are reduced and sutured to parietal peritoneum to prevent reherniation. Occasionally, such loops may be

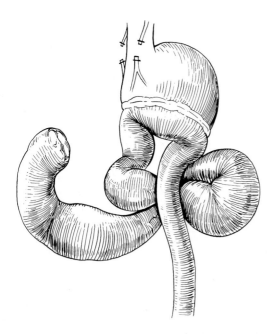

Figure 32–5. Herniation of the afferent jejunal limb posteriorly behind the efferent limb of a Billroth II reconstruction. (Redrawn from Schwartz SI, Ellis H. *Maingot's Abdominal Operations*, 9th ed. Stamford, CT: Appleton and Lange; 1989:710)

found to be nonviable and should be resected or distortion of the anastomosis owing to its positioning will suggest that it be revised and placed more proximally on the gastric remnant.

Acute Afferent Loop Obstruction. Afferent limb obstructions have generally been attributed to use of excessive length of the limb in constructing a gastrojejunostomy. The cause of the obstruction may be adhesions, twisting, internal herniation, volvulus, or kinking at the angle formed with the gastric remnant. Acute obstruction of the limb is implicated as a factor predisposing to duodenal stump leak. Recognition of the latter complication should prompt a search for the former.

Afferent limb obstruction is essentially a closed-loop obstruction. Bile and pancreatic secretions accumulate within the loop, permitting pressures within the loop, and ultimately the pancreatic duct, to rise. The obstruction leads to abdominal pain out of proportion to physical findings. Serum alkaline phosphatase levels may be elevated and the amylase and lipase levels also rise, mimicking pancreatitis. If the obstruction is unrelieved, tachycardia, leukocytosis, fever, and localized tenderness or peritoneal findings will ensue. Shock may develop. If there is any doubt about the diagnosis, ultrasound and CT scan are useful in delineating the obstructed afferent limb and excluding pancreatitis.[32,33] Endoscopy is not helpful in this setting. If the diagnosis is otherwise obvious, the abdomen should be explored after appropriate resuscitation.

Management at the time of exploration depends on the operative findings. Often, the patient is unstable. If the bowel is viable, and the cause of the obstruction is twisting or kinking, the most expeditious maneuver may be to decompress the obstructed limb through a side-to-side enterostomy with the efferent limb below the gastrojejunostomy. If volvulus or intussusception are found, the loop can be shortened or divided and anastomosed distally to create a Roux-en-Y configuration. All mesenteric defects must be closed. If gangrene is present in the distal duodenum and jejunum, it may be possible to resect the nonviable bowel and perform a duodenojejunostomy to a Roux limb. If the second and third portions of the duodenum are not viable, it probably will be impossible to avoid pancreaticoduodenectomy (Fig 32–6).

Hepatobiliary-Pancreatic Complications

Post-Operative Pancreatitis. Precise estimates of the incidence of this complication following gastrectomy are not available, but it is almost certainly <5%. Most cases result from operative trauma to the head or proximal body of the pancreas. The two circumstances in which such trauma are likely to arise are (1) in close dissection

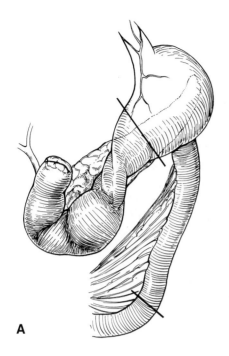

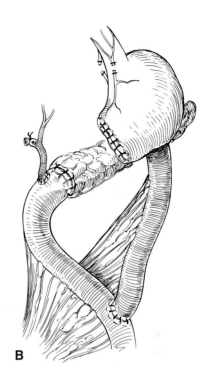

A

B

Figure 32–6. Torsion of the afferent jejunal limb producing limb necrosis. This may require pancreaticoduodenal resection. (Redrawn from Schwartz SI, Ellis H. *Maingot's Abdominal Operations*, 9th ed. Stamford, CT: Appleton and Lange; 1989:710)

of the head of the pancreas away from the duodenum, so that the latter can be closed, and (2) in the dissection of the posterior duodenal wall away from a large posteriorly penetrating ulcer crater. In this second circumstance, the pancreas usually forms the base of the ulcer crater and injury can occur to the ductal system of the pancreas. Extensive dissection can result in injury to the duct of Santorini, which constitutes the main duct in 5% of cases (pancreas divisum). Although not specifically studied for use in this setting, octreotide has been shown to reduce morbidity following pancreatic surgery or operative injury.[35,36] Given the potentially devastating consequences of pancreatitis following gastrectomy, it seems reasonable to use octreotide in the postoperative period when pancreatic substance or one of the ducts may have been injured.

An episode of pancreatitis may become manifest within the first 3 days after surgery. The presentation may be acute, including symptoms of restlessness and abdominal pain and signs of tenderness, fever, and leukocytosis, and the serum amylase and lipase will become elevated. When a Billroth II reconstruction has been performed, obstruction of the afferent loop may be an important consideration of the differential diagnosis. The importance of the distinction is that pancreatitis initially should be managed expectantly and its morbidity could be exacerbated by early operation. In contrast, an acute afferent loop obstruction is a surgical

emergency and should be operated on as soon as possible. Thus, emergency ultrasound or, preferably, CT scan should be performed to make the distinction and guide therapy. When a Billroth I reconstruction has been performed, the clinical picture points to pancreatitis.

Management consists of resuscitation, nasogastric decompression, and other general measures used in the management of acute pancreatitis. If more than three Ranson criteria are present, indicating a high likelihood of complications, broad-spectrum antibiotics are recommended. It should be noted that the value of antibiotics are difficult to establish in this specific setting. Following a severe episode of acute pancreatitis, it may be necessary to follow-up with serial CT examinations (see Chapter 7). It may also be necessary to operatively drain infected fluid collections or abscesses. However, this could lead to persistent pancreaticocutaneous fistula. Persistence of such fistulas may necessitate surgical interventions, including excision of the tract, use of Roux-en-Y diversion, or partial pancreatectomy.

Postoperative Jaundice. It is not unusual to observe mild jaundice in the early postoperative period following gastrectomy, particularly if the duodenum is severely diseased. Postoperative edema in this area can lead to partial obstruction of the common bile duct. In this setting, hyperbilirubinemia is mild and resolves quickly. Other causes of jaundice in this setting include (1) anastomotic leak and reabsorption of bile from the peritoneum, (2) biliary calculi, (3) acute pancreatitis, or (4) injury to the extrahepatic biliary ducts.

Injury to Bile Duct or Pancreatic Duct. This complication is rare, but occurs when dissecting a duodenum that has been shortened and distorted by scarring. It is not always necessary to expose the common bile duct during a dissection of the distal stomach. However, when such scarring is present, it is safe practice to perform a generous Kocher maneuver and to open the hepatoduodenal ligament in order to fully expose the distal common bile duct. When anatomy is severely distorted, passage of a T tube or red rubber catheter via a choledochotomy will serve as a reference for the common duct, preventing inadvertent ligation or transection. Alternatively, a silastic catheter can be placed via the common duct, exiting through the liver to provide a biliary stent in the postoperative period. Occasionally, an unexpected choledochoduodenal fistula will be discovered when the cholangiogram is performed.

If the common bile duct is injured during dissection, management depends on the type of injury. If the duct is transected cleanly and there has been relatively little dissection of surrounding tissues, the blood supply may be adequate to support an end-to-end anastomosis of the transected ends. A T tube should be placed via a separate longitudinal choledochotomy and its distal end placed through the anastomosis as a stent. If there are any doubts about the blood supply to the duct, a safer reconstruction would be an end-to-side choledochoduodenostomy or choledochojejunostomy to a Roux limb.

As noted above, in the course of dissecting a deep penetrating ulcer from the head of the pancreas, the duct of Santorini may be encountered. In this circumstance, the duodenum is extensively mobilized and advanced to cover the ulcer bed (Fig 32–7). The ends of the open duodenum are sutured to the surrounding pancreas, which is usually quite firm and capable of holding sutures, owing to chronic inflammation. The area is drained well, using closed-suction drainage. It is not unreasonable to administer octreotide postoperatively in this setting.

One rare but devastating complication is the disruption of the ampulla of Vater, separating it partially or completely from the head of the pancreas and pancreatic ductal system.[37] Again, the complication occurs because of severe shortening and distortion of the duodenum due to scarring. In this setting, the general principles of management would include (Fig 32–8) (1) bringing up a Roux limb of jejunum to suture to the head of the pancreas, incorporating the pancreatic portion of the bile duct and main pancreatic duct, (2) T tube stenting of the biliary duct and, if possible, stent-

ing of the pancreatic tube using a pediatric feeding tube, and (3) wide drainage. It may be helpful to tack the Roux limb to the anterior abdominal wall, in case an interventional radiologist requires access to the anastomoses in the future. A resection of the pancreatic head and duodenum is probably not necessary unless the avulsion was accompanied by extensive tissue damage.

Miscellaneous Complications

Necrosis of the Gastric Remnant. Ischemic necrosis of the gastric remnant is a rare complication of gastric resection. It is most likely to occur if, in the course of the operation, the left gastric artery has been divided close to its origin and if a splenectomy has been performed. In this setting, the blood supply to the gastric remnant depends on inconstant phrenic arterial branches. Ischemic necrosis also can occur following highly selective vagotomy with antrectomy, a procedure not commonly performed. In this setting, the left gastric artery has been detached during the vagotomy and the blood supply of the gastric remnant depends on the splenic artery. If the spleen is absent or injured during the procedure, a near total gastrectomy should be performed in order to avoid ischemic necrosis.

The symptoms of such necrosis are severe abdominal pain and shock-like presentation that develop within 24 to 72 hours after the initial operation. Injection of the nasogastric tube using water soluble contrast will reveal the leak, and the patient should be brought to surgery immediately. If a viable cuff of gastric tissue is present, a side-to-end anastomosis is performed to a Roux-en-Y limb of jejunum. If not, a total gastrectomy with Roux-en-Y reconstruction is performed. If the necrosis extends to the distal esophagus and the inflammatory reaction in the area is intense, it may be necessary to ligate the distal esophagus or perform tube drainage. A cervical esophagostomy is performed and a feeding jejunostomy placed. If the patient survives, a subsequent reconstruction can be performed with an esophagojejunostomy or a colonic interposition (Fig 32–9).

Gastrostomy Complications. Although not performed as commonly as before, gastrostomy tubes are occasionally used in the management of patients who would not tolerate nasogastric suction or who have severe pulmonary dysfunction, esophageal reflux, or motility disorders. Attention to technique will avoid complications such as bleeding, separation of the stomach from the abdominal wall, placement of the tube into the transverse colon, or leakage with peritonitis. Attention must be given to the method by which the tube is secured to the abdominal wall or the tube may migrate and obstruct the pylorus. Also, attention must be given to care of the tube insertion site, since the breakdown of skin and the

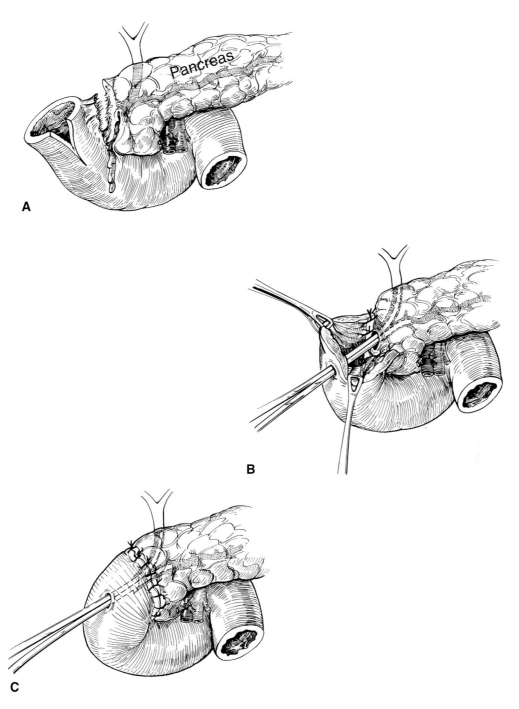

Figure 32–7. The opened duodenum is mobilized, the posterior wall spatulated, and the duodenum is advanced and sutured over the area of injury to the biliary/pancreatic ducts. External drainage is achieved with closed-suction systems. (Redrawn from Schwartz SI, Ellis H. *Maingot's Abdominal Operations,* 9th ed. Stamford, CT: Appleton and Lange; 1989:715)

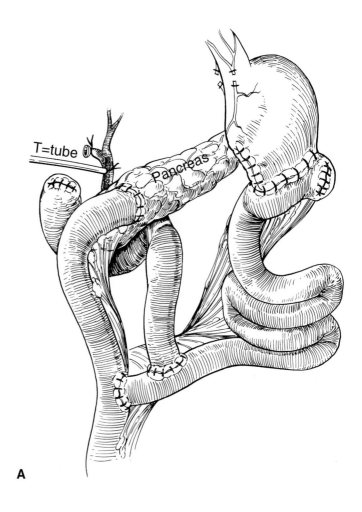

A

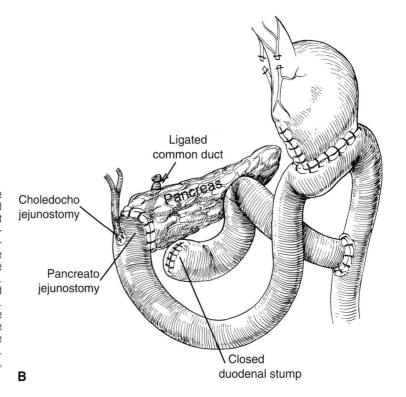

Figure 32–8. Alternatives in managing ampullary disruption. **A**. The jejunal segment leading from the closed duodenal stump is divided several cm beyond the ligament of Treitz. The distal jejunal segment then is anastomosed end-to-side to the gastric remnant. Approximately 60 cm distal to the gastrojejunostomy the bowel is again divided and the distal divided end is anastomosed to the head of the pancreas, incorporating the injured pancreatic duct. Two separate end-to-side jejunojejunostomies are required to restore continuity. **B**. Alternatively, the jejunum is divided beyond the ligament of Treitz and the distal divided end of jejunum is anastomosed to the injured area. A gastrojejunostomy is carried out distal to this anastomosis and the short afferent jejunal segment is anastomosed end-to-side to restore continuity. In both cases, the area is drained well. A decompressive tube gastrostomy and tube feeding jejunostomy are both well advised. (Redrawn from Schwartz SI, Ellis H. *Maingot's Abdominal Operations*, 9th ed. Stamford, CT: Appleton and Lange 1989:713–714)

B

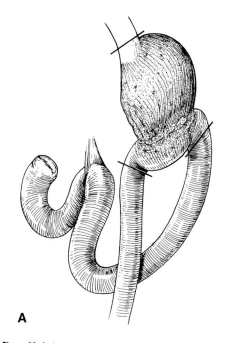

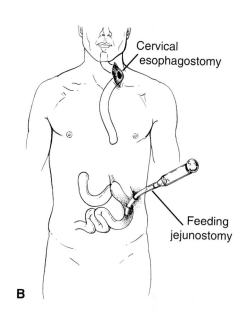

Figure 32–9. Approach in case of necrosis of the entire gastric remnant following Billroth II reconstruction. The gastric remnant is resected. Esophagostomy and tube feeding jejunostomy are performed. Restoration of continuity is performed at a later date. (Redrawn from Schwartz SI, Ellis H. *Maingot's Abdominal Operations,* 9th ed. Stamford, CT: Appleton and Lange; 1989:708)

widening of the tract may contribute to the failure of the site to heal when the gastrostomy tube has finally been removed.

Inadvertent Gastroileostomy.
This complication is not as rare as might be thought. The complication occurs because of inadequate exposure, the surgeon's haste, and failure to consider the possibility of mistaking ileum for more proximal jejunum. The symptoms are sometimes subtle and may not develop until postoperative week 2. In most cases, however, a problem is obvious as soon as the patient begins to eat. Foul eructation and profuse diarrhea with electrolyte disturbance occur, leading rapidly to malnutrition and weight loss. The diagnosis is made by barium swallow and upper GI series. Management consists of reoperation, takedown, and gastrojejunostomy (Billroth II or Roux-en-Y reconstruction).

Omental Infarction.
This is a rare complication, occurring when omentum incarcerates and strangulates in the retroanastomotic space or other internal traps. The symptoms are sudden pain and evolution of local tenderness, fever, and leukocytosis in 1 to 3 days. The evolution of symptoms and signs is not unlike that of appendicitis. Exploration of the abdomen usually is undertaken as the result of the fear of a more serious postoperative complication.

Intra-Abdominal Abscess.
This complication is not rare, but seems to occur more commonly after total gastrectomy for carcinoma. Spillage of colonized luminal contents may be responsible, although leakage from the esophagojejunal anastomosis usually is involved. The symptoms are those of gradually worsening upper abdominal pain and tenderness, anorexia, fever, and leukocytosis. The abscess is readily imaged by CT and drained under CT guidance. A severely loculated collection, interloop, or multiple abscesses should be drained surgically. Closed-suction drains are usually adequate. Pleural effusion is not uncommon as a sympathetic response to a subphrenic abscess. One technique for obtaining extraperitoneal access to a subphrenic cavity involves resection of the twelfth rib, with entry into the cavity.

LATE POSTGASTRECTOMY COMPLICATIONS

Syndromes of Ulcer Recurrence

Stomal Ulceration/Recurrent Ulcer.
It is highly unusual to encounter recurrence of type I gastric ulcer disease following gastrectomy. Except in rare situations (such as a Kelling-Madlener procedure for bleeding from a highlying gastric ulcer) the ulcer, and the area of increased ulcer susceptibility are excised with the distal stomach. In contrast, recurrence is a well-recognized consequence of any procedure performed for duodenal ulcer-

ation that includes vagotomy and drainage, or partial gastrectomy with Billroth I reconstruction. Although duodenal ulcers can recur following vagotomy, antrectomy, and Billroth II reconstruction, a recurrence in the duodenum is most unusual (see Chapter 30). Ulceration at the gastrojejunal anastomosis, however, can occur on either the gastric side or the jejunal margins of the stoma. Recurrence rates associated with each of the standard procedures are discussed in foregoing chapters. Table 32–5 lists contributing factors to postoperative duodenal ulcer recurrence and their management. The most common cause for recurrent peptic ulceration has been attributed to an incompletely performed vagotomy. Other contributing factors include (1) retained antrum following Billroth II reconstruction, (2) G-cell hyperplasia, gastrinoma with or without an associated syndrome of multiple endocrine neoplasia, (3) gastric stasis, and (4) regular or recent increase in use of nonsteroidal antiinflammatory agents. Occasionally, recurrence of peptic ulceration and bleeding can be induced by portal-caval shunting.

Previously, recurrence of a duodenal ulcer after a definitive operation was managed by proceeding to a more definitive procedure. Thus, if the patient had undergone a vagotomy alone, the vagi were reapproached and an antrectomy was performed. If the patient had undergone vagotomy and antrectomy, it was assumed that the vagi had been incompletely severed and completion vagotomy was attempted. A transthoracic approach might be attempted in this setting. If recurrence could not be controlled, total gastrectomy with Roux-en-Y reconstruction was performed. In each case, acid secretion and serum gastrin levels were evaluated in order to

exclude the possibility of gastrinoma, retained antrum, or G-cell hyperplasia.

The optimal approach for managing recurrent duodenal ulcers is not clear-cut. The approach depends on the original indications for surgery, the original procedure performed, and the way in which the recurrence presents. If perforation or bleeding refractory to medical management are present, surgery has to be performed to close the perforation or to stop the bleeding. The approach will then be similar to that outlined above.

The availability of powerful antisecretory medications has decreased the need to reoperate because of recurrent pain that is persistent or refractory to medical management. In such cases, the first step is endoscopy to confirm the recurrence. The next step should be exclusion of hypergastrinemia. For such evaluations, all antisecretory medications (histamine H2 receptor blockers or omeprazole) must have been discontinued for at least 24 hours. The literature does not support the routine use of acid-secretion studies in order to support the diagnosis of hyperchlorhydric hypergastrinemia.[38,39] All antisecretory operations and medications cause elevations of serum gastrin, but rarely above 200 or 300 pg/mL. In contrast, any serum gastrin level above 1000 pg/mL is diagnostic for gastrinoma or retained antrum. Between these two ranges, provocative testing using intravenous infusion of calcium/secretin may be indicated.[40] A rise in serum gastrin of at least 100 pg/mL after infusion of 2 U/kg of secretin is diagnostic of Zollinger-Ellison syndrome. Although secretin can elicit increases of serum gastrin levels in normal individuals and those with G-cell hyperplasia or retained antrum, the observed rise is rarely above 40 pg/mL. When such nonphysiologic hypergastrinemia has been documented in response to stimulation, a number of imaging studies may be helpful. CT scan using intravenous contrast, magnetic resonance imaging (MRI), or endoscopic ultrasound will demonstrate a gastrinoma, if it is >1 cm in diameter. The possibility of a duodenal gastrinoma should always be kept in mind. If the gastrinoma is identified, the possibility of hyperparathyroidism should be investigated by measurement of serum calcium.

If the secretin test is negative, G-cell hyperplasia and retained antrum may have to be considered more strongly in the differential diagnosis. A standard high-protein meal may be useful in confirming a diagnosis of G-cell hyperplasia in patients with an intact gastric antrum. Such a meal usually stimulates increases in serum gastrin about 300% above baseline fasting levels.[41] Radionuclide scanning with ^{99m}Tc may be similarly useful for determining the presence of retained antral tissue that has been excluded from the stream of chyme by a Billroth II reconstruction. Gastric mucosa prefer-

TABLE 32–5. FACTORS CONTRIBUTING TO POSTOPERATIVE RECURRENCE OF DUODENAL ULCER

Factor	Approach to Management
Ulcerogenic drugs/smoking	Discontinue smoking/medications; measure salicylate levels in patients with postoperative gastric ulcers to exclude surreptitious abuse
Hypergastrinemia	
Zollinger-Ellison tumor	Surgery to remove tumor in pancreas or duodenum; total gastrectomy if disease is metastatic and ulcer diathesis not medically manageable
Retained antrum following Billroth II gastrectomy	Surgery to remove antral segment and revise duodenal stump
G-cell hyperplasia	Antrectomy
Hypercalcemia/Nyperparathyroidism	Parathyroidectomy
Gastric Outlet Obstruction	Dilatation or revision of gastric outlet
Incomplete vagotomy	Completion of vagotomy—transabdominal or thoracic approach.

entially takes up the radionuclide. The excluded antral tissue is localized in the epigastrium/right upper quadrant and can be detected 15 to 20 minutes after bolus intravenous injection of the ^{99m}Tc.[42]

With other factors excluded, the evaluation of postoperative duodenal ulcer recurrence focuses on the possibility that the previously performed vagotomy is not complete. Congo-red testing may be useful, as discussed in an earlier chapter.[39,43] The mainstay of evaluation should be acid secretion studies, if symptoms are refractory to medical management and reoperation is under strong consideration. Perhaps the best method for evaluating gastric acid secretion after vagotomy is to measure acid output under baseline conditions and during stimulation by a sham meal (SAO). After return of acid output to baseline levels, peak acid output (PAO) is measured in response to stimulation by maximal doses (12 μg/kg subcutaneously) of pentagastrin. If PAO secretion rates are above 2 mmol/hr, the ratio SAO:PAO of 0.1:1.0 can be used to confirm the completeness of vagotomy. Very low levels of PAO make the test unreliable, but also make an incomplete vagotomy unlikely.[39,43]

In cases where endoscopy confirms the presence of a recurrent ulcer, medical management usually will suffice to control symptoms. A number of studies have suggested that recurrences can be healed, in 80% of cases, by aggressive antisecretory management and that further recurrences can be prevented, in 70% of patients in this group, by maintenance therapy.[39] Omeprazole would be the medication of choice in this setting. It should be remembered that the long-term effects of maintenance therapy with omeprazole are not fully understood.[44]

With regard to surgical therapy in such cases, the procedure should be tailored to the circumstances. Before surgery, endoscopy should be performed to verify the location of the ulcer and witnessed, if not performed, by the surgeon. When hypergastrinemia and factors other than incomplete vagotomy have been excluded, acid secretion (SAO/PAO) studies should be performed to document a hypersecretory state. In addition, solid-phase radionuclide gastric emptying studies can document delayed gastric emptying and upper GI series should be performed to determine if there is associated deformity of the gastric outlet. A radionuclide-labeled HIDA scan may help to identify the presence of bile reflux.

If the patient has previously undergone vagotomy without antrectomy, then it is reasonable to perform an antrectomy and to approach the vagi again, using a supraceliac approach or transthoracic approach. If excessive morbidity may be anticipated from this approach and acid secretion studies have documented incomplete vagotomy, a transthoracic, possibly thoracoscopic, approach may be safer.[45] Mechanical deformity

and obstruction of the gastric outlet may contribute to postoperative recurrence, and should be corrected. However, correction of mechanical outlet problems without re-vagotomy or antrectomy is not likely to lead to permanent healing of the recurrence. If there is a reasonable likelihood that gastric motility is impaired, it is probably best to resect most of the stomach and leave a small gastric cuff.

The role of Roux-en-Y reconstruction in management of postoperative ulcer recurrence is not clear. As discussed below, alterations is gastric emptying can follow this reconstruction, leading to gastric stasis and the "Roux stasis" syndrome. This reconstruction will eliminate alkaline reflux into the gastric remnant, which may be documented preoperatively, as discussed above. In this case, construction of a Roux gastrojejunostomy is warranted. If there is any likelihood of gastric emptying disturbance in the preoperative work-up, it is prudent to generously re-resect the distal stomach, leaving only a small gastric remnant. The jejunal side of the Roux-en-Y reconstruction is highly susceptible to marginal ulceration. Great care should be taken to make sure the re-vagotomy is complete.[39,43]

Gastrojejunocolic Fistula. This complication has virtually disappeared. Previously, it complicated as many as 5% of cases in which simple gastrojejunostomy or inadequate gastric resections without vagotomy had been performed. Currently, the appearance of such a fistula following a definitive ulcer procedure should lead to a search for carcinoma or Crohn's disease. In the absence of such pathology, high levels of NSAID use also may be suspected. Anecdotal reports have suggested that some patients may take these medications surreptitiously and are not always willing to volunteer information regarding the extent of their use.[46] Levels of salicylates can be measured in most hospitals, but it may be difficult to test for metabolites of other medications. Nevertheless, documentation of such surreptitious use is important, in order to prevent recurring problems.

The symptoms are those of gastrocolic fistula: fecal vomiting, halitosis, weight loss, diarrhea.[47] Occasionally, such fistulas will present in association with other complications of ulcer disease, such as bleeding, perforation, or gastrointestinal obstruction. The diagnosis of fistula is made by barium contrast studies and CT scan. Upper and lower endoscopy are indicated to exclude other pathology. Surprisingly, upper endoscopy does not always permit visualization of the fistula, although the ulcer leading to it will be appreciated.

Initially, management consists of bowel rest, parenteral nutrition, administration of intravenous antibiotics and antisecretory agents (H2 blockers). Case reports suggest that some of these fistulas may heal with expectant management; most will require surgery. A full preoperative bowel preparation should be performed. If the fistula develops following gastrojejunostomy alone, the recommended procedure is vagotomy, hemigastrectomy, and Billroth II reconstruction. A limited colectomy as part of the en bloc resection is usually the most prudent way to handle the colon. Although carcinoma may have been undetected in the preoperative evaluation, it cannot be totally excluded until the fistula has been removed. If the fistula has resulted from inadequate gastrectomy without vagotomy, a vagotomy now is performed with more generous removal of the gastric remnant en bloc with the colon. If a vagotomy and antrectomy have previously been performed, it may be best to perform a subtotal gastrectomy en bloc with the colon and Roux-en-Y reconstruction.

Mechanical Disorders

Chronic Afferent Loop Obstruction. The chronic afferent loop syndrome implies a chronic obstruction of afferent loop emptying into the efferent limb. It usually occurs after Billroth II reconstruction when the afferent loop is unusually long. As discussed earlier, longer afferent limbs are predisposed to kinking, twisting, or volvulus. The obstruction is low grade, causing symptoms as the loop distends with bile and duodenal secretions. When intraluminal pressures within the loop become high enough, the obstruction is released, forcing the accumulated secretions into the gastric remnant. The symptoms accompanying these events are upper abdominal pain followed by projectile bilious vomiting. Two important questions to the patient relate to these episodes of emesis: (1) is food mixed with bile in the vomitus, and (2) is the pain relieved by vomiting? If food is mixed with bile and pain is unrelieved after vomiting, an afferent loop obstruction is much less likely than the syndrome of alkaline reflux gastritis.

As with the more acute version of this complication, CT scan or ultrasound may be more useful in making the diagnosis of a chronically dilated afferent loop in the right upper quadrant than barium studies. Once the diagnosis is confirmed, surgery should be performed to correct the anatomic disturbance. The efferent loop can be shortened, suspended, and pexed to parietal peritoneum, or anastomosed in side-to-side fashion to the efferent loop. The latter approach may be used when it is hazardous to expose the entire afferent loop, but carries with it the risk for bacterial overgrowth.

Chronic Efferent Loop Obstruction and Internal Hernia after Billroth II Reconstruction. Chronic obstruction of the efferent loop presents essentially as small bowel obstruction. Adhesive bands or internal hernias may account for the obstruction. If the symptoms are persistent, but low-grade in intensity, the diagnosis usually can be made by upper GI barium studies. Using CT scan, a chronically dilated, thick-walled and relatively fixed loop of bowel will be seen. Endoscopy is not always helpful in this situation.

One trap for internal hernia is created in the retroanastomotic space, posterior to a Billroth II reconstruction performed in the antecolic position. One approach to preventing acute kinking of the afferent or efferent loop behind an antecolic anastomosis is to anchor these loops to surrounding structures or to the parietal peritoneum. With regard to Billroth II reconstruction, two traps may be created posteriorly, above or below the anastomosis; however, internal hernia seems to occur much less frequently after retrocolic than after antecolic positioning. Experienced surgeons have taught that it is prudent to fashion a gastrojejunostomy from "left to right," in other words, in the isoperistaltic position. The afferent loop should lie to the left of the stomach and be tacked to the greater curvature, whereas the efferent loop, coming off to the patient's right, can hang dependently.

Jejunogastric Intussusception. This is a rare long-term complication following Billroth II reconstruction. If not suspected, the clinical picture can be quite nonspecific and the possibility of intussusception may not even be considered. The dominant symptom is pain, occasionally, but not regularly, associated with nausea and vomiting. Usually, it is the efferent limb rather than the afferent limb which is the intussusceptus. A firm mass may be palpable in the epigastrium. An emergent CT scan or water soluble upper GI contrast study may reveal a coiled-spring appearance within the gastric remnant. Between episodes of intussusception with entrapment, endoscopy may visualize the jejunal segments as they migrate in and out of the gastric remnant. If such a condition is strongly suspected to have caused acute symptoms, surgical intervention is indicated. The efferent limb can be anchored to the parietal peritoneum or a new gastrojejunostomy, possibly using a Roux-en-Y reconstruction, can be fashioned.

Late Gastroduodenal Obstruction. Following a Billroth I anastomosis for duodenal ulcer, inflammation around the duodenum and postbulbar area may lead to chronic scarring and distortion of the gastroduodenal anastomosis. The patient presents with symptoms of obstruction of the gastric outlet, including gastric fullness and discomfort relieved by vomiting of nonbile-stained and partially digested food. The patient also may present with symptoms indicating recurrence of the ulcer diathesis. On upper GI study by barium or endoscopy, the stomach is dilated and the outlet stenotic. Such stenoses are not usually amenable to endoscopic dilatation, but there is little harm in attempting this. Surgery is indicated for persistent and worsening symptoms. The simplest solution for this problem is to perform a gastrojejunostomy placed on the greater curvature proximal to the anastomosis. There is no necessity, and much potential harm, in trying to approach the anastomosis directly.

Pathophysiologic Disorders

General Physiological Derangements. Most chronic sequelae of gastrectomy are attributable, at least partly, to alterations in gastric motility or mucosal function. In health, the motor functions of the stomach are (1) to accept and store a bolus of ingested food, (2) to reduce larger particles of food to smaller ones and, (3) to provide "gated" emptying of smaller food particles into the small intestine, a process known as *sieving,* where they are digested into macromolecules and nutrients that can be absorbed. The tone of the proximal stomach decreases when a bolus of food is swallowed (receptive relaxation) and when the bolus actually passes into the stomach (accommodation). These responses are distinct and both are mediated by the vagi. The grinding action of the distal stomach actually is initiated by pacemakers located in muscularis of the proximal stomach. Peristaltic contractions mix and propel the food particles and gastric secretions toward the pylorus. Vagal inputs to the stomach coordinate these contractions and the timing of pyloric relaxation, so that larger particles are repelled but smaller ones can pass into the duodenum (sieving). The pylorus not only prevents passage of larger particles into the small intestine but must prevent reflux of duodenal content into the stomach. The small intestine also plays a role in regulating gastric emptying, mainly through neurohumoral mechanisms.

Gastric surgery may interfere with some or all of these motor functions. Nonselective vagotomies impair the reservoir function of the proximal stomach and coordination of pyloric emptying. Even the highly selective vagotomy (HSV) impairs receptive relaxation and accommodation, diminishing the ability of the stomach to act as a reservoir and accelerating the emptying of liquids to an earlier phase of the digestive process. Any procedure that resects or bypasses the pylorus abolishes the sieving of particles, and differential emptying of liquids and solids. In addition, it permits reflux of intestinal contents into the stomach.

Mucosal functions that are altered by gastric surgery include (1) colonization of gastric lumen by coliforms and anaerobes, owing to loss of pyloric integrity and alkalinization of the lumen, (2) loss of barrier properties owing to assault by detergent-like actions of intestinal contents and bile, (3) disturbances of neurohumoral function caused by vagotomy, loss of endocrine mass in the antrum, and nonphysiologic reconstructions, such as Billroth II or Roux Y procedures, and (4) decreases in divalent cation absorption owing to the loss of gastric

acid and loss of intrinsic factor necessary for vitamin B_{12} in the distal ileum. One important consideration in evaluation of a patient with postgastrectomy syndromes is that more than one disorder may be present. All of the potential physiological derangements outlined above must be borne in mind while taking a history and performing physical and diagnostic examinations.

Alkaline Reflux Gastritis. This may be the most frequently recognized long-term complication of gastrectomy and it may be the one for which remedial surgery is most commonly performed.[48] Five to fifteen percent of patients undergoing gastric surgery ultimately will complain of symptoms consistent with this diagnosis.[7] In the presence or absence of gastric acid, the detergent-like effects of bile can cause injury to the gastric mucosa and the esophageal mucosa.[49,50] This disorder is most commonly associated with the Billroth II reconstruction; Billroth I reconstruction and pyloroplasty are less commonly associated. Although regurgitation of bile is required, the ability of the gastric remnant to clear the refluxed bile also may be a contributing factor.[51]

The symptoms include burning epigastric pain, nausea, and bilious vomiting that does not relieve the pain. This latter symptom is distinguished from the pain of the afferent loop syndrome, which is relieved after the vomiting of bilious material. The vomitus also contains food, another distinguishing feature. The volume of refluxed material may not correlate with severity of symptoms. The diagnosis requires (1) upper GI endoscopy and biopsies, which should demonstrate bile in the gastric remnant and histologic evidence of mucosal inflammation and "intestinalization" of gastric glands, (2) CT scan and upper GI barium contrast studies, which should demonstrate no evidence of afferent loop dilatation or obstruction. In addition, it is generally recommended that gastric emptying studies with solid-phase radionuclide be performed. If reconstructive surgery is anticipated, it is important to anticipate the possibility of severe alterations in gastric remnant emptying. Radiolabeled HIDA scans also may be useful in evaluating the volume of bile reflux and any alterations in clearance from the gastric remnant.[52] Finally, Warshaw has suggested that instillation of 0.1 N NaOH may reproduce the patient's symptoms.[53]

Medical management of this disorder is not usually effective. Agents that bind bile salts, such as cholestyramine, have not proven very effective.[54] Other agents such as the H2 receptor blockers and prokinetic agents such as metaclopramide have not been effective either. Because defective bile clearance is thought to play a role, it is reasonable to speculate that more consistent prokinetic agents such as cisapride, domperidone, or erythromycin might be useful adjuncts in managing symptoms. No objective data are available for these latter agents.

Surgical management of a well-documented case of alkaline reflux gastritis is indicated, if symptoms are persistent and disabling to the extent of interfering with work and lifestyle. For patients who have undergone Billroth II reconstruction, the operation of choice is a conversion to a Roux-en-Y configuration. Alkaline contents should be diverted 45 to 60 cm beyond the gastric remnant (Fig 32–10). As discussed above, the vagotomy must be complete in order to avoid ulceration of the especially acid-sensitive Roux limb. If there are any concerns about the completeness of the previous vagotomy, acid secretion studies (SAO/PAO) may be indicated. If there are concerns about delayed gastric emptying before surgery, it is prudent to perform an extensive gastrectomy, leaving only a small gastric pouch.

For patients who have undergone Billroth I reconstruction, two options may be considered: the first is conversion to a Roux-en-Y gastrojejunostomy and the second is to consider the interposition of an isoperistaltic 20 cm jejunal loop between the gastric outlet and duodenal stump (Fig 32–11). The general experience with this operation is limited, but excellent results have

been reported with objective documentation of decreased levels of bile reflux.[55] This operation offers a theoretical advantage of not excluding duodenal electrical activity and avoiding gastric stasis associated with the Roux reconstruction (Roux syndrome, see below). In the Vanderbilt and Mayo Clinic experiences, 75% to 80% of patients with alkaline reflux gastritis benefited from the Roux procedure and it remains the standard operation for this condition.[17,48]

Early Dumping Syndrome. About 15% of patients develop dumping symptoms following vagotomy and drainage. Up to 50% of patients undergoing vagotomy and antrectomy with Billroth II anastomosis experience these symptoms in the first 6 months following surgery. Although all procedures that involve vagotomy and/or bypass or resection of the pylorus are associated with a risk for the syndrome, the lowest risk is associated with highly selective vagotomy and Roux-en-Y reconstructions. Dumping syndromes are separated into early and late forms, based on the interval between ingestion of a meal and the development of symptoms. Early dumping usually is observed within 20 minutes after a meal. Gastrointestinal symptoms of dumping include abdominal pain, fullness, nausea, vomiting, and explosive diarrhea. Cardiovascular manifestations include sweating, dizziness, weakness, palpitations and flushing.

The term dumping is traced back to Mix who, in 1922, used barium contrast studies to observe rapid emptying from the stomach through a gastrojejunostomy in a patient with symptoms described above.[56] Experimental studies have suggested that sudden emptying of carbohydrate-rich liquid in the small intestine can lead to shifts of fluid from the microvasculature to the lumen.[57] Disturbances have been observed in the levels of gastrointestinal hormones such as serotonin, gastric inhibitory polypeptide, vasoactive intestinal polypeptide, and neurotensin after ingestion of food and in the interval in which symptoms are observed.[7, 17] The symptoms of early dumping are certainly exacerbated by ingestion of foods containing carbohydrates and high levels of simple sugars and correlated with rates of gastric emptying.[7,58] Based on these considerations, it seems likely that HSV carries the lowest risk for dumping because the pylorus remains intact. The Roux reconstruction also carries a low risk for dumping because it is associated with impaired gastric emptying.

The diagnosis is made on clinical grounds. However, solid-phase radionuclide gastric emptying scans can provide supportive information by demonstrating rapid gastric emptying. Normal or slow gastric emptying times virtually exclude the diagnosis of early dumping. Endoscopy and barium studies help to define the anatomy and provide clues that the dumping syndrome may be mixed with other postgastrectomy syndromes such as al-

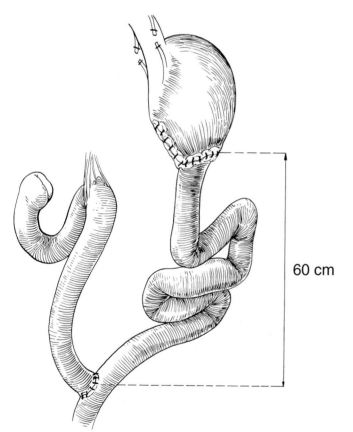

60 cm

Figure 32–10. Roux-en-Y diversion used for management of alkaline reflux gastritis and esophagitis. (Redrawn from Schwartz SI, Ellis H. *Maingot's Abdominal Operations,* 9th ed. Stamford, CT: Appleton and Lange; 1989:716)

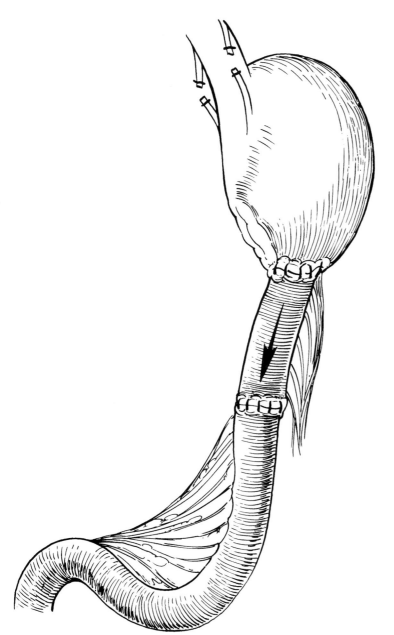

Figure 32–11. Henley loop (isoperistaltic jejunal transfer). Although described using a 10 cm segment of jejunum, longer segments (20 to 30 cm) may give better results in the management of alkaline reflux, dumping, or Roux stasis syndrome.

kaline reflux gastritis or afferent loop syndrome. A provocative test for dumping consists of ingestion of 300 to 350 mL of 15% to 25% glucose solution and should reproduce symptoms.[59,60]

Medical management consists of dietary modifications, including (1) increased frequency and decreased volume of meals, (2) avoiding concentrated carbohydrates, and (3) taking liquids 30 minutes after solids. One recently described adjunct to treating dumping symptoms involves the long-acting somatostatin analogue, octreotide.[59–61] Responses were good or excellent in the majority of cases when octreotide was given subcutaneously in doses of 50 to 100 μg, anywhere from 15

min to 2 hours before the provocative meal.[61] A recommended regimen would include 50 to 100 μg given before breakfast and then twice more at regular intervals between the first and last meal of the day. Presumably, the dominant contribution of somatostatin is to suppress the exaggerated release of vasoactive and motility-altering hormones elicited by ingestion of the test meal.[61]

Symptoms of dumping often improve in the first 6 months after surgery, but, in 1% of patients, symptoms persist and become disabling. The impact of octreotide therapy in this group has not been fully assessed, but surgery may be considered if symptoms persist, if the patient cannot tolerate octreotide or has a high requirement for octreotide. A number of operative solutions have been tried. One strategy is to reconstruct the pylorus, if the patient has had pyloroplasty. Another is to convert a gastrojejunostomy to a gastroduodenostomy, thereby reestablishing physiologic gastroduodenal flow. A third approach is to insert an isoperistaltic 10 cm jejunal segment (Henley loop) between the gastric remnant and the duodenum (Fig 32–11) or to place a double-limb pouch, 10 cm long, between the duodenum and the gastric remnant (Fig 32–12). None of these solutions has been consistently successful in >50% of cases.[6,17] Owing to the inconsistency of these approaches, conversion to a Roux-en-Y configuration has emerged as the relatively simplest solution to early dumping symptoms. In a recent series at the University of Florida, 22 patients underwent this procedure for early persistent dumping symptoms; 17 improved substantially.[62]

Late Dumping Syndrome. The symptoms of late dumping include the vasomotor symptoms observed in early dumping, but without the gastrointestinal symptoms. Late dumping appears to be attributable to release of enteroglucagon in response to high carbohydrate loads in the small intestine. Enteroglucagon sensitizes the pancreatic β cell so that the meal induces exaggerated and prolonged secretion of insulin.[63] Despite the early increase in blood glucose levels right after a meal, the persistence of the hyperinsulinemia causes hypoglycemia and vasomotor symptoms.

The diagnosis is made on clinical grounds. However,

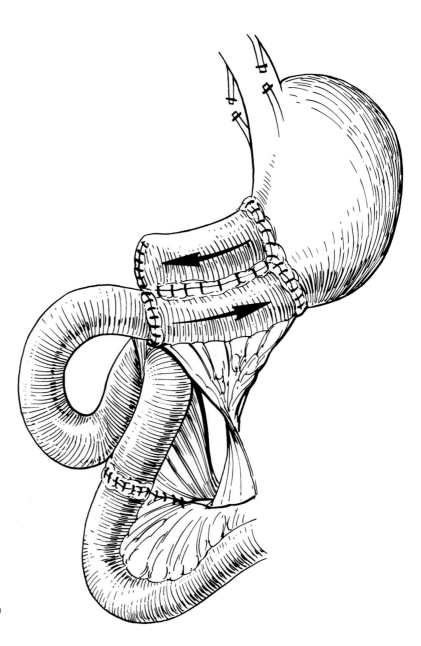

Figure 32–12. The double-limb pouch has proven effective in 50% to 60% of cases.

it is important to document hyperinsulinism and exclude the possibility of insulinoma. Treatment involves dietary modification. Carbohydrate content of each meal is reduced and hypoglycemic attacks can be managed by snacks between meals. Paradoxically, in patients with severe symptoms, insulin can be given before meals as a way of suppressing the early postprandial hyperglycemia that causes the exaggerated response of enteroglucagon later on. Octreotide may also be useful.

Chronic Gastric Atony. A decrease of gastric motor activity is not uncommon in the early period after vagotomy and can certainly be influenced by the type of reconstructive procedure. The symptoms of impaired emptying are epigastric fullness and pain, nausea after eating, and vomiting of partially digested food hours after ingestion. Liquids, which are usually tolerated better than solids, may provide the mainstay of nutrition. The clinical picture may be complicated by the formation of a bezoar.

As discussed in the section on postvagotomy complications, even the HSV procedure has an associated risk of gastric atony, usually in the range of 1% to 3%. Less selective vagotomies are associated with higher rates of gastric atony. Underlying conditions that may increase the risk of this complication include preoperative gastric outlet obstruction, diabetes and its associated autonomic neuropathy, adrenal disorders, and hypothyroidism.

Medical therapy with prokinetic agents such as cisapride or erythromycin has been of some value. Operative revision often is required if symptoms persist for longer than 6 months to 1 year without any improvement. Vagal innervation cannot be restored, so that the reservoir that harbors static contents must be eliminated. This forms the basis of the most consistently successful therapy to date, namely, resection of virtually the entire gastric remnant with Roux-en-Y gastrojejunostomy. Results with this approach are slightly above 50% for marked or complete relief of symptoms, and 25% for no improvement.[6,8]

Roux Stasis Syndrome. An important subgroup of patients with chronic postgastrectomy gastric atony is identified in those who actually undergo Roux-en-Y gastrojejunostomy as the primary reconstruction or for some other postgastrectomy complication. About 30% of this patient group will develop symptoms of gastric atony after vagotomy and Roux-en-Y reconstruction.[64-66] Both the vagotomy and the Roux-en-Y configuration contribute to the high incidence of gastric atony in this group of patients. Although emptying of the gastric remnant is the most prominent consequence, transit through the limb itself is impaired.[67] Thus, it is not uncommon to observe delayed transit through the Roux limb even after completion gastrectomy.[66] There are no reliable criteria for predicting which patients will develop the Roux stasis syndrome.[66]

Medical management is not usually successful in this subgroup and completion gastrectomy becomes the operative procedure of choice. In this procedure, the length of the Roux limb is adjusted to about 40 cm. While success rates hover around 50% for major improvement and 25% for some improvement, the procedure leaves a significant number of patients unimproved. Alternative approaches that are under consideration include (1) intestinal pacing,[68] (2) conversion to a 20 to 40 cm Henley loop configuration,[55,69] and (3) various procedures that would re-establish electrical, but not necessarily mechanical, connection of the Roux limb to more proximal intestine and pacesetting potentials.[70]

Specific Malabsorption and Nutritional Disturbances

Nutritional consequences of gastric surgery result from alterations in food intake as well as impairment of food digestion or nutrient absorption. Decreases in food intake or alterations in composition of meals result from the patient's desire to avoid nausea or dumping symptoms and may contribute significantly to malnutrition. However, there are specific disorders of digestion and malabsorption caused by removal of all or part of the stomach and nonphysiological rearrangement of the upper GI tract. These disorders include (1) maldigestion of complex protein, fat, and carbohydrate with steatorrhea and, occasionally, azotorrhea, (2) abnormal feelings of satiety, (3) deficiency of iron and vitamins B_{12} and folate, and (4) osteomalacia.

Maldigestion. The normal values for 24 hour fecal fat excretion ≤6% of dietary fat intake and for fecal nitrogen excretion, ≤2 g. The most severe disturbances are associated with total gastrectomy, which is associated with a mean fecal fat excretion level of 16% and fecal nitrogen excretion of about 2 gm.[71] The other types of gastrectomy, with or without vagotomy are not, on average, associated with such high levels of fecal fat or protein excretion. However, such disturbances may occur in any individual who has undergone even a vagotomy/pyloroplasty or vagotomy/gastroenterostomy. Patients who have undergone Billroth II reconstruction seem to be at higher risk for such disturbances than those who have undergone Billroth I reconstruction.

Although more difficult to document, gastric resection also leads to disturbances in carbohydrate digestion and absorption. Flatulence, a symptom of such malabsorption, is reported by most patients undergoing these procedures. Breath hydrogen levels are abnormally high in such patients.[72] However, the implications of such analyses can be confused by bacterial overgrowth in the intestine, also a known consequence of gastric surgery and bypass of the pylorus. Gastric surgery also may unmask previously unsuspected or clinically mild lactose intolerance.[71] The characteristic symptoms after ingestion of milk products or ice cream include cramps, flatulence, and explosive diarrhea caused by the rapid entry of lactose into the colon.

The increased levels of fecal excretion of complex carbohydrate, fat, and protein that follow gastric surgery are not associated with alterations in mucosal function. Therefore, they are due to maldigestion, that is, inadequate mixing with pancreatic enzymes and bile. Such mixing is normally affected by rates and timing of secretion of pancreatic juice and bile and by the rate at which food enters the duodenum from the stomach. In addition, intestinal transit regulates the mixing of enzymes, bile, and complex nutrients and should guarantee sufficient contact with the mucosa to ensure absorption. The loss of the pylorus and of vagally mediated receptive relaxation and accommodation contribute to accelerated gastric emptying. In addition, the loss of vagal efferents to the pancreas and biliary tract elicit significant reductions in the volume of pancreatic juice[73,74] and alterations in biliary motility. Detailed studies of nutrient absorption have indicated that these factors combine to push the sites of nutrient absorption further downstream, from the usual site (100 to 150 cm of jejunum) to the ileum.[71] However, in most cases, digestive capacity and mucosal absorptive capacities are not overwhelmed and maldigestion is not clinically apparent, except through symptoms described above.

Disturbances in Sensations of Satiety. It is generally thought that early satiety after gastric surgery is a consequence of the smaller volume of the gastric remnant. Experience with gastric partitioning procedures for morbid obesity, however, indicates that more than 90% of gastric capacity must be reduced before high levels of satiety are observed. Thus, diminished gastric capacity caused by gastric resection does not generally explain the higher levels of satiety with smaller volumes of food. Animal studies have suggested that there are sensory afferents that relay satiety signals from the mucosa. Such signals may be triggered by sensation of specific nutrients or perhaps luminal distention. Some observations have suggested that such signals may be triggered more intensely in the distal intestine.[71,75] Thus, it seems plausible that the factors that tend to accelerate movement of nutrients to the distal intestine might cause early satiety. This is consistent with observations that highly selective vagotomy is less commonly associated with postcibal fullness than other gastric surgical procedures. This procedure also causes the least intense disturbances of gastric emptying, pancreatic secretion, biliary motility.

Anemias and Iron Deficiency. Hypochromic and microcytic anemia is common following gastric resection and is at-

tributable to iron deficiency. Dietary iron is found predominantly in its ferric (Fe^{3+}) form, which, compared with the ferrous (Fe^{2+}) form, is much less soluble in the pH range from 4.0 to 7.0. The ferrous ions in the diet usually are found trapped in heme molecules (hemoglobin, myoglobin, cytochromes) and are liberated after interaction of the heme with pancreatic proteases. For efficient absorption, the Fe^{3+} form must be converted by its interaction with gastric acid to the Fe^{2+} form. Curiously, iron deficiency is not commonly found in individuals who are hypochlorhydric but have not undergone gastric surgery. Thus, loss of acid secretion alone does not account for decreased iron absorption. On the other hand, the absorption of Fe^{2+} is carried out most efficiently in the duodenum and the efficiency of absorption decreases distally in the intestine. Thus, gastric resection and Billroth II reconstruction would bypass the most efficient Fe- absorbing region. In general, however, absorptive capacity for iron adapts, even after Billroth II reconstructions. Thus, iron deficiency is usually attributable to the combination of the loss of acid secretion and the bypass of more proximal and efficient areas of iron absorption in the duodenum.

Deficiency of vitamin B_{12} is accompanied by macrocytic anemia, with neurological symptoms and pernicious anemia. Pernicious anemia inevitably follows total gastrectomy within 2 to 5 years, unless vitamin replacements are given. After as much as 75% gastrectomy, the incidence of pernicious anemia is <1% and is exceedingly rare after lesser gastric resections. Subclinical decreases in serum and tissue B_{12} levels are observed after partial gastrectomy.[71] Folate levels also may decline, owing to the loss of B_{12}. However, even if vitamin B_{12} levels are not profoundly depressed, folate levels may be impaired owing to selection of foods that are folate-poor and to poorer absorption of folate in an acid-free environment. Folate is most abundant in high-fiber vegetables and organ meats, foods that tend to cause postcibal symptoms in postgastrectomy patients.

The relatively mild imbalances in serum iron, B_{12}, and folate levels that are caused by gastric surgery do not need to be monitored routinely, except when the patient has undergone total or near total gastrectomy. In these latter patients, a reasonable approach to follow-up would include blood counts every three months until stable levels had been reached in year 2 or 3 following surgery and then every 6 months thereafter. Dietary supplementation of iron and folate and a vitamin B_{12} injection two or three times a year would be recommended for these patients, with yearly assessment of iron, B_{12} and folate levels. For patients who have undergone lesser procedures, dietary instruction, and simple multivitamin supplementation of the diet should be sufficient, with yearly assessment of the complete blood count and indices.

Bone Disease. Demineralization of bones is normal in the older populations, but clearly accelerated by gastric resection.[71] The process is more pronounced after total gastrectomy than partial resections but not apparently influenced by the type of reconstruction (Billroth I or Billroth II). Vagotomy without gastric resection is not associated with acceleration of demineralization.[76] Osteoporosis and osteomalacia both contribute, but it is the latter that is attributable uniquely to the surgery. The diagnosis can be supported by findings of elevated alkaline phosphatase, depressed serum calcium (after correction for serum albumin), and decreased serum levels of 25-hydroxy vitamin D with elevated 1,25 dihydroxy vitamin D. Serum PTH levels also are elevated. Pathologic fractures, especially vertebral fractures, have been reported to be three times more common in postgastrectomy patients than in matched control subjects.[71]

The causes of the osteomalacia remain unclear. Reductions in dietary calcium intake probably contribute. Such decreases may result from the unwillingness of the patient to take calcium-rich foods such as dairy products that cause postcibal symptoms. The best treatment may be prevention and would include dietary supplements with calcium. Some physicians give vitamin D supplements. Nevertheless, such preemptive treatments have not been studied prospectively. A recommended approach to follow-up would include bi-yearly measurements of serum calcium and alkaline phosphatase. Bone densitometry, hand films, or bone biopsies are not routinely warranted.

Miscellaneous Complications

Small Gastric Remnant. As discussed above, early satiety is a recognized consequence of gastric resections and may not be solely due to a small gastric remnant. However, following gastric resections of >80% of the stomach, early satiety and postcibal epigastric pain and vomiting can be attributed to the greatly diminished size of the gastric reservoir. This "small gastric remnant syndrome" can be accompanied by weight loss, malnutrition, and mixed anemias. Rapid gastric emptying, as assessed by radionuclide gastric emptying studies, is not associated. Medical management is often successful and includes increasing the frequency of meals and decreasing their volume. Vitamin supplements should be provided, if the patient has not already been taking them. Pancreatic enzyme supplements may ameliorate symptoms.[7] When symptoms are refractory and severe, it may be appropriate to consider resection of the gastric remnant, conversion to a Roux-en-Y configuration and construction of a Hunt-Lawrence pouch (Fig 32–13).

Bezoar Formation. Bezoars are mixtures of hair (trichobezoar), fruit, and undigested vegetable matter (phytobezoar). They tend to occur more frequently in patients with Billroth I reconstructions or small reconstructed gastric outlets. The accumulation of such materials and their failure to pass beyond the gastric remnant may reflect underlying motility disorders. Perhaps 10% to 15%

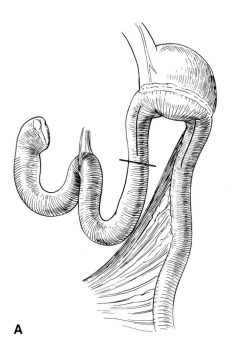
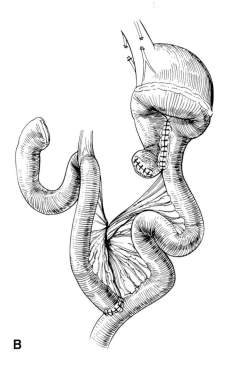

A   **B**

Figure 32–13. The Hunt-Lawrence pouch in management of small gastric remnant syndrome. Operation is restricted to highly selected cases.

of patients with motility disorders (gastric stasis, Roux stasis) develop bezoars. Occasionally such bezoars can become obstructing or they can cause early satiety and contribute to malnutrition.

Endoscopy visualizes the bezoar and provides the most expeditious way to break it up.[77,78] Several sessions involving irrigation and fragmentation may be required to remove it and the recurrence rate is quite high.[77,78] Occasionally, surgery may be necessary to remove a bezoar from the gastric remnant. If the bezoar passes into the intestine and causes obstruction, surgery cannot be avoided.[78] Such procedures should not be undertaken simply to remove the bezoar. Patients with large and highly symptomatic bezoars almost always will have an associated emptying disorder of the gastric remnant. In such cases, it is prudent to treat the patient as having a syndrome of gastric atony. If surgery is contemplated, a completion gastrectomy with Roux-en-Y reconstruction may provide the only reasonable approach.

Carcinoma of the Gastric Remnant. Following gastric resection, the overall incidence of carcinoma in the gastric remnant appears to be between 1% and 5%.[44] Whether this incidence reflects a truly increased risk for development of gastric carcinoma remains controversial. In a study of 6459 Swedish patients who had undergone various gastric operations, the overall risk of developing gastric carcinoma was not greater than that in age- and sex-matched controls.[79] However, specific subgroups had higher than predicted incidences of carcinoma, including (1) those who had Billroth II reconstruction, (2) surgery performed for gastric ulcer, and (3) interval of >20 years since surgery. Toftgaarg also found that the risk of gastric carcinoma rose after a latency period of 15 years following surgery.[80] In a population-based study in Olmstead County, Minnesota, however, these observations were not supported.[81] Despite some continued ambiguity about the nature of the risk, the reported incidence of gastric carcinoma in such patients seems high enough to warrant yearly endoscopic surveillance, starting 12 to 15 years after gastrectomy. Such lesions usually are advanced, unless they are detected before symptoms have developed. Completion gastrectomy is the preferred approach for such lesions.

REFERENCES

1. Sakurai H, McElhinney AJ. Perforation of the esophagus: experience at the Bronx VA Hospital 1969–1984. *Mt Sinai J Med* 1987;54:487

2. Hom S, Sarr MG, Kelly KA, et al. Postoperative gastric atony after vagotomy for obstructing peptic ulcer. *Am J Surg* 1989; 157:282

3. Johnston GW, Spencer EFA, Wilkinson AJ, et al. Proximal gastric vagotomy; follow-up at 10–20 years. *Br J Surg* 1991;78:20

4. Wilbur BG, Kelley KA. Effect of proximal gastric, complete gastric and truncal vagotomy on canine gastric electrical activity, motility and emptying. *Ann Surg* 1973; 178:295

5. Goldstein HM, Cohen LE, Hagen RO, et al. Gastric bezoars: a frequent complication in the postoperative ulcer patient. *Radiology* 1973;107:341

6. Eckhauser FE, Knol JA, Raoer SA, et al. Completion gastrectomy for postsurgical gastroparesis syndrome: preliminary results with 15 patients. *Ann Surg* 1988;208:345

7. Eagon JC, Miedema BW, Kelly KA. Postgastrectomy syndromes. *Surg Clin North Am* 1992;72:445

8. Karlstrom L, Kelly KA. Roux gastrectomy for chronic gastric atony. *Am J Surg* 1989;157:44

9. Dagradi AE, Stempien SJ, et al. Terminal esophageal spasm after vagotomy. *Arch Surg* 1962;85:955

10. Donahue PE. Early postoperative and postgastrectomy syndromes. *Gastroenterol Clin North Am* 1994;23:215

11. Balison JR, Woodward ER. Effects of hiatus hernia repair and truncal vagotomy on human lower esophageal sphincter pressure. *Ann Surg* 1973;177:544

12. Conklin JL, Christensen J. Motor functions of the pharynx and esophagus. In: Johnson LR (ed), *Physiology of the Gastrointestinal Tract*, 3rd ed. New York, NY: Raven; 1994:903

13. Dodds WJ, Stewart ET, Kishk SM, et al. Radiologic amyl nitrite test for distinguishing pseudo-achalasia from achalasia. *AJR Am J Roentgenol* 1986;146:21

14. Triadafilopoilos G, Aaronson M, Sackel S, et al. Medical treatment of esophageal achalasia. *Dig Dis Sci* 1991;36:260

15. Steele RJ, Munro A. Successful treatment of gastric stasis following proximal gastric vagotomy using endoscopic balloon dilatation. *Endosc* 1989;21:120

16. Kennedy T, Magill P, et al. Proximal gastric vagotomy, fundoplication, and lesser curve necrosis. *BMJ* 1979;1:455

17. Sawyers JL. Management of postgastrectomy syndromes. *Am J Surg* 1990;159:8

18. Allan JG, Gerskowitch VP, Russell RI. The role of bile acids in the pathogenesis of postvagotomy diarrhea. *Br J Surg* 1974;61:516

19. Allan JG, Russell RI. Cholestyramine in treatment of postvagotomy diarrhea—double blind controlled trial. *Br Med J* 1977;1:674

20. Mackie CR, Jenkins SA, Hartley MN. Treatment of severe postvagotomy/postgastrectomy symptoms with the somatostatin analogue octreotide. *Br J Surg* 1991;78:1338

21. Cuschieri A. Surgical management of severe intractable postvagotomy diarrhoea. *Br J Surg* 1986;73:981

22. Ihasz M, Griffith CA. Gallstones after vagotomy. *Am J Surg* 1981;141:48

23. Thompson D, Wild R, Merrick MV, et al. Cholelithiasis and bile acid absorption after truncal vagotomy and gastroenterostomy. *Br J Surg* 1994;81:1037

24. Burch JM, Cox CL, Feliciano DV, et al. Management of the difficult duodenal stump. *Am J Surg* 1991;162:522

25. Welch CE, Rodkey GV. A method of management of the duodenal stump after gastrectomy. *Surg Gynecol Obstet* 1954;98:376

26. Welch CE, Rodkey GV, von Ryll Gryska P. A thousand operations for ulcer disease. *Ann Surg* 1986;204:454

27. Mulvihill S, Pappas TN, Passaro E Jr, Debas HT. The use

of somatostatin and its analogues in the treatment of surgical disorders. *Surgery* 1986;100:811

28. Torres-Garcia AJ, Arguello JM, Balibrea JL. Gastrointestinal fistulas: pathology and prognosis. *Scand J Gastroenterol* 1994;207(suppl):39

29. Ysebaert D, Van Hee R, Hubens G, et al. Management of digestive fistulas. *Scand J Gastroenterol* 1994;207(suppl):42

30. Cullen JJ, Sarr MG, Ilstrup DM. Pancreatic anastomotic leak after pancreaticoduodenectomy: incidence, significance, and management. *Am J Surg* 1994;168:295

31. Nubiola-Calonge P, Badia JM, Sancho J, et al. Blind evaluation of octreotide (SMS 201-995), a somatostatin analogue, on small-bowel fistula output. *Lancet* 1987;2:672

32. Conter RL, Converse JO, McGarrity TJ, Koch KL. Afferent loop obstruction presenting as acute pancreatitis and pseudocyst. *Surgery* 1990;108:22

33. Hopens T, Coggs GC, Goldstein HM, Smith BD. Sonographic diagnosis of afferent loop obstruction. *AJR Am J Roentgenol* 1982;138:967

34. Gale ME, Gerzof SG, Kiser LC, et al. CT appearance of afferent loop obstruction. *AJR Am J Roentgenol* 1982; 138:1085

35. Pederzoli P, Bassi C, Falconi M, Camboni MG. Efficacy of octreotide in the prevention of complications of elective pancreatic surgery. *Br J Surg* 1994;81:265

36. Montorsi M, Zago M, Mosca F, et al. Efficacy of octreotide in the prevention of pancreatic fistula after elective pancreatic resections: a prospective, controlled, randomized clinical trial. *Surgery* 1995;117:26

37. Erlich EW, Howard JM. Ampullary disconnection during gastrectomy. *Ann Surg* 1969;170:961

38. Adami H, Enander L, Enskog L, et al. Recurrences 1 to 10 years after highly selective vagotomy in pre-pyloric and duodenal ulcer disease: frequency, pattern, and predictors. *Ann Surg* 1984;199:393

39. Thirlby RC. Postoperative recurrent ulcer. *Gastroenterol Clin North Am* 1994;23:295

40. Metz DC, Pisegna JR, Fishbeyn VA, et al. Control of gastric acid hypersecretion in the management of patients with Zollinger-Ellison syndrome. *World J Surg* 1993;17:468

41. Friesen SR, Tomita T. Pseudo-Zollinger-Ellison syndrome: hypergastrinemia, hyperchlorhydria without tumor. *Ann Surg* 1981;194:481

42. Lee C, P'eng F, Yeh PH. Sodium pertechnate ^{99m}Tc antral scan in the diagnosis of retained gastric antrum. *Arch Surg* 1984;119:309

43. Thirlby RC, Patterson DJ, Kozarek RA. Prospective comparison of Congo Red and sham feeding testing to determine vagal; innervation of the stomach. *Am J Surg* 1992; 163:533

44. Soybel DI, Modlin IM. Implications of sustained suppression of gastric acid secretion. *Am J Surg* 1992;163:613

45. Thirlby RC, Feldman M. Transthoracic vagotomy for postoperative peptic ulcer. *Ann Surg* 1985;201:648

46. Perrault J, Fleming CR, Dozois RR. Surreptitious use of salicylates: a cause of chronic recurrent gastroduodenal ulcers. *Mayo Clin Proc* 1988;63:337

47. Soybel D, Kestenberg A, Brunt EM, Becker JM. Gastrocolic fistula as a complication of benign gastric ulcer. *Br J Surg* 1989;76:1298

48. Kelly KA, Becker JM, van Heerdon JA. Reconstructive gastric surgery. *Br J Surg* 1981;68:687

49. Silen W. Horizons in gastrointestinal research. *Surgery* 1972;72:91

50. Schweitzer EJ, Bass BL, Batzri S, Harmon JW. Bile acid accumulation by rabbit esophageal mucosa. *Dig Dis Sci* 1986; 31:1105

51. Mackie C, Hulks G, Cuschieri A. Enterogastric reflux and gastric clearance of refluxate in normal subjects and in patients with and without bile vomiting following peptic ulcer surgery. *Ann Surg* 1986;204:537

52. Ritchie WP Jr. Reflux gastritis as a surgical problem. In: Sawyers JS, Williams LF (eds), *Difficult Problems in General Surgery*. Chicago, IL: Year Book Medical; 1989:79

53. Warshaw AL. Intragastric alkaline infusion: a simple, accurate provocative test for diagnosis of symptomatic alkaline reflux gastritis. *Ann Surg* 1981;194:297

54. Meshkinpour H, Elashoff J, Stewart H et al. Effect of cholestyramine on the symptoms of reflux gastritis. *Gastroenterology* 1977;73:441

55. Sousa JES, Troncon LEA. Andrade JL, et al. Comparison between Henley jejunal interposition and Roux-en-Y anastomosis as concerns enterogastric biliary reflux levels. *Ann Surg* 1988;208:597

56. Mix CL. "Dumping stomach" following gastrojejunostomy. *Surg Clin North Am* 1922;2:617

57. Roberts KE, Randall HT, Farr HW, et al. Cardiovascular and blood volume alterations resulting from intrajejunal administration of hypertonic solutions to gastrectomized patients. *Ann Surg* 1954;140:631

58. Donovan IA, Gunn IF, Brown A, et al. A comparison of gastric emptying before and after vagotomy with antrectomy and vagotomy with pyloroplasty. *Surgery* 1974;76:729

59. Primrose JN, Johnston D. Somatostatin analogue SMS 201-995 (octreotide) as a possible solution to the dumping syndrome after gastrectomy or vagotomy. *Br J Surg* 1989;76:140

60. Mackie CR, Jenkins SA, Hartley MN. Treatment of severe postvagotomy/postgastrectomy symptoms with the somatostatin analogue octreotide. *Br J Surg* 1991;78:1338

61. Lamers CB, Bijlstra AM, Harris AG. Octreotide, a long-acting somatostatin analog. In the management of postoperative dumping syndrome. *Dig Dis Sci* 1993;38:359

62. Vogel SB, Hocking MP, Woodward ER. Clinical and radionuclide evaluation of Roux-Y diversion for postgastrectomy dumping. *Am J Surg* 1988;155:57

63. Shultz KT, Neelon FA, Nilsen LB, et al. Mechanism of postgastrectomy hypoglycemia. *Arch Int Med* 1971;128:240

64. Herrington JL, Scott HW, Sawyers JL. Experience with vagotomy and antrectomy and Roux-en-Y gastrojejunostomy in surgical treatment of duodenal, gastric and stomal ulcers. *Ann Surg* 1984;199:590

65. Britten JP, Johnson D, Ward DC, et al. Gastric emptying and clinical outcome after Roux-en-Y diversion. *Br J Surg* 1987;74:900

66. Gustavsson S, Ilstrup DM, Morrison P, et al. Roux stasis syndrome after gastrectomy. *Am J Surg* 1988;155:490

67. Perino LE, Adcock KA, Goff JS. Gastrointestinal symptoms, motility, and transit after Roux-en-Y operation. *Am J Gastroenterol* 1988;83:380

68. Cullen JJ, Kelly KA. The future of intestinal pacing. *Gastroenterol Clin North Am* 1994;23:391

69. Ramus NI, Williamson RCN, Johnston D. The use of jejunal interposition for intractable symptoms complicating peptic ulcer surgery. *Br J Surg* 1982;69:265

70. Schirmer BD. Gastric atony and the Roux syndrome. *Gastroenterol Clin North Am* 1994;23:327

71. Meyer JH. Nutritional outcomes of gastric operations. *Gastroenterol Clin North Am* 1994;23:227

72. Bond JH, Leavitt MD. Use of pulmonary hydrogen measurements to quantitate carbohydrate absorption: study of partially gastrectomized patients. *J Clin Invest* 1972;51:1219

73. Mayer EA, Thomson JB, Jehn D, et al. Gastric emptying and sieving of solid food and pancreatic and biliary secretions after solid meals in patients with truncal vagotomy and antrectomy. *Gastroenterology* 1982;83:182

74. Mayer EA, Thomson JB, Jen D, et al. Gastric emptying and sieving of solid food and pancreatic and biliary secretions after solid meals in patients with nonresective gastric surgery. *Gastroenterology* 1984;87:1264

75. Doty JE, Gu YG, Meyer JH. The effect of bile diversion on satiety and fat absorption from liquid and dietary solid sources. *J Surg Res* 1988;45:437

76. Blichert-Toft M, Beck A, Christiansen C, et al. Effects of gastric resection and vagotomy on blood and bone mineral content. *World J Surg* 1979;3:99

77. Cifuentes Tebar J, Robles Campos R, Parrilla Paricio P, et al. Gastric surgery and bezoars. *Dig Dis Sci* 1992;37:1694

78. Chisolm EM, Leong HT, Chung SC, Li AK. Phytobezoar: an uncommon cause of small bowel obstruction. *Ann R Coll Surg (Engl)* 1992;74:342

79. Lundegardh G, Adami HO, Helmick C, et al. Stomach cancer after partial gastrectomy for benign disease. *N Engl J Med* 1988;319:195

80. Toftgaard C. Gastric cancer after peptic ulcer surgery. *Ann Surg* 1989;210:159

81. Schafer LW, Larrson DE, Melton LJ, et al. The risk of gastric cancer after surgical treatment of benign ulcer disease. *N Engl J Med* 1983;309:1210

33

Morbid Obesity

Harvey J. Sugerman

Morbid obesity has been defined arbitrarily in the past as 100 pounds above ideal body weight (IBW), using tables derived by the Metropolitan Life Insurance Company.[1] A 1991 National Institutes of Health Consensus Panel on Gastric Surgery for Severe Obesity[2] concluded that it would be preferable to refer to the problem as clinically severe obesity, rather than using the pejorative term "morbid," and that the weight for this criteria be a body mass index, or BMI, >35 kg/m^2. Approximately 4 million Americans[2] have a BMI between 35 and 40 kg/m^2 and another 1.5 million have a BMI >40 mg/kg^2. For an average adult male, a BMI of 40 mg/kg^2 is roughly equal to 100 lbs over IBW.

■ PATHOPHYSIOLOGY

The causes of morbid obesity are unknown but probably include genetic factors, abnormalities of neural and/or humoral transmitters to the hypothalamic hunger and/or satiety centers, dysfunction of the hypothalamic centers themselves, and pyschologically induced oral dependency drives. Morbidly obese adults have been found to have a lower basal energy expenditure. It has been our experience that patients who have lost weight following a gastric procedure for obesity will begin to regain weight if their caloric intake excess 1100 calories per day. This is a difficult dietary restriction to maintain for life and is probably the reason that dietary weight reduction programs have not had long-term successful outcomes. A genetic predisposition to obesity has been noted in several studies. In adopted children, the severity of obesity was more concordant with the natural than the adoptive parents.[3] Furthermore, monozygotic twins have much more similar weights, including marked overweight, than dizygotic twins, even if they grow up in different environments.[4] When identical twins were placed in a controlled environment and asked to eat 1000 calories per day above their normal basal caloric intake, there was a great variability as to weight gain; however, the twins gained weights as pairs, some a great deal, others little.[5] Other studies have shown that children born to overweight mothers had a significantly lower basal energy expenditure and more rapid weight gain than children from normal weight mothers.[6]

■ COMORBIDITY OF SEVERE OBESITY

Severe obesity is associated with a large number of associated problems that gave rise to the term "morbid obesity" (Table 33–1). Several of these problems are underlying causes for the earlier mortality associated with obesity and include coronary artery disease, hypertension, impaired cardiac function, adult-onset diabetes mellitus, obesity hypoventilation and sleep apnea syndromes, venous stasis and hypercoagulability leading to an increased risk of pulmonary embolism, and necrotizing panniculitis. Morbidly obese patients also can die as a result of difficulties in recognizing the signs and

TABLE 33–1. MORBIDITY OF SEVERE OBESITY

CENTRAL OBESITY
Metabolic Complications (Syndrome X)
  Noninsulin Dependent Diabetes (adult onset/Type II)
  Hypertension
  Dyslipidemia
    Elevated triglycerides
    Hypercholesterolemia
  Cholelithiasis, Cholecystitis
Increased Intra-abdominal Pressure
  Stress Overflow Urinary Incontinence
  Gastroesophageal Reflux
  Venous Disease
    Thrombophlebitis
    Venous Stasis Ulcers
    Pulmonary Embolism
    Obesity Hypoventilation Syndrome
    Nephrotic Syndrome
    Hernias (Incisional, Inguinal)

PSEUDOTUMOR CEREBRI

RESPIRATORY INSUFFICIENCY OF OBESITY (PICKWICKIAN SYNDROME)
  Obesity Hypoventilation Syndrome
  Obstructive Sleep Apnea Syndrome

CARDIOVASCULAR DYSFUNCTION
  Coronary Artery Disease
  Increased Complications after Coronary Bypass Surgery
  Heart Failure subsequent to:
    Left Ventricular Concentric Hypertrophy—Hypertension
    Left Ventricular Eccentric Hypertrophy—Obesity
    Right Ventricular Hypertrophy—Pulmonary Failure
  Prolonged Q-T Interval with Sudden Death

SEXUAL HORMONE DYSFUNCTION
  Amenorrhea, Hypermenorrhea
  Hirsutism
  Stein-Leventhal Syndrome
  Infertility
  Endometrial Carcinoma
  Breast Carcinoma

OTHER CARCINOMAS: COLON, KIDNEY, PROSTATE

INFECTIOUS COMPLICATIONS
  Difficulty Recognizing Peritonitis
  Necrotizing Pancreatitis
  Necrotizing Subcutaneous Infections
  Wound Infections, Dehiscence

DEGENERATIVE OSTEOARTHRITIS
  Feet, Ankles, Knees, Hips, Back

PSYCHOSOCIAL IMPAIRMENT

DECREASED EMPLOYABILITY, WORK DISCRIMINATION

symptoms of peritonitis.[7] There is an increased risk of uterine, breast, and colon cancer. Premature death is much more common in the severely obese individual; there is a 12-fold excess mortality in morbidly obese men in the 25 to 34 years of age group.[8]

A number of obesity-related problems may not be associated with death but can lead to significant physical or psychological disability. These include degenerative osteoarthritis, pseudotumor cerebri (benign intracranial hypertension), cholecystitis, skin infections, chronic venous stasis ulcers, stress overflow urinary incontinence, gastroesophageal reflux, sex hormone imbalance with dysmenorrhea, hirsutism, infertility, the nephrotic syndrome, and idiopathic cirrhosis. Many morbidly obese patients suffer from severe psychological and social disability, including marked prejudice regarding employment.

CENTRAL (ANDROID) VERSUS PERIPHERAL (GYNOID) FAT DISTRIBUTION

It has been noted that visceral obesity has much greater metabolic problems than peripheral obesity, and are commonly referred to as android versus gynoid obesity because of their relative prevalence in men and women, respectively. It appears that visceral fat is metabolically much more active than subcutaneous fat, so that there is a greater rate of glucose production, type II diabetes, and hyperinsulinism leading to increased sodium reabsorption and hypertension.[9] There is also a greater production of cholesterol, with an increased incidence of gallstones and hypercholesterolemia, primarily in the form of low-density lipoprotein, leading to a higher than normal incidence of atherosclerotic cardiovascular disease. The increased visceral fat has been related to an increased waist:hip ratio or, in more common terms, as the "apple" versus "pear" distribution of fat. Computerized axial tomographic (CAT) scans, however, have noted a much better correlation between anterior-posterior abdominal diameter and visceral fat distribution than with the waist:hip ratio.[10]

A recent study documented an increased bladder pressure in morbidly obese women that was associated with a high incidence of stress and/or urge overflow urinary incontinence.[11] It is quite probable that much of the comorbidity of severe obesity is related to an increased intra-abdominal pressure secondary to a central distribution of fat (Table 33–1). The intra-abdominal pressure can be predicted most easily from the anterior-posterior abdominal diameter rather than the waist:hip ratio, which could be normalized in severely obese individuals who may have both a central and peripheral distribution of fat. In addition to overflow urinary incontinence, this increased intra-abdominal pressure could be responsible for the increased venous stasis disease and venous stasis ulcers. Likewise, it may explain the gastroesophageal reflux, the nephrotic syndrome secondary to increased renal venous pressure, incisional and inguinal hernias, and obesity hypoventilation syndrome secondary to a high-riding diaphragm and restrictive lung disease. This also can lead to increased intrapleural pressures that can then cause increased intracardiac pressures. As a result, severely obese patients with obesity hypoventilation syndrome may require high cardiac filling pressures to maintain an adequate cardiac output (vide infra).

CARDIAC DYSFUNCTION

Morbid obesity may be associated with cardiomegaly and impaired left, and/or right ventricular function. Severe obesity is usually associated with a high cardiac output and a low systemic vascular resistance leading to left ventricular hypertrophy. Obesity also is associated frequently with hypertension, which leads to concentric left ventricular hypertrophy. This combination of obesity and hypertension, with left ventricular eccentric and concentric hypertrophy, may lead to left ventricular failure.[12] Correction of morbid obesity improves cardiac function is these patients.[13] Morbid obesity also is associated with an accelerated rate of coronary atherosclerosis. These patients often have hypercholesterolemia and a decreased high-density to low-density lipoprotein ratio. Obese women with a BMI >29 kg/m^2 have a significantly increased incidence of myocardial angina and/or infarction.[14] In addition to the direct cardiac effects, respiratory insufficiency associated with morbid obesity can result in hypoxemic pulmonary artery vasoconstriction which, in severe cases, may lead to right, or biventricular, heart failure associated with tricuspid valvular insufficiency.[15,16] Correction of the respiratory insufficiency with surgically induced weight loss will correct the elevated pulmonary artery and wedge pressures within 3 months to 1 year after surgery.[16] Other respiratory-induced problems include severe obstructive sleep apnea syndrome, which may be associated with pro-

longed sinus arrest, premature ventricular contractions, and sudden death.

PULMONARY DYSFUNCTION

Respiratory insufficiency of obesity is associated with either obesity hypoventilation syndrome (OHS), obstructive sleep apnea syndrome (SAS), or a combination of the two, commonly called the Pickwickian syndrome.[15–17]

Obesity Hypoventilation Syndrome

OHS probably arises primarily from the increased intra-abdominal pressure in patients with central abdominal obesity, which leads to a high-riding diaphragm. As a result, the lungs are squeezed, producing a restrictive pulmonary defect. A heavy, obese thoracic cage also may contribute to the pathophysiology secondary to a decreased chest wall compliance. These patients have a markedly deceased expiratory reserve volume, leading to alveolar collapse and arteriovenous shunting at end-expiration. They also have smaller reductions in all other lung volumes (Fig 33–1), and hypoxemia and hypercarbia while awake (Fig 33–2) and a blunted ventilator response to CO_2. Although chronic hypoxemia leads to pulmonary artery vasoconstriction, these patients often have both markedly elevated pulmonary artery pressures and pulmonary capillary wedge pressures (Fig 33–3), suggesting both right and left ventricular failure. In some patients, these pressures may be spurious, since there is often a marked increase in pleural pressures secondary to the high-riding diaphragm and increased intra-abdominal pressure. As a result, the transatrial and transventricular pressures may be, in fact, normal. Thus, morbidly obese patients with OHS may not respond well to diuresis and may need these elevated pressures to maintain an

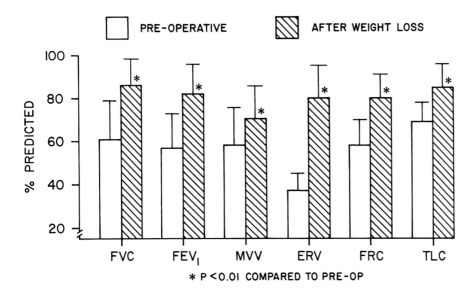

Figure 33–1. Spirometry and lung volumes in morbidly obese patients with obesity hypoventilation syndrome and their improvement following surgically induced weight loss. (From Sugerman et al. Gastric surgery for respiratory insufficiency of obesity. *Chest* 1986;90:82)

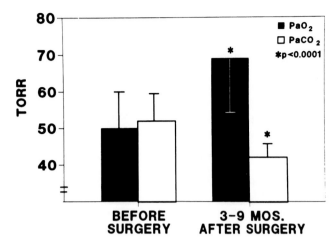

Figure 33-2. Significantly improved PaO_2 and $PaCO_2$ in 18 patients 3 to 9 months after gastric surgery–induced loss of $42 \pm 19\%$ excess weight. (From Sugerman HJ, Baron PL, Fairman RP, et al. Hemodynamic dysfunction in obesity hypoventilation syndrome and the effects of treatment with surgically induced weight loss. *Ann Surg* 1988;207:604)

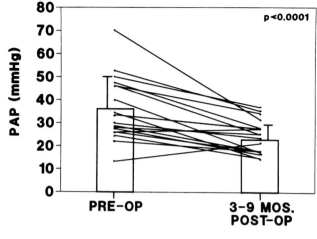

Figure 33-3. Increased pulmonary artery pressure in patients with obesity hypoventilation syndrome and its improvement following surgically induced weight loss. (From Sugerman HJ, et al. Hemodynamic dysfunction in obesity hypoventilation syndrome and the effects of treatment with surgically induced weight loss. *Ann Surg* 1988;207:604)

adequate cardiac output. As a result of the increased inferior vena caval and pulmonary artery pressures, they are at risk for a fatal pulmonary embolism.[15,16]

Obstructive Sleep Apnea Syndrome

The obstructive SAS is associated with severe obesity and is the result of both depression of the normal genioglossus reflex, possibly secondary to a large, heavy tongue, and deposition of fat within the hypopharynx with narrowing of the airway.[15–18] These patients snore loudly while asleep and suffer from severe daytime somnolence with tendencies to fall asleep while driving or at work. The daytime somnolence is probably secondary to impaired stage III, IV, and REM sleep during usual sleeping hours. The diagnosis of obstructive SAS is suggested by a history of severe daytime somnolence, frequent nocturnal awakening, loud snoring, and morning headaches, and is confirmed with sleep polysomnography. This technique documents cessation of airflow during sleep associated with persistent respiratory efforts. This syndrome may be associated with sudden death and should always be considered in trauma victims who have fallen asleep while driving. In a recent series from the Medical College of Virginia, 12.5% of the patients who underwent gastric surgery for morbid obesity had respiratory insufficiency.[17] Of the affected individuals, 51% had sleep apnea syndrome alone, 12% had obesity hypoventilation syndrome alone, and 37% had both. Of these, 64% were men, in contrast to only 14% of the entire group of patients who underwent surgery for obesity. Patients with respiratory insufficiency were significantly more obese than those without pulmonary dysfunction. However, obesity is not the only factor causing respiratory embar-

rassment, since many patients who underwent surgery for morbid obesity and did not have a clinically significant pulmonary problem weighed more than the patients with respiratory insufficiency. Most of the obese patients with respiratory dysfunction had an additional pulmonary problem, such as sarcoidosis, heavy cigarette use, recurrent pulmonary embolism, myotonic dystrophy, or idiopathic pulmonary fibrosis. Obstructive SAS and OHS are associated with a high mortality and serious morbidity; weight reduction will correct both.[15–18]

DIABETES

Obesity is a frequent etiologic factor in the development of Type II adult onset noninsulin dependent diabetes mellitus (NIDDM). Morbidly obese patients can be very resistant to insulin owing to the marked down regulation of insulin receptors. Most of these patients no longer require insulin following gastric surgery–induced weight loss.[19] The tendency toward hyperglycemia manifested by obese patients is another risk factor for coronary artery disease as well as for fatal subcutaneous infections. Gastric surgery induced–weight loss is associated with complete resolution of the diabetes in the vast majority of patients and this effect is long-lasting.[20,21]

VENOUS STASIS DISEASE

Morbidly obese patients have an increased risk for deep venous thrombosis, venous stasis ulcers, and pulmonary embolism. Low levels of antithrombin III may increase their risk of blood clots. The increased weight within the abdomen raises the intra-abdominal pressure and, therefore, the inferior vena caval pressure. As a result, there is an increased resistance to venous return, increasing the tendency to deep venous thrombosis. A similar mechanism may be responsible for the increased risk of pulmonary embolism in patients with right heart failure secondary to hypoxemic pulmonary artery vasoconstriction. Venous stasis ulcers are common in morbidly obese patients. These can be incapacitating and extremely difficult to treat; weight reduction may be the critical factor, as pressure stockings, Unna boots, and wound care are often ineffective.

DEGENERATIVE JOINT DISEASE

The increased weight in the morbidly obese leads to early degenerative arthritic changes of the weight-bearing joints, including the knees, hips, and spine. Many orthopedic surgeons refuse to insert total hip or knee prostheses in patients weighing over 250 pounds because of an unacceptable incidence of prosthetic loosening. Weight reduction following gastric surgery for obesity should permit subsequent successful joint replacement. In some instances, the decrease in pain following weight loss obviates the need for joint or intervertebral disc surgery.

OTHER OBESITY-RELATED CONDITIONS

Morbidly obese patients frequently suffer from gastroesophageal reflux. Women often have problems with stress overflow urinary incontinence.[11] Both of these problems are probably related to an increased intraabdominal pressure. Psuedotumor cerebri, also known as benign intracranial hypertension, may be associated with morbid obesity. Women often suffer from sexual dysfunction owing to excessive levels of both the virilizing hormone, androstenedione, and the feminizing hormone, estradiol. These may produce infertility, hirsutism, ovarian cysts (Stein-Levinthal syndrome), hypermenorrhea, and endometrial carcinoma. There is also a significantly increased risk of breast, prostate and colon carcinoma in the morbidly obese, as well as an increased risk of hernias, nephrotic syndrome and idiopathic cirrhosis.

■ DIETARY MANAGEMENT OF MORBID OBESITY

There are a number of dietary programs for weight reduction that include hospital-supervised programs, psychiatric behavioral modification programs, commercial organizations, commercial diets, protein-sparing fast programs, and diet pills provided by unscrupulous physicians. Unfortunately, no dietary approach has achieved uniform long-term success for the morbidly obese. Although many individuals can lose weight successfully

through dietary manipulation, the incidence of recidivism in the morbidly obese approaches 95%.[25] A National Institutes of Health Consensus Conference in 1992 concluded that dietary weight reduction with or without behavioral modification or drug therapy had an unacceptably high incidence of weight regain in the morbidly obese within two years after maximal weight loss.[26]

■ SURGICAL MANAGEMENT OF MORBID OBESITY

SURGICAL ELIGIBILITY

Patients are considered eligible for surgery by most insurance companies if they weigh 100 pounds or more than the 1983 Metropolitan Life Insurance Company IBW tables.[1] Some insist that they be both 100 lbs and twice IBW. The 1991 NIH Consensus Conference on Gastrointestinal Surgery for Severe Obesity concluded that "patients whose BMI exceeds 40 kg/m^2 are potential candidates for surgery if they desire substantial weight loss, because obesity severely impairs the quality of their lives. . . . In certain instances, less severely obese patients (those with a BMI between 35 and 40 kg/m^2) may also be considered for surgery. Included in this category are patients with high-risk comorbid conditions such as life-threatening cardiopulmonary problems (for example, severe sleep apnea, Pickwickian syndrome, and obesity-related cardiomyopathy) or severe diabetes mellitus. Other possible indications for patients with a BMI between 35 and 40 kg/m^2 include obesity-induced physical problems that interfere with lifestyle (for example, joint disease that would be treatable, and for the obesity and body-size problems precluding or severely interfering with employment, family function, and ambulation)."[2]

JEJUNOILEAL BYPASS

The first popular surgical procedure for morbid obesity was the jejunoileal bypass. This operation produced an obligatory malabsorptive state through bypass of a major portion of the absorptive surface of the small intestine. The procedure connected a short length of proximal jejunum (8 to 14 inches) to the distal ileum (4 to 12 inches) as an end-to-end or end-to-side anastomosis. The end-to-end procedures were associated with a better weight loss, but required decompression of the bypassed small intestine into the colon. The jejunoileal bypass was associated with a number of early and late complications. The most serious postoperative complication was cirrhosis, the result of either protein-calorie malnutrition and/or absorption of endotoxin from bacterial overgrowth in the bypassed intestine, a clinical example of bacterial translocation. A rheumatoid-like arthritis also occurred as a result of absorption of bacterial products from the bypassed intestine; antigen-antibody complexes to bacterial antigens were found in the joint fluid of affected individuals. Rapid weight loss, as well as malabsorption of bile salts, increased the risk of cholelithiasis owing to the decrease in cholesterol solubility. Hypocalcemia was frequent due to chelation of calcium with bile salts, leading to severe osteoporosis. Multiple kidney stones developed as a result of increased oxalate absorption from the colon, where it is normally bound to calcium. Intractable, malodorous diarrhea with associated potassium and magnesium depletion, metabolic acidosis, and severe malnutrition were common, as was vitamin B_{12} deficiency. Bacterial overgrowth in the bypassed intestine also led to vitamin K deficiency, interstitial nephritis with renal failure, pneumatosis intestinalis and bypass enteritis associated with occult blood in the stools and iron-deficiency anemia. Many of these problems, which are associated with bacterial overgrowth in the bypassed intestine, can be treated with metronidazole.

Some physicians feel that all jejunoileal bypass procedures should be reversed since cirrhosis may develop insidiously in the absence of abnormal liver function tests.[26] Most believe that medical therapy should be tried first. If the medical problems are severe and do not respond to metronidazole or progressive liver and/or renal dysfunction occurs the jejunoileal bypass can be reversed. Because these patients will invariably regain their lost weight,[27] conversion to a gastric procedure for obesity should be considered unless the patient is too ill (eg, severe cirrhosis with portal hypertension). Randomized prospective studies have shown that the gastric bypass operation is associated with a comparable weight loss and a significantly lower complication rate than jejunoileal bypass.[28] Because of the significant complication rate, the jejunoileal bypass should no longer be performed.

GASTRIC PROCEDURES FOR MORBID OBESITY

In 1966, Mason and Ito reported the results of weight loss using a gastric bypass (GBP) with division of the stomach into a small upper pouch connected to a loop gastroenterostomy.[29] The concept for this procedure was based upon the observation of weight loss that often followed subtotal gastrectomy for duodenal ulcer disease. There was concern that peptic ulcers would develop in the bypassed stomach or duodenum and, although these have occurred, the incidence is very low. Serum gastrin levels and acid secretion from the bypassed stomach are low.[30] The technique for GBP was simplified with the use of stapling instruments. The concept of gastroplasty then was proposed as a safer, easier method for restricting food intake. In gastroplasty, the stomach is only stapled, leaving a small opening to permit the normal passage of food into the distal stomach and duodenum.

Gastroplasty

Gastroplasties have been performed with either horizontal or vertical placement of the staples. Horizontal gastroplasty usually required ligation and division of the short gastric vessels between the stomach and spleen and carried the risk of devascularization of the gastric pouch or splenic injury. Horizontal gastroplasties included a single application of a 90 mm stapling device without suture reinforcement of the stoma between upper and lower gastric pouches or a double application of staples with either a central or lateral polypropylene-reinforced stoma. In one study, the failure rates (loss of less than 40% of excess weight) for these three horizontal gastroplasty procedures were 71%, 46%, and 42%, respectively.[31] Because of this high failure and complication rate, the horizontal gastroplasty is no longer indicated for the surgical treatment of obesity. The vertical banded gastroplasty (VBGP) is a procedure in which a stapled opening is made in the stomach, with a stapling device, 5 cm from the cardioesophageal junction (Fig 33–4).[32] One application of a 90 mm "bariatric" stapling device with four parallel rows of staples are made between this opening and the angle of His, a strip

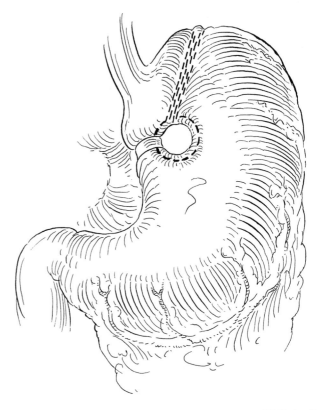

Figure 33–4. Vertical banded gastroplasty. (Redrawn from Sugerman HJ, Starkey JV, Birkenhauer R. A randomized prospective trial of gastric bypass versus vertical banded gastroplasty for morbid obesity and their effects on sweets versus non-sweets eaters. *Ann Surg* 1987;205:613)

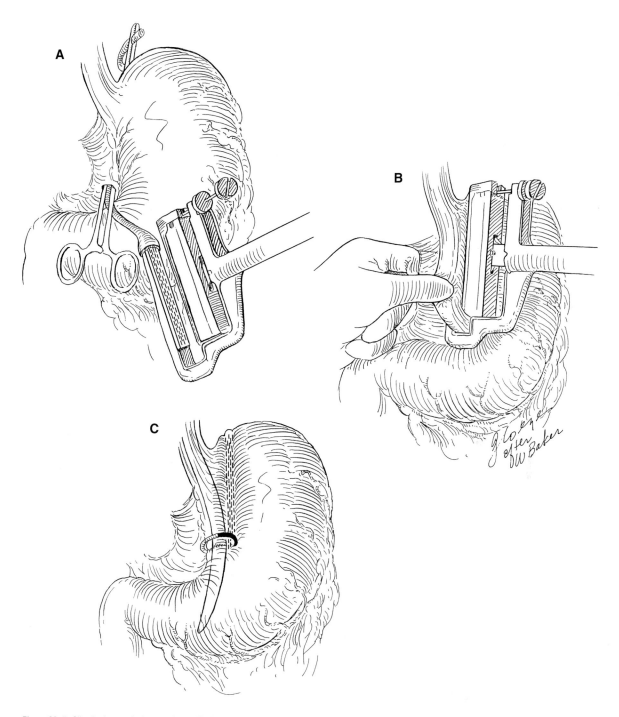

Figure 33–5. Silastic ring vertical gastroplasty. (Redrawn from Willibanks OL. Longterm results of silicone elastomer ring vertical gastroplasty for the treatment of morbid obesity. *Surgery* 1987;101:606)

of polypropylene mesh is wrapped around the stoma on the lesser curvature and sutured to itself but not to the stomach, creating a 5 cm circumference outlet of the small upper gastric pouch. Use of a 4.5 cm circumference stomal outlet was not found to produce a better weight loss; in fact, many patients developed maladaptive eating behavior with this small outlet, drinking high calorie liquids, as meat and chicken would often get caught in the small stoma.[33] Erosion of the mesh into the stomach has been an unusual complication of this procedure. Pouch enlargement is much less likely to occur with a vertical staple line in the thicker, more muscular part of the stomach (as contrasted to the horizontal gastroplasties), and the stomal diameter is fixed with the mesh band. The Silastic ring gastroplasty is a similar procedure that uses a vertical staple line and a Silastic tubing–reinforced stoma (Fig 33–5).[34]

Gastric Banding. Gastric banding is another form of gastroplasty in which a polypropylene or silastic band is placed around the stomach just below the gastroesophageal junction. In several series, gastric banding has had markedly variable weight loss results.[35,36] Furthermore, the operation can be associated with kinking of the banded stoma, obstruction, and intractable vomiting. An adjustable, inflatable band has been developed and may have more acceptable results; however, confirmatory data are not yet available.[37] There is currently a Food and Drug Administration study of laparoscopic adjustable gastric banding underway in the United States. More than 2 000 of these procedures have been performed in Europe.

Gastric Bypass

Compared with the current standard, the original gastric bypass procedure had a much larger proximal gastric pouch and anastomotic stoma. This often was associated with an inadequate weight loss. The current gastric bypass that is performed at the Medical College of Virginia is constructed by placing three superimposed 90 mm staple lines in a vertical direction, creating a small gastric pouch (15 to 30 mL) with a 45 cm Roux-en-Y limb, and the stoma restricted to 1 cm (Fig 33–6). A recent series of VBGP procedures reported a 35% incidence of staple line disruption when using the TA-90B (Auto-suture, Inc, US Surgical Corporation, Norwalk, CT) bariatric stapler with four parallel rows of a 90 mm stapler.[38] Because of the risk of staple line dehiscence, some surgeons transect the stomach, whereas others oversew the staple line. With three superimposed 90 mm staple lines, we have have <1% incidence of staple line breakdown.

Gastroplasty Versus Gastric Bypass

Randomized prospective trials have documented a significantly better weight loss with gastric bypass than various types of horizontal gastroplasty procedures, in

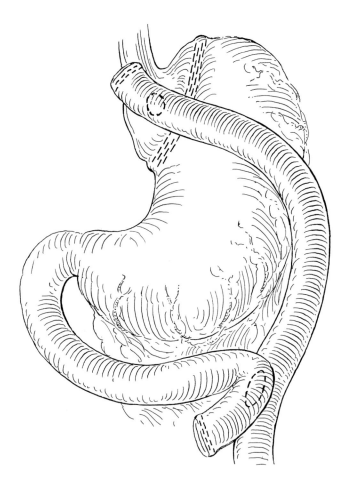

Figure 33–6. Roux-Y gastric bypass. Current technique with small (15 to 30cc) proximal gastric pouch and 1 cm stoma. (Redrawn from Sugerman HJ, Starkey JV, Birkenhauer R. A randomized prospective trial of gastric bypass versus vertical banded gastroplasty for morbid obesity and their effects on sweets versus non-sweets eaters. *Ann Surg* 1987;205:613)

which the poorer results were thought to be secondary to technical causes, such as stomal or pouch enlargement or staple line disruption.[39,40] The VBGP was developed by Mason with the hope that these technical problems would be solved and that the weight loss would be comparable to gastric bypass without the potential gastric bypass risks of iron and vitamin B_{12} deficiencies.[32,33] In a randomized prospective trial,[41] the GBP was compared with VBGP and a significantly better weight loss was again noted with the GBP procedure (Fig 33–7). On the average, the GBP patients lost two-thirds of their excess weight during the 3 years after surgery, as compared with about 40% for VBGP. When patients were divided into eating pathology based upon preoperative dietary interview, it was found that sweets eaters had a markedly decreased weight loss after VBGP as compared with GBP (Table 33–2). There was no significant difference in weight loss between sweets and nonsweets eaters in the GBP group. The more favorable weight loss results in sweets eaters after GBP appeared to

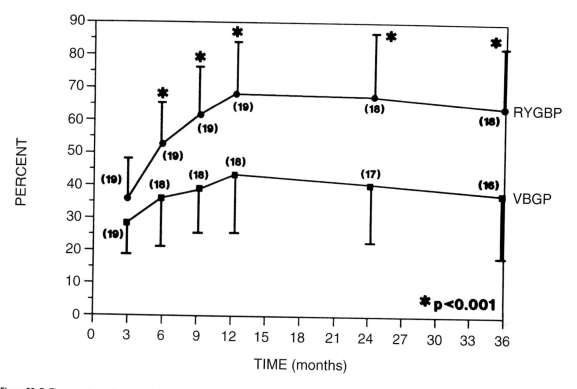

Figure 33–7. The percentage of excess weight loss ± standard deviation over 3 years following random assignment of gastric bypass (RYGBP) as compared to vertical banded gastroplasty (VBGP). Values in parentheses indicate number of patients. (From Sugerman HJ, Starkey JV, Birkenhauer R. A randomized prospective trial of gastric bypass versus vertical banded gastroplasty for morbid obesity and their effects on sweets versus non-sweets eaters. *Ann Surg* 1987;205:613)

be the result of the development of dumping syndrome symptoms with the ingestion of simple carbohydrates, although it is certainly possible that some carbohydrate malabsorption also could be responsible after bypass of the duodenum and upper jejunum. In another study, it was noted that GBP patients had an intolerance of both sweets (including high-calorie beverages) and milk products, owing to lactose intolerance. This study also suggests that food preference differences are partially responsible for the lower calorie intake and greater weight loss after GBP, as these patients now avoid ice cream and milk shakes, major problems for many VBGP patients.[42] Most GBP patients claim that they have lost their craving for sweets. It is difficult to know if this is merely a conditioned response to the fear of dumping-syndrome symptoms, which they have either experienced or about which they have heard, or if it is a true loss of the desire to eat sweets. Regardless of cause, these patients are usually grateful that they no longer want to eat high-calorie sweets. Randomized studies from Sweden[43] and Canada[44] also noted significantly better weight loss with GBP than with VBGP. Another randomized study from Australia also noted a better weight loss with GBP than with a vertical gastroplasty[45]; however this gastroplasty stoma was restricted with two polypropylene sutures rather than a mesh or silastic band and may not be com-

TABLE 33–2. PERCENT DECREASE IN EXCESS WEIGHT IN SWEETS EATERS VS NONSWEETS EATERS WITH GBP VS VBGP

	Sweets Eaters	Nonsweets Eaters
GBP		
	(1) 69±17 <12>	67±17 <7>
	(2) 62±19 <11>	75±19 <7>
	(3) 59±17 <11>	71±21 <7>
	$P < 0.001$	NS
VBGP		
	(1) 36±13 <12>	57±18 <6>
	(2) 35±14 <11>	53±22 <6>
	(3) 32±18 <11>	50±21 <5>
	$P < 0.05$	NS

(From Sugerman HJ, Starkey JV, Birkenhauer R. A randomized prospective trial of gastric bypass versus vertical banded gastroplasty for morbid obesity and their effects on sweets versus non-sweets eaters. Ann Surg *1987;205:613*

parable to either the VBGP or silastic ring gastroplasty. A study from the Mayo Clinic also casts doubts about the effectiveness of the VBGP.[46]

Physiology of Gastric Bypass. A group of nondiabetic morbidly obese patients were given a protein-fat meal on one day and 100 gm oral glucose on the second day, before and 6 to 9 months after VBGP and GBP. All of the GBP, but none of the VBGP patients, claimed that the oral glucose meal produced one or more of the following symptoms: severe nausea, light-headedness, flushing, and diarrhea. This was associated with a much greater release of enteroglucagon after a glucose meal in GBP than VBGP patients.[47] When challenged before or after either GBP or VBGP with the protein-fat or glucose meals, no differences were noted in serum levels of 5-hydroxytryptamine, vasoactive inhibitory peptide, or cholecystokinin.[47] Several other studies have evaluated the responses of these and other intestinal peptides after various challenge meals following horizontal gastroplasty and GBP.[48–57] In general, gastroplasty has little effect on gut peptide responses, whereas GBP is associated with significant changes in these substances. GBP patients had significantly reduced insulin and glucose concentrations compared with preoperative concentrations, there were no significant changes in either glucose or insulin response after VBGP (Figs 33–8 and 33–9).

This is probably not secondary to the greater weight loss in the GBP group, since a similar result was noted in a study by Sirinek and associates at only two months after GBP, with the loss of only 21% of preoperative weight.[45]

Selective Assignment of Patients to Gastroplasty or Gastric Bypass. After completion of our randomized study, we elected to selectively assign sweets eaters (82%) to GBP and non-sweets eaters (18%) to VBGP.[58] With selective assignment, weight loss with VBGP improved significantly from $41 \pm 19\%$ loss of excess weight at two years after surgery to $55 \pm 19\%$ (Fig 33–10). Nevertheless, GBP still had a significantly better weight loss than VBGP, with the loss of $71 \pm 21\%$ of excess weight at two years after surgery. Similar results also have been noted in a study from New Jersey where the authors attempted to selectively assign patients who frequently ingested sweets and sweet milk products (eg, milk shakes, ice cream) and still found a significantly better weight loss in their GBP than their VBGP groups.[59] In both our randomized and selective studies, there were no significant differences in preoperative weights between VBGP and GBP groups, nor were there significant differences in age, sex, or race.[41,58] In our selective study, patients of African-American origin did not lose as much weight as white patients. Patients without insurance and Medicaid lost as much weight as did those with private insurance (Fig 33–11).[58] Thus, we do not be-

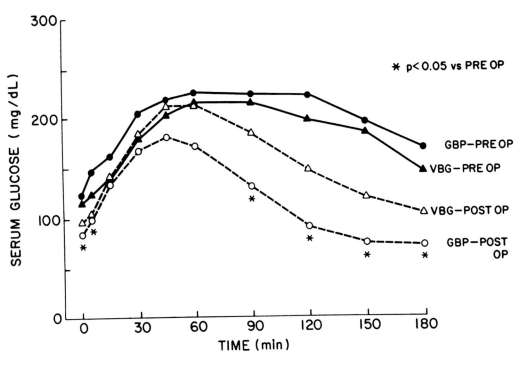

Figure 33–8. Comparison of the blood glucose response to a glucose meal in morbidly obese subjects before and after GBP (n=9) and VBGP (n=7). (From Kellum J, et al. Gastrointestinal hormone responses to meals before and after gastric bypass and vertical banded gastroplasty. *Ann Surg* 1990;211:763)

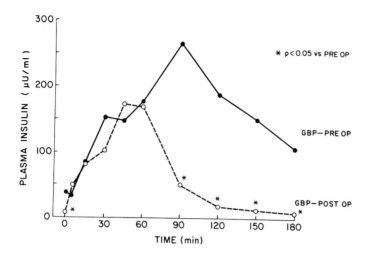

Figure 33–9. Comparison of the insulin response to a glucose meal in morbidly obese subjects before and after GBP (n=5). *denotes P<0.05 versus preoperative value. (From Kellum J, et al. Gastrointestinal hormone responses to meals before and after gastric bypass and vertical banded gastroplasty. *Ann Surg* 1990;211:763)

lieve the poorer weight loss in blacks was the result of economic factors, but probably the result of cultural dietary differences. We only rarely perform a gastroplasty procedure at the Medical College of Virginia and reserve it for young menstruating females who deny ingestion of significant amounts of simple carbohydrates. All but two of the patients in the randomized trial have had their VBGP converted to GBP; the two unconverted patients have failed the VBGP procedure, weighing as much or more than they did prior to their bariatric procedure.

Long-Term Follow-Up after Gastric Surgery for Obesity. Long-term GBP follow-up data have only recently become available. In one study with 90% follow-up, Yale noted that GBP patients lost an average of 60% of their excess weight at 5 years after surgery[60] (Fig 33–12). We noted a similar result at 5 years with 80% follow-up, with maintenance of more than 50% loss of excess weight and a decrease in BMI from 49±10 to 33±8 up to 9 years af-

ter GBP[61] and up to 6 years after conversion from VBG to GBP (Table 33–3).

General Complications Associated with Bariatric Surgery

Abdominal Catastrophe. It may be very difficult to recognize an abdominal catastrophe in morbidly obese patients.[7] They may complain of abdominal pain, and yet, on abdominal examination, have no evidence of peritoneal irritation (no guarding, tenderness, or rigidity). Symptoms include shoulder pain, pelvic or scrotal pain, back pain, tenesmus, urinary frequency, and, of great importance, marked anxiety. Signs of infection (fever, tachypnea, and tachycardia) may be absent. Patients with peritonitis often have clinical symptoms and signs suggesting a massive pulmonary embolus: severe tachypnea, tachycardia, and sudden hypotension. Such acute pulmonary failure is probably secondary to sepsis-induced adult respiratory distress syndrome (ARDS). Thus, peritonitis must be sus-

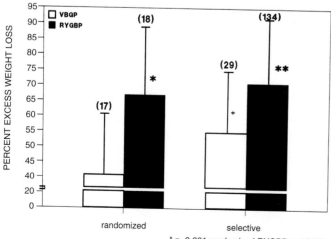

* p<0.001 randomized RYGBP vs VBGP
** p<0.01 selective RYGBP vs VBGP
+ p<0.05 selective VBGP vs randomized VBGP

Figure 33–10. Percentage of excess weight loss 2 years after selective assignment of "Sweets Eaters" to Roux-Y gastric bypass (RYGBP) and "Nonsweet Eaters" to vertical banded gastroplasty (VBGP) as compared with random assignment. Values in parentheses indicate number of patients. (From Sugerman HJ, Londrey GL, Kellum JM, et al. Weight loss with vertical banded gastroplasty and Roux-Y gastric bypass for morbid obesity with selective versus random assignment. *Am J Surg* 1989;157:93)

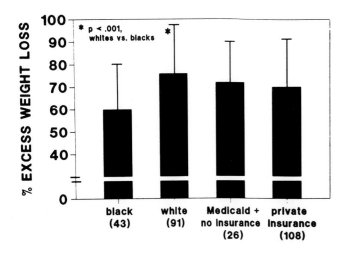

Figure 33–11. Significantly better weight loss in Caucasian patients who undergo GBP than black patients. (From Sugerman HJ, Londrey GL, Kellum JM, et al. Weight loss with vertical banded gastroplasty and Roux-Y Gastric bypass for morbid obesity with selective versus random assignment. *Am J Surg* 1989;157:93).

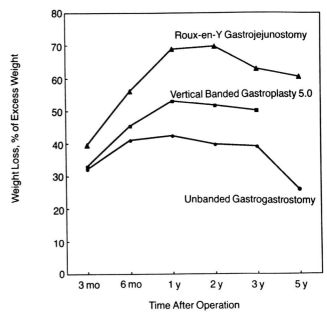

Figure 33–12. Long-term weight loss in gastric bypass, vertical banded gastroplasty and gastrogastrostomy patients. (From Yale CE. Gastric surgery for morbid obesity. *Arch Surg* 1989;124:941

pected in any morbidly obese patient with acute respiratory failure. Because a high index of suspicion of peritonitis is required to detect the condition in morbidly obese patients, radiographic contrast studies using water soluble agents such as diatrizoate meglumine (Gastrografin) may be indicated, even when there are few clinical signs. If a perforated viscus is suspected, an exploratory laparotomy may be necessary, despite normal findings on radiographic contrast study.

Complications After Gastric Bypass

Acute Gastric Distention.
Following gastric bypass surgery for clinically severe obesity, the distal, bypassed stomach occasionally will develop massive gaseous distention that can lead to a gastric perforation or disruption of the gastrojejunostomy. The primary symptom of this complication is the development of hiccups and a feeling of bloatedness. Massive gastric dilation can lead to severe left shoulder pain, and shock. The problem is usually secondary to edema at the Roux-en-Y anastomosis, but can be secondary to a mechanical problem. The diagnosis is made with an urgent upright abdominal radiograph that reveals the markedly dilated, air-filled, bypassed stomach. Occasionally, the dilated, bypassed stomach is filled with fluid and the diagnosis may be more subtle and difficult. In a few patients, when the dilation is primarily the result of air, the problem can be relieved with percutaneous transabdominal skinny needle decompression with subsequent passage of gastric, biliopancreatic juices

and gas through the Roux-en-Y anastomosis. Should the dilation recur, or the patient be in serious difficulty, an emergent laparotomy with insertion of a gastrostomy tube should be performed and the jejunojejunostomy evaluated. Patients with extensive adhesions from prior abdominal surgery should have a gastrostomy tube inserted at the time of gastric bypass surgery to prevent this potentially lethal complication.

Internal Hernia.
Following gastric bypass for morbid obesity, the patients are at risk for developing an internal hernia with a closed-loop obstruction, bowel strangulation. There are three potential locations for these internal hernias: the Roux-en-Y anastomosis; through the opening in the transverse mesocolon through which the retrocolic Roux limb is brought; and the Petersen hernia, located behind this Roux limb, before it passes through the mesocolon. The primary symptom of an internal hernia is periumbilical abdominal pain that usually is cramping consistent with visceral colic. Internal hernias may be very difficult to diagnose. An upper gastrointestinal (UGI) radiographic series is often normal. This may be devastating for the patient, should bowel infarction occur from a closed-loop with obstruction strangulation. One should always carefully inspect the plain abdominal radiograph for the abnormal placement or "spreading" of the Roux-en-Y anastomotic staples. The safest course of action may be to subject the patient with recurrent attacks of periumbilical pain to an abdominal surgical exploration.

TABLE 33–3. WEIGHT-LOSS DATA IN PATIENTS FOLLOWED FOR ≥5 y SINCE GASTRIC BYPASS SURGERY[a]

	Weight	Ideal Body Weight	BMI	Weight Loss	Excess Weight Loss
	kg	*%*	*kg/m²*	*%*	*%*
Preoperative (n=114)	136±30	213±46	49±10		
1 y (n=114)	94±26	147±38	34±8	31±12	62±26
2 y (n=114)	90±24	141±35	32±8	34±11	67±24
3 y (n=114)	90±23	142±34	32±8	33±11	66±23
4 y (n=114)	93±25	146±36	33±8	31±10	62±22
5 y (n=114)	95±25	149±37	34±8	30±10	60±23
6 y (n=88)	95±25	149±36	34±8	30±11	59±22
7 y (n=47)	92±21	148±31	34±7	28±12	57±25
8 y (n=15)	93±16	153±24	34±5	26±9	51±17
9 y (n=3)	85±26	148±34	33±8	28±13	56±26

[a]X±SD. Significant (P<.0001) decreases in all weight parameters were noted between preoperative and each year 1 through 9; significant (P<.01) increases were noted between the year 2 and years 5 through 8 for percent weight loss and percent excess weight loss. (*Amer J Clin Nutr* 1992;55:560S–6)

Overall Complication Rate After GBP. Complications in our series included a 1.2% incidence of anastomotic leak with peritonitis, 4.4% severe wound infection (defined as serious enough to delay hospital discharge), 11.4% minor wound infections and seromas (easily treated at home), <1% incidence of gastric staple–line disruption with the use of three superimposed rows of a 90 mm stapler, 15% stomal stenosis, 13% marginal ulcer, 7% incisional hernia, and 10% cholecystitis necessitating cholecystectomy.[61] Forty percent of our GBP patients with a normal intraoperative gallbladder ultrasound developed gallstones, with sludge developing in another 10% within 6 months of surgery.[62,63] Gallstone formation can be decreased to 2% with 300 mg cusodeoxycholic acid pu orem bid for 6 months after gastric bypass. The operative mortality in our series of 672 gastric bypass procedures was 0.4%. Patients with respiratory insufficiency of obesity had a 2.2% operative mortality, in contrast to a 0.2% mortality in those without pulmonary dysfunction.[17]

The data from both our randomized prospective trial[41] and selective study[58] do not support the contention that VBGP is safer than GBP. Although the GBP has an additional anastomosis, complications, including leaks and peritonitis, occur with both operations. One of the criticisms of GBP is the difficulty in evaluating the distal gastric pouch and duodenum. This has been achieved in 75% of patients in one study,[64] with retrograde passage of an endoscope into the duodenum and stomach, and by others with percutaneous distal disten-

sion gastrography.[65] To our knowledge, bleeding from either the distal gastric pouch or duodenal ulcer has occurred in only 1 of our >1200 GBP patients. One of our patients developed a gastric perforation in his proximal gastric pouch after high-dose nonsteroidal anti-inflammatory medication. Gastric mucosal metaplasia of the bypassed stomach was noted in 5% of patients following retrograde endoscopy,[64] which has raised a concern regarding the risk of carcinoma arising in the bypassed stomach. Thousands of these procedures have been performed since 1967 and only case of cancer in the bypassed stomach has been reported. We have had a second case.

Micronutrient Deficiencies After GBP. These are another potential problem following gastric surgery for obesity. Both VBGP and GBP patients should be advised to take a multivitamin daily for life. When compared with VBGP, GBP has significantly lower hemoglobin and serum iron concentrations.[41,58,66–68] This is primarily a problem in menstruating women, since there were no significant differences between hemoglobin and iron concentrations in the nonmenstruating GBP patients, when compared to the VBGP group.[58] All menstruating females who undergo GBP should be treated prophylactically with supplemental oral ferrous sulfate, 325 mg/day. As many as six iron tablets per day may be required with heavy menstrual bleeding; on occasion, intramuscular Imferon injections or, rarely, hysterectomy, may become necessary.[58] Vitamin B_{12} deficiency is a greater risk with GBP than VBGP.[41,58,66–68] This can be prevented with supplemental oral vitamin B_{12}, 500 mcg/day.[69] A few patients may require, or prefer, monthly B_{12} injections, and can be taught to self-administer them. There is a concern that GBP can lead to other divalent cation deficiencies. We have not found problems with serum levels of magnesium or zinc, 5 to 9 years after GBP. However, calcium deficiency may occur, leading to osteoporosis, which may take many years to become manifest and may not be reflected in normal serum calcium levels; therefore, we recommend that our patients take oral calcium supplements. Rarely, polyneuropathy or Wernicke-Korsikoff encephalopathy have been noted after gastric obesity surgery.[70,71] These have occurred only in association with intractable vomiting and severe protein-calorie malnutrition and are thought to be secondary to acute thiamine deficiency. Should a patient develop severe and protracted vomiting after either VBGP or GBP, it is incumbent upon the physician to provide intravenous multivitamin supplements, especially thiamine, prior to instituting nutritional repletion.

Failed Weight Loss

One of the greatest problems with all gastric procedures for morbid obesity is the risk of failed weight loss or

TABLE 33–4. EFFECT OF CONVERSION FROM VBGP TO GBP OWING TO DEVELOPMENT OF MALADAPTIVE EATING BEHAVIOR

	No. Patients	Weight (lbs)	% Excess Weight Loss
Preop VBGP	13	288±13	
Preop GBP	13	261±7	15±5
1 yr after GBP	10	187±13[a]	70±6[a]
2 yrs after GBP	8	187±19[a]	75±8[a]
3 yrs after GBP	6	186±20[a]	71±10[a]
4 yrs after GBP	6	202±25[a]	60±14[a]
5 yrs after GBP	3	212±40	62±18
6 yrs after GBP	2	180±8	75±5

[a]P<.001 GBP vs pre-VBG or at conversion to GBP

weight regain. We,[58] and others,[46] have found that 20% of our VBGP patients have difficulty with solid foods and develop a maladaptive eating behavior with the frequent ingestion of high-calorie liquid carbohydrates. Yale noted that 10% of his VBGP patients failed the procedure for this reason.[60] We have converted 49 VBGP patients to GBP. The average loss of excess weight after VBGP was 31±5% and reached 67±2% at 2 years after conversion to GBP, a value not different from our primary GBP group (Table 33–4).[41,58,61] Four patients became sweets eaters and had lost only 15±5% of excess weight at >1 year after VBGP, without any radiographically demonstrated problems with the procedure; 1 year after conversion to GBP, they lost an average of 78±11% of excess weight.

GBP patients also can suffer from inadequate weight loss. Some patients will develop stomal dilation after the procedure. Naslund[72] was not able to document a correlation between stomal size and weight loss for GBP, whereas there was a relationship between these variables and weight loss after horizontal gastroplasty. In our experience, failure of GBP is the result of either the loss of dumping-syndrome symptoms in a small percentage of patients or, more commonly, the frequent ingestion of high-fat junk foods, such as potato or corn chips, microwave popcorn, or peanut-butter crackers.[58,61] These foods crumble easily and empty quickly from the pouch, so that the patient does not feel full. Patients need dietary instruction to eat foods, low in calories and high in fiber, that will stay in the small gastric pouch longer and provide a feeling of early satiety without a large number of calories (eg, raw carrots, broccoli, cauliflower, apples and oranges). Neither we, nor others,[73] have found reoperation to make the pouch or stoma smaller to be beneficial to the GBP patient who has failed the procedure. These patients must be made aware prior to surgery that the

operation is designed to help them help themselves. It can be easily beaten and they must continue to work for the rest of their lives with appropriate food choices and exercise. It has been our experience that patients who begin to eat more than 1,100 calories per day will begin to gain weight. If they only gain one-half pound per month, this becomes six pounds per year or 60 pounds in ten years. Bariatric surgical patients need lifelong counseling to optimize the results of their surgery.

BILIOPANCREATIC DIVERSION

The unacceptable incidence of complications following the jejunoileal intestinal bypass has already been discussed. In recent years, investigators from Italy have proposed a combined gastric restrictive and intestinal malabsorptive procedure, known as the biliopancreatic diversion.[74] This procedure does not have a blind intestinal limb, and only occasionally produces complications from bacterial overgrowth in the bypassed small bowel. In this operation, a subtotal gastrectomy is performed leaving a proximal gastric pouch of about 200 mL for superobese (>225% IBW) patients and 400 mL for the others; the distal 250 cm of small intestine is anastomosed with a large (2 to 3 cm) stoma to the proximal gastric remnant and the proximal, bypassed small intestine is reanastomosed to the distal ileum, 50 cm from the ileocecal valve. In this manner, the quantity of food ingested is partially restricted and then passes down the intestine mostly undigested and unabsorbed until it reaches the bile and pancreatic juices in the terminal 50 cm of ileum (the common absorptive intestinal channel) where digestion and absorption take place. These patients usually have four to six steatorrheic stools per day which are malodorous and float, reflecting fat malabsorption. In addition to the iron-deficiency anemia and vitamin B_{12} deficiency seen with the standard GBP, these patients are at risk for severe protein deficiency and fat-soluble vitamin deficiencies. These may lead to osteoporosis secondary to calcium and vitamin D malabsorption, night-blindness and skin eruptions secondary to vitamin A deficiency, as well as a prolonged prothrombin time. We, and others, have found this procedure to have a very high incidence of these complications.[75–78] The nutritional complications of this operation may be less severe in Italian patients whose diet is high in complex carbohydrates (eg, pasta), as compared to the high fat content of the American diet (eg, fried foods, potato and corn chips). A number of Italian patients, however, have required rehospitalization for total parenteral nutrition or extension of the "common absorptive channel" from 50 to 150 cm.[77,78] Although one California group reported favorable results, they also stated that fat-soluble vitamin supplementation was mandatory, osteoporosis and iron deficiency may be severe, and 4.1% required reversal for uncorrectable protein-calorie malnutrition.[79]

We have treated a few patients who failed the standard GBP by converting them to the partial biliopancreatic procedure with a 50 cm common absorptive ileal channel, which we have called a "distal gastric bypass," since we did not resect the distal stomach. Unfortunately, this also was associated with an unacceptable incidence of severe malnutrition and fat-soluble vitamin deficiencies.[80] This modification differs from the standard partial biliopancreatic diversion, since the gastric pouch was only 50 cc rather than 200 to 400 cc as originally recommended.[74] More recently, a few superobese patients with significant comorbidity who had failed a standard GBP have been converted to a biliopancreatic bypass with a 150 cm common absorptive intestinal channel, with resumed weight loss. In this group, prophylactic fat-soluble vitamins and pancreatic enzymes prevented vitamin or protein deficiencies. However, when superobese patients were randomized between a standard GBP and a distal GBP (modified partial biliopancreatic diversion), 25% of the distal GBP patients required conversion to a proximal GBP owing to severe protein-calorie malnutrition. Those who did not require conversion had a significantly better weight loss at 3 to 5 years after surgery than the patients randomized to a standard proximal GBP, but they required more nutritional supplementation in order to avoid fat-soluble vitamin deficiencies or osteoporosis.[80] One study suggested that a "long-limb" gastric bypass increases the average weight loss in superobese patients from 50% to 66% loss of excess weight, the amount normally seen in the average patient after GBP, without evidence of additional nutritional deficiencies.[81]

SELECTIVE ASSIGNMENT OF PATIENTS TO DIFFERENT OBESITY PROCEDURES

We had hoped that we could selectively assign patients to the different operations available for the treatment of morbid obesity based on preoperative dietary assessment: VBGP for patients who only ate large quantities of food (gorgers), GBP for patients addicted to sweets, and a malabsorptive biliopancreatic bypass (or distal GBP) for patients who ate small amounts of high-fat junk foods all day long (nibblers). Unfortunately, even with selective assignment, VBGP patients still lost significantly less excess weight than GBP and frequently did not correct their obesity-related comorbidity.[58] Distal GBP patients had an unacceptable incidence of malnutrition and fat-soluble vitamin deficiencies.[80] Thus, we currently recommend a standard GBP in almost all patients. We reserve the VBGP for young menstruating females who are clearly not sweets eaters and have no significant comorbidity, a "long-limb" GBP for superobese patients, and the distal GBP for superobese patients who fail a standard GBP and have significant comorbidity (diabetes, sleep apnea, obesity hypoventilation, venous stasis ulcers, pseudotumor cerebri, etc). The distribution of types of surgical procedures for morbid obesity performed at our center during the past 10 years is shown in Fig 33–13. This documents the progressive decrease in the number of gastroplasty procedures and increase in frequency of GBP as a result of the randomized and selective studies,[41,58] as well as our transient flirtation with malabsorptive distal-GBP.[80]

GASTRIC BYPASS TECHNIQUE

Following induction of general anesthesia, two grams of Ancef are administered, thigh-length intermittent venous compression boots are placed, a urinary catheter and nasogastric (NG) tube are inserted, and the abdomen is prepped and draped. An upper midline abdominal incision is made from the xiphoid to the umbilicus and the fat is spread apart manually. This identifies the linea alba with minimal blood loss from the large subcutaneous veins usually present in these patients. The peritoneal cavity is entered and the properitoneal fat spread and cauterized, as is the falciform ligament. A Polytrac retractor (Pilling Co., Philadelphia, PA) is placed with two large Mayo-Richardson retractors laterally, a bladder blade at the umbilicus, and a finger retractor over a wet laparotomy pad, bringing the left lobe of the liver superiorly. The triangular ligament of the left lobe of the liver does not need to be incised. The abdomen and pelvis are manually explored.

The gastrohepatic omentum is incised and the opening enlarged superiorly with electrocautery, care taken to avoid transection of an aberrant left hepatic artery originating from the left gastric artery, in 25% of cases. The esophagus is bluntly mobilized, encircled with a 1/2 inch penrose drain, and retracted superiorly by wrapping the Penrose drain around the liver retractor arm, bringing the gastroesophageal junction into the wound. The Roux-en-Y anastomosis then is constructed, prior to stapling the stomach, to ensure that the jejunum will reach the gastric pouch without tension. Should excessive tension be noted, the GBP can be aborted and the less effective, but safer (under these circumstances) VBGP constructed. This would be precluded if the stomach had been stapled for GBP.

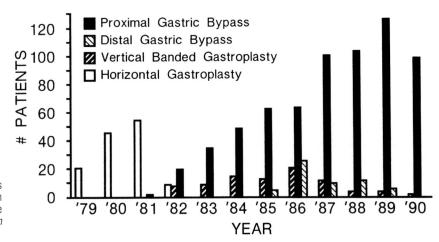

Figure 33–13. Distribution of patients with various operations for morbid obesity at the Medical College of Virginia from 1980 through 1990. (From Sugerman HJ, Kellum JM, Engle KM, et al. Gastric bypass for treating severe obesity. *Am J Clin Nutr* 1992;55:560S)

The transverse colon is retracted superiorly and the ligament of Treitz identified. Two to three feet of jejunum are advanced until an area with the longest mesentery is identified; the jejunum then is transected with a GIA stapler (Auto-Suture Inc, US Surgical Co, Norwalk, CN). A three to four inch segment of jejunum is resected with another firing of the GIA stapler and ligation of the mesentery to minimize tension on the Roux limb. The mesentery is further opened posteriorly, as much as possible. A 45 cm segment of jejunum then is measured for the average obesity patient, or 150 cm if the patient is superobese, using a pre-cut umbilical tape. A functional end-to-side stapled jejunojejunostomy is constructed with a third firing of the GIA stapler, closing the opening with a 55 mm horizontal stapler. The mesenteric window is closed with a running, 2-0 polyglycolic acid suture. Openings are made by bluntly passing two fingers through the transverse mesocolon lateral to the middle colic vessels and then through the greater omentum. The Roux limb is brought through the retrocolic opening with a large Babcock clamp. If it lies easily next to the gastroesophageal junction, the gastric bypass procedure can be completed and a 3-0 silk suture is placed with the needle left on for subsequent placement into the proximal gastric pouch. If there is excessive tension, the Roux limb is resected, the GBP abandoned, and a VBGP constructed.

An opening is made next to the lesser curvature of the stomach and medial to the neurovascular bundle, between the first and second branches of the left gastric artery, 2 to 3 cm below the gastroesophageal junc-

tion. A plane is developed behind the stomach to the angle of His, at the site of the Penrose drain, along the left side of the gastroesophageal junction. A large, red rubber tube is passed through the large opening in the gastrohepatic omentum to the angle of His; the tube then is brought through the opening along the lesser curvature of the stomach with a large right angle clamp. One must be certain that the tube is below the left gastric artery or the esophagus will be stapled shut. It is extremely important that the nasogastric tube be withdrawn at this time into the esophagus above the Penrose drain to avoid stapling it into the stomach. The anvil of a PI-90 (Surgeon's Choice, 3-M Corporation, Minneapolis, MN) stapler is inserted into the red rubber tube and brought across the stomach, taking care to avoid injury to the back wall of the stomach. A small amount of the anterior gastric wall, only enough to perform the gastrojejunal anastomosis, is brought above the stapler with a sponge stick. The stapler is closed, inspected to assure that there is no gastric fold within it, and fired. The stapler is released, the staple cartridge removed, a new cartridge inserted, and the stapler closed on top of the previous staple line and fired again. This process is repeated once more for a total of three superimposed applications of the PI-90 stapler. A 1 cm gastrojejunal anastomosis is constructed with a handsewn anastomosis, using 3-0 silk for the outer layer and 2-0 polyglycolic acid for the inner layer. Prior to completing the anterior row of the inner layer, a 30 French (Fr) mercury-filled esophageal dilator is passed through the anastomosis, after releasing the tension on the Penrose drain (or the posterior esophagus will be perforated). The dilator is removed after the anastomosis is completed and the nasogastric tube advanced through it. The jejunum is digitally occluded and filled under tension with about 30 cc methylene-blue to assure the absence of leaks and the integrity of the gastric staple line.

The opening in the mesocolon is closed with running 2-0 chromic catgut to include the base of the Roux mesentery, in order to prevent a Peterson hernia behind the Roux limb. A gastrostomy tube is only inserted into the bypassed stomach if the patient has had previous surgery with multiple small bowel adhesions. An intraoperative gallbladder sonogram is obtained and the gallbladder removed, if there are gallstones or sludge present. The fascia is reapproximated with running 2 polyglycolic acid suture. The subcutaneous tissues are irrigated with 1% neomycin and the skin reapproximated with surgical staples. No subcutaneous sutures or drains are used.

VERTICAL GASTROPLASTY TECHNIQUE

The exposure of the esophagus and the stomach are the same as described for the GBP. To perform the VBGP, one passes the shaft of a 28 mm EEA (Auto-Suture, Inc, US Surgical Co, Norwalk, CT) through the anterior and posterior gastric walls, 5 cm distal to the gastroesophageal junction. This can be simplified by attaching a specially tooled sharp needle to the EEA shaft. A vertical staple line is constructed to the angle of His using a 90 mm linear stapler. A specially designed bariatric stapler, which fired four parallel rows of staples, was previously recommended; however, MacLean and associates noted a 35% staple-line dehiscence using this instrument.[38] He currently recommends transecting the stomach. However, we have found a <1% staple-line disruption rate when three superimposed applications of the 90 mm stapler in the GBP procedure were used and would suggest its use for the VBGP. Prior to applying the stapler, Mason recommends measuring the pouch capacity at 15 to 30 mL at 50 cm above the oral pharynx. The outlet of the pouch is restricted with a 1.5 cm wide band of polypropylene mesh that is sutured to itself at a circumference of 5 cm. It is important that the mesh not be sutured to the stomach or this may lead to a high incidence of mesh erosion into the gastric lumen. The greater omentum then is placed over the band and sutured to the lesser curvature of the stomach to avoid adhesions of the band to the liver, which leads to kinking and obstruction of the gastric pouch outlet.

The silastic ring gastroplasty is performed in a manner similar to the GBP except that the vertical staple line is constructed with a special notched 90 mm stapler along the lesser curvature of the stomach (Fig 33–5). At the inferior margin of the staple line, a prolene suture is passed through the stapled anterior and posterior gastric walls and inserted into a piece of silastic tubing and tied to itself, creating a 4.5 cm banded outlet stoma. In both gastroplasty procedures, it is important to document the absence of leaks with the injection of methylene blue under pressure.

EFFECT OF GASTRIC SURGERY–INDUCED WEIGHT LOSS ON COMORBIDITY

Weight loss completely corrects the NIDDM in over 90% of patients,[19–21] the hypertension in 80%,[82] and the headaches associated with cerebrospinal fluid pressure elevation in pseudotumor cerebri.[23] The obstructive sleep apnea syndrome resolves with weight loss (Fig 33–14).[15–18] Reduced lung volumes (Fig 33–1), hypoxemia, and hypercarbia (Fig 33–2) seen in the obesity hypoventilation syndrome also return toward normal, in most patients, following weight loss and remain improved for more than 5 years.[15–18] Elevated pulmonary artery and pulmonary capillary occlusion pressures will improve significantly after weight loss correction of abnormal arterial blood gases (Fig 33–3).[16] The loss in weight usually corrects female sexual hormone abnormalities and increases fertility.[83] The profound weight loss significantly reduces urinary bladder pressures (Fig 33–15), probably as a result of a decrease in intra-abdominal pressure, with resolution of both urge and stress incontinence in 90% of women who present with this complaint (Fig 33–16).[11] This decrease in intra-abdominal pressure with weight loss is probably also responsible for the healing of chronic venous stasis ulcers associated with venous insufficiency. Both the reduction in intra-abdominal pressure, as well as a marked decrease in both acid and bile in the proximal gastric pouch, result in a significant decrease in gastroesophageal reflux symptoms after GBP. An increase in gastroesophageal reflux symptoms may be seen as a complication of VBGP, necessitating conversion to GBP.[84] Weight loss also will frequently improve low back pain, as well as joint-related pain, and may permit successful total artificial joint replacement when indicated, without the unacceptable incidence of loosening following joint replacement in the morbidly obese. Patient self-image and employability also may be significantly improved following correction of morbid obesity.

Inappropriate operations in the morbidly obese patient include bladder neck suspension for stress or urge incontinence, Nissen fundoplication for gastroesophageal reflux, ventriculoperitoneal shunt for pseudotumor cerebri, uvulopalatopharyngoplasty (UPPP) for obstructive sleep apnea syndrome, total joint replacement for degenerative joint disease of the hips or knees, laminectomy for intervertebral disc disease, or split

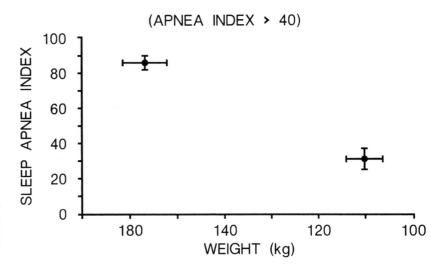

Figure 33–14. Decrease in sleep apnea index (*P*<.001) associated with decrease in weight (*P*<.0001) after gastric surgery for obesity in patients with severe obstructive sleep apnea (apnea index >40). (From Sugerman HJ, Fairman RP, Sood RK, et al. Long-term effects of gastric surgery for treating respiratory insufficiency of obesity. *Am J Clin Nutr* 1992;55:597S)

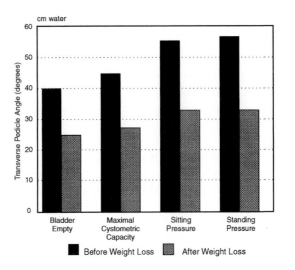

Figure 33–15. Significant (*P*<.001) decreases in bladder pressures 9 to 18 months following GBP induced weight loss of 88±17 kg. (From Bump RC, Sugerman HJ, Fantl JA, et al. Obesity and lower urinary tract function in women: effect of surgically induced weight loss. *Am J Obstet Gynec* 1992;167:392)

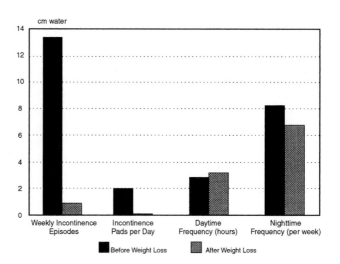

Figure 33–16. Significant (*P*<.01) decrease in frequency of urge and/or stress overflow urinary incontinence 9 to 18 months following surgically induced weight loss of 88±17 kg and associated decrease in bladder pressures. (From Bump RC, Sugerman HJ, Fantl JA, et al. Obesity and lower urinary tract function in women: effect of surgically induced weight loss. *Am J Obstet Gynec* 1992;167:392)

thickness skin graft for venous stasis ulcer. All of these problems might be better served first by performing a gastric bypass procedure. Should the problem persist after weight loss, then the "more standard" procedure could be undertaken with a greater likelihood of success. One of these operations, the Nissen fundoplication, may have to be taken down in order to perform either a VBGP or GBP, which would significantly increase the morbidity of the weight reduction procedure.

Published data support the efficacy of gastric surgery for severe obesity with BMI >35 kg/m². There are no studies showing dietary management, with or without behavioral modification programs, to have significant success for these unfortunate patients more than 1 to 2 years after initial weight loss. GBP has been shown to be significantly more effective for weight loss than any gastroplasty procedure, including VBGP, which often fails to correct the patients' comorbidity.[87] On the average, patients lose two-thirds of their excess weight within 2 years following GBP. Long-term results show the loss of approximately 60% of excess weight at five years and more than 55% up to 10 years after surgery. The GBP may be associated with vitamin B_{12} deficiency and iron deficiency anemia in menstruating women. There is a concern that it could lead to calcium deficiency and osteoporosis. It may also be "beaten" by the frequent nibbling of high-fat junk foods. Thus, it is important that patients be followed for life with dietary expertise to evaluate micronutrients and eating patterns following weight reduction surgery. Significant weight loss is associated with correction of severe, life-threatening comorbidity such as respiratory insufficiency of obesity, diabetes, hypertension, and cardiac dysfunction. It also will frequently alleviate problems associated with major debility, such as degenerative joint disease, pseudotumor cerebri, venous stasis ulcers, gastroesophageal reflux, and urinary incontinence. Until there is a better medical approach for these unfortunate individuals, gastric surgery for the correction and control of severe obesity is the only proven treatment; this was recognized in the 1991 National Institutes of Health Consensus Development Conference.[2]

REFERENCES

1. Metropolitan Life Insurance Company. New weight standards for men and women. *Stat Bull Metrop Ins Co* 1959:40:1
2. NIH Conference. Gastrointestinal surgery for severe obesity: Consensus Development Conference Panel. *Ann Int Med* 1991;115:956
3. Stunkard AJ, Sorensen TA, Hanis C, et al. An adoption study of human obesity. *N Engl J Med* 1986;314:193
4. Stunkard AJ, Harris JR, Pedersen NL, et al. The body-mass index of twins who have been reared apart. *N Engl J Med* 1990;322:1483
5. Bouchard C, Tremblay A, Despres J-P, et al. The response to long-term overfeeding in identical twins. *N Engl J Med* 1990;322:1477
6. Roberts SB, Savage J, Coward WA, et al. Energy expenditure and intake in infants born to lean and overweight mothers. *N Engl J Med* 1988;318:461
7. Mason EE, Printen KJ, Barron P, et al. Risk reduction in gastric operations for obesity. *Ann Surg* 1979;190:158
8. Drennick EJ, Bale GS, Seltter F, et al. Excessive mortality and causes of death in morbidly obese men. *JAMA* 1980; 243:443
9. Kissebah A, Vydelingum N, Murray R, et al. Relation of body fat distribution to metabolic complications of obesity. *J Clin Endocrinol Metab* 1982;54:254
10. Kvist A, Chowdhury B, Grangard U, et al. Total and visceral adipose tissue volumes derived from measurements with computed tomography in adult men and women: predictive equations. *Am J Clin Nutr* 1988;48:1351
11. Bump RC, Sugerman HJ, Fantl JA, et al. Obesity and lower urinary tract function in women: effects of surgically induced weight loss. *Am J Obstet Gynecol* 1992;167:392
12. Messerli FH, Sundgaard-Riise K, Reisin ED, et al. Disparate cardiovascular effects of obesity and arterial hypertension. *Am J Med* 1983;74:808
13. Alpert MA, Terry BE, Kelly DL. Effect of weight loss on cardiac chamber size, wall thickness and left ventricular function in morbid obesity. *Am J Cardiol* 1985;55:783
14. Manson JE, Colditz GA, Stampfer MJ, et al. A prospective study of obesity and risk of coronary heart disease in women. *N Engl J Med* 1990;322:882
15. Sugerman HJ, Fairman RP, Baron PL, et al. Gastric surgery for respiratory insufficiency of obesity. *Chest* 1986; 90:82
16. Sugerman HJ, Baron PL, Fairman RP, et al. Hemodynamic dysfunction in obesity hypoventilation syndrome and the effects of treatment with surgically induced weight loss. *Ann Surg* 1988;207:604
17. Sugerman HJ, Fairman RP, Sood RK, et al. Long-term effects of gastric surgery for treating respiratory insufficiency of obesity. *Am J Clin Nutr* 1992;55:597S
18. Charuzi I, Ovnat A, Peiser J, et al. The effect of surgical weight reduction on sleep quality in obesity-related sleep apnea syndrome. *Surgery* 1985;97:535
19. Herbst CA, Hughes TA, Gwynne JT, et al. Gastric bariatric operation in insulin-treated adults. *Surgery* 1984;95:201
20. Pories WJ, Caro J, MacDonald KG, et al. Is type II diabetes mellitus (NIDDM) a surgical disease? *Ann Surg* 1992; 215:633
21. Pories WJ, MacDonald KG, Morgan EJ, et al. Surgical treatment of obesity and its effects on diabetes: 10-year follow-up. *Am J Clin Nutr* 1992;55:582S
22. Deitel M, Khanna RK, Hagen J, et al. Vertical banded gastroplasty as an antireflux procedure. *Am J Surg* 1988; 155:512
23. Amaral JF, Tsiaris W, Morgan T, et al. Reversal of benign intracranial hypertension by surgically induced weight loss. *Arch Surg* 1987;122:946
24. Johnson D, Drennick EJ. Therapeutic fasting in morbid obesity. *Arch Intern Med* 1977;137:1381
25. Methods for voluntary weight loss and control. NIH Tech-

nology Assessment Conference Panel. *Ann Int Med* 1992; 116:942

26. Hocking MP, Duerson MC, O'Leary PJ, et al. Jejunoileal bypass for morbid obesity: late follow-up in 100 cases. *N Engl J Med* 1983;308:995

27. Halverson JD, Gentry K, Wise L, et al. Reanastomosis after jejunoileal bypass. *Surgery* 1978;84:241

28. Griffen WO, Young VL, Stevenson CC. A prospective comparison of gastric and jejunoileal bypass for morbid obesity. *Ann Surg* 1977;186:500

29. Mason EE, Ito C. Gastric bypass. *Ann Surg* 1969;170:329

30. Mason EE, Munns JR, Kealey GP, et al. Effects of gastric bypass on gastric secretion. *Am J Surg* 1976;131:162

31. Sugerman HJ, Wolper JL. Failed gastroplasty for morbid obesity: revised gastroplasty versus Roux-en-Y gastric bypass. *Am J Surg* 1984;148:331

32. Mason EE. Vertical banded gastroplasty for obesity. *Arch Surg* 1982;117:701

33. Mason EE. VBG: effective treatment of uncontrolled obesity. *Bull Am Coll Surg* 1991;76:18

34. Willibanks OL. Longterm results of silicone elastomer ring vertical gastroplasty for the treatment of morbid obesity. *Surgery* 1987;101:606

35. Granstrom L, Backman L. Technical considerations and related reoperations after gastric banding. *Acta Chir Scand* 1987;153:215

36. Kirby RM, Ismail T, Crawson M, et al. Gastric banding in the treatment of morbid obesity. *Br J Surg* 1989;76:490

37. Kuzmak LI, Yap IS, McGuire L, et al. Surgery for morbid obesity: using an inflatable gastric band. *AORN J* 1990; 51:1307

38. MacLean LD, Rhode BM, Forse RA. Late results of vertical banded gastroplasty for morbid and super obesity. *Surgery* 1990;107:20

39. Pories WJ, Flickinger EG, Meelheim D, et al. The effectiveness of gastric bypass over gastric partition in morbid obesity: consequences of distal gastric and duodenal exclusion. *Ann Surg* 1987;196:389

40. Lechner GW, Elliott DW. Comparison of weight loss after gastric exclusion and partitioning. *Arch Surg* 1983;118:685

41. Sugerman HJ, Starkey JV, Birkenhauer R. A randomized prospective trial of gastric bypass versus vertical banded gastroplasty for morbid obesity and their effects on sweets versus non-sweets eaters. *Ann Surg* 1987;205:613

42. Kenler HA, Brolin RE, Cody RO. Changes in eating behavior after horizontal gastroplasty and Roux-en-Y gastric bypass. *Am J Clin Nutr* 1990;52:87

43. Agren G, Naslund I. A prospective randomized comparison of vertical banded gastroplasty (VBG), loop gastric bypass (GBY) and gastric banding (GB). Presented at the 4th International Symposium on Obesity Surgery; London, England: August, 1989

44. MacClean LD, Rhode BM, Sampalis J, et al. Results of the surgical treatment of obesity. *Am J Surg* 1993;165:155

45. Hall JC, Watts JM, O'Brien PE, et al. Gastric surgery for morbid obesity: the Adelaide study. *Ann Surg* 1990; 211:419

46. Nightingale ML, Sarr MG, Kelly KA, et al. Prospective evaluation of vertical banded gastroplasty as the primary operation for morbid obesity. *Mayo Clin Proc* 1991;66:773

47. Kellum JM, Kuemmerle JF, O'Dorision TM, et al. Gastrointestinal hormone responses to meals before and after gastric bypass and vertical banded gastroplasty. *Ann Surg* 1990;211:763

48. Sirinek KR, O'Dorisio TM, Hill D, et al. Hyperinsulinism, glucose-dependent insulinotropic polypeptide, and the enteroinsular axis in morbidly obese patients before and after gastric bypass. *Surgery* 1986;100:781

49. Schrumpf E, Bergan A, Djoseland O, et al. The effect of gastric bypass operation on glucose tolerance in obesity. *Scand J Gastroenterol* 1985;20(S):24

50. Meryn S, Stein D, Strauss EW. Fasting- and meal-stimulated peptide hormone concentrations before and after gastric surgery for morbid obesity. *Metabolism* 1986;35:798

51. Meryn S, Stein D, Strauss EW. Pancreatic polypeptide, pancreatic glucagon and enteroglucagon in morbid obesity and following gastric bypass operation. *Int J Obes* 1986; 10:37

52. Sirinek KR, O'Dorisio TM, Howe B, et al. Neurotensin, vasoactive intestinal peptide, and Roux-en-Y gastrojejunostomy. *Arch Surg* 1985;120:605

53. Amland PF, Jorde R, Kildebo S, et al. Effects of a gastric partitioning operation for morbid obesity on the secretion of gastric inhibitory polypeptide and pancreatic polypeptide. *Scand J Gastroenterol* 1984;19:857

54. Miskowiak J, Andersen B, Stadel F, et al. Meal stimulated levels of pancreatic polypeptide (PP) and vasoactive intestinal peptide (VIP) in gastroplasty for morbid obesity. *Regul Pept* 1985;12:231

55. Miskowiak J, Andersen B, Stadil F, et al. Serum gastrin and blood glucose levels in gastroplasty for morbid obesity. *Scand J Gastroenterol* 1984;19:669

56. Shulkes A, Allen RD, Hardy KJ. Meal stimulated neurotensin release following gastric partitioning for morbid obesity. *Aust NZ J Surg* 1983;53:149

57. Miskowiak J, Andersen B, Stadil F, et al. Plasma secretin before and after gastroplasty for morbid obesity. *Scand J Clin Lab Invest* 1984;44:363

58. Sugerman HJ, Londrey GL, Kellum JM, et al. Weight loss with vertical banded gastroplasty and Roux-Y gastric bypass for morbid obesity with selective versus random assignment. *Am J Surg* 1989;157:93

59. Brolin RE, Kenler HA, Robertson LB, et al. Weight loss and dietary intake after vertical banded gastroplasty and Roux-en-Y gastric bypass. Presented at the Annual Meeting of the Society for Surgery of the Alimentary Tract; Boston, Massachusetts: May, 1993

60. Yale CE. Gastric surgery for morbid obesity. Complications and long-term weight control. *Arch Surg* 1989; 124:941

61. Sugerman HJ, Kellum JM, Engle KM, et al. Gastric bypass for treating severe obesity. *Am J Clin Nutr* 1992;55:560S

62. Shiffman ML, Sugerman HJ, Kellum JM, et al. Gallstone formation after rapid weight loss: a prospective study in patients undergoing gastric bypass surgery for treatment of morbid obesity. *Am J Gastroenterol* 1991;86:1000

63. Shiffman ML, Sugerman HJ, Kellum JM, et al. Gallstones in patients with morbid obesity. Relationship to body weight, weight loss and gallbladder bile cholesterol solubility. *Int J Obes* 1993;17:153

64. Flickinger EG, Sinar DR, Pories WJ, et al. The bypassed stomach. *Am J Surg* 1985;149:151

65. Cardella JF, Linner JH, Drew RL. Percutaneous distal distension gastrography: new technique for evaluation of distal stomach in patients with gastric bypass. *Semin Int Radiol* 1988;5:241

66. MacLean LD, Rhode GM, Shizgal HM. Nutrition following gastric operations for morbid obesity. *Ann Surg* 1983; 198:347

67. Amaral JF, Thompson WR, Caldwell MD, et al. Prospective hematologic evaluation of gastric exclusion surgery for morbid obesity. *Ann Surg* 1985;201:186

68. Halverson JD. Micronutrient deficiencies after gastric bypass for morbid obesity. *Am Surg* 1986;52:594

69. Boylan LM, Sugerman HJ, Driskell JA. Vitamin E, vitamin B-6, vitamin B-12, and folate status of gastric bypass surgery patients. *J Am Diet Assoc* 1988;88:579

70. Kramer LD, Locke GE. Wernicke's encephalopathy. *J Clin Gastroenterol* 1987;9:549

71. Feit H, Glasberg M, Ireton C, et al. Peripheral neuropathy and starvation after gastric partitioning for morbid obesity. *Ann Int Med* 1982;96:453

72. Naslund I, Nickbom G, Christoffersson E, et al. A prospective randomized comparison of gastric bypass and gastroplasty. *Acta Chir Scand* 1986;152:681

73. Schwartz RW, Strodel NE, Simpson WS, et al. Gastric bypass revision: lessons learned from 920 cases. *Surgery* 1988;104:806

74. Scopinaro N, Gianetta E, Civalleri D, et al. Partial and total biliopancreatic bypass in the surgical treatment of obesity. *Int J Obes* 1981;5:421

75. Liszka TG, Sugerman HJ, Kellum JM, et al. Risk/benefit considerations of distal gastric bypass. *Int J Obes* 1988; 12:604 (Abstract)

76. Cates JA, Drenick EJ, Abedin MZ, et al. Reoperative surgery for the morbidly obese: a university experience. *Arch Surg* 1990;125:1400

77. Gianetta E, Friedman D, Adams GF, et al. Etiological factors of protein malnutrition after biliopancreatic diversion. *Gastroenterol Clin North Am* 1987;16:503

78. Scopinaro N, Gianetta E, Friedman D, et al. Surgical revision of biliopancreatic diversion. *Gastroenterol Clin North Am* 1987;16:529

79. Holian DK, Clare MW. Biliopancreatic diversion for malignant obesity. *Contemp Surg* 1991;39:26

80. Sugerman HJ, Kellum JM, Rothrock MK, et al. Proximal vs distal gastric bypass in the superobese patient: a randomized study. Presented at the Annual Meeting of The Society for Surgery of the Alimentary Tract; Boston, Massachussetts: May 18, 1993

81. Brolin RE, Kenler HA, Gorman JH, et al. Long-limb gastric bypass in the superobese. A prospective randomized study. *Ann Surg* 1992;215:387

82. Foley EF, Benotti PN, Borlase BC, et al. Impact of gastric restrictive surgery on hypertension in the morbidly obese. *Am J Surg* 1992;163:294

83. Deitel M, Toan BT, Stone EM, et al. Sex hormone changes accompanying loss of massive excess weight. *Gastroenterol Clin North Amer* 1987;16:511

84. Kim CH, Sarr MG. Severe reflux esophagitis after vertical banded gastroplasty for treatment of morbid obesity. *Mayo Clin Proc* 1992;67:33

85. MacLean LD, Rhode BM, Forse RA. A gastroplasty that avoids stapling in continuity. *Surgery* 1993;113:380

34

Stomach and Duodenum: Operative Procedures

David I. Soybel ▪ *Michael J. Zinner*

▪ HISTORICAL PERSPECTIVE

The earliest recorded operations on the stomach were performed for penetrating injuries.[1] In the late 1800s,[2] experimental studies in the surgical laboratories of Billroth confirmed the feasibility of removing the pylorus, a concept developed by Michaelis in the early part of that century. In 1881, Rydygier performed the first successful pylorectomy and, in 1884, he performed the first gastroenterostomy. Both of these operations were performed for benign peptic ulcer disease. In 1881, Billroth performed the first successful pylorectomy for malignancy. In this case, the duodenum was anastomosed to the lesser curvature of the stomach and the greater curvature was oversewn. The patient initially did well, but died of disseminated abdominal carcinomatosis four months later. In 1885, Billroth performed a resection of a large pyloric carcinoma, using an anterior gastrojejunostomy for the reconstruction. In subsequent years, Billroth, his students, and others devised several approaches to gastroduodenal and gastrojejunal reconstruction,[2,3] some of which will be detailed below. Following popularization of gastrojejunostomy for reconstruction after gastric resection or palliation of unresectable gastric malignancy, surgeons were confronted with early complications such as bleeding, anastomotic leak, intestinal obstruction, and late complications, such as stomal ulceration, bilious vomiting, afferent and efferent limb obstructions, and dumping.[4] At present, these problems remain unsolved.

Pyloroplasty was initially devised by Heineke for treatment of congenital hypertrophic pyloric stenosis, and results were poor. Jaboulay's side-to-side anastomosis of the distal greater curvature and duodenum, in 1892, and the Faience extension of this anastomosis to include the pylorus itself were subsequently refined by Kocher. Kocher improved the technical ease of the operation by including a mobilization of the duodenum from its lateral peritoneal attachments. The first pyloromyotomy was performed for this lesion in 1912 by Ramstedt.

In the early part of the 20th century, a dramatic rise was observed in the incidence of duodenal ulceration. A period of intense clinical and laboratory investigation from 1920 to 1940 led to the recognition that surgically performed vagotomy could reduce gastric acidity under resting conditions and in response to luminal and humoral stimuli. The use of vagotomy for patients with complications of ulcer disease was pioneered by Latarjet, who reported 24 such cases in 1922. Latarjet himself recognized that vagotomy might lead to delayed gastric emptying and had added a drainage procedure, gastrojejunostomy. Confusion regarding the role of delayed gastric emptying in the pathogenesis of peptic ulcers, however, led many surgeons away from vagotomy and drainage as a treatment for recurrent peptic ulceration.

It remained for Dragstedt and his colleagues at the University of Chicago to resurrect this concept in the 1940s.[6] Subsequently, Farmer and Smithwick, and others introduced the combination of truncal vagotomy and hemigastrectomy, an operation that also removed the gastrin-producing antral mucosa.[2] In the 1950s, Harkins' group in Seattle began to evaluate forms of vagotomy that left intact the celiac and hepatic branches (proximal selective vagotomy) alone, or in combination with preservation of vagal motor branches to the antrum (highly selective, HSV, or parietal cell vagotomy, HSV).[7,8] These modifications arose from an appreciation of the contributions of antral motility to proper digestion, as well as improved understanding of specific postvagotomy complications such as dumping and diarrhea. The popularization of HSV is largely attributable to the efforts of Johnston, Goligher, Amdrup, and others, who, in the 1960s and 1970s, demonstrated the feasibility of obtaining ulcer recurrence rates as low as that of conventional truncal vagotomy (TV) without the incidence of dumping and diarrhea that was associated with TV with drainage or gastrectomy.[9,10]

It is worth noting that surgeons have done more than develop new and interesting operative approaches to acid peptic disease. They played a major role in advancing current concepts of pathophysiology of ulcer disease and recurrence, and in understanding the physiological consequences of ulcer treatments, both medical and surgical. To understand the importance of the technical details in the execution of antisecretory operations, it is necessary to fully appreciate the anatomy of the vagus nerve and the gastric microvasculature, as well as the physiology of acid secretion, mucosal barrier function, and gastric motility.

■ VAGOTOMY

TESTS OF VAGAL CONTROL OF ACID SECRETION

Historically, vagal control of acid secretion has been assessed by measuring acid secretion in response to various stimuli. Acid secretion can be measured directly by placement of a tube into the stomach, through which gastric juice is aspirated. Acid secretion also can be assessed semiquantitatively, using pH sensitive dyes that coat the mucosa and turn color when acid is being secreted from the gastric glands. Although the former analytic methods permit accurate and quantitative assays of secretory capacity before and after operation, the latter colorimetric methods can provide relatively rapid means of assessing secretory capacity of the stomach during the operation itself. As discussed below, a colorimetric method may even be considered an essential part of any selective or highly selective vagotomy operation.

Analytic Assessment of Gastric Acid Secretion

Under fluoroscopic control and in the supine, semirecumbent position, a radiopaque 18-French (Fr) sump should be positioned in the gastric antrum. Optimal position of the tube is obtained if at least 16 mL can be recovered from a test infusion of 20 mL of normal saline. In patients who have undergone partial gastrectomy, blockade of the gastric outlet may be indicated, if there is significant bile contamination of gastric aspirates. Measurements of acid secretion are obtained after a overnight fast and must be performed at the same time of day, with a standard protocol. A commonly used protocol would include aspiration of gastric contents at 15 min intervals: 2 to 4 discarded "equilibration" periods, 4 baseline periods, followed by 4 periods of stimulation. The volume of the gastric aspirate from each period is measured and then its titratable acidity is measured by adding known quantities of 0.1 N NaOH until the pH has returned to 7.0. Currently, two forms of stimulation are used. First, pentagastrin (12 μg/kg) may be given as a subcutaneous injection. Vagotomy is known to decrease the sensitivity of the parietal cell to gastrin stimulation. Second, a "sham-feeding" protocol can be used to stimulate the cephalic, vagal-mediated phase of acid secretion by allowing the patient to see, smell, and chew an appetizing meal (steak and potatoes in some parts of the United States, tofu and tomato juice in others).

The indices that are used for comparison include (1) basal acid output (BAO), defined as the number of millimoles (mmol) of H^+ secreted in the baseline 1 hr period; (2) peak acid output (PAO), defined as the rate of H^+ secretion in the two periods of highest response after pentagastrin (6 μg/kg sc in prevagotomy patients, 12 μg/kg in postvagotomy patients); (3) sham feeding-stimulated acid output (SAO), defined as the sum of four consecutive periods after sham feeding. Table 34–1 gives the range of BAO, PAO, and SAO found in the normal population. Table 34–2 illustrates how the different indices of gastric acid secretion are altered by various antisecretory operations. One very sensitive index appears to be the ratio SAO/PAO. If this is less than 0.1, a complete vagotomy seems assured.[11,12]

TABLE 34–1. NORMAL ACID OUTPUT VALUES IN HEALTHY ADULTS (mmol/hr)

	BAO	MAO	PAO	BAO/PAO
Men	0–12	7–53	11–64	0.0–0.3
Women	0–7	2–38	5–45	0.0–0.3

BAO=basal rate; MAO=maximal rate; PAO=peak rate of acid output as defined in text. (Adapted from Goldschmiedt M, Feldman M. Gastric secretion health and disease. In: Sleisenger MH, Fordtran JS (eds), *Gastrointestinal Disease, 5th ed.* Philadelphia, PA: WB Saunders; 1993.)

TABLE 34–2. EFFECTS OF DIFFERENT OPERATIONS ON GASTRIC ACID OUTPUT

	Reduction after Operation (%)			
	BAO	*SAO*	*PAO*	*Food*
Truncal Vagotomy	60	95	65	65
Selective Vagotomy	60	95	55	—
Highly Selective Vagotomy	80	95	60	50
Antrectomy & Vagotomy	80	95	80	—
Antrectomy	80	55	50	—

BAO=basal, SAO=sham feeding stimulation, PAO + Peak, secretagogue-induced stimulation.
(Adapted from Thirlby RC. Studies of gastric secretion. In: Scott HW, Sawyers JL (eds), *Surgery of the Stomach, Duodenum and Small Intestine, 2nd ed.* Boston, MA: Blackwell Scientific; 1992.)

Colorimetric Methods Congo-Red

Congo-red is a nontoxic dye that turns from red to black in the presence of a pH below 3.0. When normal gastric mucosa is sprayed with an alkalinized solution containing Congo-red, it will turn black within minutes. After vagotomy, the Congo-red–stained mucosa will remain red, except in areas not yet denervated. Thus, its use has been advocated in patients undergoing highly selective vagotomy. At present, the Federal Drug Administration, in the United States, permits use of Congo-red in humans under specifically approved protocols.[13]

VAGAL REGULATION OF GASTRIC MOTILITY AND EMPTYING

As stated by Professor David Johnston in a previous edition of this book, ". . . Only when one fully understands the physiologic rationale of highly selective vagotomy will one be sufficiently motivated to do it well." This statement was made, not in reference to the innervation of parietal cells that secrete HCl, but to the neural regulation of gastric motor function and emptying. The vagus dominates the motor activity of the normally functioning stomach in three ways. First, it mediates receptive relaxation and gastric accommodation; that is, the relaxation of the gastric fundus when intraluminal pressures in the proximal esophagus and stomach are increased by the presence of chyme. Second, the vagus mediates increases in antral myoelectrical activity that result from distension of the proximal stomach by chyme. Third, the vagus appears to mediate coordination of pyloric emptying with antral myoelectrical activity, in response to changes in proximal gastric motor activity and, perhaps, in response to changes in composition and pH of duodenal content.[14]

It should be recognized that while truncal or selective vagotomy interrupts the vagal pathways to the antrum and pylorus, all three forms of vagotomy (truncal, selective, highly selective) abolish receptive relaxation

and gastric accommodation. It has been claimed that, in the absence of pyloric scarring or stenosis, that vagotomy only temporarily impairs gastric emptying. This rationale has been used to justify combinations of selective and relatively nonselective approaches, such as a posterior truncal and anterior highly selective (or anterior seromyotomy) vagotomy. Such arguments become important in thinking about the feasibility of laparoscopic approaches to the vagus and the need for, and choice of, drainage procedures. Nevertheless, caution is advisable in recommending mixtures of approach or dispensing with drainage procedures after truncal or selective vagotomy. The assumptions that the antral/pyloric coordination will return after truncal vagotomy or that gastric emptying after pyloromyotomy is as good as that after pyloroplasty are currently being tested, but have been disputed.[15] In addition, the full spectrum of complications following such mixtures of approach remains relatively uncharacterized and has not been studied in properly controlled trials.[16–18] It remains the surgeon's primary responsibility to ensure that the quality of care provided by newer laparoscopic approaches is comparable to that which has already been achieved with conventional surgical approaches.

OPERATIVE APPROACHES TO THE VAGUS (OPEN)

Patient Position, Incisions, and Exposure

To perform a complete vagotomy, access to the upper part of the stomach and lower esophagus is crucial. It is helpful for the operating surgeon, standing on the patient's right, to wear a headlight. When access to the duodenum is required, as in gastrectomy, excellent exposure is available through a chevron incision. However, in most patients, either thin or obese, a midline incision carried up along the xiphoid will be adequate. In the obese, extension of the incision below the umbilicus facilitates exposure. Placing the patient in a position of reverse Trendelenburg is helpful. A nasogastric (NG) tube is placed with its tip at the most dependent portion of the greater curvature. The NG tube helps to keep the position of the esophagus in mind. A self-retaining retractor is required. We use a Bookwalter retractor that provides excellent accessories for securing wide exposure to the upper abdomen and, by means of well-placed Mickulicz pads, for holding the small bowel and transverse colon in the lower abdomen (Fig 34–1). Some surgeons advocate routine mobilization of the left lobe of the liver by dividing the left triangular ligament. This mobilization is not always necessary and, when the lobe is floppy, can impede exposure. If this maneuver is performed, the lateral segment of the left lobe is held upward and to the right by a Richardson or Herrington-type retractor accessory. Care must be taken to place sponges or a pack between the retractor attachment and

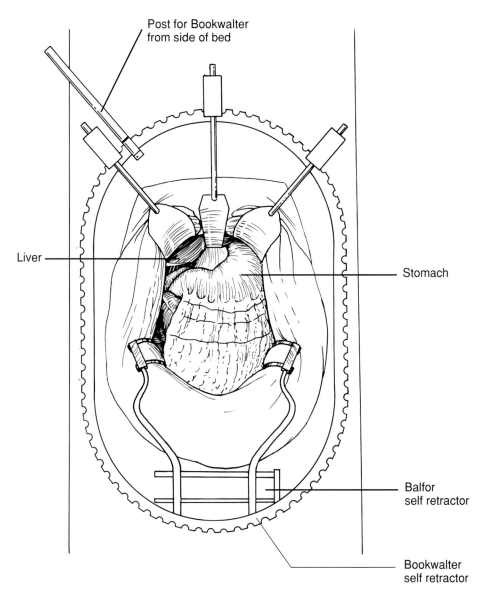

Figure 34–1. Use of the Bookwalter retractor for exposure of the upper abdomen.

liver, and not to put much tension on the liver. Otherwise, fracture of the liver parenchyma and bleeding will result.

TV

TV is performed in conjunction with some form of drainage procedure. In the elective setting, it is used in conjunction with antrectomy for definitive management of refractory symptoms of duodenal ulcer, pyloric channel ulcer (gastric ulcer type II), or gastric ulcers combined with duodenal (Dragstedt) ulcers. In the current era of highly effective antisecretory therapies such as omeprazole, and anti-*Helicobacter* antibiotics, the main indication for TV and antrectomy is in the setting of pyloric outlet obstruction with a long-standing history of ulcer symptoms or complications such as bleeding

and perforation. TV and pyloroplasty is reserved for emergency operations for complications such as bleeding or perforation. Occasionally, TV plus gastroenterostomy will be an appropriate compromise when the duodenum is too scarred to permit a safe antrectomy and duodenal closure. The anatomy of the vagal trunks and nerves of Latarjet is shown in Figs 34–2 and 34–3.

Using a Mickulicz pad or carefully applied Babcock clamps, the assistant places downward traction on the greater curvature of the stomach, thereby placing traction on the gastroesophageal junction and lower esophagus. The first step is to incise the peritoneal covering of the gastroesophageal junction. The peritoneum is opened horizontally, from the angle at the lesser curve to the cardiac notch at the greater curvature. The surgeon's thumb and right index finger are used in a blunt

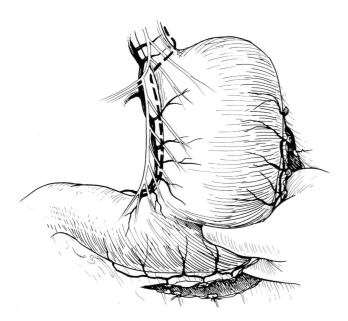

Figure 34–2. The distribution of the anterior vagus is shown. The *dotted line* indicates the line of dissection. Note that it goes around the incisura to within about 6 cm of the pylorus. The gastrocolic omentum has been partially divided to permit access to the posterior nerve of Latarjet and to allow the stomach to be grasped and used as a retractor. Note that the gastroepiploic arteries are carefully preserved (Redrawn from Johnston D. Vagotomy. In: Schwartz SI, Ellis H. *Maingot's Abdominal Operations.* 8th ed. Norwalk, CT, Appleton-Century-Crofts, 1982. After RN Lane)

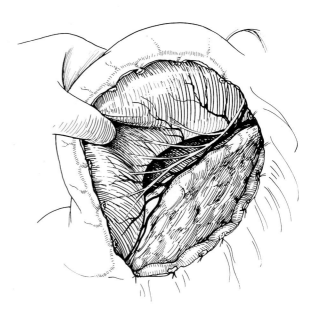

Figure 34–3. The posterior wall of the stomach and posterior nerve of the Latarjet are shown. The terminal Y fork of the nerve is preserved and all the other branches to the stomach are divided leaving about 5 cm of the distal portion of the stomach innervated. (Redrawn from Johnston D. Vagotomy. In: Schwartz SI, Ellis H. *Maingot's Abdominal Operations,* 8th ed. Norwalk, CT: Appleton-Century-Crofts, 1982. After RN Lane)

dissection to encircle the esophagus. When teaching this maneuver, it is not uncommon for the trainee to confuse the right crus of the diaphragm with the esophagus itself or even the posterior vagal trunk. Extra time spent at this juncture to correctly identify all structures is in the teaching aspect of the operation. A Penrose drain is passed around junction in order to place more effective downward traction on the gastroesophageal junction. When encircling the esophagus, the surgeon stays wide of the esophagus in order to prevent inadvertent entry into the lumen and to include the vagal trunks. In the course of this maneuver, the posterior vagal trunk usually will be palpated as a taut cord.

A single anterior vagal trunk usually is identified in the anterior midportion of the esophagus, 2 to 4 cm above the gastroesophageal junction (Fig 34–4). At this level, however, it is not uncommon for vagal fibers to be distributed among two or three smaller cords. These cords are palpable as much as they are visible and can be separated from surrounding esophageal muscle fibers using a nerve hook. These trunks are individually lifted up and 2 to 4 cm segments of each are separated from surrounding tissues. A medium-size clip is applied at the most superior end and a clamp is applied inferiorly. The 2 cm length of nerve is resected and a clip is applied below the clamp. Small bleeders are cauterized precisely. If it has not been done already, the esophagus should be

more widely mobilized for a distance of 4 to 5 cm above the gastroesophageal junction. Smaller, individual vagal fibers that ramify from the main trunks toward the lesser curvature and the cardiac notch then can be identified and cut or cauterized. The "criminal nerve" of Grassi, discussed in more detail in the section describing parietal cell vagotomy, also may be identified here, wrapping around the cardiac notch from its origin at the posterior trunk. The posterior vagal trunk itself usually will have been identified along the right edge of the esophagus. If the anterior vagus already has been divided, the esophagus is more mobile. This mobility allows the surgeon to place downward traction on the gastroesophageal junction, which causes the posterior vagus to "bowstring" and makes it easier to identify. A 2 to 4 cm segment is separated from surrounding tissues, its margins marked with clips, and resected. Major branches of the anterior vagus and the posterior vagal trunk should be sent to pathology for examination in frozen sections. Care should be taken to note the results of the pathologist's frozen section diagnosis in the dictated operative note.

Selective Vagotomy

Selective vagotomy (SV) is not commonly practiced in the United States, but has found favor with European surgeons who prefer not to cut the posteriorly derived vagal branch that innervates the small intestine and

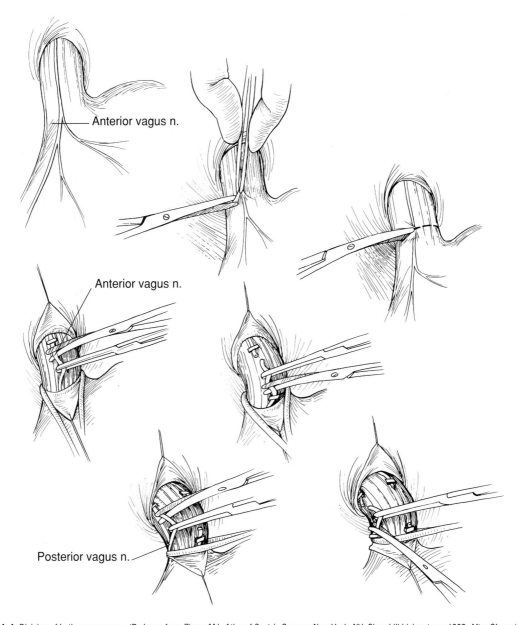

Anterior vagus n.

Anterior vagus n.

Posterior vagus n.

Figure 34–4. Division of both vagus nerves. (Redrawn from Zinner MJ. *Atlas of Gastric Surgery.* New York, NY: Churchill Livingstone; 1992. After Gloege)

pancreas and the anteriorly derived vagal branch that supplies the gallbladder and liver. There is evidence that preservation of such branches can avoid alterations in gallbladder motility that might lead to stasis and stone formation.[19] However, it is not clear whether preservation of the small intestinal and pancreatic nerves protects against some symptoms of the dumping syndrome.[16,20–22] SV involves interruption of both nerves of Latarjet and therefore does not avoid the need for a drainage procedure. Thus, the main indication for SV may be in patients undergoing elective antrectomy with vagotomy for refractory ulcer symptoms or obstruction.

Exposure to the vagus, gastroesophageal junction and esophagus are obtained in the same way that the surgeon would perform TV. Anteriorly, the nerve of Latarjet is identified by following the anterior vagal trunk as it descends from the esophagus to the lesser curvature of the stomach. Frequently, the descending branch of the left gastric artery is in close proximity to the site where the hepatic/gallbladder branches take off toward the liver in the gastrohepatic (lesser) omentum. A segment of the nerve of Latarjet is severed between clips and sent for examination on frozen section. The most expeditious way to perform this maneuver is to cross-clamp the portion of the lesser omentum that

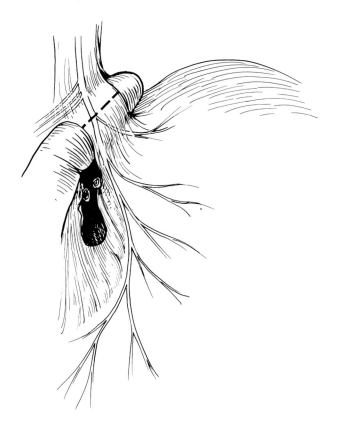

Figure 34–5. Selective vagotomy. The descending branch of the left gastric artery has been divided and the anterior gastric branches of the anterior vagus are about to be divided. (Redrawn from Griffith CA. Selective gastric vagotomy. In: Nyhus LM, Wastell C (eds), *Surgery of the Stomach and Duodenum,* 3rd ed. Boston, MA: Little, Brown; 1977:275. After Gloege)

contains the artery and nerve, ligating and dividing these structures together (Fig 34–5). The dissection continues upward along the lesser curvature, gastroesophageal junction, and esophagus. Division and ligation of blood vessels and nerves in this bundle avoids the hepatic/gallbladder branches and denervates the cardia, as was described for TV. This dissection opens up the plane for dissection and ligation of the posterior nerve of Latarjet.

Highly Selective Vagotomy

Generally accepted indications for highly selective vagotomy (HSV) include: elective management of intractable symptoms of duodenal ulcer disease, emergency treatment for perforated duodenal ulcer, and emergency treatment of perforated gastric ulcer when the ulcer is to be excised in a wedge rather than be resected in continuity with the distal stomach. HSV also has been advocated for management of bleeding gastric or duodenal ulcers, but this has not been widely practiced. Finally, there is published experience in pyloric outlet obstruction using HSV in combination with finger or endoscopic balloon dilatation,[22,23] but long-term persis-

tence or recurrence rates of obstructing symptoms are not known.

A number of variations of the technique have been described and will not all be reviewed here. However, it is worth cataloguing the decisions that the surgeon must make in preparing for and performing this operation. The first decision is whether to use Congo-red dye for intraoperative testing of the completeness of vagotomy. It may be difficult, and sometimes contraindicated, to perform endoscopy in the setting of acute bleeding or perforation. If the test is to be used, the endoscopic equipment and reagents should be assembled in the operating room before the operation begins. Conceptually, then, the operation is divided into four phases: (1) exposure and gastric mobilization; (2) dissection of the anterior leaf of the lesser omentum; (3) dissection of the posterior leaf of the lesser omentum; and (4) dissection of vagal fibers traveling to the stomach along the distal esophagus.

Exposure and Gastric Mobilization. Exposure to the vagus nerves, esophagus and gastroesophageal junction is obtained as described above. A wide bore (18-Fr) NG tube should be placed by the anesthesia team. A number of authors have emphasized the importance of the stomach as a retractor in this operation. We recommend mobilization of the distal part of the gastrocolic omentum (Fig 34–3). The dissection should be carried outside the gastroepiploic arcade, in order to avoid loss of any blood supply to the greater curvature. Congenital adhesions between the stomach and peritoneum overlying the pancreas are divided sharply. The goal of this dissection is to obtain sufficient mobility of the stomach so that it can be rotated upward and to the patient's right, thus permitting visualization of the posterior leaf of the lesser omentum and the posterior nerve of Latarjet through the lesser sac. The nerve can be seen running close to the descending branch of the left gastric artery. Vagal fibers can be seen running transversely toward the lesser curvature.

Dissection of the Anterior Leaf of the Lesser Omentum. The anterior leaf of the lesser omentum now is dissected. The next decision point is to define the distal margin of the dissection of the branches of the nerve of Latarjet (Fig 34–6). An important landmark is the incisura angularis. The "crow's foot" is the neurovascular bundle that innervates the junction of the corpus and antrum, and has three characteristic branches from which its name derives. These nerves contain motor branches to the antrum and secretory branches to the oxyntic mucosa. Thus, leaving this bundle intact makes the antisecretory operation less complete, but fully severing it may lead to disturbances of gastric emptying. Two approaches for defining the distal margin of the dissection have been

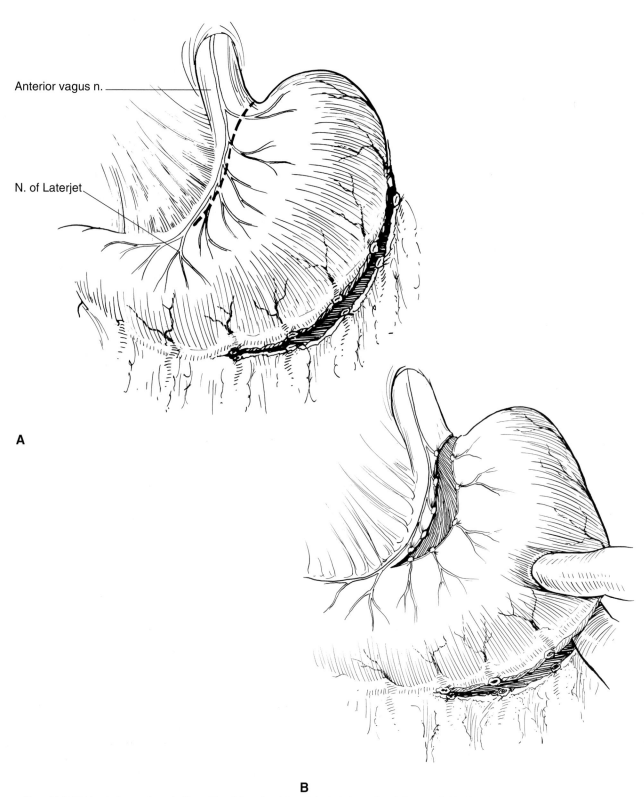

A

B

Figure 34–6. Highly selective vagotomy. **A.** Planned line of dissection of the anterior leaf of gastrohepatic ligament. **B.** The dissection is carried out, beginning just proximal to the crow's foot and extending upward, to the left of the gastroesophageal junction. (Redrawn from Zinner MJ, *Atlas of Gastric Surgery*. New York, NY: Churchill Livingstone; 1992. After Gloege)

advocated. First, one may arbitrarily begin the dissection at a predetermined 6 to 7 cm proximal to the pylorus, a distance that usually corresponds to the most proximal of the three branches of the crow's foot. Alternatively, one may identify this most proximal branch and begin the dissection there. It is helpful to begin the dissection a few centimeters proximal to the agreed-upon distal margin, since strong traction during subsequent parts of the operation may cause traction injury on the antral motor branches and vessels that accompany them. These last few centimeters are dealt with last.

The assistant provides downward and leftward traction on the greater curvature, thus placing tension on the anterior nerve of Latarjet as it runs along the lesser curvature. The hepatic fibers usually are visualized without difficulty in the upper part of the lesser omentum. It is helpful to "score" the serosa of the lesser curvature, from the incisura to the cardia and then transversely across the gastroesophageal junction. The incision is performed with dissecting scissors or a #15 knife, not electrocautery. This maneuver thus widens the gap between the nerve and the gastric wall. Individual branches of the nerve and their accompanying blood vessels run transversely from the lesser omentum onto the lesser curvature. These structures are ligated in continuity with 3-0 silk ligatures before division. (We avoid the use of hemostats in this dissection.) This part of the operation is performed gently and should not cause blood loss. The dissection proceeds along the lesser curvature until the gastroesophageal junction is reached. The left and anterior aspect of the esophagus is now uncovered and, for the moment, the dissection stops.

Dissection of the Posterior Leaf of the Lesser Omentum.
The posterior leaf of the lesser omentum then is dissected. Care should be taken in setting up the exposure for this part of the operation. In one approach, the stomach is rotated upward and to the patient's right (Fig 34–3). Alternatively, the posterior leaf can be reached by working through the anterior leaf as illustrated in Fig 34–7. Using the thumb and fingers, the gastroesophageal junction is "rolled" counterclockwise so that the posterior wall moves to the right and the anterior wall moves to the left. The nerve branches and their accompanying vessels then are ligated in continuity and divided. The dissection should not be carried to <6 cm from the pylorus. To avoid the main left gastric vessels, this approach to the dissection should be carried about two-thirds of the distance along the lesser curvature. After reaching the left gastric vessels, the surgeon returns to the anterior approach, ligating and dividing the remainder of the posterior leaf through the window in the anterior leaf.

Dissection of the Distal Esophagus.
The goal of this dissection is to clear the distal esophagus of all nerve fibers for a distance of approximately 5 cm above the gastroesophageal junction. The importance of this part of the dissection is well documented.[24] It should be noted that the prior dissection of the lesser omentum has allowed the main vagal trunks to move upward and to the patient's right, thereby minimizing the risk of damaging the main trunks in this part of the dissection. Nevertheless, the operative technique requires that this dissection stay close to the lesser curve and esophagus. Any dissection toward the tissues to the right (ie, toward the main vagal trunks) should be avoided.

This part of the procedure begins with dissection of the left side of the esophagus (Fig 34–8). Denuding the surface can be performed gently, using a finger or "peanut" dissector to isolate the adventitia that contains nerves, vessels, and lymphatics. This dissection is where the "criminal nerve" of Grassi is likely to be encountered. Tissues are ligated in continuity and divided. This dissection should also clear the 2 or 3 cm of the cardia, just distal to the gastroesophageal junction, and small fibers running to the greater curvature will be divided here. It is not usually necessary to divide any of the short gastric arteries.

The anterior aspect of the esophagus is now cleared of vagal fibers (Fig 34–9). Gentle traction and lift of fibers will isolate them for division between ligatures or by cautery. We prefer ligation in continuity with fine (4-0 or 5-0) silk, to avoid injury to the esophageal muscle. The posterior aspect is now reexposed with downward traction of the gastroesophageal junction and a counterclockwise rotation of the distal esophagus. Working through the window of the anterior leaflet, the upward branches of the left gastric artery are visualized as they pass to the cardia and gastroesophageal junction. They are ligated in continuity and divided. The dissection continues upward along the cardia and gastroesophageal junction, until it is possible to encircle the lower esophagus with a Penrose drain. Downward traction on the gastroesophageal junction is provided by this drain, and additional nerve fibers are seen in the adventitia. Smaller fibers are cauterized while held away from the esophageal muscularis, whereas larger ones are ligated with clips or fine silk and divided. Throughout this dissection, the positions of the nerves of Latarjet and the main trunks should be checked.

The final part of the operation involves completion of the most distal dissection to the crow's foot and checks for hemostasis. A number of authors have, in the past, suggested that reperitonealization of the lesser curvature be performed. The rationale for this maneuver is that the devascularization that is part of the HSV may lead to small areas of necrosis of the gastric wall and

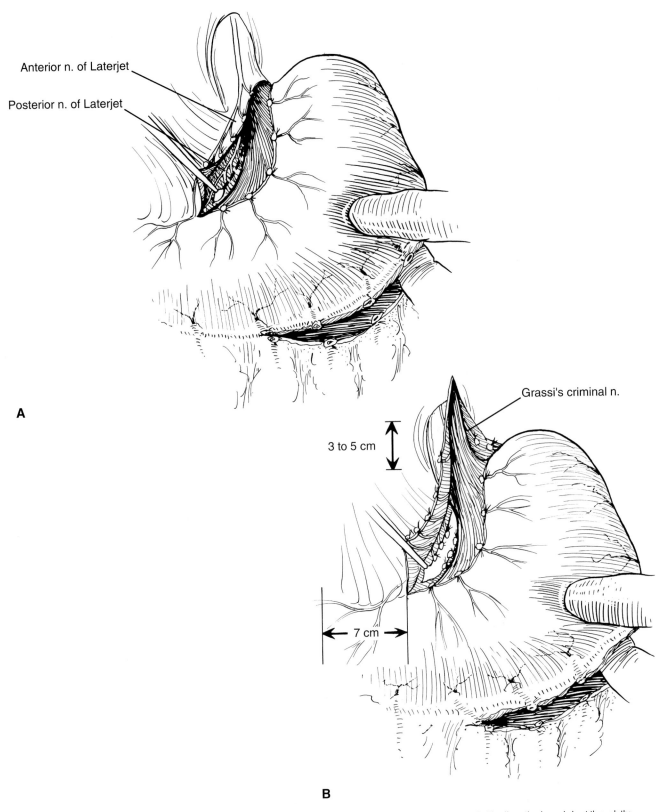

Figure 34–7. Parietal cell vagotomy. **A.** The line of dissection of the posterior leaf of gastrohepatic ligament is illustrated. **B.** The dissection is carried out through the window created by prior dissection of the anterior leaf. (Redrawn from Zinner MJ. *Atlas of Gastric Surgery.* New York, NY: Churchill Livingstone; 1992. After RN Lane)

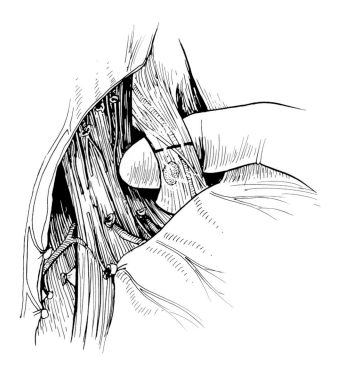

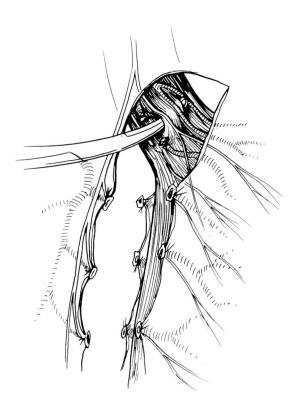

Figure 34–8. The serosa has been cut to the left of the esophagus, and fatty areolar tissue to the left of the esophagus, containing nerve fibers, blood vessels, and lymphatic vessels, is hooked up by the right index finger. The angle of His and the adjacent esophagus and a 2 to 3 cm portion of fundus of the stomach are thoroughly cleared. In this way, small nerve fibers running to the proximal 3 cm portion of fundus ("criminal" nerves of Grassi) are eliminated. (Redrawn from Johnston D. Vagotomy. In: Schwartz SI, Ellis H. *Maingot's Abdominal Operations.* Norwalk, CT: Appleton-Century-Crofts; 1982. After RN Lane)

Figure 34–9. Anterior gastric branches of the anterior vagal trunk running downward on the anterior surface of the esophagus are gently lifted by the hemostat and either ligated or clipped before being divided, or destroyed with diathermy. (Redrawn from Johnston, D. Vagotomy. In: Schwartz SI, Ellis H. *Maingot's Abdominal Operations.* 8th ed. Norwalk, CT: Appleton-Century-Crofts; 1982. After RN Lane)

localized perforations. Such leaks have been reported in about 0.2% of patients.[25] Also, it has been argued that reperitonealization might impede reestablishment of vagal nerve connections to the gastric wall.[26] The reperitonealization would thus protect against such leaks. The reperitonealization can be performed by inversion of the serosa of the lesser curve with running or continuous 3-0 Maxon or Novafil suture. Alternatively, a vascularized pedicle of omentum can be used to cover the deserosalized lesser curvature. Bleeding complications have been reported with this latter method, but it minimizes tension within the gastric wall.

Reoperative Approaches to the Vagus Nerves

Approximately two-thirds of patients with duodenal or pyloric channel ulcer recurrence after an initial antisecretory operation (TV, SV, HSV, etc) have evidence of intact vagal innervation.[11,27] Although many such recurrences are amenable to medical regimens, a small fraction ultimately may be considered for reoperation, especially if surgery is required to control an acute complication such as bleeding or perforation following a period of ulcer-related symptoms. Prior surgery will have made the standard approaches to the lesser curvature

and gastroesophageal junction hazardous and often caused dense adhesions to a previously mobilized left lobe of the liver. Thus, two approaches to the vagus, both nonselective, may be considered for completion of the failed vagotomy, especially if it was performed in conjunction with antrectomy. It should be stressed that when such a reoperation is contemplated, especially in a nonemergent setting, it is prudent to obtain some form of acid secretion profile to document the hypersecretory state. Also, because of the nonselective nature of the completion vagotomy, an antrectomy or drainage procedure must be performed.

In the setting where standard access is difficult owing to prior surgery, Barroso and associates have utilized a transabdominal suprahepatic approach to the vagi.[28] A high midline incision is used, with mechanical retractors to elevate the subcostal margin. A 18-Fr NG tube is placed. The triangular, left coronary, and falciform ligaments and adhesions are divided, permitting downward retraction of the left lobe. Using the NG tube, the esophagus and hiatus are located. The esophagus and vagi are dissected at the level of the diaphragm. In some cases, the diaphragm at the hiatus is incised anteriorly for a distance of 3 to 5 cm, exposing the esophagus at

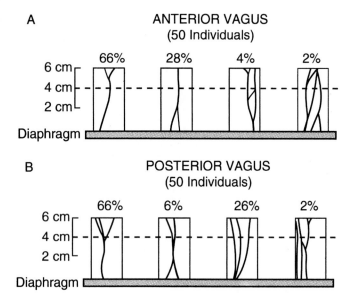

Figure 34–10. Anatomy of the anterior (**A**) and posterior (**B**) vagus nerves above the diaphragm in 50 cadavers. Incidence of each anatomic group indicated by percentage. (Redrawn from Jackson RG, Anatomy of the vagus nerves in the region of the lower esophagus and stomach. *Anat Rec* 1949;103:1)

the lower mediastinum. The trunks are easily identified and ligated in the unoperated area of the lower thoracic esophagus. The hiatus is closed with interrupted nonabsorbable sutures.

A transthoracic approach to this region has also been used,[29] and, with the advent of thoracoscopy, may become increasingly attractive for this limited set of patients. The operation is performed through the left chest, entered via the eighth intercostal space. A NG tube is positioned with its tip in the stomach. After division of the inferior pulmonary ligament, the base of the left lung is retracted upward and laterally. The mediastinal pleura overlying the esophagus is incised for a distance of 8 cm. The esophagus then is mobilized and encircled with a Penrose drain. Vessel loops are used to retract individual vagal trunks as they are identified. The supradiaphragmatic anterior vagus may have multiple branches at the level of the diaphragm, but rarely are there multiple trunks at a level 4 cm above the diaphragm.[30] In contrast, the posterior vagus has multiple branches above the level of the diaphragm, but is a single trunk at this level more than 90% of the time (Fig 34–10). Thus, the best opportunity for a complete vagotomy lies 4 cm above the diaphragm for the anterior trunk and at the diaphragm for the posterior trunk. A circumferential dissection of the 6 cm of esophagus just above the diaphragm is carried out, with technique similar to that performed during HSV. Tube thoracostomy is required for 2 to 3 days postoperatively.

OPERATIVE APPROACHES TO THE VAGUS (LAPAROSCOPIC)

As noted above, the advent of laparoscopic approaches has led surgeons to reconsider traditional approaches to peptic ulcer disease. The advantages of minimally invasive approaches revolve largely around the minimal postoperative discomfort and rapid recovery, with a potential benefit in reduced cost of surgery versus cost of long-term medication.[31] At the same time, rapid advances have occurred in our understanding of the role of *H pylori* and mucosal growth, and angiogenesis factors in ulcer healing and recurrence. In addition, limitations in access and suturing techniques have increased the difficulty of access to the lesser sac and of performing drainage procedures. These considerations have led surgeons to question the rationale for drainage procedures whenever truncal vagotomy has been performed. A number of approaches have evolved to address these difficulties and been given credibility in the laparoscopic experience. One such approach has been to combine truncal vagotomy with pyloric dilatation or seromyotomy. Another has been to combine a posterior truncal vagotomy and anterior highly selective vagotomy or with an anterior seromyotomy. The important elements of the laparoscopic approach to the vagi are discussed here.

Patient Position and Port Placement

The patient is placed on the operating room table with legs in stirrups and apart (Fig 34–11). Video monitors are placed on either side, at the head, often, the surgeon works best when standing between the legs, with the camera operator on the right and first assistant on the patient's left. The scrub nurse/technician and instrument table are placed at the patient's right foot. A large esophageal tube or even a gastroscope is placed in the stomach to facilitate visualization of the distal esophagus. Frequent aspiration of the gastric contents are crucial to maintain total collapse of the stomach and the best visualization. We recommend an open technique to gain access to the peritoneum, insufflating to a pressure of 14 mm Hg. Five ports are placed in the following locations: (1) 12 mm (laparoscope port) at the superior edge of the umbilicus or placed 5 cm above and lateral to the rectus on the right; (2) 5 mm (irrigation/suction and dissection) in the subxiphoid position, just to the right of the midline; (3) 10 mm (retraction and grasping forceps) midway between the umbilicus and xiphoid, to the right of the rectus and possibly as far as the midclavicular line; (4) 10 mm (grasping forceps) midway between the umbilicus and xiphoid, almost to the anterior axillary line on the left; and (5) 12 mm (operating port) just lateral to the rectus about 3 cm above the umbilicus. A number of sur-

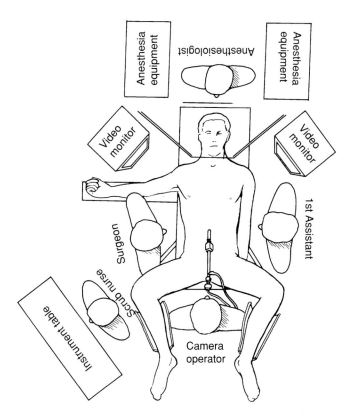

Figure 34–11. Sites for trocar placement in laparoscopically assisted vagotomy. (Redrawn from Bailey RW, Zucker KA, Flowers JL. Vagotomy. In: Ballantyne GH (ed), *Laparoscopic Surgery*. Philadelphia, PA: WB Saunders; 1994)

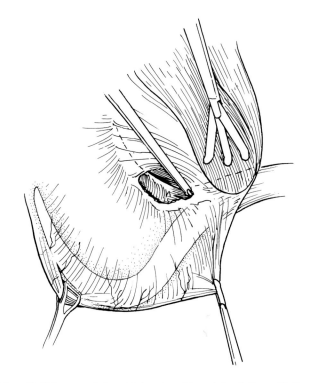

Figure 34–12. Laparoscopically assisted vagotomy. The gastrohepatic ligament is dissected anteriorly without injury to the vagi. (Redrawn from Katkhouda N, Mouiel J. Laparoscopic treatment of peptic ulcer disease. In: Brooks DC (ed), *Current Techniques in Laparoscopy*. Philadelphia, PA: Current Medicine;1994)

geons prefer the angled 30° laparoscope for this operation, but this is not always more useful.

Laparoscopic truncal vagotomy

The left lobe of the liver is retracted using a probe placed via the subxiphoid port or the 10-mm fan retractor placed via the higher right-side port (Fig 34–12). Visualization is improved when tissues from the hiatus are dissected away from the esophagus and lesser curvature. One can encounter a coronary hepatic vein or accessory hepatic artery in this dissection. These do not always need to be sacrificed. The right crus of the diaphragm usually is seen here and can be retracted with one of the blades of the liver retractor (Fig 34–13). A Babcock clamp is used to retract the anterior greater curvature (distal to the cardia) to the patient's left. A hook coagulator or dissecting forceps is used to incise the lesser omentum, entering the lesser sac just above the take-off of the hepatic branch of the anterior vagus. A plane is developed between the right crus and the esophagus and continued posteriorly. Continued dissection along the wall of the esophagus reveals the posterior trunk, which is ligated between clips and divided (Fig 34–14). The excised nerve seg-

ment is sent for frozen-section examination. The next step is identification of the anterior vagal trunk(s). The phrenoesophageal membrane usually has been entered and the incision is extended toward the left, first by scoring the membrane with scissors and then bluntly pushing away the membrane with a cotton dissector. The visualization of major anterior trunks is often easier in the laparoscopic approach, owing to magnification and excellent video optics. These branches also are ligated and divided between clips (Fig 34–15), with frozen-section confirmation of the nerve segment. Smaller anterior branches are identified and cauterized after being held away from the esophageal wall. It is possible to dissect tissues on either side of the esophagus for a distance of 5 to 6 cm, thereby ensuring division of any major nerve branches to the lesser curve and cardia. The main difficulty can occur in visualizing the angle of His and possibly missing major vagal branches, including the "criminal nerve." With the use of a traction forceps placed through the subxiphoid port, and a cotton dissector placed via the left grasping forceps, it is possible to expose the left edge of the gastroesophageal junction and cauterize or clip any branches.

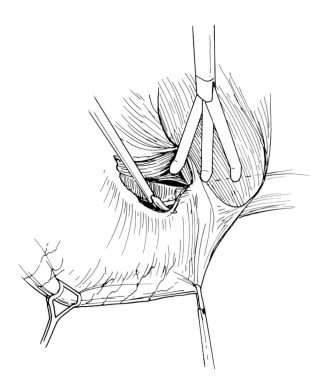

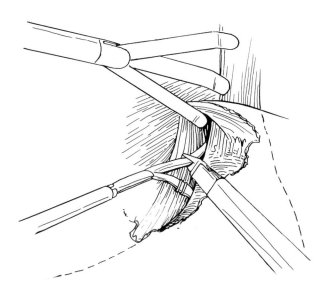

Figure 34–14. Laparoscopically assisted vagotomy. The anterior trunk is ligated between clips and divided. (Redrawn from Katkhouda N and Mouiel J. Laparoscopic treatment of peptic ulcer disease. In: Brooks DC (ed), *Current Techniques in Laparoscopy*. Philadelphia, PA: Current Medicine; 1994)

Figure 34–13. Laparoscopically assisted vagotomy. The crus of the diaphragm is retracted to the patient's right. The anterior vagal trunk is exposed at the gastroesophageal junction. (Redrawn from Katkhouda N and Mouiel J. Laparoscopic treatment of peptic ulcer disease. In: Brooks DC (ed), *Current Techniques in Laparoscopy*. Philadelphia, PA: Current Medicine; 1994)

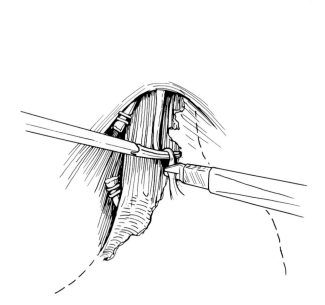

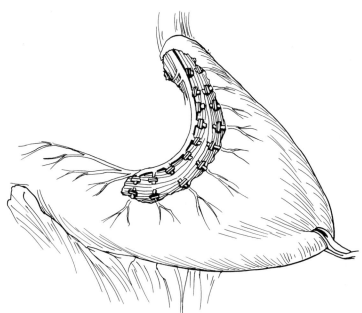

Figure 34–15. Laparoscopically assisted vagotomy. Ligation and division of posterior vagus between clips. (Redrawn from Katkhouda N and Mouiel J. Laparoscopic treatment of peptic ulcer disease. In: Brooks DC (ed), *Current Techniques in Laparoscopy*. Philadelphia, PA: Current Medicine; 1994)

Figure 34–16. Laparoscopically assisted parietal cell vagotomy. Dissection of anterior leaf of gastrohepatic ligament. (Redrawn from Katkhouda N and Mouiel J. Laparoscopic treatment of peptic ulcer disease. In: Brooks DC (ed), *Current Techniques in Laparoscopy*. Philadelphia, PA: Current Medicine; 1994)

Anterior proximal vagotomy or seromyotomy

A laparoscopic dissection of the posterior leaf is feasible.[32] However, the combination of posterior truncal vagotomy and an anterior selective operation is appealing, since it avoids the difficult maneuver of working through the lesser sac in order to visualize the posterior lesser omentum and nerves accompanying the ascending left gastric artery branches. For highly selective vagotomy, is begun at the crow's foot, approximately 6 cm from the pylorus. Retraction of the greater curvature is performed using a Babcock clamp (Fig 34–16). With the magnification available through the scope, the proximal branch of the crow's foot is often, but not always, relatively easy to identify. The anterior leaf of the lesser omentum is approached by dividing and ligating the neurovascular bundles between clips. Electrocautery is used sparingly and, preferably, not at all. The serosa overlying the gastroesophageal junction is scored as in the open procedure. Dissection of the distal 5 cm of esophagus and cardiac branches is carried out as described above for truncal vagotomy.

The goal of an anterior seromyotomy, as described originally by Taylor and others, is to sever the neurovascular bundles dividing the serosa and muscularis that transmit these nerves to the mucosa.[33,34] The anterior surface of the stomach is retracted and placed on stretch using the right and left grasping ports. The outline of the seromyotomy is scored using a coagulator hook or spatula, on the anterior surface of the stomach, 1 cm from the visible border of the lesser curve. Moving caudad and parallel to the lesser curvature, a line is traced from the gastroesophageal junction to the first branch of the crow's foot or, arbitrarily, 6 cm from the pylorus. The hook coagulator is most suitable for performing the seromyotomy, using monopolar current for electrocoagulation. The hook cuts through successive layers of the gastric wall, of the serosa, outer oblique muscle fibers, middle longitudinal fibers, and inner circular fibers. The two grasping ports, then are used to place traction on the two edges of the gastric wall, exposing the deep circular fibers that may split as much from traction as from cautery. The darker submucosa/mucosa layer pops through the muscularis. This layer is inspected for any evidence of full-thickness cautery injury or perforation. With a complete seromyotomy, the gap between the cut edges should be about 6 to 8 mm.

A number of decent-sized vessels may be encountered in the dissection. Prolonged cauterization may provide hemostasis but risks a full-thickness burn and subsequent perforation. The hook can be used to isolate these vessels and lift them for clipping in continuity. Recent advances in design of needle holders may make it possible to suture these vessels in continuity before division by scissors. The integrity of the mucosa should be verified by moderate expansion of the stomach using the NG tube for insufflation. Some authors use methylene-blue solution (1 vial per 200 cc), placed intragastrically, for this maneuver. The seromyotomy then is closed using a continuous suturing technique. A tongue of omentum may be mobilized and secured over the seromyotomy as a patch, secured with sutures placed through either edge of the seromyotomy.

■ DRAINAGE PROCEDURES

In the context of bilateral truncal or selective vagotomies, the purpose of a drainage procedure is to preserve the pylorus but bypass or render it ineffective. The options for drainage include (1) gastroenterostomy; (2) pyloric dilatation; (3) pyloromyotomy; and (4) pyloroplasty. Generally, these techniques are used when TV or SV are performed, but also may be used with HSV in order to treat obstruction resulting from acid-peptic scarring. We will discuss techniques for performing gastrojejunostomy in the subsequent discussion of gastric resection.

PYLORIC DILATATION

In open procedures, the simplest technique reported for performing pyloric dilatation is to perform a small gastrotomy, approximately 3 to 4 cm in length, proximal to the pylorus. A finger is introduced through the pylorus, forcing it to widen. The gastrotomy then is closed with a single layer of 3-0 silk interrupted sutures. A second technique, advocated for use in laparoscopic cases, is to use a balloon. The balloon, 15 mm in length, may be positioned endoscopically and inflated to 45 psi for 10 min. Other dilators are available for positioning over a wire and inflation to higher pressures, which may prevent pyloric spasm. Advocates of pyloric dilatation after laparoscopic TV or SV have suggested that a drainage procedure is not required as often as previously thought or may only be necessary in the early postoperative phase and not permanently.[35,36] Thus, it is argued, dilatation can be repeated postoperatively and in the outpatient setting. Most surgeons, however, subscribe to the need for some form of formal drainage procedure after SV or TV.

PYLOROMYOTOMY

Pyloromyotomy is performed using the same techniques as described in the setting of hypertrophic pyloric stenosis in the infant (Fig 34–17). An incision is made to score the anterior surface of the stomach from 1 to 2 cm proximal to 1 cm distal to the pyloric ring. The

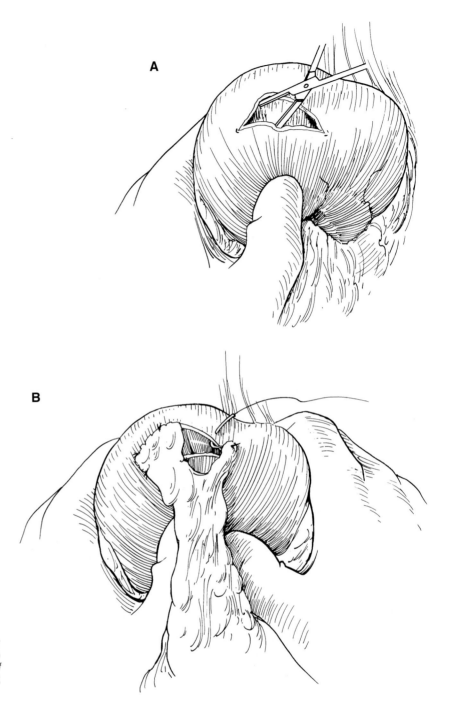

Figure 34–17. Pyloromyotomy. **A.** Dissection of seromuscular layers, avoiding entry into bowel. **B.** Omental patch is used to cover the dissected area. (Redrawn from Welch CE. *Surgery of the Stomach and Duodenum.* Chicago, IL: Year Book Medical; 1973)

separation of pyloric muscle fibers is accomplished mainly with a fine-tip hemostat and the knife. Cautery is avoided and only used in the muscularis, not the submucosa. When this procedure is performed in the setting of esophagogastrectomy, the pylorus is usually soft and unscarred. In the setting of chronic duodenal ulcer disease, the pylorus is often scarred and it is difficult to obtain the gentle, meticulous separation of muscle layers that is required and, at the same time, to avoid entering the mucosa. Laparoscopic versions of this proce-

dure also have been advocated in the setting of laparoscopic TV or SV.[37]

PYLOROPLASTY

The most expeditiously performed pyloroplasty is the Heineke-Mickulicz procedure (Fig 34–18). This is difficult to perform if the pyloric region is very scarred. The operation usually is performed in the setting of emergency surgery for bleeding or perforation of a gastric or

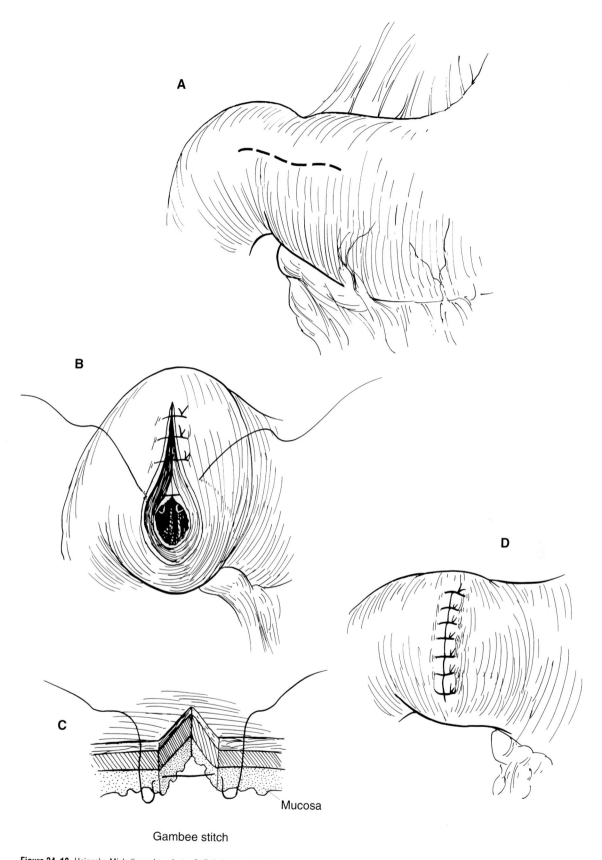

Figure 34–18. Heinecke-Mickulicz pyloroplasty. **A.** Full-thickness incision extends from 2 cm proximal to 1 to 2 cm distal to the pyloric ring. **B.** The incision is closed vertically. **C.** Illustration of Gambee stitch. **D.** Finished pyloroplasty. (Redrawn from Zinner MJ. *Atlas of Gastric Surgery*. New York, NY: Churchill Livingstone; 1992. After Gloege)

Mucosa

Gambee stitch

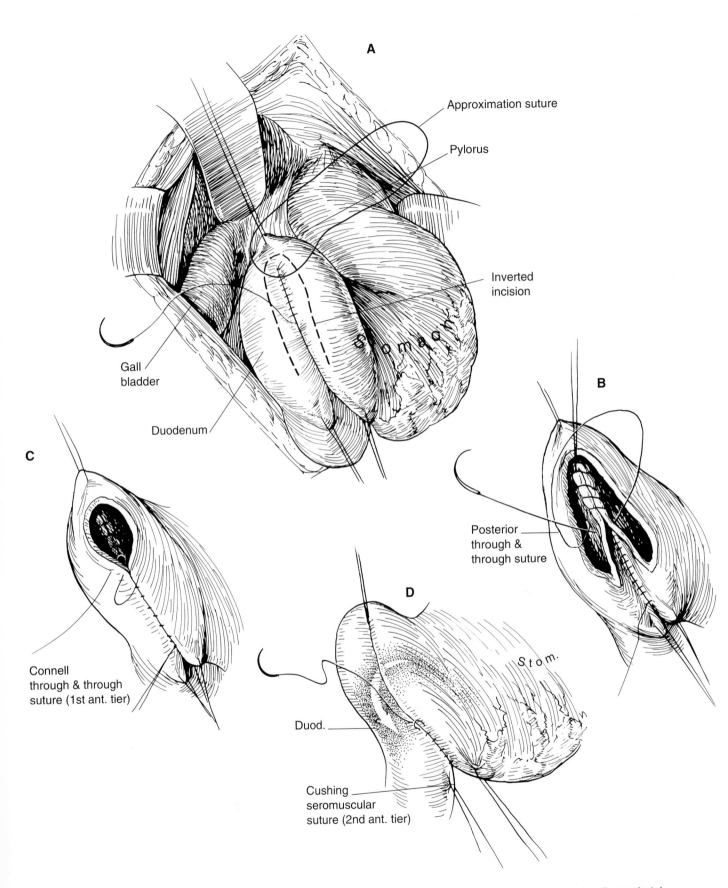

Figure 34–19. Finney U shaped pyloroplasty. **A.** The distal stomach and proximal duodenum are aligned with traction strands and their adjacent walls approximated with a Cushing suture; the inverted U shaped incision into the lumens of the stomach and duodenum is indicated. **B.** Suture of the posterior septum of stomach and duodenum. **C.** The first anterior tier of sutures (Connell) is placed. **D.** The operation is completed with a reinforcing tier of Cushing sutures. (Redrawn from Zuidema GD (ed). *Shackelford's Surgery of the Alimentary Tract* vol II 3rd ed. Philadelphia, PA: WB Saunders; 1991)

duodenal ulcer. A vagotomy is performed, usually after bleeding has been controlled. If the indication is a bleeding or perforated duodenal or pyloric channel ulcer, the incision for the pyloroplasty may include the ulcer or be used to gain access to the ulcer. The incision is, therefore, the planned pyloroplasty incision.

It is not always necessary to perform a Kocher maneuver; however, duodenal mobilization is usually helpful in relieving any tension on the intended suture line. Unless the duodenal bulb is unusually mobile, we recommend this as the initial step. In this maneuver, the peritoneum along the right border of the duodenum is incised from the lateral border of the common bile duct to the junction of the second and third portions of the duodenum. After duodenal mobilization, 3-0 silk stay sutures are placed, untied, superior and inferior to the site of the intended incision, which then is made on the anterior surface in a longitudinal direction, using electrocautery, from 2 cm distal to the pyloric muscle to 3 cm proximal to the pylorus. The closure of the pyloroplasty is performed vertically, in order to minimize narrowing of the lumen. In our experience, a single-layer closure is preferable as a means of avoiding too much narrowing of the lumen. The Gambee stitch (Fig 34–18) is a single-layer inverting suture used in this setting. The suture, usually performed with 3-0 or 2-0 silk, begins on the outside and (1) is placed full thickness (serosa to mucosa) on the same side; (2) is brought, on the same side, back through the mucosa to the submucosa; (3) is carried through the submucosa to the mucosa on the opposite side; (4) is brought full thickness from mucosa to serosa on that side. When the pylorus is scarred and the tissue inflexible, it is often helpful to tie the sutures after they have been placed, rather than as they are being placed. The stay sutures then are removed, after completion of the pyloroplasty. A tongue of vascularized omentum may be brought up to cover the closure and it is sutured to the gut wall with 3-0 vicryl suture.

The Finney pyloroplasty can be used when scarring has involved the pylorus and duodenal bulb and would not permit a tension-free, patulous Heineke-Mickulicz pyloroplasty. The Finney pyloroplasty is, in essence, a side-to-side gastroduodenostomy (Fig 34–19). In beginning this operation, dense adhesions often are encountered surrounding the pylorus and duodenal bulb. These must be lysed systematically. The Kocher maneuver then is performed, carrying the mobilization distally. Complete mobility of the duodenum and freedom from surrounding adhesions are essential to this operation.

A 2-0 silk stay suture is placed on the upper anterior surface of the pyloric ring. Another stay suture is placed on the greater curvature of the stomach approximately 10 cm proximal to the pylorus, and a third stay suture is placed approximately 10 cm distal to the pylorus. Trac-

tion cranially on the pyloric suture and caudally on the other two sutures brings the anterior surfaces of the stomach and duodenum into apposition. The apposed surfaces are sutured together using interrupted 3-0 silk Lembert seromuscular sutures. Using electrocautery an inverted U shaped incision is made beginning on the gastric side just distal to the traction suture, travelling longitudinally through the pylorus, then distally to a point just proximal to the traction suture. If the ulcer is present on the anterior surface of the duodenal bulb, it is excised. The posterior inner layer between the stomach and duodenum then is sutured closed with a continuous over-and-over 3-0 vicryl or chromic catgut suture. This closure is begun at the superior edge, is carried caudally, then converted into a Connell inverting technique as the suture is brought around the inferior edge to begin closing the anterior portion of the inner layer. The anterior outer layer then is closed using interrupted 3-0 Lambert sutures. Some surgeons use 3-0 Maxon or PDS suture material for single-layer continuous closure of the gastroduodenostomy. An omental patch may be used to cover the closure, as additional insurance against a suture line leak.

■ GASTRIC RESECTIONS

The common indications for gastric resections include peptic ulcer disease and tumors of the stomach. Safe performance of gastric resection requires an understanding of the following: (1) the physiology of vagal innervation and gastric emptying; (2) the surface and vascular anatomy of the stomach; (3) the principles of reconstruction following resection, specifically the Billroth I (B-I) gastroduodenostomy, the Billroth II (B-II) gastrojejunostomy, and the Roux-en-Y configuration; (4) the principles of surgical stapling techniques as well as hand-sewn suturing techniques; and (5) the specific early and late postoperative complications that arise from different gastric resections and different forms of reconstruction. Degrees of resection are correlated to the surface anatomy, as shown in Fig 34–20. This discussion is divided into three sections. The first will describe techniques for performing wedge resections and closure of the gastric wall for ulcers, polyps, or tumors derived from neuroendocrine or submucosal tissues. Carcinomas are not amenable to wedge resection and should be removed, for cure or palliation, by formal regional resection. The second section will describe techniques for distal gastric resections, focusing on antrectomy or hemigastrectomy (with or without vagotomy) for peptic ulcer disease and when the major decision involves the choice of B-I or B-II reconstruction. The third section will describe techniques used in management of gastric carcinoma, focusing on proximal, subtotal or to-

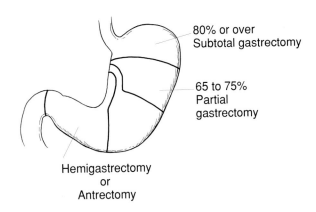

80% or over
Subtotal gastrectomy

65 to 75%
Partial
gastrectomy

Hemigastrectomy
or
Antrectomy

Figure 34–20. Amount of stomach removed in antrectomy or hemigastrectomy: 60% to 75% for partial gastrectomy and 80% for subtotal gastrectomy. Note that most of the lesser curvature of the stomach is excised in all these resections.

tal resection, and the techniques of regional node dissection.

WEDGE RESECTION OF THE STOMACH

Exposure is gained through an upper midline incision, carried from the xiphoid to the umbilicus. A Bookwalter or other mechanical retractor is highly desirable, especially for lesions located on the lesser curvature or in the proximal stomach. The technique of wedge resection depends on the location of the lesion. When a gastric tumor, such as a carcinoid or leiomyoma, is located on the greater curvature of the stomach it is important to note the proximity to the pylorus or gastroesophageal junction. Wedge resection may not be possible if the lesion lies too close (within 2 cm) to these borders, since the closure might narrow the lumen and cause partial obstruction to the flow of chyme. Formal resection then may be necessary. If proximity to these borders is not a problem, omental adhesions to the tumor are left in contact with the lesion. Further away from the tumor, the portion of the omentum that is adherent is divided between clamps and will come with the specimen. Branches of the gastroepiploic arteries that supply the gastric wall adjacent to the tumor are ligated in continuity with 3-0 silk ligatures and divided. The gastroepiploic artery need not be divided, unless it is adherent to the surface of the tumor. At a distance of 2 cm from the base of the tumor, the serosa of the gastric wall is scored using the cautery, describing a circle. The cautery then is used to deepen the incision through the muscularis. As the muscularis is divided, submucosal bleeders will pop through, requiring precise cauterization to secure hemostasis. When the tumor and surrounding gastric wall have been excised, the gastrotomy is closed longitudinally in two layers. The inner layer is a full-thickness hemostatic layer sewn continuously using 3-0 chromic

or vicryl suture and the outer layer uses interrupted seromuscular 3-0 silk Lembert sutures. An omental patch is not necessary, unless there are specific concerns about the blood supply to the closure. When situated favorably, such lesions are also amenable to laparoscopic resection.[38,39]

When tumors are located on the lesser curvature, or it is necessary to perform a gastrotomy in order to stop ongoing bleeding from a gastric ulcer, the excision can be performed from the mucosal side of the lesion (Fig 34–21). Once the inside borders of the lesion have been identified, it is important to obtain optimal exposure of the lesion from the serosal aspect. It may be necessary to sacrifice one or both nerves of Latarjet or the left or right gastric arteries and this determination can only be made from the outside of the stomach. If the lesion is located on the lesser curvature and cannot be removed without sacrifice of both nerves of Latarjet, a pyloroplasty should be performed. In such cases, our preference is that the resection is extended to include the distal stomach and a B-I or B-II reconstruction (see below). One variation on this latter approach for high-lying bleeding or perforated gastric ulcers is Pauchet's operation, a modification of an operation originally described by Shoemaker. This procedure involves removal of the antrum and a tongue of the corpus that extends upward to include the ulcer (Fig 34–22).[40]

DISTAL GASTRIC RESECTIONS AND RECONSTRUCTIONS

Vagotomy and Antrectomy

An antrectomy for duodenal or pyloric channel ulcer removes about 35% of the distal stomach and must include all of the nonacid-secreting portion. The incision is made in the upper midline and a Bookwalter or mechanical retractor is helpful. An NG tube is positioned under the surgeon's guidance, with its tip in the midportion of the stomach. Truncal vagotomy is performed first, as described earlier. The incisura is a reasonable landmark for the proximal margin of resection on the lesser curvature, while the terminal portions of the right gastroepiploic artery indicate the margin on the greater curvature.

The distal stomach is mobilized in the following fashion: first, the lesser sac is entered by incising the gastrocolic ligament. These attachments are sometimes avascular but usually are divided between clamps and ligated with 3-0 silk ligatures. The stomach may thus be lifted upward, revealing the posterior gastric wall. Congenital adhesions from the posterior wall and pancreas capsule are divided sharply. The dissection is carried distally along the greater curvature (Fig 34–23), dividing the small branches of the gastroepiploic artery to the gastric wall. The dissection reaches the main right gastroepiploic artery, which sometimes has to be di-

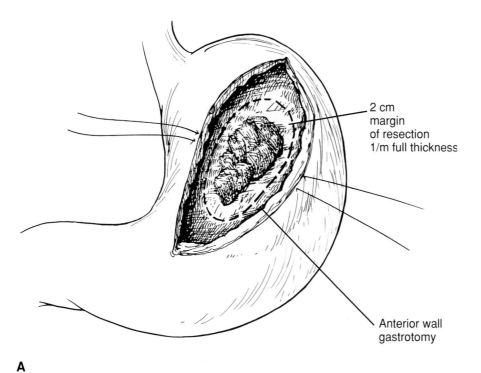

2 cm
margin
of resection
1/m full thickness

Anterior wall
gastrotomy

A

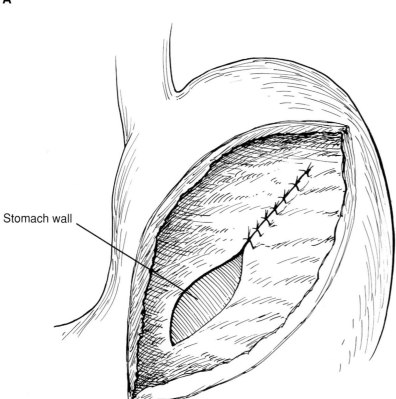

Stomach wall

Figure 34–21. Small tumors or polyps not amenable to endoscopic polypectomy can be excised with surrounding wedge of normal gastric wall. **A.** A 2-cm margin is advisable. **B.** The gastrotomy can be closed in 1 or 2 layers, using 2-0 nonabsorbable sutures sewn in interrupted fusion.

B

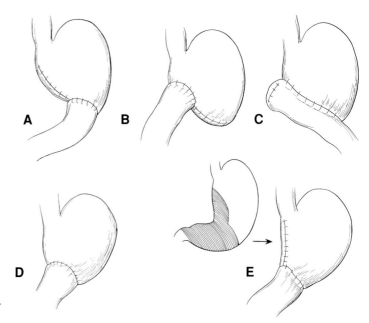

Figure 34–22. Billroth I operations: **A.** Billroth I; **B.** Horsley; **C.** von Haberer-Finney; **D.** von Haberer; **E.** Schoemaker.

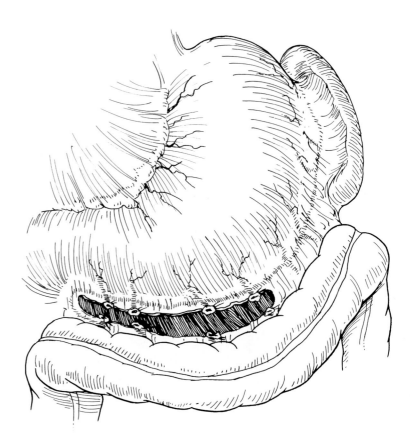

Figure 34–23. Billroth I operation. **A.** Use of the ligate-divide-stapler, LDS II. This instrument, employing a disposable cassette, applies two stainless steel clips and cuts between, thus reducing operating time and effort significantly. *Continued*

A

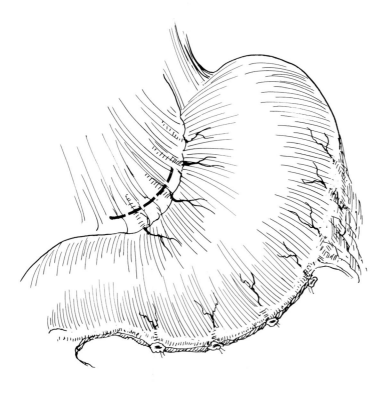

B

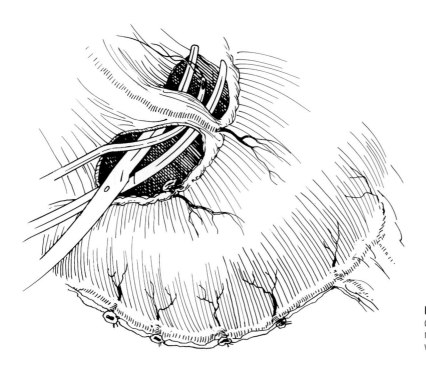

C

Figure 34–23, cont'd. B. Extent of dissection of lesser curve. **C.** Division of vessels entering the lesser curve in much the same way as when performing proximal gastric vagotomy.

vided between Kelly clamps and ligated with 2-0 ligatures. When possible, the dissection should be carried between the gastric wall and the artery, thereby preserving the main gastroepiploic artery as additional collateral blood supply to the suture lines and coming anastomosis. When the dissection reaches the pylorus, small bleeders should be divided between fine hemostats and ligated with fine silk ligatures. The dissection should be meticulous and gentle, since pancreatic tissue lurks in this area and inflammation can be activated in this dissection. The dissection should be carried about 1 cm past the pylorus, if a B-I reconstruction is anticipated. If a B-II is anticipated, the dissection need only be carried far enough to comfortably place the transverse linear stapler past the pylorus or to oversew the duodenum by a hand-sewn technique.

The assistant's left hand is used to lift the distal stomach forward and inferiorly. The more flimsy tissues of the lesser omentum are divided along the lesser curvature, using the electrocautery. Starting at the incisura and working toward the pylorus, the tissues of substance are divided between clamps and ligated with 3-0 silk ligatures. This dissection generally will include the descending branch of the left gastric artery. When the right gastric artery is reached, it is divided and ligated

with 2-0 silk ligatures. At this point (Fig 34–24), we prefer to divide the stomach. This is accomplished with the 90 mm GIA stapler (Ethicon name) or the gastric TA-90mm (Ethicon names). If the latter stapler is used, the stomach distal to the staple line is occluded with a crushing intestinal clamp, and the gastric wall is divided. The clamp then is used as a handle for manipulating the distal stomach. The final portion of the dissection involves gentle dissection of the posterior duodenal wall from the pancreas. Since this dissection may involve separation of pancreas elements from the posterior duodenal wall, cautery is used minimally or not at all, and tissues are separated gently with fine hemostats and ligated with 4-0 silk. If B-I anastomosis is anticipated, the duodenum is divided using the electrocautery, just distal to the pyloric ring. If B-II anastomosis is anticipated, the transverse TA-30 mm stapler is placed flush with the pyloric ring. After firing the stapler, a knife is used to sever the pylorus from the staple line. The specimen then is removed to a sterile table. The staple line can be inverted with 3-0 silk Lambert sutures or covered with an omental patch, if there is a concern about vascular supply or tension on the staple line. The specimen then can be opened and turned inside-out to reveal the gastric mucosa. The proximal

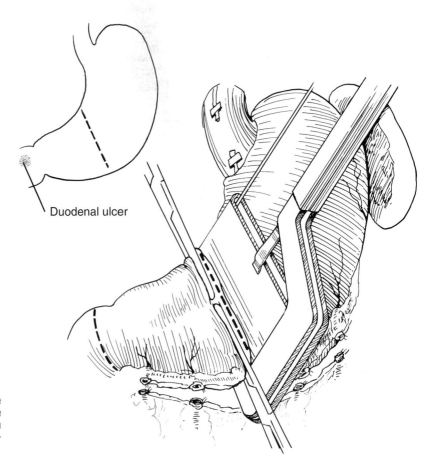

Duodenal ulcer

Figure 34–24. Billroth I operation. Division of stomach beyond the incisura. The gastric 90 stapler facilitates this maneuver. Note the truncal vagotomy has already been performed. (Redrawn from Zinner MJ. *Atlas of Gastric Surgery*. New York, NY: Churchill Livingstone; 1992. After Gloege)

border of the resection should contain transverse and obliquely oriented rugae characteristic of the acid-secreting gastric corpus and distinguishable from the longitudinally oriented antral folds. This maneuver verifies complete removal of the antrum.

B-I Reconstruction. When distal gastrectomy is performed for type I gastric ulcer, B-I anastomosis is preferable. A B-I anastomosis can be used safely for duodenal or pyloric channel ulcer, if scarring of the duodenal bulb and pylorus are minimal. If this form of reconstruction is planned, a Kocher maneuver should be performed prior to the distal gastrectomy. This will help to minimize tension on the anastomosis. As shown in Fig 34–25, the lower portion of the gastric staple line is removed, as shown in the figure, or by excision of gastric wall just posterior to the staple line. The length of the staple line to be removed is the width of the duodenal stump. The gastroduodenostomy is performed in two layers (Fig 34–26). The posterior layer of interrupted 3-0 silk Lembert seromuscular sutures is placed first. The inner 3-0 vicryl sutures are placed next to each other, sewn away from each other in over-and-over fashion until the sutures are brought around the edges to the anterior aspect. Connell sutures are used to invert the inner anterior layer. The anterior outer layer is closed with interrupted 3-0 silk Lambert sutures. The junction of the sewn anastomosis and the superior portion of the gastric staple line has been called the "angle of sorrow" owing to the complication of leakage where these suture/staple lines meet. A number of authors recommend inversion of the upper staple line by 3-0 silk Lembert sutures and a special covering suture for this junction. A second strategy is to cover this area with a tongue of omentum.

A B-I anastomosis also may be performed using mechanical stapling techniques. As shown in Fig 34–27, the duodenum is transected just distal to the pylorus with the knife and a purse-string suture is positioned circumferentially around its edge. The anvil of the circular stapler, usually a size 25 mm, is secured in the duodenal stump by the purse-string. The circular stapler is inserted through an anterior gastrotomy and fired through the posterior wall of the stomach (Fig 34–28). It is very important that the margin of the stapled suture line be placed 3 cm proximal to the stapled gastric closure, to provide maximum blood supply to both staple lines. The anterior gastrotomy then is closed with a TA-55 stapler or sutured closed in two layers.

B-II Reconstruction. When scarring or undue tension preclude B-I anastomosis following distal gastrectomy, a B-II gastrojejunostomy is indicated. Before describing our technique, it is worth pointing out the decisions that one will make in performing this reconstruction.

Closure of the Duodenal Stump. The first set of decisions focuses on the technique used for closure of the duodenal stump. Careful attention should be given to mobilizing the duodenal stump and obtaining a secure tension-free closure. If the duodenum is relatively free of scar or inflammation, this presents no problem and the TA-55 stapler may be used for closure as described above. If heavily scarred, dissection of the duodenum and performance of the antrectomy may be abandoned in favor of a safer vagotomy and gastroenterostomy.

If one is committed to the antrectomy and scarring prevents mobilization of the pylorus and duodenal bulb, one may rarely find a need to perform a Bancroft procedure, in which the most distal portion of the pyloric channel and antrum are left in situ after resection of the more proximal antrum (Fig 34–29). The mucosa of the retained segment is stripped,[41] removing all gastrin-secreting tissue that could cause a retained antrum syndrome. In the classic approach for this procedure, the greater and lesser curvatures are mobilized without dissecting too far into the tissues surrounding the pylorus. About 7 to 8 cm from the pylorus, the seromuscular coat of the antrum is incised circumferentially down to the level of the submucosa. Using sharp dissection, the muscle coat is separated from underlying mucosa. This dissection can be facilitated by submucosal injection of 1:100 000 epinephrine solution, as has been described for the mucosal proctectomy in ileal pouch–anal anastomosis procedures.[42] When the pyloric channel opening is reached, a fine purse-string absorbable suture (3-0 chromic catgut or vicryl) picks up small bites of submucosa at the pyloric ring. Transfixion and ligation of the mucosa is tempting, but should be avoided, as this would lead to mucosal ischemia and subsequent perforation. A small margin of mucosa is left to be invaginated into the pylorus as the purse-string is gently closed and tied. The proximal margins of the seromuscular cuff are excised, leaving just enough to close over the purse-string. Omentum is used to cover this closure, if possible.

One other important circumstance to be prepared for is the closure of the duodenum distal to a posteriorly perforated or deeply penetrating ulcer. In this setting, the ulcer crater is left in situ (Fig 34–30). In other settings, the anterior wall of the duodenum can be sutured to the ulcer base, with care being taken to suture ligate any exposed vessels. The suture line can be protected by a vascularized tongue of omentum.

Position of the Jejunal Loop: Antecolic or Retrocolic. The second decision in performing a B-II reconstruction is whether to bring the loop of jejunum behind (retro) or in front of (ante) the transverse colon. In performing the gastrectomy for benign disease, there is no clear evidence that this makes any difference and we prefer the retro-

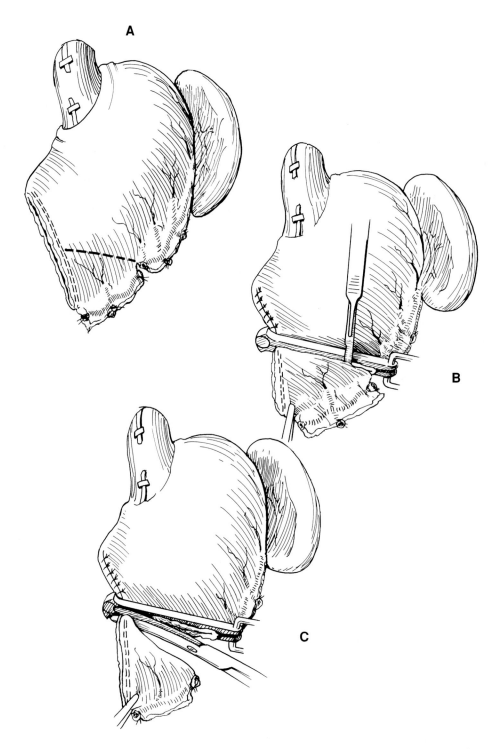

Figure 34–25. Billroth I operation. Division of lower portion of suture line. (Redrawn from Zinner, MJ. *Atlas of Gastric Surgery.* New York, NY: Churchill Livingstone; 1992. After Gloege)

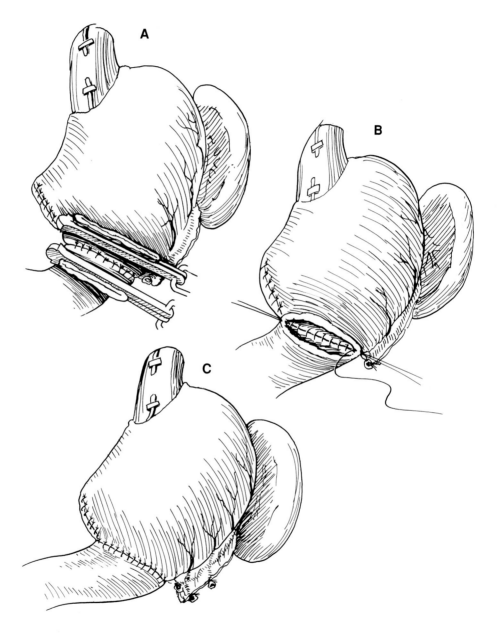

Figure 34–26. Billroth I operation. Construction of the gastroduodenostomy is performed end-to-end, in two layers. (Redrawn from Zinner MJ. *Atlas of Gastric Surgery.* New York, NY: Churchill Livingstone; 1992. After Gloege)

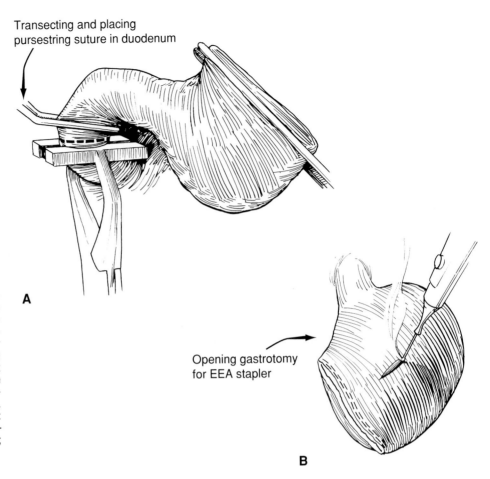

Transecting and placing
pursestring suture in duodenum

A

Opening gastrotomy
for EEA stapler

B

Figure 34–27. A. A Dennis clamp can be placed across the proximal duodenum, and the purse-string device can be placed at the selected site of duodenal division. **B.** A gastrotomy is made with the cautery on the anterior surface of the stomach, carefully avoiding large vascular arcades. This should be done at least 3 cm proximal to the row of staples. The gastrotomy should be large enough to accommodate the end-to-end stapling device easily. (Redrawn from Siegler HF. Gastric resection: Billroth I. In: Sabiston DC Jr (ed), *Atlas of General Surgery.* Philadelphia, PA: WB Saunders; 1994. After R Gordon)

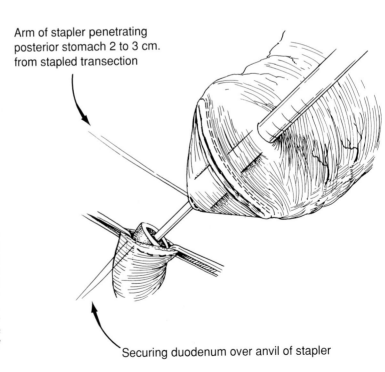

Arm of stapler penetrating
posterior stomach 2 to 3 cm.
from stapled transection

Securing duodenum over anvil of stapler

A

Figure 34–28. A. The gastrotomy edges should be grasped with two Babcock clamps and the end-to-end stapling device, minus the anvil, should be passed into the lumen of the stomach. The center rod should be gently pressed against the posterior wall of the stomach approximately 4 cm from the gastric line, and cautery should be used to permit passage of the rod through the posterior wall of the stomach. A purse-string suture will ensure that the stomach does not tear at the site of center rod penetration. The selected anvil size should be applied, and the open end of the duodenum should be grasped with Allis clamps. The duodenal wall should be gently pulled over the anvil, and the purse-string suture should be snugly tied around the center rod. *Continued*

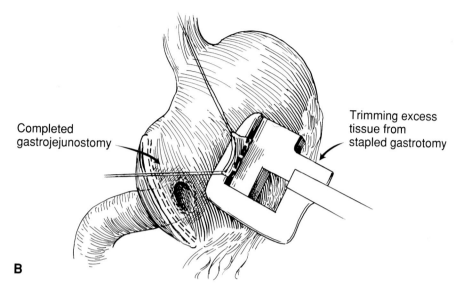

Completed gastrojejunostomy

Trimming excess tissue from stapled gastrotomy

Figure 34–28, cont'd. B. The cartridge and the anvil should then be approximated, being certain that no extraneous tissues are caught between the anvil and the circular cartridge. The instrument should be fired, and the anastomosis should then be carefully observed by direct visualization to ensure that hemostasis is adequate. The surgeon should then remove the anvil and check the circular tissue from both the duodenum and the stomach to be certain that the tissue doughnuts are intact. If the doughnuts are defective, external Lambert sutures will need to be applied to secure a complete anastomosis. The gastrotomy is closed by grasping each end with Allis clamps and incorporating the entire thickness of the stomach wall through the jaws of the 55-mm stapler. (Redrawn from Siegler HF. Gastric resection: Billroth I. In: Sabiston DC Jr (ed), *Atlas of General Surgery*. Philadelphia, PA: WB Saunders; 1994. After R Gordon)

B

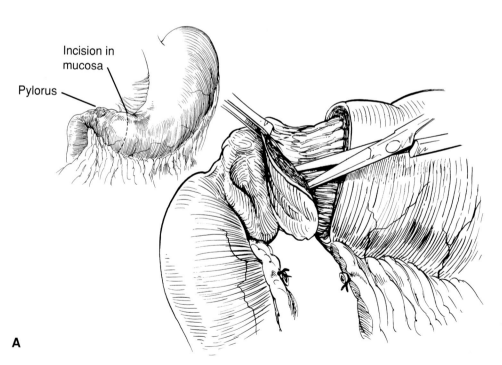

Incision in mucosa

Pylorus

Figure 34–29. Bancroft procedure. (Redrawn from Kirkham JS. Partial and total gastrectomy. In: Schwartz SI, Ellis H. *Maingot's Abdominal Operations*. Norwalk, CT: Appleton-Century-Crofts, 1982) *Continued*

A

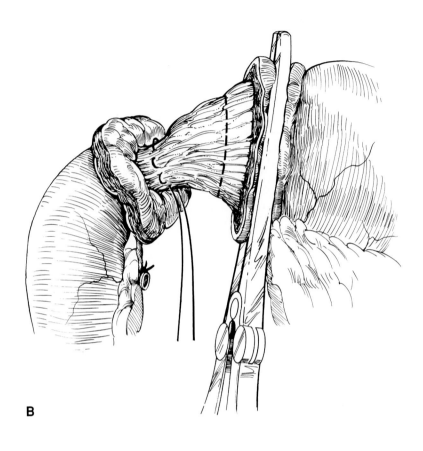

B

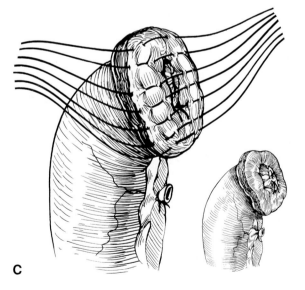

Figure 34–29, cont'd.

C

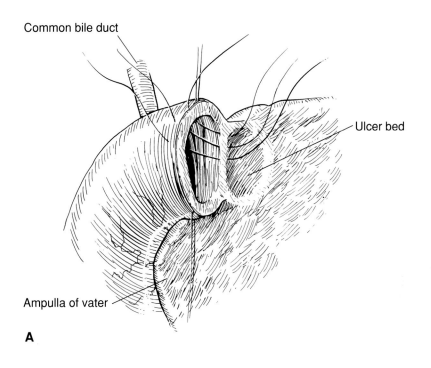

Common bile duct

Ulcer bed

Ampulla of vater

A

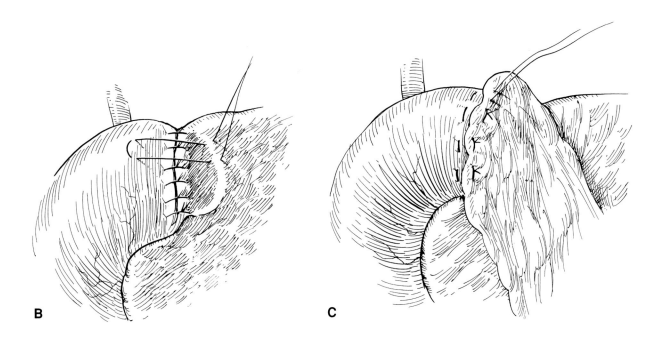

B

C

Figure 34–30. Closure of a chronic, ulcer-scarred duodenal stump. (Redrawn from Zinner MJ. *Atlas of Gastric Surgery*. New York, NY: Churchill Livingstone; 1992. After Gloege)

colic position. For malignant disease, it has generally been held that the retrocolic position may be predisposed to obstruction owing to enlargement of lymph nodes or serosal implants in the transverse mesocolon. Whether or not this predisposition exists, positioning the jejunal limb in front of the colon requires a somewhat longer mesentery. As long as the anastomosis will not be under tension, the antecolic position will permit emptying as effective as that through a retrocolic anastomosis. If a retrocolic position is chosen, the window in the transverse mesocolon should be wide enough to permit both the afferent and efferent limbs of the jejunum to slide comfortably through. When this window is closed following construction of the anastomosis, it is preferable to tack the mesentery above, on the gastric side, rather than on the jejunal side. This will prevent kinking and obstruction of the jejunal limbs and positions the anastomosis below the mesentery.

Length of the Afferent Limb. The third decision is the choice of the segment of jejunum used for the anastomosis. In general, the segment should be as close to the ligament of Treitz as possible and still reach the stomach without tension. This generally leaves 10 to 20 cm of the proximal jejunum as the afferent limb. The shorter this length, the less likely the possibility of an afferent limb syndrome developing. The incidence of other complications such as alkaline reflux gastritis, dumping or postvagotomy diarrhea should not be influenced by the length of the afferent limb.

Anastomotic Position on the Stomach and Technique. Fig 34–31 schematically illustrates a number of described variations on the B-II reconstruction. We will describe one hand-sewn and one stapled technique for anastomosis. As shown in Fig 34–32, the inferior portion of the gastric staple line is excised with electrocautery, taking a small

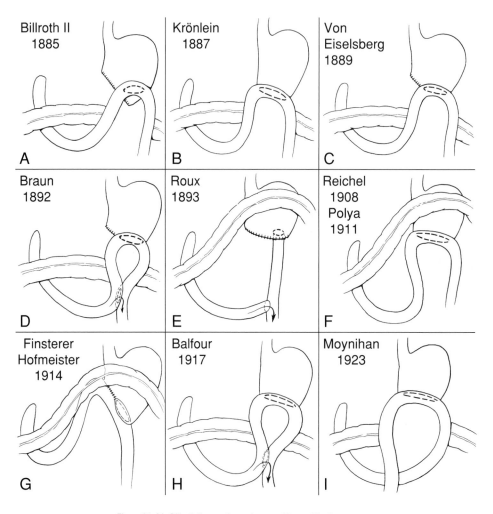

Figure 34–31. Billroth II operation and some of its modifications.

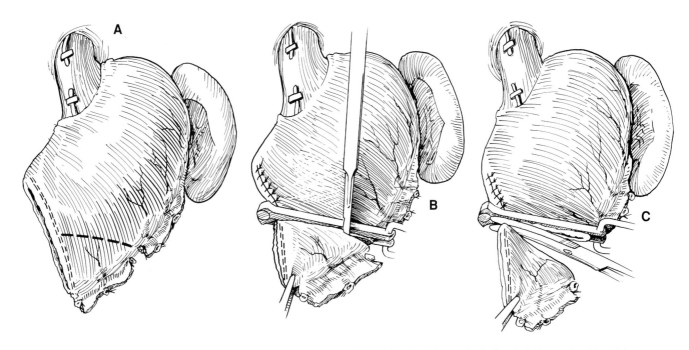

Figure 34–32. Billroth II operation. The antrum is resected as in Billroth I operation. The distal portion of the resection line is excised. (Redrawn from Zinner MJ. *Atlas of Gastric Surgery*. New York, NY: Churchill Livingstone; 1992. After Gloege)

wedge of stomach behind the staple line. The superior portion of the staple line can be reinforced with 3-0 silk Lembert sutures at this time or can be reinforced later by tacking the afferent limb of jejunum, just beyond the anastomosis, to the gastric wall. The proximal jejunal limb is brought, untwisted, through a window in the transverse mesocolon (Fig 34–33). Traction seromuscular sutures (2-0 or 3-0 silk) are placed at both corners of the anastomosis. The gastrojejunal anastomosis is performed in two layers (Fig 34–34), between the most caudal part of the stomach and the jejunal limb. The outer layer is comprised of 3-0 silk Lembert seromuscular sutures. The inner layer is performed in the posterior row by running two 3-0 vicryl sutures in opposite directions around the corners and then in Connell fashion for the anterior row. Placement of the anastomosis on the posterior gastric wall, about 2 to 3 cm from the gastric staple line also will provide a suitably dependent position for drainage of gastric content. The window in the transverse mesocolon is closed, as illustrated in Fig 34–35.

Figs 34–36 and 34–37 illustrate the technique for stapled gastroenterostomy. As before the jejunal limb is placed in the retrocolic position. Traction sutures are placed on the gastric wall posterior to the anastomosis, bringing the jejunal limb into apposition. The 55 mm GIA-type stapler is fired after its two limbs are placed through a small gastrotomy and small enterotomy, respectively. The open end of the anastomosis is then closed with a TA-55 stapler. It should be noted that

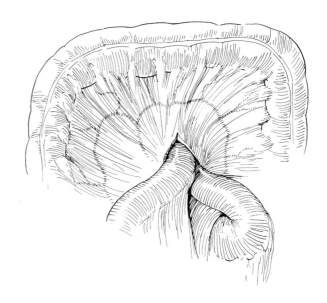

Figure 34–33. Billroth II operation. The jejunal segment, located 10 to 20 cm beyond the ligament of Treitz, is brought through a window in the retrocolic mesentery. (Redrawn from Zinner MJ. *Atlas of Gastric Surgery*. New York, NY: Churchill Livingstone; 1992. After Gloege)

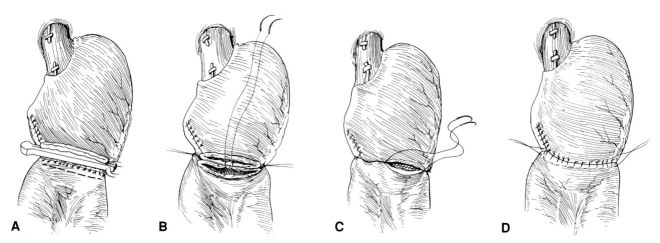

A   **B**   **C**   **D**

Figure 34–34. Billroth II operation. The gastrojejunal anastomosis is constructed in 2 layers, as described in the text. (Redrawn from Zinner MJ. *Atlas of Gastric Surgery.* New York, NY: Churchill Livingstone; 1992. After Gloege)

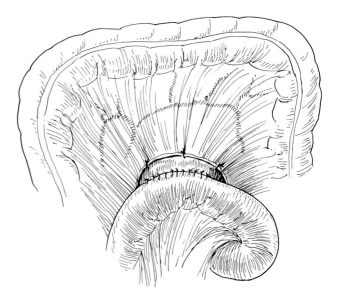

Figure 34–35. Billroth II operation. The retrocolic window in the mesentery is closed in order to avoid herniation of other viscera. The mesentery is linked to gastric wall, positioning the anastomosis below the closure. (Redrawn from Zinner MJ. *Atlas of Gastric Surgery.* New York, NY: Churchill Livingstone; 1992. After Gloege)

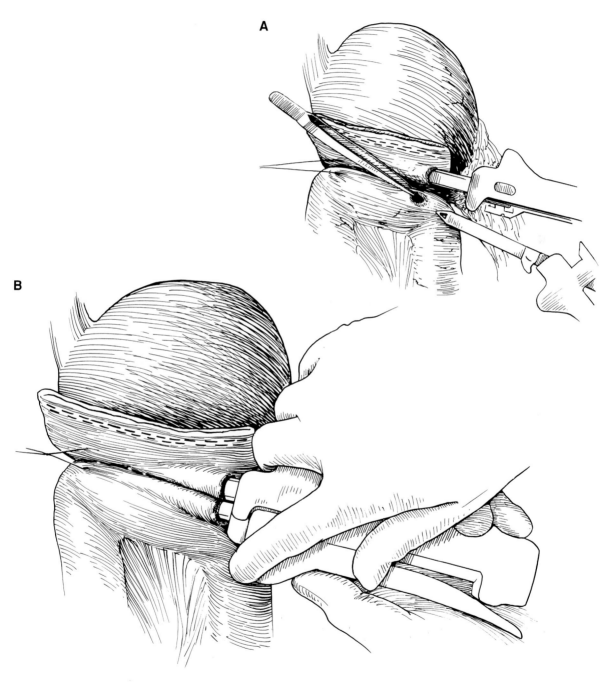

Figure 34–36. Stapling technique for Billroth II gastrojejunostomy. (After W Baker)

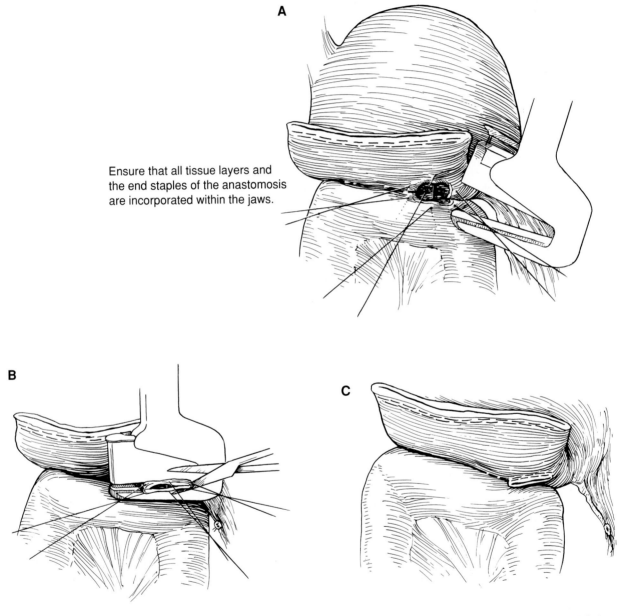

Ensure that all tissue layers and
the end staples of the anastomosis
are incorporated within the jaws.

Figure 34–37. A. Billroth II operation. **B and C.** The transverse stapler is used to close the common opening over the gastrojejunal anastomosis. (After W Baker)

these staple lines, especially that from the TA-55, are difficult to reinforce without undue tension. The blood supply of the gastric and intestinal walls are ample and reinforcement with Lembert sutures generally is not necessary.

SUBTOTAL AND TOTAL GASTRIC RESECTIONS

The main indications for subtotal (70% to 80%) gastric resection is carcinoma of the antrum or pylorus or primary gastric lymphoma. However, in cases of ulcers that lie very proximal on the lesser curvature, the proximity to the gastroesophageal junction prevents excision without significant narrowing of the gastric inlet. Similarly, the main indication for total gastric resection is a bulky carcinoma of the body or distal fundus and, rarely, otherwise unmanageable symptoms of an unresectable gastrinoma. Indications for near-total (>90%) gastric resection include the uncommon settings of the Roux stasis syndrome and gastroparesis unresponsive to medical management, as well as carcinoma or lymphoma of the body of the stomach. The approaches for subtotal and near total gastrectomy will be discussed only briefly, focusing on issues of exposure and techniques for resection of the stomach itself and reconstruction. The principals of resection for gastric carcinoma will be presented subsequently in conjunction with the discussion of radical total gastrectomy for carcinoma.

Subtotal/Near-Total Gastric Resections

In principal, a subtotal gastrectomy is simply an extended antrectomy or hemigastrectomy. A few technical issues are worth noting. First, the exposure provided by a midline incision is usually not as adequate as that provided by a chevron incision. Second, the left gastric artery always is ligated and divided in this dissection and, once the level of gastric transection has been determined, the branches of the left gastroepiploic artery and short gastric arteries are ligated in continuity and divided up to this predetermined level. Third, in opting for a near total gastric resection, a 1 to 2 cm cuff of gastric wall is left behind and is the margin for the anastomosis. For this operation, it is desirable to preserve the uppermost one or two short gastric vessels, in order to ensure the adequacy of the blood supply for the gastric side of the anastomosis. Finally, although it is often possible to reconstruct with a standard gastrojejunostomy, we prefer a Roux-en-Y reconstruction since this minimizes tension on the suture line and, theoretically, reduces the risk of anastomotic obstruction by persistence or recurrence of tumor.

Total Gastrectomy for Carcinoma

The goals of total gastrectomy for carcinoma are (1) clear margins on both esophageal and duodenal sides;

(2) removal of local/regional lymph node–bearing tissues, including those surrounding the right and left gastric arteries, right gastroepiploic artery, and short gastric arteries; (3) removal of the omentum en bloc with the stomach; and (4) removal of the lymphatic tissues overlying the pancreatic capsule. We favor a Roux-en-Y reconstruction with a direct esophagoenterostomy rather than a jejunal pouch, although the techniques for both forms of reconstruction will be described. It remains unclear whether more radical forms of lymphadenectomy truly improve outcomes in terms of local recurrence or long-term survival. The Japanese experience with smaller and earlier forms of gastric carcinoma suggests that more radical approaches could alter outcomes, but this has not been observed in European or North American patient groups.[43]

Fig 34–38 illustrates the en block resection. Generally, an upper midline or chevron incision will provide good exposure. A thoracoabdominal incision (Fig 34–39) is rarely necessary, but can provide better exposure when the patient's habitus suggests a deep hiatus. This latter incision also should be considered when preoperative endoscopy suggests that the tumor is close enough to the cardia so that the distal thoracic portion of the esophagus might be included with the resection. If this latter approach is chosen, the abdominal portion of the incision is performed first, in order to assess resectability. The patient is placed in a left thoracotomy position. The incision is carried from the line of the eighth rib obliquely toward the umbilicus. If resection appears feasible, the incision is extended over the eighth rib to the posterior angle. Occasionally, the seventh rib will provide better exposure. A separate rib retractor, for the chest, and a self-retaining retractor without a ring, for the abdominal portion, provide the best retraction. The diaphragm is divided toward the hiatus, but the muscle does not always have to be divided completely. Thus, it may be possible to spare the neurovascular bundle. Significant bleeding is encountered and requires suture ligation with 2-0 or 0-0 vicryl.

In the abdominal approach, the Bookwalter retractor is used. Extra care in positioning retractors on the left lobe of the liver, diaphragm, and small intestine, for optimal exposure of the hiatus is time well spent. The dissection is begun by dividing the omentum from the transverse colon (Fig 34–40). This relatively avascular plane can be separated using the elecrocautery. Deviation from this plane will injure the colon or require tedious ligation and division of omental blood vessels. The lesser sac then is entered, allowing assessment of the retroperitoneum, with regard to local tumor extension and lymph node involvement. The distal portion of the gastrectomy then is performed. The origin of the right gastric artery at the common hepatic artery is identified, ligated in continuity with 2-0 silk ligatures and di-

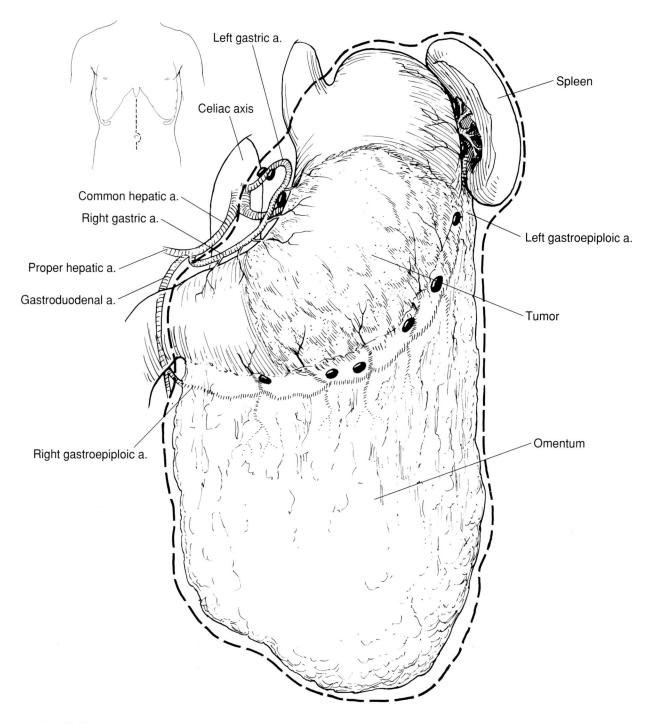

Figure 34–38. Anatomy relevant to resections for gastric carcinoma. (Redrawn from Zinner MJ. *Atlas of Gastric Surgery*. New York, NY: Churchill Livingstone; 1992)

Left gastric a.

Celiac axis

Spleen

Common hepatic a.

Right gastric a.

Left gastroepiploic a.

Proper hepatic a.

Gastroduodenal a.

Tumor

Right gastroepiploic a.

Omentum

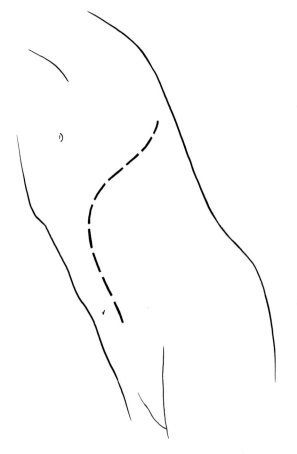

Figure 34–39. Thoracoabdominal incision for radical total gastrectomy for carcinoma of the stomach. The incision is carried along the 7th or the interspace.

observed (Fig 34–42). If tumor is invading this plane, a decision must be made regarding inclusion of the body and tail of the pancreas in the specimen. In our view, the arguments for this radical approach are weak. However, the plane made by the peritoneum overlying the pancreas is a natural plane and there may be sense in taking this peritoneum with the en bloc specimen. This layer can be dissected off the anterior face of the pancreas and swept gently as a front toward the left gastric vessels and splenic hilum. If a curative resection appears to be feasible, but would require removal of the body and/or tail of the pancreas, we do not see this as a contraindication to resection. The origin of the left gastric artery then is identified at the celiac axis, ligated in continuity using 2-0 silk and divided (Fig 34–43). The stump of the artery is suture-ligated as well. From the celiac axis side, the tissue surrounding the artery contains lymphatics and is swept toward the lesser curvature. When the tumor is located in the more proximal body and corpus, the case for inclusion of the spleen with the en bloc specimen has not been persuasive.[44–46] Inclusion of the spleen is indicated if there are obvious tumor bearing nodes or if there is direct invasion of the splenic hilum. Through the lesser sac, the tail of the pancreas is identified. The splenic artery and vein are separated, suture ligated and divided individually. At this point, the short gastric vessels are then part of the en bloc specimen and are not dissected or divided.

vided. Lymphatic-bearing tissues are swept toward the gastric side. The right gastroepiploic artery is identified, usually by palpation and traced as far to the right as possible. It is usually possible to trace the artery to its origin at the gastroduodenal artery, which is similarly ligated in continuity and divided. Using the electrocautery, the lesser omentum is incised near the liver and its tissues are swept toward the lesser curvature, from the duodenum to the esophagus. Any small vessels are ligated with 3-0 ligatures. The dissection is carried onto the peritoneal surface of the esophagus. The duodenum may be divided at this time, using the GIA stapler, or a TA-55 stapler that is fired twice, once on the duodenum and once directly on the pylorus. The duodenum is divided just distal to the pyloric ring (Fig 34–41).

With the distal portion of the stomach divided, full access to the left gastric artery is obtained posteriorly through the lesser sac. This approach optimizes visualization of the celiac axis and its branches. With the assistant retracting the stomach upward and anteriorly, a number of congenital adhesions between the posterior gastric wall and the peritoneum overlying pancreas are

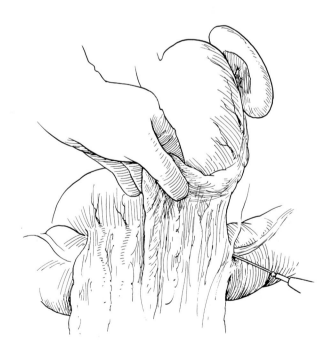

Figure 34–40. Resection for gastric carcinoma. The gastrocolic mentum is detached from the transverse colon using electrocautery. (Redrawn from Zinner MJ. *Atlas of Gastric Surgery.* New York, NY: Churchill Livingstone; 1992. After Gloege)

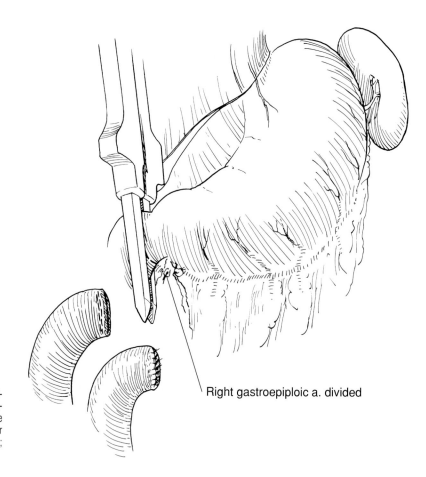

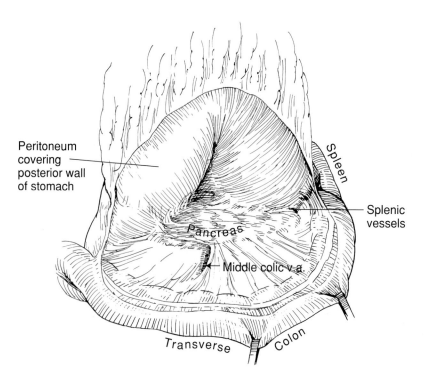

Figure 34–41. Resection for gastric carcinoma. The duodenum is divided beyond the pylorus. Either the linear cutter or transverse stapling instruments are appropriate. If feasible, the duodenal staple line is reinforced using 3-0 silk Lambert sutures. (Redrawn from Zinner MJ. *Atlas of Gastric Surgery*. New York, NY: Churchill Livingstone; 1992. After Gloege)

Right gastroepiploic a. divided

Peritoneum covering posterior wall of stomach

Spleen

Splenic vessels

Pancreas

Middle colic v. a.

Transverse Colon

Figure 34–42. Resection for gastric carcinoma. With the lesser sac fully visualized, the thin layer of tissue overlying the pancreas is exposed and can be removed with the en bloc specimen.

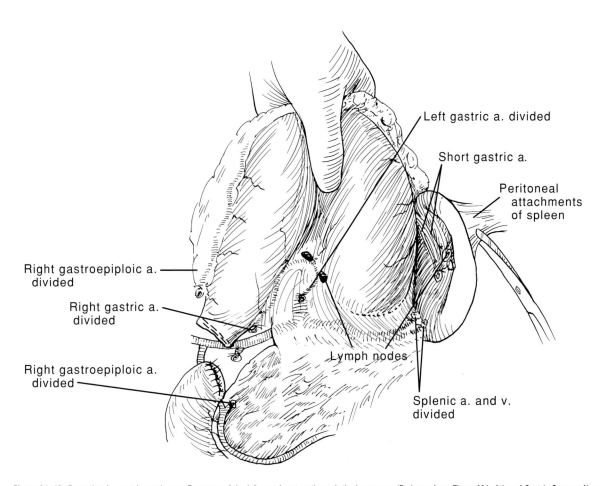

Left gastric a. divided

Short gastric a.

Peritoneal
attachments
of spleen

Right gastroepiploic a.
divided

Right gastric a.
divided

Right gastroepiploic a.
divided

Lymph nodes

Splenic a. and v.
divided

Figure 34–43. Resection for gastric carcinoma. Exposure of the left gastric artery through the lesser sac. (Redrawn from Zinner MJ. *Atlas of Gastric Surgery*. New York, NY: Churchill Livingstone; 1992. After Gloege)

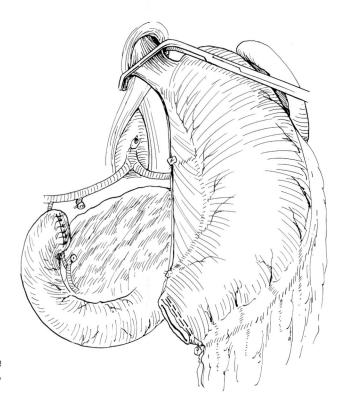

Figure 34–44. Gastric resection for carcinoma. The esophagus is transacted just above the gastroesophageal junctions. (Redrawn from Zinner MJ. *Atlas of Gastric Surgery*. New York, NY: Churchill Livingstone; 1992. After Gloege)

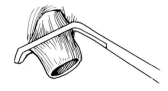

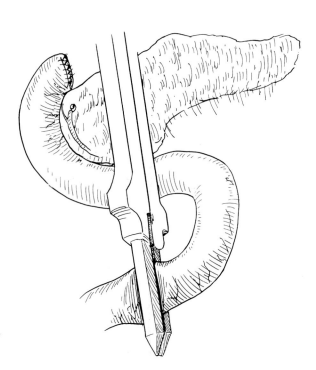

Figure 34–45. Gastric insert for carcinoma. Construction of Roux-en-Y limb begins with division of jejunum 15 cm beyond the ligament of Treitz. (Redrawn from Zinner MJ. *Atlas of Gastric Surgery*. New York, NY: Churchill Livingstone; 1992. After Gloege)

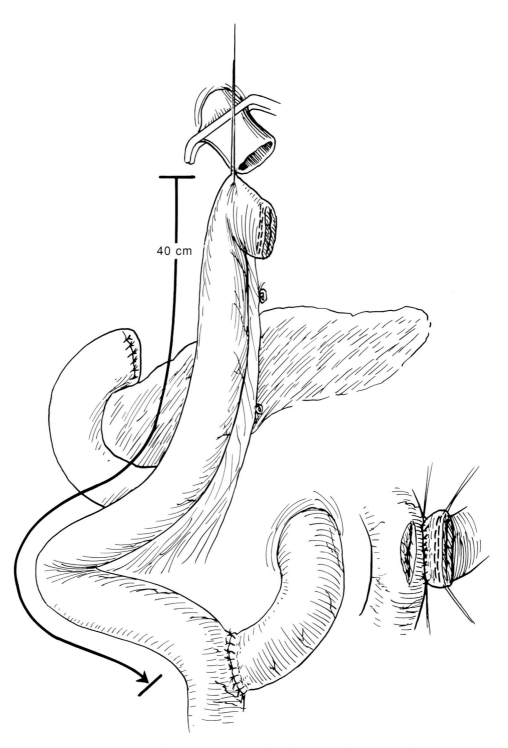

Figure 34–46. Construction of the Roux-en-Y anastomosis. The enteroenterostomy is performed in two layers. The length of the Roux limb measures 40 cm. (Redrawn from Zinner MJ. *Atlas of Gastric Surgery*. New York, NY: Churchill Livingstone; 1992. After Gloege)

40 cm

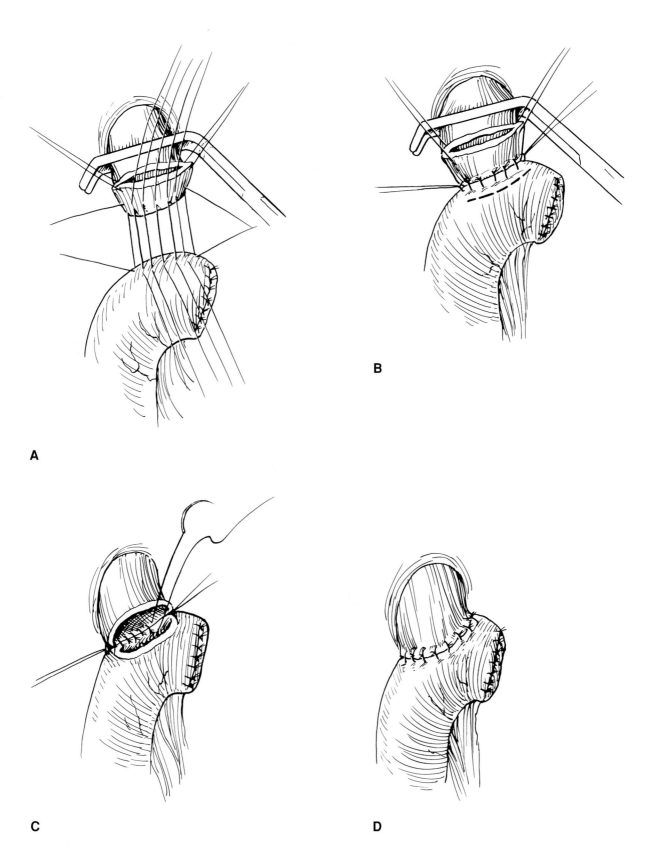

A

B

C

D

Figure 34–47. Roux-en-Y reconstruction following total gastrectomy. The anastomosis is prepared using two layers of interrupted 3-0 silk sutures. (Redrawn from Zinner MJ. *Atlas of Gastric Surgery*. New York, NY: Churchill Livingstone; 1992. After Gloege)

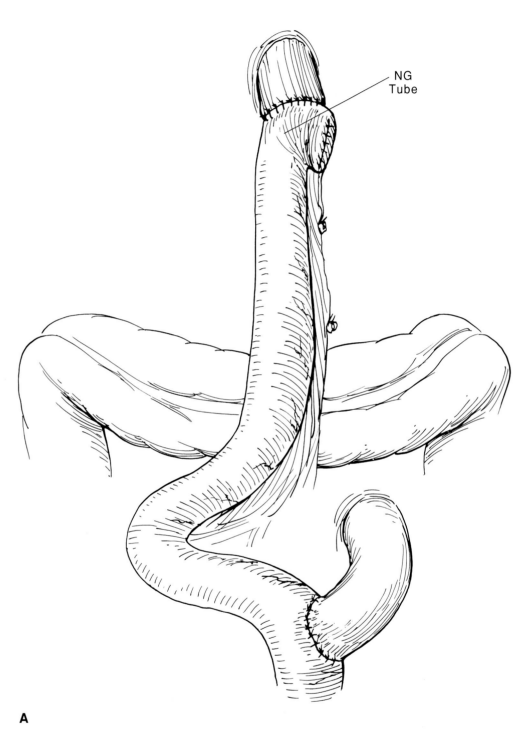

A

Figure 34–48. A. Roux-en-Y reconstruction completed. (Redrawn from Zinner MJ. *Atlas of Gastric Surgery.* New York, NY: Churchill Livingstone; 1992).

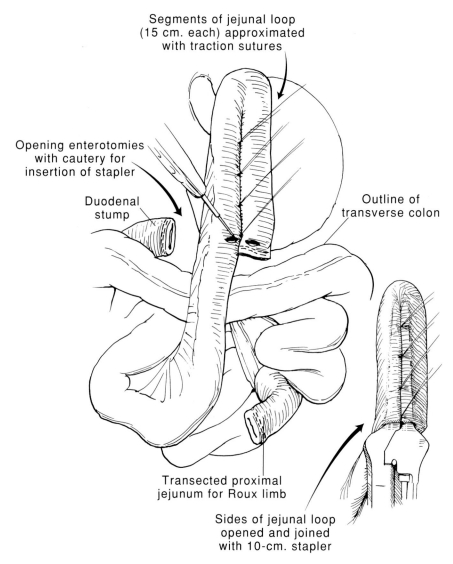

Segments of jejunal loop
(15 cm. each) approximated
with traction sutures

Opening enterotomies
with cautery for
insertion of stapler

Duodenal
stump

Outline of
transverse colon

Transected proximal
jejunum for Roux limb

Sides of jejunal loop
opened and joined
with 10-cm. stapler

B

Figure 34–48, cont'd. B. Total gastrectomy—stapler version. Formation of the jejunal pouch. (Redrawn from Siegler HF. Total gastrectomy: stapler. In: Sabiston DC Jr (ed), *Atlas of General Surgery,* Philadelphia, PA: WB Saunders; 1994. After R Gordon)

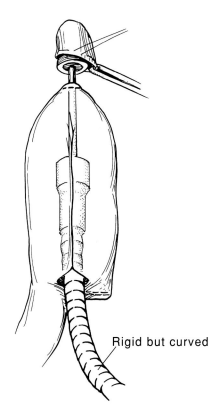

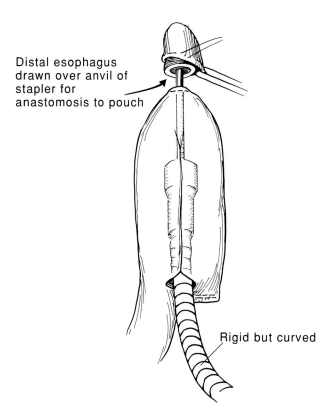

Distal esophagus
drawn over anvil of
stapler for
anastomosis to pouch

Rigid but curved

Rigid but curved

Figure 34–49. Total gastrectomy. The circular stapler is positioned via the enter-otomies. The center rod is pushed through the antimesenteric border of the jejunum using the cautery to prevent tearing. (Redrawn from Siegler HF. Total gastrectomy: stapler. In: Sabiston DC Jr (ed), *Atlas of General Surgery*. Philadelphia, PA: WB Saunders; 1994)

Figure 34–50. Total gastrectomy. Cartridge and anvil are approximated and circular stapler is fired. (Redrawn from Siegler HF. Total gastrectomy: stapler. In: Sabiston DC Jr (ed), *Atlas of General Surgery*. Philadelphia, PA: WB Saunders; 1994)

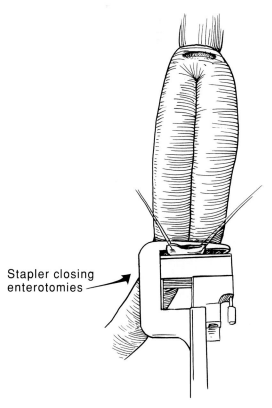

Stapler closing
enterotomies

Figure 34–51. Completed pouch and esophagojejunal anastomosis. The enterotomy is closed with the transverse 55-mm stapler. (Redrawn from Siegler HF. Total gastrectomy: stapler. In: Sabiston, DC Jr (ed), *Atlas of General Surgery*. Philadelphia, PA: WB Saunders; 1994)

The posterior aspect of the esophagus then comes into view as the stomach and spleen are lifted upward. Posteriorly, the front of peritoneal tissue can be dissected bluntly until the superior border of the pancreas is reached. The peritoneum is continuous with the peritoneum investing the gastric side of the gastroesophageal junction. If this layer has not been included with the dissection, the peritoneum must be divided here, exposing the gastroesophageal junction posteriorly. Fig 34–44 demonstrates the stomach completely mobilized except for its attachment to the esophagus. A noncrushing clamp is placed on the mobilized esophagus and the specimen is resected. To minimize spillage of luminal contents, a second clamp is placed on the gastric side or the TA-55 stapler may be fired below the line of resection and above the gastroesophageal junction.

Our preferred technique for reconstruction is a simple Roux-en-Y, with an end-to-side esophagojejunal anastomosis with the Roux limb. Using the GIA stapler, a section of jejunum is divided 10 to 15 cm beyond the ligament of Treitz (Fig 34–45). The Roux limb is brought, antecolic, up to the esophagus. An enteroenterostomy is constructed between the jejunum on the duodenal side of the Y and the jejunum, 40 to 45 cm distal to the Roux limb staple line (Fig 34–46). The enteroenteral anastomosis can be performed using hand-sewn two-layer technique or stapling technique. The esophagojejunal anastomosis is performed using interrupted 3-0 silk sutures for both inner and outer layers, as shown in Fig 34–47. The completed reconstruction is shown in Fig 34–48. This figure emphasizes the antecolic position of the anastomosis when the operation is performed for malignant disease. Areas of potential internal herniation in the mesentery are closed with absorbable 3-0 sutures.

A jejunal pouch also may be constructed, with the idea of anastomosing the esophagus in end-to-side fashion with the antimesenteric border of the pouch. The technique is illustrated in Figs 34–48 through 34–51 and can be performed expeditiously using surgical staplers. The pouch is constructed with the goal of providing a reservoir function. Alternatively, a number of surgeons expressed a preference for leaving an island of undivided intestine at the bend in the pouch. This should, theoretically, optimize the blood supply to the anastomosis. The circular stapler can be passed through the open end of the Roux limb, in order to perform the end-esophagus to side-jejunum anastomosis. The liner stapler then can be fired in such a way as to leave the island of undivided intestine. One important point is that the pouch can be made too long, giving rise to stasis and ineffective clearance of food from the pouch into the intestine. The pouch should not be more than 15 cm in length.

REFERENCES

1. Finney JMT. The development of surgery of the stomach with special reference to the part played by American surgeons. *Ann Surg* 1929;90:829
2. Herrington JL. Historical aspects of gastric surgery. In: Scott, HW Jr, Sawyers JL (eds), *Surgery of the Stomach, Duodenum and Small Intestine*, 2nd ed. Boston, MA: Blackwell Scientific; 1992:1–28
3. Absolon KB. The surgical school of Theodor Billroth. *Surgery* 1961;50:702
4. Mikulicz-Radecki J. Small contributions to the surgery of the intestinal tract. *Trans Am Surg Assoc* 1903;21:124
5. Stabile BE, Passaro E. Duodenal ulcer: a disease in evolution. *Curr Prob Surg* 1984;21:79
6. Waisbren SJ, Modlin IM, Lester R. Dragstedt and his role of therapeutic vagotomy in the United States. *Am J Surg* 1994;167:345–359
7. Harkins HN, Schmitz EJ, Harper HP, et al. A combined physiologic operation for peptic ulcer. *West J Surg* 1953; 61:316
8. Griffith CA, Harkins HN. Partial gastric vagotomy: an experimental study. *Gastroenterology* 1957;32:96
9. Johnston D, Wilkinson A. Selective vagotomy with innervated antrum without drainage procedure for duodenal ulcer. *Br J Surg* 1969;69:626
10. Goligher JC, Hill G, Kenny T. Proximal gastric vagotomy without drainage for duodenal ulcer: results after 5–8 years. *Br J Surg* 1978;65:145
11. Feldman M, Richardson C, Fordtran JS. Experience with sham feeding as a test for vagotomy. *Gastroenterology* 1980; 79:792
12. Thirlby RC. Studies of gastric secretion. In: Scott HW Jr, Sawyers JL (eds), *Surgery of the Stomach, Duodenum and Small Intestine*, 2nd ed. Boston, MA: Blackwell Scientific; 1992:124–143
13. Charles M, Andrus MD. St. Louis University Department of Surgery, St Louis, MO (Protocol personally communicated 1994.)
14. Mayer EA. The physiology of gastric storage and emptying. In: Johnson LR (ed), *Physiology of the Gastrointestinal Tract*. New York, NY: Raven; 1994:929–976
15. Johnston D. Vagotomy. In: Schwartz, SI (ed), *Maingot's Abdominal Operations*, 8th ed. Norwalk: Appleton-Crofts; 1985:797–820
16. Morris DL, Harrison JD, Jorgensen JO, et al. Posterior truncal vagotomy and stapling of anterior stomach wall in 30 patients with duodenal ulcer: acid inhibition, gastric emptying, and endoscopic dye spraying. Prospects for endoscopic vagotomy. *Surg Laparosc Endosc* 1993;3:375
17. Fich A, Neri M, Camilleri M, et al. Stasis syndromes following gastric surgery: clinical motility features of 60 symptomatic patients. *J Clin Gastroenterol* 1990;12:505
18. Paimela H, Hallikainen D, Ahonen J et al. The prognostic significance of radiologically determined gastric emptying before proximal gastric vagotomy. *Acta Chir Scand* 1986;152:611
19. Pechlivanides G, Xynos E, Chrysos E, et al. Gallbladder emptying after antiulcer gastric surgery. *Am J Surg* 1994; 168:335

20. Saik RP, Greeburg AG, Peskin GW. Pros and cons of parietal cell versus truncal vagotomy. *Am J Surg* 1984;148:93

21. Cheadle WG, Baker PR, Cuschieri A. Pyloric reconstruction for severe vasomotor dumping after vagotomy and pyloroplasty. *Ann Surg* 1985;202:568

22. Rossi RL, Dial PF, Georgi B, et al. A five to ten year follow-up study of parietal cell vagotomy. *Surg Gynecol Obstet* 1986;162:301–306

23. Wang CS, Tzen KY, Chen PC, Chen MF. Effects of highly selective vagotomy and additional procedures on gastric emptying in patients with obstructing duodenal ulcer. *World J Surg* 1994;18:131

24. Hallenbeck GA, Gleysteen JJ, Aldrete JS, Slaughter RL. Proximal gastric vagotomy: effects of two operative techniques on clinical and gastric secretory results. *Ann Surg* 1976:8:435

25. Johnston D. Operative mortality and post-operative morbidity in highly selective vagotomy. *BMJ* 1975;4:545

26. Grassi G. Highly selective vagotomy with intraoperative acid secretion test of vagal section. *Surg Gynecol Obstet* 1975:140:259

27. Butterfield DT, Whitfield PF, Hobsley M. Changes in gastric secretion with time after vagotomy and the relationship to recurrent duodenal ulcer. *Gut* 1982;23:1055

28. Barroso FL, Caltabiano A, Ornellas A. Transabdominal suprahepatic approach to repeat vagotomy after proximal gastric vagotomy. *Surg Gynecol Obstet* 1990;171:167

29. Thirlby RC, Feldman M. Transthoracic vagotomy for post-operative peptic ulcer: effects on basal, sham feeding, and pentagastrin-stimulated acid secretion, and on clinical outcome. *Ann Surg* 1985;201:648

30. Jackson RG. Anatomy of the vagus nerves in the region of the lower esophagus and stomach. *Anat Rec* 1949;103:1

31. Oddsdottir M, Soybel D. Peptic ulcer disease. In: Ballantyne, GH (ed), *Laparoscopic Surgery*. Philadelphia, PA: WB Saunders; 1994:137

32. Dallemagne B, Weerts JM, Jehaes C, et al. Laparoscopic highly selective vagotomy. *Br J Surg* 1994;81:554

33. Taylor TV, Lythgoe JP, MacFarland JB, et al. Anterior lesser curve seromyotomy and posterior truncal vagotomy and pyloroplasty in the treatment of chronic duodenal ulcer. *Br J Surg* 1990;77:1007

34. Katkhouda N, Heimbucher J, Mouiel J. Laparoscopic posterior vagotomy and antreior seromyotomy. *Endosc Surg Allied Technol* 1994;2:95

35. Bemelman WA, Brummelkamp WH, Bartelsman JWFM. Endoscopic balloon dilatation of the pylorus esophagogastrectomy without a drainage procedure. *Surg Gynecol Obstet* 1990;170:424

36. McDermott EW, Murphy JJ. Laparoscopic truncal vagotomy without drainage. *Br J Surg* 1993;80:236

37. Pietrafitta JJ, Schultz LS, Graber JN, Hickok DF. Laser laparoscopic vagotomy and pyloronyotomy. *Gastrointest Endosc* 1991;37:338

38. Clancy TV, Moore PM, Ramshaw DG, Kays CR. Laparoscopic excision of a benign gastric tumor. *J Laparoendosc Surg* 1994;4:277

39. Llorente J. Laparoscopic gastric resection for gastric leiomyoma. *Surg Endosc* 1994;8:887

40. Donahue PE, Nyhus LM. Surgical excision of gastric ulcers near the gastroesophageal junction. *Surg Gynecol Obstet* 1982;155:85

41. Bancroft FW. A modification of the Devine operation of pyloric exclusion for duodenal ulcer. *Am J Surg* 1932;16:223

42. Becker JM, Kelly KA, Haddad AC, Zinsmeister AR. Proximal gastric vagotomy and mucosal antrectomy: a possible approach to duodenal ulcer. *Surgery* 1983;94:58

43. Wanebo HJ, Kennedy BJ, Chmiel J, et al. Cancer of the stomach. A patient care study by the American College of Surgeons. *Ann Surg* 1993;8:583

44. Robertson CS, Chung SC, Woods SD, et al. A prospective randomized trial comparing R1 subtotal gastrectomy with R3 total gastrectomy for antral cancer. *Ann Surg* 1994; 220:176

45. Brady MS, Rogatko A, Dent LL, Shiu MH. Effect of splenectomy on morbidity and survival following curative gastrectomy for carcinoma. *Arch Surg* 1991;126:359

46. Adachi Y, Kamakura T, Mori M, et al. Role of lymph node dissection and splenectomy in node-positive gastric carcinoma. *Surgery* 1994;116:837

INDEX

Note: Page numbers in italics indicate figures; those followed by t indicate tables.